AF616406

# CLINICAL UROLOGIC PRACTICE

EDITOR

**Barry S. Stein, MD**

Professor and Chairman of Urology
Brown University School of Medicine
Surgeon-in-Chief, Department of Urology
Rhode Island Hospital
Providence, Rhode Island

ASSOCIATE EDITORS

**Anthony A. Caldamone, MD**

Associate Professor of Urology
Brown University School of Medicine
Chief of Pediatric Urology
Rhode Island Hospital
Providence, Rhode Island

**Joseph A. Smith, Jr., MD**

Professor and Chairman, Department of Urology
Vanderbilt University School of Medicine
Nashville, Tennessee

Norton Medical Books
W • W • Norton & Company
New York • London

Printed in the United States of America

Drug Dosage

The authors and publisher have exerted every effort to ensure that drug selection and dosage set forth in this text are in accord with current recommendations and practice at the time of publication. However, in view of ongoing research, changes in government regulations, and the constant flow of information relating to drug therapy and drug reactions, the reader is urged to check the package insert for each drug for any change in indications and dosage and for added warnings and precautions. This is particularly important when the recommended agent is a new and/or infrequently used drug.

Library of Congress Cataloging-in-Publication Data

Clinical urologic practice / editor, Barry S. Stein; associate
editors, Anthony A. Caldamone, Joseph A. Smith, Jr.
p. cm.—(Norton medical books)
1. Urology. 2. Urinary organs—Diseases. I. Stein, Barry S.
(Barry Stephen), 1948– . II. Caldamone, Anthony A. III. Smith,
Joseph A., 1949– . IV. Series.
[DNLM: 1. Urologic Diseases. WJ 100 C6405 1995]
RC871.C597 1995
616.6—dc20
DNLM/DLC
for Library of Congress 94-22583
CIP

ISBN 0-393-71023-8

W.W. Norton & Company, Inc., 500 Fifth Avenue, New York, N.Y. 10110
W.W. Norton & Company Ltd., 10 Coptic Street, London WC1A 1PU

1 2 3 4 5 6 7 8 9 0

# CONTENTS

# CONTRIBUTORS

**Gerald L. Andriole MD**
Associate Professor, Division of Urology, Washington University School of Medicine, St. Louis, MO

**Stephen F. Bardot MD**
Head, Urologic Oncology, Ochsner Clinic, New Orleans, LA

**Mark F. Bellinger MD**
Director of Pediatric Urology, The Children's Hospital of Pittsburgh; Associate Professor of Surgery, The University of Pittsburgh, Pittsburgh, PA

**Ralph C. Benson Jr MD**
Center for Urological Treatment and Research, Nashville, TN

**Richard Bihrle MD**
Associate Professor, Department of Urology, Indiana University School of Medicine, Indianapolis, IN

**William Bihrle III MD**
Senior Staff, Department of Urology, Lahey Clinic Medical Center, Burlington, MA

**David A. Bloom MD**
Chief, Department of Pediatric Urology, Associate Professor, Department of Surgery, University of Michigan Hospitals, Ann Arbor, MI

**George J. Bosl MD**
Genitourinary Oncology Service, Division of Solid Tumor Oncology, Department of Medicine, Memorial Sloan-Kettering Cancer Center, New York, NY

**Reginald C. Bruskewitz MD**
Professor, Department of Surgery, Division of Urology, University of Wisconsin Hospital and Clinics, Madison, WI

**Anthony A. Caldamone MD, FAAP**
Associate Professor of Urology, Brown University School of Medicine; Chief of Pediatric Urology, Rhode Island Hospital, Providence, RI

**Edward W. Campbell Jr MD**
Associate Professor, Division of Urology, The University of Maryland School of Medicine, Baltimore, MD

**Carla D. Chiapella MD**
Department of Urology, Rhode Island Hospital; Division of Urology, Brown University School of Medicine, Providence, RI

**Jong Woo Choe MD**
Division of Urology, The University of Maryland School of Medicine, Baltimore, MD

**E. David Crawford MD**
Professor and Chairman, Division of Urology, University of Colorado Health Sciences Center, Denver, CO

**William J. Cromie MD, FAAP**
Associate Professor of Surgery and of Pediatrics, and Chief, Section of Pediatric Urology, Albany Medical College of Union University, Albany, NY

**John J. Cronan MD**
Associate Director, Department of Diagnostic Imaging, Rhode Island Hospital; Clinical Associate Professor, Department of Radiation Medicine, Radiology, Brown University School of Medicine, Providence, RI

**William C. DeWolf MD**
Urologist-in-Chief, Beth Israel Hospital, Harvard Medical School, Boston, MA

**David A. Diamond MD**
Associate Professor of Urology and Pediatrics, University of Massachusetts Medical Center, Worcester, MA

**John P. Donohue MD**
Distinguished Professor and Chairman, Department of Urology, Indiana University School of Medicine, Indianapolis, IN

**Marlene J. Egger PhD**
Associate Professor, Division of Epidemiology, Biostatistics and Prevention Research, Department of Family and Preventive Medicine and Utah Regional Cancer Center, University of Utah School of Medicine, Salt Lake City, UT

**Brian A. Feagins MD**
Urology Resident, Division of Urology, Department of Surgery, University of Texas Southwestern Medical Center, Southwestern Medical School, Dallas, TX

**Jennifer Fischbach MD**
Radiation Oncology, LDS Hospital; Cottonwood Hospital, Salt Lake City, UT

**Robert C. Flanigan MD**
Professor and Chairman, Department of Urology, Loyola University Medical Center; Chief of Urology, Hines Veteran's Administration Hospital, Maywood, IL

**Richard S. Foster MD**
Assistant Professor, Department of Urology, Indiana University School of Medicine, Indianapolis, IN

**Jackson E. Fowler Jr MD**
Professor and Chairman, Division of Urology, University of Mississippi Medical Center, Jackson, MS

**Kumaresan Ganabathi MD, FRCS**
Fellow in Female Urology and Urodynamics, Kaiser permanente Medical Center, Los Angeles, CA

**John P. Gearhart MD**
Associate Professor, Departments of Pediatric Urology and Pediatrics, The Johns Hopkins University School of Medicine; Director, Division of Pediatric Urology, James Buchanan Brady Urological Institute; Department of Urology, The Johns Hopkins Hospital, Baltimore, MD

**M. David Gibbons MD**
Associate Professor, Departments of Urology and Pediatrics, Georgetown University; Director, Department of Pediatric Urology, Georgetown University Children's Medical Center, Washington, DC

**Bruce R. Gilbert MD, PhD**
Clinical Assistant Professor of Surgery (Urology), The New York Hospital—Cornell Medical Center, New York, NY

**Christopher W. Graham MD**
Chief Resident in Urology, Georgetown University Medical Center, Washington, DC

**Laurence F. Greene MD, PhD***
Clinical Professor of Surgery/Urology, University of California, San Diego, School of Medicine, La Jolla; VA Medical Center, San Diego, CA

**Philip Hanno MD**
Professor and Chairman, Department of Urology, Temple University School of Medicine, Philadelphia, PA

**William C. Hulbert Jr MD, FAAP**
Associate Professor, Departments of Urologic Surgery and Pediatrics, Associate Chief of Pediatric Urology, University of Rochester Medical Center; Associate Chief, Department of Urology, Rochester General Hospital; Chief of Pediatric Urology, University of Rochester Children's Disability Center, Rochester, NY

* Deceased

**Stephen C. Jacobs MD**
Professor and Chairman, Division of Urology, The University of Maryland School of Medicine, Baltimore, MD

**Gerald H. Jordan MD**
Associate Professor, Department of Urology, Eastern Virginia Medical School; Director, Adult Reconstructive Surgery, The Devine Center for Genitourinary Reconstructive Surgery, Sentara Norfolk General Hospital, Norfolk, VA

**Susan M. Jones Kalota MD**
Chief Resident of Surgery/Urology, University of California, San Diego, School of Medicine, San Diego, CA

**Louis R. Kavoussi MD**
Assistant Professor, Division of Urology, Harvard Medical School; Head, Section of Endourology, Brigham and Women's Hospital, Boston, MA

**Michael A. Keating MD**
Assistant Professor of Urology, Indiana University School of Medicine; Attending Pediatric Urologist, The James Whitcomb Riley Hospital for Children, Indianapolis, IN

**A. Richard Kendall MD**
Professor of Urology, Temple University School of Medicine, Philadelphia, PA

**Thomas E. Kingston MD**
Division of Urology, Brown University School of Medicine, Providence, RI

**Michael O. Koch MD**
Associate Professor, Department of Urology, Vanderbilt University Medical Center; Chief, Department of Urology, Nashville Veteran's Affairs Hospital, Nashville, TN

**John N. Krieger MD**
Professor of Urology, University of Washington School of Medicine, Seattle, WA

**Richard F. Labasky MD**
Assistant Professor of Surgery, Division of Urology, University of Utah School of Medicine, Salt Lake City, UT

**Gary E. Leach MD**
Chief of Urology and Director of Urodynamics Laboratory, Kaiser permanente Medical Center; Associate Clinical Professor of Urology, University of California, Los Angeles, CA

**Ronald W. Lewis MD**
Professor, Department of Urology, Mayo School of Medicine; Consultant in Urology, Mayo Clinic, Rochester, MN

**Larry I. Lipshultz MD**
Professor of Urology, Baylor College of Medicine, Houston, TX

**Kevin R. Loughlin MD**
Associate Professor of Urological Surgery, Director, Urological Research, Brigham and Women's Hospital; Division of Urology, Harvard Medical School, Boston, MA

**Leon S. Malmud MD**
Herbert M. Stauffer Professor of Diagnostic Imaging, Temple University Hospital and School of Medicine, Philadelphia, PA

**Michael Malone MD**
Senior Staff, Department of Urology, Lahey Clinic Medical Center, Burlington, MA

**Gianantonio Manzoni MD**
Section of Pediatric Urology, Department of Urology, Regional Hospital of Varese, Varese, Italy

**Alan H. Maurer MD**
Director, Division of Nuclear Medicine, Temple University Hospital and School of Medicine, Philadelphia, PA

**W. Scott McDougal MD**
Chief of Urology, Massachusetts General Hospital; Professor of Urologic Surgery, Harvard Medical School, Boston, MA

**Emilio Merlini MD**
Section of Pediatric Urology, Department of Pediatric Surgery, ''C. Arrigo'' Children's Hospital, Alessandria, Italy

**Robert A. Mevorach MD**
Fellow, Department of Pediatric Urology, University of California, San Francisco, CA

**Lori M. Minasian MD**
Fellow, Genitourinary Oncology Service, Division of Solid Tumor Oncology, Department of Medicine, Memorial Sloan-Kettering Cancer Center, New York, NY

**James E. Montie MD**
Chairman, Department of Urology, Cleveland Clinic, Ft. Lauderdale, FL

**Robert J. Motzer MD**
Assistant Attending Physician, Genitourinary Oncology Service, Division of Solid Tumor Oncology, Department of Medicine, Memorial Sloan-Kettering Cancer Center, New York, NY

**Michael J. Naslund MD**
Assistant Professor, Division of Urology, The University of Maryland School of Medicine, Baltimore, MD

**Andrew C. Novick MD**
Professor and Chairman, Department of Urology and Head, Section of Renal Transplantation, Cleveland Clinic Foundation, Cleveland, OH

**Michael A. O'Donnell MD**
Department of Urology, Beth Israel Hospital, Boston, MA

**C. Lowell Parsons MD**
Professor of Surgery/Urology, University of California, San Diego, School of Medicine, San Diego, CA

**Dennis S. Peppas MD**
Fellow, Department of Pediatric Urology, Instructor, Department of Urology, The Johns Hopkins Hospital, The Johns Hopkins University School of Medicine, Baltimore, MD

**Robert O. Peterson MD, PhD**
Associate Professor, Department of Pathology, Temple University Hospital, Temple University Medical School, Philadelphia, PA

**David M. Pfeffer MD**
Staff Urologist, Culpeper Memorial Hospital, Culpeper, VA; Fauquier Hospital, Warrenton, VA

**Johannes Pohl MD**
Professor of Urology, Klinik und Poliklinik für Urologie, Westfalische Wihelms Universtat, Münster, Germany

**Michel A. Pontari MD**
Assistant Professor of Urology, Department of Urology, Temple University Hospital, Philadelphia, PA

**Glenn M. Preminger MD**
Professor, Department of Urologic Surgery, Duke University Medical Center, Durham, NC

**Ronald Rabinowitz MD, FAAP, FACS**
Professor, Departments of Urologic Surgery and Pediatrics, Associate Co-Chairman, Department of Urology, Chief of Pediatric Urology, University of Rochester Medical Center; Chief, Department of Urology, Rochester General Hospital; Associate Chief of Pediatric Urology, University of Rochester Children's Disability Center, Rochester, NY

**John F. Redman MD**
Professor and Chairman, Department of Urology, University of Arkansas for Medical Sciences, College of Medicine, Little Rock, AR

**Jerome P. Richie MD**
Chief of Urology, Division of Urology, Brigham and Women's Hospital; Harvard Medical School, Boston, MA

**Mark S. Ridlen MD**
Director of General Diagnosis, Department of Diagnostic Imaging, Rhode Island Hospital; Clinical Assistant Professor, Department of Radiation Medicine, Radiology, Brown University School of Medicine, Providence RI

**Robert A. Riehle Jr MD**
Medical Director, Albany Memorial Hospital, Albany, NY

**Randy M. Rockney MD, FAAP**
Assistant Professor, Departments of Pediatrics and Family Medicine, Brown University, Providence; Memorial Hospital of Rhode Island, Pawtucket, RI

**Stephen N. Rous MD**
Professor of Surgery (Urology), Dartmouth Medical School, Lebanon, NH; Section of Urology, Dartmouth-Hitchcock Medical Center; Chief of Urology, Veterans Affairs Medical Center, White River Junction, VT; Adjunct Professor of Urology, Medical University of South Carolina, Charleston, SC

**Randall G. Rowland MD, PhD**
Professor, Department of Urology, Indiana University School of Medicine, Indianapolis, IN

**William T. Sause MD**
Clinical Professor, Department of Radiology, University of Utah; Director, Department of Radiation Therapy, LDS Hospital; Cottonwood Hospital, Salt Lake City, UT

**Howard I. Scher MD**
Genitourinary Oncology Service, Division of Solid Tumor Oncology, Department of Medicine, Memorial Sloan-Kettering Cancer Center, New York, NY

**Carson D. Schneck MD**
Department of Anatomy, Temple University School of Medicine, Philadelphia, PA

**Michael J. Schutz MD**
Assistant Professor of Urology, University of Arkansas for Medical Sciences, Little Rock, AR

**E. James Seidmon MD**
Associate Professor of Urology, Department of Urology, Temple University Hospital, Philadelphia, PA

**Mark Sigman MD**
Assistant Professor, Division of Urology, Brown University School of Medicine, Providence, RI

**Larry T. Sirls MD**
Fellow in Female Urology and Urodynamics, Kaiser permanente Medical Center, Los Angeles, CA

**Joseph A. Smith Jr MD**
Professor and Chairman, Department of Urology, Vanderbilt University School of Medicine, Nashville, TN

**Robert E. Steckler MD**
First Author Fellow, Division of Urology, The Hospital for Sick Children, Toronto, Ontario, Canada

**Barry S. Stein MD**
Professor and Chairman of Urology, Brown University School of Medicine, Providence; Surgeon-in-Chief, Department of Urology, Rhode Island Hospital, Providence, RI

**Raju Thomas MD, FACS**
Associate Chairman for Clinical Affairs, Associate Professor and Chief, Division of Endourology, Lithotripsy and Stone Disease, Tulane University School of Medicine, New Orleans, LA

**E. Darracott Vaughan Jr MD**
James J. Colt Professor of Urology, The New York Hospital—Cornell Medical Center, New York, NY

**Robert E. Vlach Jr MD**
Chief Resident, Department of Surgery, Division of Urology, University of Wisconsin Hospital and Clinics, Madison, WI

**Julian Wan MD**
Assistant Professor, Department of Urology, SUNY—Buffalo, Children's Hospital of Buffalo, Buffalo, NY

**Christopher Ying MD**
Department of Nephrology, Lahey Clinic Medical Center, Burlington, MA

**August Zabbo MD**
Chief, Section of Urology, Department of Veteran's Affairs Medical Center; Assistant Professor, Division of Urology, Brown University School of Medicine; Department of Urology, Rhode Island Hospital, Providence, RI

**Philippe E. Zimmern MD, FACS**
Staff Urologist and Codirector of the Urodynamics Laboratory, Kaiser permanente Medical Center; Assistant Clinical Professor of Urology, University of California, Los Angeles, CA

# PREFACE

In a crowded field, why should there be another hardcover textbook of urology? We have created this new book, *Clinical Urologic Practice*, in the expectation that busy residents and practicing physicians, whether urologists or not, need a convenient but complete reference covering the entire sweep of the profession, packaged in one volume.

To this end we have the usual chapters on anatomy and physiology, current imaging technologies, infectious diseases, problems of the genito-urinary tract, carcinomas of the prostate and other regions, medical and surgical therapies, and pediatric urology. We should point out some of the more innovative chapters to be found in *Clinical Urologic Practice*, those for instance on "Molecular Biology of Urologic Cancer," "Laparoscopic Urologic Surgery," and "Biostatistical Concepts." We should also mention what is *not* to be found: lengthy descriptions of actual surgical procedures, which are ever-changing and better relegated to the many available atlases. Clinical relevance has been the watchword of this project from its inception. Our fifty-seven contributing authors are all experts in their assigned topics. They have made sure to provide the most up-to-date coverage, including very recent literature references, of just the information the busy urologist needs, no more, no less.

## The History of Clinical Urologic Practice

The field of urology has moved as fast as any area of medicine in recent years, with new methods of diagnosis and treatment being discovered at a rapid pace. An attempt to keep up with the explosion of information in urology was made for many years by Drs. Richard Kendall and Lester Karafin, editors of *Goldsmith's Practice of Surgery* looseleaf urology volumes. After Norton Medical Books took over publication of the looseleafs, retitling them *Practice of Urology*, a major effort was mounted to revise and replace the chapters we inherited. Within three years three quarters of the material was new or updated, and that work has not been wasted. Today the rest of the chapters have been revamped to meet the needs of the late 1990s, and *Clinical Urologic Practice* can take its rightful place as the authoritative urological reference for residents and practicing urologists.

## Currency and Completeness

With the revisions and replacements of the last batch of chapters, they now average under two years old. Our intention is to continue the active revision process, reviewing each topic and commissioning new authors and new chapters as necessary to maintain the freshness of the references and the currency of the clinical insights. At the same time, we intend to maintain the balance between comprehensive breadth and adequate depth of the subject. Only you the reader can tell us whether we have succeeded.

Barry S. Stein, MD
Anthony A. Caldamone, MD
Joseph A. Smith, Jr., MD
November 1994

# Clinical Urologic Practice

# 1

# Surgical Anatomy of the Upper Genitourinary Tract

*Barry S. Stein, Carson Schneck, and A. Richard Kendall*

## ABDOMINAL WALL MUSCULATURE

### ANTEROLATERAL ABDOMINAL WALL

The most superficial of the 3 layers of the anterolateral abdominal wall muscles is the external abdominal oblique (Fig. 1). Its origin is from the lower eight ribs, and its aponeurotic insertion is medially into the linea alba by way of the rectus sheath and inferiorly into the pubis and anterior half of the iliac crest. The fibers of the external oblique are directed medially and downward. Below the line of the umbilicus and anterior superior iliac spine, the muscle continues as an aponeurosis, which turns under inferiorly to form the inguinal (Poupart's) ligament.

The internal oblique is the middle of the three layers and takes origin from the lumbodorsal (thoracolumbar) fascia, iliac crest, and inguinal ligament. It is directed upward and medially to the lower ribs (T10–T12), and to the rectus sheath, as well as downward toward the pubic crest.

The innermost layer, the transversus abdominis, takes origin from the iliac fascia, inguinal ligament, iliac crest, lumbodorsal fascia, and from the lower six costal cartilages. The direction of the fibers is horizontal. The insertion ends in an aponeurosis, which fuses with the rectus sheath.

Deep to the transversus abdominis muscle, is the transversalis fascia, which functions as the inner fascia of the abdominal wall and fuses with the iliac fascia, diaphragmatic fascia, and parietal pelvic fascia.

The rectus abdominis muscles are paired midline abdominal muscles, taking origin from the xiphoid process and the costal cartilages of the fifth to seventh ribs. They insert on the pubic crest and symphysis pubis. Each is contained within the strong rectus sheath, formed anteriorly in part by the aponeurosis of the external oblique. Above the arcuate line (linea semicircularis), the internal oblique sends fibers to both the anterior and posterior rectus sheath. The aponeurosis of the transversus abdominis and transversalis fascia contribute to the posterior rectus sheath. Below the arcuate line all three aponeuroses form the anterior sheath, and the posterior sheath is formed strictly by the transversalis fascia.

The pyramidalis muscle, when pres-

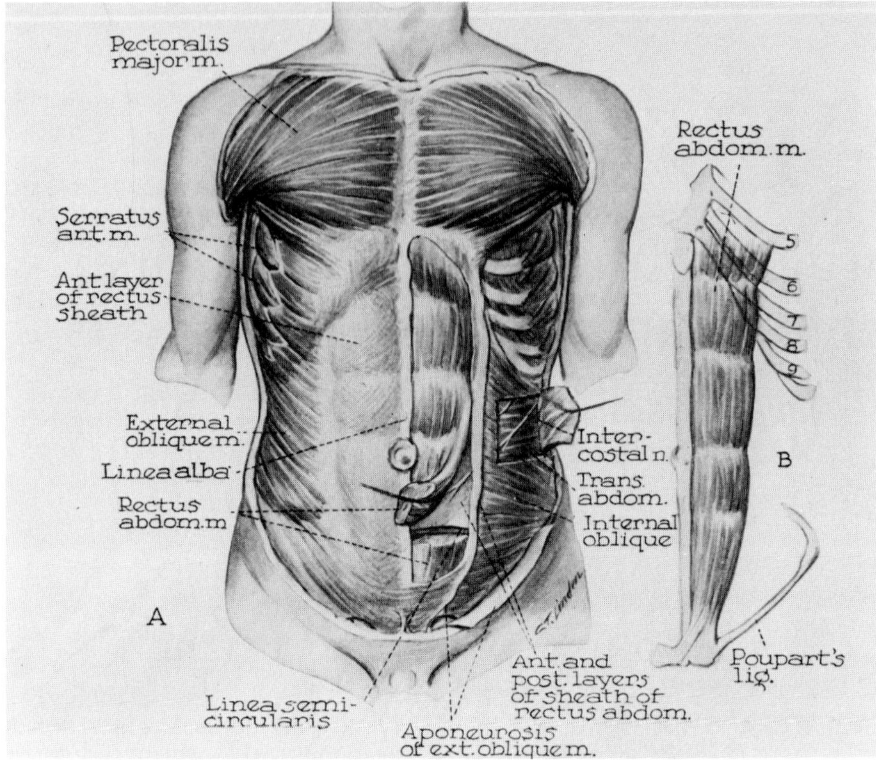


**Fig. 1.** Anterolateral abdominal wall muscular relationships. (Thorek P: Anatomy in Surgery, 2nd ed. Philadelphia, JB Lippincott, 1962)

ent, is triangular in shape and lies anterior to the rectus muscles in their pelvic portion.

## POSTEROLATERAL ABDOMINAL WALL MUSCULATURE

The latissimus dorsi along with the external oblique forms the most superficial muscle layers in the flank (Figs. 2 and 3). Latissimus dorsi takes origin from the seventh to twelfth thoracic vertebrae, the lumbar, and sacral spinous processes as well as the supraspinous ligament. It inserts on the floor of the intertubercular sulcus of the humerus.

The lumbar triangle of Petit (lumbar trigone) is the area bounded by the external oblique, latissimus dorsi, and iliac crest. In this area, the abdominal wall is relatively thin since it is only formed by the aponeuroses of origin of the internal oblique and transversus abdominis muscles and the transversalis fascia. Hence this is an area of potential hernia and a region where blood or purulent material originating in the retroperitoneal region can most readily track to the surface.

The intermediate muscle group of the flank consists of serratus posterior inferior, the internal oblique, and the sacrospinalis (erector spinae) muscles. Serratus posterior inferior lies deep to latissimus dorsi and takes origin from the lower thoracic and upper lumbar vertebrae. Its insertion is to the lower four ribs. Sacrospinalis is an extensive muscle group taking origin at the sacrum and ilium, extending toward the head with intermediate attachments to the ribs and vertebrae. The sacrospinalis is enclosed by the lumbodorsal fascia, which is converted to an aponeurosis by the attachments of the latissimus dorsi, internal oblique, and transversus abdominis muscles. This fascia has a posterior layer

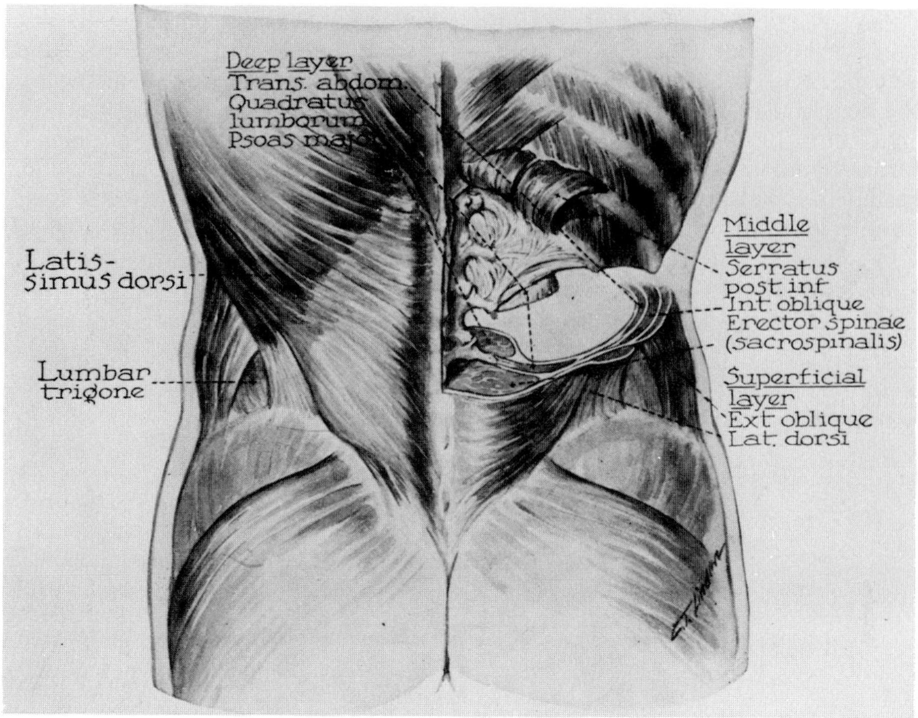


**Fig. 2.** Posterolateral abdominal wall muscular relationships. (Thorek P: Anatomy in Surgery, 2nd ed. Philadelphia, JB Lippincott, 1962)

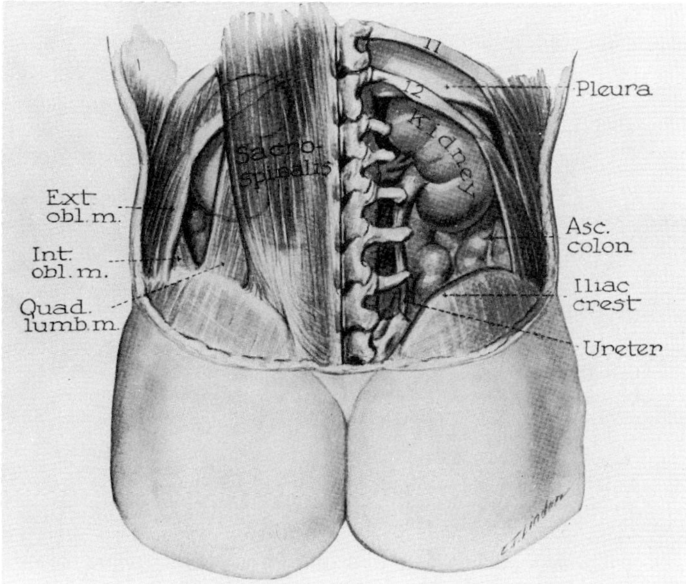


**Fig. 3.** Posterolateral muscular relationships—deep muscles. (Thorek P: Anatomy in Surgery, 2nd ed. Philadelphia, JB Lippincott, 1962)

attaching to the spinous processes and an anterior layer attaching to the transverse processes of the lumbar vertebrae.

The deep muscles of the flank consist of quadratus lumborum, psoas major, and transversus abdominis (Figs. 18, 25, 32, and 33). Quadratus lumborum takes its origin from the iliac crest and the lower lumbar transverse processes, and inserts on the inferior aspect of the 12th rib and upper lumbar transverse processes. It is bounded posteriorly by the anterior layer of the lumbodorsal fascia, which attaches to the transverse processes of the lumbar vertebrae and anteriorly by the continuation of the

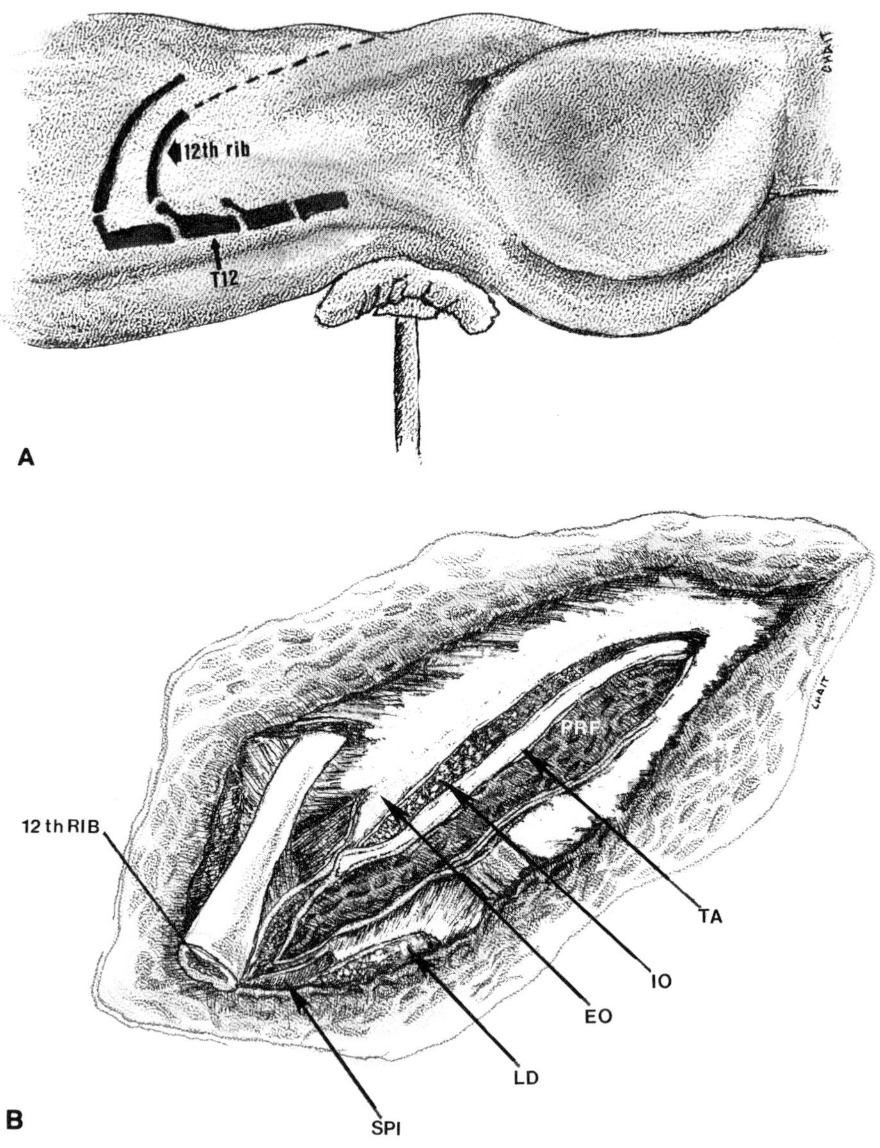


**Fig. 4A.** Incision (*interrupted line*) for 12th rib extraperitoneal approach to the kidney. **B.** Muscular relationships underlying this approach. The 12th rib has been resected. *PRF*, pararenal fascia. *TA*, transversus abdominis muscle. *IO*, internal oblique muscle. *EO*, external oblique muscle. *LD*, latissimus dorsi. *SPI*, serratus posterior inferior. (After Cockett ATK, Kushiba K: Manual of Urologic Surgery. New York, Springer–Verlag, 1979)

transversalis fascia over the quadratus lumborum and psoas major muscles. The psoas major takes origin from the lumbar vertebrae, and inserts on the lesser trochanter of the femur.

## SKIN INCISIONS

Figure 4*A* shows the location of the skin incision for the flank, extrapleural twelfth rib approach. In Figure 4*B* the relationship of the above-described abdominal muscles to the incision is depicted. Note the relationship of the anterior abdominal wall muscles (external oblique, internal oblique, and transversus) to serratus posterior inferior and latissimus dorsi. The lumbodor-

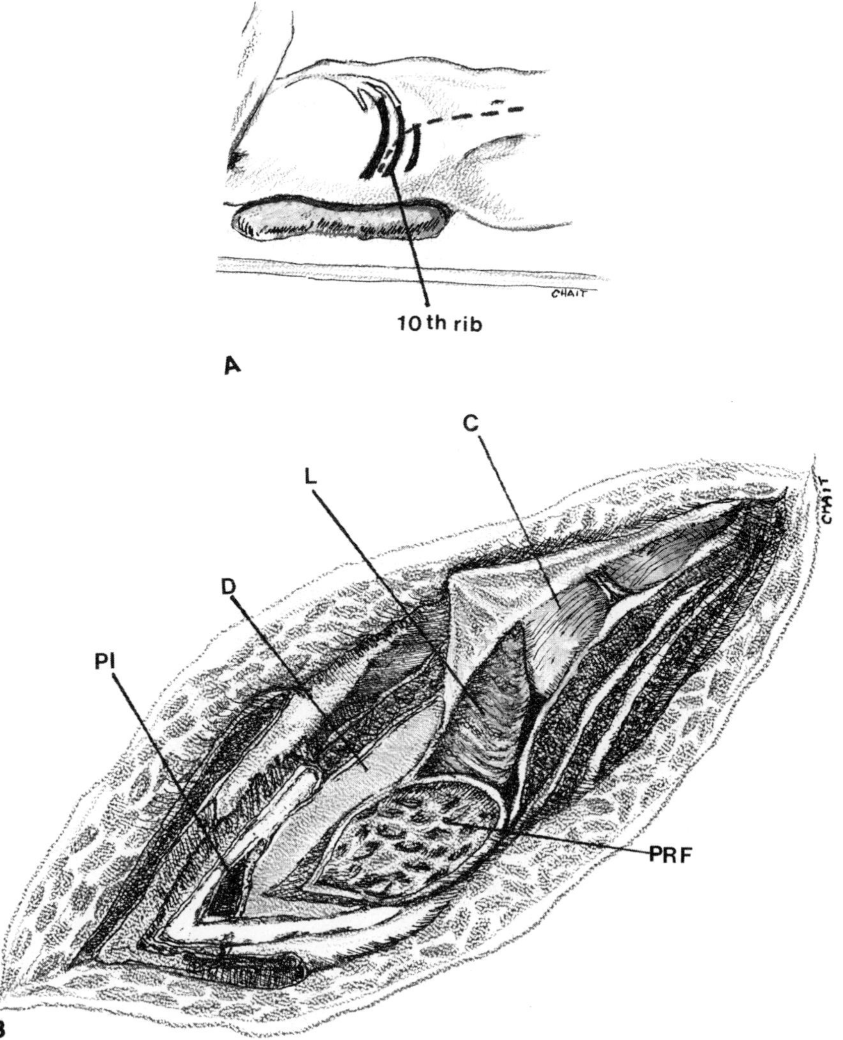


**Fig. 5A.** Skin incision (*interrupted line*) for thoracoabdominal approach. **B.** Muscular and peritoneal relationships underlying incision for thoracoabdominal approach. *PRF*, pararenal fascia. *Pl*, pleura. *D*, diaphragm. *L*, liver. *C*, colon. (After Cockett ATK, Kushiba K: Manual of Urologic Surgery. New York, Springer–Verlag, 1979)

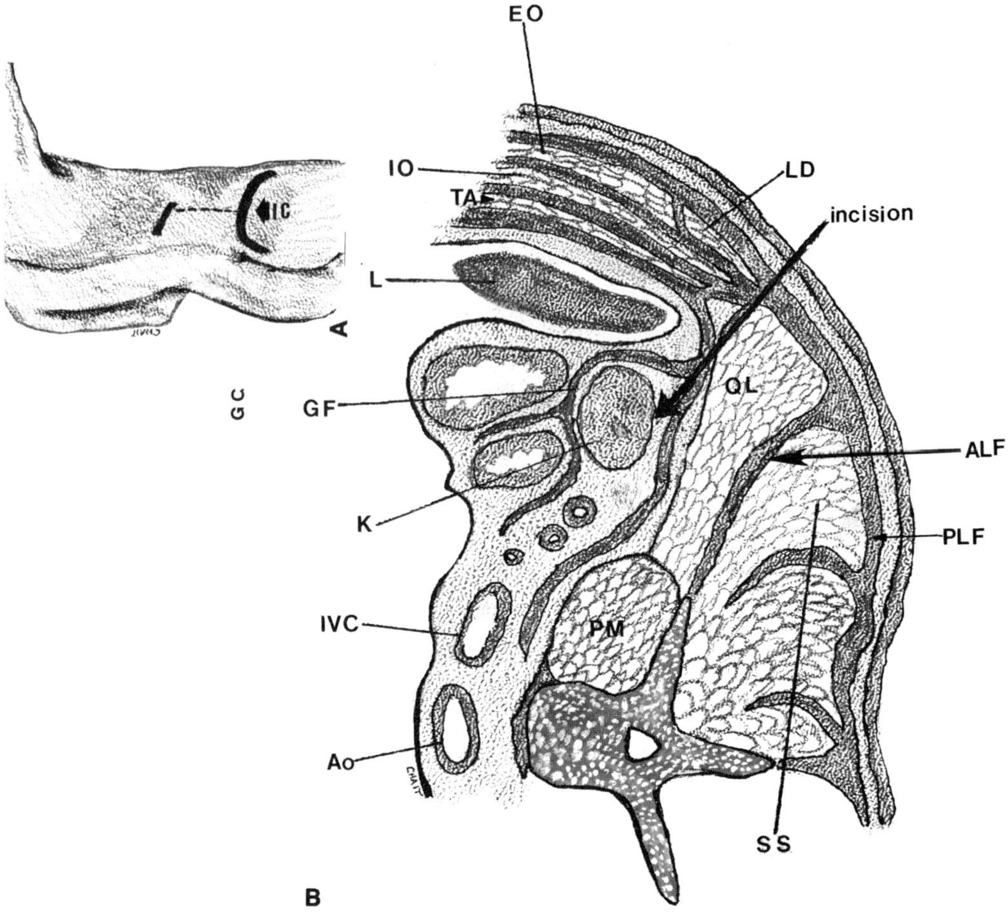

**Fig. 6A.** Skin incision (*interrupted line*) for posterior approach to the kidney. **B.** Muscular relationships encountered in this approach. *ALF*, anterior layer of lumbodorsal fascia. *PLF*, posterior layer of lumbodorsal fascia. *SS*, sacrospinalis muscle. *QL*, quadratus lumborum muscle. *PM*, psoas major muscle. *LD*, latissimus dorsi muscle. *EO*, external oblique muscle. *IO*, internal oblique muscle. *TA*, transversus abdominis muscle. *L*, liver. *GF*, Gerota's fascia. *K*, kidney. *IVC*, inferior vena cava. *Ao*, aorta. (After Cockett ATK, Kushiba K: Manual of Urologic Surgery. New York, Springer–Verlag, 1979)

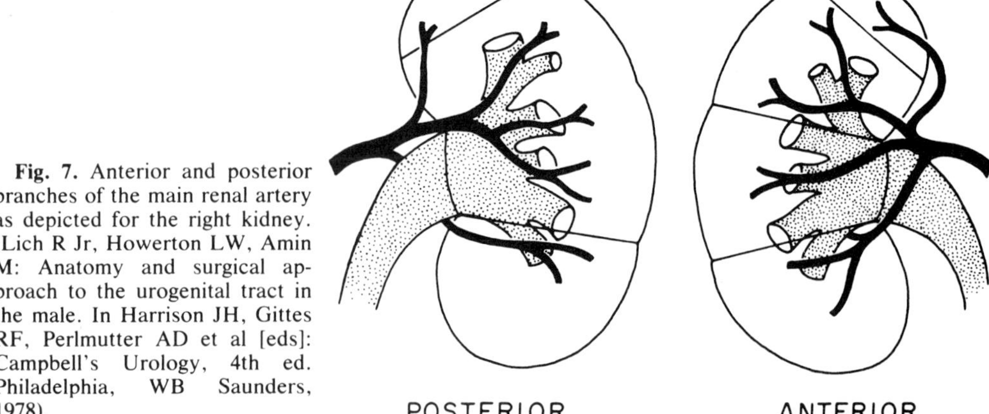


**Fig. 7.** Anterior and posterior branches of the main renal artery as depicted for the right kidney. (Lich R Jr, Howerton LW, Amin M: Anatomy and surgical approach to the urogenital tract in the male. In Harrison JH, Gittes RF, Perlmutter AD et al [eds]: Campbell's Urology, 4th ed. Philadelphia, WB Saunders, 1978).

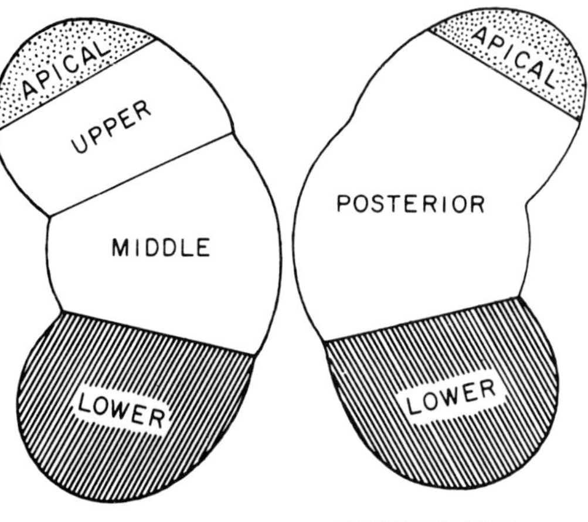


**Fig. 8.** Areas of the kidney supplied by the branches of the main renal artery as depicted for the left kidney. (Lich R Jr, Howerton LW, Amin M: Anatomy and surgical approach to the urogenital tract in the male. In Harrison JH, Gittes RF, Perlmutter AD et al [eds]: Campbell's Urology, 4th ed. Philadelphia, WB Saunders, 1978)

sal fascia has been incised, and the pararenal fat can be seen. The standard flank incision would reveal the identical muscle pattern.

The thoracicoabdominal approach, with the skin incision between the ninth and tenth ribs is shown in Figure 5*A*. The relationship of the anterior abdominal muscles, flank muscles, pleura, and peritoneal contents can be seen in Figure 5*B*.

The posterior approach may be useful for pretransplant nephrectomy, renal biopsy, and pyelolithotomy. The patient can be placed in the prone or lateral position. The skin incision is depicted in Figure 6*A*. Figure 6*B* shows diagrammatically the method of entry to the retroperitoneal space from this approach.

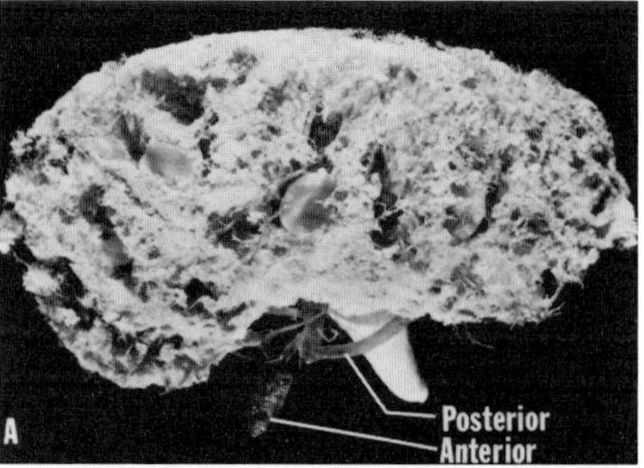


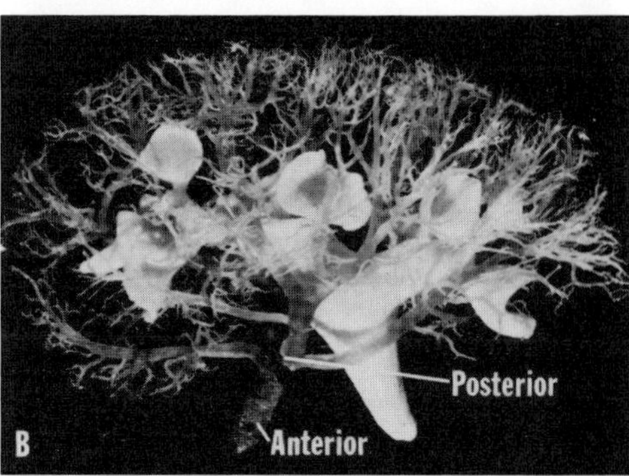


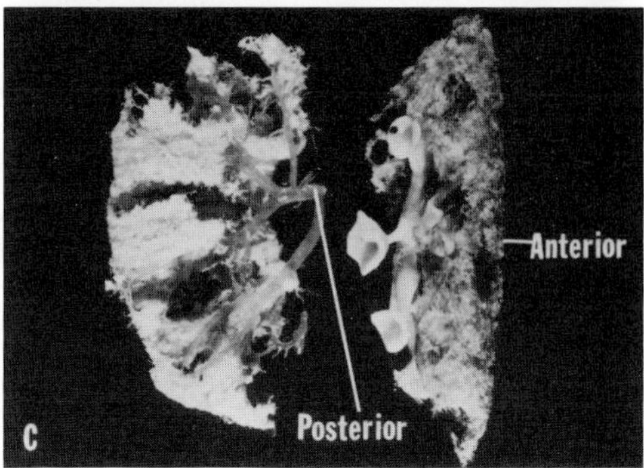


**Fig. 9.** Arterial casts of the renal vasculature depicting the supply from the anterior and posterior branches. (Boyce WH: Renal calculi. In Glenn JF [ed]: Urologic Surgery, 2nd ed. Hagerstown, MD, Harper & Row, 1975)

## RETROPERITONEAL ANATOMY

The anatomical structures of the retroperitoneum are explored closely by using photographs of dissections, followed by cross-sectional and longitudinal sagittal anatomical sections with correlated computed tomography (CT) and sonograms. These pages have been planned as an atlas so that they may be removed from the book and used as a guide to be followed while reading the text. Figure 24 depicts the levels of the cross-sectional anatomy while Figure 31 depicts the levels of the longitudinal sections. Figure 11 is a diagrammatic illustration of the retroperitoneal organs and their relationship to the intraperitoneal organs. This is useful for comparison to the photographs for purposes of orientation.

## ADRENAL GLANDS

The paired adrenal glands are triangular structures weighing 3 g to 6 g each which lie superior and anteromedial to the kidneys. The adrenal glands lie within their own investment of the perirenal fascia. Contrary to their depiction in many texts and atlases, the adrenal glands are more nearly situated in the sagittal plane than the coronal plane (see Figs. 17 and 26). The right adrenal gland is triangular in shape. The inferior aspect of the right adrenal gland lies on the upper pole of the right kidney. Its ante-

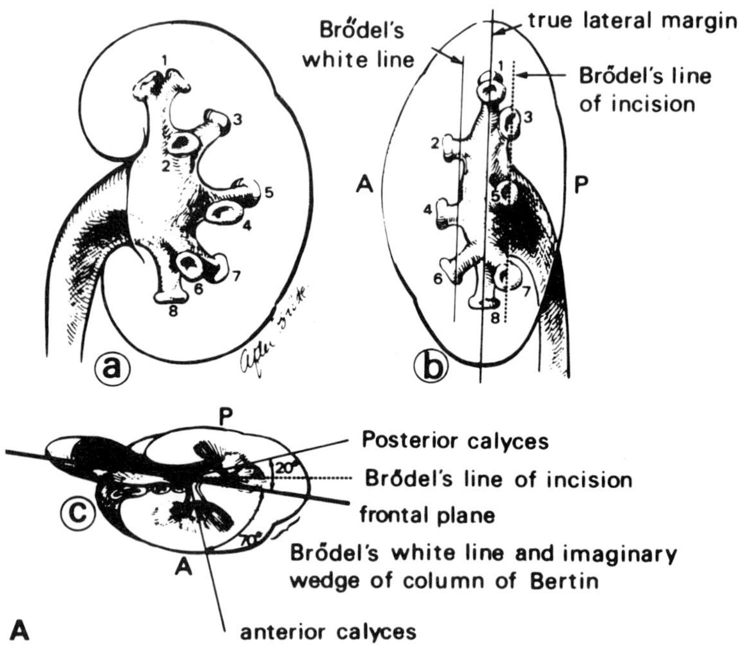


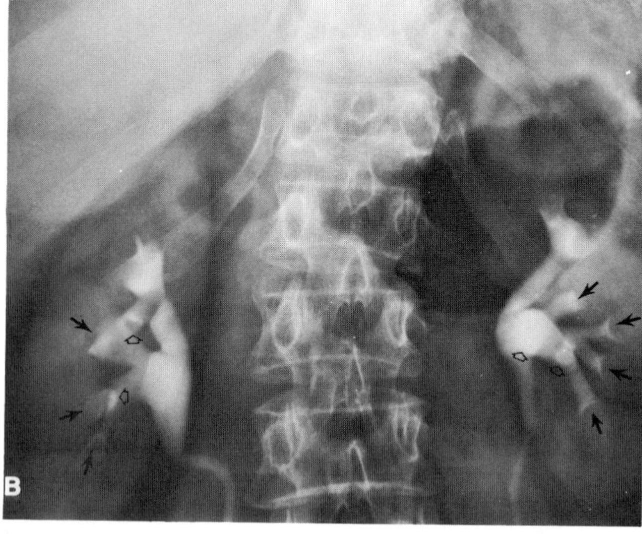


**Fig. 10A.** Left kidney depicting the orientation of the anterior and posterior calyces. (Kaye KW, Goldberg ME: Applied anatomy of the kidney and ureter. Urol Clin North Am 9:3, 1982) **B.** Intravenous urogram demonstrating anterior and posterior calyces. The anterior calyces (*solid arrows*) are seen in the lateral plane while the posterior calyces (*open arrows*) are viewed on end.

rior border is related to the inferior vena cava and its upper pole bounded by the bare edge of the liver and the diaphragm posteriorly. Its lateral surface is covered by the peritoneum and related to the right lobe of the liver, while its medial surface is related to the right crus of the diaphragm (see Figs. 17 and 26). The left adrenal gland is semilunar in shape and typically more related to the anteromedial than the superior aspect of the left kidney, since it is tethered inferiorly by the entry of its vein into the left renal vein (Figs. 20 and 22). The left adrenal gland lies in the posterior wall of the lesser sac (omental bursa). It is crossed on its lateral aspect by the splenic artery and vein and the pancreas, and it is related medially to the left crus of the diaphragm (Figs. 19, 20, 23, 25, 26, and 35). The arterial supply to the adrenal glands may be by way of three networks of arteries, the superior artery arising from the inferior phrenic artery, the middle artery which arises from the aorta directly, and the inferior artery which may branch from the renal artery. The right adrenal vein empties directly into the inferior vena cava (Fig. 17), while the left adrenal vein empties into the renal vein, as described above. The lymphatic drainage is to the para-aortic nodes.

## KIDNEY

The kidneys are bean-shaped paired organs weighing between 90 g and 220 g. The right kidney is usually situated 1 cm to 2 cm caudad to the left because of the large volume of the liver above. The kidneys show three degrees of obliquity which are not widely appreciated. First, their concave, hilar border where the renal vessels and renal pelvis enter and leave is directed anteromedially (Figs. 14, 17, 22, 27, and 28). This is because the kidneys are suspended into the paravertebral gutters by their vascular pedicles. Therefore, they are resting on the oblique side slopes of the midline longitudinal ridgeline of the posterior abdominal wall. This ridgeline is formed by the lumbar spine and psoas major muscles and capped by the aorta and inferior vena cava. Hence, each kidneys' concave hilar border is directed anteromedially, the convex border is situated posterolaterally, and the surfaces face anterolaterally and posteromedially. Second, the inferior pole of each kidney is situated lateral to the superior pole because the psoas major muscle upon which the kidney rests medially increases its mass as it descends (Fig. 12). Finally, the inferior pole is anterior to the superior pole since the musculature of the paravertebral gutters, which forms the kidney bed, forms an inclined plane directed forward about 45° as it is followed downward to the pelvic inlet (Figs. 16, 32, and 33).

The right kidney is bounded superiorly and anteromedially by the right adrenal gland and also superiorly by the right lobe of the liver (Figs. 17, 26, and 32). Below the adrenal gland, it is bounded anteromedially by the inferior vena cava (Figs. 12, 17, and 27). Lateral to the inferior vena cava, the second portion of the duodenum has an intimate relationship with the renal hilus. At lower levels the ascending colon and hepatic flexure contact the anterolateral surface (Figs. 15, 29, and 32). The peritoneum covers the right kidney anteriorly below the right coronary ligament where the right subhepatic space or the hepatorenal pouch of Morrison intervenes between the liver and kidney (Figs. 15, 27, and 32). The muscular bed of the right kidney is composed of the diaphragm superiorly, the psoas major muscle medially, the quadratus lumborum directly posteriorly and the transversus abdominis posterolateral (Figs. 18 and 33). Four nerves run through the right renal fossa: posteriorly, the subcostal, iliohypogastric, and the ilioinguinal nerves, which course over the quadratus lumborum; and medially, the genitofemoral nerve descends along the psoas major. The iliohypogastric and ilioinguinal nerves may be conjoined until they reach the level of the true pelvis. Three of these are visualized in Figure 18.

The left kidney lies higher than does the right. Above the renal vessels, the left kidney is bounded anteromedially by the left adrenal gland (Figs. 21, 22, and 25). The upper part of the left kidney's anterolateral surface is usually related medially to the splenic artery and vein and the pancreatic body and tail and laterally to the spleen (Figs. 19, 20, 25, 26, and 36). The lower part of its anterolateral surface is covered by the splenic flexure of the colon and the descending colon laterally, and the aorta and fourth part of the duodenum medially (Figs. 19, 20, 27, 28, and 36). Posteriorly, the muscular bed of the left renal fossa is similar to that of the right (Figs. 23, 28, and 36).

Both kidneys are covered by a strong fibrous capsule, which is surrounded by the perirenal fat. The perirenal fat is invested by a double fascial layer known as the *renal (Gerota's) fascia*. This fascia is weak in its anterior half, but strong posteriorly. It extends cranially from the area of the diaphragm, inferiorly to the true pelvis. The leaves fuse laterally, the posterior leaf extends medially to join with the ligaments of the vertebral column while the anterior sheath extends medially to the great vessels. The left and right renal fasciae do not meet. The adrenal gland is bounded inferiorly by its own sheath of fascia so that it has its own separate investment. The fat outside the renal fascia is known as the pararenal fat. The right anterior pararenal space is bounded anteriorly by the posterior leaf of the peritoneum and posteriorly by the anterior leaf of the renal fascia. This space on the right side contains the second part of the duodenum, head of the pancreas, and right hepatic flexure of the colon (Figs. 27, 28, and 29). The left anterior pararenal space includes the pancreatic body and tail, the splenic flexure of the colon, and the descending colon (Fig. 26). The posterior pararenal spaces lie between the posterior renal fascia anteriorly and the transversalis fascia posteriorly. This space normally contains only fat and may expand to accommodate fluid or purulent drainage.

The renal arteries, usually singular in number to each side, arise directly from the aorta just caudad to the superior mesenteric artery. The right renal artery either arises inferior to the left or passes in an inferior direction following its take off from the aorta. In approximately 25% of the population, accessary renal arteries each arising from the aorta may exist (Fig. 21). These may arise anywhere from the aorta and on occasion have been reported as arising from iliac arteries. The main renal artery divides shortly after exiting the aorta into an anterior and posterior branch. The anterior branch immediately subdivides into four branches that supply the apical, upper, middle, and lower segments of the kidney (Figs. 7 and 8). The posterior branch courses posterior to the renal pelvis and supplies the posterior segment of the kidney. The anterior branches supply the entire anterior surface of the kidney and wrap around to supply approximately 1 cm of the lateral aspect of the posterior surface of the kidney. This area between the supply of the anterior and posterior branches is the avascular plane of the kidney, utilized for anatrophic nephrolithotomy (Fig. 9).

The right renal artery passes posterior to the inferior vena cava en route to the right kidney (Figs. 17, 27, and 34). Posterior to the right renal artery are the psoas major muscle, right crus of the diaphragm, and right sympathetic chain. Anterior to the right renal artery is the inferior vena cava and right renal vein. The duodenum and pancreatic head commonly also overlie the right renal artery. The left renal artery is shorter than the right and courses posterior to the left renal vein. It is bounded posteriorly by the left crus of the diaphragm, left psoas major muscle, and left sympathetic trunk (Figs. 19, 21, and 35). The body and tail of the pancreas and splenic artery and vein may also overlie the left renal artery (Figs. 20 and 35).

The right renal vein, owing to its kidney's proximity to the inferior vena cava, is shorter than the left and generally has no collateral vessels emptying directly into it (Figs. 12, 13, 17, 28, and 33). The right gonadal and adrenal veins enter directly into the inferior vena cava

(Figs. 12 and 17). The left renal vein, longer than the right, passes posterior to the superior mesenteric artery and anterior to the aorta (Figs. 12, 13, 20, 21, 27, and 35). This forms the so-called *nutcracker* effect on the left renal vein. The left adrenal and gonadal veins empty directly into the left renal vein (Figs. 12, 13, 20, and 22). The adrenal vein may empty either proximally or distally to the entry of the gonadal vein. In some cases, an anomalous lumbar vein may empty directly into the left renal vein or into the gonadal vein just before it drains into the left renal vein. This may cause troublesome bleeding if it is avulsed (Figs. 13 and 22).

The lymphatic drainage of the kidneys is to their respective para-aortic locations. Due to the embryologic origin of the testes, the drainage of the testes is to the para-aortic region and the area between the great vessels (Fig. 14).

The sympathetic nerves that control ejaculation take origin from the ventral nerve roots of T-11 through L-1. They course down the lateral aspects of the great vessels to form the hypogastric nerves. Damage to these nerves during retroperitoneal lymphadenectomy will lead to a lack of ejaculation (Figs. 15 and 20).

## THE UPPER COLLECTING SYSTEM

The collecting tubules enter by way of the renal pyramid into the calices. The number of calices in a normal kidney varies greatly, but there are generally six to eight. One or more calices may drain into an infundibulum that leads to the renal pelvis. The calices are divided into two main groups, those directed anteriorly and those directed posteriorly. There is a 90° difference in the plane formed by the anterior and posterior calices. Brodel's line of incision for anatrophic nephrolithotomy passes through the plane composed of the posterior calices (Fig. 10A). Since the kidney is suspended by its vasculature in the renal fossa, as previously described, a coronal plane of the body is not a true coronal plane of the kidney and its collecting system. Relative to the coronal plane of the body, the anterior calices would appear to be directed laterally, while the posterior calices would point directly posterior. Thus, on an intravenous urogram (Fig. 10B) the anterior calices would appear to be extending laterally while the posterior calices would be seen on end.

The renal pelvis exits the hilus of the kidney posterior to the renal arteries and veins (Figs. 13, 14, and 22). The pelvis tapers to form the ureter, which courses medially to lie on the psoas major muscle. The ureter then courses directly inferiorly to the true pelvis, passing posterior to the gonadal artery and vein, but crossing anterior to the iliac artery and vein (Figs. 12, 14, 17, and 30). There are three areas of physiologic narrowing of the ureter, the first at the level of the uteropelvic junction, the second where the ureter crosses anterior to the bifurcation of the common iliac vessels, and the third where the ureter courses through the muscular wall of the bladder.

The ureteral arteries originate from the renal, gonadal, and inferior vesical arteries, which have extensive anastomosing branches over the course of the ureter. The venous drainage parallels the arterial supply, while the lymphatic drainage to the upper ureter is to the aortic and para-aortic nodes, similar to those draining the kidney.

The authors gratefully acknowledge Churhill Livingstone Inc. for its permission to use figures that appeared in Ultrasound in Inflammatory Disease, edited by Joseph AE, Cosgrove DO, volume 11 in Clinics in Diagnostic Ultrasound.

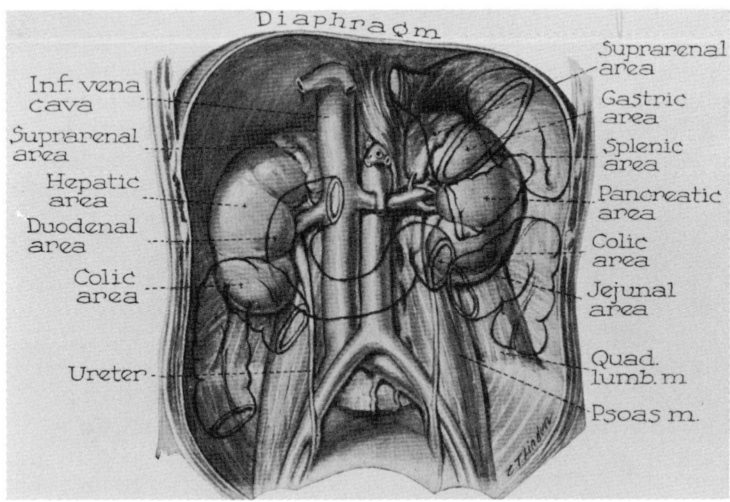


**Fig. 11.** Diagram of the relationships of the retroperitoneal and intraperitoneal structures. (Thorek P: Anatomy in Surgery, 2nd ed. Philadelphia, JB Lippincott, 1962)

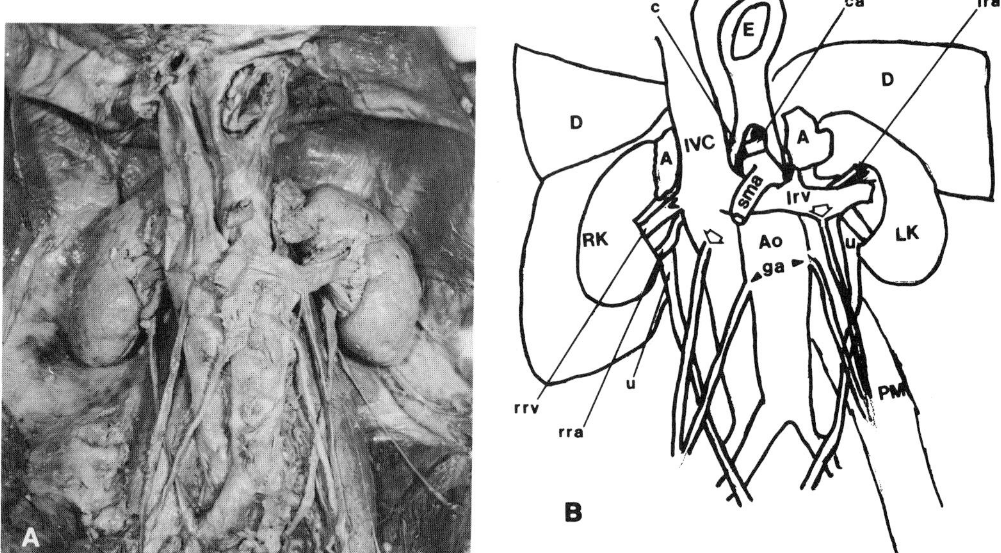


**Fig. 12A,B.** This dissection and the line drawing of the posterior retroperitoneal space depict the relationship of the kidneys (*RK*, *LK*) and adrenals (*A*) to the aorta (*Ao*) and the inferior vena cava (*IVC*). Both left and right renal arteries (*lra*, *rra*) and veins (*lrv*, *rrv*) are well visualized. Both gonadal arteries (*ga*) are seen, as are both gonadal veins (*open arrows*). The ureters (*u*) cross posterior to the gonadal vessels and anterior to the iliac vessels. The left renal vein (*lrv*) can be clearly seen crossing between the superior mesenteric artery (*sma*) and the aorta. The crura (*c*) of the diaphragm (*D*) can be seen just cranially to the celiac axis (*ca*) and pass posterior to lie under the renal arteries.

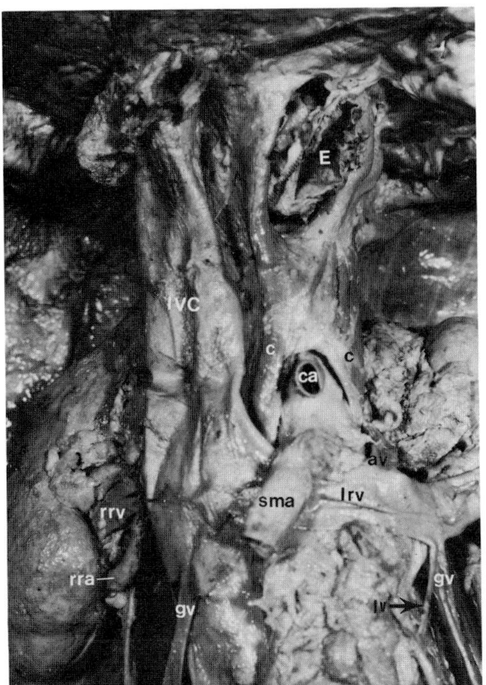


**Fig. 13.** Closer view of the great vessels at the level of the dissection identical to that shown in Figure 12. The right (*rrv*) and left renal vein (*lrv*) can be seen exiting the inferior vena cava (*IVC*), and the branches of the left renal vein are well depicted. The first branch is the adrenal vein (*av*) followed by the gonadal vein (*gv*). An anomalous lumbar vein (*lv*) can be seen joining with the gonadal vein just prior to its entry into the left renal vein. The right gonadal vein can be seen entering the inferior vena cava directly. The esophagus (*E*) is noted superiorly. The superior mesenteric artery (*sma*) is also shown.

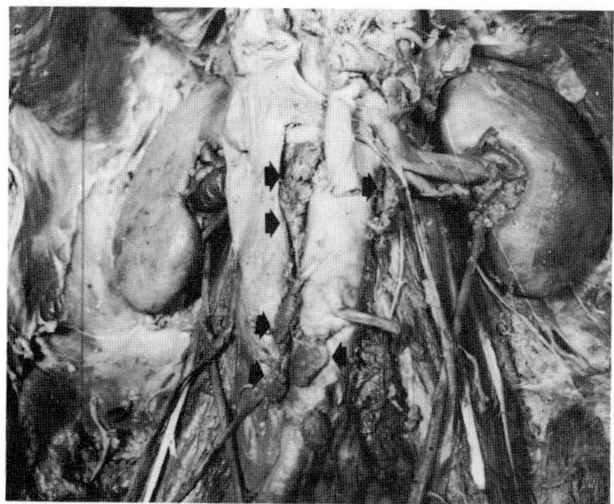

**Fig. 14.** In this specimen the lymphatic drainage is well seen. Arrows point to enlarged lymph nodes between the aorta and inferior vena cava, as well as in the left para-aortic region.

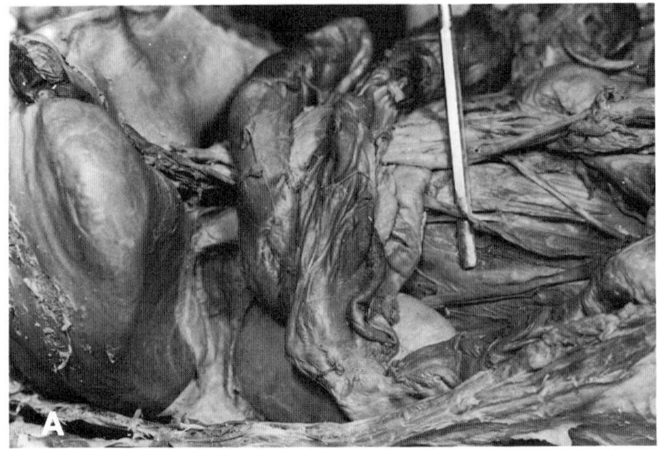


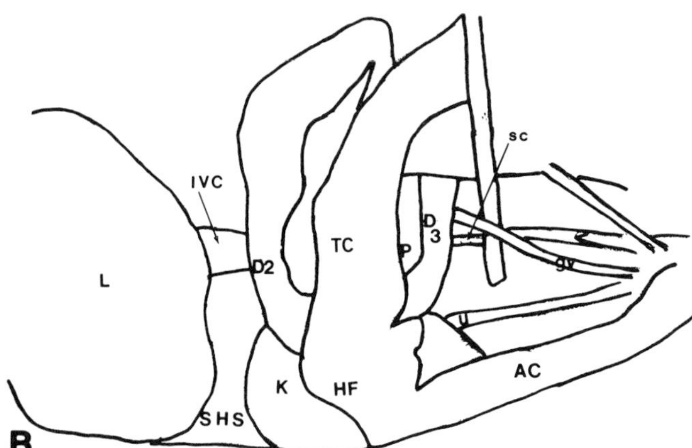


**Fig. 15A, B.** Relationships in the right renal fossa. The right lobe of the liver (*L*) and the coronary ligament bounding the right subhepatic space (pouch of Morrison, labeled *SHS*) is seen. The second part of the duodenum (*D2*) and the head of the pancreas (*P*) can be seen draping over the anteromedial aspect of the kidney (*K*), while the hepatic flexure (*HF*) can be seen overlying the superior aspect of the lower pole of the kidney. The probe is under the gonadal vein (*gv*) and above the sympathetic chain (*sc*) on the right side which can be seen lying deep to the probe. Also shown are ureter (*u*), the third part of the duodenum (*D3*), the ascending colon (*AC*), the transverse colon (*TC*), and inferior venacava (IVC).

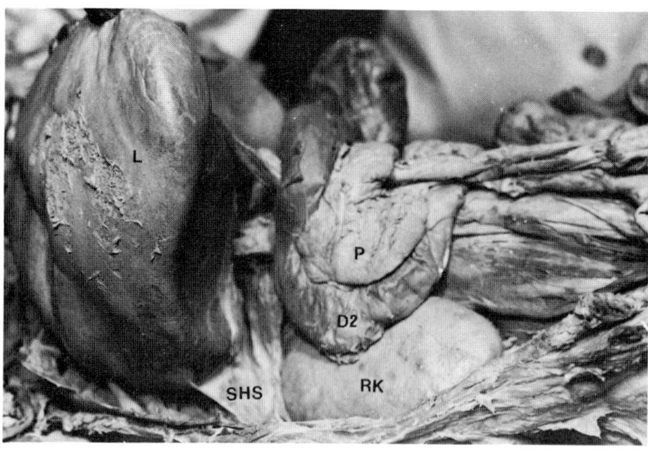


**Fig. 16.** In this figure, the right colon has been reflected. This affords a better view of the right subhepatic space (*SHS*) and the relationship of the second part of the duodenum (*D2*) and the head of the pancreas (*P*) to the right kidney (*RK*). The liver (*L*) is also shown.

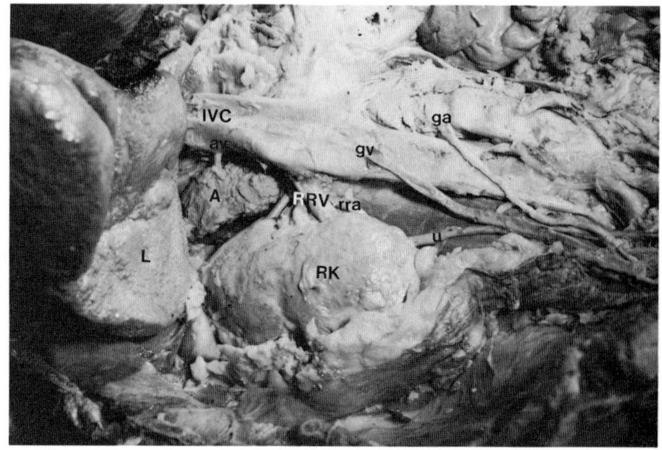


**Fig. 17.** All intestine has been reflected. The adrenal (*A*) can be seen lying in the sagittal plane suspended by the adrenal vein (*av*), which drains directly into the inferior vena cava (*IVC*). As seen, it lies in a superomedial location relative to the right kidney (*RK*). The right kidney can be seen to have an anteromedial and posterolateral border as it hugs the right paravertebral gutter suspended by its vascular pedicle. The lower pole of the right kidney can be seen lying anterior to the upper pole owing to the incline of the paravertebral musculature. The relationships of the renal vessels (*RRV*, *rra*) are well demonstrated, and the right gonadal artery (*ga*) and vein (*gv*) can be seen coursing over the right ureter (*u*). *L* is the liver.

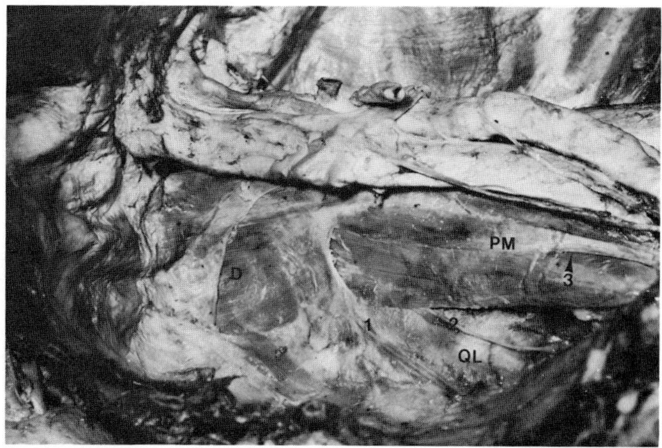


**Fig. 18.** The right renal fossa with all contents except the great vessels removed. The diaphragm (*D*) can be seen in the superior aspect of the renal fossa, while the psoas major (*PM*) constitutes its medial aspect. The quadratus lumborum (*QL*) extends posterior and lateral. While the transversus abdominis is not demonstrated in this figure, it forms the posterolateral wall of the right renal fossa. The subcostal nerve (*1*), the conjoined ilioinguinal and iliohypogastric nerves (*2*), and the right genitofemoral nerve (*3*) are seen.

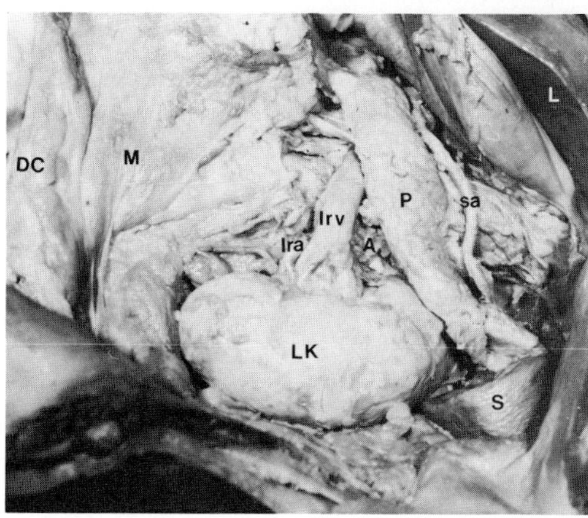


**Fig. 19.** In this view of the left renal fossa, the descending colon (*DC*) and its mesentery (*M*) have been retracted. The relationships of the left kidney (*LK*) to the adrenal (*A*) and a high tail of the pancreas (*P*), and spleen (*S*) are well seen. The left edge of the liver (*L*) can be seen in the top of the figure. The left renal artery (*lra*) can be seen lying posterior to the left renal vein (*lrv*). The splenic artery (*sa*) is also seen.

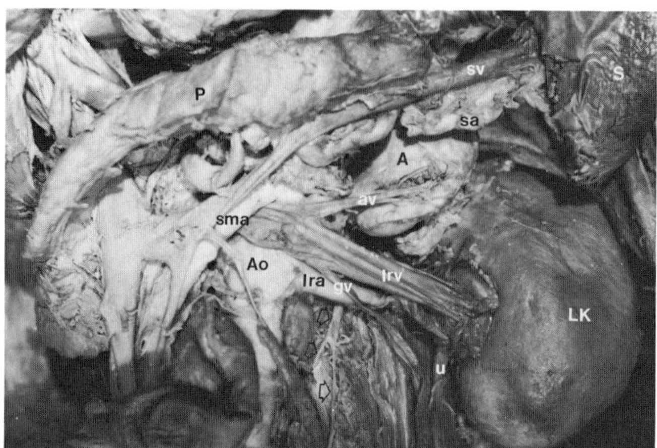


**Fig. 20.** The pancreas (*P*) has been elevated to demonstrate the relationships of the splenic vessels to the left retroperitoneal space. The splenic artery (*sa*) can be seen overlying the superior aspect of the left adrenal gland (*A*) and the upper pole of the left kidney (*LK*). The adrenal vein (*av*) and gonadal vein (*gv*) can be seen clearly branching from the left renal vein (*lrv*). The left renal artery (*lra*) can be seen lying just inferior to the renal vein. The left renal vein courses between the aorta (*Ao*) and superior mesenteric artery (*sma*) as shown, creating the "nutcracker" effect. The arrows point to the sympathetic chain as it courses posterior to the left renal artery.

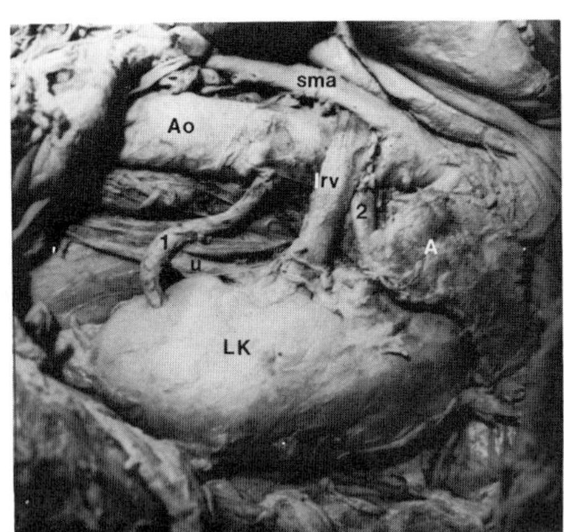


**Fig. 21.** In this figure, two renal arteries are present. The lower artery (*1*) supplies the basilar lower segment of the left kidney, while the main renal artery (*2*) supplies the remainder of the kidney. From a more lateral aspect, the "nutcracker" effect on the left renal vein (*lrv*) is again seen. (See previous figures for explanation of other labels.)

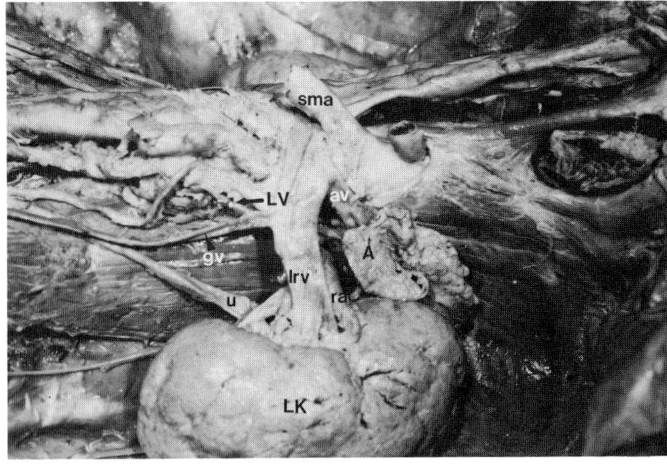


**Fig. 22.** In this section with intestine, pancreas, and spleen removed, the relationships of the left kidney (*LK*) and its vasculature are well depicted. The gonadal vein (*gv*) and adrenal vein (*av*) can be seen entering the left renal vein (*lrv*). In this case, an anomalous lumbar vein (*LV*, *arrow*) joins the gonadal vein just prior to its entering the renal vein. The ureter (*u*) can be seen lying posterior to the gonadal vein. The renal artery (*ra*) is shown.

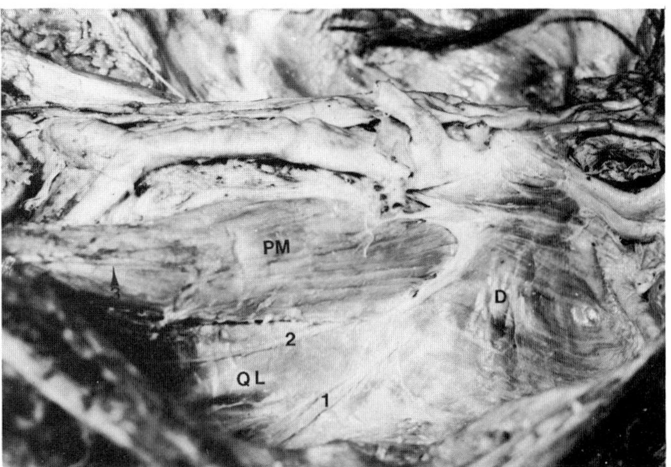


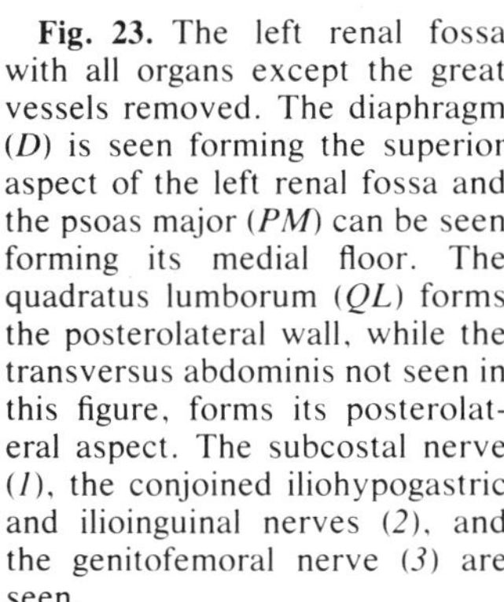
**Fig. 23.** The left renal fossa with all organs except the great vessels removed. The diaphragm (*D*) is seen forming the superior aspect of the left renal fossa and the psoas major (*PM*) can be seen forming its medial floor. The quadratus lumborum (*QL*) forms the posterolateral wall, while the transversus abdominis not seen in this figure, forms its posterolateral aspect. The subcostal nerve (*1*), the conjoined iliohypogastric and ilioinguinal nerves (*2*), and the genitofemoral nerve (*3*) are seen.

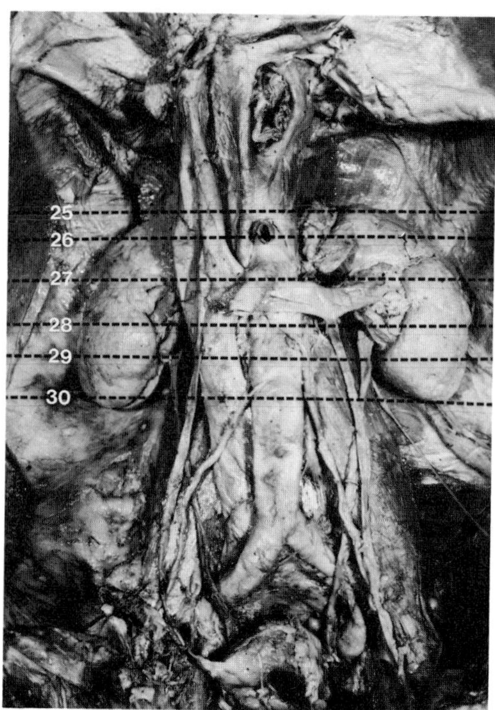


**Fig. 24.** In this view of the retroperitoneal space, dotted lines have been added to depict the approximate levels of the cross sectional anatomy to be demonstrated in Figures 25 through 30. This figure shows orientation.

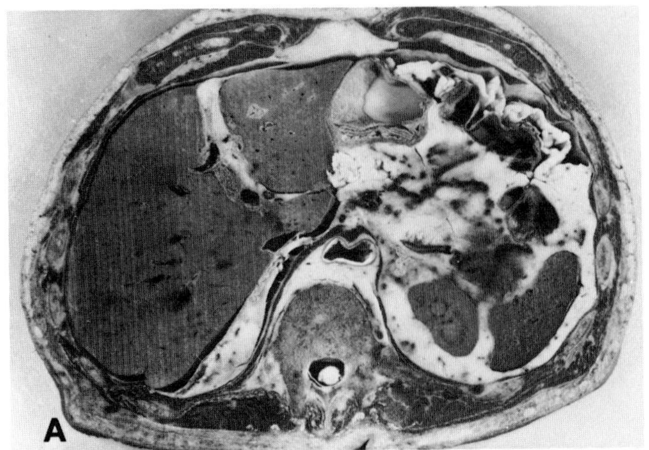


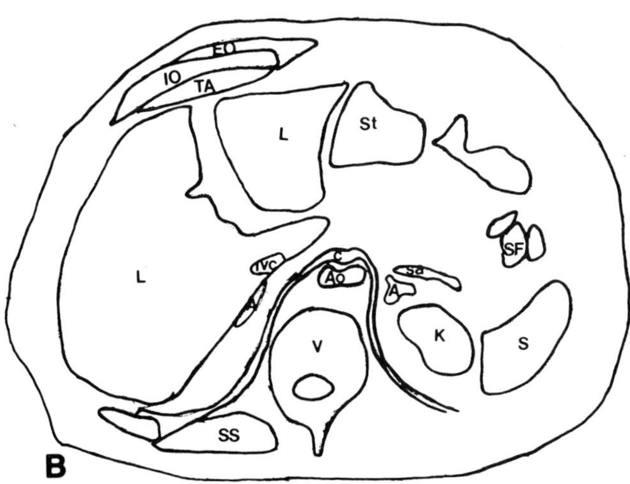


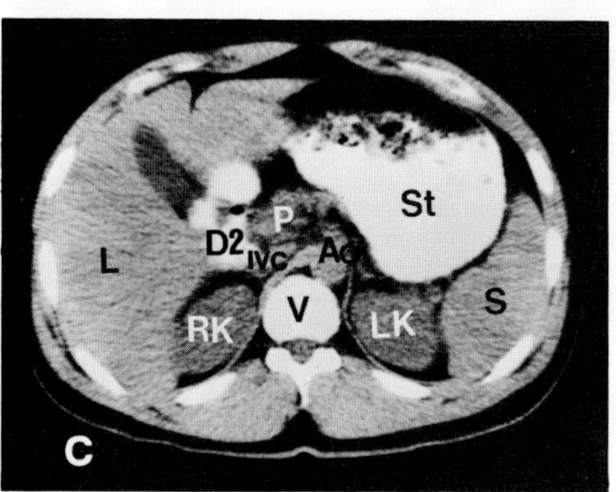


**Fig. 25A,B.** Cross section and line drawing through the upper pole of the left kidney. At this level, both adrenal glands (*A*) can be seen. The relationship of the left crus (*c*) of the diaphragm, left upper pole of the kidney (*K*), left adrenal gland(*A*), spleen (*S*), and splenic artery (*sa*) can be seen, as can the liver (*L*). In addition, a good demonstration of the arterolateral (*EO*, external oblique; *IO*, internal oblique; *TA*: transversus abdominis); and posterolateral (*SS*, sacrospinalis) abdominal wall muscles are seen. The aorta (*Ao*) and inferior vena cava (*ivc*) are shown. **C.** Computed tomography scan at a slightly lower level than that of the cross sectional anatomy. The relationship of the upper poles of both kidneys (*RK*, *LK*) to the liver (*L*), spleen (*S*), inferior vena cava (*ivc*), aorta (*Ao*), second part of duodenum (*D2*), stomach (*St*), and pancreas (*P*) are well shown.

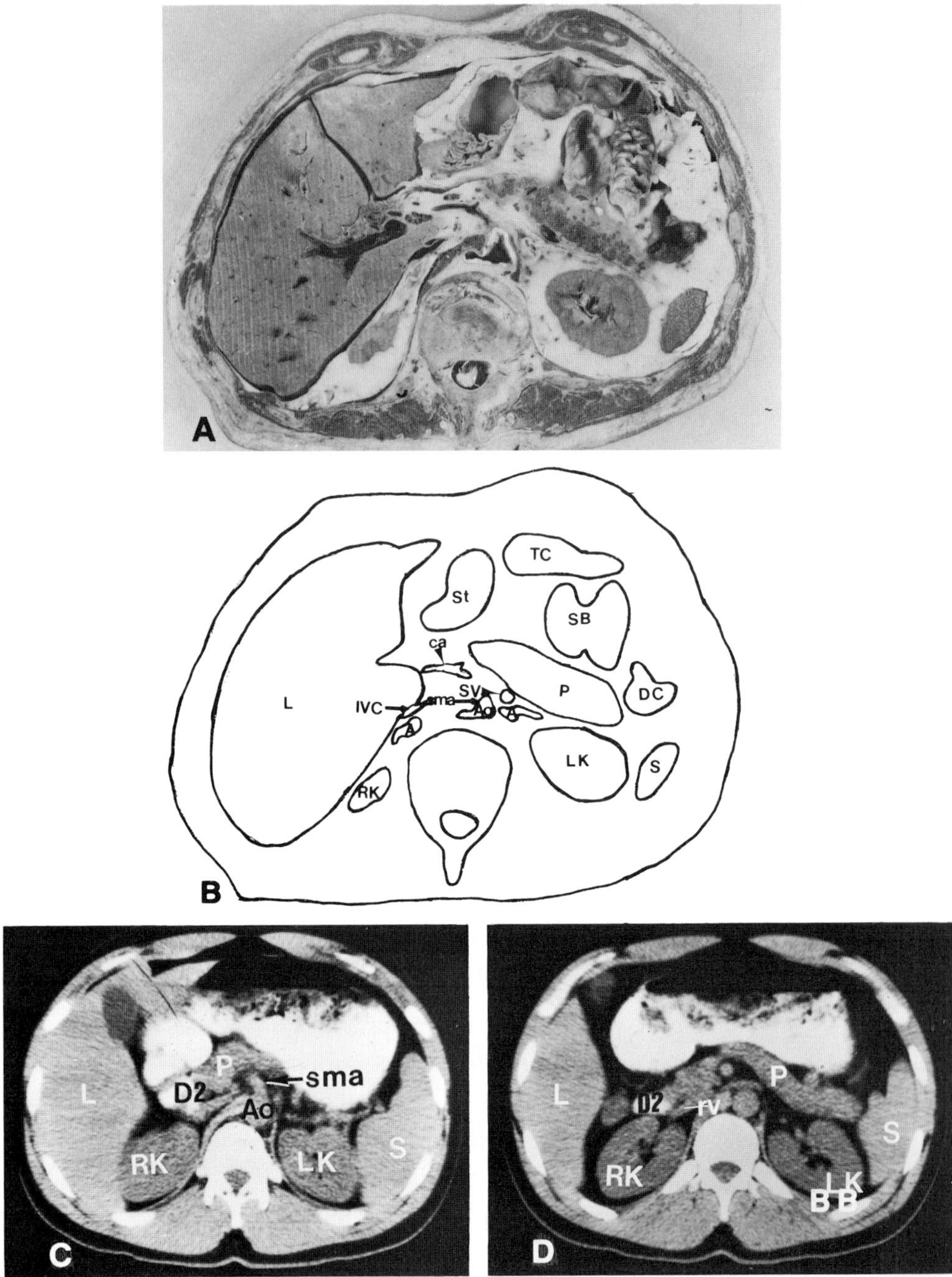


**Fig. 26A,B.** Cross sectional view to the upper pole of the right kidney. At this level both adrenal glands (*A*) are still well seen. The celiac axis (*ca*) can be seen exiting the aorta (*Ao*). The relationship of the splenic vein (*sv*) to the left adrenal and pancreas (*P*) is well seen at this level. The tip of the spleen (*S*) is barely visible, but the descending colon (*DC*) can now be seen. Portions of the transverse colon (*TC*), stomach (*St*), and small bowel (*SB*) are present. Also shown are left kidney (*LK*), liver (*L*), and superior mesenteric artery (*sma*). **C.** CT scan at approximately the same level showing the relationships of the great vessels to both kidneys (*LK*, *RK*), liver (*L*), spleen (*S*), second part of the duodenum (*D2*), pancreas (*P*), and superior mesenteric artery (*sma*, *arrow*). **D.** CT scan at a slightly lower level demonstrating the right renal vein (*rrv*) and its relationships to the second part of duodenum (*D2*) and right kidney (*RK*), and the tail of the pancreas (*P*) and spleen (*S*) to the left kidney (*LK*). **E.** Transverse ultrasonic view at approximately the same level. The relationships of both kidneys to the great vessels can be seen. Splenic vein (*SV*) is shown coursing posterior to the pancreas (*P*) and anterior to the superior mesenteric artery (*sma*) to join the portal vein (*PV*).

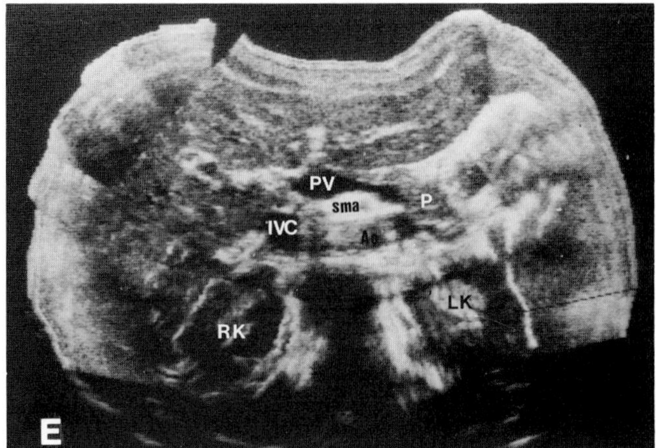


**Fig. 26.** (*Cont'd*)

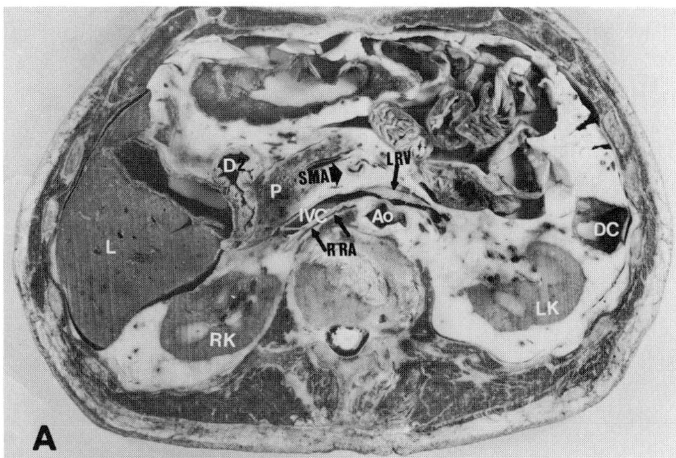


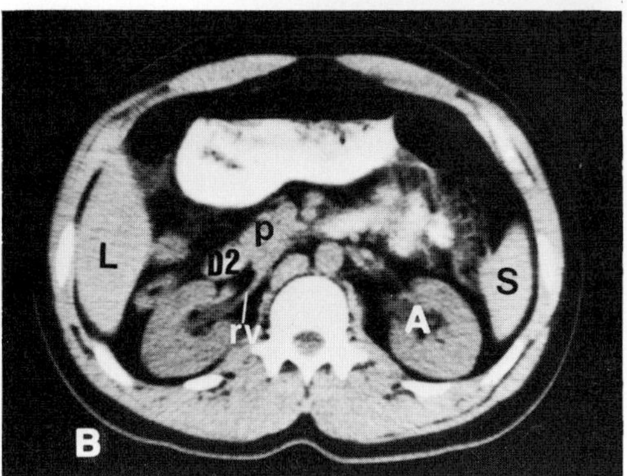


**Fig. 27A.** Cross sectional view through the mid sections of both kidneys. In this view the relationship of the right kidney (*RK*) to the liver (*L*), second part of the duodenum (*D2*), and pancreas (*P*) is well demonstrated. The right renal artery (*RRA*) can be seen coursing posterior to the inferior vena cava (*IVC*). The left renal vein (*LRV*) can be seen crossing between the aorta (*Ao*) and superior mesenteric artery (*SMA*) to enter the inferior vena cava (*IVC*). The relationship of the left kidney (*LK*) and descending colon (*DC*) is well demonstrated. **B.** CT scan view of the same area.

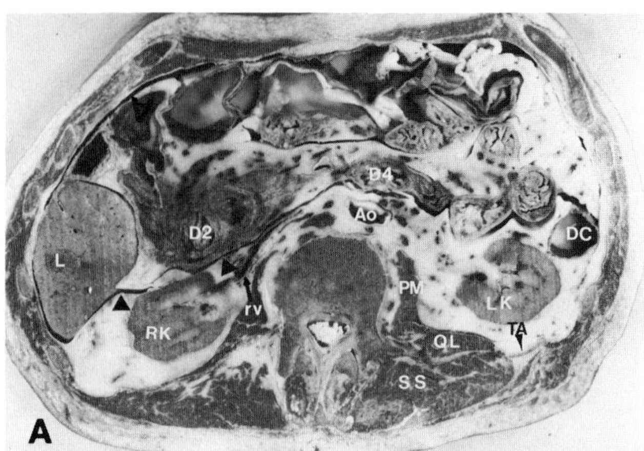


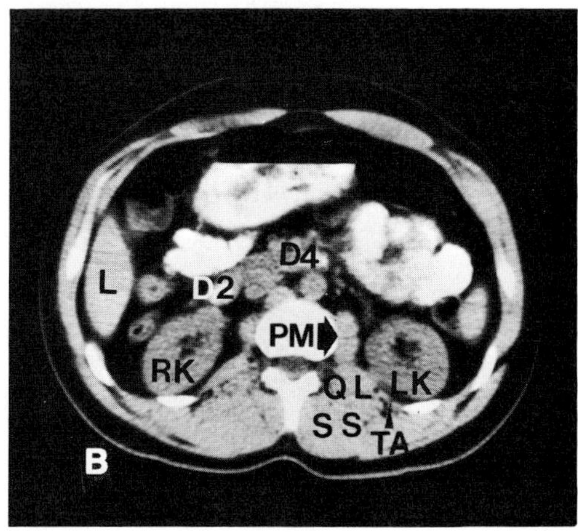


**Fig. 28A.** A lower cross section through both kidneys. In this view the relationships of the right kidney (*RK*) are again stressed, the right renal vein (*rrv*) can be seen entering the inferior vena cava (*ivc*). The relationships of the right kidney to liver (*L*) and second part of duodenum (*D2*) are demonstrated. The triangles point to the anterior leaf of Gerota's fascia. The relationship of the muscle bed of the left kidney (*LK*) is well demonstrated in this section. The psoas major (*PM*) can be seen forming the medial aspect of the bed of the kidney, while the quadratus lumborum (*QL*) lies directly posteriorly. The transversus abdominis (*TA*) is seen on the posterolateral aspect. The sacrospinalis (*SS*) can be seen lying deep to quadratus lumborum. In addition, both the second and fourth parts of duodenum (*D4*) are seen. **B.** CT scan of the same level again demonstrating the muscular bed of the kidney and second and fourth parts of duodenum.

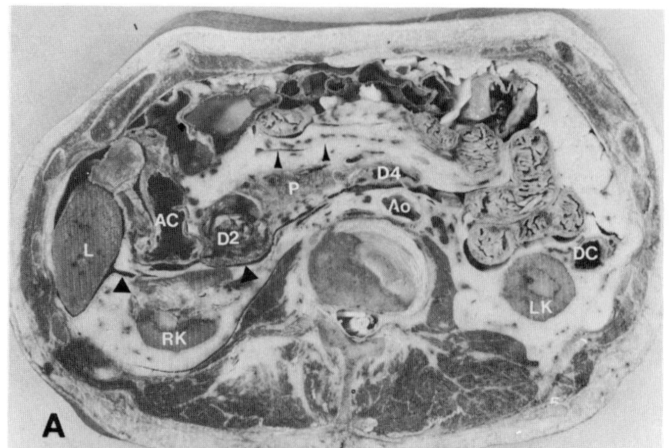


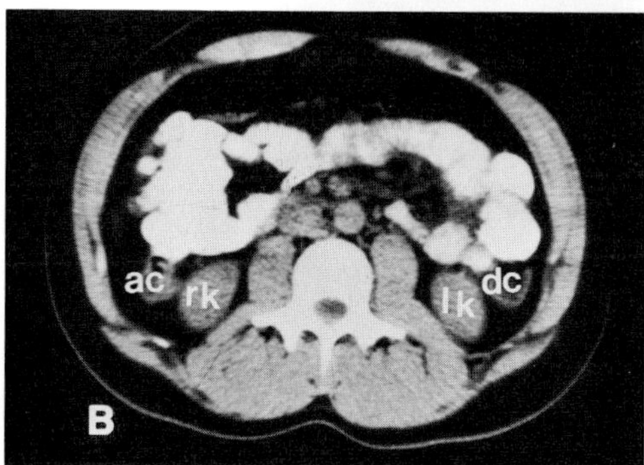


**Fig. 29A.** Cross sectional view through the lower poles of both kidneys (*LK*, *RK*). The right anterior Gerota's fascia is again noted by the triangles. The right pararenal space can be well seen in this view containing the ascending colon (*AC*), second part of duodenum (*D2*), and pancreas (*P*). It is bounded posteriorly by the anterior leaf of Gerota's fascia and anteriorly by the posterior peritoneum (*arrow heads*). The left pararenal space contains only descending colon (*DC*) as seen. The liver (*L*) and fourth part of the duodenum (*D4*) can also be seen. **B.** CT scan of the same level.

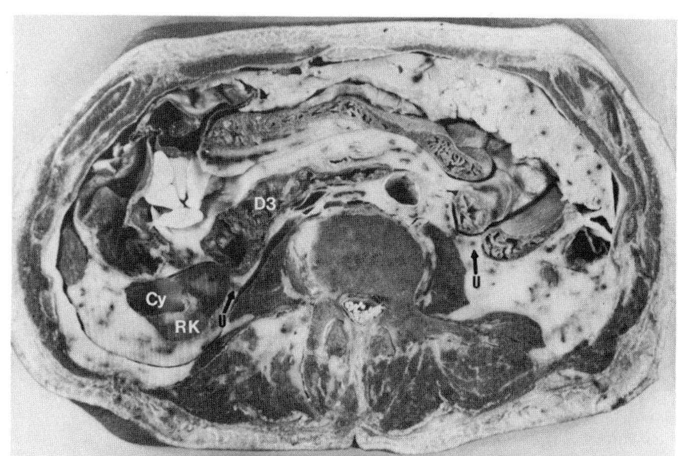


**Fig. 30.** Cross sectional view to the lower pole of the right kidney (*RK*). The left kidney at this time is no longer seen. An incidental simple cyst (*Cy*) is noted. At this level both ureters (*U*) can be seen, the left ureter coursing more anterior than the right, owing to its earlier exit from the kidney. The third part of duodenum (*D3*) can be seen.

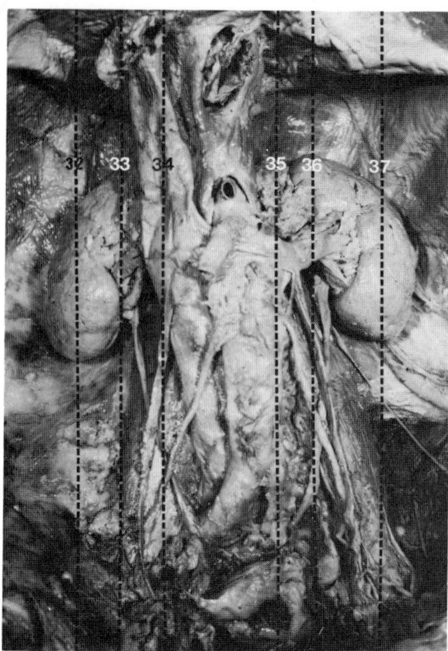


**Fig. 31.** Demonstrates the levels of the longitudinal sagittal sections for orientation.

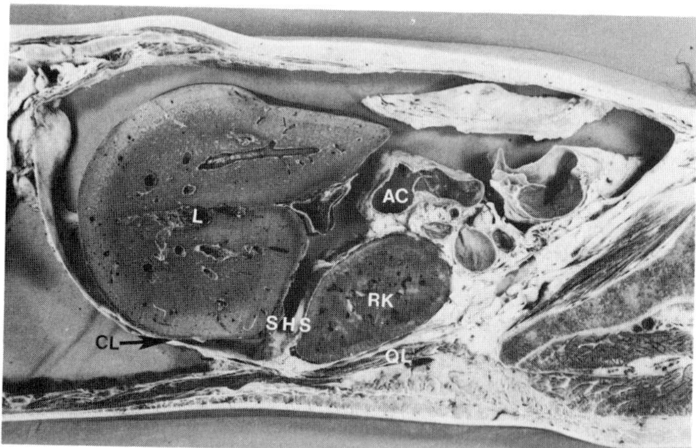


**Fig. 32.** Section through the lateral aspect of the right kidney (*RK*). The relationship of the right kidney and the liver (*L*) and coronary ligament (*CL*) forming the right subhepatic space (*SHS*) is well seen. The ascending colon (*AC*) and quadratus lumborum (*QL*) also appear.

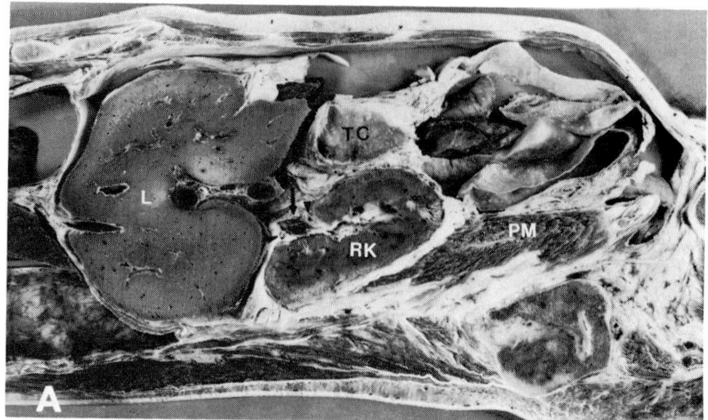


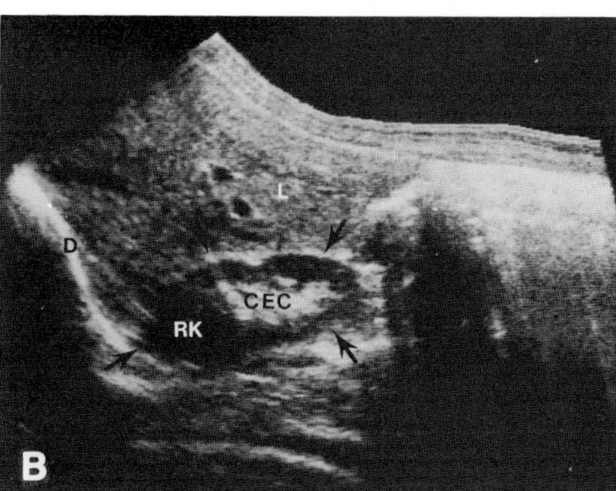


**Fig. 33A.** Longitudinal section through the medial aspect of the right kidney (*RK*). The arrow points to the right renal vein while the arrow heads point to the anterior and posterior branches of the right renal artery. The kidney can be seen lying on the psoas major (*PM*) muscle. The transverse colon (*TC*) is also apparent. In this view it is easy to see why the inferior pole of the right kidney lies more anterior than the upper pole, owing to the incline of the paravertebral muscles. **B.** Longitudinal ultrasound demonstrating the right kidney (*RK*). The outline of the kidney is documented by arrows. The light area in the middle of the renal shadow is the central echo complex (*CEC*), which represents the collection system. Its relationship to the right lobe of the liver (*L*) and diaphragm (*D*) is visualized.

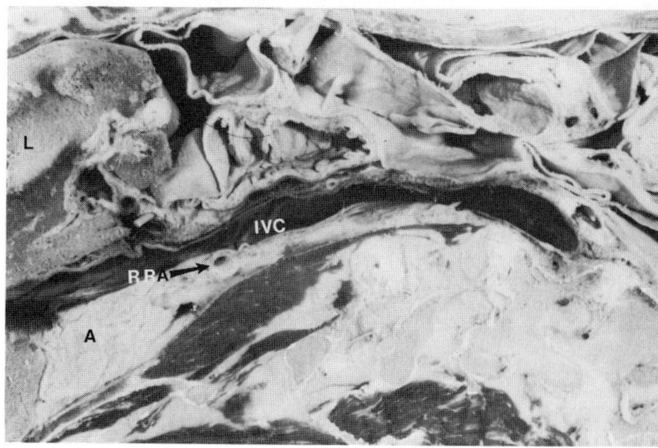


**Fig. 34.** Longitudinal section through the inferior vena cava (*IVC*). This demonstrates the relationship of the right renal artery (*RRA*) as it courses posterior to the inferior vena cava. Also the relationship of the right adrenal (*A*) to the posterior aspect of the vena cava is well seen. The liver (*L*) can be seen.

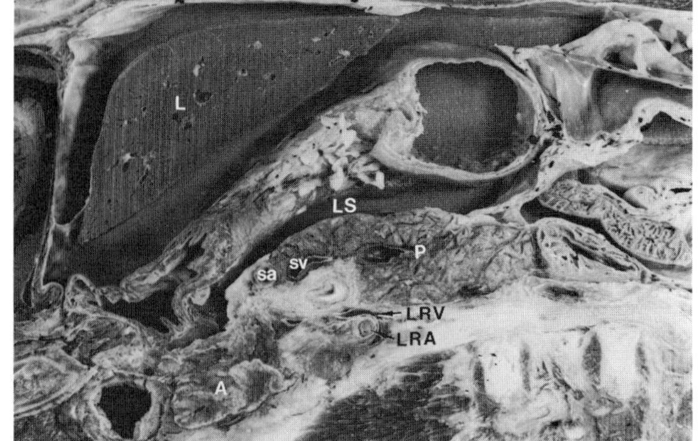


**Fig. 35.** Longitudinal view to the level of the left adrenal gland (*A*). The relationship of the left adrenal gland and the lesser sac (*LS*), splenic artery (*sa*) and splenic vein (*sv*), left renal artery (*LRA*) and left renal vein (*LRV*), liver (*L*), and pancreas (*P*) are well seen.

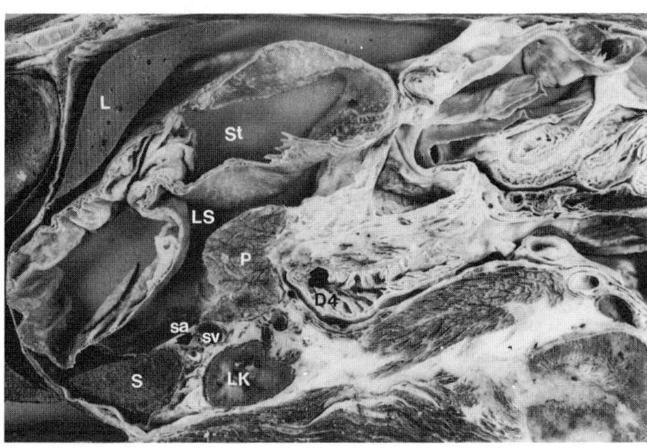


**Fig. 36.** Longitudinal section through the medial aspect of the upper pole of left kidney (*LK*). The relationships of the upper pole of the left kidney to the spleen (*S*), splenic artery (*sa*) and splenic vein (*sv*), lesser sac (*LS*), pancreas (*P*), stomach (*St*), liver (*L*), and fourth part of duodenum (*D4*) are well seen.

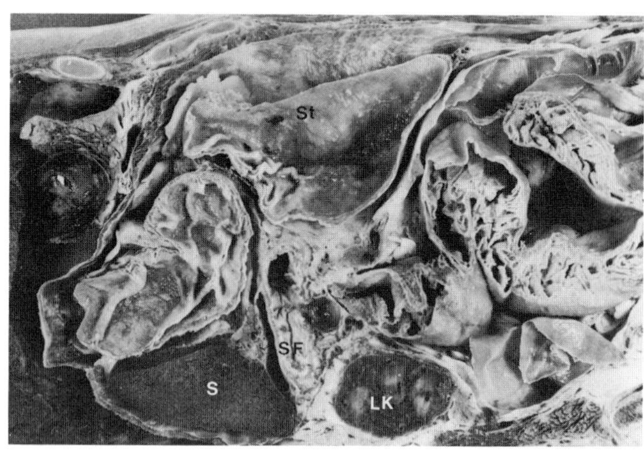


**Fig. 37.** Longitudinal view through the lateral aspect of the left kidney (*LK*). The relationship of the spleen (*S*), splenic flexure (*SF*), and left kidney are demonstrated. The stomach (*St*) is shown.

## REFERENCES

1. Thorek P: Anatomy in Surgery, 2nd ed., Philadelphia, JB Lippincott, 1962
2. Lich R Jr, Howerton LW, Amin M: Anatomy and surgical approach to the urogenital tract in the male. In Harrison JH, Gittes RF, Perlmutter AD et al (eds): Campbell's Urology, 4th ed. Philadelphia, WB Saunders, 1978
3. Boyce WH: Renal calculi. In Glenn JF (ed): Urologic Surgery, 2nd ed. Hagerstown, MD, Harper & Row, 1975
4. Cockett ATK, Kushiba K: Manual of Urologic Surgery, New York, Springer-Verlag, 1979
5. Kaye KW, Goldberg ME: Applied anatomy of the kidney and ureter. Urol Clin North Am 9:3, 1982

# 2

# Surgical Anatomy of the Lower Genitourinary Tract

*John F. Redman*

## INTRODUCTION

Over the past decade there has been a resurgence of interest in the applied anatomy of the lower genitourinary tract. New discoveries, as well as clinical interpretations and dissections of some of the more complex areas of anatomy, have come about through investigations of methods for extirpative surgery for cancer of the prostate and bladder, procedures to alleviate female stress incontinence, and operations to restore erectile function in the male. Imaging techniques, such as ultrasound examination, computed tomography, and magnetic resonance studies, in a nonconventional way have aided in the understanding of pelvic and lower tract anatomy. Endoscopic scrutiny during laparoscopic surgery no doubt will further pique an interest in the anatomy of the pelvis.

Attention to anatomic detail can make operations more technically satisfying and decrease morbidity. Each procedure should be considered an opportunity to increase one's ability to recognize anatomic structures through a developing incision, an exercise which may be enhanced by pre- and postoperative review of textbook anatomy.

Since the lower genitourinary tract is located caudal to the umbilicus and surrounded by the bony pelvis, a description of the lower tract anatomy will begin with the anatomy of the osteomuscular structures that form the pelvis.

## THE BONY PELVIS

A cursory examination of the bony pelvis would suggest that it is one intact osseous structure, when, in fact, it is formed of four bones: the paired coxals (innominates), the sacrum, and the coccyx (Fig 1). The large flared coxals are further divided into three parts which join in the acetabulum: the ilium, the ischium, and the pubis. The pubic portion of the coxals joins in the midline, ventrally separated by cartilage, which is termed the symphysis pubis.

The pelvis is unique, in that cranially it is bowl- or basin-shaped, while caudally it forms a ring. The bowl-shaped portion is referred to as the greater or false pelvis, while the ring-shaped portion is termed the lesser or true pelvis. The linea terminalis separates the two portions, and can be traced from the pectineal line to the pubis, and to the arcuate line of the ileum onto the upper border of the first sacral vertebra (Fig 2).

The pelvis is further characterized by a large foramen, the obturator foramen, that lies in the caudal aspect of the coxal bone, and by the ligaments and fibrous condensations termed ligaments. The sacrotuberous ligament (which extends from the ischial tuberosity to the lateral aspect of the sacrum and coccyx) and the sacrospinous ligament (bridging from the ischial spine to the dorsolateral aspect of the sacrum) divide the space between the sacrum and

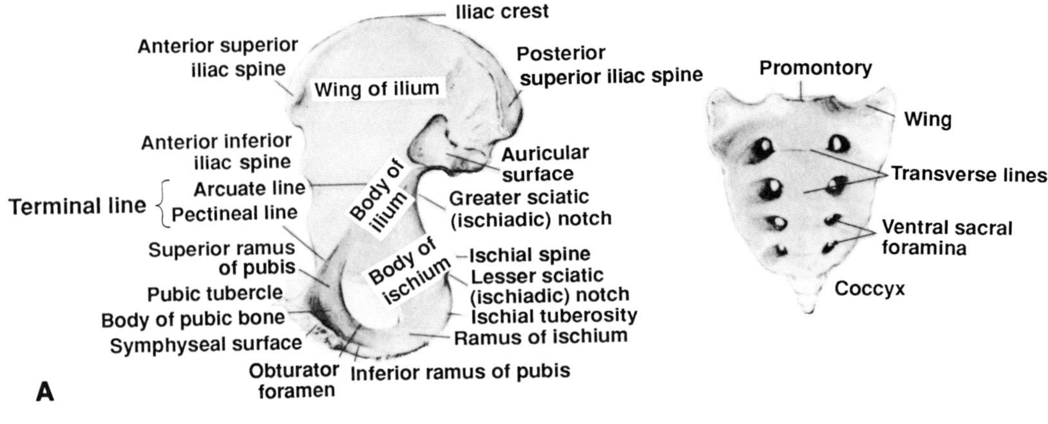


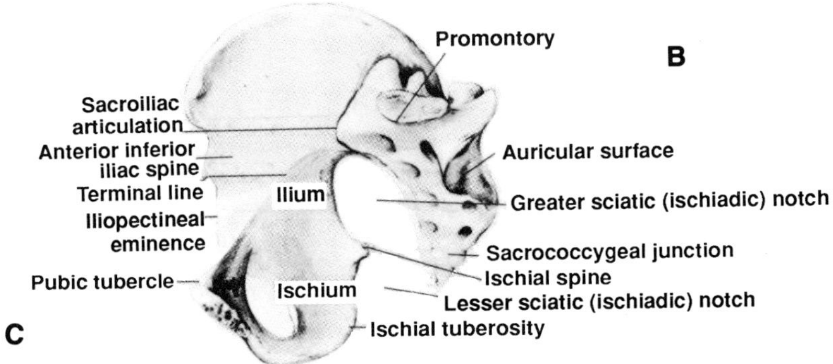


**Fig 1.** A, Coxal bone, medial aspect; B, sacrum, anterior aspect; C, articulated right coxal bone, sacrum, coccyx, left oblique view. [From Danforth DN, Scott JR, *Obstetrics and Gynecology,* 5th ed (Philadelphia: JB Lippincott Co; 1986), with permission.]

**Fig 2.** View of the pelvis from above showing bones, articulations, ligaments and foramina. [From Jones HW, et al, *Novak's Textbook of Gynecology,* 11th ed (Baltimore: Williams & Wilkins Co; 1988), with permission.]

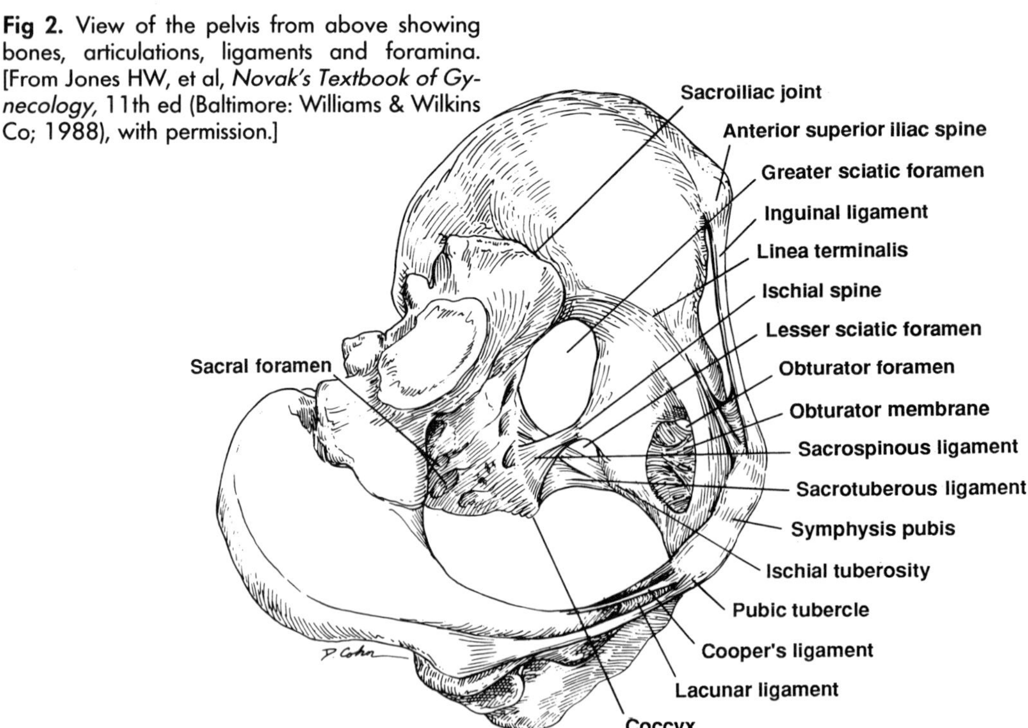

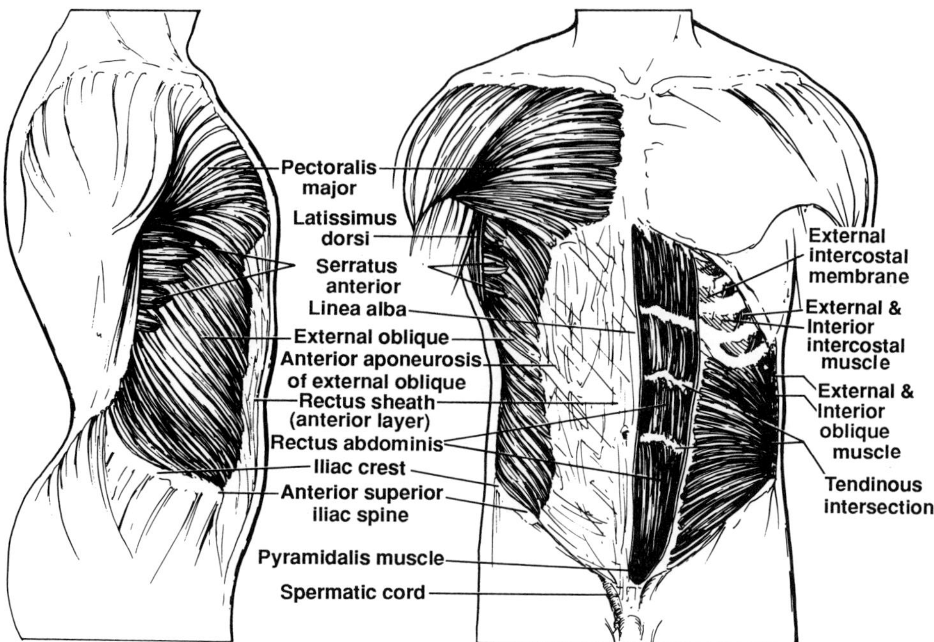


**Fig 3.** Superficial musculature of the anterior abdominal wall. [From Gillenwater JY, et al, eds, *Adult and Pediatric Urology,* 2nd ed (Chicago: Mosby-Year Book, Inc; 1991), with permission. Original drawing by Young.]

the coxal bone into two foramina, the greater and lesser sciatic foramina. The free edge of the external oblique aponeurosis, extending from the pubic tubercle to the anterior superior iliac spine, is termed the inguinal ligament, while the periosteum covering the pectineal line of the pubis is termed Cooper's ligament.

## LOWER ABDOMINAL WALL AND PELVIC MUSCULATURE

### Lower Anterior Abdominal Wall Musculature

When viewed anteriorly, the bony pelvis resembles a widened V; this V is bridged by muscle. The pelvic viscera are, therefore, contained in roughly a three-sided osseous structure covered by a ventral musculofascial wall. The muscles include the ventrally oriented rectus abdominis and the laterally oriented flat muscular sheets: the external oblique, the internal oblique, and the transversus abdominis muscles. Of particular interest to surgeons is the arrangement of the medial aponeurosis of these muscles as they form the rectus sheaths.

The most superficial of the lateral lower abdominal wall muscles is the external oblique muscle (Fig 3). Its fibers course obliquely downward to their insertion point on the anterior half of the iliac crest. The broad, flat aponeurosis of the external oblique muscle begins medially and is located approximately midway between the midline of the abdomen and the anterior axillary line. This aponeurosis joins in the formation of the anterior rectus sheath melding with the aponeurosis of the internal oblique muscle, and joins with its mate in the midline to form the linea alba. The inferior free border of the aponeurosis, the inguinal ligament, bridges from the pubic tubercle to the anterior superior iliac spine. It is attached laterally to the iliopsoas fascia and medially to the pectineus fascia, bridging the femoral vessels.

The internal oblique muscle is situated between the external oblique and transversus abdominis muscles. Its fibers course obliquely craniolaterally (Fig 4). The mus-

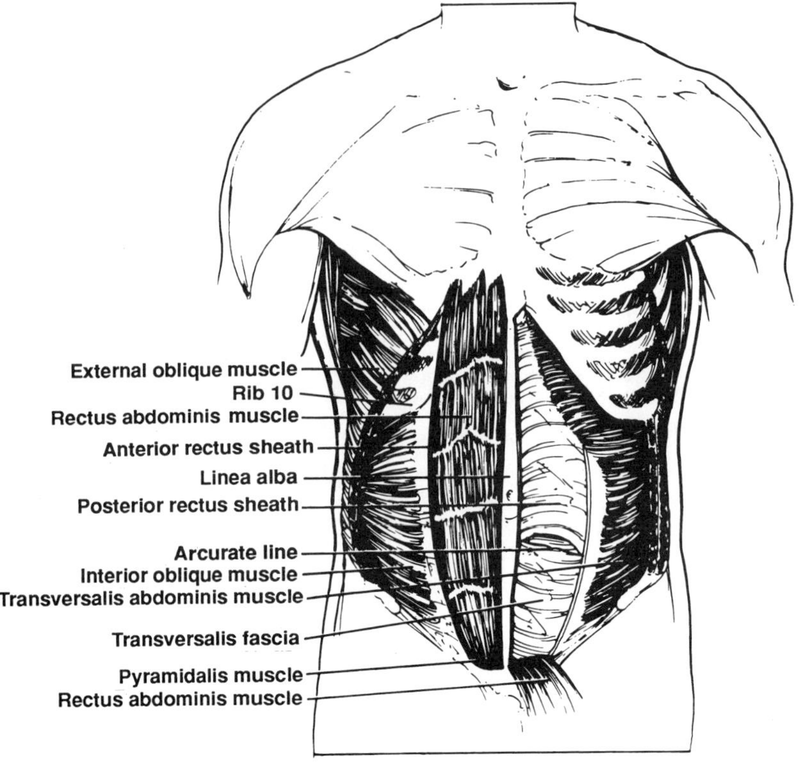


**Fig 4.** Line drawing showing relationships of internal oblique, transversus abdominis, and rectus abdominis muscles. [From Gillenwater JY, et al, eds, *Adult and Pediatric Urology,* 2nd ed (Chicago: Mosby-Year Book Inc; 1991), with permission. Original drawing by Young.]

cle originates from the iliopsoas fascia, the anterior two thirds of the intermediate line of the iliac crest, and the posterior lamina of the lumbodorsal fascia. Its aponeurosis uniquely forms the sheath of the rectus abdominis. The internal oblique aponeurosis is more curvilinear than is that of the external oblique, and is wider at its cranial aspect. Cranial to the arcuate line (semilunar line of Douglas), which is located approximately 4 cm caudal to the umbilicus, the aponeurosis of the internal oblique muscle splits, with the ventral half joining the aponeurosis of the external oblique to form the anterior rectus sheath and the dorsal half joining the aponeurosis of the transversus abdominis muscle to form the posterior rectus sheath (Fig 5). Caudal to the arcuate line, the aponeurosis of the internal oblique muscle fuses with the aponeurosis of the external oblique muscle and the transversus abdominis muscle, and all aponeuroses pass ventral to the rectus abdominis to form the anterior rectus sheath. It should be noted that the arcuate line is not always discrete, in that the aponeurosis of the internal oblique muscle may abruptly pass ventral to the rectus abdominis muscle, while the aponeurosis of the transversus abdominis muscle continues to pass dorsal to the rectus for a variable distance before taking a ventral position, sometimes forming one or more additional arcuate lines.

The transversus abdominis muscle lies beneath the internal oblique. In the lower abdomen it originates from the iliopsoas fascia, the anterior two thirds of the inner lip of the iliac crest, and the anterior lamina of the lumbodorsal fascia. Its aponeurosis in the lower abdomen lies almost immediately beneath that of the transversus abdominis. Cranial to the arcuate line, the aponeurosis passes dorsal to the rectus abdominis muscle to fuse with the dorsal lamina of the aponeurosis of the internal oblique muscle to form the posterior sheath. Caudal to the arcuate line, it crosses ventral to the rectus, joining in the formation of the anterior rectus sheath. Only the dorsal investing fascia of the transversus abdominis muscle and aponeurosis (transversalis fascia) cover the dorsal aspect of the rectus abdominis muscle caudal to the arcuate line.

**Fig 5.** Cross-section in the lumbar region showing the lower abdominal musculature and fusion of the anterior abdominal muscular aponeuroses below the arcuate line; inset shows composition of rectus sheath above the arcuate line. [From Gillenwater JY, et al, eds, *Adult and Pediatric Urology,* 2nd ed (Chicago: Mosby-Year Book Inc; 1991), with permission. Original drawing by Young.]

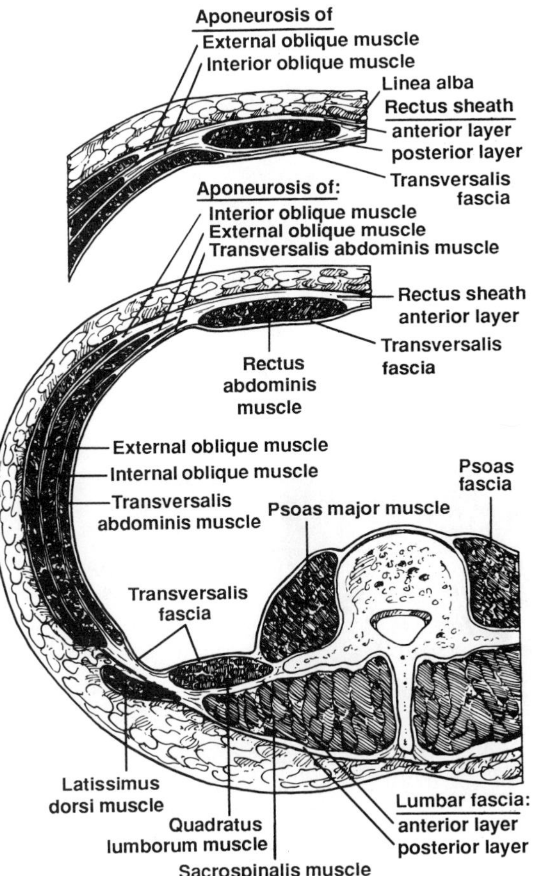


The rectus abdominis muscles are paired, vertically oriented, broad straps which narrow from the level of the umbilicus to their tendinous attachment on the pubis. Superficially, the lateral margin of the recti can be identified through the skin in lean subjects by longitudinal depressions termed semilunar lines, which can be an aid in incision placement. The recti are invested cranial to the arcuate line by the anterior and posterior rectus sheaths. Caudal to the arcuate line, the recti are covered dorsally by the dorsal investing fascia of the transversus abdominis muscle, the transversalis fascia.

The pyramidalis muscles are triangular-shaped muscles whose bases arise from the pubis. They are located just ventral to the rectus abdominis and are contained within its sheath. Generally one muscle is larger than the other.

## Pelvic Musculature

The wall and floor of the pelvis are comprised of muscle. The iliacus, psoas, piriformis, and obturator internus muscles either originate from or pass through the pelvis before reaching insertion points on the femur (Fig 6). The other muscles of the pelvis are the levator ani and coccygeus (Fig 7).

The prominent musculature of the dorsal aspect of the pelvis, which may be visualized on operatively entering the pelvis anteriorly, consists of the iliacus and the psoas muscles. The iliacus muscle arises from and covers the iliac fossa. Caudally and medially it joins with the psoas muscle, and together they pass beneath the inguinal ligament to form a tendon, which inserts into the lesser trochanter of the femur. The psoas major muscle originates from the lateral aspects of the lumbar vertebra and parallels the lateral margin of the sacrum before joining the iliacus muscle. In the pelvis, the glistening tendon of the psoas minor muscle courses ventrally over the ventral surface of the psoas minor.

Although much of the musculature of the pelvis is not directly visualized intraoperatively, the obturator internus and levator ani muscles are easily identified as the pelvic viscera are swept away from the pelvic

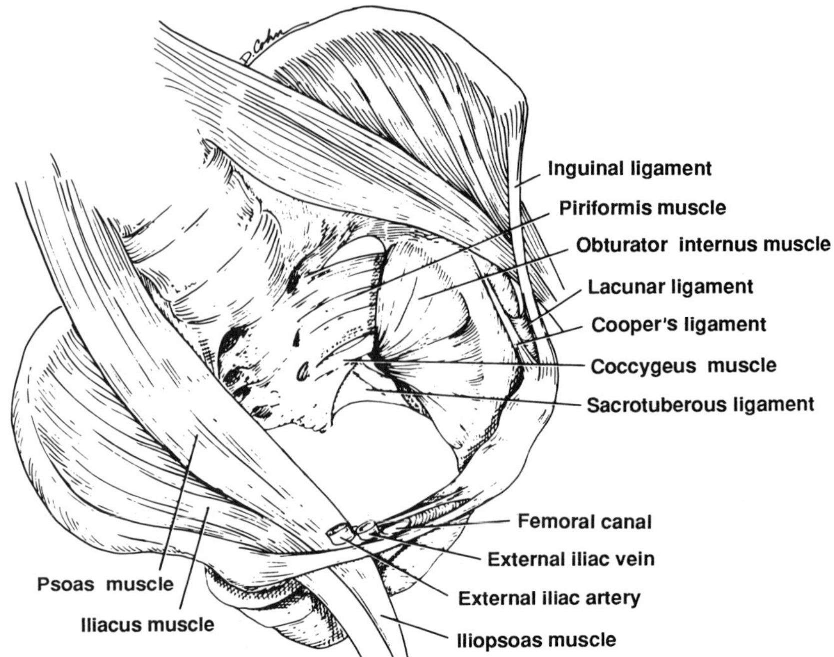


**Fig 6.** Musculature of the true and false pelvis. [From Jones HW, et al, *Novak's Textbook of Gynecology,* 11th ed (Baltimore: Williams & Wilkins Co; 1988), with permission.]

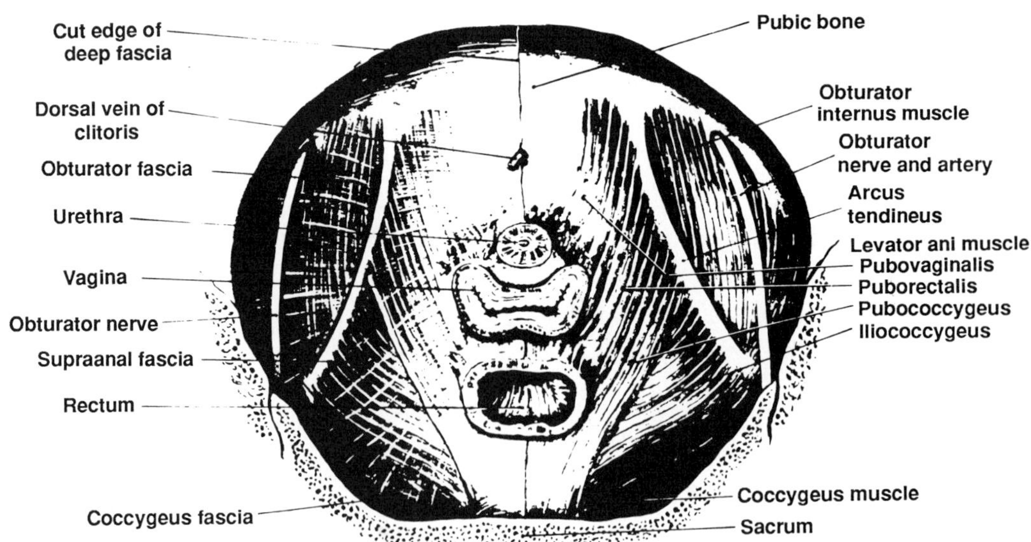


**Fig 7.** Musculature of female pelvic floor as visualized from above. [From Crafts RC, *A Textbook of Human Anatomy,* 3rd ed (New York: John Wiley & Sons Inc; 1985), with permission.]

sidewall. However, only a portion of the obturator internus muscle is visualized in the pelvis. It is a triangular-shaped muscle which arises from the inner aspects of the coxal bone and forms the primary anterior covering of the true pelvis. The apex of the muscular triangle passes through the lesser sciatic foramen to ultimately insert on the greater trochanter of the femur. A thickening of the fascia of the obturator internus muscle bridges from the ischial spine to the superior pubic ramus and gives rise to the levator ani muscle, which covers the bulk of the obturator internus muscle. Therefore, only that part of the obturator internus lateral to the arcus tendineus is visible in the pelvis. The piriformis muscle, which is also triangular in shape, originates from the lateral aspect of the sacrum and forms the posterior covering of the true pelvis. It exits the pelvis through the greater sciatic foramen and has an insertion point on the greater trochanter of the femur. Of significance to the pelvic surgeon is the fact that the sacral plexus is largely located on the ventral aspect of the piriformis muscle.

The major portion of the pelvic diaphragm is formed by the levator ani muscle. Through it passes the visceral tubes: the urethra, vagina, and rectum. The levator ani has three primary components: the pubococcygeus, the iliococcygeus, and the puborectalis muscles. The anterior portion of the levator ani (the pubococcygeus and puborectalis) are closely associated, with the pubococcygeus lying lateral to the puborectalis. Both originate from the posterior surface of the pubic ramus and the arcus tendineus and insert into the anococcygeal raphe and onto the lateral and anterior portion of the coccyx.

The iliococcygeal portion of the levator ani muscle is less thick than the remainder of the levator ani. The iliococcygeus arises from the arcus tendineus and inserts on the anorectal raphe and the tip of the coccyx. The coccygeus, which is triangular-shaped, arises from the ischial spine and the sacrospinous ligament and inserts onto the anterior caudal aspect of the coccyx and sacrum. The muscle is situated as part of the pelvic floor between the iliococcygeus and piriformis.

## PELVIC VASCULATURE, LYMPHATICS, AND INNERVATION

### Pelvic Vasculature

**Pelvic Arteries.** The arterial vasculature of the pelvis derives from three primary vessels: the common iliac, inferior mesenteric, and gonadal arteries. A fourth but smaller source vessel is the middle sacral artery, which arises from the caudal-most aspect of the bifurcation of the aorta and courses over the fifth lumbar vertebra, the sacrum, and the coccyx.

The major blood supply to the pelvis is given by the paired common iliac arteries and their branches, which arise at the bifurcation of the aorta anterior to the body of the fourth lumbar vertebra (Fig 8). Coursing caudally and laterally, the common iliac arteries divide between the fifth lumbar vertebra and the sacrum into internal and external iliac arteries.

The external iliac is the direct extension of the common iliac. It progresses caudally and laterally along the medial aspect of the psoas before passing beneath the inguinal ligament; at that point it is termed the femoral artery. The internal iliac artery splits into two primary branches just before passage under the inguinal ligament: the inferior epigastric and deep circumflex iliac arteries. The inferior epigastric artery arises medially, and passes medial to the internal ring before coursing along the ventral aspect of the abdominal wall. It penetrates the transversalis fascia at the abdominal wall, and passes along the ventral-lateral aspect of the rectus abdominis muscle which it supplies with blood. Two small branches are also derived from the inferior epigastric artery: a pubic branch, which runs along the posterior surface of the pelvis, and a cremasteric branch, which penetrates the transversalis fascia of the inguinal canal to supply the cremasteric muscle. The inferior epigastric artery may also be the origin of an abberant obturator artery. From the lateral aspect of the internal iliac artery, just opposite the inferior epigastric artery, arises the deep circumflex iliac artery, which courses laterally to run between the transversus abdominis and the

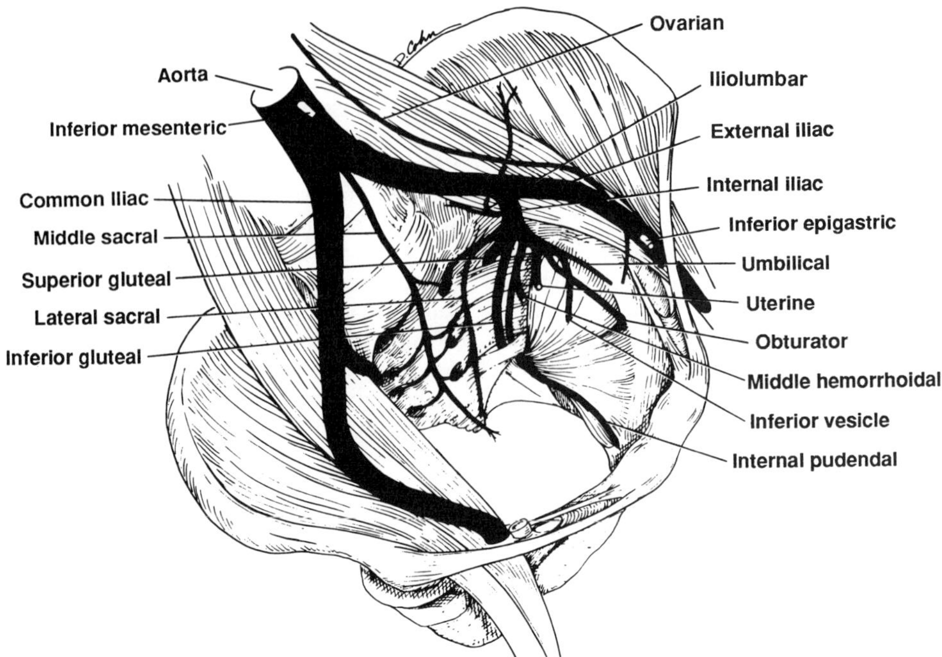


**Fig 8.** Arterial vasculature of the female pelvis. [From Jones HW, et al, *Novak's Textbook of Gynecology,* 11th ed (Baltimore: Williams & Wilkins Co; 1988), with permission.]

internal oblique muscle, to which it supplies blood.

The principal blood supply to the pelvis is derived from the internal iliac artery. Although a general pattern of distribution of the vasculature can be presented, it is well to know that a great range of variation exists. Shortly after arising from the common iliac artery, the internal iliac vessel divides anterior to the greater sciatic foramen to form a posterior and an anterior division.

The posterior division gives rise to three branches, which supply the pelvis and the gluteal region: the iliolumbar, the lateral sacral, and the superior gluteal. The first branch, the iliolumbar artery, courses posteriorly and then craniolaterally. A large branch, the iliac artery, crosses dorsal to the common iliac artery and psoas muscle to emerge and course laterally on the cranial aspect of the iliacus muscle along the iliac crest. The lateral sacral vessel, as its name indicates, courses along the anterolateral aspect of the sacrum. The superior gluteal artery passes posteriorly through the greater sciatic foramen to supply the gluteal muscle. Hence the admonition, in ligation of the internal iliac artery to control pelvic hemorrhage, that the ligature should be placed distal to the take-off of the posterior division to preserve the superior gluteal artery.

The anterior division of the internal iliac artery gives rise to parietal and visceral branches. The parietal branches constitute the inferior gluteal, obturator, and internal pudendal arteries. The visceral branches are the umbilical, inferior vesical, middle hemorrhoidal, uterine, and vaginal arteries. The inferior gluteal and the internal pudendal arteries are the terminal vessels of the anterior division of the internal iliac. The inferior gluteal is the larger of the two vessels and passes between the sacral nerves and exits the pelvis caudal to the piriformis muscle to supply the gluteal muscles. The inferior pudendal artery exits the pelvis between the piriformis and the coccygeus muscles, crosses the ischial spine and then runs in a sheath of obturator fascia along the obturator internus muscle's medial surface (Alcock's canal) accompanied by the internal pudendal vein and nerve to provide the primary vasculature of the perineum. In Alcock's canal the vessel lies caudal to the levator ani muscle, which is separated by a fat-filled space between the levator ani and the obturator internus muscles that is termed the ischiorectal fossa. Arising medially from the internal pudendal artery is the inferior hemorrhoidal artery, which passes through the fatty tissue of the fossa to supply the levator ani, the anal canal, the external sphincter, the anus, and the perineal skin. The internal pudendal artery terminates as a perineal artery which gives rise to, in the male, the posterior scrotal arteries and, in the female, the posterior labial arteries (Fig 9), and in both sexes vasculature to the ischiocavernosus, bulbospongiosus, and transversus perineal muscles. The internal pudendal artery enters the urogenital diaphragm and in the male gives rise to the artery of the bulb of the penis, a urethral artery, and the deep and dorsal arteries of the penis. In the female it gives rise to the artery of the bulb of the vestibule and the clitoral artery, both deep and dorsal.

The obturator artery is usually the first branch of the anterior division; it runs caudally along the pelvic sidewall, and exits through the obturator foramen. A pubic branch is common.

The umbilical artery is the first branch of the anterior division of the internal iliac artery. Antenatally, the umbilical artery traverses from the internal iliac to the umbilicus; it becomes obliterated in infancy and in early childhood only the proximal segment remains patent from just lateral to the bladder to the umbilicus. The obliterated segment becomes a dense, white, fibrous structure termed the lateral umbilical ligament and is held to the bladder by retroperitoneal connective tissue. Surgically, the lateral umbilical ligament is noteworthy as an intraperitoneal anatomic landmark. It can be a guide to the retroperitoneal ureter, which passes dorsal to it, and can also serve as a guide to the internal iliac artery, from

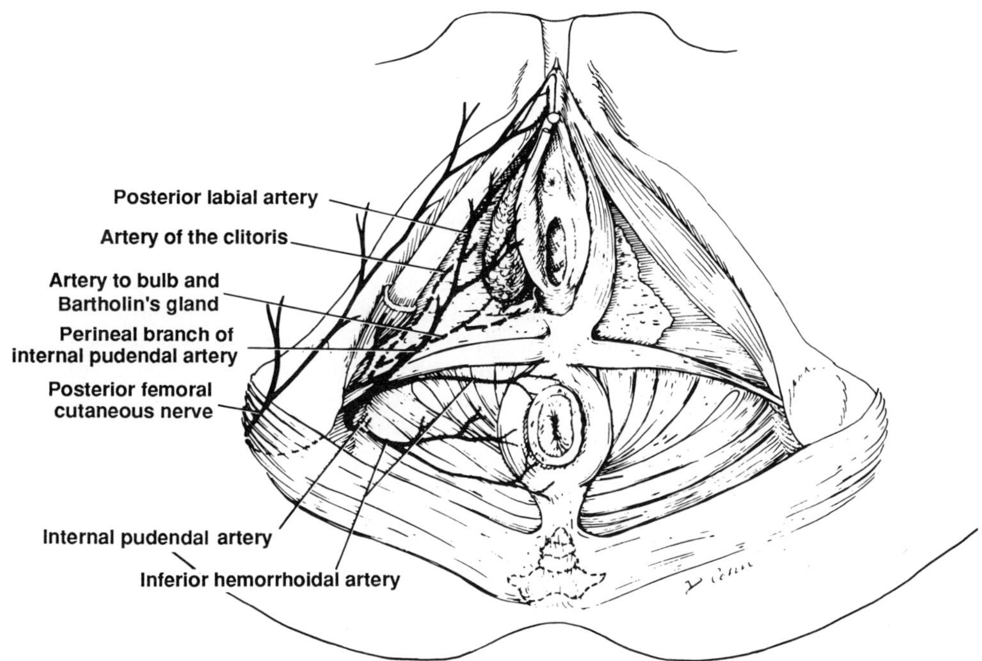


**Fig 9.** Arterial vasculature of the female perineum. [From Jones HW, et al, *Novak's Textbook of Gynecology,* 11th ed (Baltimore: Williams & Wilkins Co; 1988), with permission.]

which it arises. The umbilical artery may be the origin of the artery of the vas deferens and the superior vesical artery.

The inferior vesical artery arises just caudal to the obturator artery and, in the male, supplies vasculature to the posterior and caudal portion of the bladder, the seminal vessels, and gives rise to the prostatic arteries. The artery of the vas deferens may also derive from the inferior vesical artery. In the female, the inferior vesical artery may arise as a branch of the uterine artery or as a separate branch of the anterior division. The middle hemorrhoidal artery, which vascularizes the mid-portion of the rectum, arises either separately or with the interior vesicle artery.

In the female, the uterine artery arises from the anterior division at the approximate site from which the inferior vesical arises in the male. It courses caudally and medially on the levator ani to the base of the broad ligament, where it then passes ventral to the ureter (approximately 2 cm from the cervix). At the level of the cervix, it gives rise to the vaginal artery, which progresses caudally. The vaginal artery may at times arise as a separate branch of the anterior division. The uterine artery proceeds circuitously along the lateral body of the uterus and the broad ligament, anastomoses with the ovarian artery, and forms a vascular arcade giving branches to the ovary, the uterine tube, and the broad ligament.

The gonadal arteries—the internal spermatics and ovarians—arise from the medial ventral aspect of the abdominal aorta just caudal to the origin of the renal arteries and course caudally and laterally. These arteries are contained within the intermediate stratum of retroperitoneal connective tissue. In the male, the internal spermatics pass obliquely and then ventral to the ureter and, along with the gonadal veins and vas deferens, pass through the internal ring and down the inguinal canal. In the female, the ovarian artery enters the infundibuliform ligament and passes ventral to and in close proximity with the ureter after supplying the ovary. After supplying the ovary, it continues in the mesovarium, caudal to the uterine tube, to supply the uterine tube. The ovarian artery then runs medial to the cornu of the uterus, where it anastomoses with the uterine artery.

The inferior mesenteric artery arises from the ventral midline of the aorta, approximately 3 cm proximal to its bifurcation. After giving rise to the left colic and sigmoidal arteries, it continues into the pelvis as the superior hemorrhoidal artery. Within the wall of the rectum, the superior hemorrhoidal artery anastomoses with the middle hemorrhoidal artery from the internal iliac and the inferior hemorrhoidal artery from the internal pudendal.

**Pelvic Veins.** The primary venous drainage of the pelvis is through the internal iliac vein and its tributaries. The tributaries basically follow the course of the respective arteries of the same name. The venous drainage differs from the arterial supply in that, generally, multiple veins exist in an area served by one artery. Further, the pelvic organs are surrounded by extensive networks, or plexuses, of veins. Prominent pelvic plexuses are the vesical, prostatic, rectal, uterine, and vaginal.

The vesical plexus is most pronounced anteriorly and caudally. In the male, it receives drainage from the prostatic plexus and drains by vesical veins into the internal iliac. In the female, it receives the dorsal vein of the clitoris and then drains into the vaginal plexus. The prostatic plexus (Santorini's plexus) is located anteriorly and laterally within the retroperitoneal connective tissue covering the prostate. The deep dorsal vein of the penis trifurcates over the prostate and, with the prostatic venous drainage, drains blood from both the penis and the prostate through the vesical plexus and prostatic veins to the internal iliac (Fig 10). The uterus and vaginal plexuses are extensive, and communicate with each other and, ultimately, the vesical and rectal plexuses to drain to the internal iliac.

The gonadal veins are unique in that, after forming from the pampiniform plexus just cranial to the respective gonad, they course cranially to drain obliquely into the inferior vena cava on the right and to the caudal aspect of the renal vein on the left, entering at a right angle.

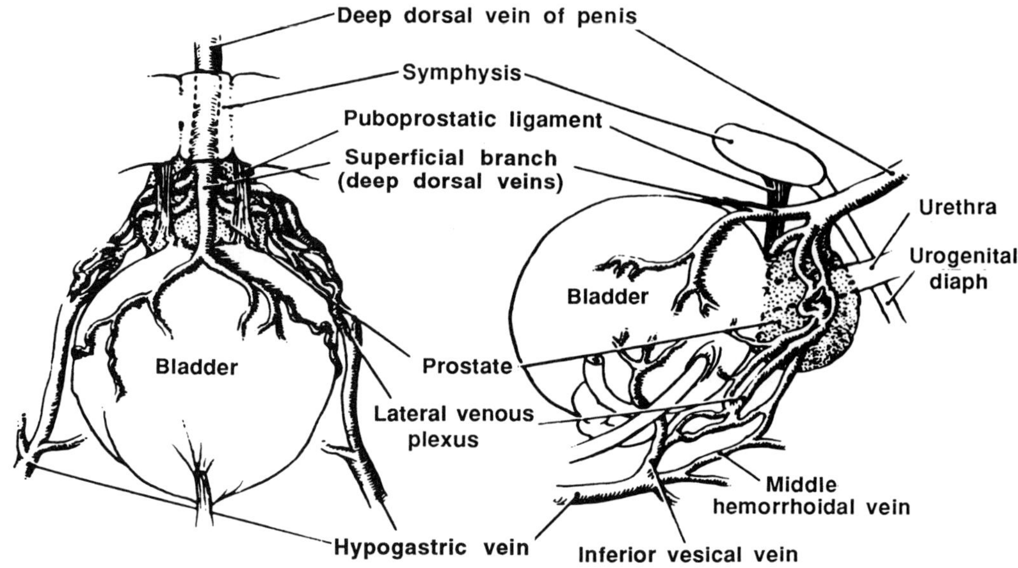


**Fig 10.** A, Trifurcation of dorsal vein of penis as viewed from above; B, lateral view. [From *J Urol* (1979;121:199), with permission.]

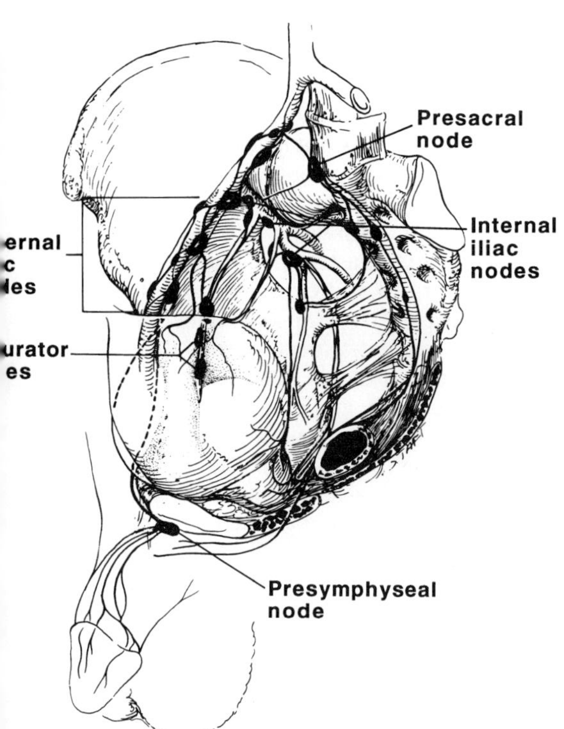


**Fig 11.** Nodal chains of lymphatic system in the male pelvis. [From Walsh PC, et al, eds, *Campbell's Urology,* 5th ed (Philadelphia: WB Saunders Co; 1986), with permission.]

## Pelvic Lymphatics

It is a general rule that the lymphatic vessels, for the most part, retrace the course of the arterial supply of the organ from which they arise. The lymphatic channels are interspersed by lymph nodes; the nodal chains thus formed are known by the names of the arterial vessels they accompany. These nodal chains are the internal, external, and common iliac; the inferior and superior gluteal; the superficial and deep inguinal; and the sacral and para-aortic (Fig 11). The specific lymphatic drainage of the pelvic organs is of particular interest to the surgeon who contemplates extirpative surgery for neoplasms.

The lymphatic drainage of the bladder per se is to the external iliac chain; however, regional nodes receiving drainage from the bladder include nodes located along the internal iliac, common iliac, and lateral sacral chains. The anterior bladder wall is drained by lymphatics which follow the lateral umbilical ligament. The anterior superior bladder wall drains to the middle chain of the external iliac group which is located between the iliac artery and vein and to the internal chain of the external iliac group which is adjacent to the obturator nerve. The anterior medial wall lymph drainage is to the middle chain of the external iliac group. The posterior bladder wall has four main lymphatic channels. Channels from the superior, middle, and lower portion of the bladder wall (exclusive of the base) drain to the middle and internal group of the external iliac chain, while the base drains to nodes located near the bifurcation of the common iliac.

Lymphatic vessels in the prostate drain primarily into the internal iliac group that receives the lymphatic vessels which follow the prostatic artery from the superior lateral aspect of the prostate. The posterior surface of the prostate also drains to the internal iliac and obturator groups as well as to presacral and external nodes.

The penile skin and prepuce is drained by lymphatic vessels which follow the superficial penile vasculature and terminate in the superficial lymph nodes. The glans and corpora are drained by lymphatic vessels which accompany the deep dorsal vein. These vessels drain to the deep inguinal lymph nodes and ultimately to the external iliac group. The anterior urethra in the male is drained by lymphatic vessels which terminate in the superficial and deep inguinal nodes; this drainage is subsequently received by the external iliac group. The membranous urethral lymphatic drainage is similar to that in the female urethra, that is, through the internal iliac, obturator, and external iliac chains.

The scrotal and vulvar lymphatic vessels drain in homologous fashion to the superficial and deep inguinal lymph nodes.

The vaginal lymphatic drainage differs by region. The lower third of the vagina's lymphatic vessels are similar to the vulva, and drain to superficial and deep inguinal nodes. The middle third of the vagina is drained by lymphatic vessels that accompany the vaginal artery to terminate in internal iliac nodes. Lymphatic vessels accompanying the uterine artery drain the upper part of the vagina to terminate in the external and internal nodal chains. Cervical drainage is to internal and external iliac nodes, as well as rectal and sacral nodes. The lymphatic drainage of the uterus is regional. Most of the body of the uterus is drained by lymphatic channels which terminate in the external iliac chain. The upper body and fundus of the uterus, along with the uterine tube, are drained by lymphatics which accompany the ovarian vessels and terminate in the lateral and para-aortic lymph-node group. At the juncture of the round ligament, the uterus is drained by the lymphatics of the round ligament, which terminate in the superficial inguinal nodes.

The gonadal lymphatic drainage is similar in each sex; the lymphatics accompany the gonadal vessels and terminate in the lateral and para-aortic lymph node group. These nodes are located between the renal vessels and the aortic bifurcation.

### Pelvic Innervation

The pelvis receives innervation from somatic and visceral nerves. The somatic nerves are all branches of the lumbosacral plexus (Fig 12). The lumbar plexus is located in the psoas muscle and arises from the ventral primary division of the first four lumbar nerves. Six branches are of surgical interest: the iliohypogastric, ilioinguinal, lateral femoral cutaneous, femoral, genitofemoral, and obturator.

The iliohypogastric nerve is first identified generally as it emerges from the craniolateral aspect of the psoas. It then courses over the ventral aspect of the quadratus lumborum and enters the abdominal wall, running caudally and medially between the external and internal oblique muscles and then over the inguinal canal to supply sensory innervation to the skin of the craniolateral thigh, pubis, anterior scrotum, and labia majora. The ilioinguinal nerve parallels the course of the iliohypogastric nerve, and emerges from the lateral aspect of the psoas just caudal to the iliohypogastric; the ilioinguinal nerve endows a similar spectrum of sensory innervation. The lateral femoral cutaneous nerve passes

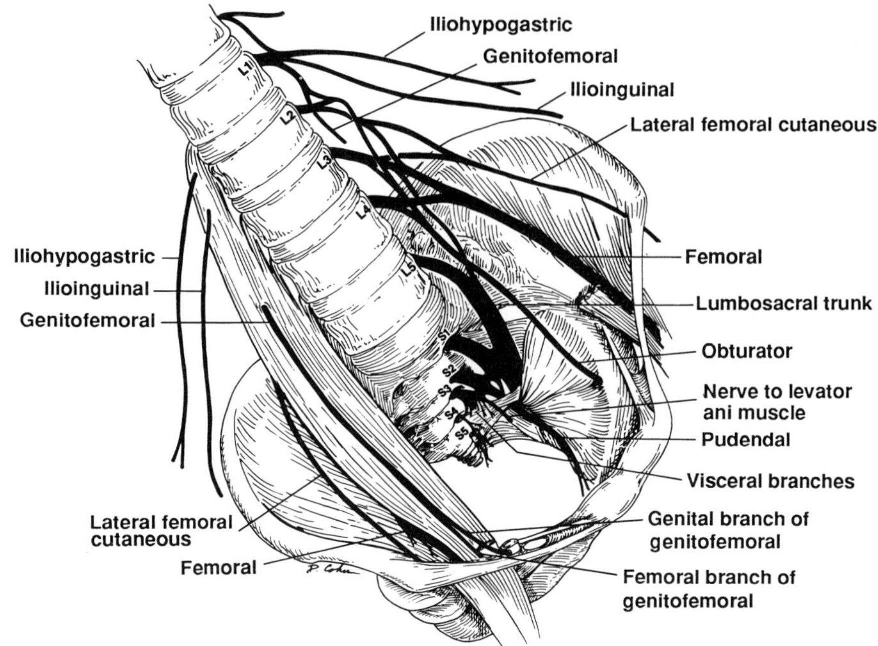


**Fig 12.** Lumbosacral plexus and branches. [From Jones HW, et al, *Novak's Textbook of Gynecology,* 11th ed (Baltimore: Williams & Wilkins Co; 1988), with permission.]

from the lateral aspect of the psoas muscle just cranial to the iliac crest and then courses over the iliacus muscle before passing beneath the inguinal ligament at the anterior superior iliac spine to supply sensory innervation to the lateral thigh. The femoral nerve is a large nerve, which emerges from the lateral aspect of the psoas muscle, which it parallels as it runs over the iliacus muscle to course beneath the inguinal ligament lateral to the femoral artery. The genitofemoral nerve emerges from the psoas muscle at about the level of the lateral femoral cutaneous nerve, and runs along the ventral surface of the psoas muscle, parallel with the external iliac artery. It divides into a genital and femoral branch at varying points of its course. The genital branch passes through the internal ring and accompanies the external spermatic vessels, supplying sensory innervation to the cremasteric muscle, the scrotum, and the labia majora. The femoral branch passes beneath the inguinal ligament to innervate the skin of the anterior thigh. The obturator nerve is the only branch of the lumbar plexus to emerge from the medial border of the psoas muscle. This nerve passes over the obturator internis muscle, but does not lie on the muscle per se. Accompanied by the obturator vessels, it courses through the obturator foramen to innervate the adductor muscle of the thigh and the skin of the medial aspect of the thigh.

The sacral plexus is located in the pelvis, lies on the piriformis muscle, and is formed from the ventral primary division of the fourth and fifth lumbar nerves and the first through third sacral nerves. Although 12 primary nerves are formed from the sacral plexus, only three are of true interest to the pelvic surgeon: the posterior femoral cutaneous, pelvic splachnics, and the pudendal nerves.

The posterior femoral cutaneous nerve is not generally noted. However, at the caudal border of the gluteus maximus, just lateral to the ischial tuberosity, it gives rise to a perineal branch that courses medially along the ischiopubic ramus to innervate the skin of the scrotum and vulva. The pelvic splanchnic nerves (nervi erigentes), which carry preganglionic parasympathetic fibers and sensory fibers, course medially to join the inferior hypogastric plexus in supplying all of the pelvic viscera. The pudendal nerve exits the pelvis through the greater sciatic foramen. Inferior to the piriformis muscle, it courses over the ischial spine to enter the ischiorectal fossa and follows the pudendal vessels in Alcock's canal along the obturator internis muscle. The pudendal nerve gives the primary innervation to the perineum, which it supplies through three branches: the inferior hemorrhoidal, the perineal, and the dorsal nerve of the penis and clitoris. The inferior hemorrhoidal nerve exits from Alcock's canal and, passing medially to the anus, innervates the external anal sphincter and the perianal skin. The perineal nerve also arises from Alcock's canal and gives innervation to the external anal sphincter; the transverse perineal, ischiocavernosus and bulbocavernosus muscles; the urogenital diaphragm; the skin; and the vulva. The dorsal nerve of the penis or clitoris travels within the urogenital diaphragm to reach those organs.

The visceral nerves are contained within the intermediate stratum of retroperitoneal connective tissue and provide afferent and efferent innervation to the pelvic viscera and vasculature (Fig 13). The innervation is conveyed through nerve plexuses which are also, in some instances, referred to as nerves. The primary plexuses carrying innervation to the pelvis are the superior and inferior hypogastric plexuses. The gonads and uterine tubes are supplied by nerves which proceed from the pre-aortic plexuses with the gonadal vessels.

The superior hypogastric plexus, which

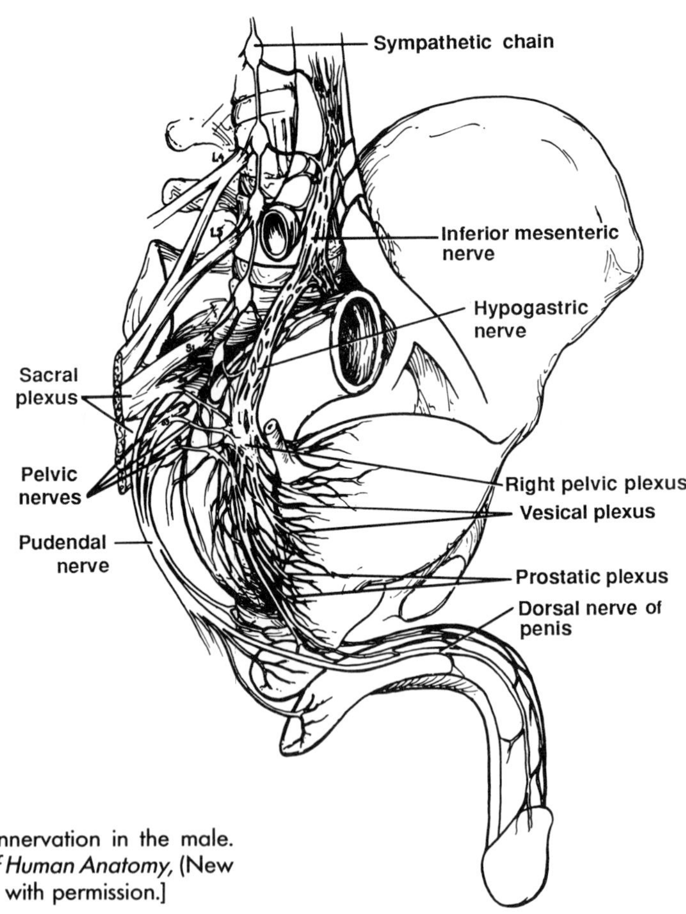


**Fig 13.** Pelvic visceral innervation in the male. [From Toldt C, *An Atlas of Human Anatomy,* (New York: MacMillan; 1948), with permission.]

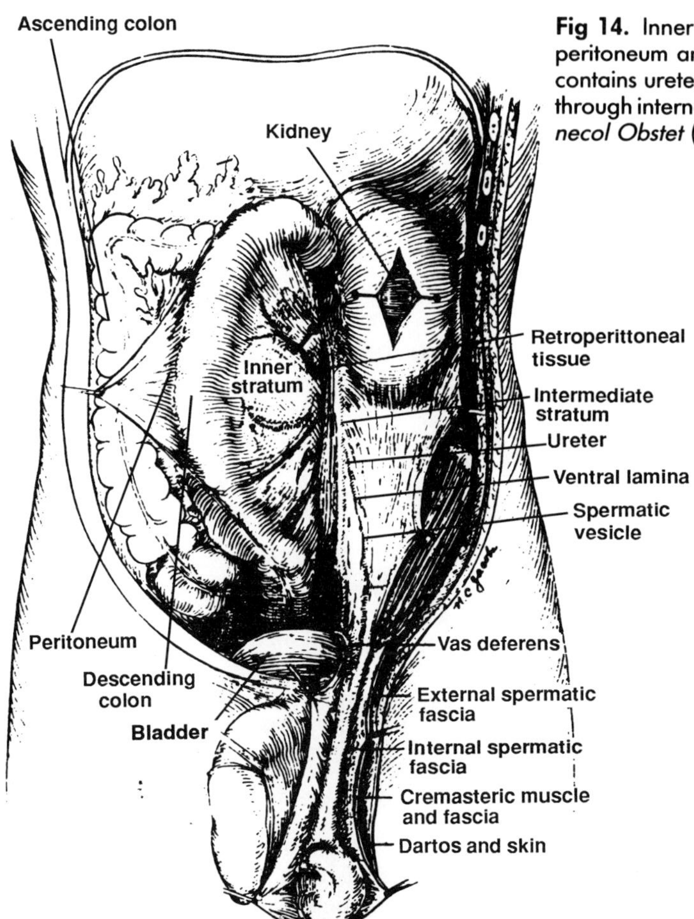


**Fig 14.** Inner stratum covering dorsal aspect of peritoneum and mesentery; intermediate stratum contains ureter and gonadal vessels and extends through internal ring into scrotum. [From *Surg, Gynecol Obstet* (1946;83:586), with permission.]

is a continuation of the aortic plexus, is located over the bifurcation of the aorta and sacral promontory. Just caudal to the sacral promontory, it bifurcates into plexuses, termed the right and left hypogastric nerves, which course caudally and laterally along the pelvic side wall. They then diverge on either side of the rectum and join with the pelvic splanchnic nerves to form the inferior hypogastric (pelvic) plexus. The inferior hypogastric plexus gives rise to three smaller plexuses: the middle hemorrhoidal, the vesical, and the prostatic or uterovaginal (Frankenhauser's). The prostatic plexus, located in the retroperitoneal connective tissue on the dorsal aspect of the prostate, courses anteriorly through the urogenital diaphragm as cavernous nerves of the penis. The uterovaginal plexus passes through the broad ligament to the uterus and vagina.

## RETROPERITONEAL CONNECTIVE TISSUE AND THE PERITONEUM

The lower genitourinary tract is located primarily within the retroperitoneum; for this reason it is imperative to have knowledge of the retroperitoneal connective tissue. Cleavage planes and organ pedicles are more easily identified if the retroperitoneal layers are dissected as such. A practical schema is that in which the retroperitoneal connective tissue is considered to consist of three layers or strata: an outer, inner, and intermediate (Fig 14). The inner stratum forms the supporting connective tissue of the peritoneum. The outer stratum consists of the investing fascia of the muscles of the abdominal and pelvic walls, which are collectively termed transversalis fascia. The intermediate stratum is fat-laden connective tissue that forms the pack-

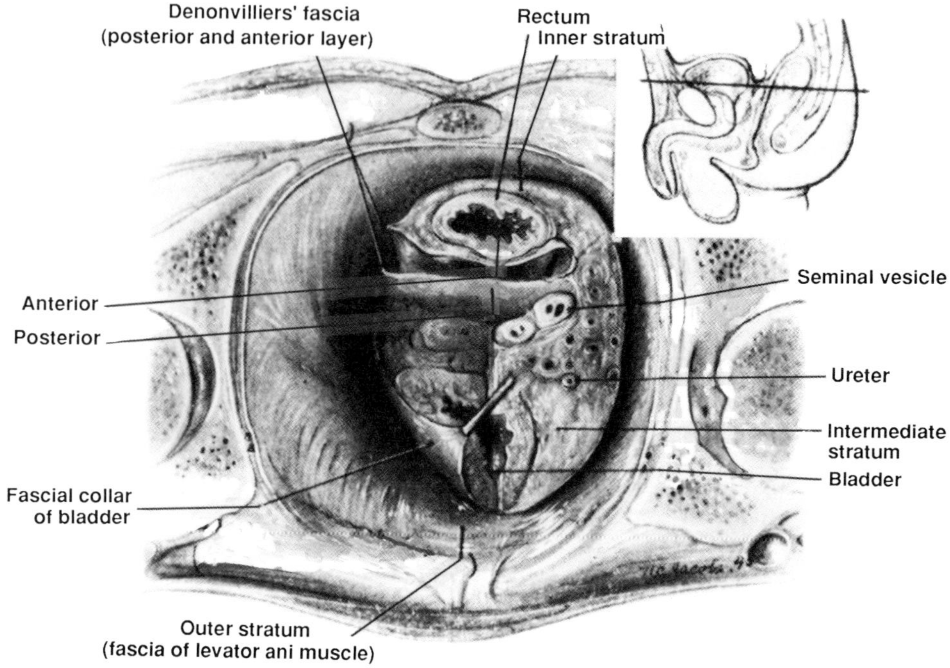


**Fig 15.** Cross-section through male pelvis (see inset) showing relationships of pelvic viscera to retroperitoneal connective tissue. [From *Surg, Gynecol Obstet* (1946;83:589), with permission.]

ing material between the inner and outer stratum. The thickness and fat content varies; the layers are thicker in the dorsal pelvis but are so scant anteriorly, especially in the midline, that the transversalis fascia adheres to the peritoneum. Anatomic texts frequently apply the term endopelvic fascia to the intermediate stratum. Exposure of the pelvic side wall can therefore be accomplished retroperitoneally by sweeping the intermediate stratum from the outer stratum (transversalis fascia) to visualize the lateral aspects and the pedicles of the bladder, the lower ureter, and the iliac vessels (Fig 15). This exposure is impeded by the tethering which occurs at the level of the internal ring by the adherence of the peritoneum and the gonadal vessels, or round ligament proceeding through the ring. With freeing of the vessels from the intermediate stratum or cutting of the round ligament, the exposure of the pelvic and abdominal side wall may continue. A further useful concept is that of fused fascial planes, which arise when two layers of serosa become adherent in the developmental process (such as with the application of the ascending and descending colon to the abdominal side wall); the serosa disappears, leaving only the inner stratum and a resultant potential cleavage plane.

Fibrous condensations of the intermediate stratum form "ligaments" and pedicles which include the lateral vesical pedicles, and, in the female, the uterosacral, cardinal, and pubocervical ligaments (Fig 16). The double-leafed peritoneal extension from the uterus to the pelvic side-wall is termed the broad ligament; the retroperitoneal connective tissue contained within this ligament is termed the parametrium.

The female urethra is attached to the pubic symphysis by condensations of extraperitoneal connective tissue termed pubourethral ligaments. Similarly, the prostate is attached by the puboprostatic ligaments.

Within the peritoneal cavity, the pelvic structures are overlain by peritoneum and exhibit varieties of recesses and bands; this presentation is particularly notable at lap-

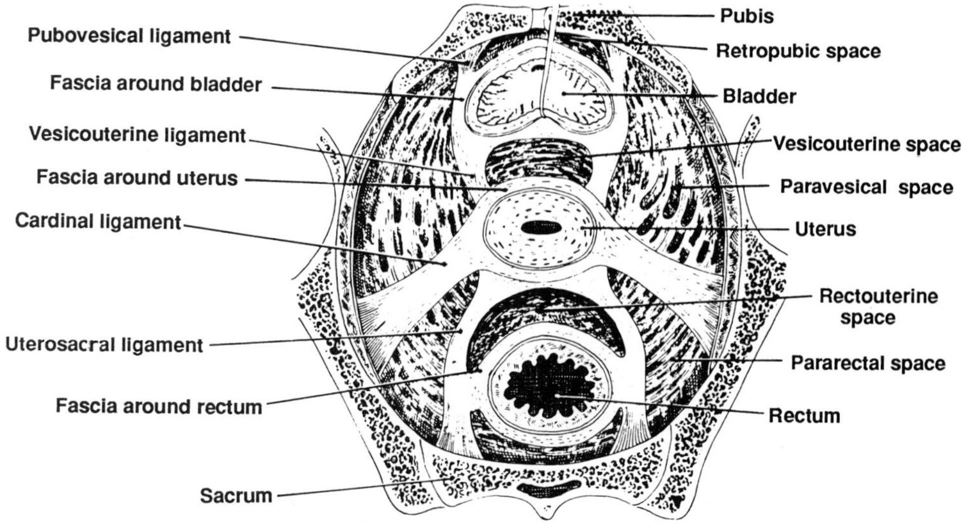


**Fig 16.** Schematic drawings of condensations ("ligaments") of intermediate stratum of retroperitoneal connective tissue in the female pelvis. [From Crafts RC, *A Textbook of Human Anatomy,* 3rd ed (New York: John Wiley & Sons Inc; 1985), with permission.]

aroscopy. Between the bladder and the rectum in the male and the bladder and the uterus in the female is a deep recess, the rectovesical and rectouterine pouch, respectively. The apparent bands bridging from the bladder to the sacrum in the male and from the uterus to the sacrum in the female are termed the vesicosacral and uterosacral folds, respectively.

## SPECIFIC REGIONS OF SURGICAL INTEREST

A discussion of applied anatomy of the lower urinary tract of necessity should include a description of three specific regions: the perineum, the inguinal canal, and the anterior femoral region.

### The Perineum

The perineum embodies a diamond-shaped area which covers the caudal outlet of the bony pelvis (Fig 17). The anterior-posterior boundaries are the pubic symphysis and coccyx, while the lateral boundaries are defined by the ischial tuberosities. A line drawn to connect the ischial tuberosities would divide the diamond into an anterior (urogenital) and posterior (anal) triangle. The perineal body (central perineal tendon) is located in the mid-portion of the bases of the triangles and is the central fixation point of the perineum.

The urogenital triangle may be distinguished by the presence of the external genitalia, which overlies or penetrates the urogenital diaphragm. Anatomically, the urogenital triangle is usually further divided for discussion into components termed the superficial and deep spaces of the perineum. The superficial perineal space is located between the membranous layer of the subcutaneous connective tissue and the perineal membrane (inferior fascia of the urogenital diaphragm). The deep space lies deep to the perineal membrane, between the perineal membrane and the investing fascia of the muscles of the so-called urogenital diaphragm.

In the superficial perineal space in the male is located: the corpora spongiosa covered by the bulbospongiosus muscle, the corpora cavernosa of the penis covered by the ischocavernosus muscle, and the superficial transversus perinei muscles along with perineal vasculature and nerves. In the female are found the homologous structures, that is, the bulbospongiosus muscles covering the vestibular bulbs and the is-

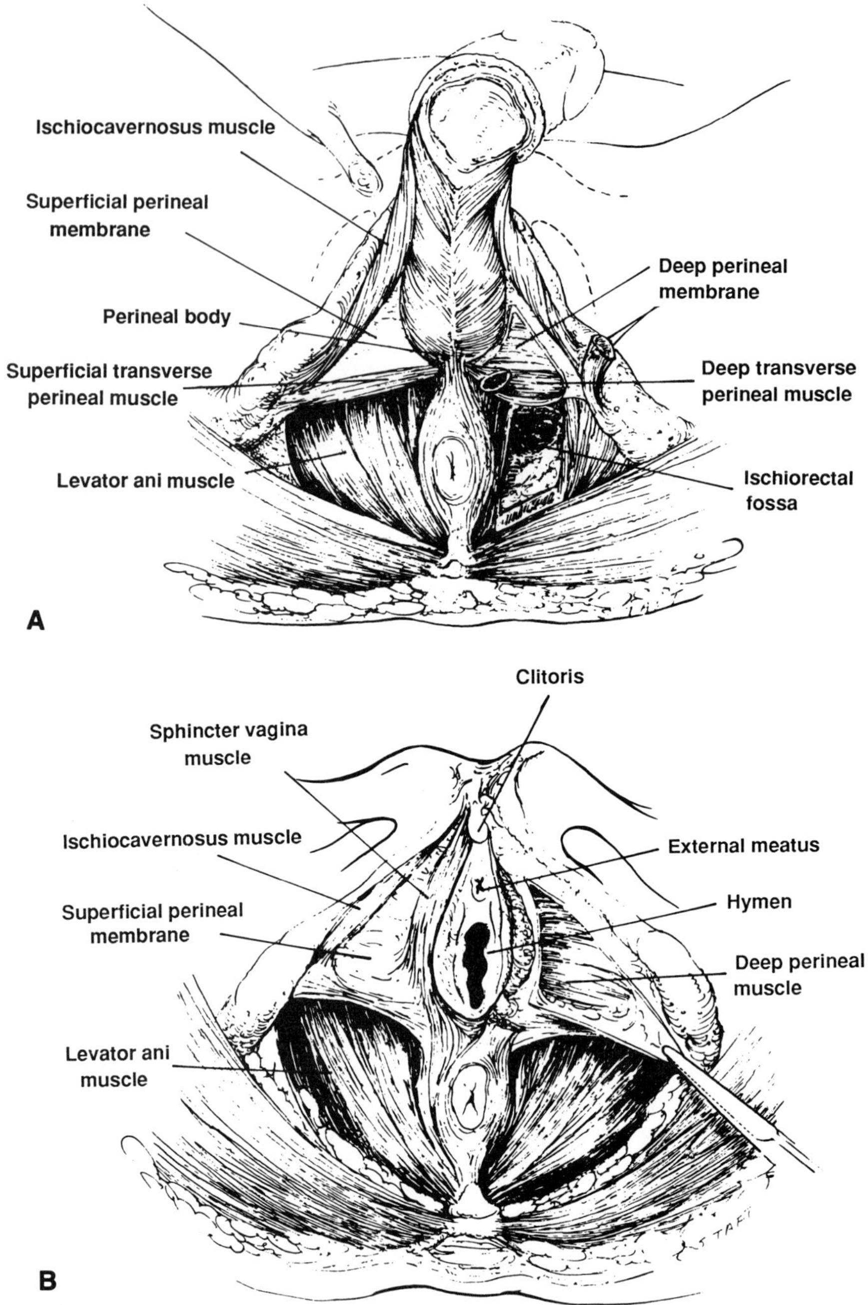


**Fig 17.** A, male perineum; B, female perineum. [From Walsh PC, et al, eds, *Campbell's Urology,* 5th ed (Philadelphia: WB Saunders Co; 1986), with permission.]

chiocavernosus muscles covering the crura of the corpora cavernosus of the clitoris.

In the male, the deep space of the perineum contains the deep transverse perineal muscles posteriorly and the sphincter urethrae anteriorly. Since the sphincter urethrae muscle and the deep fascia cranial to it continue into the pelvic cavity alongside the urethra, a "sandwich-like" urogenital diaphragm does not actually exist. The

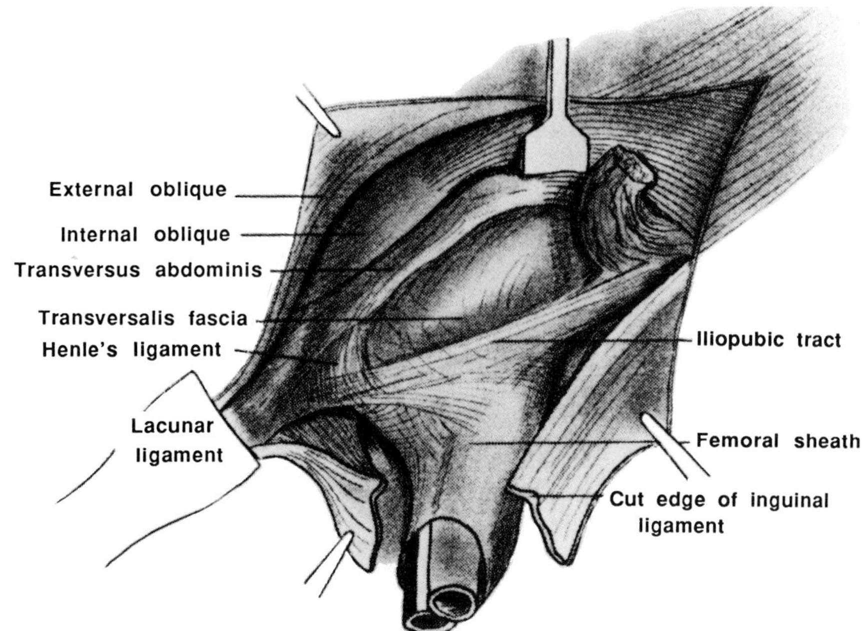


**Fig 18.** Floor of inguinal canal. [From *Surg, Gynecol Obstet* (1946;82:482), with permission.]

paired bulbourethral glands (Cowper's), along with the continuation of the internal pudendal artery and dorsal nerves of the penis, are contained within the deep space. In the female, the muscular structures are the same, with the exception that the deep transverse perineal muscle is perforated by the vagina.

The anal triangle contains the centrally located anus, surrounded by the external anal sphincter, which is anchored anteriorly by the perineal body and posteriorly by the coccyx. On either side of the external anal sphincter lies the ischiorectal fossa, which is bounded craniomedially by the levator ani and laterally by the obturator internis muscles. Traversing the ischiorectal fossa are the inferior hemorrhoidal vasculature and nerves. The fatty tissue of the ischiorectal fossa is overlain with the superficial fascia, which in the perineum, is known as Colles fascia.

## The Inguinal Canal

On cross-section, the inguinal canal is roughly triangular shaped, with anterior, posterior, and inferior sides. Anteriorly it is formed by the external oblique aponeurosis, which in the middle third of the anterior side becomes the superficial inguinal ring. The posterior side is formed by the transversus abdominis aponeurosis and transversalis fascia. The transversalis fascia of the inguinal canal is reinforced by three fibrous structures: the iliopubic tract, the aponeurosis of the transversus abdominis muscle, and Henle's ligament (Fig 18). The iliopubic tract is a fibrous thickening of transversalis fascia which parallels the inguinal ligament, while Henle's ligament is a thin, lateral expansion of the rectus sheath. The inferior side of the triangle is formed by the lower border of the inguinal ligament.

## The Femoral Triangle

The femoral, or Scarpa's, triangle is bounded on its base by the inguinal ligament, medially by the abductor longus muscle, and laterally by the sartorius muscle (Fig 19). The floor of the triangle is formed by three muscles from medial to lateral: the pectineus, psoas, and iliacus muscles. Traversing the triangle from cranial to caudal, emerging from beneath the inguinal ligament and lying on the muscular

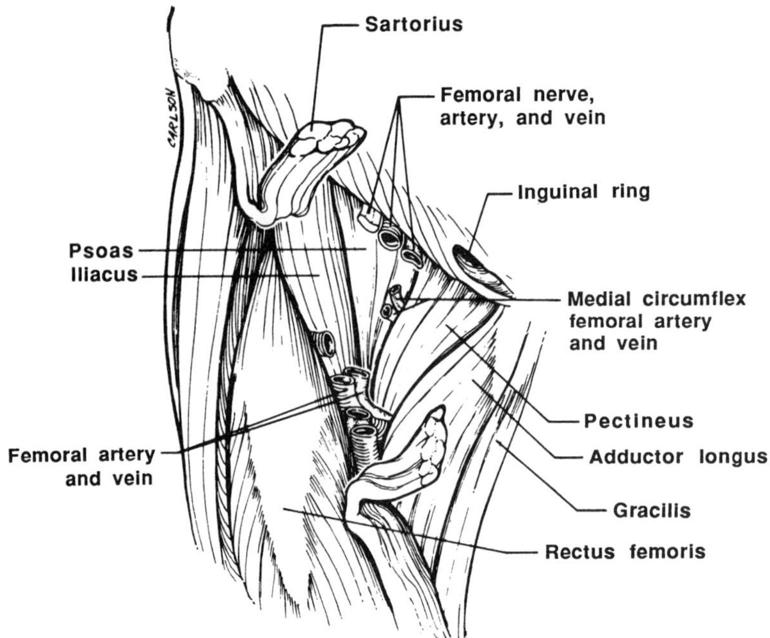


**Fig 19.** Floor of the femoral triangle. [From Johnson DE, Ames FC, *Groin Dissection* (Chicago: Year Book, 1985), with permission.]

floor are, from medial to lateral: the femoral vein, artery, and nerve. The femoral vessels are contained within the femoral sheath, which is formed anteriorly by the transversalis fascia. Superficial vessels arise from the femoral vessels and course over the anterior abdominal wall. These include: the superficial external pudendals, the superficial inferior epigastrics, and the superficial circumflex iliacs. The femoral triangle is overlain by fascia lata, which are perforated by an opening termed the fossa ovalis, through which emanates the superficial vessels and which receives the greater saphenous vein. The lymph nodes deep to the fascia lata are termed the deep inguinal nodes and those superficial to the fascia, the superficial nodes.

## ORGANOLOGY

This section will cover the gross anatomy and relationships of the pelvic organs. General information in regards to vasculature, lymphatic drainage, and innervation of each of the pelvic organs is discussed above.

### The Bladder

**Gross Anatomy.** Generally the bladder is thought of as spherical, which indeed it is, in the distended or full state. However, when empty, it may be described as tetrahedral in shape with four angles and four surfaces. The angles are formed by the two ureterovesical junctions, the urachovesical junction and the urethrovesical junction. The surfaces are: a superior, two inferolateral and a posterior (fundus or base). The juncture of the bladder with the fibrous remnant of the urachus, termed the median umbilical ligament, is the apex, whereas the junction of the bladder with the urethra is the neck. The interior of the bladder is characterized by mucosa which, when the bladder is distended, appears smooth, although the syncytial quality of the underlying bladder musculature can still be discerned through the thin mucosa. The base of the bladder is distinguished by an always smooth mucosal triangle, the trigone, in which the angles are formed by the ureteral orifices and the internal urethral orifice (Fig 20). An incision through the blad-

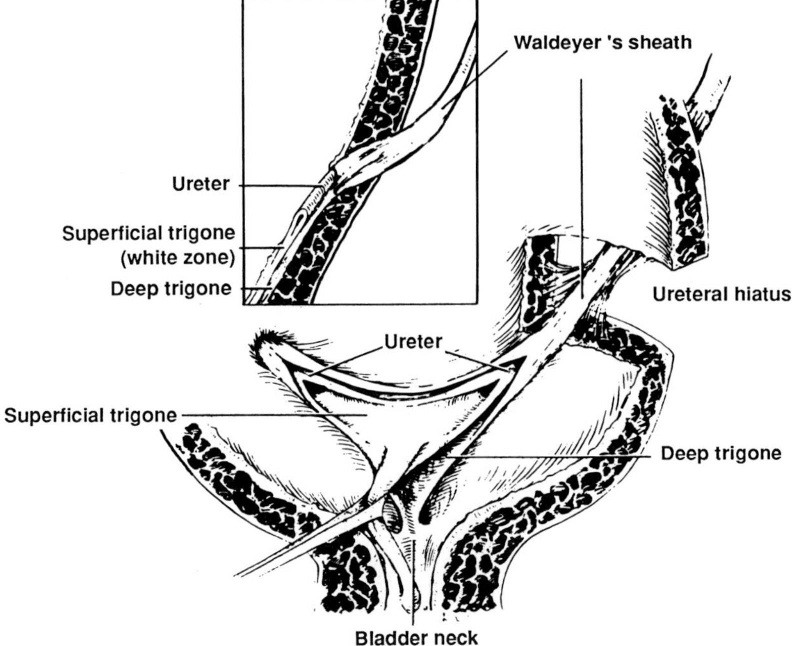


**Fig 20.** Normal ureterovesico-trigonal complex. [From Walsh PC, et al, eds, *Campbell's Urology,* 5th ed (Philadelphia: WB Saunders Co; 1986), with permission.]

der wall reveals it to be made of muscle of varying thickness, with no particular evidence of layering despite the description that the bladder has three muscular layers (Fig 21). Distinct layers are noted only at the vesical neck.

**Relationships.** In general, when full, the bladder sits low in the pelvis behind the pelvic symphysis. In infants, the bladder extends high above the symphysis; with increasing age, the bladder gradually assumes the adult position. The bladder is encased in intermediate stratum of retroperitoneal connective tissue that both supports the bladder through varying condensations and also contains the vasculature, including the extensive vesical venous plexus. Serosa (peritoneum) covers the posterior and superior surface of the bladder. When viewed intraperitoneally, the median umbilical ligament can be seen extending to the umbilicus contained within the retroperitoneum and extending from the lateral aspects of the superior surface of the bladder. Also continuing to the umbilicus are lateral (sometimes termed medial) umbilical ligaments, which represent the obliterated umbilical arteries.

Condensations of intermediate stratum of retroperitoneal connective tissue form so-called ligaments of the bladder. Dorsolaterally, condensations extend from the arcus tendinous of the pelvis to the bladder, forming a vascular pedicle termed the lateral pedicle or ligament of the bladder. Dense condensations of this connective tissue anchor the neck of the bladder to the pelvis and are termed puboprostatic ligaments. In the female, similar condensations are known as the pubovesical ligaments.

Anteriorly, the potential space that exists between the connective tissue surrounding the bladder and the transversalis fascia is termed the prevesical space (space of Retzius). Posteriorly in the male, the bladder is separated cranially from the rectum by the rectovesical pouch (cul-de-sac of Douglas). Caudally, the base of the bladder is in apposition to the rectum; however, at its neck it is separated by the ampulla of the vasa and the vasa deferentia (Fig 22). In

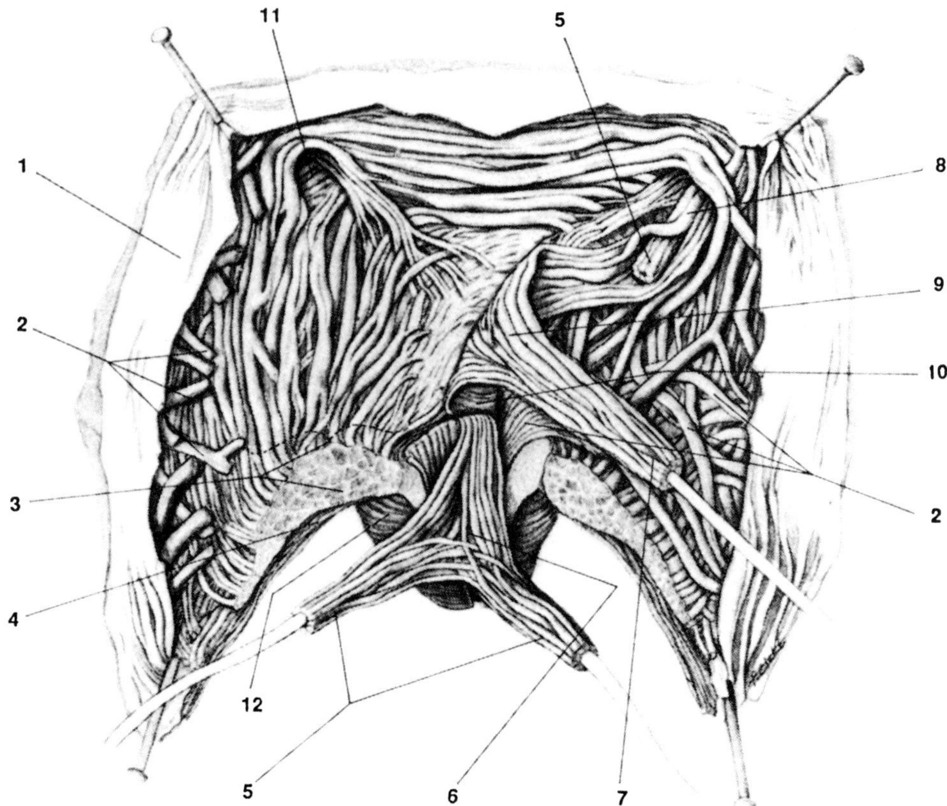


**Fig 21.** Muscle layers around the bladder neck as seen from the inside of a male bladder: 1, remaining edge of the bladder mucosa; 2, inner longitudinal layer with mesh-like arrangement of fibers that continue in the urethra; 3, middle circular fibers condensed anteriorly and fanning out dorsocranially; 4, outer longitudinal coat; 5, intravesical ureter cut and reflected downward; 6, superficial trigone dissected and reflected; 7, intramural ureter with Waldeyer's sheath; 8, Waldeyer's sheath; 9, deep trigone (direct continuation of Waldeyer's sheath); 10, apex of deep trigone ending at the internal meatus; 11, the ureteral hiatus; 12, the prostate. [From *Br J Urol* (1966;38:55), with permission.]

the female, the bladder is separated from the uterus cranially by the vesicouterine pouch (cul-de-sac of Douglas), but caudally it is in apposition to the cervix and vagina. In the male, the musculature of the bladder melds with that of the prostate, on which it rests.

## The Lower Ureter

**Gross Anatomy.** The ureters, which are contained within the intermediate stratum of retroperitoneal connective tissue, enter the pelvis overlying the mid-portion of the psoas muscles. They are contained within a specialization of the retroperitoneal connective tissue termed the ureteric sheath or fascia. Although their course into the pelvis is relatively constant, they are dynamic muscular structures and have a fair degree of mobility which is needed for their rhythmic peristalsis. In addition, the width of the ureter may change dramatically with peristalsis. A particular area of ureteral widening, termed the pelvic spindle, is formed between the point where the ureter crosses the iliac vessel and the point where it crosses dorsal to the lateral umbilical ligament. The area of the ureter from the crossing of the iliac to the bladder is termed

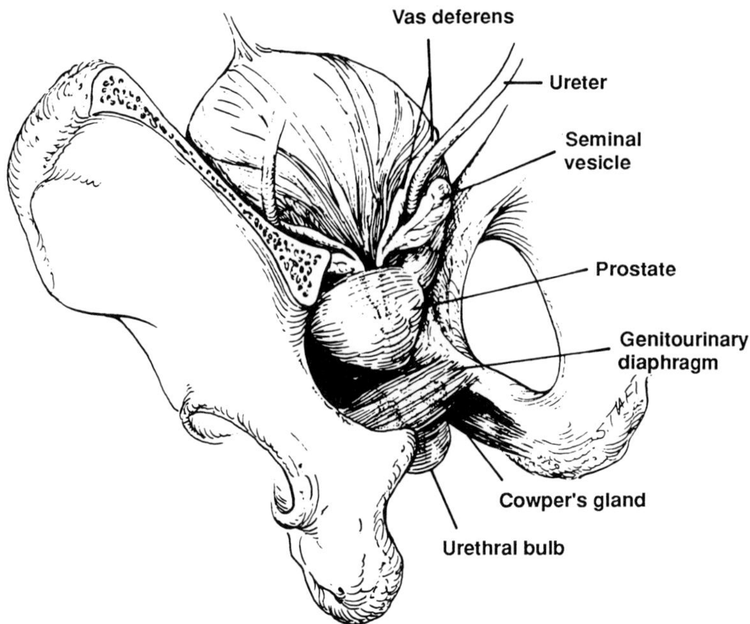


**Fig 22.** Posterior view of bladder and its relationships to the seminal vesicles and vasa. [From Walsh PC, et al, eds, *Campbell's Urology,* 5th ed (Philadelphia: WB Saunders Co; 1986), with permission.]

the pelvic ureter. The terminal portion of the ureter, the ureterovesical junction, has three segments. The portion of the ureter just adjacent to its entry into the bladder wall is termed the juxtavesical ureter. That portion that traverses the bladder wall is the intravesical ureter, while the .8- to 1-cm segment that lies beneath the submucosa is the submucosal segment. The ureteral musculature continues into, and joins in the formation of the trigone of, the bladder. Duplication of ureter is not uncommon and triplication may also occur. When multiple ureters exist, they are usually separate on entering the pelvis but are closely joined in a common sheath as they approach the bladder, even though within the bladder the orifices may be separated considerably. Invariably, the lower orifice will be found to drain the upper renal pole-collecting structures.

The pelvic ureter receives abundant vasculature from a variety of vessels including longitudinal vasculature which arises from the aorta. Arterial supply is derived from the common and internal iliac, the gonadals, the superior and inferior vesicles, and the middle hemorrhoidal vessels.

**Relationships.** The ureter is relatively easily seen, as it enters the pelvis contained within the intermediate stratum of retroperitoneal connective tissue just dorsal to the peritoneum. Of critical importance in surgery of the female is knowledge of the relationship of the gonadal vessels which cross ventral to the ureter approximately at the point of entrance of the ovarian vessels into the infundibuliform ligament en route to the ovaries. As the ureter crosses the iliacs, it reaches its most medial position; indeed, at this point the ureters are within 5 to 6 cm of each other. They then course laterally into the hollow of the pelvis before turning medially toward the bladder. From the point where the ureter passes dorsal to the lateral umbilical ligament to its juxtavesical segment, the ureter is largely hidden from view within the pelvis (except in extremely lean subjects).

In the male, the vas deferens crosses ventral to the ureter, usually at about the po-

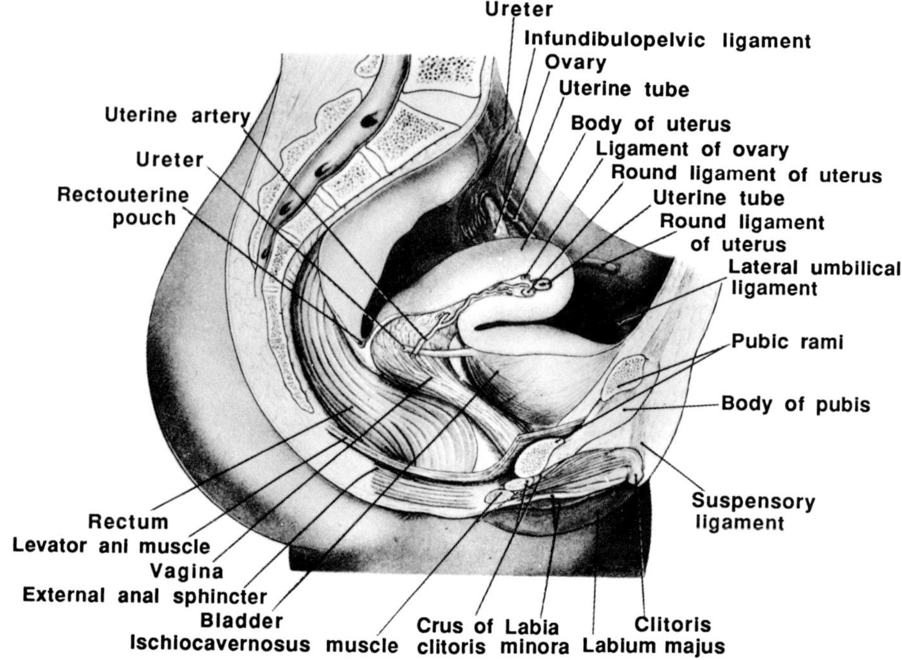


**Fig 23.** Lateral view showing relationships of uterus, cervix, ureter, and uterine artery. [From Hamilton WF, *A Textbook of Human Anatomy,* 2nd ed (St. Louis: CV Mosby Co; 1976), with permission.]

sition of the crossing of the lateral umbilical ligament. In females, the ureter passes through the caudal aspect of the broad (Mackenrodt's) ligament, in which it is surrounded by the uterine venous plexus. Imperative to the pelvic surgeon is the knowledge that the ureter is accompanied by the uterine artery for 2.5 cm as the artery passes ventral to it (Fig 23). The ureter also courses approximately 1.5 cm from the side of the supravesical portion of the cervix.

## Prostate

**Gross Anatomy.** The prostate resembles a chestnut, both in configuration and size. It has also been described as an inverted, compressed cone with a blunt tip. A fibrous tissue capsule covers the gland. The cranial aspect of the prostate, the base of the cone, is termed the base, while the caudal aspect is termed the apex. The prostate is traversed by three tubular structures: the posterior urethra, and the paired ejaculatory ducts. When sectioned in the coronal midline, the urethra will be noted to form a 35° angle in the mid-portion of the gland. Further, the urethra roughly indicates a separation of the prostate into a thicker dorsal or posterior glandular portion and a thinner ventral or anterior fibromuscular portion. The ejaculatory ducts traverse the dorsal prostatic substance, from its base to a point just distal to the mid-portion of the prostate, where a small hillock is located; this structure is known as the verumontanum (colliculus seminalis). Within the urethra, a ridge may be noted, which extends from the vesical neck to the membranous urethra; this is termed the urethral crest. The verumontanum marks the approximate midpoint of the crest, and in its midpoint a small depression is located, the utricle (vagina masculina) (Fig 24). On either side of the utricle, just dorsal to the verumontanum, the openings of the ejaculatory ducts are located. On either side of the urethral crest is a depression, termed the

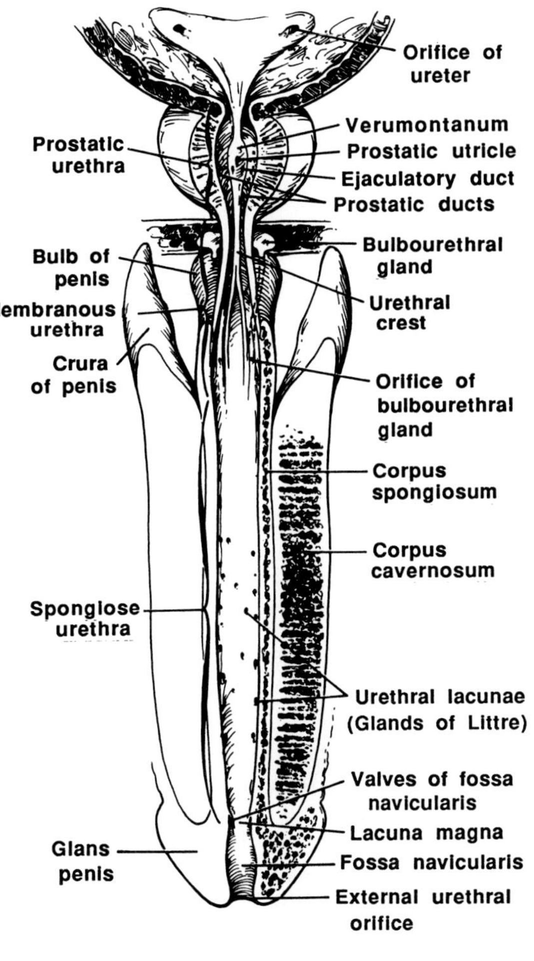


**Fig 24.** Anterior and posterior urethra in the male. [From Clemente CD, *Anatomy—A Regional Atlas of the Human Body,* 2nd ed (Baltimore: Williams & Wilkins Co; 1981), with permission.]

prostatic sinus, which is perforated by the openings of the ducts of the prostatic glands. A majority of the ducts are located distal to the verumontanum.

Prostatic lobes were described by Lowsley in the 1930s, based on fetal and newborn prostatic material. The lobar terminology is frequently, though erroneously, used to describe the enlargements produced by benign prostatic hyperplasia, which may occur in the so-called lateral and median lobes. The detailed work of McNeal, who described four distinct regions of the glandular prostate, became more than a scholarly work with the burgeoning use of transrectal prostatic ultrasound examinations. The four regions or zones are the peripheral, central, transitional, and periurethral (Fig 25). The peripheral zone constitutes approximately 75% of the volume of the glandular prostate while the central zone accounts for 20%. Four percent of the glandular prostate is formed by the transitional zone, which is composed of two small areas

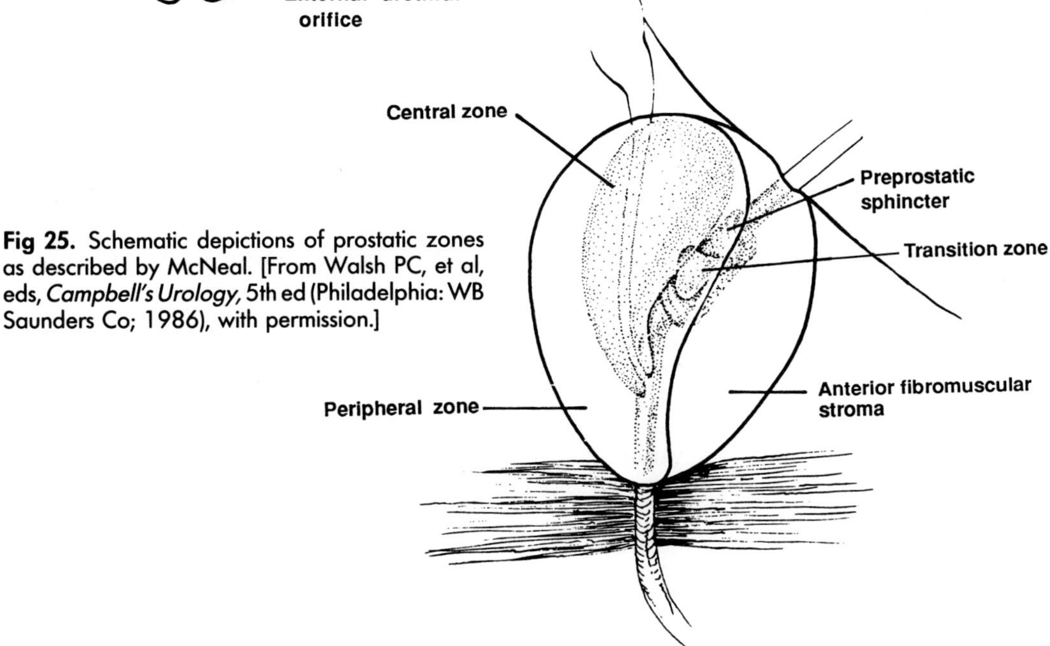


**Fig 25.** Schematic depictions of prostatic zones as described by McNeal. [From Walsh PC, et al, eds, *Campbell's Urology,* 5th ed (Philadelphia: WB Saunders Co; 1986), with permission.]

of glandular tissue lateral to the proximal segment of the prostatic urethra and to the rings of smooth muscle that surround the dorsal aspect of the urethra, or the pre-prostatic sphincter.

The arterial vasculature of the prostate generally originates via the prostatic artery, a branch of the inferior vesicle. After supplying vasculature to the base of the bladder and the seminal vesicles, this artery approaches the prostate on its dorsolateral aspect. Within the prostate, the prostatic artery divides into a peripheral capsular group and a central urethral group. The urethral vessels enter at the prostatovesical junction perpendicular to the urethra, and enter the internal urethral orifice at the 7 to 11 o'clock and 1 to 5 o'clock areas of its circumference. The apex of the prostate also receives arterial blood from the middle hemorrhoidal and internal pudendal arteries.

The venous drainage of the prostate occurs via capsular veins, which drain to the prostatic venous plexus (Santorini's plexus) and ultimately to the vesical plexus and internal iliac veins (Fig 10). The prostatic plexus also communicates (without valves) with the extradural venous plexus (Batson's plexus), which is believed to be a route for skeletal metastasis of prostatic carcinoma.

**Relationships.** The base of the prostate is intimately related to the base of the bladder, with the superficial trigone of the bladder extending to the verumontanum and the bladder's vesical musculature blending with that of the prostate. The apex of the prostate is likewise intimately related to the urogenital diaphragm, with the prostatic capsule and closely adherent extraperitoneal connective tissue being attached to the superior investing fascia of the deep transverse perineal muscle. Anteriorly, the prostate lies beneath the pubis and is covered by intermediate stratum of retroperitoneal connective tissue through which course the dorsal veins of the penis and the associated arborizations. The prostate is firmly held to the pubis anteriorly by the dense fibrous condensations of the retroperitoneal connective tissue termed the puboprostatic ligaments. On the lateral aspects of the prostate, the levator ani muscle is closely associated. The inner investing fascia of the levator (endopelvic fascia), forms an investing fascial collar around the apex of the gland.

Posteriorly, the prostate rests for the most part on the ventral aspect of the rectum, from which it is separated by connective tissue. The nature of the connective tissue has engendered a considerable number of dissertations. The most common term given to the connective tissue is Denonvillier's fascia, which is described as a residuum of the former double-leafed rectogenital septum. However, Jewett and associates have stated that they were unable to demonstrate any structure that fit the textbook description of Denonvillier's fascia.[1] One description is that the cleavage plane that exists between the prostate and the rectum is represented by the inner stratum covering the anterior surface of the rectum and the intermediate stratum of retroperitoneal connective tissue which lies over the posterior aspect of the prostate. A layer of connective tissue can also be identified which is contiguous with that covering the perivesical fat that extends caudally to cover the anterior and posterior surfaces of the seminal vesicles. At the posterior apex of the prostate, a firm muscular attachment of fused fibers of the levator ani may be found which is contiguous with the lower anterior rectal wall, or the rectourethralis muscle (Fig 26). On the lateral aspects of the prostate posteriorly, the retroperitoneal connective tissue contains the capsular vasculature of the prostate, the innervation of the prostate, and the corpora cavernosa (Fig 27).

At the prostato-vesicle junction, the bases of the seminal vesicles are in apposition to the posterior cranial aspect of the prostate.

## MALE EXTERNAL GENITALIA

The male external genitalia will, for purposes of organization, include the anatomy of the penis and anterior urethra; the scrotum and spermatic cords; and the testis, epididymis, and vas deferens.

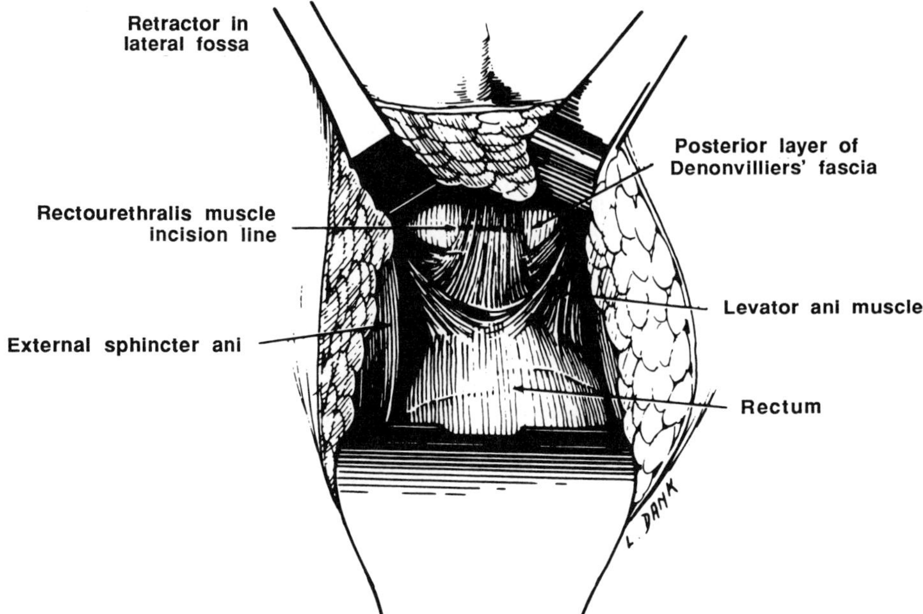


**Fig 26.** Rectourethralis muscle with relationships of rectum and prostate. [From Glenn JF, Boyce WH, eds. *Urologic Surgery,* 2nd ed (Hagerstown, MD: Harper & Row; 1975), with permission.]

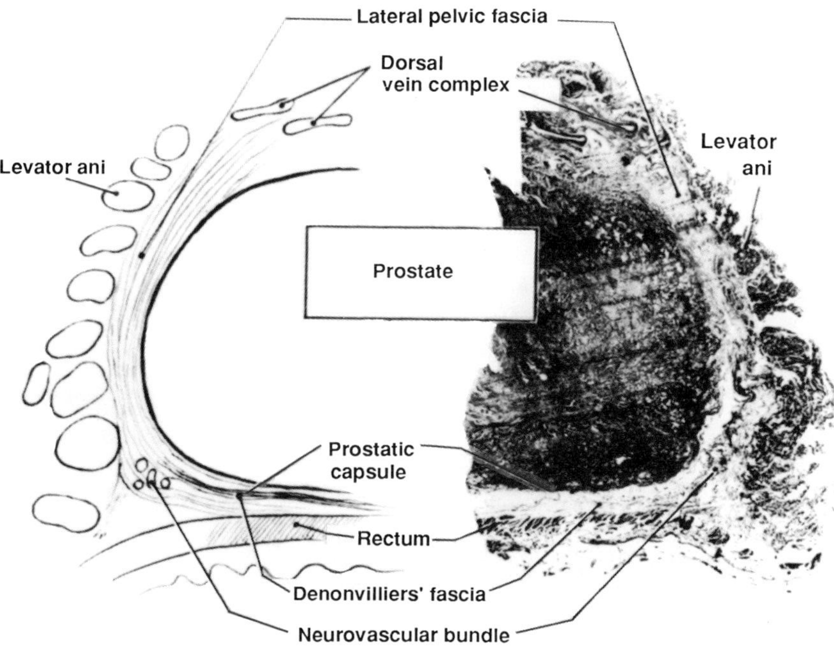


**Fig 27.** Cross-section of adult prostate showing position of neurovascular bundle. [From *Prostate* (1983;4:477), with permission.]

## Penis

**Gross Anatomy.** The penis is usually described as having two portions, a pendulous part and a perineal part. Other terminology for the pendulous segment are the corpus or body. The perineal segment is referred to as the radix or root. The pendulous portion is capped by the glans, or balanus, which is a direct extension of the corpus spongiosum. The penis is primarily composed of three erectile bodies: the paired corpora cavernosa and the ventral midline corpora spongiosa which terminate distally as the glans. Although the corpora cavernosa are considered to be paired cylindrical structures, in the pendulous portion they are intimately connected with each other by an incomplete midline septum. The corpora cavernosa diverge proximal to the pubic symphysis, and the crura of the penis, as they are now known, firmly attach to the pubic rami and the medial border of the ischium. The corpus spongiosum containing the urethra is also cylindrical, and is characterized by—in addition to the glans—the bulb-like expansion in the perineum known as the bulb of the penis. The configuration of the pendulous portion of the penis, along with the coverings, are better understood on examination of a cross-section of the penis (Fig 28). The two paired cylinders of the corpora cavernosa create a dorsal and a ventral groove. In the dorsal groove is found the neurovascular bundle, while ventrally the groove supports the corpora spongiosa. On cross-section it is also noted that the corporal bodies are composed of a vascular, sponge-like tissue and are contained within a dense, grayish covering, the tunica albuginea. The corpora, as well as the neurovascular bundle, are surrounded by Buck's fascia, an extension of the investing fascia of the bulbocavernosus muscle. Superficial to Buck's fascia, the pendulous portion of the

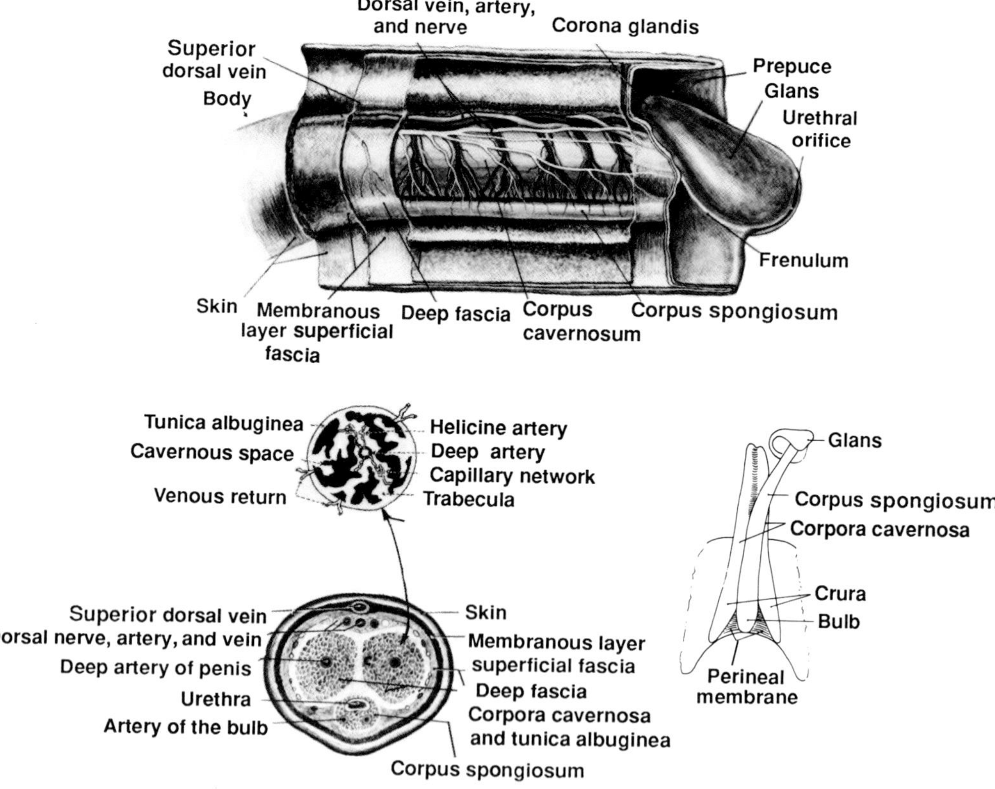


**Fig 28.** Gross anatomy of penis. [From Crafts RC, *A Textbook of Human Anatomy,* 3rd ed (New York: John Wiley & Sons Inc; 1985), with permission.]

penis is covered by superficial membranous fascia, the dartos tunic, which is contiguous with the dartos tunic of the scrotum. The skin of the penis forms a double-leafed structure that covers the glans, termed the foreskin or prepuce, which is characterized on the ventral aspect of the glans by a midline tether termed the frenulum. The dorsolateral base of the glans penis, which projects over the body of the penis, is referred to as the corona, while the groove thus created is termed the retroglandular sulcus or neck of the penis. The urethral meatus presents at the ventral tip of the glans.

**Relationships.** The perineal portion of the penis, the root, is largely covered by muscle (Fig 17A). The crura of the corpora cavernosa are covered by the ischiocavernosus muscle and aponeurosis from their origin on the ischium to the level of their divergence. The corpora spongiosa is covered by the bulbospongiosus muscle, which joins in the midline to form a fibrous septum. The penis is attached to the arch of the pubis and the anterior abdominal wall by fibrous tissue bands. Attachment to the anterior abdominal wall is achieved via a midline thickening of Scarpa's fascia, the fundiform ligament. Just inferior to the fundiform ligament, the root of the penis is attached to the symphysis pubis by a fibrous extension of Buck's fascia known as the suspensory ligament of the penis. The fascia of the ischiocavernosus and bulbospongiosus muscles meld with the inferior fascia of the urogenital diaphragm, with the fascia of the bulbospongiosus also attaching to the perineal body.

**Vasculature.** The penis is vascularized by four paired branches of the internal pudendal artery (Fig 29). The first one or two branches to supply the penis are the bulbourethral arteries, which may arise as sep-

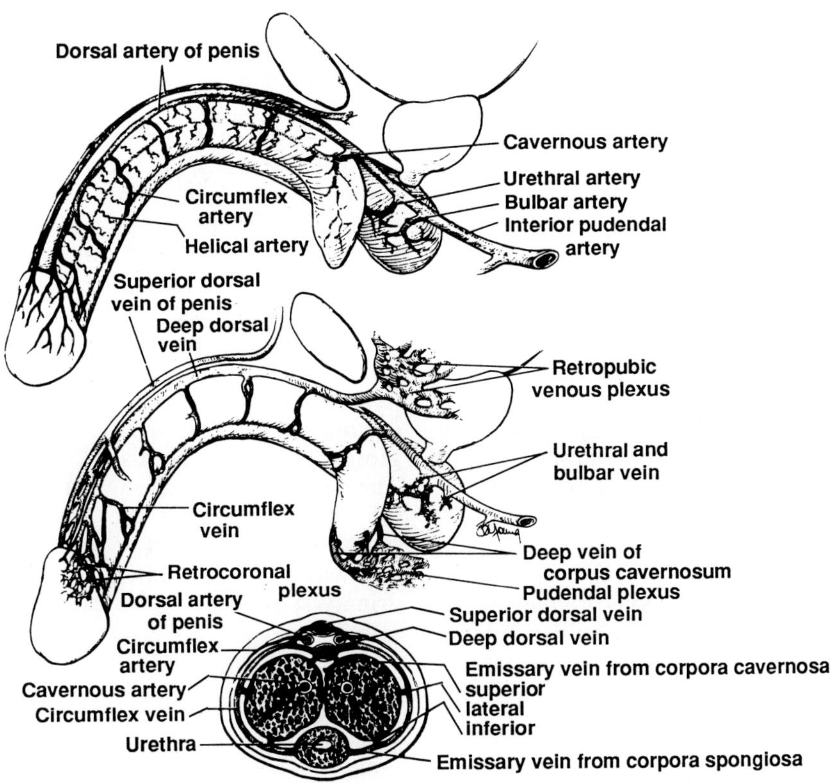


**Fig 29.** Arterial and venous vasculature of penis. [From Gillenwater JY, et al, eds, *Adult and Pediatric Urology,* 2nd ed (Chicago: Mosby-Year Book Inc; 1991), with permission. Original drawing by Young.]

arate urethral arteries or as arteries to the bulb. They enter the corpora spongiosa just distal to the urogenital diaphragm and traverse the corpora spongiosa. The second branch is the deep (corporal or profunda) branch, which courses centrally in the spongy tissue of the corpora cavernosa after entering the corpora at the proximal inferior medial aspect. The third branch is the dorsal artery of the penis, which courses over the corpora cavernosa ventral to Buck's fascia to supply the glans penis. At regular intervals along its course, it gives off circumflex branches that enter the tunica albuginea of the penis.

Recently, the venous drainage of the penis has been the object of increased study because of its clinical implications in the management of "venous leak," an etiologic factor in male sexual dysfunction. Although venous drainage of the penis has been generally described, it is recognized that numerous anastomotic communications exist. Three primary venous drainage systems are recognized (Fig 29). The superficial dorsal vein of the penis lies dorsal to Buck's fascia and drains the penile skin and glans penis, with outflow to the saphenous and pudendal veins. The deep dorsal penile vein lies ventral to Buck's fascia and arises from the retrocoronal plexus of veins. It is then joined by circumflex veins along the root, which in turn drain dorsal and ventral emissary veins from the corposa cavernosa. Proximal to the corona and distal to the pubic symphysis, the deep dorsal and deep superficial veins anastomose. The deep dorsal vein passes beneath the pubic arch, where it trifurcates over the prostate—in part flowing to Santorini's plexus and in part to the vesical plexus. Exiting the proximal corpora cavernosa and draining to the pudendal plexus are large, short veins—the deep veins of the corpora cavernosa. The primary venous drainage of the corpora spongiosa is via the bulbar and urethral veins, which also drain to the pudendal plexus.

## Anterior Urethra

The anterior urethra, as opposed to the posterior or prostatic urethra, is comprised of the membranous and the spongiose urethra (Fig 24). The spongiose urethra is arbitrarily divided into two segments. The segment extending from the membranous urethra to the divergence of the corpora cavernosa is the bulbous urethra, while the remaining portion from the divergence to the tip of the glans is the pendulous urethra. The urethra is characterized by two relative dilatations. The dilatation just distal to the membranous urethra is termed the intrabulbar fossa, while the dilatation within the glans is termed the fossa navicularis. The lumen of the anterior urethra, characterized by recesses and orifices, is most narrow at the urethral meatus. Within the fossa navicularis are noted variably sized recesses on the anterior wall termed lacunae magna. Primarily on the anterior wall of the pendulous urethra are numerous small recesses termed urethral lacunae, while on the posterior aspect are noted additional small orifices of the mucosal and submucosal glands (glands of Littre). Also on the floor of the bulbous urethra, approximately 2 to 3 cm distal to the membranous urethra, are the paired orifices of the ducts of the bulbourethral glands (Cowper's glands). On the floor of the membranous urethra is located the urethral crest (crista urethralis), a ridge that is contiguous with the verumontanum within the posterior urethra. The ridge bifurcates and then continues into the bulbous urethra. Exaggerations of these bifurcating folds present as posterior urethral valves.

**Relationships.** The bulbous and pendulous urethra are encased by the corpora spongiosa, which is thinnest at its dorsal aspect. The membranous urethra, from the apex of the prostate through the urogenital diaphragm, is covered on its anterior and lateral aspects by the fibers of the external urinary sphincter.

## Scrotum

The scrotum is characterized by transverse rugations of its skin and a midline raphe, which is contiguous from the perineum to the ventrum of the penis. The raphe marks the position of the median septum

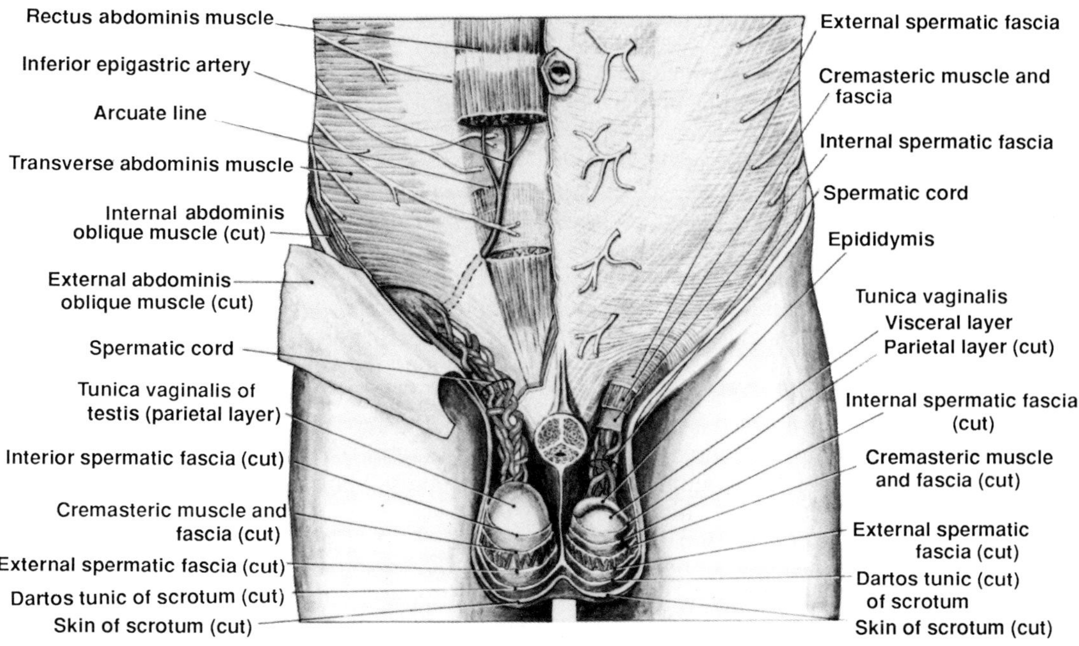


**Fig 30.** Contributions to the spermatic cord from the anterior abdominal wall musculature and fascia. [From Crafts RC, *A Textbook of Human Anatomy,* 3rd ed (New York: John Wiley & Sons Inc; 1985), with permission.]

which separates the scrotum internally into two separate compartments. The rugations of the scrotum are produced by the dartos tunic containing smooth muscle fibers, and are representative of the superficial membranous fascia (Fig 30). The dartos tunic of the scrotum is contiguous with the dartos tunic of the penis and Colles' fascia of the perineum. The dartos is closely adherent to the thin scrotal skin, which becomes contracted or loose depending on the involuntary contractions of the muscle. Deep to the dartos tunic are three layers, which are derivatives of the anterior abdominal wall and which are contiguous with the coverings of the spermatic cord. These are the external spermatic fascia, the cremasteric muscle and fascia, and the internal spermatic fascia. The external spermatic fascia is a derivative of the fascia of the external oblique aponeurosis. The cremasteric muscle is limited to widely separated, looping bands of muscle interspersed by cremasteric fascia, while the internal spermatic fascia is contiguous with transversalis fascia. The tunica vaginalis is also generally considered to be a layer of the scrotum. It forms a parietal and visceral layer which covers the anterior two thirds of the testis and epididymis and is a remnant of the patent processus vaginalis peritonei.

## Spermatic Cord

The spermatic cord is a distinct structure which extends from the internal inguinal ring to the scrotum, with the layers of external spermatic fascia, cremasteric muscle and fascia, and transversalis fascia being derived from the anterior abdominal wall (Fig 30). They surround the internal spermatic vessels and vas deferens. Exceptions are that the external spermatic fascia begins at the external ring with the relatively abrupt termination of the external oblique aponeurosis. A further exception is that within the inguinal canal the cremasteric muscle is heaviest over the cranial aspect of the cord, while along the posterior and inferior aspect the layer is represented primarily by cremasteric fascia. When incised along the inguinal ligament, this fascia allows the complete separation of the cremasteric muscle and fascia from the internal spermatic fascia, without leaving a prominent sail of cremasteric muscle along the inguinal floor in hernia repair. Within the confines of the investing internal spermatic fascia is located the internal spermatic artery, the pampiniform plexus, and the vas deferens. A patent processus vaginalis, if present, will be found anterior and medial to the spermatic vasculature. The vasculature, vas deferens, and serosal sac, if present, will all be contained within the fat-laden intermediate stratum of retroperitoneal connective tissue which is contiguous with that found within the retroperitoneum. Exaggerations of this fat are usually termed cord lipomas.

## Testis

**Gross Anatomy.** The testes are paired, elongated, ovoid organs with a volume in the adult of 25 to 30 mL. Suspended from the spermatic cord in separate compartments of the scrotum, the testes are oriented so that the long axis is vertical, and the mediastinum or port of entry of the vasculature is located posteriorly. Each is covered by a dense, grayish-white capsule, the tunica albuginea, through which can be seen the underlying vessels of the tunica vasculosa. Arising from the tunica albuginea are trabeculae or septa, which divide the testicle into approximately 250 lobules. These lobules contain the yellowish seminiferous tubules (Fig 31). Emanating from the upper pole of the testis, near the attachment of the epididymis, is a small hydatid with a narrow stalk, known as the appendix testis.

**Relationships.** The testis is intimately invested on its anterior two thirds by the visceral tunica vaginalis, a fluid-filled space existing between that and the parietal layer of tunica vaginalis. The posterior aspect of the testes is covered by the epididymis and the retroperitoneal connective tissue which accompanies the vasculature of the testis

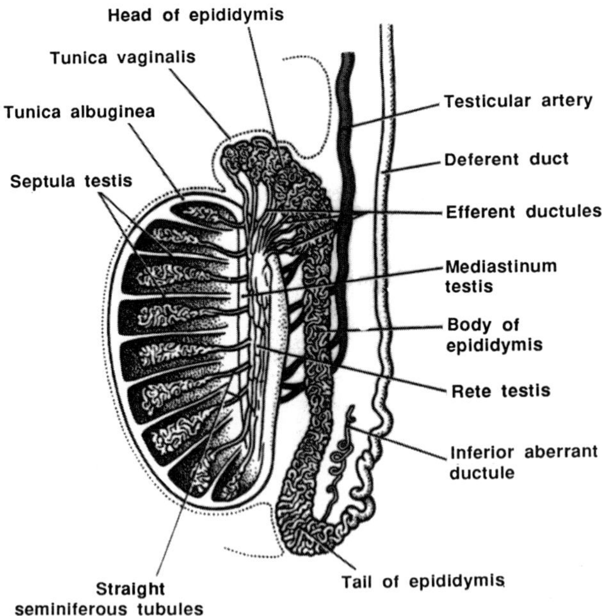


**Fig 31.** Schematic illustration of longitudinal section of tubules with epididymis and vas deferens. [From Williams, et al, *Gray's Anatomy,* 36th ed (Philadelphia: WB Saunders, 1980), with permission.]

and epididymis. The head of the epididymis covers the most cranial aspect of the upper testicular pole.

### Epididymis and Vas Deferens

**Gross Anatomy.** The epididymis is formed from the efferent ductules which emanate from the mediastinum of the testis and the efferent ductules forming from the rete testis, which communicate with the seminiferous tubules (Fig 31). The efferent ductules emanating from the testis are straight, but they become enlarged and convoluted forming relative small masses termed the lobules of the epididymis. Each of the ducts ultimately drains into a common duct, the epididymal duct, which itself is extremely convoluted. Near the lower pole of the testis, the epididymal duct turns sharply to pursue a cranial course, which becomes the convoluted portion of the vas deferens.

The epididymis is described as having three parts: a head (globus major), a body, and a tail (globus minor). Within the head are found the efferent tubules and their terminal lobules, while the body is comprised of the convoluted epididymal duct. The convolutions of the duct of the epididymis and convoluted portion of the vas can be clearly seen through the serosal and adventitial coverings of the epididymis. As the convoluted portion of the vas deferens reaches the level of the head of the epididymis, the muscular wall becomes thick and the vas becomes a firm structure; at this point visualization of the contained lumen of the ductus deferens is no longer possible. Contained within the spermatic cord and accompanying the internal spermatic vasculature, the vas proceeds through the internal inguinal ring just lateral to the inferior epigastric vessels and then diverges from the internal spermatic vessels to cross ventral to the ureter and dorsal to the lateral umbilical ligament to course posterior to the bladder. Posterior to the base of the bladder, the vas dilates into a fusiform structure termed the ampulla of the vas. Just prior to entering prostatic tissue as the narrow ejaculatory duct (a convoluted diverticulum), the seminal vesicle emanates from the lateral aspect of the vas. It is a grayish opalescent structure measuring from 3–4 cm to 1–1.5 cm.

## FEMALE GENITALIA

The female genitalia include the internal and external genitalia. The internal genitalia include the ovaries, uterine tubes, uterus, and vagina. The mons pubis, labia majora and minora, clitoris, vaginal vestibule, bulb of the vestibule, and greater vestibular glans constitute the external genitalia.

### Internal Genitalia

#### Ovary

*Gross Anatomy.* The ovaries are paired, ovoid organs which are grayish-pink in coloration. In nulliparous women, the ovary has a vertical orientation and is described as having an inferior and superior pole (or extremity) and a medial and a lateral border. It is also described as having a mesovarium (anterior) and free (posterior) border. The ovary is smooth prior to the age of ovulation but increasingly becomes irregular in contour over time due to scarring. The surface is covered by germinal epithelium which is contiguous with the peritoneum.

*Relationships.* The ovary essentially is suspended within the peritoneal cavity. It is attached at its superior pole by the suspensory ligament to the pelvic sidewall and also by the ovarian fimbria to the uterine tube (Fig 32). The suspensory ligament, also known as the infundibular ligament, contains the ovarian vessels. At its inferior pole, the ovary is attached by the ligament of the ovary to the lateral margin (cornu) of the uterus. The anterior border of the ovary is connected to the posterior aspect of the broad ligament by the mesovarium, a two-leafed peritoneal fold which carries vasculature and innervation to the ovarian hilum. The lateral border depresses the pelvic sidewall at the bifurcation of the common iliac artery to form the ovarian fossa. The medial border is covered by the uterine tube.

### Uterine Tube

*Gross Anatomy.* The uterine tubes (fallopian tubes or oviducts) are paired tubular structures which arise from the craniolateral aspect of the uterus (Fig 32). The tubes, which are 10–14 cm in length and 1–2 cm in outer diameter, are divided for description into four segments or divisions: a uterine (interstitial) part, an isthmus, an ampulla, and an infundibulum. The uterine part traverses the uterine wall and is 1–2 cm in length, with an ostium measuring only 1–1.5 mm in diameter. The segment immediately adjacent to the uterus is the isthmus, which is 3–4 cm in length and 1–2 mm in internal diameter. It is also the straightest and narrowest segment of the tubes. The widest and most tortuous segment is the ampulla, which is 4–6 cm in length, and which has an internal diameter of 6 mm. The terminal end of the tube is known as the infundibulum because of its funnel or trumpet shape. This section is fringed along the margin of the funnel by 20 to 25 frond-like projections termed fimbriae. The ovarian fimbriae join the superior pole of the ovary. The diameter of the infundibular ostium, which opens into the peritoneal cavity, is 3 mm.

*Relationships.* The uterine tubes course in the free edges of the broad ligaments and are covered both anteriorly and posteriorly by peritoneum. The exception is the infundibulum, which is free of the broad ligament and which opens into the peritoneal cavity. This course takes it caudal to, and along the inferior pole of, the ovary and the mesovarian border to the superior pole, where it turns posteriorly and then downward so that the fimbriated end lies adjacent to the surface of the ovary.

### Uterus

*Gross Anatomy.* The uterus is a pear-shaped or piriform, thick-walled organ with two parts, the upper corpus or body, and the cervix. On opening the uterus it is noted that the uterine cavity has a triangular shape, with the apex of the triangle placed

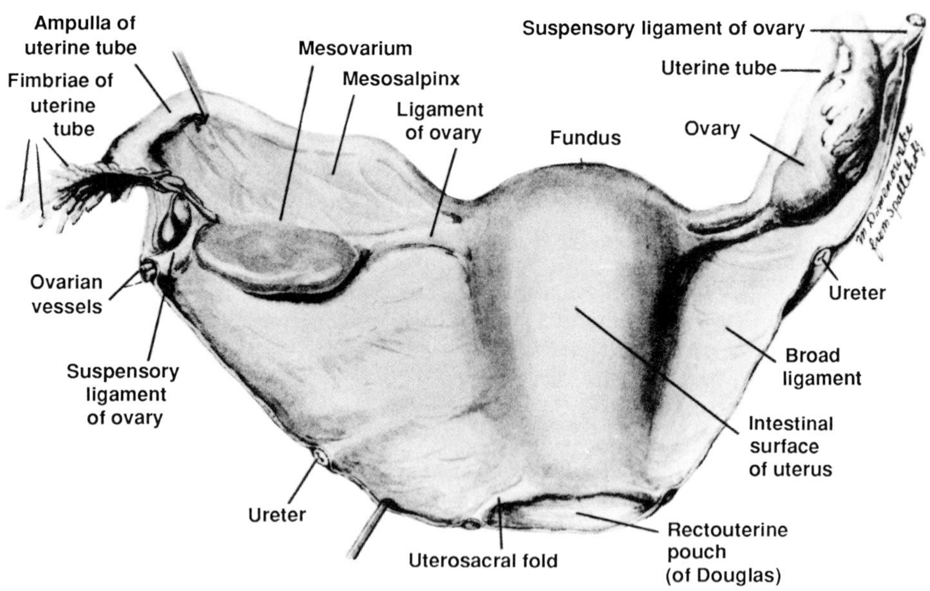


**Fig 32.** Uterus, uterine tubes, and ovaries; posterior aspect showing ligament and suspensory ligament of ovary. [From Danforth DN, Scott JR, *Obstetrics and Gynecology,* 5th ed (Philadelphia: JB Lippincott Co; 1986), with permission.]

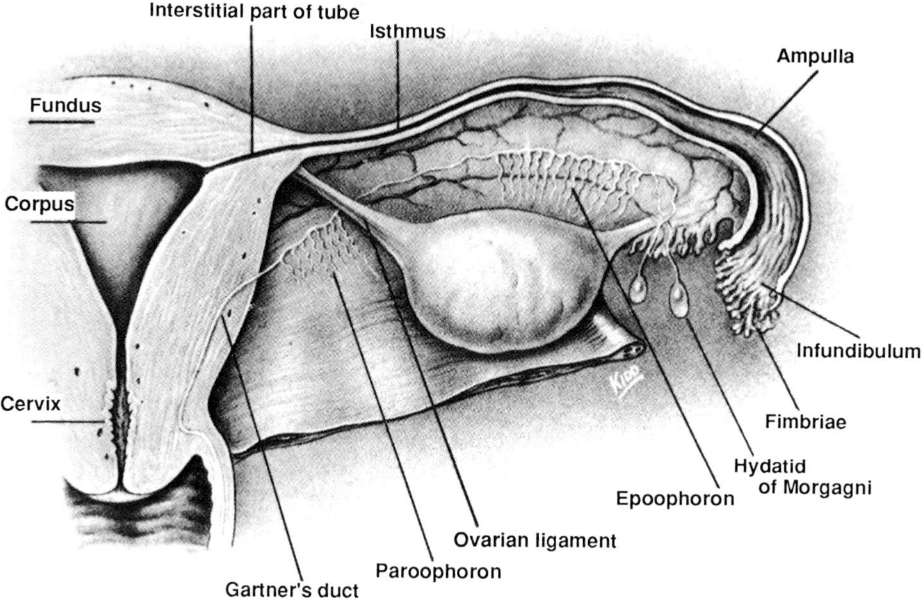


**Fig 33.** Uterus sectioned showing uterine cavity and relationships. [From *Jeffcoate's Principles of Gynaecology,* 5th ed (London: Butterworth & Co; 1987), with permission.]

caudally, that is, at the internal os of the uterus (Fig 33). The basilar angles are formed by the orifices of the uterine tubes; the positions of these orifices are termed the cornu. The dome-shaped portion of the uterus, which lies above the uterine cavity and above the cornua, is the fundus. Externally, at the junction of the internal os, the uterus narrows. This section is known as the isthmus, and marks the junction of the cervix and the corpus. The muscular wall of the uterus is termed the myometrium, while the endometrium is the mucosal lining of the uterine cavity. The perimetrium is the term for the peritoneum covering the corpus and supervaginal cervix. The cervix portion of the uterus is described as having two parts: the vaginal part, which extends into the vagina, and the supervaginal part.

***Relationships.*** The uterus is primarily an intraperitoneal organ. Posteriorly, the uterus is in apposition to the rectum, but these structures are separated by the recto-uterine pouch (Fig 23). Similarly, anteriorly the uterus is separated by the utero-vesical pouch. The lateral aspects of the uterus are supported by the broad ligaments. In relation to the vagina, the uterus is anteflexed, that is, it lies with its long axis at a right angle to the long axis of the vagina. The cervix, therefore, is in apposition to the posterior wall of the vagina. Normally, 20% of women will have a uterus which is retroflexed.

## Vagina

***Gross Anatomy.*** The vagina may be described as a distensible, fibromuscular canal. For most of its length on cross-section it has a configuration of the letter H, with the mid-portion of the anterior and posterior walls in apposition. The most noticeable feature of the vaginal lumen per se is the transverse folds termed rugae. On the anterior and posterior walls are two median longitudinal ridges, known as the vaginal columns. The terminal portion of the anterior vaginal column is termed the urethral carina. Four arches, termed fornices, are formed as the cervix enters the anterior wall of the vagina. The two lateral recesses, on either side of the cervix, are the lateral fornices. A shallow anterior fornix and a deep posterior fornix are also present, as the length of the posterior wall is at least 2 cm longer than that of the anterior wall. The opening of the vagina is termed the introitus, while the membrane partially covering the introitus, most noticeable in children, is the hymen.

***Relationships.*** The vagina slants dorsally and cranially with a ventral curve (Fig 23). It is in apposition to the bladder and urethra on its anterior aspect, and is separated from them by intermediate stratum of retroperitoneal connective tissue. A plane between the vagina and bladder may be achieved surgically. However, a separation of the urethra and the vagina is quite difficult, due to the denseness of the connective tissue. The vesical trigone generally is located over the middle one third of the vagina. The relationships of the vagina posteriorly may be considered in fourths. The cranial one fourth is separated from the rectum by the rectouterine pouch of peritoneum (the cul-de-sac of Douglas). In the middle two fourths, the vagina is separated from the rectum by only the fusion fascial plane of connective tissue, the rectovaginal septum. The caudal one fourth is in apposition to the perineal body (the central tendon of the perineum). Laterally, the cranial one third of the vagina is surrounded by intermediate stratum of retroperitoneal connective tissue. On the lateral and caudal aspects the lateral fornices are 1–2 cm medial to the ureters and to the uterine artery, which crosses dorsal to them. At the junction of the middle and lower thirds, the vagina passes through the pubococcygeus muscles, while the caudal one third passes through the urogenital diaphragm and bulbocavernosus muscle.

### External Genitalia

The external genitalia, which are contained within the superficial perineal space, include the mons pubis, labia majora and minora, clitoris, vestibule, bulb of the vestibule, and greater vestibular glands (Figs 17B, 34). In the female, all of the structures

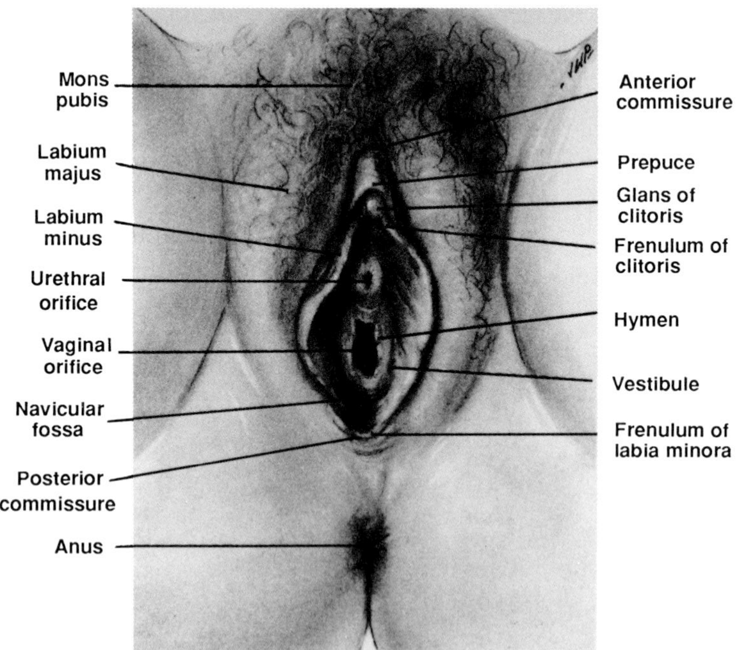


**Fig 34.** Superficial anatomy of the vulva and perineum. [From Danforth DN, Scott JR, *Obstetrics and Gynecology,* 5th ed (Philadelphia: JB Lippincott Co; 1986), with permission.]

occupying the superficial perineal space are collectively termed the vulva. The mound of fat overlying the pubis is termed the mons pubis. The labia majora, the homologue of the scrotum, externally form the lateral aspects of the vulva and, for the most part, cover the thin labia minora which lie between them. The space between the labia minora, from the clitoris to the perineum, is termed the vestibule. The posterior joining of the labia minora is known as the fourchette. Cranially the labia minora join again to cover the glans clitoris as a prepuce. Within the vestibule, just posterolateral to the introitus, is found the orifices of the ducts of the greater vestibular glands (Bartholin's glands). Skene's glands (periurethral glands) drain by ducts which open into the vestibule on either side of the urethral meatus. The labia majora overlie the bulbospongiosus muscles, which in turn cover the vestibular bulbs, the homologues of the corpora spongiosa in the male. The crus of the clitoris, covered by the ischiocavernosus muscles, are attached to the pubic rami and are capped by the glans clitoris. The clitoris itself is joined to the symphysis pubis by the suspensory ligament of the clitoris.

**Female Urethra.** Extending from the vesical neck to the urethral meatus, the female urethra is approximately 3 to 4 cm in length. The lumen is characterized by a posterior longitudinal mucosal fold (termed the posterior urethral crest), small recesses (lacunae), and periurethral mucosal glands. The most distal of the periurethral glands are Skene's glands, whose ducts open adjacent to the urethral meatus. The urethra consists of vascular spongy submucosal tissue which is overlain by muscular coats and fibroelastic tissue.

***Relationships.*** From the vesical neck to the urogenital diaphragm the urethra is surrounded by intermediate stratum of retroperitoneal connective tissue whose condensations form the support of the urethra. Anterior to the urethra is located the pubis, to which the vesical neck and the proximal urethra are connected by condensations of retroperitoneal connective tissue termed the pubovesical ligaments. Similar condensations, termed the pubourethral ligaments, connect the pelvis with the mid-urethra. The dorsal vein of the clitoris passes between the urethra and the arch of the pubis en route to the vesical plexus. Posteriorly, the urethra and anterior vaginal wall are so intimately related that no distinct cleavage plane exists. Near the junction of the urethra and the pelvic floor, a fascial collar is formed around the urethra and the vagina by the investing fascia of the pubococcygeus muscle. Following the urethra's passage through the urogenital diaphragm, it terminates to become the urethral meatus in the vestibule.

### Rectum and Anal Canal

***Gross Anatomy.*** The rectum and anal canal form the terminis of the large bowel. The junction of the rectum and the sigmoid colon occurs at approximately the level of the third sacral vertebral body. The rectum follows the curve of the coccyx; 4–5 cm ventral to the tip of the coccyx, the rectum passes through the urogenital diaphragm to become the anal canal, which turns dorsally at a right angle (Fig 23).

***Relationships.*** The cranial two thirds of the rectum are covered by peritoneum. The cranial one third is covered on its anterior and lateral surfaces by peritoneum, while the mid-third is covered only on its ventral aspect. The lateral aspects of the rectum are invested by intermediate stratum of retroperitoneal connective tissue. In the female, the rectum is separated from the uterus anteriorly by the rectouterine pouch; in the male it is separated anteriorly from the posterior aspect of the bladder by the rectovesical pouch. The covering stratum of the rectum per se is inner stratum, since the rectum in its entirety was at one time covered by peritoneum. In its terminal third, which is free of a peritoneal covering, the ventral surface of the rectum is in apposition in the male to the posterior wall of the bladder, the seminal vesicles, vasal ampulla, and the prostate (Fig 35). The cleavage plane that exists between the rectum and these structures is between the

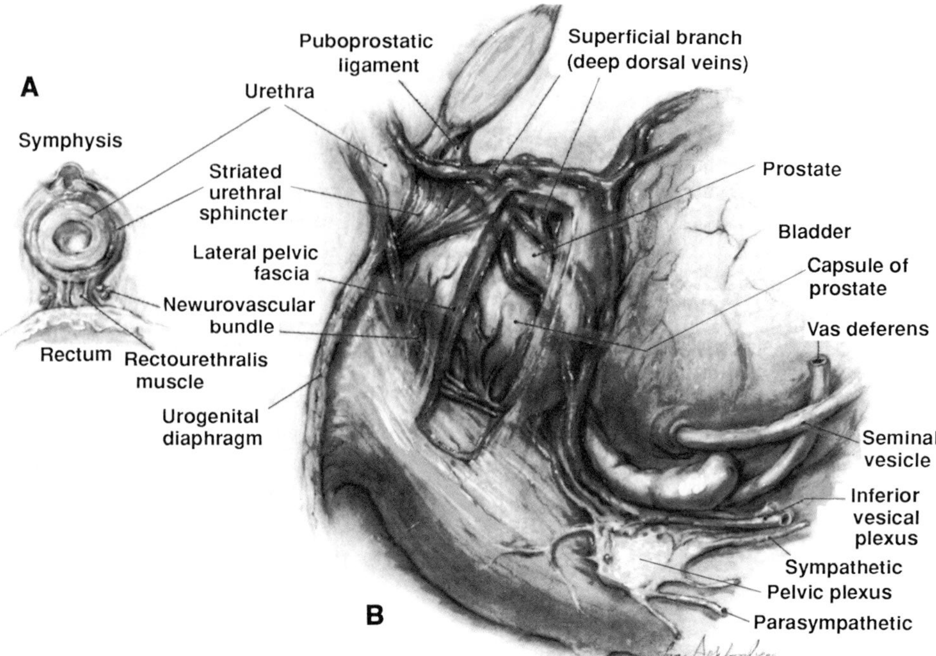


**Fig 35.** A, Cross-section of the urethra just distal to the apex of the prostate; B, anatomical relationship of prostate to the pelvic fascia and rectum. [From Marshall FF, *Operative Urology* (Philadelphia: WB Saunders, 1991), with permission.]

inner stratum of connective tissue covering the rectum and the intermediate stratum covering the bladder, seminal vesicles, and prostate. The connective tissue layers thus form the laminae (anterior and posterior) of Denonvilliers' fascia. In the female the rectum is in apposition to the vagina, from which it is separated by a fusion fascial plane, the rectovaginal septum. After the rectum passes through the levator ani muscles, it becomes the anal canal which passes through the external and internal sphincter to terminate as the anus.

## REFERENCE

1. Jewett JH, Eggleston JC, Yawn DH. Radical prostatectomy in the management of carcinoma of the prostate: probable cause of some therapeutic failures. *J Urol.* 1972;107:1034.

## SUGGESTED READING

Danforth DN, Scott JR. *Obstetrics and Gynecology*. 5th ed. Philadelphia: JB Lippincott Co; 1986.

Gosling JA. The structure of the female lower urinary tract and pelvic floor. *Urologic Clin North Am.* 1985;12:207–214.

Hamilton WF. *A Textbook of Human Anatomy*. 2nd ed. St. Louis: CV Mosby Co; 1976.

Jones HW, Wentz AC, Burnett LS. *Novak's Textbook of Gynecology*. 11th ed. Baltimore: Williams & Wilkins Co; 1988:40–67.

McVay CB. *Surgical Anatomy*. 6th ed. Philadelphia: WB Saunders Co; 1984;II.

Redman JF. Anatomy of the genitourinary system. In: Gillenwater JY, Grayback JT, Howards SS, Duckett JW, eds. *Adult and Pediatric Urology*. Chicago: Year Book Medical Publishers Inc; 1987.

Redman JF. Surgical anatomy of the lower urinary tract. In: Bushbaum HJ, ed. *Gynecologic and Obstetric Urology*. 3rd ed. Philadelphia: WB Saunders Co. In press.

Tanagho EA. Anatomy of the lower urinary tract. In: Walsh PC, Gittes RE, Perlmutter AD, Stamey TA, eds. *Campbell's Urology*. 5th ed. Philadelphia: WB Saunders Co; 1986:46–74.

Williams PL, Warwick R. *Gray's Anatomy*. 36th ed. Philadelphia: WB Saunders Co; 1980.

# 3

# Renal Physiology

*Bruce R. Gilbert*
*E. Darracott Vaughan, Jr.*

## INTRODUCTION

Although the kidneys receive 20% of the cardiac output, they constitute only one half of 1% of the total body mass. The 180 L of glomerular filtrate produced each day are finely processed to maintain the internal milieu with exquisite precision.

The nephron, the functional unit of the kidney, consists of a glomerular capillary network, a proximal convoluted tubule, a loop of Henle, a distal convoluted tubule, and a collecting duct. There are approximately two to three million nephrons within two adult human kidneys; at rest only one tenth of this amount is required to maintain homeostasis. Therefore, a large reserve exists. The precise quantification of this reserve enables decisions regarding therapy to be made when renal dysfunction occurs. This chapter will review normal renal physiology and will examine the impact of alterations in renal function on urology. We will also discuss the limitations of various quantitative methods, while presenting several "bedside techniques" for the assessment of renal function.

## DEVELOPMENTAL PHYSIOLOGY

Three bilateral excretory systems develop during embryologic growth. The earliest is the *pronephros,* which is composed of approximately 7 tubules. The proximal ends of these tubules form nephrostomes which enter into the coelomic cavity, while the distal ends coalesce to form the pronephric duct which empties into the cloaca. The pronephros appears to be nonfunctional in mammals. At about the fourth week of development, the second system, the *mesonephros,* develops caudal to the first. The mesonephros consists of a glomerular structure, a proximal tubular segment, and a distal tubular segment. This structure produces some tubular fluid, at least transiently. In the female this structure regresses by the third month of gestation. In the male, the mesonephric tubules and duct (the former pronephric duct) develop into the efferent ductules of the epididymis, the duct of the epididymis, the ductus deferens, the seminal vesicle, and the ejaculatory duct. The third system, the *metanephros*, originates from two different embryologic tissues at about the eighth week of fetal life[1]: the glomerulus and tubules arise from the mesenchyme of the nephrogenic ridge.[2] The excretory portion (collecting duct, calyces, pelvis, and ureter) arise from a specialized structure of the mesonephric duct, the ureteric bud. The nephrons in the metanephros appear to be functional as early as the 11th to 12th week of fetal life. It appears that morphologic and functional maturation of nephrons starts in the deep nephrons and then extends to the superficial nephrons.

The morphologic and functional effects

of renal senescence begin in the cortical regions and progress toward the medullary portions of the kidney—the opposite of nephron maturation. In humans, the kidney loses over 20% of its weight between the 4th and 8th decade. While the greatest loss occurs in the cortex, the medullary portion is also involved, and displays a generalized fibrosis similar to that seen with chronic hypertension. However, even without hypertension, arteriolar hyalinization and glomerular sclerosis results in the loss of 50% of glomeruli by the eighth decade.[1]

## RENAL HEMODYNAMICS

### Functional Organization of the Renal Circulation

The renal circulation is designed to simultaneously accomplish bulk filtration, reabsorption, and precise selective regulation of the constituents of normal urine. From an enormous blood flow of about a liter per minute, only about 1 mL of urine is formed per minute. The energy requirement of this process is about 10% of basal oxygen consumption, yet the efficiency of the kidney is reflected in its low arteriovenous oxygen difference.[2]

Originally, the renal circulation was quantified by clearance techniques measuring total renal blood flow. More recently, micropuncture and microangiographic techniques have advanced the understanding of the renal microcirculation.[3,4] It is now known that the kidney is not composed of a single homogeneous circulation but is rather made up of several distinct microvascular networks. These include the glomerular microcirculation, the cortical peritubular microcirculation, and the microcirculation that nourishes and drains the inner and outer medulla.[2]

The gross anatomy of the renal vasculature has previously been described. The interlobular arteries taper as they pass through almost the entire renal cortex, and each gives rise to about 20 afferent glomerular arterioles that supply one or more of the 1.5 million glomeruli of the human kidney. The vascular pathways in the glomerulus change under different physiologic conditions, and there is intermittent flow within glomeruli which may play a role in regulation of glomerular filtration rate (GFR). The discovery that the glomerular mesangium contains contractile elements that respond to angiotensin II (AII) and other vasoactive substances supports this hypothesis.[5] As they extend beyond the glomerulus the efferent arterioles form dense peritubular capillary plexuses that nourish the proximal or distal convoluted tubules situated in the cortex. Alternatively the arterioles pass into the medulla (especially from juxtamedullary glomeruli) and divide into bundles of vasa recta that parallel medullary rays.[4] Microdissection and injection studies have recently shown that, except for the initial portion of the peritubular capillaries in the outer cortex, the efferent peritubular capillary network and the nephron arising from each glomerulus are dissociated.[6] There are distinct outer and inner medullary capillary networks. In the inner medulla, the degree of organization of vascular–tubular relations correlates with concentrating ability.[7]

The major changes in hydraulic pressure across the renal vascular bed are shown in Figure 1. The role of physical factors in the regulation of GFR will be discussed later.

**Measurement of Renal Blood Flow.** Measurements of the clearance of organic iodides, Diodrast, and para-aminohippurate (PAH) are used to estimate renal blood flow (RBF), and are based on application of the Fick principle. At low plasma concentrations these substances are almost totally secreted by the renal tubules; there is no extrarenal metabolism, storage, or production. Accurate utilization of the technique requires normal renal function and extraction, and assumes a renal venous concentration approaching zero. Since the extraction is probably never complete, the term "effective renal plasma flow" (ERPF) has been used. In disease states, venous sampling with actual determination of PAH extraction ($E_{pah}$) is required to calculate true renal plasma flow.

Accordingly, clearance of PAH ($C_{pah}$) is calculated by the formula $U_i \times Q_u =$

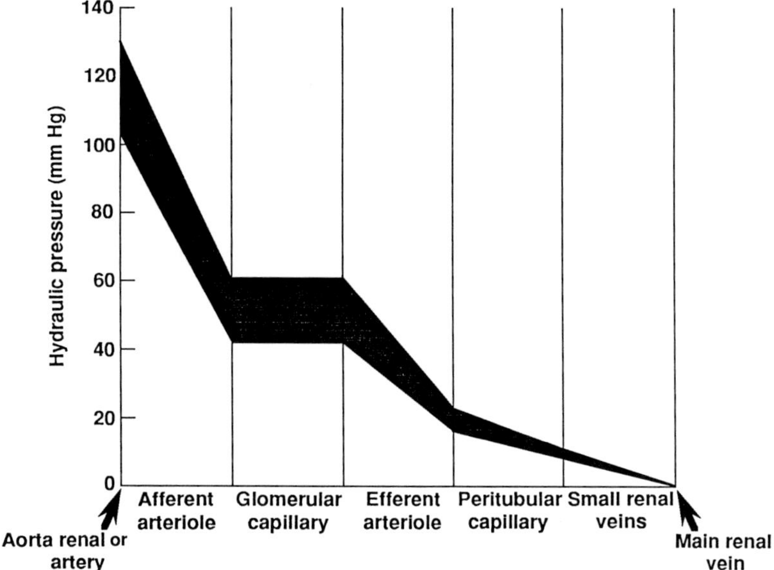


**Fig 1.** Diagram showing changes in the magnitude of intravascular hydraulic pressure from renal artery to renal vein in the Munich-Wistar rat. Steepest axial hydraulic pressure drops occur along the afferent and efferent arterioles; no significant pressure drop has been detected along glomerular capillary vessels. Thus, the cortical capillary exchange beds of the glomerular and peritubular networks operate at markedly different hydraulic pressures. Since the transglomerular hydraulic pressure difference exceeds the local oncotic pressure difference, fluid is lost from these capillaries by filtration. In the peritubular network, the transcapillary oncotic pressure difference exceeds the prevailing hydraulic pressure difference, thereby favoring fluid absorption into these capillaries.

$(A_i - V_i) \times RPF$ where:

$U_i$ = concentration of indicator in urine (mg/mL)
$Q_u$ = purine flow rate (mL/min)
$A_i$ = concentration of indicator in arterial elasma (mg/mL)
$V_i$ = concentration of indicator in venous plasma (mg/mL)
RPF = renal plasma flow rate (mL/min)

Rewriting this equation,

$$RPF = \frac{U_iQ_u}{A_i - V_i}$$

Since extraction is assumed to be almost complete in the clinical setting (that is, $V_i = 0$) and $A_i$ is kept constant, the equation for $C_{pah}$ becomes:

$$RPF = \frac{U_iQ_u}{A_i} \text{ or } \frac{U_{pah} \times V}{P_{pah}}$$

where $U_{pah}$ = urine concentration of PAH and $P_{pah}$ = plasma concentration of PAH.

Of note, $U_iQ_u$ = excreted load of the indicator (mg/min) and $V = Q_u$ (urine flowrate).

The conversion of renal plasma flow rate to blood flow is achieved by dividing RPF by the plasma fraction of whole blood as estimated by the hematocrit (HCT).

$$RBF = \frac{RPF}{1 - HCT}$$

The complexity of determination of RBF by the $C_{pah}$ technique and the requirement of normal renal function have led to a search for alternative techniques. Single-injection techniques using a variety of radionuclides followed by measurement of the rate of disappearance of the isotope tag from the blood or by noninvasive monitoring are discussed elsewhere (Volume 1, Chapter 6). Radionuclide monitoring techniques allow calculation of differential RBF from each kidney, which often provides critical clinical information.

**Distribution of Renal Blood Flow.** Total RBF estimated by $C_{pah}$ technique is 1200 mL/min/1.73 $m^2$; this value has been confirmed by a variety of methods. In infants up to 1 year of age, RBF is about one half of the adult flow; it reaches the adult level at about 3 years of age.[8] RBF falls after age 30, and has declined to about one half of maximum by age 90.[9] When related to renal mass, RBF is remarkably similar in various species, and is usually about 4 mL/g/min.

Although it is well documented that the perfusion rate in different regions of the kidney is not uniform, there remains considerable disagreement about regional blood flow measurements obtained by different methods under differing experimental conditions. Moreover, no clear correlation exists between distribution of renal blood flow and renal function. The utilization of inert gas washout, radioactive microspheres, or nondiffusible indicators is beyond the scope of this review.[3,10] This area remains under investigation and may be relevant to the understanding of the pathophysiology of acute renal failure.[11] The attractive hypothesis that there is a causal relationship between the distribution of RBF and sodium handling awaits confirmation.

The renal cortex receives about 90% of the total renal blood flow (5 to 6 mL/min in the outer cortex), while flow in the outer medullary is only about 1 mL/min. However, medullary flow, "sluggish" relative to the cortex, is still greater per gram than flow to the liver, brain, or resting muscle.

## Glomerular Filtration Rate

The elaboration of urine begins at the glomerulus with the formation of a nearly protein-free ultrafiltrate of plasma which enters Bowman's space. As the filtrate passes through the tubules, substances may be removed (reabsorption) or added (secretion). Clearance is "a quantitative description of the rate at which the kidney excretes various substances relative to their concentration in plasma."[12] It is calculated as follows:

$U_x$ = concentration of x in a timed urine collection (mg/mL)
$V$ = volume of urine per unit time (mL/min)
$P_x$ = concentration of x in plasma (mg/mL)
$U_xV$ = rate of urinary excretion of x = excreted load (mg/min)
$C_x$ = $U_xV/P_x$ = the (plasma) clearance of x (mL/min)

$C_x$ is the volume of plasma containing x that would have to be completely cleared of x per unit time to supply an amount of x for urinary excretion at the measured rate. Clearance does not necessarily mean that an *actual* volume of plasma is, in fact, completely cleared of x. Rather, it refers to a "*virtual volume*" of plasma that would provide the measured amount of x.

A substance that is freely filtered and undergoes neither reabsorption nor secretion will have a clearance equal to the GFR. The clearance of inulin, a carbohydrate polymer of fructose, measured during a constant infusion, is the standard for measurement of GFR. A clearance greater than that of inulin indicates that a substance also undergoes tubular *secretion*; a clearance less than that of inulin implies tubular *reabsorption*.

Rewriting the clearance equation for x = inulin, we have:

$$C_{inulin} = U_{inulin}\,V/P_{inulin}$$

Because of the difficulty in measuring inulin clearance, the clearance of endogenous creatinine is used for clinical purposes as an estimate of GFR. Its plasma concentration remains stable during a 24-hour period, and its rate of excretion does not vary with urine flow. Thus, creatinine clearance ($C_{cr}$) can be calculated during a 24-hour collection of urine, with a plasma sample obtained at any time during the collection period. In normal man, filtered creatinine does not undergo tubular reabsorption; some tubular secretion does occur. At the plasma creatinine concentration that prevails at normal GFR, the ratio $C_{cr}/C_{inulin}$ is close to 1, implying negligible secretion. At progressively lower GFRs, however, tubular secretion plays an increasingly important part in creatinine excretion. At GFRs below 30 mL/min, $C_{cr}$ may overestimate $C_{inulin}$ by 50% to 80%. Because this represents small absolute differences at low GFRs, $C_{cr}$ is satisfactory as an estimate of GFR in patients with chronic renal insufficiency.

Kidney weight is more closely correlated with body surface area than with either height or weight. In order to compare renal function in persons of different sizes, GFR is frequently described per standard unit of body surface area, 1.73 $m^2$.[12]

Often the need arises to accurately predict $C_{cr}$ without waiting for the results of 24-hour urine testing. For example, the dose of various potentially toxic drugs may need to be quickly adjusted when beginning therapy. Several investigators have devised formula to predict $C_{cr}$ utilizing serum creatinine, body weight, age, and sex as variables. The most widely used of these is that described by Crockcroft and Gault.[13] Estimated GFR is given by the following equation:

$$\frac{(140\text{-age})(\text{weight})}{72\ S_{cr}}\ \text{mL/min}$$

(multiply the equation by 0.85 for women)

where:

1. $S_{cr}$ is serum creatinine (mg/dL)
2. Age is in years
3. Weight is in kg

The major prerequisite for use of this formula is that renal function be at steady state (as defined by a stable serum creatinine). The group studied by Crockcroft and Gault consisted of 249 patients ranging in age from 18 to 92 years old whose measured mean $C_{cr}$ ranged from 37.4 to 114.9 mL/min. The correlation coefficient between measured and calculated $C_{cr}$ was 0.84; this value is not significantly different than the correlation between two consecutive measurements of $C_{cr}$ obtained from the same individual.

**Factors Affecting Glomerular Filtration.** Micropuncture studies of individual nephrons in the Munich-Wistar rat and the squirrel monkey, which possess glomeruli on the renal cortical surface, have permitted direct measurement of the factors that determine single-nephron glomerular filtration rate (SNGFR).[14–16] Assuming that all nephrons behave in a manner similar to those accessible to micropuncture, the regulation of whole-kidney GFR can be understood in terms of changes in one or more of the forces that regulate SNGFR. The symbols designating these forces, used in the following discussion, are summarized in Table 1.

The principal driving force for glomerular filtration is the hydrostatic pressure at the glomerular capillary ($P_{gc}$). This pressure is a consequence of the forces that maintain systemic blood pressure—cardiac output and systemic vascular resistance. $P_{gc}$, which favors ultrafiltration, is opposed by the hydrostatic pressure in Bowman's space of the renal tubule ($P_t$). The differ-

**TABLE 1. Factors Governing SNGFR**

| | |
|---|---|
| Pgc | Hydrostatic pressure in the glomerular capillary |
| Pt | Hydrostatic pressure in the tubule (and its proximal extension, Bowman's space) |
| $\Delta P$ | Net transglomerular hydrostatic pressure |
| $\pi gc$ | Oncotic pressure of glomerular capillary plasma |
| $\pi t$ | Oncotic pressure of tubular fluid |
| $\Delta\pi$ | Net transglomerular oncotic pressure |
| Puf | Effective ultrafiltration pressure ($\Delta P - \Delta\pi$) |
| $k_f$ or Lp | Hydraulic permeability of glomerular capillary |
| A | Glomerular surface area available for ultrafiltration |
| $K_f$ or Lpa | Glomerular ultrafiltration coefficient |

ence between these values is the transmembrane hydraulic pressure gradient ($\triangle P$):

$$\triangle P = P_{gc} - P_t$$

Complementing these hydrostatic forces are the osmotic pressures exerted by plasma proteins, known as colloid osmotic pressure or oncotic pressure. The oncotic pressure of glomerular capillary plasma ($\pi_{gc}$) tends to oppose transcapillary fluid movement; the oncotic pressure of tubular fluid ($\pi_t$) tends to favor it. The difference between these two forces at any point is the transmembrane oncotic pressure ($\triangle\pi$):

$$\triangle\pi = \pi_{gc} - \pi_t$$

Under normal circumstances, filtration of plasma proteins is negligible and $\pi_t$ is essentially zero. At any point along the length of the capillary, the effective filtration pressure ($P_{uf}$) can be calculated as follows:

$$P_{uf} = \triangle P - \triangle\pi$$

As filtration proceeds along the length of the glomerular capillary, the concentration of protein, and hence $\pi_{gc}$, rises. By the time the plasma reaches the efferent arteriole, $\pi_{gc}$ has risen to a value equal to $\triangle P$. This local equality of $\triangle P$ and $\pi_{gc}$ is known as filtration pressure equilibrium (FPE). Precisely where along the length of the capillary FPE occurs cannot be determined, but at this point SNGFR becomes zero. FPE occurs in the surface glomeruli of the Munich-Wistar rat under hydropenic conditions. Whether FPE occurs in human glomeruli remain uncertain. In addition to $P_{uf}$, SNGFR is determined by both the hydraulic permeability of the glomerular capillary ($k_f$ or $L_p$) and the total surface area available for ultrafiltration (A). The hydraulic permeability of the glomerular capillary is much greater than that of capillaries in nonrenal tissues. Because $k_f$ and A cannot at present be independently measured, they are considered together as their product, the glomerular ultrafiltration coefficient, $K_f$ or $L_pA$:

$$K_f = k_f \times A$$

The factors that determine SNGFR can thus be summarized by any of the following equations:

$$SNGFR = K_f(P_{uf})$$

$$SNGFR = K_f(\triangle P - \triangle\pi)$$

$$SNGFR = Kf\ [(Pgc - Pt) - (\pi_{gc} - \pi_t)]$$

The actions of these forces are illustrated in Figure 2.

Changes in any of the foregoing variables in health or disease will have predictable effects on SNGFR.[17,18]

**Autoregulation of Glomerular Filtration Rate and Renal Blood Flow.** Autoregulation of GFR and RBF is believed to occur mainly through variations in afferent arteriolar resistance. Parallel regulation of GFR and RBF result in response to changes in arterial pressure (Fig 3). There is less than 10% change in RBF or GFR over a wide range of perfusion pressure, from 80 to 180 mm Hg. This phenomenon was described as early as 1947, and appears to be a critical mechanism controlling renal homeostasis.[19] Only at very low arterial perfusion pressure does an increase in efferent arteriolar resistance contribute to the maintenance of $P_{gc}$, sustaining SNGFR at reduced RBF.[20]

The mechanism of autoregulation remains incompletely defined. Autoregulation is not unique to the kidney, but is most efficient in the renal and cerebral circulations. Since it is present in innervated, denervated, and isolated kidneys, it is assumed to be mediated by events intrinsic to the kidney—hence the term "autoregulation." At present it appears that more than one proposed mechanism of autoregulation—namely, myogenic, metabolic, tubuloglomerular feedback, and/or humoral systems—may be causative. There is particular interest in a juxtaglomerular apparatus, which may play a critical role, although data from experiments utilizing a variety of angiotensin and prostaglandin blockers are conflicting.[21]

Evidence from micropuncture studies supports the hypothesis that changes in the rate of fluid flow in the distal tubule elicit changes in glomerular arteriolar resistance. This phenomenon is known as *distal tub-*

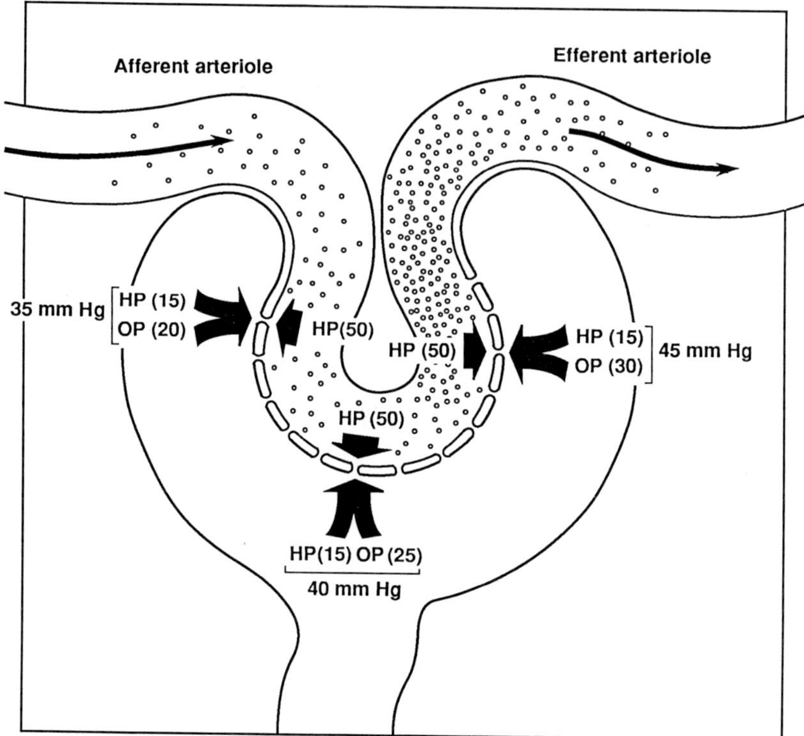


**Fig 2.** Starling forces regulating glomerular filtration. Net filtration pressure is the result of opposing hydrostatic pressure (HP) in the glomerular capillary and of the sum of hydrostatic pressure in Bowman's space and plasma oncotic pressure (OP). Net filtration pressure is maximal at the afferent arteriolar site of the capillary and approaches zero toward the efferent arteriolar site, because of increasing plasma oncotic pressure as a direct consequence of ultrafiltration.

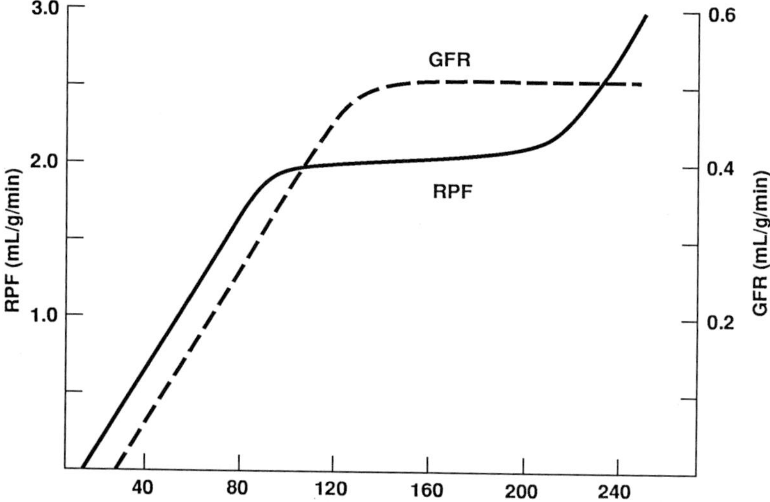


**Fig 3.** Autoregulation of renal plasma flow (RPF) and stability of glomerular filtration rate (GFR) over a similar range of mean arterial pressures. [Adapted from Shipley RE, Study RS, Changes in renal blood flow, extraction of inulin, glomerular filtration rate, tissue pressure and urine flow with acute alterations of renal artery blood pressure, *Am J Physiol* (1951;167:676), with permission.]

*uloglomerular feedback*. The morphologic association of the macula densa portion of the distal tubule and the afferent arteriole of the same nephron suggests that these structures are involved in the autoregulatory response. Considerable controversy persists, however, over (1) what aspect of distal tubular flow is perceived as the signal that engages autoregulation and (2) what are the mechanisms and sites of changes in arteriolar resistance. The initiating signal appears to be tubular-fluid chloride and its reabsorptive transport by cells of the macula densa.[22,23] Many recent studies have indicated that chloride might not be the only signal.[24,25]

Increases in distal fluid osmolality appear to result in an increase in intracellular free calcium concentration ($\{Ca^{2+}\}_i$). This increase in $\{Ca^{2+}\}_i$ might have two separate and opposite effects. First, it may enhance contraction of both the afferent and efferent arterioles. This would result in a decreased SNGFR and prevent an acute loss of fluid and electrolytes. Second, however, an increased $\{Ca^{2+}\}_i$ results in a decrease in renin release from the granules of the juxtaglomerular cells of the afferent arteriole. In the face of a continued stimulus, such as volume expansion, this would reduce local angiotensin II production and increase SNGFR, resulting in an increased excretion rate.

An alternative theory first proposed by Bayliss explains autoregulation as a consequence of variations in afferent arteriolar tone that occur as a direct result of changes in arterial blood pressure (*myogenic theory*).[26] An increase in pressure stretches the arteriolar smooth muscle and elicits contraction of the muscle layer, thus increasing afferent arteriolar resistance and regulating both GFR and RBF.[18]

The *metabolic theory* predicts that vasodilatory metabolites accumulate with a decrease in organ perfusion which results in a return to baseline blood flow rates. The major objection to this theory results from the well-known relationship between renal blood flow and renal metabolism.[27] Renal metabolism is primarily determined by the rate of sodium reabsorption, which in turn is directly related to GFR. Since GFR is known to vary with RBF, it would follow that an increase in metabolism would produce an increase of the putative vasodilator and thus RBF. This would make autoregulation by vasodilatory metabolites impossible.

Autoregulatory factors, including vasodilatory prostaglandins, kinins, adenosine, and the renin-angiotensin system have been implicated in the autoregulation of RBF and GFR.[27–32] However, controversy persists, and the role of these *humoral factors* needs better definition.

It is most likely that all of these systems contribute, in part, to the phenomenon of renal autoregulation, and future studies will probably delineate the relative contribution of each.

**Glomerular Permeability.** The fluid entering Bowman's space is nearly free of albumin and larger molecules. Restriction to glomerular filtration of certain molecules is known as glomerular permselectivity. The determinants of glomerular permselectivity include effective glomerular "pore" size and the electrostatic charge on the glomerular filtration barrier. The degree of filtration of a molecule is thus determined by its size, shape, and charge. Filtration of macromolecules such as albumin may also be affected by renal hemodynamics.

The filtration of molecules larger than inulin (molecular radius = 14 Å) is progressively restricted, and approaches zero at molecular radii of about 40 Å.[14] The molecular radius of albumin is 36 Å.

The glomerular filtration barrier is covered by sialoproteins that bear fixed negative charges. Albumin is a polyanion at physiologic pH. Hence, it is also restricted from glomerular filtration by the interaction of similar electrostatic charges. Neutral dextran, which has a molecular radius equal to that of albumin but which lacks a net negative charge, is filtered more than 100 times as easily as albumin.[33] In certain forms of renal disease, diminution in the glomerular charge barrier may increase glomerular permeability to albumin, resulting in proteinuria.

The glomerular filtration of albumin may

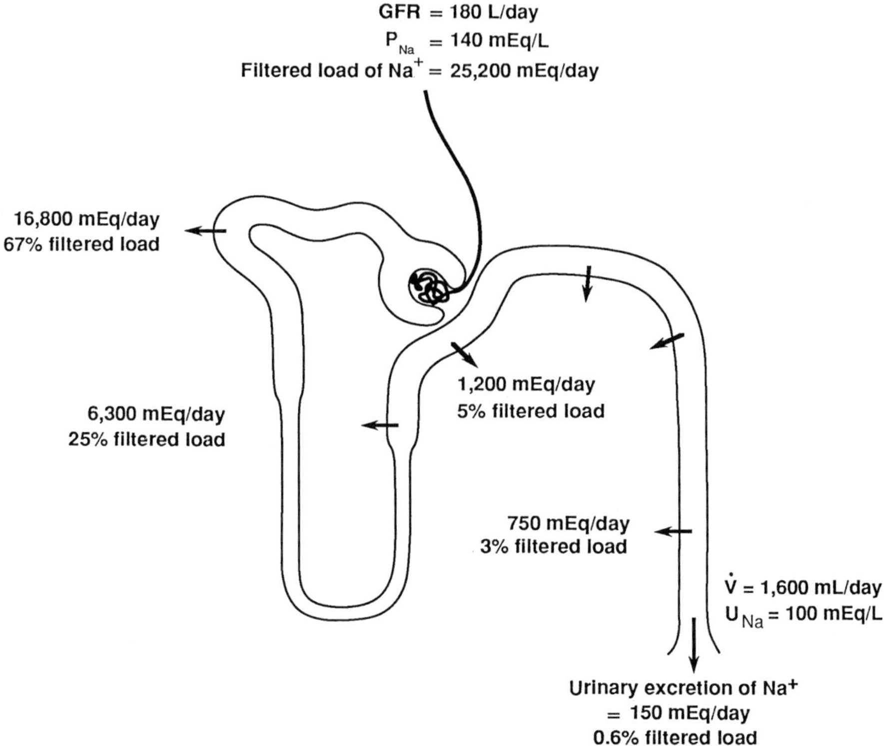


**Fig 4.** Daily renal turnover of $Na^+$ in a normal adult human. The diagram of the nephron represents the composite of the roughly 2 million nephrons of both kidneys. In steady state (equilibrium), the organism is, by definition, in balance. For $Na^+$, this means that the daily output of $Na^+$ equals the daily intake. Obviously, $Na^+$ is excreted mainly by the kidneys; the difference between the rate of urinary excretion of $Na^+$ and the daily intake is made up by extrarenal routes of excretion, such as sweat, saliva, and other gastrointestinal secretions. Under normal circumstances the extrarenal losses of $Na^+$ are negligible. GFR = glomerular filtration rate; $P_{Na}$ and $U_{Na}$ = plasma and urinary concentration of sodium, respectively.

also be increased by a reduction in renal plasma flow unaccompanied by a change in glomerular filtration rate. Such an increase in "filtration fraction" (the ratio of GFR/RPF) may lead to an increase in the concentration of albumin in the glomerular capillaries and thereby augment the gradient favoring albumin diffusion into the filtrate.

## SALT AND WATER HANDLING

Sodium (Na) and its associated anions (mostly chloride and bicarbonate) are confined to the extracellular fluid (ECF) compartment and are the principal determinants of ECF osmolality. Because water moves freely across cell membranes, and because the osmolality of ECF is kept constant, it follows that the volume of ECF is directly related to the total body content of sodium. Renal tubular reabsorption of sodium and water preserves ECF volume despite glomerular filtration of large volumes of plasma. Changes in tubular sodium reabsorption defend ECF volume against changes in the filtered sodium load produced by changes in GFR. In addition, changes in excretion maintain sodium balance at varying levels of intake. The handling of sodium by the nephron is summarized in Figure 4.

The reabsorption of sodium ion takes place against electrical and chemical (concentration) gradients and requires expenditure of metabolic energy. Such a process is described as active transport. The energy for the bulk of sodium reabsorption derives from aerobic metabolism. There is a direct, linear relationship between the rate of sodium reabsorption and oxygen consumption by the kidney.[34]

The exact mechanisms of sodium transport throughout the nephron continue to be investigated. In the proximal tubule, sodium in the tubular lumen travels down its concentration gradient, across the luminal (apical) membrane, into the tubular epithelial cell. Within the cell, the concentration is kept low by pumps in the basal and lateral membranes that extrude sodium into the peritubular space, from which it can enter the peritubular capillaries. These pumps, involving the enzyme Na,K-ATPase, represent the "active" (energy-consuming) component of sodium transport. For the most part, chloride reabsorption follows sodium extrusion as a consequence of the negative luminal potential created by outward sodium movement.

Water is reabsorbed "passively," by moving down a gradient of osmolality between tubular fluid (lower) and peritubular (higher). This gradient is established by the reabsorption of sodium and its attendant anions. Because the water permeability of the proximal tubule is high, only a small osmotic gradient is required to effect water movement.

Similar sodium-reabsorptive processes probably operate in the distal tubules and collecting ducts. Unlike these other segments, however, the thick ascending limb of the loop of Henle has a positive luminal potential. Among the mechanisms proposed to account for this is active transport of chlorine with secondary, passive sodium reabsorption.[35,36]

## Regulation of Sodium Excretion

Defense mechanisms ensure that the bulk of filtered sodium is reabsorbed in the proximal nephron segments. Renal autoregulation keeps GFR, and hence the filtered sodium load, constant. If a hemodynamic disturbance that changes GFR occurs, the filtered load of sodium changes. The proximal tubule alters its absolute rate of sodium reabsorption in parallel, so that the fractional sodium reabsorption remains constant. This phenomenon, termed glomerular–tubular balance, prevents loss or accumulation of large amounts of sodium. The mechanism by which glomerular–tubular balance is achieved remains uncertain. One hypothesis stresses the importance of physical factors.[37] Because the transglomerular passage of plasma protein is restricted, a change of GFR produces a parallel change in the protein concentration in the glomerular capillaries. This fluid passes into the efferent arteriole and thence to the peritubular capillaries. Thus, a rise in GFR would result in an increase in peritubular oncotic pressure. This tends to favor net sodium reabsorption. Decrements in peritubular oncotic pressure would have the opposite effect. The importance of peritubular protein concentration in the regulation of proximal sodium reabsorption has been challenged.[38] An alternative theory suggests that the glomerular filtrate itself contains a substance that stimulates its own reabsorption.[39] The identity of this substance is unknown.

Like with chronic dietary changes, comparatively small changes in sodium intake produce changes in urinary sodium excretion via changes in the handling of this ion by the collecting ducts. Except with extreme changes in ECF volume, such as can be produced by parenteral infusions, chronic sodium loading is usually not associated with changes in proximal reabsorption. Reabsorption by the collecting ducts is stimulated by aldosterone, the secretion of which is regulated, in part, by ECF volume through the activity of the renin-angiotensin system. Other humoral factors may also regulate sodium excretion, including substances whose production in the kidney is related to the sodium balance, such as prostaglandins, angiotensin II, dopamine, and bradykinin.

The existence of one or more "natriuretic hormones," thought to be produced in the central nervous system or at other sites in response to sodium loading, has also been proposed.[40,41] Natriuretic hormones may act on the collecting duct to inhibit reabsorption, perhaps by inhibition of Na, K-ATPase. There is growing evidence that an atrial natriuretic factor (ANF) may play a physiologic role in the regulation of salt and water balance in humans.[42–46] ANF is secreted principally by atrial myocytes in response to increased intravascular volume. It acts in concert on the veins, the kidneys, and the adrenal glands to reduce systemic blood pressure and intravascular volume, chronically as well as acutely.[47] The reduction in systemic blood pressure is the result of a reduced peripheral vascular resistance, diminished cardiac output and decreased intravascular volume. In the kidney, ANF acts on specific receptors to induce hyperfiltration, inhibition of $Na^+$ transport, and suppression of renin release. These actions result in a natriuresis, diuresis, and lowering of arterial blood pressure.[48] ANF also inhibits aldosterone biosynthesis both by inhibiting renin secretion from the renal juxtaglomerular apparatus and, more directly, by a receptor-mediated effect on adrenal glomerulosa cells. These actions also tend to lower arterial blood pressure and intravascular volume.

Changes in peritubular hydrostatic pressure in the renal interstitium can alter handling by the proximal tubule, the loop of Henle, and possibly by the collecting duct.[38,49,50] An increase in interstitial pressure resulting from a rise in arterial pressure, renal vasodilation, or alterations in filtration fraction (resulting from changes in filtration dynamics at the glomerular tuft) can increase renal Na excretion acutely. Whether such physical factors influence tubular function directly or through resultant changes in the levels of intrarenal hormones remains undetermined. Stimulation of the adrenergic innervation to the kidney increases tubular Na reabsorption, independent of changes in GFR or renal plasma flow.[51] The site at which sympathetic stimulation acts appears to be the proximal tubule.

The rate of sodium excretion is of diagnostic importance in determining the cause of oliguria. With prerenal azotemia, sodium excretion is usually less than 15 mmol/L, whereas sodium excretion is *usually* higher with renal causes (eg, acute tubular necrosis). However, prerenal factors often coexist with renal disease, thus there is considerable overlap in the urine sodium concentration ($U_{Na}$) in these two situations.[52] Therefore, only values that are clearly abnormally high or low are diagnostic. The fractional excretion of sodium ($FE_{Na}\%$), obtained by dividing the clearance of sodium by the clearance of creatinine, provides a much better index by which to differentiate renal from prerenal causes. $FE_{Na}\%$ is calculated by the following formula:

$$FE_{Na}\% = (U_{Na} * P_{Cr} * 100)/(P_{Na} * U_{Cr}) = (C_{Na}/C_{Cr}) * 100$$

where:

$U_{Na}$ = urine sodium concentration

$P_{Cr}$ = plasma creatinine concentration

$U_{Cr}$ = urine creatinine concentration

$C_{Na}$ = clearance of sodium

$C_{Cr}$ = clearance of creatinine

A value lower than 1% favors a prerenal etiology while a value greater than 1% favors a renal cause. Although fairly sensitive and specific, $FE_{Na}\%$ values of less than 1% have been reported in patients with a variety of causes of acute renal failure other than prerenal disease (eg, myoglobinuria or hemoglobinuria, radiocontrast nephropathy, renal azotemia superimposed on chronic prerenal failure as in hepatic cirrhosis).[53]

## Urinary Dilution and Concentration

In the proximal tubule, where some two thirds of the glomerular filtrate is reabsorbed, water follows NaCl reabsorption, and the tubular fluid remains isotonic to plasma (normally 270 to 285 mOsm/kg). Separation of NaCl from water reabsorption occurs in the loop of Henle, by a mechanism that generates tubular fluid that is hypotonic (dilute) as compared with plasma. In the absence of vasopressin (ADH), the final urine remains dilute, permitting the excretion of a water load. The loop of Henle also helps generate a hypertonic medullary interstitial environment. Under conditions of water deprivation (hydropenia), ADH causes fluid in the collecting ducts to equilibrate osmotically with the medullary interstitium. This results in hypertonic (concentrated) urine, and conserves water. Urine osmolality may vary normally from 50 mOsm/kg to approximately 1200 mOsm/kg.

The excretion of water relative to solute may be described quantitatively as free water clearance ($C_{H_2O}$). Not a true clearance in the sense of inulin or creatinine, $C_{H_2O}$ is the difference between the measured urinary flow rate and the "osmolar clearance," ie, the rate of urine formation that would be necessary to excrete the measured urinary osmolar load at a tonicity equal to that of plasma. The calculation of $C_{H_2O}$ is summarized below.

$$C_{H_2O} = V - C_{osm}$$

$V$ = urine flow rate (mL/min)

$C_{osm}$ = osmolar clearance (mL/min) $= (U_{osm} \times V)/P_{osm}$

$U_{osm}$ = urine osmolality (mOsm/kg)

$P_{osm}$ = plasma osmolality (mOsm/kg)

$U_{osm} \times V$ = urinary osmolar load (mOsm/min)

$$C_{H_2O} = V - [(Uosm \text{ x } V)/P_{osm}]$$

$$C_{H_2O} = V\,[1 - (U_{osm}/P_{osm})](\text{mL/min})$$

When dilute urine is produced, $U_{osm} < P_{osm}$, and $C_{H_2O}$ is positive, implying net free water excretion. When concentrated urine is produced, $U_{osm} > P_{osm}$, and $C_{H_2O}$ has a negative value, implying net free water conservation. Negative free water clearance ($-C_{H_2O}$) is symbolized as $Tc_{H_2O}$.

The formation of hypotonic tubular fluid occurs in the thick ascending limb of the loop of Henle. This segment is impermeable to water. The reabsorption of Cl and Na separates solute from water and reduces the osmolality of fluid leaving this segment to approximately 100 mOsm/kg. This process occurs irrespective of external water balance. Administration of a water load reduces systemic extracellular fluid tonicity and inhibits ADH secretion. In the absence of ADH, the cortical and medullary portions of the collecting duct remain impermeable to water. Because NaCl reabsorption can continue in these segments, urine osmolality may be further reduced to the minimum of 50 mOsm/kg. The excretion of dilute urine maintains ECF tonicity in response to a water load.

Concentrated urine is elaborated in response to hydropenia, which raises ECF osmolality and stimulates ADH secretion. In man, ADH binds to receptors on the basolateral membrane of collecting duct epithelial cells. This activates the enzyme adenylate cyclase, which catalyzes intracellular cyclic AMP (cAMP) formation. cAMP—via a cAMP-dependent protein kinase—facilitates phosphorylation of a component of the apical membrane. Through a process that also involves cel-

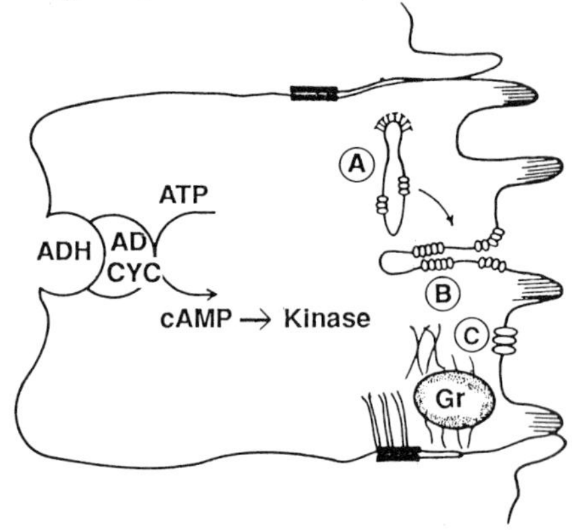


**Fig 5.** Diagrammatic view of the intercellular action of antidiuretic hormone (ADH). The hormone is bound to receptors on the basolateral membrane of the receptor cell and activates adenylate cyclase, increasing the intracellular concentration of cAMP. A series of intermediate steps take place (ADCYC), including activation of a cAMP-dependent protein kinase. Cytoplasmic tubular structures (aggrephores, A) are induced to fuse with the lumina membrane (B), and aggregates of water conducting particles are delivered to the membrane (C). Gr = subluminal granule; ATP = adenosine triphosphate. [Adapted from Hays RM, Franki N, Ding G, Effects of antidiuretic hormone on the collecting duct, *Kidney Int* (1987;31:530), with permission.]

lular microtubules, this increases the permeability of the collecting tubule of water (Fig 5). Urea permeability is also increased in the medullary portion. During hydropenia, most water reabsorption occurs in the cortical collecting tubule, where hypotonic luminal fluid leaving the loop of Henle equilibrates with the isotonic interstitium of the cortex. The isotonic fluid in the cortical collecting tubule subsequently becomes hypertonic in the medullary collecting duct, by osmotic equilibration with the hypertonic medullary interstitium.

The kidney generates medullary hypertonicity by means of the loop of Henle. According to the "countercurrent hypothesis," reabsorption of NaCl without water in the ascending limb, and its deposition in the interstitium, creates a local (horizontal) osmotic gradient. The increase in medullary tonicity causes water to leave the descending limb, raising its tonicity. The proximity of the descending and ascending limbs of the same tubules (arranged in hairpin curves) causes a constant gradient of tonicity at any given horizontal level to be multiplied along the vertical axis, creating high tonicities at the bend of the loop. This creates the progressive gradient of medullary tissue osmolality from corticomedullary junction to the papillary tip (Fig 6). Modification of the countercurrent hypothesis has been proposed to account for the importance of urea in augmenting urinary concentration.[54,55] According to the modified hypothesis, the process of urinary concentration begins with active chloride transport in the ascending thick limb. Urea and water (to which this segment is impermeable) remain behind in the hypotonic fluid. In the cortical and outer medullary collecting tubules, ADH augments water but not urea permeability. Water leaves these segments, raising the luminal concentration of urea. In the inner medullary collecting duct, ADH enhances urea permeability as well. Urea thus leaves the tubule and accumulates in the interstitium. This action raises medullary tonicity and causes water to

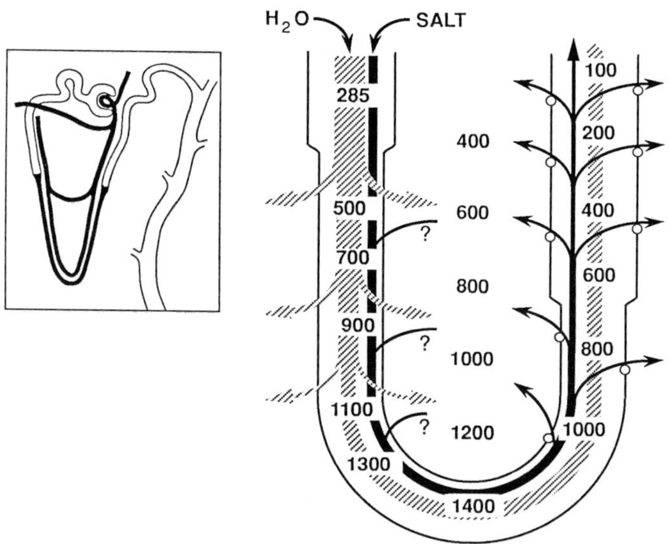


**Fig 6.** The loop of Henle, the "countercurrent multiplier." The numbers indicate the osmotic concentration in mOsm/kg $H_2O$ of the tubular fluid and the interstitial fluid. The active transport of salt, without water, out of the ascending limb increases the osmotic concentration of the medullary interstitium. The small horizontal gradient is multiplied vertically by countercurrent flow. Water is reabsorbed from the descending limb by this osmotic force. Note that tubular fluid flows out of the loop at an osmotic concentration lower than that of the entering fluid. Fractionally more solute than water has been lost to the medullary interstitium.

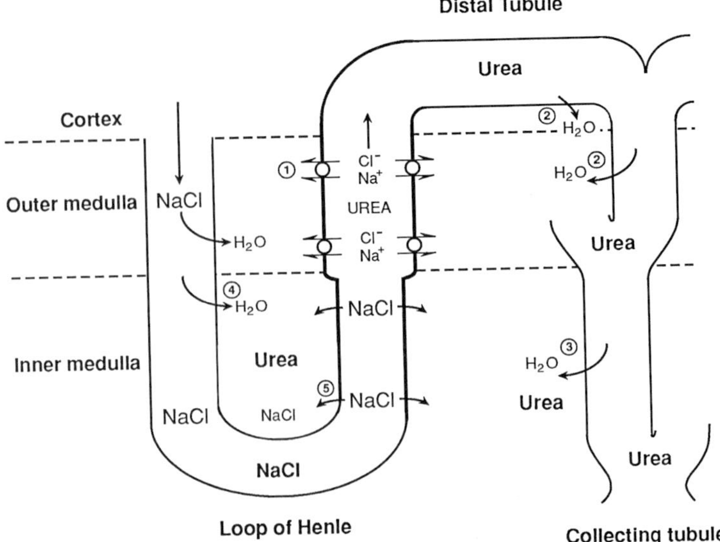


**Fig 7.** Recent modifications of the countercurrent hypothesis by Stephenson, Kokko, and Rector. Both the thin ascending limb in the inner medulla and the thick distal tubule are impermeable to water, as indicated by the thickened lining. In the thick ascending limb, active chloride reabsorption, accompanied by passive sodium movement (1), renders the tubule fluid dilute and the outer medullary interstitium hyperosmotic. In the last part of the distal tubule and in the collecting tubule in the cortex and outer medulla, water is reabsorbed down its osmotic gradient (2), increasing the concentration of urea that remains behind. In the inner medulla, both water and urea are reabsorbed from the collecting duct (3). Some urea reenters the loop of Henle (not shown). This medullary recycling of urea, in addition to trapping of urea by countercurrent exchange in the vasa recta (not shown), causes urea to accumulate in large quantities in the medullary interstitium (indicated by large type), where it osmotically extracts water from the descending limb (4) and thereby concentrates sodium chloride in descending limb fluid. When the fluid rich in sodium chloride enters the sodium chloride–permeable (but water–impermeable) thin ascending limb, sodium chloride moves passively down its concentration gradient (5), rendering the tubule fluid relatively hypoosmotic to the surrounding interstitium.

leave the descending limb of Henle's loop, which is permeable to water but not to NaCl or urea. The raises the NaCl concentration of fluid reaching the hairpin turn. The ascending thin limb is impermeable to water but not to NaCl or urea. In this segment, NaCl diffuses down its concentration gradient, into the interstitium. Urea diffuses in, but at a slower rate, leading to progressive reduction of luminal tonicity in the segment. The osmotic gradients that are established are multiplied by the countercurrent mechanism. An additional effect of this mechanism is to cause some urea to remain in the medulla, where it recycles between the collecting duct, the interstitium, and the loop of Henle. This mechanism is summarized in Figure 7.

## Acid-Base Balance

To maintain the acid-base balance of the ECF, the kidney must excrete net acid at a rate equal to the rate of extrarenal net acid production (approximately 0.3 to 1.0 mEq/kg day). The kidney maintains the pH of the ECF by regulating the plasma bicarbonate $HCO_3^-$) concentration. It does so by two processes: (1) reclamation of filtered $HCO_3^-$ and (2) generation of new $HCO_3^-$ by means of net acid excretion. The proximal tubule lowers the luminal pH from 7.3 to approximately 6.7, and thus reabsorbs the major portion of $HCO_3^-$. The collecting tubule provides the final urinary acidification with titration of ammonia, phosphate, and other titratable buffers.[56]

The normal filtered load of $HCO_3^-$ is about 4500 mEq/day. Less than 0.1% of filtered $HCO_3^-$ appears in the final urine; approximately 80% of filtered $HCO_3^-$ is reclaimed by the proximal tubule. Although the net result of this process is referred to as $HCO_3^-$ reabsorption, the $HCO_3^-$ in tubular fluid is not directly reabsorbed as such. Instead, the tubular epithelial cells add $HCO_3^-$ to peritubular blood as a consequence of proton ($H^+$) secretion. The enzyme carbonic anhydrase, with then-tubular epithelial cells, catalyzes the hydration of carbon dioxide ($CO_2$) to form carbonic acid ($H_2CO_3$). Dissociation of $H_2CO_3$ yields $H^+$ and $HCO_3^-$. The $H^+$ is secreted into the tubular lumen, where it combines with filtered $HCO_3^-$ to form $H_2CO_3$. Carbonic anhydrase is also present in the brush border, where it catalyzes the dehydration of luminal $H_2CO_3$ to $CO_2$ and water. The $CO_2$ can diffuse back into the cell, where it may be hydrated to form additional $H_2CO_3$. The $HCO_3^-$ generated within the cell diffuses into peritubular blood, possibly via specific pathways.[57] The bulk of $H^+$ secretion by the proximal tubule appears to be coupled to sodium reabsorption by a direct-exchange mechanism.[57]

The factors that can affect proximal $HCO_3^-$ reabsorption include (1) *extracellular fluid volume*—decrements in absolute or effective volume enhance $HCO_3^-$ reabsorption, whereas increments have the opposite effect; (2) *arterial* $Pco_2$—hypercapnia stimulates $HCO_3^-$ reabsorption, whereas hypocapnia inhibits; (3) *body potassium stores*—there is a slight stimulation of proximal $HCO_3^-$ reabsorption by prior potassium depletion; (4) *parathormone*—inhibits reabsorption; and (5) phosphate depletion—inhibits reabsorption.

The kidney adds new $HCO_3^-$ to blood by secreting $H^+$ in excess of that which is necessary to reclaim filtered $HCO_3^-$. This process results in net acid excretion. Under normal circumstances, net acid secretion replaces the $HCO_3^-$ consumed in buffering the strong acid by-products of metabolism, mainly sulfuric and phosphoric acids. Depending on diet, some 40 to 70 mEq of $H^+$ derived from such acids are produced daily. Net acid excretion may also increase in response to the addition of ketoacids or lactic acid in disease states, or to compensate for hypercapnia. The secreted $H^+$ is taken up by urinary buffers, principally monohydrogen phosphate ($HPO_4^=$) and ammonia ($NH_3$), which are converted to $H_2PO_4^-$ and $NH_4^+$. Net acid excretion is equal to the sum of $H_2PO_4^-$ and $NH_4^+$ excretion, minus any $HCO_3^-$ that escapes reabsorption. The $H_2PO_4^-$ is also referred to as titratable acid. This term denotes the amount of strong base required to titrate urine back to pH 7.4. A comparatively small proportion of secreted $H^+$ is unbound to buffers; it is this component that can result in a minimum urinary pH of about 4.4.

Most net acid excretion occurs in the collecting ducts, where $H^+$ is secreted by pumps that are not directly coupled to sodium reabsorption. This process also depends on intracellular carbonic anhydrase. There is no brush border carbonic anhydrase in the collecting ducts. The rate of net acid excretion can be modified by (1) *the electrical gradient between the tubule cell and the lumen*—$Na^+$ reabsorption in the collecting ducts creates a negative intraluminal potential; this favors $H^+$ secretion. The gradient is augmented by increased sodium delivery and reabsorption, especially when $Na^+$ is accompanied by a poorly reabsorbed anion. This enhancement of $H^+$ secretion by $Na^+$ reabsorption brings about an indirect coupling of these processes; (2) *mineralocorticoids*—aldosterone can directly stimulate the capacity of the $H^+$ pump.[58] In addition, by stimulating $Na^+$ reabsorption in the collecting duct, aldosterone enhances the electrical gradient that favors $H^+$ secretion; (3) *buffer availability*—$NH_3$ is produced in the kidney from glutamine. It gains access to the tubular fluid in both the proximal and the distal nephron by nonionic diffusion. Acidosis increases renal $NH_3$ production. Increased buffer availability, by taking up free $H^+$, reduces the chemical gradient against which $H^+$ is pumped; this stimulates $H^+$ secretion. The mechanism by which a change in systemic pH affects ammoniagenesis remains undefined. Ammoniagenesis can also be stimulated by

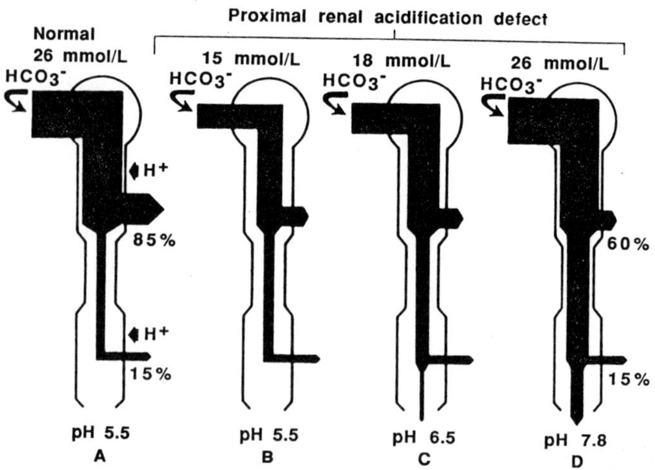


**Fig 8.** Schematic representation of the proximal renal acidification defect in Type II RTA. Effect of changes in plasma bicarbonate concentration on the delivery of bicarbonate to the distal nephron and as a consequence, on urinary pH and on excretion of bicarbonate. A, In normal subjects, at normal plasma bicarbonate concentrations, approximately 15% of the filtered bicarbonate load escapes reabsorption in the proximal tubule and is reabsorbed in the distal nephron; urinary bicarbonate excretion is nil, urinary pH is appropriately low, and net acid excretion is normal. B, In patients with Type II RTA, bicarbonate excretion might also be nil, urinary pH may be appropriately low, and net acid excretion may not be diminished at reduced plasma bicarbonate concentration (metabolic acidosis). This is because the amount of $HCO_3$ escaping reabsorption proximally and delivered to the distal nephron is not supranormal when the amount of bicarbonate presented to the proximal tubule for reabsorption is significantly reduced. C, When, however, metabolic acidosis is somewhat mitigated (by administration of $NaHCO_3$), supranormal amounts of bicarbonate are delivered out of the proximal tubule because the defective proximal tubule cannot reabsorb the modest increase in filtered load of $HCO_3$. As a consequence, bicarbonate escapes reabsorption in the distal nephron, urinary pH becomes inappropriately high, and net acid excretion is reduced. D, If the plasma bicarbonate concentration and filtered bicarbonate load are increased to normal levels, the amount of bicarbonate escaping reabsorption proximally greatly exceeds the resorptive capacity of the normal distal nephron, and massive bicarbonaturia occurs. In the illustration of Type II RTA, renal tubule reabsorption of bicarbonate ($T_{HCO3}$) at normal plasma bicarbonate concentration (26 mmol/L) is reduced by 25%. [Adapted from Morris RC, Sebastian A, McSherry E, The symposium on acid-base homeostasis, *Kidney Int* (1972;1:322), with permission.]

potassium depletion and inhibited by potassium loading. An adaptive increase in ammoniagenesis is the principal mechanism for the excretion of increased acid loads.[59]

**Defective Tubular Hydrogen Ion Secretion.** Defects in renal tubular hydrogen ion secretion, also termed renal tubular acidosis (RTA), may occur either in the proximal tubule (RTA type 2) or in the distal tubule (RTA type 1).[60]

*Proximal RTA (Type 2).* Three major processes occur in the nephron to rid the body of excess acid: sodium bicarbonate reabsorption, ammonia trapping, and titratable acid formation. Unlike in the distal tubule, in the proximal tubule the formation of titratable acid and $NH_4^+$ is negligible. The major function of the proximal tubule is the reabsorption of bicarbonate. One bicarbonate ion is reabsorbed for each hydrogen ion excreted. The proximal tubule has a high-capacity bicarbonate transport system, and it reabsorbs approximately 80% of filtered bicarbonate. In proximal RTA defects, the reabsorptive threshold (Tm) for bicarbonate is thought to be lowered (Fig 8).[61] This results in the delivery of large amounts of sodium bicarbonate to the distal kidney. The distal tubule has a relatively low capacity for bicarbonate reabsorption (however, it is a "high-gradient system" and is able to secrete hydrogen ions across a large gradient). Thus, the hydrogen ions secreted distally primarily absorb free bicarbonate producing little $NH_4^+$ bonding and titratable acid secretion. This results in an alkaline, bicarbonate-rich urine. Extracellular volume contraction occurs secondarily to this massive anion ($HCO_3^-$) loss. In an attempt to compensate for this extracellular volume contraction, chloride reabsorption is increased, resulting in a hyperchloremic metabolic acidosis. As systemic acidosis progresses, the filtered load of sodium bicarbonate diminishes, allowing only small amounts of bicarbonate to be delivered distally. Thus, below this lowered bicarbonate reabsorptive threshold (Tm), distal acidification processes can compensate for defective proximal acidification. This results in more complete bicarbonate reabsorption distally with titratable acid and $NH_4^+$ production and urine with a pH of 5.0 or less. However, the amount of bicarbonate required to maintain a normal serum level is massive, since it must equal the amount of bicarbonate excretion. In proximal RTA, potassium and calcium excretion are increased. However, since citrate excretion is relatively normal, nephrocalcinosis and renal calculi formation are rare. Clinically, the effects on children include: osteomalacia, rickets, abnormal gut calcium absorption, decreased phosphorus, and abnormal vitamin D metabolism.

**Distal RTA (Type 1).** In distal RTA defects, the distal tubule is unable to secrete hydrogen ions against a large gradient and is thus unable to produce a urine pH of less than 5.4 even when challenged.[61] Minimal urine pH in distal RTA ranges from 5.4 to 6.5, depending on the severity of the transport defect. The distal tubule normally accounts for, at most, 15% of total bicarbonate reabsorption. Since proximal reabsorption is not affected in distal RTA, the urinary bicarbonate concentration is only 5 mEq/L, even at a urine pH of 6.5. Thus daily excretion of bicarbonate is not usually greater than 10 to 15 mEq/day in patients with distal RTA.

Therefore, the acidosis of distal RTA is more easily controlled than is the acidosis of proximal RTA. Systemic acidosis results in increased bone reabsorption and, in turn, increased urinary calcium. In addition, the urine is mildly alkaline (unlike proximal RTA that maintain an almost normal urine pH) and nephrocalcinosis is common in distal RTA secondary to low solubility of the excess calcium in a mildly alkaline urine with a decreased citrate content.

Two subsets of patients with RTA have been described. The first group presents with *complete RTA* (cRTA); these patients comprise the majority of those with RTA. The patients are acidotic and usually present with the known renal manifestations of the disease (eg, nephrocalcinosis). Another group of patients presents with *incomplete RTA* (iRTA). Patients with iRTA are nonacidotic and present with nephrocalcinosis. Like patients with cRTA, these patients are also unable to increase the urinary excretion of titratable acid to a normal maxima when presented with an acid load.[62] These patients are considered to have a "milder" form of the disease. Functional renal mass and GFR is relatively well maintained, and excretion of $NH_4^+$ is sufficient to prevent frank acidosis.[63]

The acidosis of RTA is non-anion gap acidosis (anion gap being defined as the difference between the major intravascular cations, sodium and potassium minus the sum of the major anions, chloride and bicarbonate; normally between 12 and 16) associated with *hyperchloremia* and *hypokalemia* in contradistinction to the acidosis associated with ATN or reduced GFR (a hypochloremic and hyperkalemic acidosis). The hyperchloremia results from increased NaCl reabsorption stimulated by volume contraction secondary to sodium bicarbonate loss in the urine. The hypokalemia results from stimulation of the renin-angiotensin-aldosterone (secondary to volume contraction) axis as well as increased distal Na-K exchange occurring with the increased distal delivery of $NaHCO_3$.

### Potassium

Over 90% of plasma potassium undergoes glomerular filtration. Most of it is reabsorbed in the proximal tubule and the loop of Henle. The bulk of potassium in the final urine is added to tubular fluid by secretion in the late distal tubule and cortical collecting duct. Tubular epithelial cells in these segments take up potassium from peritubular fluid by a mechanism involving Na,K-ATPase.[64] This gives rise to an intracellular transport pool of potassium. Potassium secretion is favored by the negative intratubular potential created by distal Na reabsorption, and by the concentration gradient between intracellular potassium and tubular fluid. In addition to these passive forces that influence potassium secretion, an active transport mechanism may exist.[65] There is no evidence either for a coupled exchange between $Na^+$ absorption and $K^+$ secretion or for competition between intracellular $K^+$ and $H^+$ for tubular secretory pathways.

Potassium excretion is augmented by an increase in distal tubular fluid flow rate (as with saline or osmotic diuresis, diuretic drugs, or postobstructive diuresis). This promotes potassium secretion by maintaining a steep potassium concentration gradient between the cell and the tubular fluid. In addition, increased quantities of sodium are presented to distal reabsorptive sites. The negative intratubular potential created by increased sodium reabsorption also promotes potassium secretion.

Mineralocorticoids stimulate potassium secretion, possibly by stimulating Na,K-ATPase in the basolateral membrane.[65] This would increase potassium uptake and raise intracellular potassium concentration, thereby enhancing potassium secretion.

### Calcium

Only that portion of plasma calcium that is not bound to plasma proteins is filtered at the glomerulus. Ultrafilterable calcium (Ca) represents about 60% of total plasma calcium. There is subsequent tubular reabsorption of 96% to 98% of this filtered load. The bulk of calcium reabsorption occurs in the proximal tubule and the ascending limb of the loop of Henle. Additional reabsorption occurs in the distal convoluted tubule and cortical collecting duct.[66] Calcium movement along the nephron appears to be subject to two transepithelial transport processes. One is a paracellular and gradient-dependent (concentration) process that predominates in most segments of the nephron. The other is a transcellular, energy-dependent process that characterizes calcium transport in the distal nephron.[67] Recent investigations have focused on the role of a cytosolic calcium binding protein ($CaBP_r$) located in the distal tubule that might modulate calcium transport in this nephron segment.[68,69] Regulation of calcium by several known factors (eg, vitamin D, parathyroid hormone [PTH]) might be due to their effect on production of $CaBP_r$ in the distal tubule.

Calcium reabsorption in the proximal tubule occurs parallel with sodium reabsorption, with a component of calcium absorption being directly sodium-dependent.[70] Calcium reabsorption in the proximal tubule is inhibited by PTH, cyclic AMP, acetazolamide, exogenous sodium loading, and phosphate depletion. The effect on urinary calcium, however, depends on the behavior of more distal nephron sites. In the loop of Henle (as well as the distal convoluted tubule and collecting duct), calcium reabsorption is stimulated by PTH. This accounts for the hypocalciuric effect of this hormone despite its inhibition of proximal calcium absorption. Calcium reabsorption in the loop of Henle is inhibited by furosemide. When diuretic-induced extracellular volume depletion is prevented by replacement of salt and water losses, furosemide causes an increase in urinary calcium excretion.[71] This accounts for the efficacy of furosemide in the emergency treatment of hypercalcemia. Final modulation of urinary calcium excretion occurs in the distal tubule and collecting ducts. In these segments, active transport of calcium occurs, which can be dissociated from sodium reabsorption. Thus, chlorthiazide, which inhibits distal tubular sodium transport, also directly stimulates calcium absorption in this segment.[72] This may be the major explanation for the reduction in urinary calcium excretion with chronic administration of thiazides. An additional hypocalciuric effect of thiazide diuretics may result from extracellular fluid volume contraction, with consequent stimulation of calcium reabsorption in the proximal tubule.

Other factors that stimulate calcium reabsorption between the late proximal tubule and the early distal convoluted tubule include hypocalcemia, metabolic alkalosis (increased tubular $HCO_3^-$), vitamin D, and phosphate loading. Reabsorption is inhibited by hypercalcemia, metabolic acidosis, hypermagnesemia, and phosphate depletion.[66]

## Phosphate

Plasma inorganic phosphate, existing as a mixture of $HPO_4^=$ and $HPO_4^-$, is 80% to 90% ultrafilterable at the glomerulus. Of the filtered load, 80% to 97% is reabsorbed. The tubular reabsorption of phosphate can increase to nearly 100% in response to phosphorus deprivation. Most phosphate reabsorption occurs in the proximal tubule. The existence of a distal site of phosphate transport is also suspected.[73,74] PTH inhibits its phosphate reabsorption in the proximal tubule and increases urinary phosphate. This effect is associated with increased urinary excretion of nephrogenous cyclic AMP.

# EXCRETION OF ORGANIC SOLUTES

## Urea

Urea is the major end product of protein catabolism in man. It is freely filtered at the glomerulus. Water reabsorption increases the urea concentration in tubular fluid, with subsequent urea diffusion out of the tubule. At typical urine flow rates of 1 mL/min, 30% to 40% of filtered urea is reabsorbed in the proximal tubule. The medullary collecting ducts are also permeable to urea, and their permeability is enhanced by vasopressin. Reabsorption of urea in the collecting duct is enhanced by antidiuresis and inhibited by water diuresis. Urea reabsorbed in the collecting ducts contributes to the hypertonicity of medullary interstitial fluid and plays an important role in urinary concentration.

The rate of urea reabsorption is inversely related to tubular fluid flow rate. At urine flow rate of about 2 mL/min, during water diuresis, 60% to 70% of filtered urea is excreted, ie, urea clearance is 60% to 70% of the GFR. At low urine flow rates, during antidiuresis or reductions in renal blood flow, urea clearance may fall to 10% to 20% of the GFR. This accounts for the disproportionate increase in BUN compared with serum creatinine in states of "prerenal azotemia."

## Uric Acid

Uric acid is the end product of purine catabolism in man. On a low-purine diet, uric acid production from endogenous sources is about 700 mg per day. Two thirds of the uric acid load is excreted by the kidneys. Intestinal excretion, with degradation by bacterial enzymes, accounts for the rest. Because of its low pKa (5.75), it exists in plasma almost entirely as urate. The low pH attained in urine in the distal nephron favors the formation of uric acid, which is of limited solubility in water.

Current evidence favors a four-component model for renal handling of urate[75]: (1) plasma urate is freely filtered at the glomerulus; (2) filtered urate undergoes nearly complete tubular reabsorption; (3) approximately 50% of this reabsorbed urate is secreted into tubular fluid; and (4) postsecretory reabsorption reclaims about 80% of the secreted urate. Antiuricosuric agents such as pyrazinoic acid (the metabolite of the antituberculous agent pyrazinamide) inhibit the tubular secretory mechanism. Probenecid, a uricosuric agent, acts by inhibiting postsecretory reabsorption.[76] The majority of patients with gout appear to have an impairment in renal uric acid excretion, which is incompletely characterized.[77]

Urate secretion is accomplished by organic anion secretory mechanisms located in the proximal tubule. A variety of other substances share and mutually compete for this mechanism. They include oxalate, lactate, hippurate, penicillins, cephalosporins, thiazides, furosemide, and ethacrynic acid. A separate organic cation-secretory mechanism also exists. Among the substances transported by this system are creatinine, cimetidine, and trimethoprim.

### Glucose

Although glucose is freely filtered at the glomerulus, it undergoes essentially complete reabsorption in the early portion of the proximal tubule, so that urine is normally glucose-free. With progressively higher filtered loads (at higher plasma glucose concentrations), reabsorption increased, until a tubular maximum glucose reabsorption rate (TmG) is attained. Filtered glucose in excess of the TmG appears in the urine.[12]

Glucose transport is linked to proximal sodium reabsorption. When the latter is inhibited, as by ECF volume expansion, the TmG falls. These observations have given rise to the following model: Glucose in tubular fluid interacts with a carrier mechanism in the luminal membrane of the tubular epithelial cell. This carrier, which exhibits saturation kinetics, facilitates the entry of glucose into the tubular epithelial cell. Sodium is required for glucose-carrier interaction. Once transported into the cell, glucose may diffuse down its own concentration gradient from tubular epithelial cell to peritubular blood.

### Amino Acids

Circulating amino acids readily cross the glomerular filter and undergo nearly complete reabsorption by proximal tubular cells. This occurs via mechanisms in the brush border membrane. As in the case of glucose, this process appears to be carrier-mediated, Na-dependent, and energy-requiring.[78] Separate transport mechanisms in the basolateral membrane also mediate cellular uptake of amino acids from peritubular fluids.

Much attention has been focused on the tubular transport mechanisms for cystine and the cationic (dibasic) amino acids: arginine, lysine, and ornithine. Reabsorption of these amino acids is defective in classic cystinuria. Because of the insolubility of cystine, urinary stones are formed. A model for tubular handling of these amino acids must account for the following observations: (1) whereas patients with classic cystinuria have excessive excretion of all four amino acids, patients have been described with either isolated cystinuria or hyperdibasic aminoaciduria (arginine, lysine, ornithine) without cystinuria. (2) In cystinuric patients, the clearance of cystine can exceed creatinine clearance, implying tubular secretion of cystine. (3) Renal cortical tissue slices from cystinuric patients may show no defect in taking up cystine from bathing medium, compared with slices from normal subjects.

According to the currently favored model, there are separate transport systems in the basolateral and brush border membranes. In the basolateral membrane are two uptake mechanisms—one for cystine and another for arginine, lysine, and ornithine. Amino acids that accumulate within the cell may be secreted into tubular fluid. In the brush border are three separate reabsorptive mechanisms. One is shared by all four amino acids; the second is for arginine, ornithine, and lysine only; and the third is for cystine alone.[79]

### Citrate

Urinary citrate may help prevent calcium nephrolithiasis by chelating urinary calcium. Plasma citrate, present at concentrations of 0.05 mMol to 0.3 mMol, undergoes glomerular filtration and subsequent proximal tubular reabsorption. Citrate excretion in man ranges between 10% and 35% of the filtered load.[80] In addition, some of the citrate that escapes filtration is taken up by the tubular cells from postglomerular blood. Citrate that enters the cell is metabolized via the citric acid cycle to $CO_2$ and water.

Citrate excretion is profoundly influenced by systemic acid-base balance, through consequent changes in tubular cell pH. Metabolic alkalosis increases citrate excretion. A rise in cellular pH inhibits citrate metabolism, leading to a rise in intracellular citrate concentration. The latter tends to inhibit citrate reabsorption. Metabolic acidosis has the opposite effect. Distal renal tubular acidosis and administration of acetazolamide are associated with hypocitruria and relatively alkaline urine. Both conditions predispose to calcium nephrolithiasis and nephrocalcinosis.

## REFERENCES


1. Lindeman RD, Tobin JD, Shock NW. Longitudinal studies on the rate of decline in renal function with age. *J Am Geriatr Soc.* 1985; 33:278.
2. Beeuwkes RI, Ichikawa I, Brenner BM. The renal circulation. In: Brenner BM, Rector F Jr, eds. *The Kidney.* Philadelphia: WB Saunders Co; 1981.
3. Barger AC, Herd JA. Renal vascular anatomy and distribution of renal blood flow. In: Orloff J, Berliner RW, eds. *Handbook of Physiology: Section 8, Renal Physiology.* Washington, DC: American Physiological Society; 1973;249.
4. Bookstein JJ, Clark RI. *Renal Microvascular Disease: Angiographic-Microangiographic Correlates.* Boston: Little, Brown & Co; 1980.
5. Handler JS, Kreisberg JI. Biology of renal cells in culture. In: Brenner BM, Rector F Jr, eds. *The Kidney.* Philadelphia: WB Saunders Co; 1981.
6. Beeuwkes RI. Vascular-tubular relationship in the human kidney. In: Leaf A, Giebisch, eds. *Renal Pathophysiology—Recent Advances.* New York: Raven Press; 1979:155.
7. Kaissling B, et al. The structural organization of the kidney of the desert rodent *Psammomys obesus. Anat Embryol.* 1975:148:121.
8. McCrory WW. *Developmental Nephrology.* Cambridge: Harvard University Press; 1972.
9. Davies DF, Shock NW. Age changes in glomerular filtration rate; effective renal plasma flow and tubular excretory capacity in adult males. *J Clin Invest.* 1950;29:496.
10. Dworkin LD, Brenner BM. The renal circulations. In: Brenner BM, Rector F Jr, eds. *The Kidney.* Philadelphia: WB Saunders Co; 1981.
11. Brenner BM, Stein JH. Acute renal failure. In: Brenner BM, Stein JH, eds. *Contemporary Issues in Nephrology.* vol 6. New York: Churchill Livingstone; 1980.
12. Smith HW. *The Kidney: Structure and Function in Health and Disease.* New York: Oxford University Press; 1951.
13. Crockcroft DW, Gault MH. Prediction of creatinine clearance from serum creatinine. *Nephron.* 1976;16:31–41.
14. Brenner BM, Humes HD. Mechanics of glomerular ultrafiltration. *N Engl J Med.* 1977; 297:148.
15. Tucker BJ, Blantz RC. An analysis of the determinants of nephron filtration rate. *Am J Physiol.* 1977;232:F477.
16. Osgood RW, Reineck HJ, Stein JH. Methodologic considerations in the study of glomerular ultrafiltration. *Am J Physiol.* 1982;242:F1.
17. Dworkin LD, Ichikawa I, Brenner BM. Hormonal modulation of glomerular function. *Am J Physiol.* 1983;244:F95.
18. Fried TA, Stein JH. Glomerular dynamics. *Arch Intern Med.* 1983;143:787.
19. Forster RP, Maes JP. Effect of experimental neurogenic hypertension on renal blood flow and glomerular filtration rate in intact denervated kidneys of unanesthetized rabbits with adrenal glands demedulated. *Am J Physiol.* 1947; 150:534.
20. Blythe WB. Captopril and renal autoregulation. *N Engl J Med.* 1983;308:390.
21. Thurau K, Schnermann J. The juxtaglomerular apparatus. *Kidney Int.* 1982;22(suppl 12).
22. Wright FS, Briggs JP. Feedback regulation of glomerular filtration rate. *Am J Physiol.* 1977; 233:F1.
23. Schnermann J, Ploth DW, Hermle M. Activation of tubuloglomerular feedback by chloride transport. *Pflugers Arch.* 1976;362:229.
24. Bell PD, McLean CB, Navar LG. Dissociation of tubuloglomerular feedback responses from distal tubular chloride concentration in the rat. *Am J Physiol.* 1981;240:F111.
25. Bell PD, Reddington M. Intracellular calcium in the transmission of tubuloglomerular feedback signals. *Am J Physiol.* 1983;245:295.
26. Bayliss WM. On the local reactions of the arterial wall to changes in arterial pressure. *J Physiol.* 1902;28:220.
27. Spielman WS, Thompson CI. A proposed role for adenosine in the regulation of renal hemodynamics and renin release. *Am J Physiol.* 1982;242:F423.
28. Schnermann J, Briggs JP, Weber PC. Tubuloglomerular feedback, prostaglandins and angiotensin in the autoregulation of glomerular filtration rate. *Kidney Int.* 1984;25:53.
29. Maier M, Starlinger M, Wagner M. The effect of hemorrhagic hypotension on urinary kallikrein excretion, renin activity and renal cortical blood flow in the pig. *Circ Res.* 1981;48:386.
30. Levens NR, Peach MS, Carey RM. Role of the intrarenal renin-angiotensin system in the control of renal function. *Circ Res.* 1981;48:157.
31. Moore LC, et al. Renal hemodynamic regulation by the renin-secreting segment of the afferent arteriole. *Kidney Int.* 1990;38:S65.
32. Briggs JP, Schnermann J. Macula densa control of renin secretion and glomerular vascular tone: evidence for common cellular mechanisms. *Renal Physiol.* 1986;9:193.

33. Brenner BM, et al. Determinants of glomerular permselectivity: insights derived from observations in vivo. *Kidney Int.* 1977;12:229.

34. Lassen NA, Munckl O, Thaysen JH. Oxygen consumption and sodium reabsorption in the kidney. *Acta Physiol Scand.* 1961;51:371.

35. Burg MD, Green N. Function of the thick ascending limb of Henle's loop. *Am J Physiol.* 1973;224:659.

36. Warnock DG, Eveloff J. NaCl entry mechanisms in the luminal membrane of the renal tubule. *Am J Physiol.* 1982;242:F561.

37. Brenner BM, Troy JL. Post-glomerular vascular protein concentration: evidence for a casual role in governing fluid resorption and glomerular balance by the renal proximal tubule. *J Clin Invest.* 1971;50:336.

38. Knox FG, et al. Role of hydrostatic and oncotic pressures in renal sodium reabsorption. *Circ Res.* 1983;52:491.

39. De Wardener HE. The control of sodium excretion. *Am J Physiol.* 1978;235:F163.

40. De Wardener HE, Clarkson EM. The natriuretic hormone: recent developments. *Clin Sci.* 1982;63:415.

41. Genest J. Volume hormones and blood pressure. *Ann Intern Med.* 1983;98:744.

42. Laragh JH. Atrial natriuretic hormone, the renin-aldosterone axis and blood pressure-electrolyte homeostasis. *N Engl J Med.* 1985;313:1330.

43. Atlas SA, Laragh JH. Atrial natriuretic hormone: a regulator of blood pressure and electrolyte homeostasis. *Kidney Int.* 1988;34(suppl 2):S64.

44. Goetz KL. Physiology and pathophysiology of atrial peptides. *Am J Physiol.* 1988;254:E1.

45. Lang RE, Unger T, Ganten D. Atrial natriuretic peptide: a new peptide in blood pressure control. *J Hypertens.* 1987;5:255.

46. Richards AM, McDonald D, Fitzpatrick MA. Atrial natriuretic hormone has biological effects at physiological plasma concentrations in man. *J Clin Endocrinol Metab.* 1988;67:1134.

47. Brenner BM, Ballermann BJ, Gunning ME. The diverse biological actions of atrial peptides. *Physiol Rev.* 1990;70:665.

48. Ballermann BJ, et al. Vasoactive peptides and the kidney. In: Brenner BM, Rector F Jr, eds. *The Kidney.* Philadelphia: WB Saunders Co; 1981.

49. Gilbert BR, Maude DL. Influence of peritubular hydrostatic pressure on salt and water reabsorption in the isolated perfused rat kidney. *Kidney Int.* 1977;12:558.

50. Gilbert BR, Maack T, Windhager EE. Microperfusion study of the effects of colloid osmotic pressure on proximal tubule reabsorption in the isolated perfused rat kidney. *Fed Proc.* 1979; 38:112.

51. DiBona GF. Neurogenic regulation of renal tubular sodium reabsorption. *Am J Physiol.* 1977;233:F73.

52. Espinel CH, Gregory AW. Differential diagnosis of acute renal failure. *Clin Nephrol.* 1980;13:73–77.

53. Kamel KS, et al. Urine electrolytes and osmolality: when and how to use them. *Am J Nephrol.* 1990;10:89–102.

54. Kokko JP, Rector FC Jr. Countercurrent multiplication system without active transport in the inner medulla. *Kidney Int.* 1972;2:214.

55. Jamison RL, Robertson CR. Recent formulations of the urinary concentrating mechanism: a status report. *Kidney Int.* 1979;16:537.

56. Alpern RJ, Dennis DK, Rector FJ. Renal acidification mechanisms. In: Brenner BM, Rector F Jr, eds. *The Kidney.* Philadelphia: WB Saunders Co; 1991:318–379.

57. Warnock DG, Rector FC Jr. Proton secretion by the kidney. *Ann Rev Physiol.* 1979;41:197.

58. Al-Awqati Q, et al. Characteristics of stimulation of H transport by aldosterone in turtle urinary bladder. *J Clin Invest.* 1976;58:351.

59. Tennen RL. Ammonia metabolism. *Am J Physiol.* 1978;235:F265.

60. Rodriguez-Soriano J, Edelman CM Jr. Renal tubular acidosis: mechanisms, classifications and implications. *N Engl J Med.* 1969;281:1405.

61. Morris RC, Ives HE. Inherited disorders of the renal tubule. In: Brenner BM, Rector F Jr, eds. *The Kidney.* Philadelphia: WB Saunders Co; 1991:1596–1656.

62. Wrong O, Davies HEF. The excretion of acid in renal disease. *Q J Med.* 1959;28:259.

63. Wrong OM, Feest TG. The natural history of distal renal tubular acidosis. *Contrib Nephrol.* 1980;21:137.

64. Wright FS, Giebisch G. Renal potassium transport: contributions of individual nephron segments and populations. *Am J Physiol.* 1978; 235:F515.

65. Giebisch G, Stanton B. Potassium transport in the nephron. *Ann Rev Physiol.* 1979;16:537.

66. Sutton RAL. Disorders of renal calcium excretion. *Kidney Int.* 1983;23:655.

67. Bronner F. Renal calcium transport: mechanisms and regulation—an overview. *Am J Physiol.* 1989;257:F707.

68. Huang YC, Christakos S. Modulation of rat calbindin-$D_{28}$ gene expression by 1,25 dihydroxyvitamin $D_3$ and dietary alteration. *Mol Endocrinol.* 1988;2:928.

69. Varghese SS, et al. Analysis of rat vitamin D-dependent calbindin D28k gene expression. *J Biol Chem.* 1988;263:9776.

70. Suki WN. Calcium transport in the nephron. *Am J Physiol.* 1979;237:F1.

71. Costanzo LS. Mechanism of action of thiazide diuretics. *Semin Nephrol.* 1988;8:234.

72. Costanzo LS, Windhager EE. Calcium and sodium transport by the distal convoluted tubule of the rat. *Am J Physiol.* 1978;235:F492.

73. Knox FG, et al. Phosphate transport along the nephron. *Am J Physiol.* 1977;233:F261.
74. Dennis VW, Stead WW, Myers JL. Renal handling of phosphate and calcium. *Ann Rev Physiol.* 1979;41:257.
75. Levinson DJ, Sorenson LB. Renal handling of uric acid in normal and gouty subjects: evidence for a 4-component system. *Ann Rheum Dis.* 1980;39:173.
76. Fanelli GM Jr. Urate excretion. *Ann Rev Med.* 1977;28:349.
77. Rieselbach RE, Steele TH. Influence of the kidney upon urate homeostasis in health and disease. *Am J Med.* 1974;56:665.
78. Schafer JA, Barfuss DW. Membrane mechanisms for transepithelial amino acid absorption and secretion. *Am J Physiol.* 1980;238:F335.
79. Broadus AE, Thier SO. Metabolic basis of renal-stone disease. *N Engl J Med.* 1979;300:839.
80. Simpson DP. Citrate secretion: a window on renal metabolism. *Am J Physiol.* 1983; 244:F223.

# 4

# Genitourinary Pathology

*Robert O. Peterson and Barry S. Stein*

## KIDNEY

### NORMAL ANATOMY AND HISTOLOGY

The structural unit of the kidney, the lobe, is composed of an outer cortex overlying the medulla, which tapers to form the renal papilla which, in turn, protrudes into a calix of the renal pelvis. The cortex contains the glomeruli, segments of the proximal and distal convoluted tubules, straight segments of the loop of Henle, and the collecting tubules. The medulla can be divided into two regions: an outer and an inner zone. The outer zone is immediately subjacent to the overlying cortex at the corticomedullary junction and contains straight segments of the loop of Henle, the collecting tubules, and the blood vessels of the medulla (vasa recta). The inner zone of the medulla contains only collecting tubules converging to the tip of the papillae, and sparse vasculature in the interstition between the tubules. The renal papilla is covered by transitional epithelium of the calix continuous with the renal pelvis (Figs. 1 and 2).

### CYSTIC DISEASES

#### Congenital Multicystic Disease

Congenital multicystic disease is a form of renal dysplasia most commonly unilateral and presents as a palpable abdominal mass in the newborn. The dysgenesis is usually total, but examples of subtotal renal involvement have been reported. The affected kidney is composed of multiple cysts that vary in size up to several centimeters. The clustered cysts result in a loss of the normal configuration of the kidney. Frequently the renal artery and ureter are likewise dysplastic. Histologically, no renal parenchyma can be identified in the fibrous walls of the multiple cysts. On occasion, the primitive mesenchyma in the fibrous stroma intervening between the cysts may contain focal abortive tubules and foci of cartilage or muscle (Figs. 3 and 4).

#### Infantile Polycystic Disease

Infantile polycystic disease is an autosomal recessive disorder that usually presents early in infancy as renal failure and often includes bile duct proliferation and portal fibrosis. The renal manifestations are always bilateral. The kidneys are markedly enlarged, although the surface of the kidney is not distorted by cystic structures. On cut surface, however, small cysts are scattered throughout the cortex and medulla, which appear linear in the area of the renal capsule and become spherical toward the medulla. Microscopically, the kidney is normally formed, and glomeruli and

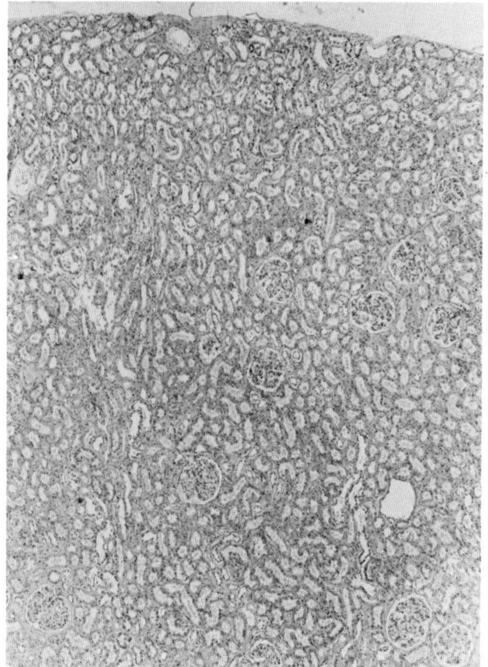

**Fig. 1.** Normal Kidney. The renal cortex is composed predominantly of segments of the proximal and distal convoluted tubules with their respective glomeruli.

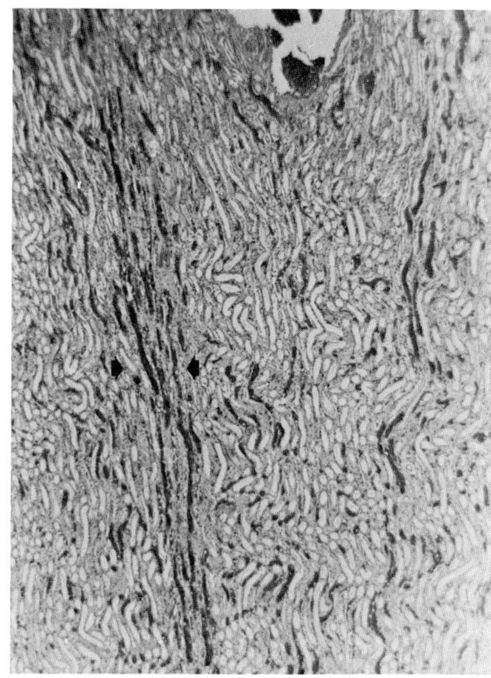

**Fig. 2.** Normal Kidney. The outer zone of the renal medulla is composed of clusters of collecting tubules and straight segment of the proximal convoluted tubules together comprising the components of the medullary rays of the cortex. The vasa recta of the medulla (*arrow*) is found between the tubular components of the medullary rays.

nephrons are often present. The cysts have their origin in the collecting ducts and are lined by low cuboidal epithelium (Figs. 5 and 6).

## Adult Polycystic Disease

Adult polycystic disease is transmitted as an autosomal dominant trait with variable penetrance, which usually presents as renal failure in the third to fifth decade of life. These patients may also have cysts of the liver and aneurysms in the circle of Willis. This bilateral disease is more common than is infantile polycystic disease. The affected kidneys are enlarged with multiple cysts apparent on the cortical surface and throughout the kidney on cut surface. Microscopically, the cysts have flattened or absent epithelial lining, vary in size, and contain fluid. The intercystic renal parenchyma contains intact glomeruli and scattered foci of interstitial fibrosis with atrophic nephrons (Figs. 7 and 8).

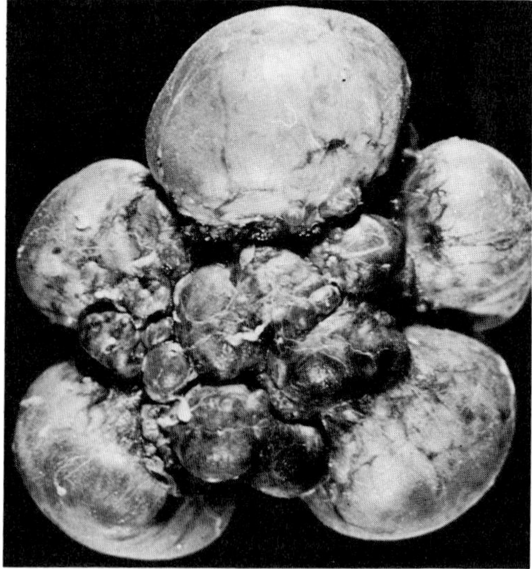

**Fig. 3.** Multicystic Disease of the Kidney. The affected kidney is composed of clustered cysts of varying size with total loss of the normal renal configuration.

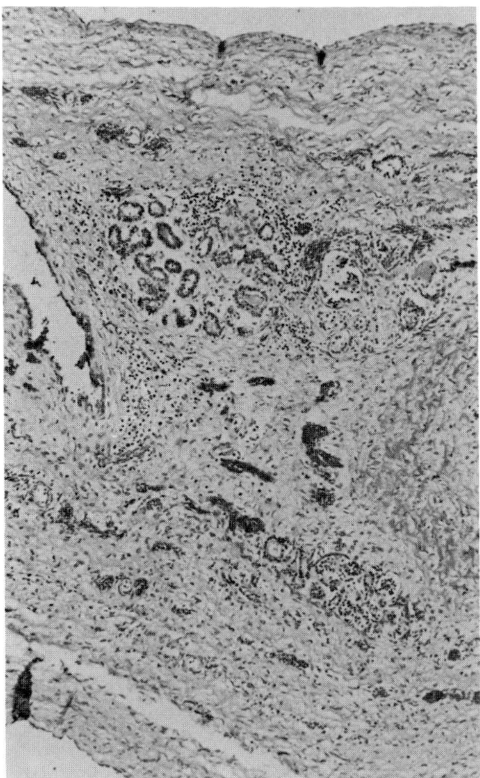

**Fig. 4.** Multicystic Disease. The walls of the cyst are composed primarily of collagenous fibrous tissue with a few scattered primitive tubules.

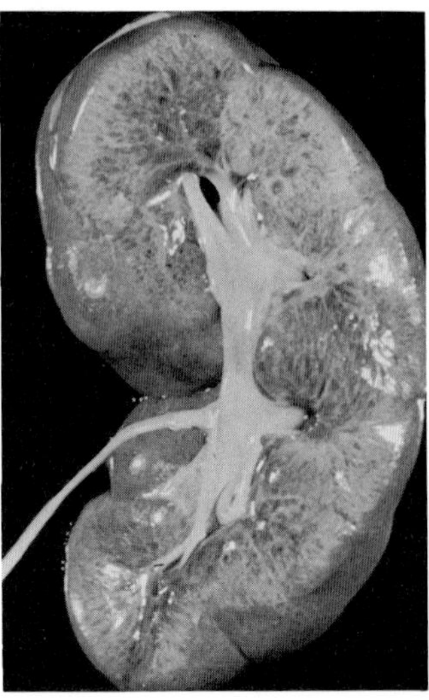

**Fig. 5.** Infantile Polycystic Disease. The characteristic widespread small cysts with retention of the overall configuration of the kidney is seen in this example of infantile polycystic disease.

## Uremic Medullary Cystic Disease

Uremic medullary cystic disease complex afflicts both patients presenting in infancy with an autosomal recessive trait known as *familial juvenile nephronopthisis* and adults who can present with a sporadic or autosomal dominant trait designated as *medullary cystic disease*. A severe tubular nephropathy is accompanied by polyuria, polydipsia, and azotemia progressing quickly to renal failure and death. A progressive atrophy of the tubules with glomerular sclerosis leads to the typical end-stage shrunken kidneys. Microscopic features include multiple cystic tubular dilatations located in the outer medulla, in association with significant intracystic and cortical fibrosis and parenchymal atrophy. Chronic inflammatory cells may be found in the intracystic areas of the cortex and medulla.

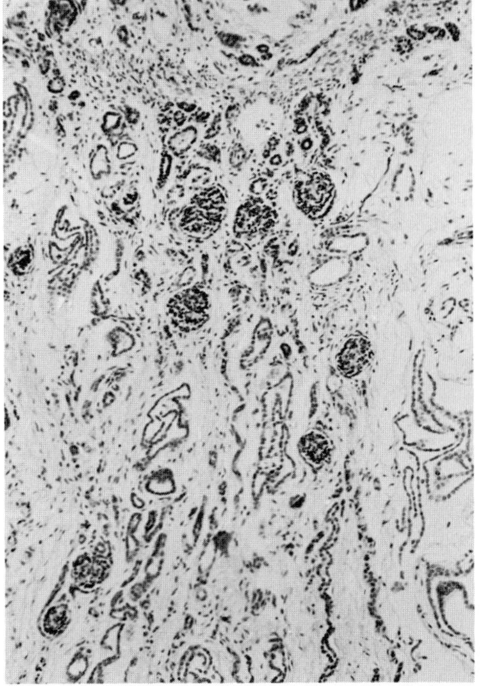

**Fig. 6.** Infantile Polycystic Disease. Normal glomeruli are present between the numerous linear cysts lined by low cubiodal tubular epithelium.

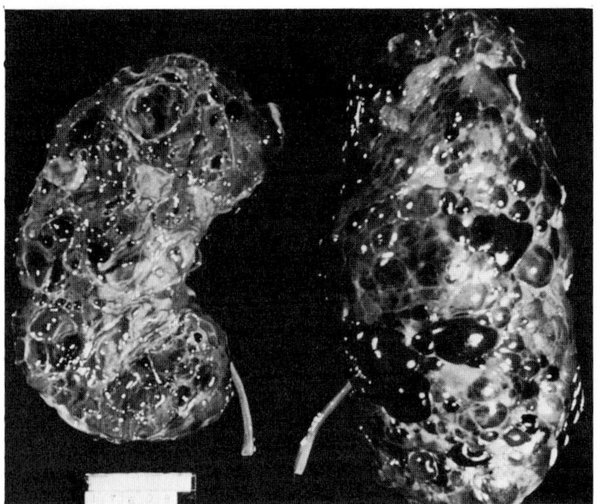

**Fig. 7.** Adult Polycystic Disease. The cortical and cut surfaces reveal the number and widespread distribution of the thin-walled cysts in this enlarged polycystic kidney.

## Simple Cyst of Kidney

The majority of kidneys with simple renal cyst are first noted at autopsy. They are variable in size and are most commonly present on the outer cortex, where they distort the contour of the kidney (Fig. 9). The histologic features of these cysts are lack of or cuboidal epithelial lining and a fibrous capsule. The remaining kidney frequently shows evidence of the changes of small vessel disease common in the elderly in whom the majority of these cysts are found. Carcinoma has rarely been described as occurring in the wall.

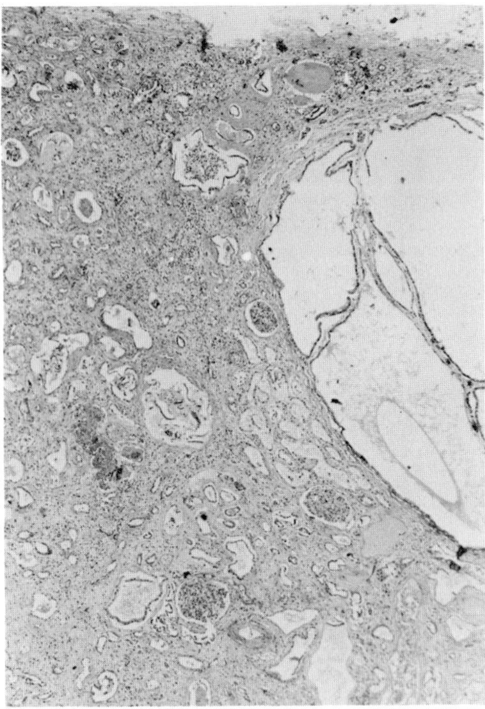

**Fig. 8.** Adult Polycystic Disease. The cysts are adjacent to areas of the renal cortex with interstitial fibrosis, tubular atrophy, and scattered histologically normal glomeruli.

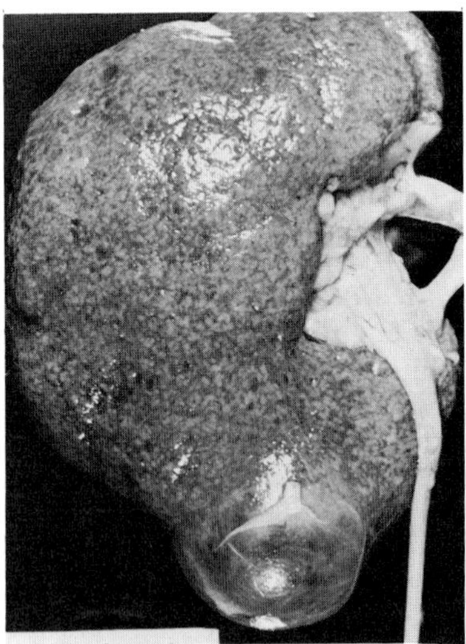

**Fig. 9.** Simple (Retention) Cyst. The single thin-walled cyst at the lower pole contained clear serous fluid. The cortical surface elsewhere shows a fine granularity characteristic of benign nephrosclerosis.

### Medullary Sponge Kidney

Medullary sponge kidney, otherwise known as *tubular ectasia*, is a disorder demonstrating cystic or dilated collecting tubules in the area of the renal papilla. Variable numbers of papillae may be involved, but in most patients it is present in at least 75% of the tubules. Most of these patients are asymptomatic but may present with calcifications in the ectatic tubules or with urinary tract infections. Histologically, the cysts are lined by variable types of epithelium, including transitional cells on occasion, and contain fluid with desquamated cells. Frequently evidence of infection is present within and around the cysts, with acute and chronic inflammatory cells seen. Focal calcification of the medullary parenchyma is not uncommon.

### Multilocular Cyst

Multilocular cyst often presents as a renal mass with a complex ultrasonographic appearance. On gross examination, a solitary mass is easily separable from the normal renal parenchyma, which is compressed around it (Plate 1). The cut surface usually reveals multiple cystic structures with fibrous septa that divide the cystic mass into multiple noncommunicating compartments. They are filled with cystic fluid which is usually clear, and the cysts may continue to grow until the mass fills the perinephric space. The histologic features include an epithelial lining of cuboidal cells overlying the wall (composed of collagenous fibrous tissue with occasional smooth muscle fibers). Atrophic changes in the adjacent renal parenchyma are observed. The septa of the cysts contain no normal renal cortical structures. Multilocular cysts are to be separated from cystic forms of Wilms' tumor, which have undifferentiated renal blastoma components in the wall of the septa of the cysts (see Polycystic Nephroblastoma). This is generally a unilateral disease but may on occasion present bilaterally.

## INFLAMMATORY DISEASES

### Acute Pyelonephritis

The hallmark and necessary criteria for the diagnosis of acute pyelonephritis are concurrent inflammation of the renal parenchyma and pelvis. Characteristically, the affected kidney in acute pyelonephritis has a random distribution of abscesses that involve both the medulla and cortex. The abscesses are rimmed by hyperemic renal parenchyma. The renal pelvis is mottled with focal areas of hyperemic mucosa alternating with areas of purulent exudate. Histologically, an acute inflammatory cell infiltrate is observed in the interstitium of the kidney and the renal pelvic mucosa in a pattern corresponding to the gross lesions. Frequently the infection results in tubular destruction with an outpouring of neutrophils into the tubules. Focal abscesses with complete destruction of a cluster of adjacent tubules are common.

Appropriate special stains will demonstrate the bacteria in such foci. The acute inflammatory cell infiltrate in the cortical interstitium is patchy with evident resistance to destruction demonstrated by the glomeruli. As the infection resolves, the inflamed areas show increasing numbers of plasma cells and lymphocytes and decreasing numbers of neutrophils. Ultimate resolution is with collagen deposition and scar formation. At all stages, there is evidence of involvement of both the renal parenchyma and renal pelvis. The result is focal distortion of the caliceal contour in a patchy distribution (Figs. 10 and 11).

### Chronic Pyelonephritis

BACTERIAL PYELONEPHRITIS. The result of recurrent or persistent bacterial infection is termed *chronic pyelonephritis*. This produces the smallest kidneys encountered at the time of autopsy. The cortical surface demonstrates marked, patchy, or confluent depressed scars, which are noted on cross section of the kidney to involve both the cortex and

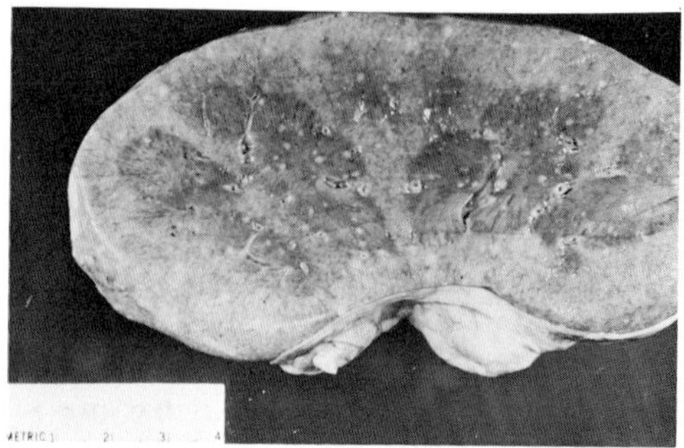

**Fig. 10.** Acute Pyelonephritis. The cut surface of the kidney reveals numerous small abscesses in the cortex and medulla.

underlying medulla with significant distortion of the underlying calix. The microscopic features include abundant interstitial fibrosis with atrophy and focal obliteration of the tubules included in the scar. The tubules may show evidence of epithelial atrophy with eosinophilic proteinaceous material in the lumen, a feature called *thyroidization*. There is an interstitial infiltrate of plasma cells, lymphocytes, and histiocytes. The glomeruli continue to show apparent resistance with preserved glomerular tufts, but periglomerular fibrosis is present. If the intrarenal arterial branches are incorporated in a pyelonephritic scar, ischemic atrophy of the regional glomeruli will result. (Figs. 12 and 13).

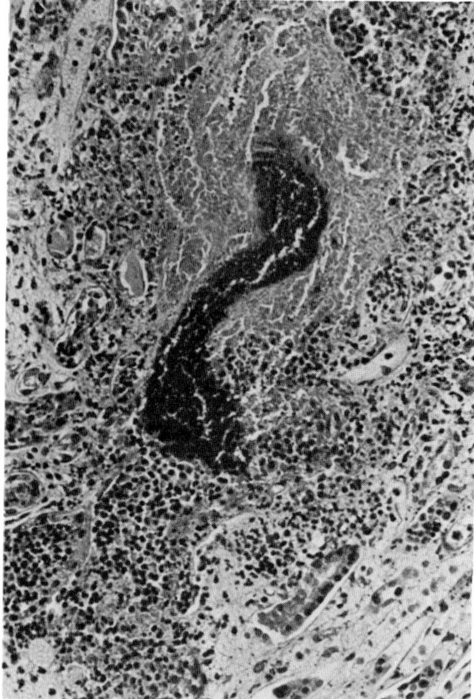

**Fig. 11.** Acute Pyelonephritis. An abscess with local tubular destruction is surrounded by numerous acute inflammatory cells in the medullar interstitium and in adjacent renal tubular segments.

XANTHOGRANULOMATOUS PYELONEPHRITIS. There is marked infiltration of histiocytes among the chronic inflammatory cells seen in the xanthogranulomatous variation of chronic pyelonephritis. This is often associated with proteus infection and calculus disease of the kidney. The histiocytes are lipid-laden, giving the nodular abscesses a yellow color on gross examination (Plate 2), and the cell cytoplasm, a foamy appearance on microscopic examination. There is considerable parenchymal destruction with abundant necrosis, sheets of histiocytes with occasional giant cells, and an admixture of lymphocytes and plasma cells (Fig. 14). The lesions can look strikingly similar to renal cell carcinoma.

MALAKOPLAKIA. Renal malakoplakia

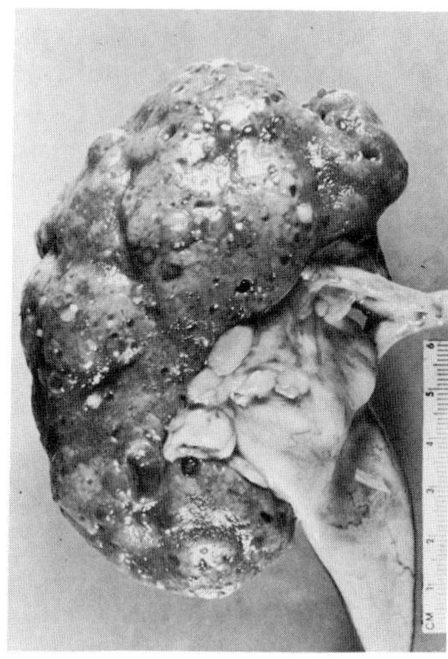

**Fig. 12.** Chronic Pyelonephritis. The cortical surface of this small kidney contains numerous irregular linear and confluent depressions resulting from inflammatory destruction of underlying parenchyma.

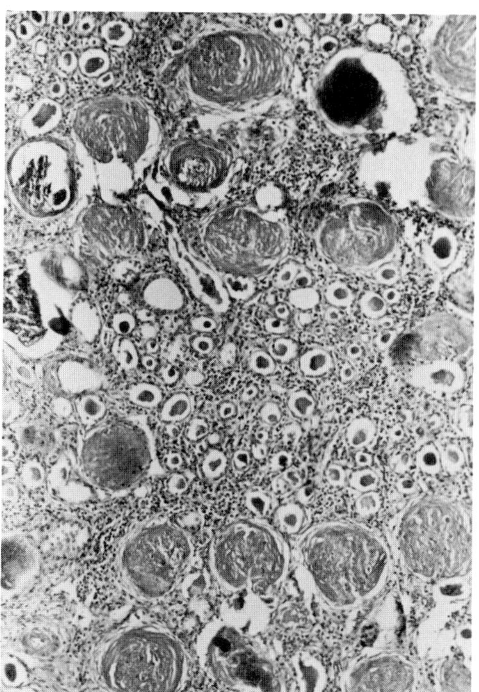

**Fig. 13.** Chronic Pyelonephritis. Numerous lymphocytes infiltrate the renal parenchyma between atrophic tubules (containing proteinaceous secretions) and many fibrotic remnants of glomeruli.

has been rarely reported. It presents as fever, flank pain, or palpable flank mass, often associated with infection of the urinary tract.

Histologically, malakoplakia is identical to the lesion seen in the bladder and a thorough discussion of this entity can be found under that topic (Figs. 15 and 63).

## Papillary Necrosis

Necrosis of the entire medullary pyramid is termed *papillary necrosis*. This can be a complication of acute pyelonephritis, especially in diabetics, or it can occur in association with analgesic abuse or sickle cell disease. When it occurs as a complication of acute pyelonephritis, it is patchy in the affected kidney. The distal papilla may appear grey-yellow. Histologically, the affected papilla shows evidence of coagulative necrosis with preservation of the tubular outlines and a striking paucity of inflammatory cells in the interstitium. In contrast, the margin of the necrotic papilla has a dense infiltrate of neutrophils. Occasional cases show sloughing of the necrotic papilla and the diagnosis may be made by examination of these (Figs. 16 and 17).

## Renal Tuberculosis

With the decrease in the incidence of tuberculosis in the general population, renal tuberculous infection has correspondingly decreased. It has been described as occurring in two gross patterns: miliary renal tuberculosis and caseous renal tuberculosis. The histologic features of the classic caseating granuloma of tuberculosis are present in both forms, the differences being that in the caseous variety the lesions are larger and there is increasing destruction of the kidney. The granulomas of the miliary form tend to be located more commonly

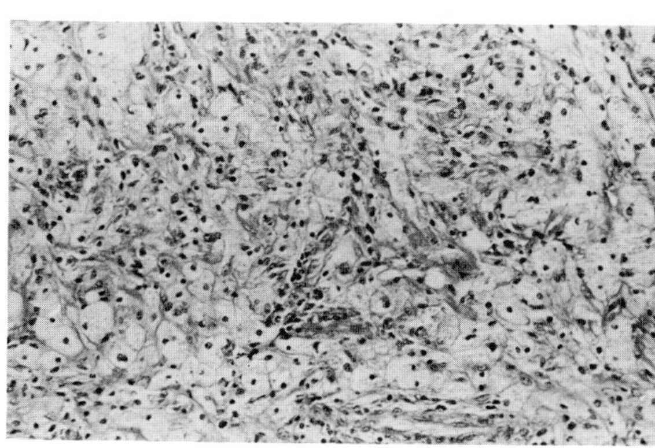

**Fig. 14.** Xanthogranulomatous Pyelonephritis. The inflammatory-cell infiltrate is chiefly composed of large foamy histiocytes with admixed lymphocytes and occasional neutrophils. The renal parenchyma has been destroyed in the region of the lesion.

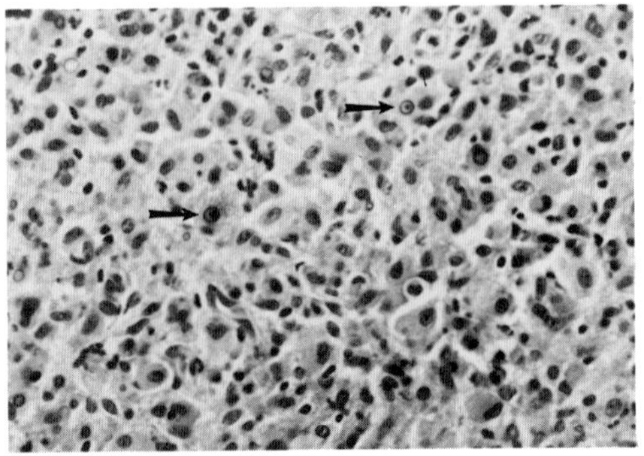

**Fig. 15.** Malakoplakia. The presence of Michaelis–Gutmann bodies (*arrows*) is demonstrated by use of the PAS stain. The predominant cells are histiocytes with fewer numbers of neutrophils and lymphocytes.

in the cortex, while those of the caseous form are more commonly in the medulla with marked distortion and frequent ulceration into the renal pelvis (Figs. 18 and 19).

## BENIGN NEOPLASMS

### Congenital Mesoblastic Nephroma

Congenital mesoblastic nephroma is the most common benign neoplasm found in the newborn. These tumors are frequently bulky, and their cut surface is whorled and fibrous. They are well demarcated on gross inspection, but histologically no capsule is present, and microscopic foci of the lesions are found in and around adjacent renal parenchyma. The neoplasm is composed of nodules of spindle cells, which have the light- and electron-microscopic features of smooth muscle or fibroblasts (Figs. 20 and 21).

### Angiomyolipoma

Angiomyolipoma are benign tumors found in patients with tuberous sclerosis, the lesions of which are frequently bilateral. Usually, however, they are unilateral and predominate in females by a three to one ratio. Grossly, these lesions grow quite large by the time of discovery, and hemorrhage into the tumor is common. These complex lesions are composed of adipose tissue, smooth muscle, and multiple vascular channels.

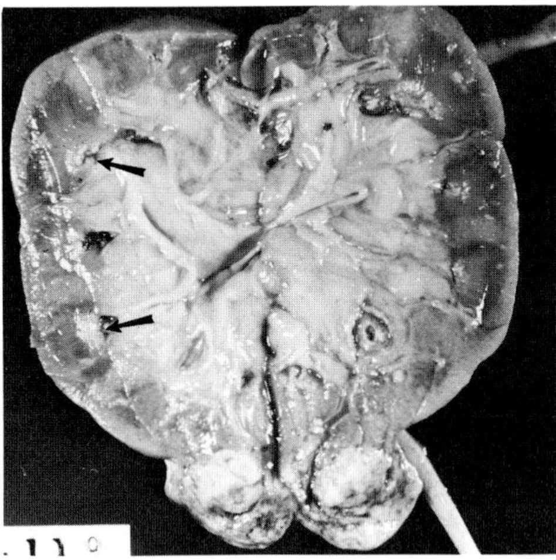

**Fig. 16.** Papillary Necrosis. The cut surface of the kidney shows multiple papillae with granular, pale tips (*arrows*). An incidental renal cell carcinoma is present in the inferior pole of the kidney.

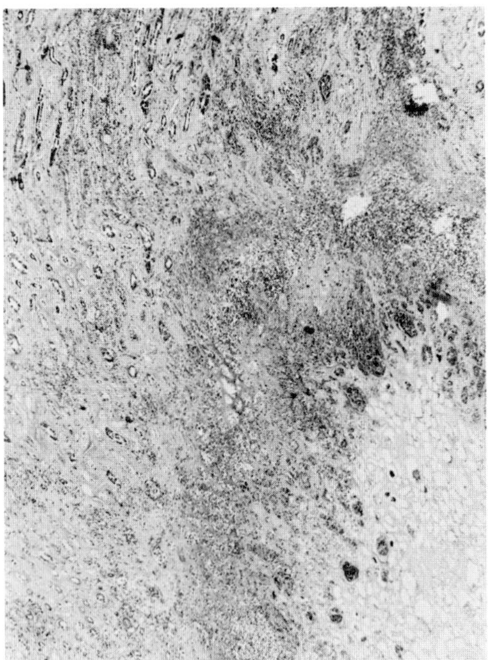

**Fig. 17.** Papillary Necrosis. The necrotic papillary tip is virtually acellular, but the tubular outlines have been preserved. The upper margin of the necrotic area has a dense infiltrate of neutrophils located in the upper medulla.

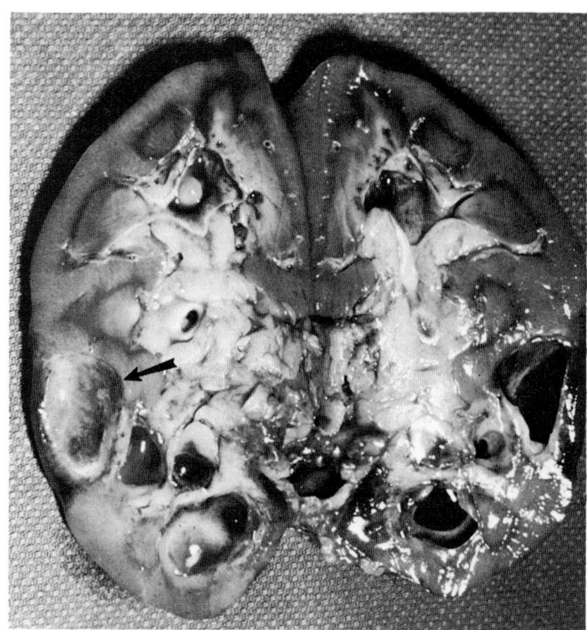

**Fig. 18.** Tuberculosis. The cut surface of the kidney reveals multiple tuberculous cavities (*arrow*) with necrosis and hemorrhage in the affected regions of the kidneys.

Microscopically, the normal renal parenchyma is replaced by the combined tissues noted above. The blood vessels vary in number, but commonly are numerous, thick-walled, and associated with disorganized bundles of smooth muscles that surround the vessels and infiltrate the scattered clusters of adipose cells. On occasion, the smooth muscle cell nuclei are pleomorphic and hyperchromatic, but the clinical behavior remains benign (Figs. 22 and 23).

## Renal Cortical Adenoma

The existence of renal cortical adenoma is accepted because of general agreement, historically perpetuated. Neoplasms larger than 3 cm have a significantly greater probability of metasta-

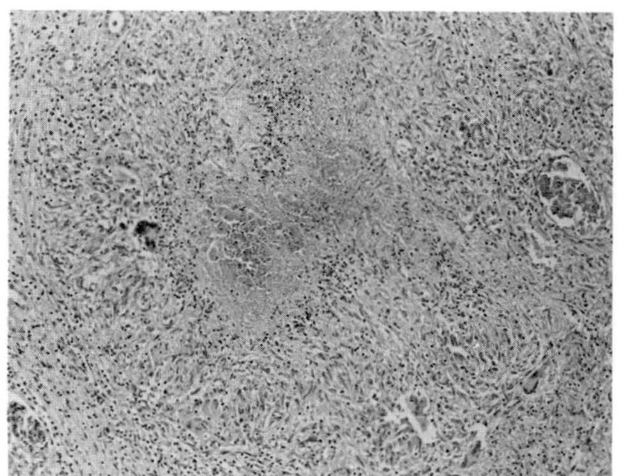

**Fig. 19.** Tuberculosis. Confluent granulomas with necrosis and scattered giant cells are present in the cortex. The associated inflammatory cells include histiocytes, lymphocytes, and occasional plasma cells. The renal parenchyma is destroyed in the affected area of the granulomatous inflammation.

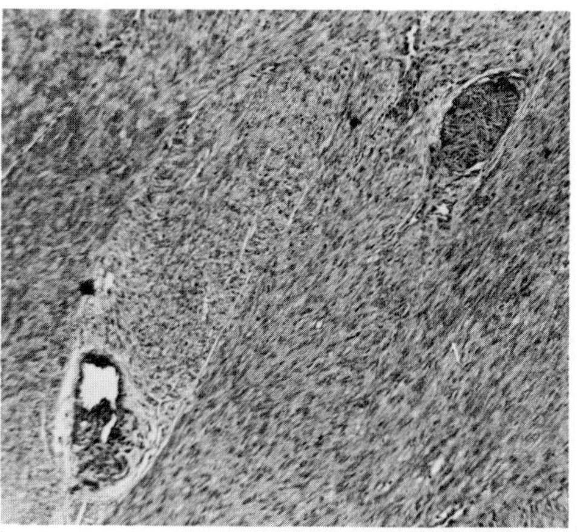

**Fig. 20.** Congenital Mesoblastic Nephroma. Bundles of spindle cells encircle a nerve within the kidney. No necrosis, nuclear atypia, or mitotic figures are present.

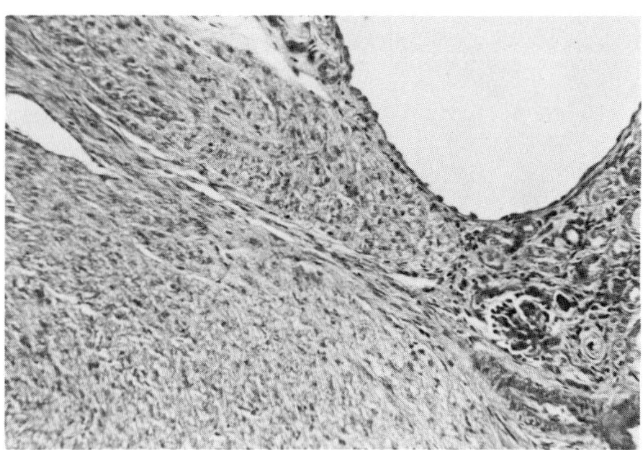

**Fig. 21.** Congenital Mesoblastic Nephroma. Spindle cells compress and infiltrate the adjacent renal parenchyma.

sizing than do smaller ones. Virtually all standard pathology textbooks now define renal cortical adenoma as a neoplastic growth less than 3 cm, and a renal cell carcinoma as a primary renal malignancy larger than 3 cm. Renal cortical adenomas, therefore, range in size from microscopic foci to 3.0 cm, have a yellow color when observed on the cortical surface of the kidney, and may be single or multiple. They are very common incidental findings at autopsy, and their frequency is even higher in kidneys harboring renal cell carcinoma. Histologically, they are discrete but lack a capsule. The tumor cells are arranged in tubules, solid nests, or occasional papillary areas. Delicate fibrous trabeculae are interspersed among the groups of tumor cells. Pleomorphism and mitotic activity are insignificant or absent. Not uncommonly, foci of hemorrhage with tumor necrosis is observed. Less commonly, these growths undergo spontaneous regression secondary to hemorrhagic necrosis, with organization and fibrosis. Corpus albicans-like structures with scattered clusters of tumor cells are observed amid deposited hemosiderin and macrophages. Electron-microscopic studies of these neoplasms confirm their origin from proximal tubular epithelium (Figs. 24 and 25).

### Oncocytoma

The oncocytoma (renal tubular adenoma with oncocytic features) is an interesting neoplasm, which has only recently been recognized. The majority of oncocytomas reported are in excess of 5 cm, and to date none have metastasized.

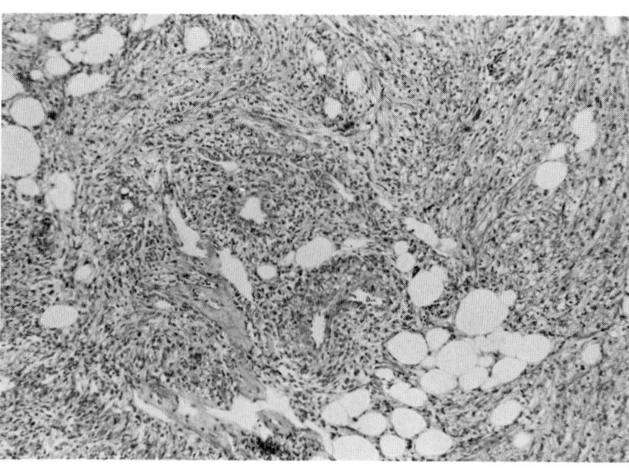

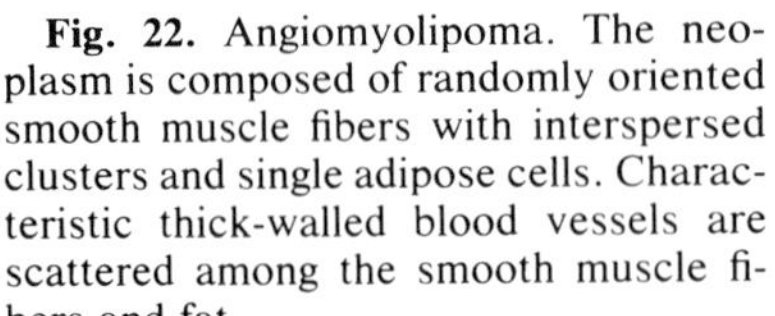

**Fig. 22.** Angiomyolipoma. The neoplasm is composed of randomly oriented smooth muscle fibers with interspersed clusters and single adipose cells. Characteristic thick-walled blood vessels are scattered among the smooth muscle fibers and fat.

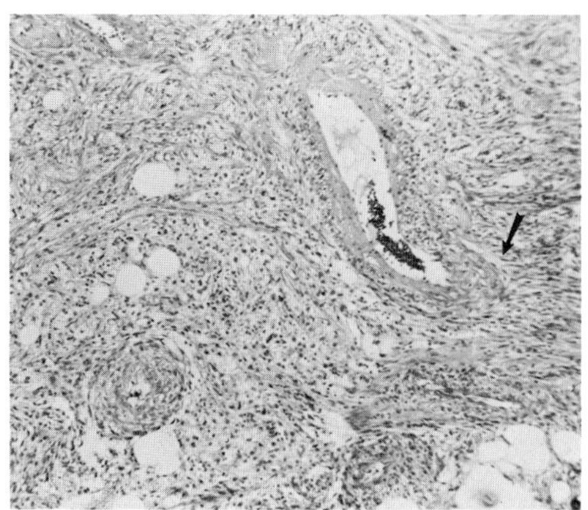

**Fig. 23.** Angiomyolipoma. The smooth muscle of the vascular walls merge with the smooth muscle cells dispersed throughout the lesion (*arrow*).

The gross appearance is characteristically well demarcated, uniformly brown-red, frequently with a central fibrous scar, but devoid of the classic variegated color, foci of hemorrhage, and necrosis of renal cell carcinoma (Plate 3). Histologically, the tumor cells are uniformly of the granular type with minimal pleomorphism and mitotic activity. Fibrous septa separate the tumor cells in cords, tubules, or nests. The absence of hemorrhage and necrosis noted in the gross description above is correspondingly true in the histologic picture. There is no invasion of the renal capsule or vein. Electron-microscopic studies confirm the renal tubular origin of these neoplasms, and the predicted numerous mitochondria of all oncocytic neoplasms is observed (Figs. 26*A*, *B* and 27 and Plate 4).

## MALIGNANT NEOPLASMS

### Wilms' Tumor

Wilms' is the most common malignant neoplasm to occur in the kidney in children but is less prevalent than leukemia, lymphoma, central nervous system tumors, and neuroblastoma in the pediatric population. There is no sex predilection, and the neoplasm is unilateral in all but 3% to 10% of reported cases. Growth to enormous size has been reported, and penetration of the renal capsule with spread into the adjacent adipose tissue is common. Invasion of the renal vein tributaries is also common. The cut surface has a gray-white encephaloid appearance, with irregular foci of hemorrhage, necrosis, and cyst formation frequent.

The classic Wilms' tumor is composed of three elements: epithelial cells, primitive renal blastema, and a stromal component (Figs. 28 and 29). The epithelial cells, which merge with the background stromal component, form abortive or dilated tubules or glomeruli. The background stroma has a varied composition of small, round cells with hyperchromatic nuclei; little or no apparent cytoplasm arranged in sheets of high cell density; or sparse spindle or stellate cells

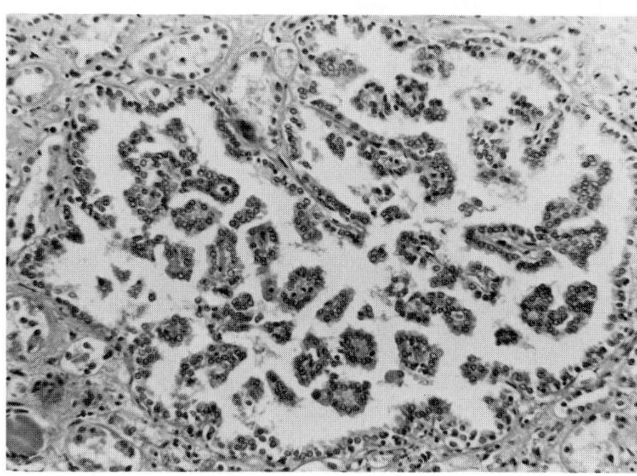

**Fig. 24.** Renal Cortical Adenoma. This cystic structure with numerous papillary projections into the lumen is lined by epithelial cells with features suggesting their renal tubular origin. No mitoses or significant pleomorphism is present.

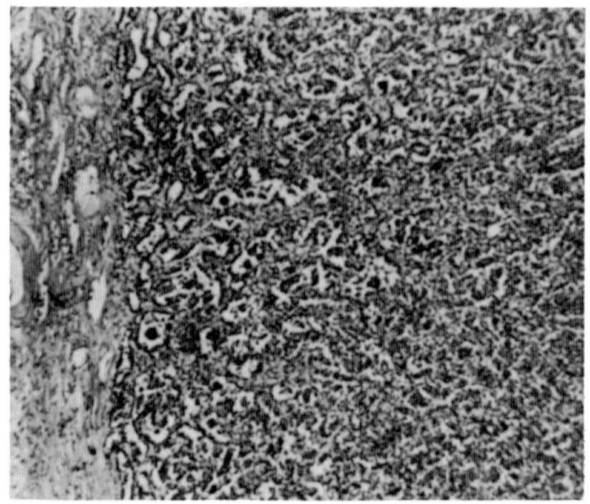

**Fig. 25.** Renal Cortical Adenoma. This cortical adenoma is composed of a complex pattern of small tubules with little intervening stroma. There is an absence of pleomorphism and necrosis, and no mitotic figures are present. The interface with the adjacent normal cortex is seen near the left margin of the photograph.

in a myxoid background. Scattered striated muscle cells are common, and some cases have been reported to contain primitive cartilage and bone. There is evidence that the degree of anaplasia of the stromal component correlates with the ultimate prognosis.

Occasionally a monophasic nephroblastoma is described, composed of only epithelial or stromal cells (Fig. 30).

## Polycystic Nephroblastoma

Polycystic nephroblastoma is regarded as a cystic variant of Wilms' tumor and manifests its presence in childhood. The renal parenchyma intervening among the cysts contains primitive renal epithelial components and spindle cell stroma similar to that found in a classic Wilms' tumor.

## Renal Cell Carcinoma

Renal cell carcinoma is the most frequent primary malignancy of the kidney in adults. It is most commonly diagnosed in the sixth and seventh decades, but it has been found at virtually any age, including, on rare occasions, in children.

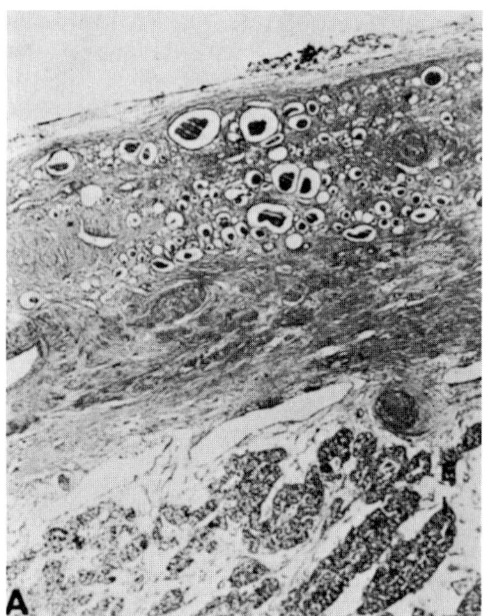


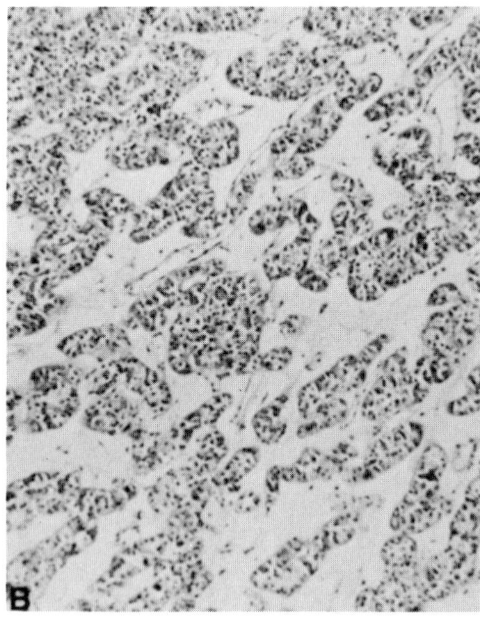


**Fig. 26.** Oncocytoma. **A.** The renal cortical structures beneath the capsule include sclerotic glomeruli and dilated tubules, the result of chronic pyelonephritis found in association with the renal oncocytoma at the bottom of the photograph. The tumor is composed of cords of oncocytic cells separated by an edematous stroma. **B.** The oncocytic cells with abundant eosinophilic cytoplasm are arranged in irregular cords with intervening edematous stroma containing thin-walled blood vessels.

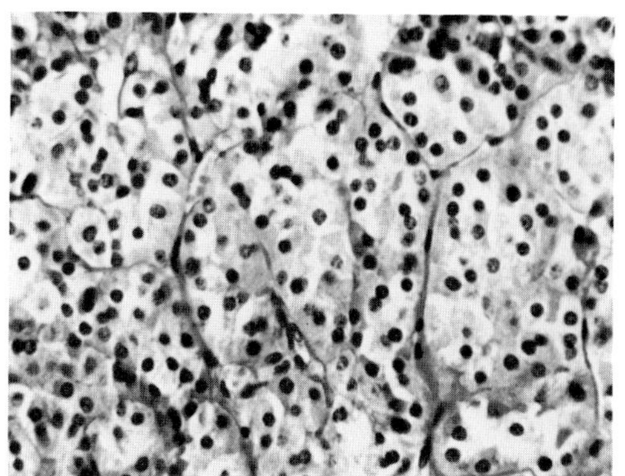

**Fig. 27.** Oncocytoma. The oncocytic cells, here showing the absence of significant nuclear pleomorphism, are arranged in nests separated by thin fibrous trabeculae.

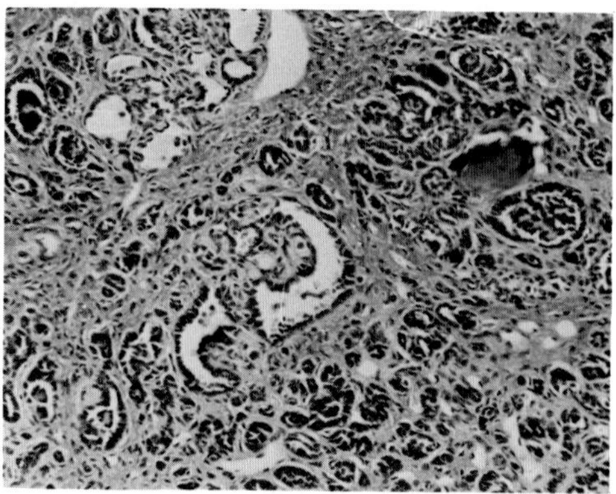

**Fig. 29.** Wilms' Tumor. Primitive tubule and glomerulus-like structures are separated by collagenous stroma containing individual spindle and polygonal cells with hyperchromatic nuclei.

The gross appearance of these neoplasms characteristically has a variegated color reflecting the tumor and secondary degenerative changes. The neoplasm is yellow-gray, admixed with areas of hemorrhage and variable amounts of necrosis frequently with cyst formation (Fig. 31 and Plate 5). The outline of each kidney is distorted, its extent dependent on the size of the tumor. On cut surface, it appears deceptively well defined, most commonly occupying one pole of the kidney. The renal capsule may appear intact and markedly expanded by the enlarging neoplasm. Tumor penetration of the capsule and into the adjacent adipose tissue within Gerota's fascia may be apparent on gross examination. The well-known tendency to invade the renal vein may likewise be observed. Distortion of the renal pelvis is common, but penetration into the pelvis is uncommon.

Histologically, several patterns of tumor organization are observed, not uncommonly within the same specimen. A tubuloalveolar pattern is most common; others frequently encountered include tubular, solid cords and sheets and papillary patterns and rarely a sarcomatous form. In the sarcomatous pattern, the

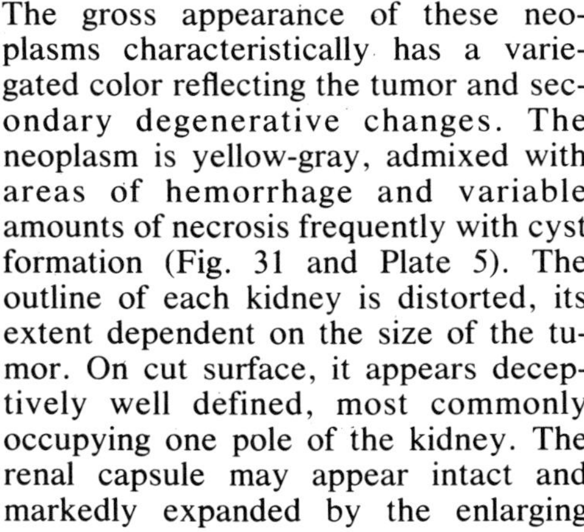

**Fig. 28.** Wilms' Tumor. The expanding neoplasm on the right is well demarcated from the normal cortex on the left. The neoplasm is composed of poorly developed tubular structures with varying amounts of intervening stroma.

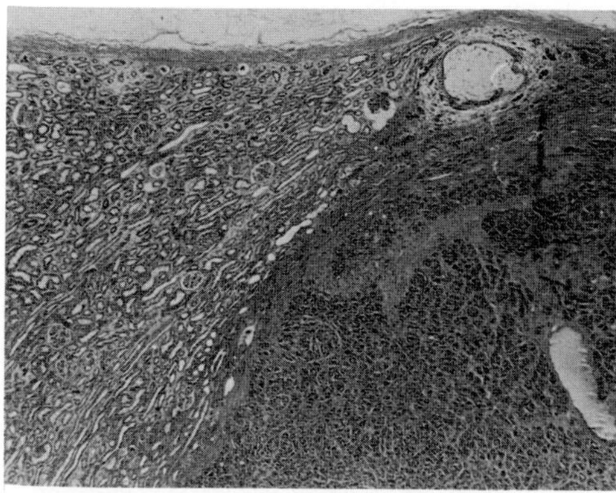

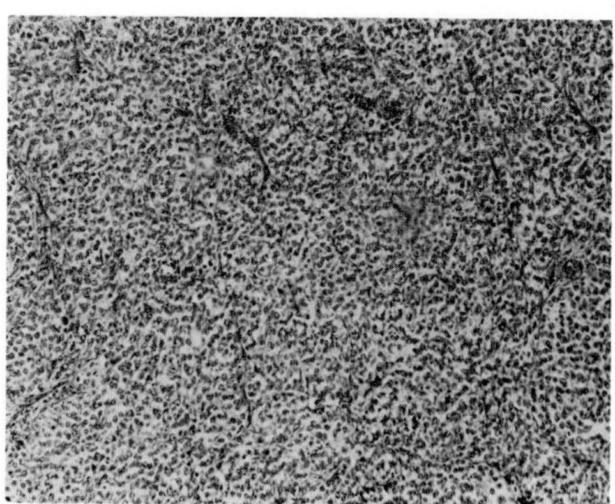

**Fig. 30.** Wilms' Tumor. An example of monophasic Wilms' tumor composed of primitive mesenchymal cells without evidence of epithelial structures.

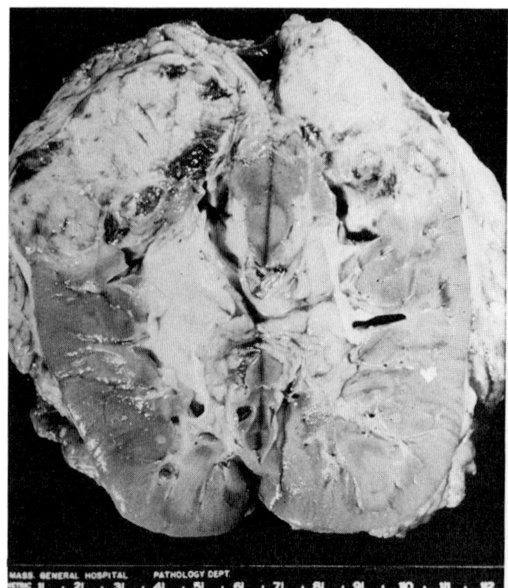


**Fig. 31.** Renal Cell Carcinoma. The tumor replaces the upper pole of the kidney, and the cut surface shows the characteristic features of focal hemorrhage and necrosis with expansion of the renal capsule and apparent compression without invasion of the adjacent renal parenchyma. Microscopic invasion of both capsule and adjacent kidney cortex was found.

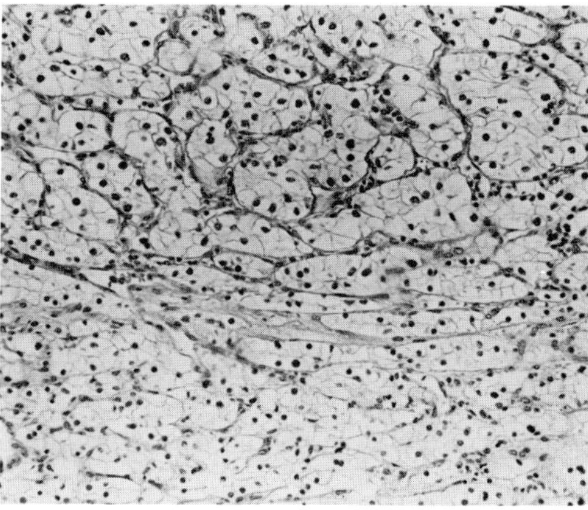

**Fig. 32.** Renal Cell Carcinoma. The tumor cells are arranged in an alveolar or nest pattern and are exclusively of the clear-cell type.

cells are spindle-shaped and grow in disorganized sheets. The most common cytologic feature present in the other histologic patterns is a mixture of epithelial cells that have either an eosinophilic cytoplasm (granular cell type) or a clear vacuolated cytoplasm (clear cell type). Tumors that appear entirely composed of either granular cells or clear cells are seen, but mixtures of the two cell types are the most common. Reflecting the gross appearance, the amount of necrosis and hemorrhage within the tumor varies. Microscopic evaluation may disclose invasion of the renal capsule and intrarenal vein tributaries, all of which on gross examination were free of tumor. The renal parenchyma adjacent to the tumor always shows compression and microscopic invasion by the tumor. Satellite nodules of tumor cells may represent intrarenal metastases or independent primary tumors (Figs. 32–35 and Plate 6).

One variant of renal cell carcinoma, the papillary cystic type, is characterized by extensive necrosis with minimal viable tumor seen attached to the fibrous pseudocapsule of the tumor. The necrotic contents of these tumors have a variable consistency not uncommonly entirely fluid, and an evacuated cystic mass results from cutting this surface rim. The viable tumor cells present on microscopic examination are either arranged in a papillary formation or found imbedded in the collagenous fibrous pseudocapsule (Figs. 36 and 37).

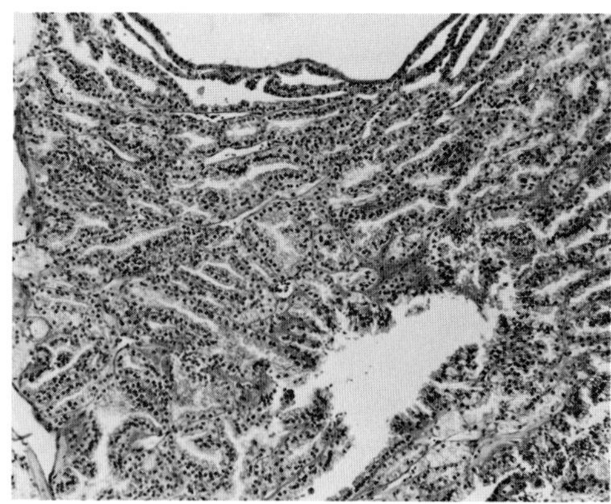

**Fig. 33.** Renal Cell Carcinoma. This renal cell carcinoma is composed predominantly of granular cells, with fewer clear cells in a tubular and microcystic pattern.

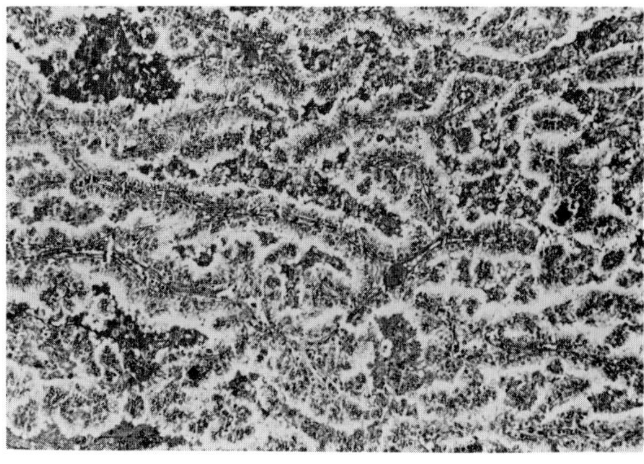

**Fig. 34.** Renal Cell Carcinoma. This neoplasm contains clear cells in a tubular-papillary pattern. Malignant cells line the thin fibrovascular septa.

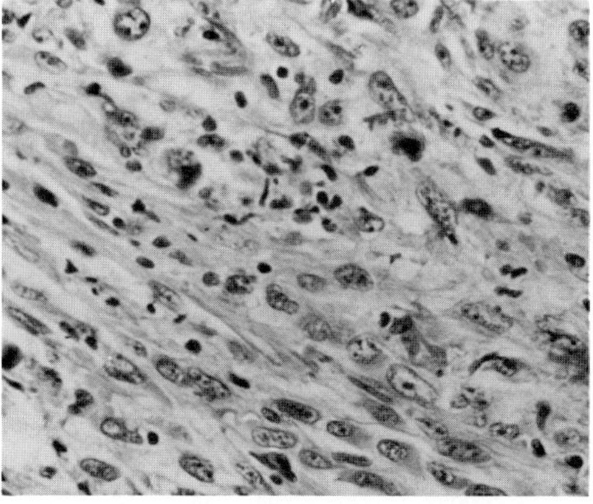

**Fig. 35.** Renal Cell Carcinoma. The sheets of elongated and spindle cells without tubular differentiation are characteristic of the sarcomatous pattern of renal cell carcinoma.

## Renal Sarcoma

All histologic types collectively are rare neoplasms of the kidney. In order of descending incidence, the renal sarcomas reported in the literature are fibrosarcoma, leiomyosarcoma, liposarcoma, rhabdomyosarcoma, and all other types. These highly lethal neoplasms have histologic features similar to those of the corresponding examples in other sites.

## Leukemic and Lymphomatous Involvement of the Kidney

The majority of patients with generalized lymphoma and leukemia examined at autopsy have gross or microscopic infiltration of the kidneys. The histologic and cytologic picture reflects the type of leukemia or lymphoma involved. Most

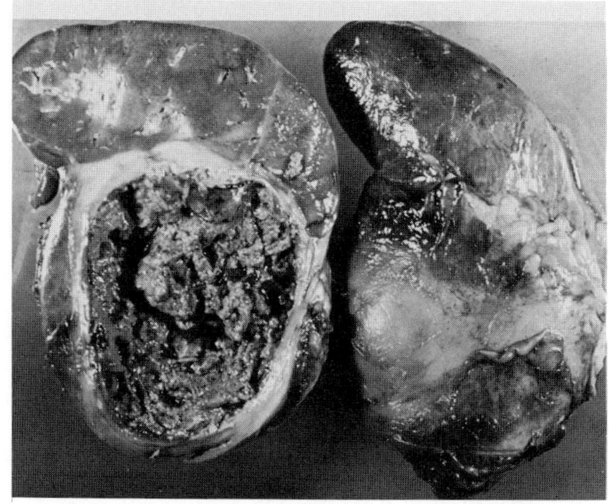

**Fig. 36.** Renal Cell Carcinoma. The large well-delineated cystic mass replacing the lower pole of the kidney contains abundant necrotic tumor. Viable tumor was limited to a narrow rim adjacent to the inner surface of the capsule. This is characteristic of the papillary cystic variety of renal cell carcinoma.

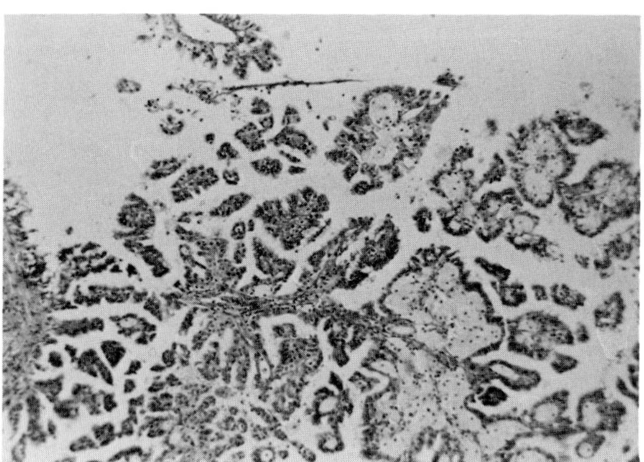

**Fig. 37.** Renal Cell Carcinoma, Papillary Cystic Type. Delicate papillary projections of the tumor extend from the wall of the cystic mass. Fragments of papillary fronds lie free in the cyst lumen. The central core of several papillae contain histiocytes (foam cells).

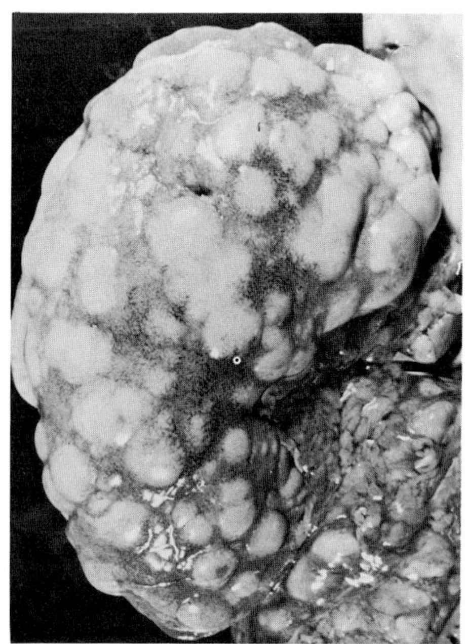

**Fig. 38.** Malignant Lymphoma. Widespread multiple nodules of lymphoma are present on the cortical surface of the kidney.

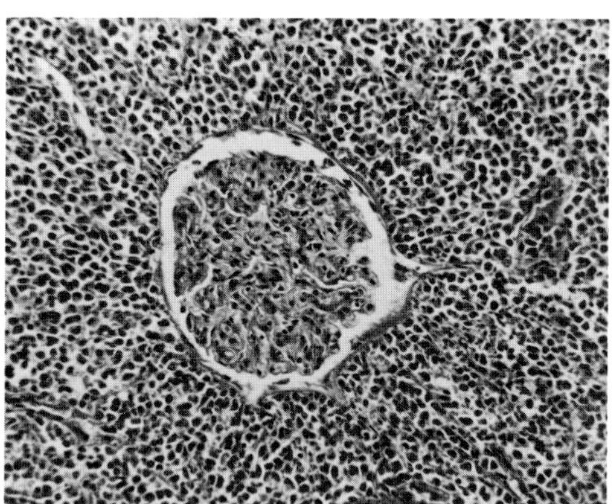

**Fig. 39.** Malignant Lymphoma in the Kidney. The interstitium of the cortex contains a massive infiltrate of lymphoma cells with destruction of renal tubules and apparent sparing of the glomerulus in the center.

leukemias and non-Hodgkin's lymphoma diffusely infiltrate the renal interstitium (Figs. 38 and 39). Less commonly, leukemias and generally Hodgkin's disease have a nodular infiltrate in the kidney.

## Metastatic Neoplasms to the Kidney

Metastatic malignant neoplasms to the kidney are not uncommon. Exclusive of leukemia and lymphomatous involvement of the kidney, the most common sites of origin are the lungs, breasts, and the gastrointestinal tract. Five to ten percent of renal cell carcinomas metastasize to the contralateral kidney. The majority of metastatic lesions to the kidney are detected only at autopsy. The histologic features reflect those present in the primary lesion (Fig. 40).

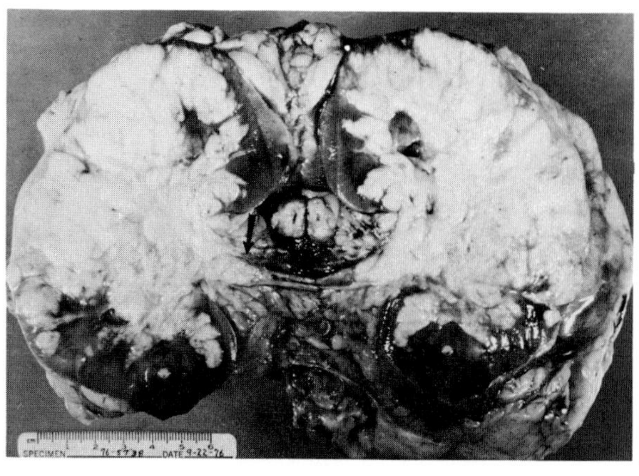

**Fig. 40.** Metastatic Squamous Cell Carcinoma. The tumor shows widespread infiltration of the kidney with invasion of the renal vein (*arrow*). The primary site of the metastatic tumor was the larynx.

# RENAL PELVIS AND URETER

## NORMAL HISTOLOGY

The urothelium lining the renal pelvis and ureter are identical to that of the bladder (Figs. 41–43). In fact, most of the pathologic entities described under Urinary Bladder have also been reported as occurring in the renal pelvis and ureter, although less frequently. Only the pathologic entities that are unique to or distinctly different in these organs are discussed in this section.

## FIBROEPITHELIAL POLYP OF THE URETER

Fibroepithelial polyps of the ureter are rare benign neoplasms referred to as fibromyxoma, myxoma, fibroma, and vascular fibrous polyps, reflecting the variations possible in the predominant stromal component. The majority of cases are located at the ureteropelvic junction. The surface of these polyps is smooth and most commonly covered with normal transitional epithelium. The bulk of the polyp is composed of vascularized collagenous fibrous tissue with or without areas of myxoid change, edema, and chronic inflammation (Figs. 44 and 45). These tumors are to be differentiated from true fibromas, leiomyomas, hemangiomas, and lymphangiomas, all of which have been reported in the ureter.

## ENDOMETRIOSIS OF THE URETER

Involvement of the ureter by endometriosis with obstruction has been reported in rare instances. Unilateral in-

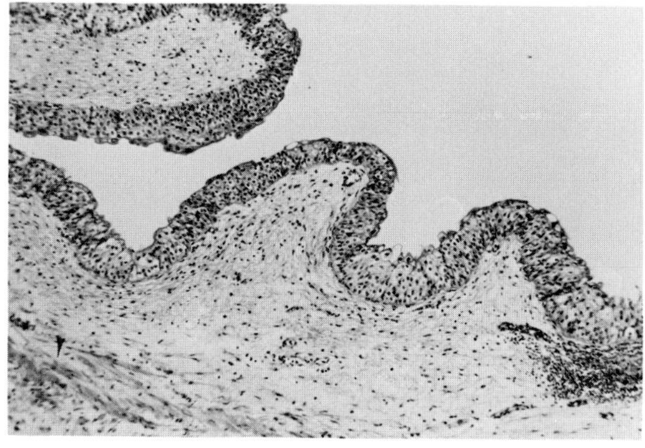

**Fig. 41.** Normal Renal Pelvis. Transitional cell urothelium covers a lamina propria composed of delicate collagen with scattered smooth muscle fibers (*arrow*).

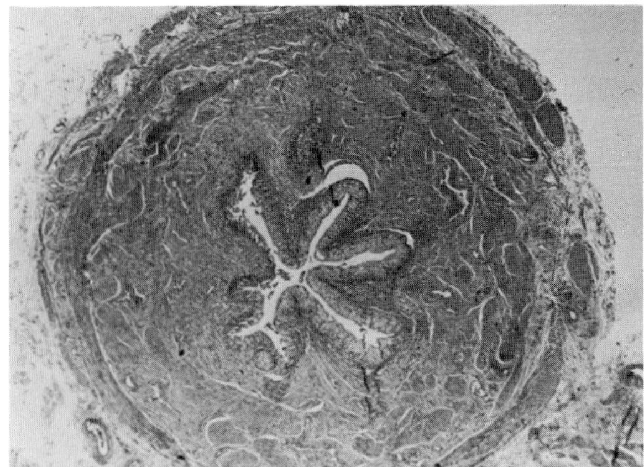

**Fig. 42.** Normal Ureter. The cross section shows the stellate lumen lined by transitional cell urothelium. The inner longitudinal muscle layer is surrounded by the outer circumferential muscle layer.

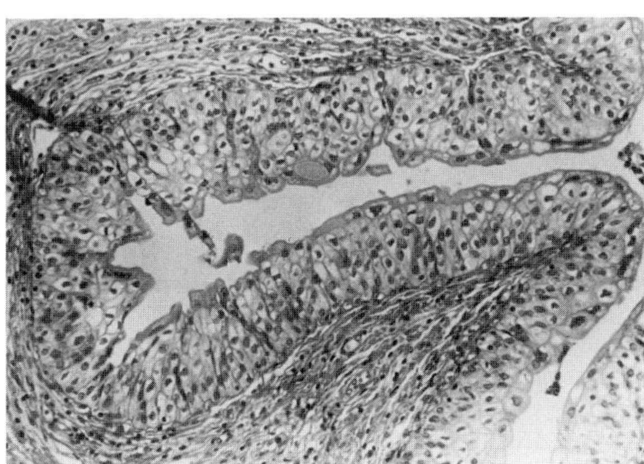

**Fig. 43.** Normal Ureter. The transitional cell urothelium rests on a lamina propria composed of fibromuscular tissue.

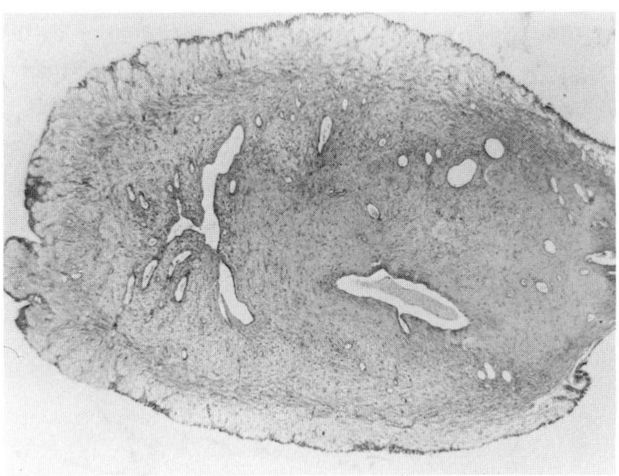

**Fig. 44.** Fibroepithelial Polyp. A thin urothelial lining covers the fibrovascular core of the polypoid structure.

volvement is most common, but bilateral ureteral endometriosis has been reported. The lower one third of the ureter is most frequently involved. Usually there is associated endometriosis of the urinary and genital tracts. Ureteral endometriosis has been classified as being either extrinsic or intrinsic. Extrinsic endometriosis of the ureter, comprising 80% of reported cases, is characterized

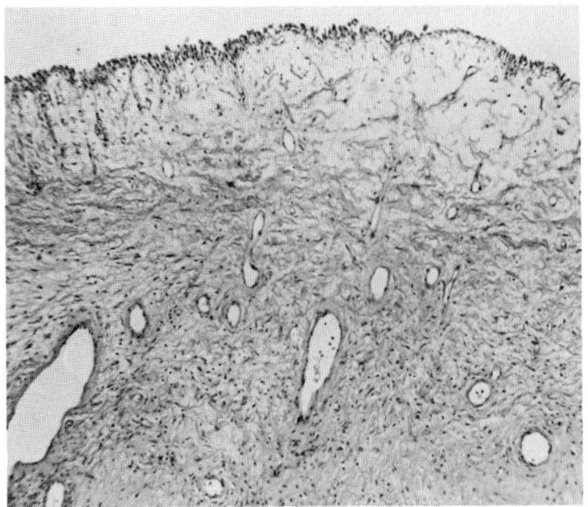

**Fig. 45.** Fibroepithelial Polyp. The fibrous tissue immediately beneath the urothelium is edematous. Several thin-walled blood vessels are present in the deeper fibrous stroma.

by involvement of the periureteral adventitia in a focal or concentric manner. Intrinsic endometriosis is characterized by involvement of the muscular layer, the lamina propria, and on occasion the mucosa of the ureter. Whether extrinsic or intrinsic, endometriosis contains endometrial stroma with or without demonstrable endometrial glands in association with collagenous fibrosis. Evidence of old hemorrhage is demonstrated by the presence of hemosiderin in the endometrial stroma. The fibrosis is in part the cause of the ureteral stricture and is the result of the inflammatory response to the local hemorrhage (see Fig. 72).

## IDIOPATHIC RETROPERITONEAL FIBROSIS

The gross lesion of idiopathic retroperitoneal fibrosis appears as a firm mass or thick plaque in the retroperitoneum surrounding the ureter. Histologically, fibrosis intermingled with chronic inflammatory cells is the prominent feature. The retroperitoneal fat is divided into nests by the expanding and infiltrating fibrous tissue. Areas of fat necrosis are frequently found along with the inflammatory cell infiltrate of lymphocytes, histiocytes, and plasma cells. Occasional giant cells may be seen in areas of fat necrosis (Fig. 46).

## MALIGNANT NEOPLASMS

### Transitional Cell Carcinoma of Renal Pelvis and Ureter

Transitional cell carcinoma occurring in the renal pelvis is associated with unique etiologic agents (*i.e.*, analgesic abuse, Balkan nephropathy) in rare cases but is histologically identical to the tumor occurring in the bladder (Figs. 47–51).

### Metastatic Neoplasms to the Ureter

Although ureteral obstruction secondary to extrinsic nodal compression is common, metastatic disease to the ureter itself is rare. The most common distant

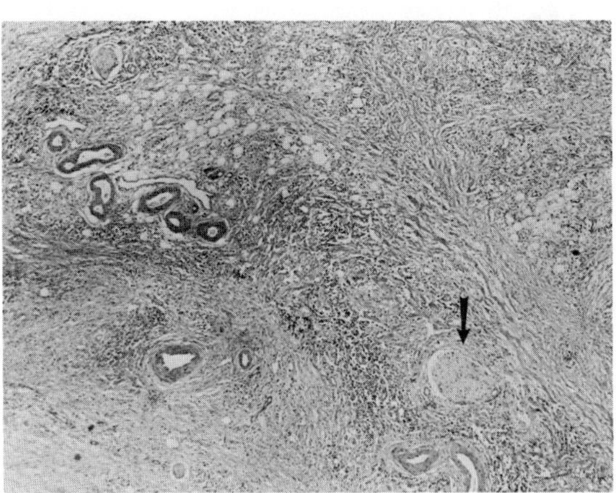

**Fig. 46.** Idiopathic Retroperitoneal Fibrosis. Collagenous fibrous tissue infiltrates the retroperitoneal fat and around a nerve segment (*arrow*) accompanied by chronic inflammatory cells including histiocytes, lymphocytes, and plasma cells.

primary sites include breast, stomach, bladder, and cervix. Ureteral obstruction by Hodgkin's disease, non-Hodgkin's lymphoma, and leukemic infiltration of the retroperitoneum and ureter have been reported (Fig. 52).

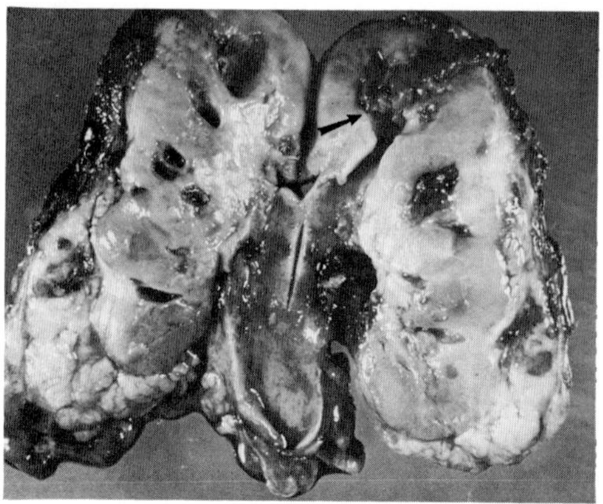

**Fig. 47.** Transitional Cell Carcinoma of the Renal Pelvis. The tumor protrudes into the pelvis and invades the kidney (*arrow*).

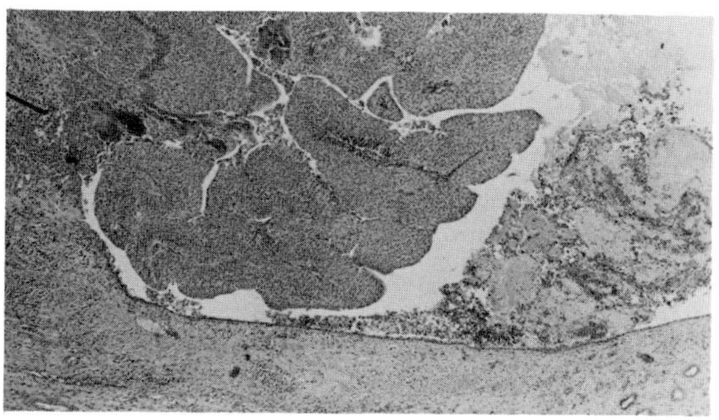

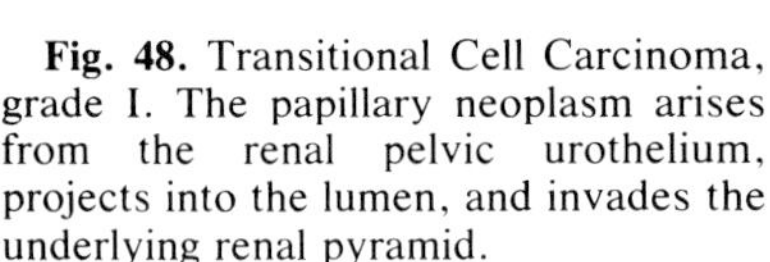

**Fig. 48.** Transitional Cell Carcinoma, grade I. The papillary neoplasm arises from the renal pelvic urothelium, projects into the lumen, and invades the underlying renal pyramid.

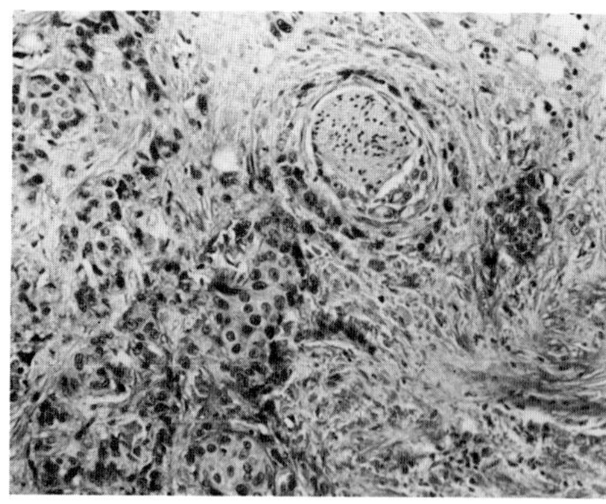

**Fig. 49.** Transitional Cell Carcinoma, grade 3. The tumor has invaded the hilar adipose tissue and shows perineural invasion.

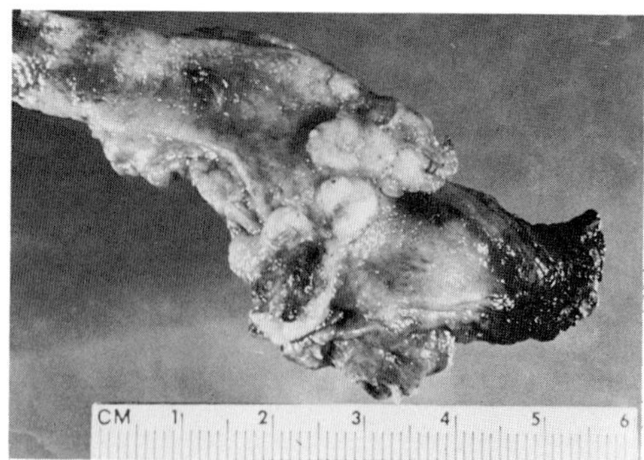


**Fig. 50.** Transitional Cell Carcinoma of the Ureter. The neoplasm is an irregular raised lesion with central ulceration.

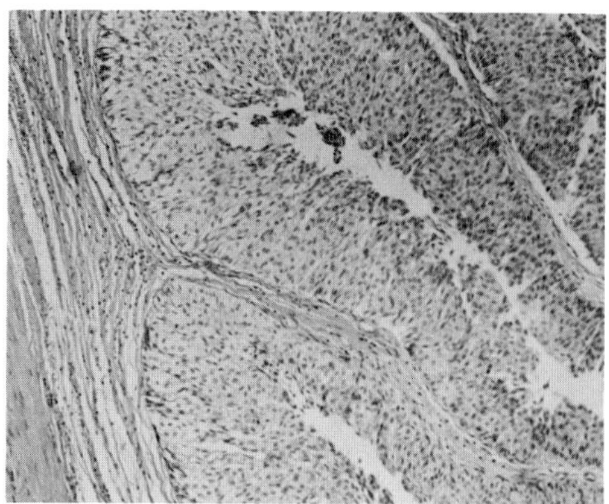

**Fig. 51.** Transitional Cell Carcinoma, grade 2. The typical papillary structure of this low-grade transitional cell carcinoma is evident. No invasion of the ureter wall is present in this section.

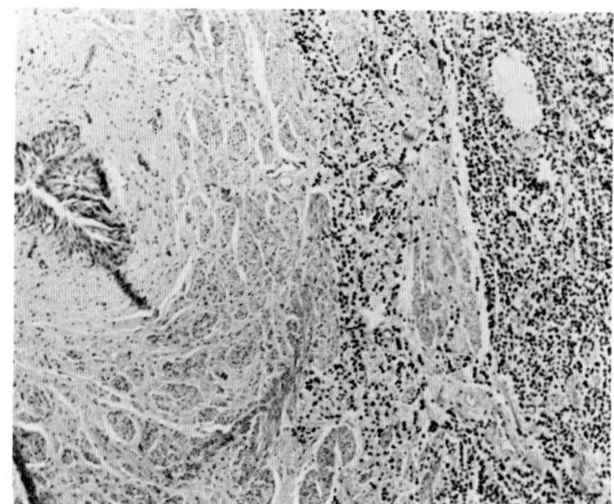

**Fig. 52.** Malignant Lymphoma Invading the Ureter. The lymphoma cells surrounding the ureter infiltrate the outer circular muscle bundles.

# BLADDER

## NORMAL HISTOLOGY

The mucosal lining of the bladder is composed of transitional cell epithelium with five to seven cell layers. The maturational process proceeds from the immature basal cells, to the intermediate cells, and finally to the superficial or "umbrella cells" on the luminal aspect of the urothelium. The lamina propria, composed of loose collagen and elastic fibers, is well vascularized. Lymphatic vessels and occasional small clusters of lymphocytes are present. External to the lamina propria is the muscularis, organized in variably oriented bundles of smooth muscle cells covered by adipose tissue. Occasional lymphoid aggregates or lymph nodes are present in the adipose tissue (Figs. 53 and 54).

## CONGENITAL AND DEVELOPMENTAL ABNORMALITIES

### Exstrophy of the Bladder

Exstrophy of the bladder is a congenital disorder characterized by incomplete closure of the anterior abdominal wall and anterior wall of the bladder and frequently a lack of fusion of the symphysis pubis. The bladder mucosa everts through the defect of the anterior wall, and the resultant abrasion by clothing and the escape of urine result in chronic inflammation of the mucosa and surrounding skin. Although the surface epithelium is initially of transitional cell type, characteristic changes in the epithelium include chronic inflammation of the mucosa, frequently with associated ulceration; squamous metaplasia of the urothelium; and glandular metaplasia with or without mucous secretion. In addition to these changes involving the mucosa and submucosa, fibrosis and mild chronic inflammatory changes are observed in the muscularis layer. These changes have been observed in infants as young as 2 weeks and are characteristically present in all affected patients older than 1 year.

Carcinoma complicating exstrophy of the bladder has been reported in approximately 40 cases. Although transitional cell carcinoma and squamous cell carcinoma have been reported, the most frequent epithelial malignancy is adenocarcinoma, often associated with cystitis glandularis (see Figs. 86 and 87).

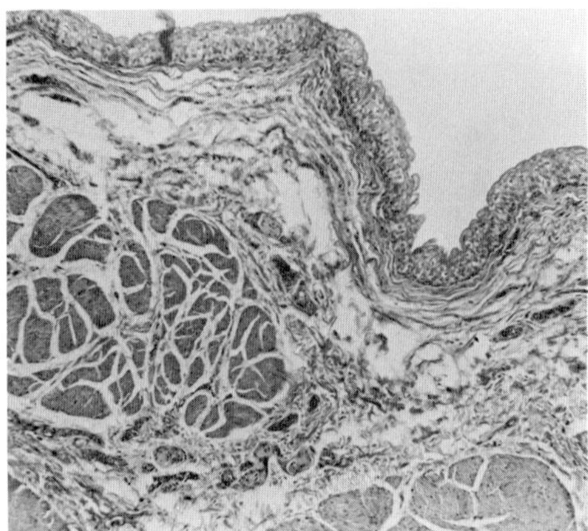

**Fig. 53.** Normal Bladder. The bladder mucosa overlies loose collagenous fibrous tissue of the lamina propria. The muscularis is organized in bundles of smooth muscle with variable orientation in the plane of section. Blood vessels, lymphatics, and nerves are present in the fibrous stroma of the lamina propria and muscularis.

## Urachus

In the adult, the urachus represents the vestigal remnant of the allantois. In fetal development, the allantois forms a communication between the cloaca and the allantoic sac in the umbilicus, where it converges with the two umbilical arteries. In later fetal and postnatal development, the bladder (derived from the anterior compartment of the cloaca) descends with the urachus, which ultimately comes to coverge with the obliterated umbilical arteries about 5 cm cephalad of the bladder. The communication of the urachus to umbilicus thereafter is normally represented by a thin ligamentum commune. In the adult, the urachus has three regions: supravesical, intramural, and intramucosal. The persistence of these remnants gives rise to urachal cysts, sinus tract, and diverticula.

The lining transitional cell epithelium retains the ability to undergo metaplastic change to squamous or mucous-producing columnar cells. Consistent with this capacity to undergo metaplastic change, subsequent neoplastic development in the urachus may take the form of transitional cell carcinoma, squamous cell carcinoma, adenocarcinoma, or mixture of the three histologic types. Of these three types, adenocarcinoma is the most commonly encountered neoplasm. As not all malignancies of the anterior abdominal wall or dome of the bladder are of urachal origin, the following criteria are necessary to make the diagnosis reliably:

The neoplasm should be located in the dome or anterior wall of the bladder.

The bulk of the neoplasm is deep within the muscularis of the bladder.

The presence of a primary malignancy of similar histology elsewhere has been eliminated.

Additional confirmatory findings include

The presence of an intact overlying mucosal surface devoid of neoplastic change and

Extension of the neoplasm cephalad from the bladder.

The diagnosis of urachal carcinoma cannot be made on histologic evidence alone (see Figs. 86 and 87).

## Diverticulum of the Bladder

Historically, bladder diverticula have been divided into two categories, congenital and acquired. The congenital diverticulum, present at birth, has all layers of the bladder wall represented, including the muscularis. Acquired diverticulum, by the nature of its forma-

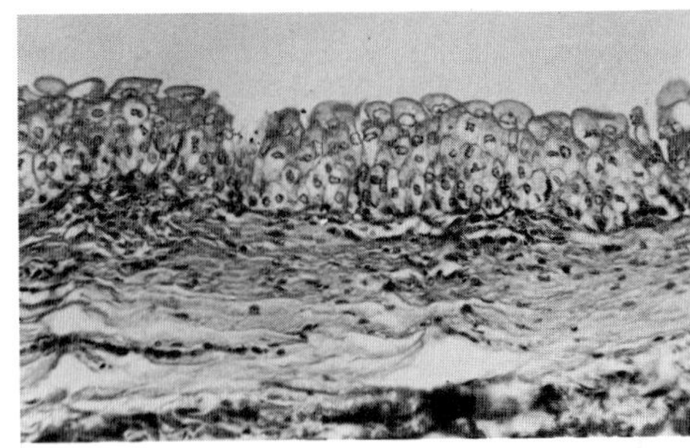

**Fig. 54.** Normal Bladder. The urothelium is composed of transitional cells five to eight layers thick. The configuration of the bladder transitional cells, here reflecting a flaccid bladder, is variable.

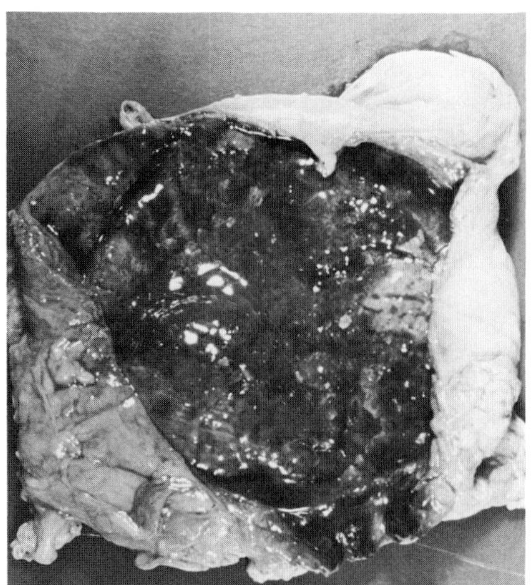

**Fig. 55.** Hemorrhagic Cystitis. The bladder mucosa is intact but reflects diffuse hemorrhage throughout the lamina propria.

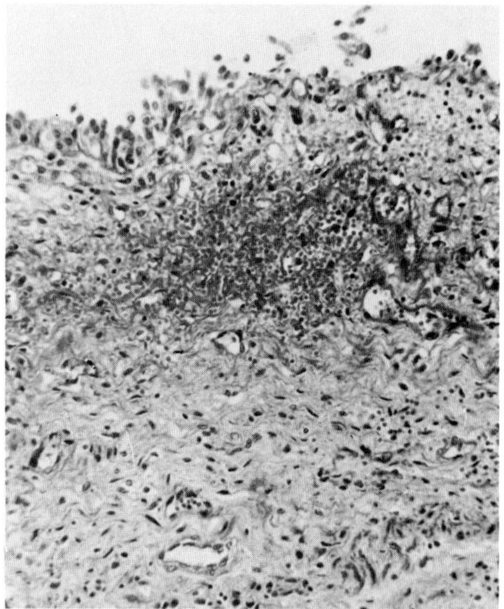

**Fig. 56.** Hemorrhagic Cystitis. Dilated and congested vessels with extensive extravasation of red blood cells within the lamina propria are the prominent features. The urothelium shows focal ulceration and extensive sloughing.

tion (*i.e.*, progression of a cellule into a diverticulum) does not contain muscle fibers in its wall.

Neoplasms arising within bladder diverticula have been reported as occurring almost exclusively in male patients. The majority of tumors reported in diverticula are transitional cell carcinomas; less frequently squamous cell carcinoma or adenocarcinoma have been reported.

## INFLAMMATORY DISEASES

### Acute Cystitis

The histologic hallmark of acute cystitis is the presence of neutrophils in the area of mucosal injury. Frequently, the mucosa is ulcerated, and the underlying lamina propria is edematous. An offending organism may be identified by special stains, but frequently no specific cause is demonstrated microscopically.

Variations of the basic theme of the acute inflammatory reaction include

Intramural hemorrhage (hemorrhagic cystitis; Figs. 55 and 56)

Ulceration with focal necrosis (suppurative cystitis)

Marked edema, of the lamina propria (bullous cystitis; Fig. 57)

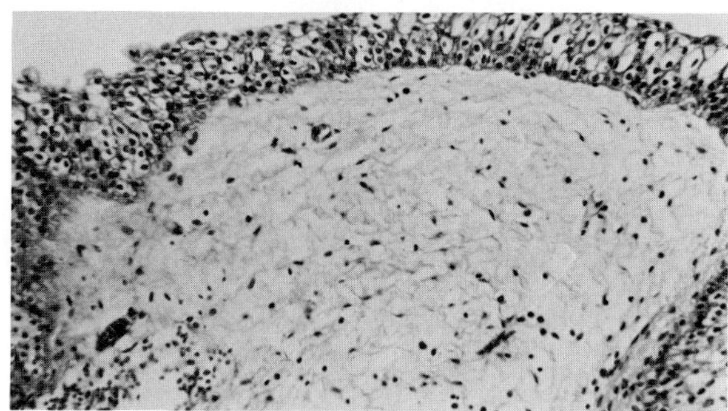

**Fig. 57.** Bullous Cystitis. The prominent edema of the lamina propria is associated with scattered chronic inflammatory cells in the interstitium.

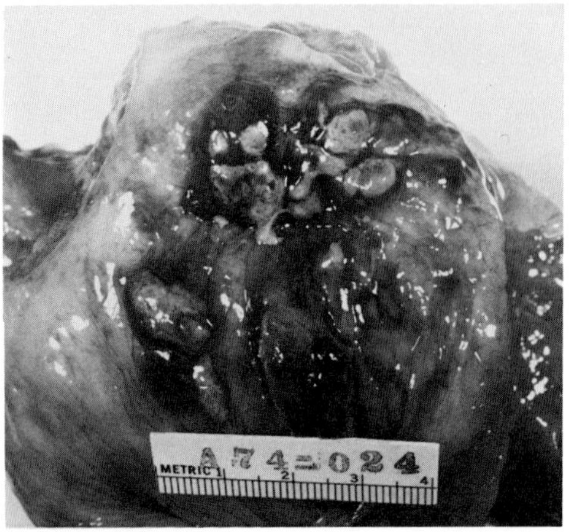


**Fig. 58.** Gangrenous Cystitis. The bladder mucosa is covered in many sites replaced by adherent inflammatory exudate.

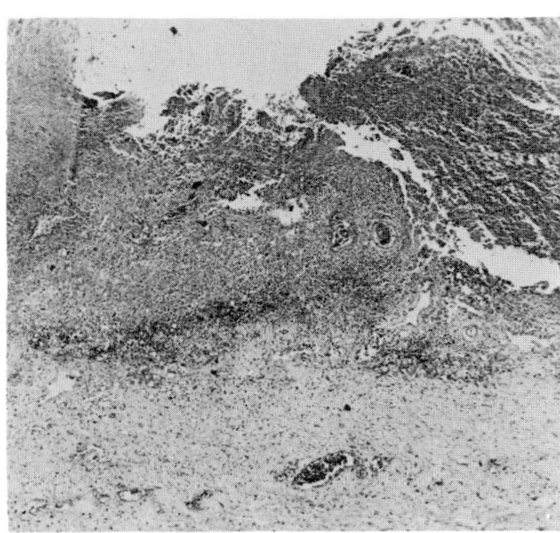

**Fig. 59.** Gangrenous Cystitis. The mucosal destruction is accompanied by a dense infiltrate of acute inflammatory cells with fibrin deposition in the superficial lamina propria.

Widespread mucosal and lamina propria necrosis (gangrenous cystitis; Figs. 58 and 59)

## Chronic Cystitis

EOSINOPHILIC CYSTITIS is an inflammatory disorder of the bladder characterized by a dense infiltration of eosinophils throughout the bladder wall. It is frequently associated with an allergic history, peripheral eosinophilia, and negative findings in urine cultures. A similar picture may also be seen in interstitial cystitis or in parasitic cystitis (Fig. 60).

EMPHYSEMATOUS CYSTITIS is a rare form of cystitis most commonly reported in women and diabetics and characterized by numerous gas-filled intramural cysts of the bladder. The cysts result from gas-forming bacteria that invade the bladder wall and are surrounded by compressed stroma of the lamina propria. Multinucleated giant cells are occasionally observed along the outer margins of such cysts.

INTERSTITIAL CYSTITIS (Hunner's Ulcer) is a disease of unknown etiology, which occurs more frequently in women. The classic urologic complaints include frequency, urgency, hematuria, and often severe suprapubic pain. Changes are progressive and may vary from mild symptoms of cystitis to mucosal ulceration and eventually to fibrosis of the bladder wall with a diminished bladder capacity. There is marked transvesical edema and a chronic inflammatory cell

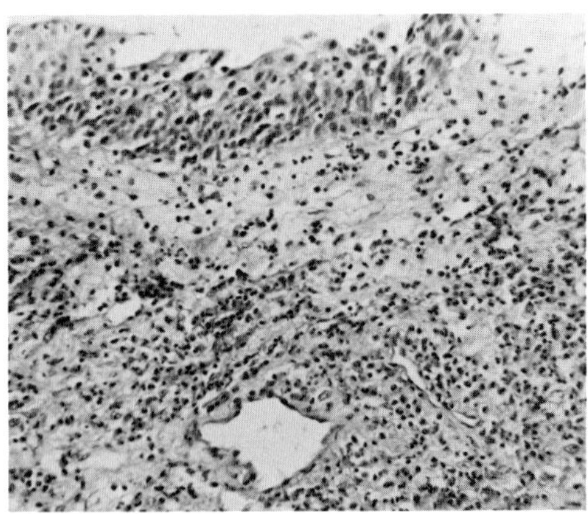

**Fig. 60.** Eosinophilic Cystitis. The lamina propria and bladder mucosal cells contain a dense infiltrate composed almost exclusively of eosinophils.

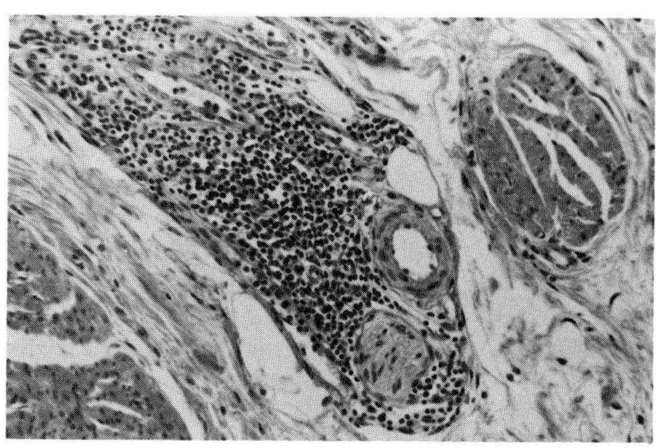

**Fig. 61.** Interstitial Cystitis. The inflammatory infiltration of lymphocytes, plasma cells, and occasional neutrophils is present deep in the muscularis of the bladder. The overlying mucosa (not in the picture) was extensively ulcerated.

infiltrate including lymphocytes, plasma cells, and particularly eosinophils. The large eosinophilic infiltrate may produce fibrosis, and it is on this basis that an allergic etiology has been suggested (Fig. 61).

CYSTITIS FOLLICULARIS is recognized only at the microscopic level by the presence of lymphoid follicles with germinal centers located beneath the mucosa of the bladder. These germinal centers may or may not have an associated nonspecific chronic inflammatory cell background in the lamina propria. Lymphoid follicles in the absence of any clinical, bacteriologic, or pathologic evidence of infection and inflammation are commonly observed. No etiology has been identified, and its biologic significance remains unsettled (Fig. 62).

MALAKOPLAKIA presents grossly as yellow-tan plaques of the vesical mucosa and microscopically as sheets of histiocytes (von Hansemann cells) with finely vacuolated cytoplasm. Numerous such histiocytes contain round to oval intracytoplasmic inclusions (Michaelis–Gutmann bodies). These inclusions are PAS-positive and commonly are calcified. Similar bodies are observed in extracellular locations in the lesions. There is commonly a background of plasma cells and lymphocytes (Fig. 63).

TUBERCULOSIS OF THE BLADDER most commonly involves the trigone and is rarely if ever the sole location of infection in the urinary tract. The histopathology of granulomatous infections here is identical to that of the classic caseating granulomas found elsewhere.

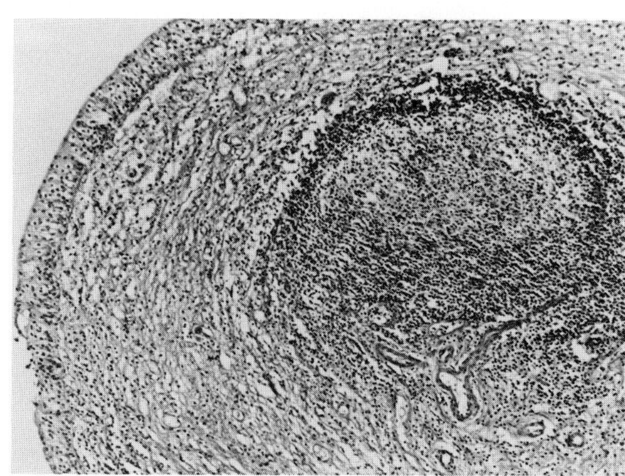

**Fig. 62.** Cystitis Follicularis. The intact urothelium overlies a lamina propria containing a lymphoid aggregate with a germinal center. Scattered lymphocytes are present throughout the lamina propria.

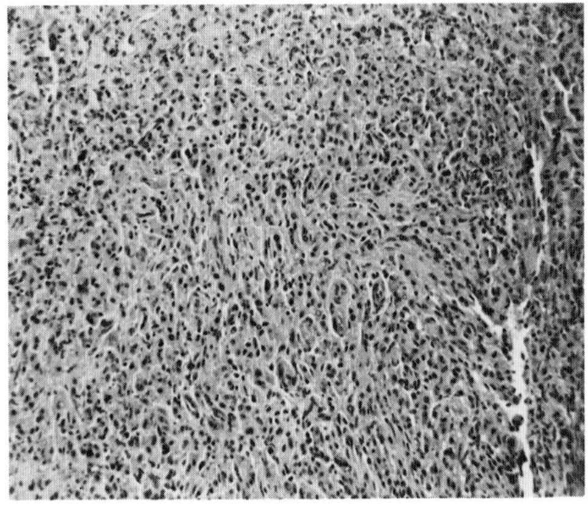

**Fig. 63.** Malakoplakia. The cellular infiltrate is composed almost exclusively of histiocytes. Numerous intracytoplasmic inclusions (Michaelis–Gutmann bodies) are present in the histiocytes.

The organisms can be demonstrated with special stains for acid-fast bacilli. Areas of granulomatous inflammation are usually present with central caseating necrosis and peripheral epithelioid multinucleated giant cells. Scattered lymphocytes and other cells of chronic inflammatory disease are usually present (Fig. 64).

FUNGAL INFECTIONS OF THE BLADDER. Chronic cystitis due to a variety of fungal organisms has been reported. The most frequent fungus is candida with a high risk observed among diabetics. These organisms may cause granulomatous reactions similar to those of tuberculosis, and the specific diagnosis rests in the demonstration of the fungus by special histologic stains or in culturing the organism.

PARASITIC CYSTITIS. Parasites may cause chronic cystitis, the most common of which is caused by *Schistosoma haematobium*. Either adult worms or deposited eggs may be found in the bladder wall. The eggs evoke a mixed inflammatory cell reaction including numerous eosinophils, neutrophils, lymphocytes, and foreign-body giant cells. In time, the ova become calcified with surrounding fibrosis of the bladder wall. Chronic schistosomal cystitis predisposes the patient to the development of malignancies of the mucosal surface. The most common malignancy is squamous cell carcinoma, but transitional cell carcinoma has been reported (Fig. 65).

RADIATION CYSTITIS. Clinical cystitis developing in patients previously irradiated is associated with histologic changes unique to this form of injury to the bladder. These changes are found in the mucosa and lamina propria, which show the histologic picture of acute cystitis, occasionally with ulceration of the mucosa. Mucosal thinning with one to five cell layers is common. The lamina propria is edematous with an accompanying mixed inflammatory cell infiltrate, scattered fibroblasts with enlarged hyperchromatic nuclei, and hyalinization of the collagenous stroma. Endothelial cells

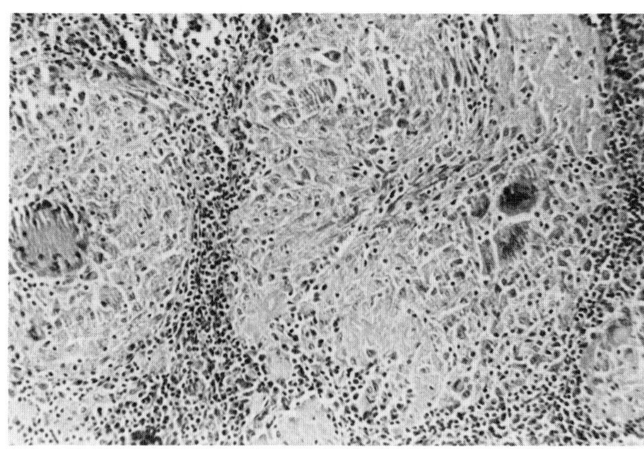

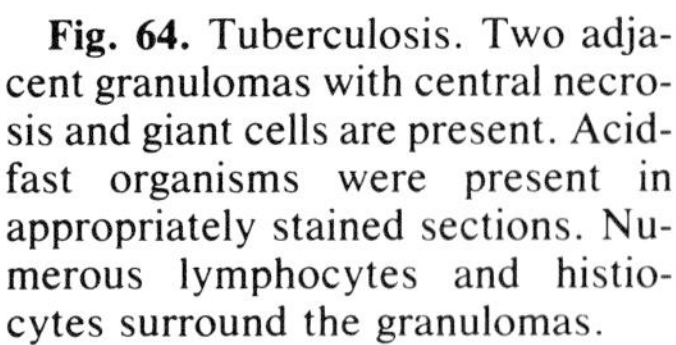

**Fig. 64.** Tuberculosis. Two adjacent granulomas with central necrosis and giant cells are present. Acid-fast organisms were present in appropriately stained sections. Numerous lymphocytes and histiocytes surround the granulomas.

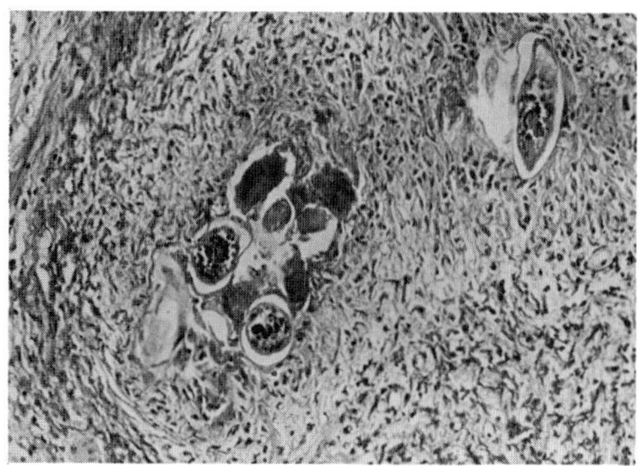

**Fig. 65.** Schistosomiasis. The ova of the schistosome organisms are surrounded by reactive fibrosis and chronic inflammatory cells.

proliferate, and subintimal accumulation of histiocytes has been described. The vessels in the lamina propria show fibrinoid necrosis and are more prone to hemorrhage than are normal vessels (Fig. 66).

PROLIFERATIVE CYSTITIS. In addition to the inflammatory conditions just discussed, a prolonged cystitis may lead to the changes of proliferative or reactive cystitis. These common epithelial proliferations have been the subject of a large number of reports in the literature. Histologically, they appear as epithelial invaginations of the lamina propria. They are most commonly observed in the bladder but are reported to occur at all levels of the urinary tract. They may be composed of solid buds of epithelial cells, similar to those seen on the surface of the bladder, or they may have glandlike spaces with or without secretions present. In the earliest stages of development, the solid buds of urothelium are in continuity with the surface. These are called von Brunn's nests (Fig. 67). With increasing growth downward into the lamina propria, the apparent continuity with the surface is lost. Frequently the central portion of the structure demonstrates degeneration of cells with the production of a lumen. This entity is called *cystitis cystica*. Step sections of a specimen containing cystitis cystica will reveal the continuity with the surface epithelium. It is common to see the transitions from von Brunn's nests to cystitis cystica in the same section. The lining cells vary from flattened urothelial cells to cuboidal or columnar cells (Fig. 68). The designation of *cystitis glandularis* has been given to the cases in which the lining is composed of mucous-secreting columnar cells. These structures are most frequently located in the trigone region of the bladder but can be found in any location. They are found in all age groups and with equal frequency in both sexes (Fig. 69).

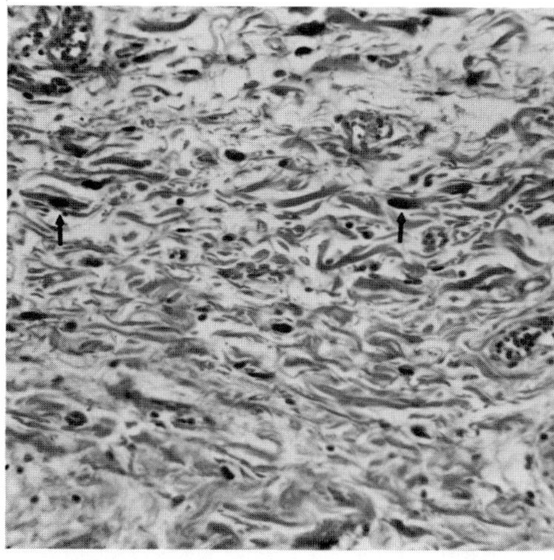

**Fig. 66.** Radiation Cystitis. The presence of numerous enlarged, hyperchromatic fibroblasts (*arrows*) with increased collagenous fibrosis in the lamina propria is characteristic of radiation injury.

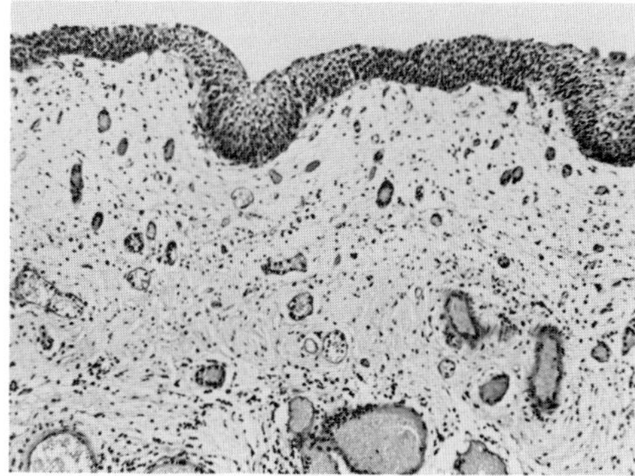

**Fig. 67.** Brunn's Nests. The lamina propria is focally penetrated by a solid bud of urothelial cells similar to the surface epithelium. Scattered chronic inflammatory cells and vascular dilatation are noted in the deep lamina propria.

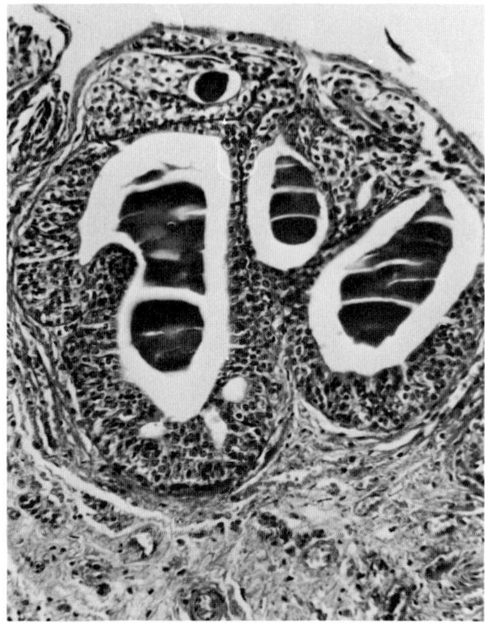

**Fig. 68.** Cystitis Cystica. Urothelial cell nests with a central lumen that contains secretions are present beneath the surface, here devoid of urothelial cells. Step sections revealed continuity of the lining urothelial cells of the cysts with the surface.

Controversy continues over the risk of neoplastic change in bladders containing these proliferative changes.

## METAPLASTIC CHANGES

The normal human transitional cell epithelium is capable of changing to squamous, glandular, or nephrogenic tissue. Squamous metaplasia is most commonly encountered in the trigone and bladder neck region and is more common in women (Fig. 70). It appears to be less frequent than cystitis cystica or von Brunn's nests. The pathogenesis of this epithelial change is unknown. Only 22% of cases reported were associated with chronic inflammation. Squamous cell carcinoma of the bladder has been reported in association with squamous metaplasia of the bladder mucosa. The frequency of malignant change of the squamous epithelium however, is quite low. The term *leukoplakia* has been used interchangeably with squamous metaplasia; however, *leukoplakia* should be used only to describe dysplastic change.

Mucous and glandular metaplasia may occur, often initiating in von Brunn's nests or on the surface epithelium, leading to the development of mucous secreting columnar cells. The epithelium may also become metaplastic to a tubular form that vaguely resembles renal tubules; hence, the name *nephrogenic adenoma*. The terms *adenomatoid metaplasia* or *nephrogenic metaplasia* have also been applied to this lesion. A history of previous urinary tract infection or instrumentation with associated chronic inflammatory changes in the wall of the bladder is common. Occasional dem-

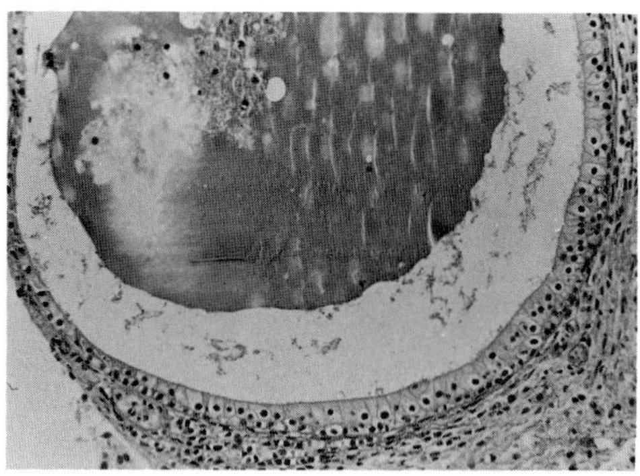

**Fig. 69.** Cystitis Glandularis. Secretions markedly distend the glandular structure lined by metaplastic mucous-secreting columnar cells of urothelial origin.

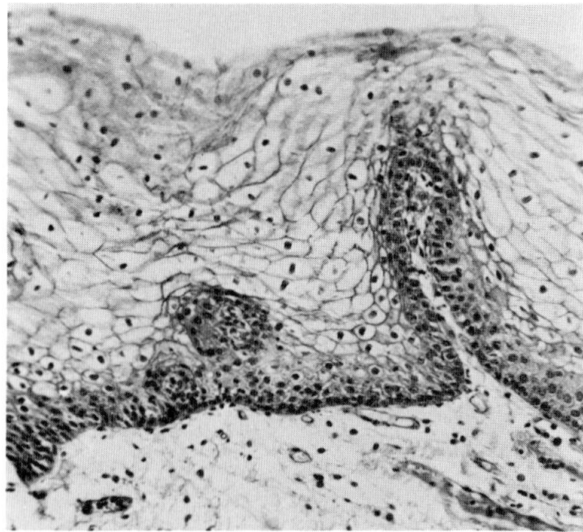

**Fig. 70.** Squamous Metaplasia. The typical transitional urothelium has been replaced by squamous epithelium. No atypia is present.

onstration of continuity of the bladder surface epithelium with the epithelial lining of the tubular structures of the lesion and occasional foci of squamous metaplasia in the tubules lend support to the interpretation of this as a metaplastic change.

The histologic features are very characteristic. Multiple, small tubular structures located in the lamina propria and lined by cuboidal, columnar, or flattened epithelium are present with a background infiltration of chronic inflammatory cells (Fig. 71). Variations on this basic pattern include foci of squamous metaplasia of the lining epithelium, PAS-positive secretions in the tubules, and focal areas of tubular dilatation with papillary projections. To date, only two cases of nephrogenic adenoma have been found to be associated with adenocarcinoma of the bladder.

## MISCELLANEOUS DISORDERS

### Amyloidosis of the Bladder

Vesical amyloidosis has been reported to occur as either an isolated bladder lesion or as a part of generalized amyloidosis. In either form, bladder amyloidosis is rare, and the pathologic features are similar to those observed elsewhere in the urinary tract. Involvement of the bladder may be diffuse or localized with an exophytic mass apparent. Ulceration of the overlying mucosa is common, and the lamina propria will show a dense deposit of very acellular, homogeneously staining pink substance. Minor degrees of lymphocyte infiltration may be seen, but inflammatory cells are not prominent in the amyloid tumor.

### Endometriosis

Endometriosis may appear to form tumorlike areas in the bladder in women 18 to 48 years of age. Approximately 50% of all reported patients have a history of pelvic surgery, which is implicated as a cause in endometriosis involving the bladder. Most commonly, the submucosal and muscular layers are the areas involved. Both endometrial glands and stroma will be seen within the bladder wall (Fig. 72*A*, *B*).

## BENIGN NEOPLASMS

### Hemangioma

Uncommonly, hemangiomas have been reported to occur in the bladder wall. Most patients are in the first two decades of life. Histologically, the vascular channels may be small and numerous (capillary hemangioma) with little intervening stroma of collagenous fibrous tissue. Inflammatory cell infiltrate is associated with ulceration of the overlying mucosa. The vascular channels may be relatively large with stroma intervening (cavernous hemangioma).

### Paraganglioma

Paraganglioma has been reported as occurring in the urinary bladder. These

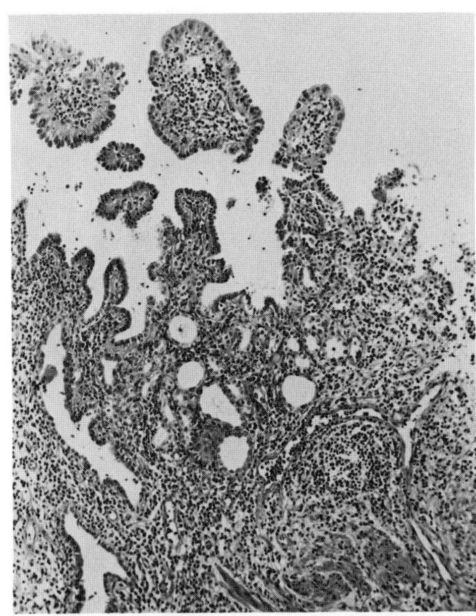

**Fig. 71.** Nephrogenic Adenoma. Papillary and simple tubular structures located in the mucosa and superficial lamina propria and lined by epithelium similar to renal tubular epithelium characterized this lesion. Numerous acute and chronic inflammatory cells infiltrate the adjacent lamina propria.

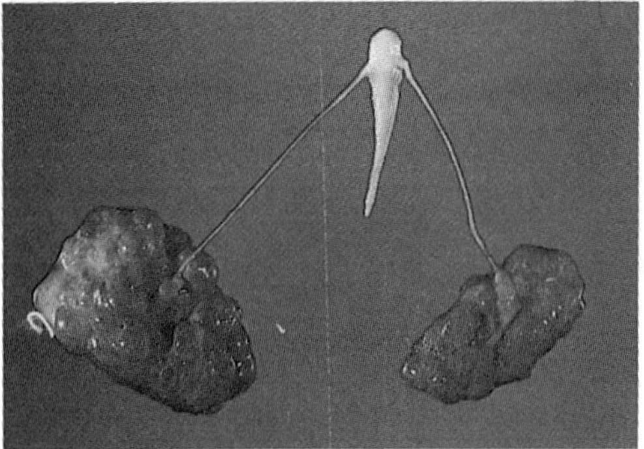

**Plate 1.** Benign Multilocular Cystic Nephroma. This rare example of bilateral multilocular cystic nephroma is associated with hypoplasia of the ureters and bladder.

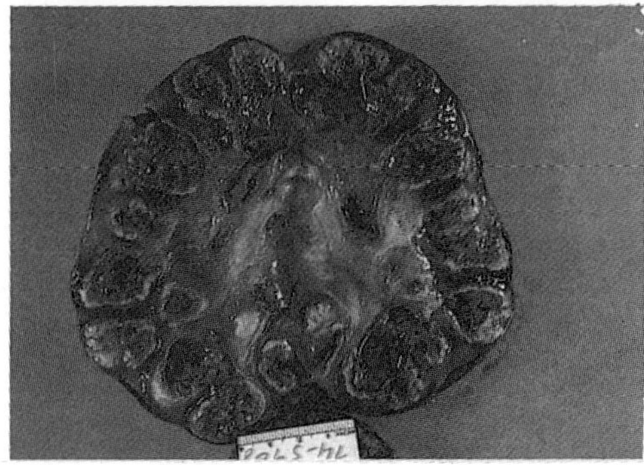

**Plate 2.** Xanthogranulomatous Pyelonephritis. The cut surface of the kidney shows distorted calyces rimmed by yellow-tan renal parenchyma containing a heavy infiltrate of histiocytes.

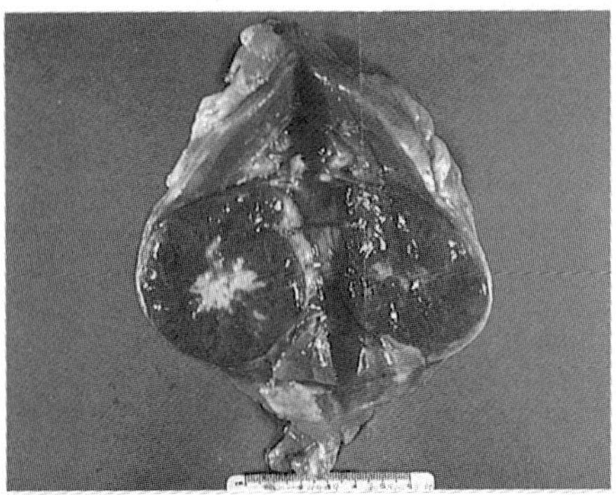

**Plate 3.** Renal Tubular Oncocytoma. The well circumscribed neoplasm has a central area of fibrosis surrounded by tumor similar in color to the normal renal parenchyma.

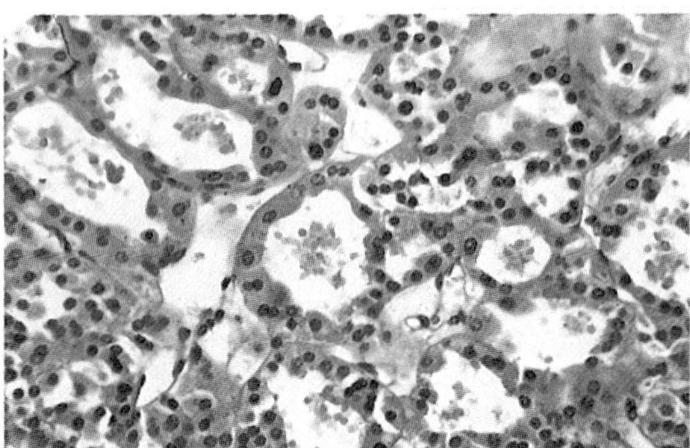

**Plate 4.** Renal Tubular Oncocytoma. The oncocytic cells are arranged in tubules. There is an absence of tumor necrosis, mitoses, and significant pleomorphism.

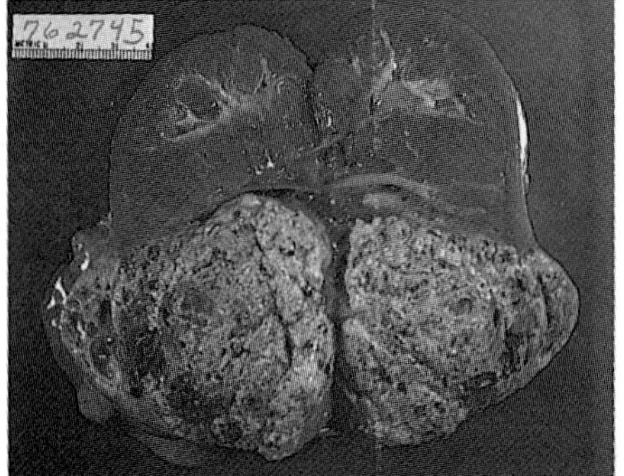


**Plate 5.** Renal Cell Carcinoma. The deceptively well-delineated renal cell carcinoma shows extensive necrosis and hemorrhage with penetration of the overlying capsule.

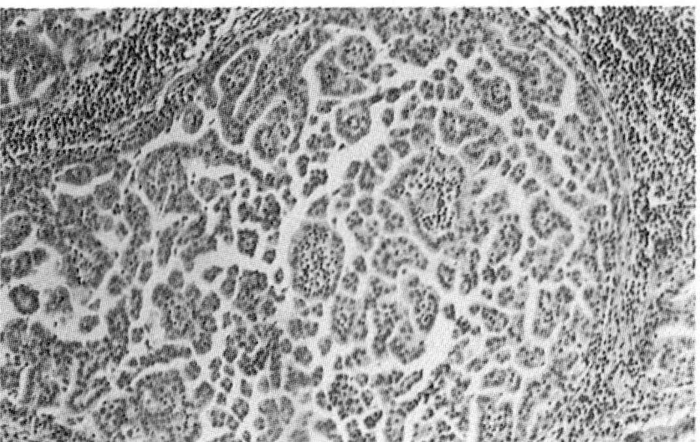

**Plate 6.** Renal Cell Carcinoma. The tumor is composed of granular cells arranged in a papillary formation.

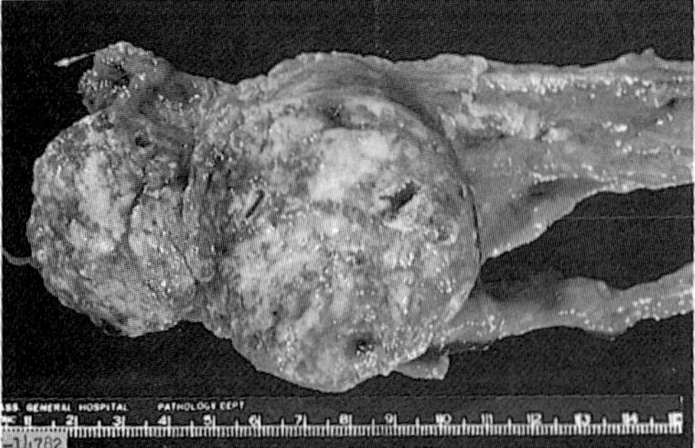


**Plate 7.** Teratocarcinoma Metastatic to Retroperitoneum. The cut surface of the tumor reveals extensive necrosis and focal hemorrhage.

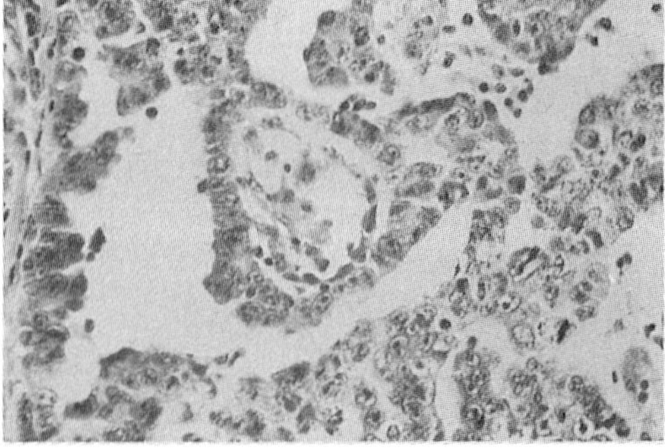

**Plate 8.** Embryonal Carcinoma of the Testis. The neoplastic cells line irregular clefts and microcysts. Occasional mitoses are present.

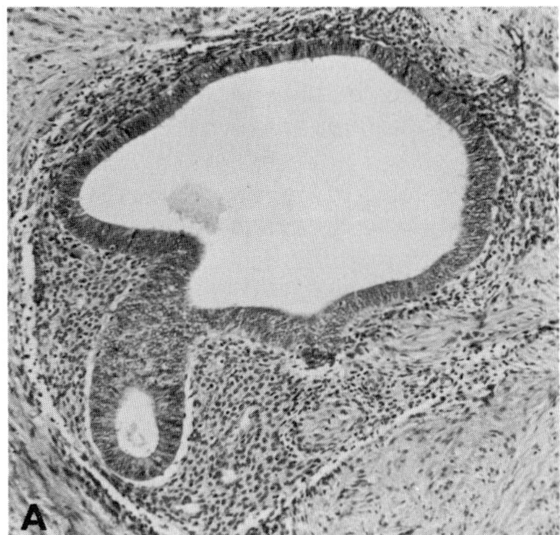


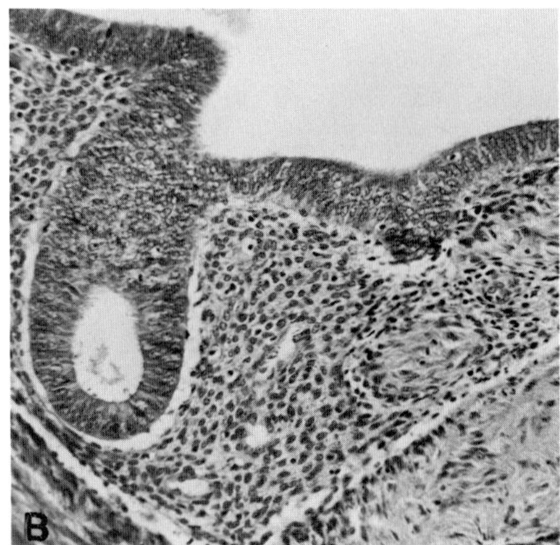


**Fig. 72A.** Endometriosis of the Bladder. Endometrial glandular epithelium with associated endometrial stromal cells within the vesical muscularis layer are diagnostic. **B.** Endometriosis of the Urinary Bladder. The endometrial gland epithelium is surrounded by typical endometrial stromal cells.

neoplasms commonly take origin in the submucosa and protrude into the bladder lumen. The overlying mucosa frequently shows ulceration. The periphery of the tumor may show clear demarcation from the adjacent normal tissue, or they may show tumor infiltration of the bladder muscle. The tumor cells are arranged in nests, separated by thin fibrovascular septa. The cells have central or eccentrically located round nuclei with eosinophilic cytoplasm. Occasional bizarre cells with enlarged hyperchromatic nuclei may be found, and mitoses are rare to absent. Some patients will show cytoplasmic granules with silver stains. There is a general concensus that the histologic potential of a paraganglioma cannot be reliably predicted from the histologic picture, the best criteria for malignancy of this tumor being the presence of metastases.

## Neurofibroma

Neurofibroma may be found in the bladder, and on histologic section obvious nerve bundles will be seen. The remainder of the tumor may consist of spindle-shaped cells with thin, elongated nuclei.

## Granular Cell Tumor

The histogenesis of granular cell tumor remains unsettled, with evidence supporting neural origin in most reports, but occasional reports provide evidence of muscle origin. These neoplasms are typically solid, intramural masses, frequently associated with ulceration of the overlying urothelium. The tumor cells are arranged in nests or cords, separated by thin fibrovascular trabeculae. The individual cells have abundant cytoplasm with eosinophilic granules. Pleomorphism, necrosis, and mitoses are not prominent features. The cytologic features of one malignant granular cell tumor of the bladder included significant pleomorphism, increased nuclear size, and hyperchromatic nuclei (Fig. 73).

## Inverted Papilloma

The inverted papilloma is a rare benign neoplasm of the urinary tract which has been reported as occurring in the renal pelvis, ureter, bladder, and urethra. The trigone of the bladder is the most common location in the urinary tract. The histopathology of this exophytic lesion is characteristic regardless of its location. The surface urothelium is composed of normally arranged transitional cells,

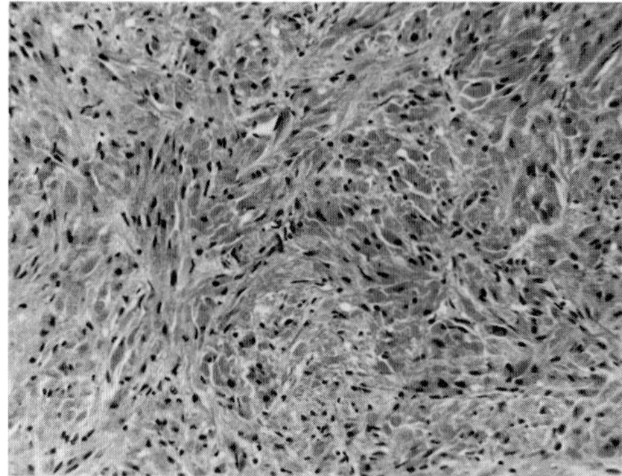

**Fig. 73.** Granular Cell Tumor. The tumor cells contain relatively small, hyperchromatic nuclei and characteristically abundant, eosinophilic granular cytoplasm.

three to seven cells thick. From this normal urothelium, cords of similar-appearing cells extend into the submucosa. Occasional gland lumina are found in these epithelial cords, some with PAS-positive mucin. The intervening stroma is composed of delicate collagen fibers with thin-walled blood vessels (Fig. 74). Occasional cases have foci of squamous metaplasia in the epithelial cords. One reported case was associated with a papillary transitional cell carcinoma arising from the surface.

### Papilloma

The papilloma of the bladder is a rare lesion which may be single or multiple. Histologically this neoplasm is characterized by thin, delicate papillary excrescences with a covering urothelium, histologically and cytologically normal. The epithelial layers are less than eight cells thick, and there is no evidence of disorganized maturation or cellular atypia (Fig. 75). Papillary growths evidencing greater epithelial disorganization, pleomorphism, and cell layers composed of more than eight cells, are regarded as transitional cell carcinoma.

## PRECANCEROUS LESIONS OF THE UROTHELIUM

As the bladder epithelium progresses to the development of overt transitional cell carcinoma, several intermediate steps have been recognized. These intermediate steps include simple hyperplasia of the urothelium and urothelial dysplasia.

Hyperplasia of the urothelium is present when the bladder lining is either focally, or in a diffuse manner, thickened beyond the normal seven cell layers. Nuclear abnormalities are inconspicuous. The biologic significance of this change is currently unsettled. It is seen in association with other forms of epithelial atypia, neoplasia, and chronic inflammation or in the absence of these changes (Fig. 76).

Urothelial dysplasia (atypia) is characterized by nuclear abnormalities associated with a thickened urothelium. These dysplastic areas involve only the epithelium and have no fibrovascular stalk. The superficial cell layer tends to be absent with increasing frequency as the atypia increases (Fig. 77).

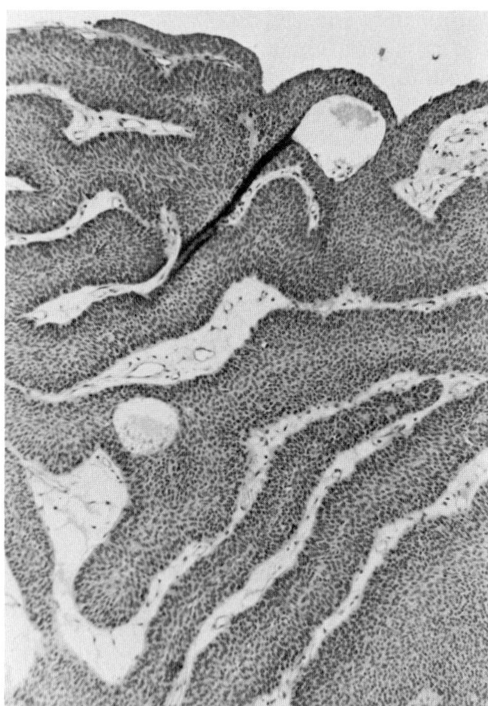

**Fig. 74.** Inverted Papilloma. Extensive invagination of the surface urothelium in cords with focal gland formation is characteristic of this lesion. The urothelium within the cords evidences no atypia and is similar to the cells on the surface.

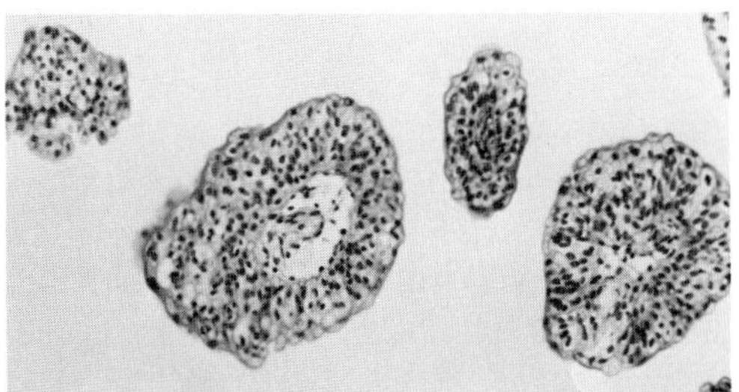

**Fig. 75.** Papilloma. The thin papillary structures have a central fibrovascular core covered by transitional epithelium with normal cytologic features. The number of cell layers is not greater than normal bladder urothelium.

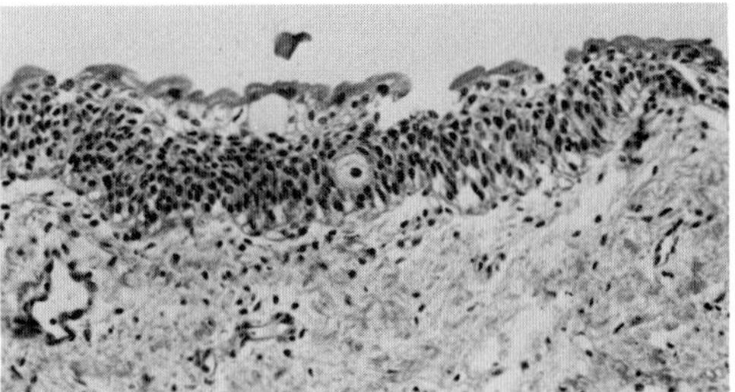

**Fig. 77.** Dysplasia of Bladder Urothelium. Scattered atypical nuclei with loss of polarity and variability of size and shape are present. The superficial layers, with the exception of focal interruptions, are preserved. The basement membrane is intact.

## MALIGNANT NEOPLASMS

### Nonpapillary Carcinoma *In Situ*

Nonpapillary carcinoma *in situ* is characterized by increased cellular atypia, pleomorphism, and a superficial cell layer less apparent than that of dysplastic epithelium. The most common histologic type is composed of small cells with hyperchromatic nuclei. Another type is composed of larger cells with variable staining of the nuclei (Fig. 78). Friedell has compared the histologic and cytologic features of nonpapillary carcinoma *in situ* to that of grade III papillary carcinoma. Decreased intercellular cohesiveness is common.

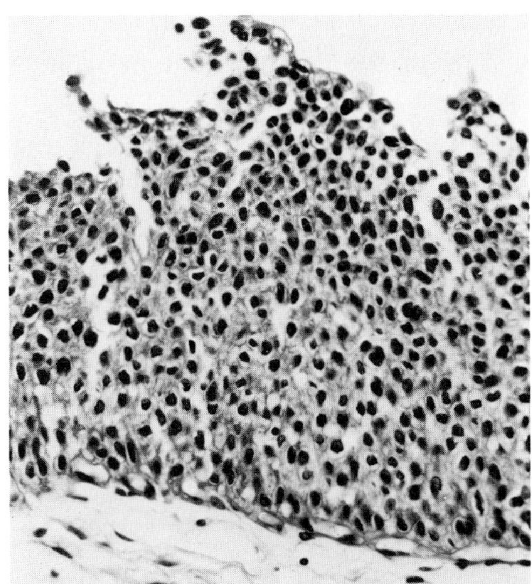

**Fig. 76.** Hyperplasia with Atypia. The epithelium is significantly thickened and contains mild atypical (dysplastic) features including focal loss of nuclear polarity and variation of nuclear size and shape.

### Transitional Cell Carcinoma

Transitional cell carcinoma is the most common neoplasm of the urinary bladder, comprising 90% of vesical carcinoma in the United States. It is most frequently located in the area adjacent to the trigone, and exophytic growth is encountered most frequently. However, these tumors may show solid or infiltrative growth characteristics. The grading system according to WHO classification is herein presented.

Papillary transitional cell carcinoma, noninvasive grade I, is defined as a papillary projection covered by thickened urothelium with only slight atypical features and rare mitotic figures. Invasion is rare and inevitably limited to the subjacent lamina propria (Figs. 79 and 80).

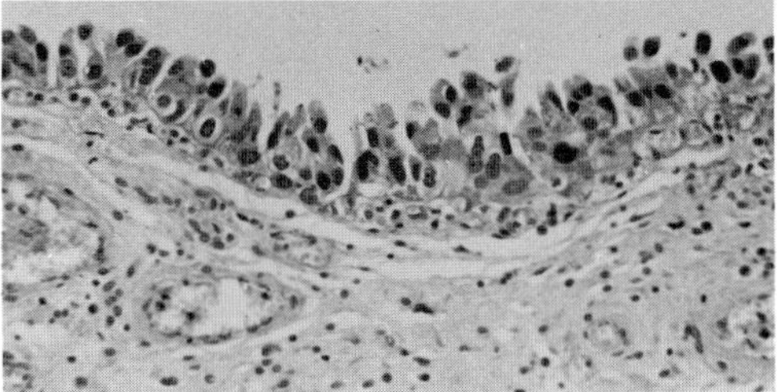

**Fig. 78.** Carcinoma-in-situ of the Bladder. The atypical urothelial cells have hyperchromatic nuclei which vary in size, shape, and orientation. Focal areas with loss of intercellular cohesion are present. The basement membrane is intact.

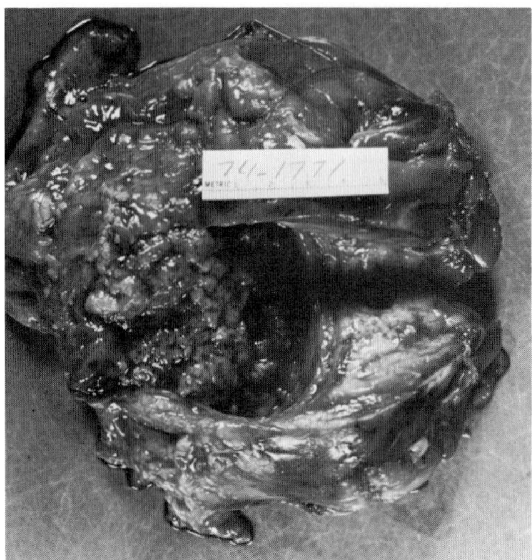


**Fig. 79.** Transitional Cell Carcinoma of the Bladder. The extensive papillary neoplasm is present in the center of this bladder specimen.

Papillary transitional cell carcinoma, noninvasive grade II, is defined as a papillary projection that tends to be shorter and blunter than are grade I lesions. Nuclear pleomorphism is common, as are large nucleoli; mitoses are not uncommon (Figs. 81 and 82). When invasion does occur, the invasive component is histologically similar to that of the surface.

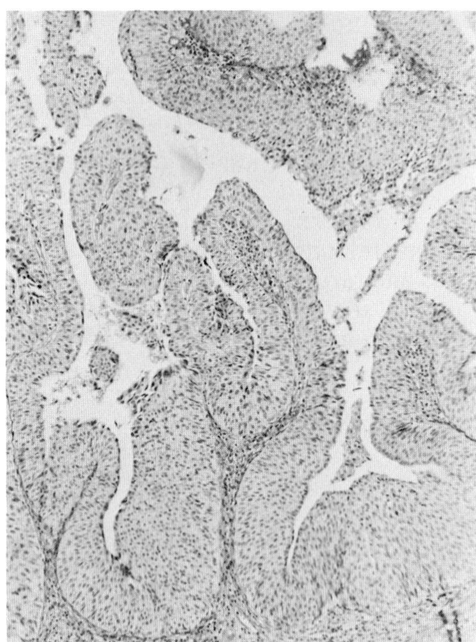

**Fig. 80.** Transitional Cell Carcinoma, grade 1. The papillary structures are covered by a thickened urothelium demonstrating only slight nuclear atypical features. Mitotic figures were rare in this neoplasm.

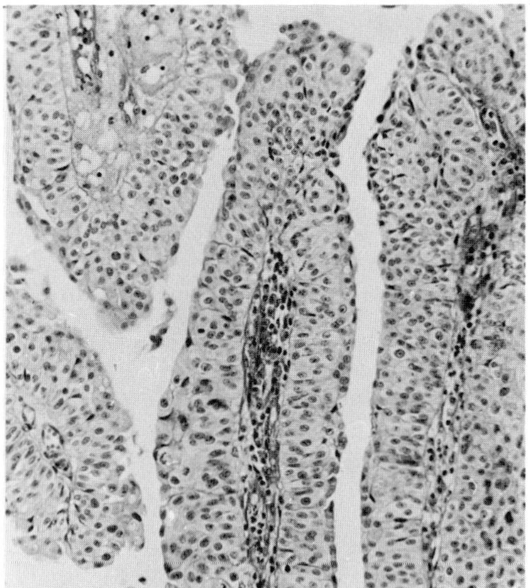

**Fig. 81.** Transitional Cell Carcinoma, grade 2. This papillary neoplasm is characterized by nuclear pleomorphism and uncommon to rare mitoses. Most tumor cells have prominent nucleoli.

Papillary transitional cell carcinoma, noninvasive grade III, is defined as possessing marked cytologic abnormalities

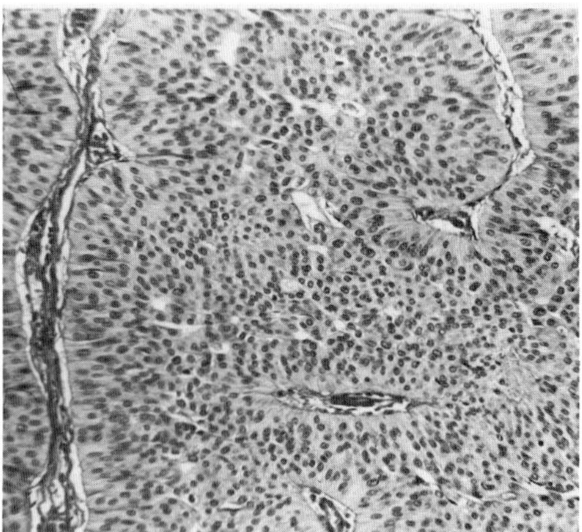

**Fig. 82.** Transitional Cell Carcinoma, grade 2. Fused papillary projections of transitional cell carcinoma with moderate variation of nuclear size and shape are present. Compare with Figure 81.

with widespread nuclear pleomorphism, chromatin clumping, irregular nuclear membranes, and occasional bizarre cells. Mitoses may be numerous, and the invasive form is histologically similar. The gross features are that of a solid tumor with a paucity of papillary structures (Figs. 83 and 84).

Invasion of the bladder wall is uncommon with low-grade neoplasms but is increasingly probable with high-grade neoplasms. The close correlation of tumor grade and stage and ultimate outcome is well recognized in these neoplasms.

## Squamous Cell Carcinoma

Although focal areas of squamous differentiation in transitional cell carcinoma, especially those of high grade, are not uncommon, tumors composed exclusively of squamous cell carcinoma in the bladder constitute only 8% of lesions in this country. Histologically, approximately two thirds of the patients have moderately well-differentiated squamous cell carcinoma, but all grades are observed (Fig. 85). Eighty-six percent to 100% of the tumors are observed to be infiltrating the bladder wall at the time of initial presentation. Squamous metaplasia has been observed in association with these neoplasms.

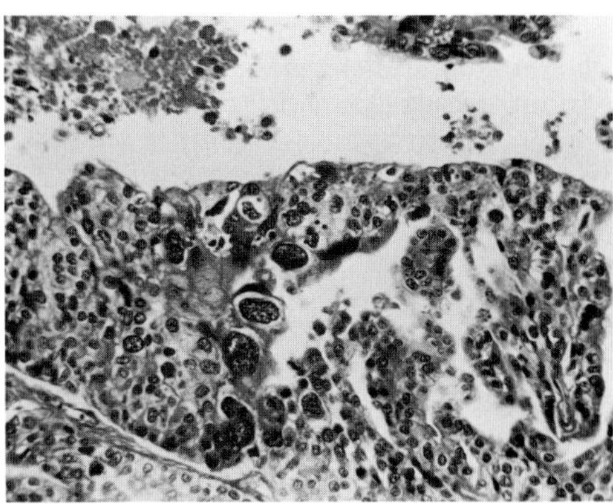

**Fig. 84.** Transitional Cell Carcinoma, grade 3. A focus of marked nuclear pleomorphism in the center is present in a background of more uniform malignant transitional cells.

## Adenocarcinoma of the Bladder

Primary adenocarcinoma of the bladder constitutes less than 2% of all primary bladder neoplasms. The majority of cases are single lesions, but multiple lesions have been observed, and they frequently are invasive at the time of initial presentation. The pathogenesis of these tumors is generally accepted to involve tumors that arise from columnar cell metaplasia (*i.e.*, cystitis cystica or glandularis); those of urachal origin; or those that form in an exstrophic bladder. The histologic pattern of these neoplasms is variable with individual cases showing a predominance of gland forma-

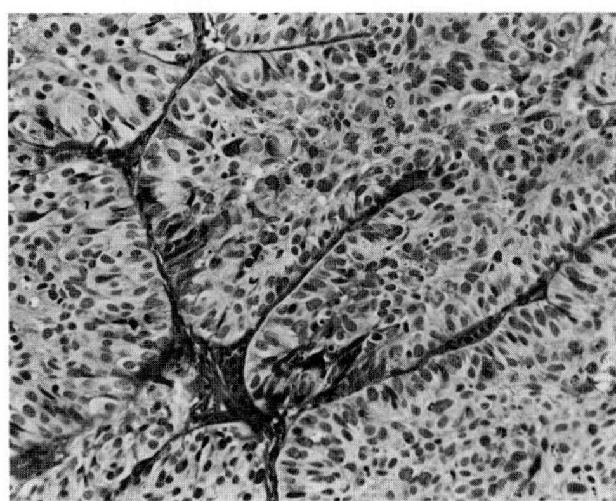

**Fig. 83.** Transitional Cell Carcinoma, grade 3. Marked nuclear pleomorphism and frequent mitoses associated with blunting and fusing of the papillae are present.

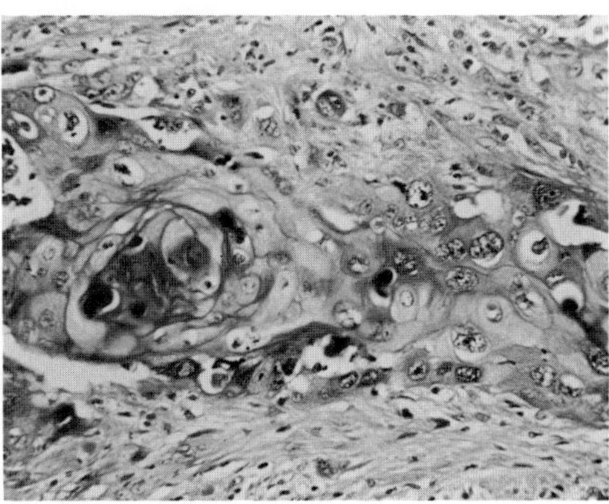

**Fig. 85.** Squamous Cell Carcinoma. Squamous differentiation as seen in this photograph was present uniformly throughout this invasive bladder neoplasm.

tion, papillary formation, or focal areas of admixed transitional cell carcinoma. Mucin production is common. The characteristic cytologic feature of these tumors is the presence of neoplastic columnar cells together with the intracytoplasmic production of mucin. There may be marked evidence of goblet cells reminiscent of colonic mucosa (Fig. 86).

Signet ring adenocarcinoma has also been reported as occurring in the bladder either primarily or mixed with transitional cell carcinoma. The signet ring cell carcinoma diffusely infiltrates the wall of the bladder, and neoplastic cells singly or in small clusters frequently in association with pools of mucin are observed. The nuclei of the tumor cells are displaced to one side by the intracellular, PAS-positive, mucicarmine-positive material (Fig. 87). Before the primary signet ring cell carcinoma can be diagnosed, appropriate diagnostic studies to eliminate another primary site with vesical metastases must be completed.

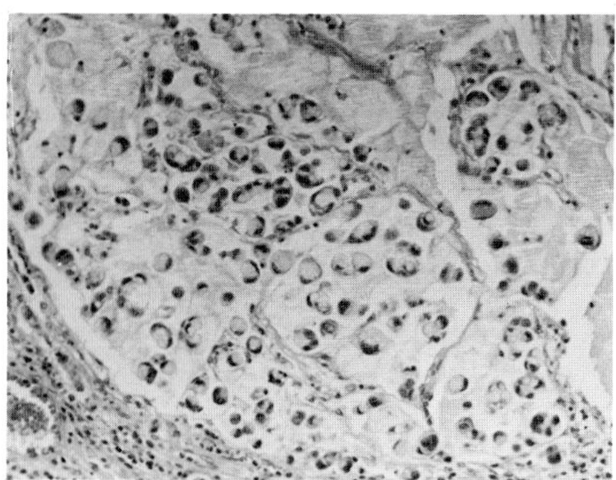

**Fig. 87.** Adenocarcinoma, Signet Ring Cell Type. The tumor cells with signet ring appearance are found in pools of extracellular mucin within the wall of the bladder.

## Rhabdomyosarcoma of the Bladder

Sarcoma botryoides (rhabdomyosarcoma of the bladder) is most common in young children but has occasionally been reported in adults. The gross appearance of this neoplasm is reminiscent of clusters of grapes. Histologically, rhabdomyosarcoma of the bladder is most commonly of the embryonal type with tumor cells in greatest density immediately beneath the mucosa. Deeper, the cells are dispersed in an edematous stroma. Cells with the diagnostic cross striations of neoplastic skeletal muscle cells are not always found (Fig. 88).

## Miscellaneous Primary Sarcomas

Miscellaneous sarcomas (*i.e.*, leiomyosarcoma, fibrosarcoma, etc.) have been described as rarely occurring in the bladder. These resemble sarcomas located in other areas.

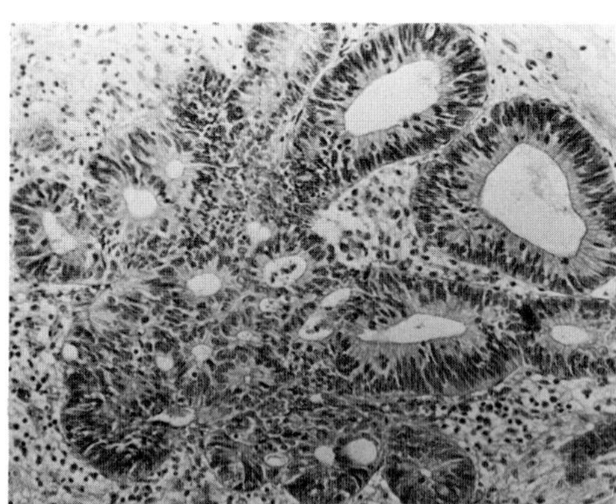

**Fig. 86.** Adenocarcinoma. A group of well differentiated glands lined by tumor cells with hyperchromatic nuclei are present. Several glands merge without intervening stroma.

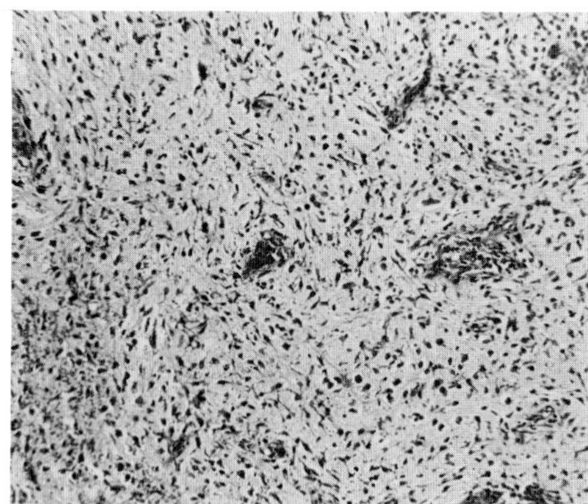

**Fig. 88.** Rhabdomyosarcoma. The stellate, round, and spindle-shaped tumor cells infiltrate an edematous stroma. Nuclei vary in size but are uniformly hyperchromatic.

### Metastatic Neoplasms to the Bladder

The involvement of the urinary bladder by direct extension from malignant neoplasms arising in adjacent organs such as cervix, endometrium, vagina, prostate, and colorectal organs, is not uncommon. Less frequent is metastatic involvement of the bladder by malignancies of distant sites, the most common of which are breast, lung, stomach, and skin.

# PROSTATE GLAND AND ACCESSORY SEX GLANDS

## NORMAL HISTOLOGY AND AGE RELATED CHANGES

### Prostate Gland

At the 11th week of fetal life, tubules begin to arise as outpouchings of the urethra, which will eventually form the lobes of the adult prostate gland. At birth, the prostate gland exhibits squamous metaplasia due to maternal estrogens and chorionic gonadotropins. This resolves rapidly, and the prostate develops into the pattern of transitional-epithelium-lined ducts within a fibromuscular stroma, seen until puberty when the prostate begins to exhibit its adult characteristics. In adulthood, the prostate gland is composed of 30 to 50 tubuloalveolar glands (acini) in a fibromuscular stroma, all enclosed in a fibrous capsule composed of collagen and elastic fibers. The excretory ducts enter the prostatic urethra. The secretory component is composed of alveoli of variable size and shape. The mucosa commonly shows papillary (''saw tooth'') projections with fibrovascular cores. The epithelium is pseudostratified columnar cells with basal nuclei, the outermost epithelial cells being oriented circumferentially. This same cell population lines the ducts throughout most of their length to the urethra, where there is a change to transitional cell epithelium (Fig. 89).

The fibromuscular stroma contains smooth muscle, elastic fibers, and collagen with random orientation. Skeletal muscle fibers are observed in the stroma of the most peripheral areas of the prostate gland. In addition, capillaries, myelinated and nonmyelinated nerves, and lymphatics are present in the stroma. Secretions are present in the alveolar and ductal lumina. Concretions with concentric laminations (corpora amylacea) are observed with increasing frequency with age. These may calcify, forming the typical prostatic calculi. From age 40 to 60, patients may have patchy atrophy throughout the prostate gland, with an increase in the collagen tissue. After patients have reached the age of 60, mucosa of the acini demonstrates widespread atrophy, associated with the diminished overall size of the acini. Scattered lymphocytes are commonly observed in the stroma and do not signify the presence of chronic prostatitis.

### Seminal Vesicles

The mucosal lining of the seminal vesicle is a complex pattern of papillary structures that frequently fuse to form anastomosing bridges. The mucosal lining cells are arranged in a pseudo-

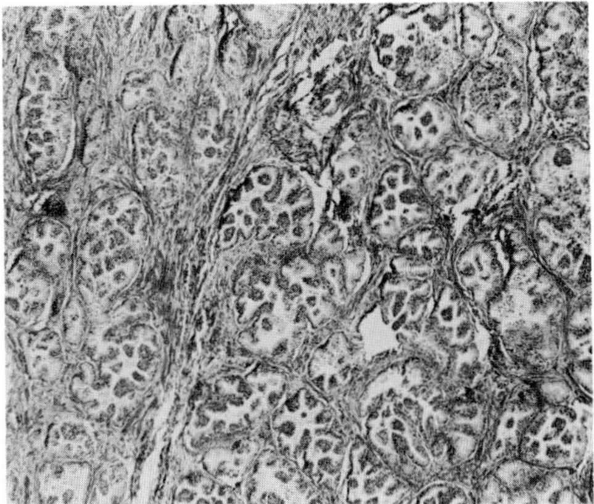

**Fig. 89.** Normal Prostate. The prostatic acini are uniformly distributed with intervening fibromuscular stroma.

stratified pattern and are composed of low columnar or cuboidal cells. The epithelium contains secretory granules with a lipochrome pigment that appears brownish-yellow. The submucosa is a mixture of circumferential smooth muscle fibers and collagen. The histologic changes observed with increasing age include

Nonuniform atrophy of the mucosa

Occurrence of scattered atypical mucosal lining cells with enlarged hyperchromatic nuclei

Increasing collagenous fibrosis with concurrent diminution in smooth muscle in the submucosa

Occasional glands with submucosal calcification associated with the collagenous fibrosis (Fig. 90)

### Cowper's Gland

Cowper's glands are tubuloalveolar glands located in the membranous urethra, the main excretory ducts of which enter on the floor of the proximal bulbous urethra. The secretory components of the gland are composed of alveoli separated by thin fibrous septa continuous with the periglandular fibrous capsule. The septation is incomplete in many areas, and adjacent alveoli fuse. The secretory cells have a varied appearance in different functional states from cuboidal to tall columnar with basal nuclei. The lumen of the alveolus is present only when the lining cells are low columnar or cuboidal, being obliterated when the lining cells assume greater size. The cytoplasm is clear or granular. Secretions are present in the lumina of both alveoli and ducts (Fig. 91).

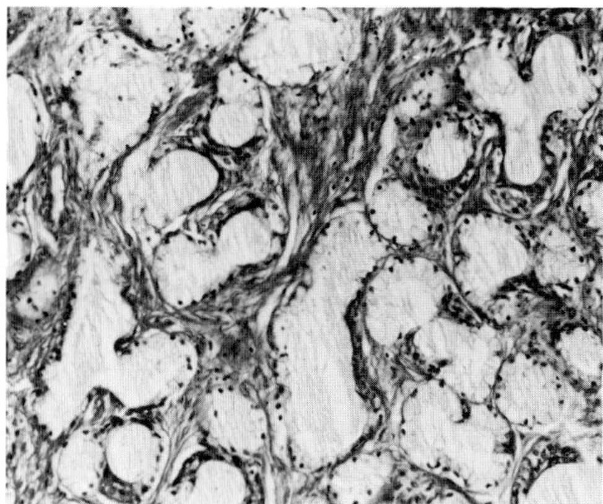

**Fig. 91.** Normal Cowper's Gland. The tubular-acinar glands are lined by mucous-secreting cells with abundant clear cytoplasm.

## INFARCTION OF THE PROSTATE

Infarction of the prostate is most commonly observed in association with prostatic hyperplasia. Histologically, coagulative necrosis of an area of the prostate, associated on occasion with frank hemorrhage into the infarct area, is observed. An acute inflammatory infiltrate is present around the margins and within the infarcted area. Healing results in the production of a fibrous scar with loss of the normal architectural components of the prostate in the affected area. Squamous metaplasia in the prostatic acini

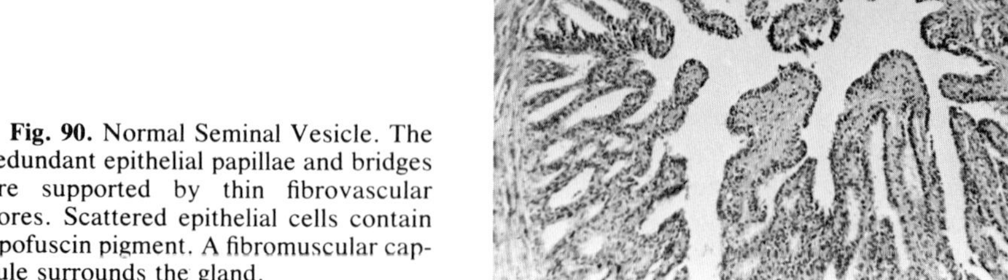

**Fig. 90.** Normal Seminal Vesicle. The redundant epithelial papillae and bridges are supported by thin fibrovascular cores. Scattered epithelial cells contain lipofuscin pigment. A fibromuscular capsule surrounds the gland.

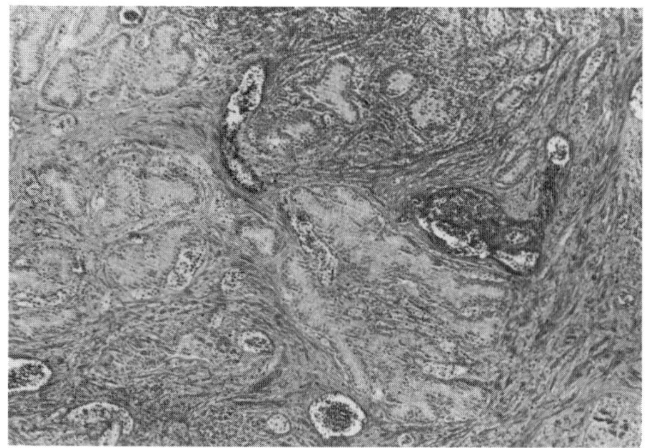

**Fig. 92.** Infarct of the Prostate. This recent infarct shows coagulative necrosis and sloughing of the glandular epithelium.

adjacent to the infarcted areas is observed on occasion (Figs. 92 and 93).

## INFLAMMATORY DISEASES

### Acute Prostatitis

The presence of acute inflammation in prostatic fragments obtained by a transurethral resection is a common incidental finding.

Acute prostatitis, which is rarely biopsied, is most commonly diagnosed by clinical means. The histopathology of acute prostatitis is that of large numbers of neutrophils and necrotic debris within the ducts and acini, as well as the adjacent stroma. Necrosis of the ductal and acinar lining epithelium is present. Microabscesses with localized destruction of prostatic glands and stroma are frequently seen; rarely these areas will coalesce to form a large abscess. With destruction of prostatic parenchyma, ultimate resolution results in fibrous scar formation (Fig. 94).

### Chronic Prostatitis

BACTERIAL PROSTATITIS. The failure of acute bacterial prostatitis to resolve results in the evolution of chronic bacterial prostatitis. The histopathology of chronic prostatitis is characterized by significant numbers of lymphocytes, plasma cells, histiocytes, and neutrophils in the prostatic stroma (Figs. 95 and 96). Localized collections of lymphocytes alone in the prostatic stroma are not regarded as abnormal, nor indicative of ongoing prostatitis.

GRANULOMATOUS PROSTATITIS. **Specific Etiology.** Granulomatous prostatitis

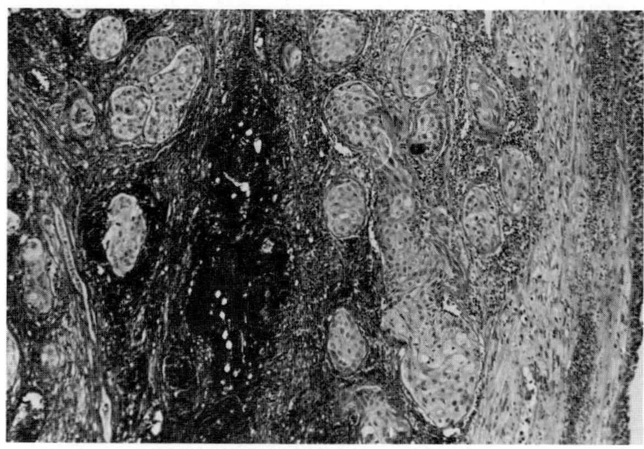

**Fig. 93.** Infarct of the Prostate. The hemorrhagic infarct on the left is associated with squamous metaplasia of the adjacent prostatic acini.

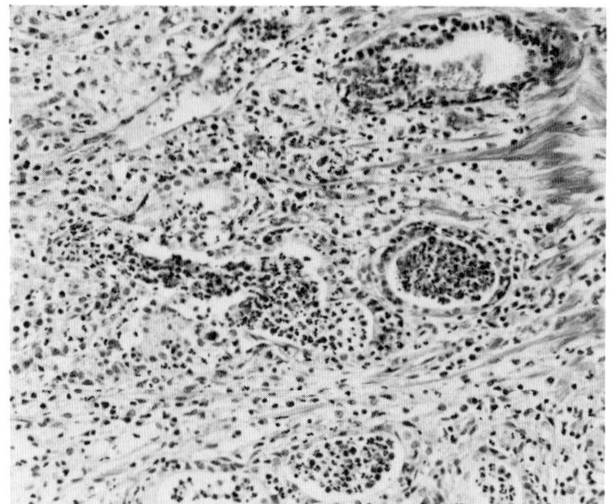

**Fig. 94.** Acute Prostatitis. Numerous neutrophils are present within the stroma and acini with focal necrosis of glandular epithelium.

may be associated with specific infections such as tuberculosis, brucellosis, cryptococcosis, coccidioidomycosis, and blastomycosis. In addition, echinococcal disease with cyst formation has been observed in the prostate. The histopathologic features, with the use of special stains to demonstrate the organisms, in combination with the clinical picture and culture of prostatic tissue secretions, will assist in the diagnosis of the specific etiology. All of these causes of chronic prostatitis will histologically resemble nonspecific granulomatous prostatitis (Fig. 97).

**Nonspecific Etiology.** Nonspecific granulomatous prostatitis constitutes no more than 1% to 4% of all specimens of prostatitis evaluated histologically. The principal clinical feature of these lesions is their tendency to mimic prostatic cancer on physical examination. Microscopically, these lesions must be differentiated from specific infective granulomas, which can be identified by special histologic stains or culture procedures.

The etiology of this disorder is unknown, but possible mechanisms include an inflammatory response to inspissated prostatic secretions, which may leak from the duct into the adjacent stroma, and bacterial products resulting from localized prostatic duct obstruction.

Histopathologic features include

Noncaseating granulomas with lymphocytes, plasma cells, and histiocytes, some of which exhibit multinucleation

Localized destruction of the prostatic ducts and acini

Resultant fibrosis in the late stages of development (Fig. 98)

In addition, an eosinophilic type of nonspecific granulomatous prostatitis has been described, which has the above features in addition to

Large numbers of eosinophils in the inflammatory exudate

Granulomas with central fibrinoid necrosis

Associated necrotizing vasculitis of prostatic vessels in many cases

Association with systemic or pulmonary allergic diathesis

MALAKOPLAKIA has been reported as occurring in the prostate. This may be found incidentally following a transure-

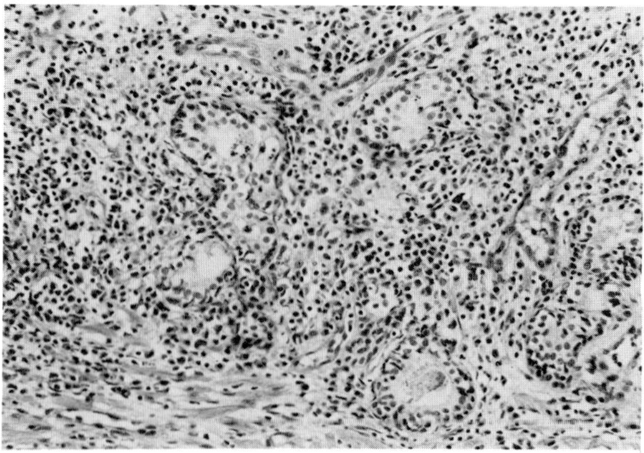

**Fig. 95.** Chronic Prostatitis. A dense infiltrate of lymphocytes is present in the stroma and within destroyed prostatic acini.

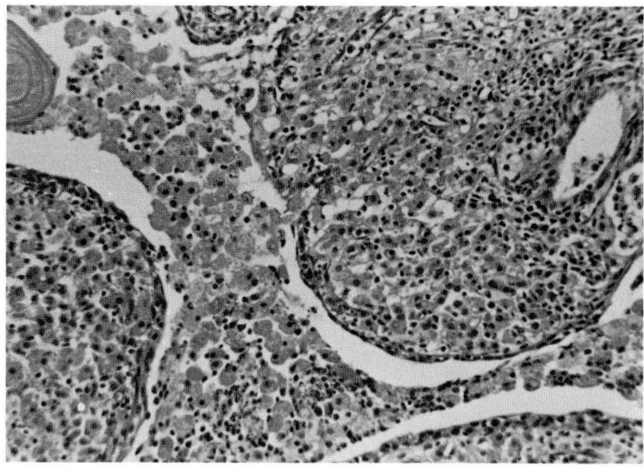

**Fig. 96.** Chronic Prostatitis. The inflammatory cell infiltrate is composed predominantly of histiocytes with fewer lymphocytes and plasma cells.

thral resection or may present as a prostatic nodule mimicking carcinoma. Histologically this is identical to malakoplakia of the bladder (see Malakoplakia of Bladder for a further description).

## BENIGN PROSTATIC HYPERPLASIA

Benign prostatic hyperplasia is a common disorder characterized by nodular hyperplasia of prostatic acini, stroma, or both, in men middle aged and older. Clinically significant enlargement is far less frequent than the overall incidence of 50% to 60% in men aged 40 or over. When the enlarged nodules, located in the lateral and middle lobes of the prostate, are of sufficient size, they are noted to compress the urethral lumen. A rim of compressed tissue (nonhyperplastic prostate) surrounds the nodules, resulting in a pseudocapsule (Fig. 99). Histologically, the hyperplasia may be predominantly acinar (epithelial), or stromal (smooth muscle and collagen), or combinations of both. The hyperplastic acini are clustered, of regular outline, and with frequent papillary projections. The lining cells are columnar to cuboidal and overlie smaller basal cells, giving the appearance of two rows of nuclei. Little or no pleomorphism is present, and mitoses are only rarely observed (Fig. 100).

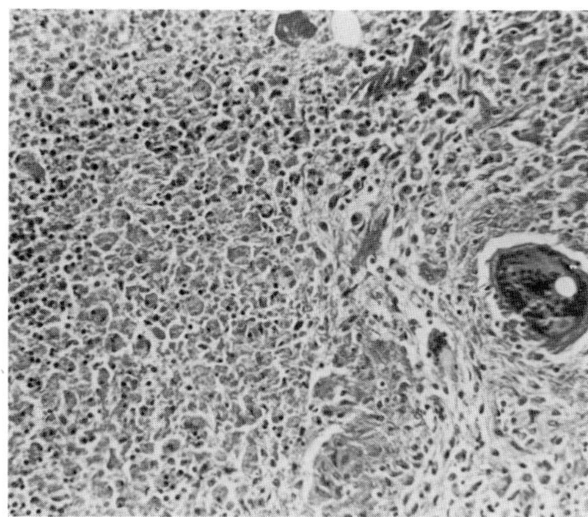

**Fig. 97.** Tuberculosis of the Prostate. A Langhans' giant cell on the right is adjacent to an area of necrosis with scattered lymphocytes and histiocytes. Special stain disclosed acid-fast organisms present in the lesion.

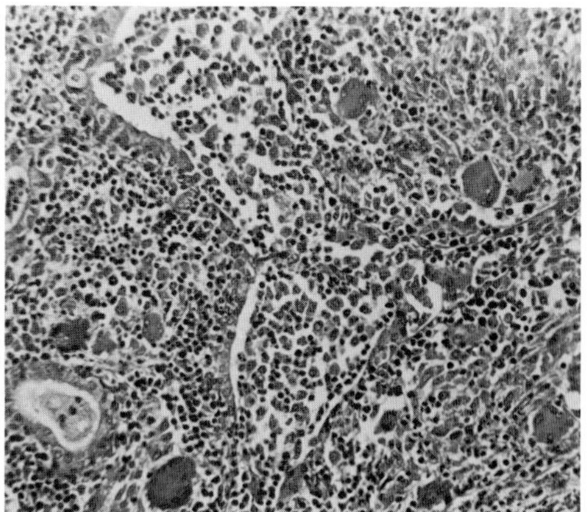

**Fig. 98.** Nonspecific Granulomatous Prostatitis. Numerous lymphocytes, histiocytes, and giant cells infiltrate the stroma with destruction of the prostatic acini. No organisms were found with the use of special stains.

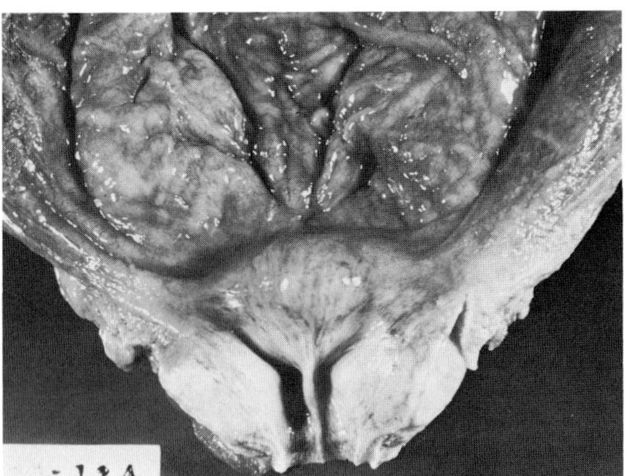

**Fig. 99.** Prostatic Hyperplasia. The enlarged prostate, partially obstructing the vesicle outlet, causes muscular hypertrophy and trabeculation of the bladder wall.

On occasion the stromal component may dominate, with obliteration of adjacent glands by the compression of the smooth muscle and collagen (Fig. 101). Frequently associated with these changes are foci of chronic inflammation, inspissated secretions, squamous metaplasia, and corpora amylacea.

## MALIGNANT NEOPLASMS

### Adenocarcinoma of the Prostate

Adenocarcinoma of the prostatic acini is the second most common malignancy by incidence and third most common cause of death in men. By histologic type, these represent 96% of all prostatic carcinomas. Prostatic hyperplasia and adenocarcinoma frequently coexist, but no role in carcinogenesis has been demonstrated for benign prostatic hyperplasia. Prostatic adenocarcinoma may occur as a single lesion, but more commonly it is multifocal. The interface with the non-neoplastic prostate may be irregular or well demarcated.

The microscopic description of prostatic carcinoma is best discussed in two separate categories: glandular patterns and cellular features. The glandular pattern may vary with the small, regular glands, lying back to back without significant intervening stroma, representing

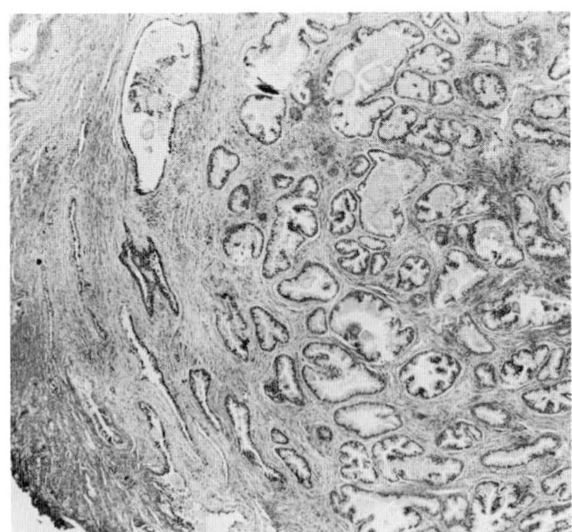

**Fig. 100.** Prostatic Hyperplasia. The columnar acinar-lining epithelium is present in two layers. Numerous papillary projections are present in the enlarged acini.

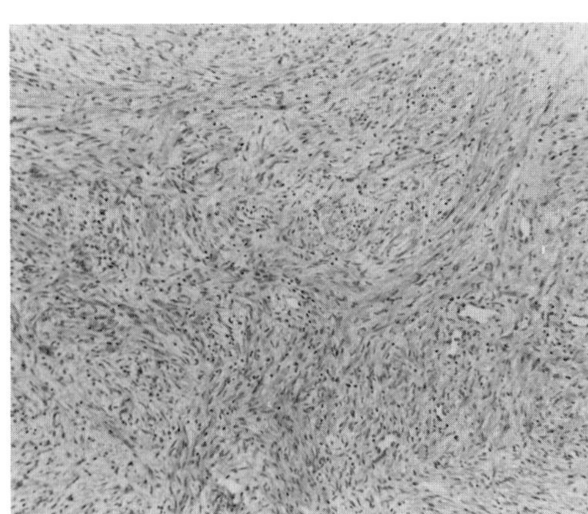

**Fig. 101.** Prostatic Hyperplasia. The stromal nodule, devoid of acini, is composed of fibromuscular tissue.

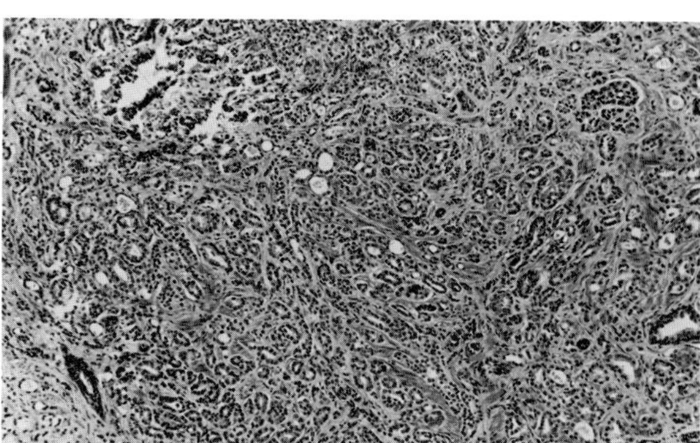

**Fig. 102.** Adenocarcinoma of the Prostate, Gleason grade 3. Small single glands and individual tumor cells infiltrate the prostatic stroma.

the most well-differentiated pattern (Figs. 102 and 103). Moderately differentiated tumors may show glandular structure that varies from large branching glands with increasing stroma among them, to the papillary infoldings or cribriform (gland-in-gland) pattern (Fig. 104). Poorly differentiated tumors may exhibit glands of irregular patterns or infiltrating sheets, cords, or nests of tumor cells without definitive gland formation (Figs. 105 and 106). More than one pattern may appear within a single prostate gland.

The cellular features include nuclear changes and cytoplasmic variations. Cell borders are well defined in the low-grade tumors. The nuclei tend to be uniform in size, shape, and staining quality in the well differentiated lesions, but these features vary as the tumor becomes less differentiated. Mitotic figures are rarely seen. The cytoplasm is usually eosinophilic but may be clear (hypernephroid pattern).

In the microscopic recognition of prostatic adenocarcinoma, very well differentiated neoplasms may be exceedingly difficult to diagnose. The low-power evaluation of the specimen for the presence of small glands, haphazard arrangement of glands, and glands lacking a double cell layer and a surrounding fibrous stroma should suggest the presence of prostatic adenocarcinoma. Unequivocal evidence of malignancy includes the presence of lymphatic, perineural space and capsular or seminal vesicle invasion.

Gleason has devised a grading system for prostatic carcinoma on the basis of the glandular pattern. Both the primary and secondary glandular patterns are graded I to V, and the numbers are added together to form a combined score. Grade I glands are very well differentiated, round to oval, uniform in size, and closely packed (see Fig. 102). Grade II glands are also well differentiated, the glands round to oval shape, but they vary slightly more than the glands in the Grade I pattern. There is also more stroma intervening between the glands (see Fig. 103). The most common pattern

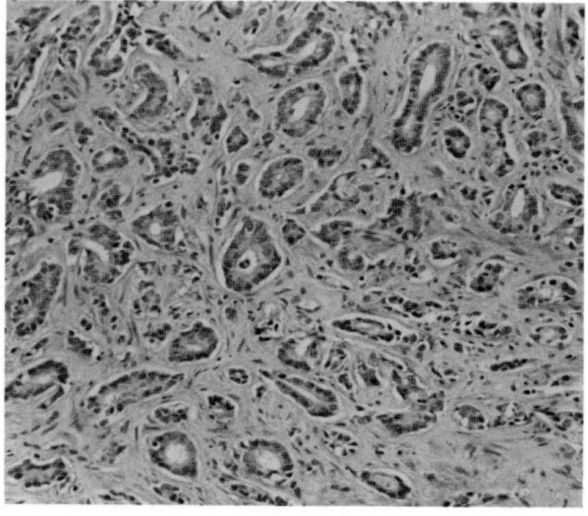

**Fig. 103.** Adenocarcinoma of the Prostate, Gleason grade 3. Neoplastic glands lined with a single layer of tumor cells are separated by stroma in which individual tumor cells are infiltrating.

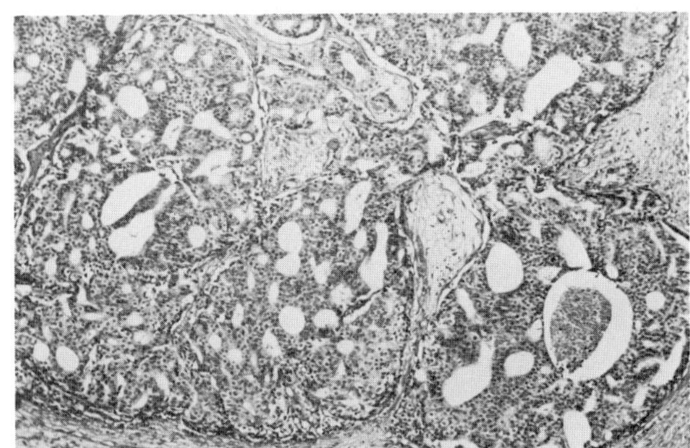

**Fig. 104.** Adenocarcinoma of the Prostate, Gleason grade 3. Tumor cells in large nests have a cribriform arrangement. One focus of tumor cell necrosis is present on the right.

is Grade III, which is moderately differentiated. Two subpatterns are recognized, the single, separate glands that can vary significantly in size and are more elongated and widely separated; the second pattern is that of the papillary or cribriform pattern (see Fig. 104). Gleason Grade IV tumors are poorly differentiated and appear as irregular masses of fused glands (see Fig. 105). These grow raggedly and infiltrate the stroma in an aggressive manner. A secondary form included in the Grade IV category is that of the "hypernephroid" or clear cell pattern. The fifth Gleason grade consists of very poorly differentiated tumors, with minimal glandular formation (see Fig. 106). These infiltrate as masses or nests of tumor cells. Also included as Grade V are the signet ring cell tumors. The patient's prognosis is inversely proportional to the Gleason grade.

Squamous metaplasia may occur in the cells of the prostate gland following estrogen treatment for prostatic carcinoma. There is vacuolization of the epithelial cells and rupture of the cells with extrusion of the nuclei. Some cells show pyknosis and atrophy (Fig. 107).

## Ductal Adenocarcinoma of the Prostate

Adenocarcinoma taking origin in the prostatic ducts has been reported in approximately 58 cases. The presentation and laboratory picture are identical to those of adenocarcinoma of the acini, including elevation of acid phosphatase level and the presence of osteoblastic bone lesions. This adenocarcinoma has been further divided into two groups:

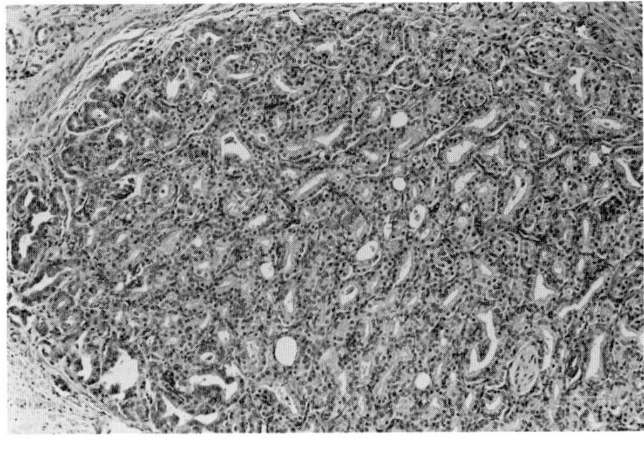

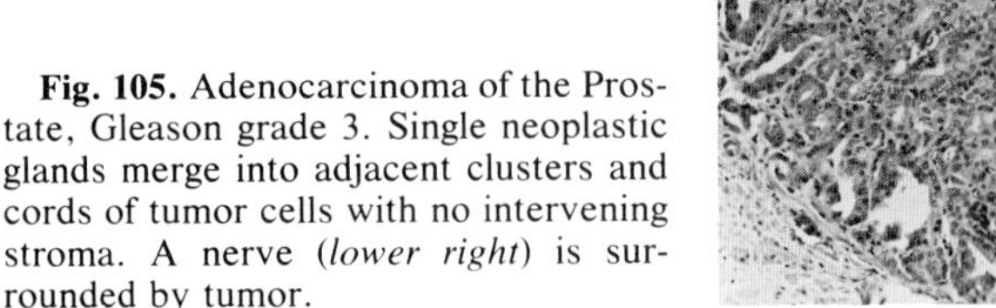

**Fig. 105.** Adenocarcinoma of the Prostate, Gleason grade 3. Single neoplastic glands merge into adjacent clusters and cords of tumor cells with no intervening stroma. A nerve (*lower right*) is surrounded by tumor.

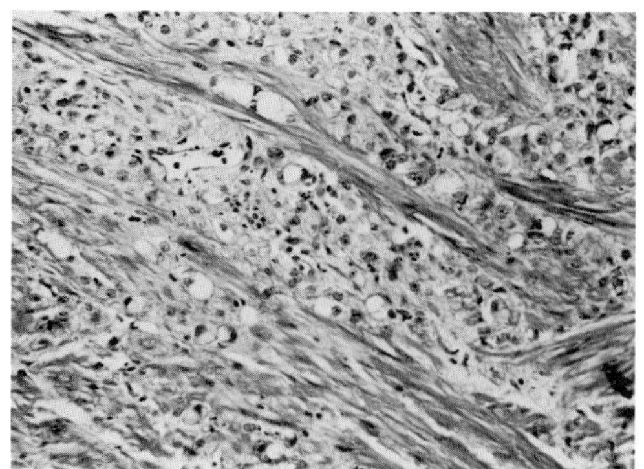

**Fig. 106.** Adenocarcinoma of the Prostate, Gleason pattern 5. The tumor cells infiltrate the fibromuscular stroma in cords and single cells with no evidence of gland formation.

adenocarcinoma of the primary and secondary prostatic ducts. The characteristics of the adenocarcinoma of the primary prostatic ducts are

A neoplasm with papillary formation located in dilated periurethral duct spaces

Columnar lining cells with basal nuclei and a moderate amount of pale cytoplasm

Tumor cells demonstrating stainable glycogen and acid phosphatase activity, with negative stains for mucin (Fig. 108)

Adenocarcinoma taking origin in the secondary prostatic ducts are characterized by a neoplastic proliferation of columnar cells with clear to eosinophilic cytoplasm, involving the smaller prostatic ducts in a low papillary, comedo, or cribriform pattern.

Both type may show intraductal extension as well as invasion of the prostatic stroma. These may be present as focal areas, admixed with a predominating carcinoma of acinar origin.

## "Endometrial Carcinoma" of Prostate

In 1967, Melicow and associates described a prostatic carcinoma composed of columnar cells with infoldings and papillary projections in a tumor located principally near the verumontanum. The overall pattern and cytologic features were interpreted as being similar to endometrial carcinoma, and the neoplasm was termed "endometrial carcinoma of the prostatic utricle." This may represent a variant of the ductal adenocarcinoma of the prostate and not a malignancy of mullerian origin. The histologic features of carcinoma that can be interpreted as endometrial include

Neoplastic glands with papillary projections, cribriform pattern, or mixture of both

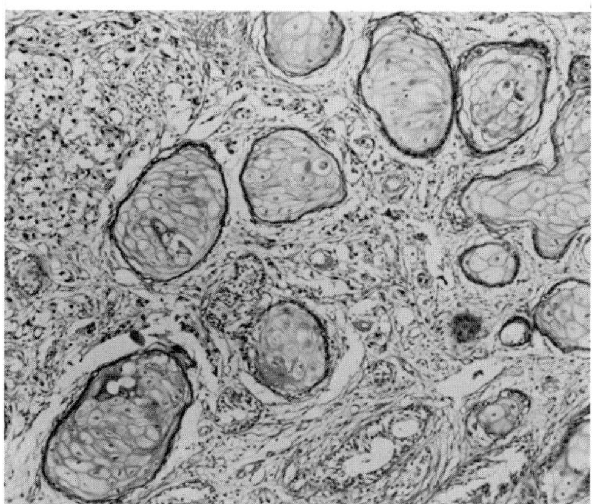

**Fig. 107.** Adenocarcinoma of the Prostate with Estrogen Therapy Effect. The poorly differentiated adenocarcinoma (Gleason pattern 5) shows uniform pyknotic nuclei infiltrating the stroma adjacent to glands with squamous metaplasia.

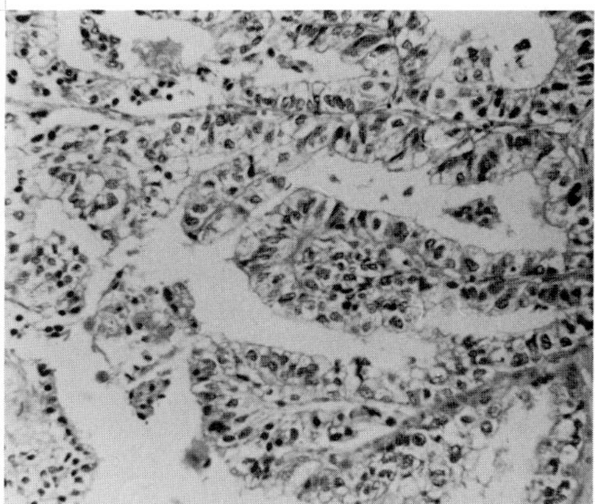

**Fig. 108.** Prostatic Duct Adenocarcinoma. Dilated prostatic ducts with neoplastic cells in a papillary configuration surround similar cells lying free in the lumen. The cytoplasm of the cells is clear, and there is loss of nuclear polarity.

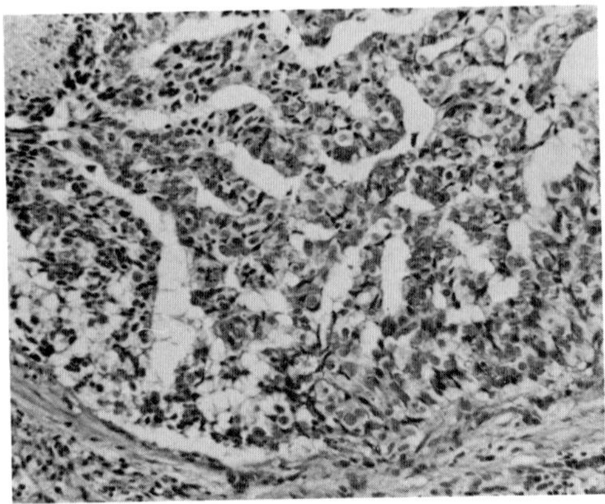

**Fig. 109.** "Endometrial" Adenocarcinoma of the Prostate. The dilated duct is filled with a papillary neoplasm showing bridging and cells with eosinophilic cytoplasm. Elsewhere the tumor formed glands lined by columnar cells with similar appearance.

Glands and papillae lined by tall columnar cells, commonly showing dark eosinophilic cytoplasm and hyperchromatic basal nuclei

Occasional tumor with subnuclear vacuolization or cilia on luminal surface

Electron microscopic and histochemical studies, although limited in number have not supported the endometrial origin of these last-described neoplasms (Fig. 109).

### Mucinous Carcinoma of the Prostate

Histologically mucinous neoplasms are composed of acini of varying size filled with extracellular mucin. The tumor cells, columnar mucous-secreting or typical signet ring, line the acini or appear to float free in pools of mucin. Merging of this pattern with the more typical pattern of adenocarcinoma of acinar origin has been observed (Fig. 110).

### Transitional Carcinoma of the Prostate

The most common histologic type of prostatic carcinoma of ductal origin is transitional cell carcinoma. When confined to the ducts, the tumor cells frequently fill and distend the ductal lumen, and papillary configurations are not present. The cytologic features are identical to those of transitional cell carcinoma in any other location of the urinary tract. Infiltration of the prostate usually takes the form of cords or individual tumor cells. Retrograde spread within the prostatic ductal system to the prostatic acini is observed. Because the tumors take origin from the most distal segment of the prostatic ducts as they enter the prostatic urethra, *in situ* spread to the urethra and, on occasion, bladder has been reported. Perineural and lymphatic invasion has been reported (Fig. 111).

### Squamous Cell Carcinoma of the Prostate

Histologically, squamous cell carcinoma is a rare neoplasm characterized by invasive nests or cords of cohesive squamous cells, showing intercellular bridges and, in some instances, squamous pearl formation. The cytologic features are those of malignant squamous cells with hyperchromatic nuclei with variable pleomorphism and mitotic activity. No instance of mixed squamous cell carcinoma and adenocarcinoma has been reported (Fig. 112).

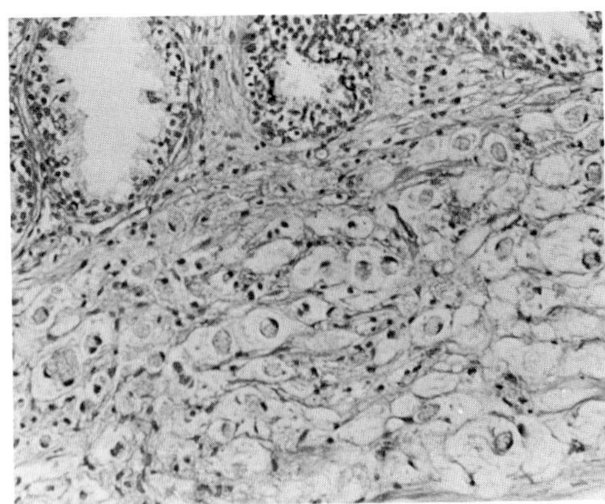

**Fig. 110.** Mucinous Adenocarcinoma of the Prostate. Signet ring cells, lying in secreted mucin, infiltrate the prostatic stroma.

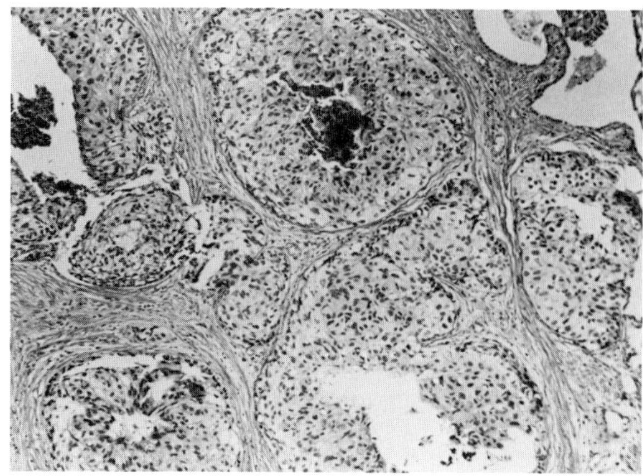

**Fig. 111.** Prostatic Transitional Cell Carcinoma. The neoplastic transitional epithelium fill many affected distal prostatic ducts. Necrotic tumor cells are present in the lumen of two ducts.

# URETHRA

## NORMAL HISTOLOGY

The male prostatic urethra is lined by transitional cell urothelium in continuity with that of the bladder. The transitional epithelium of the prostatic urethra makes a gradual change to stratified columnar epithelium in the membranous and penile portions of the urethra. In the roof of the penile urethra are scattered the mucous-secreting glands of Littre, which empty into recesses the lacunae of Morgagni. The most distal portion of the urethra outward from the fossa navicularis is lined by stratified squamous epithelium. The bulbourethral, or Cowper's, glands present in the membranous urethra are mucous-secreting glands of the tubuloalveolar type, which open into the floor of the bulbous urethra (Fig. 113).

As in the male, the transitional cell epithelium of the bladder of the female urethra is continuous with the proximal 1 cm to 1.5 cm. This gradually changes to stratified columnar epithelium, which, in turn, becomes squamous epithelium near the external urethral orifice. Mucosal invaginations with minimal penetration of the periurethral tissue (urethral lacunae) are more common in the proximal urethra. The periurethral glands of Skene, histologically similar to the glands of Littre in the male, are more prevalent in the distal urethra.

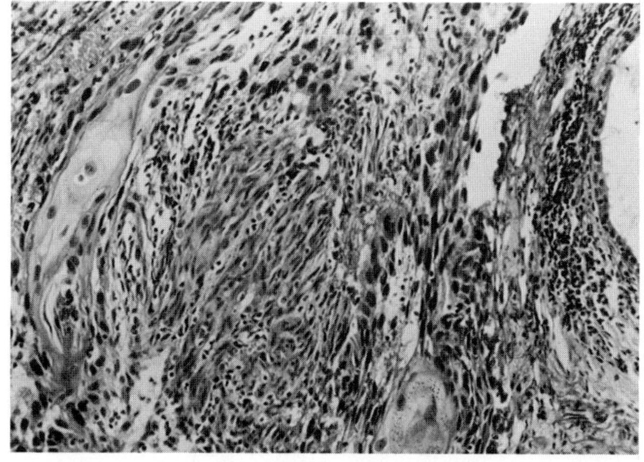

**Fig. 112.** Prostatic Squamous Cell Carcinoma. The neoplasm with uniform and prominent squamous differentiation infiltrates the prostatic stroma. Abundant lymphocytes are intermixed adjacent to the tumor.

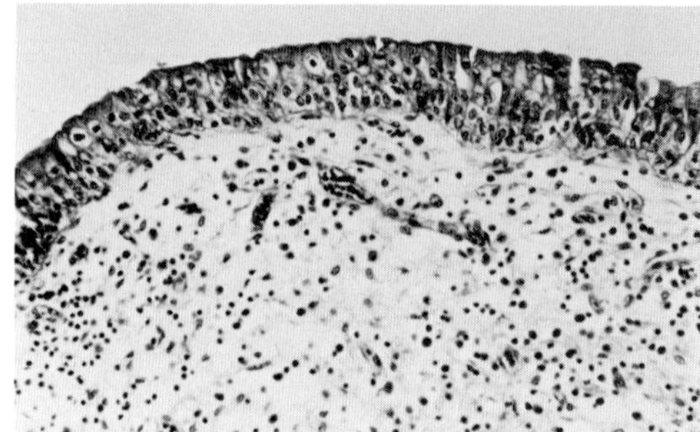

**Fig. 113.** Normal Urethra. The stratified columnar epithelium of the urethra overlies the fibrous tissue of the lamina propria. Scattered lymphocytes are present in the lamina propria.

## NON-NEOPLASTIC DISORDERS

### Urethral Diverticulum

Diverticula of the urethra, virtually limited to women, are thought to develop in association with periurethral gland inflammation and obstruction. Most cases involve women aged 25 to 45 years. Endometriosis and carcinoma have been reported in association with these diverticula.

### Adenomatous Polyp

Adenomatoid (polypoid or papillary) lesions arise from or near the verumontanum in young males. The surface and glandular structures are lined by columnar cells with the appearance of prostatic acini. Some authors regard these lesions as ectopic prostatic tissue (Fig. 114).

### Fibroepithelial Polyp

Polyps of the urethra are most commonly observed in children. The overlying epithelial surface is similar to that described for polypoid urethritis. The stroma is characterized by abundant fibromuscular connective tissue devoid of the chronic inflammatory cells and numerous thin-walled vascular channels present in polypoid urethritis.

### Urethral Caruncle

Urethral caruncle occurs exclusively in women, most frequently after menopause. Caruncles are inflammatory lesions that are found near the urethral meatus and may be associated with pain and bleeding. These usually occur on the ventral surface of the urethra and appear as protruding red masses. The etiology and pathogenesis are unsettled, but prolapse of the urethral mucosa with associated chronic inflammatory changes has been suggested.

The microscopic features of this lesion are those of acute and chronic inflammation of the mucosa and submucosa. The overlying mucosa is either squamous cell or transitional cell epithelium, frequently exhibiting ulceration, acanthosis, and hyperkeratosis. Occasionally dysplastic changes are present in the epithelium, and the lesion must be differentiated from carcinoma. The submucosa contains a variably dense infiltration of acute and chronic inflammatory cells and

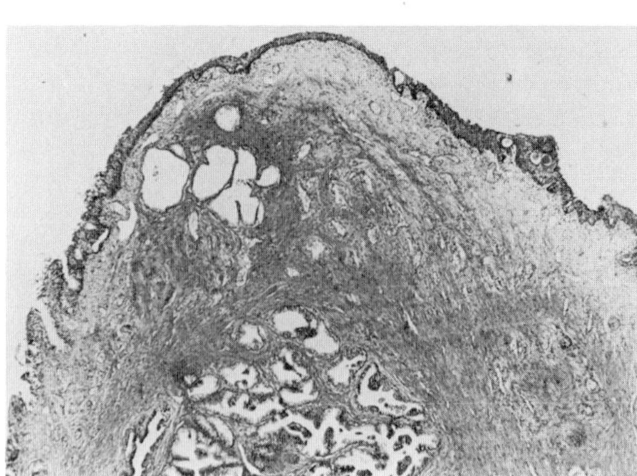

**Fig. 114.** Adenomatous Polyp (Ectopic Prostatic Tissue in the Urethra). The polypoid structure is covered with transitional cell urothelium. Multiple prostatic acinar structures are scattered throughout the fibromuscular stroma.

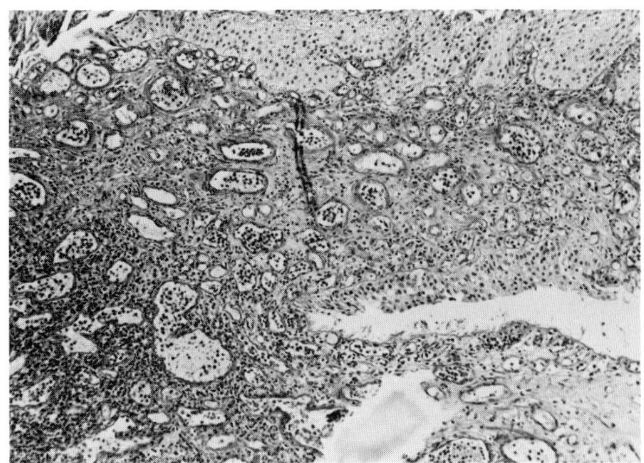

**Fig. 115.** Caruncle. The submucosa of the distal urethral segment contains numerous thin-walled blood vessels. Numerous acute and chronic inflammatory cells are present in the intervening stroma. Focal hyperplasia of the overlying mucosa is seen at the top.

increased numbers of thin-walled blood vessels. The blood vessels may be so numerous as to suggest a benign vascular neoplasm. The intervening stroma is edematous. Four major variants have been described:

Papillomatous
Angiomatous
Granulomatous
Mucinous

Although urethral malignancy has been reported in patients with a caruncle, there is no evidence that a caruncle is premalignant (Fig. 115).

### Polypoid Urethritis

Polypoid urethritis lesions are also known as inflammatory polyps and appear most often near the bladder neck. The polypoid lesions are characterized by the abundant inflammatory cells and numerous thin-walled blood vessels in an edematous fibrous stroma. The covering epithelial surfaces may show focal ulceration, hyperplasia, urethritis cystica, and squamous or mucinous metaplasia. The lesion is regarded as inflammatory in nature and not neoplastic.

### Condylomata Acuminata

Condylomata of the urethra have been reported in both men and women, but they are significantly less frequent there than on the penis or vulva (see under Penis). The histologic features of acanthosis and papillomatosis with the typical cytologic changes associated with this lesion are identical to those present in the exophytic lesions involving the penis and vulva (see Fig. 131).

### Miscellaneous Benign Lesions of the Urethra

Benign tumors of the urethra are extremely uncommon. Leiomyomata, hemangioma, and inverted papilloma have all been reported as presenting intraurethrally. Nephrogenic adenoma has also been described as occurring in the urethra. All of these lesions are identical histologically to their counterparts in other areas of the genitourinary tract.

## MALIGNANT NEOPLASMS

Carcinoma of the urethra is an uncommon lesion. It has been reported twice as often in the female urethra as in the male.

One third of male patients have a history of venereal disease and one third have a history of urethral stricture, which preceded the ultimate diagnosis. Approximately 75% to 80% of all urethral carcinoma is squamous cell type, approximately 15% transitional cell, 5% adenocarcinoma, and 1% undifferentiated. The most common locations for urethral carcinoma are the bulbomembranous urethra (55%) and the penile

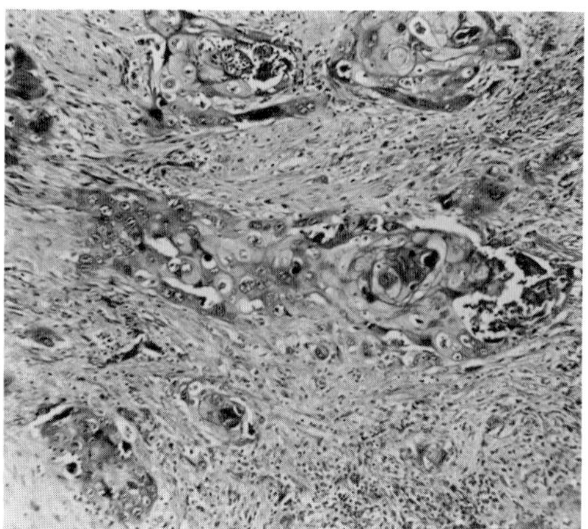

**Fig. 116.** Squamous Cell Carcinoma. Sheets and cords of malignant squamous cells invade the adjacent fibrous tissue of the urethral lamina propria.

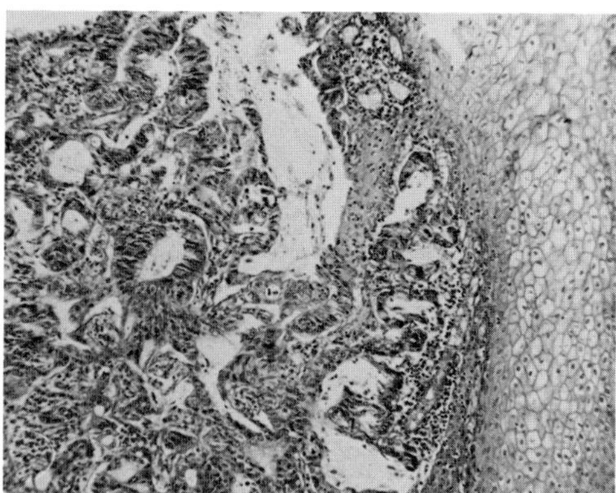

**Fig. 117.** Adenocarcinoma. Well-differentiated glands of the neoplasm cover the surface to the left of squamous cell epithelium of the distal urethra present on the right. Invasion of the underlying lamina propria by adenocarcinoma is present.

urethra (35%). Adenocarcinomas may occur secondary either to metaplasia of the urothelium or from neoplastic changes in the glands of Cowper or Littre.

In the female urethra, approximately 70% of all urethral carcinoma is squamous; 20%, adenocarcinoma; and almost 10%, transitional cell carcinoma. Undifferentiated carcinoma, malignant melanoma, cloacogenic carcinoma, and carcinoid and mesonephric carcinoma make up a total of 1% of urethral carcinoma in the female. Transitional cell carcinoma arises more commonly in the proximal urethra while squamous cell and adenocarcinoma arise more commonly in the distal urethra. Adenocarcinoma is thought to arise from Skene's ducts (Figs. 116–118).

# PENIS

## NORMAL HISTOLOGY

The lowermost layer of the epidermis of the penis is known as the *basal* layer and is composed of tall columnarlike cells. The epithelium here may project downward into the dermis, creating fingerlike projections known as the *rete pegs*. The granular layer is the second layer of skin and together with the basal layer constitutes the prickle layer. The granular layer is so named because of the appearance of the cells, nuclei of which become increasingly pyknotic and finally disappear. The outermost portion of the epidermis is the stratum corneum or horny layer. This skin is completely keratinized; the cells have no nuclei or granules; and cell boundaries are quite indistinct. The subcutaneous tissue contains sweat glands and smooth muscle but no adipose tissue or hair follicles. The corpora cavernosa penis and the corpora cavernosum urethra are composed of erectile tissue, anastomosing vascular channels, intervening collagenous fibrous tissue, scattered smooth muscle bundles, and elastic fibers (Fig. 119).

## INFLAMMATORY DISEASES

### Balanoposthitis

Balanoposthitis refers to inflammation of the glans penis (balanitis) and prepuce (posthitis). Inflammation of both may occur independently, but most commonly both are concurrently inflamed. A

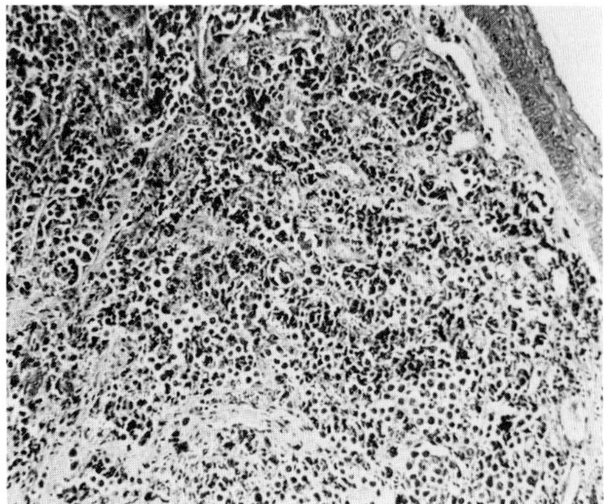

**Fig. 118.** Malignant Melanoma. The pigment-containing melanoma cells have infiltrated the lamina propria beneath adjacent normal urothelial lining of the urethra.

wide variety of causative agents have been identified, including both gram-positive and gram-negative organisms. This is common in diabetics. The histologic appearance in the majority of cases is nonspecific, and the lesion is characterized by an acute inflammatory reaction, (*i.e.*, infiltration of neutrophils with vascular dilatation and edema). Chronicity of the lesion results in the production of granulation tissue and fibrosis.

## Venereal Diseases

SYPHILIS. The disorder caused by the spirochete *Treponema pallidum*, transmitted by sexual intercourse, clinically evolves in three stages.

The characteristic lesion of primary syphilis is the chancre at the site of inoculation. The initially small papule ulcerates. The typical ulcer becomes firm with elevated margins resembling a button. The incubation period for syphilis averages 3 weeks. The diagnosis is definitively made by dark-field examination for the presence of the organism. Histologically, the inflammatory cell infiltrate has a predominance of plasma cells in association with lymphocytes and fewer neutrophils. A prominent feature is the obliterative endarteritis of the vessels in the base of the ulcer (Fig. 120).

The characteristic lesion of secondary syphilis is a diffuse maculopapular rash which, in the area of the original inoculation, may appear as an epidermal plaque, the condylomata lata. The histologic features of these lesions are similarly characterized by a predominating plasma cell infiltrate, underlying epidermal hyperplasia with papillomatosis, and acanthosis (Figs. 121 and 122).

The gumma, the lesion of tertiary syphilis, does not involve the penile skin.

CHANCROID is caused by a gram-negative coccobacillus, *Hemophilus ducreyi*. Clinically, these ulcers are shallow, soft, and quite painful to the touch. They are also associated with a painful enlarge-

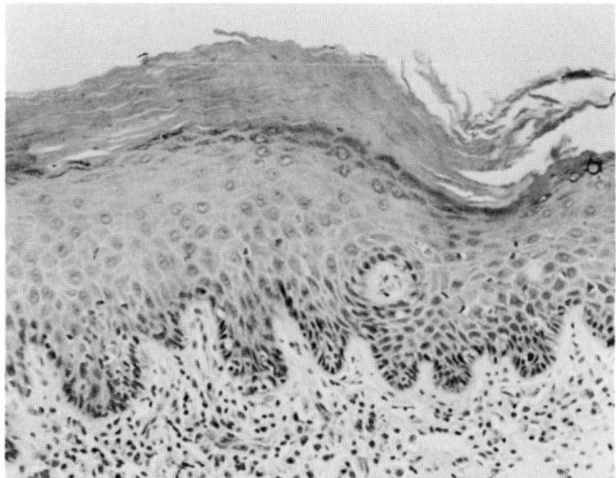

**Fig. 119.** Normal Penis. The epidermis demonstrates normal maturation to the granular layer with overlying hyperkeratosis.

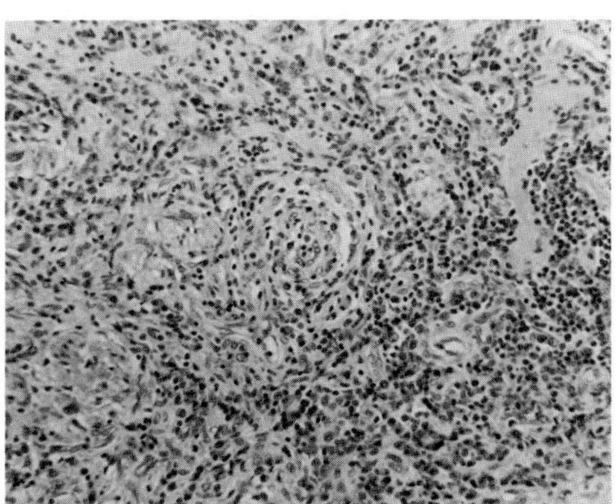

**Fig. 120.** Primary Syphilis. A dense infiltrate of plasma cells and lymphocytes surrounds and obliterates the vascular structure in the center.

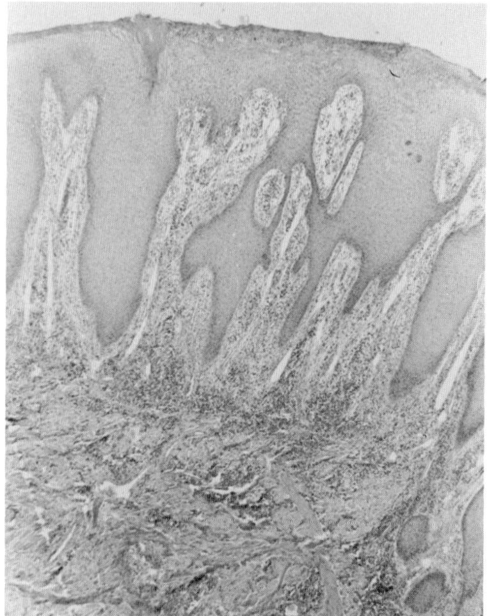

**Fig. 121.** Condyloma Lata. The epidermis shows hyperkeratosis and acanthosis. A dense infiltrate of plasma cells and lymphocytes is present in the underlying dermis.

ment of the regional lymph nodes. The incubation period is short, generally 1 to 5 days. Diagnosis is made by gram stain of the ulcer for the typical gram-negative rods. Histologically, the classic lesion has three zones. The most superficial layer of the ulcer is composed of necrotic tissue overlying the intermediate zone and composed of an acute inflammatory cell infiltrate with acute vasculitis of small vessels. The deepest zone is composed of changes characteristic of resolving acute inflammation—that is, fibroblastic proliferation and a mixed inflammatory cell infiltrate composed of lymphocytes, plasma cells, histiocytes, and neutrophils. Foci of necrosis with surrounding acute inflammatory cells are also observed in the affected regional lymph nodes in the groin (Fig. 123).

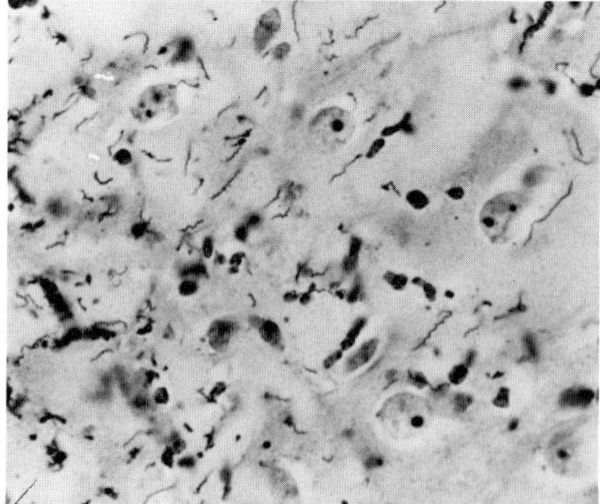

**Fig. 122.** Condyloma Lata. Spirochetes are demonstrated in the epidermis by use of the Warthin–Starry stain.

GRANULOMA INGUINALE infection is caused by the gram-negative coccobacillus *Donovania granulomatis*. Clinically, the initial lesion presents as a papule that enlarges to form an irregular ulcer, frequently with satellite lesions that may ultimately coalesce with the primary ulcer. Satellite ulcers also occur along the root of the lymphatic drainage. The incubation period is 1 to 12 weeks, and diagnosis is by biopsies and staining. Histologically, the ulcers are composed of necrotic debris on the surface with an

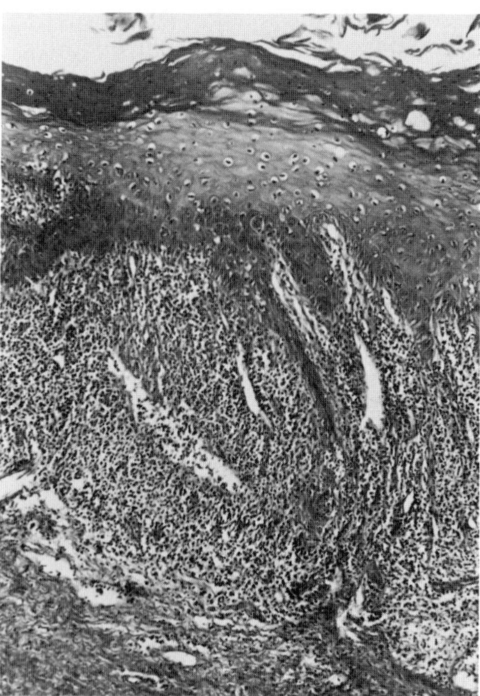

**Fig. 123.** Chancroid. A dense acute and chronic inflammatory cell infiltrate with acute vasculitis is present in the high dermis with papillomatosis of the epidermis adjacent to an ulcer. Gram stain disclosed the gram-negative rods.

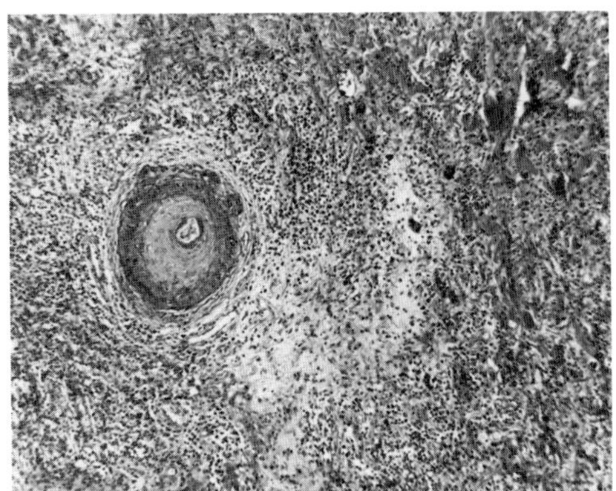

**Fig. 124.** Granuloma Inguinale. A dense acute and chronic inflammatory cell infiltrate associated with focal areas of tissue necrosis is present in the dermis.

overlying exuberant acute inflammatory cell infiltration (Fig. 124). An important histologic feature is the presence of varying numbers of histiocytes containing phagocytized bacteria called *Donovan bodies* (Fig. 125). This lesion tends to be more destructive and chronic than is chancroid. Healing is frequently associated with the production of fibrous scars in the region of the original and satellite ulcers.

LYMPHOGRANULOMA VENEREUM is the result of venereal inoculation by the L-1, L-2, or L-3 sera types of *Chlamydia trachomatis*. The incubation period is 2 days to 3 weeks. The infection is characterized by epidermal ulceration most commonly on the male penis or in the vagina or perirectal region of the female, with a prominent enlargement of regional lymph nodes. The primary lesion on the penis often will be missed. The diagnosis can be made by the lymphogranuloma venereum–complement fixation test, or by the intradermal Frei test. Fistulous connections with the skin or the rectum may exist. Histologically, the primary lesion is relatively nonspecific with epidermal necrosis, ulceration, and a prominent acute inflammatory response (Figs. 126 and 127). The deepest layers of the ulcer have the components of granulation tissue with fibrosis. Occasionally, defined granulomas with histiocytic giant cells may be present. The affected lymph nodes contain a necrotizing acute inflammatory response with prominent necrosis of the lymphatic tissue and frequently the perinodal tissue, resulting in draining sinus tracts to the overlying skin. The coalescing abscesses in the lymph nodes result in the classic "stellate abscesses" with the surrounding acute inflammatory cells and a mantle of histiocytes with occasional giant cells. Ultimate resolution results in a diffuse fibrous scarring and resultant lymphatic obstruction.

HERPES PROGENITALIS is caused by the herpesvirus type 2 and is subclinical in approximately 40% of cases. The cases occurring in men that are clinically apparent most commonly affect the prepuce and glans. The incubation period is 3 to 14 days at the time of initial infection and 12 to 24 hours for cases of reinfection. The lesions present as small vesicles that rupture, resulting in a small ulcer. Regional lymph nodes may be enlarged and tender. Culture is difficult but possible, and serologic tests are now available. Histologically, the characteristic findings of multinucleated epithelial cells with intranuclear inclusions are characteristic of herpes infection. The surrounding subcutaneous tissue contains an acute inflammatory cell infiltrate associated with stromal edema (Fig. 128).

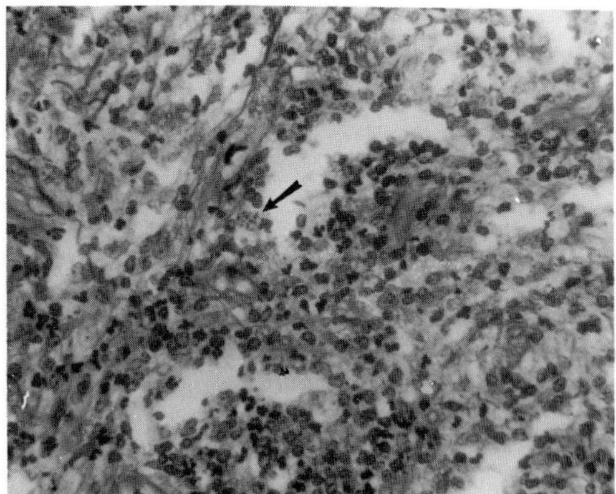

**Fig. 125.** Granuloma Inguinale. The inflammatory cells present include neutrophils, lymphocytes, plasma cells, and histiocytes with phagocytized bacteria (Donovan bodies) indicated by the *arrow*.

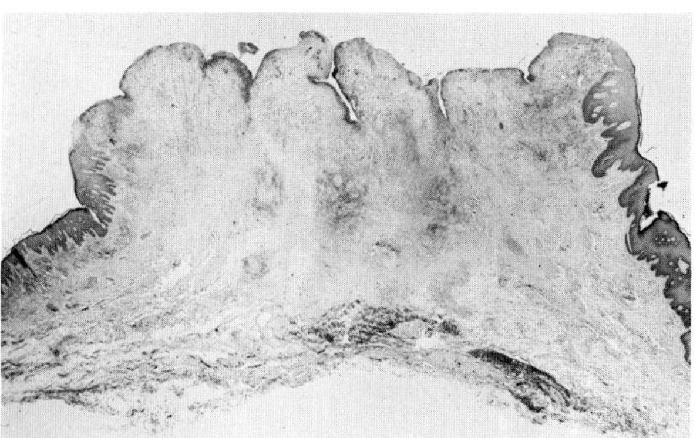

**Fig. 126.** Lymphogranuloma Venereum. The dermis and subcutaneous tissue beneath the epidermal ulcer contain all stages of healing with acute inflammation limited to the high dermis. The adjacent epidermis shows papillomatosis and acanthosis.

## MISCELLANEOUS PENILE DISORDERS

### Balanitis Xerotica Obliterans

Balanitis xerotica obliterans (lichen sclerosis et atrophicus), a disorder of the epidermis, most commonly involving the glans penis or prepuce of elderly men, is characterized clinically by small white macules to larger plaques in the epidermis. Histologically, the epidermis is thin with associated hyperkeratosis. The underlying papillary dermis has a diffuse amorphous collagenous fibrosis with associated stromal edema and lymphatic infiltration in the reticular dermis (Fig. 129).

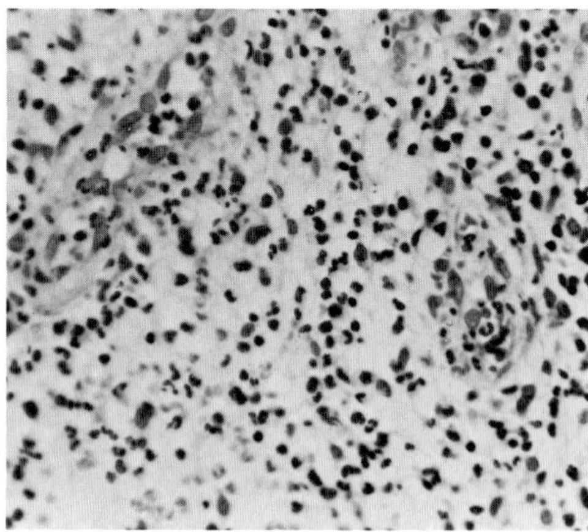

**Fig. 127.** Lymphogranuloma Venereum. The inflammatory cell infiltrate of the dermis is nonspecific with neutrophils, lymphocytes, and occasional histiocytes.

### Peyronie's Disease

A disorder of unknown etiology was first described by Peyronie in 1743. He described three patients who experienced pain and curvature of the penis at the time of erection. The penile shaft had a fibrous thickening associated with these symptoms. Numerous studies have

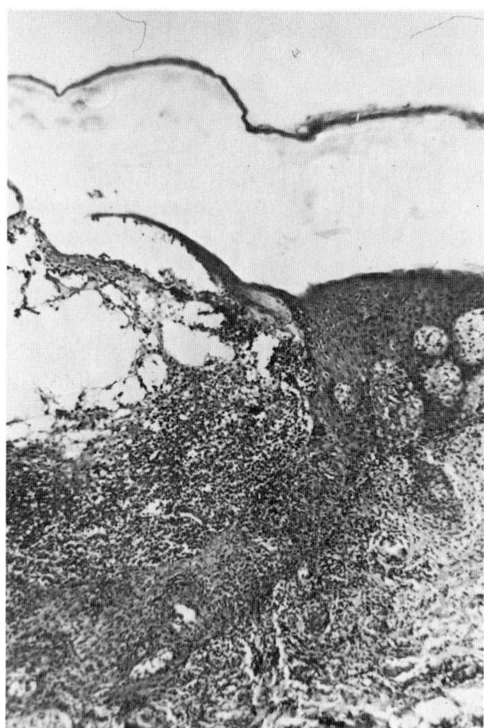

**Fig. 128.** Herpes Infection. The shallow epidermal ulcer underlying a ruptured vesicle contains squamous epithelial cells with prominent intranuclear inclusions at the margin (*inset*).

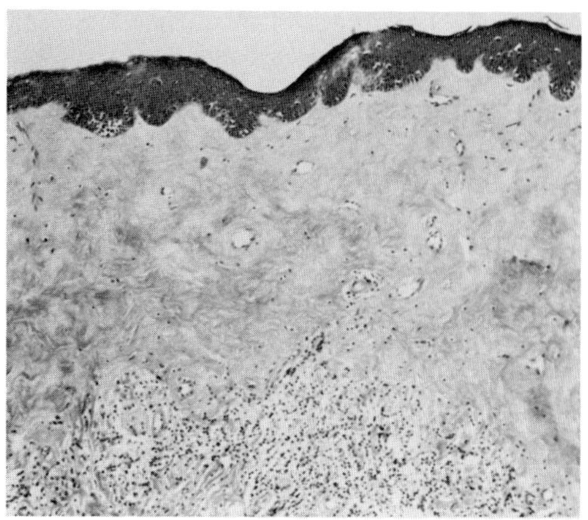

**Fig. 129.** Balanitis Xerotica Obliterans. The epidermis is thin and shows focal hyperkeratosis. The underlying dermis is composed of amorphous abundant collagen with an associated chronic inflammatory cell infiltrate beneath.

been published on the cause, clinical features, and therapy in the intervening years. In a review of 26 cases at the AFIP files, Smith reported that the early lesions were characterized by a chronic inflammatory cell infiltrate in the perivascular tissues deep to Buck's fascia. In time this feature diminishes, and variably extensive collagenous fibrosis involving Buck's fascia and infiltrating the corpus cavernosum and tunica albuginea occurs (Fig. 130).

## BENIGN NEOPLASMS

### Condyloma Acuminata of the Penis

Condyloma acuminata of the penis are wartlike exophytic lesions most commonly encountered on the glans and prepuce in uncircumcised males. The majority are millimeters to a few centimeters in size but are capable of extensive superficial growth to involve ultimately the penile shaft as well as the glans and prepuce. Evidence supports a viral etiology.

The histologic features of condyloma, regardless of their size, are epidermal acanthosis (thickening of prickle cell layer), hyperkeratosis (thickening of stratum corneum), parakeratosis (retention of nuclei in stratum corneum), and papillomatosis (upward proliferation of the dermal papillae and downward projection of rete pegs). Scattered vacuolated cells and mitoses are found in the acanthotic epidermis. The nuclei show no atypia of significance. There is a constant accompanying dermal infiltrate of chronic inflammatory cells. The proliferative process is exophytic with no tendency to downward displacement or infiltration of the underlying dermis (Fig. 131).

This lesion must be differentiated from the Bushke–Lowenstein tumor and squamous cell carcinoma. In addition, the cytologic changes induced by treatment of this lesion with Podophyllin must not be confused with carcinoma.

### Miscellaneous Benign Neoplasms of the Penis

Benign neoplasms of the penis are very rare, and the reported cases reflect a wide histogenetic spectrum. The largest series was published by Dehner and Smith, and neoplasms of vascular origin were the most common. The histopathology of these neoplasms is not different from that of the corresponding tumors in other more common locations.

### Bushke–Lowenstein Tumor

The clinical and pathologic features of Buschke–Lowenstein tumor (verrucous

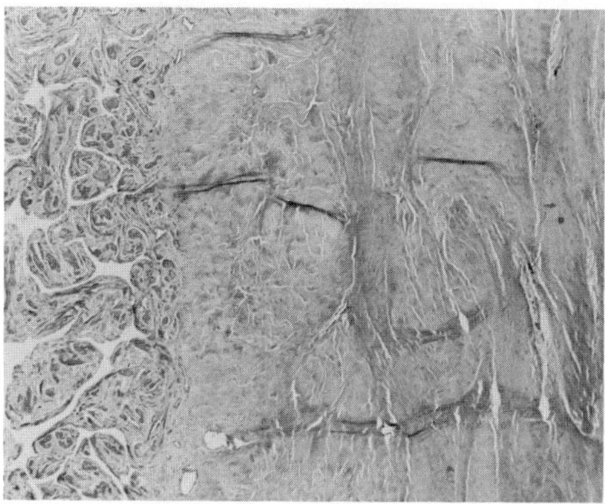

**Fig. 130.** Peyronie's Disease. The dermis is markedly thickened by dense collagenous tissue that focally infiltrates into the smooth muscle investing the corpus cavernosum at the left.

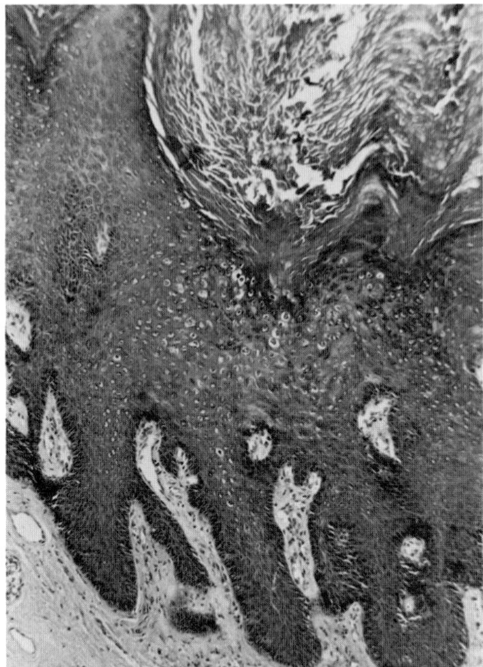

**Fig. 131.** Condyloma Acuminatum. The epidermis shows hyperkeratosis, parakeratosis, acanthosis, papillomatosis with scattered vacuolated cells.

carcinoma) as described by Lowenstein, can be summarized as follows:

A papillary growth of the glans and prepuce with tendency to recur following inadequate local therapy

Recurrences demonstrating rapid growth with occasional extensive involvement of penis

Histologic features of papillomatosis, acanthosis, hyperkeratosis, parakeratosis, and absence of atypia of epithelium at all layers and an underlying chronic inflammatory cell infiltrate

A marked tendency to infiltrate deeper tissue layers with tissue destruction

Absence of lymph node metastases accompanying the extensive local infiltrative growth

Radiotherapy not effective

Electrocoagulation or surgical excision most effective therapy

Tumors coexist with adjacent squamous cell carcinoma *in situ* or squamous cell carcinoma of usual histologic variety with the latter's propensity to metastasize to regional lymph nodes

## PREMALIGNANT LESIONS

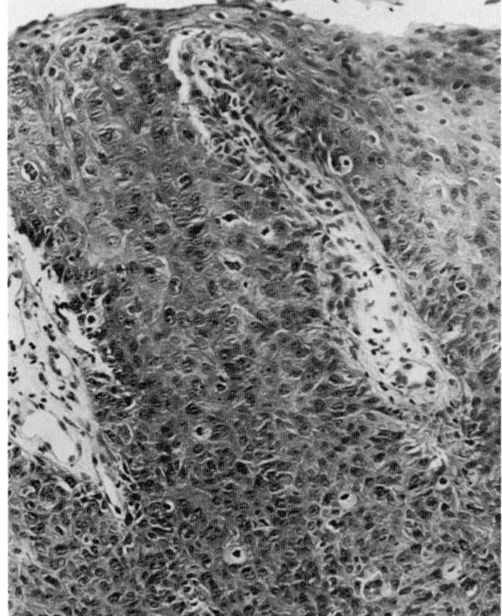

**Fig. 132.** Erythroplasia. The dysplastic cells are found at all levels of the epidermis, which shows acanthosis and papillomatosis.

### Erythroplasia of Queyrat

Erythroplasia of Queyrat (carcinoma *in situ*) is a dysplastic lesion most commonly occurring on the glans and prepuce as an ulcerated plaque. The histologic features include acanthosis, papillomatosis, and dysplastic cytologic changes, involving all layers of the epidermis. The dysplastic changes consist of atypical cells with an irregular arrangement and a loss of the polarity of normal penile skin. Scattered mitotic figures can be found. There is an underlying chronic inflammatory cell infiltrate, as is characteristic of Bowen's disease. Progression to invasive squamous cell carcinoma is reported in as many as 10% of these cases (Fig. 132).

### Bowen's Disease

Bowen's disease, which shows full-thickness dysplasia of the epidermis or

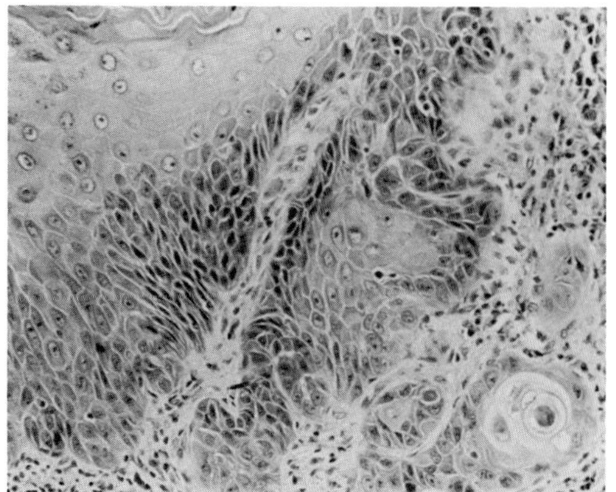

**Fig. 133.** Squamous Cell Carcinoma. This well-differentiated neoplasm shows clusters of squamous cells infiltrating the underlying dermis at the right. One squamous pearl is present at the lower right corner.

carcinoma *in situ*, is most commonly observed in the penile shaft. Histologic features of the lesion include papillomatosis, acanthosis, and dysplastic cytologic changes throughout the epidermis. An underlying chronic inflammatory cell infiltrate is present in the dermis. Progression to invasive squamous cell carcinoma has been reported in approximately 5% of cases. Some authors have reported a significant number of patients with Bowen's disease to have associated malignancies involving internal organs, but this observation has not been unanimously accepted.

## MALIGNANT NEOPLASMS

### Squamous Cell Carcinoma of the Penis

Squamous cell carcinoma of the penis constitutes 1% to 2% of all malignant tumors in the male. The frequency of the practice of circumcision in the male population is inversely related to the incidence of penile squamous cell carcinoma. Eighty percent of all cases occur after the age of 50, with the peak incidence in the seventh decade. The most common location is the glans, followed by the prepuce and shaft. The histopathology of penile squamous cell carcinoma in most cases is typical of the neoplasm elsewhere on the skin. The gross lesion is typically an irregular, firm mass involving the epidermis with associated direct invasion of the underlying penile dermis. The majority of penile squamous cell carcinomas are well differentiated with abundant evidence of keratin (pearl) formation, and intercellular bridges. Superficial spread of the tumor is common with multiple foci of dermal invasion. The epidermis adjacent to the neoplasm frequently contains dysplasia of variable severity. The infiltrating tumor is usually arranged in nests, broad bands, or an occasional thin cord of malignant squamous cells. An associated inflammatory cell infiltration of the adjacent penile tissue is common. Perineural and lymphatic invasion are not uncommon. Tumor metastases to regional lymph nodes either with or without distant metastases are the most commonly encountered evolution of this neoplasm (Figs. 133 and 134).

### Basal Cell Carcinoma

Basal cell carcinoma is a rare lesion reported to occur on the shaft, glans, and prepuce of the penis. Local invasion of the dermis is the rule, but local and distant metastases have been reported once. The microscopic appearance of this lesion is identical to that found in the same lesion elsewhere on the skin.

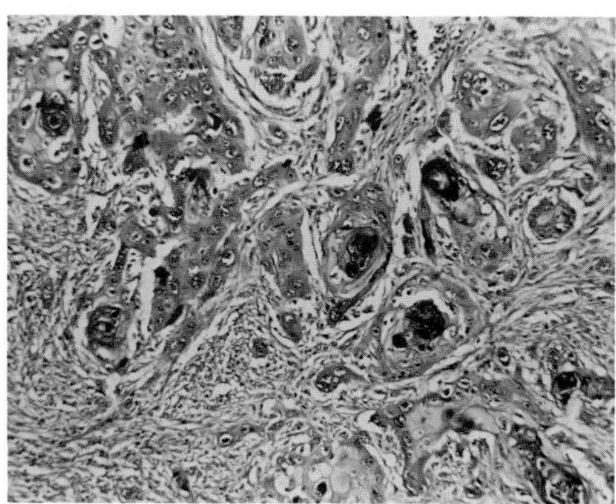

**Fig. 134.** Squamous Cell Carcinoma. Numerous bizarre squamous cells are present in these nests of invading tumor.

### Sarcoma

Various sarcomas have been described as occurring in the penis. Leiomyosarcoma, angiosarcoma, fibrosarcoma, and Kaposi's sarcoma have all been reported on the penile skin.

### Malignant Melanoma

Thirty-seven cases of malignant melanoma of the penis have been reported to date. The most frequent site of involvement is the glans. Only in one case has malignant melanoma involved the penile shaft. The microscopic features of melanoma of the penis are those observed elsewhere. Only 3 of the 37 patients have been known to survive 5 years.

### Metastatic Neoplasms of the Penis

Malignant neoplasms metastatic to the penis are uncommon. Malignancies taking origin in adjacent or regional organs (*i.e.*, prostate, bladder, rectum) constitute approximately 75% of the reported cases. The mode of metastases is frequently not apparent, but retrograde venous or lymphatic spread have been suggested.

# TESTIS

## NORMAL HISTOLOGY AND AGE RELATED CHANGES

The testis at birth contains tubules that are filled with undifferentiated cells, among which are rare cells identifiable as spermatogonia and Leydig cells, present in the interstitium as small clusters or individual cells. The identifiable Leydig cells decrease to an apparent total absence beginning at age 3 months. This histologic picture persists until 3 years of age, when the tubules begin to enlarge, becoming more tortuous with increasing numbers of identifiable germ cells. The apparent absence of Leydig cells persists through age nine.

From age nine to eleven, boys manifest continued tubular enlargement and germ cell maturation. Sertoli cells are recognizable, and Leydig cells reappear. Beyond twelve years of age, the testis shows uniform active spermatogenesis in all seminiferous tubules, which now contain a distinct lumen. This population of germ cells, Sertoli cells, and Leydig cells is that of the adult testis through the reproductive years (Fig. 135).

Spermatogenesis involves spermatogonia differentiating into primary spermatocytes, which, in turn, undergo meiotic division into secondary spermatocytes. The secondary spermatocytes undergo a second meiotic division to

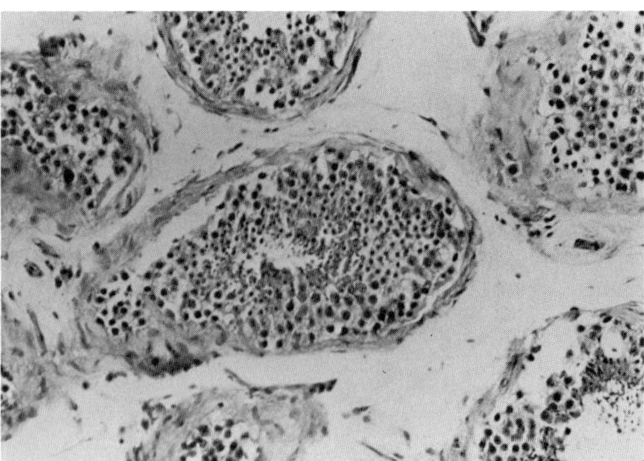

**Fig. 135.** Normal Adult Testis. Active spermatogenesis is evident in the seminiferous tubules.

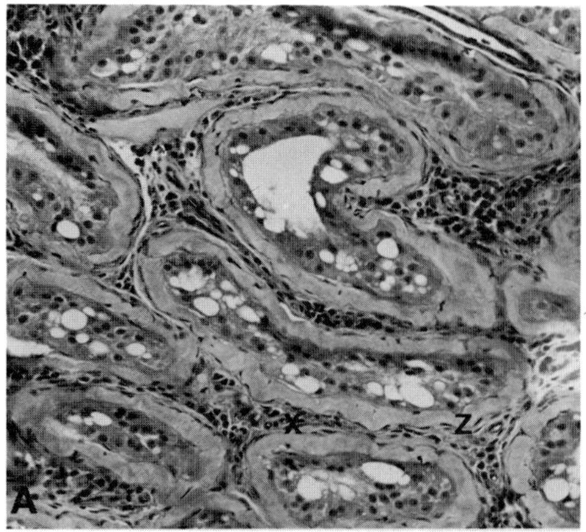


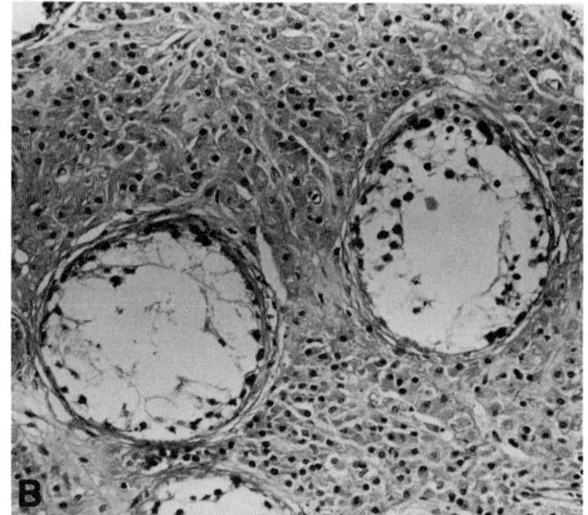


**Fig. 136.** Physiologic Atrophy. **A.** There is a marked reduction in tubular diameter, with thickening of the basement membrane and focal tubular sclerosis. Cytoplasmic vacuolization of the Sertoli cells is present. **B.** Only Sertoli cells remain in the seminiferous tubules. Leydig cell hyperplasia is present in the testicular interstitium.

spermatids, which remain attached to the luminal extension of the Sertoli cells. Upon maturation and release, spermatids become spermatozoa.

Physiologic regression of testicular germ cell production is observed with advancing age. With this decrease in germ cells is a corresponding increase in Sertoli cells and frequently an increase in the number of Leydig cells. Progression of the regressive changes is associated with tubular sclerosis and interstitial fibrosis (Fig. 136 *A, B*). This histologic picture differs from that of the tubular sclerosis characteristic of Klinefelter's syndrome, which is devoid of the peritubular elastic fibers present in the testis with physiologic regressive changes.

## CONGENITAL AND DEVELOPMENTAL DISORDERS

### Cryptorchid Testis

The histologic features of the cryptorchid testis are dependent on the age of the patient. Up to age 6 months, there is no difference between the microscopic features of a normally positioned testis and a cryptorchid testis. From this age to 3 years, the principal histologic change in the cryptorchid testis is the slightly smaller size of the seminiferous tubule. Between ages 3 and 8 years, the tubular size of the cryptorchid testis changes little compared to the significant increase in the tubular size observed in the normal testis in a boy at this age. The malpositioned testis in teenaged boys shows progressive thickening in the tubular basement membrane and peritubular fibrosis with no evidence of spermatogenesis. These changes progress to complete hyalinization of the tubules with obliteration of the last remaining Sertoli cells, which is characteristic of the cryptorchid testis removed in postpubertal adolescences and adult males. The interstitial cells may be increased, decreased, or normal in number (Figs. 137 and 138).

### Klinefelter's Syndrome

The original description of the disorder by Klinefelter included hypogonadism with gynecomastia, aspermia, and increased excretion of follicle-stimulating hormone. Subsequent studies have revealed the abnormal karyotype, characterized by an excessive number of X chromosomes. In addition, mosaic chromosome patterns have been reported (*i.e.*, XY/XXY). Histologically, the testis from prepubertal age and older is characterized by abnormally small tubules lined by Sertoli cells with few, if

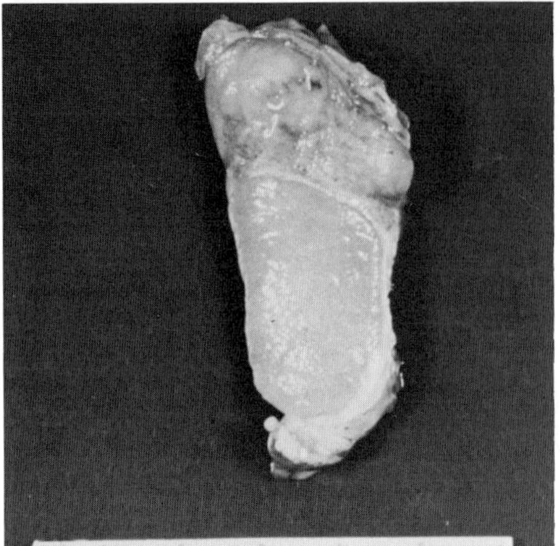

**Fig. 137.** Cryptorchid Testis. This testis from a 19-year-old man is significantly smaller than normal.

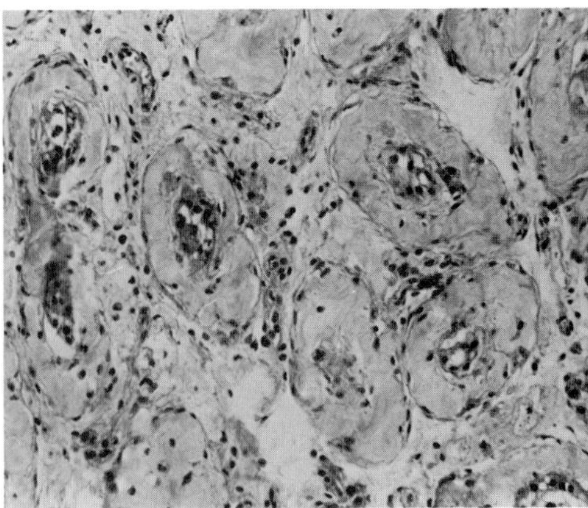

**Fig. 139.** Klinefelter's Syndrome. There is marked tubular basement membrane thickening, absence of spermatogenesis, rare Sertoli cells, and focal interstitial cell hyperplasia.

any, germ cells. Progressive hyalinization of the tubules leads ultimately to shrunken acellular cords devoid of elastic fibers at their periphery. Leydig cells (interstitial cells) are increased in number (Fig. 139). Variations of this histologic picture may be seen in the mosaic form.

## Sertoli-Cell-Only Syndrome

Infertility associated with a total absence of germ cells in the seminiferous tubules has been termed the Sertoli-cell only syndrome (germinal cell aplasia). It is regarded as a state of irreversible infertility of unknown etiology. The seminiferous tubules are populated only by Sertoli cells and are commonly reduced in size without associated interstitial fibrosis or thickening of the basement membrane (Fig. 140).

## Maturational Arrest

The most common histologic changes in the testis associated with male infertil-

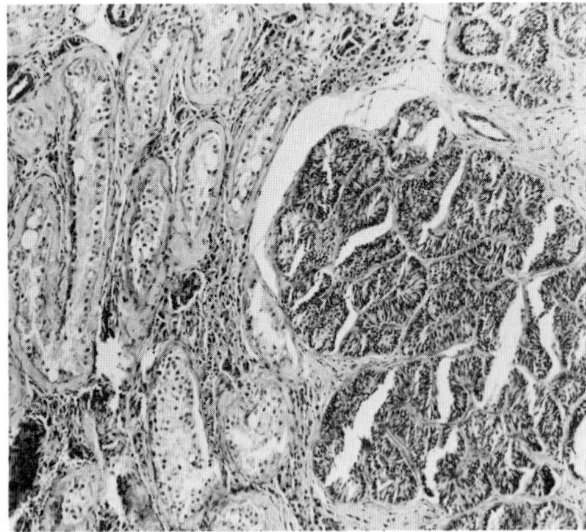

**Fig. 138.** Cryptorchid Testis. The tubular basement membrane is markedly thickened with vacuolization of the cytoplasm of the remaining Sertoli cells. A focus of Sertoli cell hyperplasia (tubular adenoma of Pick) is present on the right. The patient was 28 years old.

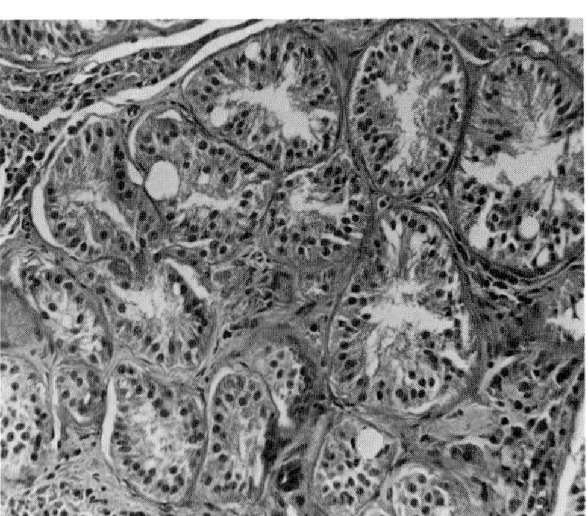

**Fig. 140.** Sertoli Cell-Only Syndrome (Germinal Cell Aplasia). The seminiferous tubules contain only Sertoli cells. The basement membrane of the tubules is not significantly thickened, and there is no interstitial fibrosis.

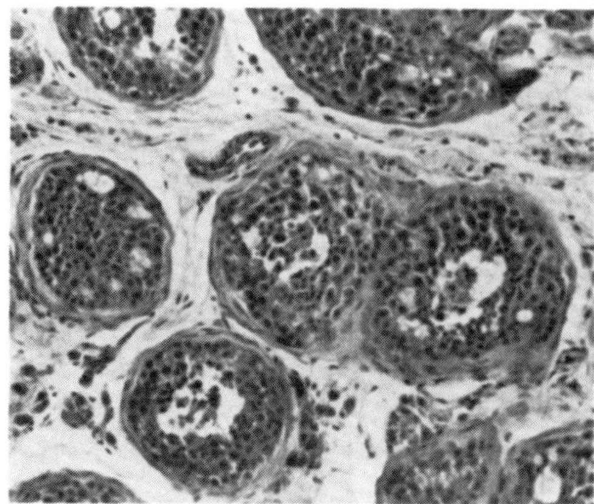

**Fig. 141.** Maturation Arrest. The tubules contain germ cells which have uniform cytologic features and a complete absence of spermatid and sperm. Scattered nests of interstitial cells are present.

ity is germ cell maturational arrest. Most commonly the arrest is uniformly present in all tubules at the spermatocyte stage with rare or absent sperm in any of the tubules. The interstitium and the interstitial cells, as well as the seminiferous tubular size, are all histologically normal (Fig. 141).

### Hypospermatogenesis

In contrast to germ cell maturation arrest, hypospermatogenesis is characterized by a uniform decrease in the number of germ cells in most or all tubules, but evident capacity of those present to mature to sperm. Thus, although there is a quantitative reduction in the germ cells, the presence of mature sperm allows histologic differentiation from maturational arrest in the testis. The interstitium and interstitial cells are normal. The ultimate form of this defect is the Sertoli-cell-only syndrome (Fig. 142).

## INFLAMMATORY DISEASES

### Mumps Orchitis

Acute mumps orchitis may occur in approximately 25% of patients with paraotitis, usually adults. Clinically the testicle will appear large and swollen and will be found in the patient who otherwise has the typical salivary gland findings. The earliest histologic changes are interstitial edema associated with vascular congestion and interstitial hemorrhage and are most commonly observed within a week. The density of lymphocyte and plasma cell infiltrate in the interstitium increases with time. Eventually, the inflammatory cell infiltrate is seen within tubules but at all times is primarily interstitial. There is obliteration of germ cells in focal tubules. The ultimate resolution is focal tubular interstitial fibrosis. A similar histologic evolution is observed in the epididymis, which is concurrently affected in the majority of cases.

### Granulomatous Orchitis

The paucity or absence of sperm in the granulomatous lesions (in contrast to

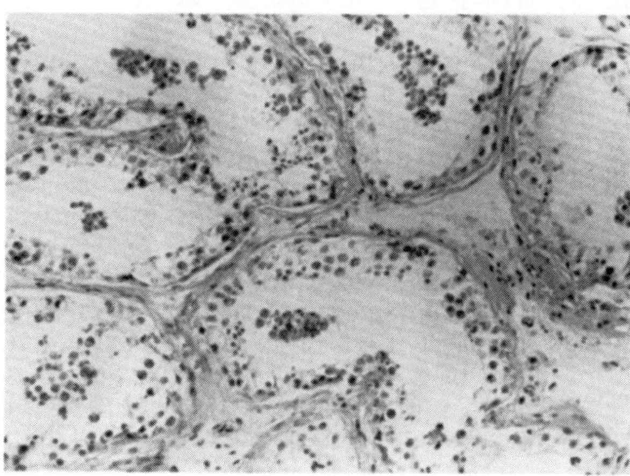

**Fig. 142.** Hypospermia. There is a marked reduction in the numbers of germ cells in this testis, which did contain some sperm in occasional tubules.

sperm granuloma of the epididymis and vas deferens) speaks against the granulomatous orchitis lesion being caused by extratubular extravasation with resultant inflammatory reaction. The histologic picture is that of noncaseating granulomas with multinucleated giant cells in a background of a dense infiltrate of lymphocytes, plasma cells, histiocytes, and occasional neutrophils. The granulomas are found both within the tubules and the interstitium. Thickening of the tubular basement membrane is not a feature of this lesion. Results of special stains tests for acid-fast bacteria and fungi are negative. Similar changes are commonly present in the epididymis.

### Malakoplakia of the Testis

The etiologic and pathogenetic considerations of malakoplakia can be found in the discussion under Bladder. This disorder is much less frequent in the testis than elsewhere in the genitourinary tract. The histologic features of malakoplakia involving the testis include a mixed inflammatory cell infiltrate with numerous histiocytes, lymphocytes, and plasma cells both within the tubules and the intertubular interstitium. PAS-positive Michaelis–Gutmann bodies, both within the histiocytes and lying free in extracellular locations, are present. In the healing stage, the affected areas of the testis undergo extensive fibrosis with tubular destruction (see Figs. 15 and 63).

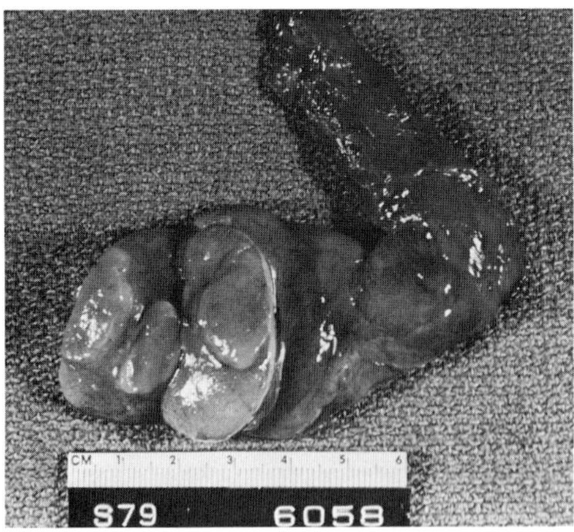


**Fig. 143.** Classic Seminoma. The cut surface shows the solid tumor confined within the testis. Hemorrhage and necrosis of the tumor are not conspicuous.

## GERM CELL NEOPLASMS

### Seminoma

The most common germ cell tumor is the seminoma, which constitutes approximately 40% of testis tumors in white adult males. Grossly the typical seminoma is a gray-white to tan mass replacing most of the testis and confined within the tunica albuginea (Fig. 143). Areas of necrosis with or without hemorrhage, and cystic change are uncommon. Histologically, there are three variants:

Classic seminoma
Spermatocytic seminoma
Anaplastic seminoma

The classic seminoma, the most frequent histologic type, is characterized by polygonal cells with clear cytoplasm and distinct cell membranes. The tumor cells proliferate in nests created by fibrovascular septa that traverse the tumor in a haphazard manner. The hyperchromatic central nuclei are variable in shape and have prominent nucleoli and granular chromatin. Occasional multinucleated cells are present, and mitoses are infrequent. Lymphocytes infiltrate the fibrovascular septa, and lymphoid aggregates with germinal centers are occasionally present. Well-formed granulomas are also present in some cases (Figs. 144 and 145).

The spermatocytic seminoma represents 5% to 10% of all cases of seminoma and usually involves older patients. These patients appear to have a better prognosis than do those with classic seminoma. The spermatocytic seminoma is composed of uniformly round nuclei with significant variation of nuclear size and staining characteristics, and eosinophilic cytoplasm. The fibrovascular septa do not have the lymphocytic infiltrate nor the granulomas observed in classic seminoma (Figs. 146 and 147).

The anaplastic seminoma is character-

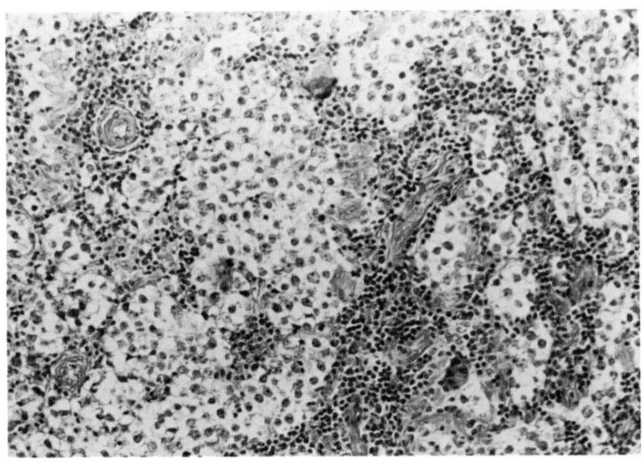

**Fig. 144.** Classic Seminoma. The seminoma cells are present in nests confined by fibrous septae containing numerous lymphocytes.

ized by significantly greater numbers of mitoses and tumor giant cells than are present in the other two histologic variants of seminoma. Lymphocytes are present in this type as are variable numbers of granulomas. Lymphatic and vascular invasion is common.

Intratubular seminoma or carcinoma *in situ* has been recently reported. Malignant cells are clearly seen limited by the basement membrane of the seminiferous tubule, although on occasion they may be seen to extend outside the tubule into the interstitial areas.

Some seminomas may contain syncytiotrophoblastic giant cells which may secrete human chorionic gonadotropin (HCG), as determined by serum levels and immunoperoxidase staining.

## Embryonal Carcinoma

Embryonal carcinoma constitutes approximately 20% of adult testis tumors. The tumor cells may secrete alpha-fetoprotein but not HCG. These malignant germ cell tumors are solid and gray-white and frequently have focal areas of hemorrhage and necrosis (Plate 7). Histologically, the most prominent feature is the dense cellularity of the tumor. The cells are arranged in sheets, cords, and occasional papillary projections, with sparse fibrous trabecular partitions scattered randomly. Indistinct cell borders, eosinophilic cytoplasm, and hyperchromatic, irregular nuclei with prominent nucleoli are characteristic. The indistinct cell borders and absence of lymphocytic

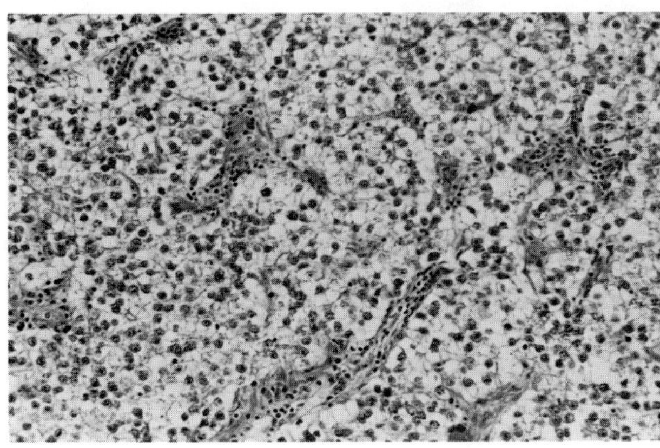

**Fig. 145.** Classic Seminoma. The cell borders of the seminoma cells are well defined, and the cytoplasm is clear. The nuclei show minimal variation of size and shape.

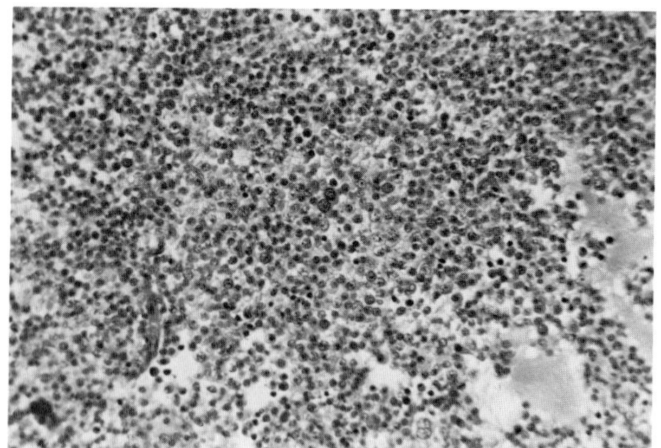

**Fig. 146.** Spermatocytic Seminoma. Scattered giant tumor cells are present in this seminoma. The nuclei are uniformly round but vary in size. The cytoplasm stains lightly eosinophilic. No fibrous septa or lymphocytes are present. Only rare mitoses were present in this tumor.

infiltrate help to distinguish this neoplasm from seminoma (Fig. 148 and Plate 8).

Occasional cases have embryoid bodies, a structure composed of microcyst with a cluster of cuboidal lining cells called the *germ cell disc*. Associated with this structure are undifferentiated cells corresponding to primitive endoderm. When such embryoid bodies constitute the bulk of the neoplasm, the tumor is called a *polyembryoma*.

## Yolk-Sac Tumor

The yolk-sac tumor (endodermal sinus tumor), or embryonal carcinoma of the infantile type, constitutes at least 60% of testicular tumors in children. It is rare to be found in its pure form in adults but may be admixed with embryonal carcinoma. Grossly this is a solid neoplasm that is gray-yellow on the cut surface. Scattered microcysts in a glistening myxoid stroma are commonly observed. Histologic features include a variable pattern of malignant epithelial cells in a sparse fibrous or myxoid stroma. The tumor cells are arranged in sheets, microcysts, and occasionally a papillary pattern. The cells lining the papillary projections or microcysts are flattened or cuboidal with hyperchromatic, irregular nuclei and cytoplasmic vacuoles and occasional clear cells. Eosinophilic, PAS-positive globules are formed within scattered tumor cells and in extracellular locations, which, on immunoperoxidase

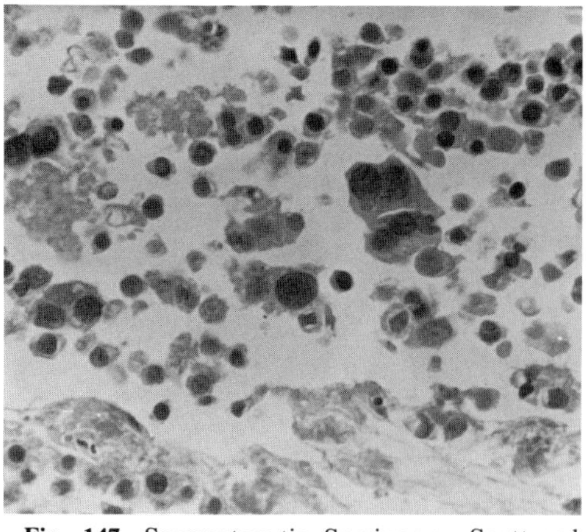

**Fig. 147.** Spermatocytic Seminoma. Scattered giant tumor cells are present in the center.

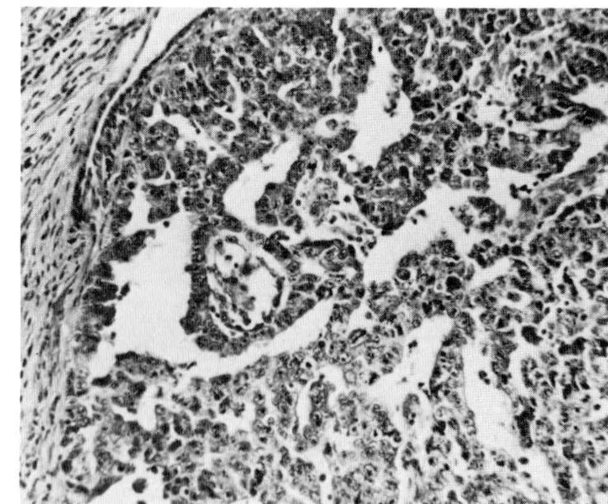

**Fig. 148.** Embryonal Carcinoma. A cystic space is lined and almost filled with carcinoma cells without distinct cell membranes. The nuclei are hyperchromatic with prominent nucleoli and lightly eosinophilic cytoplasm.

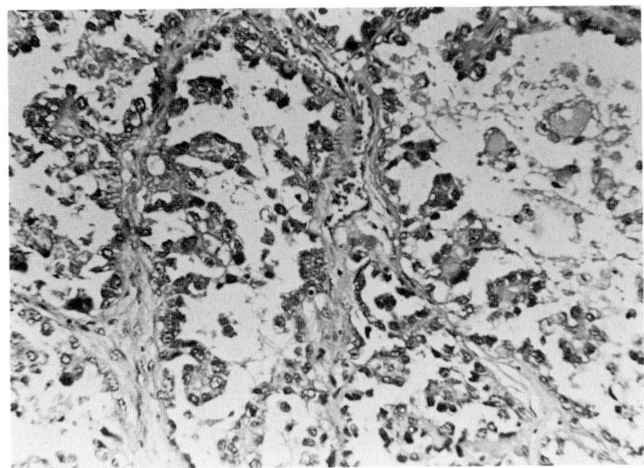

**Fig. 149.** Endodermal Sinus Tumor (Yolk-Sac Tumor). The tubular structure is lined by cells in papillary configurations. The cytoplasm is characteristically clear. One cluster of cells surrounds an extracellular eosinophilic globule.

staining, have demonstrated the presence of alpha-fetoprotein. The most characteristic feature of these neoplasms is the presence of glomeruluslike structures (Schiller–Duval bodies) with a central fibrovascular core surrounded by a layer of tumor cells all present in a microcyst (Figs. 149 and 150).

## Teratoma

"Benign" teratoma constitutes approximately 5% to 10% of adult testicular tumors and 20% to 40% of infantile testicular tumors. In children, these lesions behave in a benign manner, with metastases being reported only rarely. In adults these lesions are often associated with lymph node metastases containing embryonal carcinoma, from which the teratoma may have evolved and which may no longer be detected in the primary lesion.

On gross inspection the neoplasm contains cystic spaces and solid tan areas. Histologically these tumors contain well-differentiated organoid structures and tumor cells from all three germ cell layers: ectoderm, endoderm, and mesoderm. Exhaustive examination is required to eliminate the presence of coexistent embryonal carcinoma (Fig. 151).

## Teratocarcinoma

Teratocarcinoma neoplasms are composed of varying proportions of evident malignant germ cells of the embryonal carcinoma type admixed with areas of mature epithelial or mesenchymal components, frequently organized in abortive organoid structures (*i.e.*, bronchial or gastrointestinal mucosa). These neoplasms are more common in adults and are differentiated from teratomas by the presence of the malignant component, usually found without difficulty. On occasion a careful search is required (Fig. 152).

## Choriocarcinoma

Choriocarcinoma neoplasm is most commonly one component of a mixed germ cell neoplasm, but on rare occasions it may be present in pure form.

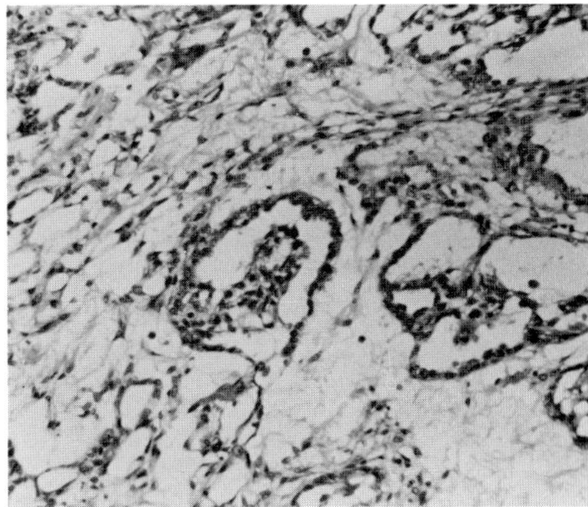

**Fig. 150.** Endodermal Sinus Tumor (Yolk-Sac Tumor). The tumor is composed of multiple dilated tubular spaces lined by flattened cells with an edematous stroma intervening. A glomerulus-like structure is present in the center.

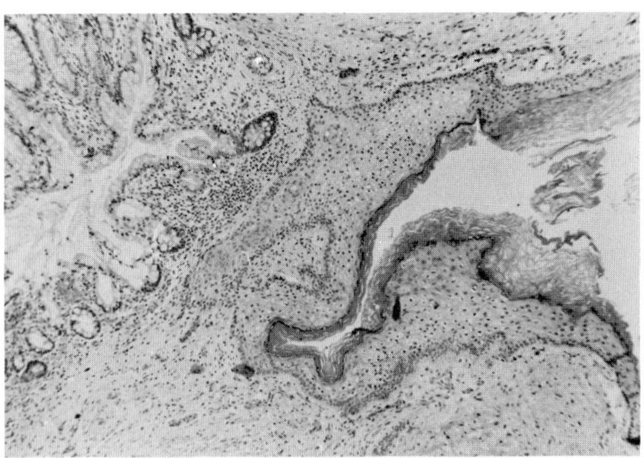

**Fig. 151.** Teratoma. A cyst lined by well-differentiated squamous epithelium is in proximity to a focus of endodermal glands with colonic features.

Virtually all of these tumors secrete HCG but not alpha-fetoprotein. The gross appearance is dependent on size and extent of contribution to a mixed neoplasm. Typical testicular neoplasms with choriocarcinomatous elements have extensive hemorrhagic necrosis. Diagnosis requires the presence of both syncytiotrophoblastic cells and cytotrophoblastic cells. The former are large, with multiple irregular, hyperchromatic nuclei and abundant eosinophilic cytoplasm with frequent vacuolization. Associated with the syncytiotrophoblasts are the smaller polygonal cytotrophoblasts, with sparse eosinophilic cytoplasm and hyperchromatic nuclei. These requisite neoplastic cells are present amid abundant hemorrhage and usually with evidence of other germ cell neoplastic components, such as seminoma or embryonal carcinoma (Fig. 153).

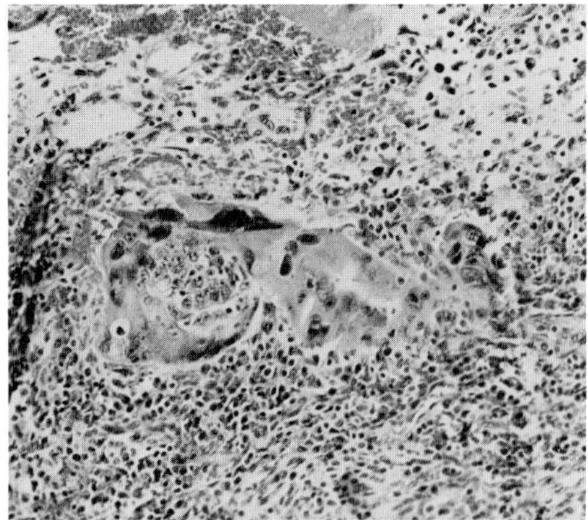

**Fig. 152.** Choriocarcinoma. The syncytiotrophoblast cells surround a cluster of cytotrophoblast cells with evident hemorrhage in the adjacent tissue.

### Gonadoblastoma

Gonadoblastoma is a rare neoplasm that usually arises in a dysplastic gonad and is composed of a mixture of germ cells with Sertoli cells or granulosa cells. Some cases contain gonadal stromal cells resembling Leydig cells. The most frequent pattern of this mixed cell population is nests or cords with intervening fibrous tissue. Amorphous calcified masses are frequently admixed in the nests of tumor cells or imbedded in the dense fibrous stroma of this neoplasm. Call–Exner bodies may be seen. This lesion is commonly associated with a germ cell tumor in the same gonad.

## GONADAL STROMAL TUMORS

### Leydig Cell Tumor

Leydig cell (interstitial cell) tumors occur in all age groups, but most commonly in children. These neoplasms may elaborate androgens or estrogens, and thus may cause precocious puberty or gynecomastia. Approximately 10% of these tumors are malignant.

On cut surface these solid lesions are yellow-tan owing to the presence of lipid within the tumor cells. Histologically the tumor cells are arranged in sheets with

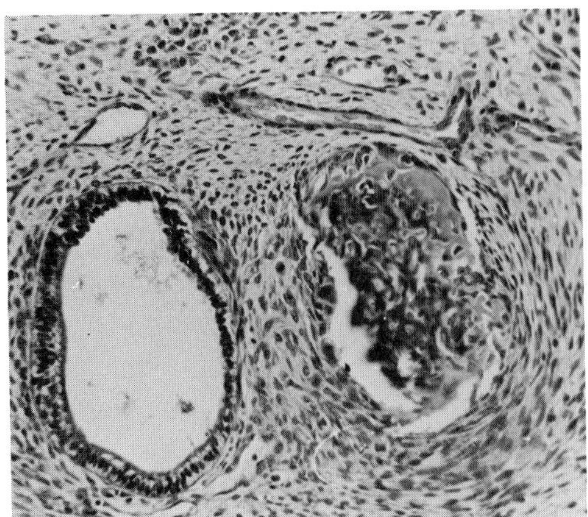

**Fig. 153.** Teratocarcinoma. A focus of malignant bone formation is adjacent to a tubular structure lined by primitive endoderm-type epithelium.

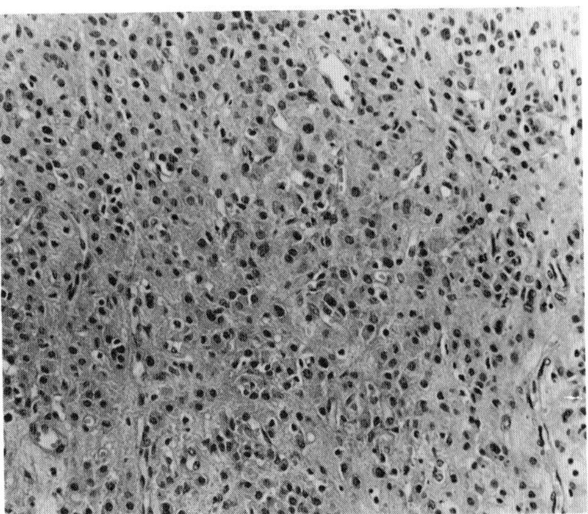

**Fig. 154.** Leydig Cell (Interstitial Cell) Tumor. The tumor cells, arranged in sheets, are moderately pleomorphic with abundant eosinophilic cytoplasm. No mitoses are present.

occasional fibrovascular septa interspersed. The cells have abundant eosinophilic cytoplasm with small clear vacuoles. Intracytoplasmic, rectangular, deeply eosinophilic inclusion bodies called *crystalloids of Reinke* may be found. The nuclei are relatively uniform with prominent nucleoli, but some cells may have large, hyperchromatic nuclei, with rare mitotic figures. The presence of interspersed seminiferous tubules in Leydig cell hyperplasia assists in distinguishing this non-neoplastic proliferation from Leydig cell tumors (Fig. 154).

Malignant Leydig cell tumors have been described only in middle-aged and elderly men. The histologic features suggesting malignancy in these tumors include increased mitotic activity and significantly more pleomorphism.

### Sertoli Cell Tumors

Ninety percent of cases of the uncommon Sertoli cell neoplasm are benign. Estrogen levels may be elevated, and 30% to 50% of these patients will present with gynecomastia. These neoplasms are derived from gonadal stroma cells and may contain Sertoli cells alone or in combination with Leydig cells or cells resembling granulosa and theca cells. The Sertoli cells, frequently arranged in cords or tubules, are polygonal or cuboidal–columnar in shape. The nucleus is vesicular and relatively large with a paucity of eosinophilic cytoplasm. The cells may be arranged in nests or sheets or may appear to be spindle-shaped. Cells with a large nucleus and abundant eosinophilic cytoplasm characteristic of Leydig cells may be found scattered among the Sertoli cells. On rare occasions the pattern of granulosa cell tumor with Call–Exner bodies may be found.

## MALIGNANT LYMPHOMA OF THE TESTIS

The most common malignancy involving the testis of patients older than 60 is malignant lymphoma. The majority of cases of testicular lymphoma represent one of the many multiple sites of systemic involvement of non-Hodgkin's lymphoma. Less commonly, testicular enlargement is the initial presentation of a patient with previously undiagnosed lymphoma. Subsequent staging procedures will disclose extratesticular involvement. Occasional reports describe patients in whom no extra gonadal lymphoma is detected and the neoplasm is interpreted as primary in the testis. Uncommonly, involvement of the testis is reported in Hodgkin's disease and myeloma. Histologically, the lymphomatous infiltrate is primary in the interstitium, with invasion of tubules and blood vessel walls observed less commonly. The cy-

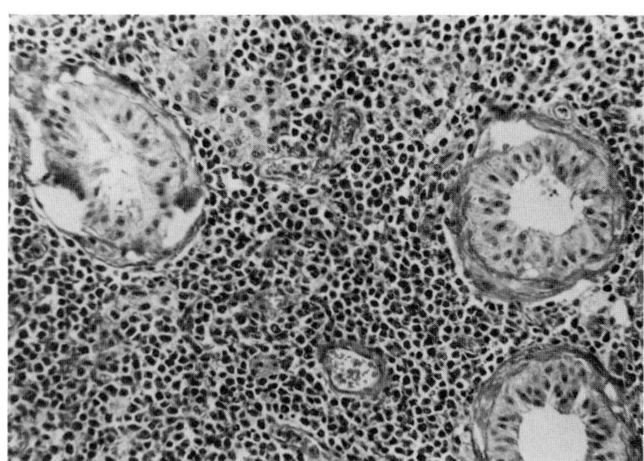

**Fig. 155.** Malignant Lymphoma in the Testis. The lymphoma cells infiltrate the interstitium. The tubules evidence decreased spermatogenesis.

tologic features and homogeneous cell infiltrate of a lymphoma distinguish this lesion from inflammatory cell infiltrates in the testis. (Fig. 155).

### METASTATIC TUMORS TO THE TESTIS

Independent of the systemic involvement of malignant lymphoma or leukemia with testicular involvement, metastatic spread to the testis is relatively rare. The most common primary sites associated with testicular metastases are prostate and lung. Rarely, malignant neoplasms of the kidney may present clinically as metastases to the testis. The histologic appearance of the tumor reflects that of the primary malignancy.

## TESTICULAR ADNEXA

### NORMAL HISTOLOGY

The epididymis is composed of multiple coiled segments of the epididymal ducts with scanty intervening stroma. The ducts are lined by tall pseudostratified columnar cells with basal nuclei. Cilia are present on the luminal surface of the cells, with mature sperm present in the lumina of the ducts. The surrounding stroma is composed of collagen with an investment of smooth muscle cells surrounding each tubule (Figs. 156–158).

### INFLAMMATORY DISEASES

#### Acute Epididymitis

When present, acute epididymitis is frequently associated with infections of the bladder, urethra, or prostate from which the organisms spread by way of the vas deferens or lymphatics. Histologically, the features of acute inflammation are present, primarily in but not limited to the ducts of the epididymis. The mucosa or the entire tubular wall may be destroyed, and focal abscesses are often present. Resolution frequently results in collagenous fibrosis (Fig. 159).

#### Chronic Epididymitis

Persistence of acute epididymitis without resolution is associated with increased numbers of lymphocytes, histiocytes, and plasma cells in the infiltrate, with a corresponding decrease in the number of acute inflammatory cells. Fibrosis of the epididymis with destruction of the tubules will result (Fig. 160).

#### Tuberculosis of the Epididymis

Tuberculosis involving the male genitalia most commonly begins in the epididymis. The histologic picture of tuber-

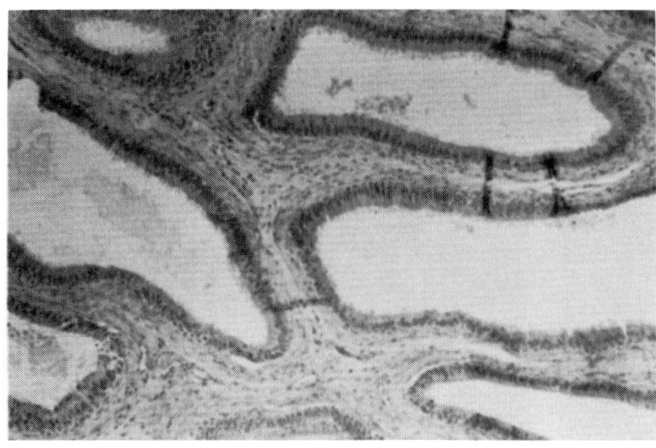

**Fig. 156.** Normal Epididymis. The ducts of the epididymis are lined by uniformly tall columnar epithelium and have a surrounding fibromuscular stroma.

culous infection of the epididymis is identical to that of these lesions elsewhere. The classic caseating granuloma with Langhans' type giant cells, palisading epithelioid histiocytes, and a margin of lymphocytes and plasma cells is observed. Special stains for the acid-fast organisms will frequently demonstrate the tubercle bacilli in the lesion. Ultimate resolution is with substantial fibrous scarring and destruction of the normal architecture of the epididymis (see Figs. 19, 64 and 97).

## Sperm Granuloma of Epididymis

The etiology of sperm granuloma of epididymis is unsettled, but whatever the initial event, sperm gain entrance to the interstitium, evoking a marked inflammatory response. Granulomatous inflammation with occasional giant cells and numerous histiocytes, showing phagocytosis of sperm fragments, in association with chronic inflammatory cells (lymphocytes and plasma cells), is the hallmark of this disorder. Local destruction or ulceration of the epididymal tubules is observed. Fragments of sperm are present throughout the inflammatory infiltrate. Variable amounts of fibrosis result from the inflammatory process. The same process may extend to involve the testis or vas deferens (Fig. 161).

## Vasitis Nodosa

Vasitis nodosa in the vas deferens is the equivalent of the sperm granuloma of the epididymis. Sperm extended into or through the wall of the vas deferens incite an inflammatory response that results in grossly apparent nodularity of this structure. Histologically, an acute and chronic inflammatory response to sperm fragments in the wall of the vas

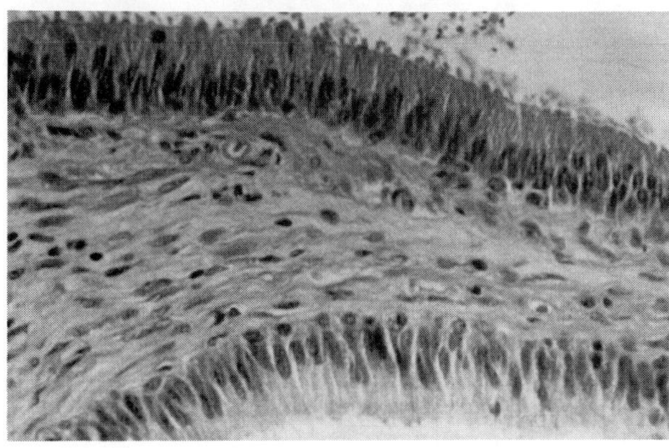

**Fig. 157.** Normal Epididymis. The ciliated pseudostratified columnar epithelium of the epididymis is invested with a layer of smooth muscle.

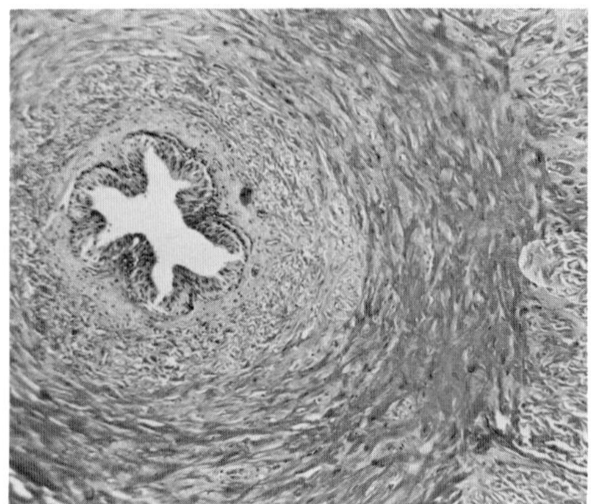

**Fig. 158.** Normal Vas Deferens. The columnar lining cells of the vas deferens rest on a basement membrane. The surrounding muscle bundles are arranged in longitudinal and circular groups.

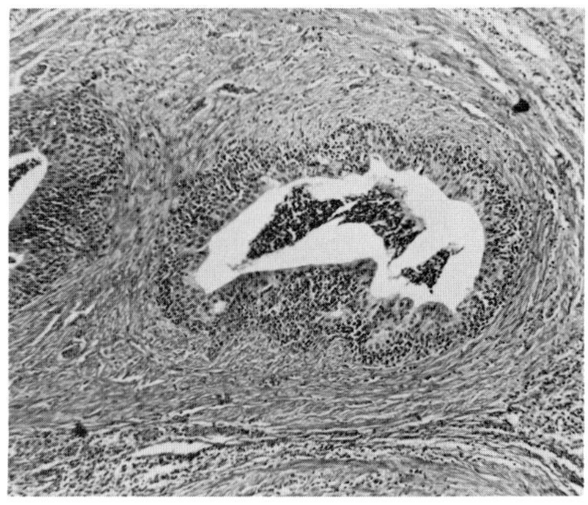

**Fig. 160.** Chronic Epididymitis. Numerous lymphocytes surround and infiltrate the wall of the epididymis.

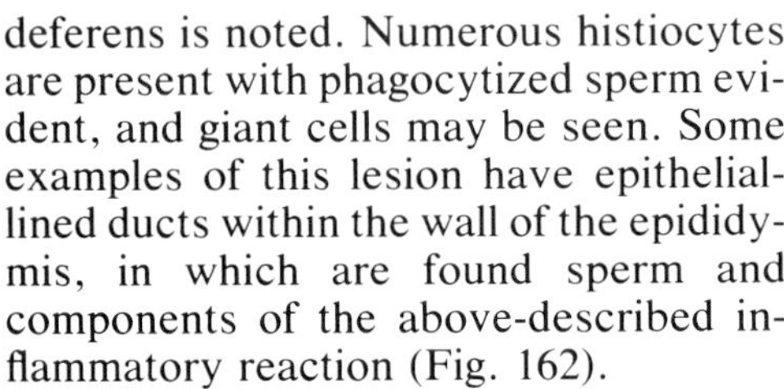

deferens is noted. Numerous histiocytes are present with phagocytized sperm evident, and giant cells may be seen. Some examples of this lesion have epithelial-lined ducts within the wall of the epididymis, in which are found sperm and components of the above-described inflammatory reaction (Fig. 162).

## BENIGN NEOPLASMS

### Adenomatoid Tumor

The most common epididymal neoplasm is the adenomatoid tumor. This is a benign tumor of mesothelial origin that usually occurs in a polar region in the epididymis. The characteristic histologic features are multiple small tubular or cystic spaces lined by flattened epithelial cells. A dense fibrous stroma intervenes between the cystic spaces, which is variable in size. There may be scattered chronic inflammatory cells throughout the stroma (Fig. 163).

### Nodular Periorchitis

Nodular periorchitis (fibrous pseudotumor), a disorder of unknown etiology

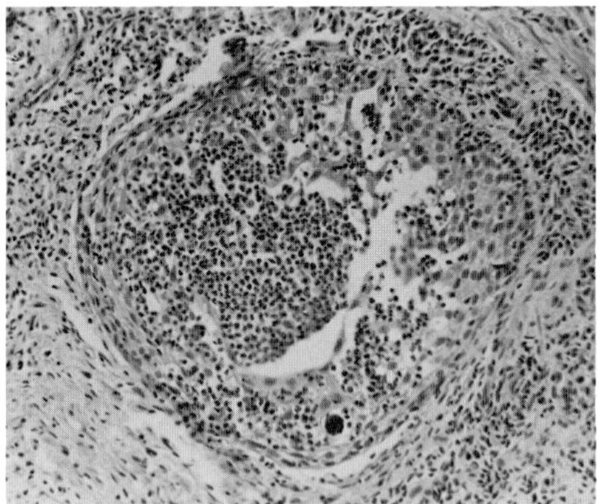

**Fig. 159.** Acute Epididymis. Numerous neutrophils are present in the lumen and the epithelium of the epididymis. The squamous metaplasia of epithelium suggests the acute inflammation is superimposed on chronic injury to the epididymis.

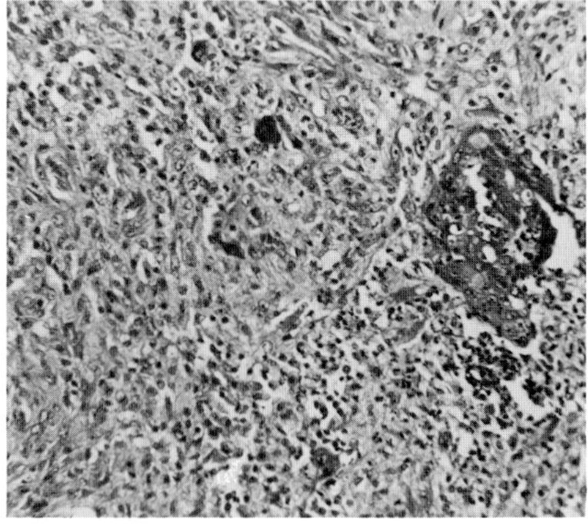

**Fig. 161.** Sperm Granuloma. The inflammatory infiltrate is composed of mixed chronic inflammatory cells including histiocytes with giant cells (*far right*). Numerous sperm fragments are present in the cytoplasm of the giant cells.

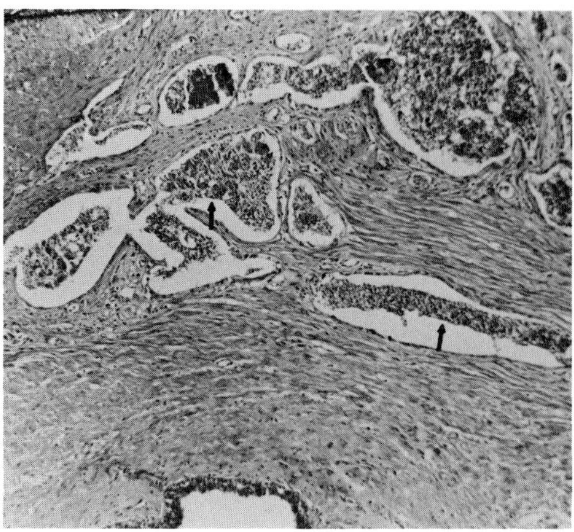

**Fig. 162.** Vasitis Nodosa. The extravasated sperm are present in the outer muscle layers of the vas deferens (*arrow*).

involving the tunica albuginea of the testis and the epididymis, is characterized by clinically apparent nodular induration of these structures. It occurs at all ages. Histologically, the early lesions are characterized by an abundant mixed inflammatory cell infiltrate and numerous thin-walled blood vessels (granulation tissue). Older lesions are characterized by increasing collagenous fibrous tissue and decreasing vascular and inflammatory cell components. Ultimately dense collagenous fibrosis with only scattered chronic inflammatory cells are present (Fig. 164).

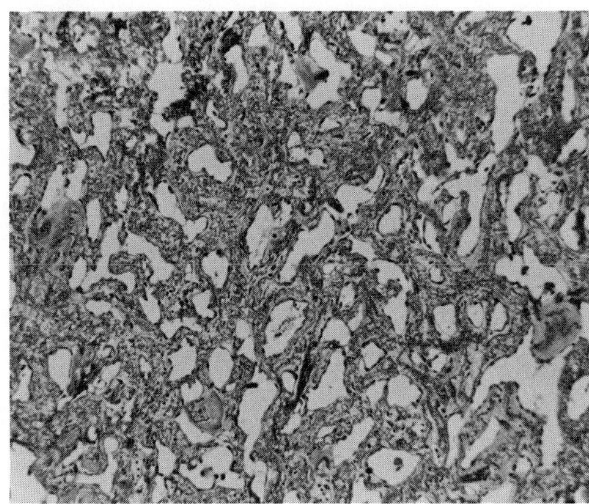

**Fig. 163.** Adenomatoid Tumor. The neoplasm contains numerous irregular cysts or tubules lined by flattened epithelium with intervening dense fibrous stroma.

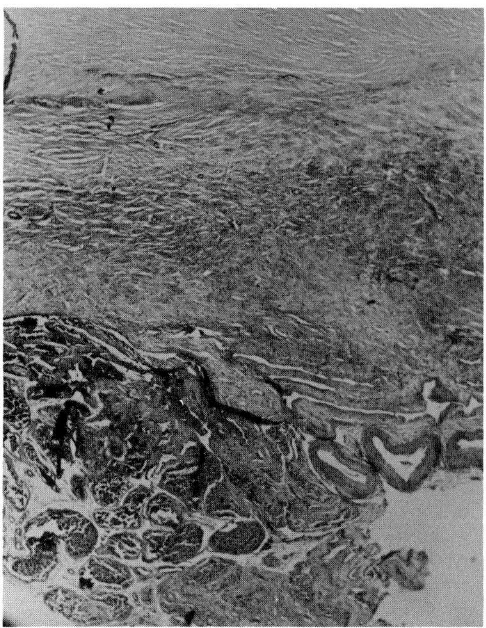

**Fig. 164.** Nodular periorchitis. The tunica albuginea is thickened by dense, acellular collagenous fibrous tissue. Minimal chronic inflammatory cells are scattered in the tunica.

## Sclerosing Lipogranuloma

Sclerosing lipogranuloma is frequently associated with a history of trauma and clinically with penile or scrotal induration. Histologically, the features are those of an acute inflammatory reaction to fat necrosis and subsequent healing with fibrosis. The histologic picture thus varies with the age of the lesion. In addition to the nonspecific acute and chronic inflammatory responses, there are histiocytes and scattered foreign body giant cells present.

## Papillary Cystadenoma

The occurrence of bilateral cystadenomas has been reported as being associated with Lindau's disease. All cases reported to date have been benign. Histologically, the ducts show dilatation with papillary proliferation of the lining epithelium, which, in turn, shows varying amounts of secretory activity. The secretory material both intracellulary and extracellularly in the lumen of the duct is PAS positive. The intervening

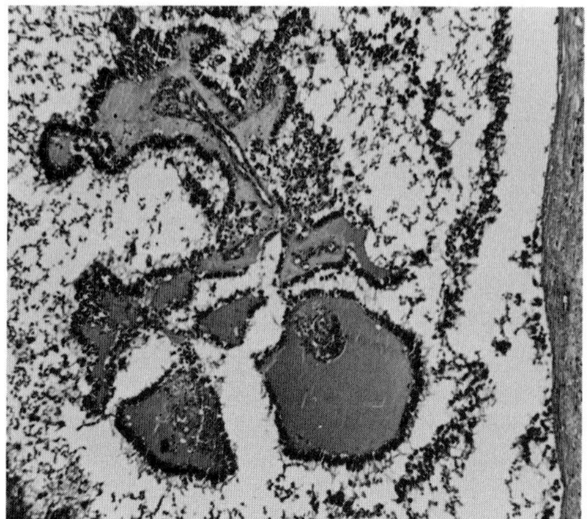

**Fig. 165.** Papillary Cystadenoma. The cystic dilatation of the epididymis contains papillary infoldings lined by epithelial cells with cleared cytoplasm and absence of atypical features. PAS-positive secretory material is present in the duct lumen.

stroma between ducts contains dense fibrous tissue (Figs. 165 and 166).

### Miscellaneous Benign Lesions of the Spermatic Cord

Benign neoplasms of the spermatic cord most frequently are lipomas, fibromas, and leiomyomas (Fig. 167). The age range of the affected patients is wide, but most cases present as painless masses in adulthood. Less commonly, granular cell tumor, adrenal rest, lymphangiomyoma, or benign germ cell tumors (adult cystic teratoma) have been reported. The histology of each of these common neoplasms, which rarely take origin in the spermatic cord, is identical to that for examples in more common sites.

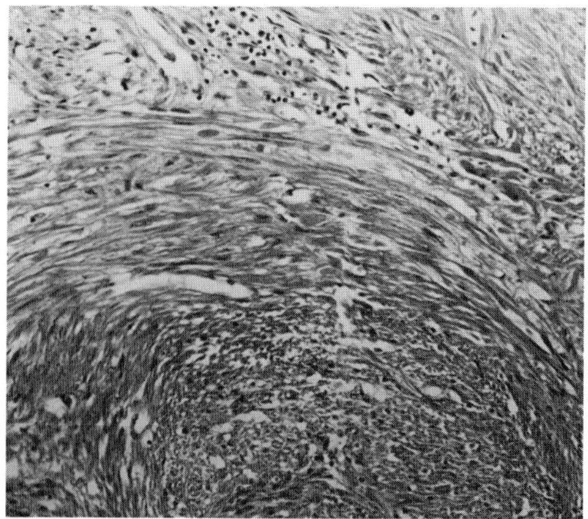

**Fig. 167.** Spermatic Cord Leiomyoma. Bundles of smooth muscle cells interlace one another. The nuclear features and absence of mitotic figures are typical of the benign smooth muscle tumor.

## MALIGNANT NEOPLASMS

### Malignant Mesothelioma

The malignant mesothelioma is often a very large tumor that appears to arise near the epididymis and extend up the

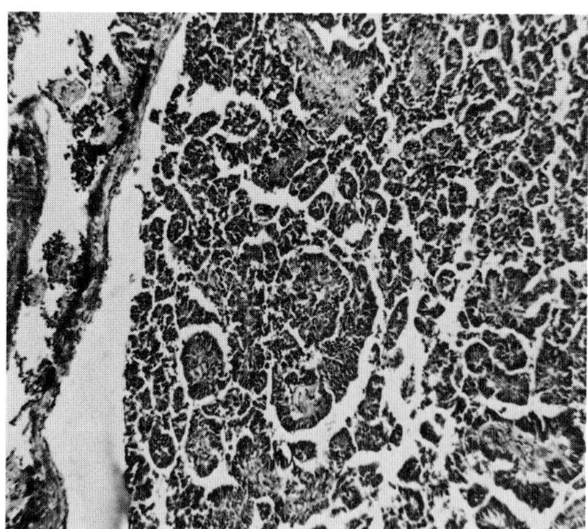

**Fig. 166.** Papillary Cystadenoma. The papillary projections are more numerous than present in the example in Figure 165. There was no evidence of invasion of adjacent epididymis by the neoplasm.

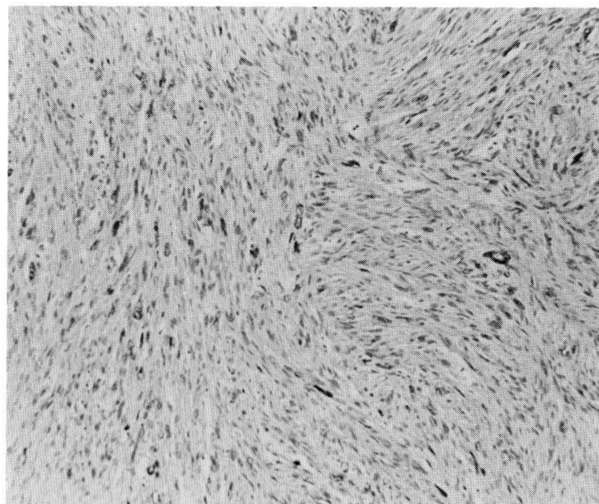

**Fig. 168.** Spermatic Cord Leiomyosarcoma. The bundles of spindle cells with random orientation constitute the pattern of the neoplasm. Scattered individual cells contain enlarged, hyperchromatic nuclei. Mitoses were common.

cord. The tunica vaginalis is often studded with numerous nodular lesions, the testis itself is uninvolved. This is an epithelial-like tumor with solid areas as well as tubular, acinar, or papillary structures. The cells usually contain abundant pink cytoplasm, and the nuclei are rather pleomorphic. The lining mesothelial cells of the tunica are hyperchromatic and hyperplastic and represent the site of origin of the neoplasm. These tumor nodules tend to recur locally.

### Embryonal Rhabdomyosarcoma

Embryonal rhabdomyosarcoma is a malignant tumor of the spermatic cord that occurs most commonly in childhood. These tumors are highly pleomorphic; the cells are often spindle shaped with very hyperchromatic nuclei. Cross striations, when present, are very helpful diagnostically but may be very difficult to see. Rhabdomyoblasts, rounded cells with intensely pink cytoplasm and an eccentric nucleus, may be present.

### Miscellaneous Malignant Neoplasms of the Spermatic Cord

A wide range of malignant neoplasms have been reported to occur in the spermatic cord. The most common of these malignancies in decreasing order of incidence are fibrosarcoma, leiomyosarcoma, and liposarcoma (Fig. 168). The majority of the other types are various soft tissue sarcomas, with rare epithelial malignancies, most commonly germ cell neoplasms. As with the benign neoplasms of the spermatic cord, the sarcomas reported are primarily malignancies that affect older men. Histologically, these malignancies are identical to those described elsewhere in the body.

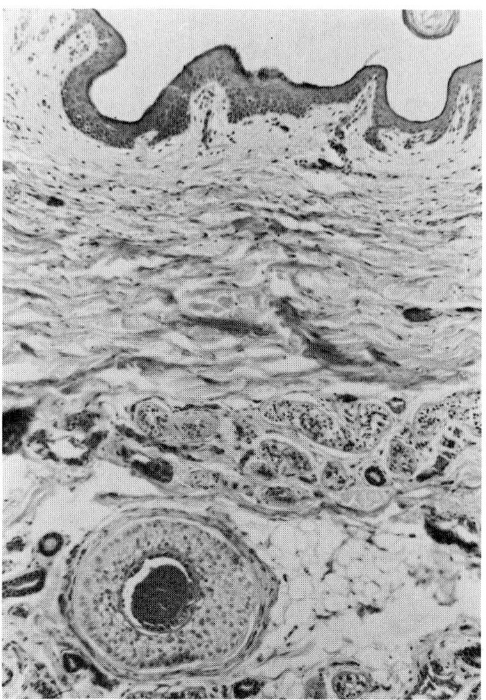

**Fig. 169.** Normal Scrotum. The thin scrotal epidermis overlies the dermis that contains the skin appendage structures, including a hair shaft and sweat glands.

Mesenchymal neoplasms of the spermatic cord include

- Leiomyoma[177]
- Leiomyosarcoma[178,179]
- Lipoma[170]
- Liposarcoma[180]
- Rhabdomyosarcoma[175,181]
- Fibrosarcoma[176,178]
- Malignant fibrous histiocytoma[182]
- Granular cell tumor[183]
- Pheochromocytoma[184]

# SCROTUM

## NORMAL HISTOLOGY

The epidermis of the scrotum is thin and composed of squamous epithelium with numerous ridges. The skin appendages include hair, sebaceous glands, and sweat glands. The dartos tunic composed of smooth muscle is deep to the dermis. Fat and muscle are present between the dartos and the tunica vaginalis (Fig. 169).

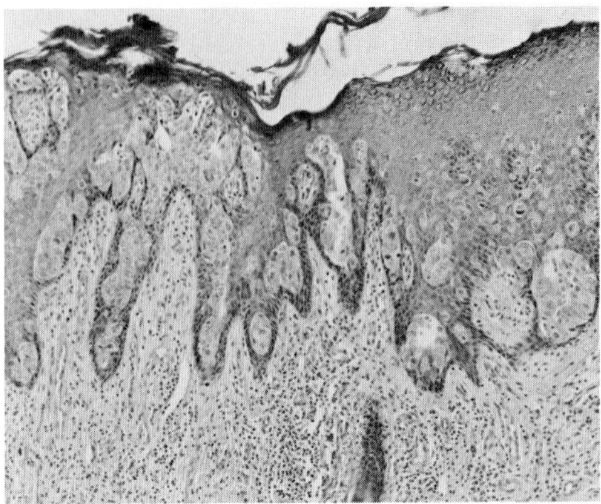

**Fig. 170.** Paget's Disease. The enlarged Paget cells are present both in nests adjacent to the basement membrane and single cells scattered throughout the epidermis.

### Paget's Disease of the Scrotum

Paget's disease is a neoplasm originally described and most commonly found in the nipple of the breast, but it also occurs in the perineal region including the scrotum. The lesion appears as an erythematous, moist plaque involving the scrotum with possible extension to the perianal and penile skin.

Microscopically nests of Paget cells are found most commonly immediately above the basement membrane of the epidermis. Scattered nests and individual cells are randomly located throughout the epidermal layer. The Paget cell has a nucleus with a distinct nuclear membrane and vesicular. nucleoplasm. The cytoplasm is abundant and stains lightly with routine H & E stains. The cytoplasm is strongly PAS positive (Fig. 170).

### Squamous Cell Carcinoma

Squamous cell carcinoma of the scrotum, the first malignancy associated with occupational exposure to a carcinogen, occurs less frequently now than when described by Pott in the 18th century. The histologic features are those typical of well-differentiated squamous cell carcinoma of the skin (described in the section on the penis).

# IMMUNOHISTOPATHOLOGY

## TESTIS

The prototype tissue for all subsequent immunohistopathology in the genitourinary tract was the study of testicular tumors for the presence of alpha-fetoprotein (AFP) and human chorionic gonadotropin (HCG). Blood levels of both have been useful markers for determining the persistence of disease after orchiectomy and for following the course of disease after further treatment, such as retroperitoneal lymphadenectomy or chemotherapy.

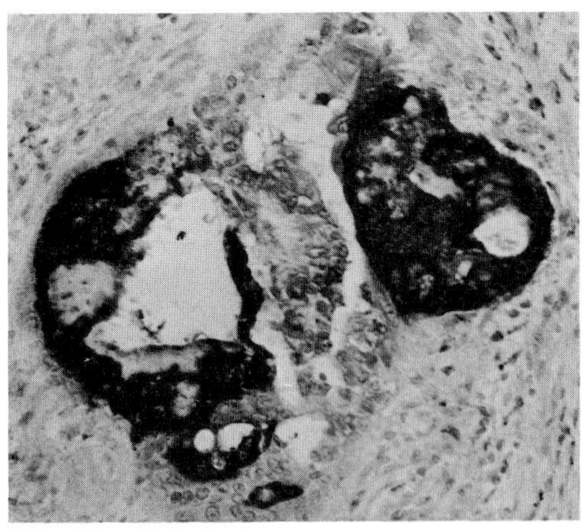

**Fig. 171.** Syncytiotrophoblastic giant cells stained for HCG by immunoperoxidase technique.

Tissue localization of these markers may be very helpful in two groups of patients. The first group are those who had orchiectomy performed prior to drawing serum levels of HCG or AFP. It may be helpful in these patients to determine whether the tumor contained these markers by immunoperoxidase staining. This may aid considerably in the interpretation of postoperative serum marker levels.

The second group of patients in whom

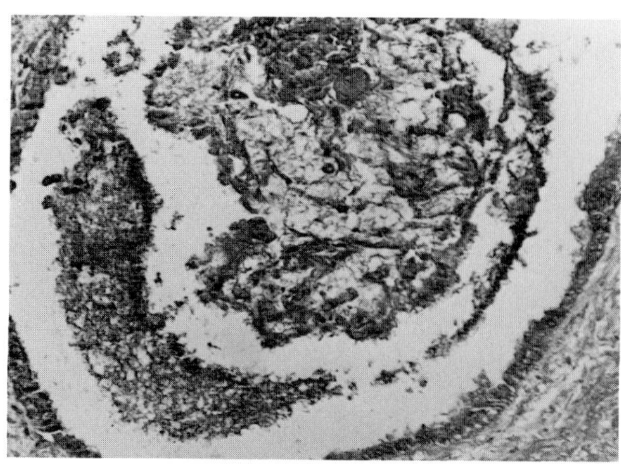

**Fig. 172.** Embryonal carcinoma stained for alpha fetoprotein by immunoperoxidase technique.

tissue levels of these markers may be helpful are those patients with seminoma and elevated serum HCG levels. If the source of the HCG can be shown to be syncytiotrophoblastic giant cells (STGC) within the seminoma, then the treatment for these patients may be different from those in whom elevated serum HCG levels cannot be localized to STGC (Fig. 171).

All immunoperoxidase staining was performed by the peroxidase–antiperoxidase method of Sternberger, the details of which have been well described elsewhere.

Alpha-fetoprotein has been detected in the glands of yolk-sac carcinoma and embryonal carcinoma (Fig. 172). Seminoma has not been described as containing alpha-fetoprotein by immunoperoxidase or serum determinations.

## PROSTATE

Immunoperoxidase localization of two distinct prostatic antigens—human prostate specific antigen (PSA) and prostatic acid phosphatase (PAP)—has been described. They have been of use when attempting to determine the unknown primary site of a metastatic lesion (Fig. 173*A*,*B*). The presence in the tumor of detectable PSA or PAP definitively identifies the prostate as the primary site. There are no reported false-positive results; however, false-negative results, especially in poorly differentiated adenocarcinoma, occur in 20% of cases. All

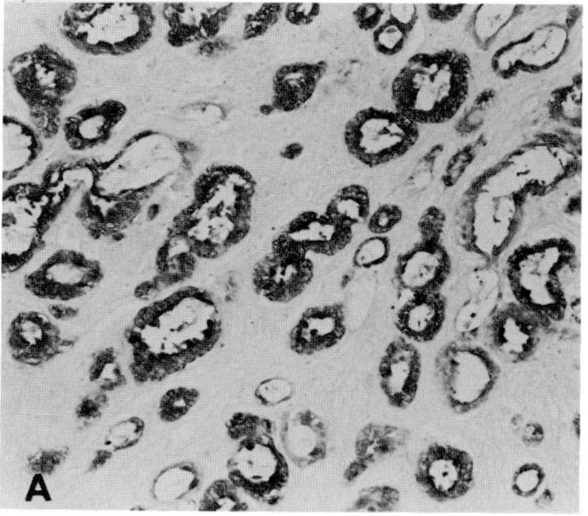


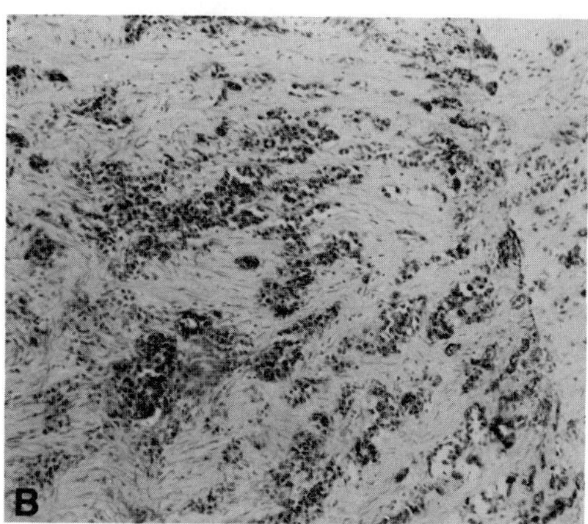


**Fig. 173A.** Prostatic adenocarcinoma stained for human prostate-specific antigen by immunoperoxidase technique. **B.** Prostatic adenocarcinoma stained for prostate acid phosphatase by immunoperoxidase technique.

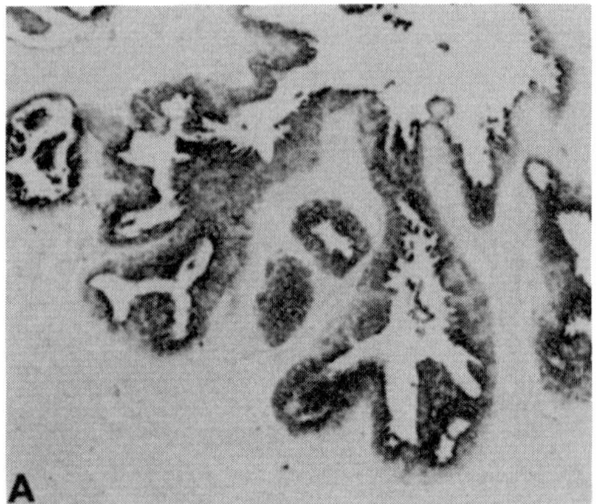


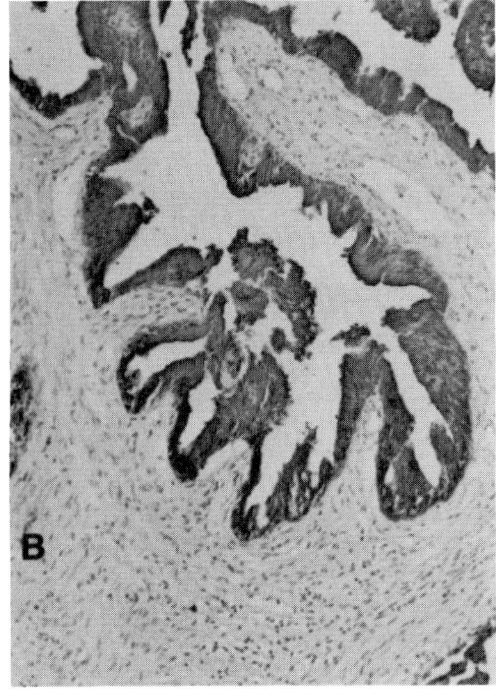


**Fig. 174A.** Benign prostatic hyperplasia stained for human prostate-specific antigen. **B.** Benign prostatic hyperplasia stained for prostatic acid phosphatase.

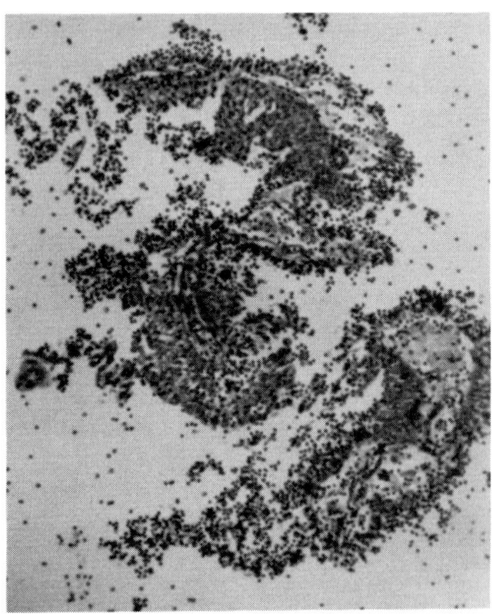

**Fig. 175.** Grade I transitional cell carcinoma of the bladder positive for blood group antigens by the specific red cell adherence test.

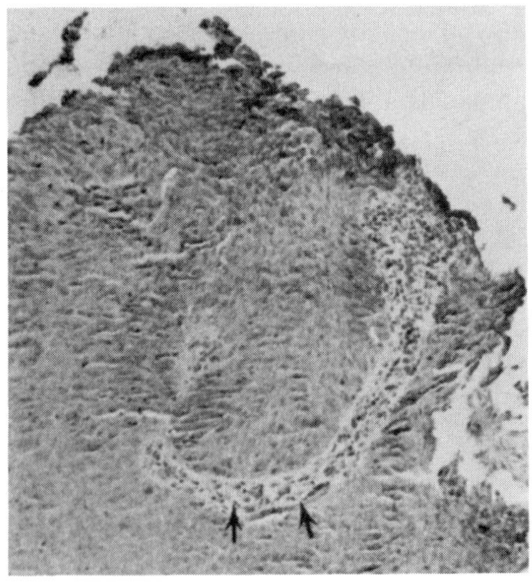

**Fig. 176.** Grade I-II transitional cell carcinoma of the bladder positive for blood group antigens by immunoperoxidase technique (note lack of staining in stalk-arrows).

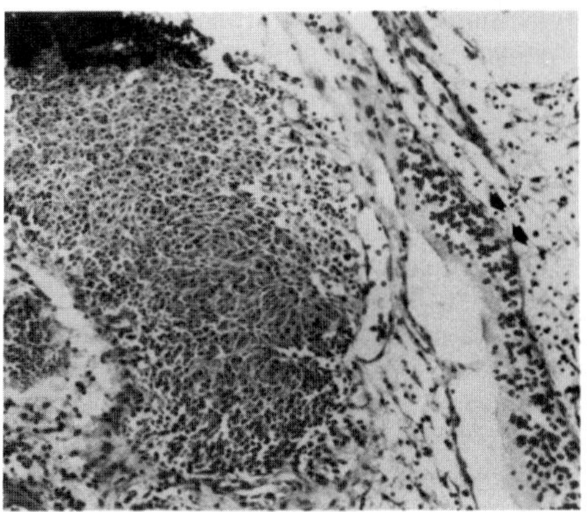

**Fig. 177.** Invasive Grade II-III transitional cell carcinoma lacking blood group antigens by red cell adherence. Note positive blood vessels (*arrows*).

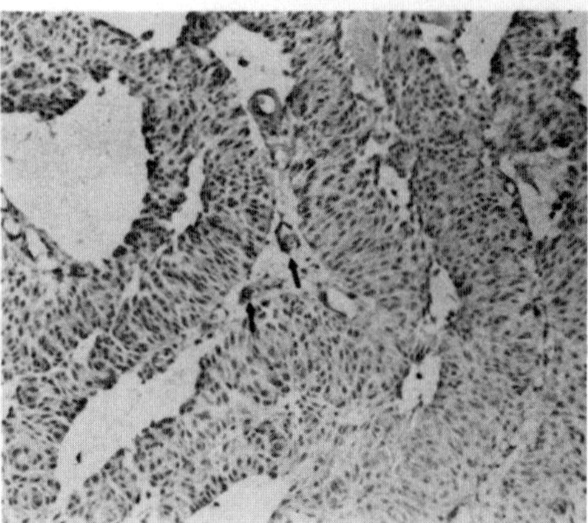

**Fig. 178.** Grade II transitional cell carcinoma negative for blood group antigens by immunoperoxidase techniques. Note positive blood vessels (*arrows*).

cases of benign prostatic hyperplasia examined have exhibited detectable PSA and PAP levels (Fig. 174*A*,*B*).

## BLADDER

The detection of blood group antigens (BGA) on the surface of transitional cell carcinomas has been helpful in identifying the subgroup of patients with low-grade superficial disease who are more likely to develop invasive disease. The measurement of BGA in patients of blood type A, B, and AB is performed by the technique of Davidsohn with modifications as described by Weinstein and colleagues, utilizing human antisera and the appropriate red blood cells. In patients with blood group 0, the technique is performed utilizing Ulex Europeus extract as the first layer in an immunoperoxidase technique, as previously described. This has increased the sensitivity and specificity of the test for those of blood type 0 and may also be useful for other blood types.

Normal bladder epithelium demonstrates the presence of such blood group antigens, and this pattern is maintained in patients with low-grade transitional cell carcinoma of the bladder whose clinical course is that of recurrent superficial disease without subsequent invasion (Figs. 175 and 176). In patients in whom BGA are lacking, subsequent development of invasive disease occurs in 60% to 70% of cases (Figs. 177 and 178).

# ADRENAL GLAND

## NORMAL STRUCTURE

The normal adrenal gland is composed of the outer cortex of mesodermal derivation, taking origin from the urogenital ridge, and the inner adrenal medulla derived from the neural crest. The weight of the organ is 2g to 4g at birth, increasing to 4g to 6g in adults. The right and left adrenal glands are of equal weight. The adrenal glands of men are equal in weight to that observed in women.

The composition of the adrenal cortex varies with age. During fetal development, the cortex is composed principally of a provisional cortex and a thin rim of subcapsular cells arranged in small nests (Fig. 179). Following birth, the provisional or fetal cortex undergoes atrophy, and the three cortical zones in the adult

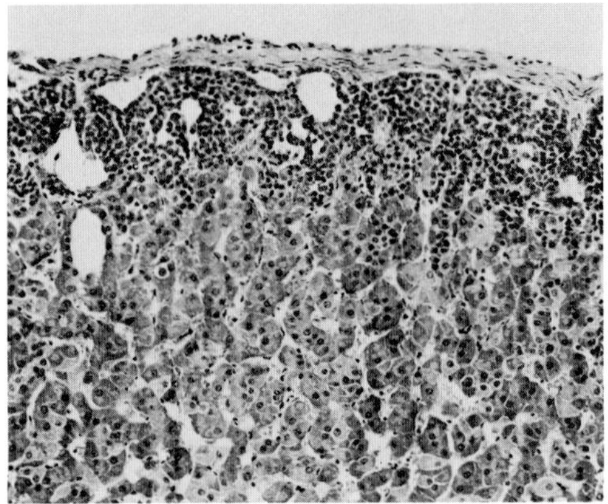

**Fig. 179.** Normal Fetal Adrenal Gland. The fetal adrenal is composed primarily of a thin rim of small cortical cells that separate the capsule from the provisional or fetal cortex composed of large cells with abundant eosinophilic cytoplasm.

adrenal cortex develop. By 1 year of age, the zona glomerulosa, fasciculata, and reticularis can be readily identified (Fig. 180*A*,*B*).

The zona glomerulosa constitutes approximately 15% of the adult adrenal cortex. The cells are arranged in small nests, in contrast to the cords of cells within the zona fasciculata. The zona glomerulosa is the cytologic source of the mineralocorticoids. The zona fasciculata, the source of the glucocorticoids and androgens, constitutes approximately 80% of the adrenal cortical cell population. It is composed of well-defined cells that have either a clear or eosinophilic cytoplasm. The clear, or light, cells of the fasciculata involve lipid storage while the eosinophilic cytoplasm contain fewer stored steroids. The innermost layer of the adrenal cortex, the zona reticularis, has synthetic functions identical to those of the zona fasciculata. The zona reticularis is less well organized than the linear cords of the zona fasciculata. The entire zona constitutes approximately 10% of the adrenal cortex. The cells of fasciculata and reticularis zones are under the control of adrenocorticotropic hormone (ACTH),

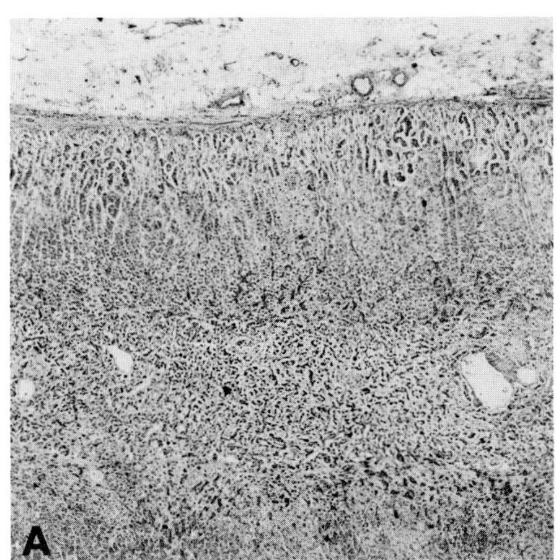



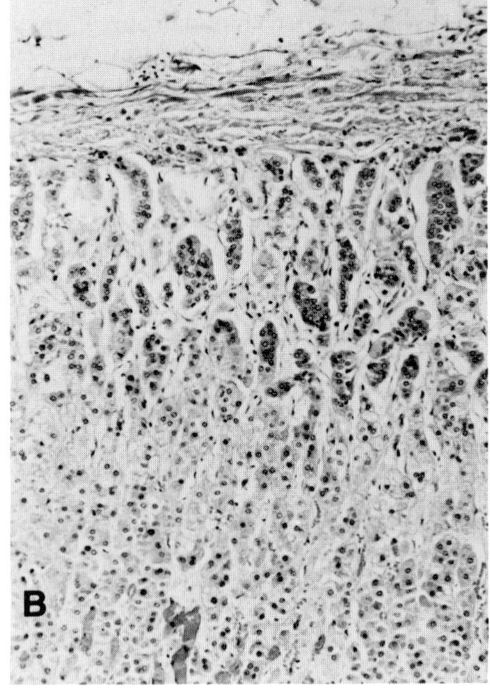



**Fig. 180A.** Normal Adult Adrenal Gland. The capsule overlies the three cortical zones—glomerulosa, fasciculata, and reticularis. Adrenal veins and arterial branches are present within the medulla. **B.** Normal Adult Adrenal Cortex. The zona glomerulosa cells in nests are smaller than the cells of the zona fasciculata arranged in cords.

synthesized by the basophil cells of the anterior pituitary gland.

Electron-microscopy studies of the normal adrenal cortex reveal differences among the different zones, but all show prominent golgi apparatus and smooth endoplasmic reticulum (ER).

The adrenal medulla contains cells of the chromaffin system of neurectodermal origin. The cells are arranged in groups and nests of varying size throughout the medulla. In addition, the adrenal veins with prominent longitudinal muscular coats are present. The use of chromate fixatives produces oxidation of the catecholamines, resulting in readily observed brown cytoplasmic granules.

## MALDEVELOPMENT

Bilateral agenesis of the adrenal gland is quite rare and incompatible with survival. Unilateral agenesis is uniformly accompanied by a compensatory enlargement (hyperplasia) of the contralateral adrenal gland.

The embryologic development of the adrenal cortex from the urogenital ridge accounts for the common findings of heterotopic tissues in proximity to the gonads (both testes and ovaries). In addition, ectopic adrenal tissue is not uncommon in the capsule of the kidney, in the retroperitoneum adjacent to the renal capsule, and, in rare reported cases, in the mesentery of the appendix, broad ligament, and hernia sacs.

A form of metaplasia observed most commonly as an incidental finding at autopsy are heterotopic hematopoietic elements. These are commonly found in association with adipose tissue and, on occasion, ectopic bone. When found incidentally, the condition is referred to as *myeloid metaplasia*. On occasion these ectopic tissues can attain a size allowing clinical detection. Such a tumor is called a *myelolipoma*. One such reported case was associated with Cushing's syndrome.

### Adrenal Hemorrhage

The majority of cases of adrenal hemorrhage, a potentially life-threatening lesion, are observed within the first few days of birth. Clinical evidence of adrenal insufficiency with or without an abdominal mass suggests the presence of adrenal hemorrhage in the newborn. Infants with a history of hypoxia and septicemia are observed to be at a higher risk for developing adrenal hemorrhage. The disorder may involve both adrenals, or it may be unilateral. When unilateral, the right adrenal gland is more commonly involved than the left.

The involved adrenal is markedly enlarged, and on cross section the presence of hemorrhage is readily apparent (Fig. 181). In this age group, the affected adrenal gland has gross features similar to those of neuroblastoma, from which it must be differentiated.

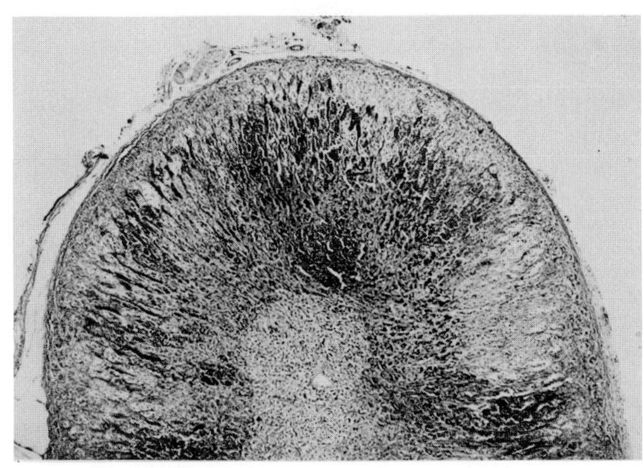

**Fig. 181.** Adrenal Hemorrhage. The intra cortical hemorrhage is most prominent in the inner cortex—the zona reticularis and zona fasciculata.

Cysts of the adrenal gland are thought by many investigators to represent resolving hematomas with fibrosis and peripheral calcification in patients who survived a past episode of an adrenal hemorrhage.

### Nodular and Diffuse Hyperplasia

Hyperplasia of the adrenal cortex may be congenital or acquired. The congenital form of hyperplasia is associated with inborn errors of steroid metabolism, resulting in one of six identified distinct clinical disorders, the most common being virilizing and salt-losing syndromes (adrenogenital syndromes). In contrast, the majority of cases of acquired hyperplasia observed at autopsy are asymptomatic, without associated hyperfunction of the adrenal cortex. The hyperplasia is always bilateral, although it may be more prominent in one gland than in the other. The frequency of hyperplastic nodules without associated clinical manifestations increases with age.

Hyperplasia of the adrenal cortex, when associated with clinical hyperfunction, reflects elevated circulating ACTH, either of pituitary origin or from ectopic sources such as extrapituitary malignant neoplasms. The most commonly associated clinical syndromes with adrenal hyperplasia are Cushing's syndrome and Conn's syndrome.

Microscopically, the hyperplasia of the adrenal cortex may be nodular or diffuse and affects the zona fasciculata and reticularis in most cases (Fig. 182*A*,*B*). Conn's syndrome may be associated with a hyperplasia primarily affecting the zona glomerulosa. Evidence of hyperplasia in the contralateral adrenal gland may be minimal or readily apparent. The hyperplastic cortical cells are enlarged, with variable proportions of clear and dark cells intermixed. Variation of nuclear size is common. Hyperplastic nodules do not have surrounding capsules.

## NEOPLASMS

### Adrenal Cortical Adenoma

The vast majority of nodules greater than 1 cm in size observed at autopsy are nonfunctional. Their frequency in reported autopsy series is approximately 2% of all adults. These nodules are usually discrete and yellow, measuring 1 cm to 5 cm in diameter. Rarely, they are larger, and increased size is associated with areas of necrosis, cystic degeneration, and, on occasion, calcification. The adenoma commonly, but not invariably,

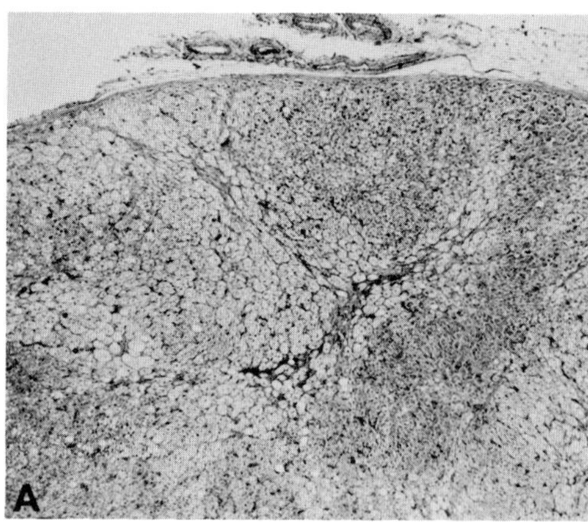


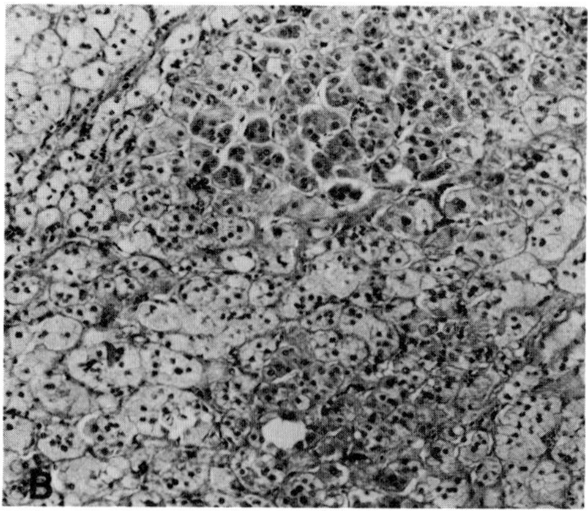


**Fig. 182.** Adrenal Cortical Hyperplasia. **A.** The hyperplastic adrenal cortex has a disorganized appearance and is composed of interspersed areas of clear and dark cells. **B.** Clear cells with abundant vacuolated cytoplasm are interspersed among smaller dark cells with eosinophilic cytoplasm.

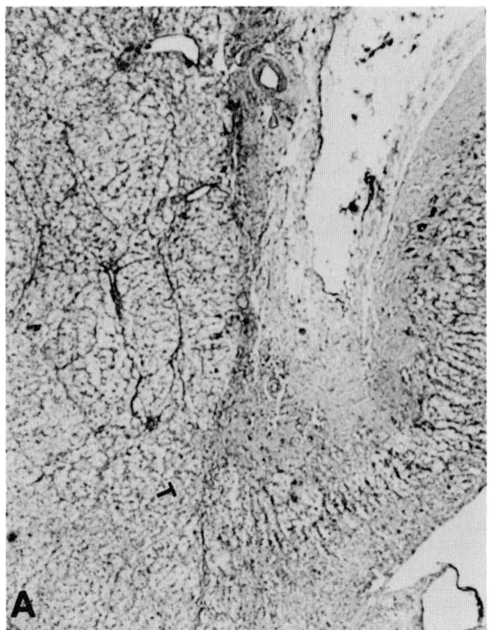


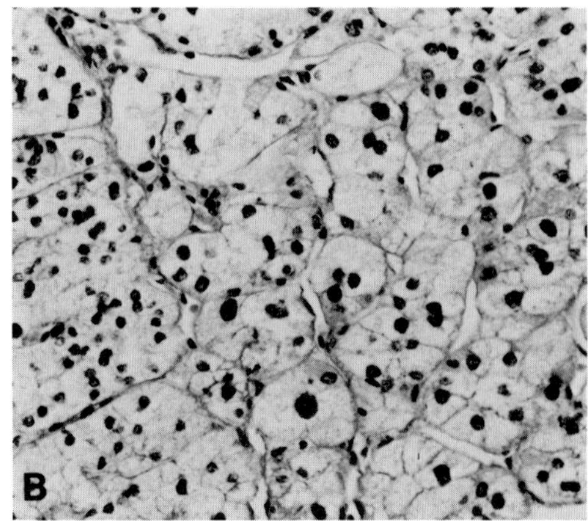


**Fig. 183.** Adrenal Cortical Adenoma. **A.** A thin fibrous pseudocapsule separates the adrenal adenoma on the left from the normal adrenal cortex on the right. **B.** The cells have abundant cytoplasm and are arranged in poorly defined nests with interspersed thin-walled vessels. Variation of nuclear size is readily apparent.

has a surrounding capsule. When present, it is frequently incomplete. The clear cell type is the most commonly encountered histologic form. Variability of nuclear size is common. Mitoses are rare to absent (Fig. 183*A*,*B*).

The size criteria of cortical nodules regarded as adenomas varies from more than 3mm to more than 1cm. Nodules of smaller dimensions, frequently multiple and bilateral, are regarded as examples of nodular hyperplasia. The contralateral adrenal is either normal or atrophic, depending on the functional status of the adrenal adenoma. When the adenoma is functional, the clinical syndromes reported are adrenogenital, Cushing's, or Conn's syndrome. Differentiation of larger masses (in excess of 5 cm) from those that will behave as carcinoma must be cautious. There is general agreement that there is no criterion short of the demonstration of metastasis that allows the separation of adrenal cortical adenoma of large size from adrenal carcinoma.

A recently described variant of adrenal cortical adenoma, termed *pigmented adenoma,* has been reported. The majority are incidental findings at autopsy and without apparent function. The black color of the adenoma is attributed to lipofuscin pigment. Histologically, the cells bear greatest resemblance to those of the zona reticularis. Rare cases have been reported with virilization, Cushing's syndrome, and Conn's syndrome.

### Adrenal Cortical Carcinoma

Adrenal cortical carcinoma is an uncommon adrenal malignancy that may show clinical functional activity or present as a nonfunctional abdominal mass. The majority of nonfunctional carcinomas are observed in elderly men; functional carcinomas are more frequent in young women.

These carcinomas are usually unilateral, solid, and show infiltrating margins within the retroperitoneal adipose tissue. The cut surface of the tumor shows multiple areas of necrosis and focal hemorrhage. Histologically these neoplasms

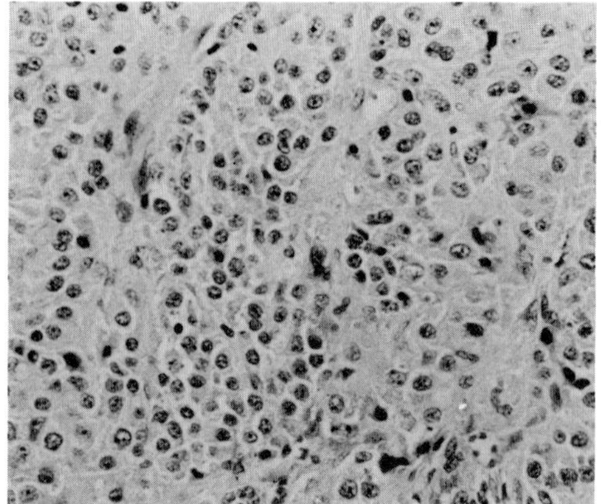

**Fig. 184.** Adrenal Cortical Carcinoma. The tumor cells grow in sheets without any recognizable organization. Scattered tumor cells contain hyperchromatic irregular, enlarged nuclei. No mitoses are present. The tumor metastasized to the liver and regional lymph nodes.

are characterized by great variation of pattern, cell size, and nuclear-staining characteristics (Fig. 184). Bizarre cells are commonly present, frequently with multiple nuclei. Mitoses are commonly observed. Some cases show incomplete encapsulation while others exhibit no apparent capsule and readily observable local invasion of adjacent tissue. None of the cytologic and histologic features of these neoplasms are reliable criteria for the diagnosis of malignancy. Unfortunately, the only reliable criterion of malignancy is the presence of distant metastases. Metastases are most common in the liver, regional lymph nodes, and lungs.

## Pheochromocytoma

Pheochromocytomas are paragangliomas the site of origin of which is the adrenal medulla. Although the majority of pheochromocytomas are not hormonally functional, these tumors may secrete epinephrine, norepinephrine, or both of these catecholamines. Although pheochromocytomas are most commonly encountered in the adrenal medulla, they may also be observed in the extra-adrenal retroperitoneum, the mediastinum, and the urinary bladder. Pheochromocytomas are a component of the multiple endocrine adenopathies, type II, in combination with medullary carcinoma of the thyroid and hyperparathyroidism. These tumors are also reported in association with neural disorders, such as neurofibromatosis and cerebellar hemangioblastomas.

These neoplasms occur most commonly in adults; however 10% occur in children. The majority of pheochromocytomas occur unilaterally, the right being involved twice as frequently as the left. They are highly variable in size, ranging from a few grams to in excess of 2 kg.

Multiple areas of hemorrhage, necro-

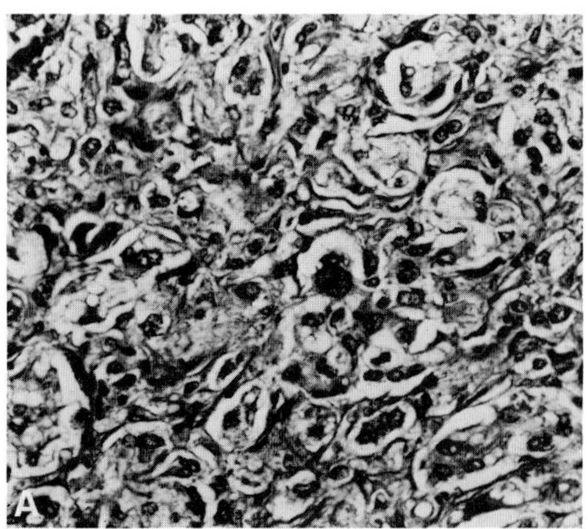



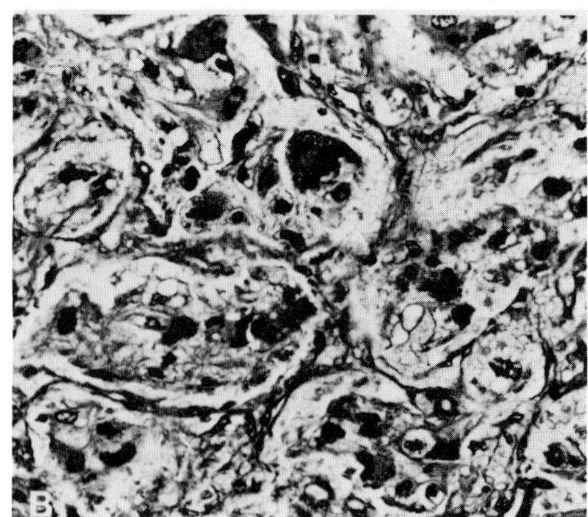



**Fig. 185.** Pheochromocytoma. **A.** The tumor cells in nests and cords are very pleomorphic. Scattered, enlarged, and bizarre nuclei are present. **B.** The nests of neoplastic cells are separated by thin fibrovascular septa. The variability of the nuclear size and cytoplasm density is apparent.

sis, and cyst formation are observed throughout the tumor, resulting in a soft, red to yellow, tumor mass. The most characteristic histologic feature is the pattern of cells in nests called "zellballen" (Fig. 185*A*,*B*). These nests of cells are separated by thin fibrovascular trabeculae. The cells show moderate variation in size and shape with round to oval nuclei with prominent nucleoli. Scattered bizarre cells may be seen but have no reliable association with clinical malignancy. The cytoplasm of the tumor cells is finely granular and eosinophilic. As with adrenal cortical carcinoma, experience has demonstrated that there are no reliable histologic features capable of predicting malignant behavior. When metastases are observed, they are most frequently found in bones, especially the ribs and vertebral column. In excess of 80% of these tumors have a benign clinical course.

### Neuroblastoma

Neuroblastomas are interesting neoplasms that originate in the adrenal medulla and less commonly in the extra-adrenal retroperitoneum. They are virtually confined to the children. Seventy-five percent of cases are observed in children less than 5 years of age. These lesions may be observed as early as birth. The age at diagnosis is correlated with the biologic course of the neoplasm: the younger the age at diagnosis, the better the survival rate of the afflicted patients. Tumors diagnosed in patients older than 2 years of age are consistently aggressive malignancies. Spontaneous regression has been reported in occasional cases. Some neoplasms manifest complete hemorrhagic necrosis with calcification. Alternatively, spontaneously arresting tumors demonstrate maturation to ganglioneuromas.

These neoplasms are generally highly hemorrhagic with multiple areas of necrosis. The necrosis and hemorrhage account for their uniformly soft composition. Infiltration into the adjacent retroperitoneal tissue is common. Histologically the tumor is characterized by a densely cellular proliferation of small round cells with minimal cytoplasm and indistinct cell borders. The necrosis and hemorrhage observed grossly are manifested at the histologic level also. The cells proliferate in nests, sheets, or both patterns (Fig. 186*A*,*B*). Occasional true rosettes characterized by tumor cells surrounding a circumscribed area of neurofibrils are a diagnostic feature. These rosettes are highly variable in number, and occasional cases appear to be devoid of these structures. Some cases contain

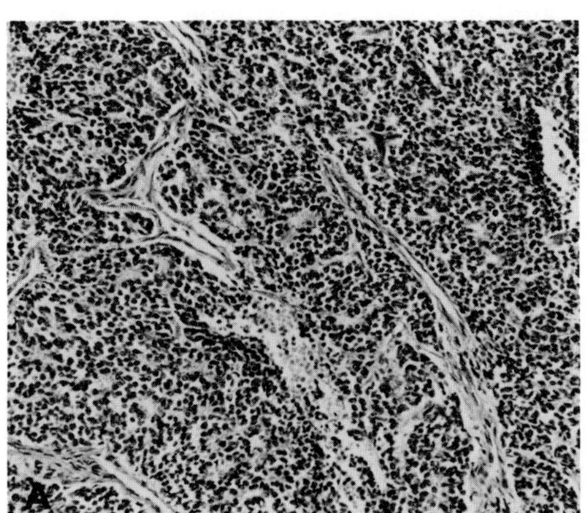

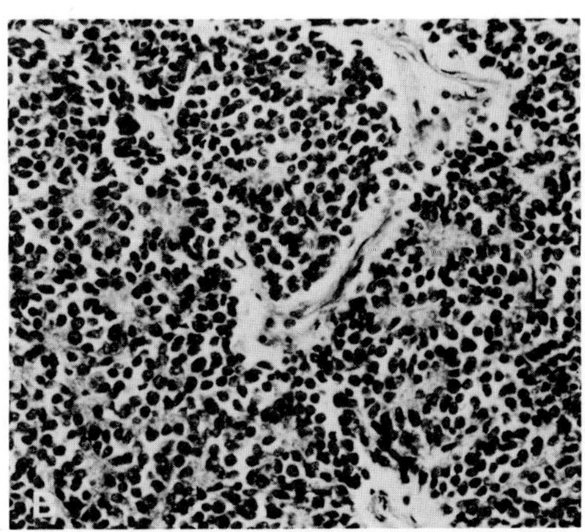

**Fig. 186.** Neuroblastoma. **A.** The tumor is highly cellular and arranged in large nests and sheets with scattered fibrovascular trabeculae. Occasional clusters of cells suggest rosette formation. **B.** Tumor cells arranged around a central acellular fibrillar area constitute the diagnostic rosettes of neuroblastoma. The nuclei are uniform in size and hyperchromaticity and virtually devoid of cytoplasm.

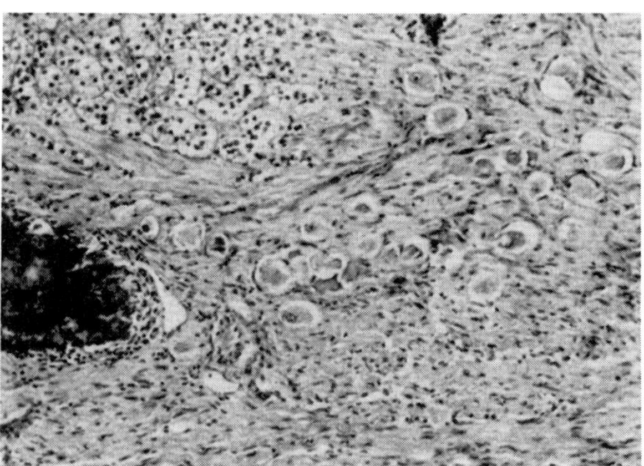

**Fig. 187.** Ganglioneuroma. The neoplastic ganglion cells are scattered in a background of fibrous tissue and occasional nerve fibers. A focus of tumor necrosis with calcification is present on the left.

nests of mature cells with more cytoplasm. In addition, some cases show focal maturation of neuroblasts to ganglion cells.

Clinically, 70% of patients demonstrate metastases at the time of initial presentation. The metastases are most common in the liver, lung, and bones. Cases with predominance of bone metastases, especially to the base of the skull and the region of the orbit, are referred to as *Hutchinson-type tumors*. Cases with predominance of liver metastases are regarded as *Pepper-type tumors*.

The entire spectrum of neoplasms involving neuroblasts and cells representing neuroblast maturation are represented by neuroblastomas, the most malignant form, and ganglioneuromas, showing the greatest extent of maturation and associated with a clinically benign course. Between these two neoplasms are ganglioneuroblastomas.

## Ganglioneuroma

Ganglioneuromas are benign neoplasms most commonly seen in the mediastinum and retroperitoneum and only rarely in the adrenal gland. They represent the most mature form of neuroblastoma-type tumors. Unlike neuroblastomas, they occur most commonly in adults.

These neoplasms appear entirely encapsulated. They are solid, gray-white neoplasms. Mature ganglion cells are present in groups or individually randomly scattered throughout the neoplasm (Fig. 187). Hemorrhage and necrosis are distinctly uncommon. There are no cells with the morphology of immature neuroblasts.

## Ganglioneuroblastoma

As indicated above, ganglioneuroblastoma tumors are intermediate in their differentiation between neuroblastomas and ganglioneuromas. As with ganglioneuromas, they are most commonly found in the mediastinum and retroperitoneum and, only uncommonly, within the adrenal. They tend to occur in children with only uncommon cases reported in adults.

These neoplasms are characteristically discrete and solid and only occasionally manifest hemorrhage and necrosis. Histologically, these neoplasms show all stages of neuroblast maturation with variable mixtures of immature neuroblasts and variably mature ganglion cells. The immature ganglion cells show variation in nuclear size and number with prominent nuclei.

The biologic behavior of these uncommon neoplasms is reported also to be intermediate between neuroblastomas and ganglioneuromas.

# REFERENCES

## KIDNEY

1. Bennington JL, Beckwith JB: Embryology and anatomy of the upper urinary tract. In Bennington JL, Beckwith JB: Tumors of the Kidney, Renal Pelvis and Ureter, 2nd series, Fascicle 12, pp 1-24. Washington, DC, Armed Forces Institute of Pathology, 1975
2. Filmer RB, Taxy JB: Cysts of the kidney, renal dysplasia and renal hypoplasia. In Kelalis PP, King LR (eds): Clinical Pediatric Urology, Ch 19, pp 680-733, Philadelphia, WB Saunders, 1976
3. Bloom DA, Brosman S: The multicystic kidney. J Urol 120:211, 1978
4. Lieberman E, Salinas–Madrigal L, Gwinn JL, et al: Infantile polycystic disease of the kidneys and liver. Medicine 50:277, 1971
5. Lambert PP: Polycystic disease of the kidney. Arch Pathol Lab Med 44:34, 1947
6. Segal AJ, Spataro RF, Barbaric ZL: Adult polycystic kidney disease: A review of 100 cases. J Urol 118:711, 1977
7. Strauss MB: Clinical and pathological aspects of cystic disease of the renal medulla. Ann Intern Med 57:373, 1962
8. Khorsand D: Carcinoma within solitary renal cysts. J Urol 93:440, 1965
9. Berger BW, Kwart AM, Nime F, Catalona WJ: Transitional cell carcinoma in a pyelogenic cyst. J Urol 118:858, 1977
10. Abeshouse BS, Abeshouse GA: Sponge kidney: A review of the literature and a report of 5 cases. J Urol 84:252, 1960
11. Banner MP, Pollack HM, Chatten J, Witzleben C: Multilocular renal cysts: Radiologic-pathologic correlation. AJR 136:239, 1981
12. Robbins SL: Diseases of the interstitium [of the kidney]. In SL Robbins: Pathology, 3rd ed, Ch 24, pp 1018-1026. Philadelphia, WB Saunders, 1967
13. Malek RS, Greene LF, DeWeerd JH, Farrow GM: Xanthogranulomatous pyelonephritis. Br J Urol 44:296, 1972
14. DeRidder PA, Koff SA, Gikas PW, Heidelberger KP: Renal Malacoplakia. J Urol 117:428, 1977
15. Stanton MJ, Maxted W: Malacoplakia: A study of the literature and current concepts of pathogenesis, diagnosis, and treatment. J Urol 125:139, 1981
16. Baggenstoss AH, Greene LF: Healed tuberculosis of the kidney. J Urol 45:166, 1941
17. Bennington JL, Beckwith JB: Tumors of the upper urinary tract. In Bennington JL, Beckwith JB: Tumors of the Kidney, Renal Pelvis and Ureter, 2nd series, Fascicle 12, pp 25-242. Washington, DC, Armed Forces Institute of Pathology, 1975
18. Colvin RB, Dickersin GR: Pathology of renal tumors. In Skinner DG, deKernion JB (eds): Genitourinary Cancer, Ch 4, p 84. Philadelphia, WB Saunders, 1978
19. Blonde RP, Brough AJ, Izant RJ: Congenital mesoblastic nephroma of infancy. A report of 8 cases and the relationship to Wilms' tumor. Pediatrics 40:272, 1967
20. McCullough DL, Scott R, Seybold HM: Renal angiomyolipoma (Hamartoma): Review of the literature and report of 7 cases. J Urol 105:32, 1971
21. Bennington JL: Cancer of the kidney—etiology, epidemiology and pathology. Cancer 32:1017, 1973
22. Lieber MM, Tomera KM, Farrow GM: Renal oncocytoma. J Urol 125:481, 1981
23. Christ ML: Polycystic nephroblastoma. J Urol 98:570, 1968
24. Weimar G, Culp DA, Loening S, Narayan A: Urogenital involvement by malignant lymphoma. J Urol 125:230, 1981
25. Wagle DG, Moore RH, Murphy GP: Secondary carcinomas of the kidney. J Urol 114:30, 1975

## RENAL PELVIS AND URETER

26. Bennington JL, Beckwith JB: Tumors of the renal pelvis and ureter. In Bennington JL, Beckwith JB: Tumors of the Kidney, Renal Pelvis and Ureter, 2nd series, Fascicle 12, pp 243-336. Washington, DC, Armed Forces Institute of Pathology, 1975
27. Stuppler SA, Kandzari SJ: Fibroepithelial polyps of the ureter. Urology 5:553, 1975
28. Davides KC, King LM: Fibrous polyps of the ureter. J Urol 115:651, 1976
29. Grossman IW, Kopilnick MD: Peripelvic renal fibroma: Radiologic, pathologic and ultrastructural study of a unique lesion. J Urol 105:174, 1971
30. Kao VC, Graff PW, Rappaport H: Leiomyoma of the ureter. Cancer 24:535, 1969
31. Litzky GM, Seidel RF, O'Brien SE: Leiomyoma of the renal pelvis. J Urol 105:171, 1971
32. Galbraith WW: Pedunculated vascular tumor of the ureter. Br J Urol 22:195, 1950
33. Roemer CE, Pfister RC, Brodsky G, Sacknoff EJ: Primary leiomyosarcoma of ureter. Urology 16:492, 1980
34. Fujita K: Endometriosis of the ureter. J Urol 116:664, 1976
35. Fitch WP, Robinson JR, Radwin HM: Metastatic carcinoma of the ureter. Arch Surg 111:874, 1976
36. Babaian RJ, Johnson DE, Ayala AG, Sie ET: Secondary tumors of the ureter. Urology 14:341, 1979

## BLADDER

37. Koss LG: Tumors of the urinary bladder. In Atlas of Tumor Pathology, 2nd series, Fascicle 11. Washington, DC, Armed Forces Institute of Pathology, 1975
38. Culp DA: The histology of the exstrophied bladder. J Urol 91:538, 1964
39. Rudin L, Tannenbaum M, Lattimer JK: Histologic analysis of the extrophied bladder after anatomical closure. J Urol 108:802, 1972
40. Loening SA, Jacobo E, Hawtrey CE, Culp DA: Adenocarcinoma of the urachus. J Urol 119:68, 1978
41. Mekras GD, Block NL, Carrion HM, Ishikoff M: Urachal carcinoma: diagnosis by computerized axial tomography. J Urol 123:275, 1980
42. Kelalis PP, McLean P: The treatment of diverticulum of the bladder. J Urol 98:349, 1967
43. Peterson LJ, Paulson DF, Glenn JF: The histopathology of vesical diverticula J Urol 110:62, 1973
44. Abeshouse BS, Goldstein AE: Primary carcinoma in a diverticulum of the bladder. J Urol 49:534, 1943
45. Rubin L, Pincus MB: Eosinophilic cystitis: The relationship of allergy in the urinary tract to eosinophilic cystitis and the pathophysiology of eosinophilia. J Urol 112:457, 1974
46. Hunner GL: A rare type of bladder ulcer in women: Report of cases. Trans South Surg Gynecol Assoc 27:247, 1914
47. Smith BH, Dehner LP: Chronic ulcerating interstitial cystitis (Hunner's ulcer). Arch Pathol 93:76, 1972
48. Kretschmer HL: On the occurrence of lymphoid tissue in the urinary organs. J Urol 68:252, 1968
49. Sarma KP: On the nature of cystitis follicularis. J Urol 104:709, 1970
50. Kerr JFR, Gaffney TJ, McGeary HM, et al: Malacoplakia: An electron-microscope and chemical study. J Pathol 107:289, 1972
51. Gupta RK, Schuster RA, Christian WD: Autopsy findings in a unique case of malacoplakia. A cytoimmunohistochemical study of Michaelis–Gutmann bodies. Arch Pathol Lab Med 93:42, 1972
52. Stanton MJ, Maxted W: Malacoplakia: A study of the literature and current concepts of pathogenesis, diagnosis, and treatment. J Urol 125:139, 1981
53. Khafagy MM, El-Bolkainy MN, Mansour MA: Carcinoma of the bilharzial urinary bladder. Cancer 30:150, 1972
54. Morse HD: The etiology and pathology of pyelitis cystica, ureteritis cystica and cystitis cystica. Am J Pathol 4:33, 1928
55. Reece RW, Koontz WW: Leukoplakia of the urinary tract: A review. J Urol 114:165, 1979
56. Molland EA, Trott PA, Paris AMI, Blandy JP: Nephrogenic adenoma: A form of adenomatous metaplasia of the bladder. Br J Urol 48:453, 1976
57. Imaitori SC, Magoss IV: Nephrogenic adenoma of bladder. Urology 16:310, 1980
58. Malek RS, Greene LF, Farrow GW: Amyloidosis of the urinary bladder. Br J Urol 43:189, 1971
59. Abramovici I, Chwatt S, Nussenson M: Massive hematuria and perforation in a case of amyloidosis of the bladder: Case report and review of the literature. J Urol 118:964, 1977
60. Moore TD, Herring AL, McCannel DA: Some urologic aspects of endometriosis. J Urol 49:171, 1943
61. Fein RL, Horton BF: Vesical endometriosis: A case report and review of the literature. J Urol 95:45, 1966
62. Hamsher JB, Farrar T, Moore TD: Congenital vascular tumors and malformations involving urinary tract: Diagnosis and surgical management. J Urol 80:299, 1958
63. Campbell EW, Gislason GJ: Benign mesothelial tumors of the bladder; A review of the literature and report of case of leiomyoma. J Urol 70:733, 1953
64. Leestma JE, Price EB: Paraganglioma of the urinary bladder. Cancer 28:1063, 1971
65. Pugh RCB: Pheochromocytoma of the bladder. Br J Urol 30:432, 1958
66. Torres H, Bennett MJ: Neurofibromatosis of the bladder: Case report and review of the literature. J Urol 96:910, 1966
67. Mouradian JA, Coleman JW, McGovern JH, Gray GF: Granular cell tumor (myoblastoma) of the bladder. J Urol 112:343,1974
68. Ravich A, Stout AP, Ravich RA: Malignant granular cell myoblastoma involving the urinary bladder. Ann Surg 121:361, 1945
69. Pieknos EJ, Iglesias F, Jablokow UR: Inverted papilloma of bladder. Urology 2:178, 1973
70. Cummings R: Inverted papilloma of the bladder. J Pathol 112:255, 1974
71. Melicow MM: Histologic study of vesical urothelium intervening between gross neoplasms in total cystectomy. J Urol 68:261, 1952
72. Eisenberg RB, Roth RB, Schweinsberg MH: Bladder tumors and associated proliferative mucosal lesions. J Urol 84:544, 1960
73. Koss LG: Mapping of the urinary bladder: Its impact on the concept of bladder cancer. Hum Pathol 10:533, 1979
74. Utz DC, Farrow GM, Rife CC et al: Carcinoma in situ of the bladder. Cancer 45:1842, 1980
75. Friedell GH, Parija GC, Nagy GK, Suto EA: The pathology of human bladder cancer. Cancer 45:1823, 1980
76. Prout GR: Current concepts: Bladder carcinoma. N Engl J Med 287:86, 1972

77. Jewett HJ: Cancer of the bladder: Diagnosis and staging. Cancer 32:1072, 1973
78. Cummings KB: Carcinoma of the bladder: Predictors. Cancer 45:1849, 1980
79. Bessette PL, Abell MR, Herwig KR: A clinicopathologic study of squamous cell carcinoma of the bladder. J Urol 112:66, 1974
80. Kramer SA, Bredael J, Croker BP et al: Primary non-urachal adenocarcinoma of the bladder. J Urol 121:278, 1979
81. Austin GE, Stafford J: Signet ring carcinoma of bladder. Urology 12:458, 1978
82. Tefft M, Jaffe N: Sarcoma of the bladder and prostate in children. Cancer 32:1161, 1973
83. Hays DM: Pelvic rhabdomyosarcoma in children: Diagnosis and concepts of management reviewed. Cancer 45:1810, 1980

## PROSTATE AND ACCESSORY SEX GLANDS

84. Andrews GS: Histology of human foetal and prepubertal prostates. J Anat 85:44, 1951
85. Mostofi FK, Price EB: Tumors of the prostate. In Mostofi EK, Price EB: Tumors of the Male Genital System, 2nd series, Fascicle 8, pp 177-262. Washington, DC, Armed Forces Institute of Pathology, 1973
86. Norris HJ, Yunis E: Age changes of seminal vesicles and vasa deferentia in diabetics. Arch Pathol Lab Med 77:40, 1964
87. Abeshouse BS: Infarct of the prostate. J Urol 30:97, 1933
88. Drach GW: Problems in diagnosis of bacterial prostatitis: Gram-negative, gram-positive and mixed infections. J Urol 111:630, 1974
89. Moore RA: Tuberculosis of the prostate gland. J Urol 37:372, 1937
90. Schmidt JD: Non-specific granulomatous prostatitis: Classification review and report of cases. J Urol 94:607, 1965
91. O'Dea MJ, Hunting DB, Greene LF: Nonspecific granulomatous prostatitis. J Urol 118:58, 1977
92. Melicow MM: Allergic granulomas of the prostate gland. J Urol 65:288, 1951
93. Towfighi J, Sadeghee S, Wheeler JE, Enterline HT: Granulomatous prostatitis with emphasis on the eosinophilic variety. Am J Clin Pathol 58:630, 1972
94. Stanton MJ, Maxted W: Malacoplakia: A study of the literature and current concepts of pathogenesis, diagnosis and treatment. J Urol 125:139, 1981
95. Moore RA: Benign hypertrophy of the prostate. J Urol 50:680, 1943
96. Waisman J, Mott LJM: Pathology of neoplasms of the prostate gland. In Skinner DG, deKernion JB (eds): Genitourinary Cancer, Ch 17, p 310, Philadelphia, WB Saunders, 1978
97. Gleason DF, Mellinger GT, Veterans Administration Committee Urologic Research Group: Prediction of prognosis for prostatic adenocarcinoma by combined histologic grading and clinical staging. J Urol 111:58, 1974
98. Dube VE, Farrow GM, Greene LF: Prostatic adenocarcinoma of ductal origin. Cancer 32:402, 1973
99. Catalona WJ, Kadmon D, Martin SA: Surgical considerations in treatment of intraductal carcinoma of the prostate. J Urol 120:259, 1978
100. Melicow MM, Pachter MR: Endometrial carcinoma of prostatic utricle (uterus masculinis). Cancer 20:1715, 1967
101. Zaloudek C, Williams JW, Kempson RL: "Endometrial" adenocarcinoma of the prostate. Cancer 37:2255, 1976
102. Uyama T, Moriwaki S: Papillary and mucus-forming adenocarcinomas of prostate. Urology 13:432, 1979
103. Greene LF, O'Dea MJ, Dockerty MB: Primary transitional cell carcinoma of the prostate. J Urol 116:761, 1976
104. Mott LJM: Squamous cell carcinoma of the prostate: Report of 2 cases and a review of the literature. J Urol 121:833, 1979

## URETHRA

105. Mostofi FK, Price EB: Tumors and tumor-like lesions of the male urethra. In Mostofi FK, Price EB: Tumors of the male genital system, 2nd series, Fascicle 8, pp 263-276. Washington, DC, Armed Forces Institute of Pathology, 1973
106. Davis BL, Robinson DG: Diverticula of the female urethra: Assay of 120 cases. J Urol 104:850, 1970
107. Palaqiri A: Urethral diverticulum with endometriosis. Urology 11:271, 1978
108. Marshall S, Hirsch K: Carcinoma within urethral diverticula. Urology 10:161, 1977
109. Stueber PJ, Persky L: Solid tumors of the urethra and bladder neck. J Urol 102:205, 1969
110. Randall A: A study of the benign polyps of the male urethra. Surg Gynecol Obstet 17:548, 1913
111. Elbadawi A, Malhoski WE, Frank IN: Mucinous urethral caruncle. Urology 12:587, 1978
112. Marshall FC, Uson AC, Melicow MM: Neoplasms and caruncles of the female urethra. Surg Gynecol Obstet 110:723, 1960
113. Schinella R, Thurm J, Feiner H: Papillary pseudotumor of the prostatic urethra: Proliferative papillary urethritis. J Urol 111:38, 1974
114. Gartman E: Intraurethral verruca acuminata in men. J Urol 75:717, 1956
115. Wani NA, Bhan BL, Guru AA, Garyali RK:

Leiomyoma of the female urethra: A case report. J Urol 116:120, 1976

116. Manuel ES, Seery WH, Cole AT: Capillary hemangioma of the male urethra: Case report with literature review. J Urol 117:804, 1977
117. Trites AEW: Inverted urothelial papilloma: Report of 2 cases. J Urol 101:216, 1969
118. Bhagavan BS, Tiamson E, Wenk RE, et al: Nephrogenic adenoma of bladder and urethra. Presented at the National American Urologic Meeting, 1981
119. Sullivan J, Grabstald H: Management of carcinoma of the urethra. In Skinner DG, deKernion JB (eds): Genitourinary Cancer, Ch 23, p 419. Philadelphia, WB Saunders, 1978
120. Levine RL: Urethral cancer. Cancer 45:1965, 1980
121. Boldvan JP, Farah RN: Primary urethral neoplasms: Review of 30 cases. J Urol 125:198, 1981
122. Kaplan GW, Bulkley GJ, Grayhack JT: Carcinoma of the male urethra. J Urol 98:365, 1967
123. McCrea LE: Malignancy of the female urethra. Urol Surv 2:85, 1952
124. Katz JI, Grabstald H: Primary malignant melanoma of the female urethra. J Urol 116:454, 1976

## PENIS

125. Robbins SL: Pathology, 3rd ed, Ch 30, pp 1267-69. Philadelphia, WB Saunders, 1967
126. Fiumara NJ: A guide to lesions of the penis. Hosp Med 6:22, 1970
127. Slachta GA, Conger KB: Inflammatory diseases of the male genital tract. In Kendall AR, Karafin L (eds): Practice of Surgery—urology, vol 1, Ch 15. Philadelphia, Harper & Row, 1981
128. Rheinschild GW, Olsen BS: Balanitis xerotica obliterans. J Urol 104: 860, 1970
129. Smith BH: Peyronie's disease. Am J Clin Pathol 45:670, 1966
130. Mostofi FK, Price EB: Tumors and tumor-like lesions of the penis. In Mostofi FK, Price EB: Tumors of the Male Genital System, 2nd series, Fascicle 8, pp 277-294. Washington, DC, Armed Forces Institute of Pathology, 1973
131. Dehner LP, Smith BH: Soft tissue tumors of the penis. Cancer 25:1431, 1970
132. Lowenstein LW; Carcinoma-like condylomata acuminata of the penis. Med Clin North Am:789, 1939
133. Boxer RJ, Skinner DG: Condylomata acuminata and squamous cell carcinoma. Urology 9:72, 1977
134. Hanash KA, Furlow WL, Utz DC, Harrison EG: Carcinoma of the penis: A clinicopathologic study. J Urol 104:291, 1970
135. Merrin CE: Cancer of the penis. Cancer 45:1973, 1980
136. Fegen JP, Beebe D, Persky L: Basal cell carcinoma of the penis. J Urol 104:864, 1970
137. Abeshouse BS, Abeshouse GA, Goldstein AE: Sarcoma of the penis, A review of the literature, a report of a new case, and a brief consideration of melanoma of the penis. Urol Int 13:273, 1962
138. Bracken RB, Diokno AC: Melanoma of penis and urethra. J Urol 111:198, 1974
139. Abeshouse BS, Abeshouse GA: Metastatic tumors of the penis: A review of the literature and a report of 2 cases. J Urol 86:99, 1961

## TESTIS

140. DeLa Balze FA, Bur GE, Scarpa–Smith F, Irazu J: Elastic fibers in the tunica propria of normal and pathologic human testis. J Clin Endocrinol Metab 14:626, 1954
141. Nistal M, Paniaqua R, Diez–Pardo JA: Histologic classification of undescended testes. Hum Pathol 11:666, 1980
142. Klinefelter HF, Reifenstein EC, Albright F: Syndrome characterized by gynecomastia, aspermatogenesis without A-leydigism, and increased excretion of follicle-stimulating hormone. J Clin Endocrinol Metab 2:615, 1942
143. Levin HS: Testicular biopsy in the study of male infertility. Hum Pathol 10:569, 1979
144. del-Castillo EB, Trabucco A, dela Balze FA: Syndrome produced by absence of the germinal epithelium without impairment of the Sertoli or Leydig cells. J Clin Endocrinol Metab 7:493, 1947
145. Ishida H, Isurugi K, Aso Y, et al: Endocrine studies in Sertoli-cell-only syndrome. J Urol 116:56, 1976
146. Charny CW, Meranze DR: Pathology of mumps orchitis. J Urol 60:140, 1948
147. Elicker ER, Evans AT: Granulomatous orchitis. J Urol 113:199, 1975
148. Waisman J, Rampton JB: Malacoplakia of the testis and epididymis. Arch Pathol Lab Med 86:431, 1968
149. Mostofi FK, Price EB: Tumors of the testis. In Mostofi FK, Price EB: Tumors the Male Genital System, 2nd series, Fascicle 8, pp 1-176. Washington, DC, Armed Forces Institute of Pathology, 1973
150. Friedman NB: Pathology of testicular tumors. In Skinner DG, deKernion JB (eds): Genitourinary Cancer, Ch 24, p. 430. Philadelphia, WB Saunders, 1978
151. Talerman A: Spermatocytic seminoma. J Urol 112:212, 1974
152. Kademian M, Bosch A, Caldwell WL, Jaeschke W: Anaplastic seminoma. Cancer 40:3002, 1977
153. Andres TL, Trainer TD, Leadbetter GW:

Atypical germ cells preceeding metachronous bilateral testicular tumors. Urology 15:307, 1980

154. Javadpour N, McIntire KR, Waldmann TA, Bergman SM: The role of alpha-fetoprotein and human chorionic gonadotropin in seminoma. J Urol 120:687, 1978

155. Javadpour N: The National Cancer Institute experience with testicular cancer. J Urol 120:651, 1978

156. Lindsey CM, Glenn JF: Germinal malignancies of the testis: Experience, management and prognosis. J Urol 116:59, 1976

157. Hopkins TB, Jaffe N, Colodny A et al: The management of testicular tumors in children. J Urol 120:96, 1978

158. Exelby PR: Testicular cancer in children. Cancer 45:1803, 1980

159. Kedia K, Fraley EE: Adult teratoma of the testis metastasizing as adult teratoma: case report and review of the literature. J Urol 114:636, 1975

160. Talerman A, Delemaire JFM: Gonadoblastoma associated with embryonal carcinoma in an anatomically normal male. J Urol 113:355, 1975

161. Rajfer J, Mendelsohn G, Arnheim J et al: Dysgenetic male pseudohermaphroditism. J Urol 119:525, 1978

162. Morin LJ, Loening S: Malignant androblastoma (Sertoli cell tumor) of the testis. A case report with a review of the literature. J Urol 114:476, 1975

163. Marshall FF, Kerr WS, Kliman B, Scully RE: Sex cord-stromal (gonadal stromal) tumors of the testis. A report of 5 cases. J Urol 117:180, 1977

164. Sussman EB, Hajdu SI, Lieberman PH, Whitmore WF: Malignant lymphoma of the testis: A clinico-pathologic study of 37 cases. J Urol 118:1004, 1977

165. Jackson SM, Montessori GA: Malignant lymphoma of the testis: Review of 17 cases in British Columbia with survival related to pathologic subclassification. J Urol 123:881, 1980

166. Pienkos EJ, Jablokow VR: Secondary testicular tumors. Cancer 30:481, 1972

## TESTICULAR ADNEXA

167. Mostofi FK, Price EB: Tumors and tumor-like conditions of testicular adnexal structures. In Mostofi FK, Price EB: Tumors of the Male Genital System, 2nd series, Fascicle 8, pp 143-176. Washington, DC, Armed Forces Institute of Pathology, 1973

168. Glassy FJ, Mostofi FK: Spermatic granulomas of the epididymis. Am J Clin Pathol 26:1303, 1956

169. Civantos F, Lubin J, Ryulin AM: Vasitis nodosa. Arch Pathol Lab Med 94:355, 1972

170. Beccia DJ, Krane RJ, Olsson CA: Clinical management of non-testicular intrascrotal tumors. J Urol 116:476, 1976

171. Oertel YC, Johnson FB: Sclerosing lipogranuloma of the male genitalia. Arch Pathol Lab Med 101:321, 1977

172. Marcus JB, Lynn JA: Ultrastructural comparison of an adenomatoid tumor, lymphangioma, hemangioma and mesothelioma. Cancer 25:171, 1970

173. Price EB: Papillary crystadenoma of the epididymis. Arch Pathol 91:456, 1971

174. Ferenczy A, Fenoglio J, Richart RM: Observations on benign mesothelioma of the genital tract (adenomatoid tumor). Cancer 30:244, 1972

175. Skeel DA, Drinker HR, Witherington R: Rhabdomyosarcoma of the spermatic cord: Report of 3 cases with review of the literature. J Urol 113:279, 1975

176. Banowsky LH, Shultz GN: Sarcoma of the spermatic cord and tunics: Review of the literature, case report and discussion of the role of retroperitoneal lymph node dissection. J Urol 103:628, 1970

177. Spark RP: Leiomyoma of epididymis. Arch Pathol Lab Med 93:18, 1972

178. Arlen M, Graystald H, Whitmore WF: Malignant tumors of the spermatic cord. Cancer 23:525, 1969

179. DeLuise VP, Draper JW, Gray GF: Smooth muscle tumors of the testicular adnexa. J Urol 115:685, 1976

180. Sogani PC, Grabstald H, Whitmore WF: Spermatic cord sarcoma in adults. J Urol 120:301, 1978

181. Beall ME, Young IS: Spermatic cord rhabdomyosarcoma case report. J Urol 117:806, 1977

182. Cole AT, Staus FH, Gill WB: Malignant fibrous histiocytoma: An unusual inguinal tumor. J Urol 107:1005, 1972

183. Chung HD: Granular cell tumor of the spermatic cord: A case report with light and electron microscopic study. J Urol 120:379, 1978

184. Soejima H, Ogawa O, Nomura Y, Ogata J: Pheochromocytoma of the spermatic cord: A case report. J Urol 118:495, 1977

## SCROTUM

185. Vermillion CD, Page DL: Paget's disease of the scrotum: A case report with local lymph node invasion. J Urol 107:281, 1972

186. Perri AJ, Feldman AE, Kendall AR, Karafin L: Paget's disease of the scrotum. Urology 6:94, 1975

## IMMUNOHISTOPATHOLOGY

187. Lange PH, McIntire KR, Waldmann TA, et al: Alpha-fetoprotein and human chorionic gonadotrophin in the management of testicular tumors. J Urol 118:593, 1977

188. Javadpour N: The National Cancer Institute experience with testicular cancer. J Urol 120:651, 1978

189. Fowler JE, Taylor G, Blum J, Stutzman RE: Experience with serum alpha-fetoprotein and human chorionic gonadotrophin in nonseminomatous testicular tumor. J Urol 124:365, 1980

190. Lange PH, Nochomovitz LE, Rosai J et al: Serum alpha-fetoprotein and human chorionic gonadotrophin in patients with seminoma. J Urol 124:472, 1980

191. Javadpour N, McIntire KR, Waldmann TA, Bergman SM: The role of alpha-fetoprotein and human chorionic gonadotrophin in seminoma. J Urol 120:687, 1978

192. Sternberger LA, Hardy PH, Cuculis JJ, Meyer HG: The unlabeled antibody-enzyme method of immunohistochemistry. J Histochem Cytochem 18:315, 1970

193. Bosman FT, Giard RWM, Kruseman ACN et al: Human chorionic gonadotrophin and alpha-fetoprotein in testicular germ cell tumours: A retrospective immunohistochemical study. Histopathology 4:673, 1980

194. Papsidero LD, Wang MC, Valenzuela LA et al: A prostate antigen in sera of prostatic cancer patients. Cancer Res 40:2428, 1980

195. Nadji M, Tabei SZ, Castro A et al: Prostate-specific antigen: An immunohistologic marker for prostatic neoplasms. Cancer 48:1229, 1981

196. Nadji M, Tabei S, Castro A et al: Prostatic origin of tumors, and immunohistochemical study. Am J Clin Pathol 73:735, 1980

197. Stein BS, Vangore S, Petersen RO, Kendall AR: Immunoperoxidase localization of prostate-specific antigen. Am J Surg Pathol 6:553,1982

198. Stein BS, Petersen RO, Kendall AR: Prostatic tissue tumor markers (abstr). Presented at the 77th Annual Meeting, Kansas City, American Urological Association, May 1982

199. Davidsohn I: Early immunologic diagnosis and prognosis of carcinoma. Am J Clin Pathol 57:715, 1972

200. Weinstein RS, Alroy J, Farrow GM et al: Blood group isoantigen deletion in carcinoma in situ of the urinary bladder. Cancer 43:661, 1979

201. Stein BS, Kendall AR: Blood group antigens and bladder carcinoma: A perspective. Urology 20:229, 1982

202. Catalona WJ: Practical utility of specific red cell adherence test in bladder cancer. Urology 18:113, 1981

203. Coon JS, Weinstein RS: Detection of ABH tissue isoantigens by immunoperoxidase methods in normal and neoplastic urothelium. Am J Clin Pathol 76:163, 1981

## ADRENAL

204. Studzinski GP, Hay DCF, Symington T: Observations on the weight of the human adrenal gland and the effect of preparations of corticotropin of different purity on the weight and morphology of the human adrenal gland. J Clin Endocrinol Metab 23:248, 1963

205. Long JA, Jones AL: Observations on the fine structure of the adrenal cortex of man. Lab Invest 17:355, 1967

206. Greenwald P: Embryonic and postnatal development of the adrenal cortex, particularly the zona glomerulosa and accessory nodules. Anat Rec 95:391, 1946

207. Culp OS: Adrenal heterotopia. A survey of the literature, and report of a case. J Urol 41:303, 1939

208. Nelson AA: Accessory adrenal cortical tissue. Arch Pathol 27:955, 1939

209. Gutkowski WT, Gray GF: Ectopic adrenal in inguinal hernia sacs. J Urol 121:353, 1979

210. Parsons L, Thompson JE: Symptomatic myelolipoma of the adrenal gland. Report of a case and review of the literature. N Engl J Med 260:12, 1959

211. Aygat F, Fosslin E, Kent R, Hudson HC: Myelolipoma of the adrenal gland. Urology 16:415, 1980

212. Bennett BD, McKenna TJ, Hough AJ et al: Adrenal myelolipoma associated with Cushing disease. Am J Clin Pathol 73:443, 1980

213. Khuri FJ, Alton DJ, Hardy BE et al: Adrenal hemorrhage in neonates: Report of 5 cases and review of the literature. J Urol 124:684, 1980

214. Ghandur–Mnaymneh L, Slim M, Muakassa K: Adrenal cysts: Pathogenesis and histological identification with a report of 6 cases. J Urol 122:87, 1979

215. Dobbie JW: Adrenocortical nodular hyperplasia: The aging adrenal. J Pathol 99:1, 1969

216. Russell RP, Mosi OT, Richter ED: Adrenal cortical adenomas and hypertension. A clinical pathologic analysis of 690 cases with matched controls and a review of the literature. Medicine 51:211, 1972

217. Commons RR, Callaway CP: Adenomas of the adrenal cortex. Arch Intern Med 81:37, 1948

218. Macadam RF: Black adenoma of the human adrenal cortex. Cancer 27:116, 1971

219. Garrett R, Ames RP: Black pigmented adenoma of the adrenal cortex. Report of 3 cases including microscopic study. Arch Pathol 95:349, 1973

220. Lipsett MB, Hertz R, Ross GT: Clinical and pathophysiologic aspects of adrenocortical carcinoma. Am J Med 35:374, 1963
221. Hunos AG, Hafdu SI, Brasfield RD, Foote FW: Adrenal cortical carcinoma. Clinicopathologic study of 34 cases. Cancer 25:354, 1970
222. O'Hare MJ, Monaghan P, Neville AM: The pathology of adrenal cortical neoplasia: A correlated structural and functional approach to the diagnosis of malignant disease. Hum Pathol 10:137, 1979
223. Beer E, King FH, Prinzmetal M: Pheochromocytoma with demonstration of pressor (adrenalin) substance in blood preoperatively during hypertensive crises. Ann Surg 106:85, 1937
224. Colkins E, Dana GW, Seed JC, Howard JE: On piperidyl-methyl-benzodioxane (933-F), hypertension, and pheochromocytoma. J Clin Endocrinol Metab 10:1, 1950
225. Nibbelink DW, Peters BH, McCormick WF: On the association of pheochromocytoma and cerebellar hemangioblastoma. Neurology 19:455, 1969
226. Overholt RH, Ramsay SH, Meissner WA: Intra-throacic pheochromocytoma. Dis Chest 17:55, 1950
227. Mahoney EM, Harrison JH: Malignant pheochromocytoma: Clinical course and treatment. J Urol 118:225, 1977
228. Fortner J, Nicastri A, Murphy ML: Neuroblastoma: Natural history and results of treating 133 cases. Ann Surg 167:132, 1968
229. Kay S: Hyperplasia and neoplasia of the adrenal gland. Pathol Annu 11:103, 1976
230. Misugi K, Misugi N, Newton WA: Fine structural study of neuroblastoma, ganglioneuroblastoma and pheochromocytoma. Arch Pathol 86:160, 1968
231. Wilson LMK, Draper GJ: Neuroblastoma, its natural history and prognosis: A study of 487 cases. Br Med J 2:301, 1974

**ACKNOWLEDGMENT**

We would like to thank Mr. Otto Lehmann for his dedication to photographic excellence, and Miss Dorothy Beyer for typing this manuscript "today." We would also like to thank Dr. Dale Huff, St. Christopher's Hospital for Children, for providing us with certain pediatric cases, and Dr. Wayne Johnson for permission to use the photomicrograph of chancroid of the penis previously published in Dermal Pathology (Johnson WC: Venereal diseases and treponemal infections. In Graham JH, Johnson WC, Helwig EB (eds): Dermal Pathology, p. 372. Hagerstown, Maryland, Harper & Row, 1972)

# 5

# Radiologic Examination of the Urinary Tract

*Mark S. Ridlen and John J. Cronan*

## INTRODUCTION

Uroradiology has felt a major impact from technologic advances in the past 15 years. Ultrasound, computed tomography (CT), and magnetic resonance imaging (MRI) have substantially altered the diagnostic imaging process undergone by the urologic patient. Interventional radiology has developed new diagnostic and therapeutic procedures which provide additional options for the urologist.

The purpose of this chapter is to provide an overview of uroradiology which can be read in one session. Multi-volume texts have been written on this subject; this chapter is not intended to supplant them, but rather to provide a concise, readable introduction to uroradiology. We begin with a modality-oriented format in order to briefly discuss the imaging characteristics of the most commonly encountered techniques in uroradiology. Subsequently, we analyze these modalities and discuss their applicability to frequently encountered disease processes.

Over the past two decades, the subspecialty of uroradiology has evolved and expanded to address the growing complexity of diagnostic imaging as applied to urology. A close working relationship between the urologist and the uroradiologist is very beneficial for patient care and provides optimal utilization of resources within the radiology department.

Uroradiology is a dynamic field. We anticipate further revisions in imaging concepts, which will be generated by continued scientific and technologic breakthroughs.

## IMAGING MODALITIES

### Plain Film of the Abdomen (KUB/ Scout Film)

The urologist should be familiar and comfortable with the interpretation of the plain film, as it remains the most frequently obtained film in the urologic evaluation and is an essential preliminary portion of the intravenous urogram (IVU). The field of view that is evaluated extends from the diaphragm to the pubic symphysis and contains the kidneys, ureters, and bladder; it is commonly referred to as a KUB. A plain film of the abdomen done as the initial film for an IVU is known as a scout film. Soft-tissue structures such as the kidney, liver, and psoas muscles should be evaluated for enlargement or distortion. Air within the bowel should be gauged, as the presence of increased air may indicate an obstruction. Calcifications must be diligently noted when they are present within the collecting system or along the course of the ureters or bladder. Since most urinary-tract stones

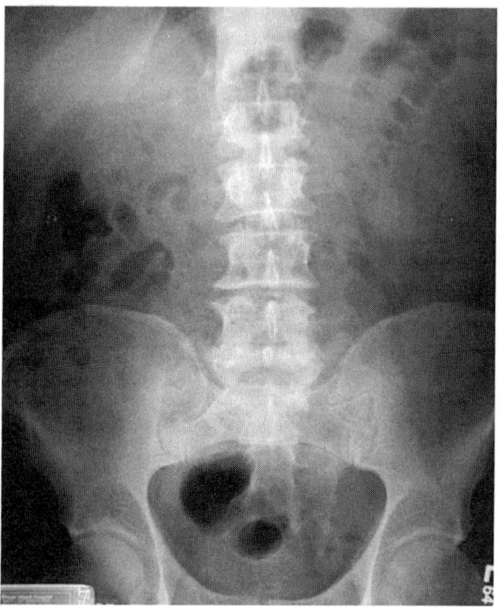

Fig 1. Normal KUB film.

(approximately 90%) are calcified, the urogram will demonstrate them, but often they are detected only after careful review (Fig 1).

## Contrast Material

Whether injected intravenously (IV) or instilled via a retrograde catheter placed directly into the collecting system, contrast material is indispensable for the practice of uroradiology. The basic unit of standard contrast material consists of three atoms of iodine attached to a benzene ring. The high iodine content causes this material to block conventional x-rays. As a result, areas of significant contrast-material accumulation produce "white" areas on standard x-ray films. When contrast material is injected IV, it is removed from the blood by glomerular filtration in the kidneys and accumulates in the urine.

In a normal adult patient with normal renal function, a total of 15 to 20 g of iodine must be injected to produce an adequate urogram. Because the concentration of iodine varies among different types of contrast material solutions, the volume of contrast material will vary. Contrast material has a very mild toxic effect upon the kidneys; when utilized in patients with renal insufficiency and diabetes, it may produce acute renal dysfunction.[1]

Adverse reactions to IV contrast injections are not unusual.[2,3] Mild reactions, which include mild nausea, vomiting, and urticaria and sneezing, occur in approximately 3% to 4% of patients. Moderate reactions consisting of severe vomiting, mild bronchospasm, and hypotension occur in approximately 1% of patients. Severe, life-threatening reactions, including cardiac arrest, pulmonary edema, and severe bronchospasm, occur in approximately 0.01% of patients; the incidence of death is 1 in 100,000 patients. Those patients with a prior history of allergic reactions to a variety of substances are at higher risk of experiencing an adverse reaction.

Standard contrast agents have relatively high osmolality and are ionic compounds. Newer nonionic contrast agents with lower osmolality have been developed and have been shown to produce fewer mild and moderate reactions. However, the incidence of death associated with newer agents appears to be about the same as that of the more established ionic compounds.[4] In addition, these new agents are approximately ten times more expensive than the standard agents; this factor has hindered their widespread use.

## Intravenous Urogram (IVU)

After the scout film is reviewed, an IVU may be performed by injecting 1.1 to 2.2 mL/kg (up to 150 mL) of iodinated contrast material IV. This iodinated contrast material will opacify the renal parenchyma, the collecting system, and the bladder.

There is some variation in the film sequence during an IVU, but most uroradiologists agree that initial films should be coned down over the kidneys to provide greater renal detail during the nephrographic or parenchymal phase—which occurs within the first 3 minutes—to facilitate evaluation of the renal tissue for masses. The normal parenchymal phase demonstrates a kidney with smooth contours and sharp margins. A bulge on the superolateral border of the left kidney can often be seen, and has been labeled a dromedary hump or

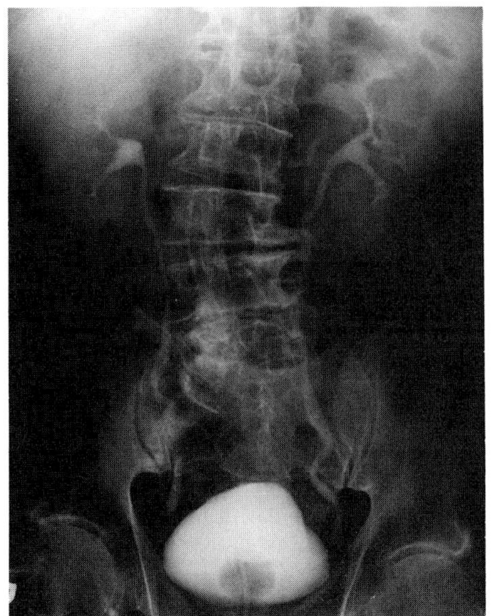

Fig 2. Normal intravenous urogram (IVU) (with indwelling Foley catheter).

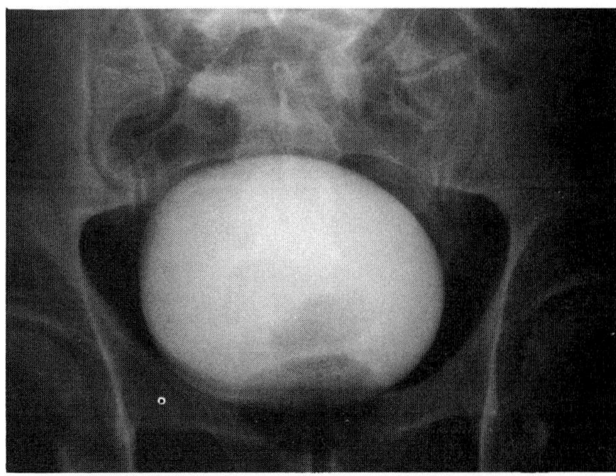

Fig 3. Normal bladder as visualized by IVU.

a splenic bump. This pseudomass represents thickened normal cortical tissue, and should not be mistaken for a pathologic process. Often small indentations along the renal contour are apparent in young patients; these parenchymal indentations represent fetal lobulation. Smooth contour and regular spacing confirms their benign nature—this normal variation should not be confused with renal parenchymal scarring.

Approximately 3 to 5 minutes after contrast material is injected, opacification of the collecting system is achieved. At this time, a large field of view should be utilized to visualize both the intrarenal collecting systems and the ureters (Fig 2). The ureters are often not seen in their entirety on a single film because of ureteral peristalsis; this should not cause concern. An intraluminal mass or extrinsic obstruction of the ureter will typically cause a fullness or columnation of the ureter. A coned-down view of the bladder should also be obtained routinely; oblique views should be utilized when indicated by clinical history (Fig 3). Evaluation of a bladder film obtained post-void provides information regarding bladder function and potential areas of outlet obstruction. The post-void bladder film may be the only film that demonstrates intravesical pathology (Fig 4). A post-void film with both obliques may also be necessary to fully evaluate the ureterovesical junction, especially when small calculi are suspected in the distal ureter.

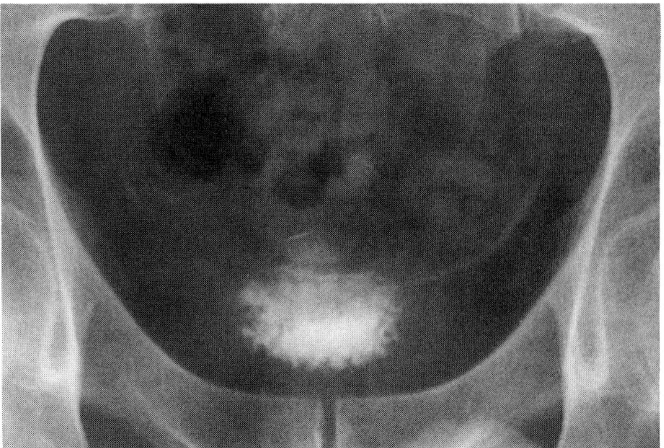

Fig 4. Normal post-void bladder film.

The renal calyces, surrounded by parenchyma, should have a cupped configuration without blunting. Cupped, non-blunted calyces and infundibula indicate that obstruction is not present. The calyces and infundibula drain into the renal pelvis,

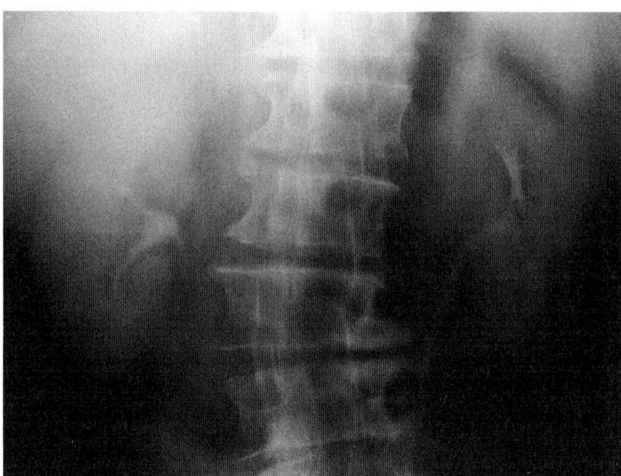

Fig 5. Normal tomogram.

which can be quite variable in appearance. The renal pelvis may be intrarenal or extrarenal; in the latter case it can be fairly large, and a prominent extrarenal pelvis may be confused with ureteropelvic-junction obstruction.

In patients over 40 years of age, tomograms should be routinely employed in nonemergency cases to better evaluate the renal parenchyma for masses. During tomography, both the x-ray tube and the film cassette are moved and structures above or below the plane of focus are blurred, thereby providing greater detail for structures within the focal plane (Fig 5). Studies have shown that only approximately one third of the renal masses visualized by tomography were also detected with conventional radiography. Hence, tomography is essential in the population at risk for renal mass development. Specific definition of the category of the renal mass (cystic or solid) detected by tomography requires ultrasound or CT.

In older patients, fat can accumulate in the renal sinus and produce nonpathologic stretching and compression of the collecting system. The appearance of renal pelvic lipomatosis on urogram may suggest a renal mass; such masses may be better defined with CT.

The ureters descend from the renal pelvis just lateral to the lumbar vertebral bodies. The ureters are at their most anterior point when they cross the iliac vessels. The iliac vessels may produce some mild extrinsic ureteral compression, which can result in nonpathologic distension of the ureter proximal to that point, particularly with the patient supine. Prone or upright films can then be obtained after alleviating ureteral distension. A distended bladder should have smooth borders and be oval or spherical in shape.

## Cross-Sectional Imaging

**Ultrasound.** No area of uroradiology has shown greater growth during the last decade than ultrasound. This technique is noninvasive, and it does not require the needle puncture or contrast injection which are essential for the performance of IVU or CT. Ultrasound does not use ionizing radiation and it has no known side effects.

An ultrasound transducer generates short pulses of sound waves which travel from the transducer into the body. In the short interval between the transmission of sound waves, the transducer also functions as a receiver for sound waves, known as echoes, that return after bouncing off various structures within the body. By quantitating the amount of echoes returning, as well as the time required for return, images can be created. Because this process can be repeated several times per second, a "real-time" image that is not disrupted by patient motion or transducer movement may be produced with modern ultrasound equipment (Fig 6). Transducers that produce a higher frequency of sound (5–10 MHz) are most useful for examining superficial structures that are closer to the transducer. Lower frequencies (2–5 MHz) may be utilized to examine structures that are at a greater depth beneath the skin.

Specialized transducers have been developed that allow intracavitary evaluation of certain body regions (eg, the vagina, rectum, and bladder), achieving better resolution than that obtained with transcutaneous scanning. With respect to urology, the most important intracavitary probe is the transrectal probe, which is placed directly into the rectum in order to evaluate the prostate gland and seminal vesicles.

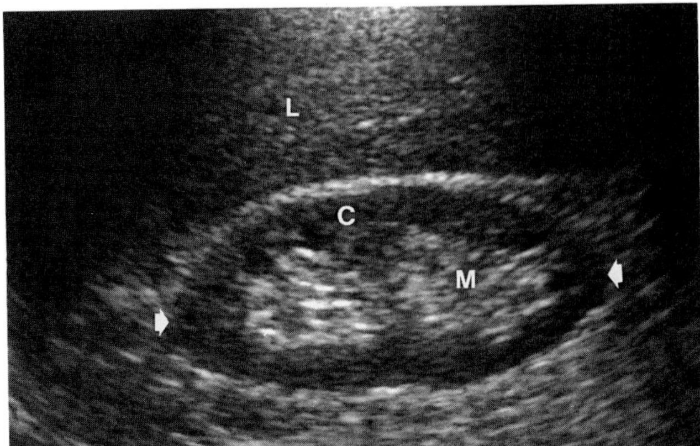


**Fig 6.** Normal renal ultrasound; sagittal image with arrows at each pole. Cortex (C) is readily differentiated from medulla (M). L = liver.

Doppler ultrasound permits assessment of motion which occurs within the field of view. The direction and speed of movement are recorded; pulsed Doppler permits this to be recorded in a small area within the field, while color Doppler assesses the entire field for motion and superimposes this information on the gray-scale image of nonmoving structures. Recent application of Doppler principles to ultrasound has proven to be very useful in the evaluation of vascular structures, including the inferior vena cava, renal veins, varicoceles, and arterial structures.

**Computed Tomography.** Computed tomography (CT) uses conventional x-rays along a proscribed arc at each level or section to be studied. A computer algorithm converts this information into an image which is composed of numerous very small picture elements, called pixels. Each pixel represents a tissue density in Hounsfield units (HUs), with a numerical range from −1000 to +1000 based on the degree of x-ray beam attenuation. Water has a value at or near zero HUs. Soft tissues are in 50–100 HU range. Bone and dense calcification provide reflection in the 700–1000 HU range. Fat translates to less than −100 HUs. CT provides exquisite delineation of the abdominal and retroperitoneal anatomy. As a survey technique, it provides a panoramic view of the urinary tract and surrounding structures. Obtaining high-quality CT images requires the utilization of intravenous contrast material.

**Magnetic Resonance Imaging.** This is the newest tool used for assessment of the genitourinary tract. It does not yet have a definitive role in urology, but with further experience it likely will have greater importance. Image acquisition is quite complex. Hydrogen atoms have a single proton and electron. When a patient is placed in the strong magnetic field of the scanner, the mobile hydrogen atoms tend to orient their magnetic poles along the north south axis in the magnetic field. A radiofrequency (RF) pulse is then sent through the patient, and alters the axis (or "tips" the hydrogen atoms) within the magnetic field. A radiosignal will then be emitted from the atom as it reorients to the original position along the main north–south axis. Detectors in the MRI unit receive this signal, and computer analysis converts the information into an image, based on the strength and location of signal.

The signal intensity recorded varies according to tissue characteristics and various technologic parameters, including the time interval between RF pulses. Specific tissue characteristics are related to differences in T1 and T2 relaxation times, which are related to the quality of the signal emitted from the hydrogen atom after the RF pulse. The contrast difference between tissues is related to inherent differences in the T1 and T2 values for each specific tissue type.

MRI has the ability to acquire images in virtually any geometric plane, which is an advantage over CT. Cortical bone and dense calcifications do not emit significant signal, because the hydrogen atoms in these compounds are in a fixed molecular position and are therefore not affected by the magnetic field. Elements that have a greater molecular weight than hydrogen are not significantly affected by the magnetic field strengths currently employed in image production.

Using MRI, moving blood may easily be differentiated from clotted blood or solid tissue. Rapidly flowing arterial blood does not allow the hydrogen atoms to orient properly and therefore does not produce significant signal but instead creates a signal void. Slower flowing venous blood may produce a mild signal. In cases where it is important to determine the patency of renal veins, specialized pulse sequences that clearly define moving blood can be utilized.

There is considerable variation in image quality from different types of MRI scanners because of differences in magnetic field strength and computer software. The specific equipment parameters necessary for optimal genitourinary tract imaging have not yet been established.

## DIAGNOSTIC PROCEDURES

### Cystography/Voiding Cystourethrography (VCUG)

Cystography permits assessment of bladder size, position, and integrity. After the bladder is filled, urethrography can be performed while the patient voids; contrast material can be used to visualize the urethra. Initially, a 15% iodinated contrast agent is instilled into the bladder through a urethral catheter. The usual method is to attach the catheter to a bottle of contrast material and fill the bladder by gravity under intermittent fluoroscopic observation. Direct injection from a syringe can also be employed; this technique is most often used in the trauma setting.

A successful VCUG requires filling the bladder until the patient reports moderate discomfort and feels that he/she can voluntarily void. Appropriate filming of the bladder is obtained at this point. The urethral catheter is then removed and the patient is instructed to void under fluoroscopic observation. Multiple spot-films are taken during voiding to document urethral anatomy (Fig 7). Finally, an overhead film is obtained after voiding has been completed to identify subtle cases of reflux that may not have been observed with fluoroscopy.

Radionuclide cystography is often performed on a follow-up basis in children who have been shown to have vesicoureteral reflux by a standard VCUG. The sensitivity of radionuclide cystography is at least the same for reflux greater than grade I and is achieved using a markedly reduced radiation dose. The radionuclide cystogram is limited in its ability to provide precise anatomical resolution, which prevents utilization of this technique as a screening test for reflux.

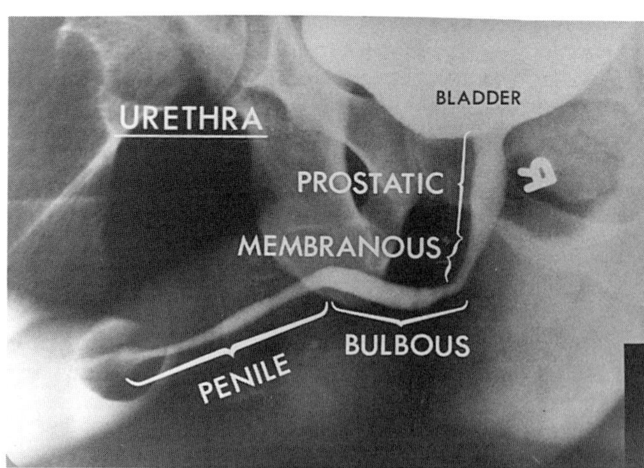


**Fig 7.** Normal voiding cystourethrogram (VCUG).

## Dynamic Retrograde Urethrography

This is the procedure of choice for the retrograde evaluation of the urethra. A 12 to 14 F Foley catheter is inserted approximately 3 cm into the urethra. The Foley balloon is then slowly inflated in the fossa navicularis. Under fluoroscopic observation, water-soluble contrast material is hand-injected into the urethra through the catheter. Multiple spot-films are obtained during injection, with the patient in an oblique position. An alternative method is the use of the Brodney clamp. In this technique, a mechanical device is clamped over the distal penis and contrast is injected through an external meatal plug (Fig 8). During a retrograde urethrogram, the posterior urethra is frequently not sufficiently distended to allow adequate evaluation. Therefore, a voiding cystourethrogram is often necessary to evaluate the posterior urethra.

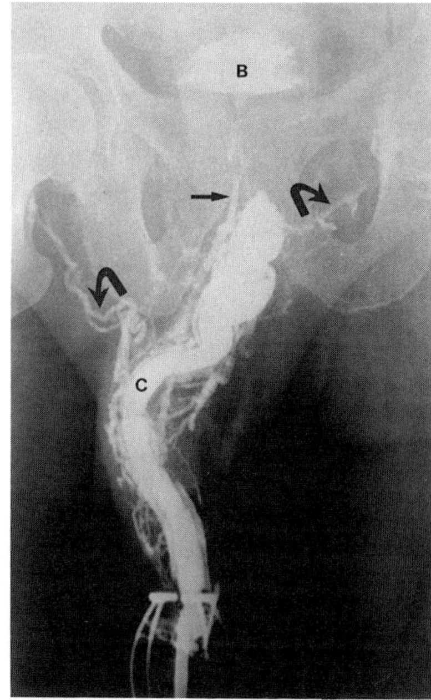


**Fig 8.** Retrograde urethrogram; overdistension produced extravasation into the venous plexus (curved arrows) and a corporal body (C). Fluoroscopic observation eliminates this degree of extravasation. Contrast material reaches the bladder (B) through the urethra (straight arrow).

## Ileal Conduit Examination (Loopagram)

Morphologic evaluation of the lumen of an ileal conduit is achieved by the retrograde injection of contrast material. In a patient with a nonobstructed, refluxing system, the ureters and collecting system of the kidneys may also be visualized. During the ileal conduit examination, a Foley catheter is inserted into the stoma and the catheter balloon is inflated a short distance inside the conduit. Under fluoroscopic observation, contrast material is instilled into the conduit by hand injection or the gravity–drip method. The material will fill the ileal loop, and usually refluxes freely into the ureters and renal collecting systems. This study can provide good visualization of the ileal conduit and renal collecting system, and allows detection of mechanical obstructions of the ileal-ureteral anastomoses as well as conduit strictures.

## Cavernosonography

Cavernosonography opacifies the corpora cavernosa permitting evaluation for penile fracture, Peyronie's disease, priapism, and impotence. Following skin anesthetization, a small needle is inserted into one of the corporal bodies, and contrast material is hand-injected under fluoroscopic observation. Both corporal bodies usually fill with a single injection because of interconnecting venous anastamoses. In the past, assessment of penile integrity following direct trauma was difficult because of the cumbersome nature of this test. Now, however, an MRI scan of the penis can be used to satisfactorily evaluate the penile shaft for fracture.

Cavernosonography may also be utilized to assess vascular impotence—specifically, that secondary to a venous leak.[5] In this situation, the technique requires placing a needle into each corporal body, one to inject contrast material or saline and the other to monitor intracorporal pressure. Initially, 40 to 60 mg of papaverine hydrochloride is injected intracorporally. Normal saline is then infused, at a rate of 30–50 mL/min. Penile erection must occur to obtain valid results. Once erection occurs, saline injection is stopped and the corporal pressure is then monitored. A venous leak may be suspected when the pressure falls rapidly. If the pressure falls, then contrast material is injected to identify the site of venous leakage after a second erection has been achieved.

Color Doppler ultrasound has shown promising results in the evaluation of impotence as well.

## Interventional Radiology

**Arteriography.** In uroradiology, diagnostic arteriography is most often performed to evaluate the renal arteries, to assess vascularity within a known or suspected mass/lesion within the kidney, or to identify an arteriovenous malformation. In this procedure, a catheter is placed into the aorta (and sometimes directly into the renal artery system), usually through a femoral artery approach. In selected cases, it may be necessary to use a brachial artery approach to the aorta and, rarely, direct access to the aorta may be used.

The initial injection of contrast material into the arterial system is performed after the tip of the catheter has been inserted in the aorta, above the level of the renal arteries. Rapid injection of the contrast material provides good visualization of the aorta, as well as of the renal artery origins, including any accessory renal arteries. On occasion, the tip of a specially designed catheter is then maneuvered into the renal artery. Selective injections of contrast material into the renal artery are then performed and these produce detailed images of the arterial structure of the kidneys. Following the arterial injection, delayed films also demonstrate the patient's renal vein.

If a focal renal artery stenosis is identified, angioplasty can be performed. In this procedure, a specialized catheter with a deflated balloon at the tip is maneuvered across the stenosis. The balloon is then inflated under fluoroscopic observation with the goal of eliminating the stenosis. An arteriogram should be performed after the dilatation is completed to assess the degree of success.

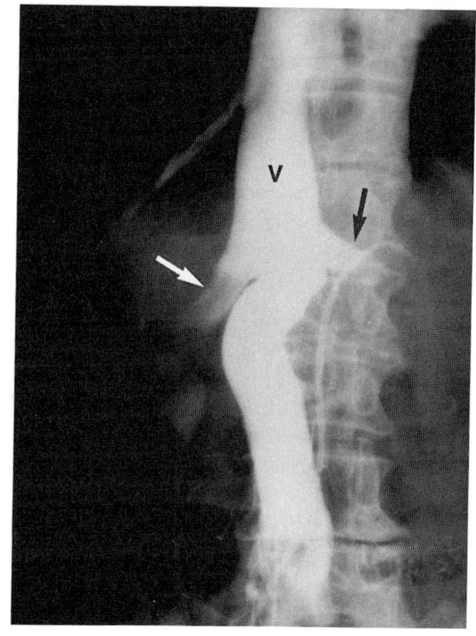


**Fig 9.** Normal inferior vena cavagram. The IVC (V) is filled with contrast material and shows normal reflux into renal veins (arrows).

**Venography.** Very few indications exist for direct opacification of the vein. Most often, venography is performed to assess the presence of clot or tumor in the inferior vena cava (Fig 9). Performance of venography requires the introduction of a catheter into the venous system, usually through a femoral-vein approach. This is a very sensitive test to determine the presence of blood clot or tumor thrombus within the inferior vena cava. Venography is usually performed when the results of CT or MRI examinations are equivocal in the staging of a renal cell carcinoma.

In the evaluation of renal vascular hypertension, a catheter can be placed directly in the renal veins to obtain blood samples for measurement of renin levels. This technique can also be performed when suspicion of an aldosteronoma exists. Following positioning of a catheter in the adrenal vein, blood samples can be obtained to identify a hyperfunctioning adrenal tumor.

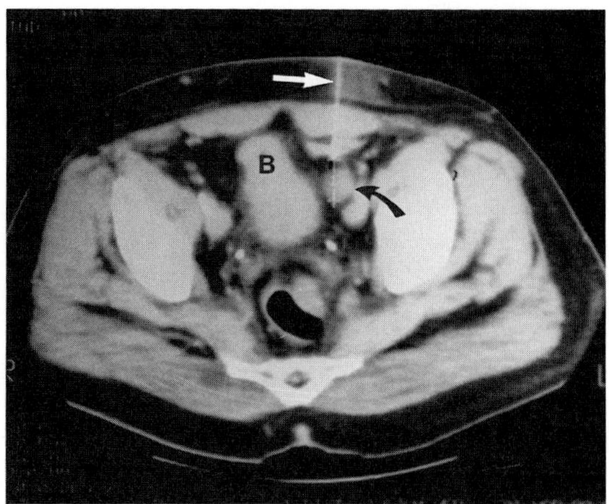


**Fig 10.** Percutaneous CT-guided needle biopsy; needle (white arrow) has been placed with its tip just anterior to an enlarged pelvic lymph node (curved arrow). B = bladder.

**Percutaneous Biopsy.** While cross-sectional imaging utilizing ultrasound or CT has greatly improved our ability to detect masses, histologic confirmation of the nature of a mass still usually requires a tissue sample. Pathologic diagnosis of an abnormal soft-tissue mass can readily be obtained by performing a percutaneous needle biopsy, usually under CT or ultrasound guidance (Fig 10). Using 20- or 22-gauge biopsy needles, tissue recovery rates are very high and the complication rate of the biopsy procedure is very low.[6]

Because the adrenal glands are frequently the site of metastatic deposits, a percutaneous biopsy of an adrenal mass is often performed to confirm the advanced stage of a primary tumor. Biopsy of enlarged lymph nodes in the abdomen and pelvis is often performed for the same indication. While nephrectomy is the standard approach to a renal mass that is suspected to be a renal cell carcinoma, a percutaneous biopsy can be performed if the diagnosis is in doubt.

**Renal Cyst Puncture.** If a renal cyst does not seem to be simple, but is still likely to be benign, then a cyst puncture can be performed.[7] However, improvements in ultrasound and CT have decreased the number of indications for this procedure. In this technique, a needle is placed into the cyst under ultrasound or CT guidance. Fluid is then aspirated and sent for cytologic evaluation. Optionally, contrast material may be injected into the decompressed cyst. Air may also be injected into the cyst, following contrast instillation, to achieve a "double-contrast" effect. With these techniques, the wall of the cyst can then be evaluated for any nodularity or irregularity which would suggest malignancy.

**Percutaneous Nephrostomy.** Performance of this procedure requires that percutaneous puncture of the renal collecting system be performed, usually under fluoroscopic guidance. Aspiration of urine following needle placement confirms the location of the needle tip within the collecting system (Fig 11). A flexible guidewire is then placed into the collecting system. The tract is then dilated in order to accept placement of a large-gauge catheter into the renal pelvis.

A percutaneous nephrostomy is most often performed to relieve a more distal urinary tract obstruction, or to provide access for a nephroscope. A ureteral stent can also be placed through a nephrostomy tract to bypass obstruction. Ureteral strictures can be dilated via the nephrostomy tract with the use of balloon catheters; the best results in patients with ureteral strictures are obtained when the disease is benign, but dilatation can also be performed for palliative purposes.[8]

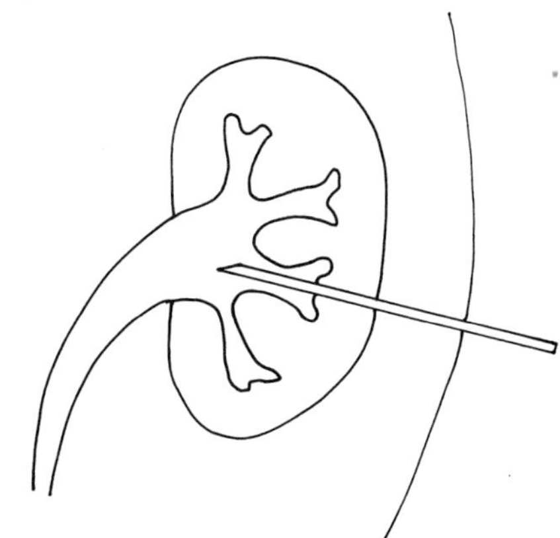

**Fig 11.** Needle placement for percutaneous nephrostomy.

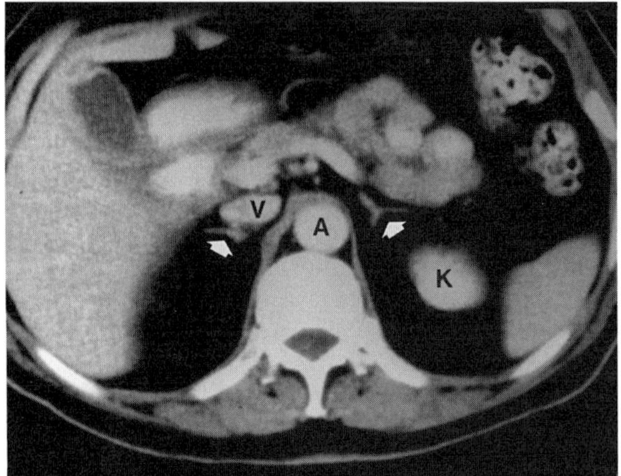


Fig 12. CT of normal adrenal glands (arrows); note relationship to IVC (V), aorta (A), and left kidney (K).

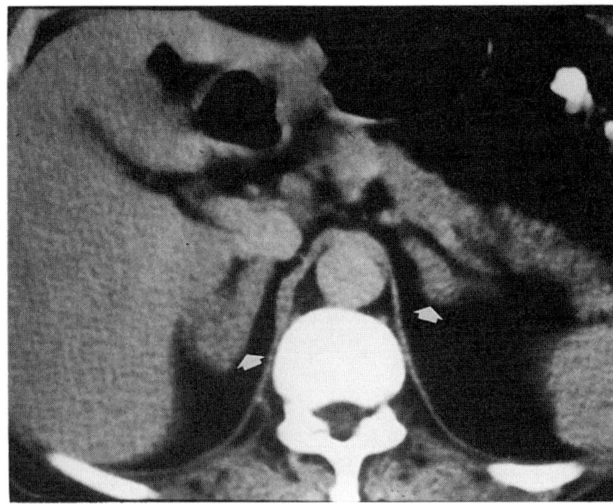

Fig 13. CT of adrenal hyperplasia; note uniform symmetrical enlargement of the glands (arrows).

## APPLICATION OF IMAGING MODALITIES

### Adrenal Gland

Both adrenal glands are located in the extreme superoposterior area of the retroperitoneal space, on either side of the vertebrae, at the level of the eleventh or twelfth rib. The glands are fixed to the inner surfaces of the superoanteromedial aspect of Gerota's fascia. The adrenal glands usually have an inverted Y appearance (Fig 12), and are best visualized using CT or MRI.

**Hyperplasia.** Most cases (80%) of endogenous Cushing's syndrome are the result of bilateral adrenal hyperplasia (Fig 13).[9] The majority of these cases are secondary to adrenocorticotropin hormone (ACTH) production from a pituitary adenoma; ectopic production of ACTH from a variety of other neoplasms is causative in the remainder. The adrenal glands are enlarged and have a ''full'' contour when hyperplastic.

### Adrenal Masses

**Adrenal Adenoma, Non-Hyperfunctioning.** Benign adenoma represents the most common type of mass in the adrenal glands. These neoplasms do not cause elevated hormone levels and are often found incidentally during CT exams. The typical appearance is of a rounded homogeneous mass which is less than 5 cm in diameter (Fig 14). Benign adenomas on T1- and T2-weighted MRI images usually do not demonstrate high signal intensity. Rather, their appearance is usually similar in intensity to liver signal (Fig 15).[10] Clinically, adrenal adenomas may be confused with metastatic lesions, and detection of an adrenal mass in a patient with a known primary malignancy may require biopsy.

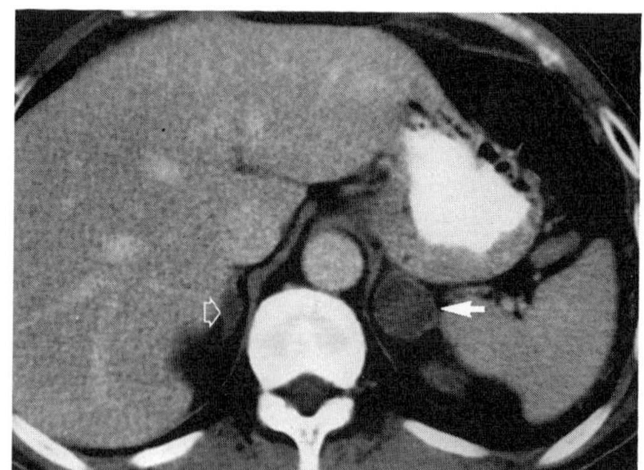

Fig 14. CT of adrenal adenoma; round mass (solid arrow) represents a typical adenoma. A small portion of a right adrenal adenoma (open arrow) is also seen.

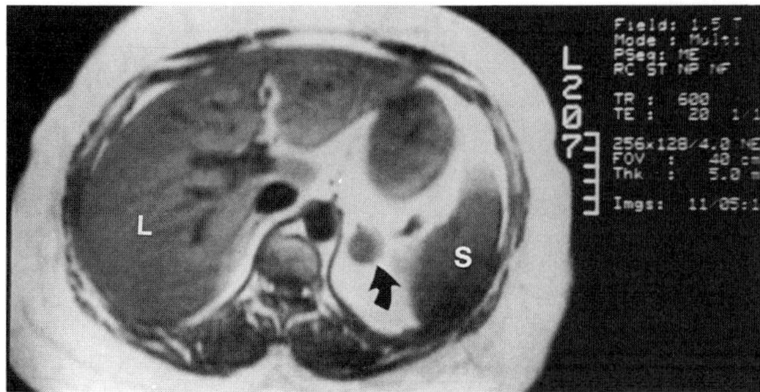


**Fig 15.** MRI of adrenal adenoma (arrow); T1-weighted image shows that this small neoplasm has a similar signal intensity to the liver (L), which should persist on the T2-weighted image. S = spleen.

**Adrenal Adenoma, Hyperfunctioning.** Primary aldosteronism, known as Conn's syndrome, is the result of excessive aldosterone production. Benign hypersecreting adrenal adenomas account for nearly 80% of such cases, while bilateral adrenal hyperplasia produces the remaining 20%.[11] These lesions are often under 1 cm in size and may be difficult to detect. Because of the need to confirm the presence of a lesion in a single adrenal gland or bilaterally, direct venous sampling is often employed for hormone analysis, especially in cases where the CT is negative or equivocal.[12] A catheter is placed via a femoral vein approach. The catheter tip is maneuvered into the vein draining each adrenal gland. Small samples of blood from each adrenal vein and the inferior vena cava below the adrenal veins are analyzed and compared to help localize a radiographically occult lesion.

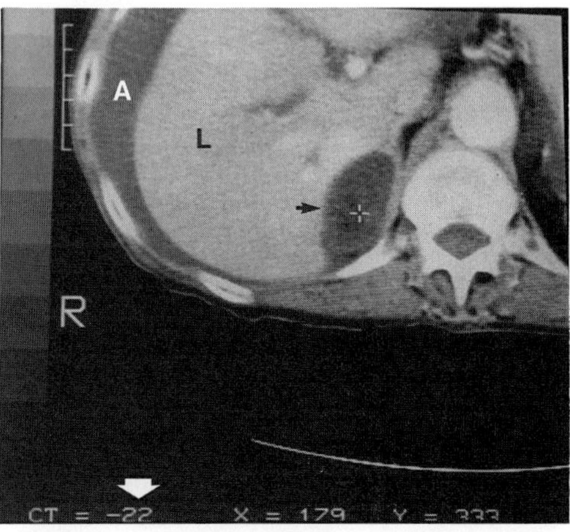


**Fig 16.** Myelolipoma; abdominal CT performed to assess ascites (A) shows an incidental right adrenal mass (black arrow). Density measurement (white arrow) of −22 HUs confirms the presence of fat.

**Myelolipoma.** These are benign tumors consisting of adipose and hemopoietic cells. Ultrasound usually is not diagnostic for myelolipoma, but can demonstrate an echogenic adrenal mass. CT is the best modality to determine the diagnosis, since HUs can be obtained to prove the fat content (Fig 16).[13]

**Hemorrhage.** Adrenal hemorrhage presents as a nonspecific soft-tissue mass involving the adrenal glands. Serial CT or MRI studies usually demonstrate a fairly rapid evolution of acute hematoma. Hemorrhages are the result of trauma or anticoagulation therapy, or may be spontaneous, although underlying systemic illness often exists in patients who experience hemorrhage.

**Adrenal Cysts.** Adrenal cysts are usually incidental findings, since most are asymptomatic. Curvilinear calcifications may be observed on plain films, and both CT and ultrasound can demonstrate a fluid-filled mass within the adrenal gland. However, the walls of these cysts may be thick, and therefore percutaneous aspiration and biopsy may be necessary to confirm the diagnosis.

**Malignant Neoplasms.** Primary adrenal carcinoma is a fairly rare malignancy (Fig 17). More commonly, malignant neoplasms metastasize to the adrenal glands. The malignant mass can sometimes be differentiated from a benign neoplasm by the

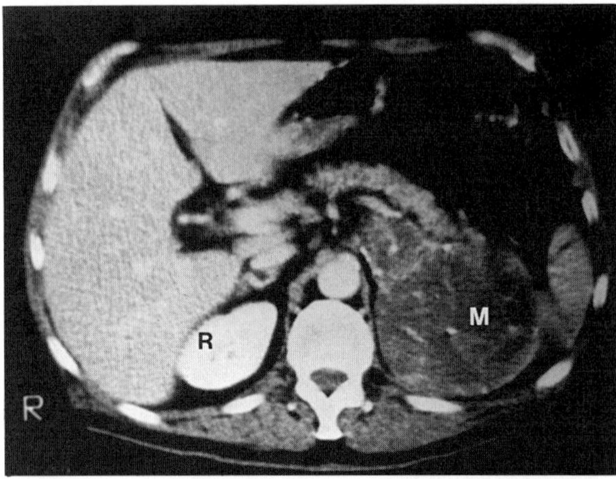


**Fig 17.** Primary adrenal carcinoma; large left adrenal mass (M) is a typical example, since these lesions are usually larger (>5 cm) and more inhomogeneous than those produced by metastasis. R = right kidney.

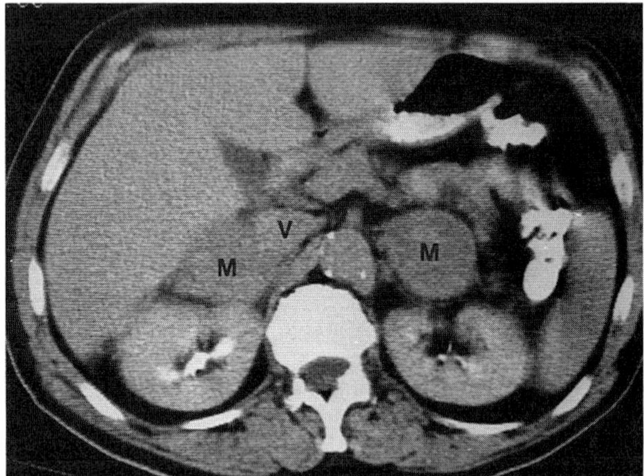


**Fig 18.** Adrenal metastases; bilateral adrenal masses (M) from a primary lung carcinoma. Right-sided lesion partially encases the IVC (V).

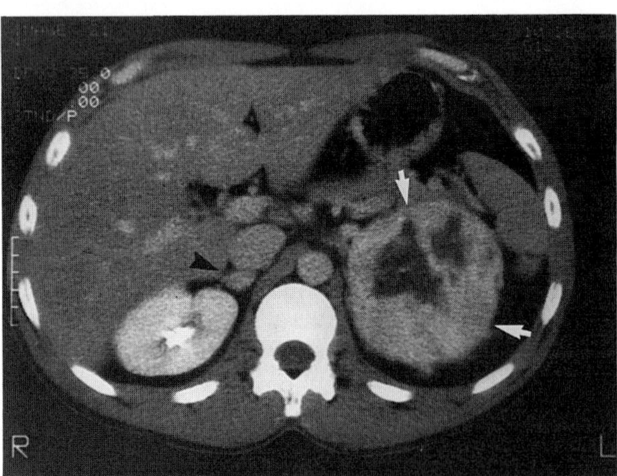


**Fig 19.** Pheochromocytomas; bilateral masses (left = white arrows, right = black arrowhead) in a patient with von Hippel-Lindau disease.

presence of irregular or lobulated margins, inhomogeneity including areas of necrosis, and large size (> 3 cm) (Fig 18).[14] In equivocal cases, percutaneous biopsy can be performed to establish the diagnosis.

**Pheochromocytoma.** In adults, 90% of pheochromocytomas will be located in the adrenal medulla (Fig 19). Extra-adrenal pheochromocytomas are usually subdiaphragmatic and located along the sympathetic nerve chain in the retroperitoneum (Fig 20). However, pheochromocytomas can occur anywhere from the base of the skull to the urinary bladder and gonads. A higher percentage of extra-adrenal pheochromocytomas occur in children (approximately 30%).

CT is the modality of choice to evaluate suspected pheochromocytomas.[15] The initial evaluation should be directed to the assessment of the adrenal glands, but if no abnormality is present in the glands, then a more extensive exam should be performed. At this time, MRI should be reserved for those patients with negative or equivocal CT exams. Ultrasound may detect larger lesions in the adrenal glands and retroperitoneum, and may be used as an initial diagnostic test in children.

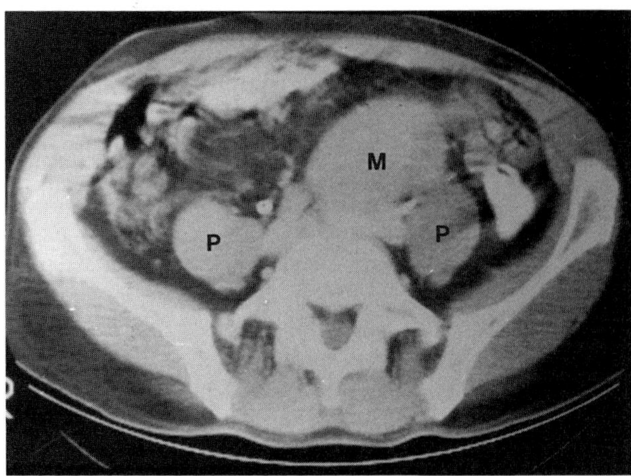


**Fig 20.** Extra-adrenal pheochromocytoma; retroperitoneal mass (M) situated between the psoas muscles (P).

If an invasive procedure such as a percutaneous biopsy is performed on a known or suspected pheochromocytoma, pretreatment with appropriate medications should be given to avoid a hypertensive episode.

## Kidney

The normal kidneys are paired organs located in the retroperitoneal space just lateral to the psoas muscles. The long axis of the kidneys roughly parallels the lateral margin of the psoas muscle so that the apex of the lower pole of the kidney is 1–3 cm more lateral than the apex of the upper pole. Because of the presence of the liver in the upper abdomen on the right, the right kidney is usually 1–2 cm more caudal in position than the left kidney. The superior margins of the kidneys usually lie near the level of T12 or L1.

Normal kidneys range in size from 9.0 to 14.0 cm.[16] In order to compensate for differences in patient stature, the height of the L2 vertebral body and its adjacent inner space can be multiplied by three in order to estimate the expected normal size for an individual patient. The left kidney may be slightly larger than the right kidney. Discrepancies in size greater than 2 cm may indicate underlying pathology and should suggest the need for further evaluation.

## Renal Masses

One of the principal functions of uroradiology is to differentiate benign renal masses from malignant masses that require surgery. In practical terms, this often means differentiating benign cysts from solid masses. Using established criteria, this function can be performed with a high degree of accuracy. We will review the characteristics of cysts vis-à-vis solid masses.

**Cysts.** A simple cortical cyst is the most common renal mass; one or more such cysts are present in approximately 50% of people greater than 50 years of age.[17] Benign cysts are usually asymptomatic and are discovered as an incidental finding during a variety of imaging modalities.

***Plain Films.*** Cysts are usually not visible on plain films. Occasionally, large cysts or those that alter the renal contour can be suggested but the diagnosis cannot be made with plain films alone. Thin calcification in the wall of the cyst is present in 1% of cases but it is a nonspecific finding that does not alter the evaluation.[18]

***Intravenous Urogram.*** A cyst produces a well-defined, hypodense mass in the renal parenchyma that is not enhanced during urography. When a cyst extends beyond the normal margin of the kidney, there is a sharp interface with the parenchyma called a ''beak'' sign (Fig 21). Even with the use of tomography, only 30% to 40% of renal masses smaller than 3 cm—either cystic or solid—will be identified.[19] A hy-

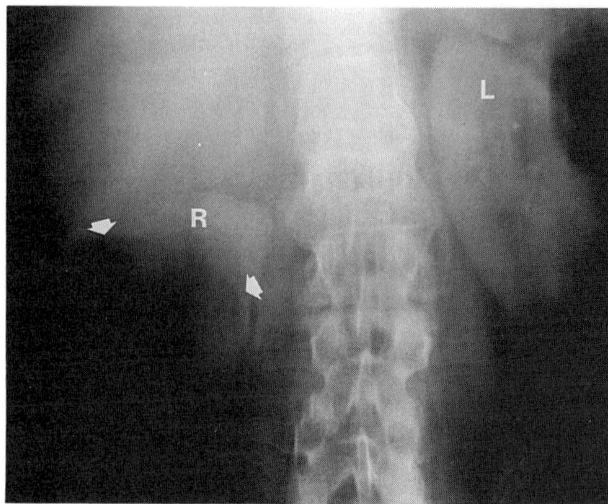


Fig 21. Benign renal cyst; tomogram reveals a hypodense round mass (arrows) in the lower right kidney (R). Left kidney (L) is normal.

povascular solid mass may mimic a benign cyst during urography. Therefore, the diagnosis of a cyst should be confirmed by another imaging modality; ultrasound is usually the most cost-effective method.

***Ultrasound.*** A simple renal cyst produces a well-defined, anechoic mass within the parenchyma. The posterior wall is sharply marginated and there is good through-transmission of sound waves (Fig 22). If a mass does not fulfill all these cystic requirements, then a CT scan should be obtained for further evaluation. Ultrasound will occasionally detect very thin septations within a cyst that are not visible by any other imaging modality. If these septations do not have focal areas of thickening, then the cyst, although minimally complicated, can still be considered benign.

A

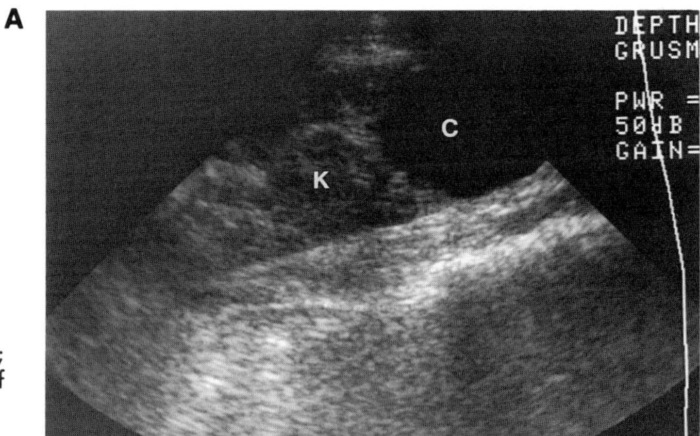


B

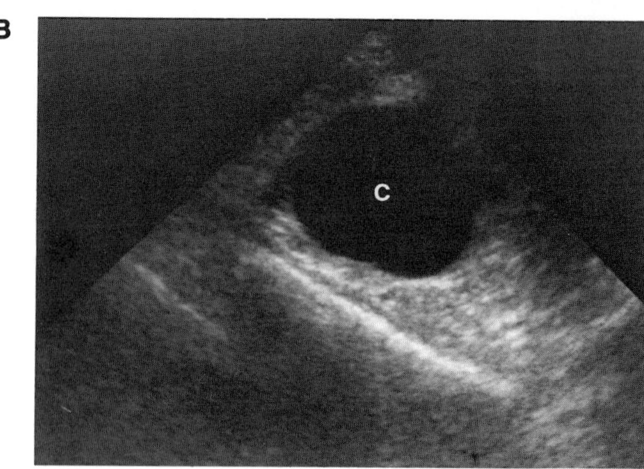


Fig 22. Ultrasound of benign renal cyst; A, sagittal and B, transverse images of a typical round, anechoic cyst (C). K = kidney.

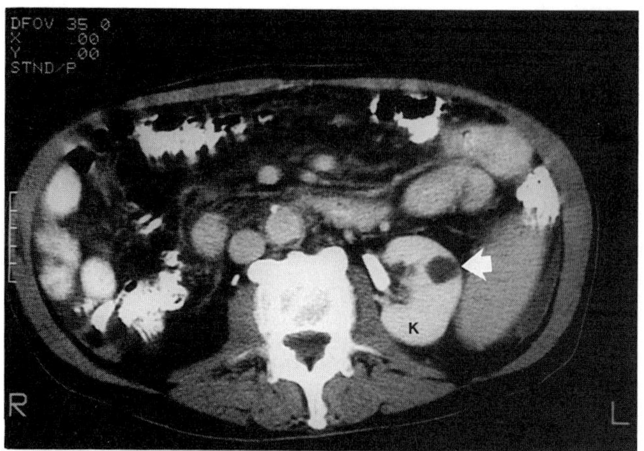


A

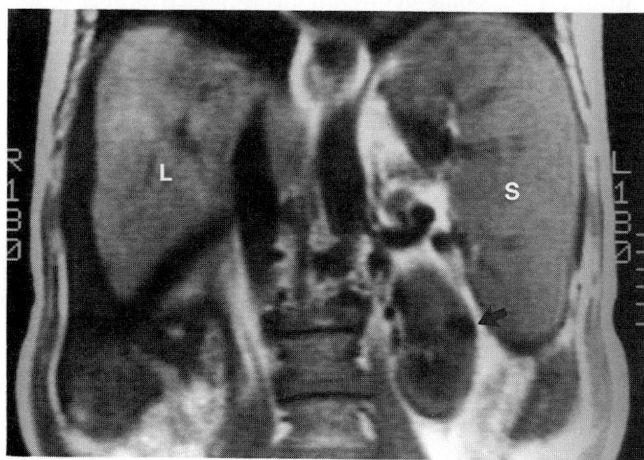


B

**Fig 23.** Benign renal cyst; A, CT demonstrates a typical hypodense cyst (white arrow) in the left kidney (K); B, coronal T1-weighted image in the same patient clearly identifies the cyst (black arrow) as a hypointense lesion. L = liver. S = spleen; C, axial T2-weighted image demonstrates the hyperintensity of the cyst (black arrow) on this pulse sequence. Kidney margin indicated by white arrows.

***Computed Tomography.*** If CT is performed specifically to evaluate a renal mass, kidney images should be obtained both before and after IV contrast material is injected. The CT findings that reveal the presence of a renal cyst are similar to those previously mentioned under urography and ultrasound (Fig 23A). A renal cyst should be homogenous, show no enhancement after injection of contrast material, and have a water density and a paper thin wall. CT possesses an advantage over ultrasound because of its excellent spatial resolution and the ability to measure the density of a mass in HUs. In a properly calibrated CT unit, the density of a simple cyst should be between 0 to 15 HUs. Lesions measuring between 15 and 30 HUs are very likely to be benign, but deserve further evaluation,

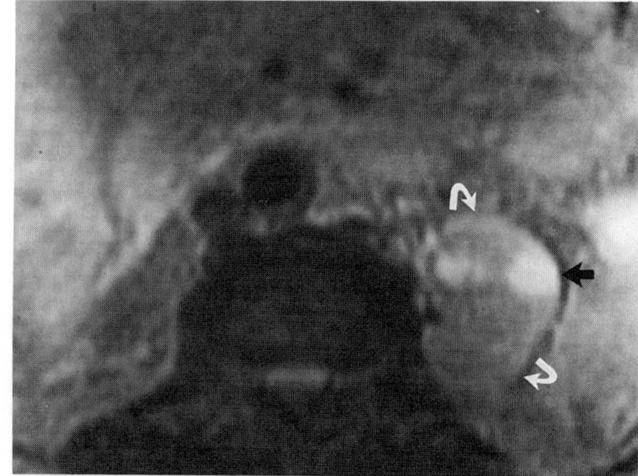

C

possibly with follow-up examinations. Lesions greater than 30 HUs should probably be evaluated histologically.[20]

The hyperdense cyst is an exception to the 30 HU rule. These are benign lesions that are well defined and homogeneous, but which have densities greater than 60 HUs. The density of such cysts is greater than surrounding normal parenchyma before IV contrast material is administered and does not enhance. Consideration of this diagnosis is necessary if one is to avoid surgery.[21]

*Magnetic Resonance Imaging.* Simple cysts have a low signal intensity with T1 images and a high signal intensity on T2 images because of their high water content.[22] MRI is especially useful in those patients with contraindications to the use of IV contrast material and when the nature of a mass remains uncertain after ultrasound (Fig 23B,C).

*Complicated Cysts.* Not all cystic lesions meet the criteria for a simple cyst.[23] If a mass is still considered likely to be benign, percutaneous cyst puncture and aspiration can be performed. Aspiration provides material for pathologic evaluation as well as the possibility of evaluating the lesion following injection of contrast material. Large cysts can cause pain by stretching the renal capsule; percutaneous cyst aspiration and decompression often provides symptomatic relief. If a cyst and/or symptoms recur, a sclerosing agent can be injected into the cyst during a second procedure.

*Renal Sinus Cysts.* Benign cysts in the renal hilum usually originate from cortical tissue. They may produce extrinsic compression of the collecting system and can even obstruct an infundibulum. Because of their location, they can be mistaken for hydronephrosis by ultrasound, but the diagnosis is easily made using CT.[24] Renal sinus cysts and renal sinus lipomatosis produce similar compression of the collecting system during urography; fortunately, both ultrasound and CT readily differentiate the sinus fat from cysts (Fig 24).

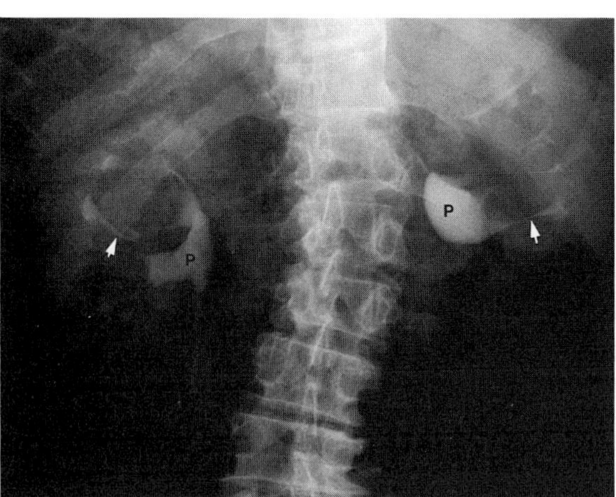

A

**Fig 24.** Renal sinus cysts; A, IVU demonstrates smooth extrinsic compression of both renal pelves (P) and stretching of the infundibula (arrows); B, CT confirms the presence of multiple simple cysts (C) within the renal sinus.

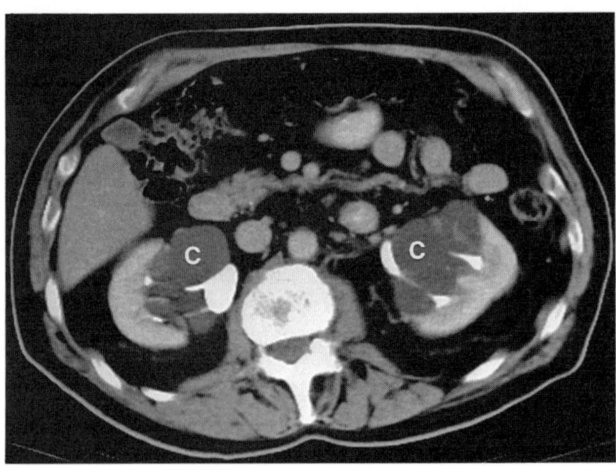


B

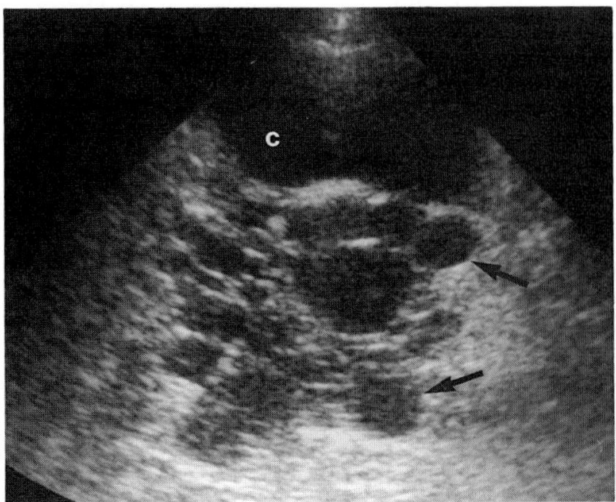


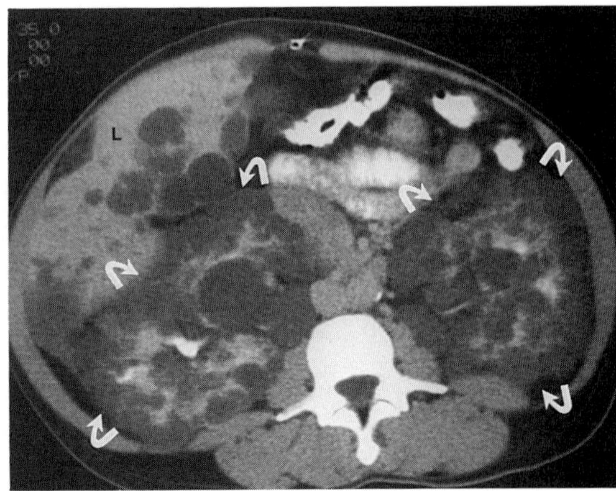


A B

**Fig 25.** Adult polycystic kidney disease; A, ultrasound identifies a large cyst (C) and multiple smaller cysts (arrows). A few echoes are often seen within the cysts because of the numerous tissue interfaces. B, CT demonstrates enlarged kidneys (defined by arrows) which contain numerous cysts. Cysts are present in the liver (L) as well, which is a common finding.

***Hydatid Cysts.*** Curvilinear calcifications in the wall of the cysts on a plain film may be the result of hydatid disease. The thick rim of hydatid disease, which is visible by urography, ultrasound, and CT, differentiates the mass from a simple cyst. Daughter cysts may be seen during ultrasound and CT.

***Medullary Cystic Disease.*** In this cystic disease multiple small cysts, less than 2 cm in diameter, exist in the renal medulla. Ultrasound is the best method to identify these cysts. The kidneys have a normal contour but the cortex is thin; in addition, the cortical-medullary differentiation is poor. Urography is often contraindicated in this setting, because of the potential of inducing renal failure. CT may not demonstrate the medullary cyst as well as ultrasound.

**Polycystic Renal Disease**

***Infantile Polycystic Kidney Disease.*** In patients with this disease, the kidneys are markedly enlarged and function poorly; ultrasound assessment of the polycystic kidney demonstrates an echogenic organ due to numerous interfaces caused by very small cysts throughout the kidney. Individual cysts are too small to be seen as discrete lesions.

***Polycystic Kidney Disease of Childhood.*** Ultrasound is the imaging modality of choice in children with polycystic disease. The kidneys are mildly enlarged and contain cysts, primarily in the medullary regions.

***Adult Polycystic Kidney Disease.*** Urography may inadvertently be performed in adult patients with polycystic disease, when the diagnosis is not suspected and the patient presents with a nonspecific complaint such as flank pain. In adults, the kidneys are enlarged and the renal margins are difficult to define; the cortex is inhomogeneous due to the presence of numerous cysts. Both CT and ultrasound clearly demonstrate numerous bilateral cysts of variable size (Fig 25). Hepatic cysts are also present in a majority of patients with this disease. Hemorrhage into the cysts is common, and can produce flank pain and, possibly, hematuria. Hemorrhage results in a hyperdense cyst as revealed on CT and an echogenic lesion as revealed by ultrasound. The cysts can also become infected, and percutaneous drainage may be necessary.

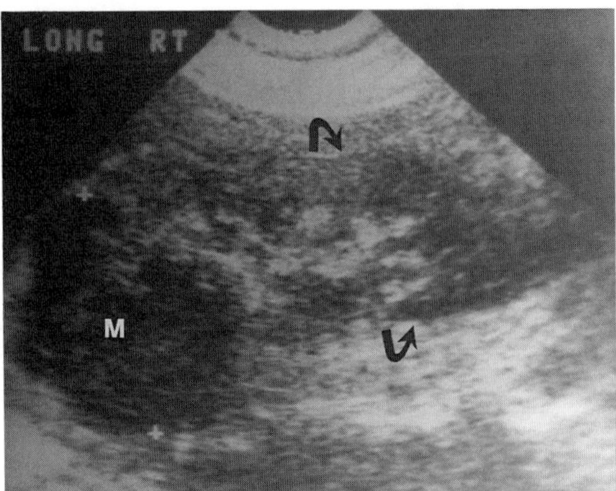


**Fig 26.** Adenocarcinoma as revealed by ultrasound; hypoechoic mass (M) with numerous internal echoes and irregular margins in the upper pole of the kidney (curved arrows).

## Neoplasm

**Adenocarcinoma.** If a renal mass does not appear to be a benign cyst, then the diagnosis of adenocarcinoma must be considered highly likely.

*Plain Films.* Approximately 15% to 20% of renal adenocarcinomas contain calcifications.[25] Course, irregular calcifications within the center of a mass may indicate carcinoma, while pure peripheral, curvilinear calcifications are more likely to represent benign cysts.

*Intravenous Urogram.* Since hematuria and flank pain are common presenting symptoms of a hypernephroma, IVU is often performed as the first imaging procedure. Urography identifies the majority of large tumors, but detects less than 50% of tumors that are less than 3 cm in diameter.[26] Therefore, if urography and cystography are negative, then performance of renal ultrasound or CT should be considered for further evaluation. Most adenocarcinomas that are visible at urography have some enhancement, but it is usually less than that of the normal renal cortex. A bulge beyond the normal margin of the kidney and distortion of the collecting system are common findings associated with a parenchymal renal mass.

*Ultrasound.* A solid mass revealed by ultrasound contains numerous internal echoes. The majority of adenocarcinomas detected by ultrasound are hypoechoic when compared to the normal cortex (Fig 26). A small percentage of carcinomas are predominantly cystic in nature; internal echoes, as well as thickening and irregularity in the walls, usually distinguish necrotic or cystic renal cell carcinomas from benign cysts.

*Computed Tomography.* CT is the most sensitive and specific imaging method to evaluate a patient for the presence of renal neoplasm. As stated previously, CT is particularly useful when images are obtained before and after IV contrast material is administered (Fig 27). However, it is very difficult to differentiate cystic from solid masses by CT unless IV contrast material is utilized.[27] Adenocarcinoma appears as a well-defined hypovascular lesion, with a density between 60 and 100 HUs.

*Magnetic Resonance Imaging.* MRI is not a cost-effective method for diagnosis of renal neoplasm, except perhaps for those patients in whom the use of IV contrast material is contraindicated. At the present time, MRI is most useful for staging a suspicious mass/lesion that has been identified by another imaging modality. Renal ade-

A

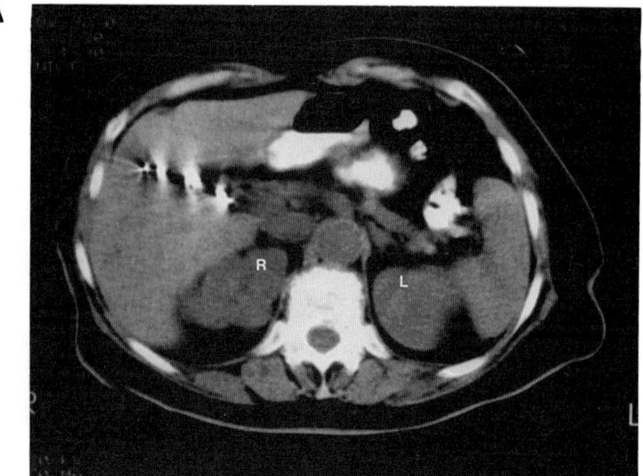


**Fig 27.** Adenocarcinoma as revealed by CT; A, before injection of IV contrast material, no mass lesions are visible. R = right kidney, L = left kidney. B, after injection of IV contrast material, a mass (arrow) is clearly visible in the right kidney.

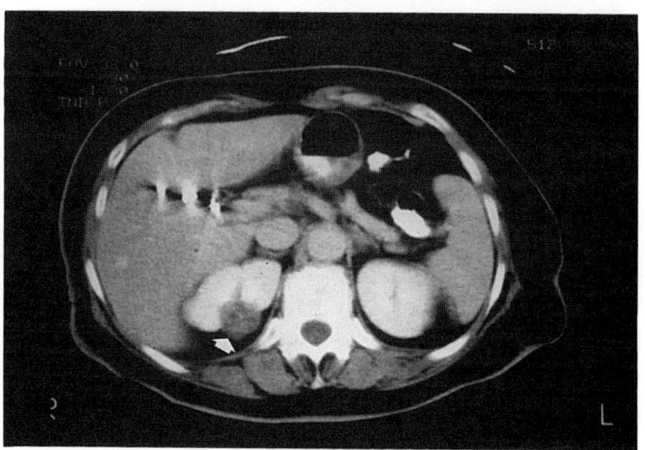

B

nocarcinoma appears as a well-defined mass on MRI.[28] This type of tumor has a variable signal intensity which is related both to the vascularity and degree of necrosis (Fig 28). As with the other cross-sectional imaging tools (ultrasound and CT), MRI cannot precisely define the histologic nature of a solid mass.

***Angiography.*** Angiography should not be employed on a routine basis to evaluate a solid renal mass. While most adenocarcinomas demonstrate some neovascularity, many are cystic or necrotic; in the latter cases angiography is nondiagnostic. Angiography is often obtained to define the blood supply of the kidney. Primary angiographic elucidation of the mass is useful if a hemi-nephrectomy is contemplated, to determine if a renal mass is properly positioned and the blood supply is favorable.

Arterial embolization of a renal tumor via a percutaneous catheter can be performed for symptomatic palliation and for the control of significant hematuria in patients with contraindications to surgery (Fig 29). Embolization may also be useful for those patients in whom blood loss during surgery must be kept to an absolute minimum.[29]

***Staging.*** Even with color Doppler, ultrasound is not yet sufficient to adequately stage adenocarcinoma of the kidney (Fig 30). CT is the best, most cost-effective modality at the present time to properly stage this type of carcinoma; CT is accurate in more than 90% of cases.[30] Extension

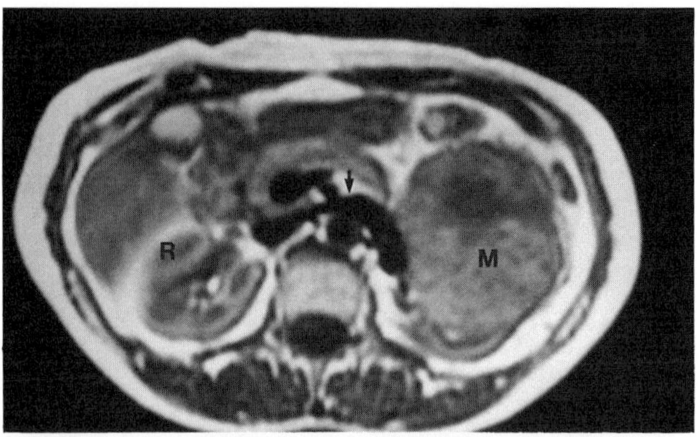


A

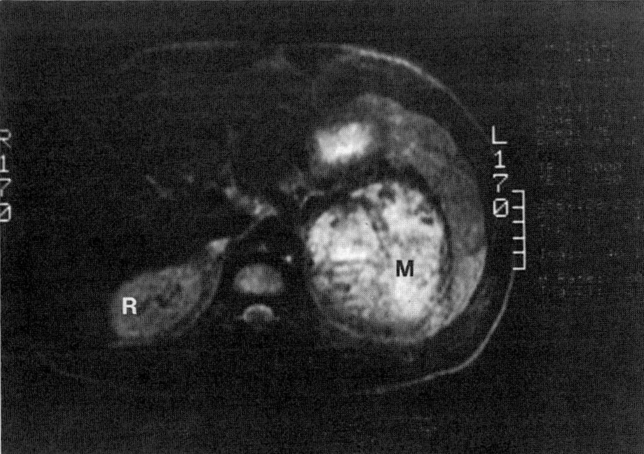


B

**Fig 28.** Adenocarcinoma as revealed by MRI; A, T1-weighted image identifies a large mass (M) in the left kidney. Lack of signal in the left renal vein (arrow) indicates freely flowing blood, right kidney (R) is normal; B, T2-weighted image demonstrates increased, but inhomogeneous, signal in the mass.

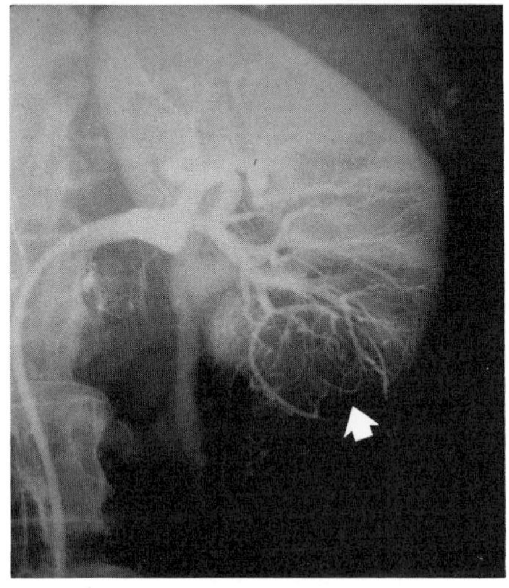

A

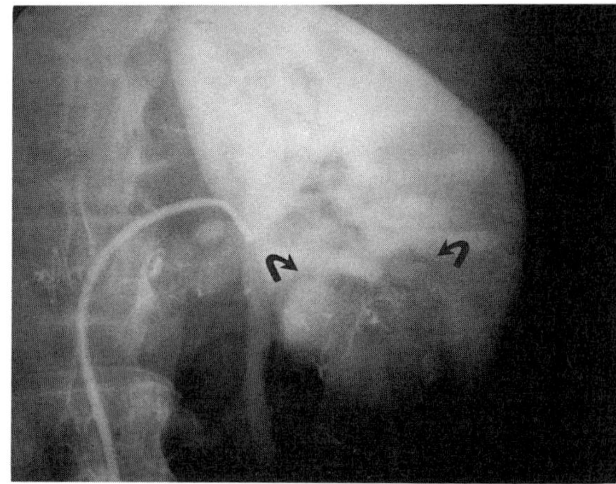

B

**Fig 29.** Adenocarcinoma; A, arteriogram demonstrates neovascularity (arrow) in the lower pole of the kidney; B, after embolization, contrast is absent in the lower pole, indicating vascular thrombosis.

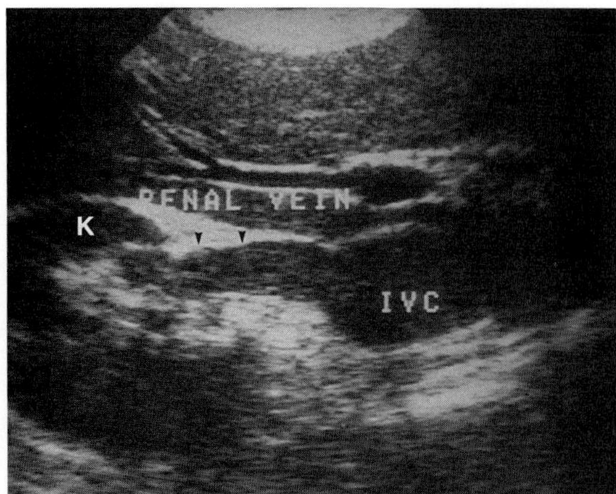


**Fig 30.** Renal vein thrombus; transverse ultrasound image demonstrates echogenic material in the renal vein (arrowheads) with some extension into the IVC. The renal neoplasm is not seen on this image. K = kidney.

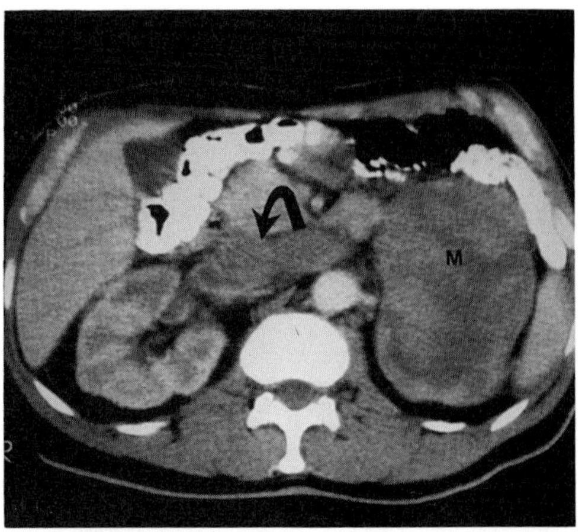


**Fig 31.** Venous thrombus; CT demonstrates a large mass (M) in the left kidney. The left renal vein (curved arrow) and the IVC are enlarged, indicating the presence of thrombus.

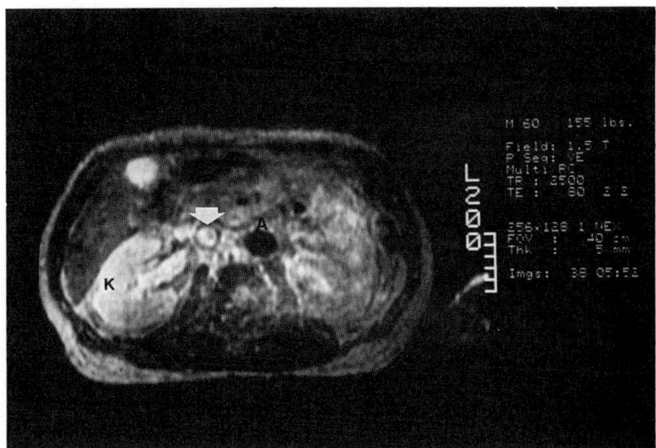


**Fig 32.** Thrombus as visualized by MRI; T2-weighted image demonstrates thrombus in the IVC (arrow). Note flowing blood in the aorta (A). The renal neoplasm is not seen on this image. K = kidney.

through the renal capsule, regional lymph node involvement, and vascular invasion are all readily identified by CT (Fig 31). MRI is at least as accurate as CT for disease staging but is more expensive. MRI offers the distinct advantage of allowing evaluation of blood flow within vessels and can identify tumor thrombus or clot in the renal vein and inferior vena cava with a high degree of accuracy (Fig 32), and can usually obviate the need for cavography. The utilization of MRI in disease staging will likely continue to increase over the next few years. Arteriography and cavography can be performed to evaluate the renal vein and inferior vena cava, respectively, in those cases where tumor involvement cannot be adequately evaluated by other modalities (Figs 33, 34).

## Other Solid Renal Masses

**Angiomyolipoma.** These benign hamartomas can be definitively diagnosed using CT, because they contain variable amounts of fat; density measurements below $-20$ HU are virtually pathognomonic. The use of small areas of measurement, even single pixels, is often necessary, since some of these tumors contain very small amounts

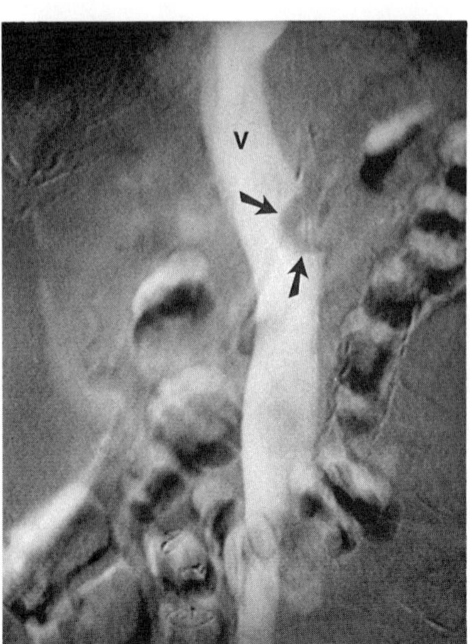


**Fig 33.** Thrombus as seen with a cavagram; thrombus (arrows) extends into the IVC (V).

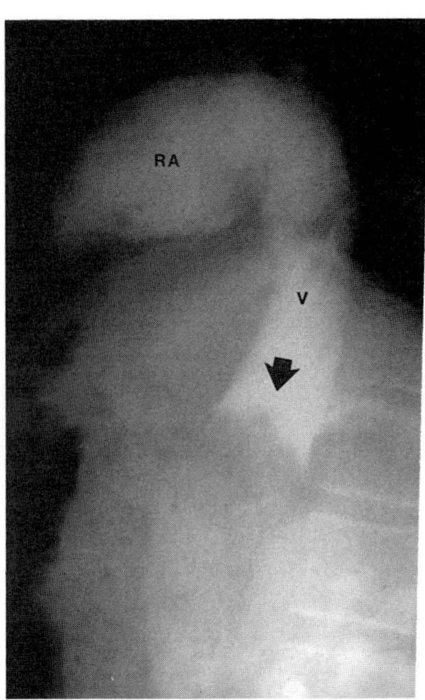


**Fig 34.** Lateral view of a cavagram delineates a large thrombus occluding the IVC (V). A jugular approach was required to define the superior extent of the thrombus. RA = right atrium.

of fat and larger areas of measurement will mask the fat content because of volume averaging.[31]

Angiomyolipomas are also often very visible on ultrasound because of their fat content. However, CT is usually necessary to confirm the diagnosis. The contralateral kidney must also be carefully studied, since these lesions can occur multiply, particularly in patients with tuberous sclerosis. Angiomyolipomas may spontaneously hemorrhage; in such cases, transcatheter embolization of the angiomyolipoma can be performed to control the bleeding (Fig 35).

**Adenoma.** These benign neoplasms cannot accurately be differentiated from adenocarcinomas by current imaging methods. Arbitrary differentiation based on size alone also does not appear to be valid.

**Oncocytoma.** This uncommon neoplasm is also very difficult to differentiate from an adenocarcinoma. A central scar has been described in this tumor, but this is not a pathognomonic finding.[32] Surgical removal is necessary to establish the diagnosis (Fig 36).

**Wilm's Tumor/Mesoblastic Nephroma.** In children, ultrasound is the best method to identify renal masses. Because of the paucity of retroperitoneal fat in children, CT often does not provide as much additional useful information for disease staging in children as in the adult. However, CT may be helpful in the evaluation of the lungs, liver, and contralateral kidney. Imaging characteristics cannot differentiate between a Wilm's tumor and a mesoblastic nephroma, but it is often possible for the physician to make the distinction because the age of onset is usually different between these two masses.

## Metastatic Disease to the Kidneys

Metastases to the kidneys are not uncommon, and bilateral lesions are fre-

A

B

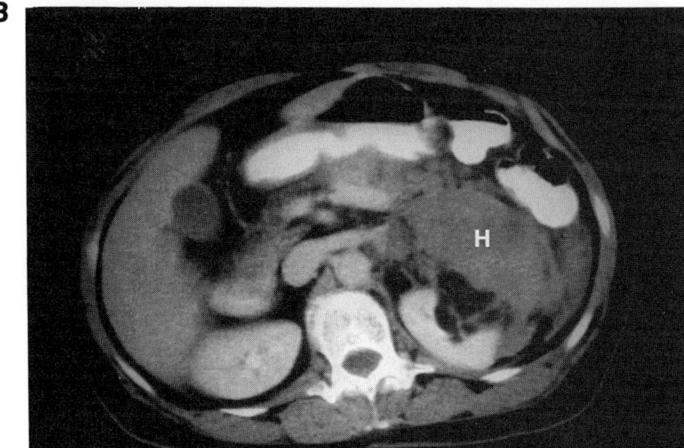


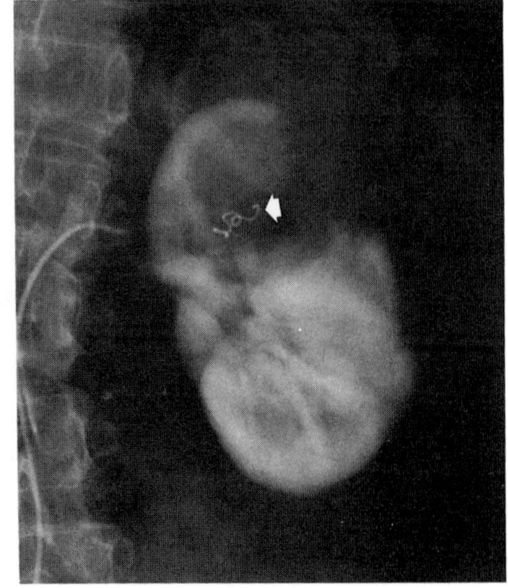

C

**Fig 35.** Angiomyolipoma; A, fat-density mass (arrows) in the left kidney (K); B, the neoplasm spontaneously hemorrhaged (H) several months later; C, because of persistent bleeding, embolization was performed with a coil (arrow).

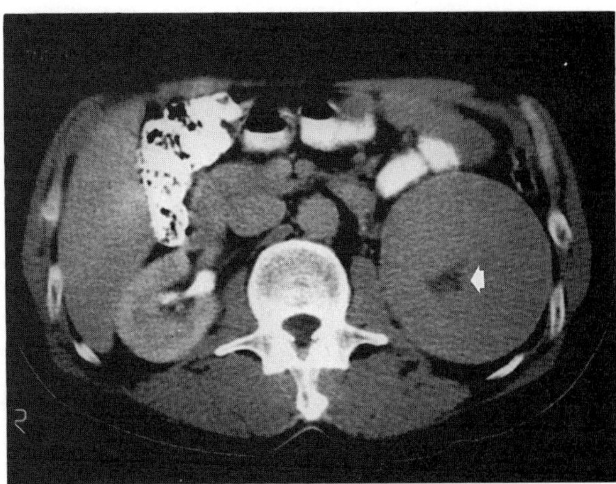

**Fig 36.** Oncocytoma; 10 cm mass in the upper pole of the left kidney with a central scar (arrow).

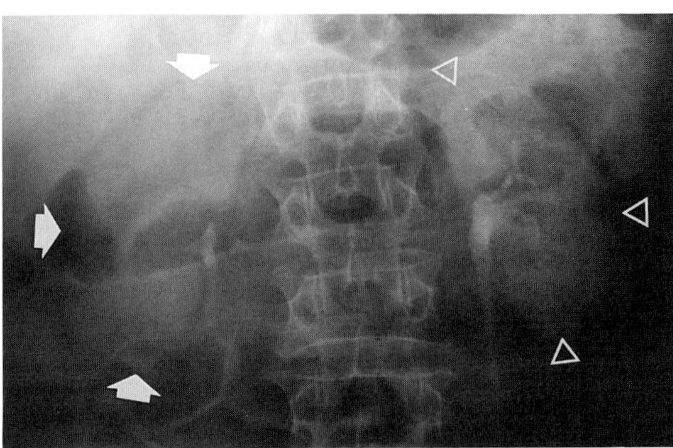

**Fig 37.** Acute pyelonephritis; non-visualization of the collecting system in the right kidney (arrows) secondary to edema. Compare to normal left kidney (open arrowheads).

quently found. Carcinomas from other organs usually produce focal solid renal masses. Renal involvement by lymphoma, particularly non-Hodgkin's lymphoma, may produce either diffuse renal enlargement or a focal mass. Leukemia usually produces a diffuse infiltration and enlargement of the kidney.

In patients with a known or suspected primary malignancy that is prone to metastasize to the kidney, percutaneous biopsy of a solid renal mass should be considered, to establish a histologic diagnosis before a nephrectomy is performed.

## Inflammation

Diagnostic imaging modalities should not be routinely used in patients with renal inflammatory disease. Only if the patient does not respond to antibiotics should imaging be performed, to rule out an abscess or renal obstruction.

**Acute Pyelonephritis.** Nearly 75% of IVUs and sonograms are normal in patients with acute pyelonephritis.[33] When radiographic findings are present, they are usually related to the generalized edema that results from inflammation. Such edema produces diffuse renal enlargement, delayed excretion of contrast material into the collecting system, and compression of the intrarenal collecting system. The radiographic findings become more prominent when infection is most severe (Fig 37). Abnormal ultrasound findings in patients with pyelonephritis are rare but, when present, consist of a hypoechoic renal cortex and generalized enlargement of the kidney when present. CT is not generally performed in the initial diagnostic evaluation of patients with acute pyelonephritis. However, CT may prove useful if the patient does not respond to appropriate antibiotic therapy, as it can reveal the presence of striations in the renal cortex that are typical of pyelonephritis.

**Acute Focal Bacterial Nephritis.** This infectious process is also known as acute lobar nephronia. Acute focal bacterial nephritis produces localized enlargement of the involved portion of the kidney that may be seen on IVU. The adjacent calyces are often compressed as well, and the nephritis may appear to be a focal renal mass. The ultrasound examination in patients with focal bacterial nephritis demonstrates a hypoechoic, poorly marginated mass within the cortex, near the cortical medullary junction.[34] The CT appearance, following injection of IV contrast material, consists of a hypodense, wedge-shaped mass (Fig 38).[35] If the infection spreads to the entire kidney (acute diffuse bacterial nephritis), then the abnormal parenchymal appearance can involve the entire kidney (Fig 39).

**Renal Abscess.** When bacterial nephritis progresses to the extent that tissue necrosis and liquefaction occur, a renal abscess is formed. Radiographic findings include an ill-defined area of decreased cortical en-

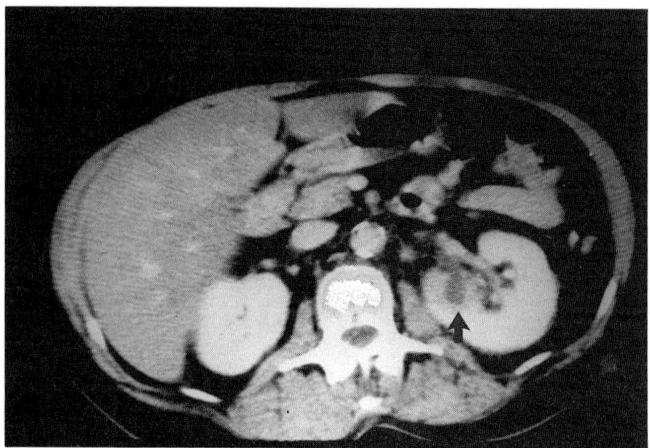

**Fig 38.** Acute focal bacterial nephritis; a previous IVU was normal, but CT defined a hypodense area (arrow) in the left kidney.

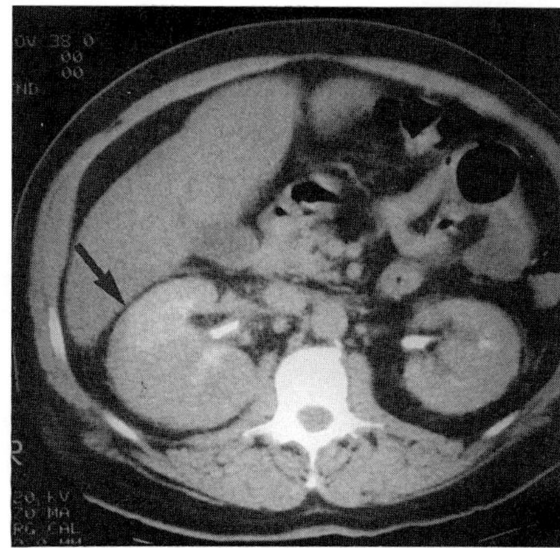

**Fig 39.** Acute bacterial nephritis; diffuse enlargement and irregular enhancement (arrow) of the right kidney. *Klebsiella* organisms were cultured.

hancement and distortion of the collecting system on IVU, and are similar to those seen with focal bacterial nephritis or malignancy. Therefore, evaluation with ultrasound or CT is indicated if a renal abscess is suspected. An abscess as revealed by ultrasound is represented by an extremely hypoechoic lesion which contains low-level internal echoes secondary to necrotic debris. It should be noted that CT is the best modality to fully delineate the extent of a renal abscess. The abscess is low density and does not exhibit contrast enhancement; the presence of gas within the abscess as demonstrated by CT almost assures the diagnosis, although this is not commonly observed.

When a focal renal abscess is suspected, diagnostic percutaneous aspiration with subsequent catheter placement for drainage can be performed under CT guidance as definitive therapy.

**Perinephric Abscess.** A renal abscess can erode through the renal capsule and extend into the perinephric space. This type of abscess can also usually be readily identified using ultrasound or CT. Gerota's fascia is a common site for perinephric abscess, and will appear thickened on CT examination in the presence of an abscess. Percutaneous catheter drainage can be used successfully to treat a perinephric abscess.

Percutaneous catheter drainage as the primary treatment modality is successful in approximately two thirds of patients with renal and/or perinephric abscesses.[36] If an underlying cause of the abscess, such as a renal calculus or vesicoureteral reflux, can be identified, then surgical treatment is often performed to correct the underlying abnormality and to prevent recurrence of the abscess. In those cases, percutaneous drainage can still be employed as a temporary method prior to surgery (Fig 40A,B).

**Pyonephrosis.** Pyonephrosis results when urine within an obstructed collecting system becomes infected. Since pyonephrosis can rapidly destroy renal function and lead

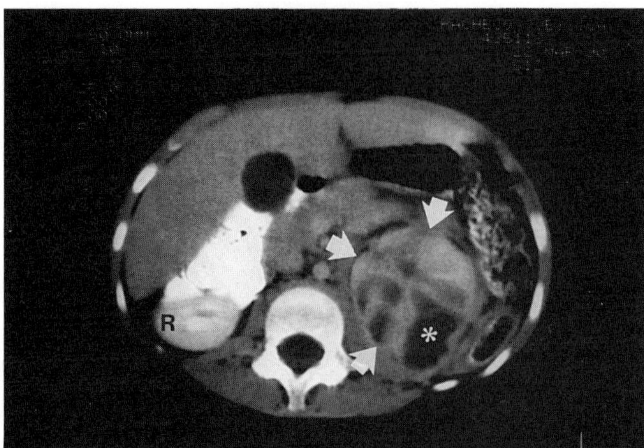


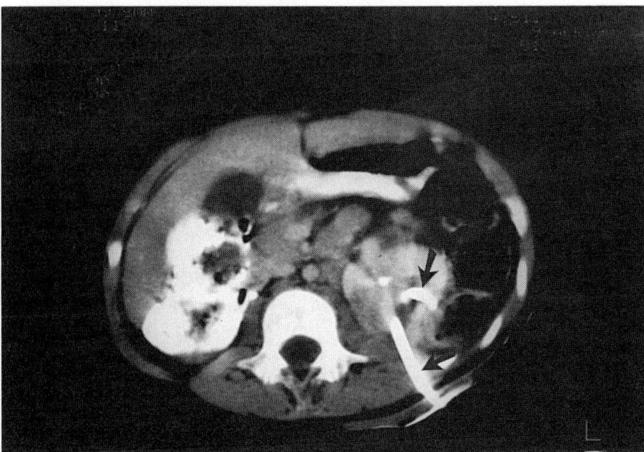


**Fig 40.** Renal abscess; A, enlarged left kidney (arrows) with focal areas of necrosis (*). R = right kidney. B, therapeutic percutaneous drain (arrows) was subsequently placed, after the diagnosis was confirmed by needle aspiration.

to life-threatening sepsis, the diagnostic evaluation should commence immediately whenever pyonephrosis is suspected. Urography often demonstrates nonspecific urinary-tract obstruction; and nearly 50% of such cases are the result of calculus disease.[37] Approximately one third of the cases will not exhibit any contrast excretion, which is an ominous sign of renal damage.[38]

Ultrasound is the best method to noninvasively evaluate pyonephrosis. Hydronephrosis may be readily identified, and low-level echoes within the collecting system are present secondary to the debris that accumulates in infected urine.

When the results of both clinical and diagnostic imaging examinations are suspicious for pyonephrosis, percutaneous aspiration with a skinny needle should be performed to confirm the diagnosis. Once the diagnosis is confirmed, a percutaneous nephrostomy tube should be placed; this can usually be done at the same setting. The underlying cause of the urinary tract obstruction can then be identified and treated when appropriate.

**Chronic Pyelonephritis.** The term chronic pyelonephritis is actually a misnomer, since this condition represents the residual changes from a previous episode of renal infection rather than a chronic infection. Thus, the term chronic atrophic pyelonephritis has been proposed as a more accurate description.[39] Since the majority of

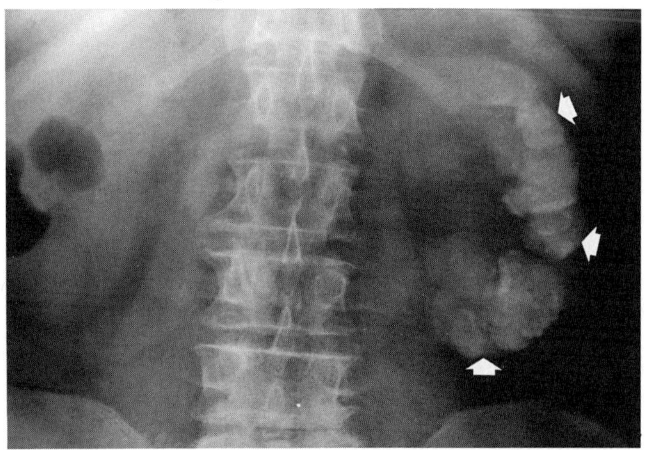

**Fig 42.** "Putty" kidney; note extensive cortical calcifications (arrows) from renal TB.

these cases occur secondary to vesicoureteral reflux, the term reflux nephropathy may also be used.

Urographic findings of chronic pyelonephritis primarily consist of one or more blunted or deformed calyces with overlying areas of cortical scarring. Ultrasound and CT may reveal cortical scarring but do not define the calyceal changes as well as urography (Fig 41).

**Renal Tuberculosis.** Renal tuberculosis usually results from hematogenous dissemination following a primary pulmonary infection. However, the chest x-ray is normal in approximately 50% of the cases.[40] Additionally, renal involvement is usually unilateral.

Urography is the procedure of choice to evaluate the urinary tract in a patient with known or suspected tuberculosis. The plain film should be carefully examined for abnormal calcifications overlying the urinary tract (Fig 42). The visible bones should also be examined for evidence of tuberculous involvement. The classic presentation of renal tuberculosis is multiple infundibular strictures with resultant dilatation of the overlying calyces. In cases where renal function is so compromised that urography does not provide adequate diagnostic information, CT may be very useful to examine the kidney morphology and determine the exact location of any renal calcifications. Retrograde pyelography can also be performed to evaluate the ureter and the renal collecting system. A completely nonfunctioning kidney can develop from tuberculosis; this is known as an autonephrectomy.

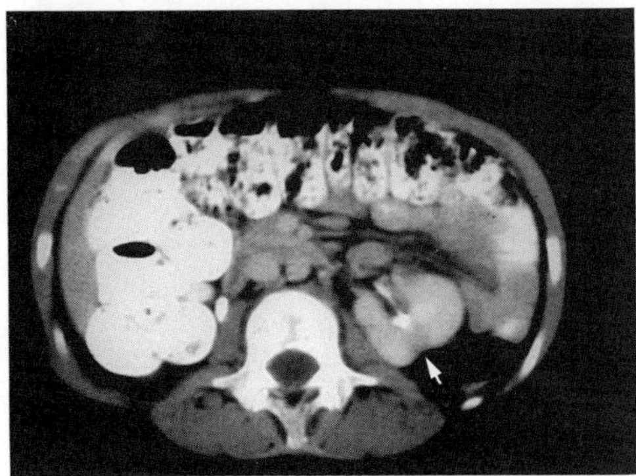

**Fig 41.** Chronic pyelonephritis; note small cortical scar (arrow) from previous infection.

## Urolithiasis and Urinary Tract Obstruction

**Plain Film of the Abdomen (KUB).** Because nearly 90% of urinary tract calculi are radiopaque, the plain film of the abdomen and pelvis is usually the first imaging test that reveals possible urinary tract obstruction.[41] One must keep in mind that overlying bowel content and osseous structures can easily obscure a urinary tract calculus, particularly those less than 5 mm in diameter. Large calculi in the renal pelvis with extension into the infundibula and calyces are known as staghorn calculi. Venous calcifications, known as phleboliths, are very common in the lower pelvis. These small rounded calcifications can occasionally be difficult to differentiate from distal ureteral calculi. Oblique films are often useful in the evaluation of a possible urinary tract calculus to determine if the abnormal calcification remains in the same plane as the urinary tract itself.

**Intravenous Urography.** The urogram is the most sensitive imaging test to assess patients with suspected stone disease. It can usually determine the cause, level, and degree of obstruction.

The earliest sign of ureteral obstruction is columnation of contrast material within the collecting system down to the point of obstruction (Fig 43). Columnation indicates that the collecting system proximal to the obstruction is distended and filled with contrast material. Normal ureteral peristalsis is absent or diminished with ureteral obstruction; as the degree and duration of the obstruction increases, the proximal dilatation of the ureter and collecting system increases (Fig 44). With increasing degrees of obstruction there is also a concomitant delay in the excretion of contrast material from the kidney, and this results in the so-called delayed nephrogram. In patients with obstruction, the renal cortex becomes very opaque, as contrast material is collected within the renal tubules because increased pressure within the collecting system impedes drainages into the renal tubules.

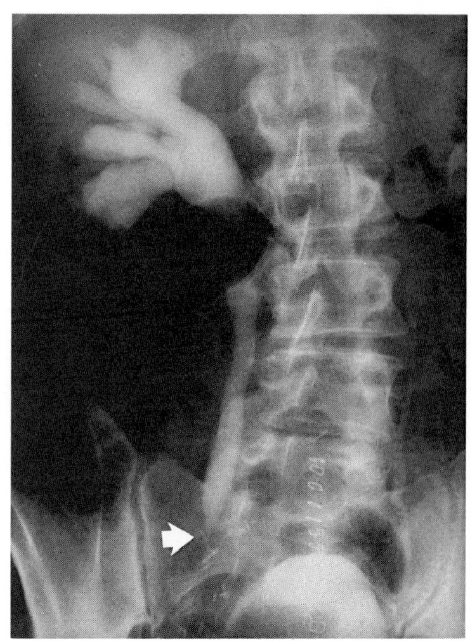

**Fig 44.** Complete ureteral obstruction; surgical clip (arrow) was inadvertently placed across the right ureter, resulting in marked dilatation of the ureter and collecting system.

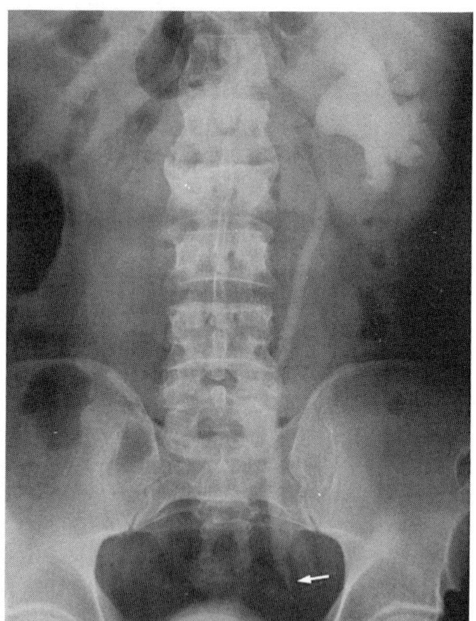

**Fig 43.** Ureteral columnation; persistent complete filling of a mildly dilated left ureter caused by a distal calculus (arrow) which is partially obscured by contrast.

Renal backflow occurs in those with urinary tract obstruction and results in retrograde flow of urine. Different types of backflow are pyelovenous, pyelotubular, pyelosinus, and pyelolymphatic. However, renal backflow is most often visualized in urologic tests as a result of overdistension of the collecting system during a retrograde pyelogram (Fig 45).

**Retrograde Pyelography.** Retrograde pyelography is invasive, and requires ureteral catheterization. This technique can opacify

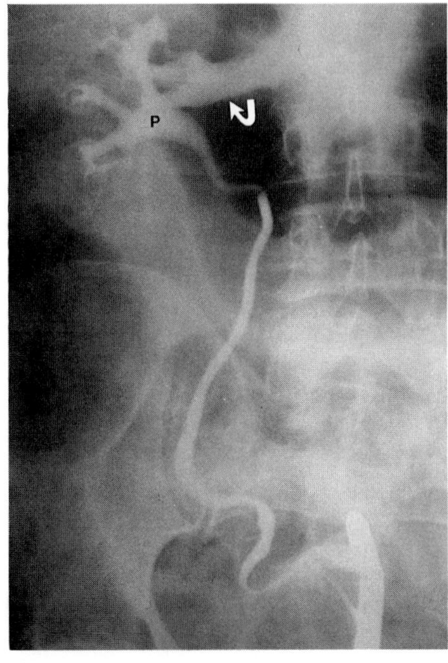


A

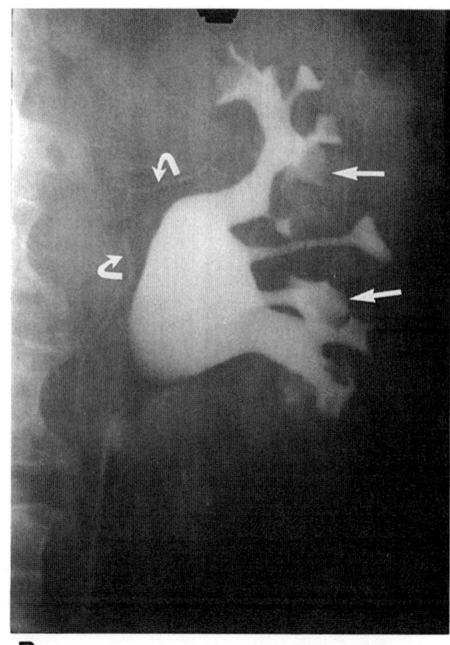

B

**Fig 45.** Iatrogenic backflow; A, pyelovenous backflow. Contrast material from a retrograde ureteropyelogram flows into the renal vein (curved arrow). P = renal pelvis. B, pyelotubular (straight arrows) and pyelolymphatic (curved arrows) backflow.

the collecting system, establish the site and etiology of obstruction, and better delineate filling defects. Retrograde pyelography provides no assessment of renal function. A retrograde pyelogram is often performed in instances where a level of obstruction is identified by urography but the etiology of the obstruction cannot be determined. Retrograde pyelography is also performed in patients in whom standard urography is contraindicated. A retrograde pyelogram is potentially a precursor to interventional urologic treatment of stone disease via baskets, lasers, and scopes.

**Ultrasound.** Assessment of renal obstruction by ultrasound depends on the presence of dilatation of the collecting system, or hydronephrosis; ultrasound does not assess the physiology of the kidney in those with obstruction. Ultrasound can be normal in up to 50% of patients with acute ureteral obstruction and should be reserved for use in those who require better visualization of the kidney and renal pelvis after urography has been performed.[42] Ultrasound is useful in demonstrating the hydronephrosis associated with chronic obstruction as well as in determining any change in hydronephrosis after a therapeutic procedure has been performed (Fig 46). Hydronephrosis does not absolutely equate with obstruction, and direct visualization of the collecting system should be considered, especially when the etiology of the obstruction is unknown.

**Computed Tomography.** CT can be employed to further evaluate a specific site of obstruction.[43] In the evaluation of the collecting system, CT can differentiate between a stone that is radiolucent on plain radiographs and a soft tissue mass (Fig 47). CT is excellent in providing a panoramic assessment of the retroperitoneum to establish the cause of obstruction, particularly when the obstruction is extrinsic.

**Antegrade Pyelography.** Percutaneous placement of a skinny needle into the col-

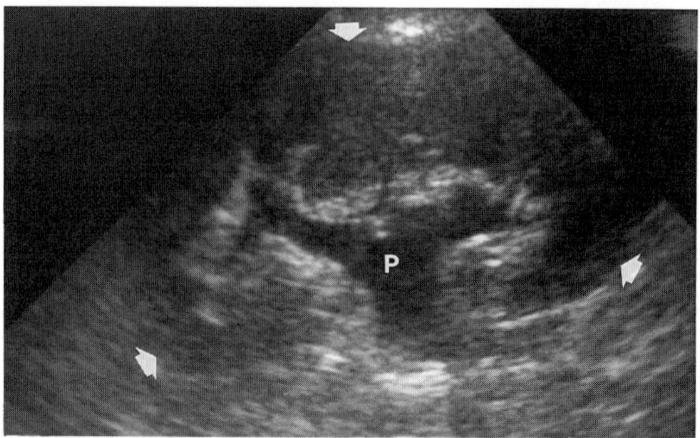


A

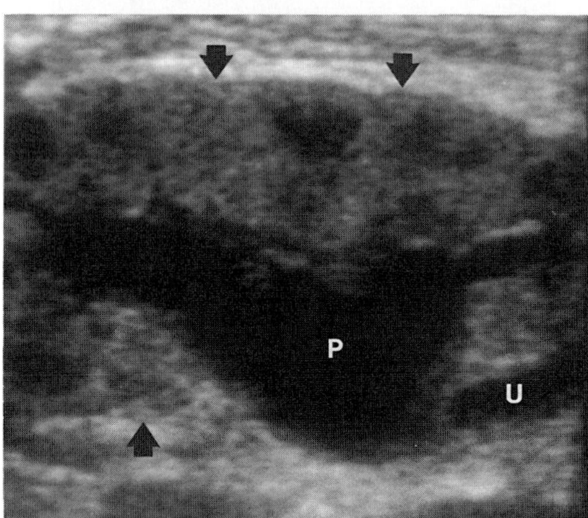


B

Fig 46. Hydronephrosis as revealed by ultrasound; A, mild hydronephrosis involving the renal pelvis (P) and infundibula. Renal margins are defined by arrows. B, moderate hydronephrosis with a dilated ureter (U), edematous pyramids result in focal hypoechoic areas in the cortex (defined by arrows).

lecting system of the kidney permits contrast material to be injected, and allows definition of the level of obstruction. Like the retrograde pyelogram, antegrade pyelography provides excellent opacification

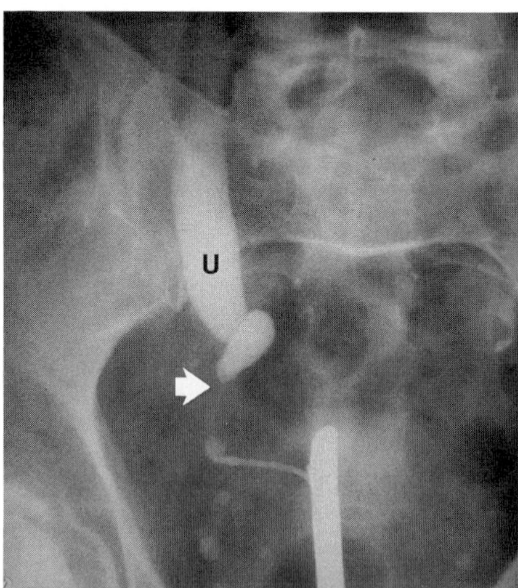


A

B

Fig 47. CT evaluation of site of obstruction; A, previous IVU had identified a ureteral obstruction. A retrograde pyelogram determined the point of obstruction (arrow) but not the etiology. U = ureter. B, non-contrast CT identified a small calculus (arrow) that was not radiopaque on plain radiographs.

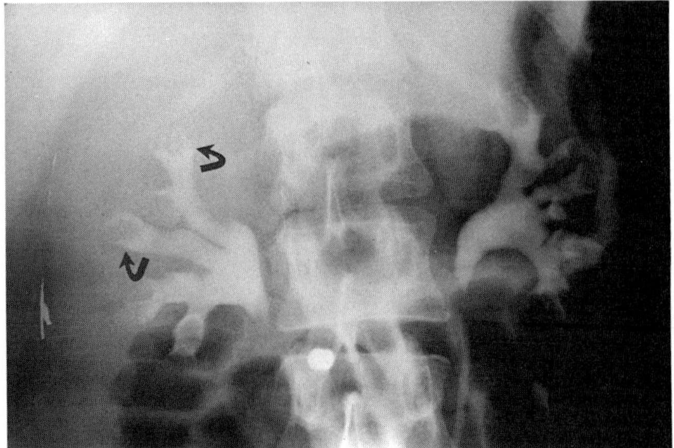

**Fig 48.** Papillary necrosis; contrast material in the collecting system outlines calyces, which are enlarged and irregular, secondary to tissue loss in the papillae, resulting in the "lobster claw" sign (arrows).

of the collecting system. Additional interventional procedures can then be performed to relieve the obstruction, either on a temporary or permanent basis.

## Renal Pelvis and Calyceal System

**Papillary Necrosis.** Ischemia in the renal papilla can result from a variety of causes, including analgesic nephropathy and sickle cell disease. This results in papillary necrosis which is best visualized with urography or retrograde pyelography. Abnormal collections of contrast material are present in the renal papillae and these collections are of variable shape and size (Fig 48). Occasionally, the entire papilla will slough. Acute urinary tract obstruction can result from a sloughed papilla, which produces a negative filling defect in the renal pelvis or ureter at urography.

**Calyceal Diverticulum.** A well-defined, smooth diverticulum may extend from a calyx into the cortical medullary portion of the kidney, with a narrow connection from the main portion of the diverticulum to the calyx. Calyceal diverticula usually occur in the upper or lower poles of the kidneys. A larger diverticulum in the central portion of the kidney is usually called a pyelogenic cyst. Neither calyceal diverticula nor pyelogenic cyst usually produce clinical symptoms, unless stones or infection develop within the diverticulum. Calyceal diverticula are most often identified by urography but can also be observed with ultrasound and CT (Fig 49).

**Medullary Sponge Kidney.** The plain film may be normal but small punctate calcifications can be seen in the medullary portion of the kidneys. During urography, small linear strands are present in the renal papillae which are the result of dilatation of the collecting ducts. The diagnosis of medullary sponge kidney is usually made after a small calculus has formed in one of the dilated tubules and then slipped into the main collecting system, producing ureteral obstruction. The obstruction usually obscures the dilated tubules on the infected side, but the diagnosis can be made from evaluation of the contralateral kidney, since both kidneys are involved.

## Renal Pelvis Neoplasm

**Transitional Cell Carcinoma.** Transitional cell carcinoma is most often identified as a filling defect in the renal pelvis during urography or retrograde pyelography. This type of tumor may be smooth or irregular, flat or papillary. The primary role of CT is to stage the tumor by determining local extension and lymphadenopathy.[44] In selected cases, CT and ultrasound can be used to identify a nonopaque calculus, which can mimic a soft-tissue mass at urography (Fig 50). Squamous cell carcinomas cannot accurately be distinguished from transitional cell carcinomas by imaging methods.

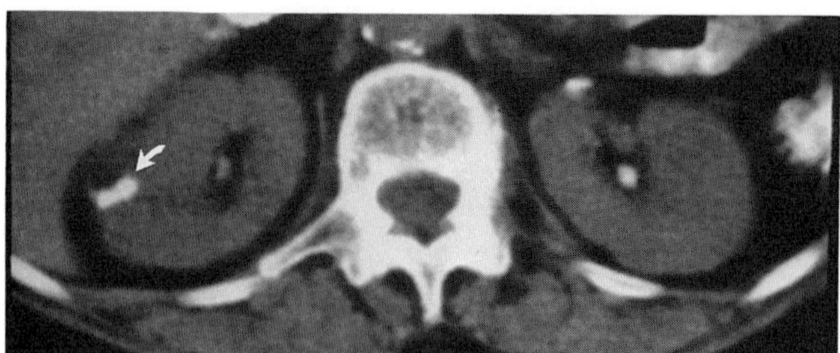


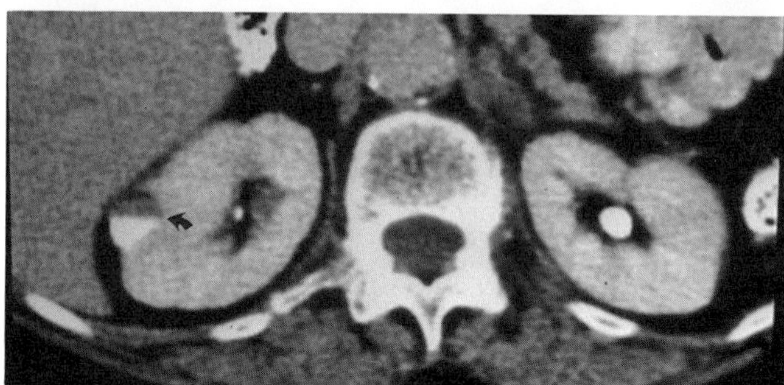


**Fig 49.** Calyceal diverticulum containing a calculus; A, noncontrast CT demonstrates calcification (arrow) in a peripheral cortical lesion; B, after IV contrast, a urine-contrast level (arrow) forms, indicating communication with the collecting system.

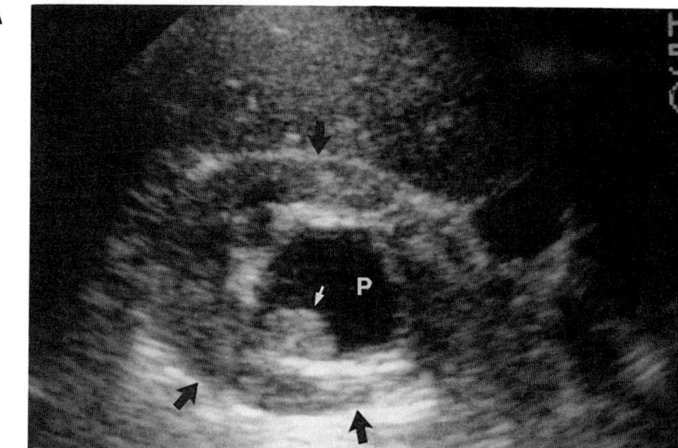


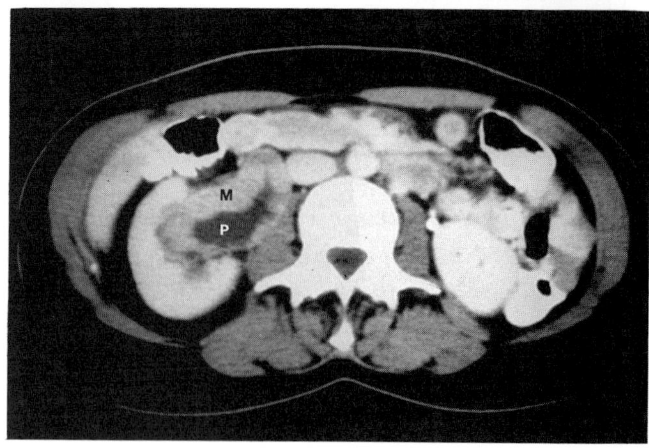


**Fig 50.** Transitional cell carcinoma; A, ultrasound demonstrates a soft tissue mass (white arrow) protruding into the renal pelvis (P). Renal margins defined by black arrows; B, CT defines the mass (M) as a markedly thickened wall. The dilated pelvis (P) is the result of tumor-produced obstruction.

## Ureter

The ureter can be readily examined in a physiologic manner during an IVU. Because of peristalsis, it is usually not possible to see all portions of the ureters simultaneously. With the help of extra views, such as those with the patient in prone or upright positions, the ureters can usually be adequately examined. To better delineate an abnormality, or in those cases where the ureter is not adequately defined, retrograde ureterography may be utilized.

**Neoplasms.** Transitional cell carcinoma is the most common primary ureteral neoplasm. These tumors typically involve the distal third of the ureter. A small focal dilatation of the ureter just distal to the lesion can produce a so-called "wine goblet" or "champagne glass" configuration visible on a retrograde ureterogram. When a filling defect is found in a ureter, great care must be taken to assess the remainder of the urinary tract, since these tumors are often multicentric (Fig 51).

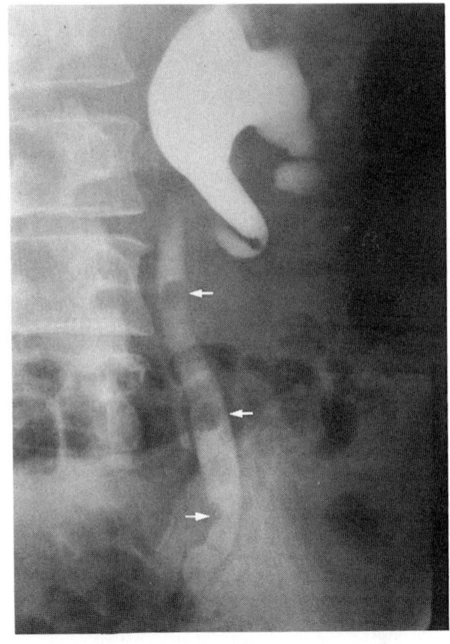

**Fig 51.** Multicentric transitional cell carcinoma; retrograde pyelogram delineates multiple filling defects (arrows) in the ureter.

CT can be useful to determine periureteral invasion as well as lymphadenopathy and more distant metastases. A CT-guided biopsy of a soft tissue lesion involving the ureter can be helpful to establish the diagnosis, and may assist in preoperative planning (Fig 52).

A ureteral transitional cell carcinoma can produce complete obstruction. However, the etiology of a ureteral obstruction may not be apparent and CT may aid in establishing the diagnosis. A non-contrast CT performed at the level of ureteral obstruction can rule out the diagnosis of a stone and strongly suggest the presence of tumor. The CT scan can aid in determining the intraluminal or extraluminal nature of a mass. A percutaneous nephrostomy tube can then be placed, which provides relief and allows an antegrade ureterogram to be

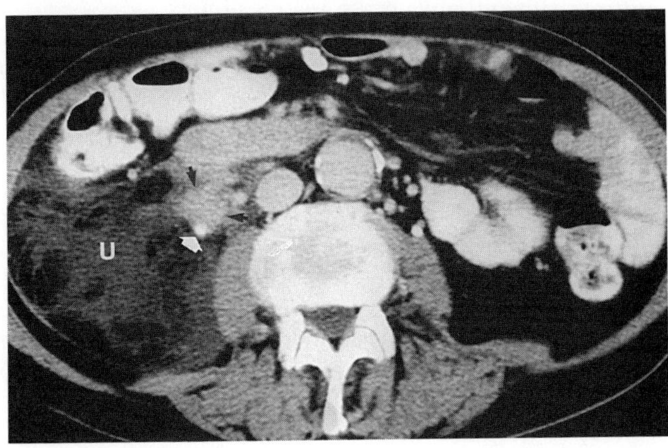


**Fig 52.** Transitional cell carcinoma; CT demonstrates a mass (black arrows) arising from the ureter (white arrow). Indistinct margins indicate periureteral invasion. Extravasated urine (U) is secondary to ureteral obstruction.

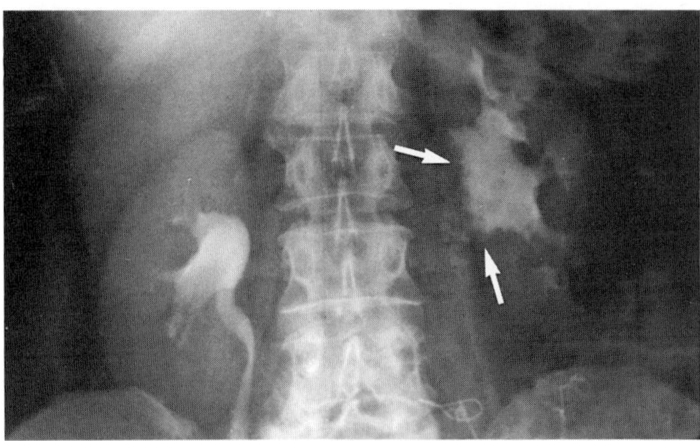

**Fig 53.** Ureteritis cystica; numerous filling defects (arrows) are present in the renal pelvis and proximal ureter.

performed to delineate the obstruction. If necessary, a retrograde ureterogram can also be performed to further define the size and nature of the lesion.

Again, it should be emphasized that imaging tools cannot establish the precise histologic nature of a mass. While transitional cell carcinoma is the most common ureteral tumor, other ureteral neoplasms, both benign and malignant, while rare, may produce similar filling defects in the ureter, and it is necessary to obtain a pathologic specimen to establish the diagnosis. Metastatic tumors to the ureter are not uncommon, with the majority being the result of direct extension.

## Inflammation

**Pyelitis/Ureteritis Cystica.** Chronic urinary tract infection can lead to the formation of multiple subepithelial cysts in the ureter, renal pelvis, and bladder. Nearly 50% of the cases are bilateral.[45] The cysts are usually 5 mm or less in diameter (Fig 53). These cysts are easily visualized with IVU or retrograde pyelography.

**Tuberculosis.** Approximately 15% of patients with renal tuberculosis will have identifiable ureteral lesions.[46] Most of these lesions are strictures that produce concomitant proximal dilatation. Areas of inflammation, prior to stricture formation, can produce an irregular lumen. Multiple levels of ureteral involvement are common (Fig 54).

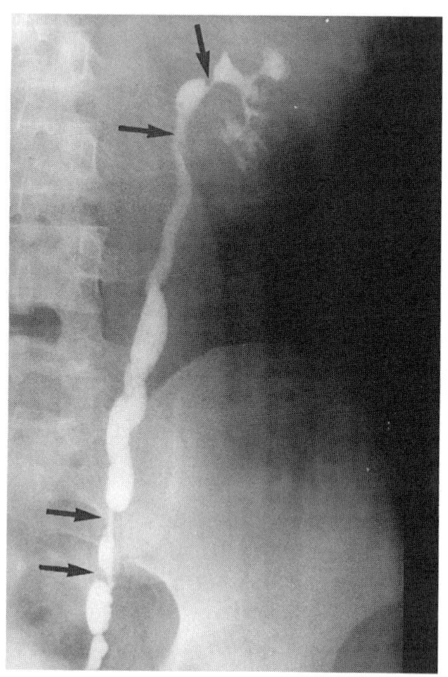

**Fig 54.** Tuberculosis; multiple ureteral strictures (arrows) with proximal dilatation as seen with retrograde ureterography.

Other inflammatory conditions in the abdomen or pelvis can affect the urinary tract by direct extension. These conditions include inflammatory bowel disease, diverticulitis, pelvic inflammatory disease, and endometriosis (Fig 55A,B). With extensive ureteral involvement, CT is the best modality for evaluating extent of disease.

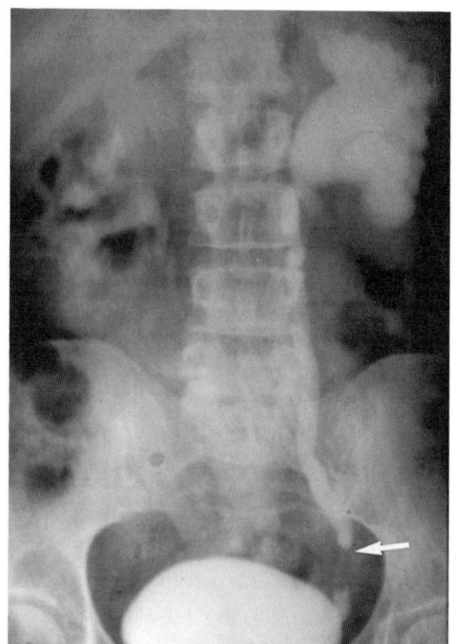


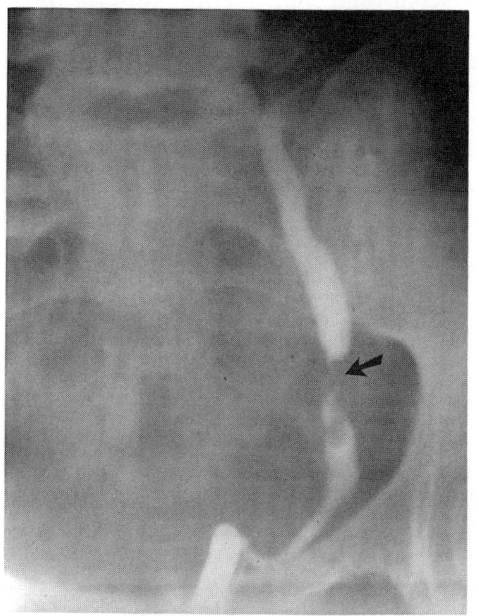


**Fig 55.** Distal ureteral obstruction; A, as observed (arrow) with IVU; B, retrograde pyelogram defines the stricture (arrow), which at surgery was found to be the result of endometriosis.

## Dilated Ureter

**Acute Obstruction.** The pathophysiology of acute ureteral obstruction is more fully discussed in the kidney section. Most ureteral obstructions are caused by calculi, which are likely to obstruct at the ureteropelvic junction, at the pelvic brim because of crossing iliac vessels, and at the ureterovesical junction. In certain cases, the cause of focal ureteral obstruction cannot be determined, even after a stent has been placed. Contiguous CT images through the ureter, without injection of IV contrast material, can identify a small calculus which is not opaque on conventional radiographs.

**Primary Refluxing Megaureter.** Megaureter is another term to describe a dilated ureter. In primary refluxing megaureter, the dilatation is the result of reflux that occurs because the ureteral orifice is abnormal. Secondary refluxing megaureter is usually the result of an abnormal bladder.

**Primary Obstructed Megaureter.** In patients with an obstructed megaureter, a focal, intrinsic, adynamic segment of the distal ureter causes a physiologic obstruction. In such cases, the distal ureter often has a beaked appearance. The majority of cases are unilateral, but approximately one third are bilateral. Additional urinary tract anomalies, including ureteral duplication, are not uncommon in patients with a primary obstructed megaureter.

**Primary Nonrefluxing–Nonobstructed Megaureter.** This type of dilatation is usually part of the Eagle-Barrett syndrome. However, high flow urine states may also cause nonrefluxing–nonobstructed megaureter.

## Miscellaneous Conditions

**Retroperitoneal Fibrosis.** In this condition, a fibrous mass develops in the retroperitoneum, below the level of the kidneys. The majority of cases (70%) are idiopathic, and the condition predominates in males, with a ratio of three to one.[47] Of the known causes, methysergide use is the most well known. However, any insult to the retroperitoneum, including surgery, can be a precipitating factor. Encasement of the ureter by the fibrous mass can produce a partial obstruction. Malignant retroperitoneal fibrosis—usually due to metastatic disease to the retroperitoneum—can produce a similar appearance of a focal mass obstructing the ureter.

On IVU, the classic appearance of benign retroperitoneal fibrosis is medial deviation and encasement of the ureters with proximal dilatation. Both ureters are usually involved, but the presentation may be asymmetric. Ultrasound, CT, and MRI demonstrate a well-marginated retroperitoneal mass; CT usually demonstrates a prominent enhancement after injection of IV contrast material. Fibrosis usually does not displace major vessels; however, lymphoma does. Percutaneous biopsy may be necessary to exclude the diagnosis of malignant retroperitoneal fibrosis (Fig 56).

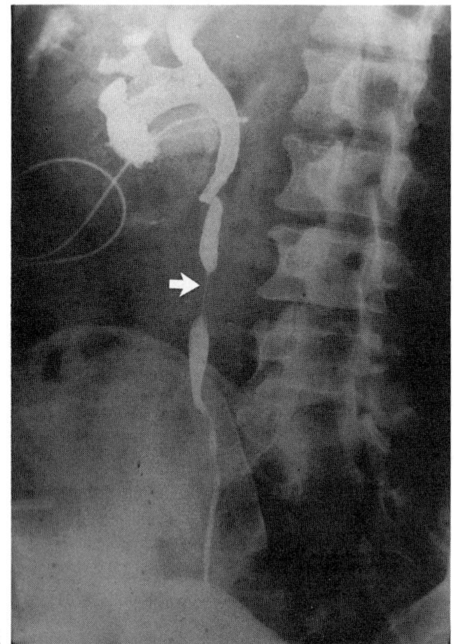


## Bladder

### Filling Defects

*Bladder Calculi.* Approximately 75% of bladder calculi are composed of material containing calcium; these can usually be identified on plain radiographs, particularly if the calculi are larger than 1 cm.[48] Although cystine stones do not contain calcium, their sulfur content confers mild radiopacity. Intravesical contrast can easily obscure smaller bladder calculi. If stones are suspected on the plain film or by the clinical history, then great care must be used, including the use of oblique films, to evaluate the bladder.

Pure uric acid and urease stones are radiolucent and not identifiable on plain films. They produce a negative filling defect in the contrast-filled bladder. Freely movable bladder calculi usually occur in the midline; however, the stones may be adherent to the wall from prior inflammatory episodes or may be displaced to one side by neoplasm. Stones may also lie within a bladder diverticulum or in a ureterocele. Bladder calculi, even those that are radiolucent on plain radiographs, are readily visualized on both CT and ultrasound. Real-time sonography is optimal for determining whether a stone is mobile, as

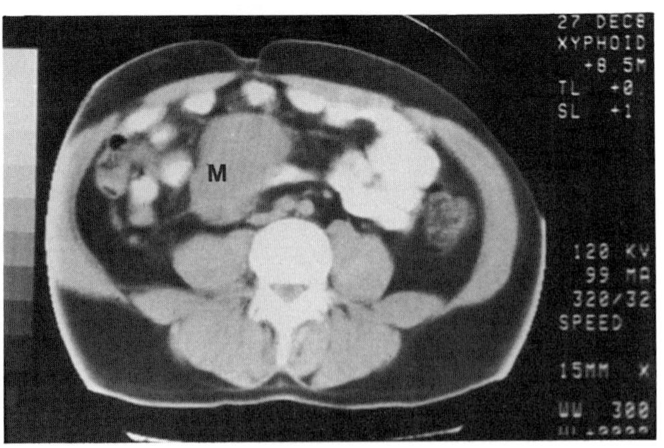


**Fig 56.** Retroperitoneal fibrosis; A, ureteral stricture (arrow) produced an obstruction which had been treated with a percutaneous nephrostomy; B, CT reveals the cause of the obstruction—a large soft tissue mass (M), which was then biopsied, and found to consist of focal fibrous tissue.

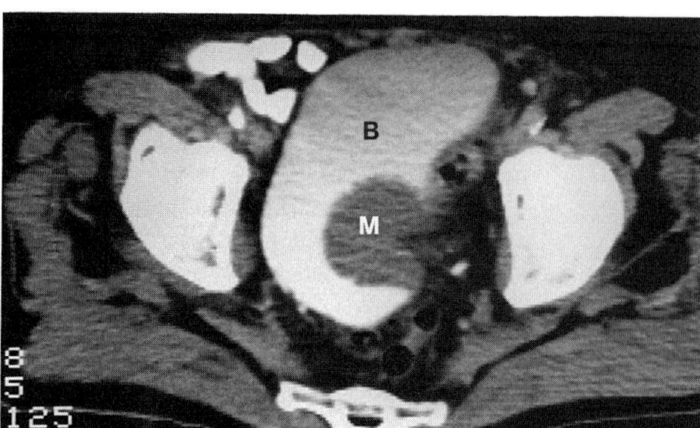


**Fig 57.** Transitional cell carcinoma; mass (M) protruding into the lumen of the bladder (B), indistinct margins indicate perivesical invasion.

it assesses movement during variation of patient position.

***Blood Clot.*** Clotted blood from a kidney, ureteral, or bladder lesion can form an irregular filling defect in the bladder which is radiolucent and freely movable until it enlarges sufficiently to fill the bladder. Whenever a blood clot is present, there is often a history of hematuria that suggests the diagnosis. However, a large clot may obscure the presence of a smaller bladder neoplasm during cystographic visualization.

***Foreign Bodies.*** Most foreign bodies that are inserted by the patient are radiopaque. Some catheter fragments and other objects are radiolucent; ultrasound is useful in instances where there is suspicion of the presence of a nonopaque foreign body.

***Bladder Tumors.*** The vast majority of bladder tumors do not calcify. Approximately 60% of bladder tumors are identified by urography, although the percentage increases to 80% when the tumors are larger than 1.5 cm. Cystography will only identify an additional 5% of tumors not seen by coned-down bladder films obtained at urography.[49] Excretory urography should be performed in all cases of bladder cancer to evaluate for synchronous lesions elsewhere in the urinary tract. IVU is also useful to identify ureteral obstruction, which may be caused by bladder trauma.

Both ultrasound and CT can readily identify bladder tumors if the bladder is distended. However, neither of these modalities is reliable in differentiating stage B1 from B2 lesions. Both CT and ultrasound are usually accurate at determining invasion of perivesical fat (Stage C), and CT provides a better evaluation of the pelvis and retroperitoneum in assessing possible lymph node involvement (Fig 57).[50] A potential pitfall of bladder assessment by CT is that edema resulting from a biopsy performed during cystoscopy can mimic invasion. Although MRI has become a useful method for staging bladder cancer, it has also not yet achieved sufficient accuracy to differentiate B1 from B2 lesions.

Diagnostic imaging cannot accurately differentiate transitional cell carcinoma from other malignant lesions. In addition, benign tumors may have an appearance similar to that of malignant lesions which have not invaded the perivesical fat.

## Inflammation

**Cystitis.** Infectious cystitis results in thickening and irregularity of the bladder wall as observed during urography. Typically, the entire wall is involved, which helps to differentiate cystitis from neoplasm. Imaging cannot differentiate acute from chronic infectious cystitis or the myriad of other causes of inflammation such as radiation or chemotherapy. Blood from a proximal urinary tract source can collect in the bladder, resulting in mucosal irritation, termed hemorrhagic cystitis (Fig 58). Emphysematous cystitis is a rare condition that

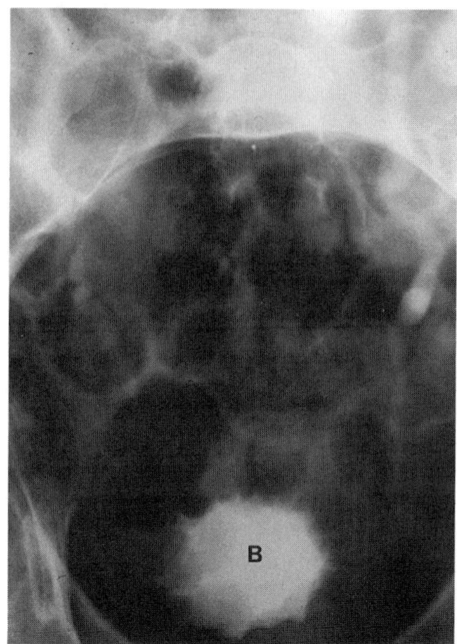


**Fig 58.** Hemorrhagic cystitis producing an irregular contracted bladder (B) margin.

results in linear collections of gas in the bladder wall. This type of cystitis is usually due to *Escherichia coli* infection, and almost always occurs in patients with diabetes mellitis.

Tuberculosis of the bladder can result in small wall calcifications similar to those seen elsewhere in the urinary tract.

Inflammatory conditions in the pelvis, primarily pelvic inflammatory disease and bowel inflammations, can produce secondary edema of the bladder wall, which is usually more localized than is that noted with primary cystitis. Such conditions are best visualized using CT.

### Miscellaneous

***Bladder Diverticulum.*** Multiple sacculations and diverticula of the vesicle wall usually result from bladder outlet obstruction. The diverticula usually occur in the lateral walls and the dome of the bladder. A wide-necked diverticulum causes rapid bladder filling and emptying while a narrow-necked diverticulum causes slow filling/emptying. It is not unusual for this latter type of diverticulum to be found only after voiding is completed. The stasis which develops from narrow-necked diverticulum can result in stone formation and infection; chronic infection can lead to carcinoma.

A congenital weakness in the bladder wall adjacent to the ureterovesical junction can produce a large solitary diverticulum termed a Hutch diverticulum. The size and position of the Hutch diverticulum may distort the ureterovesical junction enough to cause ipsilateral vesicoureteral reflux.

***Pelvic Lipomatosis.*** This describes a benign process of unknown etiology in which a large amount of fat accumulates in the bony pelvis. Pelvic lipomatosis is usually asymptomatic, but can result in increased urinary frequency due to restricted bladder volume. The bladder is elongated and the floor of the bladder can be elevated by the fatty deposits. CT has been the definitive diagnostic procedure because it readily identifies fat.[51] MRI is probably equally accurate, but is less cost-effective.

***Fistulas.*** Most bladder fistulas result from an underlying inflammatory process, such as diverticulitis or Crohn's disease, or neoplasm in either the bowel or the bladder. To find the site of the fistula, it is usually best to start with a study that imitates the normal directional flow in the fistula, ie, a barium study for pneumaturia. CT is often used to visualize the area around the bladder and assess for pathology which would lead to fistula function.

***Urethral Stricture.*** Strictures are best assessed using a combination of dynamic retrograde urethrography and VCUG in order to accurately evaluate the length and characteristics of a stricture. In addition to the focal area of urethral narrowing (of variable length) which characterizes a stricture, there are other radiographic findings that may be present. These include dilatation of the urethra proximal to the stricture, pseudodiverticulum formation, fistulas, and urethral stones (Fig 59).

Most strictures are either postinfectious, inflammatory, or iatrogenic in origin. Gon-

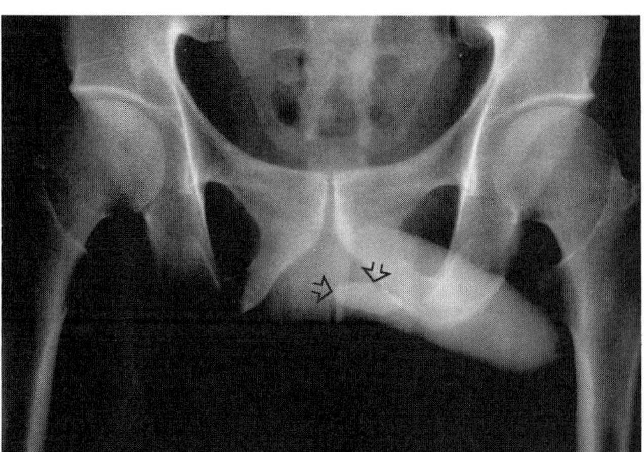

**Fig 59.** Urethral calculus (arrows) on a plain film.

orrhea is the predominate infectious agent; it produces strictures primarily in the bulbous urethra (Fig 60). These strictures can be several centimeters in length. Iatrogenic strictures tend to occur at the penoscrotal junction and at the membranous urethra, which is fixed by the urogenital diaphragm.

*Urethral Mass Lesions.* Neoplasms (both benign and malignant) and inflammatory polyps can produce discrete filling defects in the urethra. A majority of squamous cell carcinomas have been reported to be associated with previous urethral strictures. Carcinomas can mimic benign strictures. In addition, condylomata acuminata of the glans penis may spread into the urethra, form squamous papillomas, and produce multiple filling defects. If this disease is suspected, then retrograde urethrography and catheter placement should not be performed, to avoid further spread of the disease. In this case, the urethra can be evaluated by a voiding urethrogram at the conclusion of an IVU.

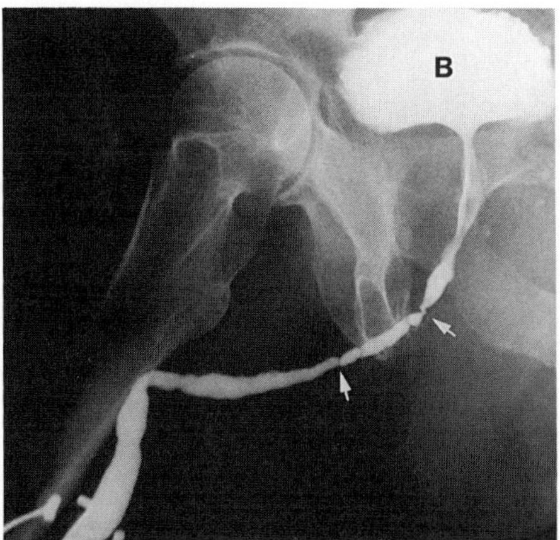


**Fig 60.** Multiple post-gonorrheal urethral strictures (arrows) on a retrograde urethrogram. B = bladder.

## Female Urethra

The female urethra is usually evaluated during VCUG. If a urethral diverticulum is suspected, then the urethra should be evaluated with the use of a double-balloon catheter. With such a catheter, balloons are positioned at either end of the urethra and contrast material is injected into the urethra through a hole between the balloons. This produces high intraluminal pressure, which is often necessary for the filling of diverticula (Fig 61).

## Scrotum

Ultrasound is the primary imaging modality for the scrotum and its contents. The testes are easily visualized as oval homogenous structures. The head of the epididymis is located superior and slightly lateral to the testes (Fig 62); the body and tail of the epididymis descend posterolaterally and then ascend posteromedially as the vas deferens. The principal function of imaging is to determine whether scrotal pathology is intratesticular or extratesticular. Ultra-

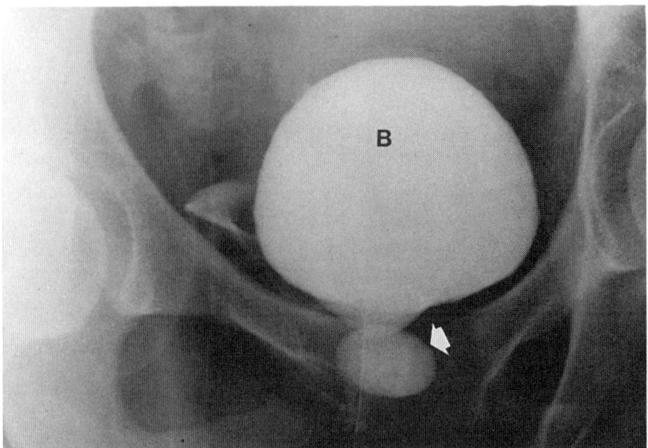


**Fig 61.** Urethral diverticulum (arrow). B = bladder.

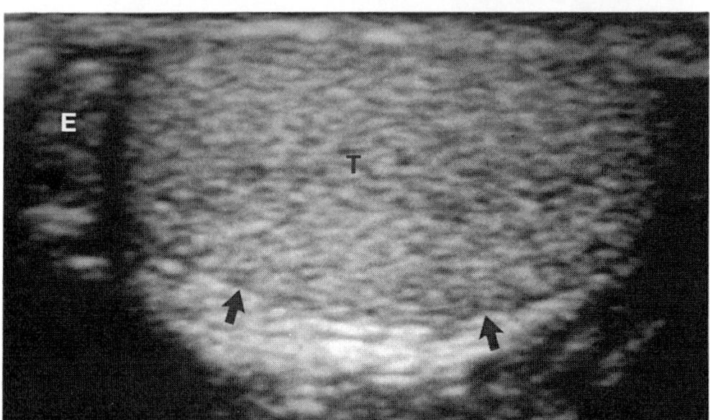


**Fig 62.** Normal sagittal ultrasound of a testis (T, defined by arrows) and the head of the epididymis (E).

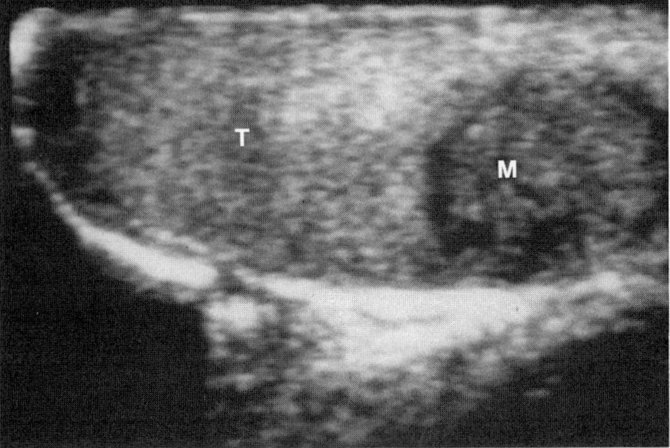


**Fig 63.** Seminoma; hypoechoic mass (M) in the lower pole of testis (T).

sound can make this distinction accurately in 90% to 95% of the cases.[52]

**Mass Lesions.** Most intratesticular lesions will be malignant. In men between 15 and 45 years of age, 95% of the tumors are of germ cell origin (Fig 63). Testicular neoplasms have a variety of appearances. Ultrasound cannot accurately differentiate the tumor cell type (Fig 64), but is useful to confirm the physical findings and to assess the contralateral testicle for an unsuspected lesion which occurs in 3% to 5% of patients.[53] Spermatic cord involvement can

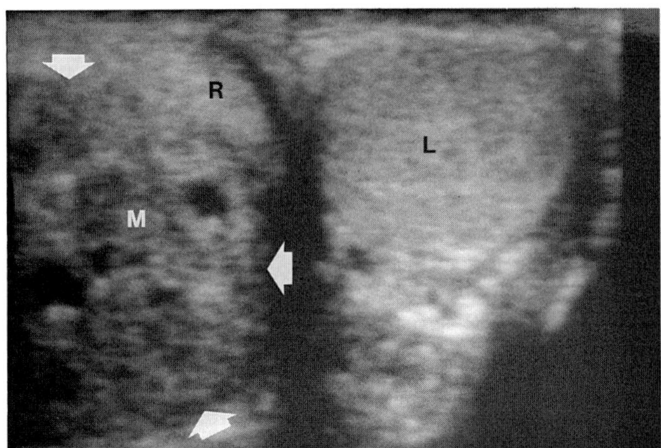


**Fig 64.** Teratocarcinoma; large inhomogeneous mass (M, defined by arrows) in the right testicle (R); compare with normal left testicle (L).

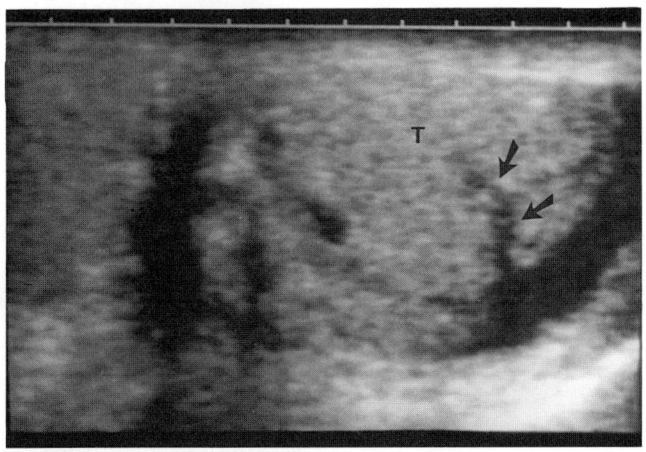


**Fig 65.** Testicular fracture; fracture line (arrows) within a testicle (T) following trauma.

also be identified. In 5% to 15% of patients, the presenting signs and symptoms of a testicular lesion will be secondary to metastatic disease. Ultrasound is important in the identification of the occult testicular neoplasm, especially since the physical examination can be entirely normal.[54] In patients over 50 years of age, metastatic tumors and lymphoma are more common as the etiology of a testicular mass than germ cell tumors.

***Trauma.*** Traumatic testicular rupture can be identified by ultrasound in over 95% of the cases.[55] This is important, since the physical examination in these patients is often difficult and a prompt diagnosis is necessary to salvage traumatized testicles by surgical intervention. Distinct fracture planes are not usually visible, but inhomogeneity in the substance of the testicle or indistinct margins are indications for surgical exploration (Fig 65). Hematoceles are not uncommon following trauma; they usually have an inhomogeneous echogenic appearance on ultrasound, and may contain septations and layers of fluid and debris. However, it is the appearance of the testes that is the most important portion of the examination and that indicates the need for surgery.

***Hydroceles.*** Hydroceles are usually readily diagnosed by physical examination and transillumination. Primary hydroceles are idiopathic and benign in nature (Fig 66). Ultrasound can be employed to evaluate secondary hydroceles which may result from tumor, infection, or trauma, and which may require treatment.

***Torsion.*** Testicular torsion must be differentiated from epididymitis. Fortunately, with the advent of color Doppler ultrasound, the diagnosis of testicular torsion can be made promptly.[56] A nuclear medicine scan of the scrotum is useful to confirm the ultrasound findings or in cases where the ultrasound findings are equivocal.

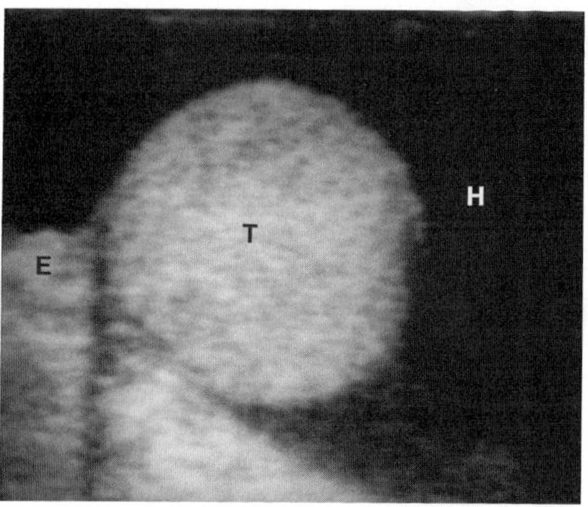


**Fig 66.** Hydrocele; large fluid collection (H) surrounding a normal testicle (T) and epididymis (E).

***Inflammation.*** Epididymitis is a common diagnosis which is often made on the basis of clinical findings. Ultrasound has a role in the evaluation of epididymitis where the physical exam is difficult, to evaluate for orchitis (which appears in 10% to 20% of the cases of epididymitis), and to differentiate the clinical findings of epididymitis from torsion, which can be difficult (Figs 67, 68). When orchitis develops, the testicle may be diffusely enlarged or may have altered echogenicity. Focal areas of necrosis may be present (Fig 69). A reactive hydrocele often occurs with epi-

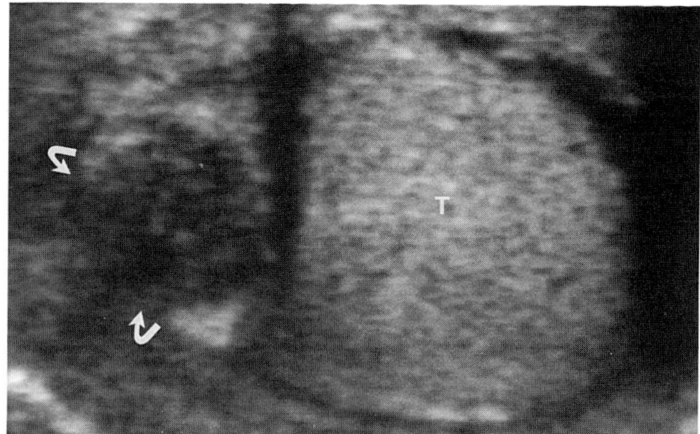


**Fig 67.** Epididymitis; ultrasound identification of a focal hypoechoic area (arrows) in the head of the epididymis. T = normal testicle.

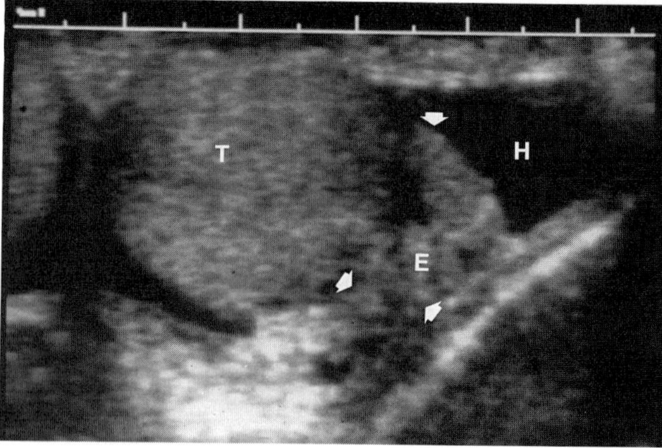


**Fig 68.** Epididymitis; enlarged body of the epididymis (E, defined by arrows) with a reactive hydrocele (H). T = normal testicle (T).

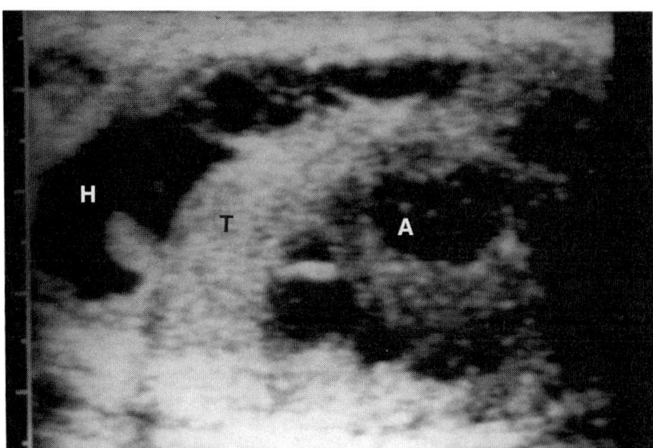


**Fig 69.** Testicular abscess; ultrasound demonstrates a focal area of tissue necrosis (A) within the testicle (T); reactive hydrocele (H) is also present.

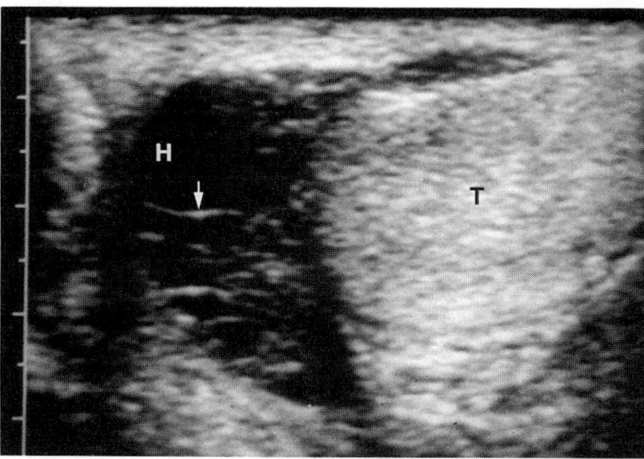


**Fig 70.** Infected hydrocele (H) with numerous septations (arrow) which was secondary to epididymitis. T = normal testicle.

didymitis; multiple septations within a hydrocele indicate that the inflammatory process has spread into the fluid, resulting in a pyocele (Fig 70).

***Varicocele.*** Varicoceles are composed of dilated veins surrounding the testicle, usually in the pampiniform plexus. Approximately 85% of varicoceles occur in the left hemiscrotum; 10% are bilateral.[57] Varicoceles, even those which are occult on physical examination, have been associated with infertility. Color Doppler ultrasound can demonstrate unequivocal evidence of a varicocele. Initially, it may be difficult to detect very slow-flowing blood within a varicocele, but when the patient is asked to perform the Valsalva maneuver or stand, the movement of blood is usually quite evident (Fig 71).[58]

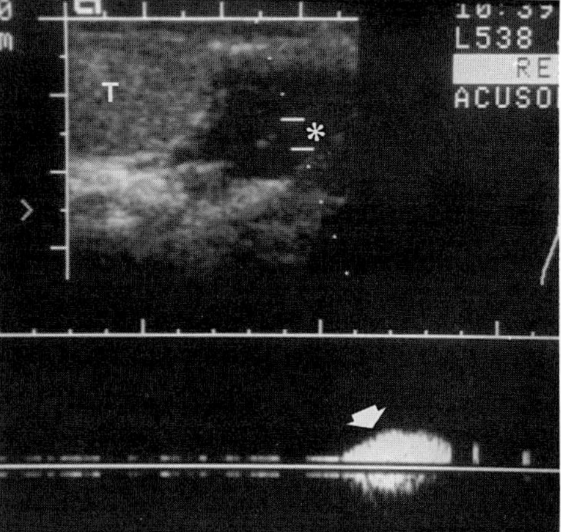


**Fig 71.** Varicocele; pulsed Doppler ultrasound gate (*) is placed within a serpiginous mass adjacent to the testicle (T). Blood flow is documented (arrow) during a Valsalva maneuver.

***Undescended Testicle.*** Nearly 90% of undescended testes are located in the inguinal canal. Ultrasound is the first modality that should be employed to locate the undescended testes.[59] If ultrasound is unsuccessful in locating the testes, then CT or MRI should be used to determine the location.

## Prostate and Seminal Vesicles

**Plain Film.** Calcifications in the prostate gland are frequently noted on plain films of the pelvis. However, they do not provide any significant clinical information.

**Ultrasound.** The advent of transrectal ultrasound has proven to be a major advance in the evaluation of the prostate gland and seminal vesicles. The use of transrectal ultrasound on a purely screening basis is still controversial, and is generally not recommended. Transrectal ultrasound clearly has a role in evaluating the prostate of patients with physical signs and symptoms or laboratory evidence suggesting the presence of prostate carcinoma.

**Fig 72.** Prostate ultrasound; transverse transrectal image with the gland defined by arrows. Enlarged urethra (U) with a clear communication to the bladder is a common finding following transurethral prostatectomy. B = bladder.

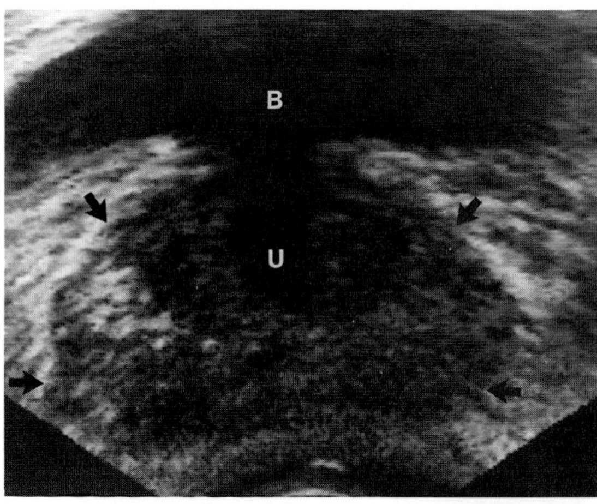


Transrectal ultrasound provides good definition of the internal architecture of the gland and delineates its margin; it also allows evaluation of the seminal vesicles (Fig 72, 73). Inhomogeneity and coarse calcifications in the central zone are frequently encountered in patients with benign prostatic hypertrophy. Small carcinomas in the peripheral zone are usually hypoechoic (Fig 74).[60] Biopsy of these lesions can be accurately performed using ultrasound guidance. Extension through the capsule and seminal vesicle invasion can also be assessed.[61]

When a prostate abscess is suspected clinically, transrectal ultrasound can be used to identify the abscess; diagnosis can be confirmed using ultrasound guided needle aspiration.

Transabdominal ultrasound is also useful to determine the post-void bladder volume in patients with symptoms of bladder outlet obstruction.

**Computed Tomography.** CT is another valuable tool to stage local and distant prostate metastases (Fig 75).[62] Enlarged lymph nodes in the abdomen and pelvis can readily be identified using CT. Not all lymph node enlargement is secondary to metastatic disease; therefore, percutaneous biopsy under

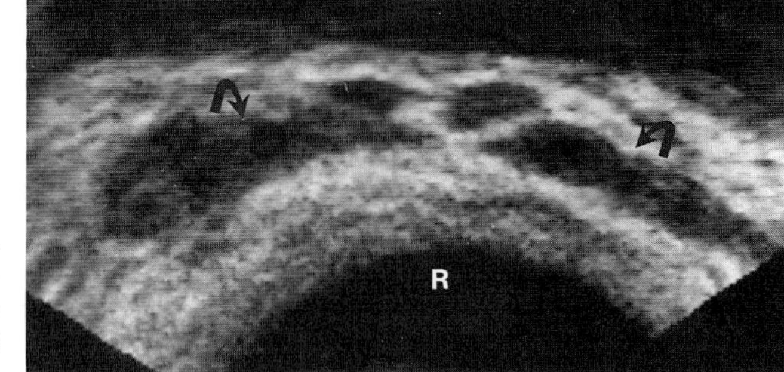


**Fig 73.** Seminal vesicles; transverse ultrasound image demonstrates normal glands (curved arrows), which are separated from the rectum (R) by echogenic fat.

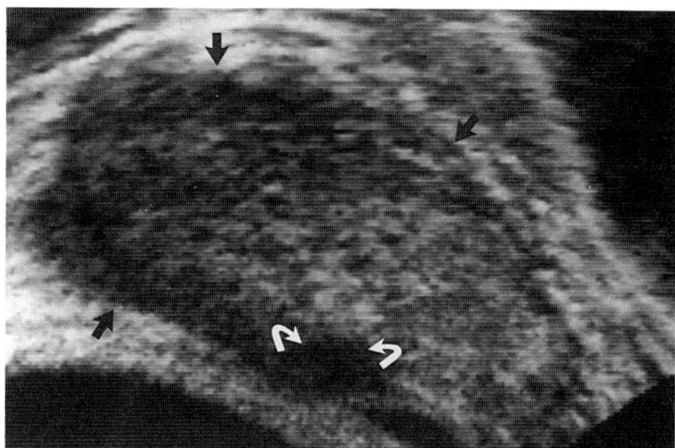

**Fig 74.** Prostate carcinoma; sagittal transrectal ultrasound image of the gland (straight arrows) reveals a focal hypoechoic lesion (curved arrows) in the peripheral zone which was later biopsied.

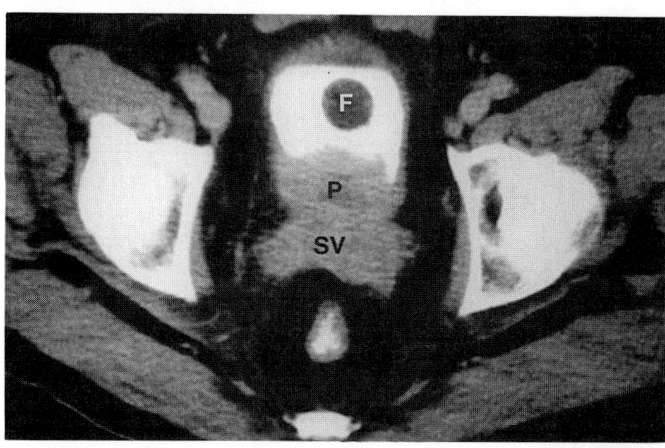


**Fig 75.** Prostate carcinoma; CT demonstrates invasion of the seminal vesicles (SV), which are enlarged and irregular, as well as the base of the bladder by a prostatic mass (P). F = Foley catheter.

CT guidance can be performed to prove the diagnosis.

**Magnetic Resonance Imaging.** Endorectal coils are currently being developed that will provide images with at least equal quality to those obtained using transrectal ultrasound. Because of the higher cost of MRI, transrectal ultrasound should remain the initial imaging modality following digital rectal examination to confirm the presence of prostate carcinoma. MRI should be reserved for assessing stage C and D disease in patients with proven prostate carcinoma since its staging capability is superior to transrectal ultrasound.

**Nuclear Medicine.** The standard bone scan remains the modality of choice in the evaluation of metastatic prostate carcinoma to the bone. Plain films should be obtained to examine any suspicious areas noticed on the bone scan.

## Urinary Tract Trauma

The assessment of urinary tract trauma has undergone tremendous change during the past decade, as CT has challenged the urogram as the primary tool for evaluating the urinary tract. In many centers, CT is utilized as the primary method of assessing upper urinary tract trauma.

**Plain Film of the Abdomen (KUB).** A KUB examination is routinely obtained in patients with blunt or penetrating trauma to the abdomen and pelvis. The bones should be closely examined for evidence of fracture in order to focus attention to adjacent areas of the urinary tract. Foreign bodies and abnormal collections of gas are also important findings.

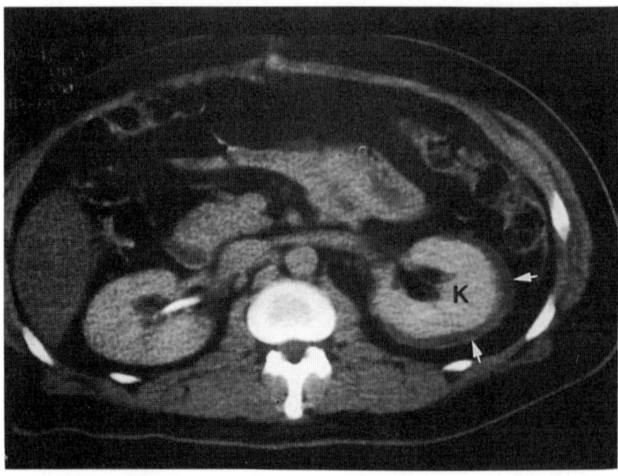


Fig 76. Subcapsular hematoma; small collection of blood (arrows) surrounds an intact left kidney (K).

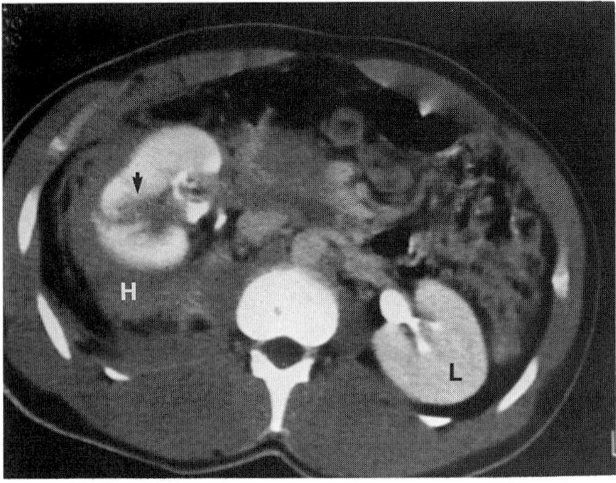


Fig 77. Fracture of kidney; trauma CT demonstrates a fracture plane (arrow) in the right kidney, with a large perinephric hematoma (H). Normal left kidney (L).

**Intravenous Urography.** Urography is the most common method to initially evaluate the upper urinary tract. Non-visualization of a kidney may be indicative of a significant vascular injury; arteriography or CT should be performed emergently in such patients. Following blunt abdominal trauma and gross hematuria, or microhematuria and shock, an IVU should be performed to search for significant renal injury. Radiographic findings include focal areas of decreased enhancement, a delayed nephrogram, a filling defect from a blood clot within the renal pelvis, and extravasation of contrast from the kidney or collecting system.

In patients with penetrating trauma and hematuria, the urogram is a less sensitive test than in patients with blunt trauma. Further evaluation of these patients should be considered, probably with CT.

**Computed Tomography.** CT is an excellent method to evaluate the kidneys for traumatic injury.[63] In addition, when there is concern for injury to organs other than the kidney, CT should be performed. Renal contusions, lacerations, and subcapsular and perinephric hematomas are readily identified (Figs 76–78). Vascular pedicle injuries are also identifiable (Fig 79). Finally, the ureters are visualized well using CT examination.

In many trauma centers, CT of the abdomen and pelvis is part of the standard protocol, following the initial assessment of the patient in the trauma room. CT supersedes the need for urography in patients and is often performed because of concern for nonrenal pathology such as liver or spleen lacerations.

**Cystography.** In a patient with suspected bladder trauma, cystography must be performed. Opacification and distention of the urinary bladder are insufficient during urography for adequate evaluation of bladder tears. Cystography is usually performed in a retrograde fashion through a Foley catheter. If this is not feasible in the trauma setting, then a cystogram can be performed following a suprapubic puncture. Cystography is very accurate in the diagnosis of significant bladder injury,[64] and will differentiate intraperitoneal from extraperitoneal bladder rupture (Fig 80A, B). Simple bladder contusions can also be identified.

**Urethrography.** Following trauma, if blood is observed at the urethral meatus, retrograde urethrography should be performed prior to placement of a catheter into the urinary bladder. Urethral tears, although

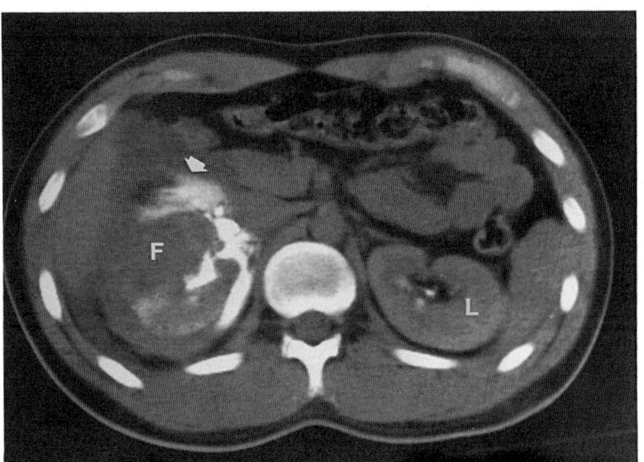


**Fig 78.** Large right renal fracture (F) with diastasis of the upper and lower poles; extravasation of contrast (arrow) is present. Normal left kidney (L).

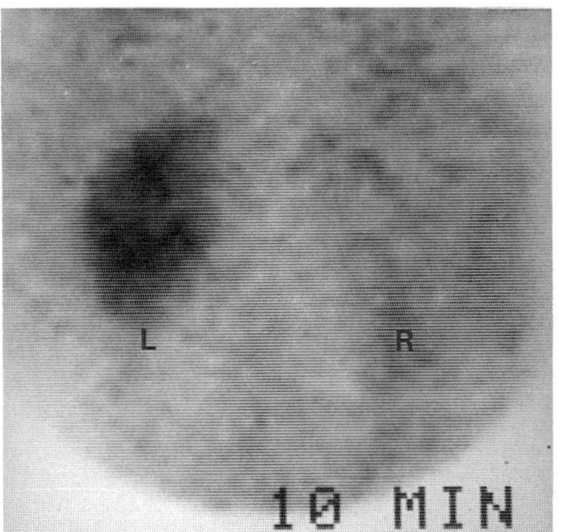


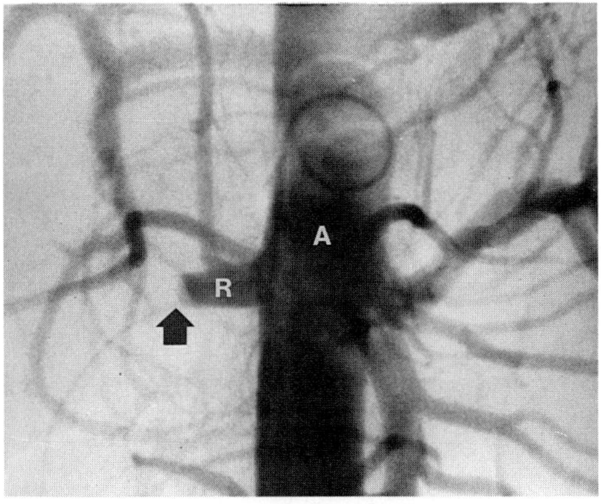


A B

**Fig 79.** Renal pedicle injury; A, posterior image from a nuclear medicine renogram demonstrates normal activity in the left kidney (L) but no activity in the expected location of the right kidney (R); B, arteriogram reveals abrupt termination (arrow) of the right renal artery (R) as a result of intraluminal thrombus. Note circular catheter tip in aorta (A); C, subsequent CT demonstrates a hypodense, infarcted kidney (arrows).

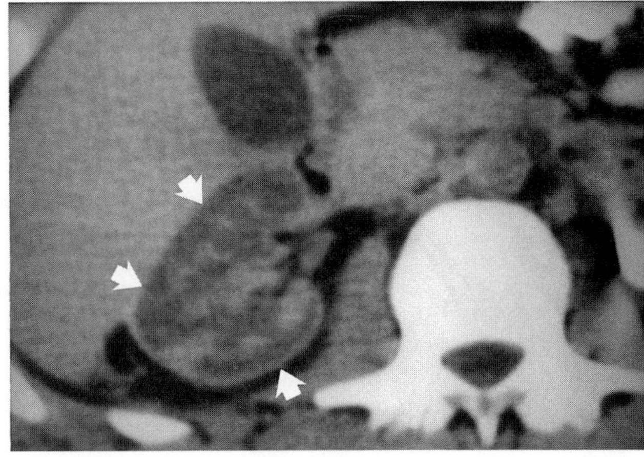

C

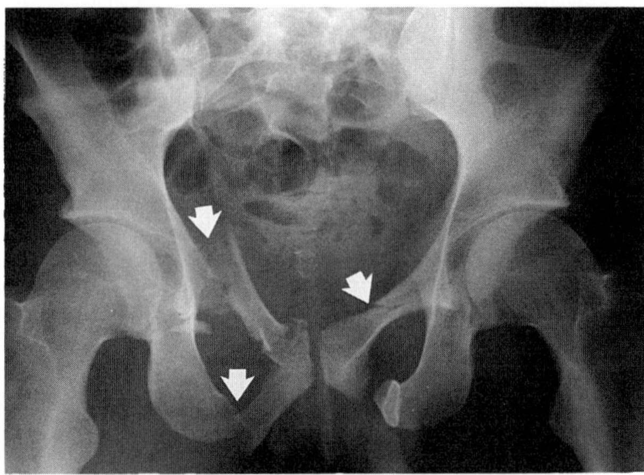

A

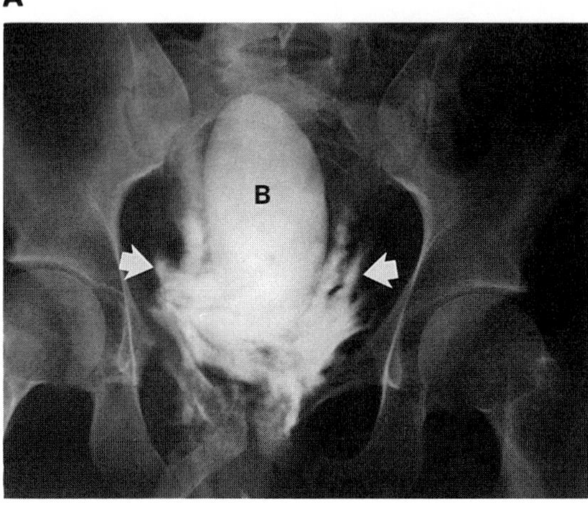


B

Fig 80. Bladder rupture; A, multiple pelvic fractures (arrows) indicate the need for cystography; B, cystogram demonstrates extraperitoneal extravasation of contrast (arrows) from the bladder (B).

usually incomplete, are readily identified by extravasation of contrast material outside the urethral lumen. The location of the tear, above or below the urogenital diaphragm, can usually be determined. If a Foley catheter is inadvertently passed into the bladder prior to the evaluation of the urethra, a second smaller tube can be placed alongside the Foley catheter to assess for extravasation. Alternatively, when the Foley catheter is removed at a later date, a VCUG should be immediately obtained.

## Renal Arterial Thrombosis and Embolism

Thrombosis of a renal artery usually is the result of severe atherosclerotic disease. Since this is a chronic process, renal atrophy commonly occurs which may be either unilateral or bilateral. Thrombosis may also occur as a result of blunt abdominal trauma. Intimal dissection during arteriography is another cause of arterial thrombosis.

Emboli, most often from the left atrium or left ventricle, may lodge within the aorta or in the renal arteries. Both local renal artery thrombosis and emboli from distant sources can obstruct the blood supply to the entire kidney or individual segments. This is readily apparent on contrast-enhanced CT scans, where the infarcted portion of the kidney is markedly hypodense (Fig 81). If the process is acute, then the size of the kidney will be within normal limits. The renal capsular arteries often have a collateral blood supply; therefore,

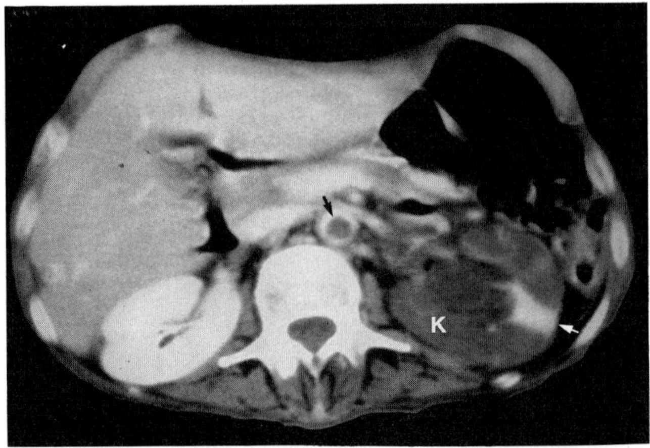


**Fig 81.** Arterial thrombosis and renal infarction; thrombus in the aorta (black arrow) has resulted in infarction of most of the left kidney (K). Only a small segment (white arrow) exhibits enhancement, indicating adequate perfusion.

an infarcted kidney may have a thin rim of peripheral enhancement providing an insufficient amount of blood supply to maintain renal function.

## REFERENCES


1. Dawson P. Contrast agent nephrotoxicity. An appraisal. *Br J Radiol.* 1985;58:121–123.
2. Cohan RH, Dunnick NR. Intravascular contrast media: adverse reactions. *Am J Radiol.* 1987; 149:665–670.
3. Ansell G, Tweedie MCK, West CR, et al. The current status of reactions to intravenous contrast media. *Invest Radiol.* 1980;15(suppl):32–39.
4. Katayama H, Yamaguchi K, Kozuka T, Takashima T, Seez P, Matsuura K. Adverse reactions to ionic and nonionic contrast media: a report from the Japanese committee on the safety of contrast media. *Radiology.* 1990;175:621–628.
5. Benson CB, Vickers MA, Arumy J. Evaluation of impotence. *Semin Ultrasound, CT, MR.* 1991;2:176–188.
6. Livraghi T, Damascelli B, Lombardi C, Spanoli I. Risks in fine needle abdominal biopsy. *J Clin Urol.* 1983;11:77.
7. Amis ES Jr, Cronan JJ, Pfister RC. Needle puncture of renal cystic masses: a survey of the Society of Uroradiology. *Am J Radiol.* 1987; 148:297–299.
8. Leroy AJ. Percutaneous nephrostomy: techniques and instrumentation. In: Pollack HM, ed. *Clinical Urography.* Philadelphia: WB Saunders Company; 1990:2725–2738.
9. Williams GH, Dluhy RG. Diseases of the adrenal cortex. In: Wilson JD, Braunwald E, Isselbacher KJ, et al, eds. *Harrison's Principles of Internal Medicine.* 12th ed. New York: McGraw-Hill; 1991:1713–1735.
10. Reinig JW, Doppman JL, Dwyer AJ, Johnson AR, Knop RH. Adrenal masses differentiated by MRI. *Radiology.* 1986;158:81–84.
11. Dunnick NR: The adrenal gland. In: Taveras JM, Ferruccci JT, eds. *Radiology: Diagnosis, Imaging, Intervention.* Philadelphia: JB Lippincott; 1988:chap. 82.
12. Dunnick NR, Doppman JL, Gill JR Jr, Strott CA, Keiser HR, Brennan MF. Localization of functional adrenal tumors by computed tomography and venous sampling. *Radiology.* 1982; 142:429–433.
13. Dieckmann K, Hamm B, Pickartz H, et al. Myelolipoma: an unusual surgical lesion of the adrenal gland. Adrenal myelolipoma: clinical, radiologic and histologic features. *Urology.* 1987;29:1–8.
14. Dunnick NR, Heaston D, Halvorsen RA Jr, Moore AV, Korobkin M. CT appearance of adrenal cortical carcinoma. *J Comput Assist Tomogr.* 1982;6:978–981.
15. Welch TJ, Sheedy PF, van Heerden JA, Sheps SG, Hattery RR, Stephens DH. Pheochromocytoma: value of computed tomography. *Radiology.* 1983;148:501–503.
16. Simon AL: Normal renal size and absolute criterion. *Am J Radiol.* 1964;92:270–273.
17. Kissane JM. Congenital malformations. In: Hepinstall RH, ed. *Pathology of the Kidney.* Boston: Little, Brown, & Company; 1974:69–119.
18. Dunnick NR, McCallum RW, Sandler CM. *Textbook of Uroradiology.* Baltimore: Williams & Wilkins; 1991:96–111.
19. Curry NS, Schabel SI, Betsill WL Jr. Small renal neoplasm: diagnostic imaging, pathologic fea-

tures, and clinical course. *Radiology*. 1986; 158:113–117.

20. Bosniak MA. The current radiological approach to renal cysts. *Radiology*. 1986;158:1–10.
21. Dunnick NR, Korobkin M, Silverman PM, Foster WL. Computed tomography of high density renal cysts. *J Comput Assist Tomogr*. 1984; 8:458–460.
22. Marotti M, Hricak H, Fritzsche P, Crooks LE, Hedgcock MW, Tanagho EA. Complex and simple renal cysts: comparative evaluation with MR imaging. *Radiology*. 1987;162:679–683.
23. Rosenberg ER, Korobkin M, Foster W, Silverman PM, Bowie JD, Dunnick NR. The significance of septations in renal cysts. *Am J Radiol*. 1985;144:593–595.
24. Amis ES Jr, Cronan JJ. The renal sinus, an imaging review and proposed nomenclature for sinus cysts. *J Urol*. 1988;139:1151–1157.
25. Babaian RJ, Lucey DT, Fried FA. Significance and evaluation of calcifications associated with renal masses. *Urology*. 1978;12:108–111.
26. Demos TC, Schiffer M, Love L, et al. Normal excretory urography in patients with primary kidney neoplasms. *Urol Radiol*. 1985;7:75–79.
27. Hartman DS, Davis CJ, Johns T, Goldman SM. Cystic renal cell carcinoma. *Urology*. 1986; 128:45–49.
28. Hricak H, Thoeni RF, Carroll PR, Demas BE, Marotti M, Tanagho EA. Detection and staging of renal neoplasms: a reassessment of MR imaging. *Radiology*. 1988;166:643–649.
29. Wallace S, Charnsangavej C, Carrasco CH, Swanson DA. Embolization of malignant renal tumors. In: Pollack HM, ed. *Clinical Urography*. Philadelphia: WB Saunders Company; 1990:3003–3017.
30. Johnson CD, Dunnick NR, Cohan RH, Illescas FF. Renal adenocarcinoma: CT staging of 100 tumors. *Am J Radiol*. 1987;148:59–63.
31. Bosniak MA, Megibow AJ, Hulnick DH, Horii S, Raghavendra BN. CT diagnosis of renal angiomyolipoma: the importance of detecting small amounts of fat. *Am J Radiol*. 1988;151:497–501.
32. Quinn MJ, Hartman DS, Friedman AC, et al. Renal oncocytoma: new observations. *Radiology*. 1984;153:49–53.
33. Davidson AJ, Taler LB. Urographic and angiographic abnormalities in adult onset acute bacterial nephritis. *Radiology*. 1973;106:249–256.
34. McCoy RI, Kurtz AB, Rifkin MD, et al. Ultrasound detection of focal bacterial nephritis (lobar nephronia) and its evolution into a renal abscess. *Urol Radiol*. 1985;7:109–111.
35. Lee JKT, McClennan BL, Melson GL, Stanley RJ. Acute focal bacterial nephritis: emphasis on gray scale sonography and computed tomography. *Am J Radiol*. 1980;135:87–92.
36. Cronan JJ, Amis ES, Dorfman GS. Percutaneous drainage of renal abscesses. *Am J Radiol*. 1984;142:351–354.
37. Yoder IC, Pfister RC, Lindfors KK, Newhouse JH. Pyonephrosis: imaging and intervention. *Am J Radiol*. 1983;141:735–740.
38. Yoder IC, Lindfors KK, Pfister RC. Diagnosis and treatment of pyonephrosis. *Radiol Clin North Am*. 1984;22:407–414.
39. Kay CJ, Rosenfield AT, Taylor KJW, et al. Ultrasonic characteristics of chronic atrophic pyelonephritis. *Am J Radiol*. 1979;132:47–51.
40. Kollins SA, Hartman GW, Carr DT, et al. Roentgenographic findings in urinary tract tuberculosis: a 10 year review. *Am J Radiol*. 1974;121:487–493.
41. Prien EL. The analysis of urinary calculi. *Urol Clin North Am*. 1974;1:229–238.
42. Kamholtz RG, Cronan JJ, Dorfman GS. Obstruction and the minimally dilated renal collecting system: US evaluation. *Radiology*. 1989;170:51–53.
43. Pollack HM, Arger PH, Banner MP, Mulhern CB, Coleman BG. Computed tomography of renal pelvic filling defects. *Radiology*. 1981; 138:645–651.
44. Gatewood OMB, Goldman SM, Marshall FF, Siegelman SS. Computed tomography of transitional cell carcinoma of the kidney. In: Siegelman SS, Gatewood OMB, Goldman SM, eds. *Computed Tomography of the Kidneys and Adrenals*. New York: Churchill Livingstone; 1984:219–225.
45. Nay C, Friedenberg RM. Diseases of the ureter. In: Ney C, Friedenberg RM, eds. *Radiographic Atlas of the Genitourinary System*. 2nd Ed. Philadelphia: JB Lippincott Company; 1981:1181–1227.
46. Murphy DM, Fallon B, Lane V, O'Flynn JD. Tuberculous stricture of the ureter. *Urology*. 1982;20:382–384.
47. Koep L, Zuidema GB. The clinical significance of retroperitoneal fibrosis. *Surgery*. 1977; 81:250–255.
48. McCallum RW, Colapinto V. *Urological Radiology of the Adult Male Lower Urinary Tract*. Springfield, IL: Charles C Thomas; 1976:260–265.
49. Hillman BJ, Silvert M, Cook G, et al. Recognition of bladder tumors by excretory urography. *Radiology*. 1981;138:319–323.
50. Weinerman M, Arger PH, Pollack HM. CT evaluation of bladder and prostate neoplasms. *Urol Radiol*. 1982;4:105–114.
51. Friedman AC, Hartman DS, Sherman J, Lautin EM, Goldman M. Computed tomography of abdominal fatty masses. *Radiology*. 1981; 139:415–428.
52. Carroll BA, Gross DM. High-frequency scrotal sonography. *Am J Radiol*. 1983;140:511–515.
53. Berthelsen JG, Shaakkeback NE, von der Maase H, Sorensen BL, Mogensen P. Screening for carcinoma in situ of the contralateral testis in

patients with germinal testicular cancer. *Br Med J*. 1982;285:1683–1686.

54. Glazer HS, Lee JKT, Melson GL, McClennan BL. Sonographic detection of occult testicular neoplasms. *Am J Radiol*. 1982;138:673–675.
55. Founier GR, Laing FC, McAninch JW. Scrotal ultrasonography and the management of testicular trauma. *Urol Clin North Am*. 1989;16:377–385.
56. Ralls WR, Larson D, Johnson MB, et al. Color doppler sonography of the scrotum. *Sem Ultrasound, CT, MR*. 1991;12:109–113.
57. Clarke BG. Incidence of varicocele in normal men and among different age groups. *JAMA*. 1966;198:1121–1122.
58. Demas BE, Hricak H, McClure RD. Varicoceles: radiologic diagnosis and treatment. *Radiol Clin North Am*. 1991;29:619.
59. Wolverson MK, Houttuin E, Heiberg E, Sundaram M, Shields JB. Comparison of computed tomography with high resolution real-time ultrasound and the localization of the impalpable undescended testes. *Radiology*. 1983;146:133–136.
60. Chang P, Friedland GW. Hypoechoic lesions of the prostate: clinical relevance of tumor size, digital rectal examination, and prostate specific antigen. *Radiology*. 1990;175:581–582.
61. Benson CB, Doubilet PM, Richie JP. Sonography of the male genital tract. *Am J Radiol*. 1989;153:705–712.
62. Hricak H, Dooms GC, Jeffrey RB, et al. Prostate carcinoma: staging by clinical assessment, CT, and MR imaging. *Radiology*. 1987;162:331–336.
63. Bretan PN, McAninch JW, Federle MP, Jeffrey RB. Computerized tomographic staging of renal trauma: 85 consecutive cases. *J Urol*. 1986; 136:561–565.
64. Sandler CM, Hall JT, Rodriguez MB, Corriere JN. Bladder injury in blunt pelvic trauma. *Radiology*. 1986;158:633–638.

# 6

# Nuclear Medicine in Urologic Practice

*Alan H. Maurer and Leon S. Malmud*

Continuing technical advances in medical imaging have resulted in significant changes in the "routine" approach to urologic studies. Ultrasound, x-ray computed tomography, and magnetic resonance tomography all permit excellent anatomic definition of the genitourinary structures, but nuclear medicine still remains most uniquely suited to quantitative assessment of renal function and urinary tract flow. With the appropriate choice of agents, accurate definition of cortical morphology also can be obtained, and more precise definition of renal masses is now possible due to advances in nuclear medicine tomographic imaging.

In general, nuclear medicine studies are noninvasive and relatively inexpensive. They involve minimal radiation exposure and have no adverse side effects. They are being used increasingly where serial studies of renal function are indicated, particularly when interventional procedures (eg, angioplasty) or therapeutic intervention (eg, in cases of transplant rejection) are planned. The recent availability of high resolution, portable cameras also permits bedside studies in patients with trauma. The rapidity with which testicular perfusion studies can be performed to diagnose testicular torsion has led to their increased use on an emergency basis.

## Basics of Nuclear Medicine Imaging

In order to understand the unique role nuclear medicine can play in evaluating renal physiology and function, it is important to understand the differences between nuclear medicine imaging and more anatomic studies obtained with either x-rays or ultrasound. Like conventional radiographs, nuclear medicine uses ionizing radiation to produce images. Pharmaceuticals with known biologic behavior are used, and their distribution in the body is followed by combining the pharmaceutical with a radioisotope. This results in a radiopharmaceutical that emits gamma rays (similar to x-rays). Unlike radiographs, however, where an x-ray beam is passed through the organ of interest and then permitted to strike a photographic film, the radiopharmaceutical is usually injected intravenously and localizes in a specific target organ. Instead of striking a piece of film, the gamma rays are detected as a flash of light (or scintillation) within the crystal of the camera. The location of the flash of light is recorded on film or in a computer.

Early studies with renal radiopharmaceuticals used simple probes, which were placed over the kidneys to record "time-activity" curves that depicted the concentration and excretion of the radiopharmaceutical (Fig 1A). These probe curves were commonly referred to as "renograms." Today, most nuclear medicine facilities exclusively use scintillation cameras with crystals capable of recording gamma rays emitted from large areas within the body. The scintillation camera enables the physician to follow the radiopharmaceutical initially from the time it is intravascular permitting evaluation of renal blood flow. By continuing to image the kidneys and surrounding organs; the filtration and excretion of the radioisotope; the size, shape, and location of the kidneys; and the flow into the urinary tract all can be evaluated with one study.

By interfacing scintillation cameras with computers, curves of renal blood flow and renal and urinary tract clearances all can be generated to produce quantitative information about blood flow, renal function, and urinary flow (Fig 1B).

The most commonly used radioisotope

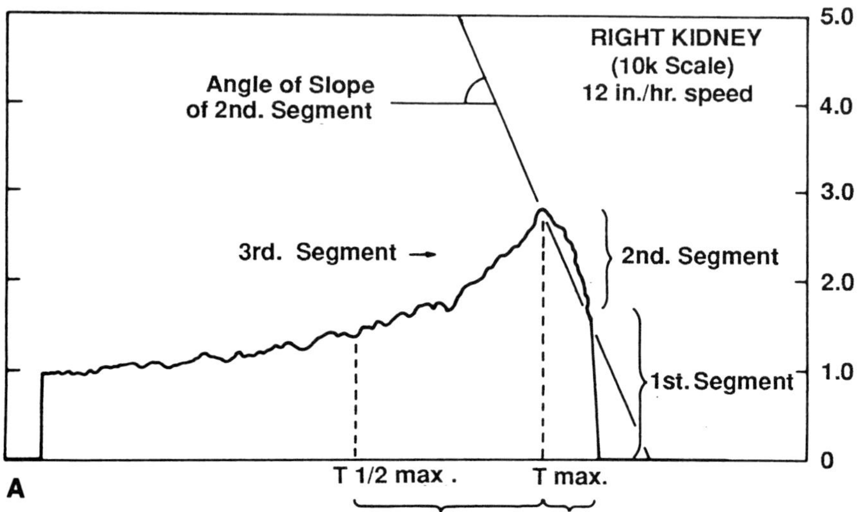


**Fig 1.** A, Normal renogram curves. Previously, probes were used to generate renogram curves; they plotted the activity in the kidney as a function of time from the right side of the graft to the left. As shown in this theoretical curve, the first segment reflects renal blood flow, the second the extraction efficiency, and the third excretion (From *Semin Nucl Med* 1974;4:133). B, These renogram curves were generated from a scintillation camera and computer. Curves from the left and right kidney are shown, with activity as a function of time displayed from left to right.

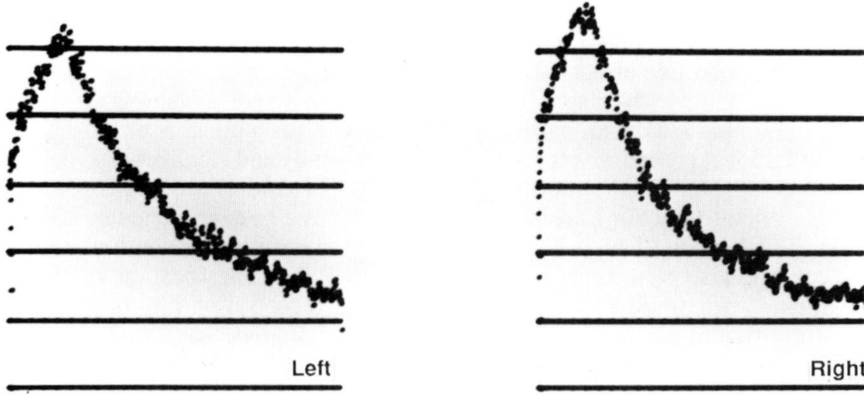

**TABLE 1. Radiation Doses in Normal Adults**

| Agent | Physical Half-life | Radiation Dose: Whole Body | Kidneys* | Bladder† | Gonads‡ | Units |
|---|---|---|---|---|---|---|
| $^{99m}$Tc DTPA | 6 h | 0.016 | 0.042 | 0.555 | 0.016 (testis)<br>0.019 (ovary) | rads/mCi |
| $^{99m}$Tc DMSA | 6 h | 0.015 | 1.40 | 0.008 | 0.006 (testis)<br>0.011 (ovary) | rads/mCi |
| $^{99m}$TcMAG3 | 6 h | 0.0067 | 0.014 | 0.48 | 0.026 (ovary)<br>0.016 (testis) | rads/mCi |
| $^{131}$I Hippuran | 8 d | 0.022 | 0.016 | 0.057 | 0.022 (testis)<br>0.026 (ovary) | rads/μCi |
| $^{123}$I Hippuran | 13.3 h | 0.006 | 0.024 | 0.40 | 0.010 (testis)<br>0.020 (ovary) | rads/mCi |

* Radiation dose could vary depending on the level of renal function; these are estimates.
† Bladder dose can be greatly reduced by hydrating the patient and encouraging frequent voiding.
‡ In general, ovaries receive a slightly higher dose because of their location.

today is technetium-99m ($^{99m}$Tc). It has a physical half-life of only 6 hours. This rapid decay results in a low radiation exposure for patients. It emits only gamma rays with an energy of 140 KeV. This low energy is ideally suited for the thin crystals used in current scintillation cameras.

Before the availability of $^{99m}$Tc, renal pharmaceuticals were labeled with isotopes such as mercury-197 (physical half-life of 27.8 days) or $^{131}$I (physical half-life of 8 days) (Table 1). Because of the long half-life associated with these isotopes and increased radiation, the dosages were administered in small quantities making imaging more difficult.

Since certain iodine compounds can give valuable information about renal function, $^{123}$I has recently been developed for use; it emits a low energy gamma ray (photon energy = 159 KeV) and has a relatively short half-life (13.3h).

## Single Photon Emission Computed Tomography (SPECT)

Most nuclear medicine imaging today, as performed with a conventional scintillation camera, provides a two-dimensional picture of the radiopharmaceutical distribution within the body. Since the radiopharmaceuticals are actually distributed throughout a three-dimensional structure, a two-dimensional or "planar" image loses the anatomic detail of internal structures even when multiple views are obtained. Improvements in anatomic resolution and lesion detection are limited by superimposition of activity in the surrounding background and structures that overlie the organ of interest.

Tomographic reconstructions can now be obtained, using a rotating form of the scintillation camera. These cameras are modified to rotate 360° around the subject (Fig 2). Similar to x-ray computed tomography (CT), filtered back projection is used for reconstruction. Improved anatomic resolution and the ability to make precise measurements of organ volumes, absolute tracer concentration (activity/unit volume), and flow (concentration/time) are now obtainable.

The technique of SPECT now permits tomographic nuclear medicine images to be acquired. The ability to perform tomographic reconstructions with metabolically active radiotracers provides both better anatomic resolution and improved quantification of *in vivo* physiologic processes.[1]

## Radiopharmaceuticals

Over the last 20 years, many radiopharmaceuticals have been proposed for use in renal imaging. Of the $^{99m}$Tc renal agents

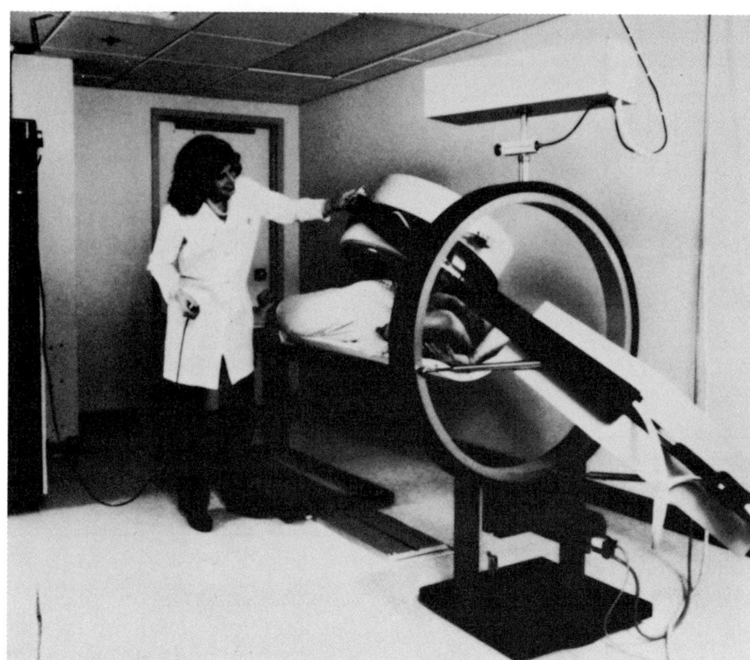

**Fig 2.** SPECT rotating scintillation camera. A standard scintillation camera is mounted on a ring, which permits 360° rotation around the patient. By acquiring 360° of data, tomographic reconstructions in sagittal, coronal, and transaxial planes can be generated.

available, four are currently in clinical use.

$^{99m}$Tc-dimercaptosuccinic acid (DMSA) was initially developed as a chelating agent for the treatment of heavy metal poisoning. The renal uptake of $^{99m}$Tc-DMSA is similar to that of mercury, with predominant localization in the renal cortex. DMSA results in excellent images of the functioning renal cortex. This ability to demonstrate cortical anatomy is useful for confirming renal "pseudo tumors" and for quantitating functional renal mass (Fig 3).[2]

$^{99m}$Tc-diethylene-triamine pentacetic acid (DTPA) is an agent used for measuring glomerular filtration (GFR).[3] It is almost entirely cleared by glomerular filtration. In man, approximately 4% to 5% of the administered dose is not excreted, and is retained in various tissues, probably due to non-chelated DTPA. Approximately 5% is protein bound. When compared to inulin, clearance estimates of GFR using DTPA are always slightly lower; but good correlations are obtained for GFR in most clinical studies. $^{99m}$Tc DTPA can be used to assess renal blood flow, function, and urinary flow. With computer acquisition, quantitative split renal function can be measured. Because of rapid cortical clearing, DTPA is not used for anatomic imaging (Fig 4). DTPA, however, does permit assessment of blood flow and function using a single radiopharmaceutical. It is also useful for performing the diuretic renogram (eg, "Lasix washout") test for obstruction.

$^{99m}$Tc-glucoheptonate (GHA) is handled by the kidneys in a more complex fashion than either DMSA or DTPA. About 75% of GHA is excreted by a combination of glomerular filtration and tubular secretion. The remainder binds to the renal tubular cells by an unknown mechanism. GHA, therefore, has some properties similar to DMSA and others to DTPA. Because its clearance is not characterized by any one mechanism, GHA cannot be used for accurate quantification of renal function. It is used when one test is desired to evaluate anatomy (25% is bound to the renal cortex),

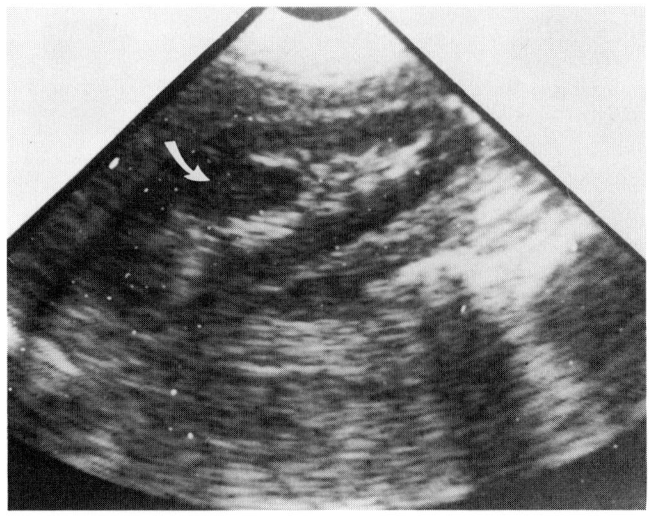

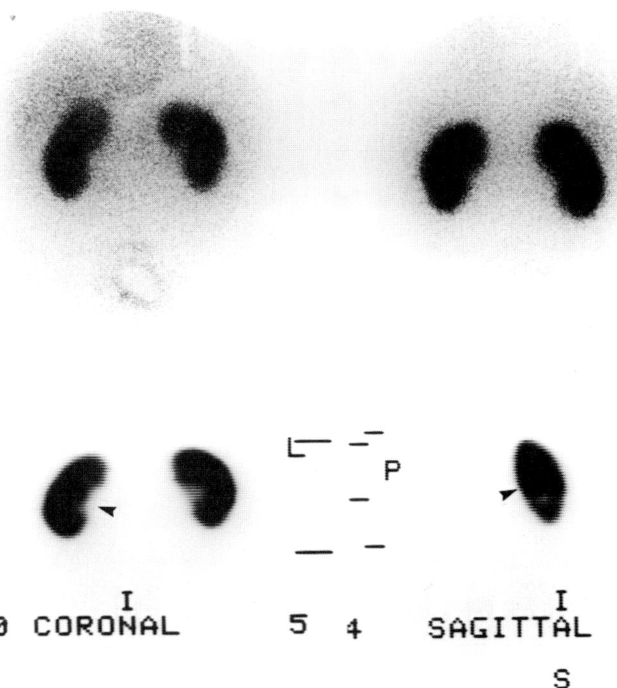


**Fig 3.** A, Cortical imaging with DMSA. The ultrasound study of this patient shows a mass of echogenicity equal to the renal cortex, which projects into the central renal pelvis (arrow); B, conventional planar (2-dimensional) images obtained with DMSA outline the functioning renal cortex and do not demonstrate a "cold" lesion in the kidney. The abnormality seen on ultrasound, therefore, has normal cortical tissue and probably represents a benign column of Bertin. The planar images, however, do not clearly demonstrate the redundant tissue projecting into the renal pelvis. C, Tomographic reconstruction, using a rotating gamma camera and SPECT, more clearly demonstrates the redundant cortical tissue (arrows) projecting into the renal pelvis characteristic of a column of Bertin.

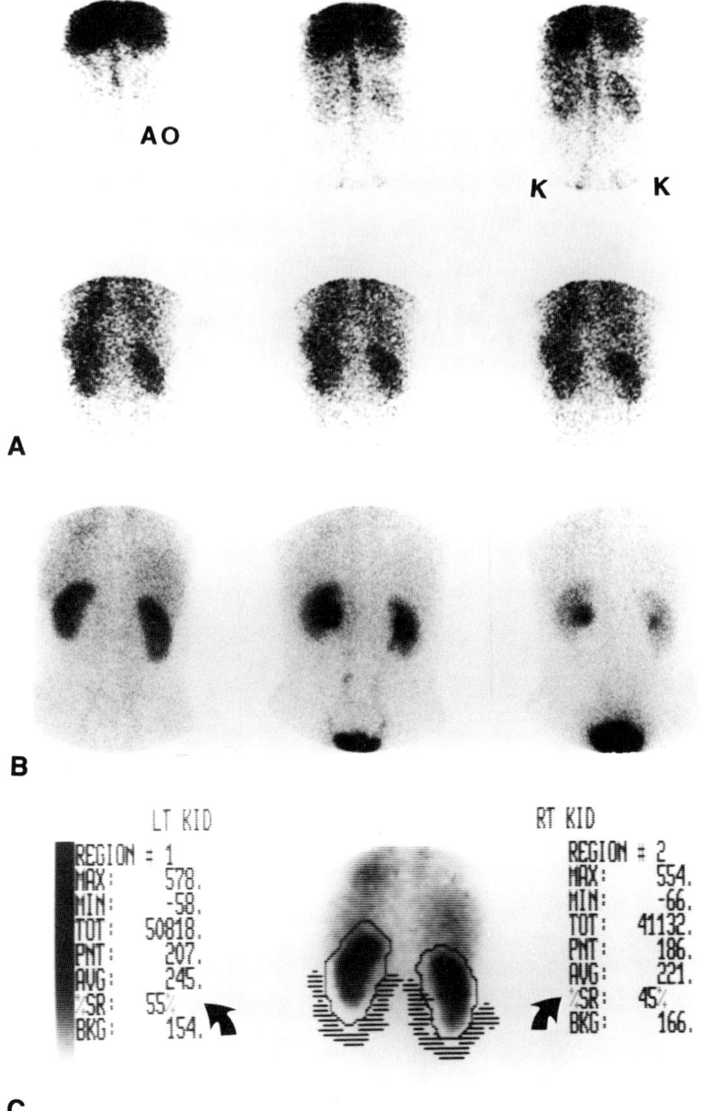


**Fig 4.** A, DTPA renal blood and functional study. Following an IV injection of DTPA, rapid, sequential images of perfusion to both kidneys can be obtained in the posterior projection (the radionuclide angiogram). In these sequential 2-second images, the abdominal aorta (AO) is seen early. This is followed by prompt and symmetric blood flow to both kidneys (K). B, Renal function images; sequential images are then obtained over the course of 20 minutes. At approximately 1-minute post-injection (left), these posterior images of the kidneys initially show the cortical phase. The tracer is then rapidly excreted into the renal pelvis 5 to 10 minutes after injection (middle). At this point, the outlines of the kidneys are not well delineated. The ureters and bladder can be seen. By 20 minutes following injection (right), most of the activity has left the renal parenchyma and is seen in the bladder. Because of its rapid clearance, DTPA is not well suited for identifying mass lesions in the kidneys. However, lesions can commonly be seen with appropriate early imaging. C, Quantitation of split renal function. If the early, 1- to 2-minute, images following injection of DTPA are acquired with a digital computer, quantification of the cortical phase can be used to give an estimate of the percent of GFR being provided by each kidney. In this case, the left kidney is providing 55% and the right 45% of total clearance (arrows).

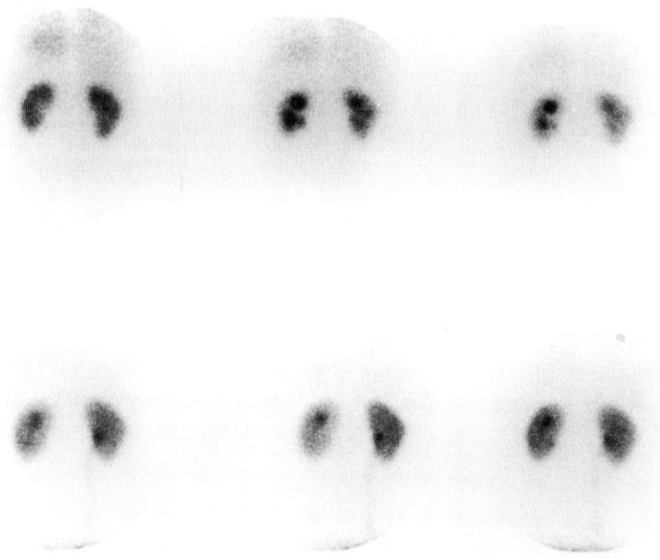

**Fig 5.** A, Similar to DTPA, early images of glucoheptonate will first show cortical activity followed by excretion. By 20 to 30 minutes following injection, however, there is persistent activity retained within the renal cortex; B, Delayed cortical phase images with GHA. Approximately 90 minutes following injection, most of the GHA has been excreted by the kidney. Because of binding within the renal cortex, adequate images for precise anatomic definition can be obtained.

and when a qualitative estimate of blood flow and function is sufficient (Fig 5).

Since its early introduction, $^{131}$I-orthoiodohippuric acid (OIH) has remained a popular agent for studying renal function. It is a structural analog of para-aminohippurate (PAH). The kidney has a 90% extraction efficiency for OIH, and this agent can be used to calculate effective renal plasma flow (ERPF).[4] It also gives accurate measurements of relative renal function, particularly when renal function is impaired. Eighty percent is cleared by tubular secretion and the remaining percent by glomerular filtration. $^{131}$I-OIH is readily available and inexpensive, but because of the long physical half-life of $^{131}$I, it must be given in small amounts. In order to block potential thyroid uptake of unbound $^{131}$I, 3 to 5 drops of Lugol's solution is given orally to the patient prior to the study.

$^{131}$I-OIH anatomic images are of poor quality, since less activity is given and the high energy of $^{131}$I is not well suited for imaging with conventional nuclear medicine cameras (Fig 6).

Changes in renal function can be monitored using a radiopharmaceutical that reflects either GFR or ERPF. With a normal filtration fraction of 20%, an agent cleared by tubular secretion such as OIH will clear the body almost five times faster than an agent cleared by glomerular filtration. Tubular agents, therefore, yield images of higher quality, particularly when renal function is impaired. For this reason $^{123}$I-OIH was developed to replace $^{131}$I-OIH, the usage of which was limited by its poor physical properties. However, the high costs associated with a $^{123}$I-label limit the amount of $^{123}$I-OIH that may be given to obtain good images. In addition, $^{123}$I-OIH must be ordered on a daily basis and, due to its short half-life, used only on the day delivered. Because of these shortcomings, efforts have been directed toward developing a $^{99m}$Tc-labeled renal agent with clearance properties similar to OIH.

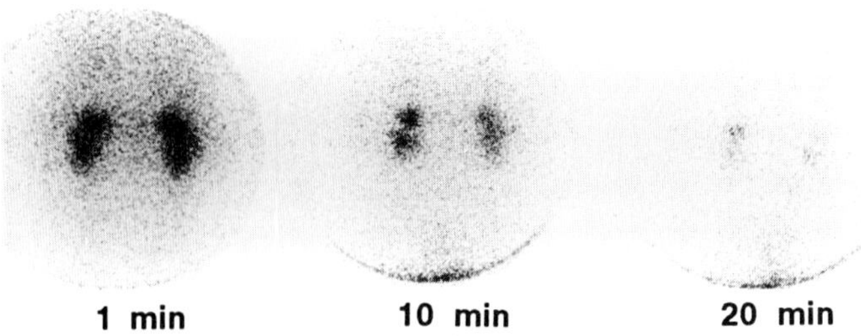


**Fig 6.** Normal $^{131}$I-hippuran study; these posterior studies of the kidneys were obtained following intravenous injection of $^{131}$I-hippuran. Because of the high energy of the gamma ray emitted and the small amount of activity injected, the hippuran images have poor anatomic definition compared to either DTPA or GHA. The study does demonstrate very rapid clearance of the radiotracer by the kidneys. The renogram curves in Fig 1A were generated from this patient.

Recently a $^{99m}$Tc-agent, $^{99m}$Tc-mercaptoacetyltriglycine (MAG3) has been developed and approved for routine clinical use in the United States. This agent has pharmacokinetic properties similar to OIH, its initial renal uptake and excretion are also very similar to OIH. Plasma clearance of MAG3 is about 50% that of OIH, due to increased binding of MAG3 to plasma proteins, but the net rate of excretion—which is the product of concentration (2X OIH) times clearance (½ OIH)—is therefore similar to that of OIH. Studies of quantification of differential renal uptake and plasma clearances show good correlation of MAG3 with OIH.[5,6]

MAG3 image quality is markedly superior to that achieved with $^{131}$I-OIH and larger doses (of up to 10 mCi) can be given so that both flow studies (eg, a radionuclide angiogram) and function studies can be obtained with injection of only one agent.[7] Currently, the substantially increased cost of $^{99m}$Tc-MAG3 over $^{99m}$Tc-DTPA or $^{131}$I-OIH limits its use for all patients. However, the rapid clearance and technetium label result in such excellent image quality that it is probably the agent of choice for patients with known renal impairment, particularly when one is performing studies such as a diuretic renogram or is administering angiotensin converting enzyme inhibition therapy (see below) where the response to pharmacologic intervention can be obscured if renal function is significantly depressed.

$^{99m}$Technetium sulfur colloid (SC), while usually associated with liver and spleen imaging, should also be included in any discussion of renal agents because of its role in diagnosing renal allograph rejection. SC is an aggregate of sulfur with particles of 0.01 to 1.0 μm in size. These are prepared in a colloid suspension and are usually injected intravenously. The particles are phagocytized by reticuloendothelial cells, predominantly in the liver and spleen. SC has been demonstrated to bind nonspecifically to fibrin in clots. Disseminated intravascular fibrin and platelet thrombosis, endothelial injury, vasculitis, and immunoglobin deposits are all pathophysiologic mechanisms that are believed to result in acute and chronic transplant rejection. They are believed to cause extraction of circulating SC within kidneys undergoing rejection. SC accumulation has been shown to help differentiate acute and chronic rejection from other causes of allograph dysfunction.[8]

Testicular perfusion studies, which are performed to differentiate acute testicular torsion from epididymitis, do not require renal-specific radiopharmaceuticals. The radiopharmaceutical employed need remain intravascular for only 2 to 3 minutes after injection. Since these studies should be performed as rapidly as possible, the agent must be readily available and require little or no preparation. Unlabeled $^{99m}$Tc-pertechnetate, which can be eluted directly from generators that are in daily use in any nuclear medicine department, meets these criteria. It also has excellent imaging qualities and can be given in large enough quantities so that the rapid sequential images required for a radionuclide angiogram of scrotal perfusion can be obtained easily, with minimal radiation dose to the patient.

## APPLICATION

### Renal Blood Flow

Either $^{99m}$Tc-DTPA, GHA, or $MAG_3$ can be used to visually evaluate renal blood flow. They can be administered in large enough quantities to obtain adequate images for a radionuclide angiogram (RNA). In a renal perfusion study, the patient is usually imaged supine, with the camera positioned below the patient's back. The radiopharmaceutical is injected in an antecubital vein, and images are acquired every 2 to 3 seconds for at least 60 seconds. Both camera and computer images can be used to analyze the data. The abdominal aorta is easily identified, and while individual renal arteries usually are not seen, the blood flow to each kidney is evaluated by comparing the timing and the intensity of the appearance of activity within the kidneys in relation to the aorta. An individual kidney is usually compared to the contralateral side. It is important to assess perfusion of the kidney relative to the activity seen in the aorta, since the injection may have not been adequate (a poor bolus), alternatively, flow may be decreased to both kidneys, and one may not see a difference from side to side.

Renal perfusion studies can be used to screen for renovascular hypertension. Both visual inspection and computer analysis of the slopes of the arterial phase of RNA can be used to detect decreased perfusion. (Fig 7). The test, however, is insensitive unless there is a high grade stenosis. In addition, decreased perfusion to a kidney is not specific for renal artery stenosis, as there are many other diseases that can result in unilateral decreased perfusion. In patients with contrast allergies, RNA may be the only method available. Also, in patients with known disease, serial RNAs can be used to serve as a guide to the timing of surgery to maximize preservation of renal function or to evaluate complications or success of surgery or percutaneous angioplasty. Acute thrombosis, restenosis, and segmental infarcts can be evaluated easily with this technique.

While ultrasound or CT generally are recommended for detecting renal masses, the RNA is helpful for determining whether a lesion is vascular or nonvascular (eg, neoplasm or cyst).

### Renal Artery Stenosis: The Captopril Renogram

While renal blood flow can be imaged directly with the conventional ''renal flow study'' (radionuclide angiogram), the appearance of decreased flow is neither a sensitive nor specific finding to confirm that renal artery stenosis (RAS) is the cause of a patient's hypertension. As noted previously, flow abnormalities usually cannot be appreciated until the RAS is high grade (>60–70%); however, functionally significant elevations in renin that cause hypertension can be present with less severe renal artery stenoses. Furthermore, a decrease in renal perfusion may be due to prior parenchymal disease and may not be due to a vascular cause. The introduction of the use of ACE inhibitors has significantly increased the sensitivity and specificity of renal scintigraphy for the diagnosis of RAS.

With a significant RAS there is a decrease in afferent arteriolar pressure. This stimulates pressure receptors so that renin secretion is increased by the juxtaglomerular apparatus. In an attempt to compensate for the decreased pressure in the glomerulus, renin stimulates production of angiotensin I which, in the presence of the converting enzyme, produces angiotensin II. This response increases perfusion pressure and induces postglomerular vasocon-

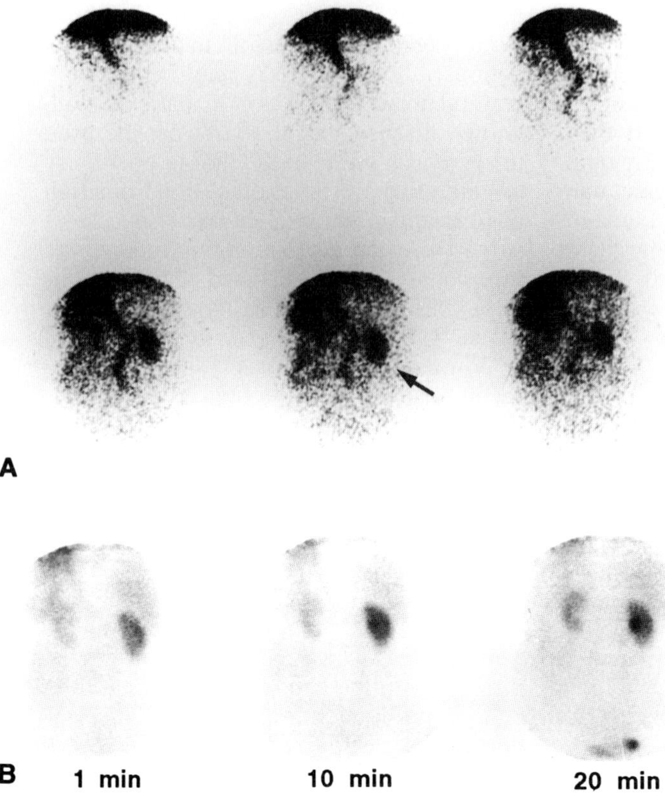


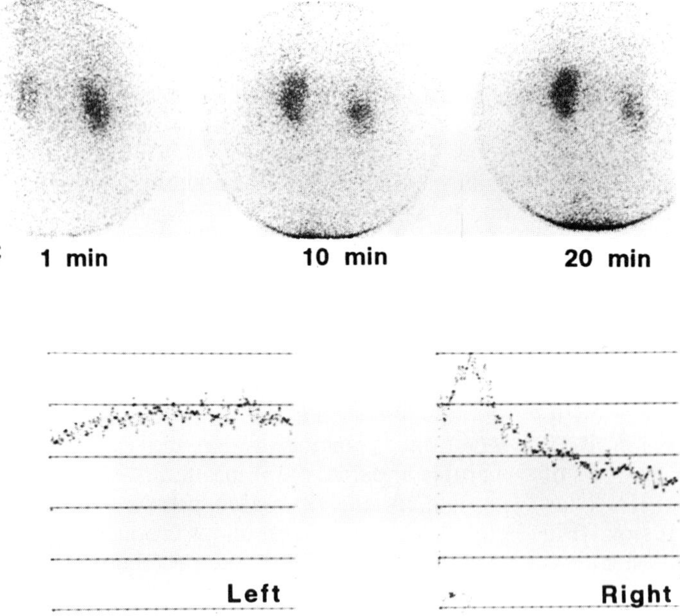


**Fig 7.** A, This radionuclide angiogram demonstrates a tortuous abdominal aorta and normal perfusion to the right kidney (straight arrow). There is very diminished and delayed perfusion to a small left kidney. B, Functional and anatomic images; these sequential images with GHA show a small and poorly functioning left kidney compared to the right. C, Hippuran study in renal artery stenosis. These sequential $^{131}$I-hippuran images confirm intact but diminished function of the left kidney. There is delayed concentration of the hippuran in the left kidney similar to the late nephrogram phase on contrast urography. D, Hippuran curves; the renogram curves generated from the hippuran study demonstrate normal concentration and excretion by the right kidney. The left kidney shows a flattened renogram curve consistent with, but not specific for, renal artery stenosis.

striction all working to restore filtration and normalize the GFR.

ACE inhibitors such as captopril or enalopril block the production of angiotensin II, resulting in a drop of afferent arterial pressure, dilatation of the afferent arterioles, and decompensation of renal function with a decrease in filtration fraction and a severe decrease in glomerular filtration.

With unilateral RAS, a compensatory increase in contralateral renal function can clinically mask the effect of an ACE inhibitor. However, the ability of radionuclide studies to measure renal function for each kidney makes it possible to detect the effect of ACE inhibition. To perform the test, the patient undergoes renography before and after receiving an oral dose of captopril. The depression of renal function after captopril administration is a very specific finding of RAS. At present, studies may be performed using either DTPA, OIH, or MAG3. Different criteria have been applied to determine what represents a significant response. At present, it is not clear which renal agent is best nor what are the optimal criteria to define positivity.[9,10]

In a study by Geyskes et al,[11] the results of captopril renography were compared to the response to corrective angioplasty. In 12 of 15 patients, captopril-induced decreased function was observed in the renograms of the affected kidneys only. After angioplasty, the renograms all normalized after repeat challenge with captopril. In this study, there was a decrease in DTPA uptake and delayed OIH excretion while OIH uptake was unaffected. These researchers' criteria demonstrated a sensitivity of 80% and specificity of 100% with this technique. Further, the results of captopril scintigraphy predicted the potential for correcting hypertension with angioplasty. There was a negative response to captopril in all 6 patients with anatomic RAS who did not respond to angioplasty. This demonstrates not only the role of captopril renography for diagnosing RAS but also its importance as a means for demonstrating the physiologic significance of questionable anatomic lesions.

### Trauma

A single agent, such as GHA, can be used to depict vascular injury, perirenal bleeding, renal vein and arterial thrombosis, arterial venous fistulae, and pseudo aneurysms. GHA also may be used at the same time to assess renal function and the status of the collecting system. Finally, extravasations can be identified. The sensitivity of radionuclide imaging in the detection of trauma is reported to be between 90% and 95%,[12] and studies can be done with portable equipment at the bedside.

### Renal Masses

Cystic lesions of the kidney are usually identified with ultrasound or CT. They appear hypovascular on RNA and are seen as parenchymal defects in the late images obtained with GHA or DMSA after concentration in the cortex. Mass lesions also will be apparent with DTPA during the first 2 to 4 minutes following injection, when most of the activity occurs within the renal parenchyma.

Renal tumors such as a hypernephroma may appear to be hypervascular during the RNA. However, since they may undergo necrosis, increased vascularity may not be present. Since renal tumors do not function as normal renal tissue, they will not concentrate GHA, DTPA, or DMSA, and cannot be differentiated from other mass lesions within the kidney such as a cyst, renal infarction, or abscess.

Since the normal kidney has many anatomic variations that may be difficult to distinguish from true mass lesions with either ultrasound, CT, or intravenous urography, radionuclide imaging has been used to separate true renal masses from "pseudo-tumors" (a benign column of Bertin). Typically, a mass is usually first detected on ultrasound. Images with either DMSA or GHA that show normal functioning tissue can confirm that no tumor is present (Fig 3). Planar imaging is usually sufficient, but recent reports indicate that SPECT imaging may be useful for better anatomic localization (Fig 3C).[13,14] Confirmation of benign renal tubular adenomas (oncocytomas) has been reported since they demonstrate normal concentration of renal radiopharmaceuticals.[15]

## Renal Obstruction

Ultrasound is generally the initial examination preferred when there is a suspected diagnosis of renal obstruction. Ultrasound, however, is a morphologic study, and the presence of a dilated collecting system does not necessarily indicate that obstruction is present. The collecting system may be dilated secondary to obstruction or other causes (eg, postoperative ectasia, atonic ureters, and prior obstruction or infection).

The ability to differentiate an obstructed system from one that is merely dilated is the key to the proper management of patients with upper urinary tract dilatation, since uncorrected obstruction will lead to further deterioration in renal function. Radionuclide renography, which monitors the accumulation of radiotracers prior to diuresis and in response to a diuretic, has become widely accepted to assess mechanical obstruction.[16]

To perform such studies, an adult patient is typically injected with 10–20 mCi of $^{99m}$Tc-DTPA. If impaired renal function due to prior obstruction is suspected, $^{99m}$Tc-MAG3 should be substituted. An RNA is first acquired at the time of injection. If there is impairment in renal function from obstruction that has been present for some time, blood flow is usually diminished to the obstructed kidney. Patients are studied in the posterior view sitting upright in order to optimize drainage from the collecting system; however, images may be obtained with the patient supine, if necessary. Images are usually acquired both on film and into a computer every 30 seconds. The data is continuously collected until visual monitoring indicates that there is a pooling of the tracer within a dilated collecting system. With intact renal function, this usually occurs within 15 to 20 minutes after injection. When accumulation within the renal pelvis appears maximal, furosemide (0.3 to 0.5 mg/kg) is administered intravenously. With an intravenous injection, the onset to a diuretic response is prompt and usually is observed within as little as 1 minute after injection. With impaired renal function, the peak effect may not be seen until 15 to 30 minutes.

In a dilated but nonobstructive collecting system, the renogram curve will show a rapid "washout" pattern (Fig 8). The furosemide accentuates the rate of tracer washout from the kidney, although in some subjects there is a transient increase in activity immediately following administration of the diuretic. In an obstructed collecting system, the kidney will demonstrate a flat response without significant washout, and in some cases progressive accumulation will continue (Fig 9).

If renal function is so poor that the kidney cannot adequately concentrate the radiopharmaceutical or respond to the diuretic, the study becomes uninterpretable. If the collecting system cannot be visualized in the first 20 to 30 minutes following injection, the ability to respond to diuresis is often too poor for valid analysis of the curves. The test is most diagnostic for complete obstruction; in partial obstruction there will be evidence for "washout." However, the curves are flattened and may be confused with poor renal function.

As radionuclide bone imaging is used increasingly both to diagnose and to monitor bone metastases from carcinoma of the prostate, there is an increased incidence of detection of unsuspected ureteral obstruction seen on bone scans. In a normal study, the $^{99m}$Tc-polyphosphate agents should show homogenous and symmetric renal activity. Occasionally the calyces, renal pelvis, and ureters may be visualized. In ureteral obstruction, there is intense accumulation of the radiotracer within the dilated collecting system. The sensitivity of the routine bone scan for detecting ureteral obstruction is low (60%) compared to routine renal studies.[17] However, since postrenal obstruction may be incidentally noted in some patients, the renal images on a routine bone scan should always be examined for possible obstruction.

Evaluation of the kidneys as a part of the routine bone scan is also helpful for making

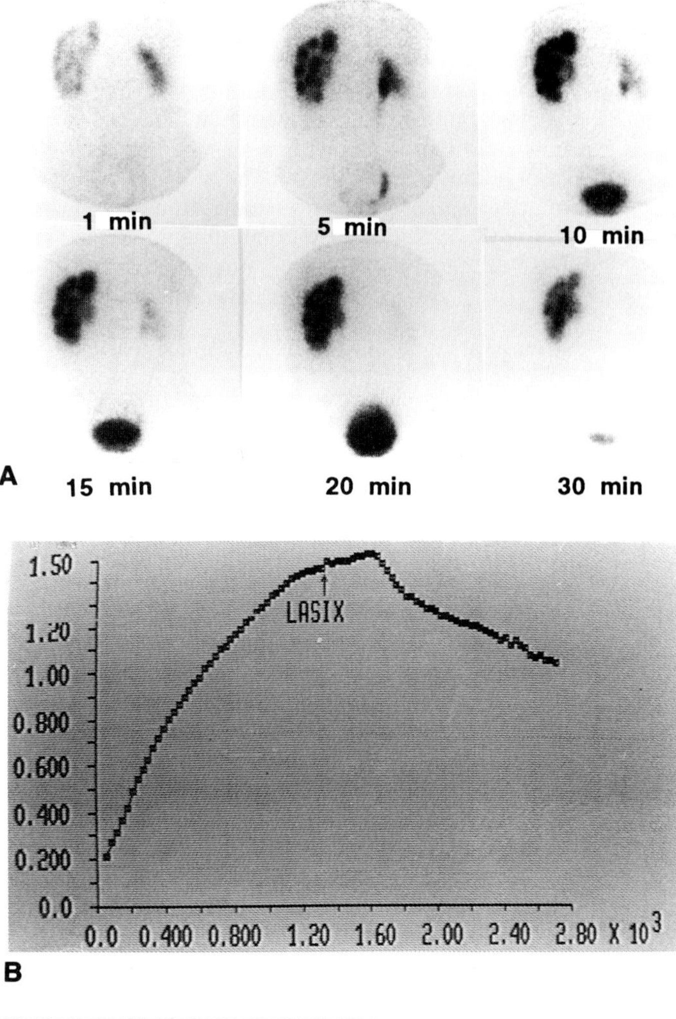


**Fig 8.** A, A 23-year-old male with prior surgery for known UPJ obstruction was referred for a diuretic renogram to evaluate possible recurrent obstruction. These serial images following IV injection of DTPA show a normal right kidney. The left kidney shows increasing "pooling" in the dilating collecting system at 20 minutes, when the patient received an IV injection of 20 mg of furosemide. There was prompt "washout" from the dilated collecting system, excluding obstruction. B, Diuretic renogram; these computer-generated curves show progressive accumulation of activity within the left kidney. Following administration of Lasix, there is an initial rise due to increased renal blood flow and clearance of the tracer, followed by a prompt emptying that corresponds to the "washout" seen in the images (Fig 8A). The renogram curves are helpful to give more objective evidence for washout, particularly when images show a questionable response.

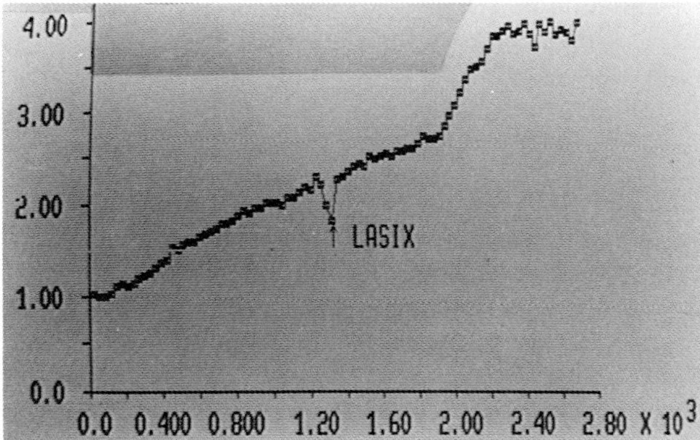


**Fig 9.** Diuretic renogram—obstructed pattern. This renogram curve, obtained in a similar manner to that described in Fig 8, shows the pattern seen with an obstructed kidney. Following Lasix administration, there is continued excretion and then a marked increase in activity within the kidney. The failure to demonstrate "washout" indicates obstruction.

the diagnosis of a "super scan." The "super scan" refers to the appearance of a better than normal looking bone scan with very intense bone uptake and no apparent metastatic lesions. This occurs with extensive, confluent metastases that cannot be individually recognized. The clue to the diagnosis lies in absent visualization of the kidneys, as the intense bone uptake leaves no tracer to be excreted.

## QUANTITATIVE STUDIES

### Measurement of Renal Function

For clinical purposes, renal function is usually measured by creatinine clearance. In addition to the technical problems associated with creatinine measurement and 24-hour urine collections, the creatinine clearance is theoretically not an accurate measurement of GFR since creatinine is excreted by the tubules as well as being filtered by the glomeruli. Also, creatinine clearance does not permit measurement of individual renal function unless bilateral ureteral catheterization is performed.

Nuclear medicine procedures are available that are rapid, accurate, simple to perform, and generally do not require complicated 24-hour urine collections. They can be easily accomplished on an outpatient basis. In addition, they permit assessment of individual renal function. This is essential for the initial evaluation and periodic follow-up of patients who have compromised and potential progressive deterioration of function in one or both kidneys.

Total renal function may be measured by several different parameters. The measurement of ERPF using the PAH method is technically difficult and requires a constant infusion of PAH intravenously as well as collection of multiple blood specimens. When a constant serum PAH concentration is reached, the rate of perfusion equals the rate of excretion by the kidneys. Carefully timed urine collections measure the amount of PAH excreted. Use of a single injection technique requires a knowledge of the blood concentration during the time of urine collection. With this method the total amount of tracer excreted in a given time divided by the average blood concentration during the time of the study gives the volume of blood cleared during that time. This method requires a complete urine collection and bladder catheterization.

A third method, which is based on compartmental analysis, is generally the one used in nuclear medicine.[18] It is based on the observation that the blood disappearance curve of renal radiopharmaceuticals can be expressed as the sum of two exponential curves. By plotting the blood clearance on semi-log paper and "curve stripping," the two exponential components can be separated (Fig 10). Each curve has an intercept (A and B) and a slope ($K_1$

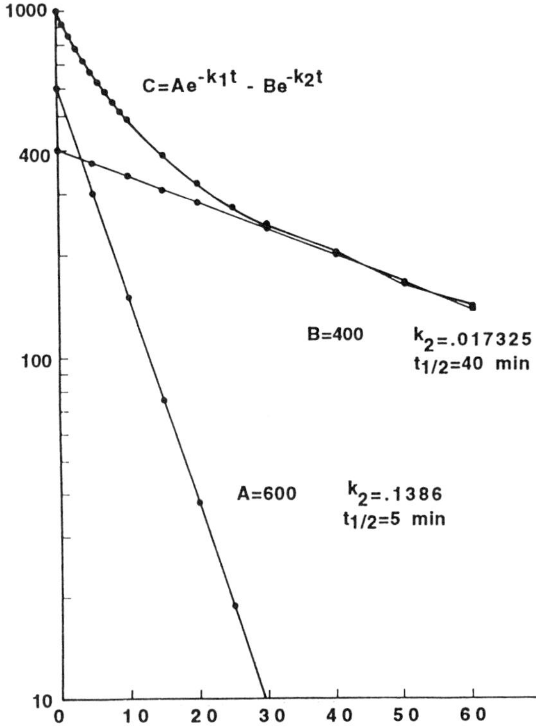


**Fig 10.** Theoretical "two-compartment" blood clearance of a renal tracer. Curve C represents the observed plasma disappearance curve with an initial value of 1,000 counts/sec/mL plasma. C is actually a composite of two monoexponential curves; A, with an intercept of 600 counts/sec and a slope of 0.1386; and B, with an intercept of 400 counts/sec and a slope of 0.017325. This administered dose had a value of 3,285,300 counts/sec; the clearance was 120 mL/min.

and $K_2$). If the dose of material injected (D) is known, then the clearance (C1) can be calculated according to the following formula:

$$C_1 = \frac{D \cdot K_1 \cdot K_2}{(A \cdot K_2) + (B \cdot K_1)}$$

This method does not require urine collection, although at least one or more blood samples are required.

Depending on the choice of radiopharmaceuticals, this technique can be used to measure either ERPF or GFR.

## Effective Renal Plasma Flow

While most physicians are familiar with GFR measurements, either ERPF or GFR can be used to monitor renal function. The results differ numerically only as a function of the radiopharmaceutical used, since the clearance measurement methods are the same. ERPF agents (OIH or MAG3) are so rapidly excreted by the renal tubules that their excretion is proportional to renal blood flow. Since ERPF agents clear approximately five times faster than GFR agents, they permit faster blood sampling and yield better image quality, especially in patients with reduced renal function.

True renal plasma flow is determined from the clearance of a compound that is almost completely cleared from the renal blood. The renal extraction ratio of any agent is the fraction of the renal arterial blood cleared by the agent given by the equation:

$$ER = \frac{A - V}{A}$$

where ER = Extraction Ratio
A = Arterial concentration
V = Venous concentration.

If the clearance of a substance and its extraction ratio are known, the total renal plasma flow can be calculated as:

$$RPF = Cl \times \frac{1}{ER}$$

where Cl = Clearance
RPF = Renal Plasma Flow.

Finally, if the renal arterial hematocrit also is known, the renal blood flow can be calculated as:

$$RBF = Cl \times \frac{1}{ER} \times \frac{1}{1 - Hct}$$

where Hct = Renal Arterial Hematocrit.

Since in practice one does not deal with compounds that are completely extracted in a single pass during perfusion of the kidney, one realistically measures an ''effective'' renal plasma flow, which usually is slightly lower than the true renal plasma flow. PAH is currently the compound of choice for chemical estimations of effective renal plasma flow. Its extraction by the normal kidney is approximately 90%, with 20% cleared by glomerular filtration and 80% by tubular secretion.

OIH or MAG3 can be used as analogs of PAH. The single biggest advantage of these agents over PAH is the simplicity of external detection with either probes or the scintillation camera, and the ease of quantifying this data using simultaneous acquisition with a computer. Several methods for calculating ERPF have been proposed. They are all based on at least a two-compartmental analysis of a biexponential plasma disappearance curve of OIH. Methods that employ both single or multiple blood samples as well as no blood samples are in use.[19]

Recent studies with $^{99m}$Tc-MAG3 show that this new agent can be used to give measurements of ERPF that correlate well with OIH.[20]

## Glomerular Filtration

The GFR is the volume of plasma ultrafiltrate produced in 1 minute in the renal glomeruli. Since GFR cannot be measured directly, various techniques, such as the clearance of exogenous creatinine and, later, inulin, have been proposed. Numerous radiopharmaceuticals have been found to correlate well with inulin. $^{99m}$Tc-DTPA is the most readily available and most commonly used radiopharmaceutical for GFR measurements. DTPA is excreted exclusively by glomerular filtration. It has a lower extraction efficiency than OIH and is extracted with about 20% efficiency. This reflects the fact that only 20% of the total renal plasma flow is handled by glomerular filtration. Differences in GFR measurements using $^{99m}$Tc-DTPA preparations by different manufacturers have been shown, and it is important that the $^{99m}$Tc-DTPA be freshly prepared.

The GFR can be calculated from biexponential or single exponential clearance curves based on compartmental analysis similar to the measurements done for ERPF.[18] Most techniques require that a ''standard'' solution be prepared. To do this, an aliquot of the dose to be given to the patient is placed in a vial. The weight of this sample is measured, and the aliquot is diluted and accurately counted. This gives the relationship between counts per minutes in the solution and weight. The syringe containing the patient's dose is also weighed before and after injection. Using such a standard, the counts measured by the camera or probe in blood or kidneys can be related to the injected dose. The GFR can then be calculated using the biexponential clearance equation above. Methods not requiring a blood sample have also been described.[21]

As with ERPF attenuation, correction for differences in renal depth, methods for choosing computer renal, and background regions of interest are technical factors that may vary from institution to institution.

## Differential Renal Function

Differential renal function is the percent of total function contributed by each kidney. Various methods are available for quantifying differential renal function. Relative renal function can be determined during the portion of the study when the plasma activity is stable and no significant amount of the radiopharmaceutical has been excreted into the collecting system. For both OIH and DTPA, this is early in the first 1 to 2 minutes before activity has been excreted into the renal pelvis. With DTPA, information concerning the distribution of GFR between the two kidneys can be obtained by measuring the amount of activity accumulated by each kidney approximately 2 to 3 minutes after injection, when only minimal amounts of tracer have left the renal parenchyma (Fig 4). The ratio of the activity in each kidney compared to total renal activity then yields the percentage of renal function provided by that kidney using the following formula:

$$\text{Percent Function (R or L)} = \frac{\text{Kidney Activity (R or L)} - \text{BKG}}{\text{(Kidney Activity (R) } (-\text{BKG}) + \text{(Kidney}} \times 100$$

where

$$\%(\text{R or L}) = \frac{[\text{Act}(\text{R or L})] - [\text{BKG}]}{[\text{Act (R)} - \text{BKG}] + [\text{Act (L)} - \text{BKG}]} \times 100$$

Different methods have been proposed for calculating split renal function using OIH. Both the area under the renogram curve at 1 to 2 minutes and the slope of the tangent to the curve at 1 to 2 minutes post injection have been used.[19]

Since DMSA concentrates selectively in renal cortical tissue, a similar calculation for renal activity will yield the relative percent of functioning cortical mass, which correlates with clearance estimates of individual renal function.[22]

DMSA provides more accurate differential function in the presence of obstruction. Since both OIH and DTPA can be retained in the renal pelvis or calyces, the activity in these areas will falsely increase the number of counts from the affected kidney.

Differential function studies can be used to predict the GFR that will remain after nephrectomy. However, one cannot predict functional recovery following surgical relief of urinary tract obstruction. The acutely obstructed kidney may demonstrate poor function and perfusion without loss of functioning nephrons. Obstruction restricts renal perfusion by raising the intrarenal pressure. Following relief of obstruction, renal function may return to normal. Thus, while measurement of differential function in the presence of obstruction gives an accurate representation of relative renal function at that point in time, it cannot be used to predict function after relief of obstruction.

### Renal Transplants

The postoperative urologic complications of renal transplant patients can be either mechanical or parenchymal. Mechanical failures can involve either complete or partial obstruction, tears in the renal collecting system, or compromise of arterial or venous blood vessels. Acute tubular necrosis and rejection are the two most important clinical considerations in patients with parenchymal failure. Nuclear imaging for the detection of complications of renal allograft surgery is common practice in most transplant centers, since it is noninvasive, has no known side effects, and has advantages over ultrasonography in that it permits assessment of all the above-noted possible complications. Nuclear imaging is not only sensitive for detecting fluid collections, but it also permits assessment of the physiological effects of such collections on renal function.[23]

Mechanical complications due to ureteral obstruction, urinary extravasation (leak), and extraurinary fluid collection (hematoma, abscess, urinoma, or lymphocele) are diagnosed in essentially the same method for grafted kidneys as for nontransplanted kidneys. Abnormalities in drainage and distortions of the urinary tract are easily seen in the nuclear images. Fluid collections appear as photopenic (areas of absent activity). Abscesses, hematomas, and lymphoceles all may appear as areas of decreased counts around the graft. When such an area is seen, a delayed image should be performed 1 to 2 hours following the early images to see if the radionuclide accumulates within the area. If this occurs, a urinoma is most likely. Additional studies, such as the use of gallium-67 or labeled white cells may be helpful to differentiate abscesses from hematomas and lymphoceles. Hematomas most often occur early, within the first 5 postoperative days. Conversely, lymphoceles seldom develop early after surgery; these collections commonly appear about 6 to 10 days after surgery.

Vascular complications are identified during the perfusion phase of the study, and, in general, appear the same as in nongrafted kidneys with the exception of renal vein obstruction. In nongrafted kidneys, little functional impairment may be present; however, function is usually absent in the grafted kidney because of the lack of collateral runoff.

Some degree of acute tubular necrosis (ATN) is initially present following transplant. Rejection, unless it is hyperacute, is not a cause of oliguria in the initial 48 hours. Therefore, maximal impairment of function with ATN is usually reached within 24 hours, and after a variable period of time should show improvement with supportive therapy. An initial diagnosis of ATN is confirmed when there is a disassociation between blood flow and function. In early ATN, the blood flow may be normal or ''supernormal'' despite severe impairment of function (Fig 11). Deterioration in renal function after 48 hours implies an additional complication and should be considered an indication of possible rejection. It should be emphasized that the perfusion and function studies with radioisotopes cannot definitely distinguish the various causes of failure (rejection, ATN, acute pyelonephritis, or renal artery or vein obstruction). The final diagnosis usually depends on evaluation of the time of functional changes together with the findings from radionuclide studies. Rejection is often diagnosed by the changing pattern in function. It is recommended that radionuclide studies be performed as soon as possible in the immediate postoperative period, and then every other day for the first 2 to 3 weeks. A pattern of gradually decreasing perfusion and function can predict the biochemical changes of rejection by as much as 2 to 3 days, and therefore enable earlier institution of antirejection therapy.

Because part of the histologic picture of rejection involves the deposition of fibrin in the glomeruli within areas of vasculitis associated with endothelial proliferation, the use of $^{99m}$Tc-SC has been successful in specifically identifying rejection as opposed to other causes of renal transplant failure. In one series of patients who were studied 14 days after transplantation, 88% of the rejections showed increased SC uptake within the transplanted kidney. In pa-

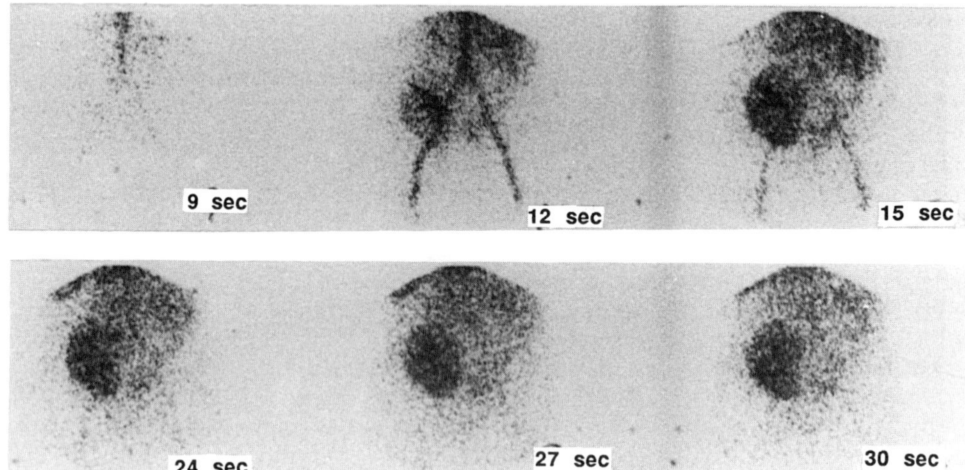


**Fig 11.** ATN in a renal transplant; 10 days following transplantation, this patient had persistent decreased renal function. The DTPA study shows intact perfusion (top) with poor clearance (bottom) of the radiopharmaceutical (no excretion to the bladder), consistent with a slowly resolving ATN.

tients with ATN and no evidence of rejection, however, 42% did show radiocolloid uptake. After 2 weeks, the incidence of SC uptake in the patients rejecting transplants progressively decreased, and thus decreased the sensitivity of the test. It is said, however, that the absence of SC uptake in the initial 14 days postoperatively is a more reliable sign to exclude rejection than is its uptake as an indicator of the presence of rejection.[24,25]

With the development of techniques for radiolabeling autologous white blood cells and platelets with $^{111}$I-oxine, several investigators have studied the accumulation of these radiolabeled cells in patients with renal transplant rejection. Because labeled platelets remain in the circulation for several days, platelet scintigraphy permits daily imaging to monitor for rejection in the week following transplantation. While high sensitivity (93%) and specificity (95%) of platelet imaging have been reported,[26] the cell-labeling techniques are time consuming and relatively expensive. This has limited their widespread use. False-positive studies have been reported with perinephric hematomas,[27] cyclosporine nephrotoxicity,[28] and in the immediate postoperative period.[29]

## PEDIATRIC STUDIES

Radionuclide studies of the kidneys and the urinary tract are particularly well adapted to pediatrics, as the problems encountered with children are usually part of a changing process that will require serial assessment. The particularly low radiation dose and the absence of side effects have increased their popularity in pediatric urology.

The same radiopharmaceuticals employed for adults are used with children, but since the renal clearance of DTPA is high, and there is no significant renal parenchymal retention, DTPA is the agent of first choice. GHA is reserved for those cases where better visualization of renal anatomy is required. DTPA can also be used for serial measurements of differential renal function and glomerular filtration rate.

In general, renal perfusion and functional studies are used in the same manner as in adults. There are, however, certain specific procedures that are used predominantly in the pediatric population.

### Radionuclide Cystography

Many pediatric patients are seen because

of urinary tract infection and suspected vesicoureteric reflux. Radionuclide cystography is the preferred method for follow-up studies in these patients because of its accuracy and low radiation burden compared with conventional x-ray techniques. The gonadal doses are decreased approximately 10-fold. Either $^{99m}$Tc-DTPA or SC may be instilled into the bladder via a catheter in conjunction with a saline infusion (direct cystography). Continuous recordings and images can be acquired using the nuclear medicine camera to observe the bladder-filling phase and the voiding phase with no additional radiation dose (Fig 12). Good correlation with micturition cystography has been found.[30] After the child voids, the residual counts can be used to quantify the amount of reflux and residual volume.

Indirect cystography following a routine DTPA study is an alternate method that avoids the need for bladder catheterization. It can only be used once the radioisotope has completely cleared the upper urinary tract and accumulated in the bladder. The child is then asked to void while reflux is assessed.

### Hydronephrosis Assessment

A dilated collecting system seen on intravenous pyelography may be due to either obstruction or nonperistaltic ureters. The assessment of hydronephrotic kidneys can be performed with radioisotope techniques even with kidneys that are poorly visualized on intravenous pyelography. Both nonobstructed and obstructed hydronephrotic kidneys may show delayed drainage on films obtained even 2 to 4 hours postinjection. In such cases, a diuretic renal scan can be employed and may be vital in making the diagnosis of a nonobstructed kidney.

In children who have had reimplantation of the ureters to correct reflux, scans taken approximately 10 days postoperatively and then serially can be used to assess kidney function and drainage.

## CONGENITAL ANOMALIES

Ectopic kidneys can be easily identified in radioisotope studies. Usually both the renal scan and ultrasound are helpful for identifying patients with a solitary kidney on the intravenous pyelogram. The renal

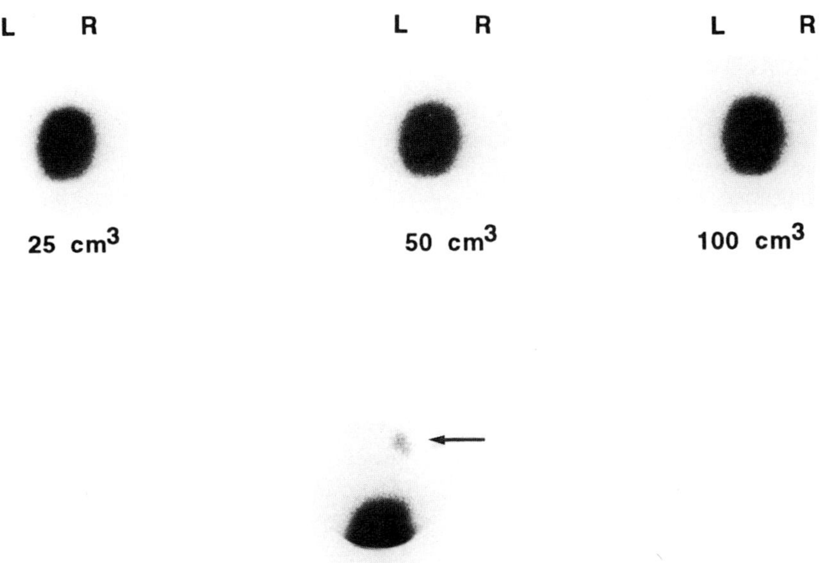


**Fig 12.** Direct radionuclide cystography; this 8-year-old female patient had a history of surgery for correction of bilateral reflux. A follow-up study at 1 year demonstrates recurrence of reflux (arrow).

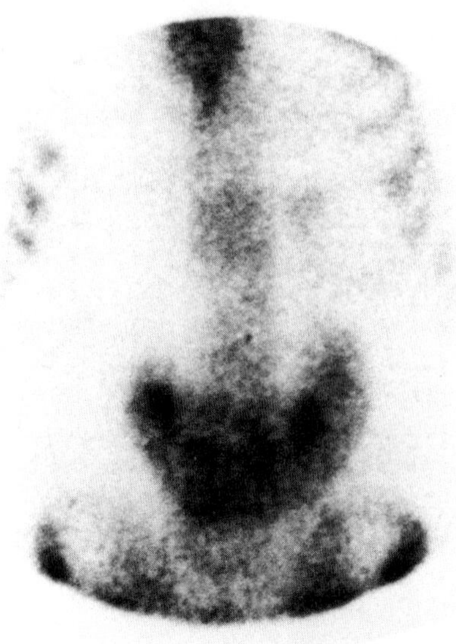

**Fig 13.** Horseshoe kidney; a horseshoe kidney was incidentally found on a bone scan performed on this 18-year-old patient. The normal concentration of the tracer in the lower pole of the kidney correctly identifies normal, functioning renal tissue.

scan is also helpful for deciding if there is functioning renal tissue joining the lower pole of a horseshoe kidney (Fig 13).[31]

## TESTICULAR IMAGING AND THE "ACUTE SCROTUM"

The "acute scrotum" is generally defined as acute, unilateral scrotal swelling with or without pain. The important differential diagnosis is between acute testicular torsion and acute epididymitis. The clinical evaluation of patients who present with the onset of acute painful swelling in the scrotum is unreliable, since scrotal tissues in testicular torsion may develop redness and edema and the scrotum will be tender to palpation as in any inflammatory process (eg, epididymitis). The history and findings of urinalysis are also often not helpful. Thus, in many cases, immediate surgical exploration is performed to improve testicular salvage.

Radionuclide scrotal imaging can eliminate the need for unnecessary surgical exploration in patients with acute epididymitis.[32] In order to be of value in evaluating patients with an "acute scrotum," the study must be available rapidly and on a 24-hour basis. For this reason, it is often not utilized, since many hospitals do not have nuclear medicine imaging available 24 hours a day. If facilities are available, the study can be performed in minutes.

The radioisotope used is $^{99m}$Tc-pertechnetate. The isotope is readily available, and no radiopharmaceutical preparation is involved. The patient is injected, and an RNA demonstrating blood flow to the scrotum is recorded. In a normal study, blood flow is seen in the iliac and femoral vessels, but no blood flow is usually seen in the area of the testicular or deferential vessels, which are small. In a normal study, therefore, no arterial perfusion to the scrotum is seen. With an inflammatory process, such as epididymitis, there is increased blood flow seen to the involved testicle. In early epididymitis, the increased blood flow will localize in a linear pattern corresponding to the epididymis. With more severe inflammation, such as epididymoorchitis, increased blood flow will be seen to the entire testicle (Fig 14).

With early testicular torsion, there is an absence of testicular blood flow. Since normally no perfusion is seen in the scrotum, the study appears normal. The appearance, therefore, of a "normal" perfusion study in a patient with an "acute scrotum" excludes an inflammatory process, and the patient should undergo surgical exploration.

Delayed scrotal images can be acquired, which will show activity in normally perfused testes. With acute testicular torsion, a "cold" testicule is seen, and later there may be a "halo" from hyperemic dartos perfusion. This finding is observed in the late phase of a "missed" testicular torsion.

While other scrotal masses (eg, hydroceles, tumors, abscesses) may be diagnosed using radionuclide imaging, the technique is primarily used to differentiate acute testicular torsion from epididymitis. The study takes only minutes to perform and should help to avoid unnecessary surgical exploration in patients with epididymitis.

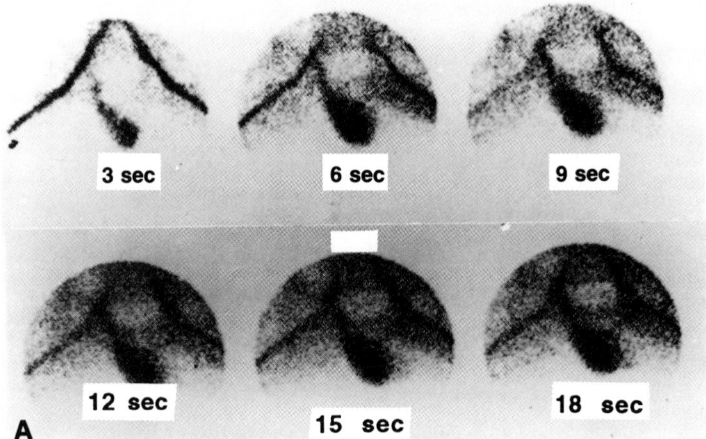


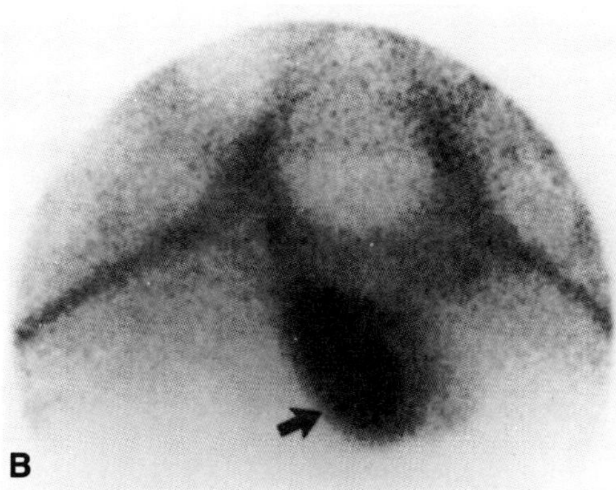


**Fig 14.** A, Testicular study showing epididymoorchitis; the radionuclide angiogram shows intense blood flow to the entire right testicle. This indicates an inflammatory process, and excludes testicular torsion in the patient who presents with acute scrotal pain. B, The delayed scrotal image shows diffuse hyperemia involving the right testicle (arrow). The absence of a "cold" testicle differentiates epididymoorchitis from a "missed" testicular torsion, which in the late phase can also demonstrate increased blood flow and hyperemia from intact perfusion to the hyperemic dartos.

## RADIONUCLIDE RADIATION THERAPY

The therapeutic use of radionuclides in urologic practice currently is limited to the palliative treatment of painful bone metastases, most commonly in patients with advanced metastatic prostate carcinoma.[33] Phosphorus-32 (P-32) is a β-particle emitter with a half-life of 14.3 days. The β particles have a limited range, and therefore deliver their ionizing radiation to a limited area. Since P-32 concentrates in normal and reactive bone, tumorcidal radiation doses can be delivered, especially to blastic skeletal metastases. Hormonal manipulations, such as the administration of testosterone, may increase the uptake of P-32 in the tumor cell itself.[34]

Hematopoietic depression due to bone marrow depression is the most serious adverse side effect, and blood counts should be monitored 6 to 8 weeks after therapy, especially in patients who already have bone marrow destruction due to tumor. Relief of pain can occur in as many as 87% of patients treated.[35]

## REFERENCES

1. Murphy, PH, DePuey EG, Sonnemaker RE, et al. Emission computed tomography: a current status report. *Nuclear Medicine Annual*. New York: Raven Press; 1980.
2. Pollack HM, Edell S, Morales JO. Radionuclide imaging in renal pseudotumors. *Radiology*. 1974;111:639.
3. Reba RC, Hosain F, Wagner HN. Indium–113m diethylenetriamine-pentaacetic acid (DTPA): a new radiopharmaceutical for study of the kidneys. *Radiology*. 1968;90:147–149.

4. Burbank MK, Tauxe WN, Maher FT, et al. Evaluation of radioiodinated hippuran for the estimation of renal plasma flow. *Proc Staff Meetings Mayo Clin.* 1961;36:372–386.
5. Taylor A, Eshima D, Christian PE, Milton W. Evaluation of Tc-99m mercaptoacetyltriglycine in patients with impaired renal function. *Radiology.* 1987;162:365–370.
6. Taylor A, Ziffer JA, Steves A, Eshima D, Delaney VB, Welchel JD. Clinical comparison of I-131 orthoiodohippurate and the kit formulation of Tc-99m mercaptoacetyltriglycine. *Radiology.* 1989;170:721–725.
7. DuCret RD, Boudreau, RJ, Gonzalez R, Carpenter R, Tennison J, Kuni CC. Clinical efficacy of Tc-99m mercaptoacetylglycine kit formulation in routine renal scintigraphy. *J Urol.* 1989;142:19–22.
8. George EA, Codd JE, Newton WT, et al. Further evaluation of 99m-Tc sulfur colloid accumulation in rejecting renal transplants in man and a canine model. *Radiology.* 1975;116:121–126.
9. Sfakianakis GN, Bourgoignie JJ, Jaffe D, Kyriakides G, Perez-Stable E, Duncan RC. Single-dose captopril scintigraphy in the diagnosis of renovascular hypertension. *J Nucl Med.* 1987;28:1383–1392.
10. Pedersen EB, Jensen FT, Eiskjoer H, et al. Differentiation between renovascular and essential hypertension by means of changes in single kidney 99mTc-DTPA clearance induced by angiotensin-converting enzyme inhibition. *AJH.* 1989;2:323–334.
11. Geyskes GG, Oei HY, Puylaert BAJ, Mees EJD. Renovascular hypertension identified by captopril-induced changes in the renogram. *Hypertension.* 1987;9:451–458.
12. Rosenthall L, Ammann W. Renal trauma. *Semin Nucl Med.* 1983;13:238–244.
13. Vitti RA, Maurer AH. Single photon emission computed tomography and renal pseudotumor. *Clin Nucl Med.* 1985;10:501–503.
14. Tarkington MA, Fildes RB, Levin K, et al. High resolution single photon emission computerized tomography (SPECT) 99m-technetium-dimercapto-succinic acid renal imaging: a state of the art technique. *J Urol.* 1990;144:598–600.
15. Caplan GE, Hartmann HR, Young R, et al. The "Hot" renal tumor. *Radiology.* 1968;91:991–992.
16. Thrall JH, Koff S, Keyes JW Jr. Diuretic radionuclide renography and scintigraphy in the differential diagnosis of hydroureteronephrosis. *Semin Nucl Med.* 1981;11:89.
17. Pollen JJ, Gerber K, Heil BJ, et al. Detection of ureteral obstructions on radionuclide bone scans. *Am J Roentgen.* 1983;141:567–570.
18. Cohen ML. Radionuclide clearance techniques. *Semin Nucl Med.* 1974;4:23–38.
19. Dubovsky EV, Russell CD. Quantitation of renal function with glomerular and tubular agents. *Semin Nucl Med.* 1982;12:308–329.
20. Russel CD, Taylor A, Eshima D. Estimation of technetium-99m-MAG3 plasma clearance in adults from one or two blood samples. *J Nucl Med.* 1989;30:1955–1959.
21. Gates GF. Glomerular filtration rate: Estimation from fractional renal accumulation of 99mTc-DTPA (Stannous). *Am J Roentgen.* 1982; 138:565–570.
22. Taylor A. Quantitation of renal function with static imaging agents. *Semin Nucl Med.* 1982;12:330–344.
23. Hattner RS, Engelstad BL, Dae MW. Radionuclide evaluation of renal transplants. *Nuclear Medicine Annual.* New York: Raven Press; 1984.
24. Frick MP, Loken MK, Goldberg ME, et al. Use of 99m-Tc-sulfur colloid in evaluation of renal transplant complications. *J Nucl Med.* 1976;17:181–183.
25. George EA, Codd JE, Newton WT, et al. Further evaluation of 99m-Tc sulfur colloid accumulation in rejecting renal transplants in man and a canine model. *Radiology.* 1975;116:121–126.
26. Tisdale PL, Collier BD, Kauffman HM, et al. Early diagnosis of acute postoperative renal transplant rejection by indium-111-labeled platelet scintigraphy. *J Nucl Med.* 1986;27:1266–1272.
27. Martin-Comin J, Roca M, Grino JM, et al. In-111 oxine labelled platelets in the diagnosis of kidney graft rejection. *Clin Nucl Med.* 1983;8:7–10.
28. Sommer BG, Innes JT, Whitehurst RM. Cyclosporine-related arteriopathy resulting in loss of allograft function. *Am J Surg.* 1985;149:756–764.
29. Desir G, Lange R, Smith E, et al. Uptake of indium-111 platelets by normal, nephrotic and transplanted kidneys. *J Nucl Med.* 1984;25:75.
30. Maizels M, Weiss S, Conway JJ, et al. Urological neurology and urodynamics. The cystometric nuclear cystogram. *J Urol.* 1979;121:203–205.
31. Grandone CH, Haller JO, Berdon WE, et al. Asymmetric horseshoe kidney in the infant: Value of renal nuclear scanning. *Radiology.* 1985;154:366.
32. Chen DC, Holder LE, Melloul M. Radionuclide scrotal imaging: Further experience with 210 new patients. *J Nucl Med.* 1983;24:841–853.
33. Joshi DP, Seery WH, Goldberg LG, et al. Evaluation of phosphorus 32 for intractable pain secondary to prostatic carcinoma metastasis. *JAMA.* 1965;193:621–623.
34. Dontai RM, Ellis H, Gallagher NI. Testosterone potentiated 32P therapy in prostatic carcinoma. *Cancer.* 1966;19:1088–1090.
35. Spencer RP. *Therapy in Nuclear Medicine.* New York: Grune & Stratton; 1978, Chap. 20, p 329.

# 7

# Evaluation of the Urologic Patient

*Susan M. Jones Kalota, Laurence F. Greene, and C. Lowell Parsons*

The specialty of urology has advanced in an explosive manner during the past two decades. Highly effective techniques both for the preservation of the normal and, more often, for the correction of the abnormal urologic function have been developed and perfected. Much of this important progress has been made in the laboratory and, as a result, a certain shifting of emphasis to this area has taken place. Yet today, perhaps more so than ever before, the clearly defined underlying principles continue to form the cornerstone of our specialty; the sequential investigation is a means to the accurate diagnosis that is so inseparable from rational treatment. Because this is particularly true in the new subspecialty of pediatric urology, a small section with special reference to the unique urologic problems of children is included.

## UROLOGIC MANIFESTATIONS

There may be complete absence of symptoms in the presence of profound pathologic changes in the urinary tract; for example, large staghorn calculi can be present in the kidneys for years without producing symptoms. Furthermore, there may be no correlation between the severity of the symptoms and the severity of the disease process that produced the symptoms. An extensive renal neoplasm might cause slight transient hematuria, whereas a minute ureteral calculus can cause the patient to be desperately ill. In addition, a wide variety of pathologic lesions may result in an identical train of symptoms; for example, the symptoms that result from vesical neoplasm, vesical calculus, benign prostatic hyperplasia, and carcinoma of the prostate may be identical. Finally, by investigating manifestations that bear no apparent relationship to the urinary tract, a lesion in the urinary tract may be discovered. Thus, a patient suffering from spontaneous fracture of a bone may be found to have metastatic carcinoma of a kidney or of the prostate gland, or, studies performed on a patient with liver dysfunction may disclose a hypernephroma.

The urologic manifestations that a patient may note can be classified into three broad categories: (1) alterations in appearance of the urine, (2) alterations of micturition, and (3) pain. Each category may be noted alone or may occur in combination. Another group of nonspecific manifestations, such as nausea, vomiting, fever, and chills, is frequently associated with disease of the urinary tract. Usually nothing characteristic about these symptoms in themselves suggests that they are due to disease of the urinary tract.

## Alterations in Appearance of Urine

Hematuria and pyuria are the most common conditions that cause alteration in the appearance of the urine and induce patients to seek medical aid. The former is not infrequently the sole sign; the latter usually is associated with other urinary signs or symptoms. It must be stressed that significant disease of the urinary tract may be present with no visible alteration in the appearance of the urine.

**Hematuria.** Normal urine may contain erythrocytes. An Addis count of normal urine collected during a 12-hour period will disclose 0 to 500,000 or possibly as many as 1 million erythrocytes. Larcom and Carter studied single-voided specimens from 3,000 healthy men applying for employment; in 2,484 instances, urinalysis did not disclose erythrocyturia. In 2% of the group, two to three erythrocytes were noted in each highpower field; in 0.7%, four to five erythrocytes were noted. These authors concluded that the presence of more than two erythrocytes in each high-power field may indicate an increased or abnormal loss of erythrocytes through the urinary tract.

From the standpoint of etiology, hematuria can be divided into three broad categories: (1) hematuria associated with, or secondary to, systemic disease; (2) hematuria secondary to diseases of structures adjacent to the urinary tract; and (3) hematuria as the result of disease primarily of the urogenital tract. Hematuria may be either microscopic or gross.

***Hematuria Associated With, or Secondary to, Systemic Disease.*** A lengthy listing of systemic diseases associated with hematuria would serve no useful purpose and it is sufficient to indicate but a few. In some cases within this category, hematuria may be the outstanding clinical symptom; for example, hematuria is present in acute glomerulonephritis with such regularity that, in the classification of Addis, the disease has been termed ''acute hemorrhagic nephritis.''

Similarly, erythrocyturia is common in diseases of the blood or blood-forming organs, such as thrombocytopenic purpura, leukemia, hemophilia, polycythemia vera, and Hodgkin's disease. Congestive failure or renal infarct secondary to disease of the heart may result in erythrocyturia. The ingestion of chemicals, such as methenamine, turpentine, cantharidin, carbolic acid, and sulfonamides, and acute and chronic diseases, such as scarlet fever, smallpox, malaria, and yellow fever, may be associated with erythrocyturia. Deficiency of ascorbic acid or vitamin K or administration of bishydroxycoumarin (Dicumarol) or heparin may result in erythrocyturia. An allergic basis is stated to be the cause of erythrocyturia following injection of tetanus antitoxin.

***Hematuria Secondary to Diseases of Structures Adjacent to the Urinary Tract.*** Hematuria in cases of this type may be due to a great variety of etiologic factors. Inflammatory conditions, such as acute appendicitis, acute salpingitis, and diverticulitis of the colon, and neoplasia involving structures adjacent to the urinary tract may be causally related to hematuria.

***Hematuria Resulting From Disease Primarily of the Urogenital Tract***

MICROHEMATURIA. Microhematuria may present a vexing problem to the urologist. The problem becomes less difficult if the patient has other urinary symptoms or if urinalysis results disclose other formed elements such as leukocytes or bacteria. Under such circumstances, the indications for complete urologic investigation are clear and the likelihood of finding the source of microhematuria is good. On the other hand, the finding of persistent microscopic erythrocyturia without other formed elements in the urine of a patient who has no urinary symptoms is perplexing. The indications for complete, extensive urologic investigation are not clear, and the likelihood of finding a significant cause for microhematuria is not good.

Urologic investigations in such patients disclose a significant lesion in 10%; in 2% the lesion is neoplastic. In half of the remaining 8% of patients, an insignificant lesion is found, and in the other half, no lesion is detected at all.

Presently, no known criteria enable the urologist to select patients for urologic studies in order not to overlook significant lesions of the urinary tract and yet not subject every patient with microhematuria to extensive investigation. The practice of carrying out complete investigations in all patients with asymptomatic microhematuria is beyond reproach. However, a compromise plan by which patients aged 50 years and older receive urographic and cystoscopic examinations has been suggested. Under this approach, urologic investigation of younger patients is limited to a plain roentgenogram of the urinary tract. Recent reports indicate that we may be able to accurately differentiate between glomerular and nonglomerular causes of hematuria. Glomerular bleeding is caused by disruption of the glomerular and peritubular capillaries, which allows erythrocytes to escape into the renal tubular lumen. As red blood cells are forced through abnormal capillaries, the cell walls are damaged, giving them a distorted, irregular shape; erythrocytes that are shed into the urinary tract from nonglomerular causes (eg, prostatic hypertrophy, renal lithiasis, urologic cancer) are isomorphic and have a uniform size and shape. This difference in morphology has been detected with scanning electron microscopy and, more simply, with the standard Coulter counter. Accurate prediction of glomerular vs nonglomerular hematuria was made in 97% of patients examined by Coulter counter analysis.

**TABLE 1. Source and Cause of Gross Hematuria in 5965 Cases**

| Source | Percent | Cause | Percent |
|---|---|---|---|
| Kidneys | 42.8 | Inflammation | 31.4 |
| Bladder | 29.7 | Neoplasia | 27.9 |
| Prostate | 14.2 | Foreign body | 20.0 |
| Ureter | 8.7 | Tuberculosis | 9.4 |
| Urethra | 4.6 | Trauma | 3.8 |
| | | Other | 7.5 |

After Doss AK. *Urol Cutan Rev.* 1947;51:676–680.

Gross Hematuria. Every patient complaining of gross hematuria requires complete urologic investigation. Table 1 shows the source and cause of hematuria in a large series of cases collected by Doss.

The age of the patient is important in a consideration of a case of gross hematuria. Gross hematuria is rare during infancy and childhood in the absence of certain systemic diseases. When it occurs, it usually is in response to infection; the infection is the result of a congenital abnormality in approximately half of the cases. Congenital obstruction at the ureteropelvic juncture may produce hydronephrosis, infection may develop, and gross hematuria may result. Neoplasms of the urinary tract are uncommon in this age group. The common malignant tumors of infants, such as Wilms' tumor or sarcoma of the bladder or prostate gland, infrequently produce gross hematuria. The former usually is detected when an abdominal mass is discovered, whereas the latter produces urinary obstruction.

In young adults and persons up to the age of 40 years, gross hematuria is most commonly a manifestation of infection, eg, pyelonephritis, cystitis, or stones. Neoplasms of the urinary tract are also relatively uncommon in this age group.

After the age of 40 years, gross hematuria as a result of neoplasms of the kidneys, ureters, or bladder becomes more frequent. In men of this age group, prostatic lesions, both benign and malignant, and urinary calculi are common causes of hematuria. Infections of the urinary tract, nevertheless, continue to represent the most common cause of gross hematuria in this age group.

A detailed description of the nature of the hematuria may help to determine the site of the lesion. In men, it should be determined whether the hematuria is present at the beginning, at the end, throughout, or independent of micturition. Initial hematuria is characterized by the appearance of blood only at the start of micturition; the urine becomes clear during voiding. This suggests an anterior urethral lesion such as urethritis, stricture, or meatal stenosis. Alternatively, initial hematuria can be produced by lesions of the prostate or prostatic urethra. In terminal hematuria, clear urine is passed until termination of micturition; then the urine becomes bloody. Terminal hematuria may result from lesions of the prostate or prostatic urethra; in some instances, the sudden contraction of the accessory muscles of micturition is responsible. Rarely, vesical neoplasms may be traumatized by the contraction of the bladder and produce terminal hematuria. In total hematuria, the urine appears bloody throughout micturition.

Total hematuria usually is produced by lesions of the kidneys and ureters. The blood enters the bladder and becomes well mixed with the urine. Lesions in the bladder likewise may result in total hematuria. Rarely, lesions of the prostatic urethra bleed into the bladder and result in total hematuria. Bleeding independent of micturition is produced by lesions situated external to the external sphincter.

The color of the urine may be of some help in diagnosis. Dark brown urine usually results from bleeding lesions in the upper part of the urinary tract, whereas bright red urine usually is associated with lesions in the lower part of the urinary tract. It may be extremely difficult to determine whether bleeding arises from the urinary or the genital tract in females; careful catheterization and examination of the urine usually settle the question.

There are several conditions in which the kidneys excrete foreign substances that result in discoloration of the urine. These conditions are hemoglobinuria, obstructive and hepatocellular jaundice, porphyria, and ochronosis. Also, ingestion of several substances can cause red-colored urine: beets and berries (beeturia); phenolphthalein, which is present in some laxatives; some food colorings; urates; and phenazopyridine (Pyridium). *Serratia marcescens* infections in infants can produce a red diaper, which may cause concern as well. This discoloration may be interpreted falsely by the patient and described to the physician as representing hematuria. Microscopic examination of a freshly voided specimen of urine enables the physician to distinguish these conditions from hematuria. Unless a secondary complication is present, erythrocytes are not present in the urine under the conditions listed, whereas they are invariably present in the urine of patients with hematuria.

**Pyuria.** Pyuria is the presence of leukocytes in the urine; the leukocytes are referred to as "pus cells." If present in sufficient numbers, leukocytes may impart a cloudy appearance to the urine.

From the patient's point of view, cloudy urine is synonymous with pyuria. However, there are other causes for cloudy urine and it is the physician's duty to exclude them. Cloudy urine may be due to the presence of amorphous phosphates and urates, bacilli, erythrocytes, chyle, or animal parasites in the urine. Pyuria can be established only by detecting, under microscopic examination, leukocytes in a freshly passed specimen of urine. Patients frequently note the formation of a cloud in their urine when it is left standing. The cloud is due to precipitation of amorphous phosphates, which appear secondary to alkalinization. It is not uncommon for freshly passed urine to be cloudy because of the presence of amorphous phosphates (disappearing with addition of acetic acid) or urates (disappearing on heating). Pyuria may not be detected if the reaction of the urine is alkaline and if examination is delayed, as leukocytes degenerate rapidly under alkaline conditions. Therefore, prompt examination of a freshly voided specimen of urine is necessary.

It is impossible to detail the myriad causes of pyuria. Pyuria may be the result of infectious, neoplastic, allergic, or traumatic disease of the urinary tract. It may be secondary to diseases in structures adjacent to the urinary tract or to general systemic diseases. It may be secondary to congenital anomalies of the urinary tract, to foreign bodies, or to the ingestion of noxious substances.

It is likewise impossible to describe in detail the various urologic procedures that may be necessary to determine the source of pyuria. The scope of the investigation will be determined by the history, by the results of physical examination, and by study of other elements in the urine. If it is noted, for example, that in addition to leukocytes the urine contains albumin, casts, and erythrocytes and that bacteria are absent, it may be assumed that the pyuria is due to nephritis, if the history and results of physical examination are in keeping with such a diagnosis. Urologic investigation for the source of pyuria in a case of this type is not necessary. On the other hand, it must be remembered that urologic disease which requires investigation may be present in the absence of pyuria. Interstitial cystitis, for example, usually is associated with normal urine.

If symptoms referable to the urinary tract are present and if significant pyuria is detected, extensive urologic investigation may be necessary. On the other hand, it may be the considered opinion of the physician that the urinary symptoms and pyuria are due to a simple infection of the urinary tract. Such infections are usually self-limited and can be eradicated rapidly and completely by suitable therapy. A minimal number of urologic studies need be undertaken under such circumstances. If pyuria persists or recurs following therapy, it must be assumed that the infection is associated with some complicating factor such as urinary obstruction, neoplasm, calculus, or tuberculosis. In such instances more complete urologic investigation is in order.

The problem becomes more complex when pyuria without symptoms referable to the urinary tract is noted. It has already been pointed out that extensive disease of the urinary tract may be present in the absence of urinary symptoms. If 10 to 20 leukocytes per high-power field are noted, examination of the urine should be repeated to determine whether this finding is persistent. If this or a greater degree of pyuria is noted, urologic studies are in order. The thoroughness with which this investigation should be undertaken varies from case to case. Thus, in the case of an adult male, if examination of the second specimen of urine discloses an absence of leukocytes and if study of the expressed prostatic secretions reveals prostatitis, it may be assumed that the pyuria resulted from prostatitis. Further urologic investigation needs to be directed only toward the prostatitis. If, on the other hand, the pyuria in this hypothetical case cannot be ascribed to prostatitis, it becomes necessary to study the remainder of the urinary tract. Such studies may entail urography, ultrasonography, cystoscopy, and bacteriologic examinations.

**Other Alterations in Appearance of Urine.** Other alterations in the appearance of the urine occur, and may attract the patient's attention. A highly concentrated urine may be deep amber in color and may resemble bloody urine. A milk-like appearance of the urine may be due to chyluria which results from an abnormal connection between lymphatic ducts and the urinary tract. The patient may note the passage of sand, gravel, or stones in the urine. Bubbles of gas in the urine, as a result of an abnormal connection between the gastrointestinal and urinary tracts or an infection of the urinary tract, may be noted. Patients may be disturbed by the odor of the urine. An ammonia odor may be detected from alkaline urine. Ingestion of certain substances (eg, asparagus) or conditions such as diabetes mellitus, urinary infections, and necrosis of malignant lesions of the urinary tract may impart odors to the urine.

## Alterations in Micturition

**Frequency.** The most common urologic complaint is frequency. Under standard conditions, a normal person urinates at intervals of 3 to 4 hours during waking hours; this is subject to variation. The factors that affect the frequency of urination may be physiologic, psychologic, or the result of urologic and general systemic disease.

Large intake of fluids results in large output of fluids and urinary frequency. It is surprising how frequently patients fail to comprehend this cause–effect relationship. Furthermore, the end products of protein metabolism are diuretic. It is clear, therefore, that urinary frequency may be a physiologic response to the type and amount of food and fluids ingested. Such factors as temperature, humidity, and recumbency affect the urinary output and, hence, the frequency of urination. A cool, moist climate, for example, is associated with decreased perspiration, increased urinary output, and increased frequency of urination.

It is common for normal persons to experience urinary frequency with passage of small amounts of urine during periods of emotional strain. Renal hyperfunction can occur as the result of emotional tension, resulting in the passage of large amounts of clear, colorless urine. Urinary frequency may be a manifestation of neurosis. High-strung, tense persons may complain of an almost constant desire to urinate. They note an imperative urge to urinate but pass only several ounces of urine; shortly thereafter they experience the same symptoms and again void a small amount of urine. It can be demonstrated that the amount of urine voided on each occasion represents but a fraction of the capacity of the bladder. Such patients frequently experience these symptoms only during waking hours and are able to sleep for intervals of 6 to 8 hours without noting the necessity to urinate. In most instances, patients who complain of severe daytime frequency and do not have nocturia are free of organic disease.

Inflammation of the urinary tract is the most common urologic cause of urinary frequency. This symptom is most striking when the inflammation involves the bladder or urethra. Mild distention of the inflamed mucosa results in a sensation of pain and a desire to urinate. A sensation of a need to urinate immediately is referred to as "urgency." Inflammation of the urinary tract which produces frequency is usually the result of bacterial action, but infection also may result from yeasts or fungi; allergic states and virus infections have also been implicated. At times, the inflammation is noninfectious in nature, as in interstitial cystitis, amicrobic pyuria, and malakoplakia. In addition, the inflammation may be factitial in nature, secondary to radiotherapy or to use of chemotherapeutic agents such as cyclophosphamide or ifosphamide.

Urinary frequency may result from irritation produced by urinary calculi. Vesical calculi produce this symptom regularly, but the presence of calculi in a renal pelvis, a ureter, the prostate, or the urethra may produce this symptom as well. The irritation that results from the presence of foreign bodies in the bladder or urethra likewise produces urinary frequency. Benign or malignant neoplasms of the bladder, prostate, or urethra are also associated with urinary frequency. In such instances, frequency is usually due to secondary infection, but it may result from urinary obstruction that causes significant post void residual or increased bladder irritability in the absence of infection.

**Dysuria.** Dysuria, or painful urination, is frequently, but not invariably, associated with urinary frequency. If dysuria is intense and associated with the passage of small amounts of urine, it is referred to as "strangury." Dysuria is usually due to voluntary contractions or involuntary spasms of an inflamed bladder; frequently it arises from inflammatory disease of the prostate gland or as a result of passage of urine through an inflamed urethra. Bacterial infections are the usual cause for inflammation of these structures, but inflammation secondary to benign or malignant neoplasms of these structures also may give rise to dysuria. Similarly, calculi situated in the lower part of a ureter, or in the bladder, prostate, or urethra, may be associated with an inflammatory reaction which manifests itself by dysuria; in women, vaginitis with local inflammation may produce dysuria.

Dysuria in the absence of inflammatory disease is usually associated with obstruction. Obstructive lesions situated at any site—from the vesical neck to the external urethral meatus—can produce dysuria; these lesions include hypertrophy of the vesical neck, congenital urethral valves, carcinoma and benign hyperplasia of the prostate gland, urethral strictures, congenital stenosis of the external urethral meatus, and phimosis.

There are few characteristic forms of dysuria which can be ascribed to a specific condition. In cases of inflammatory disease of the posterior urethra in men and of the urethral diverticula in women, the patients complain of pain during the termination of micturition. Patients suffering from interstitial cystitis relate that pain is relieved by urination.

Complete urologic investigation of patients who complain of dysuria may not uncover a cause for this symptom. In some of these patients, dysuria has been ascribed to persistence of highly acid urine, and alkalinization of the urine has been advised. In some persons, dysuria may be a manifestation of psychoneurosis. These persons interpret the normal sensations which occur with urination as pain.

**Nocturia.** Nocturia, the necessity for micturition during the night, may be the sole urinary symptom; more usually, it is associated with other urinary symptoms. Nocturia indicates that a person cannot sleep for a period of 7 to 8 hours without being awakened by the desire and necessity to urinate. It is sometimes defined as the passage of more than 500 mL of urine with a specific gravity less than 1.018 during the night. On retiring, some persons find it necessary to urinate several times before falling asleep; this should not be considered to be nocturia, inasmuch as nocturia implies being awakened from sleep by the need to urinate. The absence of nocturia, in some instances, aids in excluding organic disease of the urinary tract. Thus, it is not uncommon for a patient to complain of severe diurnal frequency and deny nocturia; it is likely that such symptoms are functional in nature.

The causes of nocturia are many and may be classified as physiologic, psychologic, urologic, and those resulting from general systemic disease. In large part, the conditions already mentioned as producing diurnal frequency cause nocturia also.

Patients frequently fail to realize that large intake of fluids results in large output of fluids. Nocturia can be expected if large amounts of fluids, particularly a diuretic agent such as coffee, are ingested during late evening hours. Similarly, a hearty meal before retiring may produce nocturia, inasmuch as the greater portion of food eaten is converted to fluids and must be excreted by the kidneys. It is not unusual for patients to state that they drink a liberal amount of water each time they are awakened by the necessity for urination; this serves to aggravate the situation.

Nocturia may occur in high-strung, tense, or neurotic persons as a manifestation of their emotional instability. They sleep poorly and are awakened by sensations of vesical distention which ordinarily would not affect more stable persons. Some experience nocturia on the basis of habit. The infant and childhood habit of urinating during the night may be carried into adult life. Persons who have suffered from enuresis are likely to experience nocturia; in an effort to prevent enuresis they have acquired the habit of nocturia. Likewise, the habitual nature of nocturia may be acquired and carried over from past illness.

Organic diseases of the urinary tract already listed as the causes of diurnal frequency also produce nocturia. Diurnal frequency and nocturia are intimately related, and it is most unusual for organic disease of the urinary tract to produce one in the absence of the other.

Generalized systemic diseases which already have been discussed as causes of diurnal frequency may also be responsible for nocturia. In patients with cardiac disease, one of the first signs of decompensation is nocturia that consists of elimination of the manifest or subclinical edema which appeared during the day. Because of the recumbent position during sleep, the venous and capillary pressures in the lower extremities are diminished and cardiac efficiency is improved. These factors reverse the process of edema formation which occurred during the day, and lead to resorption of fluid into the bloodstream and its excretion as urine during the night.

**Alterations of the Urinary Stream.** Alterations of the urinary stream are a common complaint, particularly among men. The alteration may take the form of decreased caliber of the stream with loss of normal trajectory and difficulty in emptying the bladder. It may consist of interruption of the stream or delay in initiating urination, referred to as "hesitancy." In some instances, urgency of urination rather than hesitancy may be noted.

Such alterations of the urinary stream usually are due to obstruction at a site between the vesical neck and the external urethral meatus. The nature of the obstruction may be congenital obstruction of the vesical neck, urethral valves, carcinoma or benign hyperplasia of the prostate gland, urethral stricture or carcinoma, congenital obstruction of the external meatus, or phimosis. Inflammatory disease of the bladder, prostate, or urethra, usually of bacterial origin, may alter the urinary stream. In addition, vesical neoplasms and diverticula, ureterocele, vesical and urethral calculi, urethral diverticula, cystocele, and neurogenic vesical dysfunction may result in changes in the urinary stream.

Before dismissing this subject, it must be pointed out that, normally, wide variation in the caliber of the urinary stream exists. Some persons are perturbed needlessly by the fact that their normal, narrow urinary stream is not as broad and forceful as they believe it should be. It is usually sufficient simply to reassure such persons that their stream has normal characteristics.

**Incontinence.** "Urinary incontinence," a term used broadly to indicate involuntary loss of urine, may assume a variety of forms. Detailed description of the nature of incontinence is necessary for proper evaluation of this symptom. For practical purposes, urinary incontinence may be divided into active and passive incontinence. Active incontinence implies that the patient is aware that he is going to lose urine but is unable to prevent such loss. Passive incontinence, on the other hand, implies that the patient is not aware of the loss of urine until it has occurred.

The most common form of active incontinence is stress incontinence. This symptom is experienced most frequently by middle-aged or elderly women who have borne children. They are aware that such efforts as straining, coughing, sneezing, or, in severe cases, walking, result in escape of varying amounts of urine. The incontinence results from weakness of the pelvic and perineal muscles secondary to trauma of childbirth or its attendant surgical procedures and to the aging process; cystocele is common in this group of patients. This form of incontinence, however, is not uncommon in nulliparous women. A similar form of incontinence may be noted by men as a result of injury to the external urethral sphincter following prostatic surgical procedures.

Precipitate or urgency incontinence is another common form of active incontinence. In this type, the patient is aware of an urgent need to urinate but is unable to prevent premature escape of urine; the interval between realization of the need to urinate and involuntary onset of urination is too brief to permit him to make necessary arrangements for urination. This form of incontinence is noted most frequently by patients afflicted with bacterial or abacterial inflammatory disease of the bladder, prostate, or urethra, but it may also occur in cases of benign prostatic hyperplasia or carcinoma of the prostate with or without residual urine. Precipitate urination may be a prominent feature of neurogenic bladder dysfunction.

Passive incontinence implies that the patient realizes that he is incontinent only by noting that his underclothing or perineum is wet; therefore, he is incapable of preventing loss of urine. A typical example of this form of incontinence occurs in patients with vesicovaginal or ureterovaginal fistulas. Congenital anomalies, such as exstrophy of the bladder, epispadias, and ectopic opening of a ureter in the urethra or vestibule, are associated with this type of incontinence. Passive incontinence may occur in the presence of large cystoceles or in instances in which the muscles of the urinary sphincters have been damaged. Patients who have large amounts of residual urine as a result of obstruction at the vesical neck may note incontinence of this type; in such instances it is referred to as "overflow incontinence." The onset of enuresis late in life should lead one to suspect large amounts of residual urine and overflow incontinence. Passive incontinence may accompany neurogenic bladder dysfunction and hysteria.

In each instance of urinary incontinence, it is wise to question the patient concerning other bodily functions served by the same or adjacent neural segments. Information concerning changes in bowel or sexual activity or movements of the lower extremities should be obtained.

It is apparent that knowing a patient experiences urinary incontinence is insufficient. Information concerning the characteristics of the incontinence—its onset, duration, constancy, degree, relation to other bodily functions, and other urinary signs and symptoms—must be gained if one is to evaluate this symptom properly. Such evaluation aids in determining the etiology of incontinence.

**Enuresis.** After the age of 5, persistent bedwetting during sleep is referred to as enuresis; it is probably the most common complaint related to the urinary tract in children; approximately 15% of 5-year-olds, 5% of 10-year-olds, and 1% of 15-year-olds experience enuresis. It was previously thought that emotional disorders, social maladjustment, and urinary tract obstruction were the prime causes of enuresis. However, it now appears that while this may be true of secondary enuresis, primary enuresis is more likely to be caused by a maturational lag of the CNS in the majority of patients and will resolve with time. It should be remembered that a small percentage of enuretic children may have significant urologic pathology unassociated with other urinary symptoms such as infection, neurogenic bladder, posterior urethral valves or distal urethral stenosis, and will need further diagnostic evaluation.

**Acute Retention.** Acute retention of urine indicates complete inability to urinate. Although acute retention of urine may occur at any site in the urinary tract, by common usage the term is reserved for complete retention of urine in the bladder. It is necessary to distinguish acute retention of urine from anuria; in each condition, the patient is unable to urinate. In the former condition, urine which is present in the bladder cannot be expelled; in the latter, the patient's inability to urinate results from absence of urine in the bladder. Chronic retention of urine, a less dramatic but more insidious form of retention, is discussed later.

Acute retention of urine occurs most frequently in patients with prostatism and often follows surgical procedures, particularly those involving abdominal viscera or major orthopedic procedures. Patients with benign prostatic hyperplasia generally experience obstructive urinary symptoms of increasing severity; acute retention supervenes without obvious cause, or following ingestion of cold remedies containing an α-agonist or other medications that impair bladder contractility; following ingestion of alcohol, or after exposure to cold. Patients suffering from carcinoma of the prostate may experience progressive symptoms, as related previously, but not infrequently, acute retention of urine may be the first urinary symptom which such patients note. Acute inflammatory disease of the prostate gland, such as acute prostatitis or prostatic abscess, may also produce acute retention of urine.

Acute urinary retention during the postoperative period is often due to the depressant effect of anesthetic drugs, recumbency, and the patient's failure to use the accessory muscles of urination because of the pain secondary to surgical incisions. Prostatic obstruction, which may have been subclinical before operation, may become obvious during the postoperative period. This is especially common after surgical attack on the sigmoid and rectum, in which a certain amount of pericystitis probably interferes with the proper function of the detrusor muscle. Urinary retention is common in neurogenic bladder dysfunction, following trauma to the bladder or urethra, and in cases of urethral stricture. Acute urinary retention may also be a manifestation of hysteria or psychoneurosis.

## Pain

Pain from disease of the urinary tract may be divided into local and referred pain. Local pain arising from stimulation of a nerve is perceived in the area which coincides with the distribution of the sensory fibers of that nerve. Referred pain, on the other hand, is appreciated in an area distant to its site of origin. Indeed, some of the most striking examples of referred pain are encountered in afflictions of the urinary tract; pain in the testicles due to renal calculus is common. With the exception of pain resulting from lesions of the external genitalia, most pain arising from the urinary tract is referred.

**Renal Pain.** The sensory nerve fibers to the kidneys arise from the tenth, eleventh, and twelfth thoracic and the first lumbar segments of the spinal cord supply. The renal capsule and perirenal tissue possess nerve terminals of cerebrospinal origin; the pelvis and ureter have sensory sympathetic fibers. The renal parenchyma is insensitive and may be cut, irritated, and stimulated in any manner without production of pain. However, tension on the renal capsule, pelvis, or ureter results in pain.

Pain due to renal disease may manifest itself as a dull continuous ache or sharp, intermittent colic. The dull ache of renal origin is felt in the costovertebral angle and flank. This pain results from stretching of the renal capsule such as may occur as a result of inflammatory renal disease, hydronephrosis, cyst, or neoplasm. Similar pain may be noted in the presence of calculi in the pelvis or calyces when stretching of the capsule has not occurred. Renal colic is sharp or cutting pain which starts in the costovertebral angle and extends downward along the course of the ureter; pain of this type is indicative of disease of the pelvis or ureter. Pain from renal disease may be felt at a site distant from the kidney, inasmuch as the sensory nerves of almost the entire surface of the body below the level of the diaphragm are centered in the tenth, eleventh, and twelfth thoracic and first lumbar segments of the spinal cord; as noted previously, the sensory innervation of the kidneys is similar. The testicles and labia likewise are innervated from the eleventh and twelfth thoracic segments and a few cerebrospinal fibers from the genitocrural nerve. Similarity of nerve supply of kidneys and the genitalia accounts for the association of renal colic with pain in the testicles in men and in the labia in women.

**Ureteral Pain.** The sensory nerve supply of the upper portion of the ureters is similar to that of the kidneys, and pain arising from disease of that portion of the ureters is similar to renal pain. It is impossible to dissociate renal and ureteral pain, inasmuch as ureteral disease frequently results in some degree of obstruction of the lumen, which has an effect on the ipsilateral renal pelvis and kidney. The lower portion of the ureter receives sensory fibers from the inferior mesenteric, spermatic (ovarian), and hypogastric plexuses. Pain arising from that portion of the ureter is referred to the cerebrospinal nerves which originate from similar segments of the spinal cord and is perceived in the bladder, vulva, penis, scrotum, or perineum.

**Vesical Pain.** The bladder is supplied with parasympathetic fibers which arise from the second, third, and fourth sacral segments and form the nervi erigentes (pelvic nerves) and with sympathetic fibers which arise from the presacral nerve. Pain arising from the bladder may be referred to branches of the cerebrospinal nerves which innervate the bladder, or to the cerebrospinal nerves which originate from similar segments of the spinal cord as the sympathetic nerves. Vesical pain is usually associated with micturition. A constant ache may be noted behind the symphysis, or the pain may be referred to the urethra, penis, or groin. Pain arising from disease of the trigone, urethra, or lower portion of a ureter is commonly referred to the head of the penis.

**Testicular and Epididymal Pain.** The testicles receive sympathetic sensory fibers from the eleventh and twelfth thoracic segments of the spinal cord and a few cerebrospinal fibers from the genital branch of the genitocrural nerve. Testicular parenchyma is insensitive, whereas the testicular tunics are sensitive to cutting, pulling, or squeezing. Mild pain arising from disease of the testicles or epididymis remains localized; severe pain commonly is referred to the inguinal region, to the inner aspect of the thigh, or to the lumbar or iliolumbar regions.

**Prostatic and Seminal Vesicular Pain.** Some sensory nerve fibers to the prostate originate in the eleventh and twelfth thoracic segments; the majority, however, originate in the third and fourth sacral segments of the spinal cord. The plexus of nerves about the prostate and seminal vesicles has free anastomosis with the hemorrhoidal, cavernous, hypogastric, and vesical plexuses. Consequently, pain arising from disease of these structures may be noted in the back, flank, lower part of the abdomen, perineum, or external genitalia. The close relationship between the roots of the nerves to the prostate and seminal vesicles and those of the lumbar and sacral plexuses accounts for referral of pain to the perineum and down the legs.

## Related Symptoms and Signs

**Residual Urine.** A normal bladder expels its contents completely. In disease states, variable amounts of urine may be retained in the bladder after the patient presumably has emptied it. Initially, the detrusor muscle responds to the presence of obstruction by hypertrophy to effect emptying of the bladder. If the obstruction continues, eventually the muscle is no longer able to empty the bladder; this increasing incompetence leads to residual urine, a situation analogous to the appearance of edema due to a decompensated heart. Thus, a direct measure of this decompensation is the amount of residual urine present in the bladder after voiding; volumes as great as 3,000 or 4,000 mL may be detected.

From a practical point of view, it has been the custom in most instances to overlook 60 mL or less of residual urine; the presence of larger amounts has been considered significant and worthy of further investigation and treatment. However, this is not based on good scientific or experimental evidence. Mathematical studies on the effect of the voiding mechanism alone on elimination of bacteria from the bladder have produced a formula that relates the initial and final bacterial populations to voiding intervals, bacteria doubling time, and urinary volume. By such calculations, a significant residual urine, ie, the amount that would just maintain a given infection at whatever level it is established, is 4.8 mL in a person voiding 300 mL every 3 hours. Normal residual urine is calculated to be less than 2.5 mL if intrinsic vesical defense mechanisms are not operating.

Many methods have been described for the determination of residual urine. The quantity can be determined by catheterization immediately after the patient empties the bladder. Other methods include evaluation by means of a postvoiding film as a part of the excretory urographic study or bladder ultrasound.

Urethral catheterization, the most common means of diagnosing residual urine, carries the possibility of introducing infection into the obstructed bladder, despite elaborate preventive precautions. Catheterization for this purpose is done infrequently, especially as an office procedure, and is best deferred until the patient enters the hospital, so that if a significant amount of residual urine is found, the catheter may be left in the bladder. Another disadvantage of the use of catheterization to measure residual urine—especially important in children—is that it merely measures the volume of urine left in the urinary tract after voiding. In instances in which significant vesicoureteral reflux is present, the refluxing urine returning to the bladder at the end of voiding may be measured as simple residual urine and be assumed to be the result of vesical neck obstruction. Therefore, therapeutic considerations in such a case may be misdirected to the vesical neck rather than to the ureterovesical junction.

The amount of residual urine can be estimated from the postvoiding film (a roentgenogram of the bladder obtained immediately after voiding and after the conventional series of excretory urographic studies is completed). However, the results may be misleading (1) if the patient has recently emptied the bladder and the bladder is not comfortably full for effective emptying or (2) if he is asked to urinate while lying in a recumbent position on the x-ray table. Furthermore, although useful, such estimates are at best inaccurate, because one is attempting to determine from measurements in only two dimensions.

Another rough estimate of residual urine may be obtained by ultrasonographic measurement of the bladder volume by using the formula (0.625 h × w × d). This appears to be a reasonably accurate measurement and is an easy, noninvasive procedure.

Residual urine should be regarded as a complication of obstruction of urinary outflow. The most frequent lesions that may result in residual urine are benign prostatic hyperplasia, carcinoma of the prostate gland, contracture and hyperplasia of the vesical neck, posterior urethral valves, and acute inflammatory disease of the prostate gland. Neurogenic vesical dysfunction commonly is associated with residual urine. Urethral obstruction does not, as a rule, result in residual urine unless extreme decompensation of the vesical musculature is present. In this condition, the patient usually empties the bladder completely; the presence of residual urine indicates additional obstruction at the vesical neck.

In the past, anuria, shock, and severe hemorrhage from the bladder have been ascribed to rapid decompression of a bladder distended with urine. Sufficient data have been accumulated to dispel this notion, but, from a practical viewpoint, little is gained from rapid decompression and gradual decompression is preferable. The severe postobstructive diuresis observed following rapid decompression can be controlled with intravenous (IV) fluids but can also be controlled by gradual decompression (200–300 $cm^3/h$) when good medical monitoring and IV hydration are not possible.

Most patients who have residual urine are aware of its presence because urination does not provide complete relief. Yet, there is no strict correlation between the amount of residual urine and the patient's symptoms. Similarly there is no correlation between the amount of residual urine and the nature of the obstructive lesion or of the degree of the obstruction. Chronic retention—the persistent presence of significant amounts of residual urine—may occur without the patient's knowledge. This is particularly insidious, sometimes leading to advanced uremia before its presence is detected.

**Anuria.** Anuria, the arrest of urinary output, may be classified into prerenal, renal, and postrenal types. Prerenal anuria may result from severe hypotension, congestive heart failure, thrombosis of renal vessels, and severe dehydration. Renal anuria can be produced by marked inflammatory disease of the kidneys and by toxic action of certain agents on the kidneys. Included in the latter category are such poisons as bichloride of mercury, bismuth, acetylated sulfonamide crystals, and products of mismatched transfusion. In addition, the syndrome that occurs following extensive burns or crush injuries may be placed in this group. Renal degeneration secondary to cystic disease and calculi may result in renal anuria. Postrenal anuria results from obstruction of the excretory passages of the upper part of the urinary tract. Bilateral ureteral calculi and obstructions of each ureter from extraurinary tumors are examples of conditions which may produce postrenal anuria.

**Azotemia and Uremia.** Azotemia denotes a mild degree of renal insufficiency, and there is little evidence to suggest that, in itself, it is deleterious. When azotemia becomes profound, the syndrome of uremia is likely to appear. "Uremia" identifies a complex clinical picture resulting from the failure of renal function; the term literally means "urine in the blood." Its cause remains unknown. At first, urea itself was implicated as the cause of uremia, but it now is generally agreed that an increased blood urea level does not in itself produce uremic symptoms. Numerous other metabolites have also been suspected to be the sole uremic toxin, but no single agent can be shown to account for all aspects of the clinical presentation of uremia; it is more likely that there are multiple substances playing a pathologic role in the production of the uremic syndrome.

Symptoms resulting from uremia are many; deranged renal excretory and regulatory functions may be responsible for loss as well as retention of electrolytes, water, and other substances. In addition, gastrointestinal, neuromuscular, and cardiovascular disturbances may occur. Among such clinical manifestations, those in the gastrointestinal tract are most important. Anorexia and vomiting are common in patients with uremia; occasionally, the latter may result in severe deficits of both sodium and potassium. Even though constipation may be common, diarrhea, often bloody, may occur—especially in patients with terminal stages of renal disease—due to mucosal congestion and ulceration. Neuromuscular manifestations also are common. Mental disturbances, with drowsiness intermingled with profound restlessness, may progress to lethargy and an extreme inability to concentrate; occasionally, delusions may occur, together with auditory and visual hallucinations. Some patients exhibit evidence of peripheral neuritis. Among the cardiopulmonary manifestations, pericarditis is the most characteristic and occurs in a large percentage of patients who die of uremia.

## PHYSICAL EXAMINATION

Complete and careful physical examination of the urologic patient is an absolute necessity. The results of such examination may not only indicate the nature of the urologic disease—and perhaps its extent and severity—but also may be decisive in determining the nature and mode of treatment.

### Inspection

The general appearance of the patient is important. Dry skin and coated tongue may result from dehydration; apathy, ammonia breath, and excoriations of the skin due to scratching suggest serious renal impairment. Study of bodily physique may suggest hypogonadism. Visible congenital abnormalities may indicate disease of the urinary tract (for example, congenital absence of abdominal musculature is associated almost invariably with disease of the urinary tract). Low-set ears with an abnormal fold at the top of the helix may be associated with urogenital anomalies. Similarly, acquired disease of neurogenic origin which produces visible defects may also affect the urinary tract; tabes dorsalis is an example of such disease.

Benign or malignant renal tumors may produce a visible bulge in the flank or abdomen, particularly in children or thin adults. The superficial veins of the abdomen may become dilated and clearly visible as a result of partial occlusion of the inferior vena cava due to local spread of renal neoplasms. Lagging respiration may be noted on the involved side in cases of severe perinephritis.

Inspection of the lower portion of the abdomen may disclose such congenital abnormalities as exstrophy of the bladder, patent urachus, and congenital absence of abdominal musculature. The distended bladder may be clearly visualized as an ovoid swelling situated above the pubic symphysis.

Examination of the external genitalia discloses the size and development of the penis or clitoris and may reveal various congenital anomalies such as hypospadias, epispadias, pseudohermaphroditism, hypogonadism, phimosis, stenosis of the external urethral meatus, and ectopic ureteral orifice in women. The presence and pattern of pubic hair are noted. Inflammatory lesions of the genitals, such as fistula, chancre, chancroid, balanitis, balanoposthitis, lymphopathia venereum, caruncle, urethritis, and lymphangitis, may be visible. Similarly, benign and malignant tumors of the penis or urethra may be noted.

Enlargement of the scrotum due to inflammatory lesions or to benign and malignant tumors of the testes or epididymis may be seen. An effort should be made to transilluminate all scrotal masses. This is carried out in a darkened room by placing a strong beam of light under the posterior aspect of the scrotum and examining the anterior aspect. A mass that transmits light is cystic and indicates a hydrocele or spermatocele; a hydrocele with a thick, fibrous sac and hematocele, however, may fail to transmit light. A varicocele may be visible to inspection.

### Palpation

**Kidneys.** Palpation of the kidneys is performed by placing the patient on a table in supine position with his legs drawn up to relax his abdominal muscles. The examiner stands by the patient's side and places one hand posteriorly with the fingers situated in the angle formed by the costal margin and the lumbar muscles. The other hand is placed just external to the linea semilunaris with the tips of the fingers just beneath the ribs. Gentle but firm pressure is exerted with both hands while the patient breathes slowly and deeply. At times a kidney may be palpable more readily if the patient lies in a lateral decubitus; rarely, a sitting position is best. Sharp percussion over the costolumbar angle may elicit tenderness caused by an inflamed kidney.

A kidney of normal size can be palpated in exceedingly thin patients; in such instances the lower pole of the kidney can be grasped between the hands of the examiner. Ptosis of a kidney likewise permits palpation of a kidney normal in size. The likelihood of palpating a diseased kidney depends on the size of the kidney, the obesity of the patient, and the degree of relaxation of the abdominal wall. It is usually difficult, by palpation alone, to determine the cause of enlargement of a kidney. Palpable enlargement of a kidney may occur as a result of hydronephrosis, solitary or multiple renal cysts, polycystic disease, and benign and malignant renal neoplasms.

**Bladder.** A distended bladder may be palpated as a smooth globular mass in the hypogastric region. Pressure exerted over the bladder in such instances may impart to the patient the desire for urination; pain may be noted if cystitis is present. Retention of urine may be recognized by percussion when the bladder is not sufficiently distended to permit palpation. Extravesical extension of neoplasms of the bladder to the abdominal wall may be palpable. More satisfactory palpation of the bladder can be carried out by bimanual examination as described later.

**External Genitalia.** Careful palpation of the glans penis, corpora cavernosa, and corpus spongiosum should be carried out. A fibrous plaque which produces deformity of the erect penis may be noted. The plaque is situated in the sheath of the corpus cavernosum but may involve the body of the corpus or the septum between the corpora. Thickening of the corpus spongiosum may indicate recent or ancient urethritis, periurethritis, or urethral stricture. Urethral diverticulum, represented by a soft fluctuant mass, may be noted in relation to the urethra. A milking motion of the finger along the urethra toward the external meatus may express urine or pus retained in the diverticulum. A calculus in the urethra may be palpable.

The testes may fail to descend or their descent may be incomplete so that they lie within the abdomen or in the inguinal region. The presence of this abnormality, which may be unilateral or bilateral, can be determined by palpation.

In addition to position, the size, shape, and consistency of each testis should be determined. The normal testicle is ovoid, smooth, tense, and tender to pressure. Decrease in size may result from orchitis due to mumps or hypogonadism, or from interference with blood supply to the testis during herniorrhaphy. Chronic enlargement of a testicle is due to malignant or benign tumor, tuberculosis, gumma, or chronic infection. Malignant tumors are insensitive or slightly sensitive, irregular, and firm or hard with areas of softening. Bilateral testicular tumors may occur in association with lymphosarcoma. Benign tumors are rare. Tuberculosis of a testicle is usually secondary to tuberculosis of the epididymis. Gummas of a testicle are characterized by woody hardness and excessive weight of the mass. In most instances, biopsy of the testis is necessary for correct diagnosis.

The normal epididymis lies posterior to the testicle and is flaccid and slightly sensitive to palpation. When acutely inflamed, the epididymis becomes thickened, tense, and exquisitely tender and fits over the posterior portion of the testicle like a crescent-shaped helmet. In fulminating infections, edema of the scrotum, extreme tenderness, and inflammatory hydrocele prevent differentiation of epididymis from testicle by palpation. Acute epididymitis due to nonspecific infections is usually rapid in onset, produces severe pain and tenderness, and is self-limited unless abscess formation occurs. Tuberculous epididymitis is slower in onset, mildly painful and tender, and chronic in nature. In this disease, the epididymis is usually irregularly enlarged, indurated, and nodular and usually can be distinctly differentiated from the testicle. Sinuses to the skin of the scrotum and involvement of the testicle by the tuberculous process are not uncommon.

The vas deferens is smooth and cordlike. It may become thickened, rigid, and inelastic as a result of nonspecific chronic infection. Scattered discrete nodules may be palpable if the vas is affected by tuberculosis.

Hydrocele of the testis surrounds the organ (except posteriorly), is painless, tense, or flaccid, and usually transmits light. A globular, translucent mass just above, but distinctly separate from the testis, is a spermatocele. A spindle-shaped elastic mass along the spermatic cord represents a hydrocele of the cord. The descriptive phase applied to varicocele is ''bag of worms.''

**Digital Rectal Examination.** For digital rectal examination, the patient kneels on the step of an examining table and rests his body on the table. Examiners with short index fingers prefer placing the patient in lithotomy position. The examiner's gloved finger and the patient's anus and surrounding hair should be thoroughly lubricated; adequate lubrication renders the examination less painful. The finger is introduced slowly into the anus and the tone of the anal sphincter is noted; increases or decreases in tone may result from neurogenic lesions, inflammatory diseases of the anus, or surgical treatment of disease of the anus.

The index finger is inserted into the rectum and the perineum is grasped between thumb and finger. The normal perineum is thick, smooth, and resistant. In men the bulbomembranous glands (Cowper's), if enlarged or indurated, may be palpable in the perineum on either side of the urethra. The finger is inserted higher and passes over the prostate gland. The normal prostate is flat, movable, heart-shaped, and mildly sensitive and presents a notch in its upper border and a barely perceptible groove down the center separating the lateral lobes. Acute inflammation results in enlargement, extreme tenderness, loss of normal configuration, and a sense of heat imparted to the finger. In benign hyperplasia the prostate is enlarged, broad, and flat or bulges into the rectum. The finger may not reach the upper border, but the lateral borders usually can be discerned; the gland is movable, soft or firm, and relatively nontender.

Hardness of the prostate may result from carcinoma, tuberculosis, calculi, chronic infection (particularly granulomatous prostatitis), and sarcoma. In early stages of carcinoma the prostate is nodular and not greatly enlarged; only one nodule may be present. In late cases the gland is irregular in outline, enlarged, brawny, and fixed to surrounding tissues. Often the induration extends well above the prostate and involves the seminal vesicles.

In tuberculosis the gland is normal in size or only moderately enlarged; irregularity of outline and scattered nodular areas are common. The seminal vesicles are frequently enlarged and indurated. Evidence of tuberculosis of the kidneys or epididymis aids in diagnosis. Prostatic calculi usually produce an isolated area of hardness in the prostate gland, without striking irregularity in outline of the gland. On the other hand, numerous calculi or marked associated infection may cause the entire gland to feel hard to palpation. Occasionally, friction of one calculus against another during palpation may impart the sensation of crepitus. Roentgenologic studies of the prostatic area aid in diagnosis.

Digital rectal findings noted in chronic infection of the prostate, or following prostatic surgical procedures, may be similar to findings noted in carcinoma of the prostate gland. In the former instances, however, the general configuration and outline of the gland are maintained and the presence of irregular nodules is unusual. Sarcoma of the prostate usually is associated with extreme enlargement of the gland, which may be hard or soft.

Normal seminal vesicles cannot be palpated by digital rectal examination. Distended seminal vesicles are soft, compressible, saclike structures which extend upward and outward from the base of the prostate. Induration and nodularity of the seminal vesicles occur in tuberculosis. The vesicles frequently are involved by local spread of prostatic carcinoma.

Digital rectal examination is concluded by sweeping the finger about the walls of the rectum while the patient strains. This maneuver occasionally results in detection of masses situated at a higher site in the rectum than can be detected otherwise. After its removal, the finger is examined for blood.

**Rectoabdominal Palpation.** Bimanual rectoabdominal palpation is performed in men chiefly for the purpose of determining extent of infiltration of the wall of the bladder or surrounding tissues by vesical carcinoma. Information gained from this examination may aid in deciding whether the carcinoma can be excised. The patient is anesthetized for this procedure, which usually is adjunctive to cystoscopy; following conclusion of cystoscopy the anesthesia is maintained for rectoabdominal palpation.

The examiner's finger is inserted into the rectum and the opposite hand exerts firm pressure in the hypogastrium, pushing toward the finger in the rectum. The latter palpates the prostate, seminal vesicles, and base and a portion of the posterior wall of the bladder. The abdominal hand next exerts pressure deep in the lower quadrants, enabling the rectal finger to explore the lateral walls of the bladder. A mass or fixation of extravesical tissues that can be detected between the hand and the finger usually indicates extension of carcinoma beyond the wall of the bladder. Inflammation adjacent to a vesical neoplasm may be interpreted erroneously to indicate local spread of neoplasm.

Bimanual vaginoabdominal examination can be carried out in a similar manner and for similar purposes. In addition, vaginal examination may disclose induration and thickening of the urethra in urethritis, urethral diverticulum, tenderness of the bladder in cystitis, and vesical or ureteral stone if it is situated low in the ureter.

## AUSCULTATION

Careful auscultation over the upper quadrants of the abdomen or lumbar regions may provide the first clue to the presence of vascular changes in the renal arteries or in the kidney itself. Vascular bruits are detected in the majority of patients with idiopathic fibrous and fibromuscular stenosis of the renal arteries associated with hypertension. In these cases, the characteristic bruit has an unusually high frequency in contrast to the lower frequency bruits usually noted with atheromatous lesions of the abdominal aorta. These bruits are continuous, or almost continuous, with accentuation occurring during systole. Traumatic or malignant arteriovenous fistulas in the renal region may be associated with bruits. In some cases of hypernephroma, a bruit may be audible on careful auscultation, presumably as the result of dilated sinuses within the tumor itself.

## UROLOGIC DIAGNOSIS IN CHILDREN

The spectrum of urologic disease in children is quite different from that in adults and warrants separate consideration. Congenital defects such as exstrophy of the bladder, penile chordee, and undescended testicles are obvious. But in other instances, the clinical picture may be obscured, and prolonged investigation is necessary before the exact diagnosis is made.

Urinary infection is one of the most common complaints associated with the urinary tract and occurs at least 10 times more frequently in female than in male children except during the first year of life, when it occurs more frequently in boys. The presentation is by no means stereotyped. Until the infant is 2 years of age, urinary tract infection may be responsible for feeding problems, failure to gain weight, fever, and convulsions. In children of preschool age, nondescript symptoms such as irritability, listlessness, vague abdominal pain, crying, and straining during urination are noted. Approximately two thirds of boys and one third of girls with urinary tract infections have an underlying urologic abnormality. Therefore, all children with symptomatic urinary infection should be evaluated.

Obstruction in the urinary tract is much more common in male than in female children, especially during the first year of life. Such obstruction may occur at any level from the ureteropelvic junction to the external urethral meatus. Ureteropelvic obstruction frequently causes symptoms of vague abdominal pain, vomiting, and nausea simulating gastrointestinal disease; infection of urine is fairly uncommon in such instances, unless vesicoureteral reflux also is present. Hematuria is common in hydronephrosis and may be the result of variations in intrapelvic pressure in the kidney, leading to rupture of blood vessels; it should also be stressed that approximately one third of children with malignancies in the urinary tract also have hematuria. Abdominal masses accidentally discovered are common presentations of pathologic conditions in the upper urinary tract. In the first 6 months of life, such masses are likely to be cystic, whereas after that a palpable renal or adrenal mass is more likely to be the result of tumor than of hydronephrosis. Large renal swellings tend to be silent and cystic and have all the characteristic findings of kidney enlargement in the adult. Renal tumors tend to develop more anteriorly than posteriorly; neuroblastomas of adrenal origin are deep-seated and rarely mobile. However, on palpation in the young infant, the kidney usually is situated low and is readily palpable, and the lobulation frequently present creates a confusing clinical picture. In the first 2 or 3 weeks of life, renal or adrenal masses which are readily palpable in an unstable child should suggest the possibility of renal vein thrombosis or adrenal hematoma.

In a child the bladder is an abdominal organ. Therefore, palpation of a painless distention is of no value unless the child has recently voided. If retention of urine has been confirmed, it may be the result of ulceration of the urethral meatus, concentrated urine with oxaluria, vesical diverticula, or impacted urethral calculus.

Acute urinary retention in the neonate may result from obliteration of the urethral lumen by a mucous plug, chronic retention or overflow incontinence from urethral valves in the male child, ectopic ureterocele, or neurogenic bladder dysfunction. In the young child, prostatic tumors also tend to cause chronic urinary retention and infection, whereas bladder tumors, since they are submucosal, rarely produce hematuria until ulceration and penetration of the mucosa have taken place.

Urinary incontinence in a child is a frequent complaint; in such situations a carefully taken history is of greater value than a complete urologic examination. In infants, of course, it is normal to have incontinence with regular periodic micturition with good stream. Therefore, it is important to ascertain how and when the incontinence occurred. Urgency incontinence usually is seen in the female child, the child usually being unable to restrain herself after the first sensation of bladder fullness. Dribbling incontinence results from overflow with chronic retention, neurogenic bladder in children usually secondary to myelodysplasia, or an ectopic ureter situated outside the sphincteric mechanism of the bladder. Giggle incontinence, which occurs only during periods of laughter, is an important diagnostic consideration in that it will spontaneously disappear with age and no treatment is necessary.

Other congenital anomalies may be associated with anomalies in the urinary tract; this is particularly true in those born with imperforate anus and tracheoesophageal fistula or absence of abdominal muscles.

## LABORATORY PROCEDURES

### Studies of Urine

**Routine Urinalysis** Urinalysis is necessary in the study of each urologic patient and should include (1) determination of specific gravity, osmolality, and pH; (2) studies to detect the presence of protein and reducing substances; and (3) microscopic examination for casts (cylindruria), leukocytes, erythrocytes, bacteria, and parasites.

The relationship of specific gravity to osmolality must be appreciated. The former is the measurement by which ability to concentrate the urine is routinely made in clinical settings. In most instances, it reflects osmolality fairly well. However, since specific gravity is a function of the density (weight of urine per milliliter) and osmolality reflects the number of osmotically active molecules or ions in a solution, there may be considerable difference between the two measurements in a given urine. Nonetheless, from a practical standpoint, careful determination of the urine specific gravity is one of the most important methods of assessing renal function. Clearly, the finding of a high specific gravity is strong evidence against the presence of renal insufficiency.

Since the advent of chemotherapy and antibiotic therapy, determination of urinary pH has assumed greater importance because the pH influences the efficacy of certain therapeutic agents; for example, certain sulfonamides are more effective in the presence of an alkaline rather than an acidic urine. The pH of the urine is a reflection of the ability of the kidney to maintain normal hydrogen-ion concentration in plasma and extracellular fluid. Determination of the pH is important in such conditions as hyperaldosteronism, renal tubular acidosis, metabolic alkalosis, and respiratory acidosis. The pH may be determined by simple colorimetric methods; use of sodium dinitrophenylazonaphthol disulfonate (Nitrazine paper) is a satisfactory method. The normal pH range is 4.8 to 7.5.

The dip-stick test is the easiest and most convenient method available for determining the presence of protein in the urine. However, false-positive results can occur with concentrated urine containing numerous erythrocytes, leukocytes, or vaginal secretions. Normal urine contains a small amount of protein, although the normal glomerulus for the most part bars the passage of albumin and larger plasma proteins from plasma to the glomerular filtrate. The concentration of protein in normal urine at a normal flow rate is less than 80 mg/24 h. An increase to more than 150 mg/24 h is the result of increased glomerular filtration of protein caused by glomerular damage of some kind. The degree of proteinuria varies with the type of renal disease and with the severity of the disease process. Severe proteinuria is characteristically seen with the nephrotic syndrome. It also may be found in glomerulonephritis, lupus nephritis, amyloid disease, pyelonephritis, renal neoplasms, multiple myeloma, polycystic renal disease, and numerous other diseases.

Reducing substances occur in the urine in patients with diabetes mellitus, renal glycosuria, alkaptonuria, and other diseases.

Routine urinalysis is concluded with microscopic examination of the urinary sediment obtained by centrifugation. Urinary cast formation results from precipitation of protein in the tubular lumens. Hyaline casts reflect coagulated protein, which is present in small amounts in the normal glomerular filtrate; these casts therefore are seen in urine from normal persons. Desquamated tubular epithelium leukocytes and erythrocytes combine with tubular protein to form epithelial, white cell, or red cell casts. Casts may be dissolved by an alkaline urine; therefore, a fresh specimen is needed for accurate information regarding cylindruria.

The significance of erythrocyturia and pyuria can be determined only with a knowledge of the method of collection of the urine, as described below. Finally, bacteria and parasites may be noted in examinations of unstained sediments of urine.

Urinary dip-sticks can also be used to detect levels of sugar, acetone, protein, and blood by examining color changes of the various reagents impregnated on the dip-stick. In addition, by the nature of the color change, semiquantitative analysis can be accomplished. Reagent tablets have largely been replaced by reagent strips. The labor-saving strips are reliable when used with appropriate precautions.

### Bacteriologic Studies

***Collection of Urine.*** Proper collection of the urine is necessary to permit meaningful evaluation for erythrocyturia, pyuria, and bacteriuria. Since the cornerstone of diagnosis of infection of the urinary tract is the identification of significant bacteria in the urine, it is essential to consider the techniques for collection of adequate specimens of urine for microbiologic study. The elimination of contamination is much more difficult in females than in males because of the genital anatomy and the possibility of contamination of the specimen by bacteria which normally reside in the vagina or urethra. In the male it is sufficient to retract the foreskin, wash the glans penis with an antiseptic cleansing solution, and request the patient to void. Toward the termination of urination, a sterile container is inserted into the stream; the urine so collected is studied microscopically for pyuria, erythrocyturia, and bacteriuria, either by Gram stain, culture, or both.

Three techniques are available for collection of urine from females for microbiologic studies: catheterization, midstream clean-voided collection, and needle aspiration of the bladder. Although catheterization does not eliminate entirely the problem of contamination, since the catheter will pass through the urethra (and can carry contaminants with it), it is sufficiently sterile for all practical purposes. A positive culture from a catheterized specimen is significant, since uropathogens for the most part are not normal urethral inhabitants and, if present, suggest pathology.

The ideal way to obtain a clean-catch urine specimen from a woman or girl would be to place the patient in the dorsal lithotomy position on an examination or cystoscopic table, clean the perineum (with an antiseptic solution), and collect the midstream urine while holding the labia apart. Practically, this is rarely done, either because the patient is unable to void under such circumstances or because the time and personnel are not available. Most urine specimens are collected by the patient in the bathroom. This adds a significant source of error to the examination because under these circumstances most women add vaginal secretions to the specimen. In general, when a positive culture is obtained and there is doubt as to the source of the bacteria (vagina vs bladder), one may then obtain a catheterized specimen. Interestingly, a woman with uropathogens growing in the vaginal area is more likely to have a problem with urinary infections.

It is rarely necessary to collect a urine specimen suprapubically, but if circumstances require this procedure, then it should be done as follows. First, the patient should force fluids until the bladder is full. The site of the needle puncture is the midline between the symphysis pubis and the umbilicus and directly over the palpable bladder. Unfortunately, in the female the full bladder frequently is not palpable. In such patients one must rely on the observation that suprapubic pressure directly over the bladder causes the patient to have an unmistakable desire to urinate. The site for needle puncture is shaved and the skin is cleansed with an alcohol sponge. A cutaneous wheal is raised with local anesthetic injected through a 25-gauge needle. A 3.5″ 20-gauge needle is introduced through the anesthetized skin. The progress of the needle is arrested just below the skin within the anesthetized area and then, with a quick plunging action similar to any intramuscular injection, the needle is advanced into the bladder. After the needle has been introduced, a 20-mL syringe is used to aspirate 5 mL of urine for culture and 15 mL for centrifugation and urinalysis. The obturator is reintroduced into the needle and both needle and obturator are withdrawn. A small strip dressing is placed over the needle-entry site in the skin.

Urologists frequently use a variety of so-called glass tests. Examination of the separate specimens of fractional voiding is the basis of a simple but valuable test indicating the probable source of abnormal urinary constituents. There are many variations of the glass tests, but the three-glass test is the one most commonly used. The patient is asked to void, from a full bladder, 2 to 3 oz (60 to 90 mL) of urine into a glass; this specimen will contain washings from the urethra. A similar amount is then passed into a second glass; this specimen presumably contains no urethral debris but is a sample of the bladder urine. The prostate is then massaged and the patient voids into a third glass. This specimen will contain bladder urine and the added expressed prostatic secretions. Pyuria in the first glass only indicates urethritis. If pyuria is found in the third glass only, prostatitis is to be suspected. Pyuria or erythrocyturia in all three indicates a source above the bladder neck or, less commonly, a generalized involvement of the entire urinary tract.

***Methods.*** The vast expansion of the armamentarium for treatment of infections of the urinary tract has necessitated increased bacteriologic studies. Bacteria differ in their susceptibility to various drugs; in many instances, therefore, it is necessary to identify the infecting organism in order that the most effective drug may be prescribed.

Bacteriologic studies of the urine consist of microscopic examination of a properly stained smear of urinary sediment and inoculation of various culture media with urine. Gram's method of staining the urinary sediment is most convenient for rapid orientation as to the presence and type of organisms. Almost all infections of the urinary tract, with the notable exception of gonorrhea and tuberculosis, are produced by gram-negative bacilli or gram-positive cocci (Table 2), and many simple infections can be treated adequately on the basis of this information alone. When microscopic examination of a gram-stained smear of a properly collected, uncentrifuged specimen of urine discloses even a few bacteria, infection is indicated.

Cultures are used if further identification of the organism is necessary. Blood and eosin-methylene blue agar plates are streaked using a calibrated platinum-rhodium inoculating loop. With this technique, inoculation of urine onto media is rapid, quantitation may be possible, and isolated colonies may be picked for identification procedures and antimicrobial susceptibility testing.

As a result of an effort to avoid or to eliminate urethral catheterization, emphasis has been placed on the bacterial content of a clean-voided specimen of urine. Quantitative methods of culturing urine allow accurate bacteriologic analysis from both men and women without catheterization. When the urinary tract is infected, there usually are 100,000 organisms or more per milliliter of urine; a count of $<10,000$ organisms/mL signifies external contamination. Intermediate values should be interpreted with care, and the uncertainty in this range is best resolved with a repeat culture. It must be noted, however, that antimicrobial treatment, rapid urinary flow, and urine of high acidity tend to decrease the count, whereas delay in transit to the laboratory and improper methods of collection of urine tend to increase the count. It is imperative that the specimen of

**TABLE 2. Pathogenic Organisms**

| Gram-Negative Bacilli | Gram-Positive Cocci | Gram-Negative Cocci | Fungi |
|---|---|---|---|
| Enterobacteriaceae | | | |
| *Escherichia coli* | *Streptococcus agalactiae* (Lancefield's group B) | *Neisseria gonorrhoeae* | *Candida albicans* |
| *Shigella* | | | |
| *Edwardsiella* | | | |
| *Salmonella* | *Enterococcus faecalis, E faecium* (*S faecalis, S faecium*) | | |
| *Arizona* | *Staphylococcus aureus* | | |
| *Citrobacter* | *S epidermidis* | | |
| *Klebsiella* | | | |
| *Enterobacter* | | | |
| *Serratia* | | | |
| *Proteus* | | | |
| *Providence* | | | |
| Pseudomonadaceae | | | |
| *P aeruginosa* | | | |
| Other *Pseudomonas* species | | | |
| Acinetobacter | | | |
| *A lwoffi* | | | |
| *A anitratus* | | | |

urine be properly collected and that it be examined within 2 hours, unless it has been refrigerated.

By an appropriate combination of biochemical tests, the bacteriology laboratory should be able to provide group and, in some instances, species identification of at least 90% of urinary tract isolates within 48 hours of receipt of the specimen. It may be of clinical importance, for example, to differentiate between *Proteus mirabilis* and the other three *Proteus* species indole positive (*P vulgaris, P morganii,* and *P rettgeri*) because of the former's susceptibility to ampicillin. Similarly, *Klebsiella* is ordinarily susceptible to the cephalosporins while *Enterobacter* and *Serratia* are not. Differences in susceptibility between species within the enterococcal division are not significant, so that these organisms may simply be reported as Enterococcus. The staphylococci may be speciated readily on the basis of the coagulase test.

Exact identification of the infecting organism is necessary in proper management of infections of the urinary tract which fail to respond to therapy or which recur after therapy. Furthermore, it may be desirable to determine the sensitivity of the specific organism to various chemotherapeutic and antibiotic agents, because different strains of the same bacteria may exhibit different degrees of sensitivity. Antimicrobial susceptibility studies are generally performed by the disk diffusion method or by using dilution techniques in agar or broth containing varying concentrations of antibiotics.

Certain bacteria which are capable of producing infections of the urinary tract require special methods of culture. *Neisseria gonorrhoeae* appears as a gram-negative diplococcus and can be grown in chocolate-blood agar with excess carbon dioxide in the gas phase. *Brucella,* a small gram-negative bacillary or coccoid microorganism, may be grown on beef heart infusion-blood agar. Anaerobic bacteria have rarely been implicated in urinary tract infection, and their presence may be suggested by a combination of a positive gram stain of the urine with negative routine cultures. Cultures should then be made in freshly prepared thioglycollate medium and, ideally, on blood agar media which can be incubated anaerobically. The time between collection of the urine and inoculation of media is of the essence, because it is unlikely that most anaerobes will survive for more than an hour.

Proper management of infections of the urinary tract may require information concerning the ability of the infecting organism to hydrolyze urea. Certain bacteria, referred to as "urea splitters," have the capacity to convert urea into ammonia and carbon dioxide. As a result, in infections of the urinary tract due to these bacteria, the urine is persistently and intensely alkaline, which predisposes to formation of incrustations and urinary calculi. The ability of bacteria to split urea, by virtue of urease activity, can be determined by inoculating culture media containing urea with the suspected organism and noting production of ammonia by suitable colorimetric indicators. Bacteria which commonly demonstrate urease activity include *Proteus, Klebsiella, Enterobacter, Serratia, Citrobacter, Pseudomonas aeruginosa, Ureaplasma,* and *Acinetobacter anitratus*. The organism that produces the most urease is *P mirabilis*. It should be noted that *Escherichia coli* is not associated with urease production.

Infection may exist in the urinary tract in spite of failure to demonstrate bacteria in urinary sediment by staining or to grow bacteria in routine culture media. This should lead one to suspect tuberculosis, brucellosis, or a fungal etiology of the pyuria, especially since the incidence of opportunistic infections in the urinary tract has become more frequent due to the increased use of broad-spectrum antibiotics, chemotherapeutic agents, immunosuppressive agents and the increased incidence of AIDS. Of the fungi, *Candida albicans* is the most frequently encountered yeast in urine, but *Aspergillus fumigatus, Cryptococcus neoformans, Torulopsis glabrata,* and others may also be encountered. Although the data are not clear-cut, there is some weak evidence to suggest that cell-wall–deficient bacteria—L-forms, protoplasts, spheroplasts, or variants—may rarely be responsible for persistence or recrudescence of infection.

The diagnosis of tuberculosis depends on smears of urinary sediment stained for acid-fast bacilli, or culture for *Mycobacterium tuberculosis*. The use of acid-fast smears has decreased since a report that a smear containing acid-fast bacilli indicates merely that organisms having the size, shape, and staining reaction compatible with tubercle bacilli have been noted. Neither cultural features nor virulence of organisms can be determined by this method. Therefore, more commonly the diagnosis depends primarily on the positive urine culture. At least three successive, first-voided morning urine specimens should be obtained for culture when tuberculosis is suspected.

To culture urine for *M tuberculosis,* a large specimen of urine is concentrated and freed of nontuberculous organisms by chemicals; the sediment is inoculated into a suitable medium. The cultures are observed at weekly intervals and are not discarded as negative until 8 weeks have elapsed.

When one suspects that an infection is originating in the kidneys, it is sometimes difficult to confirm the renal source of significant bacteriuria. To aid in the detection of renal bacteriuria, one can look for antibody-coated bacteria.

Evidence suggests that while simple cystitis does not elicit antibody production, renal infection elicits an antibody response specific to the infecting microorganisms. These antibodies enter the urinary tract and coat the microorganisms, and this coating of bacteria can be detected. Theoretically, then, the presence of antibody-coated bacteria suggests the presence of upper tract infection.

However, antibody-coated bacteria may also be found in the urine of patients with neurogenic bladder, prostatitis, and chronic or recurrent cystitis, thus limiting its effectiveness. While both false-positive results (eg, from vaginal bacteria or prostatic species) and false-negative results (eg, if bacteria grow in the urine prior to processing, the antibody will be diluted out) are possible in this exam, it may possibly be useful in locating the site of origin of recurrent bacteriuria if ureteral and bladder specimens are collected separately.

***Office Bacteriology.*** A number of tests have been suggested for simple, rapid screening of patients to determine the presence of significant bacteriuria, ie, 100,000 or more/mL of urine. Of the chemical methods, reduction of triphenyltetrazolium chloride (TTC [Uroscreen]) or of nitrate has been widely tested and evaluated. This test depends on the ability of bacteria to reduce soluble, colorless TTC to an insoluble red form. Similarly, the Griess nitrite test (Stat test) depends on the ability of bacteria to reduce urinary nitrates to nitrites which turn red on the addition of the test reagent. Among the objections to these tests is the fact that the color changes cannot be accurately determined in the presence of hematuria or highly colored urine. Furthermore, certain bacteria which do not reduce TTC or nitrate will be missed, and factors which slow bacterial reproduction, such as antimicrobial therapy, will adversely affect the reliability of either test.

The miniature culture plate test (Testuria) is simply a miniaturization of the standard laboratory pour plate, in which a measured area of bibulous paper is immersed in the urine, transferred to a plastic tray containing trypticase soy agar culture medium, and incubated for 18 to 24 hours. When a known quantity of urine is inoculated by this technique, the results can be quantified. A variation of this test uses glass microscope slides coated on one side with eosin-methylene blue agar and on the other with nutrient agar; the slides are dipped into the urine. Quantitation can be achieved by comparing the density of colonial growth with a photograph of slides prepared from serial dilutions of a bacterial suspension.

Another simplified technique based on classic bacteriologic methods uses a divided plastic disposable culture plate with blood agar on one side and desoxycholate agar on the other. The key to this technique is the curved-tip, eyedropper type of pipette which obviates the need for a Bunsen burner and bacteriologic loop for surface streaking the culture plate. One drop from this pipette is equivalent to 0.05 mL. Finally, the agar slant test is simply a cotton-stoppered test tube containing the classic bacteriologic agar slant which is inoculated with urine and then incubated for 12 to 24 hours; quantification of the resultant bacterial growth depends on the observer's familiarity with the test.

Many manufacturers now produce dipslides, which provide a very inexpensive and relatively reliable method for detecting bacteriuria. These consist of a microscope-type glass slide with blood agar on one side and a medium selective for gram-negative bacteria on the other, enclosed in a sterile container. The slide is removed from the container, dipped into an aliquot of freshly collected urine, and returned to the container. The dipslide is then incubated at 37°C or even at room temperature. The manufacturer provides a guide for quantitating the bacteria present. If the culture is positive, the entire apparatus may be sent to a laboratory for further identification and sensitivity testing. This procedure reduces the overall expense of standard urine culture techniques, since only the positive tests are ultimately sent to the laboratory.

Although the above-mentioned tests are relatively reliable detectors of significant bacteriuria (over 90% accuracy), it should be pointed out that these routine cultures do not detect mycobacteria. If these organisms are suspected, one must send the urine for special culture. The best urine specimen to send is the first-voided morning urine.

**Exfoliative Cytology.** Cytologic examination of exfoliated cells has gained widespread recognition and use in the diagnosis of malignant neoplasms, especially those of lung, bronchus, and female genital tract. Cytologic investigation of the urinary tract, except in certain larger centers, has lagged behind. This is based mainly on the often confusing artifactual alterations which may occur in benign cells when exposed to hypertonic urine, to inflammation, or to stones or other nonneoplastic conditions, most of which can be recognized or avoided by careful attention to the details of urine collection and processing.

There are two main techniques in widespread use for the cytologic examination of cells present in urine: 1) the sediment-smear technique, in which an aliquot of urine is centrifuged and the sediment is smeared on a slide; and 2) the filtration technique, in which the urine is passed through a transparent membrane with pores of dimensions such that any cells suspended in the urine are trapped on the membrane. The filtration techniques yield superior preparations with little distortion of cellular details when stained by the standard Papanicolaou technique (Fig 1). Such filters are commercially available.*

There are two major categories of specimens of urine: 1) a simple voided specimen, and 2) a specimen associated with some instrumentation of the urinary tract. There are important differences in the kinds and numbers of cells inherent in the two types, and for proper interpretation the cytologist must be aware of the type of specimen. For a suitable voided specimen, the first morning specimen is the least desirable due to degenerative changes that may occur in cells exposed to the urine overnight. As soon as possible after the specimen is obtained, at least 50 mL of urine is passed through a filter under light negative pressure. The filter is immediately placed in a suitable fixative solution and then stained later when convenient. For a voided specimen there should have been no instrumentation, such as catheterization or cystoscopy, and no manipulation, such as prostatic massage, for at least the prior 24 hours. Normal voided urine from the male contains few epithelial cells and rarely, if ever, clusters or clumps of such cells. The urine of females contains many more single cells but no clumps or clusters and, in the childbearing years, cyclic hormonal effects similar to those of the vaginal epithelium may be evident.

Specimens obtained during or immediately after instrumentation contain more cells than voided specimens, and there may be clumps or clusters of epithelial cells displaced from the surface epithelium by the tip of the catheter or instrument.

* Nucleopore, General Electric, Pleasanton, CA; Millipore, Millipore Corporation, Bedford, MA.

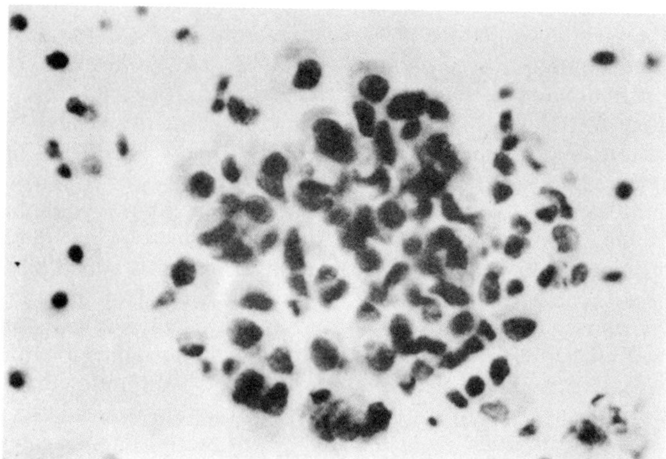

**Fig 1.** Urinary cytology. Transitional cell carcinoma, moderately undifferentiated (grade 3). (Papanicolaou stain; × 400.)

In experienced hands and under properly controlled conditions, results of cytodetection of bladder cancer are impressive. In assessing these results, it should be emphasized that many authors do not include in their data papillary transitional cell tumors in which there are no cytologic features of malignancy. Whether one regards this lesion as a benign transitional cell papilloma or a grade 1 transitional cell carcinoma, accurate urinary cytologic diagnosis is highly desirable. While the results are not as good as with cytologically malignant neoplasms, the diagnosis often may be suspected on the basis of the propensity for small fragments or fronds of the tumor to break away and pass in the urine. Voided specimens are preferred for this purpose, since a similar picture may be induced by instrumentation in the absence of a neoplasm (Fig 2). Even in patients with high-grade tumors, urine cytology may be falsely negative in 20% and falsely positive in from 1% to 12%. False-positive results are usually seen in patients with inflammation, radiation changes, or severe atypia.

Cytologic investigation of the urinary tract is of greatest value in the diagnosis of clinically unsuspected urinary tract carcinoma. It can be an important tool in the management of patients being followed after treatment of bladder carcinoma; in the

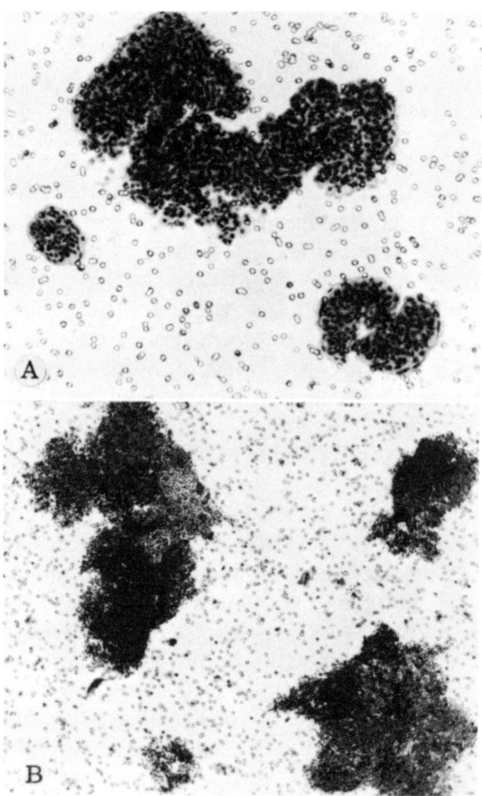


**Fig 2.** Urinary cytology. A, Papillary tumor fronds in voided urine. (Papanicolaou stain; × 110.) B, Normal epithelial cells in urine, induced by instrumentation. (Papanicolaou stain; × 50.)

asymptomatic patient, cytologic investigation may detect a malignant recurrence in an earlier, more easily treatable stage, before the lesion is cystoscopically evident. Finally, it is an important tool to the investigator interested in the evolution of premalignant changes in the bladder mucosa and the natural history of in situ and very early bladder carcinoma.

Malignant cells in urine may originate from primary carcinoma of the renal pelvis or ureters and, for practical purposes, cannot be distinguished from those of bladder cancer. In such instances, separate specimens obtained differentially from each side by means of ureteral catheterization may localize the lesion. Such specimens may be obtained either by simply collecting the urine or by lavage of the ureter or renal pelvis with isotonic saline. With either method, only cytologically malignant tumors can be diagnosed with accuracy. Urinary cytology is of limited value in the diagnosis of renal parenchymal tumors, renal cell carcinoma, or hypernephroma, because exfoliation of cells into the urinary tract occurs only when there is invasion of the renal calyceal system, usually a late manifestation of the lesion.

In the reporting of results of urinary cytologic investigation, little is gained by a complicated system of classes such as that in common use in cervical cytology. It is much more practical simply to recognize three categories of results: (1) positive for malignant cells; (2) negative for malignant cells; and (3) suspicious cells present, suggest further investigation.

## Flow Cytometry

Flow cytometry is now being performed in those with several types of urologic cancers: bladder, prostate, and renal. Its prognostic significance is not yet completely known, especially in regard to prostatic and renal cancers. In general, it has been shown in transitional cell cancer that most superficial low-grade tumors are diploid, while aneuploidy is common in high-grade tumors. Bladder washes with normal saline are generally more accurate than voided urine for detecting bladder cancer because the disruptive action of barbotage increases tumor-cell shedding and provides better-preserved cells for examination.

False-positive results can occur when inflammatory cells are present in the urine, because many of these cells have rapid DNA turnover. Other causes of artifactual changes in the urothelial cells include indwelling Foley catheters, stones, bladder instrumentation, and previous radiotherapy or intravesical chemotherapy. The first-voided morning urine should not be used, as cellular degeneration occurs in urine that has remained in the bladder for an extended period of time.

**Hormones.** A variety of hormones are excreted in the urine, and studies of the variations in the amount or nature of these hormones may be helpful in the diagnosis of various diseases. Among the more commonly used tests is the determination of urinary chorionic gonadotropin. Its presence in significant amounts may be important in confirmation of the diagnosis, indication of the extent of the disease, and prognosis in cases of neoplasm of the testis containing trophoblastic elements. A value of less than 500 mouse units (MU)/24 h is of no clinical significance.

Some of the urinary excretory products are sex hormones of the adrenal cortex and are referred to as 17-ketosteroids. In the past, evaluation of urinary 17-ketosteroids has been a major method for estimating adrenal cortical activity and has been viewed as providing an index of adrenal androgen secretion. Actually, it is a reflection of the output of steroids with androgenic activity not only from the adrenals but also from the testes and ovaries. Correlation of these hormones with androgenicity, however, is erroneous, since testosterone, the most potent of androgens, is not a 17-ketosteroid. The normal range is 7 to 22 mg/24 h for men and 5 to 8 mg for women. After middle age, the excretion gradually decreases and chronic illnesses often may decrease levels even further. High values usually accompany adrenal carcinoma and, in adrenal tumors such as those producing virilizing effects, urinary 17-ketosteroid levels are usually significantly increased. Procedures for measuring a larger fraction of urinary cortisol metabolites including 17-hydroxycorticoids and urinary 17-ketogenic steroids have been devised.

Urinary aldosterone determinations are also useful. When 24-hour urinary excretion of aldosterone exceeds 12 μg while the patient's intake of salt is normal, primary aldosteronism should be suspected. False-positive results may be obtained in sodium depletion states, which may stimulate a secretion of aldosterone.

Determination of urinary catecholamines previously was the most specific procedure available for the diagnosis of pheochromocytoma. A 24-hour urinary excretion of more than 250 μg of epinephrine (normal, 30 μg to 100 μg) is indicative of the disease. Now, diagnosis of tumors of the adrenal medulla can be established by measuring vanillylmandelic acid (VMA) in the urine; advantages of this technique are that false-positive reactions do not occur and special diets are not necessary. Normal values range between 2 and 8 mg/24 h. Increased urinary output of VMA or homovanillic acid (HVA), a metabolite of dopamine, may be found in cases of neuroblastoma. More recently, serum levels of norepinephrine (NE) and epinephrine (Epi) can be determined using highly sensitive radioreceptor assays. It is important to note that blood samples must be obtained after the patient has rested for at least 30 minutes to avoid falsely high results from stress or postural elevations of NE or Epi levels.

**Miscellaneous.** Microscopic studies of expressed prostatic secretions are usually necessary before a diagnosis of prostatitis can be established. The secretions are obtained by prostatic massage and, if the first examination yields negative results, a second examination should be performed 24 hours later. Studies of normal prostatic secretions reveal clear, translucent lecithin bodies and few, if any, leukocytes in each high-power field of the microscope. Prostatitis is suggested by the presence of numerous leukocytes (frequently in clumps), erythrocytes, and bacteria, as well as the disappearance of lecithin. At times, a diagnosis of carcinoma of the prostate can be established by the detection of malignant cells in prostatic secretion.

Studies of semen are indicated in problems of infertility and hypogonadism. Semen is collected by masturbation or interrupted coitus after a period of abstinence of 3 or 4 days. The normal variation in volume of semen is 2 to 5 mL. A count of 40 million sperm/mL of semen has been generally accepted as representing the lower limits of normal. However, fertility does not seem to be impaired until less than 20 million sperm/mL are detected. Morphologic studies of normal semen disclose that not more than 40% of sperm are abnormal in appearance. In addition, 60% of the sperm should exhibit active motions which persist for 24 hours. Sperm motility is an estimate of forward progression, which is rated on a scale from 1 to 4. A score greater than two is considered normal. Semen should also be evaluated for the presence of excess white blood cells (suggesting inflammation or infection within the genitourinary tract), the presence of excess sperm clumping (suggesting antisperm antibodies), and abnormal viscosity (which can affect sperm motility).

Present-day management of urinary calculi requires knowledge concerning the chemical composition of the calculi. This can be accurately determined by optical and x-ray crystallography. Unfortunately, such studies are not readily available and it is necessary to rely on the more common, although less accurate, chemical methods.

Measurement of urinary excretion of calcium may be helpful in management of patients with urinary calculi. Excessive excretion of calcium may be determined quantitatively from 24-hour specimens after the patient has remained on a diet containing a known amount of calcium for several days. Although the normal serum calcium concentration is well defined, urinary excretion of calcium ranges from an average of 50 mg/24 h in the child to 300 mg/24 h in the adult, over a range of dietary calcium intake of 150 to 2,000 mg/day. A large number of patients with calculus disease have hypercalciuria, but it should be stressed that the presence or absence of calculi does not depend only on hypercalciuria. Patients may excrete large amounts of calcium in the urine without forming calculi. When renal calculi are present with hypercalciuria but normal serum calcium levels, further investigations are necessary to determine the cause. There are four major categories of patients with hypercalciuria and normal serum calcium levels, those with: 1) intestinal hyperabsorption, which is the result of excessive intestinal absorption of calcium; 2) renal leak due to failure of the renal tubules to reabsorb calcium normally; 3) bone reabsorption induced by excessive parathyroid hormone production; and 4) metabolic causes of hypercalciuria.

Primary hyperoxaluria is a rare hereditary disorder characterized clinically by calcium oxalate nephrolithiasis with an increased urinary excretion of oxalate not related to dietary intake. Normal urinary excretion of oxalate is in the range 14 μg to 50 μg daily. Secondary hyperoxaluria also may occur as the result of increased oxalate ingestion or vitamin $B_{12}$ deficiency.

### Blood Chemistry

The normal ranges for the blood tests most often used in urology are shown in Table 3.

### Office Ultrasonography

Basic ultrasonography can easily be incorporated into many routine office visits. Ultrasound can be used to identify and evaluate abdominal masses, and the kidneys can be inspected for hydronephrosis, stones, or renal masses. Ultrasound can be used to evaluate postvoid residuals; increased bladder-wall thickness due to neurogenic bladder (NGB) or cystitis; masses such as tumor, stone, ureterocele; or intravesical prostatic enlargement.

The prostate can be visualized transabdominally, but is better seen transrectally. Benign and malignant lesions of the prostate can be detected. Ultrasound can also be used to provide accurate guidance for transperineal and transrectal needle biopsy of suspicious prostatic lesions. A hypoechoic lesion within the peripheral zone is suspicious for carcinoma, while benign prostatic hyperplasia frequently yields a heterogeneous pattern in the inner zones of the prostate.

Ultrasound can be particularly useful in the evaluation of a testicle that is not palpable due to a large hydrocele or when there is a question of an intratesticular vs extratesticular mass. The normal testis is echogenically homogeneous. With more elaborate equipment and extensive experience, differentiation can sometimes even be made between testicular torsion and epididymitis or epididymo-orchitis.

### Tests of Renal Function

Although the ideal, infallible test for accurate estimation of renal function has not yet been discovered, experience has demonstrated that application of certain tests now in use gives a reliable index of renal function. It must be borne in mind, however, that the various tests of renal function measure function only and not the extent of anatomic change or the potential function of a kidney; these need not go hand in hand, even when definite organic disease exists. Renal function may be greatly depressed by pathologic conditions which are primarily extrarenal, such as cardiac disease with poor compensation, intestinal obstruction, and prostatic obstruction. Successful treatment of the primary disease may be rewarded by striking improvement of renal function. Moreover, since a kidney performs multiple functions, some phases of its activities may be greatly impaired while others remain normal; different tests that do not measure the same function sometimes may give apparently inconsistent results. For this reason, it is highly desirable that two or more of the tests be used in each case.

Of the more important tests of function, the following are most useful to the urologist: (1) tests for specific gravity and osmolality (discussed under Studies of Urine); (2) estimation of retention of nitrogen; (3) excretory urography; (4) clearance tests of such substances as creatinine, inulin, para-aminohippurate; and (5) the radioisotope renogram and isotope scan (discussed under Radioisotope Techniques).

**TABLE 3. Normal Blood Values**

| Test | Range |
|---|---|
| Hemoglobin | Males, 14 to 17 g/dL<br>Females, 12 to 15 g/dL |
| Hematocrit | Males, 42% to 54%<br>Females, 38% to 46% |
| Leukocyte count | 5000 to 9000/cu mm |
| Platelet count | 130,00 to 370,000/cu mm |
| Sedimentation rate (Westergren) | <20 mm in 1 h |
| Bleeding time | 1 to 5 min (Duke)<br>1 to 6 min (Ivy) |
| Serum calcium | 8.9 to 10.1 mg/100 mL |
| Serum inorganic phosphorus | Infants, 5.5 to 6.5 mg/100 mL<br>Children, 4.5 to 5.5. mg/100 mL<br>Adults, 2.5 to 4.5 mg/100 mL |
| Sodium | 135 to 145 mEq/L |
| Potassium | 4 to 5 mEq/L |
| Chloride | 97 to 106 mEq/L |
| Carbon dioxide | 25 to 29 mEq/L |
| Urea | Males, 17 to 51 mg/100 mL<br>Females, 13 to 45 mg/100 mL |
| Glucose (fasting) | 69 to 90 mg/100 mL |
| Uric acid | Males, 4.3 to 8.0 mg/100 mL<br>Females, 2.3 to 6.0 mg/100 mL |
| Serum creatinine | Males, 0.8 to 1.2 mg/100 mL<br>Females, 0.6 to 0.9 mg/100 mL |
| Acid phosphatase | <7.9 units/L (higher in children) |
| (tartrate inhibited) | <20% |
| Alkaline phosphatase | <60 units/L (higher in children) |
| Total serum protein | 6.0 to 7.7 gm/100 mL |
| Albumin | 3.3 to 4.3 gm/100 mL |
| α-1-globulin | 0.3 to 0.4 gm/100 mL |
| α-2-globulin | 0.5 to 0.8 gm/100 mL |
| β-globulin | 0.6 to 1.1 gm/100 mL |
| γ-globulin | 0.8 to 1.6 gm/100 mL |
| Prothrombin time | 17 to 19 sec (Quick) |
| BSP retention | 5% or less in 1 h |
| Acid-base balance (Astrup) | |
| Actual pH | 7.35 to 7.42 |
| Actual $P_{CO_2}$ | 35 to 45 mm Hg |
| Standard bicarbonate | 21.3 to 24.8 mEq/L |
| Base excess | −2 to +2 mEq/L |
| Buffer base | 44 to 46 mEq/L |

**Estimation of Retention of Nitrogen.** The blood transports various nonprotein nitrogenous substances which, unless utilized by the tissues, circulate until excreted by the kidneys. Although the quantity to be eliminated varies greatly from hour to hour, through the adaptability of the kidneys the concentration in the blood is kept at a fairly constant level. When the kidneys are damaged and their capacity to excrete is thereby lessened, these substances tend to accumulate in the blood; this condition is referred to as "nitrogen retention." Estimations of the blood urea or urea nitrogen and creatinine are the procedures used most widely. Determinations of total nonprotein nitrogen have been largely abandoned because of the availability of specific measurements for individual components which have greater clinical significance.

***Blood Urea Nitrogen.*** Quantitatively, urea is the most important nonprotein nitrogenous constituent of the blood and is the chief end product of protein metabolism. Normally, it is excreted entirely by the kidneys; its blood concentration is therefore directly related to the renal excretory capacity and to the diet. Since the dietary protein intake may vary widely, the blood urea nitrogen (BUN) concentration has a wide range, varying from 5 to 23 mg/100 mL. BUN levels are increased in advanced renal diseases such as glomerulonephritis, extensive pyogenic infections, and conditions resulting in oliguria, obstructive uropathy, or tubular blockage by substances that interfere with urine excretion, such as sulfonamides, hemoglobin, myeloma, protein, and amyloid.

Consideration must also be given to the various nonrenal causes of increased BUN, referred to as prerenal azotemia. One such cause is marked hemoconcentration due to the loss of plasma water as a result of starvation, vomiting, sweating, or diarrhea. These conditions prevent adequate glomerular filtration by the prerenal deviation of water. Gastrointestinal bleeding often results in a marked increase of BUN because of the absorption of excess products of protein digestion. A slight increase may occur in severe toxic or febrile conditions in which there is marked increase in protein catabolism. Passive congestion of the kidneys due to cardiac decompensation frequently decreases the glomerular filtration rate and affects the renal plasma flow sufficiently to cause urea nitrogen retention.

***Serum Creatinine.*** Serum creatinine concentration does not adequately reflect early renal damage. As a consequence of many factors, the kidneys may be severely damaged when, by current methods and definition, the plasma creatinine level is still normal. Nevertheless, measurement of plasma creatinine has an advantage over measurement of other nitrogenous compounds in evaluating renal function in that changes in concentration of creatinine are highly specific for alterations of renal function, because rate of formation of creatinine depends almost exclusively on body muscle mass, while its elimination depends almost entirely on glomerular filtration rate. The concentration of creatinine is quite insensitive to factors such as hydration, diet, and metabolic status. This is not the case with urea or total nonprotein nitrogen.

**Excretory Urography.** Even though it is an excellent detector of morphologic derangement, the excretory urogram has several theoretic and practical limitations as a test of renal function. This is due to the fact that the mechanism of the excretion of the urographic medium is not completely understood, and it varies with different media. For example, free iodides are filtered through the glomerulus, whereas protein-bound iodides are more likely to be excreted by the proximal cells of the tubule. The transport of the new triiodinated compounds is not well localized, and a small dose is handled by different mechanisms than a larger one. Therefore, as is true of all other tests of renal function, the excretory urogram measures but one aspect of the diverse functions of the kidneys and, furthermore, such tests provide static estimation, but no information as to potential renal function.

In addition to such theoretic limitations, there are some practical considerations. For instance, with rapid movement of fluid in the collecting system, as in diuresis from overhydration, poor visualization is the result of poor density of the contrast medium and not of poor renal function. In obstructive uropathy, renal excretion may be reflexly or temporarily interrupted, an excellent example of this being renal colic from an obstructing renal stone; yet within a matter of hours after passage of the stone, the function of the kidney may return to normal. Other variable factors that may influence the value of excretory urography as a test of renal function should include the size of the patient, the state of his circulation, the presence of gas and fecal material in the bowel, and the techniques involved in making roentgenograms. Any of these could affect the final product adversely.

If sufficient medium is present in the pelvis and calyces to produce a strong contrasting shadow in the roentgenogram taken a few minutes after injection, it can be safely assumed that renal function is within normal limits. The usefulness of the excretory urogram in the investigation of renal hypertension is a matter of diverse opinion—some have found it extremely useful and others, misleading. In general, however, it is felt to be at best only minimally effective as a screening study for suspected renovascular hypertension. The major findings suggestive of this are: a unilaterally small kidney, a delayed nephrogram with a delay of contrast in the calyces and hyperconcentration of the contrast in a delayed film.

It bears repeating that, as a test of renal function, the excretory urogram is not dependable because, even with severe damage, the remarkable reserve power of the kidneys may permit enough function to excrete concentrated medium. In fact, in the opinion of some, of all tests of renal function, it is the poorest quantitative indicator, and the excretory urogram should never be accepted as the sole criterion that a kidney is capable of sustaining life after removal of the contralateral kidney.

**Clearance Studies.** The concept of blood or plasma clearance has important application in the study of renal function. Renal plasma clearance of any substance is expressed as the volume of plasma cleared of that substance by renal activity per unit time (usually one minute). Depending on the type of substance, clearance may be achieved predominantly by glomerular filtration, by cellular transport at various locations in the nephrons, or by a combination of glomerular filtration and cellular function of the nephron. Thus, renal clearance of specific solutes can be usefully related to these components of renal function.

When the function involved in the excretion of a given solute is known, the renal clearance of that solute may then become a useful measurement of that function. Clearance is indicated as follows:

$$Cx = \frac{(Ux)(V)}{Px}$$

Cx equals the volume of plasma cleared of substance x per unit of time, Ux equals the urine concentration of substance x, V equals urine volume flow per unit of time (usually one minute), and Px equals the plasma concentration of substance x.

Clearance measurement techniques may be sorted into two categories: exogenous methods and endogenous methods. In exogenous methods, clearance is assessed during a continuous infusion of the clearance substance. This infusion may augment the concentration of a material naturally present in plasma, or it may introduce a substance that normally is not present in plasma. In the endogenous method, the clearance of a substance at plasma concentrations that are naturally occurring in plasma is determined (creatinine is an example of such a substance).

***Creatinine.*** Endogenous creatinine clearance has many advantages over other methods. The rate of production of creatinine in an individual subject is quite constant. If renal excretion is constant, plasma levels remain stable. In kidney disease, the rate of excretion decreases so slowly that plasma levels are nearly constant over a 24-hour period. The rate of excretion of creatinine is primarily a function of glomerular filtration, and thus endogenous creatinine clearance closely approximates inulin clearance. Endogenous creatinine clearance has enjoyed great popularity as a clinical diagnostic test of renal function. This popularity undoubtedly has derived in part from its relative simplicity to perform, as compared with most exogenous methods.

***Inulin.*** Inulin is a soluble polysaccharide that is filtered out through glomeruli in the same concentration as it exists in the plasma. Since the substance is neither resorbed nor excreted by the tubules, all of the inulin entering the filtrate goes into the urine. Thus, the plasma clearance of inulin measures the glomerular filtration rate (GFR).

***Para-aminohippurate.*** The clearance of any substance that is completely extracted from the plasma with each passage through functional kidney tissue will measure effective renal plasma flow (ERPF). The clearance of para-aminohippurate

(PAH) is taken to represent ERPF because its renal extraction from plasma at low plasma concentration approaches 100% in normal humans. Although part of the plasma PAH filters through the glomerular membrane, it is primarily the secretory function of the proximal convoluted tubule that extracts PAH from the blood and allows the complete (or nearly complete) clearance of plasma with each circulation through active renal tissue.

**Separated Renal Function Studies.** The tests of renal function outlined previously have been used in the evaluation of function in the separate kidneys of patients with hypertension in an attempt to detect disparity that may indicate poorer functioning of one of the two kidneys or to determine the nature of any functional disturbance that is present.

For the performance of separated renal function studies, it is necessary to insert a 6 to 8 F polyethylene or Teflon catheter into each ureter so that individual samples of urine can be collected. The test of renal function performed is a matter of personal preference.

### Tumor Markers

Certain genitourinary tumors of prostatic and testicular origin are known to elaborate specific proteins that can be detected in the serum. These proteins constitute tumor markers which are useful in both the diagnosis of such malignancies and the evaluation of the success of therapy.

Testicular tumors, primarily nonseminomatous tumors, elaborate two compounds useful in the detection of malignant disease. These markers are the most sensitive available indicators of residual tumor after surgery or of the appearance of recurrent disease. α-Fetoprotein (AFP) is a glycoprotein with a half-life of 4 to 5 days. The serum level is not normally higher than 40 ng/dL. The second tumor marker is the beta subunit of human chorionic gonadotropin (β-hCG). Its half-life is 18–24 hours and its serum level in men is usually less than 1 ng/ml.

Prostatic tissue elaborates an enzyme, prostatic acid phosphatase (PAP), which has been employed as a tumor marker since the 1940s. Elevated levels of PAP occur in 70% to 85% of patients with metastatic disease, but only in 10% to 30% of patients with locally confined disease. Another marker that has recently gained wide recognition is prostatic-specific antigen (PSA), which was first described in 1979. It is elaborated by both benign and malignant prostatic tissue and appears to be volume-dependent. This makes PSA an excellent marker to measure response to therapy. Sensitivity for detection of cancer of the prostate has been as high as 95%. But with a specificity ranging from 47% to 80%, it is a poor screening method.

## RADIOISOTOPE TECHNIQUES

### Radioisotope Renogram

This test of renal function has become increasingly important and has wide clinical application, especially in the detection of hypertension of renal origin. It is relatively simple to perform and is well tolerated. The test involves the IV injection of radioiodinated substances that are subject to renal excretion. Their inflow, accumulation, and outflow through the kidney can be recorded graphically by the use of special apparatus. Sodium *o*-iodohippurate I-131 ($^{131}$I-OIH, Hippuran I 131) is best suited for the test; it has a rapid excretion rate and more than 98% is excreted by the kidney, thus preventing any false interpretation of the renogram from concomitant excretion by the liver, as is the case with iodopyracet (Diodrast) and other contrast media. At present, $^{123}$I-OIH is more commonly used to evaluate the kinetics of renal tubular function because of its shorter half-life and, therefore, the decreased risk it poses to the thyroid.

Since $^{131}$I-OIH, like PAH, measures ERPF, one would expect the initial phase of the $^{131}$I-OIH renogram to reflect some estimate of ERPF and the terminal segment to reflect a washout rate or transit time of the test substance; therefore, it would be a good index of the volume of urine excreted per unit of time. This has been found to be the case. Measurement of the ERPF can be achieved either by in vitro blood sampling techniques or by computerized gamma camera techniques that do not require blood sampling.

The patient should be normally hydrated, since dehydration or overhydration can affect the appearance of renal uptake.

The actual test begins by having the patient void. This urine is discarded after the specific gravity and osmolality have been determined, and the time at which the bladder is emptied is recorded. The patient then is seated and the detectors are placed over the most likely site of the kidneys. A short survey of background activity is obtained prior to injection of the radioactive substance. A 300 μCi dose of $^{123}$I-OIH in a small bolus (approximately 0.5 mL) is injected rapidly into an antecubital vein. The time of the injection is recorded. Immediately thereafter the detectors are placed over the area of maximal counting intensity and locked into position. The patient and the recording are carefully observed throughout the 30-minute procedure. When the recording is terminated, the patient is requested to empty his bladder again. This timed specimen is used to determine the urine volume per minute, the percentage of the radioactive dose excreted, the specific gravity, and the osmolality.

A typical normal $^{131}$I-OIH renographic curve is shown in Figure 3. From 15 to 30 seconds after the injection, a vascular spike occurs; this is followed 3 minutes later by another peak.

The first clinical application of the test was as a screening procedure in the detection of hypertension of renal origin. When the $^{131}$I-OIH renogram is sufficiently standardized and when it is used as a diagnostic aid in renovascular hypertension, interpretations are based largely on changes in ERPF and differential urine volumes (and sodium concentrations). The slope from A to B (Fig 3) seems to correlate well with PAH clearance. The slope from B to D correlates closely with urine volume and inversely with sodium resorption by the kidney per unit of time. In relatively severe stenosis of the renal artery, conventional differential clearances may reveal diminished PAH clearance values on the affected side with diminished urine/minute volume.

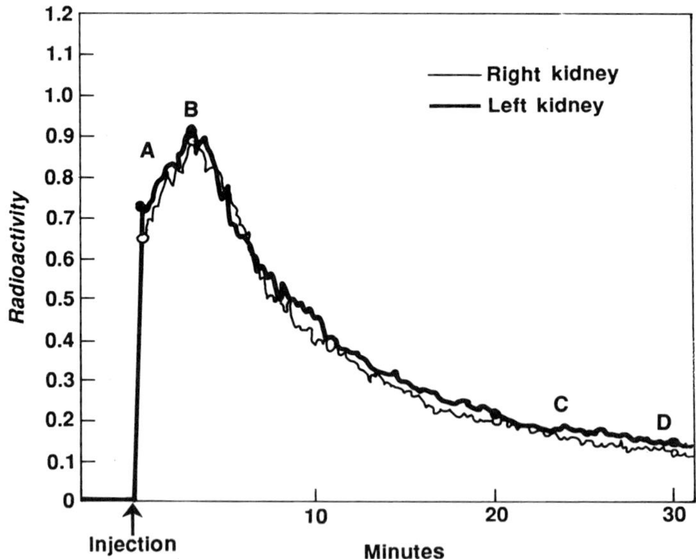


**Fig 3.** Normal isotope renogram made with $^{131}$I-OIH. Point A is a vascular spike; approximately 75% of this activity is renal. The value A to B correlates well with determinations of ERPF. The segment B to D reflects washout rate or transit time.

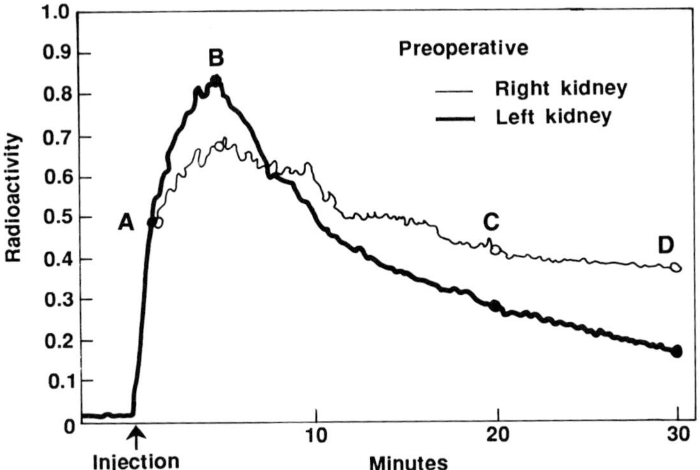


**Fig 4.** Isotope renogram of patient with severe stenosis of right renal artery. The A to B portion is depressed on affected side; B to D portion reflects retained medium. [From Emmett JL, *Clinical Urography: An Atlas and Textbook of Roentgenologic Diagnosis,* ed 2 (Philadelphia: WB Saunders; 1964).]

This is reflected in isotope renograms (Fig 4).

Both experimental and clinical investigations have proved the value of the isotope renogram as an adjunct in the diagnosis of other forms of urologic disease, such as evaluating the degree of obstructive uropathy, assessing changes in renal function, investigating the cause of azotemia, or differentiating acute ureteral obstruction from acute tubular necrosis in the early stages of postoperative anuria. In each instance, characteristic patterns are obtained.

## Renal Scintigram (Scan)*

Radioisotope photoscanning of the kidneys is a technique developed for the purpose of recording the size, shape, location, and composition of functioning renal mass. The procedure depends on the capacity of the renal substance to concentrate certain radioactively labeled agents, which can be detected by means of a scintillation scanner.

At present, this procedure is intended to be an adjunct to other methods of urologic diagnosis. It may be helpful for patients in whom conventional techniques have failed to demonstrate a space-occupying lesion or with localized areas of depressed renal function resulting from vascular changes. It may be used successfully to evaluate obstructive uropathy when azotemia or allergy prevents excretory urography. The scan is also useful in distinguishing acute tubular necrosis from rejection in the transplant recipient; it can be used to distinguish between solid renal masses and pseudotumors such as dromedary humps, fetal lobulations, and columns of Bertin. Pseudotumors will have normal renal uptake of radioactivity, in contrast to abnormal uptake observed in patients with renal masses.

Numerous radioactive agents are currently available. One of the first agents used was chlormerodrin labeled with $^{203}$Hg or $^{197}$Hg. However, these compounds have several drawbacks. Compared to other available agents, they expose the patient to unnecessarily high doses of radiation. In addition, their low photon energy produces poor-quality scintigrams. Although mer-

* A number of terms have been used to designate the display of radioactivity distribution over the body, the most recent and general of which is "scintigram." This term includes the images produced both by moving detector devices (scanners) and by stationary devices (scintillation cameras). "Scan" refers only to the output of the former.

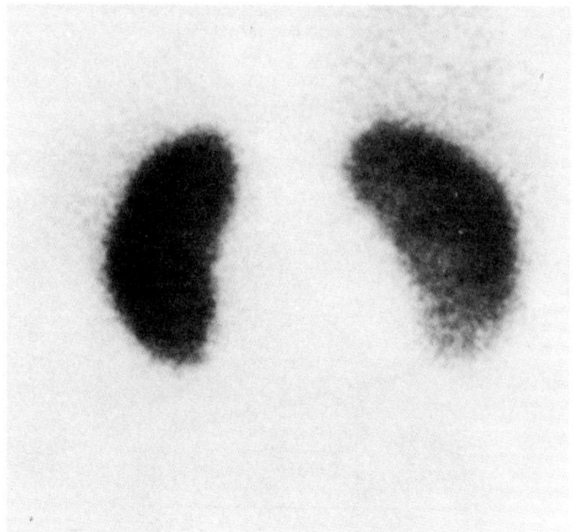

**Fig 5.** DTPA scan of normal kidney showing diffuse uptake in the renal cortex.

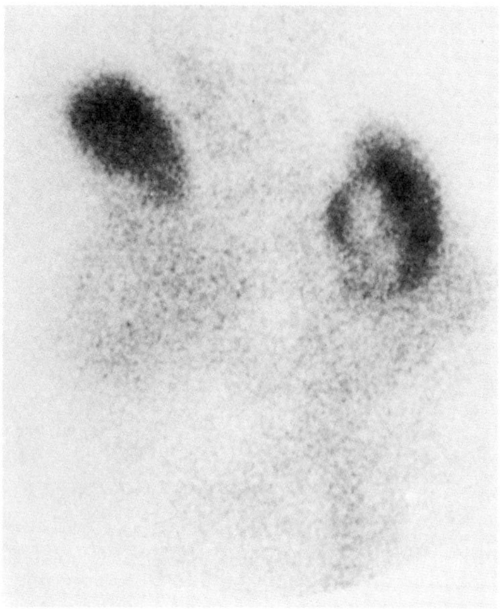

**Fig 6.** DTPA scan of kidney showing space-occupying lesion in right kidney where the cortical-labeling DTPA is not taken up.

cury is still in use, $^{99m}$Tc-labeled compounds have essentially replaced these isotopes, since technetium's shorter half-life and higher photon energy allow for much faster and superior renal imaging while delivering less radiation to the patient. A normal scan made after injection of radioactive diethylene triamine pentaacetic acid (DTPA) is shown in Figure 5. The activity is mainly peripheral, in a distribution that corresponds with the location of the renal cortex. Scans of this kind are particularly useful in delineating space-occupying lesions (Fig 6), abnormalities in shape, such as a horseshoe kidney, or renal infarcts. In addition, the quantitative assessment of the radioactive label in each kidney is a reasonably accurate method of assigning a portion of relative renal function to each kidney.

Differential measurement of renal function may be performed with {$^{131}$I}-hippurate based on the measurement of the 1- to 2-minute uptake after correction for background. Other technetium-labeled agents in current use yield better results and include DTPA, dimercaptosuccinic acid (DMSA) and glucoheptanate (GHA).

Besides $^{99m}$Tc-labeled compounds, {$^{123}$I} or {$^{131}$I}-OIH administered intravenously also provides useful information in renal scintigraphy. The rapid excretion of this compound results in the production of less morphologic detail of the cortex than that obtained with other agents, but adds important functional information, in that both the renal mass and the collecting system may be visualized (Fig 7). This indicator may be used to provide anatomic definition of patterns of delayed excretion seen on the renogram. It is particularly useful in localizing calyceal, ureteropelvic, or ureteral obstruction (Fig 8). A diuretic scintirenography with OIH or DTPA can be used to help differentiate obstruction from nonobstructive dilatation. For example, it can

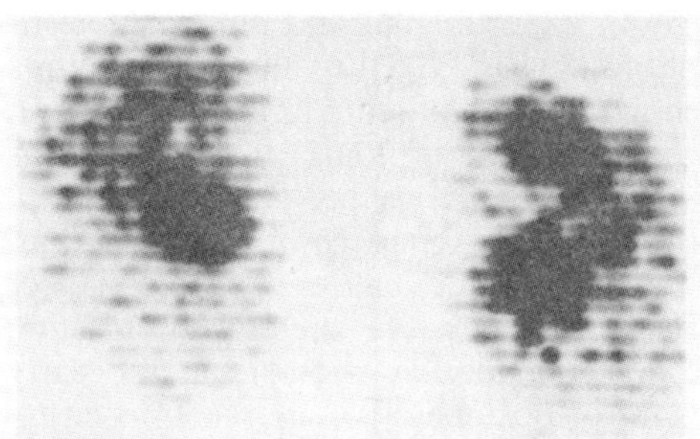

**Fig 7.** $^{131}$I-OIH scan of normal kidney.

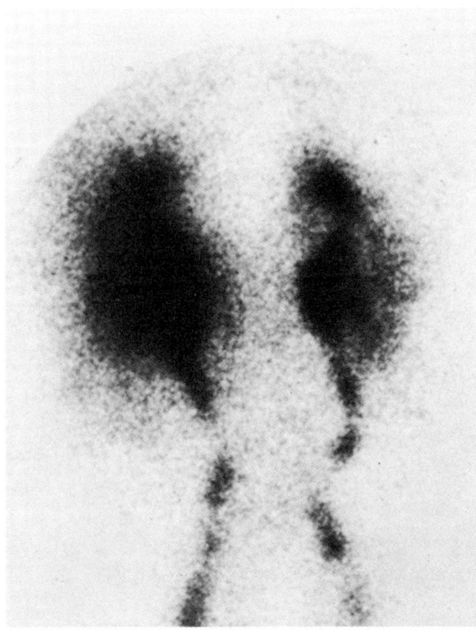

**Fig 8.** $^{131}$I-OIH scan of obstructed kidney showing retention of isotope in the renal pelvis and ureters.

be used in infants and children with reflux nephropathy, primary nonobstructive megaureter, and "prune belly" syndrome. In adults, it may help in the diagnosis of nonobstructed hydroureteronephrosis secondary to a passed renal calculus, as the sequel of chronic infection, after relieved chronic obstruction, or in high urine-flow states such as diabetes insipidus or psychogenic polydypsia. A loop diuretic such as lasix is usually given at the plateau of activity in the collecting system. At least 50% of the initial activity should be washed out of the renal pelvis within 15 minutes in a nonobstructive system. In addition, the {$^{131}$I}-OIH scan reveals the presence of infarcted kidneys and cystic kidneys, as do scintigrams obtained with DTPA, DMSA, GHA, and $MAG_{31}$ (a new $^{99m}$Tc-labelled agent with predominantly tubular secretion).

In addition to scanning the renal cortex and collecting system and assessing differential renal function, it is now possible to assess the renal arterial flow using radioisotopic techniques. Such techniques are important in the study of renal artery stenosis and of the quality of arterial flow after transplant surgery. The compounds that have been studied most extensively for this purpose are $^{99m}$Tc-DTPA and $^{123}$I-OIH (Fig 9). In this technique readings are taken immediately, at 2 seconds, and then at several more 2-second intervals after an IV injection of the radioisotope. Later, recording at 10 minutes, 20 minutes, and 30 minutes allows assessment of the renal cortex and collecting system. Adjunctive use of angiotensin-converting enzyme (ACE) inhibitors is being investigated as these agents appear to enhance the sensitivity and

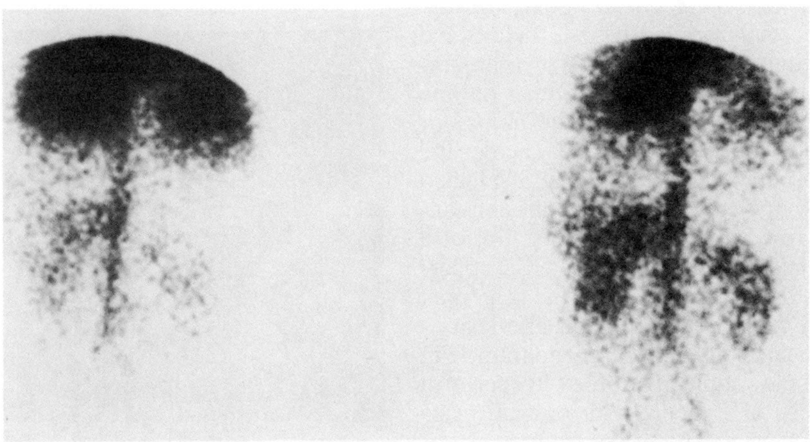

**Fig 9.** DTPA renal flow study showing flow to kidneys 2 sec after injection of DTPA. Visualized are common iliac vessels and kidneys.

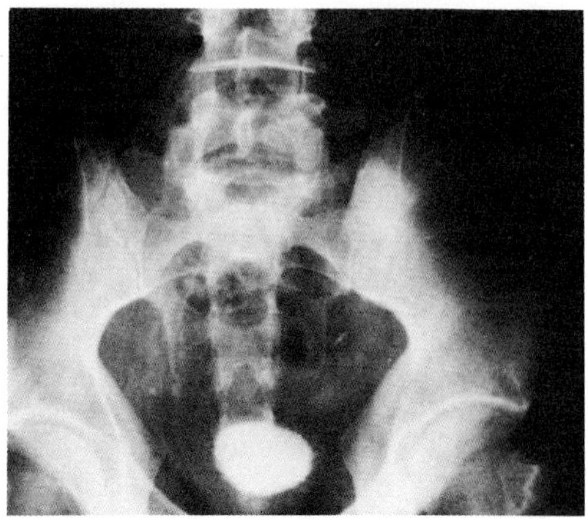
A

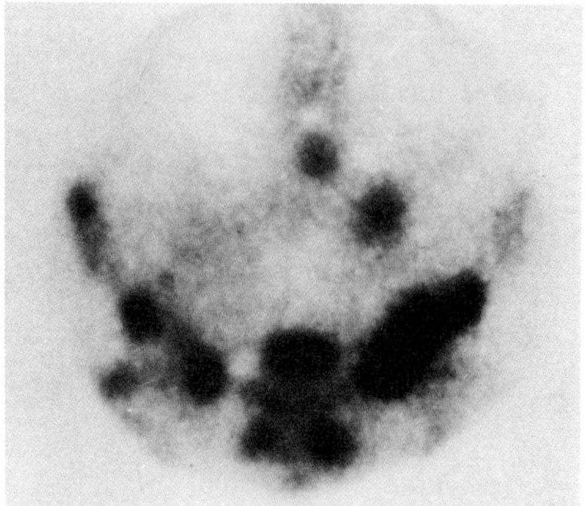
B

**Fig 10.** Prostatic carcinoma. A, roentgenogram of a patient with no apparent bony metastasis; B, multiple areas of uptake, suggesting metastasis.

perhaps the specificity of radionuclide studies of renal artery stenosis.

## Bone Scans

Radioisotope bone scans are frequently used in urologic diagnosis, particularly in a search for metastases from prostatic carcinoma. In a high percentage of cases, there is good correlation among positive bone scans, roentgenographic evidence of metastasis, and increased serum phosphatases or PSA levels. Less frequently, the bone scan will reveal a metastatic lesion not demonstrable roentgenographically (Fig 10). If, on review, the roentgenogram still appears normal or equivocal, additional roentgenographic projections or tomography of the region in question may outline the lesion. Percutaneous needle biopsy or open biopsy of the lesion usually settles the matter. The advantage of using a selected site for biopsy over the conventional general marrow biopsy for the detection of a disseminated malignant disease is apparent. In other instances, the bone scan may reveal more widespread metastatic lesions than indicated on the roentgenogram (Fig 11). It is advisable, therefore, to perform bone scans of patients with prostatic carcinoma when the roentgenogram is negative and the patient complains of skeletal pain or when excision of the primary lesion is contemplated.

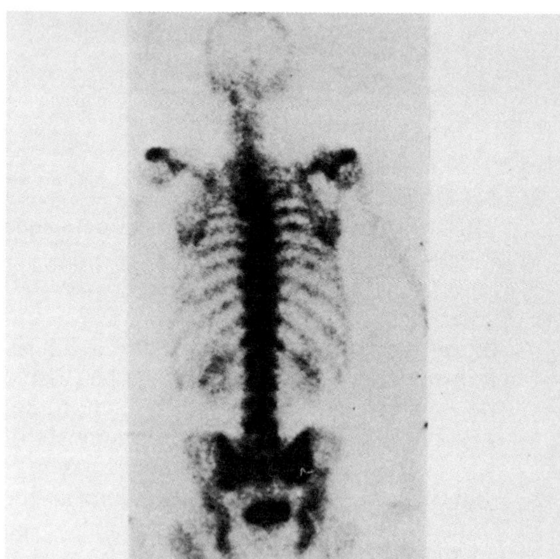

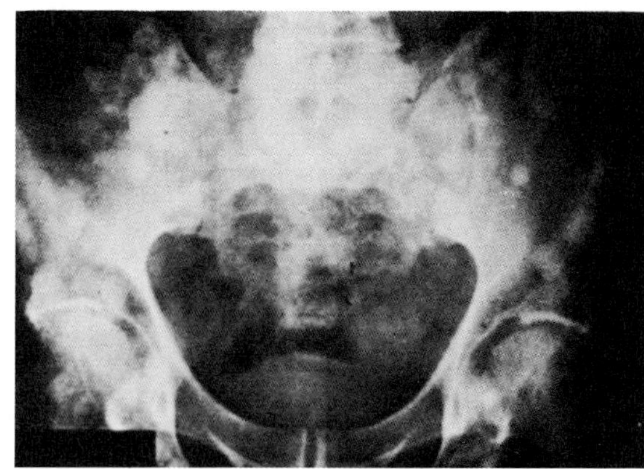

**Fig 11.** Positive roentgenogram of the pelvis, and a corresponding bone scan which shows diffuse positive uptake in the pelvis and spine, suggesting metastasis.

Infrequently, the bone scan may appear normal when the roentgenograms reveal osseous metastasis. In such instances the lesions usually are destructive, with no reactive bone formation. Such lesions cannot be demonstrated by bone scans, because increased uptake of radioisotopes in bone depends on the presence of accelerated mineral accumulation and new formation of bone rather than on destruction of bone.

For adults, 15 μCi of $^{99m}$Tc-methyldiphosphonate (MDP) is given intravenously; the scan is performed 2 hours later (Fig 12). Strontium compounds may also be employed for scanning, but one must give larger doses (100 mCi) and wait 24 to 48 hours to scan. As a result, MDP has replaced these compounds.

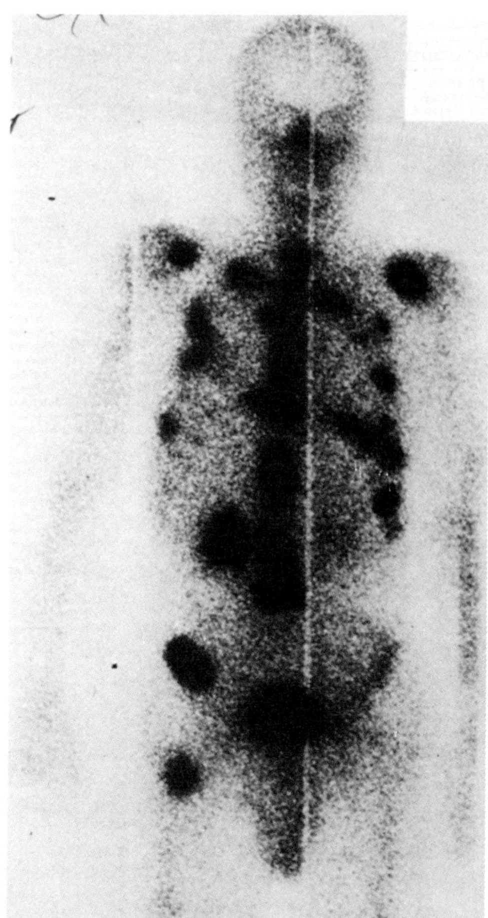

**Fig 12.** MDP scan of a patient with known carcinoma of the prostate. There are multiple areas of uptake in the spine, ribs, pelvis, and right femur.

## SPECIAL UROLOGIC PROCEDURES

### Urethral Catheterization

Obviously, unnecessary catheterization should be avoided. Urethral catheterization usually can be performed easily and safely if certain factors are kept in mind. Scrupulous cleanliness must be observed. The instruments employed must be sterile and the examiner's hands should be covered by sterile gloves. The patient's penis or the vestibule of the vagina and the labia should be thoroughly cleansed with soap and water prior to catheterization; a redundant prepuce should be retracted and the preputial space cleansed. A variety of anesthetic jellies are available which may be instilled into the urethra to ease the discomfort of catheterization. Catheterization of the urethra of an adult can be accomplished satisfactorily with a 14 or 16 F soft rubber, latex, or nylon catheter. A well-lubricated catheter is grasped with sterile gloved hands and gently passed through the urethra.

Although catheterization can be performed easily in females and in most males, it is well to consider the difficulties that may be encountered in males and the methods that may be required to overcome them. These difficulties may be the result of anatomic factors or disease processes. The anatomic factors that may interfere with catheterization are the normal curves of the urethra, the bulb of the urethra, the laxity of the floor of the anterior urethra, and the external urethral sphincter. In its course from external meatus to bladder, the urethra describes several gentle curves which may obstruct passage of the catheter. These obstructions can be obviated by holding the penis at a right angle to the body during passage of the catheter; holding the penis in this manner eliminates all curves except the gentle curve of the posterior urethra (Fig 13). A common site of obstruction to passage of a catheter is the junction of the bulb and membranous portions of the urethra. The diameter of the bulb is larger than that of the membranous urethra, and the tip of the catheter, instead of entering the membranous urethra, may become obstructed

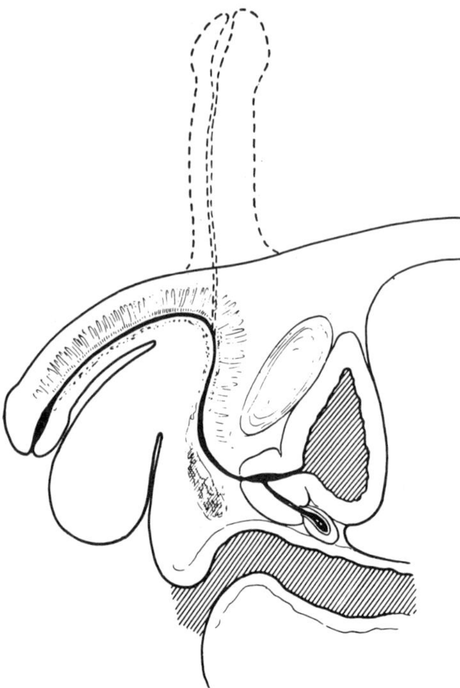

Fig 13. Normal urethral curves; all curves except the gentle curve of the posterior urethra are eliminated by holding the penis at a right angle to the body.

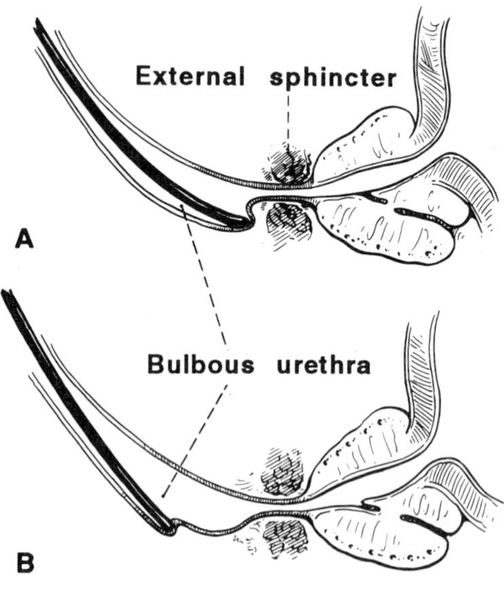


Fig 14. Catheter obstructed A, in bulb of urethra and B, by fold of urethral mucosa; these difficulties can be overcome by use of coudé catheters.

by the floor of the bulbous urethra (Fig 14, *a*). This aspect of the problem will be discussed when use of a coudé catheter is described. The floor of the urethra is lax and the passage of a catheter can be obstructed by a fold of mucosa (Fig 14, *b*). To obviate this difficulty, the tip of the catheter should be directed against the roof of the urethra, which is relatively fixed. The external urethral sphincter is in constant contraction, and may obstruct the passage of the catheter. This can be overcome by maintaining gentle, firm pressure against the sphincter with the catheter while the patient attempts to urinate.

In addition to the foregoing factors encountered in the normal urethra, the following pathologic conditions may interfere with catheterization: phimosis, congenital narrowing of the external meatus, urethral stricture, and benign and malignant hypertrophy of the prostate gland. Severe phimosis may require incision into the dorsal aspect of the prepuce (dorsal slit) in order to visualize the external meatus: circumcision will be necessary to complete the procedure. In cases of congenital narrowing of the external meatus, it is usually possible to dilate it with sounds sufficiently to permit passage of a catheter. If narrowing is extreme, meatotomy may be necessary. Measures employed to overcome difficulties in catheterization produced by urethral strictures and prostatic disease are described in later paragraphs.

The technique and maneuvers of urethral catheterization in men are as follows: The first attempt should be made with a 14 or 16 F soft rubber catheter which has a round, solid tip (Fig 15). If the catheter cannot be passed, it is likely that the tip has been obstructed by a fold of mucosa, by the floor of the bulbous urethra, by a pocket formed by hypertrophied lobes in cases of prostatic hyperplasia, or by a urethral stricture. In such instances, a coudé catheter (Fig 15, *b*) is employed; this is the most useful of all catheters. Its chief virtue lies in the fact that the tip of the catheter forms an obtuse angle with the body of the catheter. Thus, if the tip of such a catheter becomes engaged in a pocket or fold, rotation of the catheter on its long axis causes the tip to

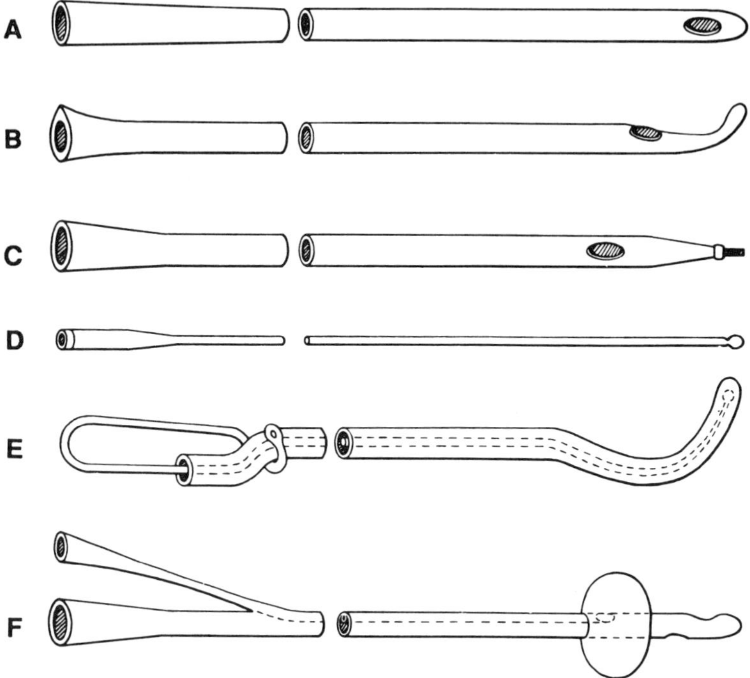


**Fig 15.** Catheters: A, soft rubber; B, coudé; C, Phillips', which attaches to D, filiform, which may be threaded over E, wire stylet; F, Foley self-retaining urethral.

disengage itself. Prior to passage of this catheter, the urethra is filled with lubricating jelly and the coudé catheter is passed with its tip directed against the roof of the urethra. A marker on the distal end of the catheter denotes the direction in which the tip is pointing. If obstruction is encountered, the catheter is rotated on its long axis, thereby avoiding pockets and folds and passing over or between enlarged prostatic lobes.

If catheterization cannot be accomplished quickly and easily, persistent attempts should be avoided, to prevent trauma. There should be no hesitancy about employing a Phillips' catheter (Fig 15, *c*) and a filiform guide (Fig 15, *d*). The filiform should be passed slowly while it is simultaneously rotated on its long axis; in this manner, pockets, folds, false passages, and prostatic lobes are avoided. At times it may be necessary to pass several filiforms in order to fill pockets and folds before one filiform can be successfully passed into the bladder. Sometimes, passage of a filiform will be aided by first filling the urethra with lubricating jelly. If a filiform can be passed successfully, a Phillips' catheter can be attached to the filiform and the catheter directed into the bladder easily. If it is impossible to pass a catheter after the filiform guide has been passed successfully, the latter should be taped in place. The presence of a filiform guide in the urethra permits patients with acute urinary retention to urinate alongside the guide. Dilatation produced by the guide usually permits passage of a Phillips' catheter the following day.

If the foregoing attempts at catheterization are unsuccessful, one might be tempted to pass rigid or metal catheters or sounds. It is likely that no more success and considerable trauma will be the result of using such instruments. It is probable that the patient has become irritable and his urethra exceedingly tender as a result of repeated unsuccessful attempts at catheterization. In such instances a hypodermic injection of morphine should be administered; after it has taken effect, further attempts can be made. It is surprising how frequently catheterization can be accomplished with ease if the patient is relaxed.

If it remains impossible yet imperative to perform catheterization, general IV or spinal anesthesia should be used. The measures described in the preceding paragraphs are repeated. If they are unsuccessful, one must resort to rigid instruments. It must be remembered that forceful use of rigid instruments may provoke great trauma, and such instruments are not safe in unskilled hands. The first rigid instrument that should be used is a soft rubber catheter that has a hollow tip and is threaded over a wire stylet (Fig 15, *e*). The wire stylet is lubricated and the catheter is threaded over it. Care must be taken to be certain that the point of the stylet is pushed well into the tip of the catheter so that it does not slip out of the eye of the catheter and injure the urethra. The stylet enclosed by the catheter is then passed into the bladder and the stylet is withdrawn. At times the physician can facilitate the passage of the catheter by placing his finger in the patient's rectum and directing the catheter.

If catheterization has been impossible, one may gently attempt to pass a sound. In instances in which passage of a filiform guide has been impossible, one is frequently surprised at the ease of passage of an 18 or 20 F van Buren sound. Likewise, because of the variations in angles of the beaks of various cystoscopes, it may be possible to pass a cystoscope when other measures fail. Before deciding that catheterization is impossible, an attempt to pass the McCarthy panendoscope under vision should be made. The physician practices urethroscopy as he attempts to make the instrument follow the urethral channel into the bladder. If the panendoscope enters the bladder, a catheter can be passed through the panendoscope and the latter withdrawn.

If drainage of the bladder for a prolonged period is necessary, this is best accomplished by the use of the Foley self-retaining bag catheter (Fig 15, *f*).

Both urethral and ureteral catheters are constructed from a variety of materials, including rubber, nylon, latex, polyvinyl, polyethylene, Silastic, and Teflon. A lower incidence of encrustations and mucous plugs and fewer foreign body reactions are claimed for the latter two types of catheters. Disposable catheters are available.

If all attempts at urethral catheterization have been unsuccessful, placement of a suprapubic catheter may be necessary. Percutaneous placement may be performed if the patient's bladder is filled to capacity, there are no anatomic abnormalities, or previous lower abdominal or pelvic surgeries, and if there are no blood coagulation disorders. There are several commercially available kits for percutaneous placement of cystotomy catheters. The kits include some sort of trocar assembly. The patient is placed in a supine position, local anesthesia is used to anesthetize the proposed tract, which will be approximately two fingerbreadths above the pubic symphysis in the midline. Localization of the bladder can be done initially with a fine spinal needle. Then, with the catheter threaded over the trocar, the bladder is punctured through the previously identified site. The catheter is then threaded into the bladder as the trocar is removed. The catheter should be secured snuggly in place with either suture or tape to ensure against its displacement.

## Passage of Urethral Sounds

Urethral sounds are used to detect and dilate urethral strictures, to determine the caliber of the urethra, and to treat inflammatory lesions of the urethra. All of the difficulties enumerated under urethral catheterization may be met.

The van Buren urethral sound (Fig 16, *a*), available in sizes 10 to 40 F, is used most commonly. The measures of cleanliness described for urethral catheterization should be used in passage of sounds. Sounds are passed with the patient lying in a dorsal recumbent position. The penis is held at right angles to the body and a well-lubricated sound is passed through the urethra until the tip of the sound enters the bulb. The weight of the sound itself usually effects its passage through the anterior part of the urethra; only slight pressure and direction are required of the physician. When the tip of the sound has reached the bulb

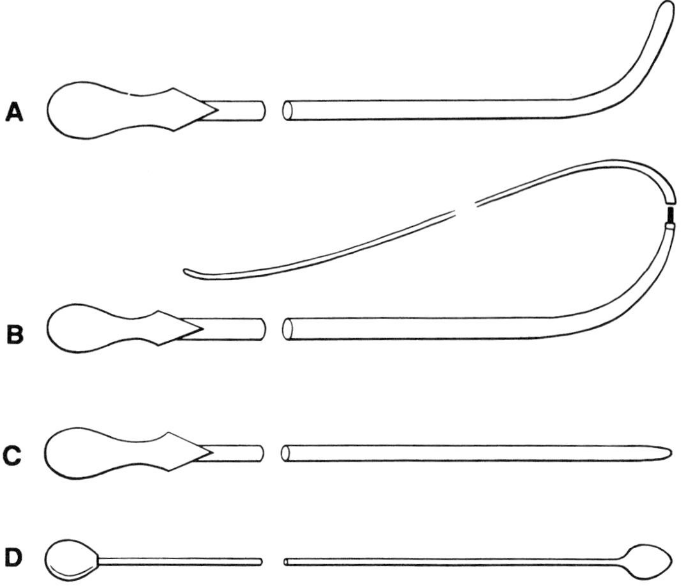


**Fig 16.** Urethral sounds: A, van Buren; B, Le Fort with detachable filiform; C, Jewett; D, Otis bougie à boule.

of the urethra, the handle of the sound is depressed so that the shaft is parallel to the plane of the body and the sound is then directed forward into the bladder. Too frequently, the beginner believes that if he performs certain described maneuvers the sound will automatically pass through the urethra. The sound has sometimes been described as an extension of the examiner's fingers and it usually is necessary to "feel one's way" through the urethra. A moderate degree of force in passage of sounds is permissible only for those who have great experience.

If passage of the van Buren sound is impossible, there should be no hesitancy about using a Le Fort sound (Fig 16, *b*). The passage of this sound is preceded by the passage of a filiform guide as described under urethral catheterization. The tip of the Le Fort sound is equipped with a thread that can be screwed to the end of the filiform. In this manner the filiform guides the passage of the sound through the urethra. The Jewett straight urethral sound (Fig 16, *c*) is available for dilatation of the urethra of females and the anterior urethra of males. Calibration of the urethra to detect urethral stricture can be accomplished best with the Otis bougie à boule urethral sound (Fig 16, *d*).

## Cystoscopy

**Indications.** Cystoscopy is performed for diagnosis and treatment of diseases of the bladder and urethra. Urethroscopy (examination of the urethra) should be an integral part of cystoscopy. As a result of the intimate anatomic and physiologic relationship between bladder and urethra, it frequently is impossible to state, prior to examination, whether disease of the bladder or of the urethra is present. Unfortunately, it is common practice to perform cystoscopy and completely disregard urethroscopy; this arises from failure to use suitable cystoscopes, as will be described later.

Cystoscopy also is performed when studies of the upper part of the urinary tract, which cannot be carried out by excretory urography, nephrotomography, or other means, are necessary. These studies may consist of tests of separated renal function, collection of specimens of urine from each kidney, and passage of ureteral catheters preparatory to retrograde pyelography.

**Preliminary Measures.** If symptoms of sufficient severity to warrant cystoscopy are present, certain measures should precede this examination. Urinalysis and a test of renal function should be performed; the latter usually consists of determination of serum creatinine or BUN levels.

In most instances, some form of roentgenographic study of the urinary tract should precede cystoscopy. Even when performed under ideal circumstances, cystoscopy and retrograde pyelography cause varying degrees of discomfort or pain. Any measure which obviates the necessity for these procedures without interfering with accurate diagnosis is desirable. The ideal plan consists of study of the upper part of the urinary tract by excretory urography and, if necessary, nephrotomography prior to cystoscopy. Such a sequence may establish the fact that the upper part of the urinary tract is normal and that cystoscopy, without retrograde pyelography, is sufficient for accurate diagnosis. On the other hand, it may show that one kidney is normal and that retrograde pyelographic study can be confined to the other kidney. Finally, it may be possible to establish a diagnosis roentgenographically, and cystoscopy may be obviated.

In some instances, however, it is neither practical nor necessary to study the upper part of the urinary tract by excretory urography or retrograde pyelography. A plain film of the region of the kidneys, ureters, and bladder is sufficient in those cases in which the urologist is convinced that the pathologic process, if present, exists in the bladder or urethra. For example, if a woman complains of symptoms suggestive of urethritis and if examination of her urine yields negative results, a plain roentgenogram of the urinary tract and a cystoscopic examination should suffice for diagnosis.

Preparation of the patient's bowel prior to cystoscopy must be considered. If cystoscopy without retrograde pyelography is to be performed, thorough evacuation of the bowel is not necessary. If retrograde pyelography is contemplated and the patient is ambulatory and has daily bowel movements, no specific measures need to be taken. Cleansing of the bowel should be carried out for patients who are bedridden or who have sluggish bowel habits. These patients are given a suitable cathartic the evening preceding examination. Preparation of the patient immediately preceding cystoscopy includes cleansing of the lower part of the abdomen, thighs, and genitalia with soap and water. Thorough cleanliness and asepsis are imperative; particular attention should be paid to the labia, vestibule of the vagina, and preputial cavity.

Some form of anesthesia should be used for cystoscopy; no degree of skill of the cystoscopist can render this examination entirely painless. A variety of proprietary anesthetic jellies that can be instilled into the urethra are available. There is no objection to preliminary administration of sedatives or analgesics; any measure that decreases the discomfort to the patient and does not prevent urethral instrumentation or obtaining desired information may be used. Intravenous injection of 10 mg of diazepam (Valium) is safe and effective. In selected cases, general or spinal anesthesia may be necessary.

**Endoscopes.** An exhaustive description of the construction, maintenance, and use of various cystoscopes can be found in *Urological and Allied Diagnostic Instruments and High Frequency Equipment,* published by American Cystoscope Makers, Inc, New York.

The Brown-Buerger (Fig 17) and Wappler cystoscopes are the instruments of choice among most urologists. By means of right-angle and retrospective lens telescopes, an excellent view of the bladder can be obtained. The use of standard accessory parts permits bilateral catheterization of the ureters and operative procedures. The introduction of fiberoptics has resulted in striking improvement in visualization of almost the entire urinary tract—from the urethra and bladder to the ureters and renal collecting system, and even to the peritoneal and extraperitoneal cavities. A number of rigid and flexible endoscopic instruments are currently available; these

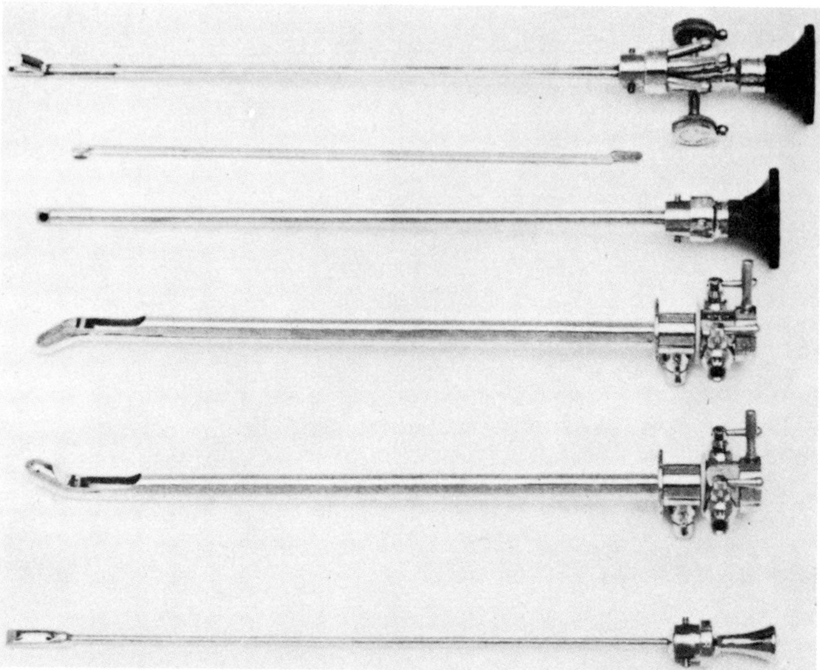

**Fig 17.** Brown-Buerger fiberoptic cystoscope.

include rigid and flexible cystoscopes in both adult and pediatric sizes, rigid and flexible ureteronephroscopes, rigid and flexible nephroscopes, and laparoscopes (Figs 18–20, 22).

The principle of fiberoptics is that light that enters the end of a glass fiber is trapped within the fiber and is transmitted to the opposite end by internal reflections. The fibers are coated with a glass of lower refractive index, and very little light is lost by diffusion. The source of light is a compact box containing a parabolic lamp with cooling and condensing attachments. The fiberoptics are placed either in the sheath or in the various types of telescopes. The disadvantage of these endoscopes is that the image may be completely obscured in the presence of active bleeding from the bladder or prostatic urethra, and the view of the posterior wall of the bladder and urethra is unsatisfactory.

The Greene cystoscope equipped with Foroblique, right-angle, and retrograde telescopes affords excellent visualization of the bladder (Fig 18). In addition, this instrument has the distinct advantage, not present in those previously described, of permitting direct-vision cystoscopy without the aid of telescopes. The view of the base of the bladder, trigone, vesical neck, and urethra, which direct vision permits, cannot be obtained with instruments in which lens systems are used, except with the McCarthy panendoscope. Ureteral catheterization is usually accomplished more easily under direct vision. Distortion of the image as a result of magnification does not occur and a clear medium is not imperative for adequate vision.

The McCarthy panendoscope and routine cystoscope permit excellent visualization of the bladder and urethra (Fig 19). With the aid of Foroblique, right-angle, and retrospective lens telescopes, the bladder and urethra can be visualized completely; the accessory parts permit ureteral catheterization and intravesical and intraurethral manipulations. Various cystoscopes for use in infants and children are available. The McCarthy infant cystoscope is probably the most widely used.

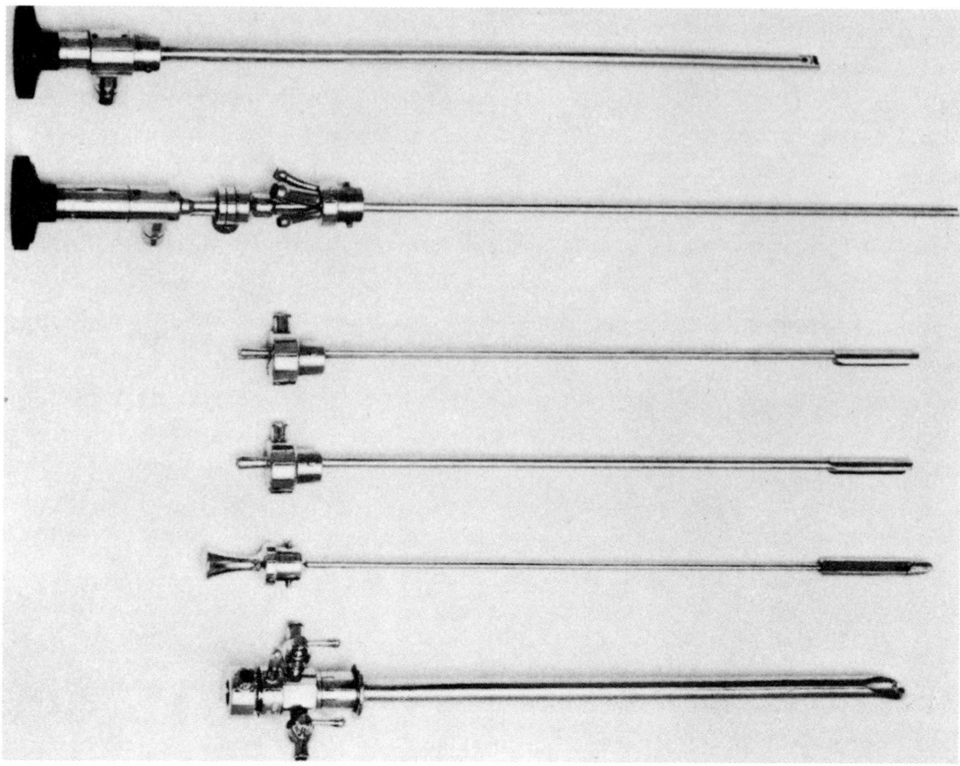

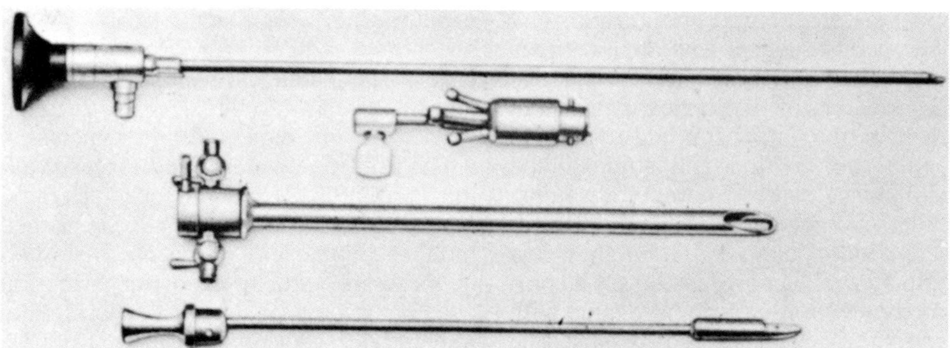

**Fig 19.** McCarthy fiberoptic panendoscope.

**Technique of Cystoscopy.** The remarks made concerning catheterization of the urethra are applicable to passage of a cystoscope. It always must be borne in mind that greater potential for injury exists when rigid instruments are passed.

Prior to cystoscopy, the patient urinates and then assumes the lithotomy position on the cystoscopic table; the physician stands between the patient's abducted legs. The external genitalia and adjacent parts of the body are cleansed as previously described, and the local anesthetic agent is instilled into the urethra and bladder. After suffi-

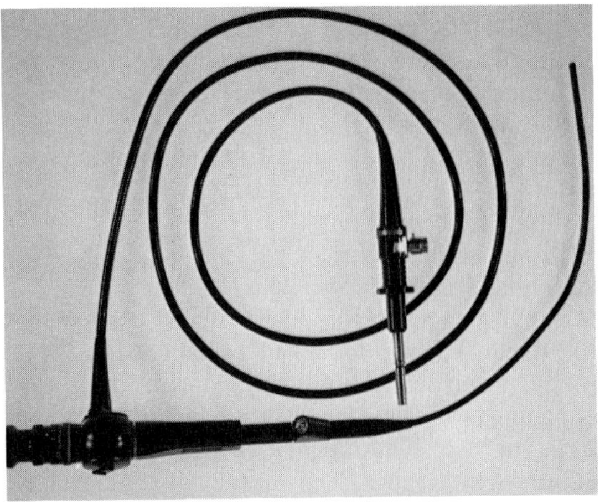

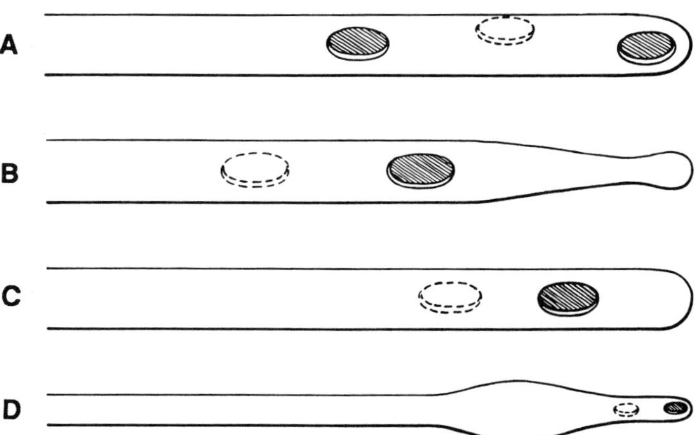


**Fig 21.** Ureteral catheters (magnified): A, whistle tip; B, olive tip; C, round tip; D, Braasch bulb.

cient time to permit the anesthetic to take effect, a well-lubricated cystoscope is passed into the bladder.

In women, the cystoscope ordinarily is introduced readily. It usually is necessary to depress the ocular end of the instrument slightly as the cystoscope is being passed. In men, the technique is more complicated. The penis is held at right angles to the body and the cystoscope is passed downward to the bulb of the urethra (in most instances the instrument reaches the bulb by its own weight). Then the ocular end of the cystoscope is depressed and, simultaneously and gently, the cystoscope is directed forward through the prostatic urethra into the bladder. In most instances, depression of the cystoscope to the horizontal plane is sufficient to permit its passage into the bladder. In most cases of prostatic hypertrophy, depression of the ocular end of the cystoscope beyond the horizontal plane may be necessary. Under such circumstances, the passage of the cystoscope may be facilitated by counter pressure: the free hand exerts upward pressure on the perineum and thereby attempts to elevate the beak of the cystoscope above the median lobe of the prostate. Counter pressure for the same purpose may be achieved by placing a finger in the patient's rectum. After passage of the cystoscope, urine that may have been retained in the bladder is withdrawn for bacteriologic studies and for determination of residual urine.

A plan of inspection of the bladder should be followed, so that, by repetition, it becomes a habit; in this manner, failure to examine the bladder and urethra thoroughly is avoided. For convenience the following method may be used. The bladder is studied both during and after distention with water. The cystoscope is rotated for inspection of the dome of the bladder, which usually can be recognized by the presence of an air bubble. The right and left lateral walls of the bladder are examined by appropriate maneuvers of the cystoscope, consisting of rotation of the cystoscope on its long axis in association with forward and backward movements. The posterior wall is examined by a pendulum or rocking movement of the cystoscope. The trigone, ureteral orifices, and vesical neck then are inspected. The urethra may be examined while the cystoscope is being removed if a Greene cystoscope or McCarthy panendoscope is being used. In men, the prostate gland and verumontanum may be examined at this time. The distinctive appearances of various lesions of the bladder and urethra are considered in detail in other chapters.

The examination of the girl's bladder and urethra presents no significant difficulties, but the narrow urethra in the male, especially in the very young, makes such an examination difficult and fraught with dangers. Since tissues in the child can be damaged easily, the greatest gentleness is necessary. A preliminary calibration of the urethra should always be done to determine the proper size of the instrument to be used. In the male child, the meatus and penoscrotal junction are the narrowest parts; whereas the former may be enlarged by gradual dilatation, the latter is relatively fixed and rigid, and rupture at this point may easily occur. Cystoscopic examination usually is done in the child in an effort to uncover congenital maldevelopment rather than a tumor or other pathologic condition. Trigonal development and the position of the ureteral orifices as well as their appearance correlate well with the degree of vesicoureteral reflux, and the presence of a periureteral diverticulum is positive proof of the incompetence of the ureterovesical junction.

## Ureteral Catheterization

Catheterization of the ureter is performed to collect urine directly from the kidney, as a preliminary step in securing a retrograde pyelogram, and for the purpose of instrumental exploration of the ureter. Catheters of sizes 4 to 6 F with various tips should be available (Fig 21). Ureteral catheterization usually is performed easily with the aid of the Brown-Buerger cystoscope. After the bladder has been examined, the examining telescope is removed and the catheterizing telescope is inserted in its place. The ureteral orifice is identified and the catheter is advanced until it appears in the visual field. The catheter is advanced still farther, so that the tip of the catheter is slightly beyond the visual field. The lid, or deflector, is now raised, bending the catheter away from the instrument. The tip of the catheter thereby comes into the field of vision and is directed into the ureteral orifice.

Catheter guides are used when the Greene cystoscope is used for ureteral catheterization. The catheter guide containing the ureteral catheter is inserted into the cystoscope and the beak of the instrument is brought as close as possible to the ureteral orifice. The tip of the catheter is placed in the orifice and the catheter is then directed up the ureter so that the tip of the catheter enters the renal pelvis. Experienced cystoscopists insert the catheter up the ureter until slight obstruction is detected; the catheter then is withdrawn slightly and, in most instances, the tip of the catheter will rest in the renal pelvis. The end of the catheter should be occluded with an ordinary straight pin in order to prevent vesical urine from entering the ureteral catheter. The pin is withdrawn after the catheter has been placed in the ureter.

Difficulty in ureteral catheterization may result from using a catheter that is too rigid,

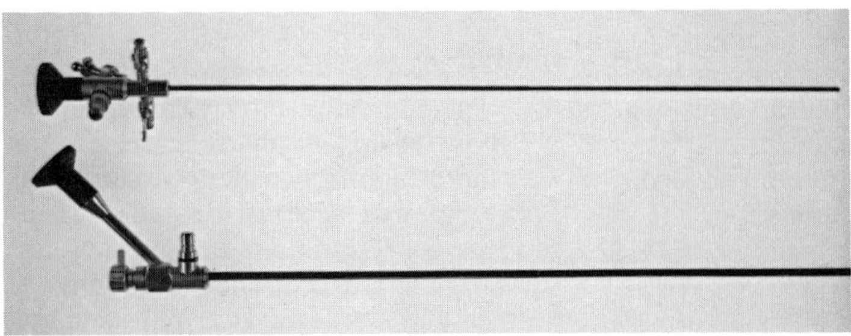

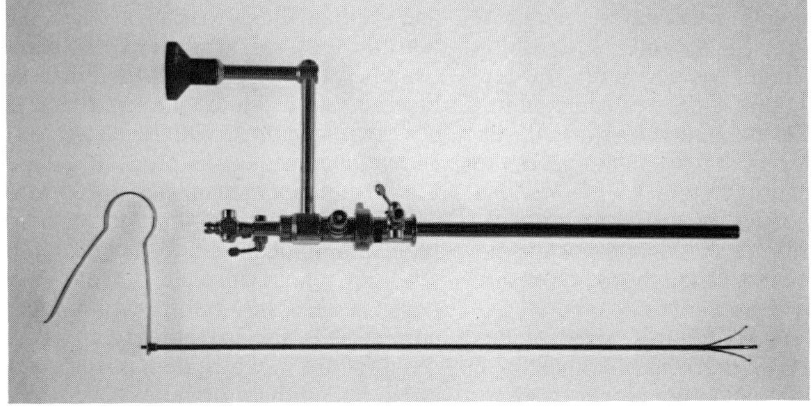

B

**Fig 22.** A, ureteroscope; B, nephroscope.

too flexible, or too large for the size of the orifice. A variety of pathologic processes may alter the size, position, and appearance of the orifice and make catheterization difficult. The passage of the catheter up the ureter may be arrested by mucosal folds, muscular spasm, or pathologic processes.

The cystoscope may be left in place while roentgenologic studies are made. This permits adjustment of the ureteral catheters if roentgenograms disclose that they have been placed improperly. On the other hand, if cystoscopy is being performed with the patient under local anesthesia, the patient is more comfortable if the cystoscope is withdrawn after passage of the catheters.

## Ureteropyeloscopy

Ureteropyeloscopy is the transurethral endoscopic inspection of the ureter and renal pelvis using a rigid or flexible ureteropyeloscope. These endoscopes (Fig 22, *a*) permit both diagnostic and therapeutic procedures to be performed. The larger rigid instruments range in size from 9 to 13.5 F, while the flexible scopes may be as small as 7 F. The larger ureteropyeloscopes have working channels that allow passage of various accessories such as stone baskets, wire graspers, and electrohydraulic, ultrasonic, or laser probes for stone disintegration. The working channel of the smaller endoscopes may allow only for irrigation or small laser fibers, but the small size of the scope theoretically lowers the risk of ureteral injury and often obviates the need for dilatation of the transmural ureter.

Diagnostic indications for ureteropyeloscopy are evaluation of filling defects, periodic surveillance of previously resected tumor, further evaluation of positive cytologies or hematuria, and evaluation of ureteral narrowing. Therapeutic options include passage of ureteral catheters, stone manipulation, treatment of urethral strictures or ureteropelvic junction obstruction, and treatment of selected ureteral or renal pelvic tumors. At present, the most common indication for ureteropyeloscopy is treatment of ureteral stones.

### Nephroscopy

In contrast to all the previously mentioned endoscopic procedures, nephroscopy is performed in an antegrade fashion through a percutaneous puncture. The percutaneous puncture is created using an imaging technique for guidance—usually ultrasound. The object is to obtain access to the renal collecting system in a manner that will allow adequate visualization of the pathology. Therefore, the location of the entry site must be well thought out to ensure the success of subsequent endeavors.

Contraindications for this percutaneous procedure are similar to those delineated in the next section on kidney biopsy, and are primarily blood clotting anomalies. Indications for percutaneous puncture of the renal collecting system are expanding rapidly, and include nephrolithotomy, dilation of ureteropelvic junction obstruction or endopyelotomy, dilation of ureteral strictures, treatment of urothelial tumors, and nephrostomy catheter placement for obstruction or perfusion chemolysis of renal calculi. Diagnostic puncture of the renal collecting system is less commonly performed, but can be used for antegrade pyelograms or Whitaker tests (pressure/perfusion studies).

The standard size of a rigid nephroscope is 24–26 F (Fig 22, *b*) and as with the previously mentioned endoscopes, flexible nephroscopes are also available. The flexible nephroscopes allow for inspection of calyces, which might be impossible with the rigid scope; however, the smaller working parts allow for fewer therapeutic maneuvers. Accessories include graspers, forceps, stone baskets, ultrasonic, electrohydraulic and laser probes, dilating balloons, and resecting elements.

## BIOPSY

### Kidney

The indications for percutaneous renal biopsy are many and relative; generally it is indicated in any patient with renal disease in whom an accurate diagnosis cannot be made by routine clinical or laboratory investigations and in whom contraindications to biopsy do not exist. With careful technique, adequate specimens can be obtained and accurate diagnosis can be made in more than 85% of cases; as expected, accuracy usually is high in patients with diffuse renal disease such as glomerulonephritis and relatively low in those with focal disease such as pyelonephritis. The procedure is particularly valuable in diagnosing obscure renal disease, such as the nephrotic syndrome, renal amyloidosis, and diabetic nephropathy, in which an exact histologic diagnosis is necessary before treatment is instituted; it is also valuable in cases of acute renal failure in which demonstration of tubular rather than glomerular involvement may indicate good prognosis after hemodialysis. Serial biopsies of the same patient can often determine the efficacy of a particular therapeutic regimen.

The urologist does not usually perform percutaneous renal biopsy, but is occasionally called on for the management of complications which might follow the procedure (which fortunately are infrequent). Perhaps the only absolute contraindication to percutaneous renal biopsy is the existence of a hemorrhagic diathesis, since bleeding occurring as hematuria, hematoma, or retroperitoneal hemorrhage represents the most serious—as well as the most frequent—complication of the procedure. When a solitary kidney is present, open biopsy with more precise hemostasis is preferable. Other, lesser contraindications include significant infection either in the renal system or systemically, suspicion of renal neoplasm or abscess, and severe hypertension (these patients tend to bleed excessively).

Many modifications of the technique are used, but the principles are identical in all.

A satisfactory plain film of the abdomen showing two renal shadows and preferably, if the renal function is adequate for visualization, an intravenous pyelogram should be obtained. Unless the disease is localized in one kidney, as indicated by the history or the physical or roentgenographic examination, attention rarely is deliberately directed to one side or the other. The right side usually is selected because of the presence of the spleen and the great vessels on the left. The midspinal line, the outline of the twelfth rib, and the prospective biopsy site in the middle or lower pole of the kidney are all drawn on the roentgenogram, and these anatomic markings are transposed to the patient's back. The patient is placed in the prone position with sandbags pressing on the abdomen so that the kidneys are in a more posterior position. It is best to measure the biopsy site laterally from the midspinal line and inferiorly from the last rib. The skin and subcutaneous tissue down to the renal capsule are infiltrated with local anesthetic, and a long 18- to 22-gauge Vim-Silverman needle is used. The needle with the obturator in place is gently inserted down to the renal capsule while the patient holds his breath. Usually, the operator is aware of perforating the capsule because an increased tissue resistance is noted at this point. The patient's gentle breathing at this time will produce a swing of the needle in an arc, due to movement of the kidney. The obturator then is removed and the Vim-Silverman needle is inserted to its full length through the cannula. The cannula is advanced over the Vim-Silverman needle and with a 360-degree rotation the entire apparatus is removed.

Percutaneous renal biopsy techniques utilizing cinefluoroscopic, ultrasonographic, or computed tomographic monitoring have been described. When the kidney has been adequately visualized, the needle is inserted under fluoroscopic or ultrasonographic control. The gray-red piece of tissue removed (the red line indicates the corticomedullary junction and the arcuate vessels) is suitably fixed. Pressure is applied for approximately 10 minutes, and the patient is kept in the prone position for at least 20 minutes.

Ideally, the patient should be confined to bed until all microscopic hematuria has subsided. The principal complication of renal biopsy is bleeding. Virtually all patients demonstrate microscopic hematuria for 24 hours, and 1 in 10 has gross hematuria. Ureteral colic due to the passage of clots may occur. Absolute bed rest and forced fluids will result in rapid cessation of the bleeding. Blood transfusions occasionally are required. Drainage of severe perinephric hematomas and, on occasion, nephrectomy have become necessary.

### Prostate

Biopsy of the prostate is indicated in all patients in whom clinical suspicion of prostate cancer exists. It can be accomplished in the following ways: 1) needle biopsy, 2) fine-needle aspiration, 3) transurethral biopsy, and 4) open perineal biopsy.

**Needle Biopsy.** Core-needle biopsy of the prostate is accomplished with a Tru-Cut needle or, more commonly now, with a Biopty needle and the automatic Biopty device (Fig 23). The biopsy may be obtained transrectally or transperineally using either digital or ultrasonic guidance.

***Transperineal Needle Biopsy.*** After proper preparation of the perineum, the needle is introduced just ventral to the anus. The needle is advanced ventral to the rectum and is always palpable by a finger placed in the rectum to direct the tip of the needle to the suspected area in the prostate. This procedure often requires local or spinal anesthetic.

***Transrectal Needle Biopsy.*** This usually is performed as an office or outpatient procedure. After cleansing enemas, the prostate is palpated with an index finger to determine the proper site for insertion of the needle; the needle is then introduced along the index finger of the right hand (Fig 24). After the site of biopsy has been selected, the Biopty gun is activated and a core of

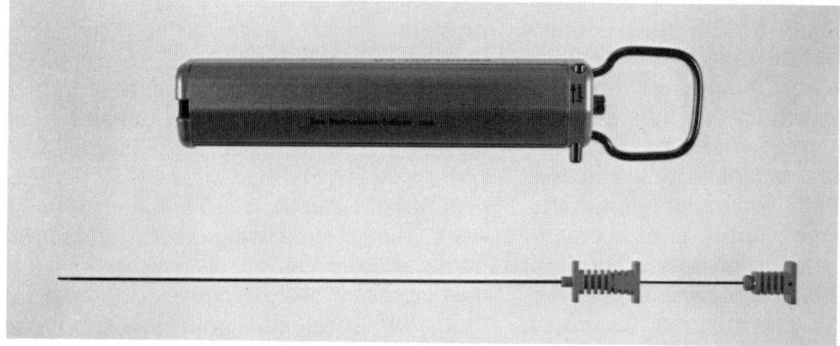

**Fig 23.** Biopty needle and the automatic Biopty device.

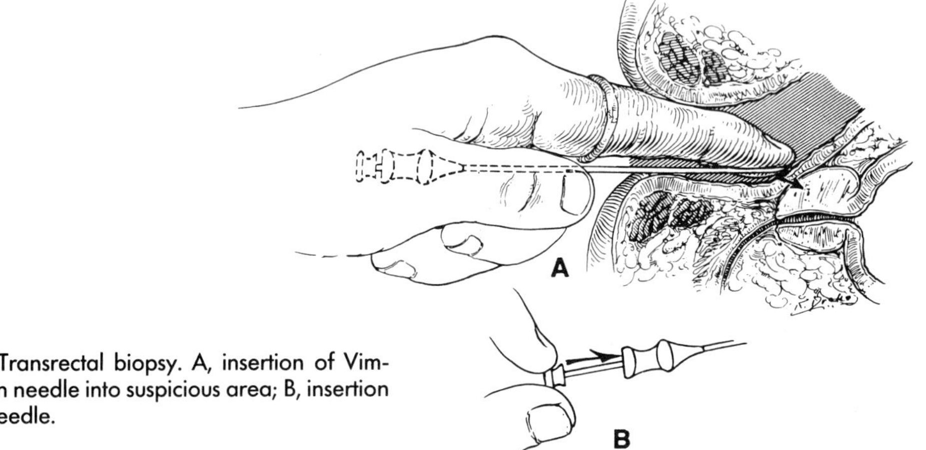


**Fig 24.** Transrectal biopsy. A, insertion of Vim-Silverman needle into suspicious area; B, insertion of split needle.

tissue is obtained. The procedure may be repeated if an unsatisfactory core is obtained or if further samples are desired. It is usually wise to biopsy both lobes of the gland, even though only one side feels neoplastic, because not infrequently the lobe that feels benign supplies the neoplastic tissue. The ease with which the transrectal needle biopsy is performed using the Biopty gun and the minimal number of associated complications have made this currently the most popular mode of prostate biopsy.

Additionally, transrectal and transperineal prostate biopsy specimens can be obtained using ultrasound guidance. A transrectal ultrasound probe is inserted transrectally to scan the prostate for hypoechoic areas within the peripheral zone. Once identified, the ultrasonic image can be used to direct the biopsy needle to the area of concern. To date, this has not been shown to be superior to digitally guided biopsy.

***Fine Needle Aspiration.*** Aspiration biopsy is performed transrectally using a Franzen needle. The nodule is identified, and a 22-gauge needle is passed through the needle guide into the nodule. Suction is applied to the syringe as the needle is moved back and forth within the nodule. Suction is stopped, the needle is withdrawn, and the sample is placed onto a microscope slide. Finally, the specimen is inspected, using cytologic techniques.

**Perineal.** Open perineal biopsies are now performed infrequently. They were previously performed in patients suspected of having localized carcinoma of the prostate immediately prior to prostatectomy. Perineal exposure of the gland and biopsy of the suspected nodule was first undertaken. Examination of frozen sections of the tissue was then performed; if the diagnosis of carcinoma was confirmed, radical prostatectomy was performed at the same setting.

**Transurethral.** Transurethral biopsy was previously the most commonly used method of establishing the diagnosis of prostate cancer. With the ease and low morbidity of needle biopsy, this is no longer the case. Additionally, performance of transurethral biopsy is generally inadequate to make the diagnosis of early prostatic cancer, as cancer tends to arise in the periphery of the gland (in contrast to benign hypertrophy which occurs periurethrally). However, in approximately 10% of patients, prostatic carcinoma will be diagnosed transurethrally only after transurethral resection of the prostate has been performed for presumed benign prostatic hyperplasia.

### Testis

Testicular biopsy is commonly used in cases in which neoplasia is suspected, in the diagnosis and evaluation of disturbances in the endocrine system, and in the study of infertility.

In the first instance, the method of biopsy is similar to that used elsewhere in the body. The examination usually is performed with the patient under general anesthesia, and the scrotum and inguinal area are prepared as for any surgical procedure. An incision sufficient to permit delivery and complete inspection of the testis is made in the inguinal area. The spermatic cord is isolated and its blood supply should be interrupted by a rubber-shod clamp. Then the testis is removed from the scrotum and, if necessary, a suitable specimen is removed and examined with frozen-section technique. If the biopsy or visualization shows a tumor, then a high ligation of the spermatic cord is done and the testis removed.

In the latter two instances, the technique varies depending on the size of the testis. If it is normal in size, the procedure may be performed by infiltrating the skin and superficial tissues with procaine hydrochloride (Novocain) or lidocaine (Xylocaine). A small incision (1 cm) is carried through the parietal layer of the tunica albuginea. A swab soaked with 10% cocaine is applied to the testis for 3 minutes and a small incision is made into the testis. The parenchyma prolapses into the incision and is excised with small scissors; the incisions in the testis and skin are closed with one stitch of plain catgut. Preservation of the testicular tubules is obtained if the tissue is fixed in Bouin's solution.

If the testicle is atrophic, biopsy is painful unless performed with the patient under general anesthesia. This is true because the parenchyma does not prolapse into the incision but must be deeply excised.

### Percutaneous Aspiration Biopsy

Recent changes in philosophy concerning "aspiration needle biopsy" of tumors has led to a rapid increase in the utilization of this technique. In this technique, the lesion to be biopsied is located by palpation (superficial lesion), or by fluoroscopic or ultrasonographic imaging (deep lesion) and the area of concern is aspirated, usually with a 22- to 23-gauge needle. The needle is removed and the contents are ejected onto a slide, fixed with 95% ethyl alcohol, and examined cytologically.

Aspiration biopsy may be applied to any area of concern in the urinary tract: subcutaneous, renal, periureteral (from pelvis of kidney to bladder), prostatic, or pelvic. This biopsy technique may be used in primary diagnosis of tumor, staging of known tumor, or diagnosis of the cause of ureteral obstruction in a patient with a known malignancy.

In the latter group with deep retroperitoneal lesions obstructing the ureter, a thin, 22- or 23-gauge needle may be passed directly through the peritoneum and into the lesion under fluoroscopic or ultrasonographic monitoring. There is no need for concern over puncturing the bowels or major blood vessels; the holes made are so small that no clinical problems have developed. The safety of this procedure has drastically reduced the need for surgical exploration, eg, to determine whether ureteral obstruction is due to metastatic tumor or to postsurgical scarring. Resultant positive aspirates eliminate the need for surgery under such conditions and allow for definite cytologic diagnosis so that one may proceed with chemotherapy. Negative aspirates, however, may be due to either tumor or scar formation and still may require surgical management.

# 8

# Urinary Tract Infections in Women: Causes, Consequences, and Clinical Management

*John N. Krieger*

## INTRODUCTION

Urinary tract infections (UTIs) occur in several identifiable female risk groups: infants, school age girls, sexually active young women, and the elderly.[1] UTIs cause major morbidity, health care expenditures, and time lost from work. For example, acute uncomplicated UTIs in young women are responsible for 6–7 million office visits per year in the U.S. and result in approximately 250,000 cases of acute pyelonephritis per year.[2,3] The entire urinary system is at risk of invasion by bacteria following infection of one of its parts. Recurrence is the rule following treatment of an initial UTI and approximately 20% of women with acute UTIs experience frequent recurrences. This chapter will summarize the epidemiology of UTIs, then focus on current concepts of the causes, clinical presentation, treatment, and differential diagnosis of UTIs in women.

## EPIDEMIOLOGY OF UTIs

The incidence and prevalence of infection differ markedly in males and females. Figure 1 presents an overview of UTIs stratified age, sex, and predisposing factors.[1] The frequency of both symptomatic and asymptomatic UTIs parallel each other. In the neonatal period UTI is much more common in boys than in girls. UTI rates depend on the population studied and clinical methods, with highest rates reported among children in newborn intensive care units.[4] For example, Ginsburg and McCracken found that male infants accounted for 75% of infants aged 5 days to 3 months hospitalized because of acute UTI.[5] After the neonatal period, the great majority of UTIs occur in females at a ratio of 10–30:1.[1] The peak age for UTI in girls occurs at the age of 3–4 years.

Among schoolchildren the prevalence of bacteriuria among girls (1%–2%) is high compared to that among boys (about 0.04%), a ratio of 30:1.[1,6,7] These data confirm the marked susceptibility of the female to urinary infection. The actual risk of a girl acquiring bacteriuria during the school years is much greater than the prevalence of 1%–2% since this rate only represents those found at one time. It is estimated that 5%–6% of girls experience at least one episode of bacteriuria during the time between entering the first grade and gradu-

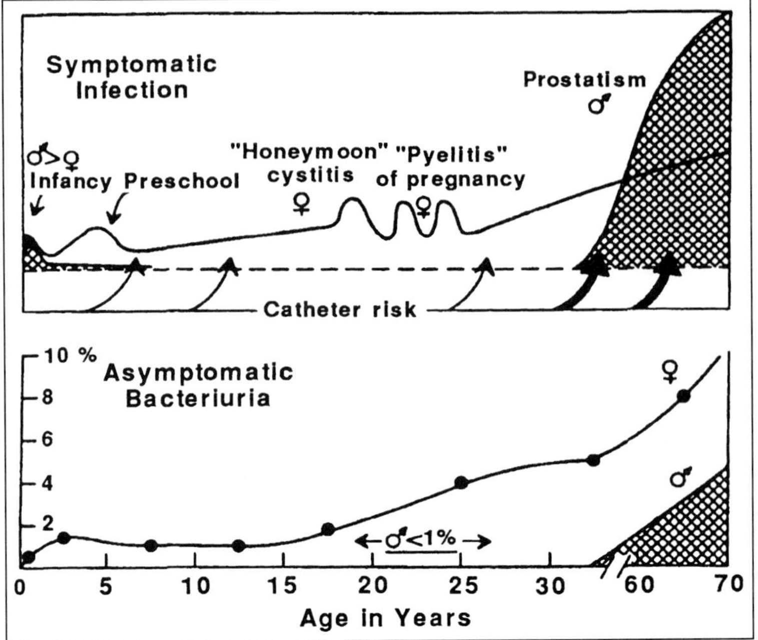


**Fig 1.** Overview of the frequency of symptomatic urinary tract infection and the prevalence of bacteriuria according to age and sex. [From Kunin CM, with permission.[1]]

ating from high school. There is an 80% recurrence rate following conventional therapy.

UTIs are far more common among adult women than in any other group and therefore deserve special emphasis. Uncomplicated UTIs in females cause considerable morbidity even though such infections rarely cause significant renal damage.[1] Most women are well acquainted with the signs and symptoms of UTI and many have been treated by their physicians for UTI at some time in the past. For example, 25%–35% of 20- to 40-year-old women will give a history of having had treatment for UTI.[1] The prevalence of bacteriuria is similar among diverse populations of adult women. For example, Evans and associates found the overall prevalence of ''significant'' bacteriuria to be 3.5%.[8] The prevalence is increased in married compared to nonmarried women, and in those who have children, and increases with parity.[1] The lowest reported prevalence of bacteriuria is in Roman Catholic nuns.[9]

The prevalence of UTI rises with age and may be 10% in women over the age of 70. The prevalence of significant bacteriuria in the elderly living in the community is higher in females than males, 6%–33% vs. 11%–13%.[10–12] Rates are extraordinarily high among residents of long-term facilities (11%–33% for men and 28%–85% for women). Uncomplicated UTIs among residents of long-term facilities may be a sentinel sign of generalized debility and may be associated with an increased death rate.[13,14]

## CAUSES OF UTIs IN WOMEN

UTI is the general term for a wide range of syndromes characterized by the presence of a positive urine culture. UTIs include a range of clinical presentations differing in significance, amount of tissue invasion, requirements for successful antimicrobial therapy, and propensity for recurrence. The varied UTI syndromes represent the outcome of a series of events: colonization of the host, development of infection, and the outcome of infection.

These events represent the interaction between virulence factors of the bacterium and host factors that determine the susceptibility to infection.[15,16] In recent years there has been considerable progress in understanding critical factors in the pathogenesis of UTIs. We will first consider bacterial virulence factors and then review our current understanding of important host factors.

## Bacterial Factors

Because *E. coli* is responsible for 90% of acute UTIs, most attention has been directed to identification of virulence factors for this organism. Bacterial strains isolated from patients with UTIs have the potential to cause pathology in the urinary tract, hence the term ''uropathogenic.'' Uropathogenic *E. coli* have a number of specific characteristics. To date, the most important of these characteristics appears to be presence of fimbrial adhesins that mediate attachment of the bacteria to host cells. (Other terms for fimbriae are pili and F antigens.)

Three classes of fimbrial adhesins appear important for attachment of uropathogenic *E. coli* to host cells: mannose-sensitive adhesins, Gal-Gal adhesins, and X adhesins.[17] Common type 1 pili (f1 serotype) bind to mannose residues on host cells.[18] The receptor for P blood group pili is Gal α(1-4)Gal, a digalactose moiety located in neutral glucophosphingolipids on epithelial and erythrocyte surfaces.[19] The X adhesins constitute a heterogeneous group of fimbrial and afimbrial adhesins that bind to receptors other than mannose or Gal-Gal. Currently identified receptors for X adhesins include NeuAca(2-3)Gal (s-pilus adhesin), glycophorin A (M-pilus adhesin), Dr[a] blood group antigen (AFA-I and AFA-III adhesins), and GalNAca(21-3)GalNAc (Forsmann binding pilus or F-pilus adhesin).[17] Other uropathogenic characteristics do not depend on adherence of the bacteria to host surfaces, such as the presence of hemolysin and aerobactin.[20]

Phenotypic expression of urovirulence traits occurs significantly more often in *E. coli* strains from patients with UTIs than in fecal strains.[21–24] Comparison of *E. coli* strains from women with uncomplicated pyelonephritis with strains from patients with cystitis and fecal strains reveals several critical differences. Certain adhesins occur more commonly in patients with more invasive infections. For example, in one study the presence of Gal-Gal and/or P adhesins was documented in over 70% of patients with acute pyelonephritis, in about 50% of patients with acute cystitis, but in only about 25% of fecal strains. Similarly, expression of hemolysin occurs significantly more often in strains from women with acute pyelonephritis or acute cystitis than in fecal isolates. The presence of genetic material coding for aerobactin occurs significantly more often in *E. coli* strains from women with acute pyelonephritis than in strains from women with acute cystitis.[3] However, comparisons of *E. coli* strains from women with initial episodes of cystitis to strains from women with recurrent cystitis reveal no apparent differences in the prevalence of these virulence factors.[20]

The current consensus of most investigators is that uropathogenic *E. coli* belong to a relatively small group of bacterial clones. These clones accumulated multiple virulence properties that enhance their ability to colonize and infect the urinary tract.[3,25,26] *E. coli* strains from women with pyelonephritis or urosepsis generally contain multiple virulence factors. Strains from women with cystitis may contain individual virulence factors, but only a minority have multiple virulence factors. Fecal isolates from asymptomatic patients are significantly less likely to contain virulence factors than strains from women with cystitis or upper UTIs. One interpretation of these findings is that virulence factors appear to be critical for establishment of upper UTIs but that these characteristics have a lesser role in establishment of lower UTIs.[3]

Bacterial virulence factors appear critical for the establishment of infections in patients with anatomically normal urinary tracts, such as most sexually active women. In contrast, patients with anatomically abnormal urinary tracts are susceptible to infection with strains that lack multiple virulence factors.[22,27] The presence of foreign bodies, reflux, stones, or use of diaphragms appears to facilitate infection with intrinsically less virulent organisms.[3,20]

### Host Factors

The urethra, efficient voiding, and absence of vesicoureteral reflux are important mechanical factors that limit ascent of bacteria within the urinary tract. Intrinsic defenses of the bladder and upper urinary tract against bacterial adherence may include other nonspecific factors, such as bladder surface glycosaminoglycans[28] and Tamm–Horsfall protein (uromucoid),[29] besides cellular and humoral immunity. There is general agreement that a discrete sequence of events occurs during acute UTIs in young women. *E. coli* causing such infections originate from fecal organisms that colonize the vaginal introitus and urethra before ascending to the bladder.[1,30] Intercourse facilitates migration of bacteria into the lower urinary tract.[30,31] Further ascent of bacteria into the upper urinary tract may result in pyelonephritis.

Several lines of evidence suggest that other host factors are of major significance in determining which women are prone to recurrent UTIs and that the defect in host factors is most likely at the cellular level. Support for this view comes from the observation that women with recurrent UTIs tend to have persistent vaginal colonization with *E. coli* compared to other women. This suggests an increased susceptibility to bacterial colonization.[32,33] Urothelial and vaginal cells from women with recurrent infections are more susceptible to adherence of uropathogenic *E. coli* than cells from women who do not have urinary infections.[34] These findings suggest that the susceptibility of host epithelial cells to attachment of *E. coli* may be critical for determining susceptibility of women to recurrent UTIs. The increased frequency of UTIs with age and sexual activity,[35] the tendency of infections to occur in clusters,[36] and the finding that most UTIs are reinfections rather than persistence of a single strain[33] also suggest the presence of an important host susceptibility factor.

**Young, Sexually Active Women.** The onset of sexual activity in women is associated with a marked increase in the frequency of UTIs. Contraceptive practice appears to be one major factor contributing to this association, particularly diaphragm/spermicide use.[3] Fihn and associates compared 114 women with bacteriuria and 85 women with dysuria who did not have UTIs.[37] Diaphragm use was associated with a twofold increase in risk for UTI when the women with UTIs and controls were matched for age, number of sexual partners, frequency of intercourse, and history of previous urinary infections. The same investigators also conducted a retrospective study comparing the incidence of UTI in 148 women who used oral contraceptives only and 165 women who used diaphragms only. The rate of infection among the diaphragm users was also twice as high as the rate of infection among oral contraceptive users. Use of the combination of a diaphragm and spermicide caused a profound disturbance of the normal vaginal flora.[3] There was a marked increase in *E. coli* colonization, with an increased vaginal pH and a decreased concentration of vaginal *Lactobacilli.* These observations suggest a major alteration in the anaerobic flora of the vagina in women who use the combination of diaphragm and spermicide.

Blood group antigens on the urothelial cell surface, particularly the Lewis blood group recessive phenotype, and nonsecretor status also increase the risk for recurrent UTIs in women.[38] In some studies, the $P_2$ blood group phenotype was also associated with an increased risk for recurrent lower UTIs[39] but other studies have not supported this association.[27,38] Although the data are incomplete, it appears that secretor status is an expression of the Lewis blood group antigens. Women who express the secretor gene express similar determinants in other secretions, such as saliva.[38] The mechanism through which secretor status influences the risk for UTI is unclear but may reflect the urothelial cells' susceptibility to bacterial attachment.[1,3,37,38,40] It is possible that secretor status could influence the risk for UTI because blood group antigens in nonsecretors are not exported to either the urothelial cell surface or vaginal secretions.[3] The absence of such antigens at this site might uncover receptors for *E. coli* resulting in increased colonization in nonsecretors.[22] To date, secretor status is the only genetic factor that appears to clearly influence susceptibility to UTIs in young women.

Other host factors that have been investigated as potential risk factors include menstrual protection, oral contraceptive use, and behavioral factors. Use of different types of menstrual protection (eg, tampons vs. napkins) does not appear to influence the frequency of bacteriuria.[9] Studies of the effect of oral contraceptives have reported conflicting results.[8,9,41,42] On balance, oral contraceptive use has little or no effect on the prevalence of bacteriuria in women under 40, but may be associated with increased rates of bacteriuria in older women.[1] Adatto and associates reported that female university students with recurrent UTIs gave a history of regular deferral of urination compared to controls without infection, but their sexual practices were remarkably similar.[43] Other workers found no difference in frequency of voiding in women with or without recurrent UTIs.[1,44] Behavioral factors, such as diet, clothing, use of bubble bath, perineal hygiene, etc., have not been shown to influence UTI rates.[42]

The following scenario summarizes current theories about host factors in the pathogenesis of acute UTI in young women.[3,33] The usual route of infection is by ascent of fecal organisms that colonize the vaginal epithelium. Colonization with uropathogens appears to be more common in women with recurrent infections. It appears that there is an increased susceptibility to vaginal colonization associated with an increased susceptibility of vaginal and urothelial cells to adhering *E. coli.* Among the most important factors that may influence the likelihood of bacterial attachment and colonization are the genetic factor of nonsecretor status and the acquired factor of diaphragm/spermicide use. The precise mechanisms by which these factors influence this susceptibility of the vaginal and urothelial cells to bacterial attachment are not yet clear.

**Elderly Women.** The most important factors responsible for the increased rate of bacteriuria in the elderly are debility and the increased frequency of diseases that interfere with normal bladder emptying.[1] These conditions include central and peripheral nervous disease associated with dementia and diabetes. Incontinence in elderly females may also be associated with an increased rate of UTI. Williams and Pannill estimate that urinary incontinence affects 5%–10% of the elderly in the community and up to 50% in institutions.[15] Stamey and Timothy showed that elderly women have decreased vaginal glycogen and a slightly higher pH.[16] Such changes may facilitate greater colonization of the periurethral zone with gram-negative enteric bacteria and an increased rate of UTI due to ascending infection of the urinary tract.

## CLINICAL EVALUATION AND TREATMENT OF UTIs IN WOMEN

This section will consider the laboratory diagnosis of UTI, and the presentation and treatment of important clinical syndromes.

### Diagnosis of UTI

Urinalysis and quantitative urine culture are the laboratory cornerstones for diagnosis of UTI and evaluation of therapy. In most clinical circumstances, adequate specimens may be obtained by the clean-catch midstream technique.[1] However, urethral catheterization or suprapubic aspiration may be necessary in obtunded patients or in selected cases where uncertainty remains after evaluation of midstream specimens.[33]

**Microbiology.** In more than 95% of cases the organisms causing UTI are Enterobacteriaceae, an *Enterococcus* species, *Staphylococcus saprophyticus,* or *Pseudomonas aeruginosa.* These organisms are different from the microorganisms that colonize the genital skin, distal urethra, and the vagina (*Staphylococcus epidermidis,* diphtheroids, lactobacilli, *Gardnerella vaginalis,* and a variety of anaerobes) that rarely cause UTI. Two general groups of pathogens causing UTI can be identified: those causing uncomplicated UTI [a relatively narrow spectrum including *E. coli, Klebsiella, Proteus,* and *S. saprophyticus* (in young women)] and those causing complicated UTI (besides the above, *Pseudomonas,* other gram-negative bacteria and enterococci).

A common problem with interpretation of urine cultures is that ~10%–20% of women harbor Enterobacteriaceae in their vaginas or periurethral areas at any time. Contamination of urine with vaginal Enterobacteriaceae or commensal flora may make the interpretation of results difficult. In general, isolation of multiple bacterial species suggests a contaminated specimen unless the patient has an indwelling catheter or a long-standing complicated infection.[45,46] Evaluation of quantitative counts and pyuria is often helpful in evaluating urine culture results.

**Quantitative Urine Cultures.** Kass and associates conducted epidemiologic studies using quantitative cultures.[47,48] They separated individuals into two populations. One population with "significant bacteriuria" consistently had large numbers of bacteria in their urine [>$10^5$ colony-forming units per milliliter of urine (cfu/mL)] and usually experienced morbidity. Two consecutive urine cultures yielding the same organism in concentrations >$10^5$ cfu/mL had a specificity of >95% and a sensitivity of >80% for predicting a clinically important UTI. The second population had few bacteria—predominantly contaminants—in their urine. These individuals experienced no morbidity and did not benefit from investigation or treatment.

Kass emphasized that a minority of patients with true infection had <$10^5$ cfu/mL in their urine. Although they can be ignored for epidemiologic studies, such patients are often important clinically. For many years, however, physicians concentrated on a diagnosis of significant bacteriuria for clinical decisions. Recent evidence has again emphasized that interpretation of urinary culture results must also consider the patient's clinical presentation.[46,49]

*S. saprophyticus* and probably fungal pathogens, such as *Candida* species, are often present in lower concentrations in the urine than are gram-negative uropathogens. For example, urine obtained by suprapubic aspiration from women with acute dysuria due to *S. saprophyticus* usually harbors only $10^2$–$10^4$ cfu/mL.[50,51]

For acutely symptomatic women criteria differ from those applied in the evaluation of patients with asymptomatic bacteriuria. In this setting isolation of markedly lower concentrations of bacteria ($10^2$–$10^5$ cfu/mL) supports the diagnosis of UTI.[33,46,49,52–54]

**Pyuria.** In women with urinary symptoms, the presence of pyuria (if documented by appropriate techniques) correlates closely with UTI. Measurement of leukocyte esterase (by dipstick) may be used for screening, but the standard method is to count the number of white blood cells (WBCs) present per high-power microscopic field (hpf) in the resuspended sediment of a centrifuged aliquot of urine. The problem with evaluation of the resuspended urine sediment is that as many as 50% of patients with significant bacteriuria will not have pyuria (ie, >5 WBC/hpf).[49,55]

Use of a counting chamber (such as a hemocytometer) increases the value of microscopic urinalysis for evaluation of pyuria.[49,55] By hemocytometer count the finding of >10 WBC/$mm^3$ of unspun urine is a much more accurate and reproducible method than examination of the centrifuged urinary sediment.[46,55] More than 96% of symptomatic men and women with significant bacteriuria and either complicated or uncomplicated UTI have ≥10 WBC/$mm^3$ in their urine. In contrast, fewer than 1% of asymptomatic, nonbacteriuric individuals have evidence of pyuria by chamber counts. Most acutely symptomatic women with pyuria but no significant bacteriuria have true UTI. The presence of bacterial uropathogens in counts >100,000 cfu/mL is evident on culture of midstream urine and may be confirmed by suprapubic aspiration. It is important to note that in children pyuria may accompany fever and, taken alone, is not very specific as an indicator of UTI.[56] Thus, in symptomatic adult patients, documentation of pyuria constitutes important evidence for UTI, provided that a rigorous technique is employed.

## Clinical Syndromes

Patients with UTIs may be classified in three categories based on clinical and laboratory findings: acute uncomplicated UTI, acute uncomplicated pyelonephritis, and complicated UTI. Because pregnancy and nursing impose special considerations for diagnosis and treatment these women are considered in a separate category. Despite some clinical overlap, specific diagnostic and therapeutic considerations are important for each syndrome.

### Acute Uncomplicated UTI (Cystitis)

**Clinical Presentation.** Acute uncomplicated UTI is a syndrome characterized by various combinations of dysuria; urinary urgency and frequency; gross hematuria; suprapubic, lower back, or abdominal discomfort; and (rarely) low-grade fever. Acute cystitis is caused by microbial invasion of the superficial mucosa of the bladder and/or urethra and the resulting inflammatory response. Essentially all patients with acute cystitis have bacteriuria in midstream urine cultures, but one third have colony counts $<10^5$ cfu/mL.[54,57] Despite the absence of classical upper tract symptoms (loin pain, costovertebral angle tenderness, and fever), at least 30% of adults with symptoms of cystitis have silent renal infection, based on localization studies.[58] Because clinical evaluation and routine laboratory studies cannot rule out covert renal infection, the clinical term ''acute uncomplicated UTI'' is used to define the group of patients—primarily healthy young women—who have no known underlying renal or urologic dysfunction but who present with symptoms of dysuria, frequency, and urgency. Most of these individuals have acute bacterial cystitis, with or without silent pyelonephritis. A significant minority of women who present with dysuric symptoms have other infections, most commonly either urethritis caused by *Chlamydia trachomatis, Neisseria gonorrhoeae,* or herpes simplex virus, or vaginitis (as discussed below). Such women can be distinguished from patients with acute uncomplicated UTI based on absence of bacteriuria.[52,54,59]

**Diagnosis.** In women with acute uncomplicated UTI, the traditional criterion of $>10^5$ cfu/mL has diagnostic specificity (99%) but low sensitivity (51%). Approximately one third of women with the clinical syndrome of acute dysuria, frequency, and urgency, with pyuria on urinalysis, and with a good clinical response to antimicrobial therapy are infected with $10^2$–$10^3$ cfu of a uropathogen/mL. In this type of patient, a diagnostic criterion of $\geq 10^2$ cfu of a uropathogen/mL provides the greatest combined sensitivity and specificity.[52,54] In routine clinical practice, a diagnostic criterion of $\geq 10^3$ cfu of a uropathogen/mL offers greater specificity (~90%) with little loss of sensitivity (~80%) for evaluation of symptomatic patients.[49,55]

**Treatment.** The goals of treatment for any UTI include sterilization of the urinary tract, resolution of clinical signs and symptoms, and prevention of reinfection.[49] In patients with uncomplicated UTI antimicrobial delivery to the site of infection is usually accomplished easily. Urinary concentrations of an antimicrobial agent often greatly exceed comparable concentrations in other sites, explaining why agents may prove effective for treatment of UTI despite ''resistance'' of the bacterial strain in standard laboratory testing (using serum levels of antimicrobial agents).[33]

Four different antimicrobial strategies are used for treatment of UTI: prolonged therapy (full-dose therapy administered for 4–6 weeks), conventional therapy (a 7- to 14-day course of treatment), short-course therapy (either single-dose therapy or multiple-dose administration over 1–3 days), and prophylactic therapy (low doses administered at regular intervals or with sexual intercourse).[46,49] Each antimicrobial regimen is designed for treatment of particular patient populations.

More data are available on treatment of acute uncomplicated UTIs in women than on treatment of any other type of UTI. Virtually every marketed oral antimicrobial agent that has a spectrum of activity against gram-negative bacteria cures UTI in >80% of patients when administered in conventional regimens, ie, full dosages for 7–14 days.[49,58] Other studies evaluated short-course therapy—both single-dose and, to a lesser extent, 3-day regimens—for acute uncomplicated UTI in women.

Single-dose treatment regimens are popular in outpatient medical and family practice settings. The following statements are applicable to single-dose therapy.[40,46,49,58,60] Single-dose therapy with many agents, including amoxicillin, trimethoprim-sulfamethoxazole, kanamycin, sulfonamides, fluoroquinolones, and tetracycline, is effective treatment for acute uncomplicated UTI in women. At present, trimethoprim-sulfamethoxazole appears most effective and represents the standard for comparison of single-dose regimens of new antimicrobial agents.[49] Single-dose treatment costs considerably less than conventional therapy and has a significantly lower incidence of adverse effects. Fewer than 5% of patients receiving single-dose therapy experience significant adverse effects.

Single-dose regimens may be less useful in urologic practice than in general medical practice. Failure to eradicate uropathogens from the vaginal reservoir represents a major limitation of single-dose therapy. Single-dose treatment appears to be associated with higher rates of early recurrence (<2 weeks after therapy) caused by the original infecting strains than conventional treatment. Such recurrences probably stem from the lesser effectiveness of single-dose therapy in eradicating vaginal *E. coli* and organisms that have invaded the kidney.

Three-day treatment has been recommended to maintain the advantages of single-dose therapy but improve cure rates. Three-day regimens appear to be more effective than single-dose regimens for preventing early reinfection, although neither single-dose treatment nor 3-day treatment is likely to be effective for renal infections. Some authorities recommend single-dose therapy in women with first or isolated episodes of cystitis and use of 3-day regimens in women with a history of multiple recent infections.[40,49,60,61]

Short-course therapy should be limited to treatment of superficial mucosal infections only. Thus, short-course regimens are inappropriate for patients with a high probability of deep-tissue infection: men; patients with overt pyelonephritis or symptoms of >7 days duration; individuals with underlying structural or functional lesions of the urinary system; immunosuppressed patients, patients with indwelling catheters, or those in whom an antimicrobial-resistant organism is likely.[46,49]

Antimicrobial prophylaxis is useful for management of women with recurrent UTIs. More than 80% of recurrent UTIs are reinfections. The remainder represent relapses due to treatment failure. Prophylactic regimens using low dosages of antimicrobials are useful for managing women with a history of three or more episodes of bacterial UTI unrelated to instrumentation in the previous 12 months. The ability of the antimicrobial regimen to prevent reinfection of the urinary tract with a new bacterial strain from the fecal and/or vaginal reservoirs depends on several factors: the success of the regimen in eradicating "uropathogens" from the gastrointestinal tract and vaginal flora, its propensity for selecting resistant subpopulations of bacteria, and the underlying susceptibility of the urinary tract to invasion by less virulent bacterial strains.[62,63] A number of agents have proven useful for prophylaxis of recurrent UTIs, including trimethoprim-sulfamethoxazole, nitrofurantoin, and cephalexin. The rate of symptom relief and microbiological suppression is >95% after 6 months. The incidence of adverse effects requiring medical intervention or discontinuation of prophylaxis is <5%.[64–66]

**Urologic Evaluation of Women with Recurrent UTIs.** Routine intravenous urograms and cystoscopy are rarely helpful for evaluating adult women who suffer from recurrent UTIs.[67–72] Fewer than 5% of sexually active young women with recurrent cystitis have significant urinary tract abnormalities detected by excretory urography and cystoscopy.[69,73] Diffuse nonspecific inflammatory changes represent essentially the only cystoscopic findings.

Generally accepted indications for uroradiologic studies include: a history of childhood UTIs; acute pyelonephritis unresponsive to appropriate antimicrobial therapy; recurrent infections caused by the same organism (particularly if associated with *Proteus* or other urea-splitting bacteria); or a history of stones, obstruction, neurologic disease, or previous urologic surgery.[1,73]

### Acute Uncomplicated Pyelonephritis

**Clinical Presentation.** Acute uncomplicated pyelonephritis is a clinical syndrome characterized by fever and chills, flank pain, costovertebral angle tenderness, and other symptoms, such as nausea and vomiting. Symptoms of lower urinary tract inflammation, such as dysuria, may be present or not. Acute pyelonephritis is usually not associated with bacteremia and hypotension, the "urosepsis" syndrome. Bacterial invasion of the kidney and the resulting inflammatory response to such invasion cause the pathophysiology of acute uncomplicated pyelonephritis. Acute uncomplicated pyelonephritis represents a deep-tissue infection occurring at an anatomic site where host defense mechanisms are relatively inefficient, because of the physicochemical environment, and where drug delivery can be difficult.[33,46] Essentially all cases occur in women, mostly between the ages of 18 and 40 years. The critical point differentiating acute uncomplicated pyelonephritis from complicated pyelonephritis is that patients with uncomplicated pyelonephritis have no history or physical findings consistent with urologic abnormalities.

**Diagnosis.** Bacteriuria is characteristic of pyelonephritis uncomplicated by obstruction, generally with counts $\geq 10^4$ cfu/mL. In studies of acute uncomplicated pyelonephritis confirmed by positive blood cultures, ~80% of patients have $>10^5$ cfu/mL; 10%–15%, $10^4$–$10^5$ cfu/mL; and the remainder, $<10^4$ cfu/mL in midstream urine cultures.[57] Thus, $\geq 10^4$ cfu of a uropathogen/mL in a patient with characteristic clinical findings is evidence of infection in patients with suspected acute uncomplicated pyelonephritis.

**Treatment.** Women with acute uncomplicated pyelonephritis have deep-tissue infection, may have bacteremia, and require intensive antimicrobial therapy. Some patients with pyelonephritis have only mild clinical illness and do not require parenteral therapy. Recent evidence suggests that a 2-week oral course of an appropriate antimicrobial agent constitutes effective treatment for acute uncomplicated pyelonephritis.[46,49,62]

Indications for parenteral therapy in acute uncomplicated pyelonephritis include gravity of the illness, associated medical conditions, concerns about the oral route of administration, because of ileus or vomiting. Standard practice is to initiate therapy with an effective antimicrobial agent intravenously until the patient is afebrile for 24–48 hr. For management of acute uncomplicated pyelonephritis, primary emphasis should be on initial control of the infection with the parenteral drug regimen. A wide variety of parenteral regimens are effective, including combinations, such as a penicillin or cephalosporin plus an aminoglycoside, and single-drug regimens, such as a third-generation cephalosporin, an expanded-spectrum β-lactam agent, a fluoroquinolone, or trimethoprim-sulfamethoxazole. These regimens have comparable efficacy provided that the infecting organism is susceptible.[49] After they are afebrile for 24–48 hr, patients should complete a 2-week course of therapy using an effective oral drug. The relative effectiveness of different oral regimens used after parenteral therapy remains undefined.

### Complicated UTI

**Clinical Presentation.** Complicated UTIs occur in the presence of functional or anatomic abnormalities of the urinary tract, in the setting of catheterization or genitourinary tract instrumentation. Such infections may or may not be associated with local urinary tract symptoms. Patients may present with any combination of symptoms of acute uncomplicated UTI (dysuria, urgency, frequency, and suprapubic pain) and/or acute uncomplicated pyelonephritis (fever, chills, flank pain) plus factors associated with complicated UTI. Whereas most UTIs in younger women are uncomplicated, UTIs in older women are often complicated. Complicated infections are often caused by bacteria other than *E. coli.* Such organisms are often relatively resistant to antimicrobial agents. Complicated UTIs are difficult to treat.

**Diagnosis.** The key to diagnosis and management is to accurately define the nature of the complicating problem. Factors that define a complicated UTI include one or more of the following: an indwelling catheter or the use of intermittent catheterization; residual urine retained after voiding; obstructive uropathy due to bladder outlet obstruction, a calculus, or other causes; vesicoureteral reflux or other urologic abnormalities, including surgically created ileal or colon loops or continent urinary diversion; azotemia due to intrinsic renal disease, even without defined structural abnormalities of the urinary tract; and renal transplantation. Presence of an abscess related to the kidney, pararenal structures, or pelvis should be considered in patients who do not respond to apparently appropriate treatment based on urine culture results. It is important to recognize that urine cultures may be sterile in the presence of an obstructed urinary tract or abscess.

**Treatment.** Accurate definition of complicating factors is critical for management. Patients with complicated UTIs often require appropriate management of urologic abnormalities besides antimicrobial therapy. Few controlled studies have compared antimicrobial regimens in the treatment of complicated UTIs because of the variety of underlying urologic disorders and variable susceptibility patterns from patient to patient. As a rule, a regimen effective against this form of UTI should suppress bacterial growth during therapy, but rates of relapse and reinfection are usually high after conclusion of therapy. Recent studies support shorter courses of therapy for all types of UTI. Continuation of this trend toward shorter courses of parenteral therapy and substitution of broad-spectrum oral therapy for parenteral therapy in patients with complicated UTI will likely be increasingly successful.[49]

### UTIs in Pregnancy and the Puerperium

**Anatomic Changes.** Changes in urinary tract anatomy that occur during gestation profoundly influence the natural history of UTIs.[74] Dilation of the renal calyces, pelves, and ureters begins during the first trimester.[75] Ureteral dilation is generally more pronounced on the right side and ends at the pelvic brim. Reduced peristalsis accompanies dilation of the upper tracts. The theories used to explain these changes involve the muscle-relaxing effects of progesterone-like hormones and mechanical obstruction by the enlarging uterus. Two other significant changes are an increase in renal length, by approximately 1 cm, and a change in relative bladder position as it becomes an abdominal rather than a pelvic organ. The net effect of these changes is a propensity to develop symptomatic upper tract infections during the third trimester.

**Incidence and Prevalence of Bacteriuria During Pregnancy.** Pregnancy does not appear to increase susceptibility to bacteriuria. In studies using a variety of methods, the prevalence of bacteriuria among pregnant women ranged from 2.5% to 11%; most investigations report a prevalence of 4%–7%.[1,76] This is similar to the prevalence of bacteriuria among other sexually active women of childbearing age. The prevalence of bacteriuria appears to be inversely related to socioeconomic status. Turck and associates found that 6.5% of 557 indigent women had bacteriuria compared with only 2% of 1170 nonindigent women.[77] This finding was confirmed in a number of other studies.[75,78,79] Sickle cell trait in black women was also associated with a twofold increased prevalence of bacteriuria of pregnancy, regardless of socioeconomic class.[80]

Recurrent bacteriuria is common among pregnant women who have bacteriuria documented at their initial prenatal evaluations. Following effective therapy, 16%–27% of women had recurrent bacteriuria before term.[81,82] In one of these studies a control group of 148 bacteriuric women received placebo therapy: 98 (66%) remained bacteriuric, 27 (18%) developed acute pyelonephritis, and 20 (14%) resolved their infections spontaneously.[81] It has been suggested that recurrent bacteriuria is independent of both the site of infection within the urinary tract and the duration of antimicrobial treatment.[83–85] Long-term (10- to 14-year) follow-up studies documented bacteriuria in 18 (29%) of 63 women treated with sulfonamide for bacteriuria during pregnancy and in 18 (25%) of 71 women treated with placebo.[86] In contrast, bacteriuria occurred in only 3 (5%) of 58 women in the original control group who did not have bacteriuria during pregnancy. These findings suggest that there is a subset of women who are prone to develop bacteriuria for biologic reasons independent of pregnancy per se.

Women who are uninfected at their initial prenatal evaluations have a low incidence of bacteriuria during pregnancy. McFayden et al. used repeated suprapubic bladder aspirates to show that only 1 of 186 uninfected women subsequently developed bacteriuria during pregnancy.[75] Similarly, Elder and colleagues used cultures of voided urine to show that only 6 (2%) of 279 uninfected women subsequently developed bacteriuria during pregnancy.[81]

**Diagnosis.** Diagnosis of UTI based on symptoms has a low predictive value for identifying bacteriuria in pregnant women. McFayden et al. found that "30% of the patients with bacteriuria had symptoms which are usually associated with urinary infection when they were first seen, but so did 25% of the uninfected control patients."[75] Thus, all pregnant women should be screened by quantitative urine cultures at their initial prenatal visit, preferably during the first trimester.[1] Subsequent efforts to evaluate and control UTIs should then concentrate on women with bacteriuria documented by the initial evaluation. The goal of screening is to prevent the serious complications associated with bacteriuria in pregnant women.

**Complications of Bacteriuria During Pregnancy.** Complications may be considered for the mother or the fetus. Various adverse effects on the mother have been reported, including development of acute pyelonephritis, anemia, toxemia, persistent bacteriuria, and chronic pyelonephritis. The strongest association is between the presence of bacteriuria in the first trimester and the development of acute pyelonephritis, usually occurring during the third trimester. Pioneering studies by Kass and associates demonstrated that 20%–40% of pregnant women who received placebo treatment for asymptomatic bacteriuria subsequently developed acute pyelonephritis.[87–89] In contrast, no cases of acute pyelonephritis occurred among women who received effective antimicrobial therapy. Other placebo-controlled studies confirmed both the association between asymptomatic bacteriuria and acute pyelonephritis of pregnancy and the markedly reduced risk for women who receive effective treatment.[76,90,91] It appears that 25%–50% of pregnant women with bacteriuria have upper urinary tract involvement.[76,83,90,92] Women who do not respond to conventional antimicrobial therapy appear more likely to have renal involvement. This subset of bacteriuric women is at especially high risk for acute pyelonephritis of pregnancy.

Pyelographic changes associated with chronic pyelonephritis were documented on postpartum evaluation of 14%–28% of women with bacteriuria during pregnancy,[75,86,90] and other abnormalities were noted frequently.[76] Zinner and Kass also suggest that approximately 1 in 3000 pregnant women with pyelonephritis eventually develops end-stage renal disease.[86] The problem is that there is no clear cause-and-effect relationship between bacteriuria of pregnancy and renal damage. It appears most likely that bacteriuria during pregnancy represents one phase in the natural history of UTIs in women,[33] and that pregnancy simply affords an opportunity to detect a chronic condition present in these women long before gestation.[76] Bacteriuria during pregnancy was associated with maternal anemia,[75,93] and an increased risk for hypertensive disease of pregnancy,[76,90] but other workers question these associations.[76,80,90,94]

Maternal bacteriuria may be associated with adverse consequences for the fetus. An association between asymptomatic bacteriuria during pregnancy and low birth weight was first reported in 1962. More than 30 other published studies examined this issue. Some confirmed the association between maternal bacteriuria and low birth weight, while others disputed it. A recent meta-analysis of pooled data from these studies concluded that asymptomatic bacteriuria was indeed associated with preterm delivery (<37 weeks of gestation) and low birth weight.[95] Bacteriuric mothers had a 54% higher risk of giving birth to low-birth-weight infants and twice the risk of giving birth to preterm infants than did nonbacteriuric mothers. Additional meta-analyses including only randomized clinical trials showed that antimicrobial treatment significantly reduced the risk of low birth weight. Several studies suggest that bacteriuria of pregnancy is associated with a high risk of fetal wastage, fetal infection, and dorsal midline fusion defects,[76] but other investigations have not confirmed these associations.

**Treatment.** The first consideration in treatment of any infection is choice of an appropriate antimicrobial drug. Knowledge that a woman is pregnant adds additional risk–benefit considerations that limit the range of therapeutic options. Table 1 summarizes our current understanding of anti-

**TABLE 1. Potential Toxicity of Antimicrobial Drugs During Pregnancy**

| Drug | Potential Toxicity: Fetal | Potential Toxicity: Material | Ref. |
|---|---|---|---|
| *Considered Safe* | | | |
| Penicillins[a] | No known toxicity | Allergy | 99, 100 |
| Cephalosporins[a] | | Allergy | 101 |
| Erythromycin base | | Allergy | 102 |
| *Used with Caution* | | | |
| Sulfonamides | Kernicterus<br>Hemolysis[a] | Allergy | 103 |
| Nitrofurantoin | Hemolysis[a] | Interstitial pneumonia<br>Neuropathy | 104 |
| Aminoglycosides | CN VIII toxicity | Ototoxicity<br>Nephrotoxicity | 105<br>106 |
| Clindamycin | | Pseudomembranous colitis<br>Allergy | 102 |
| Isoniazid | Possible neuropathy<br>Seizures | Hepatotoxicity | 107 |
| Fluoroquinolones | Cartilage toxicity | CNS reactions<br>GI sensitivity<br>Allergy | 108, 109 |
| *Contraindicated* | | | |
| Tetracycline | Tooth discoloration and dysplasia<br>Inhibition of bone growth | Hepatotoxicity<br>Renal failure | 107 |
| Erythromycin estolate | | Hepatotoxicity | 91 |
| Chloramphenicol | Gray syndrome | Marrow toxicity | 110 |
| Trimethoprim-sulfamethoxazole | Congenital anomalies<br>Folate antagonism | Vasculitis | 111 |

[a]Newer penicillins and cephalosporins have not been adequately evaluated in clinical trials.
Adopted from Krieger JN.[74]

microbial drug toxicity during pregnancy and the puerperium. Potential injury to the fetus is the greatest concern during treatment of pregnant or nursing women. Although many drugs cross the "placental barrier" and are found in breast milk, the teratogenic potential of most medications is unknown.[96] Furthermore, animal models for predicting teratogenicity are notoriously unreliable and the causes of the great majority of congenital defects are unknown.[97] Because it is difficult to distinguish the potential adverse effects of a particular drug from the natural history of the underlying disease for which the medication was prescribed, it is usually impossible to draw clinical conclusions concerning drug toxicity.[96,98]

The great majority of studies evaluating treatment of bacteriuria during pregnancy have used 7–10 days of therapy. In recent years, a number of investigators have reported favorable results using much shorter treatment courses for women with bacteriuria.[61,112–114] These findings led some authorities to recommend single-dose[96,114] or 3-day[85] therapy for pregnant women. There are valid reasons for exercising caution in accepting such recommendations. First, recent investigations of shorter therapy for bacteriuria usually excluded pregnant women. Some studies comparing single-dose and conventional therapy for pregnant women found that conventional treatment had a higher success rate.[115] Second, most treatment studies for UTIs suffer from major deficiencies in both design and interpretation.[113] Third, undue emphasis on choosing the appropriate duration of treatment is, in a larger sense, begging the real issue, ie, proper patient follow-up.

The key to treatment of any UTI, including that in a pregnant woman, is to assure elimination of bacteria from the urinary tract.[33] Sterile urine cultures obtained during or shortly after treatment are necessary to document resolution of the infection. Because recurrent UTIs are common, cultures should be obtained throughout the pregnancy following satisfactory treatment of bacteriuria. Patients who have unresolved bacteriuria during therapy deserve a thorough evaluation to determine whether the cause is microbiologic, eg, selection of resistant organisms, or anatomic, eg, presence of an infected staghorn calculus.[74]

## DIFFERENTIAL DIAGNOSIS OF UTIs IN WOMEN

The differential diagnosis of UTI in women includes the urethral syndrome and vaginitis syndromes. Clinical features of these conditions overlap and all three disorders may be associated with urinary frequency and dysuria. Additional urologic considerations include genitourinary tuberculosis; noninfectious causes of urinary tract symptoms, such as painful bladder syndrome (including interstitial cystitis); and transitional cell carcinoma in situ. These conditions are covered in other chapters.

### Low-Count Bacteriuria versus Urethral Syndrome

The traditional classification of women with acute dysuria and urinary frequency separated women with acute cystitis from those with acute urethral syndrome.[115] The differential point was whether the culture of midstream urine had $>10^5$ cfu/mL. Women with $>10^5$ cfu/mL had acute cystitis and those with fewer organisms had urethral syndrome.

During the last decade, research has shown that women with acute urethral syndrome comprise several populations.[3,52,54,116] The most common cause of acute urethral syndrome is low-count bacterial cystitis caused by *E. coli, S. saprophyticus,* and other uropathogens. These bacteria are also responsible for most cases of cystitis in women with $>10^5$ cfu/mL.

Women with acute urinary symptoms and low-count bacteriuria appear no different clinically from women with acute cystitis and $>10^5$ cfu/mL. The proportion of acute cystitis attributable to low-count bacteriuria appears to be about one third.[3] The following observations support the concept that women with low counts of uropathogens and dysuria have acute cystitis:

1. Bacteria have been isolated simultaneously in suprapubic aspirates from

women with *E. coli* in low numbers in their midstream urine.[52]

2. Ninety percent of women with low-count bacteriuria and symptoms have pyuria.[52]
3. The same organism can often be isolated 24–36 hr later from the midstream urine in higher numbers.[52,54]
4. The clinical presentation in women with low-count bacteriuria is identical to the clinical presentation of women with acute cystitis and $>10^5$ cfu/mL, including the proportion with hematuria.[52,54]
5. The response to treatment was identical in women with low-count bacteriuria and those with "significant" bacteriuria in a placebo-controlled trial.[53]

Some women who present with symptoms of dysuria and frequency actually have upper UTIs.[117,118] The distinction between upper and lower UTIs in this situation depends on localization tests, such as ureteral catheterization, the bladder washout test, or antibody-coated bacteria test. In different populations, 10%–50% of women who present with clinical findings of dysuria and frequency actually have upper UTIs (acute uncomplicated pyelonephritis).[3,117,118]

**Acute Urethritis.** In sexually active women, particularly those with multiple partners or a new partner, sexually transmitted diseases may cause an acute urethritis syndrome that mimics the clinical presentation of acute cystitis.[3,116,119] Important pathogens to be considered in this population include *Chlamydia trachomatis, Neisseria gonorrhoeae,* and herpes simplex virus. Infectious vaginitis may also produce symptoms similar to those of acute UTI. Important causes of vaginitis include *Trichomonas vaginalis, Candida* species, and the bacterial vaginosis syndrome.[3,120,121]

Our former concept that women with acute dysuria and urinary frequency could be classified as having acute cystitis ($>10^5$ cfu/mL in midstream urine) or urethral syndrome ($<10^5$ cfu/mL) has been replaced by a new algorithm.[3] Patients with what was formerly termed acute cystitis may have inapparent upper UTIs (occult pyelonephritis) or acute lower UTIs (cystitis). Similar organisms cause both clinical syndromes, with the most common being *E. coli* and *S. saprophyticus.* Patients who were formerly classified as having acute urethral syndrome may have acute cystitis, urethritis, or vaginitis. Acute cystitis syndrome is also caused by *E. coli* and *S. saprophyticus,* but with colony counts of $10^2$–$10^4$ cfu/mL. Acute urethritis is usually caused by sexually transmitted organisms, particularly *C. trachomatis, N. gonorrhoeae,* and herpes simplex virus. The most common causes of acute vaginitis are also infectious, with *T. vaginalis, Candida albicans,* and bacterial vaginosis being implicated most commonly. Figure 2 illustrates the relationships among these conditions.

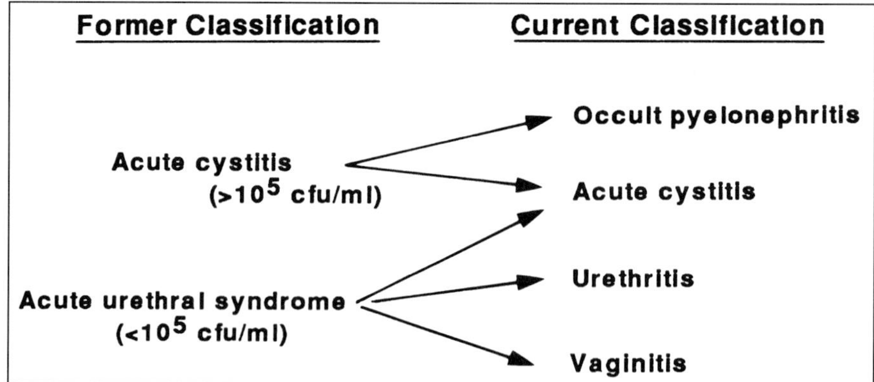


**Fig 2.** Causes of acute dysuria and frequency in sexually active women. [Adapted from Stamm WE, Hooton TM, Johnson JR, et al.,[3] with permission.]

### Vaginitis Syndromes

Because vaginitis is important in the differential diagnosis of UTIs and represents a common consequence treatment for UTIs in women, we will review the most common syndromes.

Vaginitis syndromes account for more than 10 million office visits yearly in the U.S.[122] The common complaints of excessive or malodorous vaginal discharge, vulvar pruritus, pain, and external dyspareunia may indicate vaginal infection but also may reflect the presence of cervicitis, urethritis, or cystitis. The infectious causes of vaginitis include trichomoniasis, yeast vulvovaginitis, and bacterial vaginosis.

Diagnosis of vaginitis may be complex because symptoms overlap other genitourinary syndromes, multiple etiologies exist, and vaginitis may be associated with other sexually transmitted diseases. Cultures of urine for bacteria, cervical secretions for *N. gonorrhoeae* and *C. trachomatis,* and ulcers for herpes simplex virus as well as testing for syphilis may be indicated to exclude other causes of symptoms in sexually active women.[123] Evaluation of women with possible vaginitis includes microscopic examination of vaginal discharge [with examination of fluid suspended in saline and in 10% potassium hydroxide (KOH)]; determination of vaginal fluid pH; the amine odor or ''whiff'' test (a fishy odor following addition of 10% KOH to secretions due to volatilization of amines produced by anaerobic bacterial metabolism); culture for *T. vaginalis,* which is more sensitive than microscopic examination; and culture for yeasts, which, if negative, helps to exclude the latter as a cause of symptoms.[120]

Vaginal douching and vaginal treatment with commercial products that contain *Lactobacillus* species have not proven effective for either treatment or prevention of any vaginal infection and should be discouraged. Few if any available preparations contain lactobacilli that produce hydrogen peroxide, a critical metabolite that appears to inhibit growth of other vaginal organisms. Vaginal douching with either medicated or nonmedicated preparations appears to be an independent risk factor for pelvic inflammatory disease[124] and ectopic pregnancy.[125]

**Trichomoniasis.** Trichomoniasis is caused by *Trichomonas vaginalis,* a sexually transmitted, flagellated protozoan.[126] Manifestations of vaginal trichomoniasis range from asymptomatic carriage to severe, acute inflammatory disease.[127–129] Approximately one third of asymptomatic female carriers develop symptoms within 6 months. Factors that differentiate symptomatic from asymptomatic infection are poorly defined.[130] *T. vaginalis* is frequently isolated from the urethras of male sexual partners of infected women[131] and rates of cure have usually been reported to rise when these men are treated.[132] Trichomoniasis is common in sexually active women, is often associated with other sexually transmitted diseases, and may cause chronic asymptomatic infections. Development of such chronic infection is a likely explanation for cases diagnosed in women who are not currently at risk for sexually transmitted diseases.

***Diagnosis.*** The diagnosis of trichomoniasis requires demonstration of the protozoa by microscopic examination of saline suspensions, culture, or by direct monoclonal antibody staining.[133] Most patients also have more polymorphonuclear leukocytes than epithelial cells in their vaginal secretions, a vaginal pH $\geq$4.7, and a positive amine odor test, but none of these features is required for diagnosis.

***Treatment.*** Metronidazole is the drug of choice for trichomoniasis. A single 2.0-g oral dose of metronidazole or a dose of 250 mg given three times a day for 7 days cures 85%–95% of cases, especially when male partners are treated simultaneously.[132,134] Treatment failures may be related to reexposure or resistance of *T. vaginalis* to metronidazole.[125,135,136] Other 5-nitroimidazoles (eg, tinidazole) have similar cure rates. Refractory infections should receive treatment with higher oral doses, with more prolonged courses, or with intravenous metronidazole.

**Yeast Vulvovaginitis.** Yeast vulvovaginitis, also termed candidal vulvovaginitis, is caused by *C. albicans* in 85%–90% of cases and by other *Candida* species or *Torulopsis glabrata* in 10%–15% of cases.[137,138] Most women have at least one episode of symptomatic vulvovaginal candidiasis at some point; such episodes are often associated with pregnancy, oral contraception, or antimicrobial therapy. A minority of women experience frequent relapses, perhaps related to a *Candida*-specific defect in cell-mediated immunity.[139] Many other women are asymptomatic carriers of these yeasts in their vaginas and/or rectums.[140] A protective role for the normal vaginal flora (especially *Lactobacillus* species) may reflect competition for space and nutrients.[141] Production of yeast-inhibiting bacteriocins by lactobacilli is also presumed to be important.[141] Most cases are clearly not sexually acquired, but sexual transmission may occasionally play a role in reestablishing colonization after the elimination of yeasts. Treatment of the male sexual partners of women with recurrent disease has little or no influence on the frequency of recurrent yeast vulvovaginitis.[123]

***Diagnosis.*** Three findings are required for diagnosis of yeast vulvovaginitis: symptoms and signs of a vulvar or vaginal disorder; presence of yeasts or pseudomycelia in a suspension in saline of 10% KOH by Gram stain or by culture of vaginal secretions; and exclusion of other causes of vulvovaginal symptoms.[123] Other common findings include a vaginal pH <4.5 and increased numbers of inflammatory cells in vaginal secretions, but these findings are not required for diagnosis.

***Treatment.*** Yeast vulvovaginitis has traditionally been treated with vaginal imidazoles, as topical creams or tablets, or with oral therapy for 1–14 days.[142] Short-term cure rates vary around 70%–90%. Newer oral agents (fluconazole and itraconazole), given for shorter courses, including single-dose treatment, appear to be equivalent to 5–7 days of topical treatment or oral ketoconazole. Single-dose treatment with clotrimazole (500 mg vaginally), miconazole (1200 mg vaginally), or tioconazole 5 g of 6.5% cream vaginally) also resulted in acceptable cure rates in some series. Single-dose topical therapy proved less effective in other series. Thus, most authorities recommend 3–7 days of treatment especially for severe or relapsing disease. Resistance to imidazoles and other antifungal agents is unusual in *C. albicans* and the role of drug resistance in failures of treatment or relapses remains unclear.[127]

Recurrent candidal vaginitis is occasionally associated with underlying immunodeficiency, diabetes, oral contraceptives, or estrogen therapy. For women who suffer frequent recurrences, long-term suppressive treatment (eg, 100 mg of ketoconazole daily) or patient-initiated therapy at the onset of symptoms may be effective.[139] Hepatitis and other adverse reactions are infrequent. Newer imidazoles might be tolerated even better. One recent study suggests that consumption of yogurt containing *Lactobacillus acidophilus* may provide effective prophylaxis for recurrent candidal vaginitis.[143]

**Bacterial Vaginosis.** Other terms for this syndrome include nonspecific, anaerobic, and *Gardnerella*-associated vaginitis. The term "vaginosis" is preferred because bacterial vaginosis is characterized by overgrowth of a variety of anaerobic and aerobic bacterial components of the vaginal flora, with little or no inflammation. Symptoms include vaginal malodor and increased discharge, without other evidence of vulvovaginitis. Vaginal discharge associated with bacterial vaginosis contains characteristic "clue cells," which are epithelial cells containing large numbers of adherent bacteria. There are increases in the prevalence and quantity of multiple bacterial species including *Gardnerella vaginalis, Mycoplasma hominis, Mobiluncus curtisii, Bacteroides* species, *Prevotella* species, and numerous other anaerobes. These changes in the vaginal flora are associated with reduced numbers of *Lactobacillus* species, especially those that produce KOH.[127,132,141,144,145] Polymorphonuclear leukocytes are usually absent.

Some studies suggest that bacterial vaginosis may increase the risk for development of acute pelvic inflammatory disease, premature rupture of the fetal membranes, and related complications of labor and delivery.[146,147]

Evidence regarding sexual transmission of bacterial vaginosis is conflicting. Some studies[148] suggest that the male sexual partners of women with bacterial vaginosis have had unusually high rates of carriage of *G. vaginalis,* with the same biotype, and that bacterial vaginosis develops more frequently in sexually experienced than sexually inexperienced women, often associated with a new sexual relationship.[149] Other studies suggest that treatment of male partners does not influence the rates of recurrence or relapse in women with bacterial vaginosis.[123,127]

***Diagnosis.*** The diagnosis of bacterial vaginosis requires three of the following four features: white, homogeneous vaginal discharge that smoothly coats the vaginal mucosa; vaginal pH ≥4.7; a fishy amine odor on mixing secretions with 10% KOH; and a Gram-stained preparation or saline mount showing clue cells.[120,123]

A semiquantitative system for evaluation of bacterial flora in Gram-stained smears of vaginal secretions has good reliability in research settings.[150] Tests based on products of anaerobic bacterial metabolism may be useful, but their sensitivity and specificity have not been established. Gas chromatographic analysis for short-chain fatty acids, thin-layer chromatography to identify putrescine and cadaverine, and proline aminopeptidase assays have all been used.[145,151] Quantitative cultures for anaerobic bacteria were important for defining the syndrome but are too technically demanding for routine diagnostic use.

***Treatment.*** Metronidazole (500 mg by mouth twice daily for 7 days) is the standard treatment for bacterial vaginosis. Single-dose treatment with 2.0 g of metronidazole gives similar success rates (80%–100%) at 1–2 weeks but is associated with higher relapse rates in patients followed for ≥4 weeks.[127] Clindamycin therapy may provide similar results. Two regimens employing clindamycin (300 mg intravaginally twice daily for 7 days or 5 g of 1%–2% cream instilled vaginally twice daily for 5–7 days) recently have been approved.[152,153] Oral amoxicillin, with or without clavulanic acid, has been used with variable success and is not recommended as first-line therapy.

## REFERENCES


1. Kunin CM. *Detection, Prevention and Management of Urinary Tract Infections.* Philadelphia: Lea and Febiger; 1987.
2. Cypress BK. Patients' reasons for visiting physicians: National Ambulatory Care Survey. United States, 1977–78. In: National Center for Health Statistics and Maryland H, eds. *Vital and Health Statistics. Data from the National Health Survey.* Washington, DC: U.S. Department of Health and Human Services; 1981.
3. Stamm WE, Hooton TM, Johnson JR, et al. Urinary tract infections: from pathogenesis to treatment. *J Infect Dis.* 1989;159:400–406.
4. Maherzi M, Gougnard JP, Torrado A. Urinary tract infection in high-risk newborn infants. *Pediatrics.* 1978;62:521–523.
5. Ginsburg CM, McCracken GH. Urinary tract infections in young infants. *Pediatrics.* 1982; 69:409–412.
6. Kunin CM, Deutscher R, Pachin AJ. Urinary tract infection in school children: epidemiologic, clinical and laboratory study. *Medicine.* 1964;43:91–130.
7. Edwards B, White R, Maxted H, et al. Screening methods for covert bacteriuria in schoolgirls. *Br Med J.* 1975;2:463–467.
8. Evans DA, Williams DN, Laughlin LW, et al. Bacteriuria in a population-based cohort of women. *J Infect Dis.* 1978;138:768–773.
9. Kunin CM, McCormack RC. An epidemiological study of bacteriuria and blood pressure among nuns and working women. *N Engl J Med.* 1968;278:635–642.
10. Sourander LB. Urinary tract infection in the aged—an epidemiologic study. *Ann Med Intern Fenn.* 1966;55(Suppl 45):7–55.
11. Kasviki-Charvati P, Drolette-Kefakis B, Papanayiotou PC, et al. Turnover of bacteriuria in old age. *Age Ageing.* 1982;11:169–174.
12. Bosa JA, Kobasa WD, Knight RA, et al. Epidemiology of bacteriuria in an elderly ambulatory population. *Am J Med.* 1986;80:298–314.
13. Dontas AS, Kasviki-Charvati P, Papanayiotou PC, et al. Bacteriuria and survival in old age. *N Engl J Med.* 1981;302:939–943.
14. Setia U, Serventi I, Lorenz P. Bacteremia in a long-term care facility. *Arch Intern Med.* 1984; 144:1633–1635.

15. Williams ME, Pannill FC III. Urinary incontinence in the elderly. *Ann Intern Med.* 1982;97: 895–907.
16. Stamey TA, Timothy MM. Studies of introital colonization in women with recurrent urinary infections. III. Vaginal glycogen concentrations. *J Urol.* 1975;114:268–270.
17. Denich K, Blyn LB, Craiu A, et al. DNA sequences of three papA genes from uropathogenic *Escherichia coli* strains: evidence of structural and serologycal conservation. *Infect Immun.* 1991;59:3849–3858.
18. Salit, I, Gotschlich, E: Hemagglutination by purified type 1 *Escherichia coli* pili. *J Exp Med.* 1977;146:1169–1181.
19. Kallenius G, Svenson SB, Mollby R, et al. Carbohydrate receptor structures recognized by uropathogenic *E. coli. Scand J Infect Dis.* (Suppl) 1982;33:52–60.
20. Stapleton AE, Moseley SL, Stamm WE. The role of *E. coli* virulence factors in acute cystitis. 29th Interscience Conference on Antimicrobial Agents and Chemotherapy, 1989. American Society for Microbiology. Program and Abstracts.
21. Lomberg H, Hellstrom M, Jodal U, et al. Properties of *Escherichia coli* in patients with renal scarring. *J Infect Dis.* 1989:579–582.
22. Lomberg H, Cedergren B, Leffler H, et al. Influence of blood group on the availability of receptors for attachment of uropathogenic *E. coli. Infect Immun.* 1986:919–926.
23. Johnson JR, Roberts PL, Stamm WE. P-Fimbriae and other virulence in *E. coli* urosepsis: association with patients' characteristics. *J Infect Dis.* 1987:225–229.
24. Svanborg-Eden C, Hansson S, Jodal U, et al. Host–parasite interaction in the urinary tract. *Infect Dis.* 1988:421–426.
25. Orskov F, Orskov I. Summary of a workshop on the clone concept in epidemiology, taxonomy, and evolution of the enterobacteriaceae and other bacteria. *J Infect Dis.* 1983:346–357.
26. Johnson JR, Moseley SL, Roberts PL, et al. Aerobactin and other virulence factor genes among strains of *E. coli* causing urosepsis: association with patient characteristics. *Infect Immun.* 1988:405–412.
27. Lomberg H, Hanson LA, Jacobsson B, et al. Correlation of P blood group, vesicoureteral reflux in bacterial attachment in patients with recurrent pyelonephritis. *N Engl J Med.* 1983: 1189–1192.
28. Parsons CL, Stauffer CW, Schmidt JD. Reversible inactivation of bladder surface glycosaminoglycan antibacterial by protamine sulfate. *Infect Immun.* 1988;56:1341–1343.
29. Duncan JL. Differential effect of Tamm–Horsfall protein on adherence of Escherichia coli to transitional epithelial cells. *J Infect Dis.* 1988; 158:1379–1382.
30. Nicolle LE, Harding GKM, Pureikasaitis J, et al. The association of urinary tract infection with sexual intercourse. *J Infect Dis.* 1982:579–583.
31. Buckley RM, McGuckin M, MacGregor RR. Urine bacterial counts after sexual intercourse. *N Engl J Med.* 1978:321–324.
32. Stamey TA, Timothy M, Millar M, et al. Recurrent urinary infections in adult women: the role of introital enterobacteria. *Calif Med.* 1971: 1–19.
33. Stamey TA. *Pathogenesis and Treatment of Urinary Tract Infections.* Baltimore: Williams and Wilkins; 1980.
34. Schaeffer AJ, Jones JM, Dunn JK. Association of in vitro *Escherichia coli* adherence to vaginal buccal epithelial cells with susceptibility of women to recurrent urinary tract infections. *N Engl J Med.* 1981:1062–1066.
35. Fry J, Dilane JV, Joiner CL, et al. Acute urinary infections, their course and outcome in general practice. *Lancet.* 1962:1318–1321.
36. Kraft JK, Stamey TA. The natural history of symptomatic recurrent bacteriuria in women. *Medicine.* 1977:55–60.
37. Fihn SD, Latham RH, Roberts P, et al. Association between diaphragm use and urinary tract infection. *JAMA.* 1985:240–245.
38. Scheinfeld J, Schaeffer AJ, Cordon-Cardo C, et al. Association of the Lewis blood-group phenotype with recurrent urinary tract infections in women. *N Engl J Med.* 1989:773–777.
39. Mulholland SG, Mooreville M, Parasons CL. Urinary tract infections and P blood group antigens. *Urology.* 1984:232–235.
40. Fihn SD, Johnson C, Roberts PL, et al. Trimethoprim-sulfamethoxazole for acute dysuria in women: a single-dose or 10-day course: a double-blind, randomized trial. *Ann Intern Med.* 1988;108:350–357.
41. Takahashi M, Loveland DB. Bacteriuria and oral contraceptives. Routine health examinations of 12,076 middle-class women. *JAMA.* 1974;227:762–765.
42. Foxman B, Frerichs RR. Epidemiology of urinary tract infection: 11 diet, clothing and urination habits. *Am J Public Health.* 1985;75: 1314–1317.
43. Adatto K, Doebele KG, Galland L, et al. Behavioral factors and urinary tract infection. *JAMA.* 1979;241:2525–2526.
44. Ervin C, Komaroff AL, Pass TM. Behavioral factors and urinary tract infection. *JAMA.* 1980; 243:330–331.
45. Pollack HM. Laboratory techniques for detection of urinary tract infection and assessment of value. *Am J Med.* 1983;75(18):79–84.
46. Rubin RH, Tolkoff-Rubin NE, Cotran RS. Urinary tract infection, pyelonephritis, and reflux nephropathy. In: Brenner BM, Rector FCJ, eds.

*The Kidney.* Philadelphia: WB Saunders; 1991: 1369–1429.

47. Kass EH. Bacteriuria and the diagnosis of infections of the urinary tract: with observations on the use of methionine as a urinary antiseptic. *Arch Intern Med.* 1957;100:709–714.
48. Savage WE, Hajj SN, Kass EH. Demographic and prognostic characteristics of bacteriuria in pregnancy. *Medicine* (Baltimore). 1967;46: 385–407.
49. Rubin RH, Shapiro ED, Andriole VT, et al. Evaluation of new anti-infective drugs for the treatment of urinary tract infection. *Clin Infect Dis.* 1992;15:S216–225.
50. Hovelius B, Mardh PA, Bygren P. Urinary tract infections caused by *Staphylococcus saprophyticus:* recurrences and complications. *J Urol.* 1979;122:645–647.
51. Drutz DJ, Fetchik R. Fungal infections of the kidney and urinary tract. In: Schrier RW, Gottschalk CW, eds. *Diseases of the Kidney.* Boston: Little, Brown; 1988:1015–1047.
52. Stamm WE, Wagner KF, Alexander ER, et al. Causes of the acute urethral syndrome in women. *N Engl J Med.* 1980;409.
53. Stamm WE, Running K, McKevitt M, et al. Treatment of the acute urethral syndrome. *N Engl J Med.* 1981;956–958.
54. Stamm WE, Counts GW, Running K, et al. Diagnosis of coliform infection in acutely dysuric women. *N Engl J Med.* 1982;307:463–468.
55. Stamm WE. Measurement of pyruria and its relation to bacteriuria. *Am J Med.* 1983;75:53–58.
56. Hogg RJ. A search for the ''elusive'' urinary tract infection in febrile infants. *Pediatr Infect Dis J.* 1987;6:233–234.
57. Roberts FJ. Quantitative urine culture in patients with urinary tract infection and bacteriuria. *Am J Clin Pathol.* 1986;85:616–618.
58. Fang LST, Tolkoff-Rubin NE, Rubin RH. Efficacy of single-dose and conventional amoxicillin therapy in urinary-tract infection localized by the antibody-coated bacteria technique. *N Engl J Med.* 1978;298:413–416.
59. Komaroff AL. Acute dysuria in women. *N Engl J Med.* 1984;310:368–375.
60. Johnson JR, Stamm WE. Diagnosis and treatment of acute urinary tract infections. *Infect Dis Clin North Am.* 1987;1:773–791.
61. Greenberg RN, Reilly PM, Luppen KL, et al. Randomized study of single-dose, three-day, and seven-day treatment of cystitis in women. *J Infect Dis.* 1986;153:277–282.
62. Stamm WE, McKevitt M, Counts GW. Acute renal infection in women: treatment with trimethoprim-sulfamethoxazole or ampicillin for two or six weeks: a randomized trial. *Ann Intern Med.* 1987;106:341–345.
63. Nicolle LE, Ronald AR. Recurrent urinary tract infections in adult women: diagnosis and treatment. *Infect Dis Clin North Am.* 1987;1:793–806.
64. Stamm WE, McKevitt M, Counts GW, et al. Is antimicrobial prophylaxis of urinary tract infections cost effective? *Ann Intern Med.* 1981;94: 251–255.
65. Wong ES, McKevitt M, Running K, et al. Management of recurrent urinary tract infections with patient-administered single-dose therapy. *Ann Intern Med.* 1985;102:302–307.
66. Stamm WE. Prevention of urinary tract infections. *Am J Med.* 1984;76:148–154.
67. Fair WR, McClennan BL, Jost RG. Are excretory urograms necessary in evaluation of women with urinary tract infection? *J Urol.* 1979;121:313–315.
68. Engel G, Schaeffer AJ, Grayhack JT, et al. The role of execretory urography and cystoscopy in the evaluation and management of women with recurrent urinary tract infection. *J Urol.* 1980; 123:190–191.
69. Fowler JE, Pulaski AT. Excretory urography, cystography, and cytoscopy in the evaluation of women with urinary tract infection: a prospective study. *N Engl J Med.* 1981;462–465.
70. Lieberman E, Macchia RJ. Excretory urography in women with urinary tract infection. *J Urol.* 1982;127:263–264.
71. DeLange EE, Jones B. Unnecessary intravenous urography in young women with recurrent urinary tract infections. *Clin Radiol.* 1983;34: 551–553.
72. Mogensen P, Hansen LK. Do intravenous urography and cystoscopy provide important information in otherwise healthy women with recurrent urinary tract infection? *Br J Urol.* 1983;55: 261–263.
73. Fairchild TN, Shuman W, Berger RE. Radiographic studies for women with recurrent urinary tract infections. *J Urol.* 1982;128:344–345.
74. Krieger JN. Complications and treatment of urinary tract infections during pregnancy. *Urol Clin North Am.* 1986;13:685–693.
75. McFadyen IR, Eykyn SJ, Gardner NHN, et al. Bacteriuria in pregnancy. *J Obstet Gynecol Br Comm.* 1973;80:385–405.
76. Sweet RL. Bacteriuria and pyelonephritis during pregnancy. *Semin Perinatol.* 1977;1:25–40.
77. Turck M, Goffe BS, Petersdorf RG. Bacteriuria of pregnancy: relation to socioeconomic factors. *N Engl J Med.* 1962;266:857–860.
78. Henderson M, Entwiste W, Tayback M. Bacteriuria and pregnancy outcome: preliminary findings. *Am J Public Health.* 1962;52:1187–1193.
79. Layton R. Infection of the urinary tract in pregnancy: an investigation of a new routine in antenatal care. *J Obstet Gynecol Br Comm.* 1964; 71:927–933.

80. Whalley P, Martin F, Peters P. Significance of asymptomatic bacteriuria detected during pregnancy. *JAMA.* 1965;193:879–881.

81. Elder HA, Santamarina BAG, Smith S, et al. The natural history of asymptomatic bacteriuria during pregnancy: the effect of tetracycline on the clinical course and outcome of pregnancy. *Am J Obstet Gynecol.* 1971;111:441–462.

82. Harris RE. The significance of eradication of bacteriuria during pregnancy. *Obstet Gynecol.* 1979;53:71–73.

83. Fairley KF, Bond AG, Adey FD. The site of infection in pregnancy bacteriuria. *Lancet.* 1966;1:939–941.

84. Leveno KJ, Harris RE, Gilstrap LC. Bladder versus renal bacteriuria during pregnancy: recurrence after treatment. *Am J Obstet Gynecol.* 1981;139:403–406.

85. Shortliffe LMD, Stamey TA. Urinary infections in adult women. In: Walsh PC, Gittes RF, Perlmutter AD, et al., eds. *Campbell's Urology.* Philadelphia: WB Saunders; 1985.

86. Zinner SH, Kass EH. Long-term (10 to 14 years) follow-up of bacteriuria of pregnancy. *N Engl J Med.* 1971;285:820–824.

87. Kass EH. Asymptomatic infection of urinary tract. *Trans Assoc Am Phys.* 1956;69:56–63.

88. Kass EH. The role of unsuspected infection in the etiology of prematurity. *Clin Obstet Gynecol.* 1973;16:134–152.

89. Norden CW, Kass EH. Bacteriuria of pregnancy: a critical appraisal. *Annu Rev Med.* 1968;19:432–470.

90. Kincaid-Smith P, Bullen M. Bacteriuria in pregnancy. *Lancet.* 1965;1:395–399.

91. McCormack WM, George H, Donner A, et al. Hepatotoxicity of erythromycin estolate during pregnancy. *Antimicrob Agents Chemother.* 1977;12:630–635.

92. Brumfitt W, Reeves DS. Recent developments in the treatment of urinary tract infection. *J Infect Dis.* 1969;120:61–81.

93. Brumfitt W. The effects of bacteriuria in pregnancy on maternal and fetal health. *Kidney Int.* 1975;8 (Suppl):113–119.

94. Little PJ. The incidence of urinary infection in 5000 pregnant women. *Lancet.* 1966;1:925–928.

95. Mittendorf R, Williams MA, Kass EH. Prevention of preterm delivery and low birth weight associated with asymptomatic bacteriuria. *Clin Infect Dis.* 1992;14:927–932.

96. Chow AW, Jewesson PJ. Pharmacokinetics and safety of antimicrobial agents during pregnancy. *Rev Infect Dis.* 1985;7:287–313.

97. Harbison RD. Teratogens. In: Doull J, Klassen CD, Amdur MO, eds. *Casserett and Doull's Toxicology.* New York: Macmillan; 1980.

98. Hays DP. A review of the basic principles with a discussion of selected agents. III. *Drug Intell Clin Pharmacol.* 1981;15:639–650.

99. Nation RL. Drug kinetics in childbirth. *Clin Pharmacokinet.* 1980;5:340–364.

100. Philipson A. Pharmacokinetics of ampicillin during pregnancy. *J Infect Dis.* 1977;136:370–376.

101. Yamada N, Kido K, Uchida H, et al. Application of cephalosporins to obstetrics and gynecology: transfer of cefazolin and cephalothin to uterine tissue. *Am J Obstet Gynecol.* 1980;136:1036–1040.

102. Philipson A, Sabath LD, Charles D. Erythromycin and clindamycin absorption and elimination in pregnant women. *Clin Pharmacol Ther.* 1975;19:68–77.

103. Hamar C, Levy G. Serum protein binding of drugs and bilirubin in newborn infants and their mothers. *Clin Pharmacol Ther.* 1980;28:58–63.

104. Amon K, Amon I, Huller H. Distribution and kinetics of nitrofurantoin in early pregnancy. *Int J Clin Pharmacol Ther Toxicol.* 1972;6:218–222.

105. Assael BM, Parini R, Rusconi F. Ototoxicity of aminoglycoside antibiotics in infants and children. *Pediatr Infect Dis.* 1982;1:357–365.

106. Beeley L. Adverse effects of drugs in later pregnancy. *Clin Obstet Gynecol.* 1981;8:275–389.

107. Snider DE Jr, Layde PM, Johnson MW, et al. Treatment of tuberculosis during pregnancy. *Am Rev Respir Dis.* 1980;122:65–79.

108. Walker RC, Wright AJ. The fluoroquinolones. *Mayo Clin Proc.* 1991;66:1249–1259.

109. Hooper DC, Wolfson JS. Fluoroquinolone antimicrobial agents. *N Engl J Med.* 1991;324:384–394.

110. Weiss CR, Glazka AJ, Weston JK. Chloramphenicol in the newborn infant: a physiological explanation of its toxicity when given in excessive doses. *N Engl J Med.* 1960;262:787–794.

111. Reid DWJ, Caille G, Kaufmann NR. Maternal and transplacental kinetics of trimethoprim and sulfamethoxazole, separately and in combination. *Can Med Assoc J.* 1975;112(Suppl):67S–72S.

112. Fair WR, Crane DB, Peterson LJ, et al. Three-day treatment of urinary tract infections. *J Urol.* 1980;123:717–721.

113. Fihn SD, Stamm WE. Interpretation and comparison of treatment studies for uncomplicated urinary tract infections in women. *Rev Infect Dis.* 1985;7:468–478.

114. Jakobi P, Neiger R, Mezbach D, et al. Single-dose antimicrobial therapy in the treatment of asymptomatic bacteriuria in pregnancy. *Am J Obstet Gynecol.* 1987;156:1148–1152.

115. Gallagher DJA, Montgomerie JZ, North JDK. Acute infections of the urinary tract and the urethral syndrome in general practice. *Br Med J.* 1965:622–626.

116. Berg AO, Heidrich ME, Fihn SD, et al. Establishing a cause of genitourinary symptoms in

women in a family practice. *JAMA.* 1984:620–625.

117. Fairley KF, Grounds AD, Carson NE, et al. Site of infection in acute urinary tract infection in general practice. *Lancet.* 1971:615–628.

118. Sheehan G, Harding GKM, Ronald AR. Advances in the treatment of urinary tract infection. *Am J Med.* 1984:141.

119. Curran JW. Gonorrhea and the urethral syndrome. *Sex Trans Dis.* 1977:119–121.

120. Krieger JN. Vaginitis: current concepts of etiology, diagnosis and therapy. I. General evaluation, trichomoniasis and vulvovaginal candidiasis. *AUA Update Series.* 1983;2:1–7.

121. Komaroff AL, Pass TM, McCue JD, et al. Management strategies for urinary and vaginal infections. *Arch Intern Med.* 1978:1069–1073.

122. Centers for Disease Control. Nonreported sexually transmissible diseases. *MMWR.* 1979;28:61–63.

123. McCutchan JA, Ronald AR, Corey L, et al. Evaluation of new anti-infective drugs for the treatment of vaginal infections. *Clin Infect Dis.* 1992;15 (Suppl):S115–S122.

124. Wolner-Hansen P, Eschenbach DA, Paavonen J, et al. Association between vaginal douching and acute pelvic inflammatory disease. *JAMA.* 1990;263:1936–1941.

125. Chow JM, Yonekura ML, Richwald GA, et al. The association between *Chlamydia trachomatis* and ectopic pregnancy: a matched-pair, case-control study. *JAMA.* 1990;263:3164–3167.

126. Krieger JN. Urologic aspects of trichomoniasis. *Invest Urol.* 1981;18:411–417.

127. Swedberg J, Steiner JF, Deiss F, et al. Comparison of single-dose vs. one-week course of metronidazole for symptomatic bacterial vaginosis. *JAMA.* 1985;254:1046–1049.

128. Wolner-Hansen P, Krieger JN, Stevens CE. Clinical manifestations of vaginal trichomoniasis. *JAMA.* 1989;261:571–576.

129. Rein MF. Clinical manifestations of urogenital trichomoniasis in women. In: Honigberg BM, eds. *Trichomonads Parasitic in Humans.* New York: Springer-Verlag; 1989:227.

130. Krieger JN, Wolner-Hanssen P, Stevens C, et al. Characteristics of *Trichomonas vaginalis* isolates from women with colpitis macularis (strawberry cervix) and no colposcopic evidence of colpitis macularis. *J Infect Dis.* 1990; 161:307–311.

131. Krieger JN, Verdon M, Siegel N, et al. Risk assessment and laboratory diagnosis of trichomoniasis in men. *J Infect Dis.* 1992;166:1362–1366.

132. Hager WD, Brown ST, Kraus SJ, et al. Metronidazole for vaginal trichomoniasis: seven-day versus single-dose regimens. *JAMA.* 1980;244:1219–1220.

133. Krieger JN, Tam MR, Stevens CE, et al. Diagnosis of trichomoniasis: comparison of conventional wet-mount examination with cytologic studies, cultures, and monoclonal antibody staining of direct specimens. *JAMA.* 1988;259:1223–1227.

134. Dyker JR Jr. Single-dose metronidazole for richomonal vaginitis: patient and consort. Engl J Med. 1975;293:23–24.

135. Robertson DHH, Heyworth R, Harrison C, et al. Treatment failures in *Trichomonas vaginalis* infections in females. I. Concentrations of metronidazole in plasma and vaginal content during normal and high dosage. *J Antimicrob Chemother.* 1988;21:373–378.

136. Lossick JG, Muller M, Gorrell TE. In vitro drug susceptibility and doses of metronidazole required for cure in cases of refractory vaginal trichomoniasis. *J Infect Dis.* 1986;153:948–955.

137. Oriel JD, Partridge BM, Denny MJ, et al. Genital yeast infections. *Br Med J.* 1972;4:761–764.

138. Horowitz BJ, Edelstein SW, Lippman L. *Candida tropicalis* vulvovaginitis. *Obstet Gynecol.* 1985;66:229–232.

139. Sobel JD. Pathogenesis and treatment of recurrent vulvovaginal candidiasis. *Clin Infect Dis.* 1992;14(Suppl 1):S148–S153.

140. Odds FC. Candida *and candidosis.* Baltimore: University Park Press: 1979.

141. Hillier SL, Krohn MA, Klebanoff SJ, et al. The relationship of hydrogen peroxide-producing lactobacilli to bacterial vaginosis and genital microflora in pregnant women. *Obstet Gynecol.* 1992;79:369–373.

142. Sobel JD. Vulvovaginal candidiasis in sexually transmitted diseases. In Holmes KK, Mardh P-A, Sparling PF, et al., eds. *Sexually Transmitted Diseases.* New York: McGraw-Hill; 1990:515–523.

143. Hilton E, Isenberg HD, Alperstein P, et al. Ingestion of yogurt containing *Lactobacillus acidophilus* as prophylaxis for candidal vaginitis. *Ann Intern Med.* 1992;116:353–357.

144. Eschenbach DA, Hillier S, Critchlow C, et al. Diagnosis and clinical manifestations of bacterial vaginosis. *Am J Obstet Gynecol.* 1988; 158:819–828.

145. Spiegel CA, Amsel R, Eschenbach D, et al. Anaerobic bacteria in nonspecific vaginitis. *N Engl J Med.* 1980;303:601–607.

146. Hillier SL, Martius J, Krohn M, et al. A case-control study of chorioamnionic infection and histologic chorioamnionitis in prematurity. *N Engl J Med.* 1988;319:972–978.

147. Gravett MG, Hummel D, Eschenbach DA, et al. Preterm labor associated with subclinical amniotic fluid infection and with bacterial vaginosis. *Obstet Gynecol.* 1986;67:229–237.

148. Piot P, Van Dyck E, Peeters M, et al. Biotypes

of *Gardnerella vaginalis. J Clin Microbiol.* 1984;20:677–679.

149. Amsel R, Totten PA, Spiegel CA, et al. Nonspecific vaginitis: diagnostic criteria and microbial and epidemiologic associations. *Am J Med.* 1983;74:14–22.

150. Nugent RP, Krohn MA, Hillier SL. Reliability of diagnosing bacterial vaginosis is improved by a standardized method of gram stain interpretation. *J Clin Microbiol.* 1991;29:297–301.

151. Thomason JL, Schreckenberger PC, Spellacy WN, et al. Clinical and microbiological characterization of patients with nonspecific vaginosis associated with motile curved anaerobic rods. *J Infect Dis.* 1984;149:801–809.

152. Greaves WL, Chungafung J, Morris B, et al. Clindamycin versus metronidazole in the treatment of bacterial vaginosis. *Obstet Gynecol.* 1988;72:799–802.

153. Hillier S, Krohn MA, Watts DH, et al. Microbiologic efficacy of intravaginal clindamycin cream for the treatment of bacterial vaginosis. *Obstet Gynecol.* 1990;76:407–413.

# 9

# Prostatic Infection and Inflammation

*Jackson E. Fowler, Jr.*

## INTRODUCTION

Inflammatory and infectious disorders of the prostate, and symptomatology suggestive of prostatic inflammation, are believed to affect about 50% of men at some time during adult life.[1] Clinical and laboratory investigations during the past three decades have done much to enhance our understanding of these maladies. This knowledge, when applied to the management of men with suspected prostatic inflammation, facilitates the identification of individuals with true prostatic diseases and provides a framework for rational treatment.

## CLASSIFICATION OF PROSTATITIS

A practical clinical classification of prostatitis syndromes that has been adopted by most urologists is shown in Table 1.[2] The scheme is based on the presence or absence of objective evidence of prostatic inflammation, the presence or absence of culture-documented bacterial infection of the prostate, and, to a minimal extent, the palpatory findings on prostatic examination. The logic for categorization of prostatitis syndromes along these lines is threefold.

First, men with identifiable acute or chronic bacterial infections of the prostate are differentiated from those without bacterial infection. This differentiation is critical since spontaneous resolution of bacterial infection is unlikely, the affected patient is at risk to the potentially lethal morbidity of bacteremia, and well-defined treatments are available. In contrast, the etiologies of nonbacterial prostatitis and prostatodynia are poorly defined, spontaneous resolution of the symptomatology is not uncommon, predictably effective stan-

**TABLE 1. Clinical Classification of Prostatitis Syndromes**

| Disorder | Microscopic Evidence of Prostatic Inflammation | Culture Evidence of Prostatic Infection | Abnormal Prostatic Examination |
|---|---|---|---|
| Acute bacterial prostatitis | + | + | + |
| Chronic bacterial prostatitis | + | + | — |
| Nonbacterial prostatitis | + | — | — |
| Prostatodynia | — | — | — |

(Adapted from Drach[2])

dardized treatments are not available, and serious morbidity is unlikely.

Second, the nature of the bacterial infection, acute or chronic, is specified. Patients with acute bacterial infections are at risk for life-threatening morbidity, but the prospects for cure are paradoxically great. On the other hand, the risk of immediate, serious morbidity among men with chronic bacterial infections is small but the likelihood of cure with antimicrobial therapy is less certain.

Finally, men without identifiable bacterial infection of the prostate are stratified relative to the presence (nonbacterial prostatitis) or absence (prostatodynia) of objective evidence of prostatic inflammation. Documentation of such inflammation suggests a prostatic cause for the symptomatology, whereas the lack of evidence dictates additional investigation to eliminate an extraprostatic etiology for the prostatic symptomatology.

Acute bacterial prostatitis is a distinctly uncommon infection,[3] but the relative incidence of chronic prostatitis is not well-established. In one large clinic devoted to the care of men with inflammatory prostatic symptomatology, 5% of 597 patients were found to have chronic bacterial prostatitis, 64% apparently had nonbacterial prostatitis, and 31% had prostatodynia.[4] These data are consistent with the theories of other investigators suggesting that chronic bacterial prostatitis is a relatively unusual cause of chronic prostatitis.[1,3] Prostatic resistance to bacterial infection appears to reflect the antibacterial properties of prostatic fluid that are mediated by a zinc-containing polypeptide (prostatic antibacterial factor),[5] and by spermidine.[6] A profound local immune response to bacterial infection may also contribute to the infrequency of infections.[7–9]

## ETIOLOGY AND PATHOGENESIS

### Bacterial Prostatitis

Acute and chronic bacterial infections of the prostate are caused primarily by aerobic, gram-negative enteric bacteria and, on rare occasion, enterococci.[1,3] The incidence of infection by various bacterial species and the antimicrobial susceptibilities of the organisms parallel those of bacteria that infect the urine only. *Escherichia coli* is the most common infecting agent, although infections by *Proteus*, *Pseudomonas*, and *Klebsiella* species are not unusual. Specific bacterial virulence factors that might promote infection of the prostate have not been identified.

The role of such gram-positive bacteria as *Staphylococcus* and *Streptococcus* species in inflammatory disorders of the prostate is controversial. Most investigators believe that these organisms do not produce prostatic infection.[1,3] Based on bacterial localization cultures consistent with prostatic infection, however, it has been argued that infection by these indigenous urethral bacteria are a common cause of prostatic symptomatology.[10] Methodologic considerations, and clinical data indicating that such culture results may not accurately reflect the bacteriology of the prostate, are detailed below. In addition, an anticipated local antibody response to prostatic infection has not been detected in patients with prostatic symptomatology and culture localization of *Staphylococcus epidermidis* to the prostate.[7]

### Nonbacterial Prostatitis

The cause or causes of nonbacterial prostatitis are largely unknown, as infectious etiologies have been the most widely studied. The possibility that clinically undetectable infection with gram-negative bacteria or enterococci may be operative is inconsistent with existing data concerning the nature of bacterial infection of the urinary tract, and with the characteristically favorable symptomatic response of patients with known bacterial infection of the prostate to suppressive antimicrobial therapy.

Prostatic infection by microorganisms that are difficult to identify by routine culture methodologies, such as fungi, obligate anaerobic bacteria, trichomonads, and viral agents, has been convincingly eliminated as common causes of nonbacterial prostatitis.[11–16] *Staphylococcus saprophyticus,* an agent responsible for acute urethritis in females, has been implicated as a cause of prostatic inflammation in one report.[17]

However, this organism is almost never isolated from the urine of adult males[18] and thus would appear to be an uncommon cause of nonbacterial prostatitis.

Attention has recently been focused on the possible role of *Chlamydia trachomatis* in the etiology of nonbacterial prostatitis. Although established as a common cause of nongonococcal urethritis,[19] infections by this sexually transmitted agent are not common among men older than 35 years. Moreover, most chlamydial infections are associated with a urethral discharge and respond promptly to antimicrobial therapy. These phenomena are not characteristic of nonbacterial prostatitis.

*C trachomatis* is rarely isolated from the urethra, urine, or prostatic fluid of asymptomatic men.[19–21] As such, isolation of chlamydia from these specimens implies infection. Localization of infection to the prostate, however, is not feasible, since urethral colonization invariably accompanies infection of the genitourinary organs and accurate quantitation of *C trachomatis* in culture is impossible. Serologic tests that differentiate urethral from parenchymal infections are also not available.

Data concerning the incidence of chlamydial infection among men with nonbacterial prostatitis are disturbingly variable. *C trachomatis* has been isolated from early morning urine specimens, prostatic fluid, or seminal fluid of 39 of 70 patients (56%) with "subacute or chronic prostatitis."[22] The 17% incidence of positive cultures in a comparable control population, however, is substantially greater than that found in other studies of asymptomatic men and has raised questions concerning the validity of the microbiologic methodologies.[23]

Mardh and coworkers reported a 33% incidence of serologic evidence of chlamydial infection among 79 men with "nonacute prostatitis" compared to a 3% incidence in 72 age-matched blood donors.[24] However, in a subsequent study by these investigators, *C trachomatis* could be isolated in urethral cultures from only 1 of 53 patients with "nonacute prostatitis" and from 0 of 28 expressed prostatic secretion (EPS) specimens.[25] In addition, antibody directed against *Chlamydia* was not convincingly detectable in the sera or prostatic fluid of these patients using an immunofluorescent assay.

Others also have been unable to isolate *C trachomatis* from the prostatic fluid of men with nonbacterial prostatitis,[26,27] or to detect significant prostatic-fluid antibody titers against *C trachomatis.*[28] The data from Shortliffe et al[28] are quite compelling, as the radioimmunoassay techniques employed were similar to those used for the detection of prostatic-fluid antibody directed against gram-negative bacteria in patients with chronic bacterial prostatitis.

Finally, Doble and coworkers[29] performed biopsies of abnormal areas of the prostate using transrectal ultrasound guidance in 50 men with nonbacterial prostatitis. The specimens were cultured for *C trachomatis* and assayed for the presence of *C trachomatis* antigen using immunofluorescent techniques. None of the patients had either positive cultures or positive immunofluorescent studies. This is an important contribution, as the methodologies employed obviate the potential of contamination by urethral *Chlamydia* species.

There is mounting evidence that urethral colonization by *Ureaplasma urealyticum* may result in symptomatic urethritis.[30] In contrast to *C trachomatis*, *U urealyticum* is commonly isolated from the urethral cultures of normal men. Therefore, isolation of this organism from the genitourinary fluids of men with inflammatory disorders does not necessarily imply infection. Mycoplasmas have been isolated from the seminal fluid or prostatic fluid of 46% of 79 men with symptoms of prostatitis.[13] Most of these individuals, however, had concurrent urethral colonization which may have contaminated the genital secretions.

On the basis of quantitative localization cultures, *U urealyticum* has been implicated as a cause of prostatitis in 82 (14%) of 597 patients.[4] Seventy-one (87%) of these 82 patients were rendered asymptomatic and free of *U urealyticum* colonization after treatment with tetracycline for 14 days. Because the EPS was not examined microscopically, however, objective evidence of prostatic inflammation was not reported, and categorization of the disorder as nonbacterial prostatitis or prostatodynia is not possible.

In one recent study, however, *U urealyticum* could not be localized to the prostate in any of 30 patients with inflammatory prostatic symptomatology.[31] Interestingly, positive localization culture results were found in 13 of 50 control subjects.

Meares failed to recover *U urealyticum* from the prostatic fluid or urine voided after prostatic massage in 20 men with nonbacterial prostatitis.[14] Interestingly, no species of *Ureaplasma* were cultured from the first-voided urine specimen in a single patient, a finding that may reflect the advanced age, limited sexual activity, or frequent use of antibiotics in this selected population.

Failure to differentiate between urethritis and prostatitis may account for uncertainties regarding the role of *C trachomatis* and *U urealyticum* in the pathogenesis of nonbacterial prostatitis. Urethral inflammation may result in an increased density of prostatic-fluid leukocytes due to contamination during transit through the urethra. Further, the characteristic dysuria and discharge of urethritis may be accompanied by vague perineal pains and ejaculatory discomforts, suggesting prostatic inflammation. It is advisable for both conceptual and therapeutic purposes to segregate patients with nonbacterial prostatitis by the presence or absence of urethral symptomatology, and to classify any disorder manifested by urethral symptomatology alone as urethritis rather than prostatitis.

Exploration of noninfectious processes that might result in symptomatic prostatic inflammation constitute reasonable, but as yet unrewarding, avenues of research. Inflammation mediated by prostaglandins,[1] autoimmunity,[32,33] and allergic phenomenon[34] have each been implicated in isolated reports but have yet to be supported by subsequent investigations.

## Prostatodynia

Due to the absence of objective evidence indicating prostatic inflammation, research concerning the etiology of prostatodynia has been directed primarily toward the illumination of extraprostatic sources for the apparent prostatic symptomatology. Pelvic-floor tension myalgia due to habitual contraction and spasm has been implicated as a cause of prostatodynia in one investigation.[36] Neuromuscular dysfunction of the bladder outlet and external sphincter may also be causative.[37–39]

Meares investigated 64 men with well-documented prostatodynia of at least 6 months' duration using urodynamic testing and cine-voiding cystourethrograms.[40] Sixty-two percent of the patients had symptoms of bladder outlet obstruction and 96% had decreased urinary flow rates. However, none had increased residual urine volumes in the absence of coexisting benign prostatic hyperplasia (BPH) or evidence of neurologic disease.

An increased closure pressure at the bladder outlet, the urethral sphincter, or at both sites was the only identifiable abnormal urodynamic parameter. The cine-voiding cystourethrograms generally demonstrated incomplete opening (funnelling of the bladder neck and narrowing of the prostatic urethra at the external urethral sphincter). This was seen despite the absence of external urethral sphincter contraction as measured by electromyography.

Overall, 70% of the patients were thought to have abnormal spasm of the bladder neck or urethra as the sole cause for the symptomatology, 17% were thought to have spasm in combination with tension myalgia of the pelvic floor or BPH, 9% were thought to have tension myalgia of the pelvic floor only, and 3% had no identifiable cause for the symptomatology.

The reasons for bladder outlet and urethral spasm are unclear. Meares has proposed that transient spasm of uncertain etiology may lead to urinary reflux into the prostatic ducts, and that the spasm is then perpetuated by prostatic inflammation. Hellstrom and coworkers have described three patients with prostatodynia who had elevated pressures within the prostatic urethra and intraprostatic reflux of urine demonstrated by voiding cystourethrography.[41] Reflux of urine into the prostatic ducts has also been implicated by other investigators as a cause of prostatic symptomatology.[35] This is an intriguing concept as some constituents of the urine, such as Tamm-Horsfall protein, are known to be immunogenic.

Finally, emotional instability or stress is often noted in patients with this disorder. Psychologic testing has demonstrated that patients with chronic prostatitis may suffer from psychosexual disturbances, severe anxiety, or paranoid ideation.[42–44] Response to treatments of the prostatic disorder appears to correlate inversely with the degree of psychologic disturbance.

## DIAGNOSTIC TECHNIQUES

### History and Physical Examination

A detailed analysis of the character and duration of the symptomatology, the results of prior investigations, and the response to past treatments are critical components of the history. Complete physical examination, rather than examination limited to the external genitalia and prostate, is an essential—but sometimes neglected—aspect of patient evaluation. Meticulous examination of the abdomen, perineum, and rectum may disclose an alternative explanation for the apparent prostatic symptomatology.

Acute bacterial prostatitis is usually manifested by the somewhat explosive onset of dysuria, diurnal frequency, nocturia, and urgency. These symptoms of bacteriuria are often accompanied by varying degrees of bladder outlet obstruction and low back and perineal pain due to prostatic inflammation and swelling. Fever, chills, and malaise consistent with a significant parenchymal infection are common. Some men experience a nonspecific prodrome of vague pelvic and systemic symptoms for days to weeks before consulting a physician.

On occasion, the patient may relate prior episodes suggestive of bacterial infection of the urinary tract. Such historical data raise the possibility that the current disorder constitutes an acute exacerbation of a chronic infectious process.

Fever, suprapubic discomfort, and an extremely tender, enlarged, and indurated prostate are characteristic physical findings. Rectal examination should be sufficient to rule out the presence of prostatic fluctuance suggestive of a prostatic abscess. Vigorous prostatic examination, however, should be avoided because of both patient discomfort and the risk that manipulation of the prostate will promote bacteremia. No attempt should be made to obtain prostatic fluid for microscopic or bacteriologic analysis. A marked leukocytosis is not uncommon.

The symptoms of chronic bacterial prostatitis, nonbacterial prostatitis, and prostatodynia are remarkably similar. Most patients complain of such irritative voiding symptoms as dysuria, urgency, diurnal frequency, and nocturia; ill-defined pelvic or perineal discomforts; and pain with or following ejaculation. The intensity of these symptoms is usually variable over time. Urethral discharge, which is a hallmark of urethritis, is rarely associated with prostatitis.

Palpation of the prostate usually provides little insight into the nature of the chronic prostatitis syndromes. The consistency of the prostate and the degree of discomfort accompanying digital rectal examination generally parallel those of normal men of corresponding age.

The most important historical clue to the etiology of chronic prostatic symptomatology involves documentation of prior bacteriuria. On the one hand, this infectious process is remarkably infrequent in otherwise healthy men.[45–47] On the other hand, chronic bacterial prostatitis is the most common cause of recurring urinary tract infection in males.[1] It follows that this diagnosis should be suspected if there is a history of documented bacterial infection of the genitourinary tract, and that the likelihood of chronic bacterial prostatitis is remote if past urine cultures have been sterile during symptomatic episodes.

The symptomatic response to prior antimicrobial treatment or to nonspecific therapeutic interventions is a less informative but still important historical consideration. The majority of men with chronic bacterial prostatitis will achieve complete or near complete symptomatic relief during antimicrobial therapy. This benefit results from sterilization of the urine, and is largely independent of the bacteriologic response of the prostatic infection. If treatment is not curative, the symptoms characteristically recur within several months. Therapeutic interventions with no obvious antimicrobial value, such as prostatic massage, urethral dilation, and anticholinergic therapy, are usually of no benefit.

Available evidence suggests that some patients with nonbacterial prostatitis and prostatodynia will also improve with antimicrobial therapy.[4,48,49] Unlike chronic bacterial prostatitis, however, the favorable responses are often either transient despite ongoing treatment, or long-lived despite seemingly inadequate treatment for chronic bacterial prostatitis. Men with nonbacterial prostatitis or prostatodynia frequently respond to nonspecific treatments.

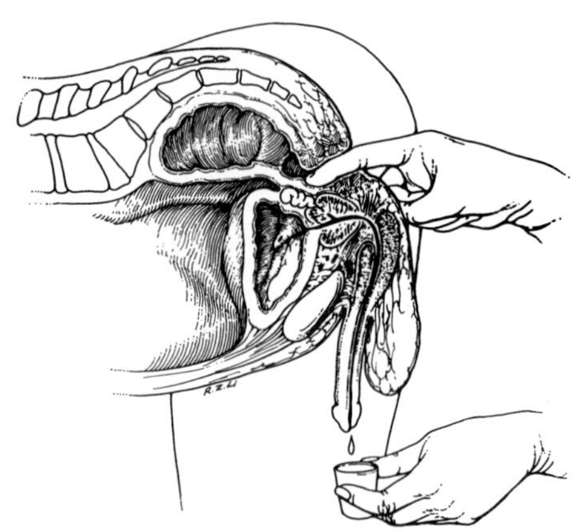

**Fig 1.** Expression of prostatic fluid by digital massage. [From Fowler JE Jr, *Urinary Tract Infection and Inflammation* (Chicago: Year Book Medical Publishers; 1989), with permission.]

## Microscopic Examination of Urine and Genital Fluids

The sediment of a centrifuged midstream urine specimen (the voided-bladder 2 or $VB_2$) from men with nonbacterial prostatitis and prostatodynia is usually unremarkable. Due to coexisting bacteriuria, acute and chronic bacterial prostatitis are usually accompanied by visible numbers of bacteria and greater than five leukocytes/high-power field (HPF) in the $VB_2$ sediment. If urethritis—rather than prostatitis—is suspected, both the first 10 mL of voided urine (the voided-bladder 1 or $VB_1$) and the $VB_2$ specimen should be examined. In urethritis, the density of leukocytes in the $VB_1$ specimen is often five to ten times greater than that in the $VB_2$ specimen.

The most important clinical material for the investigation of inflammatory prostatic disorders, EPS, is obtained by digital massage of the prostate (Fig 1). Leukocytes and lipid-laden macrophages are generally identifiable microscopically in the EPS of normal men. However, existing data suggest that greater than 10 leukocytes/HPF is unusual.[1,50–53] Therefore, an increased EPS leukocyte density, particularly if accompanied by clumping of leukocytes and more than one or two lipid-laden macrophages/HPF (Fig 2), implies prostatic inflammation. This concept is supported by the findings that: greater than 10 EPS leukocytes/HPF are often observed in specimens from men with symptoms suggesting prostatic inflammation[50,52]; the microscopic findings are usually reproducible in serial assays[54];

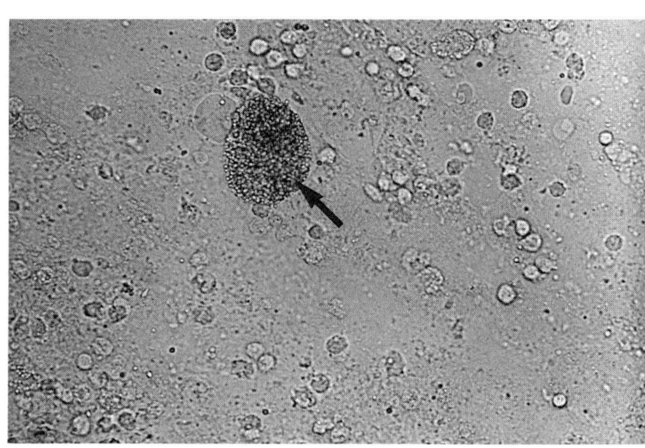

**Fig 2.** Expressed prostatic secretions from patient with *E coli* chronic bacterial prostatitis. Arrow indicates lipid-laden macrophage, which is approximately 4× larger than the accompanying leukocytes; note free fat droplet adjacent to macrophage and clumping of leukocytes (unstained, ×200). [From Fowler JE Jr, *Urinary Tract Infection and Inflammation* (Chicago: Year Book Medical Publishers; 1989), with permission.]

and alteration of the prostatic fluid lactate dehydrogenase isoenzyme 5 and 1 ratio (which is a sensitive indicator of prostatic inflammation) is generally accompanied by an increased EPS leukocyte density.[52]

Seminal fluid usually can be collected more easily and in larger volumes than EPS. Difficulties in distinguishing between leukocytes and immature sperm cells in unstained or conventionally stained samples, however, limit the practical value of microscopic analysis. Moreover, the impact of prostatic inflammation on seminal-fluid leukocyte density has not been subjected to critical analysis.

Although EPS leukocyte quantitation constitutes an objective measure of prostatic inflammation, the clinical value of this test is confounded by a variety of factors. Some investigators believe that greater than 20 EPS leukocytes/HPF should be considered as the upper limit of normal.[2,55] Normal or near normal EPS leukocyte densities may be seen in specimens from patients with culture-documented chronic bacterial prostatitis during antimicrobial therapy. Alternatively, greater than 10 EPS leukocytes/HPF are observed in approximately 5% to 10% of men with no clinical symptoms of prostatic inflammation.[50–52] Finally, the density of EPS leukocytes in normal men is related in part to the interval between ejaculation and EPS procurement,[53] leukocytes of urethral origin may contaminate EPS, immature sperm expressed from the seminal vesicles may be mistaken for leukocytes by the untrained observer, and the volume of EPS available for examination is often limited. For these reasons, the clinician must view this diagnostic test as complementary to, rather than as a substitute for, bacteriologic investigations in the evaluation of prostatic symptomatology.

## Bacteriologic Investigations

Untreated acute bacterial infection of the prostate is invariably accompanied by infection of the bladder urine. Because of the characteristic history and physical findings associated with this disorder, culture documentation of bacteriuria only is necessary for definitive diagnosis.

Culture of the urine only is not sufficient for differentiation of chronic bacterial prostatitis from nonbacterial prostatitis or prostatodynia as this specimen may be sterile in each disorder. Alternatively, documentation of bacteriuria does not necessarily imply chronic bacterial prostatitis since the symptoms of bacteriuria alone are nearly identical to those of bacteriuria associated with chronic bacterial prostatitis. Culture evidence of *prostatic infection*, therefore, is necessary to delineate both the nature of the chronic prostatitis syndromes, and the anatomic extent of urinary infections.

Quantitative culture of the first 10 mL of voided urine (the $VB_1$ specimen), a midstream urine specimen (the $VB_2$ specimen), the EPS, and the first 10 mL of urine voided immediately after prostatic massage (the voided bladder 3 or $VB_3$ specimen) is the best method for localization of bacterial infection to the prostate gland.[56] Culture of the EPS only is not sufficient for definitive diagnosis. Gram-negative bacilli colonize the distal urethra of approximately 5% of normal men and may contaminate otherwise sterile prostatic fluid.

The $VB_1$ culture identifies the urethral flora and provides an estimate of the contribution of urethral bacteria to subsequent specimens. *Staphylococcal* and *streptococcal* species, which colonize the distal urethra of about 95% of normal men, are frequently isolated from the $VB_1$ specimen and the EPS specimen. These organisms do not cause bacterial prostatitis and should be disregarded. Among men without colonization of the urethra by gram-negative bacilli, sterile urine, and an uninfected prostate, none of the culture specimens will contain gram-negative bacilli (Fig 3A). With gram-negative bacterial colonization of the urethra only, the density of isolates in the EPS is usually equal to, or less than, the density of isolates in the $VB_1$ (Fig 3B).

If there is infection of the bladder urine with or without coexisting infection of the prostate, the density of bacteria in all specimens will be equivalent and the culture study will be uninterpretable (Figs 3C,3D). To circumvent this problem, all men with bacteriuria and suspected chronic bacterial prostatitis should be treated with nitrofurantoin, penicillin, or tetracycline before

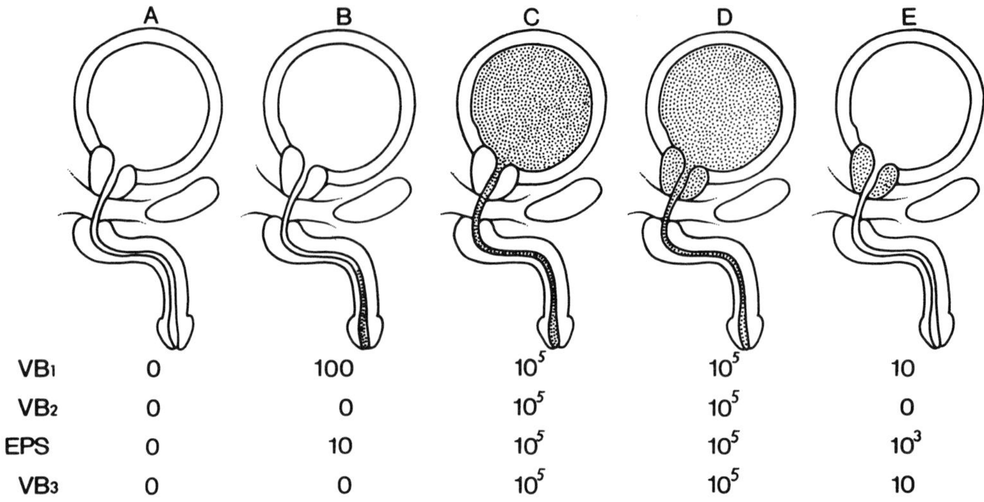


| | A | B | C | D | E |
|---|---|---|---|---|---|
| VB1 | 0 | 100 | $10^5$ | $10^5$ | 10 |
| VB2 | 0 | 0 | $10^5$ | $10^5$ | 0 |
| EPS | 0 | 10 | $10^5$ | $10^5$ | $10^3$ |
| VB3 | 0 | 0 | $10^5$ | $10^5$ | 10 |

**Fig 3.** Characteristic results of quantitative culture of $VB_1$, $VB_2$, EPS, and $VB_3$ specimens (expressed as gram-negative bacilli/mL) in A, men with no urethral colonization by gram-negative bacilli; B, urethral colonization only by gram-negative bacilli; C, bacteriuria but no prostatic infection; D, bacteriuria and coexisting prostatic infection; and E, prostatic infection with suppression of bacterial growth in the urine by antimicrobial therapy. [From Fowler JE Jr, *Urinary Tract Infection and Inflammation* (Chicago: Year Book Medical Publishers; 1989), with permission.]

bacteriologic investigation. Such therapy suppresses or eliminates gram-negative bacteria in the urethra and bladder urine but will not sterilize the prostate. Differences between the density of bacteria in the $VB_1$ and EPS cultures in patients with bacterial prostatitis, therefore, are amplified (Fig 3E). Trimethoprim, trimethoprim-sulfamethoxazole (TMP-SMX), norfloxacin, or ciprofloxacin should not be used for this purpose, as each may also suppress bacterial growth in the prostatic fluid.

If EPS is not obtainable, quantitative culture of the $VB_3$ (which should contain varying amounts of prostatic fluid) is recommended. However, the dilution of intraurethral prostatic fluid by urine is not quantifiable, and comparison of this culture specimen with the $VB_1$ specimen is less reliable for documenting prostatic infection.

Falsely positive bacterial localization cultures are unusual. The organisms responsible for prostatitis rarely colonize the urethra under normal circumstances[57] and are isolated rarely from the EPS of normal men.[1,50,58] On the other hand, bacteriuria in the absence of prostatic infection usually results in uninterpretable, rather than erroneous, culture data.

Falsely negative culture results may occur, since infection of the prostate is a focal process, and sampling errors are inevitable. For this reason, more than one culture study may be required to document infection. Treatment with trimethoprim, TMP-SMX, norfloxacin, or ciprofloxacin, which may suppress bacterial growth in both the urine and the prostatic fluid, can also lead to false-negative culture results. Knowledge of recent antimicrobial usage, therefore, is required for meaningful interpretation of the cultures.

Culture studies suggesting prostatic infection by indigenous urethral microorganisms such as *Staphylococcus* or *Streptococcus* species or diptheroids should be interpreted with caution and skepticism, as these organisms do not cause prostatic infection. Despite meticulous specimen collection and culture, up to 40% of localization studies in men with no clinical evidence of genitourinary infection will suggest prostatic infection by these bacteria.[1,58,59] Moreover, the culture results are generally not reproducible in longitudinal studies, and often suggest infection by more than one organism. These findings are inconsistent with chronic bacterial infection of the prostate.

A disproportionate susceptibility to contamination by urethral bacteria of the EPS compared to the $VB_1$ specimen is a logical explanation for these observations, since EPS is more viscous and traverses the urethra more slowly than voided urine. Treatment with antimicrobials before bacterial localization cultures in an effort to better delineate the origin of such EPS isolates is generally futile, as the organisms are difficult, if not impossible, to suppress or eradicate.[7]

The disproportionate susceptibility of EPS to contamination by the urethral flora implies that culture data indicating infection of the prostate by such potential pathogens as *C trachomatis, U urealyticum* and *S saprophyticus,* which commonly infect the urethra, may also be misleading. Recognition of these limitations of culture techniques designed to assess the extent of gram-negative bacterial infection of the male genitourinary tract is essential for meaningful investigations of the eitology and treatment of genitourinary disorders.

Culture of the seminal fluid has been advocated as an alternative method for documentation of prostatic infection if EPS is not obtainable.[60] It is reasonable to believe, and existing data suggest, that the infecting organism in chronic bacterial prostatitis is as likely to be isolated from this specimen as from an EPS specimen.[60,61] Falsely negative culture results, therefore, should be unusual. However, seminal fluid is more susceptible to contamination by the urethral flora than EPS[58] and well-defined criteria for the diagnosis of chronic bacterial prostatitis based on comparison of quantitative cultures of the seminal fluid and $VB_1$ specimens are not available. The possibility of falsely positive culture results, therefore, may be greater than that encountered using conventional techniques. Culture of the seminal fluid may be useful as a screening test for chronic bacterial prostatitis as described below, but is not recommended as a replacement for the EPS culture in definitive localization studies.

Despite the realities that chronic prostatitis is a common disorder and that identification of bacterial infection is a fundamental component of patient management, the bacterial localization culture technique has not been widely adopted in clinical practice. This appears to be due to the expense of the cultures and the time constraints of clinical practice. An alternative strategy has been proposed that should obviate these problems in the initial bacteriologic investigation of chronic prostatitis.[62] The rationale for this approach, which entails quantitative culture of the $VB_2$ to screen for bacteriuria and nonquantitative culture of the EPS to screen for prostatic infection, is based on the following considerations:

1. Isolation of urinary pathogens from the EPS specimen is necessary to establish the diagnosis of chronic bacterial prostatitis.
2. Urinary pathogens are rarely isolated from the EPS specimen in the absence of bacteriuria or chronic bacterial prostatitis.
3. Chronic bacterial prostatitis appears to be an uncommon cause of "chronic prostatitis."

It logically follows that urinary pathogens will *not* be isolated from the $VB_2$ or EPS specimens of most patients with chronic prostatitis. Confidence that these patients do not have bacterial prostatitis should parallel the confidence of diagnosis obtained with conventional bacterial localization cultures. Similarly, patients with bacteriuria will be identified with equivalent assurance, since quantitative culture of the $VB_2$ specimen is used in both study techniques. Unlike conventional bacterial-localization studies, however, recovery of urinary pathogens from the EPS specimen identifies patients who *might* have chronic bacterial prostatitis rather than patients who probably or unequivocally have chronic bacterial prostatitis. For this reason, isolation of pathogenic bacteria from either specimen necessitates subsequent bacterial localization cultures to determine the

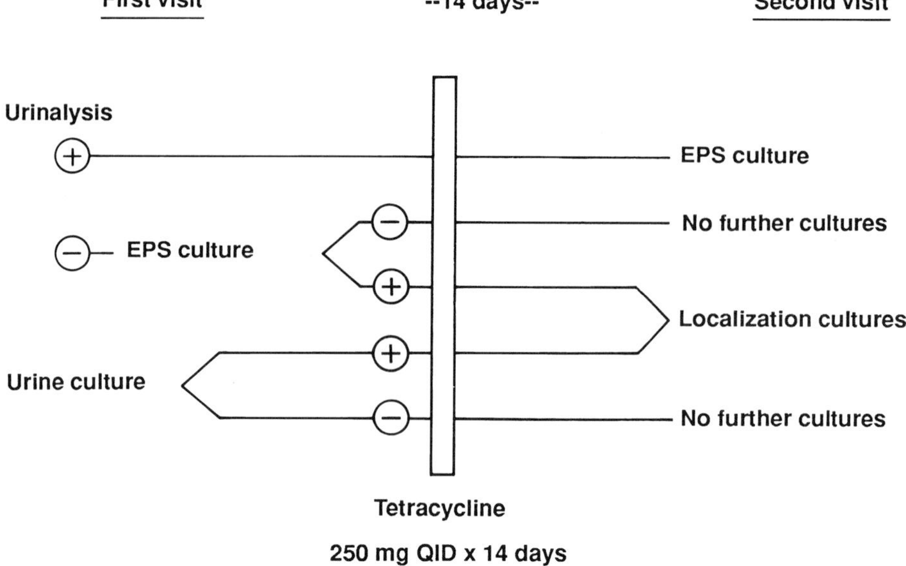


**Fig 4.** Practical approach to *initial* bacteriologic investigation of chronic prostatitis. [From Fowler JE Jr, *Urinary Tract Infection and Inflammation* (Chicago: Year Book Medical Publishers; 1989), with permission.]

source of the isolate. This duplication of effort, however, is more than compensated by the anticipated infrequency of culture-positive EPS specimens in most patient populations.

This streamlined bacteriologic strategy is easily integrated into the standard evaluation of the patient with chronic prostatitis, and special handling of EPS in the microbiology laboratory is not required. A routine that has proved practical and economical in our clinics is shown in Figure 4. The $VB_2$ is obtained before or after a careful history and examined microscopically prior to physical examination. If the urinary sediment is suggestive of bacteriuria, it is advisable to withhold collection and culture of the EPS until the next office visit. Otherwise, the EPS is procured during examination of the prostate. Retraction of the foreskin, if present, cleansing of the glans with tap water, and collection of the EPS in a wide mouth sterile container will reduce the possibilities of contamination.[1] At least one drop of prostatic fluid is almost always obtainable if patience is exercised to allow the fluid to traverse the urethra. If a limited quantity of EPS is obtained for culture, a drop which invariably remains at the meatus may be collected for microscopic analysis by applying the surface of a glass slide to the glans.

The $VB_2$ and EPS should be promptly refrigerated and cultured as soon as possible. Quantitative culture of the $VB_2$ is performed by routine techniques. At least 0.01 mL, and preferably 0.1 mL, of the EPS specimen should be streaked on the bacteriologic media that are used for routine urine cultures. Quantitation of bacterial isolates from the EPS is not necessary, since the results are not compared to the results of a $VB_1$ culture. However, all pathogenic isolates should be identified, regardless of colony count. It is critical to communicate these objectives to the microbiologist.

In the absence of identifiable alternative disorders to explain the prostatic symptoms, tetracycline (250 mg qid for 14 days) is prescribed and a return visit is arranged to coincide with the end of treatment. The rationale for this empiric treatment is twofold. First, tetracycline is a reasonable initial treatment option for nonbacterial prostatitis and prostatodynia. Second, tetracycline is active against most Enterobacteriaceae and *Pseudomonas* at concentrations achievable in the urine.[1] Therefore, if the patient has bacteriuria, this treatment will usually suppress or eradicate the infecting organism in the urethra and bladder urine, and the likelihood of interpretable localization cultures on the second visit is enhanced.

Conventional bacterial localization cultures are mandatory on the second office visit if pathogenic bacteria are isolated from the previous $VB_2$ or EPS cultures. If previously suspected bacteriuria is not documented by culture of the $VB_2$, the investigations described for the first visit are initiated.

Culture of the $VB_2$ and EPS is also well-suited for assessment of the bacteriologic response of documented prostatic infections to antimicrobial therapy, and for surveillance cultures after completion of apparently curative treatment. Culture of the seminal fluid, rather than the EPS, is probably a less useful method of screening for bacterial infection, as the likelihood of contamination is greater.

## Prostate Biopsy

Prostate biopsy for the purposes of identifying prostatic inflammation histologically, or prostatic infection by culture of the tissue, is rarely warranted. Histologic evidence of inflammation has been observed in 98% of 162 consecutive surgical prostatic specimens resected because of hyperplasia.[63] The value of culture of biopsy specimens is limited by the focal nature of the infection, which makes sampling errors inevitable and increases the likelihood of unquantifiable specimen contamination.

## Immunologic Investigation

Bacterial infections of the prostate are usually associated with detectable titers of antibody directed against the infecting organism in the serum[64] and prostatic fluid.[7,8] The presence of such antibody titers generally indicates ongoing or recent infection, and the level of antibody roughly correlates with the severity of the infection and response to treatment. Although of tremendous investigative interest, clinical application of antibody detection and quantitation has been limited by both the specificity of antibody for the infecting microorganism and the uniqueness of antigenic determinants on different gram-negative bacteria. For example, EPS antibody directed against one strain or O-serotype of *E coli* does not usually cross react, or cross reacts weakly, with another strain or O-serotype.[6] In general, therefore, the infecting organism must be available for use in the assay system.

This limitation can be circumvented to some extent if a variety of bacterial antigens representative of the spectrum of bacterial types that commonly infect the prostate are employed in the assay.[6,65,66] Similarly, since specific antigenic determinants are apparently shared by most pathogenic strains of *C trachomatis* and *U urealyticum*, assays for antibody against these agents do not require the actual infecting microorganism.

Immunoassays designed to detect microbial antigen in biologic fluids—rather than the host immune response to the antigen—constitute alternative methods for the diagnosis of infectious processes. Due largely to the advent of monoclonal antibodies, highly sensitive and specific assays for *C trachomatis* are now available and should help to clarify the role of this agent in nonbacterial prostatitis. Development of an antibody capable of recognizing the variety of gram-negative bacteria that cause chronic bacterial prostatitis, however, seems unlikely.

## Prostatic Imaging

Prostatic imaging is not recommended for routine evaluation of men with suspected chronic bacterial prostatitis. The appearance of the acutely or chronically inflamed prostate on computed tomography is similar to the appearance of the normal prostate or BPH.[67] With ultrasonography, the echogenicity of the inflamed prostate often mimics that observed with prostatic carcinoma.

## MANAGEMENT

### Acute Bacterial Prostatitis

Most men with acute bacterial prostatitis require hospitalization. An intravenous pyelogram should be obtained to rule out coexisting infected renal calculi or structural abnormalities of the upper urinary tract. Hydration, analgesics, and stool softeners are helpful supportive measures. Acute urinary retention is not infrequent, especially among men with BPH. Suprapubic urinary drainage by means of a percutaneous cystostomy is preferable to urethral catheter drainage, as the latter may be extremely uncomfortable and may exacerbate the prostatic inflammation.

If hospitalization is required, parenteral antibiotic therapy should be instituted immediately after urine and blood are obtained for culture. Combination therapy with an aminoglycoside to cover infection due to Enterobacteriaceae or *Pseudomonas*, and with ampicillin to cover infection due to enterococci, is recommended. Although these agents are not lipid-soluble and theoretically should not diffuse into prostatic fluid, clinical experience indicates that levels in the prostatic tissue fluid adequate to eradicate the infecting bacterium are usually achieved. This is due apparently to disruption by the acute inflammatory reaction of the physiologic barriers to diffusion of most antimicrobial agents into prostatic fluid.

Response to treatment is typically rapid, and oral antimicrobial therapy can usually be instituted after 3 to 4 days. Persistent fever should prompt investigations for an additional site of infection and reevaluation for possible prostatic abscess formation. Computed tomography of the prostate is particularly helpful in the diagnosis of abscesses (Fig 5). Transrectal ultrasonography may also be of diagnostic value (Fig 6).[68] Prostatic abscesses are usually associated with bacteremia, and prompt drainage by transperitoneal or transurethral incision is required.

The optimal duration of antimicrobial therapy following resolution of the acute infectious process is not known. However, all patients should be considered at risk for chronic bacterial prostatitis.[54] For this reason, and because diffusion of antimicrobials into the prostatic fluid may also be enhanced during a period of resolving

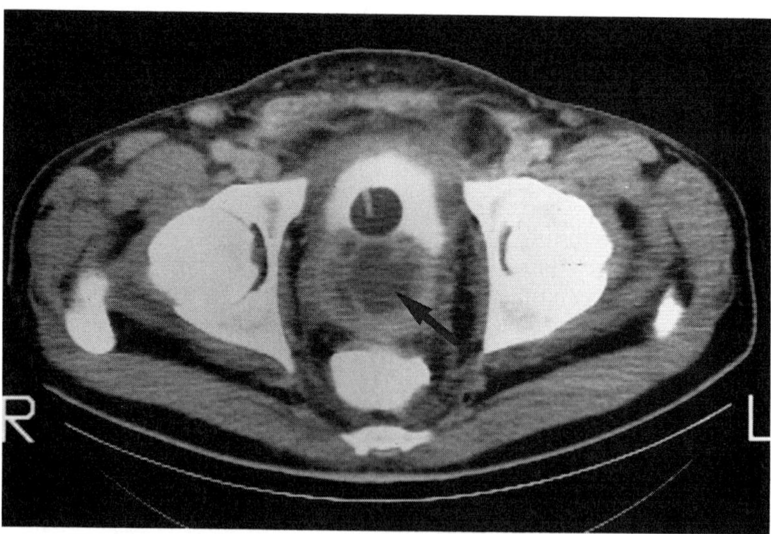


**Fig 5.** Computed tomography of the pelvis in man with *Klebsiella* prostatic abscess (arrow). [From Fowler JE Jr, *Urinary Tract Infection and Inflammation* (Chicago: Year Book Medical Publishers; 1989), with permission.]

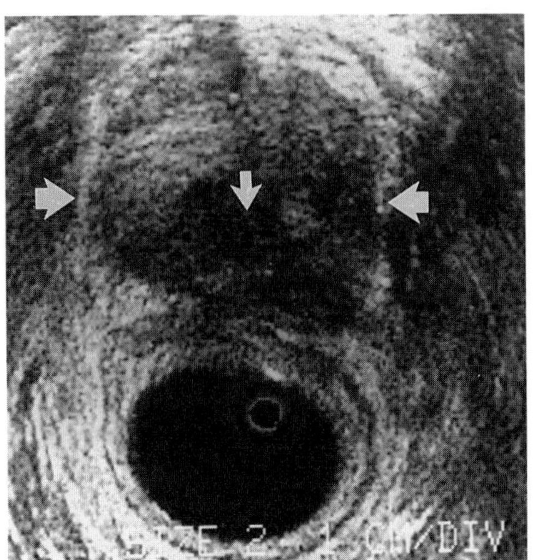

**Fig 6.** Transrectal ultrasonography of prostatic abscess shown in Fig 5; lateral arrows show prostatic capsule, middle arrow shows hypoechoic region of prostate corresponding to location of prostatic abscess. [From Fowler JE Jr, *Urinary Tract Infection and Inflammation* (Chicago: Year Book Medical Publishers; 1989), with permission.]

prostatic inflammation, full-dose oral antimicrobial therapy is recommended for one month. Trimethoprim or TMP-SMX in full oral dosages are the most logical treatment options for susceptible organisms. If the infecting organism is resistant to trimethoprim, indanyl carbenicillin is recommended. These agents are also reasonable treatment options for patients with less severe infections who seem amenable to outpatient management.

Bacteriologic documentation of treatment success or failure is an integral component of patient management. Complete bacterial localization cultures or quantitative culture of the $VB_2$ and nonquantitative culture of the EPS should be performed at 1, 4, and 12 weeks after the termination of antimicrobial therapy. Patients with persistent, culture-documented infection of the prostate should be treated for chronic bacterial prostatitis as outlined below.

Induration of the prostate often persists for months following an episode of acute bacterial prostatitis. This may result from a granulomatous reaction to the infection.

## Chronic Bacterial Prostatitis

**Treatment Objectives.** The goals of treatment of chronic bacterial prostatitis are properly categorized as *potentially curative* or *suppressive*. Potentially curative treatments are designed to eradicate the focus of infection in the prostate and, by definition, eliminate the cause of persistent bacteriuria. Suppressive therapy is designed only to suppress or eliminate bacterial growth in the urine (usually by using antimicrobial agents). This usually results in complete symptomatic relief with little risk of serious morbidity from the persistent focus of infection within the prostate.

**Potentially Curvative Antimicrobial Therapy.** Eradication of localized bacterial infections with antimicrobial therapy requires sufficient levels of an appropriate drug at the site of infection. Since infecting bacteria are isolated from the prostatic fluid of men with chronic bacterial prostatitis, it follows that, to be useful for potentially curative therapy, antimicrobial agents must achieve bactericidal levels in this fluid. However, important insights into the mechanisms that govern the diffusion of drugs across the prostatic epithelium have been provided by Stamey's investigation of the uninfected canine prostate.[1] He showed that a drug must be lipid soluble to penetrate the prostatic epithelium and that drugs that exist as bases can be concentrated in the prostatic fluid by the process of ion trapping. The clinical relevance of these observations was underscored by the finding that trimethoprim, the most active drug against chronic bacterial infections available in the 1970s, achieved higher levels than any other agent tested in the canine prostatic fluid. This is not unexpected, because trimethoprim is a lipid-soluble base. Favorable recent experiences using fluoroquinolone antibiotics for treatment of chronic bacterial prostatitis also validate the concepts put forth by Stamey because the fluoroquinolones are also lipid-soluble bases.

Reported clinical experiences with potentially curative antimicrobial therapy are uniformly limited to small study popula-

**TABLE 2. Results of Potentially Curative Antimicrobial Therapy for Chronic Bacterial Prostatitis Caused by Susceptible Gram-Negative Bacteria or Enterococci:**

| Reference | Agent | Duration of Treatment (wks) | No. of Patients | Follow-up (wks) | Percent Cured |
|---|---|---|---|---|---|
| Meares,[69] 1973 | TMP-SMX* | 2 | 13 | 12 | 15 |
| Meares,[70] 1980 | TMP-SMX | 12 | 15 | 12 | 40 |
| McGuire,[61] 1976 | TMP-SMX | 12 | 12 | 52 | 42 |
| Paulson,[72] 1978 | TMP-SMX | 12 | 14 | 52 | 79 |
| Sabbaj,[74] 1986 | TMP-SMX | 4–6 | 10 | 4–6 | 67 |
| | Norfloxacin | 4–6 | 23 | 4–6 | 92 |
| Weidner,[73] 1987 | Ciprofloxacin | 2 | 13 | 52 | 62 |
| Oliveri,[75] 1979 | Indanyl carbenicillin | 4 | 22 | 4 | 68 |
| Mobley,[76] 1981 | Indanyl carbenicillin | 4 | 12 | 4 | 67 |
| Paulson,[72] 1978 | Minocycline | 4 | 10 | 5 | 70 |
| Mobley,[77] 1974 | Erythromycin and bicarbonate | 2–4 | 26 | 26 | 88 |
| Oliveri,[75] 1979 | Cephalexin | 4 | 9 | 4 | 22 |
| Mobley,[76] 1981 | Cephalexin | 4 | 5 | 4 | 40 |

* TMP-SMX = Trimethoprim-sulfamethoxazole.

tions, and many are flawed by inadequate case definition and supporting microbiologic data. A summary of the interpretable results from clinical trials examining treatment for chronic bacterial prostatitis caused by gram-negative bacteria (or enterococci susceptible to the agent of interest) is shown in Table 2.

TMP-SMX has been most widely studied. It is probable that the sulfamethoxazole component of this combination agent is of little therapeutic value, and the efficacy of trimethoprim alone should be similar to that of TMP-SMX. Meares achieved bacteriologic cures with a 2-week course of full-dose oral TMP-SMX in 15% of 13 patients with indisputable evidence of chronic bacterial prostatitis.[69] When 15 other patients were treated by the Stanford group for a 12-week period, the bacteriologic cure rate increased to 40%.[70] The persistent infecting organisms did not develop resistance to TMP-SMX during administration.

These investigations should be considered the standard against which clinical trials of potentially curative treatment for chronic bacterial prostatitis should be measured. The diagnosis of persistent bacterial infection of the prostate was documented by multiple, confirmatory, localization cultures before treatment, the symptomatic response was clearly differentiated from the bacteriologic response, and the favorable treatment outcomes were supported by localization cultures during 3 or more months of posttreatment surveillance. For these reasons, I view the data in these reports as realistic estimates of the curability of chronic bacterial prostatitis with TMP-SMX or trimethoprim alone. Further, there is no evidence to suggest that greater diffusion into the prostatic fluid is achieved with other antimicrobials as compared with trimethoprim, and the infecting organisms in these studies were each susceptible to TMP-SMX in vivo. Therefore, the results probably constitute the best that can be achieved with any antimicrobial agent.

McGuire's report[61] that 42% of men with chronic bacterial prostatitis are curable with 12 weeks of TMP-SMX therapy is consistent with the Stanford experience, although the bacteriologic documentation of chronic infection was not as compelling as that in the Stanford studies. Drach has also reported on the efficacy of full-dose TMP-SMX.[71] His data are difficult to interpret, as apparent infections due to gram-positive organisms or to mixed gram-positive and gram-negative organisms were not clearly separated from infections caused by gram-negative organisms only. Nonetheless, he found that 9 (60%) of 15 isolates of gram-negative bacteria localized to the prostate were eradicated with this treatment.

Paulson observed a somewhat surprising 79% bacteriologic cure rate with 3 months of oral TMP-SMX therapy.[72] In this series, however, the incidence of apparent chronic bacterial infection of the prostate among the entire population of men referred for evaluation of prostatic symptomatology, 38%, was unexplainedly high, and the longevity of the infections was not established. It is possible, therefore, that a proportion of his patients had acute rather than chronic bacterial prostatitis.

TMP-SMX at full oral dosage is generally well tolerated during 12 weeks of administration, although 15% of patients may experience adverse side effects.[61,71]

Clinical experience with norfloxacin and ciprofloxacin is limited and recent, but existing data suggest an efficacy superior to that of trimethoprim. This is not unexpected, as both of these fluoroquinolones are lipid soluble and have broad antibacterial activities. Weidner and coworkers[73] treated 13 patients with well-documented chronic bacterial prostatitis with ciprofloxacin for 2 weeks. Bacterial localization cultures were obtained periodically for 1 year after treatment in almost all patients. Sixty-two percent of the patients had convincing bacteriologic cures. Sabbaj and coworkers[74] compared the efficacy of TMP-SMX and norfloxacin in the treatment of 33 patients with suggestive, but distressingly inconclusive, bacteriologic evidence of chronic bacterial prostatitis. Sixty-seven percent of the patients treated with TMP-SMX and 92% of those treated with norfloxacin had sterile prostatic or seminal fluid 4 to 6 weeks following treatment. In both studies discussed above, the side effects of treatment were minimal.

Apparent bacteriologic cure rates of 68% and 67% were reported by Oliveri[75] and Mobley,[76] respectively, with 28 days of full-dose oral indanyl carbenicillin therapy. Approximately 10% of patients experienced diarrhea during this treatment. In the former study, a "significant bacterial growth must have been present in EPS and/or seminal fluid specimens as well as in the $VB_3$ specimen" to be considered as evidence of bacterial infection of the prostate. This raises the possibility that all cases may not have satisfied the strict bacteriologic criteria for prostatic infection utilized by Meares and Stamey. In Mobley's study all patients were said to have sterile $VB_1$ cultures but infected EPS or seminal fluid cultures before the initiation of treatment, which is unusual for men with chronic bacterial prostatitis who are not receiving antimicrobial agents. In both clinical trials, evidence of treatment efficacy was determined by only one bacterial localization study that was performed 4 weeks after the end of treatment. Finally, among comparable patients in both studies treated with cephalexin, the bacteriologic cure rates were reported to be 22% and 40% respectively. These results are inconsistent with the anticipated efficacy of this lipid-insoluble drug.

Enthusiasm for indanyl carbenicillin in the treatment of chronic bacterial prostatitis has been appropriately summarized as follows: "Hopefully, a more thorough evaluation of the possible role of indanyl carbenicillin in the treatment of bacterial prostatitis will substantiate the optimism of preliminary observations."[3]

Paulson also reported a 70% bacteriologic cure rate among 10 patients treated with minocycline for 4 weeks.[72] Approximately 30% of patients, however, are unable to tolerate this regimen, primarily because of vestibular toxicity. Reservations about case definition in this study, that compared minocycline therapy to TMP-SMX, have been noted above. The data do indicate, however, that minocycline is not superior to TMP-SMX in the population studied.

Mobley's data suggesting that erythromycin combined with oral bicarbonate will effect a bacteriologic cure in approximately 90% of men with chronic bacterial prostatitis is astounding.[77] The bicarbonate was administered to alkalinize the urine, in an effort to enhance the antimicrobial spectrum of erythromycin against gram-negative pathogens.[78] However, the possibility that this regimen might alter the pH of prostatic fluid has not been confirmed and is conceptually unsound. However,

McGuire achieved apparent bacteriologic cures in 4 (44%) of 9 patients with a similar treatment.[79] The details of this study have not been published. Prolonged administration of erythromycin is frequently accompanied by gastrointestinal side effects.

Bacteriologic cures were recently reported in 4 men with gram-negative chronic bacterial prostatitis following combination treatment with rifampin and trimethoprim.[80] These data are intriguing, since rifampin provides a lipid-soluble base with a broad antimicrobial spectrum. Renal, hematologic, gastrointestinal, and hepatic toxicity may occur during therapy, and the optimal dosage and treatment schedule for prostatic infections have not been established.

Several anecdotal, but well-defined, cases suggest that chronic prostatic infections refractory to conventional oral antimicrobial therapy may be cured with a 1- to 2-week course of parenteral kanamycin.[1,81] Since aminoglycosides are not lipid soluble, these successes are unexpected. Further documentation of clinical efficacy is necessary before this regimen can be recommended for anything but a last-ditch attempt at nonsurgical cure.

The optimal duration of antimicrobial therapy to cure chronic bacterial infections of the prostate has not been established for any antimicrobial agent. Treatment with 12, rather than 2, weeks of full-dose TMP-SMX appears to increase the possibilities of cure.[70] On the other hand, the prospects for cure among patients who remain infected after 12 weeks of this treatment do not appear to increase if treatment is continued for an additional 12-week period.[61]

Clinical studies, in which localization cultures were obtained intermittently during 3 months of TMP-SMX therapy, indicate that patients with persistent infection at 4 weeks are usually not cured after the additional 8 weeks of treatment.[1,70] Those with sterile EPS cultures at 4 weeks may or may not be curable. Therefore, assessment of the bacteriologic response at this point in time—and treatment with an alternative agent or approach, if persistent infection is documented—constitutes a logical approach to therapeutic decision making.

**Potentially Curative Surgical Treatment.** Complete excision of the prostate and seminal vesicles predictably should constitute curative therapy for chronic bacterial prostatitis. The anticipated and potential morbidity of this procedure, however, limit its application in the treatment of this disorder.

Near-complete excision of prostatic tissue, by "radical" transurethral resection of the prostate (TURP), has been suggested as an alternative surgical approach. From a theoretical viewpoint, the efficacy of this treatment has been questioned, because the inflammation (and by inference, the site of infection) found with chronic bacterial prostatitis is confined in large part to the periphery of the prostate.[82,83] On the other hand, the incorporation of infecting bacteria into corpora amylacea within prostatic ducts,[1] and secondary infection of prostatic calculi,[84,85] may contribute to the relative inactivity of antimicrobial therapy. Removal of a large portion of this material during TURP, therefore, may enhance the possibilities of cure. Parenthetically, prostatic calculi can be visualized easily using transrectal utrasonography (Fig 7).

Meares has published the only interpretable results of extensive use of TURP.[86] During a 5-year period, he treated 10 men with well-documented infections who had failed at least 1 year of medical management. Appropriate parenteral antimicrobials were administered in the perioperative period, and all prostatic tissues were removed to the level of the true prostatic capsule. Four patients had radiographically identifiable prostatic calculi, but unsuspected calculi were encountered and removed in 3 other patients. The organism localized to the prostate preoperatively was recovered from 4 of 5 stone specimens that were cultured.

The postoperative morbidity was reported to parallel that seen in patients without prostatic infection. After surgery, the men were treated with an appropriate antimicrobial agent at full oral dosage for 6 to 8 weeks. Bacteriologic follow-up ranged from 6 to 66 (mean 30) months. All of the patients were thought to be cured, although two required a second TURP to remove residual infected tissues.

Meares emphasizes that radical TURP is

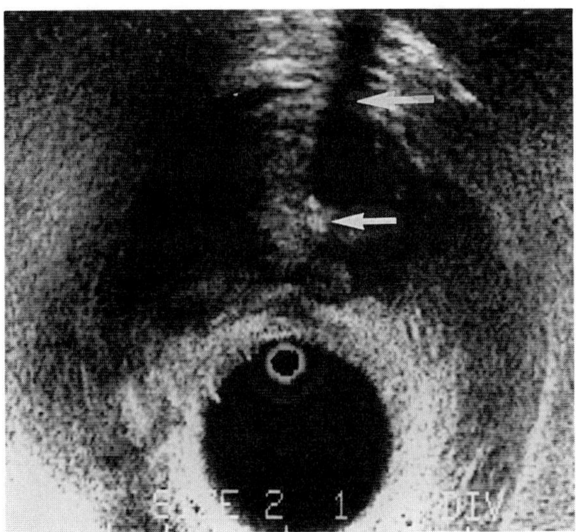

**Fig 7.** Transrectal ultrasonography in patient with prostatic calculi; lower arrow shows hyperechoic prostatic calculi and upper arrow shows posterior acoustic attenuation. [From Fowler JE Jr, *Urinary Tract Infection and Inflammation* (Chicago: Year Book Medical Publishers; 1989), with permission.]

not recommended for most patients with medically incurable chronic bacterial prostatitis, and is not appropriate for the treatment of inflammatory disorders of the prostate that are not of microbial etiology.

**Intraprostatic Antimicrobial Injection.** In an effort to obtain antimicrobial concentrations in the parenchyma and ducts of the prostate that greatly exceed those possible with systemic drug administration, direct intraprostatic injection of antimicrobial agents has been employed by a group from Belgium.[87] Twenty-nine patients with well-defined chronic bacterial prostatitis, who remained infected after a 3-week course of TMP-SMX, were injected with thiamphenicol (2.0 g) diluted in 20 mL saline on from one to three occasions. Thiamphenicol, which exists as a base, was chosen because of its broad antibacterial spectrum, lipid solubility and low protein binding. Nineteen patients (66%) had sterile EPS cultures at 1 and 6 months after treatment.

Recently, the treatment of bacterial prostatitis by injection of an aminoglycoside has been reported.[88] The injections were done with the guidance of transrectal ultrasonography, and preferentially targeted to regions thought to represent areas of infection. Fifty-nine percent of 51 patients were apparently cured. However, the duration of symptomatology before treatment ranged from 2 to 16 weeks only, and some may have had acute rather than chronic infections. Moreover, none had received conventional antimicrobial therapy before the injection procedure.

**Suppressive Antimicrobial Therapy.** Suppressive antimicrobial therapy is targeted to the bacteria which infect the urine. As such, the achievable concentration of an antimicrobial agent in the urine—rather than in the prostatic fluid—is of therapeutic importance. Most antibiotics are physiologically concentrated in urine, achieving levels 50 to 100 times greater than in serum. Since the susceptibility of most gram-negative bacteria to an antimicrobial agent is directly related to the concentration of the drug, it follows that a variety of agents that are inappropriate for the treatment of invasive infections may be effective for suppressive therapy. Standard antibiotic susceptibility testing, however, will often underestimate the number of potentially useful drugs for suppressive therapy because susceptibility is tested against drug levels achieved in the serum. For this reason, if an appropriate antimicrobial agent cannot be identified with conventional susceptibility assays, a quantitative test should be requested to determine the precise minimum inhibitory concentration (MIC) for the drugs of interest. Not infrequently, quantitative susceptibility testing will identify apparently ineffective oral agents with

MICs for the infecting organism that are five to ten times lower than the urinary concentration achieved.

Information concerning the relative efficacy of antimicrobials for suppressive therapy are not available. Logic dictates that agents employed for this purpose must be available in an oral form, and must be well tolerated during prolonged periods and active against the infecting organism at concentrations achievable in the urine. Most workers recommend low-dose trimethoprim (50 mg qd), TMP-SMX (40–200 mg qd), or nitrofurantoin (50 or 100 mg qd). A large body of data from using these agents for prophylaxis against frequent urinary reinfection in females suggests that indefinite treatment is generally well tolerated.[1] A bedtime regimen improves patient compliance, and may also enhance efficacy, since voiding during the night is less frequent than during the day, allowing the antibiotic to remain in the bladder urine for longer periods.

Tetracycline is also well tolerated at low doses over prolonged periods and may be an exceedingly useful agent in the treatment of infections caused by *Pseudomonas*.[1] Treatment with indanyl carbenicillin (500 mg daily) may be effective for infections due to highly resistant Enterobacteriaceae or *Pseudomonas*, but data concerning patient tolerance during long-term administration are not available. Experiences with low-dose norfloxacin and ciprofloxacin for suppressive treatment have not been reported, but efficacy would be expected to be excellent.

## Nonbacterial Prostatitis

Predictably effective treatments for nonbacterial prostatitis are not available. Further, since the condition is, in all likelihood, a manifestation of a variety of different inflammatory processes, and since the nature of these processes is either unknown or difficult to document in clinical practice, the prospects for meaningful treatment guidelines are remote. The chronic nature and magnitude of the individual patient's symptoms are at present the best guide to therapeutic recommendations.

Antimicrobial therapy for 2 weeks with tetracycline, minocycline, or doxycycline (which should be effective against *C trachomatis* and *U urealyticum*) is a reasonable initial approach. Erythromycin and TMP-SMX are also active against these organisms. Several reports have documented the value of these treatments in unselected populations of men with chronic prostatitis, but infectious causes for the disorders were not established.[48,49] Tetracycline therapy is recommended for all patients with clinical findings suggestive of urethritis.

Chronic antimicrobial therapy is discouraged, as evidence for an infectious cause for nonbacterial prostatitis is limited at best, the possibly erroneous concept of chronic infection is adapted by the patient, and the responsible physician may be vulnerable if serious toxicity develops. Hot sitz baths, prostatic massage, a trial of diazepam,[27] or trials of anticholinergic or anti-inflammatory agents[3] may occasionally prove beneficial. Use of oral zinc sulfate (160–140 mg qd) has been advocated, but data concerning efficacy are not available.[89]

Nonbacterial prostatitis cannot always be distinguished from prostatodynia, and both disorders may have a common etiology that leads to varying degrees of inflammation. Treatments for prostatodynia that are directed against neuromuscular disorders of the bladder outlet and external sphincter should also be considered in the management of patients with nonbacterial prostatitis.

## Prostatodynia

An important component of management of the patient with prostatodynia involves the elimination of extraprostatic causes for the symptomatology. Interstitial cystitis and carcinoma in situ of the urinary bladder—which may be indistinguishable from prostatodynia on the basis of history, physical examination, and prostatic fluid analyses—should be ruled out with cystoscopy, bladder biopsy, and cytologic examination of the urine.[90] Osteitis pubis may also masquerade as prostatodynia.[91]

Urodynamic investigations may be rewarding if voiding disturbances constitute a major component of the symptomatology. However, Meares is sufficiently confident that prostatodynia is so frequently accompanied by spasm of the bladder neck or external sphincter that he recommends therapeutic intervention without confirmatory urodynamic or fluoroscopic findings.

Contraction of the smooth muscle of the bladder outlet and external sphincter is inhibited by pharmacologic blockade of α-adrenergic receptors. The α-blocking agent prazosin (Minipress) provides symptomatic relief in some patients.[40] It should be administered initially at a dose of 1 mg daily for a period of 7 days. A bedtime regimen reduces the incidence of postural hypotension. The dose is increased to 1 mg bid during the following 2 weeks, and then to 2 mg bid. Responsive patients are treated at this dosage for a total of 6 months. Most patients who benefit, however, develop recurrent symptoms when the drug is discontinued.

Incision of the bladder neck may also be of benefit in selected patients with functional disturbances at this site. However, use of this procedure should be reserved for those who do not respond to medical management, as it usually leads to retrograde ejaculation and infertility.

Diazepam (2–5 mg tid) may help patients with suspected tension myalgia of the pelvic floor, as well as those with bladder neck or urethral spasm who do not respond completely to prazosin.[40] As with nonbacterial prostatitis, hot sitz baths and anti-inflammatory and anticholingeric agents may occasionally provide symptomatic relief.

Symptomatic improvement with α-difluoromethylornithine (α-DFMO), an inhibitor of polyamine biosynthesis, has also been reported.[92] Clinical experience with this agent in the treatment of benign disorders, however, is limited, and substantial gastrointestinal side effects have been observed. Sodium pentosanpolysulfate (Elmiron) is of no value in the treatment of prostatodynia.[93]

Counseling by trained psychologists or psychiatrists may be of tremendous benefit to patients who appear emotionally labile, who have had thorough but unrevealing urologic evaluations, and who are refractory to conventional therapy. However, the clinician must recognize that some degree of emotional disturbance is an inevitable consequence of chronic symptomatology caused by true urologic disorders that remain undefined despite repeated investigations.

For both nonbacterial prostatitis and prostatodynia, common sense, compassion, and concern for the patient's frustrations are critical ingredients for successful management. Candid conversations with the patient and, if appropriate, his wife, concerning the nature of the condition—and reassurance that the symptoms are not related to cancer, infertility, impotence, or known sexually transmissible disorders—are generally rewarding.

### Granulomatous Prostatitis

Granulomatous lesions of the prostate are identified histologically in approximately 1% of tissue specimens obtained by biopsy or by partial prostatectomy for the treatment of bladder outlet obstruction.[94,95] The process may be focal or extensive, and usually results from prostatic infection by gram-negative bacilli and/or TURP (Table 3). Collectively, infectious disorders commonly associated with granuloma formation (such as tuberculosis or blastomycosis) and systemic granulomatous diseases (such as Wegener's granulomatosis, the Churg-Strauss syndrome or sarcoidosis) are responsible for a small minority of cases. Granulomas with a prominent eosinophilic infiltrate or associated with allergic conditions and peripheral eosinophilia are exceedingly rare.

The granulomatous inflammation following bacterial prostatitis or TURP is thought to be caused by disruption of the prostatic ducts and extravasation of prostatic secretions. Tissue trauma and cautery may also be an initiating factor. Granulomas are rarely seen in the initial tissue specimen when granulomatous prostatitis follows TURP.

The granulomas following bacterial prostatitis and TURP are characterized by the presence of epithelioid and multinucleated histiocytes, lymphocytes, and plasma cells.[34] Those resulting from TURP may

**TABLE 3. Causes of Granulomatous Prostatitis**

| | Epstein and Hutchins[94] (1974) | | Stillwell et al[95] (1987) | |
|---|---|---|---|---|
| Cause | No. of Patients | (%) | No. of Patients | (%) |
| Bacterial infection | 33 | 55 | 138 | 69 |
| TURP or biopsy | 17 | 28 | 49 | 25* |
| Tuberculosis | 9 | 15 | 7 | 4** |
| Systematic granulomatous | 1 | 2 | 6 | 3 |

* Approximately 50% had recent urinary tract infection.
** Includes one patient with blastomycosis.
TURP = transurethral resection of the prostate.
(From Fowler JE Jr. *Urinary Tract Infection and Inflammation.* Chicago: Year Book Medical Publishers; 1989, with permission.)

also resemble rheumatoid nodules, with epithelioid histiocytes surrounding an area of fibrinoid necrosis.

Most patients with granulomatous prostatitis have irritative or obstructive voiding symptoms. Concurrent bacteriuria may also contribute to the symptomatology. In a report addressing the natural history of granulomatous prostatitis, 59% of patients (n = 200) had palpable induration or irregularity of the prostate suggestive of malignancy.[95] One hundred and twenty patients, without specific underlying etiologies for the disorder, were treated with antimicrobials or nonspecific therapy or were observed only. When present, irritative voiding symptoms usually resolved within a few months. However, palpable prostatic abnormalities persisted for more than 2 years in about 50% of the cases.

Prostatic cancer develops in <10% of patients with granulomatous prostatitis.[95] It is important to note that the tumors are almost always manifested locally by changes in preexisting induration or by the appearance of new abnormal findings. Although granulomatous prostatitis does not lead to prostatic malignancy, it mimics localized prostatic cancer. Biopsy is usually required to differentiate the two diseases with absolute certainty.

## INFECTIONS OF THE SEMINAL VESICLES

Although the focus of this chapter has been on prostatitis, the role of seminal vesicle infection in the pathogenesis of chronic bacterial prostatitis deserves comment. Clinically identifiable infections of the seminal vesicles are rarely seen in the absence of chronic bacterial prostatitis or epididymitis. The seminal vesicles are usually not palpable during rectal examination, and infection should be suspected if there is induration or enlargement. Isolated bacterial infection cannot be proved by culture, because prostatic secretions are invariably admixed with fluid expressed from the seminal vesicles. However, irregularity or dilatation of the lumen suggesting inflammation or infection has been demonstrated with seminal vesiculography in some patients with chronic bacterial prostatitis.[96] The seminal vesicles are clearly delineated by magnetic resonance imaging, and experience with this modality may help to clarify the incidence of seminal-vesical involvement in patients with bacterial infection at other sites in the male reproductive system.

## REFERENCES

1. Stamey TA. *Pathogenesis and Treatment of Urinary Tract Infections*. Baltimore: Williams & Wilkins; 1980.
2. Drach GW, Meares EM Jr, Fair WR, et al. Classification of benign disease associated with prostatic pain: prostatitis or prostatodynia? *J Urol.* 1978;120:266.

3. Meares EM Jr. Prostatitis syndromes: new perspectives about old woes. *J Urol.* 1980;123:141–147.
4. Brunner H, Weidner W, Schiefer H-G. Studies on the role of *Ureaplasma urealyticum* and *Mycoplasma hominis* in prostatitis. *J Infec Dis.* 1983;147:807–813.
5. Fair WR, Couch J, Wehner N. Prostatic antibacterial factor. Identity and significance. *Urology.* 1976;7:169–177.
6. Fair WR, Wehner N. Antibacterial action of spermine: effect on urinary tract pathogens. *Appl Microbiol.* 1971;21:6–8.
7. Fowler JE Jr, Mariano M. Immunologic response of the prostate to bacteriuria and bacterial prostatitis. II. Antigen specific immunoglobulin in prostatic fluid. *J Urol.* 1982;128:165–170.
8. Shortliffe LMD, Wehner N, Stamey TA. Use of a solid-phase radioimmunoassay and formalin-fixed whole bacterial antigen in the detection of antigen-specific immunoglobulin in prostatic fluid. *J Clin Invest.* 1981;67:790–799.
9. Fowler JE Jr, Mariano M. Longitudinal studies of prostatic fluid immunoglobulin in men with bacterial prostatitis. *J Urol.* 1984;131:363–369.
10. Drach GW. Problems in diagnosis of bacterial prostatitis: gram-negative, gram-positive and mixed infection. *J Urol.* 1974;111:630–636.
11. Fritjofsson A, Kihl B, Danielsson D. Chronic prostato-vesiculitis: incidence and significance of bacterial findings. *Scand J Urol Nephrol.* 1973;8:173–178.
12. Gordon HL, Miller DH, Rawls WE. Viral studies in patients with non-specific prostatourethritis. *J Urol.* 1972;108:299–300.
13. Mardh PA, Colleen S. Search for urogenital tract infections in patients with symptoms of prostatitis. *Scand J Urol Nephrol.* 1975;9:8–16.
14. Meares EM Jr. Bacterial prostatitis vs. "prostatosis": a clinical and bacteriological study. *JAMA.* 1973;224:1372–1375.
15. Nielson ML, Justesen J. Studies on the pathology of prostatitis: a search for prostatic infections with obligate anaerobes in patients with chronic prostatitis and chronic urethritis. *Scand J Urol Nephrol.* 1974;8:1–6.
16. Nielson ML, Vestergaard BF. Virological investigations in chronic prostatitis. *J Urol.* 1973;109:1023–1025.
17. Carson CC, McGraw VD, Zwadyk P. Bacterial prostatitis caused by *Staphylococcus saprophyticus. Urology.* 1982;19:6,576–578.
18. Kauffman CA, Hertz CS, Sheagren JN. *Staphylococcus saprophyticus:* role in urinary tract infections in men. *J Urol.* 1983;130:493–494.
19. Holmes KK, Handsfield HH, Wang SP, et al. Etiology of nongonococcal urethritis. *N Engl J Med.* 1975;292:1199–1205.
20. Oriel JD, Reeve P, Powis P, et al. Chlamydial infection: isolation of *Chlamydia* from patients with nonspecific genital infection. *Br J Vener Dis.* 1972;48:429–432.
21. Ulstein M, Capell P, Holmes KK, et al. Nonsymptomatic genital tract infection and male infertility. In: Hafez ESE, ed. *Human Semen and Fertility Regulation in Men.* St. Louis: CV Mosby; 1976:355.
22. Bruce AW, Chadwick P, Willet WS, et al. The role of chlamydiae in genitourinary disease. *J Urol.* 1981;126:625–629.
23. Taylor-Robinson D. The role of chlamydiae in genitourinary disease. *J Urol.* 1982;128:156. Letter.
24. Mardh PA, Colleen S, Holmquist B. Chlamydia in chronic prostatitis. *Br Med J.* 1972;4:361.
25. Mardh PA, Ripa KT, Colleen S, et al. Role of *Chlamydia trachomatis* in non-acute prostatitis. *Br J Vener Dis.* 1978;54:330–334.
26. Berger RE. Nongonococcal urethritis and related syndromes. *Monogr Urol.* 1982;3:4,97–125.
27. Thin RN, Simmons PD. Chronic bacterial and nonbacterial prostatitis. *Br J Urol.* 1983;55:513–518.
28. Shortliffe LMD, Elliott KM, Sellers RG, et al. Measurement of chlamydial and ureaplasmal antibodies in serum and prostatic fluid of men with nonbacterial prostatitis. In: *Abstracts of Annual Meeting of American Urological Association.* 1985;276A.
29. Doble A, Thomas BJ, Walker MM, et al. The role of *Chlamydia trachomatis* in chronic abacterial prostatitis: a study using ultrasound guided biopsy. *J Urol.* 1989;141:332–333.
30. Bowie WF, Wang SP, Alexander ER, et al. Etiology of nongonococcal urethritis: evidence for *Chlamydia trachomatis* and *Ureaplasma urealyticum. J Clin Invest.* 1977;59:735–742.
31. Berger RE, Krieger JN, Kessler D, et al. Case-control study of men with suspected chronic idiopathic prostatitis. *J Urol.* 1989;141:328–331.
32. Mathur S, Baker ER, Williamson HD, et al. Clinical significance of sperm antibodies in infertility. *Fertil Steril.* 1981;36:486–495.
33. Anderson RU, Ma SH. Autoimmune studies in abacterial prostatitis. In: *Abstracts of Annual Meeting of American Urological Association.* 1982:149.
34. Towfighi J, Sadeghee S, Wheeler JE, et al. Granulomatous prostatitis with emphasis on the eosinophilic variety. *Am J Clin Pathol.* 1972;58:630–641.
35. Kirby D, Lowe M, Bultitude MI, et al. Intraprostatic urinary reflux: an etiological factor in abacterial prostatitis. *J Urol.* 1982;54:729–731.
36. Segura JW, Opitz JL, Greene LF. Prostatosis, prostatitis or pelvic floor tension myalgia? *J Urol.* 1979;122:168–169.
37. Siroky MB, Goldstein I, Krane RJ. Functional voiding disorders in men. *J Urol.* 1981;126:200–204.
38. Webster GD, Lockhart JL, Older RA. The evaluation of bladder neck dysfunction. *J Urol.* 1980;123:196–198.
39. Barbalias GA, Meares EM Jr, Sant GR. Pros-

tatodynia: clinical and urodynamic characteristics. *J Urol.* 1983;130:514–517.

40. Meares EM Jr. Prostatodynia: clinical findings and rationale for treatment. In: Weidner W, Brunner H, Krause W, Rothauge CF, eds. *Therapy of Prostatitis.* Munchen, Germany: W Zucksschwerdt Verlag Gmbh; 1986:207–212.
41. Hellstrom WJG, Schmidt RA, Lue TF, et al. Neuromuscular dysfunction in nonbacterial prostatitis. *Urology.* 1974;30:183–187.
42. Rosenbloom D. Chronic prostatitis—a psychosexual approach. *Calif Med.* 1955;82:454–457.
43. Keltikangas-Jarvinen L, Ruokalainen J, Lehtonen T. Personality pathology underlying chronic prostatitis. *Psychother Psychosom.* 1982;37:37–95.
44. Nilsson JK, Colleen S, Mardh PA. Relationship between psychological and laboratory findings in patients with symptoms of non-acute prostatitis. In: Danielsson D, Juhlin L, Mardh PA, eds. *Genital Infections and Their Complications.* Stockholm, Sweden: Almquist and Wiksell; 1975;133–146.
45. Kunin CM, Zacha E, Paquin AJ. Urinary tract infections in school children: I. prevalence of bacteriuria and associated urologic findings. *N Engl J Med.* 1962;266:1287–1296.
46. Freedman LR, Phair JP, Seki M, et al. The epidemiology of urinary tract infections in Hiroshima. *Yale J Biol Med.* 1965;37:262–282.
47. Gleckman R, Crowley M, Natsios GA. Therapy of recurrent invasive urinary tract infections of men. *N Engl J Med.* 1979;301:878–880.
48. Brannan W. Treatment of chronic prostatitis. *Urology.* 1975;5:626–631.
49. Thin RN, Simmons PD. Review of results of four regimens for treatment of chronic non-bacterial prostatitis. *Br J Urol.* 1983;55:519–521.
50. Anderson RU, Weller C. Prostatic secretion leukocyte studies in non-bacterial prostatitis (prostatosis). *J Urol.* 1979;121:292–294.
51. Blacklock NJ. Some observations on prostatitis. In: Williams DC, Briggs MH, Stanford M, eds. *Advances in the Study of the Prostate.* London: William Heinemann Medical Books, Ltd; 1969:37–55.
52. Schaeffer AJ, Wendel EF, Dunn JK, et al. Prevalence and significance of prostatic inflammation. *J Urol.* 1981;125:215–219.
53. Jameson RM. Sexual activity and the variations of the white cell content of the prostatic secretion. *Invest Urol.* 1967;5:297–302.
54. Schaeffer AJ, Chmiel JS, Grayhack JS. Natural history of prostatic inflammation. In: *Abstracts of Annual Meeting of American Urological Association.* 1985:207A.
55. O'Shaughnessy EJ, Parrino PS, White JD. Chronic prostatitis: fact or fiction. *JAMA.* 1956;160:540.
56. Meares EM Jr, Stamey TA. Bacteriologic localization patterns in bacterial prostatitis and urethritis. *Invest Urol.* 1968;5:492–518.
57. Fowler JE Jr, Kessler R. Genital tract infection. In: Lipschultz LI, Howards SS, eds. *Infertility in the Male.* New York: Churchill Livingstone; 1983:283–298.
58. Fowler JE Jr, Mariano M. Difficulties in quantitating the contribution of urethral bacteria to prostatic fluid and seminal fluid cultures. *J Urol.* 1984;132:471–473.
59. Jimenez-Cruz JF, Ferrer MM, Almagro AA, et al. Prostatitis: are the gram-positive organisms pathogenic? *Eur Urol.* 1984;10:311–314.
60. Mobley DF. Semen cultures in the diagnosis of bacterial prostatitis. *J Urol.* 1975;114:83–85.
61. McGuire EJ, Lytton B. Bacterial prostatitis: treatment with trimethoprim-sulfamethoxazole. *Urology.* 1976;7:499–500.
62. Fowler JE Jr. Practical approach to bacteriologic investigation of chronic prostatitis. *Urology.* 1985;26:17–20.
63. Kohnen PW, Drach GW. Patterns of inflammation in prostatic hyperplasia: a histologic and bacteriologic study. *J Urol.* 1979;121:755–760.
64. Meares EM Jr. Serum antibody titers in treatment with trimethoprim-sulfamethoxazole for chronic prostatitis. *Urology.* 1978;11:142–146.
65. Wishnow KI, Wehner N, Stamey TA. The diagnostic value of the immunologic response in bacterial and non-bacterial prostatitis. *J Urol.* 1982;127:689–694.
66. Fowler JE Jr, Mariano M. Bacterial infection and male infertility: absence of immunoglobulin A with specificity for common *Escherichia coli* O-serotypes in seminal fluid of infertile men. *J Urol.* 1983;130:171–174.
67. Richards D, Gowland M, Brooman P, et al. Computed tomography and transrectal ultrasound in the diagnosis of prostatic disease—a comparative study. *Br J Urol.* 1983;55:726–732.
68. Lee F Jr, Lee F, Solomon H, et al. Sonographic demonstration of prostatic abscess. *J Ultrasound Med.* 1986;5:101–102.
69. Meares EM Jr. Observations on activity of trimethoprim-sulfamethoxazole in the prostate. *J Infect Dis.* 1973;129(suppl):S679–685.
70. Meares EM Jr. Long-term therapy of chronic bacterial prostatitis and trimethoprim-sulfamethoxazole. *Can Med Assoc J.* 1975; 112(suppl):22s–25s.
71. Drach GW. Trimethoprim/sulfamethoxazole therapy of chronic bacterial prostatitis. *J Urol.* 1974;111:636–639.
72. Paulson DF, deVere White R. Trimethoprim-sulfamethoxazole and minocycline-hydrochloride in the treatment of culture-proved bacterial prostatitis. *J Urol.* 1978;120:184–185.
73. Weidner W, Schiefer HG, Dalhoff A. Treatment of chronic bacterial prostatitis with ciprofloxacin. *Am J Med.* 1987;82(suppl 4A):280–283.
74. Sabbaj J, Hoagland VL, Cook T. Norfloxacin versus co-trimoxazole in the treatment of recurring urinary tract infections in men. *Scand J Infect Dis.* 1986;48(suppl):48–53.

75. Oliveri RA, Sachs RM, Caste PG. Clinical experience with geocillin in the treatment of bacterial prostatitis. *Curr Ther Res.* 1979;25:415–421.
76. Mobley DF. Bacterial prostatitis: treatment with carbenicillin indanyl sodium. *Invest Urol.* 1981;19:31–33.
77. Mobley DF. Erythromycin plus sodium bicarbonate in chronic bacterial prostatitis. *Urology.* 1974;3:60–62.
78. Sabath LD, Gerstein DA, Loder FB, et al. Excretion of erthromycin and its enhanced activity in urine against gram-negative bacilli with alkalinization. *J Lab Clin Med.* 1968;72:916–923.
79. McGuire E. Theoretical basis for treatment of prostatitis. *Urology.* 1984;24:10–11.
80. Gimarellou H, Kosmidis J, Leonidas M, et al. A study of the effectiveness of rifaprim in chronic prostatitis caused mainly by *Staphylococcus aureus. J Urol.* 1982;128:321–324.
81. Pfau A, Sacks T. Chronic bacterial prostatitis: new therapeutic aspects. *Br J Urol.* 1976; 48:245–253.
82. Blacklock NJ. Anatomical factors in prostatitis. *Br J Urol.* 1974;46:47–54.
83. McNeal JE. Regional morphology and pathology of the prostate. *Am J Clin Pathol.* 1968;49:347–357.
84. Eykyn S, Bultitude ME, Mayo ME, et al. Prostatic calculi as a source of recurrent bacteriuria in the male. *Br J Urol.* 1974;46:527–532.
85. Meares EM Jr. Infection with stones of the prostate gland: laboratory diagnosis and clinical management. *Urology.* 1974;4:560–566.
86. Meares EM Jr. Chronic bacterial prostatitis: Role of transurethral prostatectomy (TURP) in therapy. In: Weidner W, Brunner H, Krause W, Rothauge CF, eds. *Therapy of Prostatitis.* Munchen, Germany: W Zucksschwerdt Verlag Gmbh; 1986:193–197.
87. Plomp TA, Baert L, Maes RA. Treatment of recurrent chronic bacterial prostatitis by local injection of thiamphenicol into prostate. *Urology.* 1980;15:542–547.
88. Jimenez-Cruz JF, Tormo FB, Gomez JG. Treatment of chronic prostatitis: intraprostatic antibiotic injections under echography control. *J Urol.* 1988;139:967–970.
89. Marmar JL, Katz S, Praiss DE, et al. Semen zinc levels in infertile and postvasectomy patients and patients with prostatitis. *Fertil Steril.* 1975;26:1057–1063.
90. Messing EM, Stamey TA. Interstitial cystitis: diagnosis, pathology, and treatment. *Urology.* 1978;12:381–392.
91. Buck AC, Crean DM, Jenkins IL. Osteitis pubis as a mimic of prostatic pain. *Br J Urol.* 1982;54:741–744.
92. Dunzendorfer U. A-Difluoromethylornithine (aDFMO) and phenoxybenzamine hydrochloride in the treatment of chronic non-suppurative prostatitis. *Arzneimittelforschung.* 1981;31:382–385.
93. Wedren H. Effects of sodium pentosanpolysulphate on symptoms related to chronic non-bacterial prostatitis. A double-blind randomized study. *Scan J Urol Nephrol.* 1987;21:81–88.
94. Epstein JI, Hutchins GM. Granulomatous prostatitis: distinction among allergic, non-specific, and posttransurethral resection lesions. *Human Pathol.* 1984;15:818–825.
95. Stillwell TJ, Engen DE, Farrow GM. The clinical spectrum of granulomatous prostatitis: a report of 200 cases. *J Urol.* 1987;138:320–323.
96. Baert L, Leonard A, D'Hoedt M, et al. Seminal vesiculography in chronic bacterial prostatitis. *J Urol.* 1986;136:844–845.

# 10

# Sexually Transmitted Diseases

*David M. Pfeffer*

Over the last 20 years, shifts in attitudes regarding human sexuality have resulted in an increase in the incidence of sexually transmitted diseases (STDs). These diseases, each caused by a different organism and manifested by a variety of symptoms, have received increased public attention of late, in part because of the devastating effects of the acquired immunodeficiency syndrome (AIDS). The loss of inhibitions and the sexual "freedom" which many experienced during the 1960s and 1970s has now been tempered by the fear of contracting one of these diseases.

A concerted effort has been put forward by the U.S. Public Health Service—and notably by C. Everett Koop, MD, during his recent tenure as Surgeon General of the United States—to make individuals aware of the dangers of engaging in unprotected sex. It is hoped that such educational efforts, which in the past were hampered by social mores, will lead to more careful sexual practices by the individual. This, along with early detection, treatment, and contact tracing by local health departments, should begin to result in a reduction in the incidence of these diseases.

Medical professionals have made major strides toward treating patients with STDs in a nonjudgmental manner. Historically, such a manner has not always been taken, in part because of a lack of understanding regarding the natural history of these diseases and in part because effective treatment was unavailable. A significant stigma is still associated with sexually transmitted infections, and labels continue to be placed on those afflicted. To continue this progress, we as practitioners must rise to the occasion and care for infected individuals, not as criminals or deviants, but as sick patients in need of treatment.

## HISTORICAL PERSPECTIVE

STDs were documented by the ancients. Most of the early literature discussed syphilis and gonorrhea collectively, as the diseases were not recognized as separate entities until the early 1800s. Epidemics of venereal diseases occurred throughout the European continent during Medieval times; one epidemic of syphilis, which broke out shortly after Columbus returned from the New World, led to the belief that the disease was originally spread by American Indians. However, many references to STDs were documented in European literature prior to the Columbian expeditions, and this argument of the New World origin of syphilis has since been refuted (Figs 1–3).[1,2]

Philippe Ricord is credited with establishing that gonorrhea and syphilis are two separate diseases.[3] Ricord also clearly identified the three stages of syphilis in his 1838 treatise on venereal disease (Fig 4).[3]

The association between the spread of STDs and prostitution has long been recognized. In fact, the lack of understanding regarding the natural history of these dis-

1 4 8 4

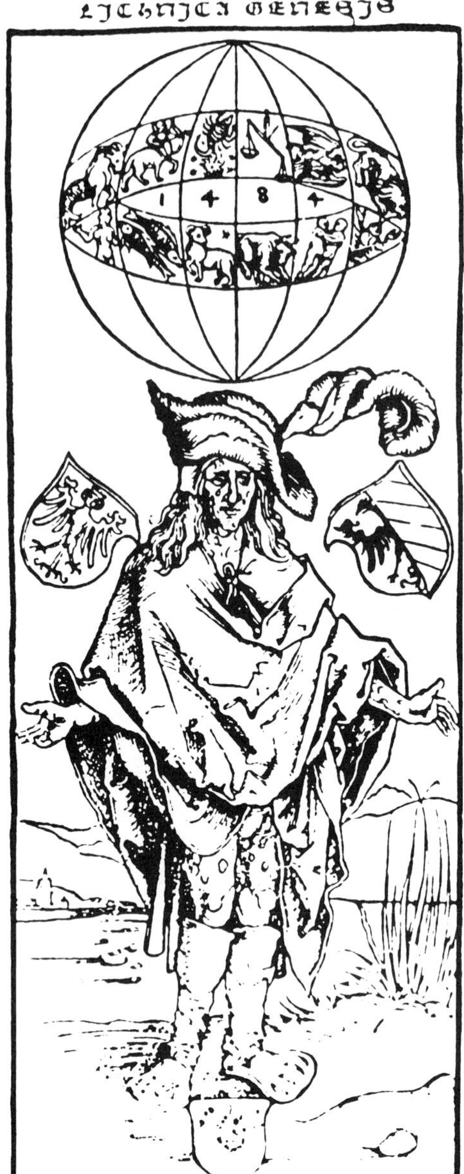

**Fig 1.** Woodcut of syphilitic from 1496 by Albert Dürer. [From Pusey W, *The History and Epidemiology of Syphilis* (Springfield, IL: Charles Thomas; 1933), with permission.]

POVR VN
PLAISIR MIL
DOVLEVR
IL SVELA
VEROLLE
FOLIE

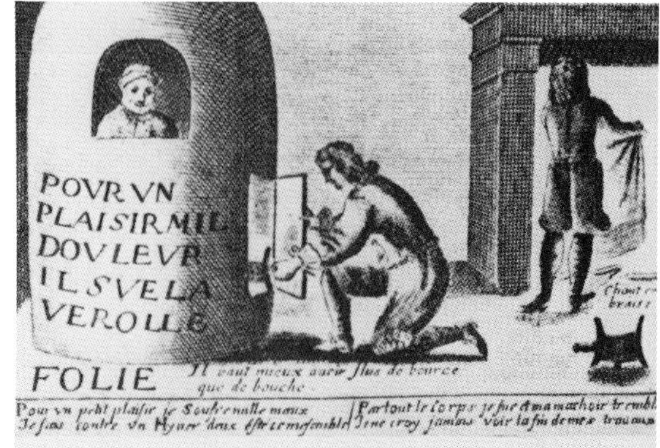

**Fig 2.** Fumigation (sweating treatment of syphilis) from the collection of engravings by Jacques Laniet of famous proverbs (Paris 1659–1663). The translation at the bottom of the woodcut reads as follows:

For one small pleasure I suffer
a thousand misfortunes
I exchange one winter for two
miserable summers
I sweat all over my body
and my jaw trembles
I do not believe I will
ever see the end of my
troubles

[From Pusey W, *The History and Epidemiology of Syphilis* (Springfield, IL: Charles Thomas; 1933), with permission.]

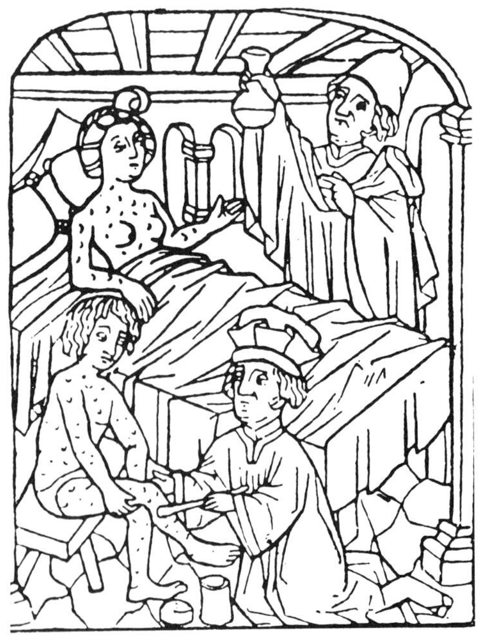

**Fig 3.** Title page from Bartholomew Steber's *Syphilis,* printed in 1497 or 1498; probably the earliest illustration of syphilis. [From Pusey W, *The History and Epidemiology of Syphilis* (Springfield, IL: Charles Thomas; 1933), with permission.]

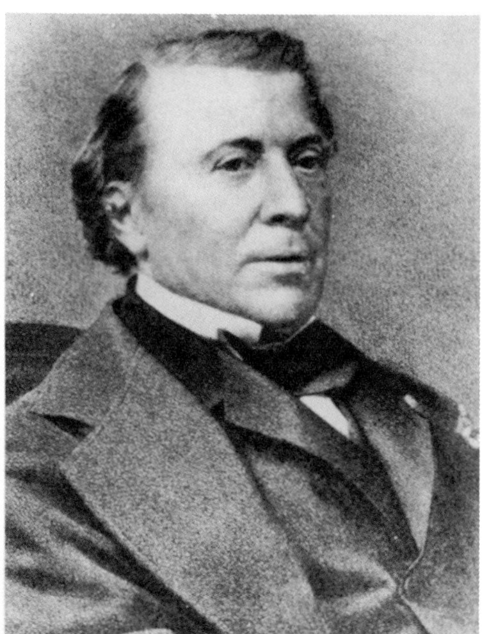

**Fig 4.** Philippe Ricord, who established the separateness of syphilis and gonorrhea. [From Pusey W, *The History and Epidemiology of Syphilis* (Springfield, IL: Charles Thomas; 1933), with permission.]

eases, as well as ineffectual treatment options, led to the examination and confinement of infected prostitutes in Europe.[4] A similar law was enacted in the U.S. city of St. Louis in 1870[5]; this law was short-lived, however, after it became apparent that the spread of STDs was not solely dependent on prostitutes.

At the turn of the century, purity crusades—organized by the "Social Hygiene Movement"—were the dominant forces behind the control of venereal diseases.[6] This movement was endorsed by lay persons as well as public health and medical personnel, and its purpose was to prevent the spread of STDs through legislative changes and education. While the movement was somewhat successful, the lack of effective treatment protocols combined with a puritanical closed-mindedness regarding sexual matters hampered any major progress.

The First International Conference on the Prevention and Treatment of Syphilis was held in Brussels in September 1899.[7] It was not until World War I, however, and the concomitant spread of STDs throughout the troops, that worldwide leaders demonstrated significant concern regarding STDs. The cost to care for infected soldiers was enormous. From the start of the war in 1914 to the summer of 1917, there were an estimated 1 million cases of syphilis and gonorrhea in France alone. In the United States, venereal disease constituted the most frequent reason for rejection of draftees: 938,232 men were rejected for military service during 1917 and 1918.[7] During the war, soldiers from the United States were educated about the perils of STDs and how to avoid them. In addition, steps were taken by the government to provide more funding for research and administration of state treatment programs through the Chamberlain-Kahn Act. In 1918, the Venereal Disease Division was created within the U.S. Public Health Service. Most states also established independent means for reporting STDs.

After World War I, the U.S. government sharply curtailed the funds available to diagnosis and treatment clinics, in part because syphilis and gonorrhea no longer posed a threat to America's military strength.

The next surge of experimentation and research was begun under Thomas Parran, MD, who became Surgeon General of the U.S. Public Health Service in 1936.[7,8,9] Parran did much to correct the misinformation regarding these diseases that was circulating at the time.

One such experiment studied the incidence and the feasibility of treatment of syphilis in the black population in the South.[10] Initial results of the study demonstrated that the prevalence of the disease among the black population was much higher than expected. This was not thought to be due to an inherent racial susceptibility, but rather to the disinclination of local physicians to treat black syphilitics and to economic factors.

The study, originally privately funded, was taken over in 1932 by the U.S. Public Health Service. The U.S. Public Health Service, in turn, changed the study into a human experiment in which 400 syphilitic black men in Macon County, Alabama, were deliberately denied any treatment in order to determine the natural course of syphilis. This study, known as the Tuskagee Study, informed these men that they were ill and promised free care and treatment. Medical treatment, however, was summarily denied despite the later development of effective antitreponemals. Men in the study were followed until their deaths, at which time an autopsy was performed. It was not until 1972, when the press and the American public became aware of this project, that it finally came to a close. Remarkably, 74 of the test subjects were still alive, although many more had succumbed to the ravages of advanced syphilis (Fig 5). An excellent account of the experiment and the individuals behind it is given by Jones in *Bad Blood,* the nickname given to syphilis among black persons in the South.[11,12]

Perhaps the major turning point in the battle against STDs was the discovery and the subsequent widespread availability of penicillin in the early 1940s. Penicillin therapy, at the time effective against both syphilis and gonorrhea, replaced the therapeutic use of arsenic and eliminated the need for inpatient care. The advent of powerful antimicrobial drugs, as well as the change in attitude of health care professionals over the last few decades has enabled the individual afflicted with an STD to now come forward for treatment without fear of being shamed or embarrassed.

## EPIDEMIOLOGY

Several important issues must be considered when examining the data concerning the incidence of STDs. First and foremost is that not all STDs need be reported to the local or state health departments. Of those that are, many cases may be incompletely reported by the health care professional involved. As recently as 20 years ago, genital herpes and condyloma acuminata were virtually unknown to the public, and data regarding their frequency are scarce prior to the 1970s. AIDS was not clearly understood to be a distinct disease entity prior to the 1980s.

For these reasons, data regarding the frequency and distribution of STDs must be viewed with at least a small degree of doubt. Still, some generalizations can be drawn. The incidence of STDs seems to be higher in men than in women. This may be due to the fact that symptoms and signs are more obvious in men than in women. Of note, the gap in the incidence of STDs between the sexes in the population of the United States appears to have narrowed somewhat over the past few years, probably because of an increased proportion of women who have engaged in premarital sex and because many people have intercourse at an earlier age than was common in the past.[13]

Over the last decade, several trends have appeared in the incidence of STDs which deserve mention. While the incidence of

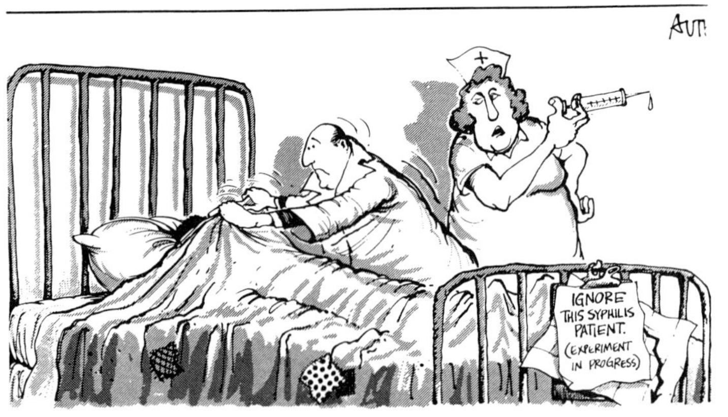


**Fig 5.** Editorial cartoon lampooning the Tuskegee Syphilis Experiment, drawn by Tony Auth in 1972 when the press and American public became aware of the study. [Courtesy of Universal Press Syndicate.]

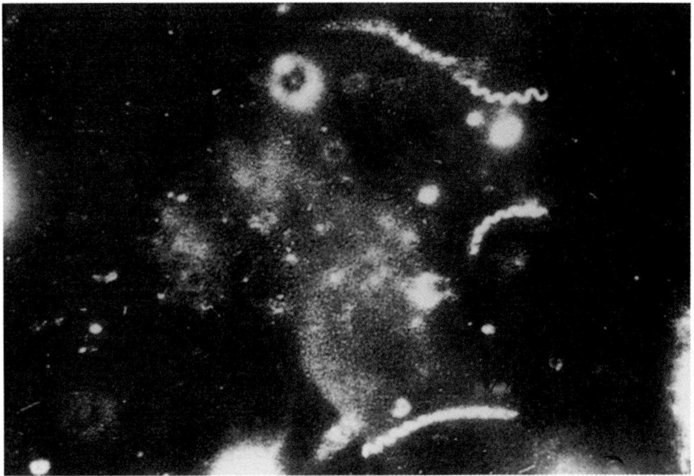

**Fig 6.** *Treponema pallidum* in the spirochete form as seen through a darkfield microscope. [Courtesy of the Centers for Disease Control, Atlanta, GA.]

gonorrhea has remained relatively constant or has slightly decreased, that of syphilis has increased steadily. In 1987, the number of cases of syphilis rose by more than 25%, the largest single-year increase in this decade.[14] Another alarming trend is that both penicillin- and tetracycline-resistant strains of *Neisseria gonorrhoeae* are now isolated from a larger proportion of cases.

Florida led the nation in the number of cases of both syphilis and gonorrhea in 1987 (the latest year for which figures are available), but this may be secondary to the development of more comprehensive reporting procedures by the state health department there. The number of office visits by patients with either human papilloma virus or genital herpes has increased from a decade ago, but may have reached a plateau in the case of herpes.

The process of contact-tracing and treatment of partners is extremely important for effective control of STDs. Whether this is done by the patients or by health department personnel is not important, as long as it is done. It may be necessary to involve the local health department to track down sexual contacts of unreliable patients, and although physician/patient relationships are considered confidential, physicians are generally protected from liability under such circumstances. In most instances, it is of paramount importance that the patient demonstrate negative posttreatment cultures prior to resuming unprotected intercourse. Otherwise, disease may be passed back and forth between sexual partners during treatment.

## SYPHILIS

Syphilis, also known as lues and called "the great imitator" because of its variable presentation, is caused by the spirochete *Treponema pallidum*. The organism was first detected by Schaudinn and Hoffmann in 1905.[15] It ranges between 6 μm and 15 μm in length and is 0.15 μm in width. It is not visible by light microscopy; darkfield examination or electron microscopy is necessary to see this spirochete (Fig 6).

Syphilis is usually acquired when *T pallidum* gains entrance through intact mucous membranes or abraded or intact skin during sexual contact. It has been estimated that the rate of infection with syphilis from an infected sexual partner is about 30%.[16] The primary dermatologic manifestation of the disease, the syphilitic chancre (Fig 7), is usually observed within 1 month of exposure. Also known as "hard" chancre, it derives this description from the firm, wood-like consistency caused by the endarteritis of the infectious process. Solitary lesions are most common, but 25% or more of patients may have multiple lesions. There may be associated inquinal adenopathy.[17]

The chancre is typically painless when touched. It teems with infective organisms

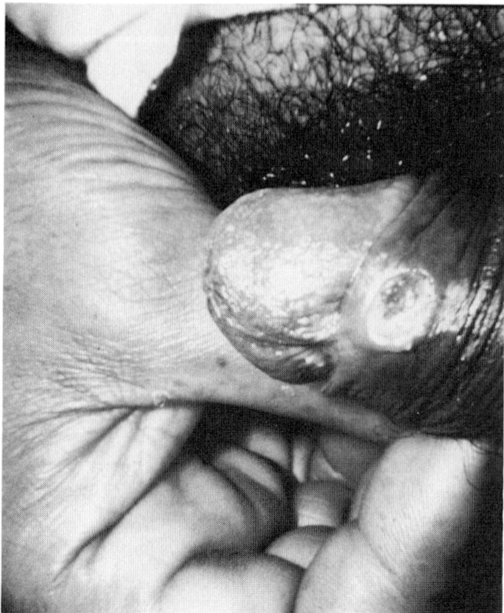

**Fig 7.** Syphilitic or "hard" chancre; this painless lesion is characteristic of the primary stage of the disease. [Courtesy of Dr Nicholas Fiumara.]

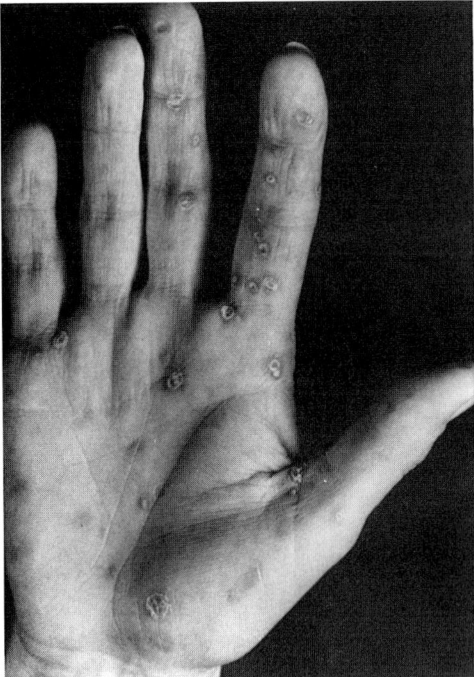

**Fig 8.** Palmar rash of secondary syphilis. [From De Graciansky P, Boulle S, *Color Atlas of Dermatology* (Chicago: Year Book Medical Publishers; 1965), with permission.]

and during this primary stage of the disease syphilis may be transmitted to between 10% and 30% of the patient's sexual contacts. The chancre may appear on the penis or labia but may also develop on the lips, mouth, or anus. It is especially important to examine the anus of homosexual patients as the anal chancre may be the only lesion noted on physical examination. If untreated, the chancre heals spontaneously in 2–6 weeks.

If undetected in the primary stage, syphilis will progress within a few weeks or months to the secondary stage. By this time, the disease is systemic and patients typically complain of malaise, low-grade fevers, headaches, and a variety of muscular aches and pains. A patchy type of alopecia, referred to as moth-eaten, may be noted by some patients, but the best-known sign of secondary syphilis is the eruption of a maculopapular, papulosquamous, or pustular rash which involves the palms and soles (Fig 8). Coloration may be varied, but is pronounced, typically with a red to brownish tinge. Another cutaneous manifestation of this stage of the disease is condyloma lata. These lesions appear as vegetating coalescent plaques, and are often observed in the anal region.

Although the rash of secondary syphilis disappears spontaneously in 4–12 weeks, the course of this stage is quite variable, and approximately 25% of patients relapse if untreated.[18]

With resolution of the cutaneous manifestations of secondary syphilis, the patient is said to have entered a latent stage (Fig 9). This is arbitrarily divided into early latency, which describes the time within 1 year of initial infection when the patient is still considered infective, and late latency, which is used when the patient is no longer considered infective. The diagnosis of latent syphilis requires a negative spinal fluid examination and a careful physical examination to rule out the possibility of active disease.

The late, or tertiary, stage of syphilis manifests itself in three ways: involvement of the bone and soft tissues, involvement of the great vessels, or involvement of the central nervous system. These manifestations may occur singly or in combination.

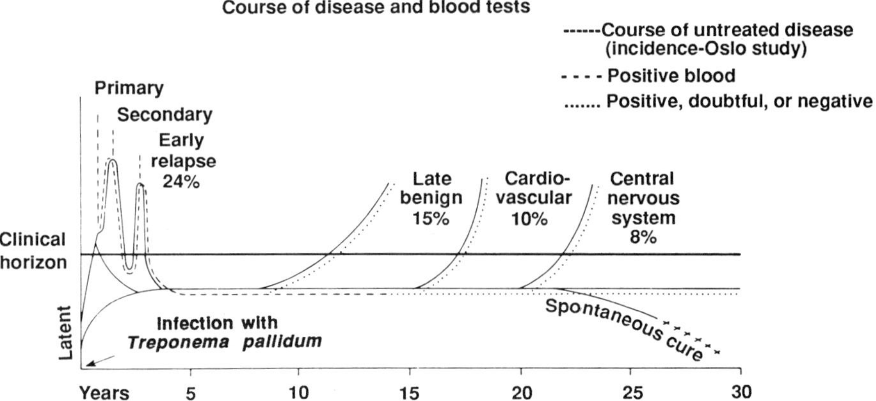


**Fig 9.** The natural history of untreated acquired syphilis. [From Habif TP, *Clinical Dermatology, A Color Guide to Diagnosis and Therapy,* 2nd ed (St. Louis: CV Mosby Co; 1990), with permission.]

Only about 35% of untreated patients progress to this stage. Late syphilitic lesions of the bone and soft tissues occur in about 10% of untreated cases. The lesions may be nodular, but the most characteristic lesion is the gumma (Fig 10), a nonspecific granulomatous inflammatory lesion with central necrosis. Long bones are more commonly affected than flat bones, and the eponym "saber shin" has been used when the tibia is affected.

Cardiovascular syphilis occurs in 10% of untreated patients, often in the middle-aged, as a result of the obliterative endarteritis of the vasa vasorum. The thoracic aorta is most commonly involved, and the endarteritis may progress to aneurysm of the root of the aorta, causing regurgitation and occlusion of the coronary arteries.

Neurosyphilis, which occurs in approximately 4% of patients with untreated syphilis, requires a reactive spinal fluid Venereal Disease Research Laboratory (VDRL) [not rapid plasma reagin (RPR)] test for diagnosis. If the infection is active, the spinal fluid will have an elevated lymphocyte count (5 cells/mm$^3$ or more) and total protein level (35 mg/dL or more). While early symptoms of neurosyphilis may present with meningeal irritation, chronic neurosyphilis invades the parenchymal tissue causing either a general paresis or tabes dorsalis from invasion of the posterior columns of the spinal cord.[19]

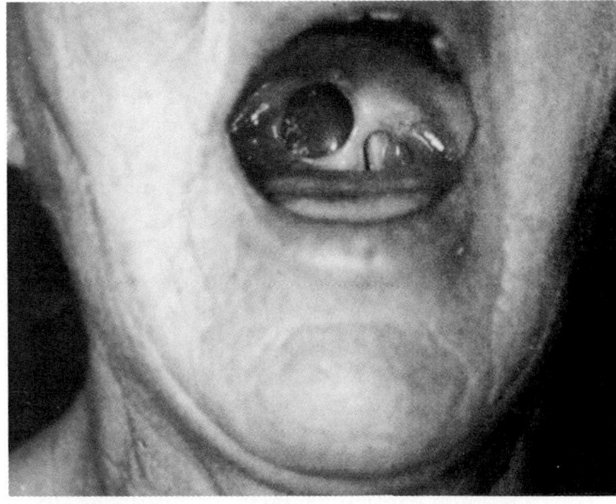

**Fig 10.** Destruction of the soft palate (gumma) from tertiary syphilis. [From Sauer G (ed), *Manual of Skin Diseases,* 5th ed (Philadelphia: JB Lippincott; 1985), with permission.]

## Diagnosis

Darkfield examination, though fraught with several problems, remains the best tool available for the diagnosis of primary syphilis. Proper techniques, and the experience of the microscopist, are two variables that dictate the sensitivity and specificity of this test. Specimens from actively weeping chancres or condyloma lata contain the highest number of organisms. The chancre should be squeezed until serum is expressed; if a crust or exudate is present on the lesion, this should be wiped clear first. The serum may then be examined under the darkfield microscope. Fluorescent treponemal antibody tests for wet mounts have been developed but are not widely used.[20] An inexperienced microscopist may identify a commensal parasite as *T pallidum* by mistake; this occurs most often with specimens obtained from the oropharynx.

Serologic tests can be divided into two classes, based on the premise that the syphilitic infection produces two types of antibodies. The nontreponemal (anticardiolipin) antibody is detected by the VDRL slide flocculation test or the RPR agglutination test; both of these tests are nonspecific, but highly sensitive. The second type of antibody produced is a specific, antitreponemal, antibody. The two most widely used tests to detect these antibodies are the Fluorescent Treponemal Antibody-Absorption (FTA-ABS) and the Microhemagglutination-*T Pallidum* (MHA-TP).

The former two tests, VDRL and RPR, are relatively inexpensive and are used primarily for screening. In addition, the patient's antibody titer as measured by VDRL or RPR can be monitored to assess the success of treatment. The other tests, FTA-ABS and MHA-TP, should be used to confirm the diagnosis of syphilis in the patient with negative results on darkfield examination and a variable VDRL titer, and to identify the patient with latent or tertiary syphilis who may have a normal VDRL titer. The FTA-ABS is positive in virtually every patient who has ever had syphilis, whether treated or not (Table 1).[21]

### Treatment

Penicillin is the preferred drug for the treatment of syphilis. Individuals who have had the disease for less than 1 year can expect a 95% cure rate from a single dosage of 2.4 million units of benzathione penicillin G (1.2 million units in each buttock). Preliminary results support the use of ceftriaxone to treat incubating and early stages of syphilis. For patients allergic to penicillin or ceftriaxone, tetracycline, erythromycin, or doxycycline may be used.[22] In general, compliance is improved with doxycycline because of its twice-daily dosing. Another alternative for the penicillin-allergic patient is skin testing and desensitization. Penicillin is the only proven therapy that has been widely used for patients with neurosyphilis, congenital syphilis, or syphilis during pregnancy.

For patients who have had syphilis for longer than 1 year, including cardiovascular or late benign disease, therapy should consist of intramuscular (IM) benzathione penicillin G 2.4 million units once a week for 3 successive weeks. Patients allergic to penicillin can be treated with doxycycline or tetracycline. A lumbar puncture may be indicated in certain patients to rule out the possibility of neurosyphilis.

Neurosyphilis is treated with aqueous penicillin G given intravenously (IV) or if outpatient compliance can be assured, procaine penicillin and probenacid for a period of 10 days to 2 weeks. Pregnant patients should be treated with the same regimens as their nonpregnant counterparts. Those allergic to penicillin should undergo desensitization. Tetracycline and doxycyline are contraindicated in pregnant patients; erythromycin should also not be used be-

**TABLE 1. Syphilis Serology Reactivity at Various Disease Stages**

| Serologic Test | Primary Syphilis (% Reactivity) | Secondary Syphilis (% Reactivity) | Latent and Late Syphilis (% Reactivity) | Neurosyphilis (% Reactivity) |
|---|---|---|---|---|
| NTA* | 70 | 99 | 70 | 52‡ |
| TA† | 76–91 | 99–100 | 95–98 | Not indicated |

* Nontreponemal antibody test (eg. VDRL, RPR)
† Treponemal antibody test (eg. FTA-Abs, ELISA)
‡ Using cerebrospinal fluid
From Bracero LA, Wormser GP. Serologic tests for syphilis. *Med Aspects Human Sex.* May 1989:74–80, reprinted with permission.

cause of the high risk of failure to cure infection in the fetus. The effectiveness of ceftriaxone in the pregnant patient has not been documented.

The patient who is sexually exposed to an individual with syphilis may remain seronegative for up to 90 days. Although syphilis cannot be diagnosed in these patients, they should be treated presumptively for the disease with the same drug schedule used for patients with early syphilis.

The Jarisch-Herxheimer reaction is a constellation of symptoms including fever, chills, arthralgias, and headache commonly seen after the treatment of syphilis. In pregnant patients, early labor may occur. This reaction is most commonly observed after treating patients with the initial stages of the disease and should not be mistaken for a penicillin or drug allergy. Under no circumstances should this reaction cause discontinuation of treatment. Patients should be forewarned that such a reaction may occur to prevent alarm. Although the underlying mechanisms are not entirely clear, the reaction may occur as a result of the liberation of treponemal endotoxins.[23]

Following treatment, all patients should be re-examined clinically and serologically at 3 and 6 months. With adequate treatment, the nontreponemal-antibody titers should decline by fourfold at 3 months in those patients with primary or secondary syphilis and at 6 months in those with latent syphilis. If symptoms persist or if titers do not fall, patients should have a cerebrospinal fluid examination and be retreated as needed.

## CHANCROID

Chancroid, or soft chancre, is an acute disease of the genitalia characterized by multiple, painful ulcerative lesions with severe, secondary suppurative lymphadenitis. Bassereau differentiated chancroid from syphilis in 1852,[24] and Ducrey later identified the causative organism,[25] which bears his name, *Hemophilus ducreyi*. Although rare in the United States, *H ducreyi* infection is frequently seen in subtropical or tropical regions. It is also more common in uncircumcised men.

### Clinical Course

*H ducreyi* has a short incubation period of between 1 and 14 days; most cases of chancroid occur 1–5 days after sexual contact with an infected individual. Typically, an erythematous lesion develops over an area of abraded skin. This progresses to a tender papule which ulcerates. The ulcer is painful, irregular, ragged in appearance, and soft to palpation (in distinction to the syphilitic "hard" chancre). It may be linear, serpiginous, or circular. The base often has a necrotic or purulent exudate, and is friable when scraped. A characteristic of chancroid is autoinnoculation. Indeed, multiple lesions occur in approximately 50% of patients of both sexes.[26] Ulcers commonly develop on or beneath the foreskin, and the frenulum is often affected—perhaps because it is easily traumatized during sex (Fig 11). Edema of the foreskin and phimosis is also common. In particu-

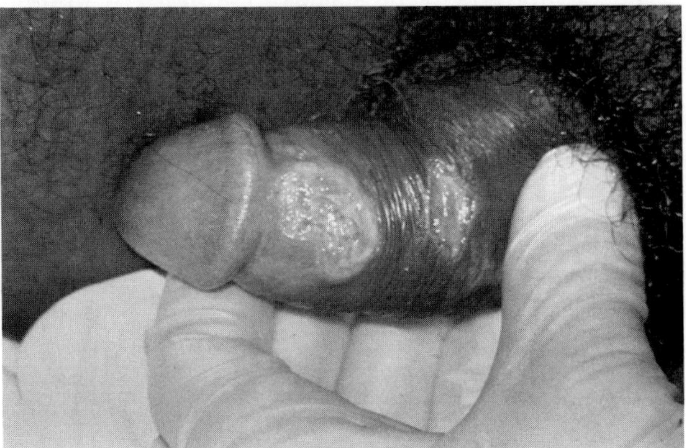

**Fig 11.** Multiple penile ulcerations of chancroid; as opposed to syphilitic chancres, these lesions are painful.

larly severe infections, the foreskin and glans may be consumed by necrosis in the infectious process, a condition called "phagedenic edema." In women, ulceration occurs primarily on the fourchette, labia, vestibule, and clitoris. Extragenital lesions have also been described, and occur on the nipples, fingers, and mouth.

Inguinal adenitis is commonly found in patients with chancroid. The nodes are painful, usually unilateral, and may be present in up to 50% of patients. The adenopathy may start out as matted tender nodes and progress to fluctuance with spontaneous rupture.

### Diagnosis

*H ducreyi* has historically been a relatively difficult organism to culture; thus, the diagnosis of chancroid is often made by exclusion, or after presumptive treatment has begun. Syphilis may coexist with chancroid, and so material expressed from the base of the ulcers should be examined by darkfield microscopy. In addition, serologic tests should be used to rule out the presence of *T pallidum.*

A smear of pus collected from infected buboes or from an ulcer after gentle cleaning with isotonic saline reveals gram-negative bacilli in chains or in a pattern often referred to as "schools of fish." Autoinnoculation techniques and the use of blood as a culture medium have been described but are not in wide use.[27,28] Lymphogranuloma venereum (LGV) and granuloma inguinale[29] remain in the differential diagnosis (as do traumatic injuries such as human bites), but can usually be ruled out by the location and the presence of multiple ulcerations as well as the short incubation period of chancroid.

At the time of this writing, no serologic test was available for use in diagnosing chancroid.

### Treatment

Fortunately, there are several antimicrobial agents that are effective in treating chancroid. Erythromycin 500 mg four times daily for at least a week may be used, as may single-dose ceftriaxone 250 mg IM.[30] Other treatment regimens include sulfamethoxazole/trimethoprim (SMX/TMP), amoxicillin/clavulonic acid, and ciprofloxacin. Resistance to trimethoprim has been reported in Southeast Asia, and should be considered in patients who have recently traveled to this area.[31]

Resolution of ulcers and adenopathy should be apparent after 1 week of appropriate antibiotic therapy. If, however, nodes remain painful and fluctuant, they should be drained through healthy adjacent skin using an 18-gauge needle (rather than by an incision) to prevent the formation of draining sinuses. Similarly, a circumcision or dorsal slit is contraindicated when the infection is active because of the risk of autoinnoculation. Cold compresses applied to ulcerated areas may provide local relief. Any person who had sexual contact with an infected patient within 10 days before the onset of symptoms should be treated, regardless of whether they are symptomatic.

## LYMPHOGRANULOMA VENEREUM (LGV)

LGV, an uncommon STD in the United States, is endemic to the tropics, especially East and West Africa.[32,33] It is caused by a biovar or serovar of *Chlamydia trachomatis,* and is similar to the strain that causes nongonococcal urethritis but is more virulent. The disease is more common in men than women,[14] and has a variety of acute and late manifestations that are often divided into three stages.

### Clinical Course

The first stage of LGV is characterized by the development of a primary genital lesion. The incubation period ranges from 3 days to 3 weeks; the lesion usually appears herpetiform in nature, but papules and ulcerations have also been described.[34] In men, lesions most commonly occur on the glans and penis. In women, lesions occur on the vagina. Small and painless, the lesion heals quickly and without scar. It often goes unnoticed by the patient.

The second stage of the disease is characterized by painful inquinal adenopathy. It is during this stage that patients often seek medical attention. The time to development of these nodes is variable, but usually is 10–30 days after infection. Patients also complain of constitutional symptoms during this stage, which may be associated with systemic infection. Fever, headache, and arthralgias are common in patients with secondary LGV.

Usually, the nodes involved are the inguinal nodes; however, if the femoral nodes are also involved, the "groove sign" becomes evident (Fig 12). This physical sign is a result of these nodal groups being separated by Poupart's ligament. It is characteristic, and indeed is often considered pathognomonic for LGV, but the "groove sign" occurs in only 15%–20% of patients infected. Only about 33% of inguinal buboes rupture spontaneously, but those that do give rise to numerous sinus tracts which drain pus—often for weeks to months. After resolution, scarring of these nodes is common.

The tertiary stage of LGV is characterized by the late rectal and genital sequelae of the disease. Rectal strictures are common, and are usually located close to the anal verge, where the lymphatic tissues lie. There have been cases of rectal cancers associated with LGV, raising the possibility that the disease in some way may cause malignant transformation.[35] Proctitis is common in homosexual men, as well as in women who engage in anal intercourse.

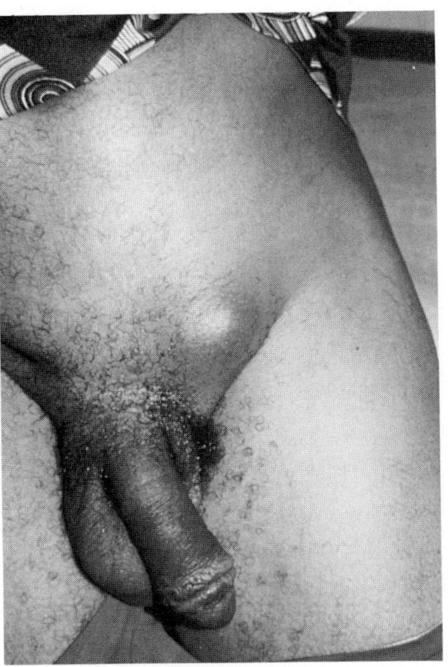

Fig 12. Inguinal lymphadenopathy characteristic of the 2nd stage of lymphogranuloma venereum.

Genital tertiary sequelae include penile and perineal fistulae as well as esthiomene and elephantiasis. Esthiomene (Greek for "eating away") refers to the ulceration of the genitalia as a result of chronically obstructed and fibrotic lymphatic tissues, and is more common in women. Similarly, elephantiasis is a result of lymphatic obstruction and may involve the penis as well as the scrotum.

## Diagnosis

The diagnosis of LGV is often made clinically. Individuals suspected of having LGV should be tested for syphilis and gonorrhea, as these diseases may coexist with LGV. The presence of lymphadenopathy should cause suspicion regarding the possibility of chancroid and genital herpes in the differential diagnosis, but the characteristic painful, self-limited ulcerations of these latter two diseases are not symptoms of LGV.

Serologic tests are available, but are not usually diagnostic. Although the Frei test is frequently mentioned, this test had low sensitivity and specificity.[36] The commercial manufacture of the Frei Antigen was discontinued in 1974, and the test is no longer available. Complement fixation titers are sensitive, but there is crossreactivity with all *Chlamydia* strains. The titers in patients with LGV are usually higher than in those with other chlamydial infections. A titer of >1:16 is common.[37] Microimmunofluorescence testing is also available, and is more sensitive than complement fixation testing. However, it too is crossreactive with other chlamydial infections.

Fluorescein-conjugated monoclonal antichlamydial antibodies provide a rapid method of detection. Chlamydial antigen is bound to the antibodies, and the preparation is visualized with the aid of a fluorescent microscope.

### Treatment

Treatment for LGV is doxycycline 100 mg, given twice daily for 21 days. Alternative regimens include tetracycline 500 mg four times daily for 21 days, erythromycin 500 mg four times daily for 21 days, or sulfisoxazole 500 mg four times daily for 21 days.[38]

Aspiration of painful buboes may be made through adjacent healthy skin. Rectal strictures are usually improved with appropriate antibiotic therapy, but dilation may be required in some instances. Elephantiasis and esthiomene may require surgical correction, but should first be treated with long-term antibiotic therapy.

## GRANULOMA INGUINALE

Granuloma inguinale is an extremely rare disease in the United States. It is also known as donavanosis and granuloma venereum. It is caused by the organism *Calymmatobacterium granulomatis*, previously known as *Donovania granulomatis* and *Klebsiella granulomatis*. Although thought to be sexually transmitted, the disease is only mildly contagious and repeated exposure is necessary for the development of symptoms.[39,40] It is most common in black persons and in tropical areas of the world.[41]

### Clinical Course

The incubation period, though variable, ranges from 1 to 12 weeks. The disease begins as a single or multiple subcutaneous nodule which breaks down to reveal bright red, usually painless, friable granulation tissue (Fig 13). If not treated, granulating areas may coalesce and spread across the body surface, resulting in scarring and gross deformity (Fig 14). Lymphadenopathy is rare and constitutional symptoms are absent. The genitalia are involved in 90% of cases, the inguinal region in 10%, and the anal region in 5%.

### Diagnosis

The diagnosis of granuloma inguinale is made on clinical grounds, but may be confirmed microscopically. A crushed tissue specimen from affected areas when stained with Wright's or Giemsa stain will reveal the presence of intracellular bipolar organisms, known as Donovan bodies.[42] The differential diagnosis includes other STDs, as well as carcinoma. A patient who is presumptively treated for granuloma inguinale with a course of antibiotics but who does not experience symptomatic resolution

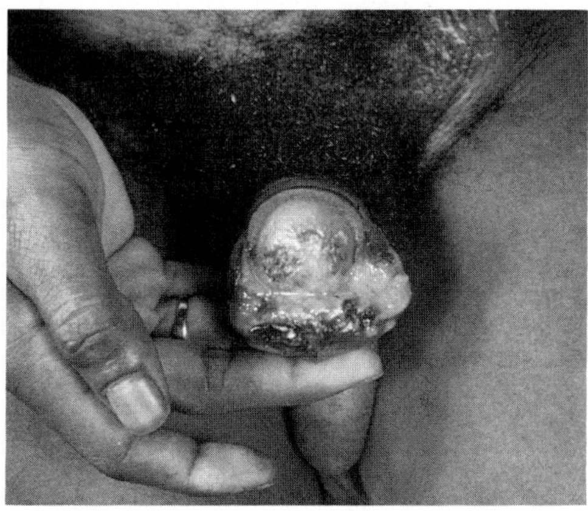

**Fig 13.** Granuloma inguinale of the penis.

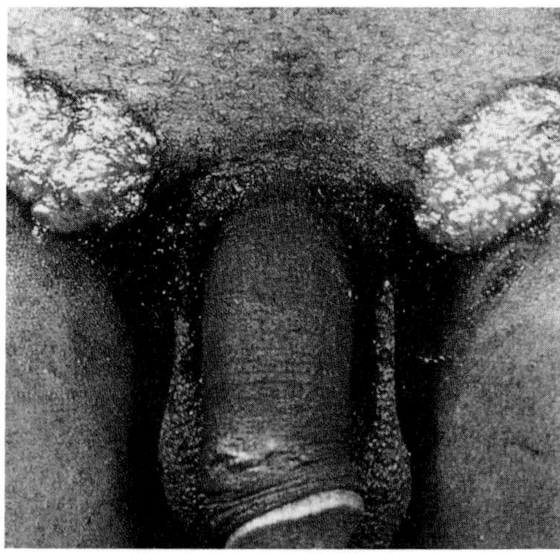

**Fig 14.** Granuloma inguinale of the inguinal region. [From Fiumara NJ, Infections of the genitals I: bacterial and fungal infections, *Infect Urol* (1989;2:79), with permission.]

should undergo biopsy to rule out the presence of cancer, which may be coexistent.

### Treatment

The mainstay of therapy in this disease is tetracycline 500 mg given four times daily or doxycycline 100 mg given twice daily. The therapy should be continued for 2 weeks or until the lesions disappear. Ampicillin and erythromycin have been used to treat tetracycline-resistant cases, but should not be used as first-line treatment.[43,44]

## URETHRITIS

Despite warnings from public health officials, urethritis continues to be an enormous health and economic burden in this country. In 1987, it was estimated that there were as many as 1.4 million cases of gonorrheal and 4.0 million cases of chlamydial urethritis. This, in addition to the 1.2 million cases of nongonococcal, nonchlamydial urethritis and 1.0 million cases of mucopurulent cervicitis, stress the magnitude of this problem.[14] These staggering numbers make it imperative for the physician to become familiar with the diagnosis and treatment of these diseases.

Bacterial organisms responsible for urethritis in the past were arbitrarily divided into gonococcal and nongonococcal infections. Although they will be discussed separately here, the reader is cautioned that the distinction is often blurred. In as many as 30%–50% of cases, these organisms may coexist.

### Gonorrhea

The term gonorrhea, meaning flow of seed (gono = semen, rheos = discharge) was coined in ancient times by Galen, who mistakenly believed the urethral discharge was composed of semen. Because of the frequent coexistence with syphilis, the two diseases were not recognized as clearly distinct until the mid-19th century. *N gonorrhoeae* is the organism responsible for gonococcal urethritis. It is a gram-negative, nonmotile diplococcus, with only one natural host: humans. Surface pili facilitate attachment of the organism to nonciliated epithelial cells and may confer resistance to phagocytosis.[45] The incubation period before onset of symptoms is variable, and ranges from 1 day to several months; symptoms usually occur 3 to 10 days after inoculation.[46] Asymptomatic infection may occur in up to 50% of women, but is less common in men. The risk of female to male transmission is estimated at 17% per episode, whereas the risk of male to female transmission is 4 times as high.[47]

Although the urethra remains the most common site of infection in the heterosexual and homosexual male, the homosexual male has a much higher incidence of anorectal and pharyngeal gonorrhea. Transmission of the disease most commonly occurs by genital or rectal contact, but infected pharyngeal secretions may cause urethritis as well.[48] Nonsexual transmission is rare, and cases of gonorrhea in children may be indicative of sexual abuse. A careful medical and social evaluation is therefore imperative in children who present with the disease.[49]

Primary symptoms in the male include dysuria and urethral discharge. The classic gonococcal discharge is described as profuse and purulent, but may be quite variable in nature (Fig 15).

In women, the primary site of infection is usually the endocervix, although secondary colonization occurs in the urethra or rectum. Most women are symptomatic, but complaints may vary, especially if the infection has gone on to infect the fallopian tubes and pelvic peritoneum.[50] Presenting symptoms may include vaginal discharge, lower abdominal discomfort, abnormal uterine bleeding, and peritonitis. Symptoms are usually more severe after menses.

The woman who seeks treatment late may present with frank pelvic inflammatory disease (PID).

**Diagnosis.** Diagnosis is made by collection of a specimen directly from the urethra 1–4 hours after the patient has last voided. Calcium alginate swabs should be used because cotton swabs are bactericidal. The swab should be inserted 2–4 cm into the urethra, rotated gently, and then used to

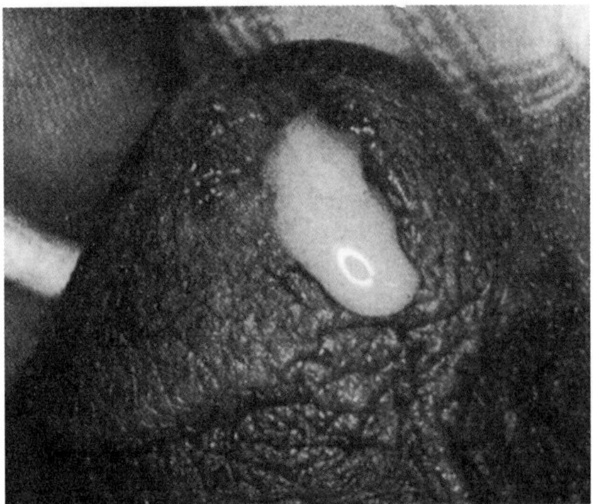

**Fig 15.** Urethral discharge characteristic of infection with *N gonorrhoeae.* [From Fiumara NJ, Infections of the genitals I: bacterial and fungal infections, *Infect Urol* (1989;2:79), with permission.]

innoculate a Thayer-Martin or New York City media plate. The organism grows best in a carbon dioxide enhanced environment, and plates should be warmed to room temperature before the swab is applied for best growth.[51]

After the culture plates have been set up, the swab should be rolled on a microscope slide. The slide is then air dried, heat fixed, and gram stained. The presence of gram-negative diplococci inside polymorphonuclear leukocytes (PMNs) is pathognomonic for gonorrhea. The sensitivity and specificity of a gram stain are 99% and 95%, respectively. The gram stain, however, should not take the place of cultures, as with the emergence of resistant strains, sensitivity testing is often necessary.[52] In addition to urethral swabs, a culture of the rectum in homosexual men is required. This specimen should be obtained from columnar epithelial cells by inserting a swab 2–3 cm into the anal canal and allowing it to rest there for 15–30 seconds before retrieval.[53] Those practicing orogenital relations require a pharyngeal swab as well, though the rate of detection of oropharyngeal infection may decrease with time after innoculation.[54]

**Treatment.** Treatment of gonorrhea has required change through the years, because of the development of resistant strains. While the vast majority of strains are still sensitive to penicillins, both penicillin- and tetracycline-resistant strains have been identified. Penicillin-resistant strains are of two different types: one type acquires its resistance from a plasmid, the other is chromosomally mediated.[55] Tetracycline-resistant gonorrhea were first identified in 1985.[56] The majority of cases of penicillinase-producing *N gonorrhoeae* are found in Florida, New York, and California.[57] In 1989, penicillinase-producing *N gonorrhoeae* (PPNG) accounted for 7.4% of isolates and tetracycline-resistant *N gonorrhoeae* (TRNG) accounted for 4.9% of isolates. The emergence of a strain of gonorrhea resistant to both tetracycline and penicillin (PPNG/TRNG) has recently been reported; this strain is said to have accounted for 0.9% of isolates in 1989. The PPNG/TRNG strains were isolated most frequently from patients in Philadelphia, where they accounted for 9.7% of isolates (Fig 16). Plasmid-mediated resistance to ceftriaxone or spectinomycin has not yet been identified. While the resistant strains are not more virulent, they do require adequate patient follow-up.[58]

Of the patients with gonococcal infections, 15% to 30% of heterosexual men and 25% to 60% of women have a coexisting chlamydial infection.[53] Treatment of gonorrhea must, therefore, take into account both the need to treat resistant gonococcal organisms as well as the need to treat *Chlamydia*. The current recommendation of the Centers for Disease Control is a 250 mg single dose of ceftriaxone given IM plus oral doxycycline (100 mg) given twice daily for 7 days. For those who cannot take ceftriaxone, the preferred alternative is spectinomycin (2 g IM) in a single dose followed by doxycycline. Neither doxycycline nor tetracycline alone is considered adequate therapy for gonococcal infections; these agents are, however, effective against the coexisting chlamydial infections. Compliance is better with doxycycline, because of the twice-daily dosing. Pregnant women who cannot take tetracycline or doxycy-

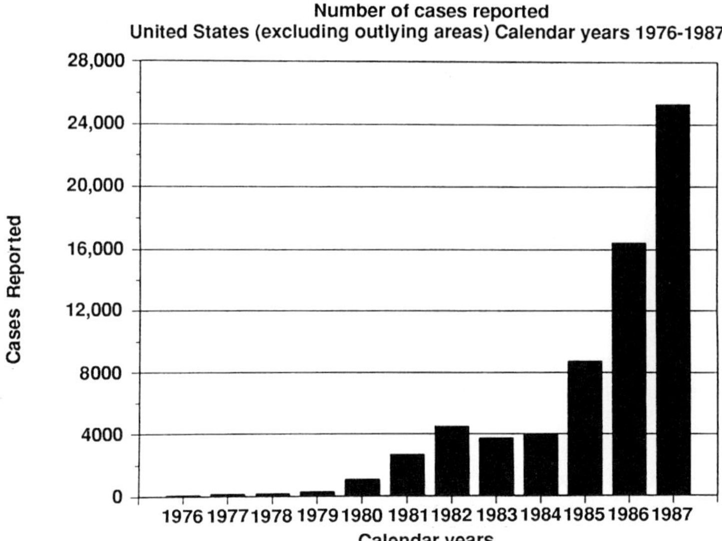


**Fig 16.** Total antibiotic-resistant strains of gonorrhea isolated per year. [Courtesy of the Centers for Disease Control, Atlanta, GA.]

cline may substitute an erythromycin preparation. Experience with single-dose ciprofloxacin (500 mg orally) and norfloxacin (800 mg orally once, or 600 mg in 2 doses) suggests that these drugs may offer an acceptable alternative.[59] They cannot, however, be used in pregnant women or children because of the possibility of causing cartilage damage.

Failure of ceftriaxone/doxycycline therapy is rare, and test-of-cure follow-up cultures are not required. However, patients treated with other regimens should be tested with repeat cultures, as should patients who return with persistent symptoms. All persons exposed to gonorrhea within the preceding 30 days should be examined, tested by culture, and treated presumptively. Infection after treatment with one of these regimens is usually due to reinfection, rather than treatment failure.[38]

Disseminated gonococcal infection occurs in fewer than 1% of patients,[51] and occurs more frequently in women than in men. Symptoms include anorexia, fever, and rash, usually followed by tenosynovitis and arthritis. The characteristic skin lesions are 5–15 mm in diameter with a pustule located on an erythematous base (Fig 17). During the first 2–3 days of this type of infection, 50% of patients will have positive blood cultures. This decreases to less than 10% of cases by the time joint effusions have developed. Typical gonococcal

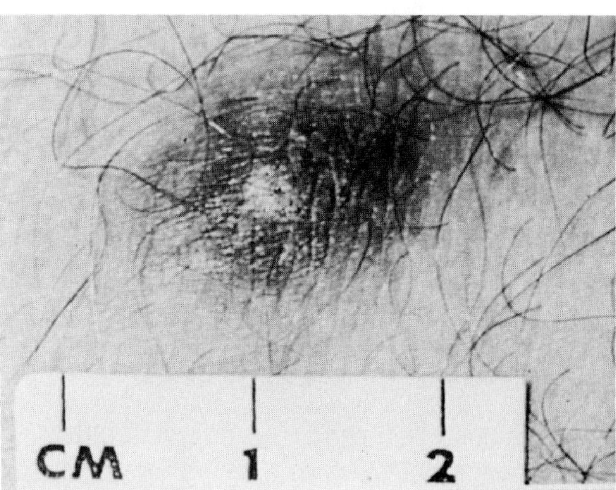


**Fig 17.** Skin lesion of disseminated gonorrhea. [From Holmes KK, et al (eds), *Sexually Transmitted Diseases* (New York: McGraw-Hill; 1984), with permission.]

arthritis is polyarticular in over 50% of cases. Examination of the synovial fluid will reveal greater than 50,000 white blood cells/mm$^3$, with 90% or more of the cells polymorphonuclear leukocytes. The arthritis requires prompt diagnosis and treatment to avoid joint destruction.[53] Treatment can be accomplished with either ceftriaxone (1 g IV or IM or q 24 h) or ceftizoxime (1 g IV q 8 h) or cefotaxime (1 g IV q 8 h). Hospitalization is recommended during initial therapy but reliable patients whose symptoms resolve and who have otherwise uncomplicated disease may be discharged after 48 hours and instructed to take ciprofloxacin 500 mg twice daily for 1 week.

Gonococcal meningitis and endocarditis are rare, and require long-term IV antibiotic therapy.

## Nongonococcal Urethritis

Nongonococcal urethritis is about twice as common as gonococcal urethritis.[60] Patients with nongonococcal urethritis (NGU) are more likely to be white, better educated, and have fewer sexual contacts than those with gonococcal urethritis.[61]

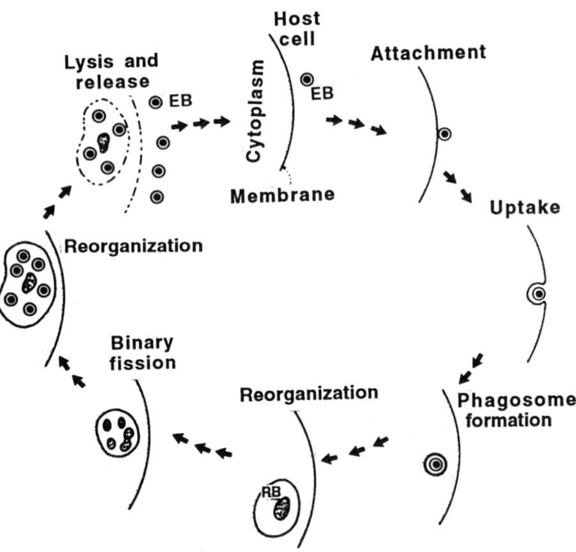


**Fig 18.** Life cycle of *C trachomatis;* EB = elementary body, the extracellular and infectious form of the organism; RB = reticulate body, the replicating and intracellular form of the organism. [From Krieger JN, Biology of sexually transmitted diseases, *Urol Clin North Am* (1984;11:15), with permission.]

The most common pathogen responsible for NGU is *Chlamydia trachomatis. Chlamydia* accounts for 50% of cases of NGU, and is the most common sexually transmitted pathogen in the United States. Fifteen serotypes of *Chlamydia* exist, three of which cause LGV. Chlamydiae are a large, diverse group of intracellular parasites that contain both DNA and RNA, divide by binary fission, but like viruses, grow only intracellularly.

The lifecycle, complete in about 48 hours, consists of an infectious particle called the elementary body. It is a metabolically inactive particle which attaches to the cell membrane and then is taken into the cell by phagocytosis. After approximately 12 hours, the elementary body reorganizes into the reproductive, metabolically active form of the bacteria known as the reticulate body. The reticulate body undergoes division and the resultant daughter cells revert to elementary bodies (Fig 18).[62]

*Ureaplasma urealyticum* may account for 20% to 30% of cases of NGU. Ureaplasma is a mycoplasm, a specific class of aerobic bacteria that represents the smallest known free-living organisms. Genital and urethral colonization by *Ureaplasma* increases with the number of previous partners, and there is evidence to suggest that this organism is not merely a commensal inhabitant.

The etiology of urethritis cannot be determined in approximately 20% of cases. Other organisms such as *Trichomonas vaginalis,* Herpes simplex virus, *Candida albicans,* and Bacteroides species have been implicated as causative agents.[63]

**Presentation.** The usual incubation period in men with NGU is 2–6 weeks. The discharge tends to be less purulent than that seen with gonorrhea, and the dysuria is less severe, but there is much overlap between the symptomatology of the two diseases. The edges of the meatus may stick together prior to voiding, a symptom that is usually most noticeable with the first-morning void. *Chlamydia* and gonorrhea may coexist in as many as 40% of cases.[64]

**TABLE 2. Urethritis**

| | Gonorrhea | Non-Gonococcal Urethritis |
|---|---|---|
| Organism | *N gonorrhoeae* | 50% *C trachomatis*<br>25% *U urealyticum*<br>25% other organisms |
| Incubation period | 3–10 d | 2–6 wks or longer |
| Discharge | Thick, purulent | Watery, mucoid |
| Dysuria | Present | Present |
| Microscopic findings | Gram-negative intracellular diplococci | Polymorphonuclear leukocytes |
| Laboratory diagnosis | Culture, Thayer-Martin, or NYC media | Fluorescent antibody stains or in-office ELISA |
| Treatment of choice | Ceftriaxone | Doxycycline |

Women infected with *Chlamydia* are often asymptomatic, yet nearly 80% of female contacts of men with proven chlamydial urethritis will have *C trachomatis* cultured from the cervix. A mucopurulent discharge from the cervix is commonly seen on pelvic examination. *Chlamydia* infection occurs more commonly in women who do not use barrier contraceptive methods, and increases with the number of lifetime sexual partners (Table 2).[65–68]

**Diagnosis.** A diagnosis is made by swabbing the urethra at least 1–4 hours after last voiding. Diagnostic monoclonal antibody kits are available and cost effective. The test usually takes fewer than 30 minutes and is read as positive when fluorescein-conjugated antibodies are noted under a fluorescent microscope. The test is about 95% sensitive and 95% specific.[69]

In-office, rapid immunoassays have recently become available which make test results available to the patient within 9 to 15 minutes. In addition to the convenience afforded to the patient, the tests are also inexpensive, at $8 to $10 per test. The tests detect the presence of *C trachomatis* antigen, so live organisms are not required to obtain a positive result. Refrigeration of some of the reagents is required, but laboratory workspace requirements are minimal. The available tests have reported sensitivities of 67% to 85% and specificities in the 97% to 99% range. Because the tests may detect antigens from nonviable organisms, test-of-cure testing, if done, should be delayed until at least 2 weeks after treatment.[70–72]

Cultures for detection of *C trachomatis* are slow, tedious to perform, and not readily available.

**Treatment.** The therapeutic regimen of choice for infection with either *Chlamydia* or *Ureaplasma* organisms is doxycycline 100 mg given twice daily for 7 days or tetracycline 500 mg given four times a day for 7 days. *C trachomatis* is not resistant to tetracycline, but 10% to 20% of *Ureaplasma* species are. The resistant *U urealyticum* are sensitive to erythromycin (500 mg 4 times daily for 7 days).

The prostate may play a role in persistent or recurrent NGU, especially when urethral cultures are negative for uropathogens. When tetracycline therapy is ineffective, a trial of erythromycin is indicated. If a second course of therapy fails, the causative organism may be *Trichomonas vaginalis;* if this organism is present, metronidazole should be started.[73] If symptoms persist, despite repeated courses of antibiotics, and an etiologic agent has not been identified, urethroscopy should be performed to rule out the possibility of a stricture or foreign body.

All sexual partners of patients with NGU should be examined and treated. The author suggests that medication *not* be given to the patient for their partner(s). In addition to decreased compliance, the potential for an adverse reaction in the sexual consort is a possibility, if a medical history is not first obtained. Optimally, treatment of both persons should be accomplished during the same time period to avoid back and forth passage of the disease.

*Chlamydia* infections in pregnant women may result in premature delivery, premature rupture of the membranes, and birth of small-for-gestational-age infants. Effective treatment during pregnancy may reduce these risks, as well as prevent transmission of the organism to the infant during passage through the birth canal.[74]

## GENITAL HERPES INFECTIONS

Although genital herpes is not a reportable venereal disease, this much publicized STD has received considerable attention in the lay press. Unlike many other STDs, genital herpes remains without a cure. In 1987, there were approximately 450,000 visits[75] to private physicians' offices for genital herpes infections. Although the disease is marked by intermittent recurrences of variable frequency, patients can learn to cope with the disease if properly informed of its natural history.

The herpes virus is a double stranded DNA virus. The five types causing infections in humans are: herpes simplex virus 1 (HSV-1), herpes simplex virus 2 (HSV-2), cytomegalovirus, varicella-zoster virus, and Epstein-Barr virus. The HSV strains are responsible for the overwhelming majority of genital herpes infections. Originally, it was believed that HSV-2 was responsible for the genital infection; however, both types of HSV are sexually transmissible, and the frequency of orogenital sex has led to an increasing incidence of HSV-1 isolated from genital lesions.[76] The importance of this incidence is its predictive value for recurrent episodes; HSV-1 infections recur in 14% to 50% of patients, while HSV-2 infections recur in 60% to 80% of individuals.[77,78] Whether this is due to differences of the latency period in the dorsal root ganglia or reinfection with different strains of the same viral type is unclear.

### Clinical Course

Infection with HSV occurs due to direct innoculation onto the skin or mucosal surfaces. Although HSV has been isolated from cloth and hot tubs, the passage of the virus by those routes has not been documented.[79,80]

Primary infections occur after an incubation period of 2–12 days, and although documented, asymptomatic primary infections are rare.[81] Systemic symptoms of fever, headache, malaise, myalgias, and lymphadenopathy may precede the development of skin lesions.[82] Urinary difficulty and frank retention are not uncommon, but resolve with the course of the infection.[83] Painful skin lesions develop as grouped vesicles on an erythematous base (Fig 19). The vesicles rupture, leaving erosions which then crust and heal, generally in 2 to 4 weeks. Viral shedding occurs on cutaneous surfaces, until a dry crust develops. On mucosal surfaces, crusts do not form, and shedding occurs until reepithelialization occurs. In men, the penis, scrotum, and thighs are most commonly affected, while in women, the external genitalia as well as the vaginal vault and cervix frequently are involved. Homosexual men who practice anal intercourse often develop rectal lesions; a severe proctitis may result.[84] Spread of lesions to extragenital sites by autoinnoculation may occur with the presence of active lesions; attention to strict hygiene should therefore be stressed.

Lesions from recurrent infections are generally less severe than those from primary infections. The cutaneous manifestations occur in a smaller area and heal

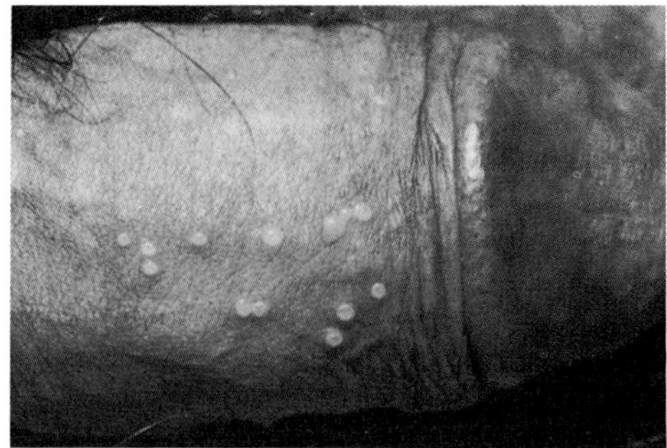

**Fig 19.** Herpes simplex infection of the penis, vesicular stage. [From Korting GW, *Practical Dermatology of the Genital Region* (Philadelphia: WB Saunders Co; 1981), with permission.]

faster. Intraurethral or intravaginal recurrent lesions may be difficult to identify. It is unclear as to what controls the reactivation of latent herpes, but scarring at the site of previous infection and immunosuppression of the patient probably plays a role.[85] A prodrome of burning or itching prior to recurrence is common.

In women, viral shedding has been shown to occur in the absence of lesions[86]; clear evidence of this has not been demonstrated in men. However, in the absence of lesions, the number of shed viral particles is low, and whether the asymptomatic patient can transmit the disease is unclear.

## Diagnosis

The presence of grouped vesicles or eroded or crusted lesions in the genital region is highly suggestive of HSV infection. Confirmation of the diagnosis can be made either with the use of viral cultures or by cytologic smears. Viral cultures are available in most laboratories. Fluid from the early vesicles provides the highest number of viral particles and should be used to innoculate the culture media.

Tzanck and Papanicolaou smears are quick and convenient alternatives to viral cultures. The Tzanck smear is performed by scraping the base of an ulcerated lesion and applying this material to a slide. Immediate fixation in absolute alcohol for 1 minute is then followed by application of Wright's or Giemsa stain for 3 minutes. The positive Tzanck smear is characterized by the presence of multinucleated giant cells. Such cells may also be seen in patients with varicella-zoster infections, but the clinical manifestations of these diseases are different from those of HSV infection.

Papanicolaou stain is more sensitive than the Tzanck smear, and in patients with HSV infections is characterized by the presence of intranuclear inclusions. Both the smear and culture tests give a higher diagnostic yield in the vesicular than the erosive stages.[87]

Serologic testing is not useful unless a rise in antibody titer is seen; however, monoclonal antibody testing holds promise as a quick and effective method of diagnosis. These tests, with high sensitivity and specificity may be available for office use in the near future. Although it is currently difficult to differentiate HSV-1 from HSV-2 genital infections, in most cases such differentiation is unnecessary, as the treatment is generally the same for both.

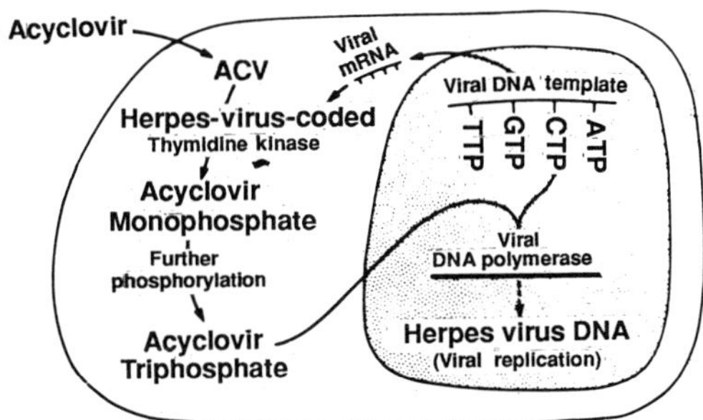


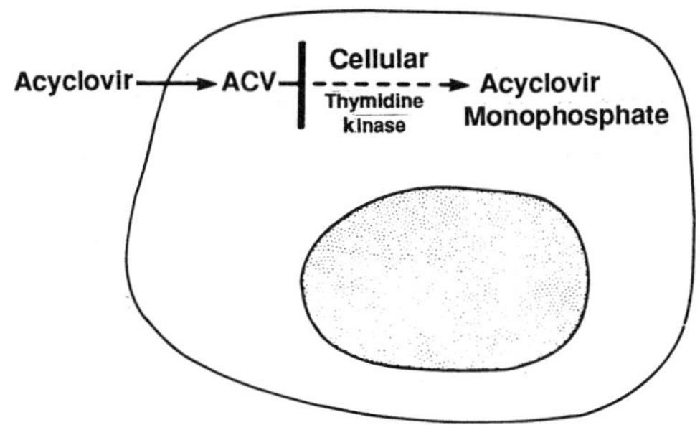


**Fig 20.** Mechanism of action of acyclovir. [From Mertz G, Corey L, Genital herpes simplex virus infections in adults, *Urol Clin North Am* (1984;11:103), with permission.]

## Treatment

Acyclovir represents the mainstay of treatment for herpes simplex viral infections. The drug, which is taken up more selectively by HSV-infected than by normal cells, is a viral thymidine kinase substrate which, when converted to its active form, inhibits viral DNA synthesis (Fig 20).[88] Although not viricidal, acyclovir helps relieve the symptoms of herpetic eruptions by shortening the healing time and decreasing the period of viral shedding. It is available in IV, topical, and oral forms.

The IV form of the drug is used in cases of severe disease (usually primary episodes), or when complications arise. It is given in a dosage of 5 mg/kg of body weight q 8 h for 5 to 7 days, or until clinical resolution occurs. If symptoms are not severe enough to merit hospitalization, then primary infections may be treated by oral acyclovir in a dosage of 200 mg given five times/day for 7 to 10 days.

Recurrent episodes may also be treated with acyclovir, in a dosage of 200 mg given orally five times/day for 5 days. It is most useful when started within 48 hours after the onset of lesions.

The other purported use for oral acyclovir is in prophylactic treatment of the patient who has frequent recurrent infections (>6 infections/year). In such cases, the use of acyclovir has been shown to prevent approximately 75% of recurrences and to lessen the number of recurrences in an additional 20% of patients. However, prophylactic acyclovir treatment is costly; if this regimen is elected, the patient's recurrence rate should be reassessed after 1 year of treatment.[38,78,80,89] Patients should also be informed that once the medication is stopped, the rate of recurrence returns to baseline. Topical acyclovir is substantially less effective than the oral drug, and may only minimally reduce the time of viral shedding during recurrences.[90,91] Cool astringent compresses may be helpful for local symptomatic relief.

Herpes infections pose special problems for the pregnant patient, because the virus has the potential to cross the placenta and affect the unborn child. Because the effects of acyclovir on the fetus have not been established, it should not be administered to pregnant patients unless the maternal infection is life threatening. The risk of passage to the neonate during a vaginal delivery should be considered if the patient has either active infection or positive cervical cultures; under such circumstances a Cesarean section is advised.

Women with genital herpes should be instructed to have a yearly Papanicolaou smear, as the HSV virus has been implicated in the pathogenesis of cervical carcinoma.

Patients with genital herpes should be advised to abstain from sexual activity during periods of active disease. Although not curable, the disease is manageable, and information to this effect should be presented to afflicted patients.

## HUMAN PAPILLOMAVIRUS (HPV) INFECTION

Condyloma acuminata, also referred to as genital or venereal warts, are caused by the human papillomavirus (HPV). HPV is a DNA virus and a member of the papovavirus group. Although the true incidence is unknown, it is extremely prevalent: approximately 2 million visits were made to private physicians' offices for evaluation of HPV infections in 1987 alone (Fig 21).[14] HPV infection may present as clinical or subclinical disease.

Clinical disease reveals itself with the typical polypoid, mulberry lesions that are usually associated with HPV types 6 or 11.[92] These lesions are usually unsightly but asymptomatic. Trauma to such lesions, however, may cause irritation or bleeding. Subclinical disease is usually caused by HPV subtypes 16, 18, 31, and 33. The subclinical, or flat, condyloma are more commonly seen in association with cervical dysplasia or carcinoma in women, and with penile intraepithelial neoplasia in men. Evidence of subclinical disease may be found in 1% to 2% of all Papanicolaou smears analyzed, although the significance of this is as yet unclear.[93]

Condyloma, clinical or subclinical, have a predilection for moist body areas. In men, the most common areas for lesions are on the penile shaft, the scrotum, the groin, and the perirectal region. Lesions are often noted under the foreskin of uncircumcised men as well as at the urethral meatus. In women, both the internal and external genitalia are usually affected, as well as the urethra and perirectal areas.

Transmission occurs primarily by sexual contact. Approximately 60% of patients who have unprotected sexual intercourse with an infected individual will develop lesions, usually within 3 months.[94,95] In addition, respiratory papillomatosis, although uncommon, may be seen in infants, presumably from acquisition of virus during birth.[96] An index of suspicion should be raised if the disease is found on the

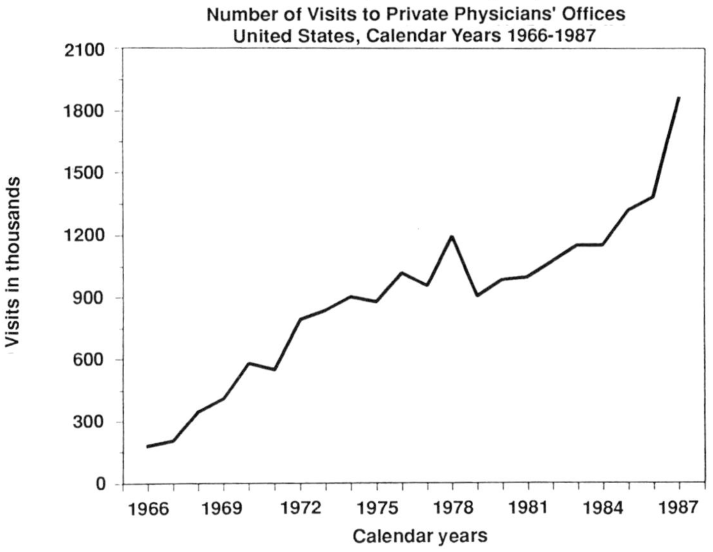


**Fig 21.** Visits to private physicians' offices in the U.S. for HPV during the years 1966–1987. [Courtesy of the Centers for Disease Control, Atlanta, GA.]

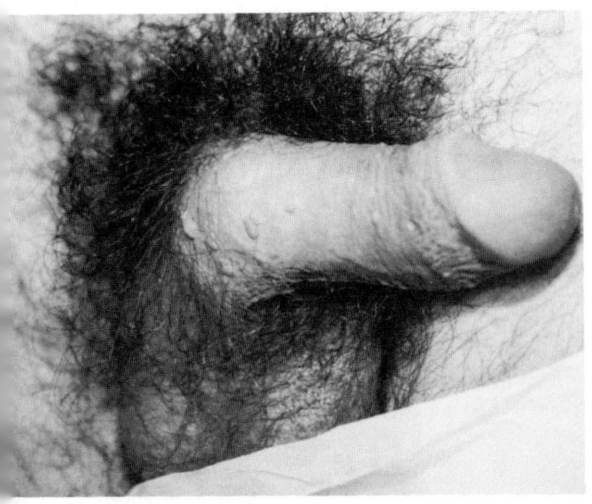

**Fig 22.** Condylomata of penile shaft.

external genitalia of children, as this may be, but is not necessarily, a sign of child abuse. Parents should be carefully questioned, as there have been several unfortunate instances where a couple has been hastily accused of abusing their child only later to be exonerated after nonsexual transmission was shown to have occurred. Nonsexual transmission of HPV occurs in at least some instances: towels, tanning beds, and hot tubs have been implicated as carriers.

## Diagnosis

Typical warty growths on the external genitalia make the diagnosis of condyloma easy (Fig 22). Large lesions on the penile shaft, with cellular changes characteristic of superficial squamous cell carcinoma, are referred to as giant condyloma of Buschke-Löwenstein. Examination of the penis, including the area beneath the foreskin and the urethral meatus should be done. The meatus may be examined either by inverting the mucosa or by using a nasal speculum to visually inspect the fossa navicularis. In addition, perirectal areas should be examined to rule out perirectal disease (Fig 23).

Subclinical disease, especially in men, presents more of a problem for both diagnosis and treatment. Subclinical disease may be detected by applying a solution of 3% to 5% acetic acid (vinegar) to the penile shaft for 5 to 10 minutes (Fig 24), followed by examination of the penis under magnification. Loupes, colposcopy, and handheld magnifying lenses have been used.[97,98] Involved areas of subclinical flat condyloma appear as white patches. It is important that the patient refrain from sex for approximately 1 week prior to magnified scanning, as inflammatory or traumatic le-

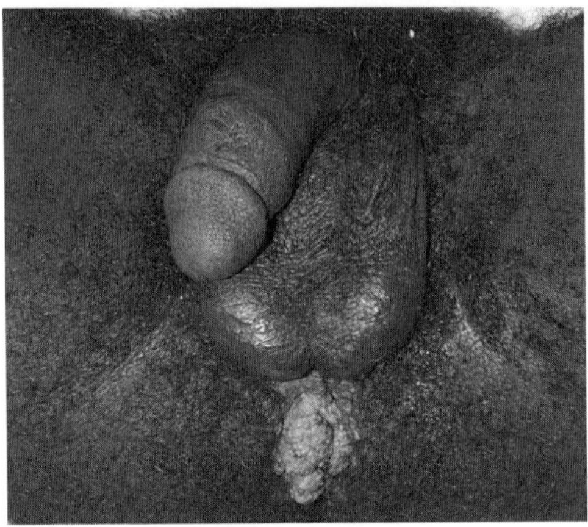

**Fig 23.** Large perianal condyloma.

sions induced by intercourse may also appear white after soaking with acetic acid. Biopsy of the acetowhite areas can be performed under local anesthesia in the office with the use of a small Baker's skin punch. Specimens should be handled in an atraumatic fashion to prevent crushing artifacts. When condyloma is present, characteristic cells called koilocytes are noted in the epidermis. The fact that these microscopic lesions contain HPV DNA has been confirmed with the use of Southern blot mapping.[99] Only 16% of lesions that produce acetowhitening but that do not have koilocytic histologic changes will harbor HPV.[100] Biopsy is, therefore, recommended when one suspects nonspecific changes.

The urethra represents a potential HPV reservoir in the male, and may be investigated with the use of the urethral brushing or urine cytology.[101] If the results of these tests are positive, urethroscopy should be performed. Although specific DNA typing of HPV is possible using Southern blot hybridization techniques, this procedure is time-consuming and costly.[102] Further, multiple types of HPV may be present simultaneously. In the clinical setting at present, therefore, Southern blot analysis for HPV does not appear to be practical.

### Treatment

There are several treatment options for grossly visible condyloma acuminata. Limited gross disease or small lesions may be treated with local applications of podophyllin, trichloracetic acid, and liquid nitrogen. Podophyllin contains podophyllotoxin, which arrests cell division in metaphase; it should be applied directly to lesions with an applicator stick. Petroleum jelly should be applied around a lesion prior to application of podophyllin, to prevent contact with normal skin areas. The patient should be instructed to leave the podophyllin in place for 3 to 4 hours before washing; if left longer, skin ulceration may occur. Although inexpensive to use, podophyllin usually necessitates multiple treatments and offers only a 25% success rate.[103] Podophyllin is contraindicated in pregnant patients, and should not be used on infants or on the vagina, cervix, or urethra. Trichloracetic acid 50% solution may be used in a fashion similar to podophyllin.

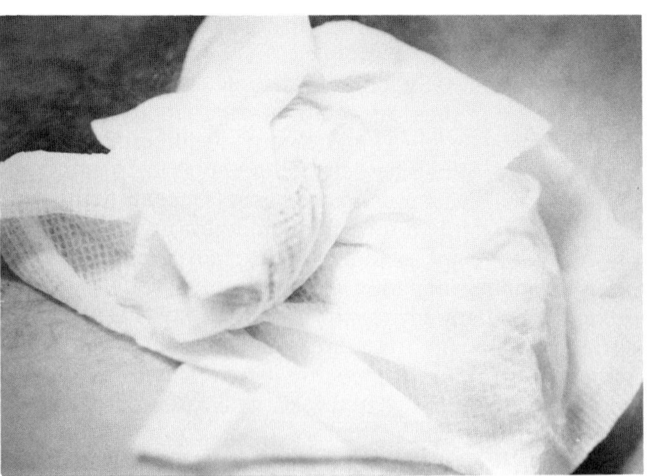

**Fig 24.** Penile wrap with 5% acetic acid for detection of subclinical human papilloma virus infection.

Immunotherapy with interferon has been attempted; intralesional injections were administered three times weekly for 3 weeks. Although somewhat effective, there are side effects which preclude the use of interferon as a first-line treatment at this time.[104,105]

Laser therapy with the $CO_2$, KTP, or Nd:YAG units are presently being used in cases of extensive or subclinical disease. Such treatments may be performed on an outpatient basis under local anesthesia. The anesthetic agent may be administered beneath the lesions with a fine-gauge needle. The laser causes coagulation necrosis, or vaporization of the lesion. Its benefit, not shared by electrocautery, is the excellent cosmetic result. In addition to treating the lesion itself, the laser beam should be applied in a defocused mode to a 3- to 5-mm rim of tissue surrounding the lesion, as virus has been demonstrated in this zone (Fig 25).[106] The presence of viral DNA has been demonstrated in the smoke of lasered condylomata; therefore, a smoke evacuator is indicated when treating lesions by laser.[107]

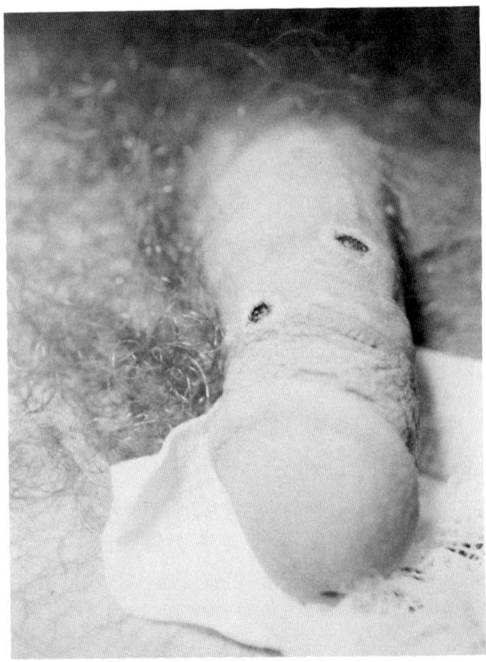

**Fig 25.** Charring effect after laser treatment of penile condyloma; note also the rim of the whitened area around each lesion which was treated with the laser in a defocused mode.

Visits should be scheduled every 2 months, until no further evidence of disease is noted. Condoms should be worn until the patient is found to be disease free. Clinical and subclinical extensive growth beneath the foreskin in an uncircumcised male is extremely difficult to eradicate with the laser or other methods; circumcision should be advised under these circumstances.

Management of condyloma of the urethra remains controversial. While meatal lesions can be treated with the laser, questions surround the treatment of patients with positive urine cytologies or brushings. In such instances, urethroscopy should be performed. If intraurethral lesions are seen, they should be treated with the KTP or Nd:YAG laser. The laser fiber can be passed through the working channel of a pediatric cystoscope to deliver the laser energy. If no lesions are noted, two options are available: a follow-up cytology after 3 to 6 months with the belief that the first cytology represented a false-positive reading, or treatment with intraurethral application of 5-fluorouracil cream twice daily for 2 weeks. Such cream is extremely caustic and may cause severe dermatitis of the hands and scrotum; patients should be warned of this and precautions should be taken.

Perirectal condyloma are commonly noted and routine examinations should include a check for their presence. The Nd:YAG and KTP lasers are preferred because of the deeper penetration these devices permit. Anoscopy should be performed as well, although condyloma rarely extend beyond the anal verge.

There is no clear-cut consensus as to what should be done regarding "the white scrotum." Although condyloma can be isolated from the acetowhite scrotum in some instances, the author's belief is that, in most instances, the acetowhitening is due to inflammatory changes and therapy probably is not indicated.

### Treatment Results

Success in eradicating HPV with the laser has been difficult to measure. Gross exophytic disease is successfully treated with a single laser treatment in 80% to 90%

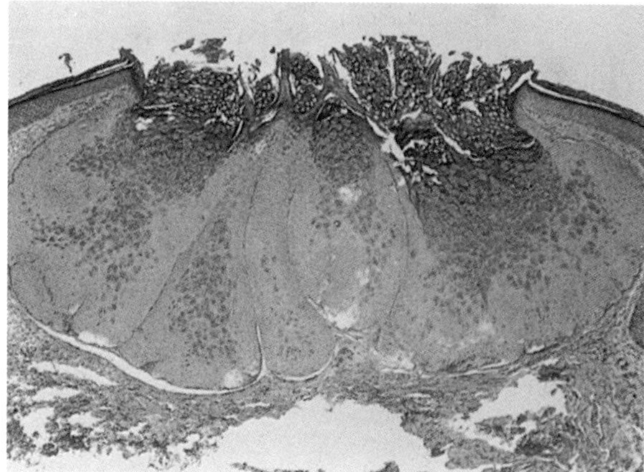

**Fig 26.** Molluscum body under low-power magnification. [From Korting GW, *Practical Dermatology of the Genital Region* (Philadelphia: WB Saunders Co; 1981), with permission.]

of cases, at least in the short term.[108,109] Subclinical infection is much more difficult to eradicate, and has a 50% recurrence rate over 20 months, despite the administration of multiple treatments.[101]

Ideally, effective therapy for HPV should reduce the risk of cervical cancer. For this reason, high-risk men whose partners' Papanicolaou smear shows severe dysplasia or carcinoma in situ should be evaluated. Patients with gross lesions should be treated. The evaluation of asymptomatic men whose female sexual consorts have had a Class II Papanicolaou smear, showing only inflammation, is probably not indicated.

A lack of specific antiviral therapy for HPV continues to make this disease difficult to treat effectively. It should be emphasized to the patient at the outset that the disease is difficult to eradicate and that multiple treatments may be required. By doing so, the patient will not be disappointed or have unrealistic expectations.

## MOLLUSCUM CONTAGIOSUM

Molluscum contagiosum is a benign viral infection of the skin. The disease is common among children and young adults. In the adult population, lesions have a predilection for the genital region, and there is good evidence that the disease is sexually transmitted.[110]

Molluscum contagiosum virus is a poxvirus which replicates in the cell cytoplasm, producing cytoplasmic inclusions and hyperplasia of infected cells. When examined microscopically, molluscum contagiosum lesions show hypertrophied epidermis with a central core of acanthosis. Viral inclusion bodies called Henderson-Paterson bodies or molluscum bodies are seen in cells of the central core (Fig 26).

The incubation period of molluscum contagiosum is generally between 2 and 6 weeks.[111] Lesions appear as flesh-colored papules, with a characteristic dimpled or umbilicated center (Fig 27). A diagnosis can be made without biopsy, based on the appearance of these lesions, in the majority of cases. The lesions generally number between one and 20; however, many more may occasionally be present.

The lesions are usually asymptomatic, and the condition may be discovered by the patient or by a physician on routine examination. A small percentage of patients develop an eczematoid reaction around the afflicted areas; this has been referred to as molluscum dermatitis.[112]

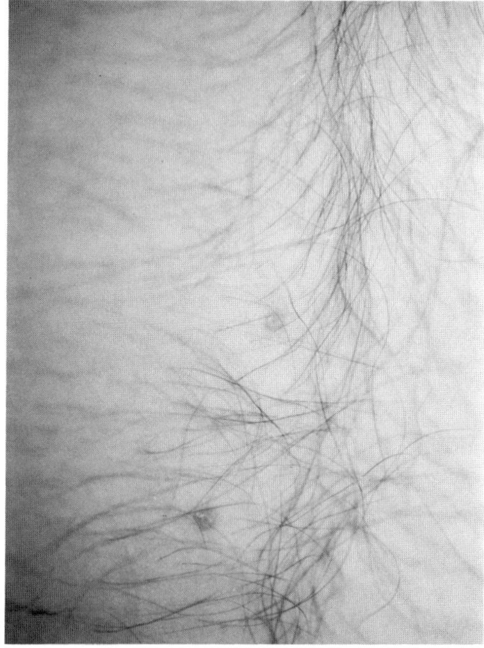

**Fig 27.** Skin lesions with central umbilicated centers characteristic of *Molluscum contagiosum.*

Molluscum contagiosum is a self-limited condition, but may take 6 months to 3 years to resolve. Treatment is advised, to reduce autoinoculation and transmission to others. Treatment by use of a sharp dermal currette to scrape out the central core is effective, and may be performed without anesthesia in cooperative patients. Topical treatments with phenol, or cryotherapy with liquid nitrogen, have also been used. When possible, sexual partners should be examined for the presence of the disease. It is important to schedule a follow-up examination after the initial treatment, as developing lesions may not be apparent at the patient's first visit.

## ACQUIRED IMMUNODEFICIENCY SYNDROME

Acquired immunodeficiency syndrome (AIDS) has rightly received considerable attention in the medical literature since the first case was reported in 1981. AIDS represents the endstage of infection with the human immunodeficiency virus (HIV). The virus has been previously referred to as HTLV-3, and is an RNA retrovirus. It has an affinity for T-helper lymphocytes, monocytes, macrophages, and colorectal cells; however, helper T cells are selectively destroyed by the virus, thereby causing an immunodeficiency.

HIV infection usually starts as an acute illness characterized by malaise and low-grade fever. After resolution of this illness, the patient becomes asymptomatic for a variable period of time, until becoming affected with AIDS related complex (ARC), in which generalized lymphadenopathy becomes evident. The final stage of the disease, AIDS, is characterized by secondary infection (most notably with *Pneumocystis carinii* pneumonia), generalized body wasting, neurologic disease, and secondary cancers. Of the latter, Kaposi's sarcoma is most commonly seen and, when found in any patient under the age of 60, is diagnostic of AIDS.[113]

### Epidemiology

It would be appropriate to say that the number of cases of AIDS has exploded in recent years. The U.S. Public Health Service estimates that between 900,000 and 1.4 million people are currently infected with HIV, and predicts that the number will continue to rise. As of June 1990, the number of cumulative cases of AIDS in the U.S. was 136,204; the death toll had reached 83,145.[114,115] Only AIDS is reportable to the Centers for Disease Control, and so the numbers of asymptomatic individuals testing positive for HIV infection and those with ARC remains unknown (Table 3, Fig 28).

**TABLE 3. Number of AIDS Cases by Year in the United States***

| | Adults (No.) | Children (No.) |
|---|---|---|
| Before 1981 | 77 | 6 |
| 1981 | 292 | 14 |
| 1982 | 1073 | 28 |
| 1983 | 2882 | 74 |
| 1984 | 5,860 | 110 |
| 1985 | 10,959 | 223 |
| 1986 | 17,810 | 302 |
| 1987 | 26,279 | 461 |
| 1988 | 31,208 | 539 |
| 1989 | 32,580 | 541 |
| **Total** | **129,020** | **2298** |

* Courtesy of the Centers for Disease Control, Atlanta, GA.

The time between infection with HIV and development of AIDS is variable, and ranges from a few months to greater than 10 years. In one study, AIDS developed in 36% of a group of homosexual and heterosexual men within 7 years after infection.[116] Most investigators now feel that, with enough time, AIDS will develop in all HIV-seropositive individuals unless some as yet unforeseen therapy is developed.[117]

HIV is believed to be transmitted in only three ways: sexual transmission by infected semen or vaginal fluids, exchange of infected blood or body secretions, and vertical transmission from infected mother to child. There continues to be no evidence of transmission to household members or close contacts other than by those methods listed above. Further, there have been no documented cases of HIV transmission from insect bites or from fomites.

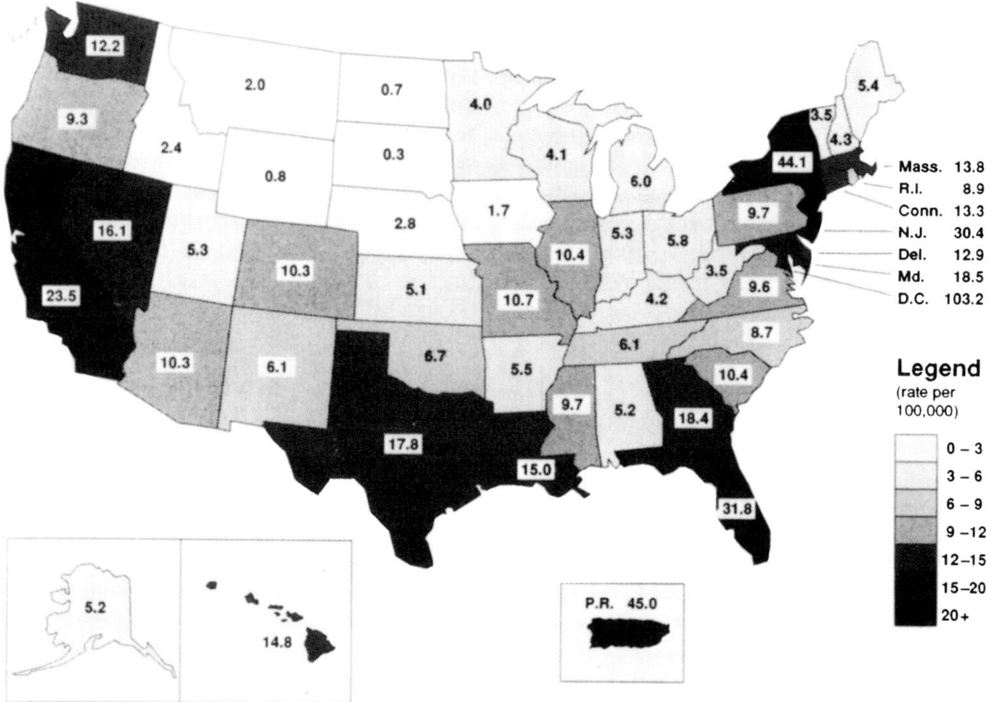


**Fig 28.** AIDS incidences per 100,000 population for cases reported August 1989 through July 1990 in the U.S. [From *HIV/AIDS Surveillance Report* (August 1990, courtesy of the Centers for Disease Control, Atlanta, GA).]

Homosexual and bisexual men make up the largest group of patients with AIDS. The next largest is the group of male IV drug abusers. In women, the disease is primarily transmitted by shared needles, although heterosexual transmission from an infected mate now accounts for an ever-increasing percentage of patients. The risk of becoming HIV-positive through blood transfusion or use of pooled blood products, although not zero, is minimal, because of routine testing and the use of heat treatment for certain blood-clotting factors. High-risk patients are asked not to donate blood because of the 4- to 12-week incubation period of the disease during which routine testing does not detect the presence of antibodies.

## Testing and Diagnosis

The Centers for Disease Control recommend that HIV testing be routinely performed when the results of such testing will contribute to the medical management of individuals or prevent further transmission of the disease.[38] Both pre- and posttest counseling are recommended, to assess and reduce the risk of HIV transmission through behavior modification and education. The reader should be aware that each state also has specific guidelines regarding HIV testing; consult the appropriate state Health Department for specific details. In most if not all states, the patient must sign an informed consent before being tested.

The screening test used to detect HIV infection is the enzyme-linked immunosorbent assay (ELISA), which detects antibodies to some HIV viral proteins. Although the specificity and sensitivity of the assay are high, it must be remembered that this test will be falsely negative during the incubation period of 4 to 12 weeks before detectable antibodies have appeared. If the initial ELISA test is positive, a repeat test should be performed in duplicate. If one of these tests is positive, then a Western-blot test should be performed. This test also measures antibodies to viral antigens.

The Western blot test is more difficult to interpret than ELISA, and results are given as positive, negative, or indeterminate. If indeterminate, the test should be repeated after 2 to 6 months. Tests are currently being developed which screen for the viral antigen rather than the antibody. They may turn out to be more specific than other tests currently available, but have not yet been licensed for general use.[118]

## Urological Manifestation of AIDS

Kaposi's sarcoma, *P carinii* pneumonia, and lymphomas are commonly seen in a patient with AIDS. Furthermore, opportunistic infections with unusual organisms such as cytomegalovirus, *Candida species*, *Toxoplasma gondii*, and *Cryptococcus neoformans* should alert the physician to the possibility of immunodeficiency and AIDS in the affected patient.

Kaposi's sarcoma, a soft-tissue tumor, can develop in any anatomic location. The lesions are reddish-purple in color and are thought to progress from a macular stage to a plaque to a nodular stage. The disease is multifocal in origin, and occurrence of new lesions is not believed to represent metastatic disease. As opposed to the more indolent form usually seen in older individuals of Italian, Jewish, and Mediterranean extraction, the new epidemic form of Kaposi's sarcoma has a more virulent course.[119] Involvement of the glans penis and penile shaft have been described and, with disease spread, urinary retention has been reported (Fig 29).[120] Systemic chemotherapy is used to treat disseminated Kaposi's sarcoma. For localized obstructing disease, external radiation is often useful.

In addition to Kaposi's sarcoma, other tumors are more common in the patient with AIDS. Lymphomas have already been mentioned, and there may be an increased incidence of testis tumors in the AIDS population, including an overrepresentation of nonseminomatous testis tumors. A higher incidence of disease is noted among black and Hispanic patients when compared with the population without the disease.[121]

Patients with AIDS have a higher incidence of infection, including urinary tract infections and STDs. In one study, pyuria was found in 52% and urinary tract infections in 20% of patients with AIDS.[122] Prostatic abscesses and epididymoorchitis have also been reported in HIV-infected patients, often secondary to infection with unusual organisms. Cytomegalovirus and *Mycobacterium* and *Salmonella* species have all been implicated as causative agents in epididymitis; orchiectomy may be required for resolution of infection or pain control.[123]

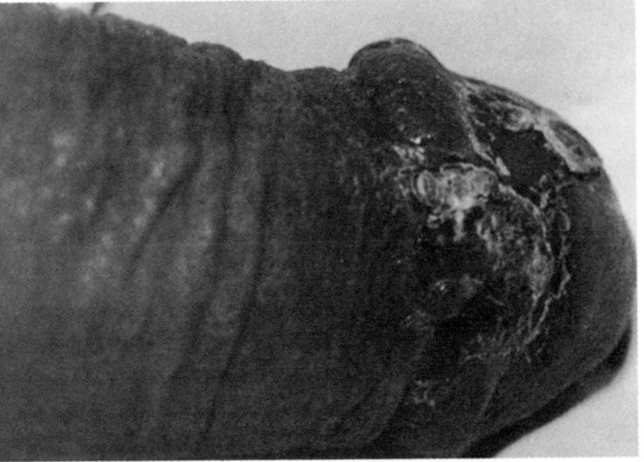

**Fig 29.** Kaposi's sarcoma of the penis in a patient with AIDS. [From Seftal AD, et al, Kaposi's sarcoma of the penis in a patient with the Acquired Immune Deficiency Syndrome, *J Urol* (1986; 136;673), with permission.]

STDs are more prevalent and pose more of a problem in the HIV-infected population.[124] Cutaneous lesions such as those caused by HSV, condyloma, and molluscum contagiosum may be slower to resolve, or may spread more extensively, depending on the degree of the patient's immunocompromised state. Syphilis in HIV-infected patients may recur even after appropriate therapy. Some authorities advise examination of cerebrospinal fluid and/or treatment with a regimen appropriate for neurosyphilis for all patients coinfected with syphilis and HIV, regardless of the clinical stage of syphilis.[125,126] All patients should receive careful follow-up. Serial titers on a VDRL or RPR test should be drawn to insure adequacy of treatment. If titers fail to decrease by fourfold over 6 months, repeated treatment is indicated.

Renal failure is commonly seen in patients with AIDS. Proteinuria and microscopic hematuria are the most common laboratory findings, and focal and segmental glomerulosclerosis are the most common lesions found when biopsy is performed.[127] The nephrotic syndrome is associated with a particularly poor prognosis, and may result in shortened survival.[122]

### Treatment

At present, only two drugs are commercially available and FDA approved for the treatment of HIV infection: zidovudine (Retrovir), also known as azidothymidine (AZT), and, most recently, didanosine (DDI).

AZT is a thymidine analogue that has been shown to inhibit replication of some retroviruses, including HIV, in vitro, by interfering with viral RNA-dependent DNA-polymerase.[128]

A double-blind, placebo-controlled trial showed that zidovudine increased the length and quality of life of patients with advanced HIV infection and AIDS.[129] The drug will only control the spread of disease; it does not cure AIDS. The current FDA-approved regimen is 100 mg q 4 h for 1 month, after which the dosage may be increased to 200 mg q 4 h, if the lower dosage was well tolerated. The most frequently reported side-effects are granulocytopenia and anemia, which occur in 3% to 12% of patients, depending on dosage.[130] Patients should, therefore, be carefully monitored during zidovudine therapy. Three percent to 5% of zidovudine recipients experience moderate to severe nausea while receiving the medication, regardless of the dosage used.

At present, it is unclear whether zidovudine offers any protective advantage to the fetus whose mother is HIV infected. Further, it is not known whether zidovudine causes fetal harm or whether it can affect reproductive capacity. Because of possible zidovudine and HIV excretion in human milk, breast feeding should be discontinued in the HIV-infected patient.

DDI was approved by the FDA in October 1991 for patients with AIDS who cannot tolerate AZT or whose health has deteriorated during zidovudine therapy. It has been approved for use in adults and children. Data is not yet available as to whether DDI therapy prolongs survival or decreases the incidence of opportunistic infections in patients with AIDS; therefore zidovudine should be used as first-line treatment. Adverse effects of DDI include pancreatitis and peripheral neuropathy; patients should be monitored for these problems. DDI should be given on an empty stomach since the absorption rate can be reduced by as much as 50% when taken with food.[131]

The risk of transmission of HIV per episode of percutaneous exposure to HIV-infected blood is approximately 0.4%[132] Studies have been undertaken in an attempt to assess the use of zidovudine for prophylaxis after occupational exposure. However, at this time, no clear-cut consensus can be drawn due to insufficient data. The worker should therefore be informed that the U.S. Public Health Service cannot make a recommendation for or against the prophylactic use of zidovudine in this setting.[130]

Research is presently being focused on the development of a vaccine against HIV, as well as the development of other antiviral agents. Progress is slow in this regard and zidovudine or DDI are currently the only treatment available to the patient with AIDS.

### Prevention

Since there is no effective treatment to eradicate the disease once an individual is infected, attention should be drawn to prevention of its spread. High-risk behavior, such as the sharing of syringes and needles, should be discouraged. Sexual spread can be controlled by abstinence or a mutually monogamous relationship. If this is not possible, condoms may reduce the risk. Women of childbearing age who are at high risk for HIV infection should receive HIV testing prior to conception.

Individuals in the health care professions should use precautions in handling the blood and body fluids of all patients, including using gloves, gowns, masks, and protective eyewear. Protective clothing is especially important in the operating room to minimize the risk of acquiring HIV infection from being splashed with infected body fluids. Needles should not be recapped, and should be disposed of safely in a properly marked container.[133] Inexperienced participants, ie, medical students, should not be part of the surgical team for an HIV-infected patient.[134]

Persons with AIDS or HIV infection cannot transmit the disease by casual contact, and should not be restricted from work or school. Inanimate objects such as telephones, water fountains, or toilets do not contribute to the spread of the disease. Household items, dishes, and eating utensils should be washed routinely in hot water and detergent, but there is no evidence that saliva can transmit infection.

Although much has been learned regarding HIV infection, fears continue to pervade the public's perception of this disease. It is the physician's responsibility not only to treat but to educate. Through education, falsehoods can be dispelled and methods of prevention stressed.

## VAGINITIS

Vaginal infections and discharge constitute a frequent source of urologic and gynecologic referrals. Vaginal complaints may prompt as many as 5 to 10 million office visits/year. Patients are often seen by urologists because of nonspecific complaints elicited by the primary care physician. Vaginal discharge or odor may be quite distressing or embarrassing to some patients who are quite relieved when asked about these symptoms. It is, therefore, important that the urologist be able to diagnose and treat these infections.

Normal vaginal discharge results from a combination of upper and lower genital tract secretions as well as normal bacterial flora. Although the flora is constantly changing, anaerobic bacteria are usually more prevalent than their aerobic counterparts by a factor of 5:1.[135] Normal secretions are odorless, clear or white, and homogenous. The normal vaginal pH is acidic, and ranges from 3.8 to 4.2; changes in the chemical environment may foster the growth of pathologic organisms.

Three of the most commonly encountered vaginal infections are bacterial vaginosis caused by *Gardnerella vaginalis, Trichomonas* (vaginitis), and *Candida* (vulvovaginitis). Each can be present in an asymptomatic state. The characteristics of each type of infection will be discussed separately (Table 4).

### Gardnerella Vaginalis

Bacterial vaginosis, or nonspecific vaginosis, is caused by the organism *G vaginalis* (previously *Hemophilis vaginalis* or *Hemophilis vaginale* or *Cornynebacterium vaginale*). It is a gram-variable coccobacillus that may be recovered from 30% to 70% of healthy asymptomatic women.[136]

**TABLE 4. Vaginitis**

| | Normal | Bacertial Vaginosis | Tricho-moniasis | Candidiasis |
|---|---|---|---|---|
| Major symptom | — | Odor | Discharge | Itch |
| Discharge present at introitus | No | Yes | Yes | No |
| Color of discharge | White | Gray | Yellow-gray | White |
| Viscosity | High | Low | Low | High |
| Location of discharge within vagina | Dependent portion | Adherent to vaginal walls | Adherent to vaginal walls | Adherent to vaginal walls |
| Mucosal erythema | None | None | Variable | Major |
| pH of environment | 3.8–4.5 | 5–6 | 5.0–6.5 | 3.8–4.5 |
| KOH Whiff Test | Negative | + + | + | Negative |
| Wet mount | Normal epithelial cells | "Clue" cells | Trichomonads | Budding filaments |

Symptoms of bacterial vaginosis only occur when the normal vaginal flora is changed. Although considered by many to be sexually transmitted, recent studies have shown no significant difference between the prevalence of clinical symptoms or isolation of the organism in groups of sexually active versus virginal adolescents.[137]

The major symptom of bacterial vaginosis is a disagreeable vaginal odor described as fishy or musty. The odor is caused by the production of polyamines by anaerobic bacteria. The discharge is thin, grey-white in color, and may be noted to be adherent to the vaginal wall on speculum exam. The patient usually does not complain of dyspareunia or dysuria, and the vulva and vaginal walls are usually not inflamed.

The diagnosis is made when three of the following four criteria have been fulfilled. First, the vaginal discharge should have a pH of greater than 4.5. While an elevated pH may be seen in *Trichomonas* infections, it is usually low in candidal infections. Second, the presence of "clue" cells should be noted on a wet mount. "Clue" cells are vaginal epithelial cells with cell borders that are granular or indistinct due to the adherence of bacteria (Figs 30,31). Third, a fishy odor is derived when a drop of vaginal discharge is mixed with one or two drops of 10% potassium hydroxide (KOH) (the whiff or sniff test). This odor is derived from the generation of volatile amines—putrescine and cadaverine—with the addition of alkali. Fourth, the characteristic discharge of bacterial vaginosis is present.[138,139] Vaginal cultures for *Gardnerella* are of low diagnostic value because of the prevalence of the organism in the asymptomatic population; therefore, treatment should not be based merely on a positive culture.

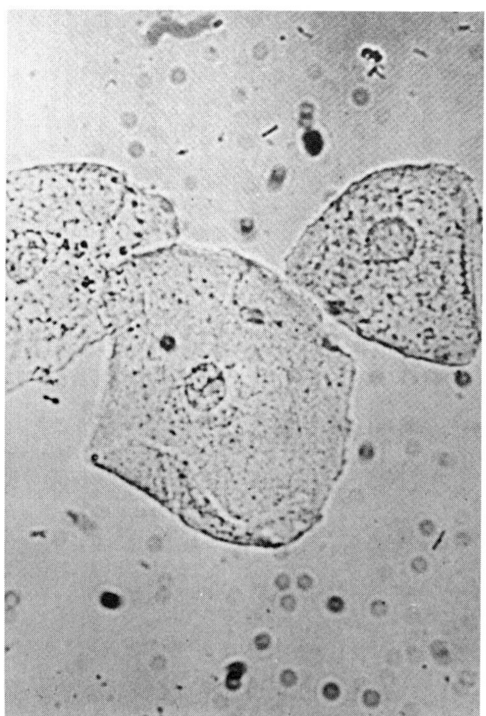

**Fig 30.** Normal vaginal epithelial cells; note the distinct cell borders. [From Holmes KK, et al (eds), *Sexually Transmitted Diseases* (New York: McGraw-Hill; 1984), with permission.]

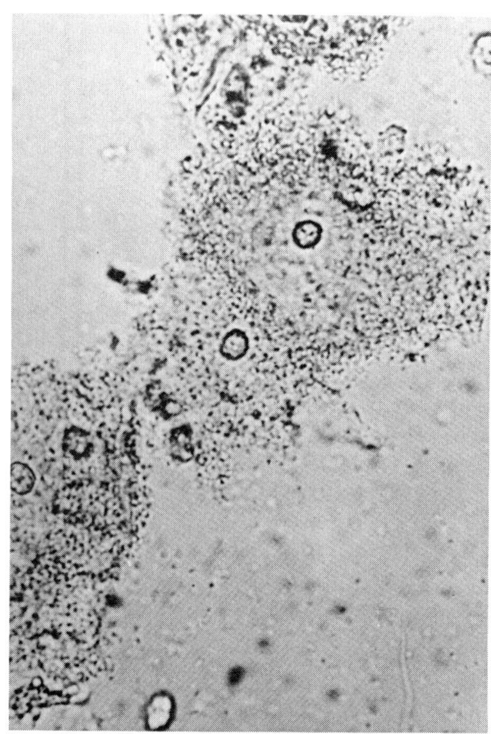

**Fig 31.** Vaginal epithelial cells with *H vaginalis* infection; note the indistinct cell borders which characterize these so-called "clue" cells. [From Holmes KK, et al (eds), *Sexually Transmitted Diseases* (New York: McGraw-Hill; 1984), with permission.]

The recommended treatment for bacterial vaginosis is metronidazole 500 mg bid for seven days. In pregnant patients or in those in whom metronidazole use is otherwise contraindicated, ampicillin 500 mg four times a day for seven days may be used; its cure rate, however, is lower.[140] Clindamycin vaginal cream has been used with good success.[141] There is no evidence to show that treatment of male partners will reduce the recurrence rate of bacterial vaginosis. Male partners, therefore, are not routinely treated. However, in cases that are difficult to eradicate, treatment of males may be of some help. Asymptomatic female carriers need not be treated.

### Trichomoniasis

Trichomonal vaginitis is caused by *T vaginalis,* a unicellular flagellate. The prevalence of trichomoniasis correlates well with sexual activity, and is highest among women with multiple sexual partners. The protozoan is isolated from between 60% to 100% of sexual partners of an individual with a positive culture. However, cases of nonsexual transmission are common, with viable organisms recovered from swimming pools, towels, and other fomites. Trichomonads can survive on toilet seats for up to 1 hour and in wet clothes for at least 3 hours. There is a high frequency of trichomoniasis in female patients presenting with other sexually transmitted disease; the converse is also true. Trichomonads are *not* part of the normal vaginal flora.

Approximately 50% of women harboring trichomonads in their vaginal secretions are asymptomatic.[142] When symptomatic, however, patients often complain of a copious vaginal discharge. The discharge may be white, gray, yellow, or greenish in color; occasionally, small bubbles may be present giving it a frothy appearance. The discharge may have a strong odor, though only 10% of women have this as a presenting complaint. Patients may complain of vaginal discomfort and irritation as the protozoan, though not systemically invasive, causes damage to epithelial cells. When erosion of the cervix by trichomonads has occurred, the term "strawberry cervix" may be used. This finding, however, is not common. The pH of the discharge is usually 5 to 6.5 (more alkaline than the usual vaginal environment).[143]

Diagnosis is made by direct microscopy of a vaginal wet mount. The wet mount is performed by taking a sample of the discharge and mixing with a small amount of normal saline. The sensitivity of direct microscopy in symptomatic women is about 75%, and the specificity is close to 100%. Asymptomatic women may have fewer resident organisms and therefore a lower sensitivity. The organisms are slightly larger than white blood cells, pear-shaped in contour, and have 3 to 5 flagella extending from one end. They are easily identified when moving, but if the wet mount is not fresh, or if the slide is cold, motion may be slow. Other studies, such as Papanicolaou smears and cultures, do not provide the accuracy of direct microscopic examination.[144–147] Once again, because of the alkaline nature of the discharge, the addition of KOH liberates amines, resulting in a positive sniff or whiff test.

Trichomoniasis is also treated with metronidazole. Either a single 2 g dose or 250 mg tid may be given for 7 days; the former is associated with higher rates of patient compliance. Patients should be warned not to drink alcohol during, and for 48 hours after, the treatment, because of the disulfiram effect.[148] The drug should not be given during pregnancy. Sexual partners should be treated simultaneously to prevent back and forth passage of the organism. Recurrence or failure to eradicate the organism is usually due to poor compliance, though resistant strains of *Trichomonas* have been reported.

### Candidal Vaginitis

Vaginal fungal infections are most commonly caused by *Candida albicans* or *Candida glabratta.* These commensal saprophytes may be isolated as part of the normal vaginal flora in approximately 25% of women. As a colonizer, *Candida* may not cause symptoms, so long as the vaginal milieu is intact. However, if the vaginal environment is disturbed, overgrowth of

*Candida* may occur. It is when this occurs that patients often are seen for evaluation and treatment.

Predisposing factors associated with candidal overgrowth include diabetes, antibiotic use, pregnancy, immunosuppression, and obesity. Antibiotics, especially those with broad-spectrum efficacy, are thought to suppress the growth of vaginal lactobacilli, thereby allowing the *Candida* to thrive. During pregnancy, the enhanced growth of *Candida* may be due to high estrogen levels.

The predominant symptom of candidal vaginitis is intense pruritis; accompanying dysuria or dysparunia may be present. A vaginal discharge of variable amount, thick and white in character but with no odor, may be present. Erythema and edema of the vaginal mucosa and vulva may be present on physical examination. On speculum examination, white patches adherent to the vaginal mucosa may be present. The pH of the discharge is usually less than 4.5.

Microscopic examination of a mixture of the vaginal discharge and a 10% KOH solution should be performed; the presence of pseudohyphae or hyphae confirm the diagnosis. Absence of these findings may occur in up to 50% of women with candidiasis.[149] If the diagnosis is suggested despite a negative smear, then culture with Nickerson's or Sabouraud's media should be performed.[150]

Treatment should be limited to symptomatic women with candidal infections, and can be accomplished by the topical or intravaginal application of antifungal agents. Clotrimazole or miconazole can be used in single, daily doses for 7 days with a cure rate approaching 90%. Boric acid gelatin suppositories or nystatin suppositories are alternatives, although they may offer inferior cure rates as compared with the imidazole agents above. *Candida* vaginitis is not considered to be an STD per se, and treatment of male contacts is usually not necessary.

Recurrence or persistence of candidal vaginitis is difficult to treat. An attempt to control predisposing factors should be made. Some have advocated prophylactic use of oral ketoconazole, with the belief that elimination of intestinal candida might help to reduce vaginal growth.[151] While this is true, recurrence rates remain high when the medication is stopped. Further, ketoconazole has its own set of associated problems, and the patient with recurrent disease might do best with short courses of refillable imidazole agents which are now available without a prescription.

## ECTOPARASITIC INFECTIONS

### Scabies

Scabies is a parasitic dermatosis caused by the human itch mite, *Sarcoptes scabiei*. The mite is small, just visible to the naked eye. The female of the species burrows into the stratum corneum, where it lives for about 1 month and lays its eggs. The burrows parallel the skin and do not extend below the stratum corneum. When egg laying is complete, the female mite dies at the end of its burrow. Ten percent of eggs will go on to become adult mites, and the hatched mites require approximately 2 weeks to mature.

The primary symptom of the disease is intense itching, which characteristically occurs nocturnally. The incubation period for previously uninfected patients is often several weeks, during which time the mites actively proliferate under the skin. This period is much shorter in previously infected individuals, and symptoms are believed to be a result of allergic sensitization to the mite or its products. The inflammatory lesions may be papules, nodules, excoriations, or vesicular (especially in children).

The diagnostic lesion, the burrow, may often be obscured by incessant scratching. The best places to look for burrows are on the hands, the extensor surface of the wrists, and the web spaces between the fingers. The burrows are several millimeters to a few centimeters in length and slightly raised. With the aid of a magnifying glass, a black speck, the female mite, can be seen at the end of the burrow.

Scabies is not exclusively an STD, but is a disease of close social contact. Family members may become affected, and the clinician should suspect scabetic infestation when several members of a family or group complain of a pruritic eruption. In addition, scabies may be transmitted from animal vectors. The disease appears to be cyclical in nature, with epidemics occurring every 30 years and lasting approximately 15 years.[152,153]

**Diagnosis.** The diagnosis of scabies is confirmed by microscopic demonstration of any stage of the mite or inspissated excrement (scybala) from typical skin lesions. Fecal pellets are more commonly seen than the organism itself. Material can be obtained by scraping the skin overlying the burrow with a scalpel coated with mineral oil. The oil prevents the loss of diagnostic material and preserves the organism. Ideally, four or five lesions should be scraped, after which the scrapings are transferred to a glass slide and examined with a microscope under low magnification. Other diagnostic methods, such as epidermal shave biopsy or dermal curettage, may also be used (Fig 32).[154]

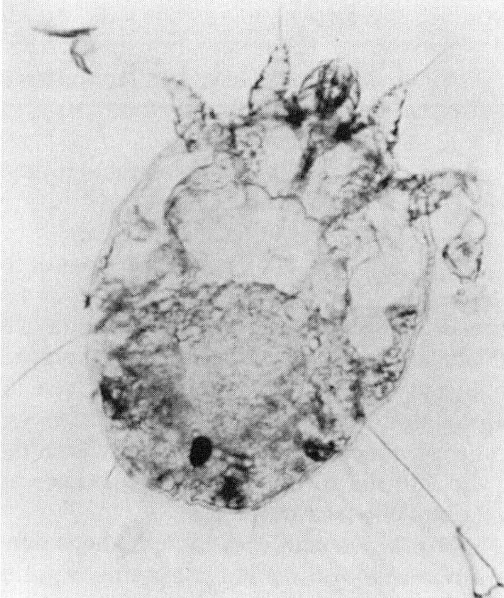

**Fig 32.** The female of the mite *Sarcoptes scabiei*. [From Sauer GC, *Manual of Skin Diseases*, 5th ed (Philadelphia: JB Lippincott Co; 1985), with permission.]

**Treatment.** There are a number of topical scabicides which can be used to eradicate the disease. Members of the patient's immediate household, as well as sexual contacts, should be treated; casual contacts need not be treated. Clothing and bed linens should be washed and dried in the hot cycle of each machine. Furniture and outerwear need not be cleaned, since the mite only survives a few days when separated from its human host.

Lindane, γ-benzene hexachloride (Kwell, Scabene) is a commonly used scabicide and is recommended for older children and adults. However, other therapies are best used in infants and small children, because of potential neurotoxicities in this group. The same is true for a pregnant or nursing patient.

Lindane is available in a cream or lotion.[155–157] The agent should be applied to all areas below the neck after bathing in tepid water. Particular attention should be paid to the genitalia, hands, and feet. It is best applied by a second individual, to assure that all portions of the body have been covered. One ounce is usually sufficient to cover the trunk and extremities of an average adult. The medication should be left in place for 8 to 12 hours, and then washed off. One treatment usually is adequate, but a second treatment 1 week later is recommended to destroy any recently hatched larva from eggs present at the initial therapy. An irritant dermatitis can occur if the medication is used too frequently.[158,159]

Crotamiton cream 10% is the preferred scabicide for infants, young children, and pregnant and lactating women. Two applications are necessary, at 24-hour intervals, with the medication washed off 24 hours after the second application. In infants and small children, the scalp and head should be included with care to avoid splashing medication in the eyes and mouth.

Topical sulfur and benzyl benzoate are other agents that have been used to treat scabies. Sulfur has staining properties and an unpleasant odor; benzyl benzoate is not commercially available in the United States.

Following effective treatment, it is not

uncommon to find that the patients continue to complain of persistent itching for 2 to 3 weeks. This pruritis is thought to be due to a hypersensitivity reaction to the dead mite or mite antigens. Topical steroids may provide relief. If the itching continues beyond this period, reexamination is indicated.

### Pediculosis Pubis

The lice that infest humans are small, wingless insects that are obligate parasites. Two species are parasitic for humans: *Phthirus pubis* (pubic or crab louse) and *Pediculosis humanus*. The latter is divided into two varieties: capitus (head louse) and corporis (body louse). The morphologic differences between head and body lice are slight and of little practical importance. The pubic or crab louse has two pairs of legs equipped with powerful claws which permit the louse to firmly hold onto pubic hair or clothing fibers and which serve as elements for locomotion.

Lice mate frequently; their eggs or nits are attached or cemented firmly to hairs at the hair/skin junction or clothing fibers. The cement is quite resilient, and the eggs hatch into nymphs in approximately 1 week. Body lice frequently lay their eggs on clothing seams.

Lice feed on human blood; to do so, they inject two cutting stylettes through the skin until a subcutaneous capillary is found. Saliva is injected and mixed with the host's blood, and may act as an irritant. Further, the body louse may act as a vector in the transmission of typhus, relapsing fever, and trench fever. Crab lice are not significant vectors of disease.

Head and body lice are acquired by personal contact or by wearing infected clothes. They may also be passed from individual to individual by sharing combs or brushes. Lice may infest beds and bed linens temporarily in parasitized individuals. Pubic or crab lice are more commonly transmitted by close, usually sexual, contact. About ⅓ of patients have other currently untreated sexual diseases. Crab lice are thought to be able to survive for only about a day when away from their host.

The most common site affected is the pubic region, but in hairy individuals the thigh, trunk, and facial hair may be involved. Eyebrow and eyelash infestation should be checked for, especially in small children.

**Diagnosis.** Diagnosis is made by the identification of the adult louse or nits. The nit can be distinguished from kinks or knots in the hair by examining the hair under a microscope. The duration of infestation can be estimated by the distance of the nit from the skin. After successful treatments, egg casings are empty on microscopic examination (Fig 33).

**Treatment.** Patients infested with lice should be treated simultaneously with their sexual contacts to prevent reinfestation. Uninfested household members need not be treated. Clothing and bed linens should be washed and dried using the hot cycle. Brushes and combs can be discarded, boiled in water, or washed in Lindane shampoo.

Lindane shampoo is an effective pediculocide. It should be lathered into affected sites for 4 minutes and then rinsed off. The lotion may also be used, but must be left in place 8 to 12 hours after application. Shaving is unnecessary, but nit removal requires the use of a fine tooth comb. Lindane should not be used on infants, small children, or pregnant and lactating women. Alternately, pyrethins and permethrin 1% cream may be applied to affected areas and washed off after 10 minutes. Treatment for involved eyelashes requires a thick application of petrolatum jelly twice a day for 8 days, followed by mechanical removal of the nits.[160–164]

## ENTERIC PATHOGENS

Certain enteric pathogens are transmitted by sexual contact. Salmonellosis, shigellosis, amebiasis, giardiasis, and hepatitis are transmitted by oral–anal contact.[165] When one considers that perhaps as many as 10% of individuals are homosexual or have participated in same-gender sexual relationships, it becomes obvious that a sig-

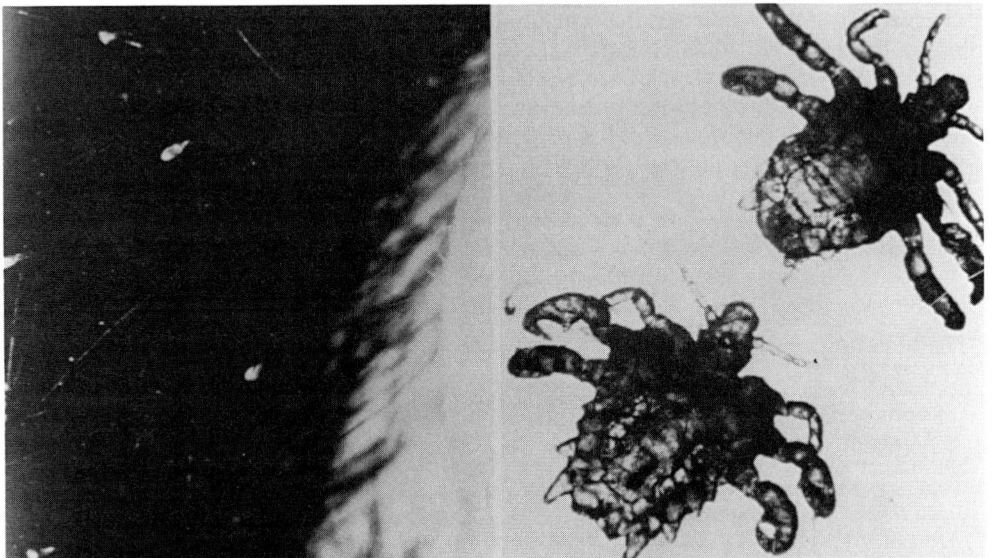

**Fig 33.** Pediculosis (crabs); on left, nits are seen attached to hair fibers, on right, the pubic louse or *Phthirus pubis* is seen magnified ×7.5. [From Sauer GC, *Manual of Skin Diseases,* 5th ed (Philadelphia: JB Lippincott Co; 1985), with permission.]

nificant number of individuals are prone to the development of these diseases.

Amebiasis and giardiasis strictly speaking are intestinal parasites. The former may cause symptoms ranging from mild diarrhea to severe proctocolitis with ulceration of the distal colon, indistinguishable from inflammatory bowel disease. *Giardia lamblia* is more typically a disease of the small intestine and symptoms usually include diarrhea, cramping, bloating, and nausea. Both organisms are commensal in a significant percentage of homosexual men.[166,167]

Diagnosis of *Entameba histolytica* is made by demonstration of the organism in the stool, on a wet mount of a rectal ulcer, or in a biopsy of a rectal mucosal lesion. If the organism is not seen, the presence of cysts or trophozoites may be sufficient to make the diagnosis. Serologic testing is also available.[168] Treatment is with metronidazole 750 mg tid for 5 to 7 days. Diiodohydroxyquin 650 mg tid for 20 days should be added if cysts are present.[169]

Giardia is more difficult to find in the stool; a small bowel biopsy may be necessary to make the diagnosis. Quinacrine hydrochloride 100 mg or metronidazole 250 mg tid are the recommended treatment regimens. In both amebiasis and giardiasis, a follow-up stool examination is recommended after treatment.[170]

Shigellosis is the most common cause of bacterial dysentery in homosexually active men. Infective symptoms start as watery diarrhea, which progress to severe abdominal cramping and the passage of small volumes of bloody mucoid stools.[171] Salmonella also causes watery diarrhea, which may contain mucus, but rarely blood. Treatment of *Shigella* is accomplished with sulfa methoxasole/trimethoprin (800 mg/160 mg) bid for 5 days or ampicillin 500 mg qid for 5 days. Salmonellosis is a self-limited disease and does not require treatment; in fact, the use of antibiotics may prolong the period of convalescent disease carriage.

Both hepatitis A and hepatitis B can be transmitted sexually.[172] Etiologic diagnosis of viral hepatitis is made by serologic testing. Most cases of acute viral hepatitis are asymptomatic or nonspecific, unless the patient presents with jaundice or dark urine. A detailed discussion is beyond the scope of this chapter; however, a vaccine is available for hepatitis B. Vaccination is recommended for all persons who have had multiple sex partners within the preceding 6 months as well as those in high-risk groups such as homosexual men, illicit IV-drug users, and prison inmates. Since the vaccine is expensive, it is cost effective to check for hepatitis B antibodies prior to vaccination in high-risk patients. The vaccination requires three injections over a 3-month period. Initially there was some controversy regarding the spread of AIDS with the vaccine; however, the long-term administration of the vaccine has not resulted in the transmission of even a single case of this disease.[173,174]

## REFERENCES


1. Clarke CW. Columbus, Charles VIII and the Serpentine Disease. *J Social Hygiene*. 1952; 38:306.
2. Rosebury T. *Microbes and Morals. The Strange Story of Venereal Disease*. New York: Viking; 1971.
3. Ricord PH. *A Practical Treatise on Venereal Disease* (1838) 2nd Ed. Doane AS, trans. New York: JS Redfield: Clinton Hall; 1944.
4. Bullough V, Bullough B. *The History of Prostitution*. New York: University Book; 1964.
5. Burnham JC. Medical inspection of prostitutes in America in the 19th century: the St. Louis experiment and its sequel. *Bull Hist Med*. 1971;45:203.
6. Pivar DJ. *Purity Crusade, Sexual Morality and Social Control, 1868–1900*. Westport, Conn: Greenwood Press; 1973.
7. Selvin M. Changing medical and societal attitudes toward sexually transmitted diseases: a historical overview. In: Holmes KK, Mordh P, Sparling PF, et al, eds. *Sexually Transmitted Diseases*. New York: McGraw-Hill; 1984:3.
8. Parran T. *Shadow on the Land*. New York: Reynal and Hitchcock; 1937.
9. Cutler JC, Arnold RC. Venereal disease control by health departments in the past: lessons for the present. *Am J Public Health*. 1988;78:372.
10. Clark T. *The control of syphilis in southern rural areas. A study by the United States Public Health Service and certain state and local departments of health in cooperation with the Julius Rosenwald Fund*. Chicago: Julius Rosenwald Fund; 1932.
11. Jones JH. *Bad Blood*. New York: Free Press; 1981.
12. Rockwell DH, Yobs AR, Moore MB Jr. The Tuskeegee study of untreated syphilis: the 30th year of observation. *Arch Intern Med*. 1964; 114:792.
13. Bell TA, Hein K. Adolescents and sexually transmitted diseases. In: Holmes K, ed. *Sexually Transmitted Diseases*. New York: McGraw-Hill Book Co.; 1984:chap 7.
14. *STD Statistics*. Atlanta, GA: Centers for Disease Control; US Dept of Health and Human Services; 1988.
15. Schaudinn FR, Hoffmann E. Vorlaüfiger Bericht uber das Vorkommen von Spirochaeten in Syphitischen Krakheitsproduckten und bei Papillomen. *Arb Gesundheitsamte*. 1905;22:527.
16. Schroeter AL, Turner RH, Lucas JB, et al. Therapy for incubating syphilis. Effectiveness of gonorrhea treatment. *JAMA*. 1971;218:711.
17. Chapel TA. The variability of syphilitic chancres. *Sex Trans Dis*. 1978;5:68.
18. Gjestland T. The Oslo study of untreated syphilis: an epidemiologic investigation of the natural course of syphilitic infection based on a restudy of the Boeck-Bruusgard material. *Acta Derm Venereol (Stockh)*. 1955;35(suppl 34):1.
19. Fiumara NJ. Late (tertiary) syphilis. In: Felman YM, ed. *Sexually Transmitted Diseases*. New York: Churchill Livingstone; 1986:39.
20. Kellogg DS. The detection of *Treponema pallidum* by a rapid direct fluorescent antibody darkfield procedure. *Health Lab Sci*. 1970; 7:34.
21. Hart G. Syphilis tests in diagnosis and therapeutic decision making. *Ann Intern Med*. 1986;64:368–376.
22. Hook EW III, Roddy RE, Handsfield HH. Ceftriaxone therapy for incubating and early syphilis. *J Infect Dis*. 1988;158:881–884.
23. Aronson IK, Keyoumars S. The enigma of the pathogenesis of the Jarisch-Herxheimer Reaction. *Br J Vener Dis*. 1976;52:313.
24. Bassereau A. *Traité des Affections de la Peau Symptomatiques de la Syphilis*. Paris: 1952:217.
25. Ducrey A. Experimentelle untersuchungen uber den Ansteckungsstoff des weichen Schankers und uber die Bubonen. *Monatsh Prakt Dermatol*. 1989;9:387.
26. Hammond GW, Slutchuk M, Scatliff J, et al. Clinical, epidemiological, laboratory and therapeutic features of an urban outbreak of chancroid in North America. *Rev Infect Dis*. 1980;2:867.
27. Sottnek FO, Biddle JW, Kraus SJ, et al. Isolation and identification of *Hemophilus ducreyi* in a clinical study. *J Clin Microbiol*. 1980; 12:170.
28. Borchardt KA, Hoke AW. Simplified laboratory technique for diagnosis of chancroid. *Arch Dermatol*. 1970;102:188.

29. Werman BS, Herskowitz LJ, Olansky S, et al. A clinical variant of chancroid resembling granuloma inguinale. *Arch Dermatol.* 1983; 119:890.
30. Bowmer MI, Nsanze H, D'Costa LJ, et al. Single-dose ceftriaxone for chancroid. *Antimicrob Agents Chemother.* 1987;31:67–69.
31. Schmid GP. The treatment of chancroid. *JAMA.* 1985;255:1757–1762.
32. Schachter J, Osaba AO. Lymphogranuloma venereum. *Br Med Bull.* 1983;39:151.
33. Osoba AO. Sero-epidemiological study of lymphogranuloma venereum in Western Nigeria. *Afr J Med Sci.* 1977;6:125.
34. Coutts WE. Lymphogranuloma venereum: a general review. *Bull WHO.* 1950;2:545.
35. Rainey R. The association of lymphogranuloma inguinale and cancer. *Surgery.* 1954;35:221.
36. King AJ, Barwell CF, Catterall RD, et al. Intradermal tests in the diagnosis of lymphogranuloma venereum. *Br J Vener Dis.* 1956; 32:209.
37. Schacter J, Smith DE, Dawson CR, et al. Lymphogranuloma venereum. Comparison of the Frei test, complement fixation test and isolation of the agent. *J Infect Dis.* 1969;120:372.
38. *MMWR.* Atlanta, Ga: Centers for Disease Control; US Dept of Health and Human Services; 1989:S-8.
39. Fritz GS, Hulder WR Jr, Dodson RF, et al. Mutilating granuloma inguinale. *Arch Dermatol.* 1975;111:1464.
40. Peck S. Granuloma inguinale. *Arch Dermatol.* 1968;98:555.
41. Hart G. Psychological and social aspects of venereal disease in Papua, New Guinea. *Br J Vener Dis.* 1974;50:453.
42. Davis CM. Granuloma inguinale. A clinical histological and ultrastructural study. *JAMA.* 1970;211:632.
43. Breschi LC, Goldman G, Shapiro SR. Granuloma inguinale in Vietnam: successful therapy with ampicillin and lincomycin. *J Am Vener Dis Assoc.* 1975;1:118.
44. Robinson H, Cohen MM. Treatment of granuloma inguinale with erythromycin. *J Invest Dermatol.* 1950;20:407.
45. Schoolnik GK, Fernandez R, Tai JY, et al. Gonococcal pili: primary structure and receptor binding domain. *J Exper Med.* 1984;159:1351.
46. Harrison WO. Gonococcal urethritis. *Urol Clin North Am.* 1984;11:45.
47. Hooper RR, Reynolds GH, Jones OG, et al. Cohort study of venereal disease, I. The risk of gonorrhea transmission from infected women to men. *Am J Epidemiol.* 1978; 108:136.
48. Soendjojo A. Gonococcal urethritis due to fellatio. *Sex Trans Dis.* 1983;10:41.
49. Neinstein LS, Goldenring J, and Carpenter S. Nonsexual transmission of sexually transmitted diseases: an infrequent occurrence. *Pediatrics.* 1984;74:67.
50. McCormick WM, Stumacher RJ, Johnson D, et al. Clinical spectrum of gonococcal infection in women. *Lancet.* 1977;1:1182.
51. Romanowski B, Harris JRW. Sexually transmitted diseases. *Clin Symp.* 1984;36:1.
52. Judson FN. Gonococcal urethritis: Diagnosis and treatment. *Arch Androl.* 1979;3:329.
53. Moy JG, Clasen ME. The patient with gonococcal infection. *Prim Care.* 1990;17:59.
54. Hutt DM, Judson FN. Epidemiology and treatment of oropharyngeal gonorrhea. *Ann Intern Med.* 1986;104:655.
55. Faruki H, Kohmescher RN, McKinney WP, et al. A community based outbreak of infection with Penicillin-resistant *Neisseria gonorrhoeae* not producing Penicillinase (chromosomally mediated resistance). *N Engl J Med.* 1985; 313:607.
56. Morse SA, Johnson SR, Biddle JW, et al. High level tetracycline resistance in *Neisseria gonorrhoeae* is due to the acquisition of the streptococcal tet M determinant. *Antimicrob Agents Chemother.* 1986;30:664.
57. *MMWR.* Atlanta, Ga: Centers for Disease Control; US Dept of Health and Human Services. 1987;36:757.
58. *MMWR.* Atlanta, Ga: Centers for Disease Control; US Dept of Health and Human Services. 1990;39:285.
59. Crider SR, Colby SD, Miller LK, et al. Treatment of penicillin-resistant *Neisseria gonorrhoeae* with oral norfloxacin. *N Engl J Med.* 1984;311:137.
60. McCutchan JA. Epidemiology of venereal urethritis: Comparison of gonorrhea and nongonococcal urethritis. *Rev Infect Dis.* 1984;6:669.
61. Thompson SE, Washington AE. Epidemiology of sexually transmitted *Chlamydia trachomatis* infections. *Epidemiol Rev.* 1983;5:96.
62. Pruessner HT, Hansel NK, Griffiths M. Diagnosis and treatment of chlamydial infections. *Am Fam Physician.* 1986;34:81.
63. Bowie NR, Wang S, Anderson ER, et al. Etiology of nongonococcal urethritis. Evidence for *C. trachomatis* and *U. urealyticum. J Clin Invest.* 1977;59:735.
64. Schacter J. Chlamydial infections. *N Engl J Med.* 1978;298:423.
65. Bell TA, Grayston, JT. Centers for Disease Control guidelines for prevention and control of *Chlamydia trachomatis* infections: summary and commentary. *Ann Intern Med.* 1986; 104:524.
66. Richmond SJ, Sparling PF. Genital chlamydial infections. *Am J Epidemiol.* 1976;103:428.
67. Brunham RC, Paavonen J, Stevens CE, et al. Mucopurulent cervicitis: the ignored counterpart in women of urethritis in men. *N Engl J Med.* 1984;311:1.

68. McCormack WM, Rosner B, McComb DE, et al. Infection with *Chlamydia trachomatis* in female college students. *Am J Epidemiol.* 1985;121:107.

69. Tam MR, Stamm WE, Handsfield HH. Culture independent diagnosis of *Chlamydia trachomatis* using monoclonal antibodies. *N Engl J Med.* 1984;310:1146.

70. Reichart CA, Gaydos CA, Brady WE, et al. Evaluation of Abbot test-pack *Chlamydia* for detection of *Chlamydia trachomatis* in STD clinic patients. *American Society of Microbiology Annual Meeting: Abstracts.* 1989:412.

71. Coleman P, Varietek V, Muschahwar IK, et al. Test pack *Chlamydia:* a new rapid assay for the direct detection of *Chlamydia trachomatis. J Clin Microbiol.* 1989;27:2811.

72. Ferris DG, Lawler FH, Harner RD, et al. Test-of-cure for genital *Chlamydia trachomatis* infection in women. *J Fam Pract.* 1990;31:36.

73. Wong ES, Hooton TM, Hill CC, et al. Clinical and microbiological features of persistent or recurrent nongonococcal urethritis in man. *J Infect Dis.* 1988;158:1098.

74. Cohen I, Veille J, Calkins BM. Improved pregnancy outcome following successful treatment of chlamydial infection. *JAMA.* 1990; 263:3160.

75. *Sexually Transmitted Disease Statistics.* US Public Health Department; 1987:53.

76. Kalinyak JE, Fleagle G, Docherty J. Incidence and distribution of herpes simplex virus types 1 and 2 from genital lesions in college women. *J Med Virol.* 1977;1:175.

77. Reeves WE, Corey L, Adams HG. Risk of recurrence after first episode of genital herpes: relation to HSV type and antibody response. *N Engl J Med.* 1981;305:315.

78. Pariser D, Pariser H, Pariser RJ. Sexually transmitted diseases 1985. Diagnosis and treatment for the clinician. *AUA Update Series.* 1985; 4:lesson 30.

79. Turner R, Shehab Z, Osborn K. Shedding and survival of herpes simplex virus from "fever blisters." *Pediatrics.* 1982;70:547.

80. Larson RE, Shapiro MA. Sexually transmitted urogenital diseases. *Emerg Med Clin North Am.* 1988;6:487.

81. Corey L. The diagnosis and treatment of genital herpes. *JAMA.* 1982;248:1041.

82. Corey L, Adams HG, Brown ZA, et al. Genital herpes simplex virus infections: clinical manifestations, course and complications. *Ann Intern Med.* 1983;98:958.

83. Riehle RA, Williams JJ. Transient neuropathic bladder following herpes simplex genitalis. *J Urol.* 1979;122:263.

84. Goodell SE, Quinn TC, Makrtichian E, et al. Herpes simplex proctitis in homosexual men: clinical sigmoidoscopic and histopathological features. *N Eng J Med.* 1983;308:868.

85. Wrzos H, Rapp F. Experimental model for activation of genital herpes simplex virus. *J Infect Dis.* 1985;151:349–354.

86. Adam E, Kaufman RH, Mirkourc RR, et al. Persistence of virus shedding in asymptomatic women after recovery from herpes genitalis. *Obstet Gynecol.* 1979;54:171.

87. Brown ST, Jaffe HW, Zaid A, et al. Sensitivity and specificity of diagnostic tests for genital infection with herpes virus hominus. *Sex Transm Dis.* 1979;6:10.

88. Furman PA, St Clair MH, Fyfe JA, et al. Inhibition of herpes simplex virus induced DNA polymerase activity and viral DNA replication by 9-(2-hydroxyethoxymethyl) guanine and its triphosphate. *J Virol.* 1979;32:72.

89. *The Medical Letter.* 1988;30:5.

90. Corey L, Nahmias AJ, Guinan ME, et al. A trial of topical acyclovir in genital herpes simplex infections. *N Engl J Med.* 1983;306:1313.

91. Reichman RC, Badger GJ, Guinan ME, et al. Topically administered acyclovir in the treatment of recurring herpes simplex genitalis: a controlled trial. *J Infect Dis.* 1983;147:336.

92. Gissman L, de Villiers EM, ZurHausen H. Analysis of human genital warts (condyloma acuminata) and other genital tumors for human papilloma virus type 6 DNA. *Int J Cancer.* 1982;29:143.

93. Howler PM. On human papilloma viruses (editorial). *N Engl J Med.* 1986;315:1089.

94. Oriel JD. Natural history of genital warts. *Br J Vener Dis.* 1971;47:1.

95. Ferenzy A. Strategies to eradicate genital HPV infection in men. *Contemp Urol.* 1990;2:19.

96. Mounts P, Shah KV. Respiratory papillomatosis: etiological relation to genital tract papillomavirus. *Prog Med Virol.* 1984;29:90.

97. Rosemberg SK. Subclinical papillomaviral infections of the male genitalia. *Urology.* 1985; 26:554.

98. Wosnitzer M. Use of office colposcope to diagnose subclinical papillomaviral and other infections of male and female genitalia. *Urology.* 1988;31:340.

99. Barrasso R, DeBrux J, Croissant O, et al. High prevalence of papillomavirus associated penile intraepithelial neoplasia in sexual partners of women with cervical intraepithelial neoplasia. *N Engl J Med.* 1987;317:916.

100. Schultz RE, Miller JW, MacDonald GR, et al. Clinical and molecular evaluation of acetowhite genital lesions in men. *J Urol.* 1990;143:920.

101. Carparniello VL, Schoenberg M, Malloy TR. Long-term followup of subclinical human papillomavirus infection treated with the carbon dioxide laser and intraurethral 5-fluorouracil: a treatment protocol. *J Urol.* 1990;143:726.

102. Zderic SA, Carpaniello VL, Malloy TR, Wein AJ. The diagnosis and management of genital infections with the human papillomavirus. *AUA Update Series.* 1988;7:lesson 34.

103. Margolis S. Therapy for condyloma acuminatum: a review. *Rev Infect Dis.* 1982;4: S829.
104. Eron LJ, Judson F, Tucker S, et al. Interferon therapy for condyloma acuminata. *N Engl J Med.* 1986;315:1059.
105. Reichman RC, Oakes D, Bonnez W. Treatment of condyloma acuminatum with three different interferons administered intralesionally. *Ann Intern Med.* 1988;108:685.
106. Ferenczy A, Masaru M, Naggi N, et al. Latent papilloma virus and recurring genital warts. *N Engl J Med.* 1985;313:784.
107. Garden JM, O'Banyon MK, Shelnitz LS, et al. Papillomavirus in the vapor of carbon dioxide laser-treated verrucae. *JAMA.* 1988;259:1199.
108. Schaeffer AJ. Use of the $CO_2$ laser in urology. *Urol Clin North Am.* 1986;13:393.
109. Rosemberg SK. Sexually transmitted papillomaviral infections, III. management of male partner. *Urology.* 1988;31:375.
110. Wilkin JK. Molluscum contagiosum venereum in a women's out-patient clinic. A venereally transmitted disease. *Am J Obstet Gynecol.* 1977;128:531.
111. Felman YM, Nikitas JA. Genital molluscum contagiosum. *Cutis.* 1980;26:28.
112. Kipping HF. Molluscum dermatitis. *Arch Dermatol.* 1971;103:106.
113. *MMWR.* Atlanta, Ga: Centers for Disease Control. Revision of the CDC surveillance case definition for acquired immunodeficiency syndrome. 1987;36(1 Suppl):3S.
114. Morgan WM, Curran JW. Acquired immunodeficiency syndrome: current and future trends. *Public Health Rep.* 1986;101:459.
115. Centers for Disease Control. *HIV/AIDS Surveillance Report.* June 1990:1–18.
116. Hessol NA, Rutherford GW, O'Malley PM, et al. The natural history of human immunodeficiency virus infection in a cohort of homosexual and heterosexual men. Presented at the Third International Conference on AIDS. Washington DC; June 1, 1987.
117. Scutchfield FD, Benenson AS. AIDS update. *Postgrad Med.* 1989;85:289.
118. Diagnostic tests for AIDS. *Med Lett.* 1988;30:73.
119. Urmacher C, Myskiowski P, Ochoa M Jr, et al. Outbreak of Kaposi's sarcoma with cytomegalovirus in young homosexual men. *Am J Med.* 1982;72:569.
120. Seftel AD, Sadick NS, Waldbaum RS. Kaposi's sarcoma of penis in a patient with acquired immunodeficiency syndrome. *J Urol.* 1986;136:673.
121. Catanese AJ, Tessler AN, Morales P. AIDS and the urologist, I: urologic manifestation of AIDS. *AUA Update Series.* 1989;8:lesson 1.
122. Kaplan MS, Wechsler M, Benson MC. Urologic manifestations of AIDS. *Urology.* 1987; 30:441.
123. Randazzo RF, Hulette CM, Gottlieb MS, et al. Cytomegaloviral epididymitis in a patient with the acquired immunodeficiency syndrome. *J Urol.* 1986;136:1095.
124. Quinn TC, Glasser D, Cannon RO, et al. Human immunodeficiency virus infection among patients in clinics for sexually transmitted diseases. *N Engl J Med.* 1988;318:197.
125. Johns DR, Tierney M, Felserstein D. Alteration in the natural history of neurosyphilis by concurrent infection with the human immunodeficiency virus. *N Engl J Med.* 1988;316: 1569.
126. Berry CD, Hooton TM, Collier AC, et al. Neurologic relapse after benzathine penicillin therapy for secondary syphilis in a patient with HIV infection. *N Engl J Med.* 1988;316:1587.
127. Sreepsada Rao TK, Fillippone EJ, Nicastri AD, et al. Associated focal segmental glomerulosclerosis in the acquired immunodeficiency syndrome. *N Engl J Med.* 1984;310:669.
128. Yarchoan R, Mitsuya H, Myers C, Broder S. Clinical pharmacology of 3′-azido-2′, 3′-dideoxythymidine (Zidovudine) and related dideoxynucleosides. *N Engl J Med.* 1989; 321:726.
129. Fischl MA, Richman DD, Grieco MH, et al. The efficacy of azidothymidine (AZT) in the treatment of patients with AIDS and AIDS-related complex. *N Engl J Med.* 1987;317:185.
130. *MMWR.* Atlanta, Ga: Centers for Disease Control; US Dept of Health and Human Services. 1990;39(RR-1):1.
131. *FDA Medical Bulletin.* Dec. 1991;21(3):5.
132. Marcus R, CDC Cooperative Needlestick Study Group. Surveillance of health-care workers exposed to blood from patients infected with the human immunodeficiency virus. *N Engl J Med.* 1988;319:1118.
133. Jagger J, Hunt EH, Brand-Elnaggar J, et al. Rates of needlesticks caused by various diseases in a university hospital. *N Engl J Med.* 1988;319:284.
134. Catanese AJ, Rowan RL, Morales P. AIDS and the urologist, part II: precautions against the HIV virus. *AUA Update Series.* 1989;8:lesson 10.
135. Bartlett JG, Polk R. Bacterial flora of the vagina: quantitative study. *Rev Infect Dis.* 1984;6:567.
136. McCue JD. Evaluation and management of vaginitis. An update for primary care practitioners. *Arch Intern Med.* 1989;149:565.
137. Bump RC, Buesching III WJ. Bacterial vaginosis in virginal and sexually active adolescent females: evidence against exclusive sexual transmission. *Am J Obstet Gynecol.* 1988; 158:935.
138. Amsel R, Totten PA, Spiegel CA, et al. Nonspecific vaginitis: diagnostic criteria and microbid and epidemiologic associations. *Am J Med.* 1983;74:14.

139. Fleury FJ. Adult vaginitis. *Clin Obstet Gynecol.* 1981;24:407.

140. Symond J, Biswas AK. Amoxicillin, augmentin, and metronidazole in bacterial vaginosis associated with *Gardnerella* vaginalis. *Genitourin Med.* 1986;62:136.

141. Sobel JD. Bacterial vaginosis: assessment and treatment. *Med Aspects of Human Sexuality.* June 1990:42.

142. McLellan R, Spence MR, Brockman M, et al. The clinical diagnosis of trichomoniasis. *Obstet Gynecol.* 1982;60:30.

143. Wisdom AR, Dunlop EMC. Trichomoniasis: study of the disease and its treatment in men and women. *Br J Vener Dis.* 1965;41:90.

144. Spence MR, Hollander DH, Smith J, et al. The clinical and laboratory diagnosis of trichomoniasis vaginalis infection. *Sex Transm Dis.* 1980;7:168.

145. Fouts AL, Kraus SJ. Trichomonas vaginalis: reevaluation of its clinical presentation and laboratory diagnosis. *J Infect Dis.* 1980;141:137.

146. Krieger JN, Tarn MR, Stevens CE, et al. Diagnosis of trichomoniasis: comparison of conventional wet-mount examination with cytologic studies, cultures, and monoclonal antibody staining of direct specimens. *JAMA.* 1988;259:1223.

147. Perl G. Errors in the diagnosis of Trichomonas vaginalis infection as observed among 1199 patients. *Obstet Gynecol.* 1972;139:7.

148. Landers DV. The treatment of vaginitis: trichomonas, yeast and bacterial vaginosis. *Clin Obstet Gynecol.* 1988;31:473.

149. Pattman RS, Sprott MS, Moss TR. Evaluation of a culture slide in the diagnosis of vaginal candidiasis. *Br J Vener Dis* 1981;57:67.

150. Eschenbach DA. Vaginal infection. *Clin Obstet Gynecol.* 1983;26:186.

151. Sobel J. Recurrent vulvovaginal candidiasis: a prospective study of the efficacy of maintenance ketoconazole therapy. *N Engl J Med.* 1986;315:1455.

152. Orkin M, Maibach HI. Evolving views of scabies and pediculosis pubis. In: Felman YM, ed. *Sexually Transmitted Diseases.* New York: Churchill Livingstone; 1986.

153. Orkin M. Today's scabies. *JAMA.* 1975; 233:882.

154. Muller G, Jacobs PH, Moore NE. Scraping for human scabies, a better method for positive preparations. *Arch Dermatol.* 1973;107:70.

155. Ginsberg CM, Lowry W, Resich JS. Absorption of lindane (gamma benzene hexachloride) in infants and children. *J Pediatr.* 1977;91:995.

156. Davies JE, Dedhia HV, Morgade C, et al. Lindane poisonings. *Arch Dermatol.* 1983; 119:142.

157. Rasmussen JE. The problem of lindane. *J Am Acad Dermatol.* 1981;5:507.

158. Orkin M, Epstein E, Maibach HI. Treatment of today's scabies and pediculosis. *JAMA.* 1976;236:1136.

159. Pariser DM, Pariser H, Pariser RJ. Sexually transmitted diseases, 1985. Diagnosis and treatment for the clinician. *AUA Update Series.* 1985;4:lesson 30.

160. Orkin M, Maribach HI. Current views of scabies and pediculosis pubis. *Cutis.* 1984;33:85.

161. Treatment of sexually transmitted diseases. *Med Lett.* 1988;30:5.

162. Noble RC. *Sexually Transmitted Diseases: Guide to Diagnosis and Therapy.* 3rd ed. Medical Examination Publishing Co; 1985;193–218.

163. DiNapoli JB, Austin RD, Englender SJ, et al. Eradication of head lice with a single treatment. *Am J Public Health.* 1988;78:978.

164. Brandenburg K, Deinard AS, DiNapoli J, et al. One percent Permethrin creme rinse vs. 1% lindane shampoo in treating pediculosis capitis. *Am J Dis Child.* 1986;140:894.

165. William DC, Felman YM, Marr JS, et al. Sexual transmitted enteric pathogens in male homosexual population. *N Y State J Med.* 1977;77:2050.

166. Allason-Jones E, Mindel A, Sargeant P, et al. Enteromoeba histolytica as a commensal intestinal parasite in homosexual men. *N Engl J Med.* 1986;315:353.

167. Sorville FJ, Strassburg MA, Seidel J, et al. Amebic infections in asymptomatic homosexual men: Lack of evidence of invasive disease. *Am J Public Health.* 1986;76:1137.

168. Patterson M, Healy GR, Shabot JM. Serologic testing for amebiasis. *Gastroenterology.* 1980;78:136.

169. Beal CB, Viens P, Grant RGC, et al. A technique for sampling duodenal contents: demonstration of upper small bowel pathogens. *Am J Trop Med Hyg.* 1970;19:349.

170. Schmerin MJ, Jones TC, Klein H. Giardiasis: association with homosexuality. *Ann Intern Med.* 1978;88:801.

171. Keusch GT. Shigella infections. *Clin Gastroenterol.* 1979;8:645.

172. Corey L, Holmes KK. Sexual transmission of hepatitis A in homosexual men. *N Engl J Med.* 1980;302:435.

173. Szmuness W, Stevens CE, Horley EJ, et al. Hepatitis B vaccine: demonstration of efficacy in a controlled clinical trial in a high risk population in the United States. *N Engl J Med.* 1980;303:833.

174. Francis DP, Hadler SC, Thompsen SE, et al. The prevention of hepatitis B with vaccine: report of the CDC multi-center efficacy trial among homosexual men. *Ann Intern Med.* 1982;97:362.

# 11
# The Adrenal Gland

*August Zabbo*

The adrenal gland consists of an anatomically and functionally distinct cortex and medulla. Adrenal hormones are essential for life; a deficiency or excess of these hormones can be responsible for some of the most dramatic clinical syndromes. The retroperitoneal position of the adrenal glands within Gerota fascia, in apposition to the superior poles of the kidneys, brings these glands into the surgical sphere of urology. Until recently, adrenal surgery has been limited to exploration and removal of pathologic glands. Exploration alone has largely been replaced by modern diagnostic imaging techniques. Along with biochemical analyses, modern imaging allows a more confident preoperative diagnosis and a directed surgical approach to adrenal pathology. Recent reports of transplanting adrenal tissue to treat neurologic conditions, such as Parkinson's disease, along with partial adrenalectomy for selected pathologic conditions, may lead to broader applications of adrenal surgery. An understanding of adrenal anatomy, physiology, pathophysiology, and surgical approaches are integral to modern urologic practice.

## EMBRYOLOGY AND ANOMALIES

The adrenal cortex and medulla have separate embryologic origins. The cortex arises from mesothelial buds near the cranial end of the mesonephros.[1] The majority of these buds join to create a mass of tissue lateral to the aorta that forms the adrenal cortex, which is identifiable in the 2-month-old fetus. The tissue from buds that do not join the main mass will involute or occasionally develop into accessory adrenal tissue, which is sometimes found near the kidneys, celiac plexus, gonadal vessels, gonads, and broad ligament.

In the developing embryo, there is an inner "fetal" zone of cortex and an outer "definitive" zone which will become the adult cortical tissue. The cortex reaches massive proportions in the fetus as compared to the adult adrenal gland because of the fetal zone's mass. The fetal adrenal gland is stimulated by adrenocorticotropic hormone (ACTH), but as the fetal zone is deficient in 3-β-hydroxysteroid dehydrogenase, it produces mainly dehydroepiandrosterone (DHEA) and DHEA sulfate, which is converted to estrogens in the placenta after initial metabolism in the fetal liver.[2] The definitive zone synthesizes the same steroid end products as the adult adrenal gland, and is the major source of fetal cortisol. At the 4th fetal month, the adrenal gland is larger than the developing kidney, but by the time of birth, it is only one third the size of the kidney.[2] In the first few weeks after birth, the adrenal gland loses half its weight secondary to regression of the fetal zone, which is complete by the end of the first year of life. By age 3, differentiation into the adult three-zone configuration of the adrenal cortex is complete.

The adrenal medulla has the same embryologic origin as the sympathetic nervous system, that is, primitive sympathetic cells of the neural crest. The cells that do not differentiate into neurons but become endocrine cells are called chromaffin cells, as they stain brown when exposed to chromic acid salts. At 6 weeks of fetal life, groups of cells similar to those forming the sympathetic chain dorsal to the aorta migrate along the central vein and enter the fetal adrenal cortex. These cells will form the adrenal medulla, which may be observed by the 8th week of gestation. Two cell types are present: sympathogonia, which will differentiate into sympathetic ganglion cells, and pheochromoblasts, which will become pheochromocytes (chromaffin cells). Other collections of pheochromocytes coalesce to form paraganglia on either side of the aorta, with the major collection occurring at the level of the inferior mesenteric artery. These cells fuse anteriorly at the bifurcation of the aorta to form the organ of Zuckerkandl, which is large in fetal life and which may provide a major source of catecholamines in the first year of life. After the first year, the organ usually atrophies. Pheochromocytes may also be found in other parts of the sympathetic nervous system, including the sympathetic fibers found in the bladder, which explains the occasional finding of a vesical pheochromocytoma. During gestation and at birth, the catecholamine content of the medulla and paraganglionic tissue is almost entirely composed of norepinephrine. But by 2 years of age, this changes so that 80% of the medullary output is epinephrine.[3]

Anomalies of the adrenal gland are rarely of clinical significance. Ectopic adrenal cortical tissue (adrenal rests) are sometimes seen in the areas of the kidneys, gonads, and gonadal vessels, or, rarely, in such sites as the lung or brain. Heterotopia indicates the inclusion of the adrenal gland within or beneath the renal capsule. Midline fusion of the adrenal gland is seen rarely. While bilateral absence of the adrenal glands would result in an unviable fetus, unilateral glandular absence is occasionally seen. It should be noted, however, because of the separate development of the kidney and adrenal, that unilateral absence of the kidney would not necessarily result in absence of the ipsilateral adrenal gland. Adrenal cysts may be congenital, or may possibly occur secondary to adrenal hemorrhage. Adrenal cytomegaly is a condition of unknown significance, in which the cells of the fetal cortex demonstrate bizarre nuclei and large amounts of eosinophilic cytoplasm.[4]

Congenital adrenal hyperplasia is caused by deficiencies of an enzyme of the steroid synthesis pathway that lead to inadequate production of the usual end products of steroid metabolism. Thus, with the lack of normal feedback inhibition, the pituitary is stimulated to produce large quantities of ACTH, which in turn results in massive enlargement of the adrenal glands and production of large quantities of steroid precursors which have dramatic clinical effects such as virilization. Twenty-one hydroxylase deficiency is the most common enzyme deficiency and when severe, results in a salt-wasting endocrinopathy. Eleven β-hydroxylase deficiency is less common, and other enzyme deficiencies are even more rare.

## ANATOMY AND SURGICAL APPROACHES

The adrenal glands lie above and medial to each kidney. They are in close proximity to the upper pole of the kidneys, with the concave posterior surface of the adrenal gland closely applied to the convex surface of the upper portion of the kidney. The right adrenal gland is also somewhat posterior to the vena cava, and the anterior surface of this gland is covered by the right lobe of the liver. On the left, the gland is just posterior to the tail of the pancreas and the splenic vessels, which may cross over its superior lateral border.

The outer adrenal cortex has a distinctly characteristic golden-yellow color and a firm consistency that differentiates it from the surrounding perirenal fat and allows surgical identification. The medulla is brownish to red, and is grossly apparent only in hyperplastic states. Normal glands weigh approximately 4–5 g with the medulla representing about 10% of the weight of the gland. The glands are frequently described as pyramidal in shape, but this is variable and the glands often have an elongated T-shaped configuration, with one branch of the T extending far cephalad, particularly on the right. The main aterial supply of the gland is derived from three sources; branches arise from the aorta, renal, and inferior phrenic arteries. Additionally, other branches from the gonadal arteries on the left side or intercostal arteries on either side may be present. From these various arteries, multiple small arterial branches pass to the anterior and posterior surfaces of the gland, where they form an extensive subcapsular plexus. One major vein drains each gland. On the right side, this is a short vein that extends directly from the gland to the vena cava, while on the left side, the adrenal vein drains into the left renal vein and is usually found directly opposite the gonadal vein. Other small veins coursing with the inferior phrenic vessels may be present.

Microscopically, the adrenal cortex may be separated into three zones: the thin outer zona glomerulosa, a relatively thick middle zona fasciculata, and an inner thin zona reticularis. The glomerulosa may be absent in some portions of the gland, and is formed by small, columnar cells arranged in clusters and arcades. This zone is the site of aldosterone synthesis.

Traditionally, the zona fasciculata was associated with glucocorticoid synthesis and the zona reticularis with adrenal sex-steroid synthesis. More recently, it has been found that this demarcation of function is not complete—there may be a qualitative difference in the responsiveness to ACTH stimulation between these two zones. This results in the relative difference in quantity of the steroids ascribed to each zone. The cells of the zona fasciculata are large, polyhedral cells filled with lipid droplets while those of the zona reticularis are smaller and contain fewer lipid droplets.

The adrenal medulla contains chromaffin cells with a generous blood and neural supply. Norepinephrine- and epinephrine-secreting cells can be differentiated by the microstructure of the granules seen on electromicrographs. The medullary cells are richly supplied with nerves derived from the T-6 through L-1 ventral rami, which reach the gland through the splanchnic nerves and celiac plexus. The majority of these nerves are preganglionic fibers which end in synapses with the secretory cells of the medulla. Thus, the medullary cells can be considered as postganglionic sympathetic neurons.

A variety of operative approaches to the adrenal glands are possible; the choice is based on the patient's body habitus and surgical history, the adrenal pathology being addressed, and, finally, the familiarity of the surgeon with the particular technique. An anterior transabdominal approach can be accomplished by using either a vertical midline incision, or preferably, a subcostal incision, as is often used for radical nephrectomy. This approach is standard in patients with pheochromocytomas, because it allows early vascular control and exploration for the presence of contralateral or ectopic pheochromocytomas. It is also useful for those with large or malignant lesions, to achieve wide exposure and allow en-bloc nephroadrenalectomy.

The thoracoabdominal approach to the adrenal gland can be used if a particularly large tumor is found (as is often the case in patients with adrenal cortical carcinomas). It is particularly useful on the right side, where the liver and vena cava may limit exposure when a subcostal incision is used. Exploration of the opposite adrenal gland is somewhat more difficult, but can be achieved with a thoracoabdominal approach.

Flank incision offers ready access to the adrenal gland, but it is somewhat more painful than the posterior approach and is thus generally reserved only for those obese patients in whom a posterior approach to a small adrenal tumor would be difficult. In such patients an 11th- or 12th-rib incision is preferred to a subcostal approach because it allows more superior exposure.

The most direct approach to the adrenal glands is via a posterior incision. On the left side, this is generally done through the bed of the 12th rib, while on the right side, the 11th or even the 10th rib can be used. This may necessitate entering the retroperitoneum transthoracically on the right side, which would require traversing the pleural cavity, retracting the lung, and incising the diaphragm. Exposure is quite limited with the posterior approach; for this reason, it should be used only for small adrenal lesions such as aldosterone-secreting adrenal adenomas. It is not appropriate for even small pheochromocytomas.

In general, in all adrenal surgery, it is best to dissect the attachments from the superior surface of the gland first. This allows for traction downward on the kidney to bring the most cephalad portion of the gland into the incision for easier dissection. Identification of the main adrenal vein and its ligation is mandatory; this may be somewhat difficult on the right side where there is a short adrenal vein draining directly into the vena cava. Complications specific to adrenal surgery include a wide variation in blood pressures, particularly during surgery for pheochromocytoma. Nelson's syndrome may occur after bilateral adrenalectomy for Cushing's disease when a pituitary tumor expands after such therapy. Adrenal insufficiency can occur after unilateral adrenalectomy, particularly when the patient has been known to have high glucocorticoid levels preoperatively (which result in atrophy of the contralateral adrenal gland). Such adrenal insufficiency should be anticipated and steroid replacement provided.

## DIAGNOSTIC IMAGING

Advances in diagnostic imaging have allowed more precise definition of adrenal pathology without the need for surgical exploration. The same advances, however, have resulted in the creation of a new clinical problem, that of the "incidentaloma," which is the finding of an unsuspected adrenal mass. Traditionally, adrenal masses were discovered by the intravenous urogram which, along with tomography, would show a suprarenal mass which may displace the kidney inferiorly. Adrenal gland calcifications observed on a plain abdominal radiograph may arise after infection of the gland with tuberculosis or histoplasmosis. Such calcifications often would be bilateral and assume an irregular or amorphous appearance. Clustered calcifications suggest past hemorrhage but are not distinguishable from calcifications secondary to granulomatous disease. Calcification is unusual in pheochromocytoma but may be present with adrenal adenomas, neuroblastomas, and malignant tumors. The calcifications associated with neuroblastoma are usually fine and punctate.

Ultrasonography may demonstrate a suprarenal mass, but this is dependent on the skill of the operator. Large adrenal masses are usually found quite readily and adrenal cysts can be definitively identified. However, small adrenal masses may be missed and, in general, identification of an adrenal mass by ultrasonography should lead to further diagnostic studies.

Computed tomography (CT) scan of the kidney is currently the most popular imaging study available to define adrenal masses. CT scan will identify greater than 90% of pheochromocytomas which are 1 cm in largest diameter. Also, in patients with Cushing's syndrome or hyperaldosteronism secondary to adrenal adenomas, CT is useful to identify the source of excess steroids. CT will also allow distinction of the fat content, providing a means to separate an adrenal myelolipoma from other adrenal pathology. Because many functional adrenal masses are small, closely spaced CT sections of the adrenal glands (0.5 cm) should be requested when these masses are being sought.

Magnetic resonance imaging (MRI) scanning is most useful for identifying intra-adrenal pheochromocytomas and neuroblastomas. It also provides excellent additional information concerning vascular and nodal involvement of malignancies. As yet, no significant improvement in diagnostic capability has been achieved using MRI as compared with CT, but such an improvement might be anticipated as techniques improve and contrast agents are developed.

Adrenal angiography is infrequently used for diagnostic purposes because of the widespread availability of CT and MRI scanning. However, there may be some cases where the diagnosis or localization of an adrenal adenoma is equivocal or where adrenal venous sampling may be of some value. Also, percutaneous biopsy of adrenal lesions, used mostly to distinguish metastatic from primary tumors, may be valuable to avoid unnecessary surgical exploration.

Radioisotope scanning is the only imaging technique that uses the endocrine activity of a tumor as its basis of detection.[5] Two different tracers are used. $^{131}$I-19-iodonorcholesterol (NP59) is a cortical-identifying agent that is capable of showing increased uptake bilaterally in Cushing's syndrome secondary to ACTH excess and unilaterally in the presence of a steroid-producing adrenal adenoma (either an aldosterone- or a cortisol-producing tumor). $^{131}$I-metaiodobenzylguanidine ($^{131}$I-MIBG) uptake is concentrated in sympathetic nerve endings. This marker is useful in searching for an extra-adrenal pheochromocytoma, metastases from a malignant pheochromocytoma, or recurrences after resection. Other neuroendocrine tumors, such as neuroblastoma, nonfunctioning paraganglioma, schwannoma, medullary thyroid carcinoma, some bronchogenic carcinomas, and carcinoid tumors can also be localized using MIBG.

## PHYSIOLOGY

### Adrenal Cortex

The major biochemical tasks of the healthy adrenal cortex are the production of glucocorticoids and mineralocorticoids, both of which are essential to life. In addition, the cortex secretes androgens; cortical androgens are insignificant when compared to those from the testes in the normal male, but constitute the major androgen supply in the female. Estrogens are produced by peripheral metabolism of adrenal steroids and are probably not of physiologic significance in either sex. The evaluation of adrenal cortical function uses biochemical analysis of various hormonal products and metabolites; an understanding of the metabolic pathways of steroid synthesis and metabolism is necessary to appreciate this laboratory evaluation.

The pathways of steroid biosynthesis in the adrenal gland are shown in Figure 1. Because the zona glomerulosa lacks 17-α-hydroxylase activity, this zone cannot produce the precursors of cortisol and the adrenal sex steroids. Its metabolic product,

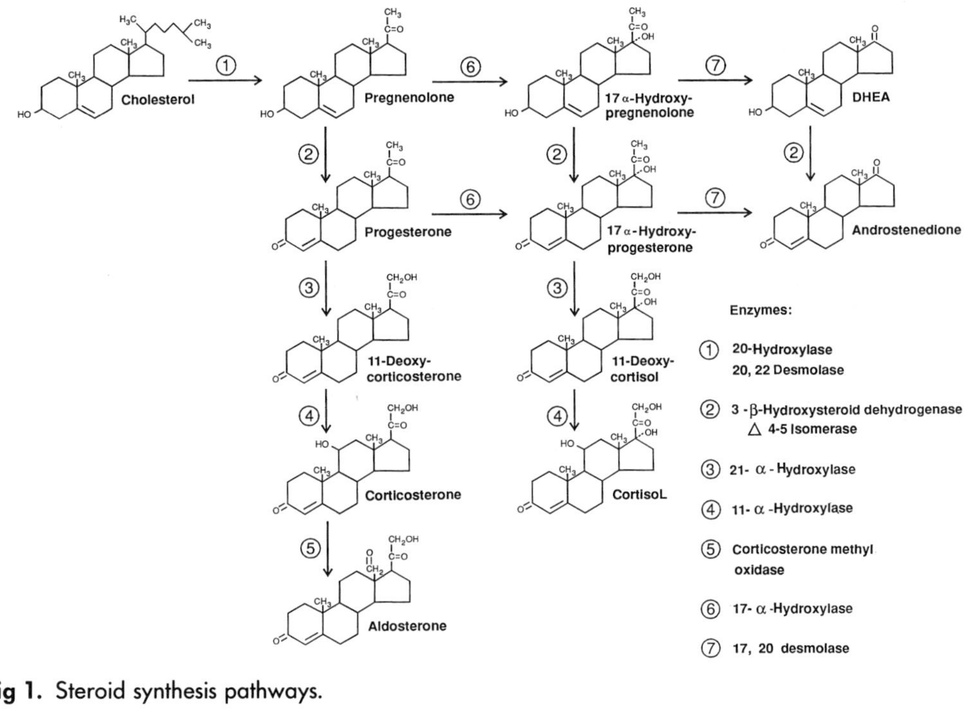

Enzymes:

1. 20-Hydroxylase 20, 22 Desmolase
2. 3-β-Hydroxysteroid dehydrogenase Δ 4-5 Isomerase
3. 21-α-Hydroxylase
4. 11-α-Hydroxylase
5. Corticosterone methyl oxidase
6. 17-α-Hydroxylase
7. 17, 20 desmolase

**Fig 1.** Steroid synthesis pathways.

then, is aldosterone, secretion of which is influenced primarily by the renin-angiotensin system and the plasma concentrations of sodium and potassium. ACTH plays a permissive role in the stimulation of the initial synthetic step of cholesterol conversion to pregnenolone, but within the zona glomerulosa this conversion occurs largely under the regulation of the renin-angiotensin system. Excess potassium stimulates aldosterone secretion, while potassium deficiency inhibits secretion. Conversely, depletion of body sodium is a potent stimulus to aldosterone secretion. Stimulation of the renin-angiotensin system results in increased aldosterone secretion. All of these factors act in concert to maintain the homeostatic balance of blood pressure and electrolytes.

Other products of the steroid biosynthesis scheme have mineralocorticoid activity, particularly deoxycorticosterone (DOC) and 18-hydroxycorticosterone. However, these products are far less potent than aldosterone. Aldosterone is 90% cleared in one pass through the liver; this rapid metabolism results in a half-life of approximately 20 minutes. The major action of aldosterone is on secretory systems, primarily the renal tubules, but its effects are also observed in saliva, sweat, and feces. The net effect of increased aldosterone levels is conservation of sodium and excretion of potassium. Aldosterone is loosely protein bound to corticosteroid-binding globulin, in contrast to the corticosteroids, which are tightly bound to this protein.

The zonae fasciculata and reticularis produce cortisol, androgens, and via peripheral conversion, estrogens. The rate-limiting step in the production of these hormones is the conversion of cholesterol to pregnenolone, which is under the influence of ACTH. There may also be some neural stimulation involved with this production.[6] Plasma lipoproteins are the major source of adrenal cholesterol, although there is some cholesterol synthesis from acetate and storage within the gland. Also produced within the zonae fasciculata and reticularis are deoxycorticosterone, 18-hydroxydeoxycorticosterone, corticosterone, and 18-hydroxycorticosterone. However, as 18-hydroxysteroid dehydrogenase is not present in the fasciculata or reticularis, aldosterone is not produced here.

Androgen production requires 17-α hydroxylation. The major adrenal androgens are dehydroepiandrosterone (DHEA), DHEA sulfate, and androstenedione. These all have weak androgenic activity but are converted peripherally to the more potent androgens, testosterone and dihydrotestosterone.

ACTH is the primary stimulant to the zonae fasciculata and reticularis and is the major regulator of cortisol and adrenal androgen production. ACTH secretion is stimulated by corticotropin-releasing hormone (CRH) from the hypothalamus. There are feedback regulatory circuits that control this hypothalamic-pituitary-adrenal axis. ACTH is necessary for steroid secretion, and, in the absence of ACTH there is markedly decreased steroidogenesis and adrenocortical atrophy.

Three mechanisms of neuroendocrine control contribute to the regulation of ACTH secretion. The first of these is the circadian rhythm, which is superimposed on episodic secretion. Cortisol secretion is generally low in the late evening and declines during the first few hours of sleep. There is a surge in ACTH and cortisol after 6–8 hours of sleep, and then cortisol declines as waking occurs. Cortisol levels decline through the day with occasional secretory episodes, which especially occur in response to eating or exercise. This rhythm can be altered by physical or psychologic stress, endocrine disorders, and such metabolic abnormalities as liver disease, chronic renal failure, and alcoholism.

Physical stress results in ACTH release and serum cortisol increases within minutes following such stresses as surgery or hypoglycemia. These stress responses originate in the central nervous system, and lead to increased hypothalamic CRH and pituitary ACTH secretion.

The final regulatory influence on ACTH and cortisol secretion is feedback inhibition. Thus, with increased glucocorticoid levels, whether they be endogenous or iatrogenically administered, ACTH levels will decrease and ultimately become unresponsive to normal stimuli.

Adrenal androgen production is also regulated by ACTH. Androgen secretion parallels that of cortisol; the existence of a separate pituitary hormone regulator for androgen secretion has not been found.

Cortisol and the adrenal androgens are bound to plasma proteins and have a half life of 70–90 minutes. Corticosteroid-binding globulin is the principal protein, binding 75% of cortisol, while albumin (which has a lower affinity for cortisol) binds approximately 15% of the circulating cortisol. Hepatic metabolism of cortisol renders the steroid inactive and water soluble. Approximately 90% of the metabolites of the adrenal steroids are then excreted in the urine.

The biologic effects of glucocorticoids are myriad, and glucocorticoid receptors are present in virtually all tissues.[7] These receptors are proteins which bind with their target hormone, enter the cell nucleus, and effect the glucocorticoid response. The major effect of glucocorticoids is on intermediary metabolism. Glucocorticoids increase hepatic gluconeogenesis by stimulating enzymes in the gluconeogenesis pathways. They also increase glycerol and free fatty acid release by lipolysis and enhance glycogen synthesis. These effects are insulin dependent. The glucocorticoids inhibit peripheral glucose uptake in muscle and adipose tissue, leading to increased serum glucose and insulin secretion. In addition, in adipose tissue, there is increased lipolysis. Paradoxically, one of the effects of glucocorticoid excess is increased fat deposition in a centrally distributed configuration. This may be due to the increased appetite caused by the steroids and the lipogenic effect of hyperinsulinemia which occurs in this state.

Multiple effects of steroids are seen in other tissues. Excessive glucocorticoid levels inhibit the formation of fibroblasts, which leads to a loss of collagen and connective tissue resulting in thin, easily bruised skin and poor wound healing. Excesses also inhibit bone formation and stimulate bone-resorbing cells. In addition, high glucocorticoid levels markedly reduce intestinal calcium absorption, which results in a secondary increase in parathyroid hormone secretion. The net effect is a negative calcium balance which may cause increased urinary calcium excretion and, possibly, urinary stone formation.

Glucocorticoids inhibit growth in children, constituting a major adverse effect of steroid therapy. The immunologic effects of glucocorticoids are well known and are used in immunosuppression, particularly in organ transplantation. Glucocorticoid administration reduces the number of circulating lymphocytes, monocytes, and eosinophiles. Glucocorticoids increase the release of polymorphonuclear leukocytes from the bone marrow, and impair the release of effector substances such as interleukins.

These steroids also increase peripheral vascular tone, possibly by enhancing the effects of other vasoconstrictors, and may increase cardiac output. Such effects are most apparent when there is steroid deficiency with its resultant refractory shock. The native glucocorticoids may also have a mild to moderate mineralocorticoid function, which results in hypertension and sodium and water retention.

Central nervous function is affected by either an excess or a deficiency of glucocorticoids as seen in Cushing's and Addisonian states, but the precise physiologic role in central nervous function is unknown.

## Adrenal Medulla

The catecholamines epinephrine and norepinephrine are the endpoints of adrenal medullary hormone production. Epinephrine is synthesized mainly in the adrenal medulla, whereas norepinephrine is found also in the central nervous system and in the peripheral sympathetic nerves. Dopamine, the precursor of norepinephrine, is found in the adrenal medulla and in noradrenergic neurons. The pathway of biosynthesis and metabolism of adrenal medullary catecholamines is shown in Figure 2. The synthetic pathway begins with tyrosine, an amino acid that may be derived from ingested food or may be synthesized from phenylalanine in the liver. Epineph-

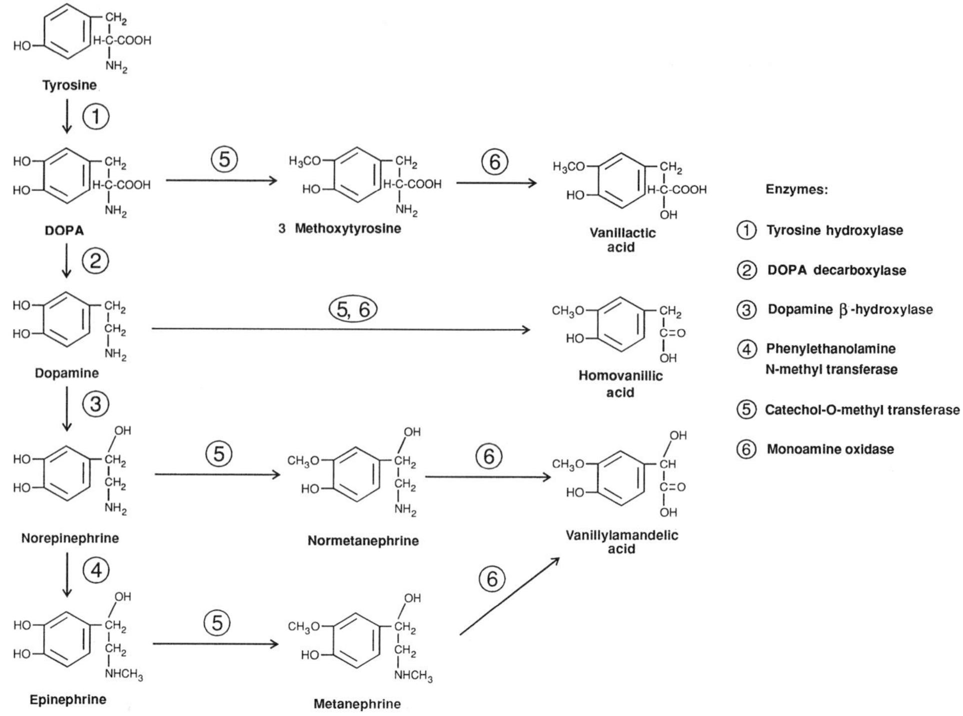


**Fig 2.** Synthesis and metabolism of catecholamines.

rine is synthesized from norepinephrine by N-methylation. This reaction is induced by high levels of glucocorticoids,[8] and probably represents the only connection between the functions of the adrenal cortex and medulla.

Catecholamines are stored in granules in the chromaffin cells that also contain ATP, neuropeptides, calcium, magnesium, and other proteins. The secretion of catecholamines is increased by stressful stimuli such as exercise, hemorrhage, surgery, hypoglycemia, anoxia, and myocardial ischemia.

Epinephrine and norepinephrine are short-acting hormones with half-lives ranging from 1 to 3 minutes. The catecholamines are bound to albumin in the circulation; free hormone is removed by several mechanisms, including reuptake by the sympathetic nerve ending or metabolism by catechol-O-methyl transferase and monoamine oxidase.

The actions of catecholamines are effected by binding to receptor molecules on the surfaces of target cells. A variety of types of adrenergic receptors, including α- and β-adrenergic as well as dopaminergic receptors (and their respective subclasses) exist. The physiologic effects of the catecholamines are well known and include increasing the rate and amplitude of cardiac contraction and increasing the irritability of the myocardium through actions on β-1 receptors. Contraction of vascular smooth muscle is mediated via α receptors. The net result of endogenous catecholamine release or exogenous injection is to increase the heart rate and cardiac output and cause peripheral vasoconstriction, all of which lead to a rise in blood pressure.

Extravascular smooth muscles are also affected by catecholamines. The hormones can induce both relaxation and contraction of the myometrium, relaxation of the bladder smooth muscle, and an increase in urethral sphincter tone. Catecholamines may also cause relaxation of tracheal smooth muscle as well as pupillary dilatation. Finally, these hormones increase oxygen consumption and lipolysis.

## LABORATORY ASSESSMENT OF ADRENAL FUNCTION

### Adrenal Cortex

Because of diurnal and other fluctuations of ACTH and adrenal steroid levels during the day, single uncontrolled plasma measurements of steroid hormones are unreliable to diagnose excessive secretion. More commonly accepted are 24-hour urine assays of excreted hormones or metabolites and specific stimulation and suppression tests. Use of a 4-hour, evening, urinary free cortisol test which may have additional advantages has also been proposed recently.[9] Plasma ACTH levels can be measured by radioimmunoassay. Measurement of ACTH is useful in differentiating Cushing's syndrome due to pituitary ACTH hypersecretion (Cushing's disease) from primary glucocorticoid-secreting adrenal tumors, which result in suppressed ACTH levels. ACTH levels are also markedly elevated in patients with the common forms of congenital adrenal hyperplasia or ACTH-producing neoplasms. Plasma cortisol can be measured by a variety of methods. Again, the utility of obtaining a single plasma cortisol concentration is limited by the normal fluctuation of levels. Thus, AM and PM levels are commonly obtained. It must be recognized that cortisol secretion increases in patients who are acutely ill, during and immediately after surgery, and following trauma. In patients with disease states causing high estrogen levels, the cortisol-binding globulin capacity is increased; thus, the assay for total cortisol shows elevated levels while the levels of the free hormone may be in the normal range.

In disease states causing excess cortisol secretion, the binding capacity of cortisol-binding globulin is exceeded, and the levels of free cortisol in the plasma are increased, as is urinary excretion of free cortisol. Free cortisol in the urine can be measured using a 24-hour urinary sample. This test is useful to detect excess cortisol secretion but not adrenal insufficiency, as the assay is not sensitive at low levels.

Prior to the availability of urinary cortisol measurements, 24-hour determinations of 17-hydroxycorticosteroids and 17-ketogenic steroids were commonly obtained. The assay of 17-hydroxycorticosteroids (Porter-Silber reaction) measures cortisol and cortisone metabolites. The tests measuring 17-ketogenic steroids provide information regarding the metabolites of cortisol and other steroids, such as pregnanetriol. 17-hydroxycorticosteroid levels are increased in obese patients, and unlike urinary free cortisol measurements, the measurement of 17-ketogenic steroids must be corrected for creatinine clearance. 17-hydroxycorticosteroids may also be increased in patients with hyperthyroidism and decreased in those with hypothyroidism, liver disease, and renal failure, and in those who are pregnant or near starvation.

Dexamethasone suppression tests are used to diagnose the presence of excess cortisol secretion, regardless of its cause. Dexamethasone is a synthetic glucocorticoid which is far more potent than cortisol and which normally suppresses pituitary ACTH release (resulting in a fall in plasma and urine corticosteroid levels). In Cushing's syndrome, the normal suppression by low-dose dexamethasone does not occur. Two forms of the low-dose dexamethasone suppression test have been described. The first involves a 1 mg dose of dexamethasone given at 11:00 PM, which is followed by obtaining a morning plasma sample for cortisol determination. Approximately 98% of patients with Cushing's syndrome will reveal abnormal suppression, with plasma cortisol levels greater than 10 μg/dL. False-positive results may occur in obese or chronically ill patients.

Alternatively, 0.5 mg of dexamethasone may be administered every 6 hours for 2 days. A 24-hour urine collection is obtained to measure levels of 17-hydroxycorticosteroids and urinary free cortisol; morning plasma cortisol levels are also determined. In patients *without* Cushing's syndrome there is a normal suppression of urinary steroid levels, and 17-hydroxycorticosteroid levels are less than 4 mg after 24 hours (or less than 1 mg/g of urinary creatinine).

A high-dose dexamethasone test may be used to differentiate primary pituitary ACTH hypersecretion (Cushing's disease) from other causes of Cushing's syndrome (such as ectopic ACTH syndrome or primary adrenal tumors) since the hypothalamic-pituitary axis in Cushing's disease is suppressible with high levels of glucocorticoids. In the overnight high-dose dexamethasone test, 8 mg is administered at 11:00 PM and the plasma cortisol level is measured at 8:00 AM the following morning. In patients with Cushing's disease, this will result in a suppression of cortisol levels by ½ the pretest level whereas levels are not suppressed in those with ectopic ACTH syndrome or cortisol-producing adrenal tumors.

A 2-day high-dose test is also available; this uses dexamethasone in doses of 2 mg given orally every 6 hours for 2 days. Measurements of 24-hour urine samples are obtained for 17-hydroxycorticosteroids and urinary free cortisol. However, with measurement of urinary levels, there is a false-negative rate of 15%–30%.

For those with adrenal insufficiency, adrenal reserve can be assessed with ACTH stimulation or metyrapone administration. ACTH testing currently is performed using synthetic human α-1, 24-ACTH (Cortrosyn). First, the baseline cortisol level is obtained. Then ACTH is administered intramuscularly or intravenously and additional plasma cortisol measurements are obtained at 30 and 60 minutes following injection. A normal response is an increase in serum cortisol levels of greater than 5 μg/dL, or to an absolute value of greater than 20 μg/dL. It is of note that aldosterone secretion is also somewhat responsive to ACTH; in patients with primary adrenal insufficiency, in whom there is usually destruction of the cortex, both cortisol and aldosterone will be unresponsive to administration of exogenous ACTH. However, in those with secondary adrenal insufficiency who have zonae fasciculata and reticularis atrophy due to insufficiency of ACTH stimulus, the zona glomerulosa (which is primarily controlled by the renin-angiotensin system but which responds secondarily to ACTH) will be present and therefore will maintain normal aldosterone response. The normal increment in plasma aldosterone levels after ACTH administration is greater than 4 ng/dL.

Metyrapone blocks cortisol synthesis at the conversion of 11-deoxycortisol to cortisol; this results in ACTH stimulation, which in turn increases plasma levels of 11-deoxycortisol. This is reflected in increased urinary 17-hydroxycorticosteroid levels. The metyrapone test is accomplished by giving a dose of metyrapone between 11 PM and 12 PM followed by blood collection, for use in plasma 11-deoxycortisol and cortisol determinations, at 8 AM the following morning. This drug should not be administered to acutely ill patients or to those in whom primary adrenal insufficiency is suspected. A normal response is an increase to greater than 7 μg/dL of serum 11-deoxycortisol, with the serum cortisol less than 10 μg/dL to ensure adequate inhibition.

Assessment of adrenal androgen production is best done by plasma assays for DHEA, DHEA sulfate, androstenedione, testosterone, and dihydrotestosterone. Excess androgen secretion results in elevated urinary 17-ketosteroids as measured by 24-hour urinary sample, but this measurement is less useful than direct measurement of the plasma androgens.

Testing for primary aldosteronism represents a diagnostic challenge. This diagnosis may be suspected in hypertensive patients with spontaneous hypokalemia or in those receiving antihypertensive agents with severe hypokalemia. A 24-hour urinary aldosterone level can be obtained and is best measured in patients after prolonged salt loading. It should be accompanied by a 24-hour urinary sodium determination to ensure adequate salt repletion.[10] Confirmatory evidence of hyperaldosteronism is provided by suppressed plasma renin activity in the presence of elevated plasma aldosterone concentration. All of these tests have significant false-positive and false-negative rates; sensitive imaging techniques are also necessary to search for an aldosterone-secreting tumor.

### Adrenal Medulla

Adrenal medullary hormones and their metabolites are elevated in patients with pheochromocytomas and other neuroendocrine tumors. 24-hour urinary measurements specific for the desired catecholamine (epinephrine, norepinephrine, or dopamine) can be obtained. More commonly, 24-hour urinary measurement of metanephrines or vanillylmandelic acid or homovanillic acid is used to substantiate the diagnosis of pheochromocytoma (Fig 2). Plasma catecholamine assays have recently become available and are valuable in diagnosing catecholamine excess; however, the assay must be done meticulously and the setting of the specimen collection must be closely controlled to avoid stimulating catecholamine release.

Occasionally, confirmation of a pheochromocytoma may require measurement of urinary or blood hormones at the time of, or immediately after, a clinical episode. In patients with infrequent episodic attacks, glucagon can be used to induce a paroxysm—the risk of such a procedure must be anticipated and the test should not be done in patients who have severe symptoms such as angina, visual changes, or arrhythmias. An alternative test to provoke paroxysms is the clonidine suppression test, which has the advantage of causing a reduction in blood pressure. After an oral dose of 300 mg of clonidine, blood pressure and plasma levels of epinephrine and norepinephrine are measured. While blood pressure is lowered in normal persons and in those with pheochromocytoma, the plasma catecholamine levels are lowered in normal subjects while the levels do not decrease in patients with a catecholamine-secreting tumor.[11]

## PATHOPHYSIOLOGY

### Cushing's Syndrome

Cushing's syndrome is the term for the constellation of symptoms and physical findings that result from excessive circulating glucocorticoids. There are many causes of Cushing's syndrome, the most common being the therapeutic use of glucocorticoids.

Cushing's disease is the most frequent spontaneous etiology of Cushing's syndrome, and is caused by excess pituitary secretion of ACTH from a pituitary microadenoma. Approximately 70% of spontaneous Cushing's syndrome patients will be found to have Cushing's disease. Ectopic secretion of ACTH, from such neoplasms as small-cell carcinoma of the lung, account for 15% of Cushing's syndrome cases. Primary adrenal tumors are causative in most of the remaining 15% of patients with Cushing's syndrome; the tumors may be benign adenomas or adrenal-cortical carcinomas. A newly recognized cause of Cushing's syndrome is excessive secretion of corticotropin-releasing hormone from either the hypothalamus or ectopic sites.[12]

The classic signs of Cushing's syndrome are well known and include centrally distributed obesity, hirsutism, oligomenorrhea, skin striae, plethora of the facies, easy bruising, acne, muscle weakness, and symptoms of diabetes such as polyuria and polydipsia. Impotence is common in men, and growth arrest is seen in children. In addition to the physical signs that are listed with the above symptoms, hypertension is also frequently observed. With the full constellation of symptoms, diagnosis is apparent. However, in patients who have less dramatic symptoms, such as a woman with obesity and hirsutism, the differential diagnosis can be more difficult.

Laboratory tests for the diagnosis of Cushing's syndrome are many and may yield equivocal results. When suspicion of Cushing's syndrome exists, repeated testing may be necessary.[12] The standard screening test is a 24-hour urinary sample for cortisol. However, because of the intermittent nature of steroid secretion, it may be necessary to repeat even this test several times. Recently it has been reported that an evening urinary free cortisol determination may be a more sensitive method for the detection of Cushing's syndrome.[9] In patients with proven excessive excretion of cortisol, measurement of the plasma ACTH level can help define the etiology of the syndrome. In patients with adrenal adenomas or carcinomas, the morning ACTH level should be suppressed to undetectable levels. In patients with ectopic secretion of ACTH, the levels are markedly increased, while in patients with Cushing's disease, the levels are in the normal to high range but are inappropriate for the high cortisol levels seen. The dexamethasone suppression test (high dose) could then be performed; patients who have ectopic ACTH secretion or adrenal tumors do not show suppression while those with Cushing's disease should show some evidence of suppressed cortisol secretion. Another means of differentiating the etiology of Cushing's syndrome is by using the metyrapone test. Metyrapone has no effect in patients with ectopic ACTH or adrenal tumors while an exaggerated response is found in patients with Cushing's disease.

If the laboratory diagnosis points to Cushing's disease as the probable cause of the syndrome, a CT or MRI scan of the pituitary gland should be done. The pituitary tumor can be so small that it may not be demonstrable. If, however, the syndrome is thought to have an adrenal origin, a CT scan of the adrenal gland may identify the adrenal pathology (adenoma, carcinoma, or adenomatous hyperplasia). Occasionally, bilateral large adrenal glands are seen, which may suggest macronodular adenomatous hyperplasia of the adrenal gland or ectopic ACTH as the causative agent. If the imaging study does not lead to a tentative diagnosis, then further workup, possibly including petrosal vein sampling for ACTH and other more invasive studies, may be necessary to arrive at a diagnosis.[12]

The treatment of Cushing's syndrome due to ectopic ACTH is directed at the source of the ectopic secretion. Often, tumors with ectopic ACTH secretion are highly malignant and are only identified at an incurable stage; if identified early, surgical extirpation of such tumors should be performed. If resection is not possible, then medical treatment of Cushing's syndrome may result in significant amelioration of symptoms. Cushing's disease is currently treated by transphenoidal pituitary microsurgery. There is a 5% to 15% recurrence rate after pituitary microsurgery and the patient may need repeat microsurgery, or possibly medical or further surgical therapy, such as bilateral adrenalectomy.

Adrenal tumors are normally treated with primary excision. Generally, adrenal cortical carcinomas are large and often at an incurable stage when detected. Their treatment is discussed more fully in the section on adrenal cortical carcinoma. In patients with adrenal adenomas, unilateral adrenalectomy should be curative.

Medical therapy for Cushing's syndrome can be accomplished with ortho,para-DDD (Mitotane) or aminoglutethimide. These compounds have significant toxicity and are generally reserved for patients with unresectable malignant disease. Metyrapone can be used therapeutically to decrease cortisol production. Excessive cortisol production results in a buildup of deoxycorticosterone and could lead to hypertension from the excess mineralocorticoid activity. Adrenal insufficiency may result from administration of metyrapone, ortho, para-DDD, or aminoglutethimide, and the patient may require replacement steroids.

## Adrenal Cortical Carcinoma

Adrenal cortical carcinoma may originate from cells in any of the three layers of the normal adrenal cortex. As such, these cancers can produce a variety of steroid precursors, end products, and metabolites, which cause variable clinical syndromes and laboratory findings of excess steroid secretion. Some adrenal cortical carcinomas are endocrinologically nonfunctioning; patients with such tumors present with symptoms related to the abdominal mass. The occurrence of adrenal cortical carcinoma is rare, approaching 2 cases per million persons.[13]

Adrenal cortical carcinoma often presents clinically as a large abdominal mass which may be associated with virilization in the female or with Cushing's syndrome. Precocious puberty may be seen in children with endocrinologically functioning tumors. A delay in time from the onset of symptoms to diagnosis has often been noted in the literature; the insidious nature of endocrinologically induced appearance changes may go unrecognized by the patient and family for some time.

Because of its rarity and the usual late diagnosis, this tumor is often discovered at a surgically incurable stage. Clinical staging may be augmented with a chest x-ray, a CT or MRI scan to check for local and intra-abdominal metastases, and a biochemical study to discover potential bone or liver metastases. The only consistently effective therapy for adrenal cortical carcinoma is total surgical extirpation.[14,15]

Perioperative steroid replacement should be routine, as the function of the contralateral adrenal gland may be suppressed. Postoperative steroid replacement should be directed by the results of functional testing. Because of the extensive nature of these primary tumors and the lack of any curative adjunctive therapy, extensive local resection—often with nephrectomy and occasionally requiring splenectomy, partial hepatectomy or pancreatectomy—may be necessary. Significant palliation of endocrinopathies can be obtained with resection of large masses, even when residual disease is present. Recurrent endocrinopathies can be treated with steroid synthesis inhibitors such as metyrapone or aminoglutethimide. The possibility of extension of adrenal cortical carcinoma into the venous system (with possible vena caval involvement) is similar to that of renal cell carcinoma; preoperative evaluation of the vascular system should be performed.

Metastatic adrenal cortical carcinoma can be treated with ortho, para-DDD (Mitotane). Response rates have generally been low[16]; higher doses of this drug (confirmed by measuring drug levels) may be more effective[17] but may also lead to significant side effects. Other chemotherapy, particularly cis-platinum-based chemotherapy, has also been used, with low response levels.

## Primary Aldosteronism

Primary aldosteronism results from the hypersecretion of aldosterone, usually secondary to an adrenal adenoma. It is an unusual cause of hypertension, occurring in less than 1% of the hypertensive population. The diagnosis of primary aldosteronism can be enigmatic but may be suspected in patients with hypokalemia and hypertension. The hypokalemia may be spontaneous or induced by diuretics and is usually resistant to standard potassium repletion therapy. The diagnosis may be confirmed by obtaining higher than normal serum aldosterone values that fail to normalize with adequate salt replacement. The diagnosis is definitive in the untreated hypertensive patient who is hypokalemic and has high urinary and serum aldosterone and a low plasma renin activity. However, this classic diagnostic pattern is not always present. In those patients in whom there are signs, symptoms, or laboratory values suggestive of primary aldosteronism, evaluation should include a 24-hour urinary aldosterone determination after salt loading. Serum aldosterone levels may remain in the same range as those seen in patients with essential hypertension, but the majority of patients with primary aldosteronism will have significantly higher 24-hour urinary aldosterone levels than those associated with essential hypertension.[10] In patients with elevated 24-hour urinary aldosterone levels, CT scanning is the next step (to lateralize the adenoma). These adenomas are frequently small, and closely spaced (0.5 cm) CT slices of the adrenal glands may be necessary to demonstrate the adenoma. Even without demonstration on CT scan, further localization procedures with adrenal vein sampling and adrenal venography may lead to diagnosis. In patients with an identified adenoma, surgery will lead to cure or at least simpler medical management of the hypertension and hypokalemia. Before surgery, patients should be placed on antihypertensive medications and potassium-sparing agents. Patients should be treated long enough to correct the metabolic abnormalities (generally several weeks). When adenoma cannot be definitively diagnosed, such drug therapy is the recommended therapeutic approach with periodic reassessment to check for appearance of an adenoma.

## Adrenocortical Insufficiency

Adrenocortical insufficiency (Addison's disease) is unusual, but may be seen after unilateral adrenalectomy, when the function of the contralateral adrenal gland has been suppressed by a tumor. Adrenocortical insufficiency is also seen in surgical patients who have been receiving chronic steroid replacement and who are not given adequate replacement doses of steroids perioperatively. The symptoms of adrenocortical insufficiency include weakness, fatigue, hypotension, hyperpigmentation, and gastrointestinal disturbances. In the surgical patient with acute adrenal crisis, hypotension and refractory shock, fever, volume depletion, weakness, hypoglycemia, and delirium may also occur.

The diagnosis of adrenal insufficiency can be confirmed by laboratory assessment of the pituitary adrenal axis, but this should not delay therapy in patients with suggestive clinical signs. To test for adrenocortical insufficiency, the ACTH levels should be measured. In those with secondary adrenal insufficiency, the ACTH levels are low while in most patients with primary adrenal insufficiency ACTH levels are high. An ACTH stimulation test will indicate the presence or absence of decreased adrenal reserve. Primary adrenal insufficiency can be caused by granulomatous infection of the adrenal glands with tuberculosis or histoplasmosis, but this is infrequently seen in the modern era.

Intravenous cortisol 100 mg every 6 hours with tapering as tolerated is used to treat acute adrenal crisis, along with correction of volume depletion and hypoglycemia. Maintenance therapy with cortisol or a synthetic steroid is usually necessary. Supplementation with a synthetic mineralocorticoid (Florinef) is necessary in patients with primary adrenocortical insufficiency.

In patients with possible pituitary adrenal suppression due to administration of exogenous glucocorticoids, or with primary or secondary adrenocortical insufficiency, steroid replacement is necessary prior to any surgery. Hydrocortisone (100 mg) may be administered when the patient is called to surgery followed by a 50 mg dose every 6 hours for the first 24 hours, with tapering reduction to maintenance doses over the next 3 to 5 days. If complications, such as fever or hypotension, develop, additional corticosteroid should be administered.

## Pheochromocytoma

Pheochromocytomas are neoplasms that stem from the chromaffin cells of the sympathetic nervous system. This disease accounts for 0.1% of patients with hypertension. The incidence is about 2 cases per million persons per year.[18] Clearly, the disease is rare, but it is nevertheless important to recognize, as paroxysms can be potentially fatal—especially in pregnant women during delivery and in surgical patients. Because of the episodic nature of the symptoms and confusion with other conditions, the diagnosis often is not made. A large review from Rochester, Minnesota showed that 76% of pheochromocytomas found in autopsy series were not diagnosed antemortem.[19]

Although the symptoms of pheochromocytoma are classically thought to occur in paroxysmal fashion, most patients with functioning tumors will have signs or symptoms most of the time. Paroxysms may be superimposed upon the chronic symptoms. Occasionally, the symptoms may be minimal and the diagnosis is made from incidental findings on an ultrasound, CT, or MRI scan.

The symptoms of a paroxysm are similar to those produced by injection of therapeutic catecholamines. The patient is aware of palpitations, usually described as forceful beating within the chest; the throbbing spreads to the lower abdomen and head, resulting in headache. Because of peripheral vasoconstriction, the limbs are cool and moist and there is facial pallor. Blood pressure measurements during paroxysms reveal moderate to severe hypertension. The symptomatic complex induces anxiety and, if the paroxysm is prolonged, may cause nausea, vomiting, diaphoresis, chest pain, and paresthesias.

Although the above-mentioned syndrome is classic, this may also be confused with other anxiety-related symptoms; sometimes paroxysms may be mistaken for hot flashes in menopausal women. Other disorders with secondary sympathetic dis-

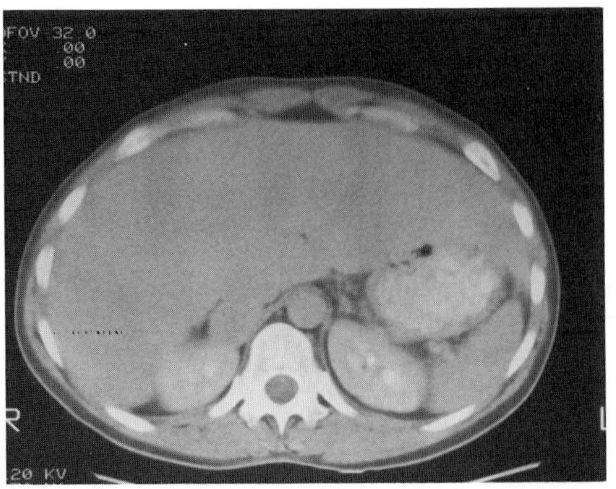


A

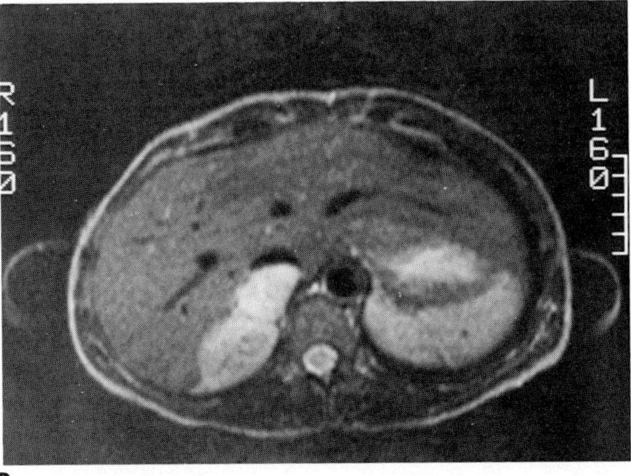


B

**Fig 3.** Von Hippel-Lindau disease. A, CT scan of 27-year-old woman showing a right pheochromocytoma; B, MRI scan of same patient showing bright right adrenal mass on T-2 weighted image.

charge, such as angina, thyrotoxicosis, or other causes of hypertension may be confused with pheochromocytoma.

Several familial syndromes are associated with the development of pheochromocytoma. These include multiple endocrine neoplasia (MEN) type IIa (Sipple's syndrome) which encompasses medullary thyroid carcinoma and a parathyroid hormone producing adenoma of the parathyroid. MEN type IIb occurs in association with mucosal neuromas and marfanoid habitus. Both of these disorders have an autosomal dominant pattern of transmission, with incomplete penetrance. Von Hippel-Lindau disease (Figs 3,4), von Recklinghausen's disease (neurofibromatosis), and Sturge-Weber disease are other familial conditions that may be associated with pheochromocytoma.

Pheochromocytomas occur most often in the adrenal gland (85%), but can also be found in extra-adrenal sites of chromaffin tissue, including the organ of Zuckerkandl and the retroperitoneal sympathetic chain. Occasionally, pheochromocytoma arising from the chromaffin cells that innervate the bladder are found; in such cases the paroxysms may be associated with urinary voiding. Tumors, when found, are usually small, but can grow to large size if the catecholamine production is low and the patient fails to report the symptoms promptly. There is no pathologic distinction on microscopy between benign and malignant pheochromocytoma, and the nature of the tumor is determined by its clinical behavior. Traditionally, it has been taught that the "rule of 10" is applied to pheochromocytomas, in that approxi-

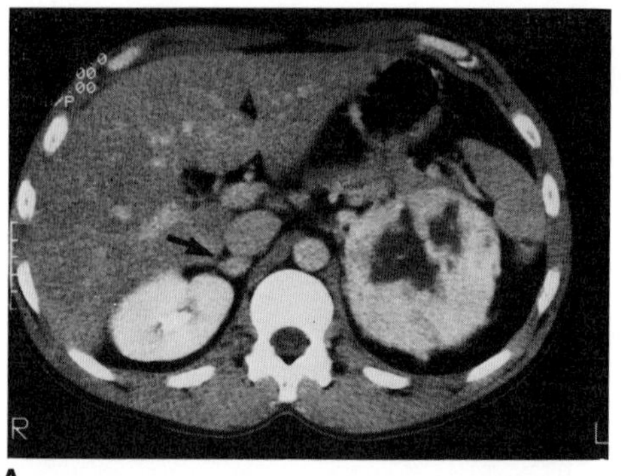


A

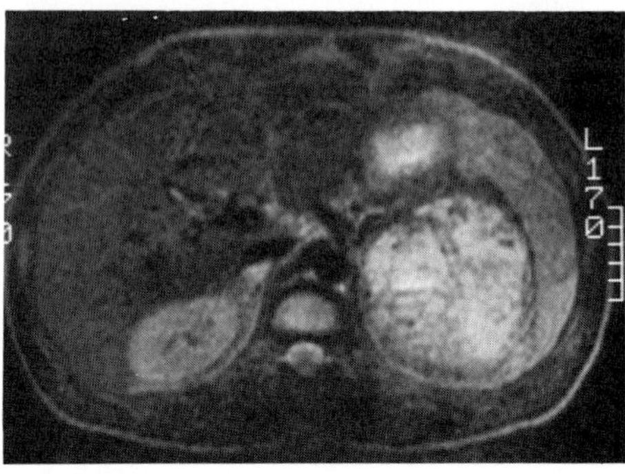

B

Fig 4. Pheochromocytoma. A, 29-year-old brother of patient in Fig 3, CT showing huge left pheochromocytoma and small right pheochromocytoma (arrow); B, MRI scan showing same tumor, with a bright adrenal mass on T-2 weighted image.

mately 10% of the tumors are bilateral, 10% are malignant, 10% are familial, and 10% are extra-adrenal. These estimates, although not exact, are reasonable; however, the incidence of malignancy may be revealed to be significantly higher if patients are followed more closely.[20] The diagnosis should be suspected in any hypertensive patient who has other suggestive symptoms or severe or difficult to control hypertension. Fifteen percent of patients found to have pheochromocytomas are not hypertensive, and other hormones, such as vasoactive intestinal peptide, calcitonin, serotonin, ACTH, and CRH may be secreted in excessive amounts along with the catecholamines.[21]

The diagnosis of pheochromocytoma may be confirmed by the finding of elevated catecholamine levels in the blood or urine. Serum catecholamine levels provide an excellent diagnostic tool. However, the assays must be done meticulously, and the setting of the test arranged carefully, with the patient fasting, supine, and relaxed. More commonly, the 24-hour urinary specimen for combined metanephrines and vanillylmandelic acid are used to screen for pheochromocytoma. Free catecholamines in the urine can also be determined, and a 24-hour urinary specimen for norepinephrine, epinephrine, and dopamine can be obtained. Patients with malignant pheochromocytomas are often deficient in dopamine betahydroxylase and phenylethylamine N-methyltransferase; such deficiencies lead to increased dopamine secretion and low urinary epinephrine levels. In addition, they also lead to large quantities of homovanillic acid in the urine. If elevated epinephrine levels are present in the urine and norepinephrine is absent, the tumor is most likely to be found in the adrenal gland. The clonidine suppression test can be used in equivocal cases to further search for biochemical evidence of pheochromocytoma.

Once the diagnosis of pheochromocytoma is made biochemically, an imaging procedure (usually CT or MRI scan) (Figs. 3,4) should be used to localize the disease. The tumor will usually be apparent on one of these studies; if not, adrenal vein sampling and/or adrenal venography may be useful to locate the tumor. When the above methods fail, MIBG nuclear scanning may be helpful in localizing a pheochromocytoma (especially for extra-adrenal tumors).[22]

The goal of initial management of a patient with pheochromocytoma is to block the excessive catecholamine secretion. Adrenergic antagonists are administered to reduce the symptoms, lower the blood pressure, and avoid such complications as myocardial infarction, cerebral vascular accident, arrhythmias, shock, renal failure, or aortic aneurysm. Also, treatment with adrenergic blockers allows reversal of vasoconstriction and expansion of the plasma volume and vascular bed. If the patient does not receive adrenergic-blocking agents prior to surgery and is not given time for the agents to take effect, there may be more dramatic fluid shifts during surgery, which lead to higher transfusion requirements and a more labile intraoperative condition. It is important to institute α-adrenergic blockade with such agents as phentolamine, prazosin, or phenoxybenzamine prior to β-adrenergic blockade. Failure to do this will lead to unopposed α-adrenergic stimulation and a hypertensive crisis. β-blockers, such as propranolol, are usually administered only to those with problematic cardiac arrhythmias. Metyrosine (Demser) is a metabolic blocker of catecholamine synthesis that can be used as a substitute for adrenergic blockade to normalize catecholamine levels. This medication, however, has the significant side effects of drowsiness and diarrhea, and several weeks of therapy is necessary to re-expand the vascular bed.

When the tumor is preoperatively known to be malignant, pharmacologic management alone is usually instituted unless there is a very large mass. There is no specific, effective chemotherapy; however, reports of using $^{131}$I-MIBG therapeutically have recently appeared.[23] In patients with benign disease, surgical excision is indicated. The patient should be prepared with adrenergic blockade prior to surgery. Alternatively, acute volume expansion and preoperative transfusion has been used with good results in some series.[24] Some surgeons would argue that preoperative blockade may prevent detection of an extra-adrenal tumor; however, given the quality of modern diagnostic imaging studies, the location of the tumor is usually not dependent on intraoperative exploration for detection. Intra-abdominal tumors should be approached surgically through transabdominal incisions; early control of the vasculature is recommended, as secretion of high levels of catecholamines may potentially occur with manipulation of the tumor. Meticulous anesthetic management is paramount, and continuous blood pressure and cardiac wedge pressure monitoring is recommended. Halothane anesthesia should be avoided, because it increases the risk of arrhythmias. There should be continual availability of agents such as nitroprusside to lower blood pressure acutely for short periods of time, if necessary. Conversely, with removal of the tumor, there may be sudden expansion of the vascular bed that causes hypotension requiring transfusion or other fluid expansion. Pressor therapy may occasionally be useful, but volume administration is usually sufficient. Follow-up should include repeat serum or urine testing for catecholamine excess to rule out recurrence or malignancy.[20]

## OTHER ADRENAL MASSES AND THE INCIDENTAL ADRENAL MASS

With the widespread availability of modern sophisticated imaging techniques, such as ultrasound, CT and MRI, unsuspected masses in the adrenal glands are not infrequently encountered. Autopsy studies show benign, clinically silent adenomas in up to 9% of subjects.[25] These "incidental" adrenal masses have been the topic of debate in the surgical and medical literature. Most authors have come to the conclusion that a certain size limit (3 to 6 cm in largest diameter) should be used as a cutoff for those lesions that should be surgically excised because of their potential for malignancy, as opposed to those that may be watched as probable benign adenomata.[26–28] Also, nearly all authors recommend biochemical screening to determine function in these masses—be it steroid or

**TABLE 1. Differential Diagnosis of Adrenal Masses**

| |
|---|
| Metastases |
| Multinodular hyperplasia |
| Adrenal adenoma |
| Adrenocortical carcinoma |
| Myelolipoma |
| Lipoma |
| Adrenal cyst |
| Lymphangioma, angioma |
| Pheochromocytoma |
| Neuroblastoma |
| Ganglioneuroma |
| Ganglioneuroblastoma |
| Granulomatous infection |
| Congenital adrenal hyperplasia |
| Adrenal hemorrhage |

catecholamine hypersecretion. Functioning masses then would also undergo surgical extirpation. Thus, a 24-hour urine specimen measuring cortisol, 17-ketosteroids, 17-ketogenic steroids, vanillylmandelic acid, and metanephrines is obtained to rule out endocrine function.

The differential diagnosis of such masses is listed in Table 1. Metastatic lesions, particularly those from primary lung, kidney, or colon carcinomas are the most common (Fig 5). Myelolipomas are benign tumors that have characteristic fat density on a CT or MRI scan. They are composed of mature fat and blood-forming elements, and the incidence at autopsy has been estimated at 0.4% to 0.8%. Simple lipomas of the adrenal gland also exist. Hemangiomas and lymphangiomas are rare findings in the adrenals. Cysts of the adrenal glands occur, and may be associated with hemorrhage and pain but are usually of no clinical consequence. Granulomatous infection, such as with tuberculosis or histoplasmosis, may result in a calcified adrenal mass. Neuroblastoma is a tumor of childhood. Those tumors showing mature ganglion cell differentiation are classified as ganglioneuroblastomas or ganglioneuromas.

Once the diagnosis of an adrenal mass has been made, differentiation is dependent on biochemical studies and imaging characteristics of the mass. Needle biopsy or aspiration of the adrenal gland may be useful to differentiate metastases from primary adrenal tumors, but often a clear histologic diagnosis of a primary adrenal tumor cannot be made from needle biopsy specimens. In addition, it should be recognized that there is the potential risk of inducing a hypertensive crisis with needle puncture of an unsuspected pheochromocytoma.

## ADRENAL GLAND TRANSPLANTATION

Autotransplantation of the adrenal gland to the caudate nucleus is a newly proposed procedure for the treatment of Parkinson's disease.[29] The theoretic advantage of transplanting adrenal cells to the caudate nucleus is to provide dopaminergic cells and restore function to the substantia nigra. The tech-

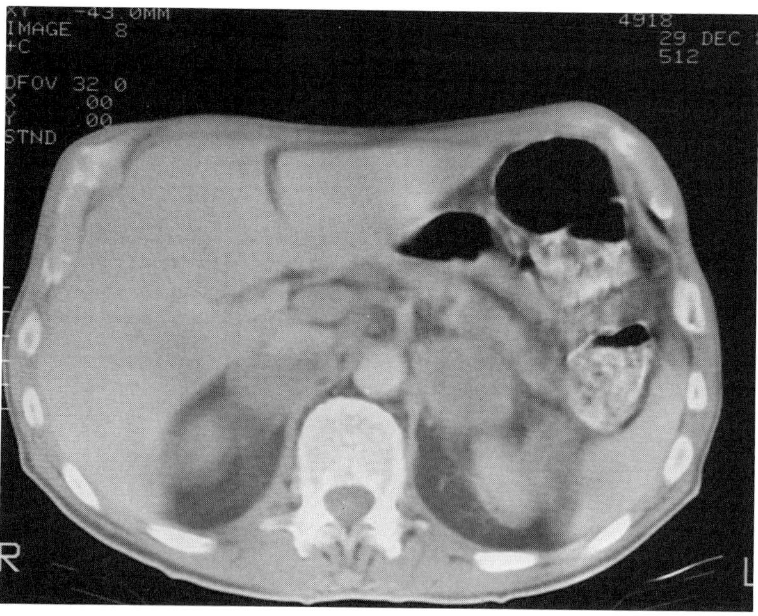


**Fig 5.** Bilateral adrenal metastases from primary lung carcinoma.

nique of harvesting of the adrenal gland has been described, and the procedure, although still considered experimental, may lead to a wider role for adrenal surgery.[30] Fetal adrenal tissue has been successfully transplanted to treat Addison's disease.[31] Autotransplantation of adrenal tissue after bilateral adrenalectomy for Cushing's syndrome to preserve some adrenal function and avoid Nelson's syndrome has met with unpredictable results. Rarely is an eucortisolic state attained; most patients remain deficient in cortisol, while a few have had hypercortisolism recur.[32]

## REFERENCES


1. England MA. *Color Atlas of Life Before Birth.* New York: Year Book Medical; 1983:152.
2. Vilke DB. The development of steroidogenesis. *Am J Med.* 1972;53:533.
3. West GB, Shepherd DM, Hunter RB. Adrenaline and noradrenaline concentration in adrenal glands at different ages and in some diseases. *Lancet.* 1951;261:966.
4. Kissane JM. *Pathology of Infancy and Childhood.* St Louis, MO: CV Mosby Company; 1975:746–783.
5. Kumar R, Ruppert D, Sayle BA, et al. Adrenal scintigraphy. *Semin Roentgen.* 1988;23:243.
6. Charlton BG. Adrenal cortical innervation and glucocorticoid secretion. *J Endocrinol.* 1990; 126:5.
7. Tyrell JB, Avon DC, Forsham PH. Glucocorticoids and adrenal androgens. In: Greenspan FS, Forsham PH, eds. *Basic and Clinical Endocrinology.* 3rd ed. Norwalk, Conn: Appleton & Lange; 1991:323–362.
8. Goldfien A. Adrenal medulla. In: Greenspan FA, Forsham PH, eds. *Basic and Clinical Endocrinology.* 3rd ed. Norwalk, Conn: Appleton & Lange; 1991:380–399.
9. Landat MH, Billaud C, Thomopoulos P, et al. Evening urinary free corticoids; a screening test in Cushing's syndrome and incidentally discovered adrenal tumors. *Acta Endocrinol.* 1988; 119:459.
10. Bravo EL. Primary aldosteronism. *Urol Clin North Am.* 1989;16:481.
11. Bravo EL, Tarazi RC, Fouad FM, et al. Clonidine suppression test: a useful aid in the diagnosis of pheochromocytoma. *N Engl J Med.* 1981;305:625.
12. Sheeler LR. Cushing's syndrome. *Urol Clin North Am.* 1989;16:447.
13. *Third National Cancer Surgery Incidence Data.* Washington, DC: National Institutes of Health; 1975. National Cancer Institute Monograph 41 NIH 75–787.
14. Bodie B, Novick AC, Pontes JE, et al. The Cleveland Clinic experience with adrenal cortical carcinoma. *J Urol.* 1989;141:257.
15. Venkatesh S, Hickey RC, Sellin RU, et al. Adrenal cortical carcinoma. *Cancer.* 1989;64:765.
16. Luton JP, Cerdas S, Billard L, et al. Clinical features of adrenocortical carcinoma, prognostic factors and the effect of mitotane therapy. *N Engl J Med.* 1990;322:1195.
17. van Slooten H, Moolenaar AJ, Van Seters AP, et al. The treatment of adrenocortical carcinoma with o'p'-DDD: prognostic implications of serum level monitoring. *Eur J Cancer Clin Oncol.* 1984;20:47.
18. Stenstrom G, Suardsudd K. Pheochromocytoma in Sweden, 1958–1981. An analysis of the National Cancer Registry Data. *Acta Med Scand.* 1986;220:225.
19. Beard CM, Sheps SG, Kurland LT, et al. Occurence of pheochromocytoma in Rochester, Minnesota, 1950 through 1979. *Mayo Clin Proc.* 1983;58:802.
20. Scott HW, Malter SA. Oncologic aspects of pheochromocytoma: the importance of follow-up. *Surgery.* 1984;96:1061.
21. Benowitz NL. Pheochromocytoma. *Adv Intern Med.* 1990;35:195.
22. Shapiro B, Cope JE, Sisson JC, et al. Iodine-131-metaiodobenzylguanidine for the locating of suspected pheochromocytoma: experience in 400 cases. *J Nucl Med.* 1985;26:576.
23. Sisson JC, Shapiro B, Beierwaltes WA, et al. Radiopharmaceutical treatment of malignant pheochromocytoma. *J Nucl Med.* 1984;25:197.
24. Stewart BH. The adrenal: surgical therapy. *AUA Updates.* 1983;2:lesson 15.
25. Grizzle WE. Pathology of the adrenal gland. *Semin Roentgen.* 1988;23:323.
26. Copeland PM. The incidentally discovered adrenal mass. *Ann Intern Med.* 1983;98:940.
27. Thompson NW, Cheung PSY. Diagnosis and treatment of functioning and nonfunctioning adrenocortical neoplasms including incidentalomas. *Surg Clin North Am.* 1987;67:423.
28. Belldegrun A, deKernion JB. What to do about the incidentally found adrenal mass. *World J Urol.* 1989;7:117.
29. Sladek JR, Gash DM. Nerve-cell grafting in Parkinson's disease; review article. *J Neurosurg.* 1988;68:337.
30. Skinner EC, Boyd SD, Apuzzo MLJ. Technique of left adrenalectomy for autotransplantation to

the caudate nucleus in Parkinson's disease. *J Urol.* 1990;144:838.

31. Yan ZB, Bing ZX, Yang WR, et al. A study of cadaveric fetal adrenal used for adrenal transplantation to treat Addison's disease: thirteen cases reported. *Transplant Proc.* 1990;22:280.

32. Lino BL, Maurizio P, Federico R, et al. The unpredictable outcome of autotransplanted adrenal gland tissue after bilateral surrenalectomy for Cushing's disease. *Surg Gynecol Obstet.* 1984;159:461.

# 12

# Renovascular Hypertension

*Andrew C. Novick*

## INTRODUCTION

The first reports in the late 1930s of surgically curable hypertension led to enthusiasm among clinicians for removing kidneys with arterial stenosis in hypertensive patients. The development of vascular surgical techniques in the 1950s made it possible to achieve successful renal revascularization in many of these cases. However, the cause-and-effect relationship between a stenotic renal artery lesion and hypertension was poorly understood, and many patients treated surgically had no improvement of blood pressure postoperatively. Continued experience in this field during the past two decades has significantly improved our understanding of the natural history and functional significance of renovascular disorders. Patients with renovascular hypertension can now be accurately identified, and successful revascularization is possible in most cases.

## CLASSIFICATION OF RENOVASCULAR DISORDERS

### Atherosclerosis

Approximately 60% of all renovascular lesions are caused by atherosclerosis.[1] This disease may be limited to the renal artery, but more commonly is a manifestation of generalized atherosclerosis involving the abdominal aorta, coronary, cerebral, and lower extremity vessels. Atherosclerotic stenosis usually occurs in the proximal 2 cm of the renal artery, and distal arterial or branch involvement is distinctly uncommon.

Due to the proximal location of these lesions, oblique aortic views are often needed to adequately visualize the area of stenosis. The lesion involves the intima of the artery, and in two thirds of the cases presents as an eccentric plaque, in the remainder the vessel is circumferentially involved with narrowing of the lumen and destruction of the intima. Dissecting hematomas frequently complicate this disease, sometimes resulting in thrombosis of the entire vessel (Fig 1).

There have been relatively few published reports on the natural history of atherosclerotic lesions in patients managed nonoperatively. The available data suggest that progressive arterial stenosis, occasionally eventuating in total occlusion, is a relatively common sequela of this disease. In 1968, Wollenweber and associates[2] reviewed 30 patients with atherosclerotic renovascular disease who had been followed with serial renal angiograms from 3 to 88 months apart; progressive renal artery stenosis was observed unilaterally in 13 patients (43%) and bilaterally in 6 patients (20%). Also in 1968, Meaney et al.[3] reported progression of atherosclerotic renal artery stenosis in 14 of 39 patients (36%) followed with serial angiography during intervals ranging from 6 months to 7 years.

More recently, Schreiber et al.[4] reviewed the outcome of atherosclerotic renovascu-

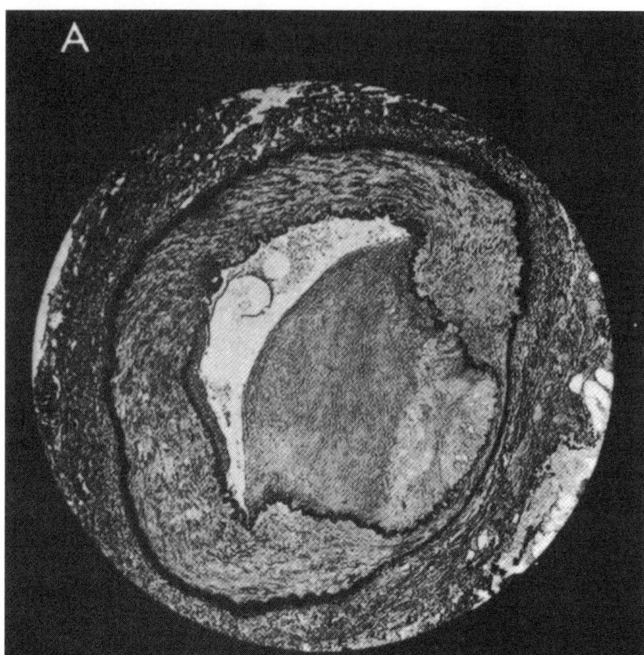


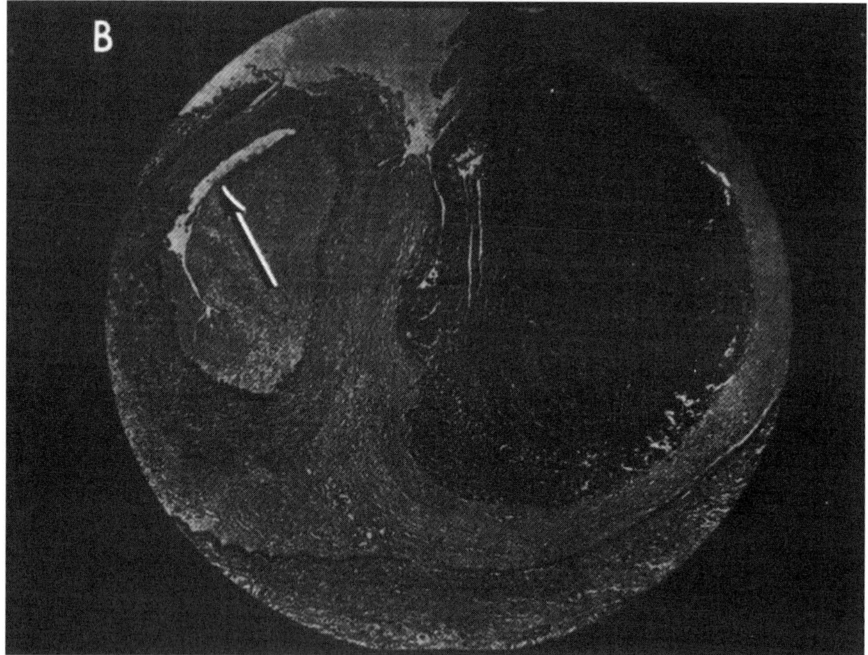


**Fig 1. A:** Cross-section of typical eccentric atherosclerotic plaque involving proximal main renal artery. **B:** Large dissecting hematoma involving media of artery initially obstructed by an atherosclerotic plaque. Note further progression of original arterial lumen *(arrow).*

lar disease in 85 patients treated medically and followed with sequential renal angiography during intervals of 3–172 months. The mean angiographic follow-up interval was 52 months and the mean clinical follow-up period in these patients was 87 months. Progressive renal artery obstruction from atherosclerosis was observed in 37 patients (44%), including 14 patients (16%) who developed complete arterial oc-

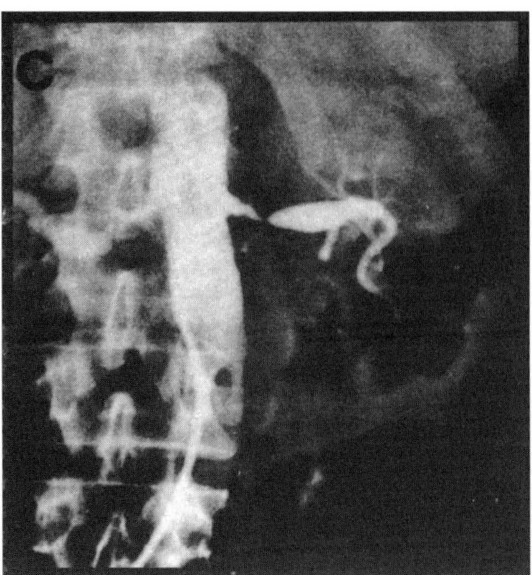

**Fig 1. C:** Aortogram demonstrating bilateral proximal renal artery stenosis from atherosclerotic plaque.

clusion. Clinical follow-up revealed that serial decreases in both overall renal function ($p < .02$) and the size of the involved kidney ($p < .001$) occurred more commonly in patients who developed progressive renovascular disease than in those who did not. However, serial blood pressure control was no different in these two groups, and therefore it is not a marker for progressive disease. This study indicates not only that atherosclerotic renal artery disease progresses in a large number of patients but also that such progression is commonly associated with clinically detectable loss of functional renal parenchyma.

## Fibrous Dysplasia

Fibrous dysplasias comprise approximately 40% of all renovascular disorders.[1] These lesions are considered to be congenital dysplasias with maldevelopment of the fibrous, muscular, and elastic tissues of the renal artery. They are subcategorized according to the layer of the arterial wall involved.[5] This classification is important since each type of fibrous dysplasia has distinct histologic and angiographic features, and each type occurs in a different clinical setting.

Primary intimal fibroplasia occurs in children and in young adults, and composes approximately 10% of the total fibrous lesions. This lesion is characterized by a circumferential accumulation of collagen inside the internal elastica lamina (Fig 2). Disruption and duplication of the elastica interna occur more often in younger patients, with dissecting hematomas as a complication in many patients. The possibility of atherosclerosis as a cause of renal artery disease in this group can be excluded clinically on lipid profiles and histologically by the absence of demonstrable lipid with special staining techniques. Intimal fibroplasia with complicating medical dissection is characterized pathologically by large dissecting channels in the outer one half of the media. These lesions are thought to develop because of defects in the internal elastica with resultant medial dissection and aneurysmal dilatation.

Angiography in primary intimal fibroplasia reveals a smooth, fairly focal stenosis unusually involving the midportion of the vessel or its branches. Dissecting hematomas may distort the area of stenosis. With nonoperative management, progressive renal artery obstruction and ischemic atrophy of the involved kidney invariably occur. Severe intimal fibroplasia may subsequently develop de novo in the contralateral renal artery. Although primary intimal fibroplasia most commonly affects the renal arteries, this may occur as a generalized disorder with concomitant involvement of carotid, upper and lower extremity, and mesenteric vessels.[6]

Medial fibroplasia is the most common of the fibrous lesions, comprising 75%–80% of the total number. It tends to occur in 25- to 50-year-old women and often involves both renal arteries. It may involve other vessels in the body, most notably the carotid, mesenteric, and iliac arteries. Microscopically, the internal elastic membrane is focal and variably thinned and lost. Within the alternating thickening areas much of the muscle is replaced by collagen; hence the term medial fibroplasia. In other areas, thinning of the media occurs to the point of complete loss, and micro-

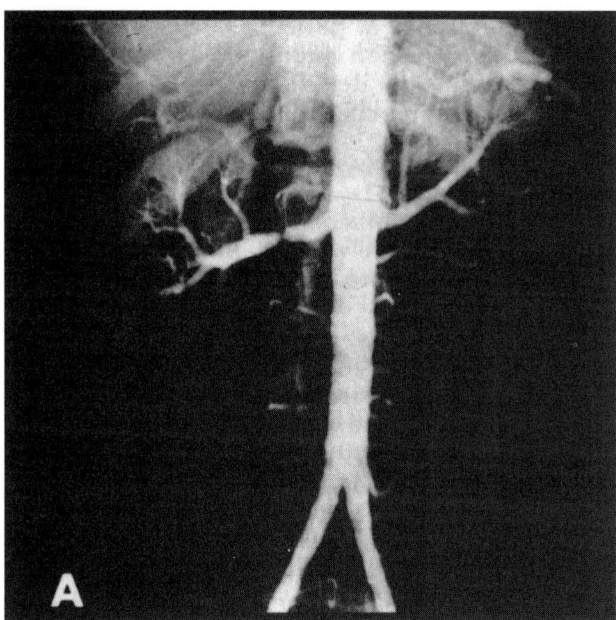


**Fig 2. A:** Aortogram in 17-year-old male demonstrates focal stenosis of mid–right renal artery from intimal fibroplasia [From Kelalis P, King L, Belman B, eds. *Clinical Pediatric Urology*. Philadelphia: WB Saunders, with permission.] **B:** Cross-section of renal artery involved with intimal fibroplasia showing circumferential accumulation of collagen compromising the lumen inside the internal elastic lamina.

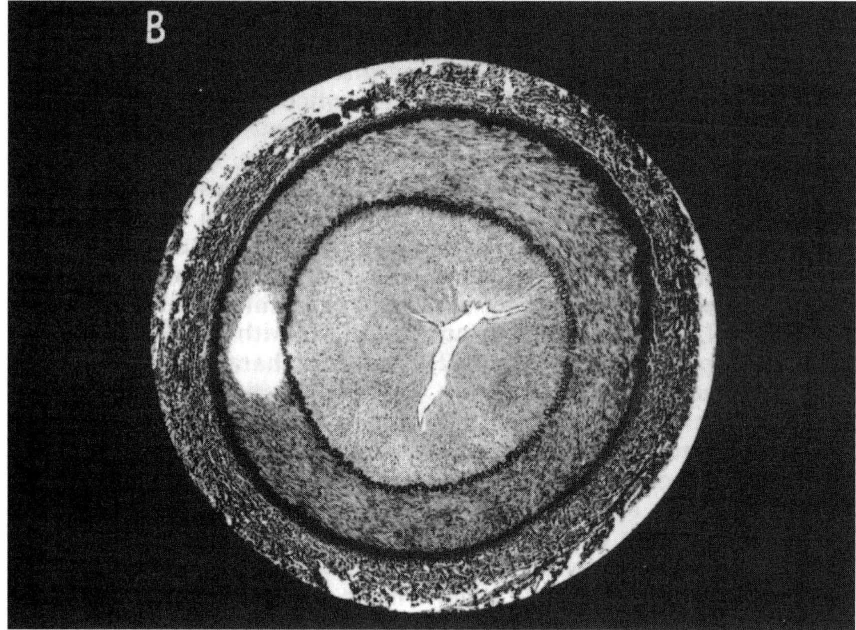


aneurysms can be seen as saccules lined by only the external elastica. In extreme cases, giant aneurysms may be found in association with medial fibroplasia.

Angiographically, medial fibroplasia demonstrates a typical "string-of-beads" appearance involving the distal two thirds of the main renal artery and branches (Fig 3). The areas of stenosis are often overshadowed by contrast medium in the microaneurysm, making the degree of actual stenosis difficult to assess. The aneurysms themselves are greater in diameter than the normal renal artery proximal to the

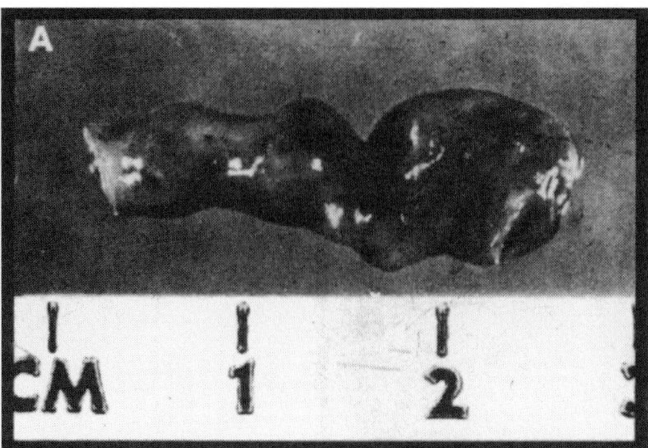


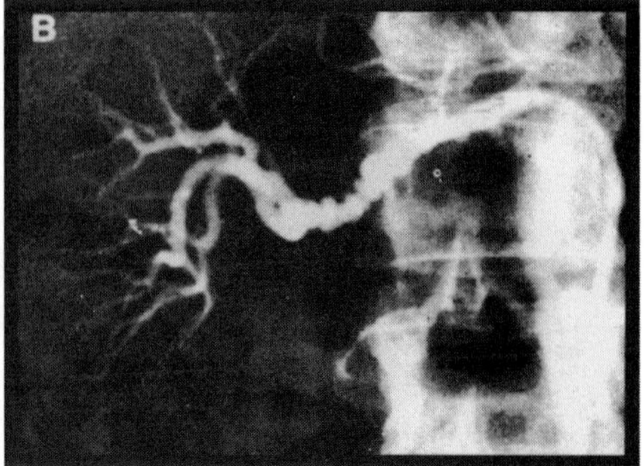


**Fig 3.** **A:** External view of resected specimen of renal artery involved by medial fibroplasia. Note small pseudoaneurysms presenting as bulges on outer surface of vessel. **B:** Right renal arteriogram in patient with medial fibroplasia demonstrates typical "string-of-beads" appearance involving the main renal artery and its proximal branches.

disease, and extreme collateral circulation is absent. These are important features in differentiating the lesion from perimedial fibroplasia. Schreiber et al.[4] studied the natural history of renal artery disease due to medial fibroplasia in 66 patients who were followed with serial angiography. Progressive renal artery stenosis occurred in 22 patients (33%) and contrary to an earlier report,[3] this occurrence was no different in patients greater than or less than 40 years of age. Significantly, there were no cases of progression to total arterial occlusion in this group. Also, clinical follow-up revealed that serial decreases in either overall renal function or the size of the involved kidney seldom occurred in patients with progressive medial fibroplasia, suggesting that the risk of losing renal function is relatively small in patients with this disease who are managed medically.

Perimedial fibroplasia occurs predominantly in 15- to 30-year-old females and has therefore been referred to as "girlie disease." Ten to fifteen percent of all fibrous lesions are perimedial fibroplasias. These tightly stenotic lesions only occur in the renal artery and consist pathologically of a collar of dense collagen enveloping the renal artery for variable lengths and thicknesses (Fig 4). The collagen is deposited in the outer border of the media and usually replaces a considerable portion of the media; in some areas it may completely replace the media. Islands of smooth muscle are occasionally seen trapped within the collagenous ring. Special stains show that the lesion is confined within the external elastica lamina and contained in all cases by intact adventitial connective tissue. The arterial lumen may be further compromised by a process of secondary intimal fibroplasia. It has been suggested that this secondary thickening of the intima is related to slowing of blood flow through a narrowed arterial segment, with resultant platelet and fibrin deposition and subsequent fibrous organization.

The arteriogram of perimedial fibroplasia may give the appearance of arterial beading, but careful observation shows that the caliber of the normal segment of the vessel is not exceeded by the "bead." This fact, along with the frequent occurrence of extensive collateral circulation, differentiates this lesion angiographically from that of medial fibroplasia. Perimedial fibroplasia produces severe stenosis and, although complicating thrombosis or dissection are relatively uncommon, progressive obstruction with ischemic renal atrophy occurs in almost all patients managed nonoperatively.

Fibromuscular hyperplasia is an extremely rare disease, comprising only 2%–3% of fibrous lesions, and tends to occur in children and young adults. This is the only renal arterial disease in which true hyperplasia of smooth muscle cells is present. The renal artery shows a concentric thick-

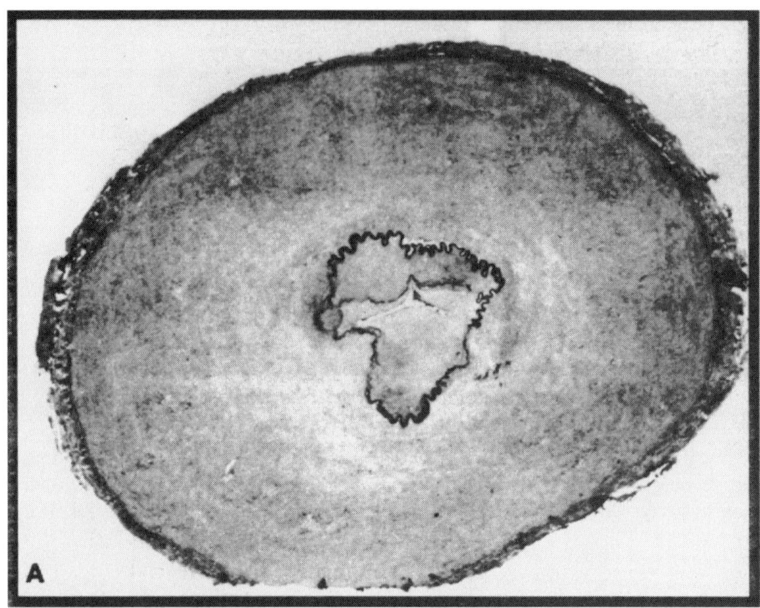


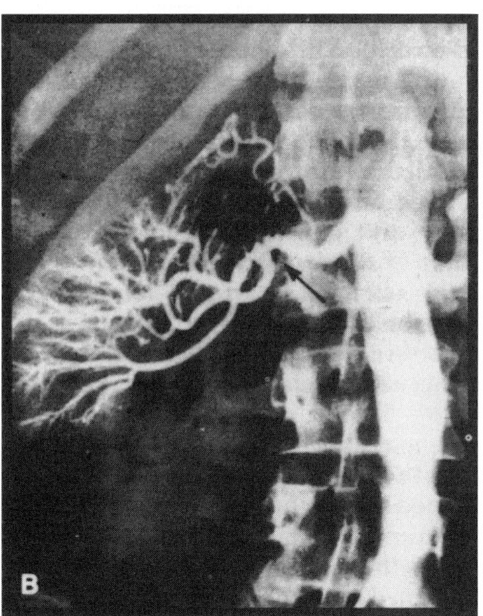


**Fig 4. A:** Photomicrograph cross-section of perimedial fibroplasia manifested as a dense fibroplasia of the outer media with loss of the elastica externa. Note the significant secondary intimal fibroplasia. **B:** Renal arteriogram in patient with perimedial fibroplasia showing irregular yet severe stenosis of the right renal artery and its proximal branches, associated with extensive collateral circulation to the kidney.

ening of its wall with a mixture of proliferating smooth muscle and fibrous tissue in variable quantity. Angiographically, fibromuscular hyperplasia presents as a smooth stenosis of the renal artery or its branches and, from a radiographic standpoint, may be indistinguishable from intimal fibroplasia. Most patients with this disease have developed progressive vascular obstruction when followed with serial angiographic studies (Fig 5).

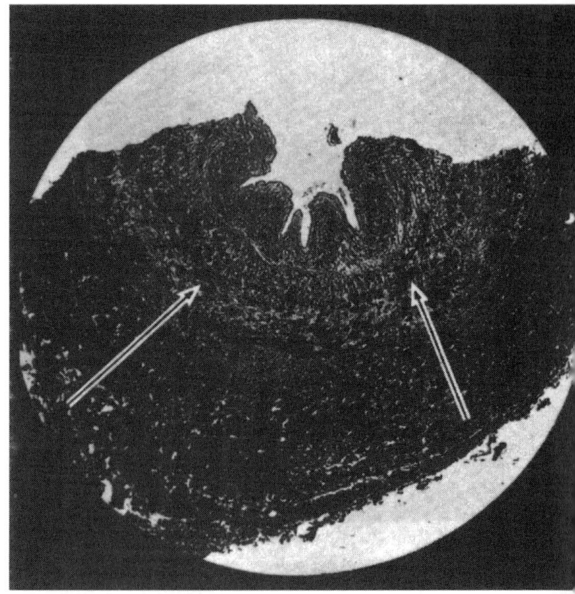

**Fig 5.** Cross-section of renal artery involved by true fibromuscular hyperplasia. Note dark-stained smooth muscle fibers interspersed with collagenous tissue in the media of this diseased vessel.

### Renal Artery Aneurysms

Renal artery aneurysms may require surgical treatment when they are the cause of significant hypertension or to obviate the risk of rupture. The latter is of greatest concern with aneurysms that are larger than 2 cm in diameter and noncalcified, particularly when they occur in premenopausal females because of the predisposition for aneurysmal rupture during pregnancy.[7] According to the classification of Poutasse,[8] there are four basic types of renal artery aneurysms: saccular, fusiform, dissecting, and intrarenal (Fig 6). Saccular aneurysms, which compose about 75% of renal artery aneurysms, are the most common. They generally occur at the bifurcation of the re-

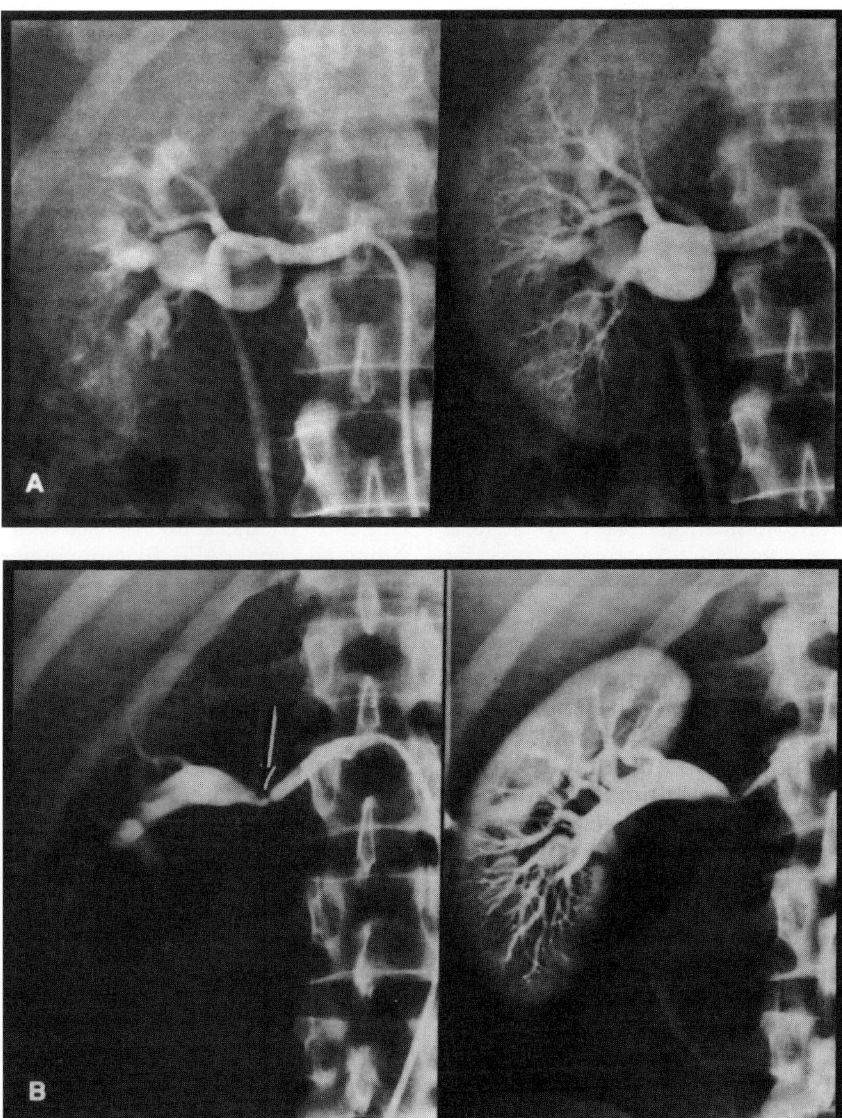


**Fig 6. A:** Right renal arteriogram shows a large saccular aneurysm at the bifurcation of the main renal artery. **B:** Right renal arteriogram shows high-grade stenosis of the main renal artery *(arrow)* from intimal fibroplasia with a poststenotic fusiform aneurysm. [A,B from Novick AC, Straffon R, eds. *Vascular Problems in Urology*. Philadelphia: WB Saunders; 1982, with permission.]

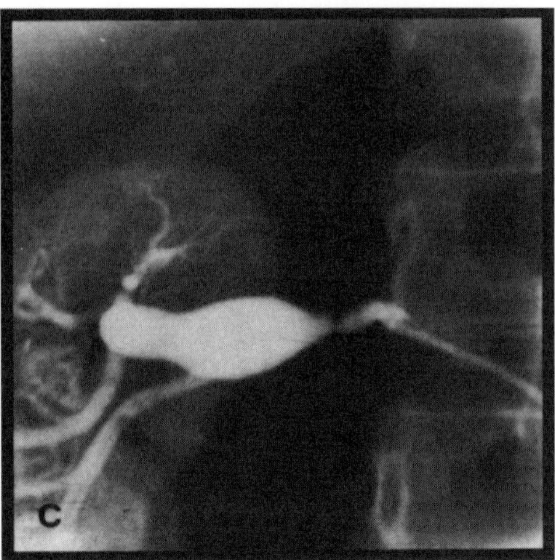


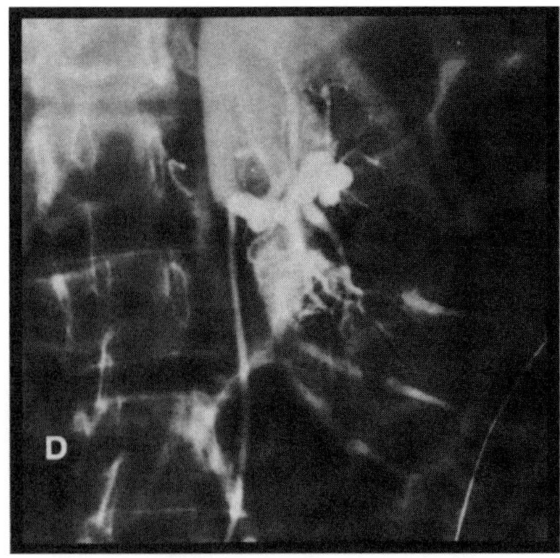


**Fig 6. C:** Right renal arteriogram shows stenosis of a primary renal arterial branch from intimal fibroplasia with a distal dissecting aneurysm. [From *Surgery* 1981;89:513, with permission.] **D:** Left renal arteriogram shows intrarenal arterial aneurysm.

nal artery, perhaps due to an inherent weakness in the wall of the artery at this point. Because of this location, branch arterial involvement is common. These aneurysms may become involved with secondary atherosclerotic degeneration and/or intramural calcification. There are several mechanisms by which saccular aneurysms may be causally related to hypertension. These include compression or displacement of renal artery branches with resulting ischemia, aneurysmal erosion into a renal vein with formation of an arterial venous fistula, mural thrombus formation within the aneurysm with peripheral renal embolization, and the association of some aneurysms with stenosing fibrous renal artery disease. It is also well appreciated that saccular aneurysms can cause hypertension in the absence of the above sequelae, most likely due to relative renal ischemia caused by the turbulent flow of blood as it passes through the aneurysmally dilated arterial segment. Saccular aneurysms may be quite variable in their location and extent. The incidence of bilateral and/or multiple renal aneurysms is approximately 25%.

Fusiform renal artery aneurysms are almost always associated with stenosing fibrous renal artery disease. The latter is the cause for the severe hypertension generally seen in these patients. Fusiform aneurysms actually represent a severe poststenotic dilatation of the renal artery. Dissecting renal artery aneurysms are most often a complication of primary intimal fibroplasia or atherosclerosis. These often become manifest clinically by the sudden onset of pain that simulates renal colic. In some patients, the dissection in the wall of the vessel may reenter the lumen more distally. In other patients, total arterial occlusion with renal infarction may ensue.

Intrarenal arterial aneurysms are of mixed origin and may be congenital, posttraumatic, iatrogenic, neoplastic, or associated with polyarteritis nodosa. Intrarenal aneurysms that occur following blunt trauma or closed renal biopsy will occasionally resolve spontaneously with expectant management. Intrarenal aneurysms do have the propensity for rupture, and surgical treatment may be indicated if their diameter is greater than 2 cm.

### Renal Arteriovenous Fistulas

Renal arteriovenous fistulas are relatively uncommon lesions that are generally discovered during the course of angiographic evaluation for suspected renal or renovascular disease.[7] The most common

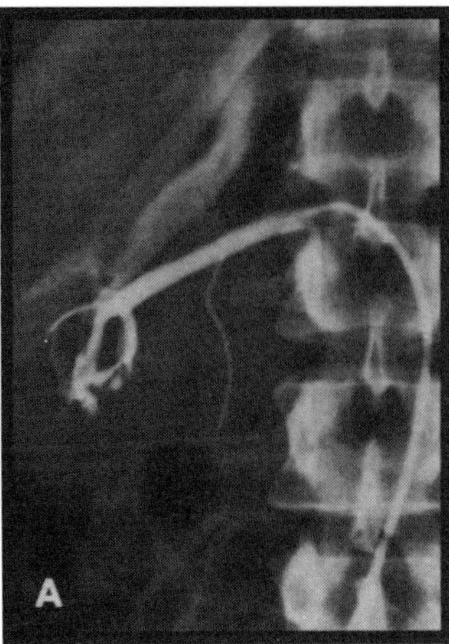


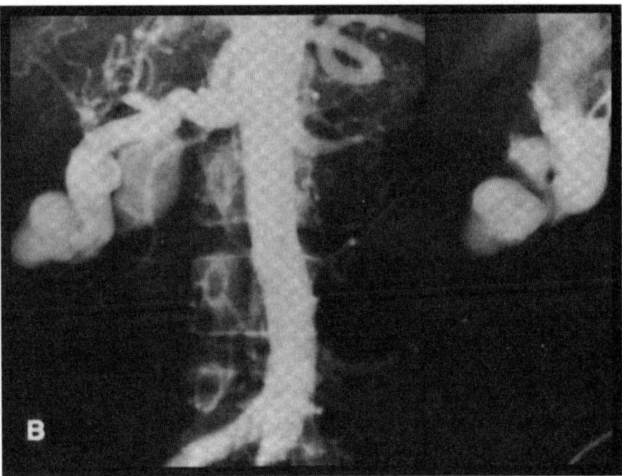


**Fig 7. A:** Selective injection of a right lower renal artery branch shows a congenital arteriovenous malformation with early filling of the venous branch. **B:** Aortogram shows a large idiopathic arteriovenous fistula involving the right kidney **(left)** with a single enlarged entering artery and exiting vein. The inferior vena cava was also visualized early in the study **(right)**. [From Novick AC, Straffon RA, eds. *Vascular Problems in Urologic Surgery*. Philadelphia: WB Saunders; 1982, with permission.]

clinical symptoms are hematuria, high-output cardiac failure, and diastolic hypertension. Congenital or cirsoid fistulas compose approximately 25% of these lesions and are the result of a developmental anomaly of the involved renal vessels (Fig 7A). The angiographic appearance is one of multiple small interconnecting arterial and venous channels with impaired distal renal parenchymal vascularity and early filling of the renal vein. Idiopathic fistulas comprise only 3%–5% of these lesions and have no apparent cause (Fig 7B). They are considered to develop as a result of venous erosion by preexisting arterial aneurysm. Acquired fistulas are the most common type, accounting for 70%–75% of all renal arteriovenous fistulas. By far the most common cause is iatrogenic trauma resulting from needle biopsy of the kidney. The majority of the latter will close spontaneously. Fistulas may also be acquired through blunt or penetrating trauma, tumor, inflammation, or prior renal surgery.

## Middle Aortic Syndrome

The middle aortic syndrome is a rare disorder, occurring in children and young adults, and characterized by nonspecific stenosing arteritis affecting the aorta and its major branches, including the renal arteries.[9] This is thought to be a form of Takayasu's disease, and an autoimmune pathogenesis is suspected. This disease can extensively involve the subdiaphragmatic aorta or, in some cases, may spare the aorta and involve primarily the renal or splanchnic vessels. The inflammatory process generally does not extend to the iliac arteries.

## Neurofibromatosis

Neurofibromatosis affecting the renal arteries is a congenital hereditary disorder characterized by café-au-lait cutaneous pigmentation, cutaneous neurofibromas, tumors of the central nervous system, skeletal disorders, and occasional gigantism. Hypertension in patients with neurofibromatosis is most often due to renal artery stenosis.[10,11] Less commonly, this may be the result of an associated pheochromocytoma or aortic coarctation. Vascular pathology occurs in the kidneys, heart, and gastrointestinal tract and consists of fibrosis and thickening of the intima, proliferation of neural tissue within the arterial wall, perivascular nodular proliferations, and occasional aneurysmal dilatation. In the kid-

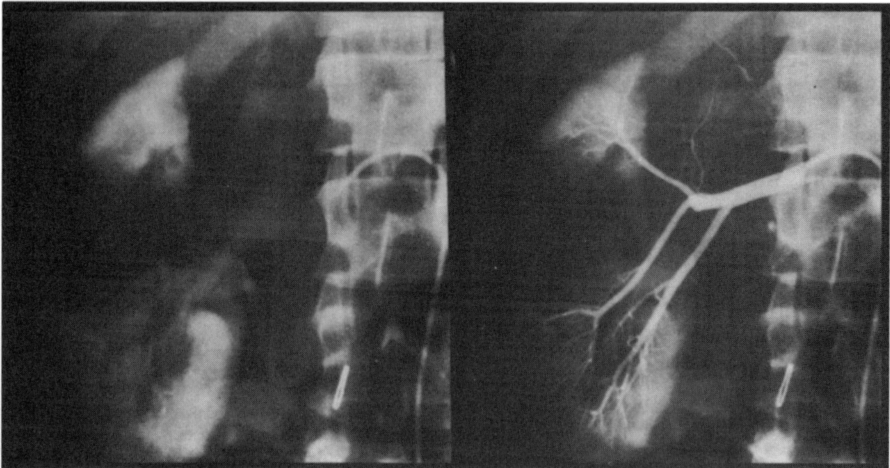

**Fig 8.** Right renal arteriogram showing thrombosis of several branches from segmental arteritis. [From Kelalis P, King L, Belman B, eds. *Clinical Pediatric Urology*. Philadelphia: WB Saunders; with permission.]

ney, arterial stenosis usually occurs at the origin or in the proximal third of the main renal artery and the angiographic appearance may be indistinguishable from that of intimal fibroplasia.

### Renal Artery Thrombosis or Embolism

Acute occlusion of the renal artery or its branches may result from thrombosis or embolism (Fig 8). Embolic occlusions may occur as a complication of rheumatic heart disease, subacute bacterial endocarditis, cardiac operations, saccular aneurysm of the renal artery, or renal artery catheterization. Thrombosis of the renal artery is somewhat less common and is associated with a variety of diseases such as intimal fibroplasia, segmental arteritis, polycythemia vera, tumors, trauma, or umbilical arterial catheterization. Blunt trauma to the renal artery may result in disruption of the intima with subsequent dissection and thrombotic occlusion.

### Extrinsic Obstruction of the Renal Artery

Extrinsic obstruction of the renal artery has been observed but is extremely rare.[12] Neural tissue, musculocutaneous fibers, and diaphragmatic crura have been suggested as etiologic factors contributing to this process. Other possible causes of extrinsic perivascular fibrosis include inflammation, trauma, tumor, or prior radiation.

### Renal Parenchymal Disease

Renin-mediated hypertension may be secondary to a variety of renal parenchymal diseases.[13,14] The incidence of hypertension in patients with chronic pyelonephritis is approximately 5%–10%. The mechanism of renin-mediated hypertension in such kidneys with segmental scars is ischemia of the relatively normal renal cortex in proximity to areas of interstitial fibrosis, within which are small vessels with intimal thickening.[15] Other renal disorders that may cause hypertension include hydronephrosis,[16,17] congenital hypoplasia or dysplasia,[18] segmental hypoplasia (Ask–Upmark kidney),[19] vesicoureteral reflux,[20] renal cell carcinoma, benign cyst, Wilms' tumor, radiation nephritis, or juxtaglomerular cell tumor.

## DIAGNOSIS OF RENOVASCULAR HYPERTENSION

The pathophysiology of renovascular hypertension is well defined. When effective blood volume or arterial blood pressure falls, renal perfusion is diminished leading to low sodium concentration at the macula densa. This leads to the secretion of renin, a proteolytic enzyme, from the adjacent juxta glomerular apparatus. Renin acts on a tetradecapeptide "renin substrate" secreted by the liver to release angiotensin I. The decapeptide angiotensin I is hydrolyzed in the lung by a converting enzyme to yield an octapeptide, angiotensin II. The latter is both a powerful pressor agent and a stimulus to the secretion of aldosterone by the adrenals. Increased aldosterone secretion leads to increased reabsorption of sodium from the distal nephron. This increased retention of sodium and water leads to an expanded blood volume, which in turn inhibits the initial signal to renal renin release.

There is no single clinical manifestation that can reliably distinguish renovascular hypertension from essential hypertension. Nevertheless, when taken in the aggregate, certain clinical manifestations are helpful in making this differential diagnosis. Patients with renovascular hypertension are much more likely to have a short duration of hypertension, advanced retinopathy, azotemia, hypokalemia, alkalosis, or a bruit auscultated in the abdomen or flank. Renovascular hypertension is much less common in blacks than in whites.[21] In general, the most helpful clues to the diagnosis of renovascular hypertension, in descending order of importance, have been as follows: (1) an abdominal bruit with both systolic and diastolic components,[22] (2) an abrupt onset or exacerbation of hypertension with rapid progression,[23] (3) onset of hypertension before age 30 or after age 55, and (4) retinal vascular changes.

The more of these clues that are present, the greater the chance of finding a lesion on renal arteriography. The prototype of the patient with renovascular hypertension due to fibrous disease of the renal artery is a 20-year-old woman whose blood pressure was normal 6 months previously and who presents with recent onset of headache, blood pressure 220/130 mm Hg, retinopathy, and a continuous bruit in the epigastrium radiating to the right upper quadrant. The prototype of the patient with atherosclerotic renovascular hypertension is a 65-year-old man who was normotensive (or had easily controlled mild hypertension) 6 months previously and who presents with a blood pressure of 250/140 mm Hg, retinopathy, with or without an abdominal bruit. In such cases, the chances of finding a renal artery lesion on angiography are excellent. Unfortunately, only a minority of patients with renovascular hypertension present with such a characteristic clinical picture. For other patients, the urologist must blend clinical judgment and experience to decide how vigorously to pursue the diagnostic search for renovascular hypertension.

When undertaking further evaluation, it is important to differentiate between renovascular disease and renovascular hypertension, since occlusive lesions of the renal artery do not always result in hypertension. The diagnosis of renovascular disease depends on angiographic demonstration of a stenotic lesion in the renal artery or its branches, whereas the diagnosis of renovascular hypertension can be confirmed only in retrospect and implies permanent relief of hypertension after revascularization or removal of the affected kidney. The simultaneous occurrence of essential hypertension and coincidental renovascular disease is, in fact, more frequent than the occurrence of true renovascular hypertension.

Several screening tests are available for pursuing the diagnosis of renovascular hypertension in patients with suggestive clinical features. The rapid sequence intravenous pyelogram (IVP) is still occasionally used as a screening test for this disease. Findings that suggest significant renal artery obstruction include delay in the function of one kidney, a decrease in renal length of more than 1.5 cm on the right or 1 cm on the left, late hyperconcentration of contrast medium in one kidney, or the presence of ureteral notching due to collateral vessels. The utility of the rapid sequence IVP as a screening test for renovascular hypertension is limited by a high rate of false-positive and false-negative studies.

Isotope renography with technetium or hippuran has not been a useful diagnostic test for renovascular hypertension due to a large number of false-positive results. However, when an angiotensin converting enzyme inhibitor such as captopril is added to the standard isotope renogram, the sensitivity and specificity increase considerably especially for unilateral renal artery stenosis.[24,25] This technique involves performing isotope renography before and 1 hr after the oral administration of 25 mg of captopril. The captopril produces an acute and reversible decrease in renal function on the side with renal artery stenosis whereas renal function on the normal contralateral side is unimpaired. Initial studies indicate excellent sensitivity and specificity of captopril renography for unilateral renal artery stenosis. This test may not be as accurate in patients with bilateral renal artery stenosis or renal artery stenosis involving a solitary kidney.

Recently, duplex ultrasound scanning of the renal arteries has become a useful noninvasive screening test for significant renal artery stenosis.[26,27] When the arterial segment is stenotic, there are alterations in laminar blood flow and the Doppler signal changes. Several Doppler criteria are used to assess the severity of the stenosis such as the ratio of renal to aortic systolic peak velocity. Duplex ultrasound scanning for renal artery stenosis is attractive because it is safe and noninvasive. The limitations are that it is highly operator-dependent and time consuming. Initial reports indicate sensitivity and specificity rates of 80%–90% in patients with renal artery stenosis. This technique will likely play a more prominent role in screening for renovascular hypertension in the future.

Renal arteriography remains the gold standard for establishing the diagnosis of renal artery stenosis. Several angiographic techniques are available including intravenous digital subtraction angiography, intraarterial digital subtraction angiography, or standard arteriography. Intravenous digital subtraction arteriography is less invasive since the contrast is injected directly into a peripheral vein. The utility of this study as a screening test is limited by frequent failure to visualize the distal main renal artery or its branches.[28,29] Recently, intraarterial digital subtraction arteriography has emerged as the preferred angiographic diagnostic test. Compared to standard arteriography, this technique is performed with a smaller catheter, requires less contrast material, and provides equally good imaging of the aorta, main renal arteries, and its branches. Developmental studies are currently in progress with magnetic resonance angiography as an even less invasive technique for imaging the aorta and renal arteries.[30] In the future, magnetic resonance angiography may replace the need for catheter arteriography with contrast in some patients.

When the diagnosis of renal artery stenosis is established upon arteriography, it is necessary to determine whether or not the lesion is functionally significant. In other words, is the lesion causing the patient's hypertension? The captopril isotope renogram test, discussed earlier in this section, may be useful in indicating the functional significance of a stenotic renal artery lesion. Differential renal vein plasma renin assays were formerly a popular test and, indeed, the diagnosis of renovascular hypertension can be made with 90% accuracy when the renin level from the stenotic kidney is two or more times higher than the renin level from the normal contralateral kidney.[31] Unfortunately, the finding of nonlateralization with this test is very unreliable, since more than 50% of such patients have ultimately proven to have renovascular hypertension.[32,33] In patients with bilateral renal artery stenosis, renal vein renin ratios may be helpful in indicating which kidney is more severely affected.

Several studies have shown that measurement of the peripheral plasma renin level is not reliable in identifying patients with renovascular hypertension. However, the utility of this test can be significantly enhanced by administering an oral dose of captopril and obtaining a repeat plasma renin measurement 1 hr later. Captopril-stimulated peripheral plasma renin activity now provides a useful noninvasive test for demonstrating the presence of renin-mediated hypertension.[34]

## INDICATIONS FOR SURGICAL THERAPY OR PERCUTANEOUS ANGIOPLASTY

Surgical renal revascularization and percutaneous transluminal angioplasty (PTA) are well established as effective methods for treating patients with severe hypertension or renal insufficiency or both resulting from renal artery disease. Multiple factors must be weighed in determining whether interventive therapy is indicated for a given patient. These include the causal relation of renal vascular disease to hypertension, the adequacy of blood pressure control with medical therapy, the natural history of untreated renal vascular disease with particular regard for the risk of impaired renal function, the medical condition of the patient, and the known results of surgical therapy and PTA in various clinical subgroups.

### Renal Vascular Hypertension

In patients with renal vascular hypertension secondary to fibrous dysplasia, the decision regarding intervention is guided by the specific type of disease as determined by angiographic findings and associated natural history.[4] Medical management of hypertension is the preferred initial treatment for patients with medial fibroplasia because loss of renal function from progressive obstruction is uncommon with this disease. Interventive treatment in the latter category is reserved for patients whose blood pressure is difficult to control with multiple drugs.

Conversely, renal artery stenosis secondary to intimal or perimedial fibroplasia generally progresses and often eventuates in ischemic renal atrophy. Early interventive therapy in these patients is therefore indicated both to preserve renal function and to facilitate blood pressure control.

In selecting patients with fibrous dysplasias for intervention, the relative efficacy of surgical revascularization vs. PTA must be considered. The results of PTA or fibrous dysplasia of the main renal artery have been excellent and equal to those obtained with surgical revascularization; therefore, angioplasty is the treatment of choice in such cases.[35–37] However, as many as 30% of patients with fibrous dysplasia have branch renal arterial involvement which increases the technical difficulty of PTA and often precludes its use; in this category, surgical renal revascularization is the primary interventive treatment.[38]

Renal artery aneurysms may require surgical treatment when they are the cause of significant hypertension or to avoid rupture.[7] The latter is of greatest concern with aneurysms that are larger than 2 cm in diameter and noncalcified, particularly when they occur in premenopausal women, because of the predisposition for aneurysmal rupture during pregnancy.

In patients with atherosclerotic renal vascular hypertension, more vigorous attempts at medical management are warranted since these patients are older and often have extrarenal vascular disease. Therefore, multiple-drug regimens that control the blood pressure are often the preferred approach. Intervention with surgery or PTA is reserved for patients whose hypertension cannot be adequately controlled or wherein renal function is threatened by advanced vascular disease. The available data indicate that PTA provides excellent results for patients with unilateral nonostial atherosclerotic renal artery lesions.[35–37,39] However, the results of PTA in the more common ostial atherosclerotic lesions have been poor, and surgical revascularization is the treatment of choice in this category.[38]

### Preservation of Renal Function in Atherosclerotic Renal Artery Disease

Knowledge of the natural history of atherosclerotic renal artery disease has made it possible to identify those patients in whom such disease poses a significant threat to overall renal function.[4] This designation applies to patients with high-grade (>75%) arterial stenosis affecting the entire renal mass, namely, where such stenosis is present bilaterally or involves a solitary kidney. In such patients, the risk of complete renal arterial occlusion is significant, and if this occurs, the clinical outcome is a critical decrease in functioning renal mass with resulting renal failure. In such patients, intervention to restore normal renal blood flow is indicated for the purpose of preserving renal function. Clinical experience has shown that these are generally older patients with diffuse atherosclerosis and ostial renal artery lesions. This description encompasses a group in which the results of PTA have been poor and where surgical revascularization provides optimum therapy[36,39–41] It has been well demonstrated that surgical revascularization can be safely and successfully performed in these older patients with diffuse extrarenal vascular disease.

In considering potential candidates for revascularization to preserve renal function, a determination must be made of the potential for salvable renal function. Total occlusion of the renal artery does not necessarily imply irreversible ischemic parenchymal damage, and it is well accepted that with gradual arterial occlusion, the viability of the kidney can be maintained through the development of collateral arterial supply.[42,43] It is also important to emphasize that revascularization to preserve renal function is generally not worthwhile in patients with severe azotemia (serum creatinine >4.0 mg/dL) because advanced underlying renal parenchymal disease inevitably is present and prevents improvement in renal function with restored perfusion. The single exception to this occurs in patients with chronic bilateral total occlusion where fortuitously the viability of one or both kidneys has been maintained through collateral supply. The degree of preoperative renal functional impairment in such patients often is severe, and the improvement following revascularization may be dramatic.[44,45] Unfortunately, this clinical presentation is rare, and a less favorable outcome of bilateral arterial occlusion on renal viability is far more common.

### Renal Vascular Disease in Children

The most common cause of renovascular disease in children is fibrous dysplasia. Other lesions in this age group include an arterial aneurysm, arteriovenous malformation, Takayasu's arteritis, neurofibromatosis, thromboembolic disease, and trauma.[46] Many renovascular lesions in children, such as intimal and perimedial fibroplasia, are known to cause progressive vascular obstruction.[4] Therefore, treatment must be directed not only at relief of hypertension but also at preservation of functioning renal parenchyma.

Medical therapy has no place in the definitive treatment of young children with renovascular hypertension since it would entail a lifelong commitment to drug therapy with the attendant risk of losing renal function from progressive disease. PTA is effective in some cases but often is not technically possible due to the small size of the diseased vessels, involvement of renal artery branches, or the presence of multiple lesions, aneurysmal disease, or perivascular scarring in cases of arteritis. For most children, surgical treatment currently offers the best prospect for both ameliorating hypertension and preserving renal function.[47]

## SURGICAL METHODS OF TREATMENT

### Preoperative Considerations

It is important to define the general medical condition of the patient since this will determine the risk of undertaking surgical treatment. Most patients with renal arterial fibrous dysplasia are young and otherwise healthy, and the operative risk is minimal in this group. In patients with atherosclerotic renovascular disease, evidence of generalized atherosclerosis should be diligently sought. Particularly important are a history of angina pectoris, congestive heart failure, myocardial infarction, transient ischemic attacks, cerebrovascular accidents, or intermittent claudication. On physical examination, careful attention should be paid to the presence of carotid bruits, focal neurologic deficits suggesting a prior cerebral infarct, third and fourth heart sounds, precordial left ventricular heave, arterial pulsations in the extremities, and the presence of an aortic aneurysm on examination of the abdomen.

The preoperative evaluation should include a thorough search for coronary artery disease because this has been the leading cause of operative mortality following surgical treatment for atherosclerotic renovascular disease.[48] In addition to a careful history, physical examination, and electrocardiogram, all operative candidates in this category should undergo a cardiac stress test. If any of the latter assessments suggest the presence of coronary artery disease, our policy is to then perform coronary cineangiography and left ventriculography. Coronary artery bypass grafting is recommended for patients with significant correctable coronary artery disease before renal revascularization.[49] Patients with either mild to moderate or advanced but compensated coronary artery disease can safely undergo renal revascularization without prior coronary artery bypass grafting. For patients with severe noncorrectable coronary artery disease, major operative intervention for renovascular disease carries a significantly increased risk and is best deferred except for the most dire of circumstances.

Cerebrovascular accident has also been a major operative complication of renal revascularization in patients with atherosclerosis, albeit a less common complication than myocardial infarction. The approach to patients whose history of examination suggests the presence of extracranial cerebrovascular disease is analogous to that employed for patients with suspected coronary artery disease. In such cases, carotid arteriography is obtained preoperatively, and if significant occlusive disease is found, endarterectomy is recommended before renal revascularization.[49]

## Nephrectomy

Although it is now possible to achieve successful renal revascularization in most cases, total or partial nephrectomy retains a role in the management of renovascular hypertension. These operations are indicated in patients with main or branch renal artery occlusion and infarction, severe arteriolar nephrosclerosis, renal atrophy (<9 cm renal length), segmental renal hypoplasia (Ask–Upmark kidney), and noncorrectable renovascular lesions such as large intrarenal aneurysms or arteriovenous malformations. Nephrectomy may also be indicated in the elderly poor-surgical-risk patient with a normal contralateral kidney, or following a failed revascularization procedure where extensive renal hilar fibrosis precludes satisfactory secondary revascularization. In properly selected patients, the results are equal to those obtained following revascularization procedures.

## Aortorenal Bypass

Although a variety of renal revascularization procedures have been employed to treat renovascular hypertension, aortorenal bypass with autogenous saphenous vein or arterial grafts is the preferred method. Excellent clinical results have been obtained with both types of bypass grafts[1]; however, long-term studies of aortorenal saphenous vein grafts have shown a large number of dilated grafts on follow-up angiography.[50] This finding has been observed more frequently in children and may reflect an enhanced susceptibility to mural ischemia of vein segments procured from younger patients. The clinical significance of these observations remains uncertain since most of these patients continue to be normotensive with excellent renal function. Nevertheless, these findings have led to preferential use of arterial autografts when they are available. The viscoelastic properties of arterial grafts, unlike the saphenous vein, match those of the renal artery and postoperative graft dilatation has not been observed. Free grafts of either the hypogastric or splenic artery may be used for aortorenal bypass with excellent results.[51,52] The hypogastric artery is generally a short vessel and is best suited for bypass of proximal or left renal artery lesions. The splenic artery provides a longer graft and is therefore preferable for bypass of distal renal artery lesions. Unfortunately, use of either of these arterial grafts may be precluded by extensive atherosclerotic involvement; in such cases, we continue to employ a saphenous vein graft. It is important to note that the spermatic or ovarian veins should never be used as bypass grafts. These veins are extremely friable and may either rupture postoperatively or undergo severe dilatation with recurrence of hypertension.

Currently, aortorenal bypass with a synthetic material is indicated only when autogenous vascular grafts are not available or when adjunctive aortic replacement is performed. Although the long-term results with Dacron grafts are satisfactory, there has been an increased tendency to thrombosis in the early postoperative period.[53] The polytetrafluorethylene graft is soft, nonelastic, easy to suture, and allows for inner fibrous healing with minimal tissue reactivity. Excellent results have been reported with such grafts in peripheral arterial reconstruction,[54] and they appear to be preferable when renal artery replacement with a synthetic material is indicated.[55]

All patients undergoing renal revascularization are hydrated with 200 $cm^3$/hr of 5% dextrose with half-normal saline intravenously for 12 hr prior to surgery. Since renovascular hypertension is associated with secondary hyperaldosteronism, potassium supplement and monitoring of serum potassium levels are needed to guard against hypokalemia. To further ensure optimal renal perfusion and an active diuresis intraoperatively, 12.5 g of mannitol is given intravenously before the operation; equivalent doses of mannitol are subsequently given just prior to revascularization, immediately following revascularization, and again in the recovery room.

When a saphenous vein graft is needed, this is obtained through an oblique groin incision made just medial to the pulsation of the femoral artery. When the surgeon procures the saphenous vein graft, care is taken not to overdistend the vein or injudiciously dissect periadventitial tissue, both of which may cause devascularization of the graft. All venous tributaries are suture-ligated with 4-0 silk, and a 4- to 6-cm segment of saphenous vein is then removed. The graft should be stored in chilled Ringer's lactate solution to which dilute heparin solution has been added. Because of the presence of valves in the saphenous vein, blood flow in the graft should always be directed toward the cephalic end, which will be anastomosed directly to the distal renal artery.

A transperitoneal subcostal incision is made, the medial end of which is curved across the midline. If needed, free grafts of either the hypogastric or splenic arteries may be readily obtained through such an incision. The hypogastric artery may be safely removed since collateral blood flow between the internal iliac systems is abundant. Endarterectomy may be performed on the hypogastric artery if mild atherosclerosis is present, but extensive disease will preclude its use as a bypass graft. When the hypogastric artery is removed, it will shrink to about two thirds of its normal length and diameter. Since the dimensions of the hypogastric artery will be restored after grafting, one must estimate the adequacy of its length for bypass grafting while it is still in its original functioning position. The splenic artery may be safely removed without sacrificing the spleen, which receives sufficient blood supply from the short gastric and gastroepiploic vessels to ensure its viability. This vessel is involved less often with atherosclerosis and a lengthy segment can generally be obtained. The splenic artery is a tortuous vessel and, upon removal, may go into muscular spasm, which reduces its lumen considerably. This can be relieved by gentle dilation of the vessel with graduated metal sounds.

The right kidney is exposed by reflecting the hepatic flexure of the colon downward and medially and using a Kocher maneuver on the duodenum; this allows access to the right renal artery, renal vein, inferior vena cava, and the aorta. The left kidney can be exposed by reflecting the splenic flexure of the colon downward and medially (Fig 9). A self-retaining ring retractor is then inserted, which provides excellent exposure and allows the operation to be comfortably performed by a surgeon and one assistant (Fig 10).

Gerota's fascia is opened laterally over the lower pole of the kidney so that the color and consistency of the kidney can be observed throughout the revascularization procedure. The aorta is then exposed widely from the level of the renal vein to the inferior mesenteric artery, ligating overlying lymphatic vessels and lumbar segmental branches as necessary to gain exposure. The renal vein is mobilized and all

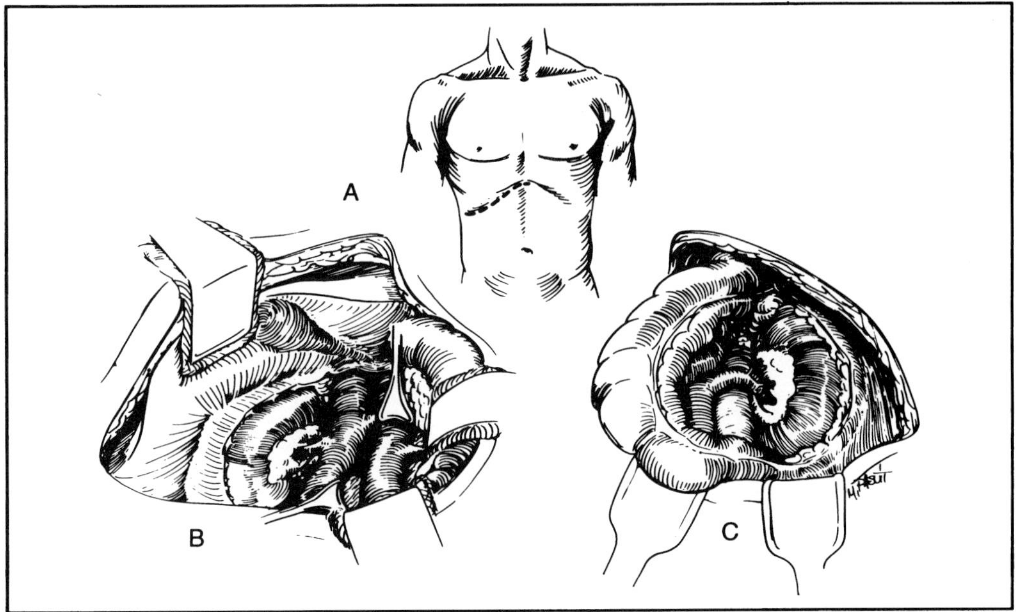


**Fig 9. A:** Subcostal incision for exposure of the right renal artery. **B:** Exposure of the right renal artery. **C:** Exposure of the left renal artery.

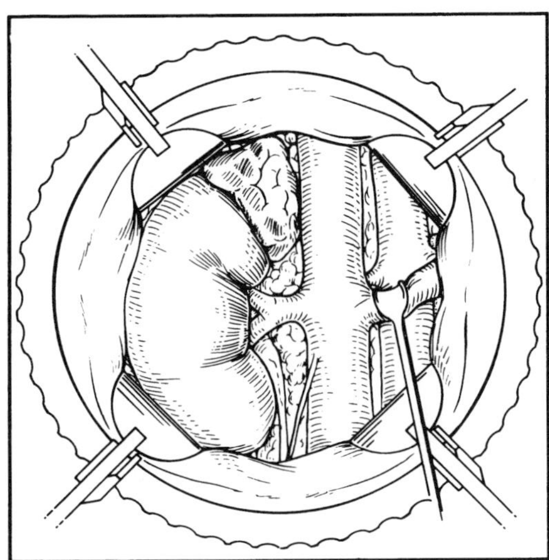

**Fig 10.** Self-retaining right retractor used in exposing the right renal artery for revascularization.

venous tributaries are secured and divided, including the gonadal and adrenal branches on the left side. The renal vein may be retracted either superiorly or inferiorly to expose the entire length of the main renal artery. After identifying the renal artery, extensive arterial dissection is delayed to avoid spasm of the vessel, which may further embarrass the blood supply to an already ischemic kidney.

An end-to-side anastomosis of the bypass graft to the aorta is done first to minimize renal ischemia time. After the surgeon applies a DeBakey clamp, an oval aortotomy is made on the anterolateral surface of the aorta. If the lateral aortic wall is only partially occluded, thereby preserving distal aortic flow, then systemic heparinization is not needed. When the DeBakey clamp totally interrupts aortic blood flow, then systemic heparinization is initiated. End-to-side anastomosis of the graft to the aorta is performed with interrupted 6-0 arterial silk sutures. The graft is then occluded proximally with a bulldog clamp and the aortic clamp is removed.

The renal artery is then dissected from its aortic origin to the primary segmental branches. On the right side, the graft is brought anterior to the vena cava in preparation for the distal anastomosis. Creation of a retrocaval tunnel requires additional dissection that can result in venous ooze with hematoma formation about the graft

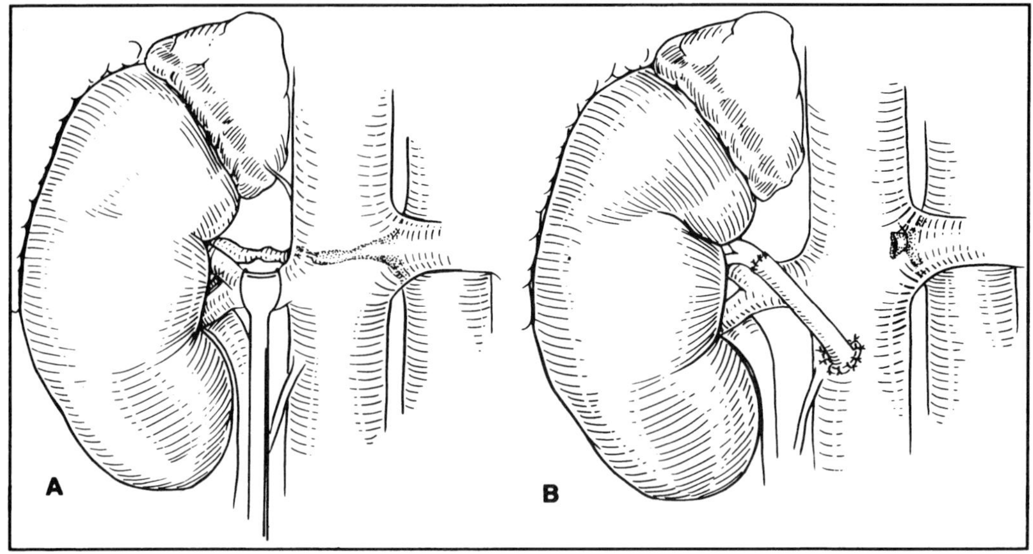


**Fig 11. A:** Exposure of right renal artery involved with extensive stenosis. **B:** Sketch of completed end-to-end right aortorenal bypass graft.

and subsequent cicatricial graft stenosis. The renal artery is ligated proximally, a bulldog clamp is placed distally, and the diseased arterial segment is completely excised and sent for pathologic examination. If the patient has not been systemically heparinized, then 10 $cm^3$ of dilute heparin solution is instilled into the distal renal artery. An end-to-end anastomosis of the graft to the renal artery is preferred since this provides better flow rates, is easier to perform, and allows removal of the diseased renal arterial segment for pathologic study. Interrupted 6-0 arterial silk sutures are employed for the distal anastomosis. Surface cooling of the kidney is not necessary since the ischemia time is minimal and usually will not exceed 15–20 min. When the anastomosis is completed, the proximal and distal bulldog clamps are released and blood flow to the kidney is restored (Fig 11).

Revascularization is more complicated when the disease extends into the branches of the renal artery or when vascular reconstruction is required for a kidney supplied by multiple renal arteries. When disease-free distal arterial branches occur outside the renal hilus, an aortorenal bypass operation can usually be done in situ. The size of the involved vessels is not a significant factor since, utilizing microvascular instruments and optical magnification, vessels as small as 2 mm diameter can be repaired in situ.[56] In patients with disease confined to a single major renal artery branch, aortorenal bypass may be done exclusively to the disease-free distal branch (Fig 12). When vascular disease extends into two primary renal artery branches, an aortorenal bypass to the conjoined branches is possible (Fig 13). However, the most useful technique for in situ revascularization of two or more renal artery branches is aortorenal bypass with a branched autogenous vascular graft.[57] Either the hypogastric artery is obtained intact with its branches or, if this is unsuitable, a branched saphenous vein graft is fashioned. This is a versatile and effective operation that minimizes renal ischemia by allowing separate end-to-end anastomosis of each graft limb to a renal artery branch (Fig 14).

## Transrenal Endarterectomy

Endarterectomy was one of the earliest methods used to treat renovascular hyper-

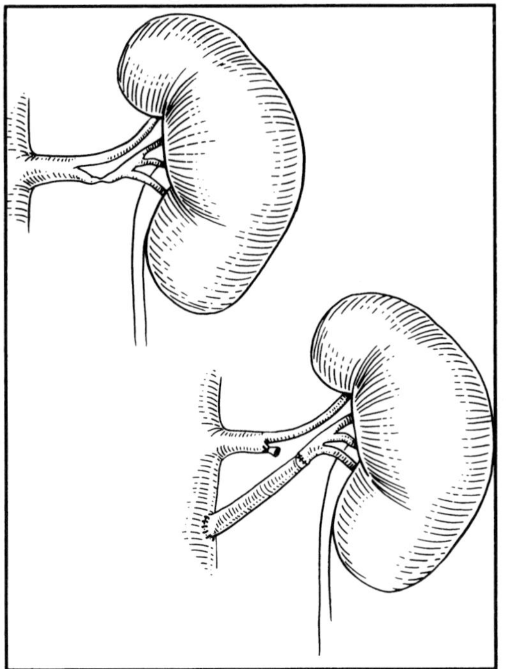

**Fig 12.** For solitary branch disease, aortorenal bypass is done exclusively to the disease-free distal branch leaving the main renal artery and remaining branches intact.

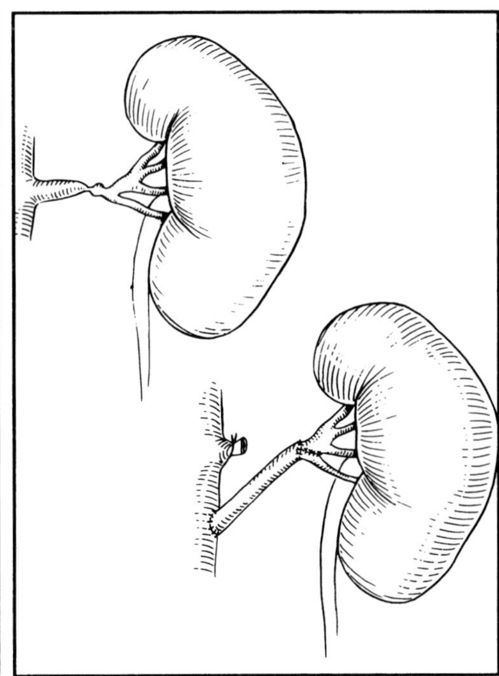

**Fig 13.** When arterial stenosis involves two primary renal artery branches, aortorenal bypass to the conjoined branches may be done.

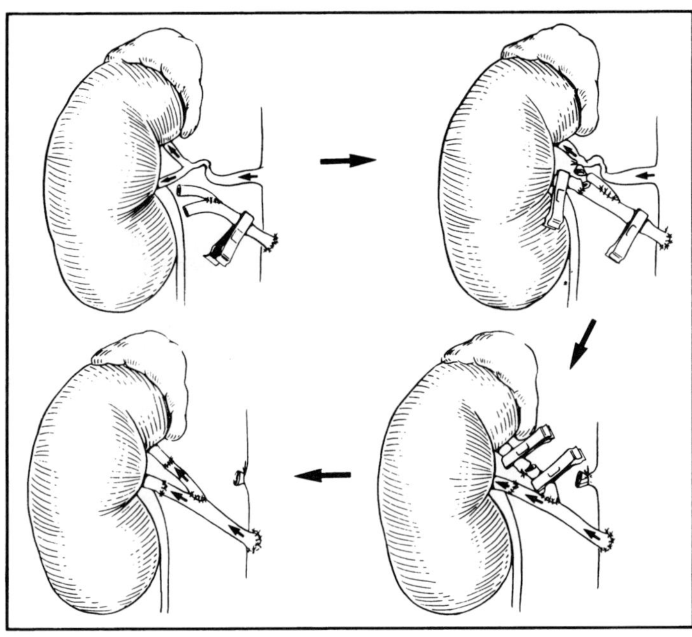

**Fig 14.** Sketch illustrating sequential vascular anastomoses involved in performing aortorenal bypass with a double-armed branched saphenous vein graft.

tension; however, with the advent of aortorenal bypass, the popularity of endarterectomy diminished considerably. Nevertheless, transrenal endarterectomy is a relatively simple procedure that continues to be effective for selected patients with renovascular hypertension.[58] Because of the lack of a suitable cleavage plane between the various fibrous lesions and the arterial wall, endarterectomy is suitable only in patients with atherosclerotic renovascular disease.

The incision and exposure are similar to that for aortorenal bypass. Transrenal endarterectomy requires only partial aortic occlusion at the origin of the renal artery (Fig 15). A longitudinal arteriotomy is made over the obstructing atherosclerotic plaque, extending proximally for 1 cm on the anterior wall of the aorta and extending distally along the renal artery to a point just beyond the plaque itself. The atherosclerotic plaque is then removed, using an endarterectomy spatula to dissect carefully between the media of the vessel and the plaque. The distal intima should be broken cleanly at a point where it is firmly adherent to the media of the artery. Any persistent distal intimal flaps are tacked down with interrupted 6-0 silk arterial sutures. A patch of autogenous saphenous vein or artery is then sutured in place with 6-0 arterial silk to ensure unobstructed closure of the arteriotomy incision. Transrenal endarterectomy also may be somewhat more difficult to perform on the right side because of the overlying vena cava and the left renal vein, or in older patients where the vessel wall may be rather thin.

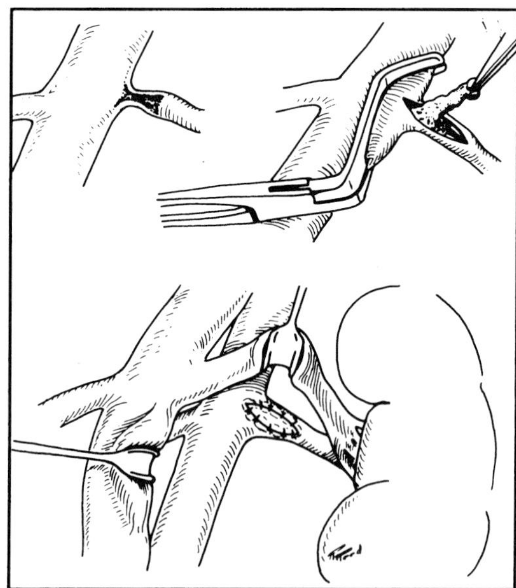

**Fig 15.** Sketch illustrating technique of left transrenal endarterectomy and patch graft angioplasty.

## Techniques in the Surgically Difficult Aorta

Severe atherosclerosis or previous operations on the abdominal aorta may preclude safe performance of aortorenal bypass or endarterectomy for some patients with renal artery disease. These patients present difficult clinical problems since they are often poor surgical risks and may possess only one functioning kidney. Intractable hypertension and failing renal function occur frequently, and thrombosis with renal infarction has been the unfortunate result in some patients. Fortunately, there are alternate methods of renal revascularization that may be safely and effectively employed in such patients (Fig 16).[59]

## Splenorenal Bypass

Splenorenal bypass provides an excellent method of performing left renal revascularization when preoperative aortography with selective celiac arteriography demonstrates a healthy splenic artery. The advantages of this procedure are that it can be carried out in untouched vascular tissues at a distance from the aorta and that it involves only a single vascular anastomosis. An extended left subcostal incision is made and the left colon and duodenum are reflected medially. The plane between Gerota's fascia and the pancreas is developed by blunt dissection, and the pancreas and spleen are gently retracted cephalad to permit access to the splenic vessels. The splenic artery may be palpated posterior and superior to the splenic vein, and that portion lying closest to the distal aspect of the renal artery is mobilized. Small pancreatic arterial branches are divided and se-

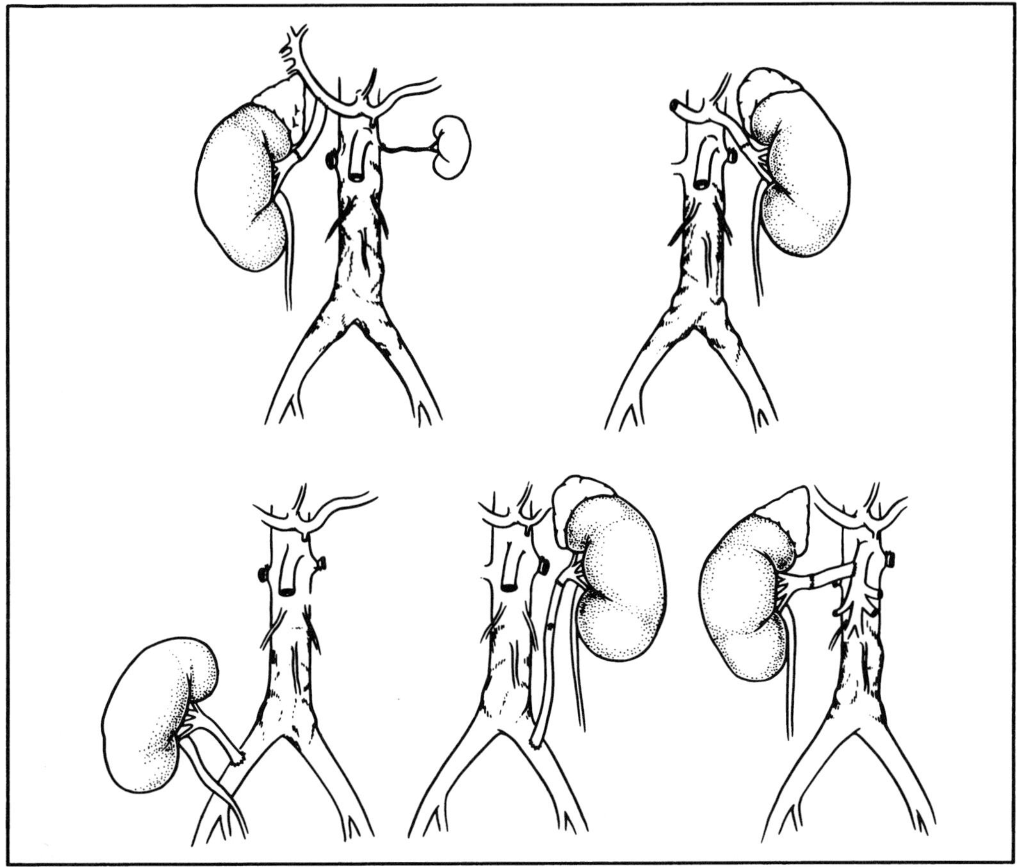

**Fig 16.** Methods of renal revascularization for patients with a surgically difficult aorta. These include hepatorenal bypass **(top left)**, splenorenal bypass **(top right)**, autotransplantation **(bottom left)**, ileorenal bypass **(bottom middle)**, and superior mesenterorenal bypass **(bottom right)**.

cured with 4-0 silk sutures. The splenic artery may be quite tortuous and should be mobilized proximally as close to the celiac axis as possible, where the vessel wall is also thicker and the luminal diameter is larger. The splenic artery is then occluded proximally, ligated distally without removing the spleen, and transected. The splenic artery may then go into muscular spasm; this can be relieved by gentle dilation with graduated metal sounds. The renal artery is mobilized and prepared as described for aortorenal bypass. End-to-end anastomosis of the splenic artery to the distal renal artery is then performed with interrupted 6-0 silk sutures (Fig 17).[60]

## Hepatorenal Bypass

The hepatic circulation is ideally suited for a visceral right renal arterial bypass operation. The liver receives 28% of the cardiac output in resting adults. It is unique in having a dual circulation from the portal vein and hepatic artery, which contribute 80% and 20% of hepatic blood flow, respectively. Hepatic oxygenation is equally derived from these two circulations. It has been well demonstrated that hepatic artery flow can be safely interrupted. When this occurs, hepatic function and morphology are maintained by increased extraction of oxygen from portal venous blood and by

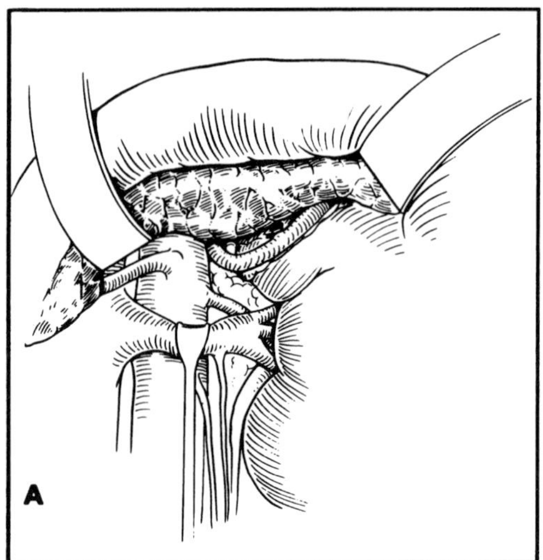


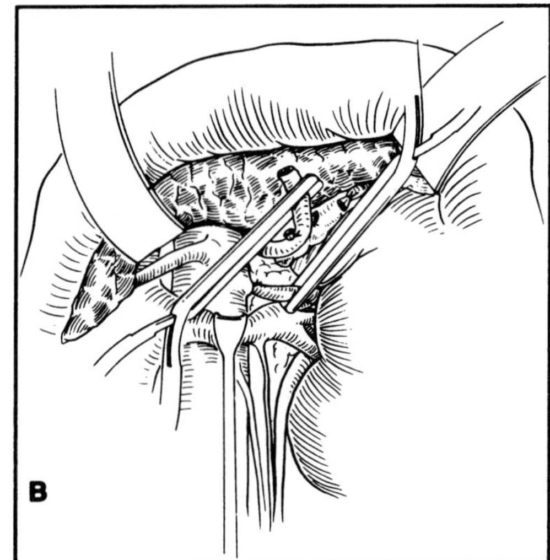


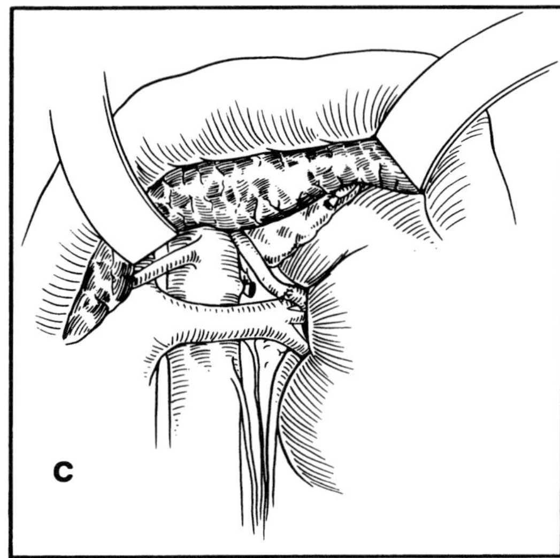


**Fig 17. A:** Exposure of the splenic artery for performance of left splenorenal bypass. **B:** The splenic artery has been mobilized and prepared after dividing small pancreatic arterial branches. The renal artery has been ligated proximally and clamped distally in preparation for end-to-end splenorenal anastomosis. **C:** Completed left splenorenal bypass operation.

the rapid development of extensive collateral arterial flow to the liver.[61]

The hepatic artery arises from the celiac axis and runs anterior to the portal vein and to the left of the common bile duct. The first major branch is the gastroduodenal artery; thereafter the hepatic artery divides into its right and left branches. In considering a hepatorenal bypass operation, one of the more clinically significant anatomic variations is origination of the right hepatic artery from the superior mesenteric artery, which occurs in about 12% of patients. The left hepatic artery arises from the left gastric artery in approximately 11.5% of patients.

Patients considered for a hepatorenal bypass operation need preoperative aortography and selective celiac arteriography with lateral views to ensure patent celiac and hepatic arteries.[62] An extended right subcostal incision is made and the common hepatic artery is readily identified anterior to the foramen of Winslow (Fig 18). This artery is then mobilized for a short distance while carefully avoiding injury to the portal vein or common bile duct. The common hepatic artery is occluded proximally and

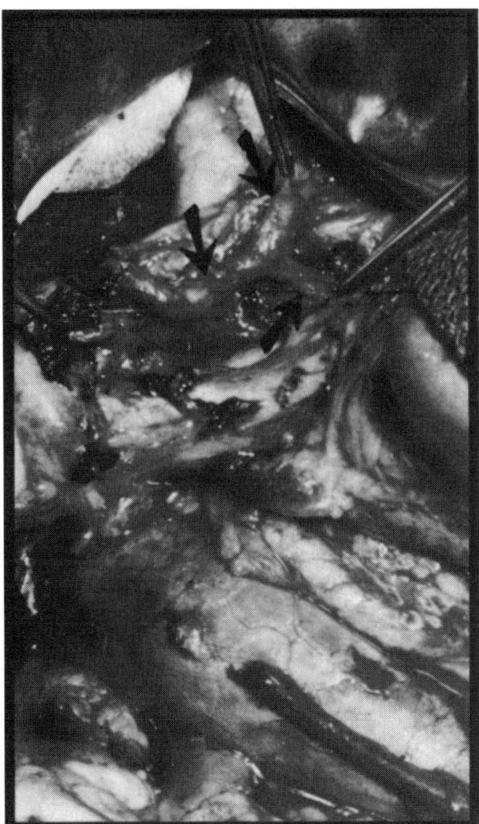

Fig 18. Operative photograph of exposed hepatic artery following careful dissection within portal triad. Large arrows superiorly indicate common hepatic artery, while arrow below shows the gastroduodenal artery arising inferiorly.

distally with bulldog clamps and an arteriotomy is made just beyond the origin of the gastroduodenal artery. The saphenous vein graft is then anastomosed end-to-side to the common hepatic artery. After completing this anastomosis, the vein graft is occluded with a bulldog clamp and hepatic arterial flow to the liver is restored. End-to-end anastomosis of the saphenous vein and distal renal artery is then performed. This technique for hepatorenal bypass preserves distal hepatic arterial flow, thereby further diminishing the risk of ischemic liver damage. In the event of an anomalous hepatic artery supply, bypass from either the right hepatic, left hepatic, or gastroduodenal arteries may alternatively be performed. Accessory hepatic arteries also occur commonly and provide an added margin of safety against possible hepatic ischemia.

### Thoracic Aortorenal Bypass

Use of the thoracic aorta for renal revascularization is a new surgical alternative in patients with severe abdominal aortic atherosclerosis when the above options are not available.[63] The thoracic aorta is often relatively disease-free in such patients and can be used to achieve renal vascular reconstruction with an interposition saphenous vein graft (Fig 19). This operation is performed through a thoracoabdominal incision, which provides excellent simultaneous exposure of the thoracic aorta and renal artery. This approach has several advantages and can be usefully applied to the management of selected older patients with severe atherosclerosis of the abdominal aorta and renal arteries.

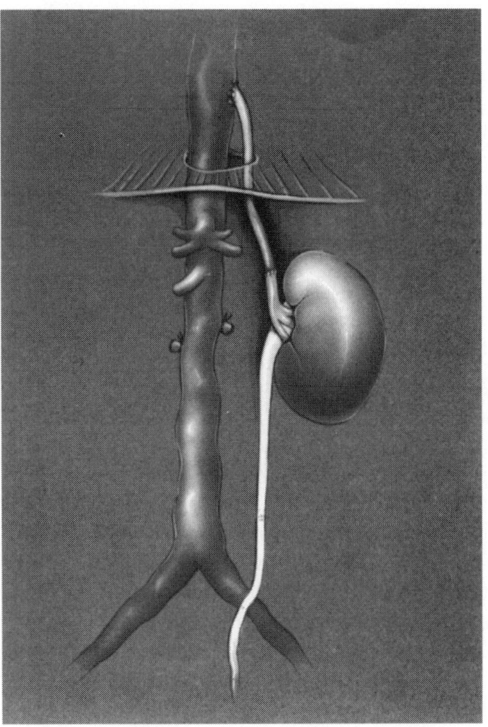

Fig 19. Sketch illustrating thoracic aortorenalbypass technique.

### Renal Autotransplantation

Renal autotransplantation may be used for revascularization of either kidney in patients with severe aortic atherosclerosis, provided there is good flow through the diseased aorta and there is no significant iliac disease. Autotransplantation is also indicated in children with renovascular hypertension and the middle aortic syndrome where the iliac vessels are generally free of disease. A midline transabdominal incision is made, the colon is reflected, the kidney and renal vessels are mobilized, and the iliac vessels are prepared. In most of these patients, the hypogastric artery is extensively diseased and autotransplantation is performed to the common iliac vessels. After ligating and dividing the renal vessels, the removed kidney is flushed by gravity flow with 500 mL chilled Ringer's lactate to which 5 mL 2% procain, 10,000 unit aqueous heparin, and 1 mL sodium bicarbonate have been added. The renal vein and artery are then anastomosed end-to-side to the common iliac vein and artery, respectively, and circulation to the kidney is restored within 30–45 min. The ureter is left intact and, although it may follow a redundant course to the bladder, normal ureteral peristalsis provides effective drainage of urine from the kidney. In such cases, care must be taken not to rotate the kidney when moving it so as to produce an obstructive torsion of the ureter.

### Iliorenal Bypass

Iliorenal bypass with a long saphenous vein graft may also be considered for patients with severe aortic atherosclerosis, good flow through the aorta, and relatively disease-free iliac arteries.[64] This operation is performed through a midline abdominal incision. In such cases, a saphenous vein graft is first anastomosed end-to-side to the common iliac artery and then end-to-end to the distal renal artery. Although both autotransplantation and iliorenal bypass are effective operations, the latter has the theoretical advantage of less operative time, a shorter period of renal ischemia, and preservation of collateral renal arterial supply. Iliorenal bypass may also be preferable for patients with significant arteriolar nephrosclerosis, since such kidneys generally flush poorly.

### Superior Mesenterorenal Bypass

In unusual cases, aortography will reveal an enlarged superior mesenteric artery that may be employed for visceral arterial bypass to either kidney. This situation is most often observed in patients with total occlusion of the infrarenal aorta. A saphenous vein graft is anastomosed end-to-side to the superior mesenteric artery and then end-to-end to the distal renal artery. This operation is infrequently indicated since in most patients the superior mesenteric artery will be either of normal caliber or will itself be involved in the disease process (Fig 20).

### Extracorporeal Revascularization and Autotransplantation

Extracorporeal microvascular repair and autotransplantation are indicated only when preoperative arteriography, with oblique views, demonstrates intrarenal extension of branch renovascular disease.[65] The advantages offered by extracorporeal revascularization include optimum exposure and illumination, a bloodless surgical field, greater protection from prolonged renal ischemia, and more facile employment of microvascular techniques and optical magnification. The operation is performed through a single midline incision extending from the xyphoid to the symphysis pubis. Before extracorporeal arterial reconstruction, the removed kidney is flushed with Collins intracellular electrolyte solution and is submerged in ice slush saline to maintain hypothermia. Under these conditions, the kidney can safely tolerate periods outside the body far in excess of those required to perform even the most complex arterial repair. Since urologic complications after ureteroneocystostomy are rare in our experience, we prefer to transect the ureter and place the kidney on a separate workbench while we perform the extracorporeal repair. Alternatively, the ureter may be left intact while working on the abdominal wall, although this is generally more cumbersome.

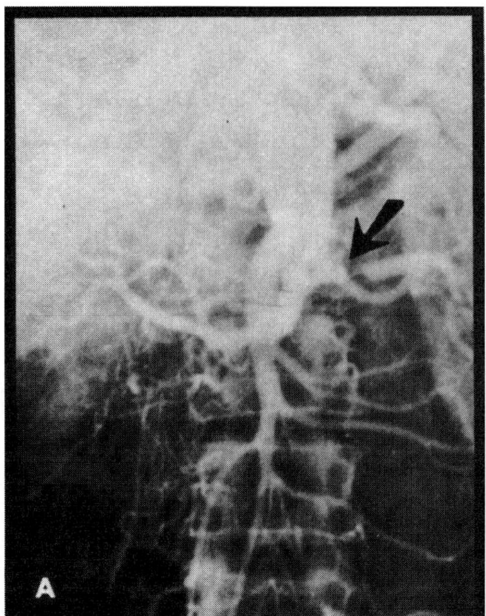


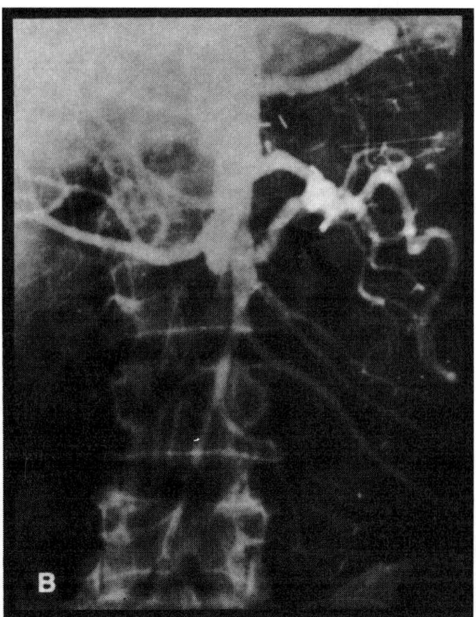


**Fig 20. A:** Preoperative arteriogram demonstrates complete aortic occlusion and high-grade left renal artery stenosis *(arrow)*. **B:** This patient underwent superior mesenterorenal bypass with a saphenous vein graft. Postoperative arteriogram demonstrates patent mesenterorenal bypass graft to the left kidney *(arrow)*.

When the surgeon performs extracorporeal microvascular branch arterial repair, a branched hypogastric arterial autograft is the optimum material for vascular reconstruction (Fig 21). If this is not available, a prefashioned branched saphenous vein graft is alternatively employed (Fig 21B). If repair of very small arterial branches is indicated, the inferior epigastric artery provides an excellent free graft for extracorporeal microvascular repair. This artery can also be employed as a branched graft,

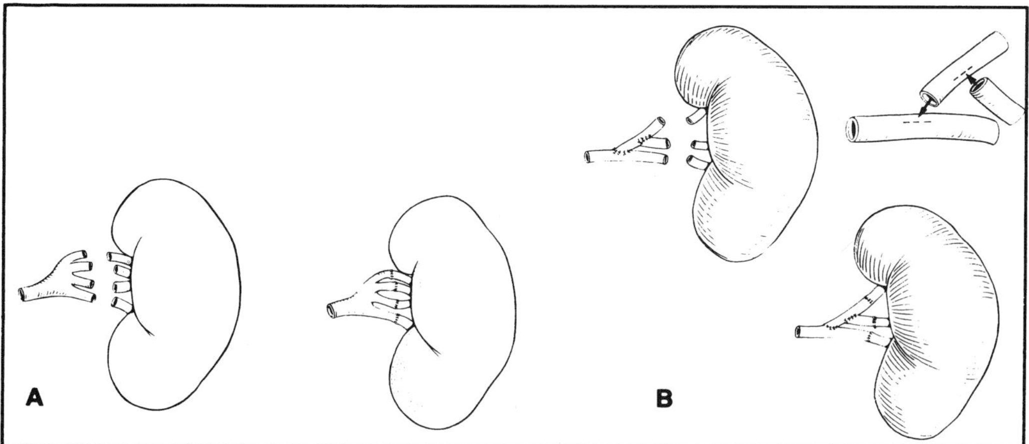


**Fig 21. A:** Extraocorporeal renal revascularization employing autogenous graft of the hypogastric artery procured intact with its branches. **B:** Extracorporeal renal revascularization employing prefashioned branched saphenous vein graft.

either by itself or in conjunction with a segment of saphenous vein. These branched autogenous vascular grafts usually allow separate end-to-end anastomosis of each graft limb to a distal renal artery branch. Other techniques that may be applicable are end-to-end anastomosis of a graft branch to two conjoined renal artery branches or direct implantation of a renal artery branch end-to-side into a limb of the graft (Fig 22).

These extracorporeal reconstructive techniques are all performed with microvascular instruments, with 7-0 to 9-0 suture material, and with optical magnification. During dissection of the renal vasculature, care is taken not to interfere with ureteral or pelvic blood supply. While revascularizing multiple arterial branches, one must anticipate the position that the various branches will assume in relation to one another upon completion of the repair. Individual branch anastomoses are then performed with careful attention to avoid subsequent malrotation, angulation, or tension. In all cases, extracorporeal repair leads to fashioning of a single main renal artery so that autotransplantation may be

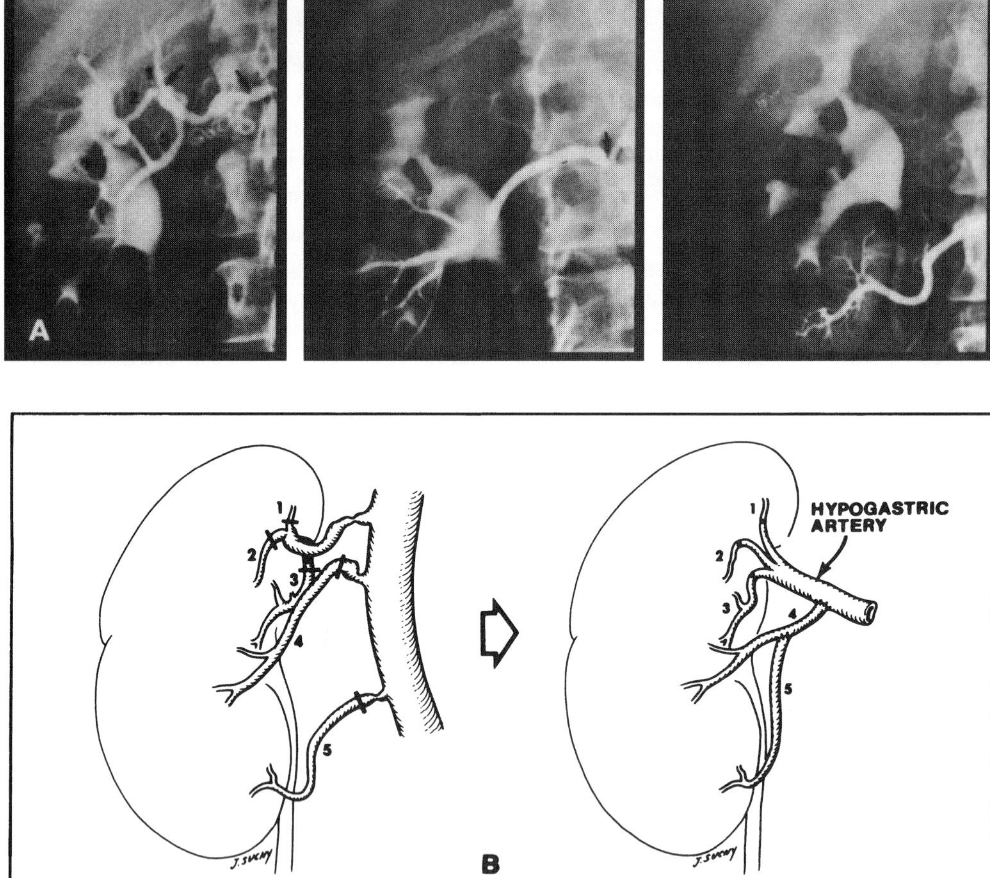


**Fig 22. A:** Preoperative arteriogram shows right kidney supplied by three renal arteries, each involved with severe proximal stenosis. Vascular disease in the upper artery extends into three distal branches. Arrows indicate sites of stenosis. **B:** Preoperative extent of renal artery disease **(left)** and completed extracorporeal repair with branched hypogastric arterial graft **(right)**.

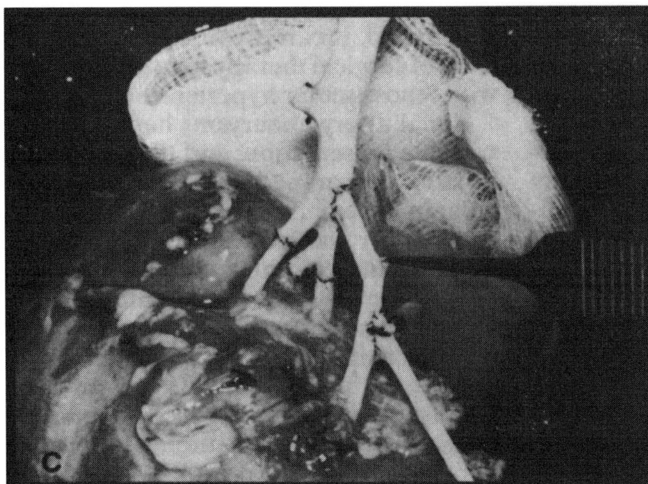


**Fig 22. C:** Operative photograph of completed extracorporeal revascularization of five segmental branches. The three diseased upper branches were repaired with branched graft to the hypogastric artery. The middle and lower renal arteries were anastomosed end to side into the graft and adjacent branch, respectively. **D:** Revascularized kidney following autotransplantation into the iliac fossa. **E:** Postoperative arteriogram of autotransplant demonstrates patency of all five revascularized segmental arteries. [From *J Urol.* 1981;126:150, with permission.]

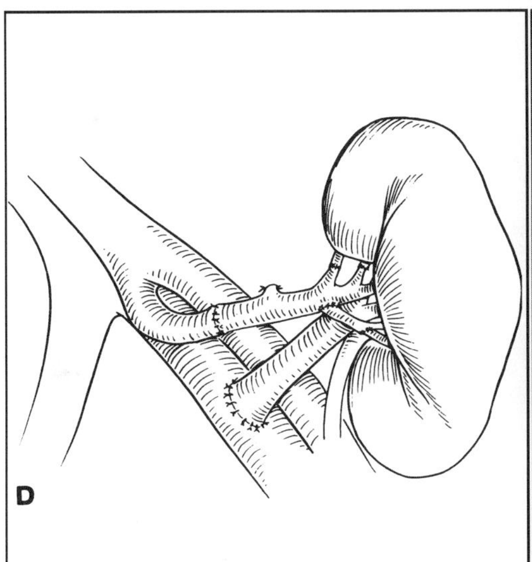


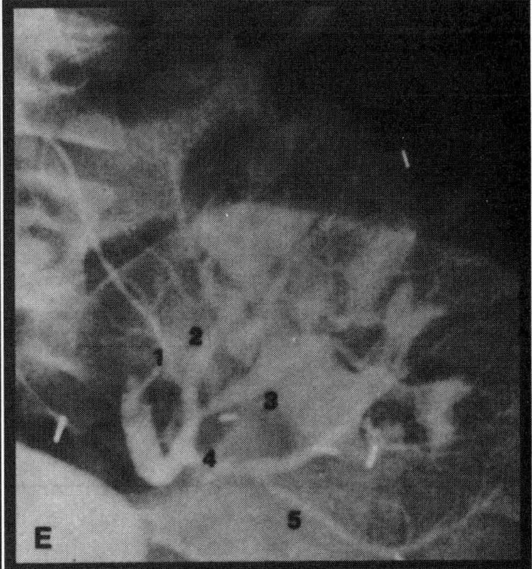


performed with one arterial anastomosis and with no increase in the critical revascularization time. The kidney is then autotransplanted to either iliac fossa, using the same technique as in renal allotransplantation, with ureteroneocystostomy as the method of restoring urinary continuity.

## Other Operations

Aortorenal reimplantation occasionally may be used to treat renovascular hypertension caused by short lesions of the proximal renal artery such as atherosclerosis or intimal fibroplasia.[66] Since an adequate amount of disease-free distal renal artery is a prerequisite for this operation, it is particularly well suited to the anatomic variant presented by an anomalous high origin of the renal artery. In performing right renal revascularization with aortorenal reimplantation, retrocaval reimplantation is done to enable maximum use of distal renal artery length; a precaval anastomosis may result in angulation of the renal artery. The advantage of aortorenal reimplantation is that it involves only a single vascular anastomosis and obviates the need for a bypass graft. Although the indications for its use

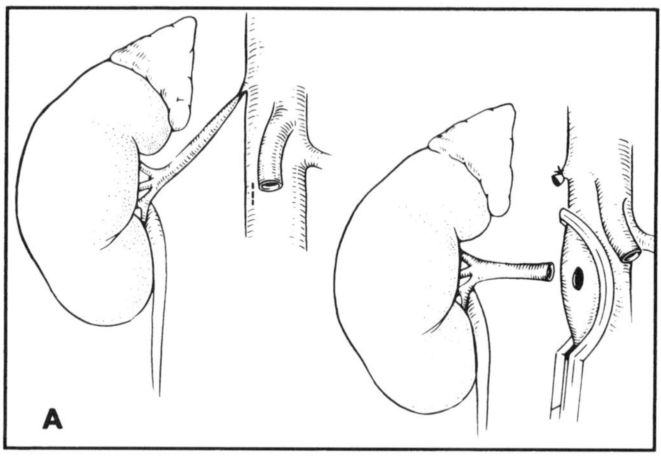


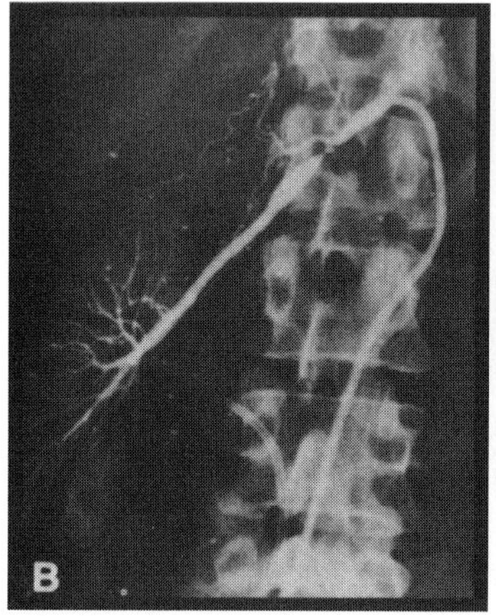


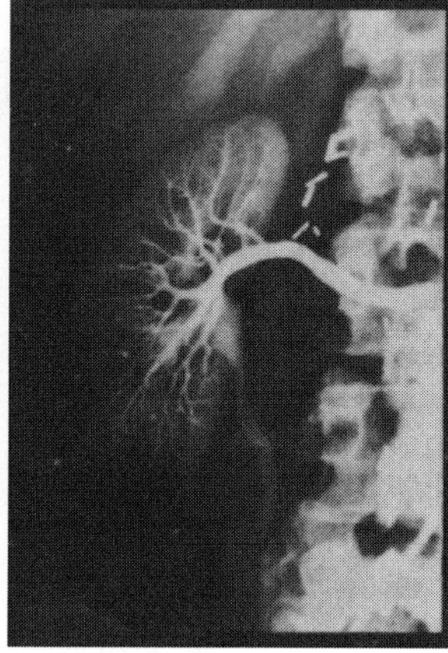

**Fig 23. A:** Direct reimplantation of the renal artery into the aorta. **B:** Preoperative selective right renal arteriogram **(left)** demonstrates proximal right renal artery stenosis from intimal fibroplasia. Postoperative arteriogram after aortorenal reimplantation **(right)** shows patent arterial repair. [From *Urology.* 1979;14:566, with permission.]

are limited, it can provide a satisfactory form of surgical therapy for a few patients with renovascular hypertension (Fig 23).

Renal artery aneurysms have a highly variable presentation, and the method of repair is determined by whether renovascular involvement is focal or diffuse. If the renal artery wall at the base of an aneurysm is intact, aneurysmectomy with either primary closure or patch angioplasty can be performed. Aneurysms with short focal involvement of the main renal artery or a branch may also be resected simply with end-to-end arterial anastomosis. When these techniques cannot be applied, or in cases of more diffuse vascular disease, an in situ or extracorporeal bypass operation with an autogenous graft is indicated (Fig 24).

Segmental resection of the renal artery and reanastomosis may also be indicated for focal, stenotic, fibrous lesions of the mid- to distal renal artery. Unfortunately, in most patients with fibrous dysplasias, vascular disease is too extensive to allow this to be done without either inadequately resecting the lesion or placing undue tension on the anastomosis. In fact, very few patients with renal artery stenosis are candidates for this operation (Fig 25).

In selected patients, where an aortic aneurysm or disabling peripheral vascular occlusive disease is present, complete excision of the aorta and replacement with a Dacron prosthesis is indicated. A side-arm bypass graft can then be interposed from the side of the Dacron prosthesis to either renal artery. This is an extensive and tech-

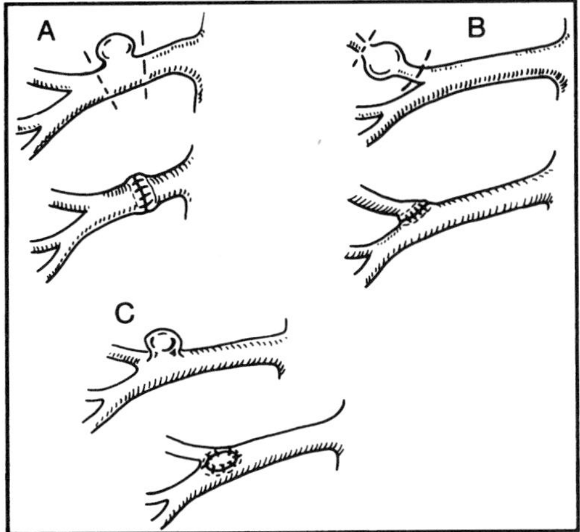


**Fig 24. A, B:** Resection and reanastomosis of the main renal artery or a proximal branch for short focal aneurysm. **C:** Aneurysmectomy and primary closure with patch angioplasty is an alternative treatment for aneurysms of the main renal artery. [From Novick AC, Straffon RA, eds. *Vascular Problems in Urologic Surgery.* Philadelphia: WB Saunders; 1982, with permission.]

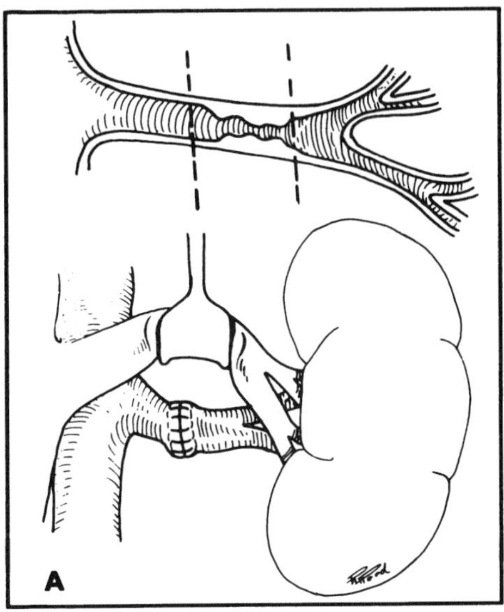


**Fig 25. A:** Segmental resection of the renal artery and reanastomosis. **B:** Selective renal arteriogram demonstrates focal stenosis of the mid–left renal artery from intimal fibroplasia **(left).** Repeat arteriogram a year after segmental resection with reanastomosis demonstrates patent arterial repair. [From Kelalis P, King L, Belman B, eds. *Clinical Pediatric Urology.* Philadelphia: WB Saunders; 1984, with permission.]

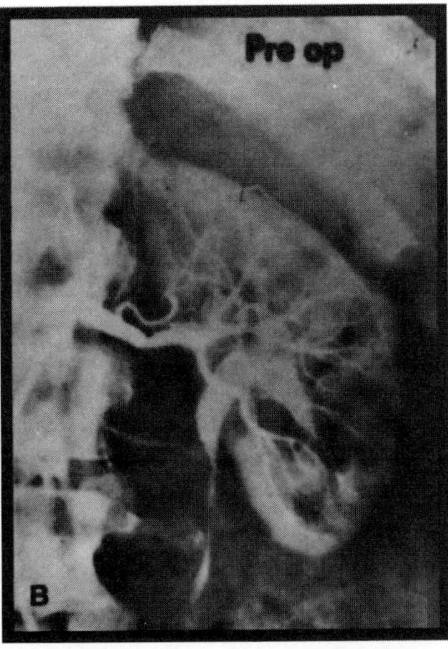


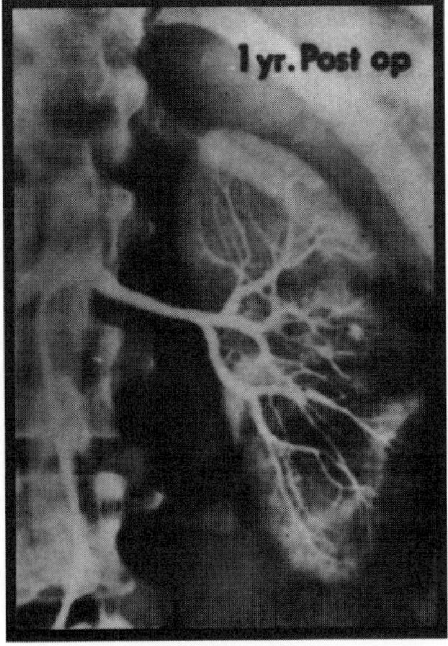

nically difficult operation that has been associated with operative mortality rates ranging from 10% to 30%.[67–69]

Transaortic endarterectomy has also been employed as a method of renal revascularization in patients with severe aortic atherosclerosis. This operation has the advantage of allowing bilateral simultaneous revascularization if both renal arteries are diseased. Nevertheless, this is also a more extensive operation that entails a lengthy and tedious dissection to mobilize and to prepare the aorta. In addition, the resultant traumatized arterial surface may predispose to reformation of thrombus. The other techniques described above for patients with a surgically difficult aorta are much less hazardous and have proven equally effective.

### Postoperative Care

Patients undergoing renal revascularization may experience wide fluctuations in their blood pressure in the early postoperative period, with either hypotensive or hypertensive episodes that may predispose to graft thrombosis or bleeding from vascular anastomotic sites. Therefore, these patients are placed in the intensive care unit for monitoring of central venous pressure, blood pressure, urine output, pulse rate, serum hemoglobin, and serum creatinine. During this period, the diastolic blood pressure is maintained between 90 and 100 mm Hg to ensure satisfactory renal perfusion. If hypertensive episodes occur, they are managed with an intravenous infusion of sodium nitroprusside. Within the first 24 hr postoperatively, a technetium renal scan is obtained to verify perfusion of the revascularized kidney. Subsequent radioisotope monitoring is performed with [$^{131}$I]orthoiodohippurate, which provides a better functional assessment of the kidney. In the absence of postoperative vasomotor nephropathy, this scan will show prompt uptake, early excretion, and complete clearance of isotope from the kidney. In many cases, serial postoperative scans will show improvement in the function of the revascularized kidney compared to a preoperative study.

If the patient's condition is stable, the nasogastric tube, central venous line, arterial line, and urethral catheter are removed 48 hr postoperatively and intensive care monitoring is discontinued. When autotransplantation with ureteroneocystostomy has been performed, urethral catheter drainage of the bladder is maintained for one week postoperatively.

## RESULTS

The results of surgical treatment for renal vascular hypertension have always been excellent in patients with fibrous dysplasia.[51,52,70–72] However, traditionally, less satisfactory results have been observed in patients with atherosclerosis.[73,74] During the past decade, refinements in establishing a preoperative diagnosis of renin-mediated hypertension and an enhanced technical efficacy of vascular reconstruction have led to improved surgical results in the latter category. There are now several reports of an 85%–90% cure or improvement rate following revascularization for atherosclerotic renal vascular hypertension.[38,75]

We reviewed the Cleveland Clinic experience with surgical revascularization in 361 patients with renal artery disease from January 1975 to December 1984.[38] The pathologic diagnosis was atherosclerosis in 241 patients, fibrous dysplasia in 104 patients, and an arterial aneurysm in 16 patients. The indication for revascularization in all patients with fibrous dysplasia or an aneurysm was to treat severe renal vascular hypertension. The indications in patients with atherosclerotic disease were treatment of renal vascular hypertension in 80 patients, preservation of renal function in 61 patients, and both control of hypertension and preservation of renal function in 100 patients.

In this series, the operative mortality rate was 2.1% in patients with atherosclerotic disease and 0% in patients with fibrous dysplasia or an aneurysm. The incidence of postoperative thrombosis or stenosis of the repaired renal artery was 4.5%. Hypertension was cured or improved postoperatively in 91.7% of patients with atherosclerotic disease and in 93% of patients with fibrous dysplasia or an aneurysm. Postoperative renal function was improved or stable in 88.8% of patients with atherosclerosis who underwent revascularization to preserve renal function.

## SUMMARY

The management of patients with renal artery disease has changed in recent years. This has occurred due to the advent of PTA as an effective method of treatment for certain patients, improved results of surgical revascularization in older patients with atherosclerosis, an enhanced appreciation of advanced atherosclerotic renal artery disease as a correctable cause of renal failure, and the development of more effective surgical techniques for patients with severe aortic atherosclerosis and branch renal artery disease. PTA has become the treatment of choice for patients with main renal arterial fibrous dysplasia and nonostial atherosclerotic lesions. Surgical revascularization remains the preferred treatment for patients with branch renal artery disease, ostial atherosclerotic renal artery disease, renal artery aneurysm, and patients in whom renal PTA has been unsuccessful. Excellent clinical results can be achieved with surgical revascularization and PTA in properly selected patients.

## REFERENCES

1. Novick AC. Surgical correction of renovascular hypertension. *Surg Clin North Am.* 1988;68: 1007.
2. Wollenweber J, Sheps SG, David GD. Clinical course of atherosclerotic renovascular disease. *Am J Cardiol.* 1968;21:60.
3. Meaney TF, Dustan HP, McCormack LJ. Natural history of renal artery disease. *Radiology.* 1968; 91:881.
4. Schreiber MJ, Pohl MA, Novick AC. The natural history of atherosclerotic and fibrous renal artery disease. *Urol Clin North Am.* 1984;11:383.
5. Harrison HG, McCormack LJ. Pathologic classification of renal artery disease in renovascular hypertension. *Mayo Clin Proc.* 1971;46:161.
6. Rybka SJ, Novick AC. Concomitant carotid, mesenteric, and renal artery stenosis due to primary intimal fibroplasia. *J Urol.* 1983;129, 798.
7. Novick AC. Renal artery aneurysm and arteriovenous malformation. In: Novick AC, Straffon RA, eds. *Vascular Problems in Urologic Surgery.* Philadelphia: WB Saunders; 1982.
8. Poutasse EF. Renal artery aneurysms. *J Urol.* 1975;113:443.
9. Kaufman JJ. The middle aortic syndrome: report of a case treated by renal autotransplantation. *J Urol.* 1973;109, 711.
10. Grad E, Rance CP. Bilateral renal artery stenosis in association with neurofibromatosis (Recklinghausen's disease): report of two cases. *J Pediatr.* 1972;80:804.
11. Tilford DL, Kelsch RC. Renal artery stenosis in childhood neurofibromatosis. *Am J Dis Child.* 1973;126:665.
12. Silver D, Clements JB. Renovascular hypertension from renal artery compression by congenital bands. *Ann Surg.* 1976;183:161.
13. Leadbetter WF, Burkland CE. Hypertension in unilateral renal disease. *J Urol.* 1938;39:611.
14. Vaughan ED, Buhler FR, Laragh JH, et al. Hypertension and unilateral parenchymal renal disease: evidence for abnormal vasoconstriction–volume interaction. *JAMA.* 1975;233: 1177.
15. Poutasse EF, Stecker JF, Ladaga LE, et al. Malignant hypertension in children secondary to chronic pyelonephritis: laboratory and radiologic indications for partial or total nephrectomy. *J Urol.* 1978;119:264.
16. Riehle RA, Vaghan EJ. Renin participation in hypertension associated with unilateral hydronephrosis. *J Urol.* 1981;126:243.
17. Belman AB, Kropp KA, Simon NM. Renal-pressor hypertension secondary to unilateral hydronephrosis. *N Engl J Med.* 1968;278:1133.
18. Meares EM, Gross DM. Hypertension owing to unilateral renal hypoplasia. *J Urol.* 1972;108: 197.
19. Rosenfeld JB, Cohen L, Garty I, et al. Unilateral renal hypoplasia with hypertension (Ask–Upmark kidney). *Br Med J.* 1973;2:217.
20. Stickler GB, Kelalis PP, Burke E, et al. Primary interstitial nephritis with reflux: a cause of hypertension. *Am J Dis Child.* 1971;122:144.
21. Simon F, Franklin SS, Bleifer KH, et al. Clinical characteristics of renovascular hypertension. *JAMA.* 1972;220:1209.
22. Eipper DF, Gifford RW, Stewart BH, et al. Abdominal bruits in renovascular hypertension. *Am J Cardiol.* 1976;37:48.
23. Hughes JS, Dove HG, Gifford RW, et al. Duration of blood pressure elevation in accurately predicting surgical cure of renovascular hypertension. *Am Heart J.* 1981;101:408.
24. Nally JV, Gupta BK, Clarke HS, et al. Captopril renography for the detection of renovascular hypertension. *Cleve Clin J Med.* 1988;55:311.
25. Geyskes GG, Oei HY, Puylaert C, Mees EJ: Re-

novascular hypertension identified by captopril-induced changes in renogram. *Hypertension.* 1987;9:451.

26. Robertson R, Murphy A, Dubbins PA. Renal artery stenosis: the use of duplex ultrasound as a screening technique. *Br J Radiol.* 1988;61:196.
27. Taylor DC, et al. Duplex ultrasound scanning in the diagnosis of renal artery stenosis: a prospective evaluation. *J Vasc Surg.* 1988;7:363.
28. Zabbo A, Novick AC. Digital subtraction angiography for non-invasive imaging of the renal artery. *Urol Clin North Am.* 1984;11:409.
29. Harvey RJ, Krumlovsky F, del Greco F, et al. Screening for renovascular hypertension. Is renal digital-subtraction angiography the preferred non-invasive test? *JAMA.* 1985;254:388.
30. Debatin JF, Spritzer CE, Grist TM, et al. Imaging of renal arteries: value of MR angiography. *Am J Radiol.* 1991;157:981.
31. Kaufman JJ. Renovascular hypertension: the UCLA experience. *J Urol.* 1979;121:139.
32. Couch NP, Sullivan J, Crane C. The predictive accuracy of renal vein renin activity in the surgery of renovascular hypertension. *Surgery.* 1976;79:70.
33. Marks LS, Maxwell MH, Varady PD, et al. Renovascular hypertension: does the renal vein renin ratio predict operative results? *J Urol.* 1976; 115:365.
34. Muller FB, Seeley JE, Case DB, et al. The captopril test for identifying renovascular disease in hypertensive patients. *Am J Med.* 1986;80:633.
35. Council on Scientific Affairs. Percutaneous transluminal angioplasty. *JAMA.* 1984;251:764.
36. Hayes J, Risius B, Novick AC, et al. Experience with percutaneous transluminal angioplasty for renal artery stenosis at the Cleveland Clinic. *J Urol.* 1988;139:488.
37. Sos TA, Pickering PG, Sniderman KW, et al. Percutaneous transluminal renal angiography in renovascular hypertension due to atheroma or fibrous dysplasia. *N Engl J Med.* 1983;309:274.
38. Novick AC, Ziegelbaum M, Vidt DG, et al. Trends in surgical revascularization for renal artery disease: ten years' experience. *JAMA.* 1987; 257:498.
39. Cicuto KP, McLean GK, Oleaga J, et al. Renal artery stenosis: anatomic classification for percutaneous angioplasty. *AJR.* 1981;137:599.
40. Novick AC, Pohl MA, Schreiber MJ, et al. Renal revascularization for preservation of kidney function in patients with atherosclerotic renovascular disease. *J Urol.* 1983;129:907.
41. Ziegelbaum M, Novick AC, Hayes J, et al. Management of renal arterial disease in the elderly patient. *Surg Gynecol Obstet.* 1987;165:130.
42. Libertino JA, Zinman L, Breslin DJ, et al. Renal artery revascularization: restoration of renal function. *JAMA.* 1980;244:1340.
43. Schefft P, Novick AC, Stewart BH, et al. Renal revascularization in patients with total occlusion of renal artery. *J Urol.* 1980;124:184.
44. Wasser WG, Krakoff LR, Haimov M, et al. Restoration of renal function after bilateral renal artery occlusion. *Arch Intern Med.* 1981;141:1647.
45. Kaylor W, Novick AC, Ziegelbaum M, Vidt D. Reversal of end-stage renal failure with surgical revascularization in patients with atherosclerotic renal artery occlusion. *J Urol.* 1989;141:486.
46. Novick AC. Renal vascular hypertension in children. In: Kelalis P, King L, Belman B, eds. *Clinical Pediatric Urology.* Philadelphia: WB Saunders; 1984.
47. Martinez A, Novick AC, Cunningham R. Goormastic: improved results of vascular reconstruction in pediatric and young adult patients with renovascular hypertension. *J Urol.* 1990;144: 717.
48. Franklin SS, Young JD, Maxwell MH, et al. Operative morbidity and mortality in renovascular disease. *JAMA.* 1975;231:1148.
49. Novick AC, Straffon RA, Stewart BH, et al. Diminished operative morbidity and mortality following revascularization for atherosclerotic renovascular disease. *JAMA.* 1981;246:749.
50. Dean RH, Wilson JP, Burko H, et al. Saphenous vein aortorenal bypass grafts; serial arteriography study. *Ann Surg.* 1974;180:469.
51. Novick AC, Stewart BH, Straffon RA. Autogenous arterial grafts in the treatment of renal artery stenosis. *J Urol.* 1977;118:919.
52. Stoney RJ, Deluccia N, Ehrenfeld WK, et al. Aortorenal arterial autografts; long-term assessment. *Arch Surg.* 1981;116:1416.
53. Kaufman JJ. Dacron grafts and splenorenal bypass in the surgical treatment of stenosing lesions of the renal artery. *Urol Clin North Am.* 1975;2: 365.
54. Haimon H, Giron F, Jacobson JH. The expanded polytetrafluorethylene graft: three years' experience with 362 grafts. *Arch Surg.* 1979;114:673.
55. Khauli RB, Novick AC, Coseriu GV. Renal revascularization and polytetrafluorethylene grafts. *Cleve Clin Q.* 1984;51:365.
56. Novick AC, Straffon RA, Stewart BH. Surgical management of branch renal artery disease: in situ versus extracorporeal methods of repair. *J Urol.* 1980;123:311.
57. Streem SB, Novick AC. Aortorenal bypass with a branched saphenous vein graft for in situ repair of multiple segmental renal arteries. *Surg Gynecol Obstet.* 1982;155:855.
58. Pechan WB, Novick AC, Stewart BH, et al. Endarterectomy and patchgraft angioplasty in treatment of atherosclerotic renovascular hypertension. *J Urol.* 1979;14:487.
59. Novick AC, Stewart BH, Straffon RA, et al. Renal revascularization in patients with atherosclerosis or a previous operation on the abdominal aorta. *Surg Gynecol Obstet.* 1977;144:211.

60. Khauli RB, Novick AC, Ziegelbaum CN. Splenorenal bypass in the treatment of renal artery stenosis: experience with 69 cases. *J Vasc Surg.* 1985;2:547.
61. Novick AC, Palleschi J, Straffon RA, et al. Experimental and clinical hepatorenal bypass as a means of right renal revascularization. *Surg Gynecol Obstet.* 1979;148:557.
62. Chibaro EA, Libertino JA, Novick AC. Use of the hepatic circulation for renal revascularization. *Ann Surg.* 1984;199:406.
63. Novick AC, Stewart R. Use of the thoracic aorta for renal revascularization. *J Urol.* 1990;143:77.
64. Novick AC, Banowsky LH. Iliorenal saphenous vein bypass: alternative for renal revascularization in patients with surgically difficult aorta. *J Urol.* 1979;122:243.
65. Novick AC. Management of intrarenal branch arterial lesions with extracorporeal microvascular reconstruction and autotransplantation. *J Urol.* 1981;126:150.
66. Noble MJ, Novick AC, Straffon RA, et al. Aortorenal reimplantation in treatment of renovascular hypertension. *Urology.* 1979;14:566.
67. Shahian DM, Najafi H, Javid H, et al. Simultaneous aortic and renal artery reconstruction. *Arch Surg.* 1980;115:1491.
68. Gomes M, Bernatz PE. Aortoiliac occlusive disease: extension cephalad to origin of renal arterial disease with considerations and results. *Arch Surg.* 1970;101:161.
69. Tarazi RY, Hertzer NR, Beven EG, et al. Simultaneous aortic reconstruction and renal revascularization: risk factors and late results in 89 patients. *Surgery.* 1987;5:709.
70. Ernst CB, Stanley JC, Marshall F, et al. Autogenous saphenous vein aortorenal autografts: a ten-year experience. *Arch Surg.* 1972;150:855.
71. Lankford NS, Donahue JP, Grim CE, et al. Results of surgical treatment of renovascular hypertension. *J Urol.* 1979;122:439.
72. Novick AC, Jackson CL, Straffon RA. The role of renal autotransplantation in complex urologic reconstruction. *J Urol.* 1990;143:452.
73. Foster JH, Maxwell MH, Franklin SS, et al. Renovascular occlusive disease: results of operative treatment. *JAMA.* 1975;231:1043.
74. Franklin SS, Young JD, Maxwell WH, et al. Operative morbidity and mortality in renovascular disease. *JAMA.* 1975;231:1148.
75. Buda JA, Baer L, Parra-Carilo JZ, et al. Predictability of surgical response in renovascular hypertension. *Arch Surg.* 1976;111:1243.

# 13

# Renal Transplantation

*William Bihrle, III, Michael Malone, and Christopher Ying*

## INTRODUCTION

The field of renal transplantation has burgeoned since the first reports of successful cadaveric and living related human transplants by Landsteiner and Hufnagel[1] and Murray et al[2] three decades ago. Advances in immunosuppression and organ preservation have made allograft transplantation the treatment of choice for end-stage renal disease (ESRD). Unfortunately, the demand for organs has far exceeded the availability as evidenced by the growing number of patients on transplant waiting lists. The absolute number of individuals with ESRD and on dialysis has increased by 47% since 1980.[3] Similarly, the size of the United Network for Organ Sharing (UNOS) list has grown from 14,000 patients in 1988 to almost 19,000 in 1991, an increase of 26% in 3 years. The number of renal transplants performed each year, however, has remained relatively static, averaging slightly less than 7000. Of these, approximately 4000 represent cadaveric transplants, a figure that highlights the serious shortage in organ availability.

This chapter is intended to provide the urologist with a brief history and an overview of the medical and surgical aspects of renal transplantation. This includes, but is not limited to, discussions, transplantation immunobiology, immunosuppression, various operative procedures, and management of complications and acute rejection.

## BRIEF HISTORY

The history of renal transplantation is really the story of advances in immunosuppression. Schwartz and Dameshek[4] demonstrated the immunosuppressive effects of 6-mercaptopurine in rabbits in 1959. Calne[5] and Zukoski et al[6] confirmed the beneficial effects of this drug on canine renal allograft survival leading ultimately to its use in human renal transplantation. For many years the combination of azathioprine and prednisone represented the mainstay of immunosuppressive therapy.

The introduction of cyclosporine in 1979 essentially revolutionized the field of transplantation. This potent immunosuppressive not only improved 1-year graft survival but permitted reduced dosages of prednisone and azathioprine, leading to a diminution in drug-related complications. In fact, randomized trials have demonstrated that the elimination of azathioprine or prednisone after triple-induction immunosuppression in renal transplantation showed no detrimental effect on graft outcome.[8] In addition, 1-year graft survival has increased from 64% to 80% since the addition of cyclosporine to the immunosuppressive regimen.[9] Recent UNOS data show 1-year graft survival of 86% and 68% with living related and cadaver donors, respectively,[10] a significant improvement since the introduction of cyclosporine.

OKT3, a monoclonal antibody introduced in 1980, has been particularly effective in the treatment of acute allograft rejection refractory to high-dose steroids.[11] FK 506, the newest immunosuppressive agent, has been primarily utilized in liver transplantation. There has been a modest experience, however, with its use in failing renal grafts unresponsive to conventional therapy.

## PATIENT SELECTION AND EVALUATION

The patient with ESRD has limited long-term management options: hemodialysis, chronic ambulatory peritoneal dialysis (CAPD), or renal transplantation. Most patients when asked to choose from this menu choose renal transplantation since it is associated with a marked improvement in the quality of life. Comparison of hemodialysis or CAPD with renal transplantation shows that transplantation is significantly more cost-effective even when expensive immunosuppressive agents and multiple, potential rejection episodes possibly requiring repeated hospitalizations are factored in.

Our policy at the Lahey Clinic is to offer renal transplantation whenever possible. Potential renal transplant patients require extensive preoperative evaluation, but the only absolute contraindications to surgery include active infection (including positive HIV serology), disseminated malignancy, or medical contraindications rendering the patient incapable of tolerating a general anesthetic and a surgical procedure. In fact, there is compelling evidence that individuals successfully treated for many types of cancer are acceptable candidates for renal transplantation.[12,13] Relative contraindications to allograft transplantation include age, advanced systemic disease, renal disease with a potentially high recurrence rate, or a noncompliant patient (immunosuppression after renal transplantation is lifelong).

Candidates for renal transplantation receive an extensive evaluation including a detailed medical and psychological history, physical examination, and routine laboratory studies as outlined in Table 1. Subsequent evaluation is based on the patient's age, evaluation results, and the primary disease process resulting in renal failure.

A history of gastrointestinal or cardiovascular disease, because of its association with increased perioperative complications, demands a more extensive evaluation. All adults undergo gallbladder ultrasound and if symptomatic gallstones are found, cholecystectomy (laparoscopic versus traditional) is performed. A history of peptic ulcer disease requires upper gastro-

**TABLE 1. Routine Laboratory and Radiologic Evaluation of Potential Renal Transplant Recipients**

| | |
|---|---|
| **Laboratory Evaluation** | |
| Blood typing | Serum cholesterol |
| Human leukocyte antigen (HLA) typing | Protein |
| Hepatitis B serology | Albumin |
| Viral serology | Triglycerides |
| CBC | VDRL |
| Electrolytes | HIV |
| Liver function tests | ECG |
| **Radiologic Evaluation** | |
| Chest x-ray | Exercise tolerance testing with thallium scan |
| Gallbladder ultrasound | Coronary angiography |
| Voiding cystourethrogram | Peripheral vascular arteriography |
| Upper GI series | Lower GI series |

intestinal series or esophagogastroscopy to exclude the presence of an active ulcer. If an ulcer is present, intensive antacid and H2 blocker therapy are begun and healing must be documented before surgery is contemplated. Asymptomatic diverticulosis requires observation only, while recurrent diverticulitis indicates the need for pretransplant colectomy.

Older patients, especially diabetics, have a propensity to develop coronary artery disease. Patients in this category undergo exercise tolerance testing (ETT) with a thallium scan. A positive ETT, or in some centers even a history of longstanding diabetes mellitus, suggests a need for more invasive diagnostics, specifically coronary angiography. Significant lesions should be treated, eg, coronary artery bypass graft (CABG) prior to renal transplantation. A higher incidence of peripheral vascular disease is found in this patient population as well. Since the iliac vessels are used for the transplant renal vessel anastomoses, noninvasive arterial and venous imaging is usually performed. Positive findings should be evaluated with arteriography or venography.

The genitourinary evaluation of the transplant candidate is designed to identify vesicoureteral reflux, obstructive uropathy, urinary tract infection, and neurogenic entities. A urine culture is routinely obtained and, if positive, prompts further investigation, including a voiding cystourethrogram (VCUG), retrograde urethrogram, or cystoscopy. If the VCUG demonstrates the presence of vesicoureteral reflux, this is best treated by nephrectomy or reimplant surgery. Radiologic or visual inspection of the lower urinary tract is helpful in the diagnosis of obstructive lesions, eg, urethral stricture or benign prostatic hyperplasia. While obvious strictures should be corrected prior to transplantation, the urologist should avoid prostatic surgery unless there is compelling evidence that the prostate is physiologically obstructing.

While there appears to be some evidence that donor-specific blood transfusions are an important adjunct in living related renal transplants, the introduction of cyclosporine A has effectively neutralized the advantage of pretransplant blood transfusions in the cadaveric transplant group.[14]

## Living Related Transplants

The severe limitation of organ availability makes the use of living related donors, although ethically challenging, an unavoidable fact of transplant life. In fact, while effective immunosuppression has narrowed the 1-year graft survival differences between the two groups, UNOS data still confer a survival benefit to well-selected, living related transplants. The living related donor is assiduously evaluated with a battery of laboratory and radiologic tests (Table 2). Obviously, the renal donor must possess two well-functioning, nondiseased kidneys, have no transmissible disease, and be physically able to tolerate a surgical procedure under general anesthesia. Above all, the donor must be psychologically committed to the concept of organ donation.

The selection of the best donor from a group of siblings and parents is based on a determination of antigen compatibility. In general, this involves an analysis of the human leukocyte antigen (HLA) system.

The code for the major histocompatibility antigens is composed of closely linked

**TABLE 2. Evaluation of a Potential Living Related Renal Donor**

| Laboratory Evaluation | |
|---|---|
| Blood typing | HIV serology |
| Human leukocyte antigen (HLA) typing | Cytomegalovirus serology |
| CBC | Creatinine clearance |
| Electrolytes | Urinalysis |
| Coagulation studies | VDRL |
| Serum cholesterol | ECG |
| Triglycerides | Serum calcium |
| Protein | Hepatitis B serology |
| Uric acid | |
| **Radiologic Evaluation** | |
| Chest x-ray | |
| Intravenous pyelogram | |
| Renal digital subtraction angiography (DSA) | |

genes on a single chromosomal complex. The major histocompatibility complex (MHC) in humans is the HLA system and occupies a segment of the short arm of the sixth human chromosome. The HLA system comprises five histocompatibility loci within the MHC. These are HLA-A, HLA-B, HLA-C, HLA-D, and HLA-DR. Approximately 9 to 35 separate antigens are controlled by each of these loci. Incompatibility with these histocompatibility antigens constitutes the immunologic barrier to renal transplantation.

The HLA chromosomal complex including the five HLA loci and their antigens is defined as a haplotype. The haplotype refers to that portion of a phenotype determined by closely linked genes of a single chromosome inherited from one parent. This is important for identifying HLA-identical siblings for potential living related donors and also in identifying zero haplotype matches with no donor potential. The HLA system is an extremely polymorphic genetic system, making it difficult to find perfectly matched cadaver kidney donors for potential recipients.

The ideal renal donor for the potential recipient, therefore, would be an identical twin. Since this is usually not possible, the siblings and parents of the patient are screened as potential donors. If multiple donors are found, then the selection of the most appropriate donor is determined.

The recipient must have a negative cross-match with the donor. Recipient serum is mixed with donor lymphocytes in complement. Lysis of donor lymphocytes means that preformed antibody to donor cells is present and the cross-match is positive. This potential donor is therefore excluded as transplantation would result in hyperacute rejection at the time of renal revascularization.

Multiple cross-match negative patients may be found and the donor with the best HLA match will be utilized. The potential donor with the least operative risk and least amount of change in life style should be selected if multiple similar HLA matches exist. Renal transplantation should be done once all evaluations have been completed and can even be done prior to the initiation of dialysis.

Patients who do not have a living related donor are placed on a regional waiting list for cadaver renal transplantation through UNOS. The basic requirements for donor recipient match are blood type compatibility and a negative cross-match as outlined above.

## RENAL PRESERVATION

Effective ex vivo preservation of cadaver kidneys for 24 to 48 hours is necessary to provide a time for sensitive cross-matching and histocompatibility testing, and to allow efficient dissemination of organs throughout the transplant network. Effective methods of short-term preservation permit transplantation of kidneys up to 3 days after procurement. Preservation of organs for longer than this period of time, while desirable for obvious reasons, is presently not technically feasible.

Short-term renal preservation is effective by one of two basic methods: continuous hypothermic perfusion[15] and cold storage.[16] While neither method is clearly superior, advances in the quality of perfusate and the practical advantages of transport with cold storage have made this form of preservation the most commonly used in this country.

In order to understand renal preservation techniques and how they have made successful renal transplantation possible, one must understand what occurs at the cellular level during warm ischemia periods, hypothermic storage, and reperfusion. During these periods there is diminished metabolic activity as well as cessation of cell membrane function leading to cell swelling and acidosis. There is also a loss of intracellular energy stores that can generate toxic free radicals that contribute to endothelial damage or reperfusion injury after revascularization. Hence, we can divide the protective effects of renal preservation into the hypothermic effect and the cold-flush perfusate effect with preservation of intracellular high-energy metabolites and free radical scavengers.[17]

## Hypothermic Effect

Hypothermia and continuous aerobic perfusion are the only theoretical means of obtaining perfusion times of months to years. Hypothermia decreases the rate at which intracellular enzymes degrade but does not stop metabolism completely, leading ultimately to loss of kidney viability.

Most enzymes of normothermic animals show a 1.5- to 2.0-fold decrease in activity for every 10°C decrease in temperature. Most organs tolerate warm ischemia of 30 to 60 minutes without complete loss of function. If you cool a kidney from 37°C to 0°C, this should extend renal preservation by 12 hours.[18] Collins demonstrated that flushing with renal perfusate extended renal preservation to as long as 30 hours.[16]

## Cold-Flush Perfusate Effect

Cold-flush perfusates have a composition that minimizes hypothermic-induced cell swelling, prevents cellular acidosis, expansion of the interstitial space, injury from oxygen-free radicals, and provides substrates for regenerating the high-energy phosphate compound adenosine triphosphate (ATP) during reperfusion. The mechanism for each will now be explained.

**Cell Swelling.** Cells are bathed in an extracellular solution high in $Na^+$ and low in $K^+$ that is maintained by the $Na^+$ pump (Na-K-ATPase). The energy required for this, ATP, is derived from oxidative phosphorylation. $Na^+$ is an impermeant outside the cell that counteracts the colloidal osmotic pressure derived from the intracellular proteins and other impermeable anions. The calculated osmotic force derived from this is about 100 to 140 mosm/kg. Hypothermic preservation suppresses the $Na^+$ pump, allowing $Na^+$ and $H_2O$ into the cell, causing swelling. Cellular swelling can be counteracted by providing 100 to 140 mosm/kg of impermeable substrate to the cell.[19] This essentially defines the composition of most perfusates, like Collins' solution, which use glucose as the impermeant.

**Cellular Acidosis.** Intracellular acidosis can damage cells and induce lysosomal instability, activate lysosomal enzymes, and alter mitochondrial characteristics. Renal preservation requires the buffering effect of alkaline cold storage solutions to minimize intracellular acidosis.

Despite the metabolically retarding effects of cold storage, ischemia occurs, stimulating glycolysis and glycogenolysis in all organs and thereby increasing the production of lactic acid and hydrogen ions as metabolic byproducts.[20]

In anaerobic glycolysis, the liver and kidney convert glucose to glucose-6-phosphate (G-6-P) via the enzyme hexokinase. G-6-P is metabolized to pyruvate and, under anaerobic conditions (cold storage), to lactic acid via the enzyme lactate dehydrogenase (LDH). If the kidney accumulates G-6-P, this suppresses further metabolism of glucose. Also, LDH in the kidney works best under aerobic conditions and is suppressed with cold storage. These are the two rate-limiting steps that suppress the production of further lactic acid and hydrogen ions as byproducts of metabolism in the kidney. This does not occur in the liver. Therefore, Collins' solution, using glucose as an impermeant, while ideal for renal preservation cannot be used for liver preservation where glucose is continually metabolized influxing intracellularly, leading to further intracellular acidosis.

**Expansion of the Interstitial Space.** Resultant expansion of the interstitial space can compress the capillary system and cause poor perfusion of perfusate at the time of renal procurement and in situ flushing. The ideal in situ flushing perfusate should allow free exchange of essential constituents while creating colloidal osmotic pressure, eg, with albumin or other colloids to prevent expansion of the interstitial space. Most cold storage perfusates do not possess these characteristics and the components of the perfusate solution go right into the interstitial space and cause edema.

**Oxygen-Free Radicals.** Oxygen-free radicals or supraoxide ($O_2^-$) can be produced during periods of ischemia when ATP is degraded to hypoxanthine. Hypoxanthine, molecular oxygen, and water then combine in the presence of xanthine oxidase (XO) and produce supraoxide free radical. Supraoxide then can induce hydroxyl ion free radical ($OH^-$) formation, which can break down cell membranes. Normally the cytochrome oxidase complex can supply enzymes such as supraoxide dismutase and catalase (SOD + CAT) to scavenge these free radicals and degrade these toxins. With ischemia this may not transpire and additional free radical scavengers (FRS) may be required.[21,22] This occurs not only with cold storage but also with reperfusion, namely, 0 to 2 hours after revascularization.[23–25] Various pharmacologic maneuvers to prevent progressive ischemic damage have been postulated including ATP Mg, $Cl_2$, and inosine,[26,27] calcium entry blockers,[28–30] prostaglandins,[31] and addition of SOD.[32] At least one group[33] believes that oxygen-free radicals may be of little significance in renal preservation as endogenous XO has a relatively low activity compared to the high endogenous activity of SOD, which scavenges supraoxide ions.

**Energy Metabolism.** Finally, an important consideration in renal preservation is that of energy metabolism. ATP degrades rapidly during hypothermic storage and forms adenosine, inosine, and hypoxanthine. Each of these end products is freely permeable to the plasma membrane. Once renal revascularization takes place, rapid regeneration of $Na^+$ pump activity and other energy-requiring steps in metabolism require ATP. Hence, ATP precursors must be available for successful renal preservation. Hypothermia slows the ischemic-induced degradation of ATP[34] and adenosine to hypoxanthine by a factor of 20, and by adding ATP $MgCl_2$ or inosine, this process may be slowed even more. This generates less hypoxanthine, which in turn generates less oxygen-free radical during reperfusion, and the cytochrome oxidase complex can more successfully degrade these free radicals.

## Perfusate Solutions

As a result of this research and a better understanding of hypothermia, ischemia, cold storage, and reperfusion injuries, Belzer et al[35] were able to develop a perfusate solution that allows 72-hour renal preservation. Table 3 shows the contrast between Collins' solution and University of Wisconsin (UW) cold storage solution. Three types of impermeant components are used in UW as opposed to only glucose in Collins' solution. Lactobionate, an impermeable anion, is used in place of glucose and prevents cellular swelling. Raffinose also is used, which gives more osmotic effect. A hydroxyethyl starch is added to prevent the expansion of the extracellular (interstitial) space. Since there is no glucose, there is no undesired production of lactic acid or hydrogen ions. There is a hydrogen ion buffer (phosphate) and precursors of ATP synthesis during reperfusion. Gluta-

**TABLE 3. Components of Collins' Solution and UW Solution**

| Solution | Amount/L |
|---|---|
| **Collins' Solution** | |
| $KH_2PO_4$ | 2.05 g |
| $K_2HPO_43H_2O$ | 9.70 g |
| KCL | 1.12 g |
| $NaHCO_3$ | 0.84 g |
| Glucose | 25.00 g |
| $MgSO_47H_2O$ | 7.38 g |
| Heparin | 5000 U |
| **UW Cold Storage Solution** | |
| $K^+$-Lactobionate | 100 mmol |
| $KH_2PO_4$ | 25 mmol |
| $MgSO_4$ | 5 mmol |
| Raffinose | 30 mmol |
| Adenosine | 5 mmol |
| Glutathione | 3 mmol |
| Insulin | 100 U |
| Penicillin | 40 U |
| Dexamethasone | 8 mg |
| Allopurinol | 1 mg |
| Hydroxyethyl starch | 50 g |

thione is depleted during ischemia and helps in dissipating free radicals. Allopurinol inhibits XO and production of oxygen-free radicals. Adenosine is needed for ATP synthesis after reperfusion.[36]

As a result of the ability of UW solution to provide superior results in multiorgan preservation to prior perfusate solutions, it has now generally replaced Collins' solution for multiorgan donors and frequently for kidney-only donors as well. UW has been compared with Euro-Collins solution in a European multicenter trial with results showing a more rapid fall in serum creatinine and an approximately 10% improvement in the rate of immediate function of renal grafts with UW.[37]

Some centers still believe that Collins' solution is as efficacious as and more cost-effective than UW solution.[38,39] When Collins' solution as we know it is used, it contains 30 mol/L of $MgSO_4$ and results in less of a creatinine elevation than Euro-Collins.[40] Data from Collins et al[41] shows an 81.8% rate of immediate function with UW solution versus 79% found in the European study. In comparing 723 kidneys preserved with Collins' solution versus 203 kidneys preserved with UW solution, the rate of immediate function was 81.2% versus 81.8%, respectively. The 1-year survival of renal grafts was 85.3% versus 82.6%, respectively, over the time period between 1988 and 1990. Hence, for kidney-only preservation, Collins' solution may be more cost-effective and provides comparable immediate function and graft survival in the cyclosporine era.

In summary, the evolution of successful renal, and especially for multiorgan, preservation has been made feasible by refinements in the perfusate. The newest solutions minimize hypothermic-induced cell swelling, lessen intracellular acidosis, minimize expansion of the interstitial space during perfusion with perfusate and reperfusion, lessen injury from oxygen-free radicals during reperfusion, and provide the precursors for regeneration of ATP during reperfusion. Further modifications of the UW solution are evolving[42] that will be more cost-effective and should not compromise graft survival. Clinical application of these components remains to be undertaken.

## PRETRANSPLANT BILATERAL NEPHRECTOMY

Most patients undergoing renal transplantation do not require pretransplant bilateral nephrectomy. The advantages of leaving native kidney in-situ include:

1. Maintenance for a moderate urinary output requiring less fluid restriction
2. Anemia of less severe proportions
3. Extirpation of native kidneys may remove the sole site of synthesis of 1,25-dihydrocholecalciferol, the active form of vitamin $D_3$
4. Avoidance of a major surgical procedure

Relative indications for bilateral nephrectomy include vesicoureteral reflux, some cases of polycystic kidney disease, and severe hypertension uncontrolled by medication or dialysis.

End-stage renal disease is a sequella of untreated severe vesicoureteral reflux. Nephroureterectomy prior to transplantation is necessary to prevent the incidence of recurrent urinary tract infections.

Patients with polycystic kidneys do not routinely require nephrectomy. The presence of chronic infections or significant hematuria requiring transfusions represents the only absolute indications for kidney removal.

Severe hypertension is a rare indication for pretransplant nephrectomy. Newer, more potent antihypertensive medications and ultrafiltration with reduction of extracellular volume will usually control hypertension. Plasma renin levels that mediate hypertension can be reduced by these newer medications, thus obviating the need for nephrectomy.

Bilateral nephrectomy for polycystic kidneys or bilateral nephroureterectomy is best performed through a midline abdominal incision from xiphoid to above the symphysis pubis. When nephrectomy is performed for hypertensively mediated small atrophic kidneys, end-stage renal disease without hydroureter, or recurrent pyelonephritis, the bilateral posterior lumbotomy approach may be used.

## IMMUNOSUPPRESSION

Effective immunosuppression is essential for renal allograft survival and function. The earliest form of immunotherapy, total body irradiation, was utilized in the late 1950s for cadaveric transplants with poor results. Empirical trials of azathioprine in combination with corticosteroids in the early 1960s demonstrated that successful kidney engraftment between nonidentical individuals was a reality.[43]

The subsequent availability of more selective immunosuppressive agents including antilymphocyte globulin, cyclosporine, and monoclonal antibody OKT3 has greatly facilitated the prevention and therapy of acute renal allograft rejection. Currently, immunosuppressive regimens incorporating judicious combinations of two or more drugs have resulted in 2-year allograft and patient survivals in excess of 85% and 95%, respectively.[44,45] Highly focused targeting of donor T-lymphocyte antigenic determinants with less global immunosuppression and attendant morbidity plus the prevention of chronic humoral rejection are goals of ongoing investigation.

### Corticosteroids

Corticosteroids remain a cornerstone of renal transplant immunosuppressive therapy. Although corticosteroids have been utilized in this setting for over 30 years, their mechanism of action is not completely understood. It is apparent that glucocorticoids act early in the cascade of antigen-stimulated T-cell proliferation. T-cell activation is dependent on contact with allograft antigen plus macrophages (accessory cells) and their products interleukin 1 (IL-1) and interleukin 6 (IL-6). Activated T cells produce interleukin 2 (IL-2) and express cell surface IL-2 receptors. Interleukin 2 is crucial as a T-cell growth factor, stimulating lymphokine secretion with consequent clonal proliferation and recruitment of cytotoxic helper T cells plus antibody-forming B cells which constitute the acute rejection response. Glucocorticoids inhibit macrophage production of IL-1 and IL-6, thereby indirectly interfering with T-cell activation and IL-2 production.[46,47] Other anti-inflammatory steroid effects include inhibition of leukocyte migration and chemotaxis.[48]

Corticosteroid therapy is typically begun intraoperatively or just prior to surgery in the form of intravenous methylprednisolone 0.5 to 2.0 mg/kg (lower doses if concomitant cyclosporine therapy is begun). In the absence of acute rejection, oral prednisone is tapered to approximate daily doses of 30 mg at 14 days, 15 mg at 3 months, and 10 mg at 6 months following transplantation. Toxicity may be reduced with alternate day dosing or steroid withdrawal 3 to 6 months postoperatively, although the risk for acute rejection is increased.[49]

High-dose or "pulse" steroid therapy (methylprednisolone 1 g IV daily on 3 consecutive days) is commonly used to treat acute renal allograft rejection. About 60% to 75% of primary rejection episodes can be reversed in this manner.[50]

**Side Effects.** Potential well-recognized corticosteroid-related side effects include enhanced susceptibility to infection, impaired wound healing, hypertension, sodium retention, hyperglycemia, gastrointestinal ulceration, and psychosis. Long-term therapy may also contribute to aseptic necrosis of bone and cataract formation. Consequently, most transplant centers have adopted immunosuppressive regimens that minimize glucocorticoid dosage in combination with cyclosporine or low-dose cyclosporine and azathioprine ("triple therapy").[51]

### Azathioprine

Azathioprine is a purine analog that is metabolized by the liver to 6-mercaptopurine. This commonly used antimetabolite inhibits synthesis of DNA and RNA necessary for the clonal proliferation of activated T lymphocytes as well as other cell lines. Azathioprine is often included in maintenance immunosuppressive regimens to prevent acute rejection but is not effective in the therapy of established rejection. Like the glucocorticoids, azathioprine is initially administered intraoperatively or just prior to the transplant procedure in doses ranging from 2 to 5 mg/kg IV. Daily white blood cell counts should be obtained to assess potential leukopenia and for dosage adjustment.[52] Azathioprine is usually withheld if the white blood cell count falls below 4000. Maintenance therapy typically consists of 1 to 2 mg/kg per day of the oral drug.

Concomitant use of allopurinol should be avoided as this xanthine oxidase inhibitor will interfere with the degradation of 6-mercaptopurine resulting in significant bone marrow toxicity. If therapy with allopurinol cannot be avoided, the dose of azathioprine should be reduced to 30% and leukocyte counts monitored closely. Decreased doses of azathioprine are also indicated in patients with liver disease.

**Side Effects.** Azathioprine has been reported to cause thrombocytopenia, red blood cell aplasia, hypersensitivity reactions, hepatotoxicity, cholestatic jaundice, and pancreatitis. A significant potential long-term complication of azathioprine use is the increased risk for lymphoproliferative disorders and skin cancer.[53]

## Cyclosporine

Cyclosporine is a fungus-derived cyclic endecapeptide first utilized in clinical renal transplantation in 1978.[54] Subsequent multicenter trials of cyclosporine and prednisone (with or without azathioprine) have demonstrated a significant 15% to 20% enhancement of renal allograft survival when compared to traditional azathioprine and prednisone regimens.[55,56]

Cyclosporine blocks activated T lymphocyte interleukin-2 messenger RNA transcription, thereby inhibiting IL-2 production. Cyclosporine and glucocorticoids act synergistically to diminish IL-2 stimulated T-cell proliferation, differentiation, and the recruitment of antibody forming B cells and macrophages.[46]

**Side Effects.** Ironically, the most concerning complication of cyclosporine therapy is nephrotoxicity. Acute or hemodynamic cyclosporine nephrotoxicity is a result of vasoconstriction, likely at the level of the afferent arteriole. This adverse effect is generally seen early during the first hours to weeks following transplantation and is reversible if the drug is discontinued or the dose minimized. Such vasoconstriction may be particularly deleterious to renal allograft function immediately following engraftment when ischemic change and acute tubular necrosis may be present. Many transplant centers withhold cyclosporine until allograft function is apparent, eg, decrease in serum creatinine to an arbitrary predetermined level. Chronic or long-term cyclosporine nephrotoxicity is clinically manifested by a gradual irreversible decline in renal function and histologically by vasculopathy (arteriolar narrowing) and interstitial fibrosis.[57] During the first weeks or months following transplantation, cyclosporine nephrotoxicity may be difficult to distinguish clinically from acute tubular necrosis or acute rejection, and these conditions may coexist. If a reduction in cyclosporine dose does not improve renal function, an allograft biopsy may be helpful.

Other cyclosporine-related side effects include hypertension, hyperkalemia, tremor, gingival hypertrophy, hirsutism, hyperuricemia, abnormal liver function, and hypomagnesemia.[58] Long-term therapy may lead to an increased risk of lymphoma.

In an attempt to avoid nephrotoxicity, lower dosage regimens for cyclosporine have evolved. Standard initial perioperative doses range from 8 to 15 mg/kg parenterally (or one third of the dose intravenously). As mentioned above, many transplant centers avoid or reduce exposure to cyclosporine in the presence of acute tubular necrosis or delayed graft function. Antilymphocyte globulin or monoclonal antibody OKT3 is used to prevent rejection until allograft function is adequate.

Available techniques for monitoring cyclosporine levels include monoclonal antibody radioimmunoassay (RIA), high-performance liquid chromatography (HPLC), and fluorescence polarization immunoassay (FPIA). Using whole-blood trough levels as a rough guide in addition to clinical parameters, the cyclosporine dose is gradually tapered to 3–6 mg/kg per day by 3 months posttransplantation. Triple therapy, or the concomitant use of azathioprine and prednisone, allows maintenance cyclosporine doses of 3 mg/kg per day or less.[49] Triple therapy is associated with a lower total exposure to corticosteroids but may not result in improved graft survival when compared to cyclosporine and prednisone alone.[59] Conversion from cyclosporine and prednisone to azathioprine and prednisone does not clearly improve allograft survival and rejection episodes may be encountered.[60]

**Drug Interactions.** Numerous cyclosporine drug interactions have been reported. Medications that can increase cyclosporine levels and potentiate immunosuppression include erythromycin, ketoconazole, diltiazem, metoclopropamide, norfloxacin, and oral contraceptives. Drugs including dilantin, phenobarbital, isoniazid, and rifampin may decrease cyclosporine levels by increasing hepatic metabolism (P450 microsomal enzyme).

### Polyclonal Immune Globulins

Polyclonal immune globulin preparations have been derived from animals inoculated with human lymphocytes or thymocytes. Resultant antilymphocyte or antithymocyte globulins (ALG or ATG) have been used to successfully reverse initial acute renal allograft rejection with an approximate 80% success rate.[61] ALG and ATG have also been incorporated as induction therapy following engraftment to prevent acute rejection until graft function is established. Polyclonal immune globulins appear to induce T-cell lymphopenia via complement-mediated lysis and clearance of lymphocytes. Potential significant adverse reactions include fever, chills, thrombocytopenia, serum sickness, anaphylaxis, and glomerulonephritis.

### OKT3 Monoclonal Antibody

OKT3 is the first commercially available monoclonal antibody for the treatment of acute renal allograft rejection. It was developed by injecting a mouse with human T lymphocytes, then producing a hybridoma of the mouse's spleen and murine myeloma cells. The hybridoma was screened and cloned to produce a pure antibody against the CD3 protein of the antigen recognition complex found on all mature T cells. When OKT3 binds to the CD3 protein, the antigen recognition complex is altered, rendering the T cell "blind" to renal allograft antigen.

In a prospective randomized trial involving 123 patients undergoing initial acute cadaveric renal allograft rejection, OKT3 was effective therapy in 89%. A significantly lower 62% rejection reversal rate was observed in patients randomized to high-dose steroid therapy.[51] The subsequent experience with OKT3 monoclonal antibody in the therapy of primary acute renal allograft rejection has suggested an effectiveness in excess of 95%.[62]

The utility of this agent in subsequent rejection episodes is mitigated by the formation of anti-OKT3 antibody which occurs in 33% to 50% of patients following initial therapy. The majority of antibody titers are low (1:100), which do not interfere with OKT3 reuse. However, high titer (≥1:1000) antibody formed in approximately 17% of responders precludes subsequent OKT3 therapy.[63] Many transplant centers have consequently reserved OKT3 monoclonal antibody for allograft rejections resistant to high-dose glucocorticoid therapy with resultant success rates as high as 96%.[64]

The standard dosage schedule for OKT3 monoclonal antibody is 5 mg IV daily for 10 to 14 days with concomitant lowering of azathioprine and prednisone doses (25 to 50 mg and 0.5 mg/kg daily, respectively). Cyclosporine has generally been withheld until the last 3 days of the OKT3 course. OKT3 antibody titers are assessed 4 weeks following initial therapy. It is apparent that the frequency and titer of idiotypic antibody formation is inversely related to the level of concomitant immunosuppression during OKT3 therapy. Continuing cyclosporine at 50% of the maintenance dose may decrease the frequency of OKT3 antibody formation to 11% without an increase in infectious sequelae.[65]

OKT3 monoclonal antibody is effective as a component of induction therapy, particularly in the setting of delayed graft function or acute tubular necrosis. Lower dosage regimens of OKT3, eg, 1 mg for 2 days followed by 2 mg for 10 days, are as effective as 5-mg doses in clearing T cells, modulating CD3 molecules, and preventing acute rejection.[66]

**Side Effects.** Typical first dose-related symptoms, including fever, chills, tremor, nausea, vomiting, dyspnea, and relative hypotension, are likely related to the release of cytokines from lysed T lymphocytes. These side effects may be ameliorated by glucocorticoid therapy in the form of methylprednisolone 500 mg intravenously 1 hour prior to the first dose of OKT3.[67] Pulmonary edema may occur in hypervolemic patients and therefore adequate diuresis or ultrafiltration is an essential prerequisite for OKT3 therapy. Opportunistic infections (particularly cytomegalovirus and herpesvirus) and lymphoproliferative disorders are potential long-term complications.

### Investigational Agents

Monoclonal antibodies directed at other components of the T-cell antigen recognition complex, eg, α β heterodimer, are currently being evaluated with favorable results.[68] Experimental evidence suggests that monoclonal antibody therapy against CD4+ or helper T cells may be clinically relevant.[69]

In an attempt to target immunotherapy at only those T lymphocytes committed to allograft rejection, thereby avoiding some of the immunosuppressive side effects of pan-T-cell antibodies (eg, OKT3), monoclonal antibodies to the IL-2 receptor have been developed. Early studies suggest that IL-2 receptor monoclonal antibodies are effective as posttransplantation prophylaxis against acute renal allograft rejection with relatively few complications.[70,71] The formation of anti-idiotypic antibody limits long-term therapy but does not preclude the subsequent use of OKT3.

FK 506 is a macrolide antibiotic that has been extensively studied in liver transplantation. This agent blocks IL-2 production by modulating an intracellular calcium messenger. T-cell proliferation is consequently inhibited in a manner similar to cyclosporine.[72] Preliminary studies of FK 506 in renal transplantation suggest allograft survival rates similar to those obtained with cyclosporine. Significant advantages appear to include decreased steroid requirement, lower incidence of hypertension, and improved serum cholesterol levels. Nephrotoxicity, tremors, paresthesias, and glucose intolerance are potential side effects.[73] Ongoing randomized trials should provide optimal dosage regimens and more accurate comparisons with cyclosporine.

Rapamycin is another macrolide antibiotic that is similar in structure to FK 506. In vitro and animal studies suggest a beneficial immunosuppressive effect potentially synergistic with cyclosporine.[74]

15-Deoxyspergualin is a bacteria-derived antitumor agent with the ability to inhibit cytotoxic T-cell proliferation. Initial clinical trials indicate that 15-deoxyspergualin is effective in reversing acute renal allograft rejection refractory to steroid therapy with relatively few side effects.[75]

A growing body of experimental and clinical evidence suggests that particular vasodilators including calcium antagonists[76,77] and prostaglandin (PGE) analogs[78] will play a significant role in renal transplant immunosuppressive therapy. These agents may enhance renal allograft function by ameliorating ischemic damage, antagonizing cyclosporine-induced vasoconstriction, and enhancing the dose–response relationship for cyclosporine.

## SURGICAL PROCEDURES FOR RENAL TRANSPLANTATION

The advent of multiple organ procurement from cadaver donors has tended to limit the urologic surgeon's involvement in this aspect of renal transplantation. However, in many situations the urologist is called on to assist in the procurement of the kidneys during multiorgan procurement procedures. In other situations, however, where only the kidneys are being procured, the urologist has primary responsibility for the surgical procedure.

Donor nephrectomy for renal transplantation can be from either a living related or cadaver donor. In either situation the operation is performed using meticulous technique. Providing the transplant surgeon with a kidney that has adequate, well-perfused lengths of artery, vein, and ureter is of critical importance. Multiple renal arteries may require leaving them on a Carrel patch and the short right renal vein may require a cuff of vena cava to facilitate an easier venous anastomosis.

### Living Related Donor Nephrectomy

Improvement in cadaver renal allograft survival has resulted in a diminution in the number of living related transplants performed annually. However, the paucity of available organs assures a role for this form of organ procurement.

The left kidney is preferred for living related donor nephrectomy because of the longer length of the renal vein. The venous anastomosis in the recipient is the deepest; the longer renal vein facilitates this anastomosis. Relative contraindications to the procurement of the left kidney include the presence of multiple left renal arteries on preoperative digital subtraction angiogram (DSA), and anatomic anomalies or other problems of the left renal pelvis or ureter.

The donor is brought to the operating room in a state of maximal hydration. The recipient operation is not begun until the donor nephrectomy is well underway, minimizing anesthesia time for the recipient. A Foley catheter is placed after induction of general anesthesia and the patient is properly positioned in the full flank position.

A supracostal 11th rib incision provides optimal exposure to the renal vessels (Fig 1A). Gerota's fascia is entered; perirenal fat is dissected from the capsule maintaining compulsive hemostasis during the dissection. Dissection along the anterior surface of the kidney reveals the renal vein (Fig 1B). After its identification it is dissected close to its origin at the vena cava. The main venous branches, gonadal and adrenal veins, are ligated and divided close to the main renal vein. Care must be taken to identify and ligate any azygos lumbar branches on the posterior surface of the renal vein. The left renal artery usually lies behind the upper border of the left renal vein (Fig 1C). The posterior aspect of the kidney is mobilized and the kidney is turned forward to dissect the renal artery to its origin at the aorta.

The ureter is immobilized in its enveloping fat and adventitia as distally as possible. It is absolutely crucial that the dissection of the ureter avoids any stripping of the ureteral vessels. Nerves and lymphatics of the kidney are ligated and divided, leaving ultimately the kidney attached only by its artery, vein, and ureter.

The ureter is transected below the pelvic brim prior to ligation of the main vessels. This allows confirmation of a brisk urinary diuresis prior to ligation of the vessels. The renal artery and vein are ligated and divided at the origin of the aorta and vena cava, respectively (Fig 1D).

Preservation of the kidney is obtained by flushing and cooling the kidney with heparinized cold (4°C) Ringer's lactate solution (Fig 1E). This usually permits 4 to 6 hours of avascular reconstruction of accessory vessels and transplantation of the kidney. The organ is flushed with 500 to 1000 $cm^3$ of perfusate solution or until a clear effluent is identified at the renal vein.

Reconstruction of vascular anomalies follow perfusion of the kidney performed as a "bench surgery" prior to transplantation. All branches are anastomosed end-to-side to the main renal artery. Two renal arteries of equal size can be spatulated and sewn to form a common lumen. The conjoined vessel is then anastomosed end-to-end to the recipient hypergastric artery or end-to-side to the recipient external iliac artery.

Multiple renal veins occur infrequently.

In general, small renal veins can be ligated without risk to the organ. Larger renal veins of comparable size should be preserved in order to avoid increased intrarenal venous pressure after revascularization. On the right, a cuff of vena cava may be taken to ensure adequate length for the renal vein. The vena cava is repaired using a 5–0 cardiovascular suture.

After delivery of the donor organ to the transplant team the stumps of the renal vessels are double-ligated with a nonabsorbable material. Hemostasis in the renal fossa is ascertained, the wound closed, and a small penrose drain left in place. Routine postoperative care is delivered with attention to urine output and overall renal function.

## Cadaver Donor Nephrectomy

Cadaver kidneys are usually procured from patients with head trauma or intracerebral catastrophes after criteria for brain death have been met. This can be defined by a neurologic diagnosis alone or with flat electroencephalograms interpreted by a neurologist. Kidneys from potential donors with chronic renal disease or systemic infection, diabetes, severe hypertension, or malignancy (excluding brain tumors) cannot be used. A serum creatinine that has increased and cannot be explained by hypovolemia or oliguria unresponsive to fluids or diuretics means that the kidney should not be used. Dopamine is the only vasoactive drug that can be utilized to support blood pressure.

The patient is placed supine on the operating table. Our preference is for a transverse incision, two finger breadths below the costal arch to the tips of the 11th ribs. A vertical incision from xiphoid to pubis in the midline may also be utilized (Fig 2A).

An incision from the hepatic flexure to the root of the small bowel mesentery is made and the intestines are packed superiorly in a Lahey bag (Fig 2B). The inferior mesenteric vein can be ligated and divided to augment exposure. The superior mesenteric artery (SMA) is dissected out and a heavy silk suture is placed around it. The abdominal aorta is then isolated between the SMA and the inferior mesenteric artery (IMA). The aorta and vena cava are dissected free and the renal vessels are identified. The ureters are isolated and divided close to the bladder and cultures are taken. The ureters are mobilized leaving a generous cuff of tissue to preserve their blood supply. The kidneys are then dissected out bilaterally.

The SMA can now be ligated so as to control the proximal aorta. The distal aorta is ligated and a cannula for perfusion is placed. The proximal aorta is clamped and the kidneys are then perfused, cooled, and preserved in situ with UW solution. The distal vena cava is then ligated and a large abdominal suction tube is cannulated into the vena cava in order to evacuate the venous blood and to ensure perfusion of the kidneys (Fig 2C).

The aorta is transected above and below the renal arteries once perfusion is complete. The vena cava is then transected and the kidneys are removed en bloc. The right renal vein is left with the cuff of vena cava. A large cuff of aorta should accompany each renal artery or multiple arteries (Fig 2D). Independent polar arteries should be taken with a patch of aorta. Polar arteries to the lower pole are of critical importance as they are usually the source of renal pelvic and ureteral blood supply. Duplex ureters are removed separately, or where they form a common ureter one or two ureteroneocystostomies may be required depending on the anatomic situation. Two separate ureters can usually be spatulated and anastomosed together prior to ureteroneocystostomy.

The spleen and multiple lymph nodes should be removed at the time of organ procurement so that their lymphocytes may be used for tissue typing. Any anomaly encountered must be documented and reported to the transplant team prior to renal transplantation.

Multiple organ procurement from cadaver donors means that the urologic surgeon involved with renal transplantation may need to have familiarity with this team approach to organ procurement. Hence, the above procurement procedure may be in

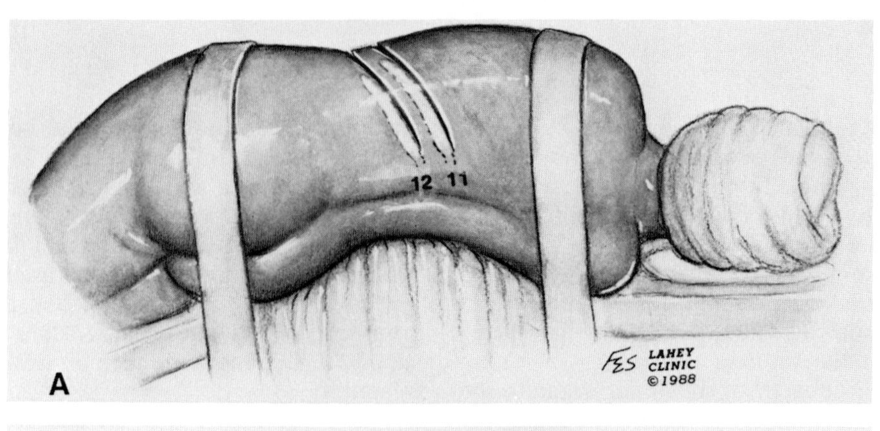
12
11
FES LAHEY CLINIC ©1988
A

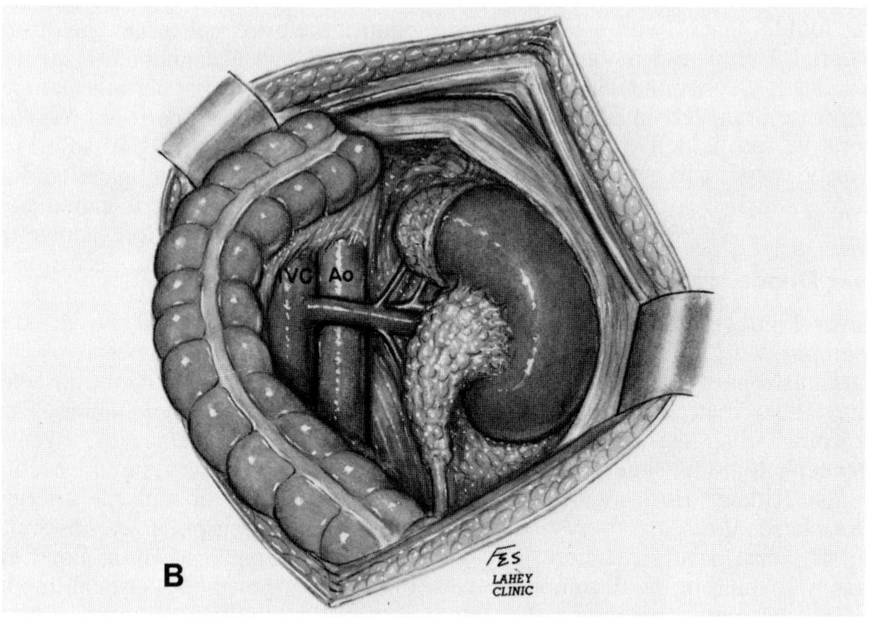
IVC
Ao
FES
LAHEY CLINIC
B

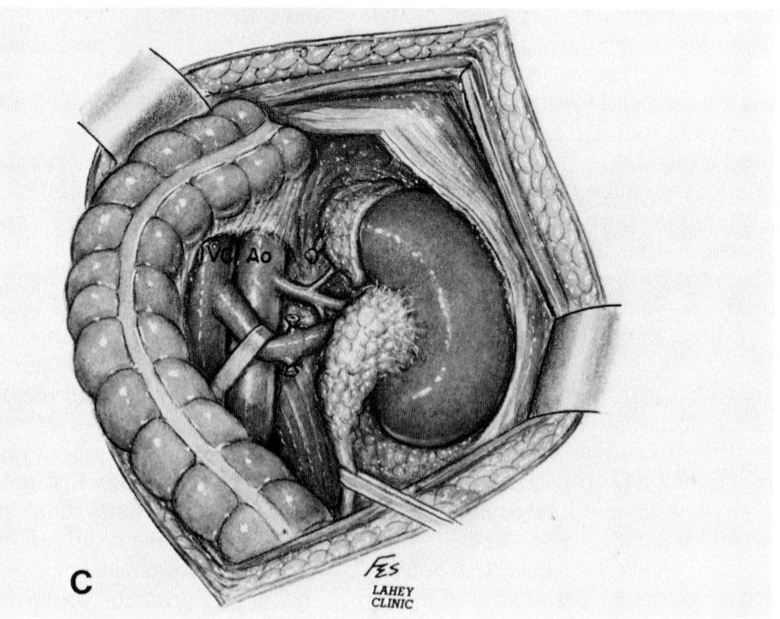
IVC
Ao
FES
LAHEY CLINIC
C

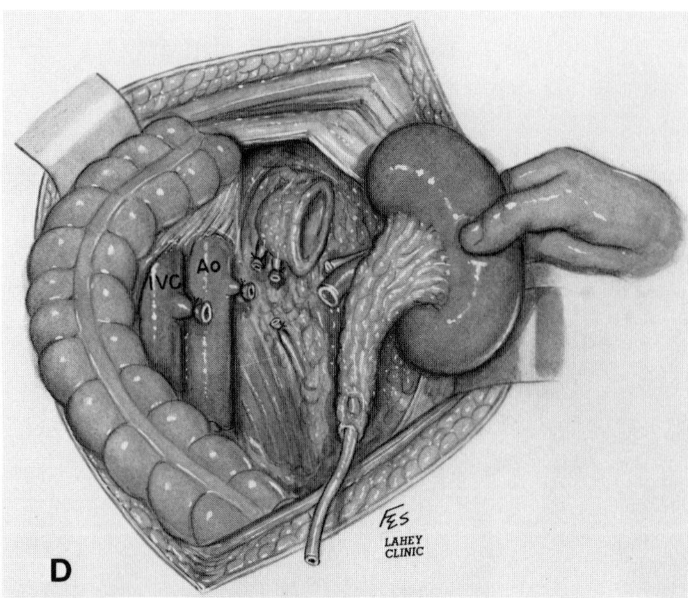


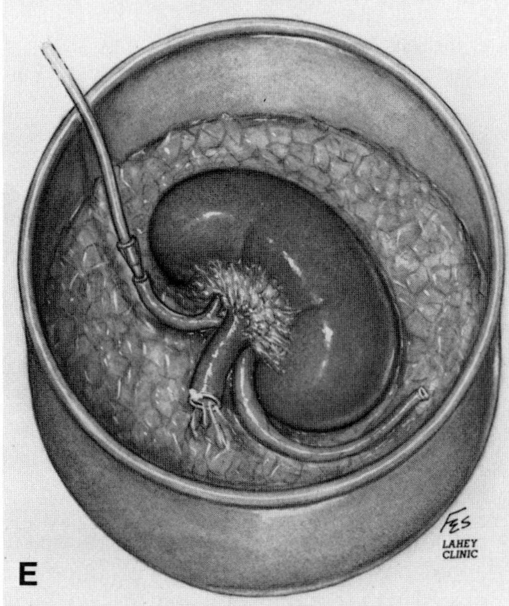


**Fig 1.** Living donor nephrectomy. **A,** patient is placed in flank position. An 11th rib supracostal incision maximizes renal exposure; **B,** dissection of left kidney demonstrates exposure of renal vein to its origin at the vena cava (IVC); **C,** after ligation of the adrenal and gonadal vessels the renal vein is mobilized to expose the renal artery; **D,** division of the renal vessels is at the origin of the aorta (Ao) and vena cava. The ureter is transected below pelvic brim. Care is taken not to maintain adventitial tissue or ureter; **E,** chilled preservation solution (Ringer's lactate, UW solution) is perfused through the renal artery.

continuity with organ procurement teams from other institutions.

## Renal Transplantation Procedure

The living related donor and recipient are admitted electively one day prior to surgery. The final serologic cross-match is done at that time. As for the unscheduled cadaver renal transplant recipient, routine blood work, chest x-ray, and electrocardiogram are obtained as well as a urine culture. Individuals who are living related donor renal recipients have more elective time to optimize renal function and electrolyte status with dialysis. Even the unscheduled recipient of a cadaver kidney may need to be dialyzed for hyperkalemia

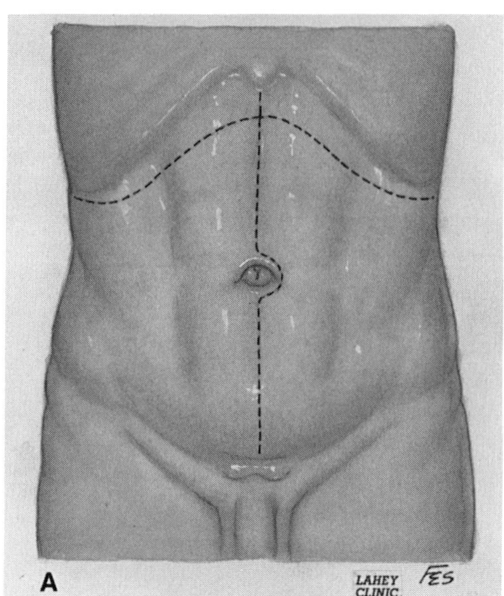


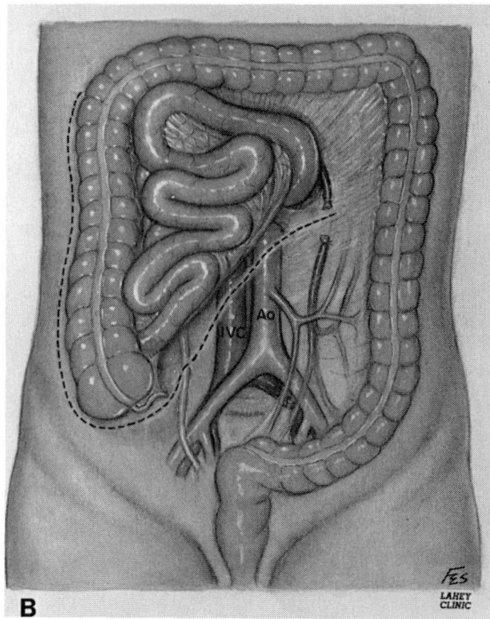


**Fig 2A,B.** Cadaver donor nephrectomy. **A,** types of incision used; each allows access to proximal aorta (Ao); **B,** the bowel is mobilized by incising the perineum from the hepatic flexure to the foramen of Winslow.

($K^+$ greater than 4.5 mEq/L) or fluid overload.

Once the preoperative evaluation is complete, the patient is brought to the operating room where a central venous line and an arterial line are placed. Good venous access is necessary for the delivery of mannitol, lasix, immunosuppressants, and vasoactive drugs that may be required during the renal transplant procedure. The patient is vigorously hydrated to maintain a central venous pressure of 10 cm $H_2O$ using normal saline intravenously. Unless there is a need for specific antibiotic prophylaxis, a cephalosporin is given, usually 1 g of kefzol.

Patients with renal failure may have certain anesthetic requirements. Choice and dose of various agents for induction are usually the same as in the general population. However, severe acidosis and electrolyte imbalance can potentiate the actions of some neuromuscular blocking agents that in turn can produce hyperkalemia.[79] Halothane and other commonly used general anesthetics are readily utilized, but all have hypotensive potential, especially in the recently dialyzed, volume-depleted patient.

Once anesthetized, the patient is positioned and a 16 French Foley catheter is inserted aseptically into the bladder. The bladder is then filled with 100 to 150 $cm^3$ of saline solution and the Foley catheter is clamped and connected to the drainage bag. This facilitates localization for incision of the bladder at the time of transplant procedure.

For renal transplantation we use a right or left lower quadrant extraperitoneal approach[80] (Fig 3A). The donor kidney is placed in the contralateral iliac fossa, which allows better alignment of the donor renal vein and recipient iliac vein.

If the contralateral iliac fossa cannot be used, the donor kidney can be placed in the ipsilateral iliac fossa. The donor kidney can be transplanted upside down, providing a better match for the donor renal vein and recipient iliac vein anastomosis.[81]

If both iliac fossae have been used and a third transplant is necessary, an intra-abdominal approach to the iliac vessels can

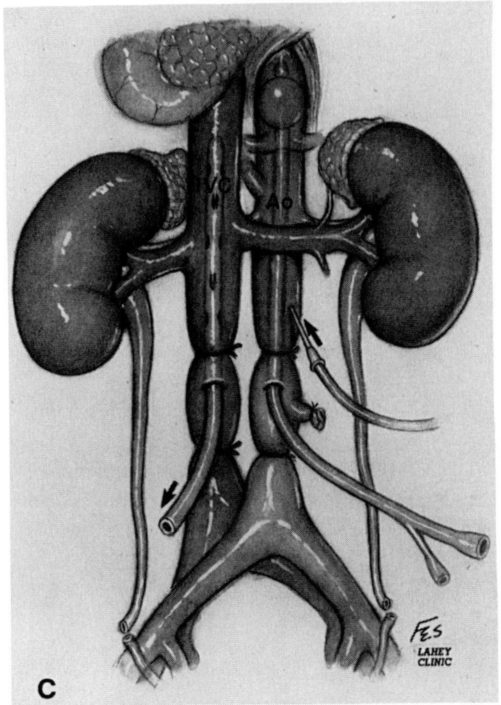


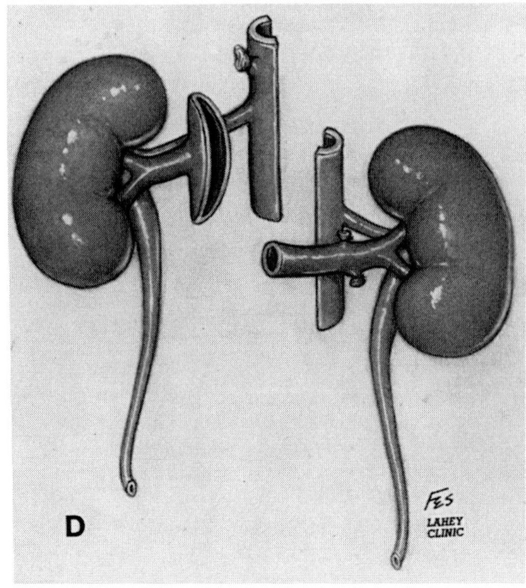


**Fig 2C,D. C,** in situ perfusion of the kidneys through an aortic cannula. The proximal aorta may be secured by ligature or inflated balloon catheter; **D,** the renal arteries are accompanied by a cuff of aorta. The right renal vein is left with a cuff of vena cava. IVC = vena cava.

be used. This is the preferred method used in pediatric renal transplant and obviates the need for dissection through scar tissue around the vessels in the iliac fossa.

A curved incision is made between the pubis and the iliac crest going through the external oblique, internal oblique, and transversus abdominis muscles. The peritoneum is exposed and the inferior epigastric artery and vein are ligated and divided. The spermatic cord is then mobilized medially in the male or the round ligament is divided in the female and the peritoneum is retracted caphalad (Fig 3B).

The iliac vessels are exposed (Fig 3C) and dissected, placing vascular loops around each vessel. Any lymphatics encountered should be ligated and divided to prevent lymphocele formation. The external iliac vein is freed beyond the point where it crosses the internal iliac artery (Fig 3D). The internal iliac artery is then dissected out if it is to be used for the arterial anastomosis.

The venous anastomosis is done first. Vascular clamps are placed on the external iliac vein for proximal and distal control and a longitudinal venotomy is made with the number 11 blade and Potts scissors (Fig 4A). An end-to-side anastomosis is made between the transplant renal vein and the recipient external iliac vein using a continuous 5–0 prolene suture (Fig 4B,C).

Next the arterial anastomosis is performed. If the donor kidney has one renal artery, either an end-to-side donor renal artery to recipient external iliac artery anastomosis or an end-to-end donor renal artery to recipient internal iliac artery anastomosis can be performed. For the end-to-side arterial anastomosis, vascular clamps are placed on the external iliac artery for proximal and distal control and a longitudinal arteriotomy is made using a number 11 blade and the Potts scissors. The anastomosis is completed using a continuous 6–0 prolene. For the end-to-end arterial anastomosis, the internal iliac artery is li-

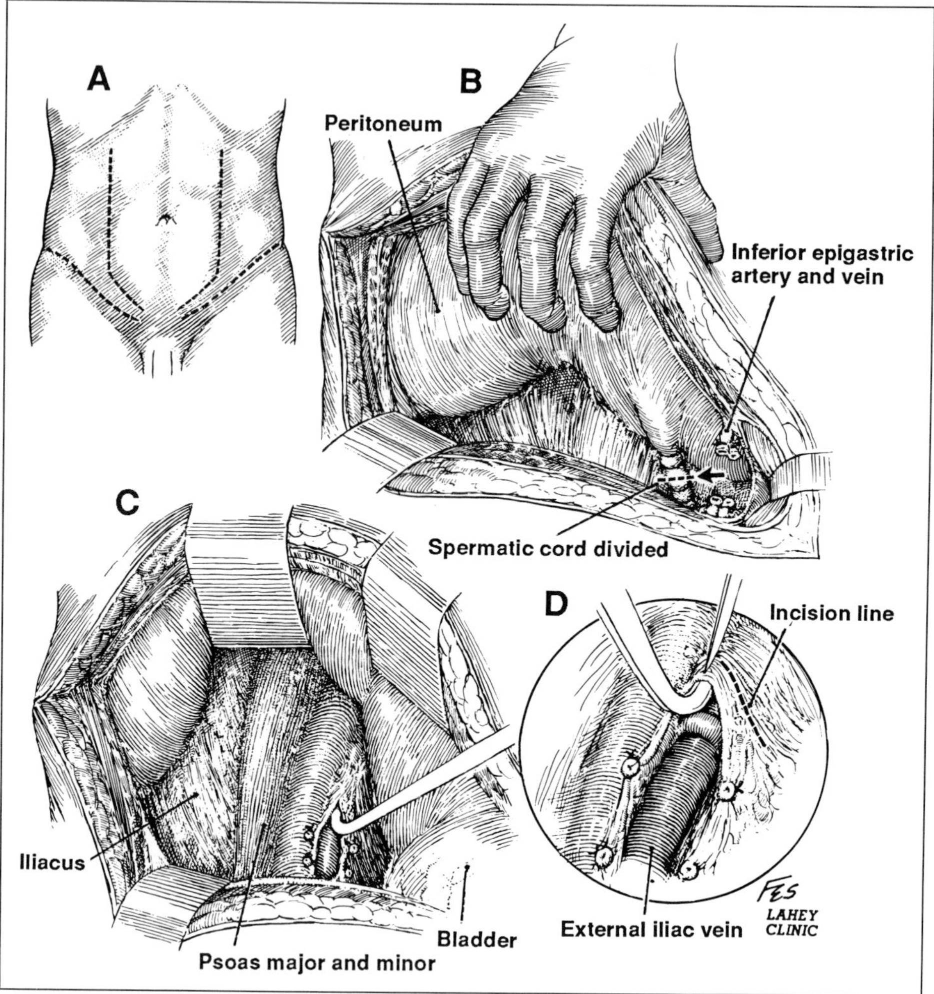


**Fig 3.** Renal transplant procedure. **A,** preferred incisions for renal transplantation; **B,** the iliac fossa is exposed by cephalad retraction of the peritoneal envelope; **C,** exposure of the iliac vessels requires ligation of lymphatic channels; **D,** the external iliac vein is dissected to the point where the hypogastric artery crosses.

gated proximal to the first branch. The hypogastric artery is usually cut at a 45° angle to make the anastomotic angle smoother. A 6–0 prolene suture placed in interrupted fashion completes the anastomosis after proximal and distal control of the iliac artery (Fig 4D).

Once both anastomoses are completed and azathioprine (5 mg/kg) and prednisone (1 to 2 mg/kg) have been infused intravenously along with 25 g of mannitol, the vascular clamps are removed and the kidney is reperfused.

Multiple renal arteries can be handled in a variety of ways. Smaller branches can be anastomosed end-to-side to the main artery on the "back table." Alternatively, the vessels may be maintained on an aortic patch that is directly anastomosed end-to-side to the external iliac artery.

In order to reestablish continuity of the urinary tract, two methods are available: the Politano–Leadbetter[82] reimplant or the extravesical Gregoir–Lich type of ureteroneocystotomy.[83,84]

The technique used for transplant ure-

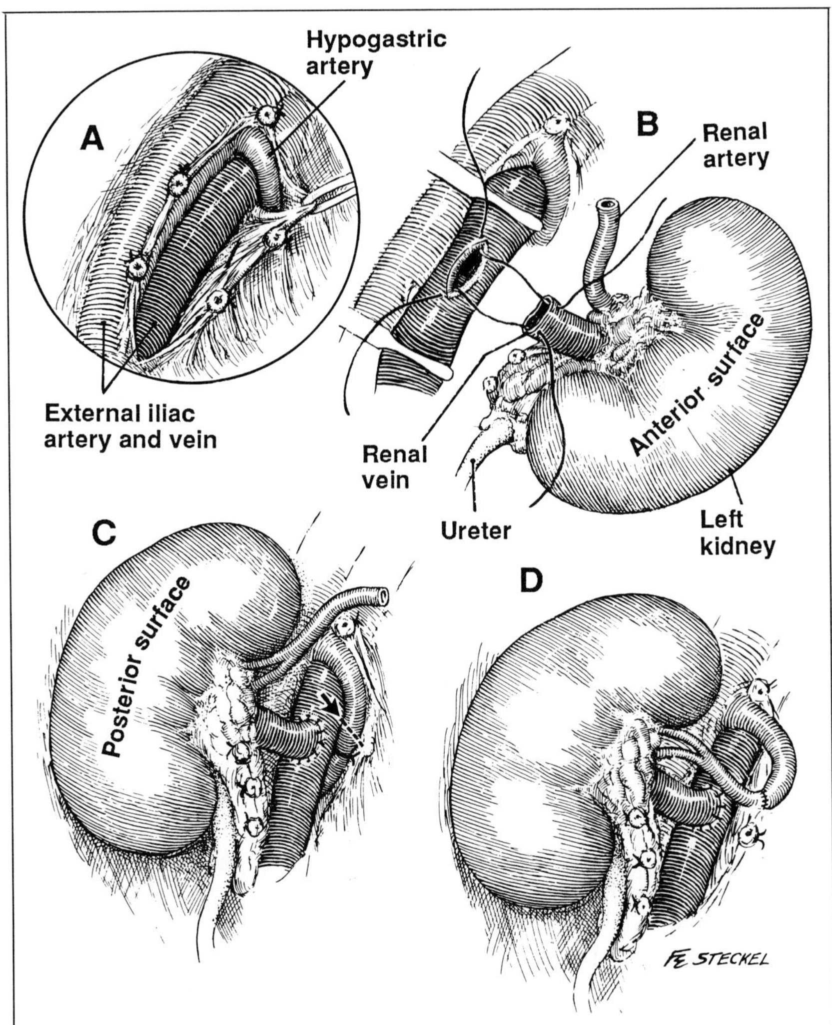


**Fig 4.** Venous and arterial anastomoses. **A,** demonstration of limits of dissection of iliac vessels; **B, C,** end-to-side venous anastomosis is completed using a continuous 5–0 prolene suture. The internal iliac artery is ligated and divided (arrow, dashed line). **D,** completed end-to-end anastomosis between the donor renal artery and internal iliac artery.

teroneocystostomy at the Lahey Clinic[85] is a modification of the Politano–Leadbetter technique.[82] Two or three cubic centimeters of saline is injected submucosally to raise a mucosal bleb (Fig 5A). A small segment of the mucosa is removed from the inferior portion of the bleb (Fig 5B). A submucosal tunnel about 3 cm in length is created by insertion of a right-angle clamp or the Strolle scissors into the opening. The right angle is rotated 180° and the detrusor muscle pierced (Fig 5C).

The distal donor ureter is brought through the submucosal tunnel (Fig 5D, E). After excision of any redundant ureter, the distal ureter is cut at a 45° angle and spatulated with a Potts scissors. The ureter is then anastomosed to the bladder mucosa using a 3–0 maxon. Two distal sutures at the 5 and 7 o'clock positions are essential to incorporating the detrusor muscle as well as mucosa to prevent ureteral disruption (Fig 5F).

The anterior bladder mucosa is closed

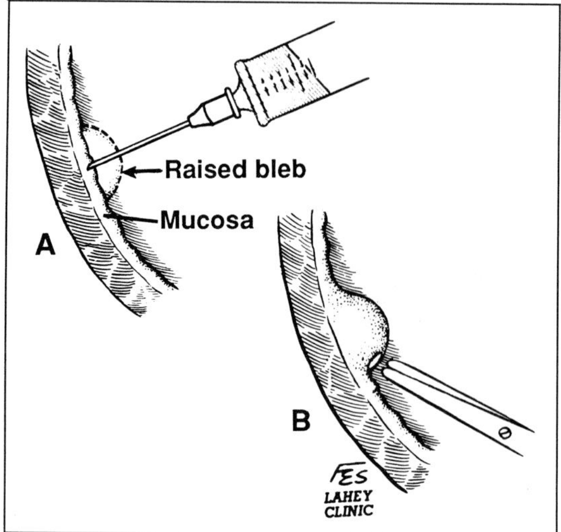


**Fig 5.** Modification of the Politano–Leadbetter technique. **A, B,** creation of a submucosal tunnel. Injection of 3 ml saline raises the mucosal layer, allowing for earlier dissection; **C,** right angle clamp along mucosal tunnel; **D, E,** the ureter is brought through the submucosal tunnel. Excess ureter is removed and the end is spatulated; **F, G,** completion of ureterovesical anastomosis using interrupted sutures.

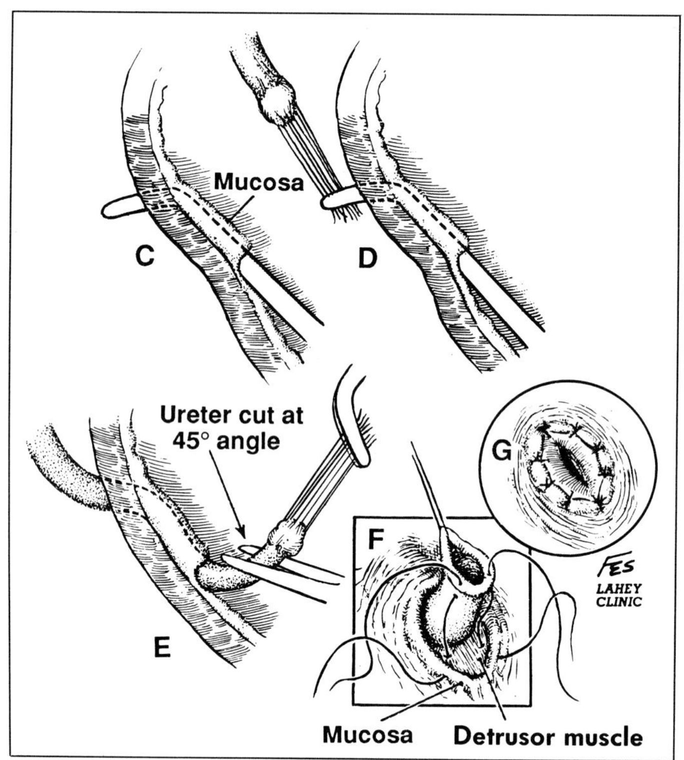


with a 2–0 continuous dexon suture and the detrusor is similarly closed with a continuous 2–0 dexon suture (Fig 5G). A Foley catheter is left in place for 7 to 10 days.

Some transplant centers use the extravesical Gregoir–Lich type of ureteroneocystotomy[83,84] (Fig 6). In this procedure, an incision is made on the dome of the bladder. The bladder muscle is carefully opened and the mucosa is allowed to prolapse. A small incision is made at the inferior portion of the bladder incision. The trans-

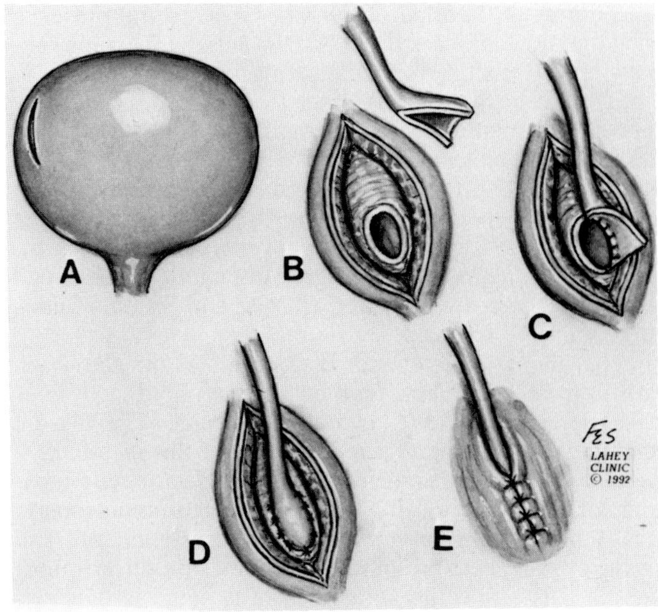


**Fig 6.** The Gregoir–Lich technique of extravesical ureteroneocystotomy.

planted ureter is anastomosed to the bladder mucosa with a 4–0 maxon suture in interrupted fashion. The ureter is placed in the trough created by the bladder muscle incision. The bladder muscles are closed over the ureter with interrupted 2–0 dexon sutures creating a submucosal tunnel.

Regardless of the method used for ureteroneocystotomy, a medial location of the collecting system is maintained. Traditional procedures of pyeloureterostomy, anastomosing the donor renal pelvis to the recipient ureter, or direct anastomosis of the bladder to the donor kidney pelvis are rarely used. However, these reconstructive techniques may be utilized in the case of an infarcted or necrotic ureter at the time of transplant or in the case of posttransplant urinary leakage.

### Transplant with Urinary Diversion

Patients with severe neurogenic disease or postinflammatory contracture may require the use of supravesical urinary diversion prior to renal transplantation. This usually involves creation of an ileal loop urinary diversion with a lower quadrant stoma prior to transplantation.

Several weeks later, the renal transplant is performed as an intra-abdominal operation. The donor kidney is placed retrocecally with an end-to-side anastomosis of the donor renal vein to the recipient iliac vein or vena cava and an end-to-side anastomosis of the donor renal vein to the recipient iliac vein or vena cava and an end-to-side anastomosis of the donor renal artery to the common iliac artery or aorta. The donor kidney ureter is then anastomosed to the ileal loop and can be stented.

## DIAGNOSIS AND TREATMENT OF REJECTION

Any comprehensive discussion of renal transplant rejection requires at least a cursory understanding of the alloimmune response, ie, insight into the mechanism of graft rejection. Simply, any transplanted organ is rejected because the host recognizes it as foreign and mounts both a cellular and humoral response resulting, if untreated, in the destruction of the graft. The trick, therefore, is twofold: (1) limit, through careful tissue typing, the dissimilarity between the donor organ and host, and (2) modify or alter through medication, radiation, etc., the host's immune response to the transplanted organ. To accomplish this it is crucial to appreciate the immunogenic cascade that occurs when antigenic stimuli are introduced to the host.

While many antigen groups can evoke an immunogenic response, it appears that a group of antigens found on the short arm of chromosome 6 and known as the MHC are the most critical. These transplantation antigens, also referred to as the HLA complex, are further divided into a class I (A, B, C) and a class II (D, DR, DP, DQ) locus. While class I (HLA-A, B, C) antigens are present in all nucleated cells, the class II locus (HLA-DR) appears limited primarily to B lymphocytes, a subpopulation of macrophages and activated T cells.

The class I antigens, through the vehicle of passenger leukocytes, specifically bind to the antigen receptor complex on cytotoxic T lymphocytes. Similarly, class II (HLA-DR) antigens are involved in the stimulation of helper T lymphocytes.

As a practical matter, the tissue-typing process involves the determination of compatibility between class I A and B antigens and class II DR antigens. The identification of these three antigens on lymphocytes is accomplished using typed monospecific antisera in a complement-mediated cytotoxicity test. Disparity or difference in the D locus is determined by the recognition that B cells or monocytes from one individual can stimulate T lymphocytes from a second individual. The resultant proliferation of T cells is known as a mixed lymphocyte culture reaction (MLC). In the presence of class I antigen incompatibility and HLA-D locus disparity an MLC reaction occurs that results in a population of cytotoxic T cells with the capacity to identify HLA-A, B, C incompatible antigens on target cells. The obvious clinical implication of this alloimmune response is to make an attempt to find donors with similar HLA antigenic specificities as the recipient. However, except in the cases of identical twins, complete antigenic compatibility is clearly illusory. In addition, the introduction of effective immunotherapy, specifically cyclosporine, seems to render compulsive histocompatibility testing somewhat moot.

Helper T lymphocytes, in the presence of class II (HLA-DR) antigen, become sensitized and release macrophage-stimulating factor. The cascade continues as the now stimulated macrophages make monokine interleukin (IL-I) which, in turn, promotes differentiation and proliferation of the helper T-cells line. Ultimately, the helper T cells produce a variety of proteins including T-cell growth factor (IL-2), B-cell growth factor (IL-4), and gamma interferon.

In general, IL-2 promotes the activation and proliferation of lymphoid cell lines including cytotoxic T cells. The class I antigens sensitize these cells in the IL-2 environment to become effector cells capable of graft destruction. Simultaneously, B lymphocytes in the presence of IL-4 become plasma cells that produce donor-specific antibodies. The stage is thus set, in the unmodified setting, for the process of graft destruction.

As indicated, destruction of the transplanted kidney occurs on a number of fronts. Direct cellular graft damage is mediated through attack on donor tissue target cells by macrophages, cytotoxic T cells, and helper cells. Donor-specific antibodies synthesized by plasma cells cause damage through both complement-mediated cell lysis and antibody-dependent cell-mediated cytotoxicity. Organ destruction is therefore a result of both activated cellular and humoral responses to an antigenic challenge.

What happens to the transplanted kidney on a cellular and macroscopic level as a result of the alloimmune response? Changes occur at both the vascular and glomerular level leading ultimately to reduced blood flow and glomerular filtration. Blood urea nitrogen increases, salt and water are retained, and parenchymal ischemia initiates the renin–angiotensin II axis resulting in peripheral vasospasm and hypertension.

## Hyperacute Rejection

Hyperacute rejection, a devastating and uniformly irreversible form of rejection, typically occurs within minutes to a few hours following transplantation. It develops in recipients with circulating class I HLA antibodies against donor cells, specifically vascular endothelium. Most of these patients have been sensitized by previous blood transfusions, multiple pregnancies, or a previously rejected graft. On a microscopic level the antigen–antibody interaction leads to complement deposition, platelet aggregation, and capillary thrombus formation. This cytodestructive and vaso-occlusive process rapidly results in cortical infarction with acellular glomeruli. Macroscopically the kidney becomes edematous and tense, dark blue or purple.

The diagnosis of hyperacute rejection is often made on the operating table at which time the organ is immediately removed. The diagnosis is suspected in patients who remain anuric after transplantation. These individuals often exhibit systemic signs, ie, fever, chills, and evidence of DIC. The Hippuran I 131 renal scan demonstrates no uptake. A digital subtraction angiogram distinguishes this entity from renal artery thrombosis by confirming arterial patency. Immediate nephrectomy is the only viable treatment option, antirejection medication having no role in this pathology.

Careful routine pretransplant crossmatching usually identifies high-risk sensitized patients, making the incidence of this disease extremely low.

### Acute Rejection

Acute rejection, the most common type of rejection, generally occurs between the first week and 3–6 months posttransplantation. It is mediated on either a cellular or humoral level with different prognosis and treatment options dependent on the rejection pattern.

**Acute Humoral Rejection.** Humoral rejection often occurs within the first week after transplantation, involves an antibody-mediated graft damage, and progresses on an accelerated basis. Vascular compromise secondary to arteriolar thrombosis results in renal ischemia.

Although acute humoral rejection and hyperacute rejection may appear clinically and pathologically similar, the latter develops immediately after transplantation and demonstrates donor-specific antibodies at the time of surgery. In acute humoral rejection the recipient has been previously sensitized to class I HLA antigens through blood transfusions or prior transplantation. A rechallenge with a large antigenic load stimulates production of donor-specific antibodies resulting in rapid graft destruction. However, in contrast to hyperacute rejection, the early form of accelerated humoral rejection can be successfully treated.

**Acute Cellular Rejection.** Acute cellular rejection, the most common form of rejection, usually occurring 7 to 10 days following transplantation, is mediated by the infiltration of T and B lymphocytes and macrophages. Clinically the patient presents with a spectrum of manifestations ranging from mild renal impairment to oliguric renal failure, hypertension, and pulmonary edema.

Typically, the patient complains of flulike symptoms, including malaise, arthralgias, anorexia, low-grade fever, hypertension, and decreased urine output. The graft is often swollen, tender to palpation, and, occasionally, painful. Laboratory evaluation reveals increased serum creatinine and urea nitrogen, and, most sensitively, a fall in creatinine clearance. In addition, the fever workup (chest roentgenogram, urine culture, etc.) is generally unremarkable.

Histologically, acute cellular rejection is characterized by a dense interstitial graft infiltrate consisting of lymphocytes, macrophages, and plasma cells. This occurs throughout the cortex and may be associated with significant interstitial edema.

**Rejection Diagnosis.** While a myriad of sophisticated laboratory tests have been proposed to diagnose and quantitate the degree of rejection, they are generally expensive and variably insensitive. As a practical matter, laboratory evaluation should aid in differentiating acute rejection from other common causes of reduced urine output, specifically acute tubular necrosis, mechanical problems (vascular and ureteral), and drug-induced nephritis. The Hippuran

I 131 scintigram fairly reliably identifies renal artery thrombosis (no uptake), acute tubular necrosis (good renal uptake, delayed excretion into bladder), and urine leaks (good uptake, pooling in perirenal space). An ultrasound of the transplant will reveal perirenal collections (urinoma, lymphocele), obstructive uropathy (ureteral obstruction), or rejection (enlarged kidney with loss of corticomedullary junction). Unfortunately, neither test definitively diagnoses acute rejection.

While the percutaneous allograft biopsy is associated with minimal risk, it is probably most revealing in diagnosing renal rejection. In general, light microscopy can help distinguish acute tubular necrosis, cyclosporine-induced nephrotoxicity, CMV glomerulopathy, and various forms of rejection (cellular versus humoral). As a practical matter, the diagnosis of acute rejection is usually made on a clinical basis, obviating the need for biopsy in all patients with acute oliguria. However, in recipients who fail to respond to antirejection therapy or where graft viability is a concern, renal biopsy becomes an important adjunctive technique.

## Chronic Renal Failure

While a comprehensive discussion of this entity is beyond the scope of this chapter, it should be noted that this disease is the major cause of graft loss in the late posttransplant period. The progression is often insidious, initially presenting as mild creatinine elevation many years after surgery. However, the deterioration in graft function, while initially subtle, is generally relentless, progressing to end-stage renal failure. Over a variable time period hypertension and proteinuria are often associated with the diminution in renal function. Treatment is primarily supportive as there is no effective antirejection regimen for this process.

## Treatment of Rejection

**Hyperacute Rejection.** The treatment of hyperacute rejection is immediate nephrectomy. Failure to promptly remove the kidney can result in a variety of potentially fatal complications, including DIC, hypertensive crisis, and adult respiratory distress syndrome.

In a word, the treatment of this problem is prevention. Sensitive cross-matching technique should identify anti-donor HLA antibodies in the recipient serum rendering the proposed surgery moot. Happily, this phenomenon has become a rarity in the modern transplant era.

**Acute Rejection.** Historically, the treatment of accelerated (humoral) acute rejection has ultimately involved nephrectomy. Response to conventional antirejection therapy, specifically steroids, is disappointing. However, OKT3 monoclonal antibody therapy has been successful in salvaging some of these units and should therefore be considered as the primary treatment for this form of rejection.

**Acute Cellular Rejection.** Acute cellular rejection, the most common form of rejection, responds well to conventional antirejection therapy. High-dose pulse glucosteroids represent the first line of treatment and appear to be effective by working at a variety of levels. Steroids have a lymphogenic effect, driving lymphocytes out of the peripheral blood. Most importantly, however, steroids inhibit the release of IL-1 by macrophages. As a result, IL-2 production by helper T cells is significantly retarded, ultimately reducing the number of effector cells. Steroids also stabilize lysosomal membranes and reduce vascular permeability.

While the dosage regimen varies, we prefer to deliver the medication in a pulsed fashion, typically methylprednisolone (1 $gm^3$ IV/day for 3 days).

OKT3, a commercially available monoclonal antibody, has become the standard second-line antirejection therapy at the Lahey Clinic. OKT3 differs from antilymphocyte globulin therapy in that it recognizes a single T-cell surface antigen, thereby avoiding injury to nonlymphoid cells. Hybridoma technology has resulted in production of a pure antibody targeted against the CD3 protein present on the surface of all mature T lymphocytes. By altering the antigen recognition complex, the T cell is unable to identify the renal allograft antigens.

OKT3 is administered intravenously, 5 mg/day for 10 days. Significant side effects include fever, myalgias, hypotension, and, at the extreme, pulmonary edema. In general, patients are premedicated with a variety of steroids, antihistamines, and antipyretics in an effort to minimize the severity of symptoms. The success rate with the use of OKT3 in steroid-resistant acute rejection is extraordinarily high, approaching 95% in some centers.

Graft irradiation and plasmapheresis are rarely employed as treatment due to a paucity of therapeutic benefit. While antilymphocyte globulin (ALG) plays a role as a primary immunosuppressant, OKT3 has generally supplanted its use in the setting of acute rejection.

## RESULTS OF RENAL TRANSPLANTATION

Both patient and graft survival following renal transplantation have increased significantly over the last decade. National Cooperative Study data indicate the following: 1-year survival for living related and cadaver transplants are 97% and 92% and 90% and 80% in 10 years.[86] One-year renal graft survival for living related and cadaver transplants are 86% and 68%, respectively, and 43% and 29% in 10 years. Analysis of long-term results in cadaveric renal transplant since the introduction of cyclosporine was analyzed by Land et al.[87] The overall results of 725 cadaveric renal transplants performed between 1982 and 1986 showed an 8-year actuarial graft survival of 39% with a half-life of all cadaveric renal transplants being 6.8 years. Patient survival during this interval was 87%. Sixty-one percent of all chronic graft losses were due to chronic rejection with only 15% being due to patient death. Other causes of renal graft loss were cyclosporin nephrotoxicity (11%), recurrent disease (6%), and noncompliance (3%).

Terasaki et al in 1989 reported data on 74,000 renal transplants from 210 centers, of which 113 centers had data from 15 to 25 years.[88] The half-life was 25 years for HLA-identical sibling donors, 13 years for parental donors, and 8 years for cadaveric donors. Cold ischemia time over 24 hours, recipient age over 55, and donor age 55 to 60 had a small effect on half-life survival. Acute tubular necrosis (ATN) had relatively little effect on 1-year survival.

The impact of HLA tissue matching in an era of exquisitely effective immunosuppression is unclear and controversial. However, there appears to be compelling evidence to suggest that six-antigen matched renal transplants fare better than other grafts, at least in a short term. Takemoto et al showed that 504 six-antigen matched renal transplants had an 87.2% 1-year graft survival as compared to only 75.8% for the contralateral transplanted kidney.[89] This advantage was reduced to 80% versus 70% at 2 years. Of interest is the fact that in this study the subset of diabetic recipients demonstrated an 89% 1-year graft survival. Finally, results from Najarian et al showed 94% and 92% 1- and 2-year survival, respectively, for nondiabetic transplant recipients.[90] The survival in diabetic renal transplant recipients was 93% and 90%, respectively, at 1 and 2 years. Compare this to the survival of ESRD patients on dialysis. Nondiabetics had a 90% and 80% 1- and 2-year survival, respectively, while diabetic patients had an 80% and 60% survival, respectively. Accruing evidence seems to clearly demonstrate that renal transplantation improves long-term patient survival as well as quality of life.

## COMPLICATIONS OF TRANSPLANTATION

### Urinary Complications

The most common causes of complications after renal transplantation are urinary obstruction and urinary leak. The incidence of these events ranges from 5% to 15%[91] with a mortality as high as 30%,[92] usually as a result of sepsis from delayed diagnosis.

While urine leak is occasionally obvious, clinical signs and symptoms of ureteral complications may be subtle, requiring various types of imaging for diagnosis.[93,94] Management approaches to various urinary complications are presented herein.

**Urinary Obstruction.** The causes of mechanical obstruction in the early postoperative period include clot in the bladder or ureter, inadvertent twisting or kinking of the ureter, compression of the intramural ureter by a tight tunnel (Politano–Leadbetter technique), infarction of a distal ureter, and compression by the spermatic cord.

In the immediate postoperative period, a clot in the bladder or ureter should be suspected as a cause of obstruction. This is easily treated by irrigating a Foley catheter to ensure patency. Suture site oozing as a source of blood clot is generally self-limiting, resolving within 24 hours. The development of anuria or oliguria following percutaneous renal biopsy should lead to the suspicion of clot in the renal pelvis or ureter. On occasion, percutaneous nephrostomy is necessary to vent the kidney until the clot lyses.

Inadvertent twisting or kinking of the ureter, compression of the ureteral tip by a tight bladder tunnel, and infarction of the distal ureter are the complications of ureteral reimplantation. Oliguria, while suggesting a mechanical obstruction, is a nonspecific sign signaling acute rejection or acute tubular necrosis as well. Ultrasound, by demonstrating hydronephrosis and caliectasis, helps to differentiate mechanical obstruction from the medical causes of oliguria and percutaneous nephrostogram defines the anatomic point of obstruction.

Ureteral obstruction identified early in the postoperative period requires immediate surgical correction. The lower pole of the transplant kidney is mobilized and the ureter identified. The ureter is reimplanted in the bladder and the original defect closed. Alternative reconstructive procedures may be required in the event of inadequate ureteral length.

Stenosis of the ureter can be encountered months to years after successful renal transplantation. This generally results from damage to the ureteral blood supply incurred during donor nephrectomy, leading to an ischemic stenosis of the distal ureter. The resulting oliguria and azotemia is differentiated from chronic rejection by renal biopsy. The combination of ultrasound and percutaneous antegrade radiography will accurately diagnose obstruction and provide definition of the location and extent of the stricture. In addition, ureteral stenting can be easily accomplished via the percutaneous route.

Therapeutic percutaneous techniques including balloon dilatation and endoscopic ureterotomy have been helpful in "bailing out" many stenotic lesions. Voegeli et al[95] reported on 14 patients who underwent percutaneous dilatation of benign ureteral strictures. Twelve patients were treated via an antegrade approach, one in retrograde fashion, and one with a combination technique. Of 14 patients, 11 (79%) had successful dilatation followed from 1 to 5 years with three reported recurrences and no renal graft losses.

**Urinary Leak.** The incidence of urinary leak varies from 0.5% to 15%.[96] The diagnosis of early urinary leak is easily made when there is drainage from the wound or the drain site. Other signs and symptoms include allograft tenderness, unexplained fever, and edema of the scrotum, labia, or thigh ipsolateral to the renal transplant. The renal transplant recipient may present with fulminant sepsis as a result of an impaired immune response.

Necrosis of the distal ureter is the most common cause of urinary leak and may not present until 1 to 3 weeks posttransplantation. This can be prevented by careful dissection of the ureter at the time of donor nephrectomy. The extravesical technique of the ureteral anastomosis to the dome of the bladder requires a shorter length of ureter resulting perhaps in a lower incidence of ureteral necrosis.[97] The complication of dehiscence of the bladder suture line is also eliminated by use of the extravesical technique.

## Calyceal-Cutaneous Fistula

The development of a calyceal-cutaneous fistula is generally felt to result from segmental infarction of the renal parenchyma in grafts with multiple renal arteries. Surgical exploration with removal of the infarcted portion of the kidney is necessary once a diagnosis is definitive. The primary closure of a calyceal system can be attempted but in the face of necrotic tissue will infrequently be successful. In the event of segmental lower pole infarction, lower pole nephrectomy may be required in order to adequately debride the involved parenchyma and ureter. Allograft salvage is obtained by anastomosing the remainder of the renal pelvis directly to the bladder. A nephrostomy tube and ureteral stent drainage will help to seal the urinary leak postreconstruction. Persistence of urinary extravasation or sepsis is an indication for transplant nephrectomy.

### Lymphoceles

Failure to ligate the lymphatic vessels along the recipient iliac vessels can lead to lymph leak. There is some evidence that open lymphatics on the donor organ may also contribute to lymph accumulation. Accumulated fluid in a close space leads ultimately to lymphocele formation. The incidence of lymphoceles postrenal transplant is less than 2%.

Extrinsic pressure on the bladder can cause urinary frequency and compression of the ureter can lead to transplant hydronephrosis. Needle aspiration under ultrasound or CT scan guidance can help distinguish lymphocele formation from a urinoma. Percutaneous catheter drainage with sclerosis may result in obliteration of the lymphocele. If this modality fails, internal drainage with a marsupialized peritoneal window is usually effective. Reports of laparoscopic lymphocele drainage and marsupialization have recently appeared in the literature. It is likely that adaptation of this technology will become the preferred treatment for this transplant complication.

### Deep Wound Infection

The incidence of deep wound infection in perinephric abscess in renal transplantation has declined. Less iliac vessel dissection, meticulous technique in the preservation of ureteral blood supply, more refined surgical technique for ureteroneocystostomy, the use of monofilament sutures, perioperative prophylactic antibiotics, and more specific immunosuppressive protocols have contributed to this phenomenon.

Ultrasound of the allograft site should be performed for unexplained fever or wound drainage. Needle aspiration will usually be diagnostic. Prompt surgical drainage is required to prevent systemic sepsis and to decrease the likelihood of infecting the vascular anastomosis, a complication requiring transplant nephrectomy.

### Nonrenal Transplant Complications Requiring Acute Surgery

Peptic ulcer disease (PUD), intestinal perforation, and pancreatitis are the main complications indirectly related to the renal transplant procedure and may require immediate surgical intervention. Immunosuppressive therapy, especially high-dose prednisone, may delay diagnosis by masking the usual signs and symptoms. Hence a high index of suspicion is required for prompt diagnosis. The incidence of PUD postrenal transplantation ranges from 3% to 16%[98] and occurs most commonly in patients with a prior history of PUD. As prevention is the best cure, this group of recipient candidates should be identified pretransplantation and vigorously treated with H2 blocker/antacid therapy.

When upper gastrointestinal bleeding is encountered, endoscopy will help to establish the source of bleeding. When upper gastrointestinal bleeding persists despite intensive H2 blocker/antacid therapy, early operative intervention is required. Gastric perforations are treated by primary repair of the defect with copious irrigation of the abdominal cavity. The etiology for perforation is presumed to be steroid-induced, but cytomegalovirus (CMV) may also play a role.[99]

Spontaneous perforation of the small intestine after renal transplantation, while rare, can occur. It is thought to be secondary to the use of steroids, and, on occasion, to CMV infection. The patient typically presents with abdominal pain and signs and symptoms of an acute abdomen. Resection of the involved small bowel segment is required.

Large bowel perforation is reported to be 1% with mortality as high as 50%.[100] It is most commonly seen in the transplant recipient with a history of diverticulitis. The individual typically presents with fever, elevated white blood cell count, and diffuse lower abdominal pain. A contrast enema or even abdominal CT scan is diagnostic. Resection of the perforated segment with colostomy and mucous fistula is the surgical treatment of choice. Reduction of immunosuppression and the liberal use of broad-spectrum antibiotics are important adjuncts.

Pancreatitis following renal transplantation is a devastating complication with reported mortality rates approaching 70%.[101] Predisposing factors include the use of prednisone and azathioprine and hyperparathyroidism. The transplant patient will present with diffuse abdominal pain, elevated white blood cell count, and an elevated amylase. Aggressive fluid replacement, nutritional support, and nasogastric suction are required. The finding of pancreatic abscess mandates immediate surgical drainage and decompression of the biliary tract. Immunosuppression is discontinued and the patient is started on broad-spectrum antibiotic coverage. Despite aggressive management and the acknowledged loss of the allograft, pancreatitis has the potential to be a fatal complication for the transplant patient.

## Vascular Complications

Historically, the incidence of vascular complications, mainly arterial thrombosis, disruption, and hemorrhage, pseudoaneurysm, and mycotic aneurysm, approached 6%.[102–104] This was mainly due to the fact that renal failure patients undergoing renal transplantation are particularly susceptible to poor wound healing and infection because of the effects of uremia and the altered host responses induced by immunosuppressive therapy. However, with a decreased incidence of perinephric infections due to meticulous surgical technique and monofilament sutures, better antibiotic therapy, and more specific immunosuppressive therapy at decreased dosages, there has been a concomitant decrease in vascular complications.

**Vascular Thrombosis.** In the setting of a single renal artery, the incidence of acute arterial thrombosis is rare. This is usually the result of a technical error with the arterial anastomosis. The salvage of the kidney is unlikely unless the diagnosis can be made intraoperatively. In the postoperative period, acute thrombosis will present as acute cessation of urine output mimicking acute tubular necrosis or acute rejection. A radionuclide scan or renal graft arteriography will provide the diagnosis but the improbability of successful revascularization necessitates transplant nephrectomy.

The transplant surgeon will occasionally encounter a donor kidney with multiple renal arteries. Thrombosis of a polar artery in this setting can be encountered and results in segmental parenchymal infarction or ureteral necrosis. A urine leak will result that might present with fever, wound tenderness, or leakage from the drain site. A pelvic ultrasound will show a perirenal graft collection and a percutaneous nephrostogram will better define the site of the leak.

Renal vein thrombosis, although uncommon, can result from expansion of the kidney with acute rejection or from placement of the kidney in a tight retroperitoneal pocket, resulting in compression of the renal vein. If thrombosis of the renal vein does occur, salvage is unlikely and the patient may need transplant nephrectomy.

Occasionally, compression of the iliac vein or iliac vein thrombosis can occur and compromise flow from the renal vein. The patient will present with a swollen leg and with a deep venous thrombosis. Noninvasive venous testing or venography will provide the diagnosis. Treatment in this case is systemic heparinization and graft preservation is likely.

**Allograft Rupture.** During an acute rejection episode, the renal allograft may acutely swell and rupture leading to hemorrhage. This usually occurs along the convex border of the kidney as a result of cortical ischemia from edema and intense cellular infiltration.[105] The patient presents with acute onset of severe pain over the renal allograft or hypovolemic shock. Immediate exploration is required and the kidney can be repaired using surgical and Avitene pledgets with large mattress (liver) sutures. If hemorrhage cannot be controlled, transplant nephrectomy may be required.

**Thrombophlebitis.** Despite the mild coagulopathy associated with renal failure, the overall incidence of pelvic vein thrombosis is over 8%.[106] With a rising hematocrit after successful renal transplantation, there seems to be a coincident risk in embolic events with a peak incidence at 4 to 5 months. Cyclosporine-treated patients may have a higher incidence of thromboembolic events.[107]

If there is a significant venous outflow obstruction from the graft, there will be a sudden fall in urine output, graft tenderness, and proteinuria. Graft function in this setting may be difficult to salvage even with prompt exploration and thrombectomy, but successful results have been reported.[108]

**Renal Artery Stenosis.** Renal artery stenosis may result from atherosclerotic disease in the recipient vessels, technical errors, arterial injury during donor nephrectomy, or immunologic injury. The stenotic area is most commonly at the renal-artery-to-iliac-artery anastomosis or just beyond it.

The incidence of hypertension posttransplant is as high as 50% to 60%[109] and the incidence of renal artery stenosis varies from 2% to 16%.[110] Routine angiography performed in 100 consecutive transplant patients showed some degree of renal artery stenosis in 23 patients.[110] However, the incidence of narrowing of the renal artery by more than 80% in association with hypertension is less than 5%.[111] This is usually associated with a high plasma renin state.

The diagnosis should be pursued in all renal transplant patients whose blood pressure cannot be controlled with traditional antihypertensive therapy and who show no evidence of acute or chronic rejection. Worsening hypertension can also be accompanied by deterioration in graft function. A bruit present in the early postoperative period is a good sign. The sudden appearance of a bruit with hypertension late after renal transplantation suggests renal artery stenosis and should be investigated. Bruits can be present in up to 88% of patients with transplant renal artery stenosis.[112]

Renal arteriography provides definitive diagnosis.[112,113] A needle biopsy of the kidney should be done to exclude chronic rejection where stenosis of the main renal artery is associated with diffuse narrowing of secondary and tertiary branches. If this is found, repair of the main renal artery stenosis will not correct hypertension.

Definitive management of significant hypertension secondary to renal artery stenosis is either surgical reconstruction[114] or percutaneous transluminal angioplasty. The surgical approach should be transperitoneal in order to get into a virgin plane of dissection. The stenosis can be resected and the transplant renal artery reimplanted into the external or internal iliac artery. A saphenous vein segment is more commonly used to bypass the stenotic area. Tilney et al[114] reported 14 of 21 patients undergoing successful repair with 3 of the 7 patients who failed to respond having chronic rejection.

Percutaneous transluminal angioplasty (PTA) is a nonsurgical option that is being utilized with increasing success.[115,116] The early experience of Molenkopf et al,[116] Dafoe et al,[117,118] and Flechner et al[119] demonstrated success rates of 76.5%, 93.8%, and 50% in 17, 16, and 2 patients with transplant renal artery stenosis, respectively. PTA was successful 76% of the time in a series of 39 patients reported by Greenstein et al.[120] There was only one renal graft loss in this series.

Contradictory to this success with PTA is the experience reported by Roberts et al[121] whereby 31 patients had 43 surgical or PTA procedures. Of the 18 surgical procedures, 72% of the patients had a cure or improvement with no renal graft losses. Of the 25 PTA procedures performed, 20% of the patients had cure or improvement with 7 renal artery injuries resulting in renal graft loss in 4 patients and emergent surgery in 3 patients to save the renal transplant. Hence, the conclusion of this study is that anastomotic stenoses of the transplant renal artery do not respond as well to PTA as to surgical reconstruction.

In the series by Deglise-Favre et al,[122] 40 patients who had characteristics and locations of transplant renal artery stenosis (TRAS) not amenable to interventional therapy, great operative risk, occurrence of complications of immunosuppression (sepsis, malignancy, hepatic dysfunction), or good control on antihypertensive drugs were followed medically. Their results showed actuarial graft survival of 100% at 1 year, 95% at 2 years, and 65% at 5 years, which did not differ from 39 TRAS patients treated with surgical reconstruction or 50 TRAS patients treated with PTA. The morbidity from 138 TRAS patients reached 7.6% and 28% for surgically versus PTA-treated lesions. Hence, patient selection into a medical treatment of TRAS provided no difference in graft failure or impaired long-term renal function.

The overall consensus of most centers would be that to attempt PTA as reoperation can be difficult. Surgical standby should always be available in the event of acute arterial injury occurring during PTA. All transplant renal artery stenoses should be deemed significant as some can occur without resultant hypertension or graft dysfunction.

## FUTURE CONSIDERATIONS

The demand for renal transplantation can logically be diminished only by elimination of the disease processes that result in ESRD. A decrease in the incidence of chronic renal failure depends in large measure on control or cure of diabetic and hypertensive neuropathy or the various glomerulopathies. Until such panaceas are found, efforts to alleviate an acute organ shortage assume the highest priority.

In an effort to expand the donor pool, some transplant centers have explored the use of living unrelated donors (friend or spouse) and ABO-incompatible donors.[123,124] Historically the transplant community has taken a dim view of living unrelated transplantation, a view based on both ethical and health-related concerns. Indeed, the incidence of donor deaths in the living related category is 0.06%,[125] arguably an acceptably low risk. It is imperative that the prospective donor undergo an extensive psychological evaluation as a prerequisite to donor nephrectomy. One-year graft survival at the University of Minnesota for living unrelated donor renal transplantation is 92%.[123]

Similarly, ABO-incompatible renal transplants can be done. An investigative protocol reported by Najarian et al involves prerenal transplant splenectomy and subsequent plasmapheresis to remove preformed antibodies. Preliminary results are said to be promising.[123]

The donor pool may be expanded by including older and younger patients as donors and through the use of kidneys from non-heart-beating donors. There is accruing evidence to suggest that, with the exception of the very young donor (less than 2 years), age does not represent a barrier to organ donation.[126–128] Non-heart-beating kidney procurement has been performed in Europe with acceptably good graft survival. In the Netherlands, for instance, this technique has increased the number of renal donors from 30 to 41 kidneys per million population.[129,130]

Advances in immunosuppression, renal preservation, and surgical technique have made renal transplantation a therapeutic option of choice for the ESRD patient. Refinements in specific immunosuppression and rejection treatment will make the transplant option safer and more durable, and, in the longer term, expand the viability of xenotransplantation. It is imperative that the urologic surgeon remain an integral member of the transplant team at both the surgical and the medical levels.

## REFERENCES

1. Landsteiner and Hufnagel: cited by Goodwin WE, Martin DC. Renal transplantation. In: Campbell MF, Harrison JH, eds. *Urology,* 3rd

ed. Philadelphia: WB Saunders; 1970:2240–2271.

2. Murray JE, Merril JP, Harrison JH. Renal hormonal transplantation in identical twins. *Surg Forum.* 1955;6:432–436.
3. Evans RW. Organ donation: facts and figures. *Dialysis Transpl.* 1990;19(5):234–237.
4. Schwartz RS, Dameshek W. Drug-induced immunologic tolerance. *Nature.* 1959;183:1682–1683.
5. Calne RY. The rejection of renal homografts: inhibition in dogs by 6-mercaptopurine. *Lancet.* 1960;1:417–418.
6. Zukoski CF, Lee HM, Hume DM. The prolongation of functional survival of canine renal homografts by 6-mercaptopurine. *Surg Forum.* 1960;11:470–472.
7. Calne RY, Rolles K, White DJG, Thiru S, Evans DB, Dunn DC, et al. Cyclosporine A initially as the only immunosuppressant in 34 recipients of cadaveric organs: 32 kidneys, 2 pancreases and 2 livers. *Lancet.* 1979; 2(8151):1033–1036.
8. Isoniemi H, Eklund B, Hockerstedt K, Korsback C, Salmela K, Von Willebrand E, et al. Discontinuation of one drug in triple drug treatment of renal allograft patients: 1-year results. *Transpl Proc.* 1990;22(4):1365–1366.
9. Opelz G. Multicenter impact of cyclosporine on cadaver kidney graft survival. *Prog Allergies.* 1986;38:329.
10. Evans RW. Executive summary: The National Cooperating Transplantation study. BHARC–100–91–020. Seattle, WA: Battelle-Seattle Research Center, 1991:17.
11. Cosimi AB, Colvin RB, Burton RC, Rubin RH, Goldstein G, Kung PC, et al. Use of monoclonal antibodies to T-cell subsets for immunologic monitoring and treatment in recipients of renal allografts. *N Engl J Med.* 1981; 305(6):308–314.
12. Mandel J, Kjellsterand CM. Long-term results of dialysis and transplantation in patients with end stage renal failure from hypernephroma. *Nephron.* 1986;44:111–114.
13. Penn I. The changing pattern of posttransplant malignancies. *Transpl Proc.* 1991;23:1101–1103.
14. Salvatierra O, Melzer J, Potter D, et al. A seven-year experience with donor-specific blood transfusions, results and consideration for maximum efficacy. *Transplantation.* 1985;40(6):654–659.
15. Belzer FO, Ashby BS, Dumphy JE. 24- and 72-Hour preservation of canine kidneys. *Lancet.* 1967;2:536.
16. Collins GH, Bravo-Sugarman MB, Terasaki PI. Kidney preservation for transplantation: initial perfusion and 30-hour ice storage. *Lancet.* 1969;2:1219.
17. Jamieson NV, Sundberg R, Lindell S, et al. An analysis of the components in UW solution using the isolated perfused rabbit liver. *Transplantation.* 1988;46:512.
18. Calne RY, Pegg DE, Pryse-Davies J, Leigh-Brown F. Renal preservation by ice cooling. An experimental study related to kidney transplantation from cadavers. *Br Med J.* 1963;5358:651–655.
19. MacKnight ADC, Leaf A. Regulation of cellular volume. *Physiol Rev.* 1977;57:510.
20. Lie JS, Ukikusa M. Significance of alkaline preservation solutions in hepatic transplantation. *Transpl Proc.* 1984;16:134.
21. Ratych RE, Chuknyski RS, Bulkley GB, et al. The primary localization of free radical generation after anoxia/reoxygenation in isolated endothelial cells. *Surgery.* 1987;102:122.
22. Baker GL, Currey RJ, Autor AP. Oxygen free radical induced damage in kidneys subjected to warm ischemia and reperfusion-protective effect of superoxide dismutase. *Ann Surg.* 1985;202:628.
23. Spragg RG, Hinshaw DB, Hyslop PA, et al. Alterations in adenosine triphosphate and energy charge in cultured endothelial and P3A8D cells after oxidant injury. *J Clin Invest.* 1985;76:1471.
24. Toledo-Pereyra LH. Definition of reperfusion injury in transplantation. *J Transpl.* 1987;43:931.
25. Parks DA, Bulkley GB, Granger DN, et al. Role of oxygen-free radicals in shock, ischemia and organ preservation. *Surgery.* 1983;94:428.
26. Belzer FO, Hoffman RM, Rice MJ, et al. Combination perfusion–cold storage for optimal kidney function and utilization. *Transplantation.* 1985;39:118.
27. Stromski ME, Cooper K, Thulin G, et al. Postischemic ATP-MGCL2 provides precursors for recent synthesis of cellular ATP in rats. *Am J Physiol.* 1986;250:F834.
28. Anaise D, Waltzer WC, Rapaport FT, et al. Metabolic requirements for successful extended hypothermic kidney preservation. *J Urol.* 1986;136:345.
29. Cheung JY, Bonventure JV, Malis CD, et al. Calcium and ischemic injury. *N Engl J Med.* 1986;314:1670.
30. Sumpio B, Bave AE. Treatment with verapamil and adenosine triphosphate MGCL2 reduces cyclosporine nephrotoxicity. *Surgery.* 1987; 101:315.
31. Bulkley GB. The role of oxygen-free radicals in the human disease processes. *J Surg.* 1983;94:407.
32. Schneeberger H, Illner WD, Abendroth D, Bulkley G, Rutili F, Williams M, Thiel M, Land W. First clinical experiences with supraoxide dismutase in kidney transplantation:

results of double-blind randomized study. *Transpl Proc.* 1989;21(1):1245–1246.

33. Southard JH, Marsh DC, McAnulty JF, Belzer FO. Oxygen derived free radical damage in organ preservation: activity of superoxide dismutase and xanthine oxidase. *J Surg.* 1987; 101:566.
34. Stromski ME, Cooper K, Thulin G, et al. Chemical and functional correlates of postischemic renal ATP levels. *Proc Natl Acad Sci USA.* 1986;83:6142.
35. Ploeg RJ, Goossens D, Camesi D, McAnulty JF, Southard JH, Belzer FO. Kidney preservation with Belzer's new pancreas preservation solution. *Transpl Proc.* In press.
36. D'Alessandro A, Southard JH, Kalayoglu M, Belzer FO. Comparison of cold storage and perfusion of dog livers on function of tissue slices. *Cryobiology.* 1987;23:161.
37. Ploeg RJ. Kidney preservation with the UW and Euro-Collins solutions. *Transplantation.* 1990;49:281.
38. Lam FT, Mavor AID, Potts DJ, et al. Improved 72-hour renal preservation with phosphate sucrose. *Transplantation.* 1989;47:767.
39. Lam FT, Ubhi CS, Mavor AID, et al. Clinical evaluation of PBS140 solution for cadaveric renal preservation. *Transplantation.* 1989; 48:1067.
40. Collins GM, Greene RD, Halasz NA. Importance of anion content and osmolarity in flush solutions for 48 to 72 hr hypothermic kidney storage. *Cryobiology.* 1979;6:217.
41. Collins GM, Bry WI, Warn R, Molenkopf F, Feduska NJ. Clinical comparison of U.W. with Collins solution for cadaveric kidney preservation. *Transpl Proc.* 1991;23:1305–1306.
42. Marshall VC, Jablonski P, Bigozas M, Howden BO, Walls K. University of Wisconsin solution for kidney transplantation: the impermeant components. *Transpl Proc.* 1991;23(1):651–652.
43. Murray JE, Merrill JP, Harrison JH, et al. Prolonged survival of human-kidney homografts by immunosuppressive drug therapy. *N Engl J Med.* 1963;268:1315.
44. Ponticelli C, Tarantino A, Montagnino G, et al. A randomized trial comparing triple-drug and double-drug therapy in renal transplantation. *Transplantation.* 1988;45:913.
45. Lewis RM, Janney RP, Golden DL, et al. Stability of renal allograft function associated with long-term cyclosporine immunosuppressive therapy—five year follow-up. *Transplantation.* 1989;47:266.
46. Strom TB, Carpenter BC. Immunobiology of kidney transplantation. In: EDS Brenner BM, Rector FC Jr, eds. *The Kidney.* Philadelphia: WB Saunders; 1991:2336.
47. Strom TB, Kelley VE. Toward more selective therapies to block undesired immune responses. *Kidney Int.* 1989;35:1026.
48. Fauci AS, Dale DC, Balow JE. Glucocorticosteroid therapy: mechanism of action and clinical considerations. *Ann Intern Med.* 1976;84:304.
49. Maiorca R, Cristinelli L, Brunori G, et al. Prospective control trial of steroid withdrawal after six months in renal transplant patients treated with cyclosporine. *Transpl Proc.* 1988;20 (Suppl 3):121.
50. Ortho Multicenter Transplant Study Group. A randomized clinical trial of OKT3 monoclonal antibody for acute rejection of cadaveric renal transplants. *N Engl J Med.* 1985;313:337.
51. Leichtman AB, Strom TB. Therapeutic approach to renal transplantation: triple therapy and beyond. *Transpl Proc.* 1988;20 (Suppl 8):1.
52. Haessleim HC, Pierre VC, Lee HM, et al. Leukopenia and azathioprine management in renal homotransplantation. *Surgery.* 1972;71:598.
53. Penn I. Cancer as a complication of clinical transplantation. *Transpl Proc.* 1977;9:1121.
54. Calne RY, White DJG, Thiru S, et al. Cyclosporine A in patients receiving renal allografts from cadaver donors. *Lancet.* 1978; 2:1323.
55. The Canadian Multicentre Transplant Study Group. A randomized clinical trial of cyclosporine and cadaveric renal transplantation. *N Engl J Med.* 1986;314:1219.
56. Ponticelli C, Minetti L, DiPalo FQ, et al. The Milan clinical trial with cyclosporine in cadaveric renal transplantation. *Transplantation.* 1988;45:908.
57. Myers BD, Sibley R, Newton L, et al. The long-term course of cyclosporine-associated chronic nephropathy. *Kidney Int.* 1988;33:590.
58. Kahan BD. Drug therapy: cyclosporine. *N Engl J Med.* 1989;321:1725.
59. Fries D, Hiesse C, Santelli G, et al. Triple therapy with low-dose cyclosporine, azathioprine, and steroids: long-term results of a randomized study in cadaver donor renal transplantation. *Transpl Proc.* 1988;20 (Suppl 3):130.
60. Hricik DE, Whalen CC, Lautman J, et al. Withdrawal of steroids after renal transplantation—clinical predictors of outcome. *Transplantation.* 1992;53:41.
61. Shield CF, Cosimi AB, Tolkoff-Rubin N, et al. Use of antithymocyte globulin for reversal of acute allograft rejection. *Transplantation.* 1979;28:461.
62. Norman DJ, Shield III CF, Barry J, et al. A US clinical study of Orthoclone OKT3 in renal transplantation. *Transpl Proc.* 1987;19 (Suppl 1):21.

63. Schroeder TJ, First MR, Mansour ME, et al. Antimurine antibody formation following OKT3 therapy. *Transplantation.* 1990;49:48.

64. Thistlethwaite JR Jr, Gaber AO, Haag BW, et al. OKT3 treatment of steroid-resistant renal allograft rejection. *Transplantation.* 1987; 43:176.

65. Hricik DE, Mayes JT, Schulak JA. Inhibition of anti-OKT3 antibody generation by cyclosporine: results of a prospective randomized trial. *Transplantation.* 1990;50:237.

66. Norman DJ, Barry JM, Bennett WM. OKT3 for induction immunosuppression and renal transplantation: a comparative study of high versus low doses. *Transpl Proc.* 1991;23:1052.

67. Chatenoud L, Legendre C, Ferran C, et al. Corticosteroid inhibition of the OKT3-induced cytokine-related syndrome-dosage and kinetics prerequisites. *Transplantation.* 1991;51:334.

68. Waid TH, Lucas BA, Thompson JS, et al. Treatment of acute cellular rejection with T10B9.1A–31 or OKT3 in renal allograft recipients. *Transplantation.* 1992;53:80.

69. Hall BM. Therapy with monoclonal antibodies to CD4: Potential not appreciated? *Am J Kidney Dis.* 1989;14 (Suppl 2):71.

70. Kirkman RL, Shapiro ME, Carpenter CB, et al. A randomized prospective trial of anti-tac monoclonal antibody in human renal transplantation. *Transplantation.* 1991;51:107.

71. Soulillou JP, Cantarovich D, Le Mauff B, et al. Randomized controlled trial of a monoclonal antibody against the interleukin-2 receptor (33B3.1) as compared with rabbit antithymocyte globulin for prophylaxis against rejection of renal allografts. *N Engl J Med.* 1990; 322:1175.

72. Erias G, Shimizu Y, van Seventer GA, et al. Effects of FK506 and cyclosporine on T-cell activation: integrin-mediated adhesion of T cells, proliferation, and maturation of cytotoxic T cells. *Transpl Proc.* 1991;23:936.

73. Shapiro R, Jordan M, Scantlebury V, et al. FK506 in clinical kidney transplantation. *Transpl Proc.* 1991;23:3065.

74. Kahan BD, Chang JY, Sehgal SN. Preclinical evaluation of a new potent immunosuppressive agent, rapamycin. *Transplantation.* 1991;52: 185.

75. Amemiya H, Suzuki S, Ota K, et al. A novel rescue drug, 15-deoxyspergualin. *Transplantation.* 1990;49:337.

76. Epstein M, Loutzenhiser RD. Renal hemodynamic effects of calcium antagonists: implications for renal transplantation. *Transpl Proc.* 1991;23:1775.

77. Palmer BF, Davidson I, Sagalowsky A, et al. Improved outcome of cadaveric renal transplantation due to calcium channel blockers. *Transplantation.* 1991;52:640.

78. Moran M, Mozes MF, Maddux MS, et al. Prevention of acute graft rejection by the prostaglandin $E_1$ analogue misoprostol in renal-transplant recipients treated with cyclosporine and prednisone. *N Engl J Med.* 1990;322:1183.

79. Koide M, Waud BE. Serum potassium concentrations after succinyl choline in patients with renal failure. *Anesthesiology.* 1972;36: 142.

80. Murray JE, Harrison JH. Surgical management of 50 patients with kidney transplants including 18 pairs of twins. *Am J Surg.* 1963;105:205.

81. Tilney NL, Kirkman RL. Surgical aspects of kidney transplantation. In: Garovoy MR, Guttman AR, eds. *Renal Transplantation.* New York: Churchill Livingstone; 1986:93–123.

82. Politano VA, Leadbetter WF. An operative technique for the correction of vesicoureteral reflux. *J Urol.* 1958;79:932–941.

83. Gregoir W, Van Regemorter G. Congenital vesicoureteral reflux. *Urol Int.* 1964;18:122–136.

84. Lich JR, Howerton LW, Davis LA. Recurrent urosepsis in children. *J Urol.* 1961;86:554–558.

85. Libertino JA, Zinman L. Technique for ureteroneocystotomy in renal transplantation and reflux. *Surg Clin North Am.* 1973;53:459–463.

86. Evans RW. Executive summary: The National Cooperative Transplantation Study. BHARC–100–91–020. Seattle, WA: Battelle-Seattle Research Center, June 1991.

87. Land W, Schneeberger H, Schleibner S, et al. Long-term results in cadaveric renal transplantation under cyclosporine therapy. *Transpl Proc.* 1991;23:1244–1246.

88. Terasaki P, Mickey MR, Iwaki Y, Cicciarelli J, Cecka M, Cook D, Yuga J. Long-term survival of kidney grafts. *Transpl Proc.* 1989; 21:615–617.

89. Takemoto S, Carnahan E, Terasaki PI. A report of 504 6-antigen-matched transplants. *Transpl Proc.* 1991;23:1318–1320.

90. Najarian JS, Matas AJ. The present and future of kidney transplantation. *Transpl Proc.* 1991;23:2075–2082.

91. Loughlin KR, Tilney NL, Richie JP. Urologic complications in 718 renal transplant patients. *Surgery.* 1984;95:297.

92. Starzl TE, Broth CG, Putnam CW, et al. Urological complications in 216 human recipients of renal transplants. *Ann Surg.* 1973;172:609.

93. Bartrum RJ, Smith EH, D'Orsi CJ, et al. The evaluation of renal transplant patients with ultrasound. *Radiology.* 1976;119:405.

94. Petrek J, Tilney NL, Smith EH, et al. Ultrasound in renal transplantation. *Ann Surg.* 1977;185:441.

95. Voegeli DR, Crummy AB, McDermott JC, Jensen SR. Percutaneous dilatation of ureteral

strictures in renal transplant recipients. *Radiology*. 1988;169:185–188.

96. Mundy AR, Podesta ML, Bewick M, Rudge CJ, Elvis FG. The urological complications of 1,000 renal transplants. *J Urol*. 1990;144: 1105–1109.
97. Thrasher JB, Temple DR, Spees, EK. Extravesical versus Politano Leadbetter–ureteroneocystostomy. A comparison of urological complications in 320 renal transplants. *J Urol*. 1990;144:1105–1109.
98. Owens ML, Wilson SE, Saltzman R, Gordon HE. Gastrointestinal complications after renal transplantation. *Arch Surg*. 1976;111:467.
99. Cohen EB, Kumorowski RA, Kauffman HM, Adams M. Unexpectedly high incidence of CMV infection in apparent peptic ulcers in renal transplant recipients. *Surgery*. 1984;97:606.
100. Church JM, Fazio VM, Braun WE, et al. Perforation of the colon in renal homograft recipients. *Ann Surg*. 1986;203:64.
101. Fernandez JA, Rosenberg JC. Post transplantation pancreatitis. *Surg Gynecol Obstet*. 1976;143:795.
102. Goldman MH, Tilney NL, Vineyard GC, et al. A 20-year survey of arterial complications of renal transplantation. *Surg Gynecol Obstet*. 1975;141:758.
103. Vidne BA, Leapman SB, Butt KM, Kountz SL. Vascular complications in human transplantation. *Surgery*. 1976;79:77.
104. Nerstrom B, Ladejoget J, Lung FL. Vascular complications in 155 consecutive kidney transplantations. *Scand J Urol Nephrol*. 1972;15 (Suppl 6):65.
105. Porter KA. Renal transplantation. In: Haptinstall RH, ed. *Pathology of the Kidney*. 3rd ed. Boston: Little, Brown; 1983:1455–1548.
106. Allen RDM, Michie CA, Murie JA, Morris PJ. Deep venous thrombosis after renal transplantation. *Surg Gynecol Obstet*. 1987;164:137.
107. VanRentergem Y, Roels L, Lerut T, et al. Thromboembolic complications in hemostatic changes in cyclosporine-treated cadaveric kidney allograft recipients. *Lancet*. 1985;1:99.
108. Clarke SD, Dennedy JA, Hewitt JC, et al. Successful removal of thrombosis from renal vein after renal transplantation. *Br Med J*. 1970; 1:154.
109. Whelton PK, Russell RP, Harrington DP, et al. Hypertension following renal homotransplantation. *Arch Intern Med*. 1978;138:233.
110. Lacombe M. Arterial stenosis complicating renal allotransplantation in man. *Ann Surg*. 1975;181:283.
111. Faenza A, Spolaore R, Poggioli G, et al. Renal artery sclerosis after renal transplantation. *Kidney Int*. 1983;23 (Suppl 14):554.
112. Smellie WAB, Vinik M, Hume DM. Angiographic investigation of hypertension complicating human renal transplantation. *Surg Gynecol Obstet*. 1969;128:963–968.
113. Flechner SM, Sandler CM, Childs T, et al. Screening for transplant renal artery stenosis in hypertensive patients using digital subtraction arteriography. *J Urol*. 1983;130:440–444.
114. Tilney NL, Rocha A, Strom TB, Kirkman RL. Renal artery stenosis in transplant patients. *Ann Surg*. 1984;199:454.
115. Grossman RA, Dafoe DC, Shoenfeld RB, et al. Percutaneous transluminal angioplasty treatment of renal transplant artery stenosis. *Transplantation*. 1982;34:339.
116. Molenkopf F, Matas A, Veith FJ, et al. Percutaneous transluminal angioplasty for transplant renal artery stenosis. *Transpl Proc*. 1983;15:1089.
117. Dafoe DC, Schoenfeld RB, Grossman RA, et al. Percutaneous transluminal angioplasty treatment of renal allograft artery stenosis. Presented at the 8th Annual Meeting of the American Society of Transplant Surgeons, Chicago, June 3–4, 1982.
118. Grossman RA, Dafoe DC, Shoenfeld RB, et al. Percutaneous transluminal angioplasty treatment of renal artery stenosis. *Transplantation*. 1981;34:339.
119. Flechner S, Novick AC, Vidt D, et al. The use of percutaneous transluminal angioplasty for renal artery stenosis in patients with generalized atherosclerosis. *J Urol*. 1982;127:1072–1075.
120. Greenstein SM, Berstandig A, McLean GK, et al. Percutaneous transluminal angioplasty: procedure of choice in hypertensive renal allograft recipient with renal artery stenosis. *Transplantation*. 1987;43:29.
121. Roberts JP, Ascher NL, Fryd DS, Hunter DW, Dunn DL, Payne WD, et al. Transplant renal artery stenosis. *Transplantation*. 1989;48:580–583.
122. Deglise-Favre AY, Hiesse CT, Lantz OT, et al. The long-term follow-up of 40 untreated cadaveric kidney transplant renal artery stenosis. *Transpl Proc*. 1991;23:1340–1343.
123. Najarian JS, Matas AJ. The present and future of kidney transplantation. *Transpl Proc*. 1991;23(4):2075–2082.
124. Berloci P, Aofani D, Bruzzone P, Renna Molajoni E, Rossi M, Pretagustini R, et al. Unrelated living donor, a valid organ source in renal transplantation under CyA Therapy? *Transpl Proc*. 1991;23(1):912–913.
125. Bay WH, Herbert LA. The living donor in kidney transplantation. *Ann Intern Med* 1987; 106:719.
126. Opelz G. Influence of recipient in donor age in pediatric renal transplantation. Collaborative Transplant Study. *Transpl Int*. 1988;1:95.
127. Rosenthal JT, Miserantino DP, Mendez R, Coyle MA. Extending the criteria for cadaver

kidney donors. *Transpl Proc*. 1990;22(2):338–339.

128. Alexander JW, Vaughan WK, Carey MA. The use of marginal donors for organ transplantation: the older and younger donors. *Transpl Proc*. 1991;23(1):905–909.

129. Vromen MAM, Leunissen KML, Persijn GG, Kootstra G. Short and long-term results with adult non-heart beating donor kidneys. *Transpl Proc*. 1988;20:743–745.

130. Kootstra G, Wijnen R, VanHoof JP, Vanderlingen CJ. 20% More kidneys through a non-heart beating program. *Transpl Proc*. 1991;23(1):910–911.

# 14

# Nephrolithiasis: Pathogenesis, Diagnosis, and Medical Therapy

*Glenn M. Preminger*

## INTRODUCTION

Considerable progress has been made in the management of nephrolithiasis over the past 10 years. This progress has been particularly noteworthy in the surgical area. Recently, the innovative surgical techniques of percutaneous nephrostolithotomy and extracorporeal shock wave lithotripsy were introduced, allowing efficacious stone removal with a significant reduction in pain and postoperative convalescence as compared to open surgical procedures. Indeed, the dramatic success of these innovative techniques has prompted some physicians to disparage the need for medical evaluation and treatment of nephrolithiasis.

However, there has been equally impressive medical progress toward pathophysiologic elucidation, diagnosis, and management of nephrolithiasis. The urinary environment of patients with stones has been found to be conducive to the crystallization of stone-forming salts because of increased supersaturation and reduced inhibitor activity. The underlying physiologic derangements predisposing to stone formation can now be detected in most patients with renal calculi. Recent clinical trials suggest that recurrent formation of renal stones may be prevented in the majority of patients using a variety of medical treatment programs. This chapter will attempt to discuss the epidemiology of renal calculi, present a comprehensive overview of the pathophysiology of nephrolithiasis, describe an in-depth diagnostic evaluation for patients with stone disease, and, finally, suggest appropriate medical therapy to prevent recurrent nephrolithiasis.

## EPIDEMIOLOGY

Renal calculi are abnormal concretions occurring in the kidneys that can be found anywhere along the collecting system of the urinary tract, which consist of crystalline components incorporated in organic matrix. Nephrolithiasis is a relatively common disorder affecting 1% to 5% of the population in industrialized countries, with an annual incidence having been reported as high as 1% in middle-aged white males. Primary bladder calculi are quite uncommon in industrialized countries except when associated with bladder outlet obstruction (most commonly prostatic obstruction), neuropathic bladder disorders, or encrustation of foreign bodies.

The most common stones seen in industrialized countries contain primarily calcium oxalate occurring alone or in combination with hydroxyapatite. Calcareous calculi account for approximately 75% of renal stones. The remaining 25% of renal calculi are noncalcareous and are composed of either uric acid, struvite, or cystine.

In several unselected population surveys, the lifetime risk for stone formation in adult white males approaches 20%, while for females it is approximately 5%–10%. In addition, the incidence of recurrent nephrolithiasis has been reported as high as 50% within 5 years from the first stone occurrence.[1] After 8 years, 63% of males were reported to form additional stones while there was an 18% recurrent stone rate in female patients.[2] Stone disease in black patients is one third to one fourth less common than in adult white males and blacks demonstrate a higher incidence of infection calculi.[3]

## METABOLIC CLASSIFICATION OF NEPHROLITHIASIS

A logical method of diagnostic differentiation is to categorize nephrolithiasis on the basis of underlying physiologic-environmental abnormalities. This classification assumes that these disturbances are pathogenetically important in stone formation.

In 1972, calcium nephrolithiasis was considered to be composed of three entities: idiopathic hypercalciuria, primary hyperparathyroidism, and normocalciuric nephrolithiasis.[4] The cause of stone formation was not disclosed in the last category, comprising 43% of the patients. However, in 1993, dramatic progress in the diagnostic separation of nephrolithiasis paralleled by advances in analytic methodology has allowed identification of physiologic or environmental causes of stones in more than 97% of patients.[5] Various diagnostic categories and their relative frequency are shown in Table 1.

Calcareous calculi (calcium oxalate or calcium phosphate) make up approximately 75% of renal calculi. Causes of calcareous stone formation include hypercalciuria, hyperoxaluria, hypomagnesiuria, and hypocitraturia. Hypercalciuria and hyperoxaluria contribute to stone formation

**TABLE 1. Classification of Nephrolithiasis**

| Classification | Percentage[a] | |
|---|---|---|
| | Sole Occurrence | Combined Occurrence |
| Absorptive hypercalciuria | 20 | 40 |
| Type I | | |
| Type II | | |
| Renal hypercalciuria | 5 | 8 |
| Primary hyperparathyroidism | 3 | 8 |
| Unclassified Ca nephrolithiasis | 15 | 25 |
| Hyperoxaluric Ca nephrolithiasis | 2 | 15 |
| Enteric hyperoxaluria | | |
| Primary hyperoxaluria | | |
| Dietary hyperoxaluria | | |
| Hypocitraturic Ca Nephrolithiasis | 10 | 50 |
| Distal renal tubular acidosis | | |
| Chronic diarrheal syndrome | | |
| Thiazide-induced | | |
| Idiopathic | | |
| Hypomagnesiuric Ca nephrolithiasis | 5 | 10 |
| Gouty diathesis | 15 | 30 |
| Cystinuria | <1 | |
| Infection stones | 1 | 5 |
| Low urine volume | 10 | 50 |
| No disturbance and miscellaneous | ≤3 | |
| | 100 | |

[a]The percentage for each diagnosis represents approximate estimates based on experience in Dallas, ranging from sole occurrence to combined occurrence with other abnormalities.

by rendering urine super-saturated with respect to stone-forming calcium salts.[6] Hyperuricosuria, in the setting of normal urinary pH (greater than 5.5), has been associated with calcium nephrolithiasis. The pathogenetic role of hypomagnesiuria and hypocitraturia in nephrolithiasis may be ascribed to the inhibitor activity of these substances.[7] Citrate lowers the urinary saturation of calcium oxalate by forming a soluble complex with calcium and lowering calcium activity. Moreover, citrate may directly inhibit crystallization of calcium oxalate and calcium phosphate.[8,9] Recently, macromolecular inhibitors have been identified that are believed to block calcium oxalate crystallization.[10,11] Low volume from inadequate fluid intake contributes to stone formation by rendering the urinary environment supersaturated with respect to stone-forming salts.[12,13]

Among noncalcareous stones, the passage of unusually acidic urine (pH less than 5.5) would favor the formation of uric acid stones because of reduced uric acid solubility in such an environment.[14] In gouty diathesis, uric acid lithiasis may coexist with calcium nephrolithiasis due to urate-induced crystallization of calcium salts. Cystine solubility is also pH-dependent. Patients with cystinuria may form cystine stones when their urinary cystine concentrations exceed the solubility limit.[15] In the presence of urinary tract infection with urea-splitting organisms, the resultant increase in ammonium ions and alkalinity may lead to struvite (magnesium ammonium phosphate) stone formation.[16]

## PHYSIOLOGIC DERANGEMENTS OF CALCIUM NEPHROLITHIASIS

### Pathophysiology of Hypercalciuria

The association of hypercalciuria with recurrent calcium nephrolithiasis has long been recognized, although the exact cause for its relationship with nephrolithiasis continues to be debated. Increased urinary calcium excretion has been demonstrated to increase the saturation of calcium oxalate and brushite as well as to reduce the inhibitor activity in urine against the crystallization of calcium salts by binding negatively charged inhibitors. One current theory considers idiopathic hypercalciuria to comprise several different entities of separate pathogenetic origins.

**Absorptive Hypercalciuria.** The basic abnormality in absorptive hypercalciuria is the intestinal hyperabsorption of calcium.[17] The consequent increase in the circulating concentration of calcium enhances the renal filtered load and suppresses parathyroid function (Fig 1). Hypercalciuria results from the combination of increased filtered load and reduced renal tubular reabsorption of calcium, a function of the parathyroid suppression. The excessive renal loss of calcium compensates for the high calcium absorption from the intestinal tract and helps to maintain serum calcium in the normal range.

Absorptive hypercalciuria occurs in three forms. In absorptive hypercalciuria type I, high urinary calcium is found during both low and high serum intakes, whereas in absorptive hypercalciuria type II, the hypercalciuria occurs only during a high calcium intake. The type II presentation is believed to be a less severe form of type I.

The third type of absorptive hypercalciuria, absorptive hypercalciuria type III, is believed to be secondary to a renal "leak"

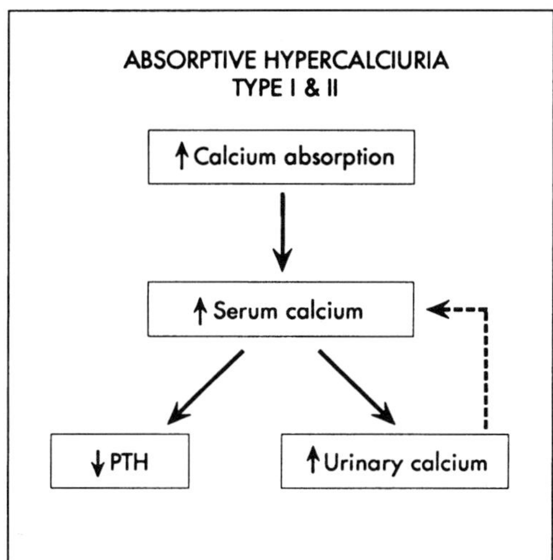


**Fig 1.** Scheme for absorptive hypercalciuria.

of phosphate as the primary event.[18,19] The ensuing hypophosphatemia is thought to stimulate the renal synthesis of 1,25-dihydroxyvitamin D [1,25-$(OH)_2$D] (Fig 1). Enhanced intestinal absorption and renal excretion of calcium would result from the increased synthesis of this vitamin D metabolite.

**Renal Hypercalciuria.** The primary abnormality in renal hypercalciuria is believed to be an impairment in the renal tubular reabsorption of calcium.[17] The resulting reduction in the serum calcium concentration stimulates parathyroid function (Fig 2). There may be excessive mobilization of calcium from bone and an enhanced intestinal absorption of calcium because of the parathyroid hormone (PTH) excess and the ensuing stimulation of the renal synthesis of 1,25-$(OH)_2$D. These effects increase the circulating concentration and the renal filtered load of calcium, often causing significant hypercalciuria.[20] Unlike primary hyperparathyroidism, serum calcium is normal and the state of hyperparathyroidism is secondary.

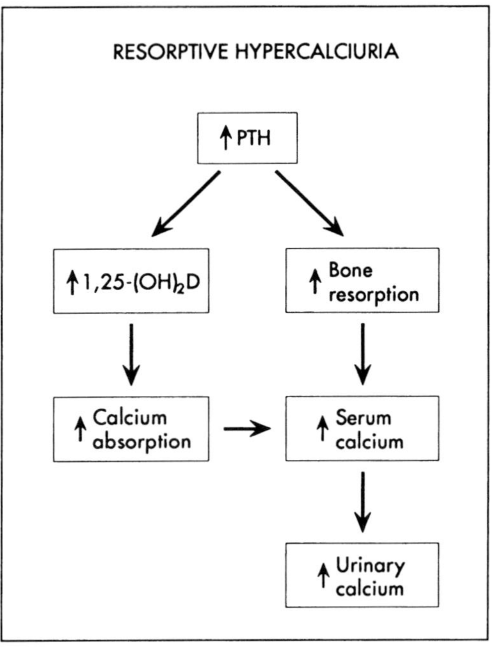


**Fig 3.** Scheme for resorptive hypercalciuria of primary hyperthyroidism.

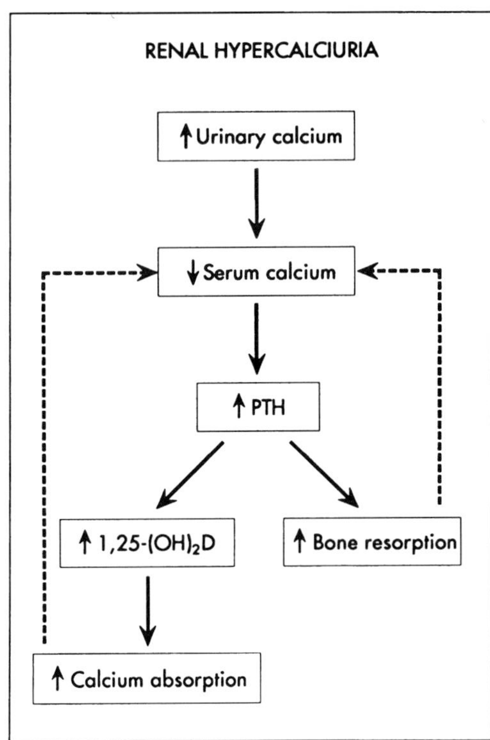


**Fig 2.** Scheme for renal hypercalciuria.

**Resorptive Hypercalciuria.** Resorptive hypercalciuria is characterized by primary hyperparathyroidism. The initial event is the excessive resorption of bone resulting from hypersecretion of PTH (Fig 3). Intestinal absorption of calcium is frequently elevated because of the PTH-dependent stimulation of the renal synthesis of 1,25-$(OH)_2$D.[21] These effects increase the circulating concentration and the renal filtered load of calcium, often causing significant hypercalciuria.[22]

**Fasting Hypercalciuria with Normal Parathyroid Function.** In some patients with normocalcemic hypercalciuric nephrolithiasis, the diagnosis of absorptive or renal hypercalciuria cannot be made with certainty.[23] This unclassified hypercalciuria is represented by fasting hypercalciuria without parathyroid stimulation. This picture points to neither absorptive hypercalciuria nor renal hypercalciuria. The lack of hyperpara-

**TABLE 2. Differential Diagnosis of Hypercalciuria**

| Test | Absorptive | Renal | Resorptive |
|---|---|---|---|
| Serum calcium | Normal | Normal | Elevated |
| Parathyroid function | Suppressed | Stimulated (secondarily) | Stimulated (primarily) |
| Fasting urinary calcium | Normal | Elevated | Elevated |
| Intestinal calcium absorption | Elevated (primarily) | Elevated (secondarily) | Elevated (secondarily) |

thyroidism suggests the diagnosis of absorptive hypercalciuria but the fasting urinary calcium is high. The fasting hypercalciuria indicates that a renal leak of calcium is present. However, secondary stimulation of parathyroid function is lacking. Unclassified hypercalciuria has been reported in as many as 50% of patients with hypercalciuria in some series.

**Differential Diagnosis of Hypercalciuria.** Different forms of hypercalciuria can be differentiated from their biochemical and physiologic pictures (Table 2). While the serum calcium is normal in absorptive hypercalciuria and renal hypercalciuria, patients with resorptive hypercalciuria have elevated circulating calcium levels. Parathyroid hormone is primarily elevated in resorptive hypercalciuria and secondarily elevated in renal hypercalciuria, whereas parathyroid activity is normal or suppressed in absorptive hypercalciuria. Fasting urinary calcium is normal in patients with absorptive hypercalciuria but is elevated in renal hypercalciuria and resorptive hypercalciuria. Finally, all three forms of hypercalciuria are accompanied by an intestinal hyperabsorption of calcium. However, this disturbance is a primary defect in patients with absorptive hypercalciuria and a secondary defect in renal hypercalciuria and resorptive hypercalciuria.

## Pathophysiology of Other Causes of Calcium Stones

**Pathophysiology of Hyperuricosuria.** Hyperuricosuria may be the only recognizable physiologic abnormality in patients with calcium nephrolithiasis (hyperuricosuric calcium oxalate nephrolithiasis).[24,25] The most common cause for hyperuricosuria in patients with hyperuricosuric calcium oxalate nephrolithiasis is probably "dietary overindulgence" with purine-rich foods.[26] When the patient gives a history of a liberal intake of meat, poultry, and fish, an estimated purine intake is much higher than in a comparable control group. This type of hyperuricosuria may be produced by an oral purine load and ameliorated by dietary purine deprivation.[24]

However, some patients with hyperuricosuric calcium oxalate nephrolithiasis (approximately 30%) have hyperuricosuria as a result of uric acid overproduction. Hyperuricosuria persists despite long-term purine deprivation. It is believed that monosodium urate is formed in the supersaturated environment of hyperuricosuric subjects (Fig 4). The monosodium urate

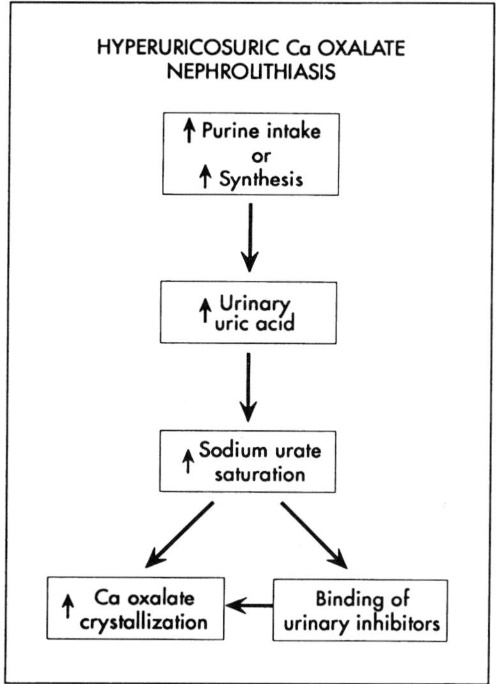


**Fig 4.** Scheme for hyperuricosuria.

(colloidal or crystalline) may then initiate calcium oxalate stone formation by direct induction of heterogeneous nucleation of calcium oxalate or by adsorption of certain macromolecular inhibitors.[27]

**Pathophysiology of Hyperoxaluria.** Urinary oxalate is derived from two major sources. Approximately 80%–90% comes from endogenous production in the liver, whereas the remainder is obtained from dietary oxalate and/or ascorbic acid. Therefore, a primary defect of in vivo oxalate synthesis, dietary overindulgence in oxalate-rich foods, or excessive vitamin C ingestion may all contribute to elevated urinary oxalate levels.[28] In actuality, however, these conditions account for a small number of patients with hyperoxaluria.

The major cause of increased intestinal absorption of oxalate (and subsequent hyperoxaluria) is ileal disease (enteric hyperoxaluria).[29,30] This disturbance may be encountered in patients with inflammatory bowel disease, gastric or small bowel resection, or jejunoileal bypass.[31] Two factors probably act in concert to cause the intestinal hyperabsorption of oxalate (Fig 5). Intestinal transport of oxalate may be primarily increased because of the action of bile salts and fatty acids on the permeability of intestinal mucosa to oxalate. The total amount of oxalate absorbed may also be increased because of an enlarged intraluminal pool of oxalate available for absorption. The intestinal fat malabsorption characteristic of ileal disease may exaggerate calcium soap formation, limit the amount of "free" calcium to complex oxalate, and thereby raise the oxalate pool available for absorption.

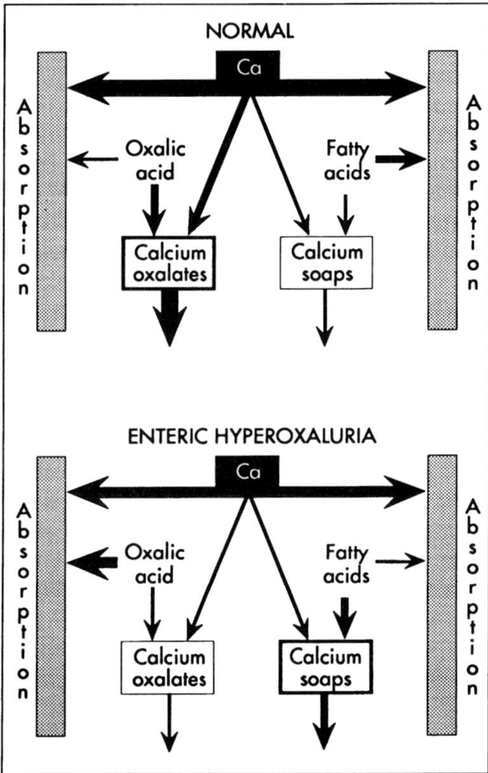


**Fig 5.** Scheme for enteric hyperoxaluria.

Enteric hyperoxaluria presents the added problem of reduced urinary output due to fluid losses from the intestinal tract. Urinary citrate may be low because of hypokalemia and metabolic acidosis.[32] Low urinary magnesium may result from impaired intestinal magnesium absorption.

The cause for the formation of calcium oxalate stones in enteric hyperoxaluria is multifactorial and includes hyperoxaluria as well as some of the other disturbances enumerated.[33] Saturation of urine with respect to calcium oxalate may be increased because of high oxalate excretion, even though urinary calcium may be low. Diminished urine volume exaggerates urinary supersaturation. Moreover, inhibitor activity against crystallization of calcium salts is reduced because of extremely low renal excretion of citrate and magnesium.

**Pathophysiology of Hypocitraturia.** The association between urinary citrate and stone formation has long been recognized, but its major diagnostic and therapeutic implications have only recently been described. Although the exact physiology of renal handling of citrate has not been elucidated, several factors influence its excretion. Citrate excretion may be enhanced by alkalosis, PTH, and vitamin D. On the other hand, citrate excretion may be impaired by acidosis, hypokalemia, and urinary tract infections. Among these factors, the acid–base status probably plays the most important role in the renal handling of citrate. For example, acidosis reduces urinary citrate both by enhancing renal tubular reabsorption and reducing the synthesis of citrate.[34] This mechanism accounts for the occurrence of hypocitraturia in renal tubular acidosis, enteric hyperoxaluria, hypokalemia (from intracellular acidosis), and a high animal protein diet (from elevated acid ash content).[35] Among patients with stones, hypocitraturia is found in all these conditions as well as with urinary tract infection.[32] It also occurs with other causes of calcium nephrolithiasis (10%–50%) and may exist as a solitary abnormality (10%).

Citrate lowers urinary saturation of calcium salts by forming soluble complexes with calcium.[36] Moreover, it directly inhibits the crystallization of calcium salts.[8,9] Thus, in the setting of low urinary citrate, the urinary environment is more supersaturated with respect to calcium salts, and nucleation and growth are promoted.

**Pathophysiology of Hypomagnesiuric Calcium Nephrolithiasis.** Magnesium has been identified as an important inhibitor of calcium nephrolithiasis. Previous clinical studies have demonstrated that treatment with magnesium oxide or magnesium hydroxide may retard recurrent calcium oxalate stone formation.[37,38] Magnesium has been demonstrated to increase the apparent solubility product of calcium oxalate and calcium phosphate.[39]

Despite its infrequent occurrence, hypomagnesiuric calcium nephrolithiasis may represent a unique cause of stone formation.[7] Besides hypomagnesiuria, this entity is characterized by hypocitraturia and low urine volume. Thus, calcium stone formation may result from combined effects of these derangements. Although its exact pathogenetic background is not known, hypomagnesiuria is probably dietary in origin.

**Pathophysiology of Gouty Diathesis.** Passage of acid urine ($pH < 5.5$) can cause both uric acid and calcium stones. Because the urinary pH is very close to or less than the dissociation constant of uric acid, the concentration of undissociated uric acid is high, leading to uric acid crystallization.[40] These uric acid crystals may induce the crystallization of calcium oxalate by the same mechanism described previously for monosodium urate in patients with hyperuricosuria. In addition, uric acid has been shown to remove naturally occurring urinary macromolecular inhibitors, thereby attenuating their activity.[41]

The term *gouty diathesis* has been used to describe the overall clinical entity of uric acid lithiasis.[40,42] The persistent feature is the passage of unusually acidic urine ($pH < 5.5$) in which uric acid is sparingly soluble. Some patients may present with gouty arthritis or hyperuricemia. Stone analysis will disclose uric acid alone or in combination with calcium oxalate/calcium phosphate. Some patients may display the above features of gouty diathesis except for the lack of uric acid on stone analysis. The stones may disclose only the presence of calcium oxalate and/or calcium phosphate. No specific cause has been detected for the unusually low urinary pH. Gouty diathesis may represent a phase of primary gout where the occurrences of hyperuricemia and gouty arthritis represent the full manifestation of the syndrome, whereas the picture of low urinary pH and uric acid/calcium nephrolithiasis without hyperuricemia or gouty arthritis reflects an early phase of classic gout.

### Pathophysiology of Noncalcareous Stones

**Uric Acid Stones.** Critical determinants for pure uric acid lithiasis are urinary pH less than the dissociation constant for uric acid (5.47) and/or hyperuricosuria. Uric acid stones are often formed in primary gout, which may be accompanied by low urinary pH and hyperuricosuria, but may also be found in secondary causes of purine overproduction, such as myeloproliferative states, glycogen storage disease, and malignancy (Table 3).[43] Chronic diarrheal syndromes (ulcerative colitis, regional enteritis, jejunoileal bypass surgery) may cause uric acid lithiasis by inducing net alkali deficit and lowering urine volume (thereby reducing urinary pH and aug-

**TABLE 3. Causes of Increased Urinary Uric Acid**

Abnormal production
- Genetic overproduction
  - Enzymatic mutation (ie, hypoxanthine-guanine phosphoribosyltransferase [HGPRT] deficiency)
- Acquired overproduction
  - Myeloproliferative disorders
  - Obesity
  - Alcohol ingestion

Abnormal excretion
- Diet high in purines
- Uricosuric drugs

menting urinary concentration of uric acid, respectively).[14,44]

**Cystine Stones.** Cystinuria is an inborn error of metabolism characterized by a disturbance in renal and intestinal handling of dicarboxylic acids, including cystine.[45] Stone formation, occurring in a minority of patients, is the result of an excessive renal excretion of cystine and its low solubility in urine. Cystine solubility is extremely pH-dependent, with lowest solubility at low range of urinary pH, gradual increase solubility with pH rising to 7.5, and rapid increase in solubility above a pH of 7.5.

The main determinant of cystine crystallization is urinary supersaturation.[46] If the urine sample is supersaturated with respect to cystine, precipitation of cystine invariably occurs. Once the urinary saturation of cystine exceeds 250 mg/L, cystine will precipitate out of solution. If one can maintain the cystine concentration under 200 mg/L, then cystine stones should not occur. Thus, there is a stronger cause-and-effect relationship between excessive cystine excretion and stone formation than for any other form of stone disease (ie, between hypercalciuria and calcium nephrolithiasis). Moreover, recent studies have demonstrated that 18%–44% of cystine stone formers will also have associated metabolic defects (ie, hypercalciuria, hyperuricosuria, hypocitraturia) which may complicate their cystine nephrolithiasis.[47]

**Infection (Struvite) Stones.** Infection of the urinary tract with urea-splitting organisms may be associated with renal stones of struvite and of calcium carbonate apatite. The critical determinant is the formation of ammonia in urine due to enzymatic degradation of urea by bacterial urease.[48] The ammonia undergoes hydrolysis to form ammonium and hydroxyl ions. The resulting alkalinity of the urine augments dissociation of phosphate to form triphosphate ions and reduces the solubility of struvite. Thus, the urinary environment becomes supersaturated with respect to struvite. Although struvite stones may form de novo from infection alone, they also occur as a complication of other causes of renal calculi such as hypercalciuria.

It is most important to note that patients with infection stones have the same percentage of underlying metabolic derangements (ie, hypercalciuria, hypocitraturia, etc.) as does the general stone-forming population.[49] Therefore, these patients should be metabolically evaluated and prophylactic treatment offered.

## DIAGNOSTIC EVALUATION OF NEPHROLITHIASIS

The goal of a diagnostic evaluation of nephrolithiasis should be to identify as efficiently and economically as possible the particular physiologic defect present in a given patient with nephrolithiasis to enable selective, rational therapy of his stone disease.[23]

Such an evaluation should be capable of identifying specific medical disorders responsible for recurrent stone disease. These include renal tubular acidosis, primary hyperparathyroidism, enteric hyperoxaluria, cystinuria, and uric acid calculi. In these relatively uncommon conditions, it is generally agreed that selective medical therapy is indicated not only to prevent further stone formation but to correct the underlying physiologic disturbance, which may lead to other metabolic or physiologic problems.

Yet, for the more common ''idiopathic'' hypercalciuric nephrolithiasis, many physicians believe that extensive diagnostic endeavors are not warranted since most of these patients will respond to thiazide diuretics. However, the term *idiopathic* should now be discarded since much is known regarding the pathogenesis of hypercalciuria. Moreover, the response to thiazide depends on the nature of hypercalciuria. Recent work has demonstrated that thiazide does not correct the specific physiologic defect responsible for hypercalciuria in patients with absorptive hypercalciuria, unlike in renal hypercalciuria.[50,51] In addition, thiazide therapy alone may cause or exaggerate hypocitraturia, contributing to calcium stone formation.[52] Therefore, an extensive diagnostic evaluation may be warranted to identify specific metabolic defects and allow individualized therapy.

Another criticism of extensive metabolic evaluation for recurrent stone formers is the complexity of these tests, making them unavailable to many practicing physicians. While many of the early diagnostic protocols were developed at research centers and utilized sophisticated procedures, newer ambulatory protocols have been devised that allow reliable diagnostic evaluation and that can be performed by a practicing physician without the use of sophisticated instrumentation. Moreover, an ambulatory evaluation can provide certain information not available from inpatient diagnostic protocols, such as the influence of customary diet and habits on stone formation.[23]

### Selection of Patients for Metabolic Evaluation

There has been much debate concerning the selection of patients as to who should undergo a diagnostic evaluation. Since stone disease is a relatively common disorder, extensive metabolic workup of all patients with nephrolithiasis combined with prolonged medical therapy would be time consuming and expensive. Although studies have shown that "single-stone formers" have the same incidence and severity of metabolic derangements as patients with recurrent stone disease,[53] some patients will not form recurrent stones despite the absence of treatment. In addition, a study of single-stone formers placed on a conservative program of high fluid intake and avoidance of dietary excess revealed a low incidence of recurrent stone disease.[54]

However, as mentioned previously, recurrent stone formation within 8 years has been reported in upward of 63% of adult males with the single-stone episode.[1] Moreover, in some patients, the initial stone episode may be a harbinger of an underlying multisystem disease such as renal tubular acidosis or renal hypercalciuria with secondary hyperparathyroidism. In such patients, specific medical therapy is justified solely to prevent extrarenal derangements such as metabolic bone disease.

One final consideration is the relatively low cost of a comprehensive medical evaluation when compared to the expense of stone removal or the care of complications secondary to stone disease.[55,56] Thus, one may consider a diagnostic evaluation to be cost-effective since it allows for the selection of effective prophylactic therapy of nephrolithiasis.

### Evaluation of Single-Stone Formers

The decision to thoroughly investigate a first-time stone former ideally should be shared by the physician and the patient.[57] While some first-time stone formers will readily accept and follow conservative therapy, others may elect to undergo a thorough evaluation. One approach is to gauge the extent of evaluation according to the estimation of potential/risk for new stone formation. Patients at high risk might be middle-aged, white males with a family history of stones, those with intestinal disease (chronic diarrheal states), pathologic skeletal fractures, osteoporosis, urinary tract infection, or gout. In these patients, an extensive evaluation is recommended. Any patients with stones composed of cystine, uric acid, or struvite should undergo a complete metabolic workup. In addition, all children with nephrolithiasis should be required to undergo a complete investigation. Because stone disease is uncommon in blacks, especially black women, one should determine the underlying etiology of nephrolithiasis in all black patients.[3]

However, the indications for performing an extensive metabolic evaluation on a first-time calcium stone former with no significant risk factors for recurrent stone disease are less clear.[58] While no reliable method exists to predict the risk of recurrent stone formation in all patients who have passed their first stone, certain factors may enable the physician to predict which of these patients are at higher risk for recurrent stone disease and therefore undergo a more extensive diagnostic evaluation.

### Abbreviated Protocol for Low-Risk Single-Stone Formers

In single-stone formers without risk, the following abbreviated protocol may be applied (Table 4). A thorough medical history should be obtained for any underlying condition that may have contributed to the stone disease. In addition, information should be gleaned concerning the patient's dietary habits including fluid consumption and excessive intake of certain foods, as well as a list of all medications taken. A multichannel blood screen can be helpful in identifying certain systemic problems. These include primary hyperparathyroidism (high serum calcium and low serum phosphorus), absorptive hypercalciuria type III (hypophosphatemia), uric acid lithiasis (hyperuricemia), and distal renal tubular acidosis (abnormalities in the serum electrolytes).

**TABLE 4. Abbreviated Evaluation of Single-Stone Formers Without Risk**

- History
  - Underlying predisposing conditions
  - Medications (Ca, Vitamin C, Vitamin D, acetazolamide, steroids)
  - Dietary excesses, inadequate fluid intake, or excessive fluid loss
- Multichannel Blood Screen
  - High calcium: primary hyperparathyroidism
  - Low phosphorus: absorptive hypercalciuria type III
  - High uric acid: gouty diathesis
  - Low K and $CO_2$, high Cl: distal renal tubular acidosis
- Urine
  - Urinalysis
    - pH >7.5: infection lithiasis
    - pH <5.5: uric acid lithiasis
    - Sediment for crystalluria
  - Urine culture
    - Urea-splitting organisms: suggestive of infection lithiasis
  - Qualitative cystine
- X-ray
  - Radiopaque stones: calcium oxalate, calcium phosphate, magnesium ammonium phosphate (struvite), cystine
  - Radiolucent stones: Uric acid, xanthine, 2-hydroxyadenine, triamterene
  - IVP: Radiolucent stones, anatomic abnormalities
- Stone Analysis

Voided urinary specimens should be obtained for comprehensive urinalysis and culture. The urinalysis should include pH determination since a pH of greater than 7.5 is compatible with possible infection lithiasis, while a pH of less than 5.5 may suggest uric acid lithiasis. The urine sediment is also examined for crystalluria since particular crystal types may give a clue as to the composition of stones the patient is forming. Urine cultures positive for urea-splitting organisms such as *Proteus, Pseudomonas,* and *Klebsiella* are suggestive of infection lithiasis. In addition, urine should be examined for the presence of cystine using a qualitative examination (nitroprusside test).

Abdominal x-rays should be obtained to document the existence of any residual stones within the urinary tract. The radiopacity of any existing stones may suggest the type of stones that are present. While magnesium ammonium phosphate and cystine stones are often radiopaque, they are not as dense as calcium oxalate or calcium phosphate stones. A plain abdominal film is also useful in identifying nephrocalcinosis (suggestive of renal tubular acidosis) and staghorn calculi (likely due to infection lithiasis). An intravenous pyelogram may be obtained to confirm the presence of radiolucent stones and also to identify any anatomic abnormalities that may be responsible for stone formation.

Finally, any available stones should be analyzed to determine their crystalline composition. The presence of uric acid or cystine crystals would suggest the presence of gouty diathesis or cystinuria, respectively. The finding of struvite, carbonate apatite, and magnesium ammonium phosphate would suggest infection lithiasis. A predominance of hydroxyapatite crystals suggests the presence of renal tubular acidosis or primary hyperparathyroidism. Stones composed of pure calcium oxalate or mixed calcium oxalate and hydroxyapatite are less useful diagnostically since they may occur in several entities including absorptive and renal hypercalciuria, hyperuricosuric calcium nephrolithiasis, enteric hyperoxaluria, hypocitraturic calcium nephrolithiasis, and low urine volume.

### Extensive Diagnostic Evaluation

A more extensive evaluation, directed at the identification of underlying physiologic derangements, should be performed in patients with recurrent nephrolithiasis as well as in stone formers at increased risk for further stone formation.[59] Patients whom one might consider at higher risk for recurrent stone disease include middle-aged white males with a family history of stones as well as those with chronic diarrheal states secondary to intestinal disease, osteoporosis, pathologic skeletal fractures, recurrent urinary tract infections, or gout. An extensive evaluation should be considered for these patients.

The extensive diagnostic approach to nephrolithiasis has evolved along with the increased availability of specialized analytic techniques. Many of the original comprehensive diagnostic procedures were developed in research centers and required an inpatient hospital admission, a constant dietary regimen prepared by a metabolic kitchen, sophisticated laboratory techniques, and trained personnel at every level.

In 1974, Pak et al. detailed an inpatient protocol for the evaluation of the pathophysiology of hypercalciuric nephrolithiasis.[4] Prior to this time, calcium nephrolithiasis was classified only as primary hyperparathyroidism, idiopathic hypercalciuria, or normocalciuric nephrolithiasis. This last category, which included stone formers without a definitive etiology, comprised almost 43% of patients. It was toward this group that the extensive metabolic evaluation was directed for further elucidation. The next major advance was the introduction of the ''fasting and calcium load'' test in 1975.[60] This test facilitated the diagnostic evaluation of hypercalciuria and was easily incorporated into an ambulatory study. In 1976, Pak et al. formulated an outpatient protocol.[61] It required collection of three 24-hr urine specimens—two while on a random diet and one while on a diet restricted in calcium and sodium. During the second of two outpatient visits, the fast and calcium load test was performed. The results of this ambulatory protocol correlate well with those of the extensive inpatient metabolic evaluation and allow additional information on environmental and dietary influences obtained from analysis of the two 24-hr urine specimens collected while on a random diet.[61]

Utilizing this basic protocol and incorporating more recent biochemical analyses (citrate, sensitive parathyroid hormone assay), it is now possible to diagnose the cause of stone formation in more than 97% of patients (Table 1).

### Description of Ambulatory Protocol

Once a patient has been identified as a recurrent stone former with a high potential risk for new stone formation, the ambulatory protocol for metabolic evaluation should be initiated.

One current version of the ambulatory evaluation involves two outpatient visits that can be completed in less than 3 weeks.[23] Most of the required laboratory analyses can be performed in a routine clinical laboratory with only a few of the specialized techniques being performed in a more sophisticated laboratory. The schedule of laboratory tests is outlined in Table 5.

Prior to and throughout the period of evaluation, the patient is instructed to discontinue any medication that is known to interfere with the metabolism of calcium, uric acid, or oxalate. These medications include vitamin D, calcium supplements, antacids, acetazolamide, and vitamin C. Current medication for stone treatment (thiazide, phosphate, allopurinol, or magnesium) should be discontinued as well. Three 24-hr urine samples are collected.

**TABLE 5. Outline of Extensive Ambulatory Protocol**

| | Blood | | | | Urine | | | | | | |
|---|---|---|---|---|---|---|---|---|---|---|---|
| | Complete Blood Count | SMA | PTH | Calcium | Uric Acid | Creatinine | Sodium | pH | Total Volume | Oxalate | Citrate | Qualitative Cystine |
| Visit 1[a] | X | X | | X | X | X | X | X | X | X | X | X |
| Visit 2[b] | | X | X | X | X | X | X | X | X | X | X | |
| Fast | | | | X | | X | | | X | | | |
| Load | | | | X | | X | | | X | | | |

[a]History and physical examination, diet history, radiologic evaluation, two 24-hr urines on random diet, and dietary instruction for restricted diet.
[b]24-hr urine on restricted diet (400 mg calcium and 100 mEq sodium a day, fast, and load test.

Two are obtained with the patient on a random diet, which is reflective of their usual dietary intake. The third 24-hr sample is collected after a week of a calcium-, sodium-, and oxalate-restricted diet. This dietary restriction is imposed to standardize the diagnostic tests, to better assess the etiology of hypercalciuria, and to prepare for the fast and calcium load test, which is performed on the second visit. Blood samples are obtained on both visits.

**First Visit.** A detailed history is taken to define the extent and activity of stone disease especially in the preceding 3 years. Parameters used to assess the aggressiveness of stone disease are the frequency of stone passage and/or the number of urologic procedures required for stone removal.

A thorough past medical history may provide clues as to the etiology of the stone disease. A history of skeletal fracture and peptic ulcer disease suggests possible primary hyperparathyroidism. Intestinal disease such as chronic diarrheal states, ileal disease, or intestinal resection may predispose the patient to enteric hyperoxaluria or hypocitraturia resulting in calcium oxalate stones. Patients with gout may form uric acid stones or calcium oxalate stones. A history of recurrent urinary tract infections may suggest infection nephrolithiasis. A physical exam should be performed but is rarely helpful unless the etiology of the stone disease has extrarenal manifestations (such as band keratopathy in hypercalcemia and tophi in hyperuricemia).

A family history for stones is taken to ascertain those etiologies that elicit a familial tendency—absorptive hypercalciuria, cystinuria, renal tubular acidosis, and primary hyperoxaluria. Medical regimens that have been instituted in the past for stone disease are discussed in detail. The failure of certain therapeutic modalities may indicate that the etiology is different from that initially suspected and that a more specific rational approach to treatment is needed.

A careful history of dietary habits, fluid ingestion, and over-the-counter (OTC) drug usage is obtained. Dietary indiscretion with regard to foods high in calcium, oxalate, and purines can aggravate existing stone disease as can inadequate fluid ingestion and frequent use of selected OTC drugs such as calcium-rich antacid tablets and high doses of vitamin C.

To this first visit, patients should bring a recent abdominal plain radiography (KUB) or intravenous pyelogram if one has been performed. If not, roentgenographic studies should be obtained. Any stone that has been passed or removed should be sent for quantitative crystallographic analysis, which will provide information on the amount and distribution of the various components.

Fasting venous blood samples drawn on the first visit should be submitted for CBC (complete blood count) and automated blood analysis (SMA) (which includes calcium, phosphorus, alkaline phosphatase, sodium potassium, chloride, carbon dioxide, creatinine, and uric acid).

Measurement of calcium, uric acid, creatinine, sodium oxalate, citrate, pH, and total volume should be performed on the 24-urine samples on two consecutive days while the patient is on a random diet. A single qualitative cystine analysis is sufficient as an initial screen for cystinuria.

The patient is then instructed to follow a restricted diet for at least 7 days prior to the second visit. Dietary restrictions include calcium (400 mg/d), sodium (100 mEq/d), and oxalate (50 mg/d). It is helpful to provide the patient with a prepared list of specific foods that are allowed and those that are to be avoided (can be obtained from author). In general, patients should abstain from dairy products and high-salt foods such as snack foods, canned soups, and processed meats.

**Second Visit.** On the second visit, a 24-hr urine specimen that has been collected on the last day of the restricted diet is submitted for analysis. It is assayed for calcium, uric acid, creatinine, sodium, oxalate, citrate, pH, and total volume. A fasting venous blood sample is again drawn for multichannel screening (as on the first visit) and also for immunoreactive parathyroid hormone.

A fast and calcium load study is performed on the morning of the second visit.[60] It is essential that the patients have adhered to the restricted diet (as outlined above) for at least 7 days prior to this testing so as to eliminate the effects of absorbed calcium on fasting calcium excretion. To assure adequate hydration, distilled water (300 mL each) is to be taken 12 hr and 9 hr prior to the calcium loading. Other than water ingestion at these time periods, the patients are to be fasting. Two hours prior to the scheduled calcium loading, patients empty their bladder completely, discard the urine, and drink an additional 600 mL of distilled water. Urine is to be collected as a pooled sample for the 2 hr prior to taking the calcium load (fasting urine). After the 2-hr fasting urine collection has been completed, a 1-g oral calcium load is administered using 250 mL of a liquid synthetic diet (Calcitest) as a carrier solution. This is prepared by first adding 500 mL of water to a can of Calcitest. Only 250 mL of the synthetic meal is used for each calcium load. Since 250 mL of the synthetic meal contains only 100 mg of calcium, 39 mL of Neocalglucon (900 mg of calcium) must be added to bring the total calcium up to 1 g. The final mixture should be taken slowly over a 5- to 10-min period. (Calcitest may be obtained from the author. Other standard meals may be substituted for Calcitest so long as the load contains 1 g elemental calcium and results in control subjects have been established.)

For the next 4 hr, urine is again collected as a pooled sample (postload urine). Both fasting and postload samples are then assayed for calcium and creatinine. Fasting urinary calcium is expressed as mg/dL glomerular filtrate (GF) since it is reflective of renal function. To obtain this unit of measurement, the urinary calcium in mg/mg creatinine is multiplied by the serum creatinine in mg/dL. Normal fasting urinary calcium is <0.11 mg/dL GF. The postload urinary calcium is best expressed as mg/mg creatinine as it is a function of a fixed oral calcium load. The normal value for this measurement is <0.2 mg calcium/mg creatinine.

## Classification of Nephrolithiasis and Diagnostic Criteria

Using the ambulatory protocol previously described, the etiology of nephrolithiasis can be classified into 13 categories reflecting specific physiologic derangements. In <3% of patients, no abnormality can be detected. These categories are listed in Table 1 along with their relative frequency. Diagnostic criteria for the 13 forms of nephrolithiasis will now be summarized; those for 12 principal presentations are compared in Table 6.

**Absorptive Hypercalciuria (AH) Type I.** This condition is characterized by normal serum calcium and phosphorus; normal or suppressed parathyroid function (normal serum immunoreactive PTH), normal fasting urinary calcium (<0.11 mg/dL GF), exaggerated urinary calcium following an oral calcium load (>0.2 mg/mg creatinine), and urinary calcium of >200 mg/d

**TABLE 6. Diagnostic Criteria**

| | Serum | | | | Urinary | | | | | | |
|---|---|---|---|---|---|---|---|---|---|---|---|
| Disorder | Ca | P | PTH | Ca Fasting | Ca Load | Ca Restricted | UA | Ox | Cit | pH | Mg |
| Absorptive hypercalciuria type I | N | N | N | N | ↑ | ↑ | N | N | N | N | N |
| Absorptive hypercalciuria type II | N | N | N | N | ↑ | N | N | N | N | N | N |
| Renal hypercalciuria | N | N | ↑ | ↑ | ↑ | ↑ | N | N | N | N | N |
| Primary hyperparathyroidism | ↑ | ↓ | ↑ | ↑ | ↑ | ↑ | N | N | N | N | N |
| Unclassified hypercalciuria | N | N/↓ | N | ↑ | ↑ | ↑ | N | N | N | N | N |
| Hyperuricosuria | N | N | N | N | N | N | ↑ | N | N | N | N |
| Enteric hyperoxaluria | N/↓ | N/↓ | N/↓ | ↓ | ↓ | ↓ | ↓ | ↑ | ↓ | N | N |
| Hypocitraturia | N | N | N | N | N | N | N | N | ↓ | N | N |
| Renal tubular acidosis | N | N | N/↑ | ↑ | N | N/↑ | N | N | ↓ | N/↑ | N |
| Hypomagnesiuria | N | N | N | N | N | N | N/↓ | N | ↓ | N | ↓ |
| Gouty diathesis | N | N | N | N | N | N | N/↑ | N | N/↓ | ↓ | N |
| Infection lithiasis | N | N | N | N | N | N | N | N | ↓ | ↑ | N |

*Note:* Fasting samples represent 2-hr collections obtained in morning following an overnight fast. Ca load samples were obtained over a 4-hr period subsequent to oral ingestion of 1 g Ca. PTH, immunoreactive parathyroid hormone; ↑, high; ↓, low; N, normal; UA, uric acid; Ox, oxalate; Cit, citrate; Mg, magnesium.

on a restricted diet of 400 mg calcium and 100 MEq sodium/day. These laboratory values reflect the characteristic features of this disorder, ie, increased intestinal calcium absorption with resultant parathyroid suppression and hypercalciuria.

**Absorptive Hypercalciuria (AH) Type II.** Biochemically, this is the same disorder as AH type I with the single exception of a normal urinary calcium (<200 mg/d) while on a restricted diet. AH type II is considered a less severe form of AH type I.

**Renal Hypercalciuria.** This condition is represented by normal serum calcium, high fasting urinary calcium (>0.11 mg/dL GF), and evidence of parathyroid stimulation (elevated serum immunoreactive PTH). These values represent a renal leak of calcium with a subsequent increase in PTH secretion. Confirmation of the diagnosis of renal hypercalciuria requires an elevated level of serum PTH. Because the hyperparathyroid state is a secondary phenomenon in response to the renal loss of calcium, it is suppressible with an oral calcium load. As a result of the secondary hyperparathyroidism, osteopenia and low bone density have been noted in some patients.

**Primary Hyperparathyroidism.** The feature of this condition is elevated serum and urinary calcium with decreased serum phosphorus in the presence of increased or inappropriately high serum PTH. Symptoms of peptic ulcer disease and bone disease may also be present.

**Unclassified Hypercalciuria (Fasting Hypercalciuria with Normal Parathyroid Function).** This condition is characterized by normal serum calcium and PTH, and high fasting calcium (>0.11 mg/dL GF). This entity presents a particular problem since it has some features of both absorptive hypercalciuria and renal hypercalciuria but lacks the distinctive characteristics needed for differentiation (Table 7). Fasting hypercalciuria supports the diagnosis of renal hypercalciuria but parathyroid stimulation is absent. The lack of secondary hyperparathyroidism is supporting evidence for AH, but fasting urinary calcium is high.

Possible explanations for this unusual presentation include inadequate dietary restriction prior to testing, insensitive PTH assay, excessive skeletal mobilization of calcium from factors other than PTH, and altered set point for PTH release or increased end-organ sensitivity to PTH. A sodium cellulose phosphate trial (to be de-

**TABLE 7. Unclassified Hypercalciuria**

| Factor | Absorptive Hypercalciuria | Renal Hypercalciuria | Unclassified Hypercalciuria |
|---|---|---|---|
| Fasting urinary calcium | Normal | Elevated | Elevated |
| Parathyroid function | Normal | Elevated | Normal |
| Primary defect | Hyperabsorption intestinal calcium | Renal leak of calcium | ?Bone mobilization/other |

scribed) may help clarify the situation by eliminating the effect of excess absorbed calcium.[62]

**Hyperuricosuric Calcium Nephrolithiasis.** Essential features include high urinary uric acid (>600 mg/d on a mean of three samples and on at least two of the three samples), normal serum calcium, normal fasting and calcium load response, normal urinary calcium and oxalate (<45 mg/d), and calcium nephrolithiasis. Urinary pH is usually >5.5.

**Hyperoxaluria.** Urinary oxalate exceeds 45 mg/d. This disorder may be primary, enteric, or diet-related. With oxalate levels >80 mg/d, the diagnosis is most likely primary hyperoxaluria or enteric hyperoxaluria. Dietary indiscretions regarding oxalate-rich foods may also result in mild to moderate hyperoxaluria (urinary oxalate 45–80 mg/d).

**Hypocitraturic Calcium Nephrolithiasis.** Hypocitraturic calcium nephrolithiasis can present as the sole physiologic abnormality or in tandem with other metabolic disorders. Hypocitraturia (urinary citrate <320 mg/d) may be a consequence of acidotic states (ie, distal renal tubular acidosis and chronic diarrheal states) or a result of thiazide-induced hypokalemia.

Distal renal tubular acidosis can present as either the complete form or the incomplete form. The complete form is characterized by a high serum chloride, low serum potassium, low serum carbon dioxide, and high urinary pH (>6.8), whereas the incomplete form presents with normal serum electrolytes but the inability to acidify urine following an ammonium chloride load. Patients with this disorder have medullary nephrocalcinosis and/or nephrolithiasis. The associated hypercalciuria, hypocitraturia, and alkaline urine are risk factors predisposing this condition to calcium phosphate stone formation (less commonly, calcium oxalate nephrolithiasis).

**Hypomagnesiuric Calcium Nephrolithiasis.** Hypomagnesiuria (urinary magnesium <50 mg/d) is the principal finding in this condition. Also noted are hypocitraturia (in approximately two thirds of patients) and low urine volume (<1 L/d in approximately 40% of patients). The majority of patients will give a history of limited intake of magnesium-rich foods such as chocolate and/or nuts, a finding suggesting that hypomagnesiuria is dietary in origin.

**Gouty Diathesis.** The constant feature of gouty diathesis is the persistent passage of unusually acidic urine (pH < 5.5). The cause of low urinary pH has not been ascertained. Some patients may present with hyperuricemia or hypertriglyceridemia. Stones formed may be uric acid alone, calcium oxalate-phosphate alone, or a mixture of the two. Occasionally, patients may alternate forming either uric acid or calcium calculi.

**Cystinuria.** Cystinuria is a genetic disorder involving a defective renal reabsorption of cystine. The diagnosis should be suspected in anyone with a childhood history of renal stones, recurrent stone episodes, and a positive family history of stone disease. Confirmation is made by a simple cyanide-nitroprusside screening test of urine and further documented by quantitative chromatography indicating urinary cystine values greater than 250 mg/g creatinine. Microscopic examination of urinary sediment will reveal characteristic cystine crystals.

**Infection Lithiasis.** Infection lithiasis is confirmed by the disclosure of magnesium ammonium phosphate on stone analysis. Urinary pH is high (>7.5), as is ammonium content. Patients who present with recurrent or persistent bacteriuria involving urea-splitting organisms (*Proteus, Pseudomonas, Klebsiella,* and certain species of *Staphylococcus*) are at risk for stone formation. The classic radiologic finding is a radiopaque staghorn calculus.

**Low Urine Volume.** Low urine volume is defined as urinary output of less than 1000 mL/d. A daily urinary volume of less than 2000 mL is considered inadequate. The most common explanation for this condition is minimal fluid ingestion but it is also seen in patients with chronic diarrheal states that result in large amounts of intestinal fluid loss. Low urine volumes contribute to stone formation by providing a concentrated environment for stone-forming substances, most notably calcium, uric acid, and oxalate.

**No Pathologic Disturbance.** No physiologic disturbance denotes normal serum calcium and PTH; normal fast and calcium load response; and normal values for urinary calcium, uric acid, and oxalate in the presence of calcium nephrolithiasis. The cause for stone formation remains unknown. It accounts for less than 3% of all nephrolithiasis.

### Simplified Metabolic Evaluation

The previously described extensive ambulatory protocol affords the physician a high diagnostic yield and is quite reliable. Therefore, this evaluation should be considered in those patients with recurrent nephrolithiasis or with a high risk for recurrent stone disease. Unfortunately, some practicing physicians have found this protocol to be time consuming and difficult to perform due to the inability to obtain certain laboratory tests. A simplified diagnostic protocol may be performed that utilizes the same standard principles and procedures as a standard outpatient evaluation yet incorporates commercially available diagnostic tests, thus making it available to all physicians.

The cornerstone of this simplified protocol has been the development of a urine preservation method that allows collection of urine without refrigeration and submission of an aliquot to a central laboratory for the analysis of various stone-forming substances[63] (StoneRisk Patient Profile, Mission Pharmacal Company, San Antonio, TX). The urinary constituents assayed include calcium, oxalate, and citrate (which may result from underlying metabolic problems) as well as total volume, sodium, and sulfate (which are influenced by environmental or dietary factors) (Table 8). From such determinations, the urinary saturation with respect to stone-forming salts can be calculated. A graphic display of this information may then be generated, highlighting the increased or reduced risk for each environmental, metabolic, or physicochemical factor (Fig 6). This automated stone risk analysis is one of many analysis packages that are commercially available in the U.S.

**Collection and Determination of Urinary Constituents.** After discontinuing any med-

**TABLE 8. Summary of Risk Factors Identified by Automated Stone Risk Profile**

| Metabolic Factors | Environmental Factors | Physicochemical Factors | Other Factors |
|---|---|---|---|
| Calcium | Total volume | Calcium oxalate | Creatinine |
| Oxalate | Sodium | Brushite | Potassium |
| Uric acid | Sulfate | Sodium urate | Ammonium |
| Citrate | Phosphorus | Struvite | |
| pH | Magnesium | Uric acid | |

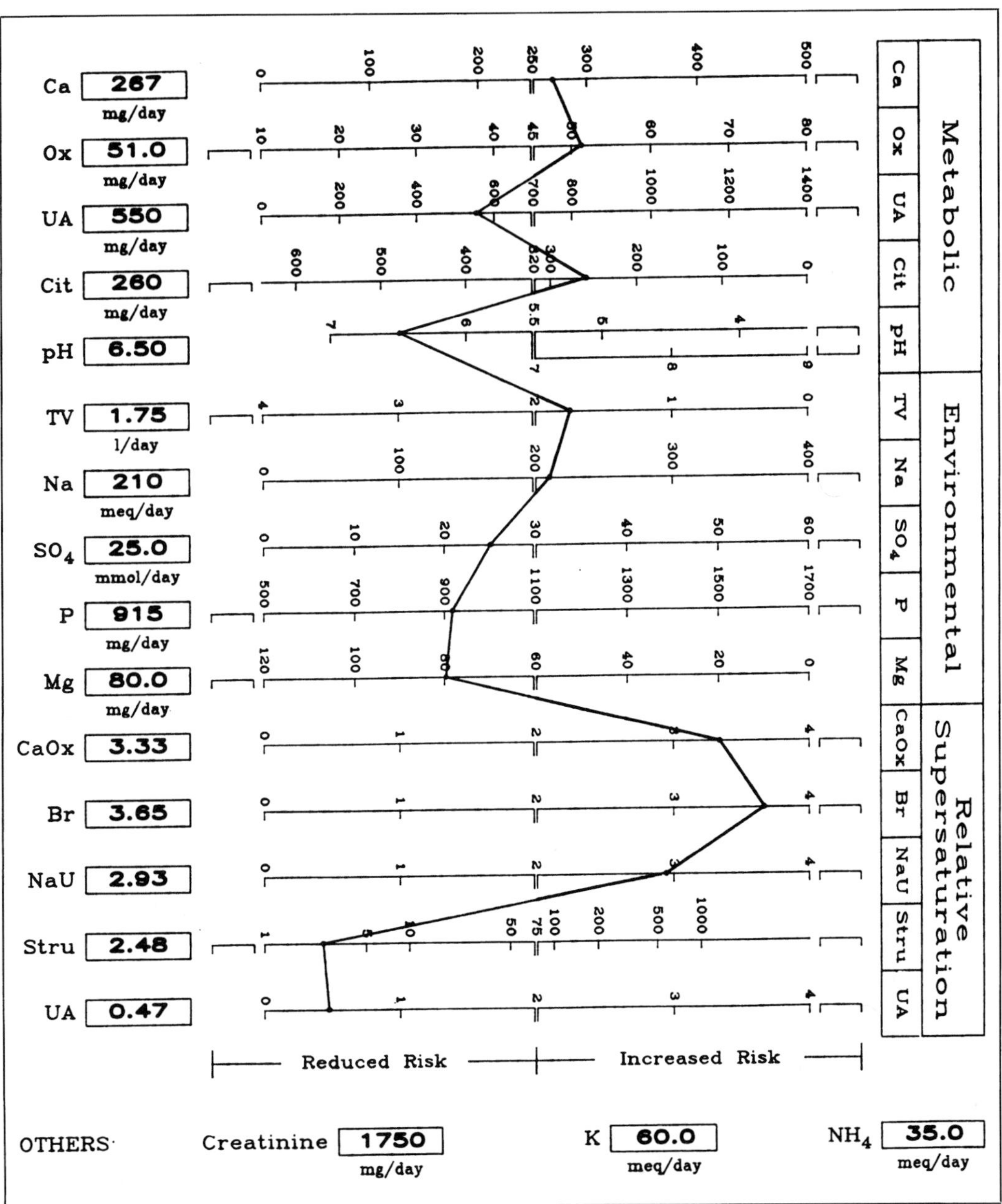


**Fig 6.** Example of an automated urinalysis profile (StoneRisk Patient Profile: Mission Pharmacal Company, San Antonio, TX).

ication that may alter the test results, one 24-hr urine collection is obtained with the patient on his or her normal diet and fluid intake. This random urine analysis should allow for screening of specific metabolic derangements and environmental influences. The first group of urinary constituents identified by the automated stone risk analysis are considered metabolic factors since alteration in the excretion of these substances may be secondary to metabolic disturbances and can lead to an increased risk of stone formation. These factors include calcium, oxalate, uric acid, citrate, and pH. The next set of risk factors for stone formation are deemed environmental factors since excretion of these substances can be controlled by the patient and are usually due to dietary habits. These factors include total volume, sodium, sulfate, phosphorus, and magnesium. Physicochemical factors are determined by various concentrations of the metabolic and environmental factors and represent the urinary saturations of calcium oxalate, brushite, monosodium urate, struvite, and uric acid.

**Interpretation of Data.** After the values of all urinary constituents and saturations have been determined, the physician receives a computerized printout that provides both a graphic and numeric display of the test results (Fig 6). These results should aid the physician in formulating a metabolic/physiologic diagnosis. However, it is usually not possible to make a definitive diagnosis of a particular metabolic derangement without further testing. For example, it is desirable to confirm the presence of hypocitraturia or hyperuricosuria by repeat measurements. In addition, while this graphic analysis will demonstrate hypercalciuria, it is not able to differentiate between the different forms of hypercalciuria. Finally, it is important to note that the ''normal limits'' cited on commercially available urine analysis packages, such as the StoneRisk Patient Profile, are not the same as those normal values that have been quoted previously where 24-hr urinary calcium of greater than 200 mg/d are considered abnormal. However, on the StoneRisk Patient Profile, the urinary calcium excretion is not considered abnormal until it is greater than 250 mg/d. Therefore, one should pay close attention to those patients who may fall in the ''gray zone'' when using a commercially available urine analysis package.

### Differentiation of Hypercalciuria (Sodium Cellulose Phosphate Screening Test)

The finding of hypercalciuria from an automated stone risk analysis requires further differentiation as to the specific etiology of the hypercalciuria.[4] This task can be met by utilizing a sodium cellulose phosphate (SCP) screening test.[62] Briefly, the procedure entails placing the patient on a low-calcium (400 mg/d) and low-sodium (100 mEq/d) diet for an entire week (Fig 6). On day 4, the patient collects a 24-hr urine for calcium and creatinine only. Beginning on day 5, the patient is given sodium cellulose phosphate at a dose of 5 g three times a day ***with meals.*** A second 24-hr urine sample for calcium and creatinine is obtained on day 7 while the patient is taking the sodium cellulose phosphate. This urine sample will allow determination of the urinary calcium excretion without the influence of excess dietary calcium. On the morning of the eighth day, a fasting urine sample is obtained.[60] (For data, see Table 9.)

Urinary calcium excretion on the 24-hr collection during day 4 (while on a low-

**TABLE 9. Outline of Sodium Cellulose Phosphate Trial**

| Day | Calcium and Sodium-Limited Diet | Sodium Cellulose Phosphate | 24-hr Urine[a] | Fasting Urine[a] | SMA, PTH |
|---|---|---|---|---|---|
| 1 | X | | | | |
| 2 | X | | | | |
| 3 | X | | | | |
| 4 | X | | X | | |
| 5 | X | X | | | |
| 6 | X | X | | | |
| 7 | X | X | X | | |
| 8 | | | | X | X |

[a]For calcium and creatinine only.

calcium and low-sodium diet) indicate that the patient's hypercalciuria can be corrected by dietary measures alone (absorptive hypercalciuria type II). The second 24-hr urine collection for calcium and creatinine as well as the fasting test will help to differentiate between absorptive hypercalciuria type I and renal hypercalciuria.[60] Restoration of normal urinary calcium while on SCP, along with a normal fasting calcium-to-creatinine ratio ($<0.11$ mg/dL GF), denotes absorptive hypercalciuria type I. However, an elevated fasting calcium-to-creatinine ratio suggests that the hypercalciuria is secondary to a renal leak of calcium. Confirmation of renal hypercalciuria is made by an elevated fasting immunoreactive PTH determination, indicative of secondary hyperparathyroidism.

The institution of an SCP screening test in the simplified diagnostic protocol may be a major improvement from the standard ambulatory evaluation. The SCP test provides improved discrimination between absorptive and renal hypercalciuria.[62] Unfortunately, in a substantial number of patients with hypercalciuric nephrolithiasis who have previously undergone the ''standard'' fasting and loading test, the differentiation between absorptive and renal hypercalciuria cannot be made with ease. The major problem in classification is the occurrence of unclassified hypercalciuria where the patients display fasting hypercalciuria without parathyroid stimulation (Table 7). The lack of parathyroid stimulation suggests the occurrence of absorptive hypercalciuria; however, the fasting urinary calcium is high. The fasting hypercalciuria indicates that a renal leak of calcium may be present. However, secondary stimulation of parathyroid function is lacking. Therefore, this picture depicts neither absorptive hypercalciuria nor renal hypercalciuria.

In the majority of these ''unclassified'' hypercalciuric patients, the occurrence of fasting hypercalciuria without parathyroid stimulation is usually due to inadequate dietary preparation prior to the determination of fasting urinary calcium. When calcium restriction is not maintained or the duration of fast is insufficient, there may be an incomplete renal clearance of intestinally absorbed calcium. Under such circumstances, patients with absorptive hypercalciuria may present with fasting hypercalciuria and those with renal hypercalciuria may not show parathyroid stimulation because of the suppressive effect of absorbed calcium. It is believed that the sodium cellulose phosphate screening test will help to better differentiate these patients with fasting hypercalciuria and normal PTH.

For example, administration of sodium cellulose phosphate during the last 3 days of the SCP screening test will effectively reduce the amount of absorbed calcium and therefore prevent the appearance of fasting hypercalciuria in those patients who truly have absorptive hypercalciuria. If, however, the hypercalciuria is due to a renal leak of calcium, the sodium cellulose phosphate is not expected to alter the finding of fasting hypercalciuria. Thus, they would have persistent fasting hypercalciuria and manifest parathyroid stimulation.

### Follow-up Utilizing an Automated Stone Risk Analysis

After appropriate medical management has been instituted, the response to therapy may be monitored by again utilizing commercially available tests. Specific tests are available for citrate and cystine as well as various combinations of calcium, uric acid, pH, sodium, and potassium. In addition, total volume determinations are included with all tests. These limited tests will enable the physician to alter medical therapy if necessary and will reinforce proper dietary and medication habits in their patients.

## TIMING OF THE METABOLIC EVALUATION

As noted previously, while the innovative techniques of percutaneous nephrostolithotomy and extracorporeal shock wave lithotripsy (ESWL) offer the stone patient an attractive alternative to conventional open surgery, they have no effect on the underlying metabolic or physiologic derangements that affect stone formation.

Therefore, a thorough metabolic evaluation accompanied with appropriately applied medical management should favorably affect the course of stone disease and significantly reduce the need for a repeat surgical procedure.[55] The question remains, however, as to the proper timing for performing a metabolic evaluation in relation to the surgical procedure.

The exact time to schedule a diagnostic evaluation is dependent on several factors including evidence of obstruction, infection, renal colic, and urgency of stone removal.[64] It has been suggested that excretion of various stone-forming substances may be impaired in the presence of urinary tract obstruction by a renal or ureteral calculus. In addition, while no definitive studies exist, one might expect similar alterations of urinary function to exist after various techniques of stone removal. Open surgical procedures, endourologic stone removal, and ESWL all exert specific types of trauma on the renal parenchyma. One might therefore expect transient alterations in renal function after such procedures. In addition, stones associated with infection may also alter various transport properties of the nephron. The presence of infection may thus give misleading results during a diagnostic evaluation.

It seems advisable, therefore, to postpone a complete diagnostic evaluation for at least a month after resolution of ureteral obstruction, infection, or after undergoing a stone removal procedure. This should allow recovery of normal renal function as well as reinstitution of the patient's regular dietary habits.

Along the same lines, a patient who is experiencing severe colic or recovering from a surgical procedure would not be expected to be following their daily routine including dietary habits and fluid intake. Therefore, a metabolic evaluation performed during an acute stone episode or with the patient still in the hospital may give misleading results (especially in relation to environmental risk factors) and not allow for a proper diagnostic evaluation. On the other hand, a patient with existing stones scheduled for elective stone removal, yet able to enjoy his or her normal lifestyle, may have a simplified metabolic evaluation performed prior to undergoing stone removal.[64]

## CONSERVATIVE MEDICAL MANAGEMENT

Certain conservative recommendations should be made for all patients regardless of the underlying etiology of their stone disease.[58] These measures include increased fluids in order to maintain a urine output >2000 mL/d.[12,65] In addition, all patients should be placed on a diet limited in oxalate and sodium. This avoidance of dietary excess should help decrease the urinary excretion of oxalate and calcium.[66] In patients with suspected absorptive hypercalciuria, a dietary limitation of dairy products may also be enforced. A restriction of animal proteins in those with "purine gluttony" and hyperuricosuria should also be encouraged.

It is anticipated that with these conservative measures alone, a significant number of patients may be able to normalize their urinary risk factors for stone formation.[54] Thus, only these conservative measures may be necessary to keep their stone disease under control. After 3–4 months on conservative management, patients should be reevaluated using either standard laboratory assays or a less comprehensive automated urinalysis package (StoneTrack, Mission Pharmacal Company, San Antonio, TX). If the patient's metabolic or environmental abnormalities have been corrected by the conservative dietary and fluid manipulations alone, then the conservative therapy should be continued and the patient followed every 6 months with repeat 24-hr urine testing. It is believed that follow-up is essential not only to monitor the efficiency of treatment but also to encourage patient compliance. If, however, a metabolic or environmental defect persists, even while on conservative therapy, then more selective medical therapy may be instituted. For example, if significant hyperuricosuria (urinary uric acid greater than 800 mg/d) persists even after dietary restriction

**TABLE 10. Physicochemical and Physiologic Effects of Pharmacologic Therapy**

| Factor | Sodium Cellulose Phosphate | Orthophosphate | Thiazide | Allopurinol | Potassium Citrate |
|---|---|---|---|---|---|
| Urinary calcium | Marked decrease | Mild decrease | Moderate decrease | No change | Mild decrease/ no change |
| Urinary phosphorus | Mild increase | Marked increase | Mild increase/ no change | No change | No change |
| Urinary uric acid | No change | No change | Mild increase/ no change | Marked decrease | No change |
| Urinary oxalate | Mild increase | Mild increase/ no change | Mild increase/ mild decrease | No change | No change |
| Urinary citrate | No change | Mild increase | Mild decrease | No change | Marked increase |
| Calcium oxalate saturation | Mild decrease/ no change | Mild decrease | Mild decrease | No change | Moderate decrease |
| Brushite saturation | Moderate decrease | Mild increase | Mild decrease | No change | No change |

of meat products, then selective medical therapy with allopurinol may be instituted.

## SELECTIVE MEDICAL THERAPY OF NEPHROLITHIASIS

Improved elucidation of pathophysiology and formulation of diagnostic criteria for different causes of nephrolithiasis have made feasible the adoption of selective treatment programs.[5,67,68] Such programs should reverse the underlying physicochemical and physiologic derangements, inhibit new stone formation, overcome nonrenal complications of the disease process, and be free of serious side effects. The rationale for the selection of certain treatment programs is the assumption that the particular physicochemical and physiologic aberrations identified with the given disorder are etiologically important in the formation of renal stones (as previously discussed) and that the correction of these disturbances would prevent stone formation. Moreover, it is assumed that such a selected treatment program would be more effective and safe than a random treatment. Despite a lack of conclusive experimental verification, these hypotheses appear reasonable and logical. For many pharmacologic treatment programs recommended for nephrolithiasis, sufficient information is now available to characterize their physicochemical and physiologic actions (Table 10).

### Absorptive Hypercalciuria

**Sodium Cellulose Phosphate.** There is currently no treatment program capable of correcting the basic abnormality of absorptive hypercalciuria type I, although several drugs are available that have been shown to restore normal calcium excretion. Sodium cellulose phosphate best meets the criteria for optimum therapy.[69] When given orally, this nonabsorbable ion exchange resin binds calcium and inhibits calcium absorption. However, this inhibition is caused by limiting the amount of intraluminal calcium available for absorption, not by correcting the basic disturbance in calcium transport.

The above mode of action accounts for the three potential complications of SCP therapy.[70] First, it may cause a negative calcium balance and parathyroid stimulation when used in patients with normal intestinal calcium absorption or with renal or resorptive hypercalciuria. Second, the treatment may cause magnesium depletion by binding magnesium as well. Third, SCP may produce secondary hyperoxaluria, by binding divalent cations in the intestinal tract, reducing divalent cation-oxalate complexation, and making more oxalate available for absorption. These complications may be overcome by using the drug only in documented cases of absorptive hypercalciuria type I, applying oral magnesium supplementation (1.0–1.5 mg magnesium gluconate twice a day, separately from SCP), and by imposing a moderate dietary restriction of oxalate.

When the above precautions are followed, SCP at a dosage of 10–15 g/d (given with meals) has been shown to reduce urinary calcium and the saturation of calcium salts (calcium phosphate as well as calcium oxalate), maintain stable bone density, and be clinically effective.[71]

**Thiazide.** Thiazide is not considered a selective therapy for absorptive hypercalciuria, since it does not decrease intestinal calcium absorption in this condition.[17] However, this drug has been widely used to treat absorptive hypercalciuria because of its hypocalciuric action and the high cost and inconvenience of alternative therapy (SCP).

Current studies indicate that thiazide may have a limited long-term effectiveness in absorptive hypercalciuria type I.[50,51] Despite an initial reduction in urinary excretion, the intestinal calcium absorption remains persistently elevated. These studies suggest that the retained calcium may be accreted in bone at least during the first few years of therapy. Bone density, determined in the distal third of the radius by photon absorptiometry, increases significantly during thiazide treatment in absorptive hypercalciuria, with an annual increment of 1.34%. With continued treatment, however, the rise in bone density stabilizes and the hypocalciuric effect of thiazide becomes attenuated. The results suggest that thiazide treatment has caused a low turnover state of bone that interferes with a continued calcium accretion in the skeleton. The "rejected" calcium would then be excreted in urine. In contrast, bone density is not significantly altered in renal hypercalciuria where thiazide has been shown to cause a decline in intestinal calcium absorption commensurate with a reduction in urinary calcium.

**Guidelines for the Use of Sodium Cellulose Phosphate or Thiazide in AHI.** Neither SCP nor thiazide corrects the basic, underlying physiologic defect in absorptive hypercalciuria. Some guidelines are offered until more selective therapy can be developed.

Sodium cellulose phosphate should be used in patients with severe absorptive hypercalciuria type I (urinary calcium greater than 350 mg/d) or those resistant to or intolerant of thiazide therapy. In patients with absorptive hypercalciuria type I who may be at risk for bone disease (growing children, postmenopausal women), thiazide may be the first choice. When thiazide loses its hypocalciuric action (after long-term treatment), SCP may be temporarily substituted for approximately 6 months followed by resumption of thiazide therapy.

Potassium supplementation should be employed when using thiazide therapy in order to prevent hypokalemia and a decrease in urinary citrate excretion. A typical treatment program might include trichlormethiazide (Naqua) 4 mg/d with potassium citrate 15–20 mEq twice a day. Amiloride in combination with thiazide (Moduretic) may be more effective than thiazide alone in reducing calcium excretion. However, it does not augment citrate excretion. Since amiloride is a potassium-sparing agent, potassium citrate should be used with caution.

In absorptive hypercalciuria type II, no specific drug treatment may be necessary since the physiologic defect is not as severe as in absorptive hypercalciuria type I. In addition, many patients show disdain for drinking fluids and excreting concentrated urine. A low calcium intake (400–600 mg/d) and high fluid intake (sufficient to achieve a minimum urine output of greater than 2 L/d) would seem ideally indicated, since normocalciuria could be restored by dietary calcium restriction alone, and increased urine volume has been shown to reduce urinary saturation of calcium oxalate.[67]

**Orthophosphate.** Orthophosphate (neutral or alkaline salt of sodium and/or potassium, 0.5 g phosphorus 3–4 times a day) has been shown to inhibit 1,25-$(OH)_2$D synthesis.[68,72] However, there is no convincing evidence that this treatment restores normal intestinal calcium absorption. Orthophosphate reduces urinary calcium probably by directly impairing the renal tubular reabsorption of calcium and by binding calcium in the intestinal tract. Urinary phosphorus is markedly increased during therapy, a finding reflecting the absorbability of soluble phosphate.[73] Physicochemically, orthophosphate reduces the urinary saturation of calcium oxalate but increases that of brushite.[74] Moreover, the urinary inhibitor activity is increased, probably owing to the stimulated renal excretion of pyrophosphate and citrate. Although contrary reports have appeared, this treatment program has been reported to cause soft tissue calcification and parathyroid stimulation.[75] It may be particularly indicated in absorptive hypercalciuria type III. Orthophosphate is contraindicated in nephrolithiasis complicated by urinary tract infection.

### Renal Hypercalciuria

Thiazide is ideally indicated for the treatment of renal hypercalciuria. This diuretic has been shown to correct the renal leak of calcium by augmenting calcium reabsorption in the distal tubule and by causing extracellular volume depletion and stimulating proximal tubular reabsorption of calcium.[67] The ensuing correction of secondary hyperparathyroidism restores normal serum 1,25-$(OH)_2$D and intestinal calcium absorption.[17] Thiazide has been shown to provide a sustained correction of hypercalciuria commensurate with a restoration of normal serum 1,25-$(OH)_2$D and intestinal calcium absorption up to 10 years of therapy.[50]

Physicochemically, the urinary environment becomes less saturated with respect to calcium oxalate and brushite during thiazide treatment, largely because of the reduced calcium excretion.[67] Moreover, urinary inhibitor activity, as reflected in the limit of metastability, is increased by an unknown mechanism. These effects are shared by hydrochlorothiazide 50 mg twice a day, chlorthalidone 50 mg/d, or trichlormethiazide 4 mg/d. Potassium supplementation (40–60 mEq/d) may sometimes be required to prevent hypokalemia and attendant hypocitraturia. Potassium citrate has been shown to be effective in averting hypokalemia and in increasing urinary citrate, when administered to patients with calcium nephrolithiasis taking thiazide.[52,76] Concurrent use of triamterene, a potassium-sparing agent, should be undertaken with caution because of recent reports of triamterene stone formation.[77,78] However, amiloride may be used with thiazide since it alone has sometimes been shown to exert a hypocalciuric action, to exaggerate the hypocalciuric action of thiazide, and to prevent hypokalemia.[79]

Thiazide therapy has also been demonstrated to raise urinary uric acid excretion in certain patients.[80] Therefore, patients on long-term therapy should be monitored for evidence of hyperuricosuria. Finally, thiazide is contraindicated in primary hyperparathyroidism because of potential aggravation of hypercalcemia.

### Primary Hyperparathyroidism

Parathyroidectomy is the optimum treatment for nephrolithiasis of primary hyperparathyroidism.[81] Following removal of abnormal parathyroid tissue, urinary calcium is restored to normal commensurate with a decline in serum concentration of calcium and intestinal absorption.[82] The urinary environment becomes less saturated with respect to calcium oxalate and brushite, and the limit of metastability (formation product ratio) for these calcium salts increases. There is typically a reduced rate of new stone formation, unless urinary tract infection is present.[83] Parathyroidectomy is contraindicated in secondary hyperparathyroidism of renal hypercalciuria and in absorptive hypercalciuria.

There is no established medical treatment for the nephrolithiasis of primary hyperparathyroidism.[84] Although orthophosphates have been recommended for the disease of mild to moderate severity, their safety or efficacy has not yet been proven. They should be used only when parathyroid surgery cannot be undertaken. Estrogen has been reported to be useful in reducing serum and urinary calcium in postmenopausal women with primary hyperparathyroidism.

### Hyperuricosuric Calcium Oxalate Nephrolithiasis

Allopurinol (300 mg/d) is the physiologically meaningful drug of choice in hyperuricosuric calcium oxalate nephrolithiasis resulting from uric acid overproduction because of its ability to reduce uric acid synthesis and lower urinary uric acid.[85] Its use in hyperuricosuria associated with dietary purine overindulgence is also reasonable since dietary purine restriction is often impractical. Physicochemical changes ensuing from restoration of normal urinary uric acid include an increase in the urinary limit of metastability of calcium oxalate.[86] Thus, the spontaneous nucleation of calcium oxalate is retarded by treatment, probably via inhibition of monosodium urate–induced stimulation of calcium oxalate crystallization.[87] Because of the potential exaggeration of monosodium urate–induced calcium oxalate crystallization, a moderate sodium restriction (150 mEq/d) is also advisable.

Potassium citrate represents an effective alternative to allopurinol in the treatment of this condition.[88] Administration of potassium citrate (at a dose of 60 mEq/d in divided doses) to patients with hypercalciuric calcium oxalate nephrolithiasis has been shown to reduce the urinary saturation of calcium oxalate (by complexing calcium) and to inhibit urate–induced crystallization of calcium oxalate.

Potassium citrate may be particularly useful in patients with mild to moderate hyperuricosuria (<800 mg/d) in whom hypocitraturia is also present. However, allopurinol is probably preferred in patients with more marked hyperuricosuria, especially if hyperuricemia coexists.

### Enteric Hyperoxaluria

Oral administration of large amounts of calcium (0.25–1.0 g four times a day) or magnesium has been recommended for the control of calcium nephrolithiasis of ileal disease.[89] Although urinary oxalate may decrease (probably from binding of oxalate by divalent cations), the concurrent rise in urinary calcium may obviate the beneficial effect of this therapy, at least in some patients.[30] Cholestyramine does not cause a sustained reduction in urinary oxalate. The replacement of dietary fat with medium chain triglycerides may be helpful in those patients who also have malabsorption.

Patients may exhibit hypomagnesiuria due to impaired intestinal absorption of magnesium. Since magnesium has been shown to complex oxalate, hypomagnesiuria may cause a significant increase in the urinary saturation of calcium oxalate. While oral magnesium supplements may correct hypomagnesiuria, they may also provoke further diarrhea. Magnesium gluconate (0.5–1.0 g three times a day) appears to be better tolerated than magnesium oxide or hydroxide. Treatment with potassium citrate (60–120 mEq/d) may correct the hypokalemia and metabolic acidosis, and in some patients increase urinary citrate toward normal (this will be discussed in greater detail in the following section).[33,90]

A high fluid intake is recommended to assure adequate urine volume. Since excessive fluid loss may be present, an antidiarrheal agent may be necessary before sufficient urine output can be achieved. Calcium citrate may theoretically have a role in the management of enteric hyperoxaluria. This treatment may lower urinary oxalate by binding oxalate in the intestinal tract. Calcium citrate may also raise the urinary citrate and pH by providing an alkali load.[91] Finally, calcium citrate may correct the malabsorption of calcium and adverse effects on the skeleton by providing an efficiently absorbed calcium compound.

### Hypocitraturic Calcium Oxalate Nephrolithiasis

In patients with hypocitraturic calcium oxalate nephrolithiasis, potassium citrate treatment is capable of restoring normal urinary citrate, lowering the urinary saturation, and inhibiting crystallization of calcium salts. Since hypocitraturia is found in a number of different conditions, each will be addressed individually.

**Distal Renal Tubular Acidosis.** Potassium citrate therapy can correct the metabolic acidosis and hypokalemia found in patients with distal renal tubular acidosis.[92] In addition, it is capable of restoring normal urinary citrate although large doses (up to 120 mEq/d) may be required in severe acidotic states. With correction of the acidosis, urinary calcium should decline into the normal range. Since urinary pH is generally high to begin with in patients with renal tubular acidosis, the overall rise in urinary pH is small.

Potassium citrate therapy will produce a sustained decline in the urinary saturation of calcium oxalate (from reduction in urinary calcium and in citrate complexation of calcium).[35] The urinary saturation of calcium phosphate does not increase since the rise in phosphate dissociation is relatively small and is adequately compensated by a decline in ionic calcium concentration.[92] In addition, the inhibitory activity against the crystallization of calcium oxalate and calcium phosphate is augmented due to the direct action of citrate.

**Chronic Diarrheal States.** Potassium citrate therapy in patients with hypocitraturia secondary to chronic diarrheal states has been shown to significantly reduce the stone formation rate and produce remission in 70% of patients.[90] The dose of potassium citrate will depend on the severity of hypocitraturia in these patients. The dosages range from 60 mEq in three or four divided doses up to 120 mEq/d.

It is recommended that a liquid preparation of potassium citrate be used rather than the slow-release tablet preparation since the slow-release medication may be poorly absorbed due to rapid intestinal transit time. In addition, frequent dose schedules (three to four times a day) for the liquid preparation are necessary since this form of the medication has a relatively short duration of biological action. A less frequent dose schedule (two to three times a day) is acceptable if the solid preparation is used because of its slow-release characteristic.

**Thiazide-Induced Hypocitraturia.** As noted previously, thiazide therapy may induce hypocitraturia due to hypokalemia with resultant intracellular acidosis.[52,76] Therefore, it should be common practice to administer potassium supplementation, preferably in the form of potassium citrate, to patients receiving thiazide for treatment of hypercalciuria. Potassium citrate has been shown to be as effective as potassium chloride in correcting thiazide-induced hypokalemia.[52] Moreover, the addition of potassium citrate to thiazide therapy significantly increases urinary citrate levels.

**Idiopathic Hypocitraturic Calcium Oxalate Nephrolithiasis.** Idiopathic hypocitraturic calcium oxalate nephrolithiasis includes hypocitraturia occurring alone in patients with calcium stones and hypocitraturia occurring in conjunction with hypercalciuria or hyperuricosuric calcium oxalate nephrolithiasis. Stones formed in this condition are predominantly composed of calcium oxalate. Potassium citrate therapy has been shown to produce a sustained increase in urinary citrate excretion from initially low values to within normal limits.[93] This resulted in a significant decline of the urinary saturation of the calcium oxalate into the normal range.

Thus it is apparent that potassium citrate can be used in a variety of conditions. Combined data from a recent long-term clinical trial utilizing potassium citrate shows no significant change in serum potassium, hematocrit, bone density, or endogenous creatinine clearance during treatment.[90] A liquid preparation of potassium citrate with a frequent dosage schedule (three to four times a day) is recommended in chronic diarrheal states. In other conditions, a solid preparation given on a twice daily schedule is generally well tolerated.

## Hypomagnesiuric Calcium Nephrolithiasis

Hypomagnesiuric calcium nephrolithiasis is characterized by low urinary magnesium, hypocitraturia, and low urine volume.[7] Therefore, management should include restoration of urinary magnesium levels with either magnesium oxide or magnesium hydroxide as well as specific treatment of the hypocitraturia with potassium citrate.[38] A preparation that contains both magnesium and citrate would be ideal in the treatment of this condition. Work is under way in the development of a potassium-magnesium citrate preparation that is currently undergoing clinical trials.[94,95]

## Gouty Diathesis

The major goal in the management of gouty diathesis, especially if the stones are predominantly of uric acid, should be threefold: increased urine volume, reduction in urinary uric acid, and maintenance of urinary pH at 6.5–7.[40,42]

Adequate urine volume is essential to decrease urinary uric acid concentration and therefore increase its solubility. Patients should be encouraged to maintain a urine output of 2500–3000 $cm^3$ of urine per day. The amount of fluid intake required to maintain this urine output is an individual variable for each patient. A reduction in urinary uric acid excretion can be accomplished in two ways. In patients where high purine intake is suspected, a low-meat (methionine) diet is recommended. In those patients where diminished meat intake either is not possible or has little effect on the urinary uric acid levels, allopurinol at a dose of 300 mg/d should be instituted.

By far, the most important modality in the management of gouty diathesis is the provision of alkali designed to raise urinary pH.[14] This is supported by a dramatic 10-fold increase in uric acid solubility by raising the urine pH from 5.0 to 7.0. In the past, urine alkalinization has been accomplished with either sodium bicarbonate or various combinations of sodium and potassium alkali therapy.[96] While sodium alkali may cause dissociation or inhibition of uric acid formation, this medication may be complicated by the development of calcium-containing stones (calcium phosphate and/or calcium oxalate).[97] Some patients have developed calcium phosphate/calcium oxalate stones after beginning sodium alkali therapy for their uric acid lithiasis.

Potassium citrate has been found to be an adequate alkalinizing agent, capable of maintaining urinary pH at approximately 6.5 at a dose of 30–60 mEq/d in two or three divided doses.[40,97,98] Moreover, some have advocated alternate day dosing with potassium citrate to treat uric acid stones.[99] Attempts at alkalinizing the urine to a pH of $>7.0$ should be avoided. At a higher pH, there is a possibility of precipitating calcium phosphate (hydroxyapatite) and therefore increasing the risk of calcium stone formation. If the urinary uric acid excretion is elevated or hyperuricemia exists, allopurinol (300 mg/d) is recommended.

## Cystinuria

The object of treatment for cystinuria is to reduce the urinary concentration of cystine to below its solubility limit (200–300 mg/L).[100] The initial treatment program includes a high fluid intake and oral administration of soluble alkali (potassium citrate) at a dose sufficient to raise the urinary pH to 6.5–7.0. When this conservative program is ineffective, *d*-penicillamine (approximately 2 g/d in divided doses) has been used.[45] This treatment has been shown to increase cystine solubility in urine via formation of a more soluble mixed disulfide. Unfortunately, penicillamine treatment produces frequent side effects including nephrotic syndrome, dermatitis, and pancytopenia.

Recent studies have demonstrated that α-mercaptopropionylglycine (Thiola) also forms a mixed disulfide bond with cystine thereby increasing the solubility of cystine.[101] This side effect profile appears to be less marked than that of *d*-penicillamine.

There have also been two recent reports of using captopril to manage cystinuria.[102,103] However, further long-term clinical trials must be performed to validate the use of this medication to treat cystine stones.

### Infection Lithiasis

If long-standing effective control of infection with urea-splitting organisms can be achieved, new stone formation may be averted and some dissolution of existing stones may be achieved. Unfortunately, such control is difficult to obtain with antibiotic therapy. If there is an existing struvite stone, it is often difficult to completely eradicate the infection because the stone often harbors the organism within its interstices.[48] For this reason, surgical removal of struvite stones is usually recommended.

In recent clinical trials, acetohydroxamic acid (AHA), a urease inhibitor, has been shown to reduce the urinary saturation of struvite and to retard stone formation.[104] When given at a dose of 250 mg three times a day, AHA has been shown to prevent recurrence of new stones and inhibit the growth of stones in patients with chronic urea-splitting infections.[105] In addition, in a limited number of patients, AHA has caused dissolution of existing struvite calculi. However, 30% of patients receiving chronic AHA therapy have experienced minor side effects and 15% developed deep venous thrombosis. Additional long-term studies must be done to determine the benefit/risk ratio of AHA.

## SUMMARY

Selective medical therapy of nephrolithiasis is highly effective in preventing new stone formation. A remission rate of greater than 80% and overall reduction in individual stone formation rate of greater than 90% can be obtained in patients with nephrolithiasis. In patients with mild to moderate severity of stone disease, virtually total control of stone disease can be achieved as evidenced by remission rates of greater than 95%.[106] The need for stone removal may be dramatically reduced by an effective prophylactic program (Fig 7).

Selective pharmacologic therapy of nephrolithiasis also encompasses the ad-

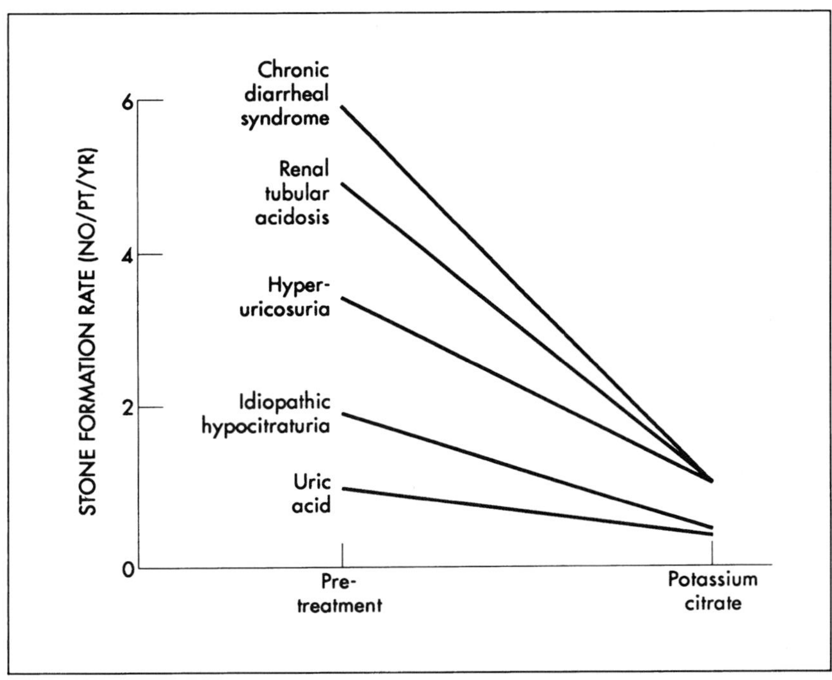


**Fig 7.** Impact of selective medical therapy on various causes of stone formation.

vantages of overcoming nonrenal manifestations that cause stone formation as well as averting certain side effects that may be caused by nonselective medical therapy. Despite these advantages, it is clear that selective medical therapy cannot provide total control of stone disease. A satisfactory response requires continued, dedicated compliance by patients to the recommended program and a commitment by the physician to provide long-term follow-up and care.

## REFERENCES


1. Ljunghall S. Incidence of upper urinary tract stones. *Min Electrol Metab.* 1987;13:220–227.
2. Ljunghall S, Danielson BG. A prospective study of renal stone recurrences. *Br J Urol.* 1984;56:122–124.
3. Sarmina I, Spirnak JP, Resnick MI. Urinary lithiasis in the black population: an epidemiological study and review of the literature. *J Urol.* 1987;138:14–17.
4. Pak CY, Oata M, Lawrence EC, Snyder W. The hypercalciurias. Causes, parathyroid functions, and diagnostic crtieria. *J Clin Invest.* 1974;54: 387–400.
5. Preminger GM. Renal calculi: pathogenesis, diagnosis, and medical therapy. *Semin Nephrol.* 1992;12:200–216.
6. Pak CY, Holt K. Nucleation and growth of brushite and calcium oxalate in urine of stone-formers. *Metabolism.* 1976;25:665–673.
7. Preminger GM, Baker S, Peterson R, et al. Hypomagnesiuric hypocitraturia: an apparent new entity for calcium nephrolithiasis. *J Litho Stone Dis.* 1989;1:22–25.
8. Meyer JL, Smith LH. Growth of calcium oxalate crystals. II. Inhibition by natural urinary crystal growth inhibitors. *Invest Urol.* 1975;13: 36–39.
9. Kok DJ, Papapoulos SE, Bijvoet OL. Excessive crystal agglomeration with low citrate excretion in recurrent stone-formers. *Lancet.* 1986;1: 1056–1058.
10. Asplin J, DeGanello S, Nakagawa YN, Coe FL. Evidence that nephrocalcin and urine inhibit nucleation of calcium oxalate monohydrate crystals. *Am J Physiol.* 1991;261:F824–F830.
11. Coe FI, Parks JH, Nakagawa Y. Protein inhibitors of crystallization. *Semin Nephrol.* 1991; 11:98–109.
12. Pak CY, Sakhaee K, Crowther C, Brinkley L. Evidence justifying a high fluid intake in treatment of nephrolithiasis. *Ann Intern Med.* 1980; 93:36–39.
13. Ljunghall S, Fellstrom B, Johansson G. Prevention of renal stones by a high fluid intake? *Eur Urol.* 1988;14:381–385.
14. Riese RJ, Sakhaee K. Uric acid nephrolithiasis: pathogenesis and treatment. *J Urol.* 1992;148: 765–771.
15. Pak CY, Fuller CJ. Assessment of cystine solubility in urine and of heterogeneous nucleation. *J Urol.* 1983;129:1066–1070.
16. Griffith DP, Musher DM, Campbell JW. Inhibition of bacterial urease. *Invest Urol.* 1973;11: 234–238.
17. Pak CY. Physiological basis for absorptive and renal hypercalciurias. *Am J Physiol.* 1979;237: F415–F423.
18. Shen FH, Baylink DJ, Nielsen RL, et al. Increased serum 1,25-dihydroxyvitamin D in idiopathic hypercalciuria. *J Lab Clin Med.* 1977; 90:955–962.
19. Shen FH, Ivey JL, Sherrard DJ, et al. Further evidence supporting the phosphate leak hypothesis of idiopathic hypercalciuria. *Adv Exp Med Biol.* 1978;103:217–223.
20. Lemann J Jr, Worcester EM, Gray RW. Hypercalciuria and stones. *Am J Kidney Dis.* 1991;17: 386–391.
21. Kaplan RA, Haussler MR, Deftos LJ, et al. The role of 1 alpha, 25-dihydroxyvitamin D in the mediation of intestinal hyperabsorption of calcium in primary hyperparathyroidism and absorptive hypercalciuria. *J Clin Invest.* 1977;59: 756–760.
22. Bilezikian JP, Silverberg SJ, Shane E, et al. Characterization and evaluation of asymptomatic primary hyperparathyroidism. *J Bone Min Res.* 1991;2:121–124.
23. Pak CY, Britton F, Peterson R, et al. Ambulatory evaluation of nephrolithiasis. Classification, clinical presentation and diagnostic criteria. *Am J Med.* 1980;69:19–30.
24. Coe FL. Hyperuricosuric calcium oxalate nephrolithiasis. *Kidney Int.* 1978;13:418–426.
25. Sarig S. The hyperuricosuric calcium oxalate stone former. *Min Electrolyte Metab.* 1987;13: 251–256.
26. Coe FL, Kavalach AG. Hypercalciuria and hyperuricosuria in patients with calcium nephrolithiasis. *N Engl J Med.* 1974;291:1344–1350.
27. Ryall RL, Grover PK, Marshall VR. Urate and calcium stones—picking up a drop of mercury with one's fingers? *Am J Kidney Dis.* 1991;17: 426–430.
28. Urivetzky M, Kessaris D, Smith AD. Ascorbic acid overdosing: a risk factor for calcium oxalate nephrolithiasis. *J Urol.* 1992;147:1215–1218.
29. Smith LH, Fromm H, Hofmann AF. Acquired hyperoxaluria, nephrolithiasis, and intestinal disease. Description of a syndrome. *N Engl J Med.* 1972;286:1371–1375.

30. Barilla DE, Notz C, Kennedy D, Pak CY. Renal oxalate excretion following oral oxalate loads in patients with ileal disease and with renal and absorptive hypercalciurias. Effect of calcium and magnesium. *Am J Med.* 1978;64:579–585.
31. Clayman RV, Buchwald H, Varco RL, et al. Urolithiasis in patients with a jejunoileal bypass. *Surg Gynecol Obstet.* 1978;147:225–230.
32. Nicar MJ, Skurla C, Sakhaee K, Pak CY. Low urinary citrate excretion in nephrolithiasis. *Urology.* 1983;21:8–14.
33. Rudman D, Dedonis JL, Fountain MT, et al. Hypocitraturia in patients with gastrointestinal malabsorption. *N Engl J Med.* 1980;303:657–661.
34. Backman U, Danielson BG, Johansson G, et al. Incidence and clinical importance of renal tubular defects in recurrent renal stone formers. *Nephron.* 1980;25:96–101.
35. Preminger GM, Sakhaee K, Pak CY. Hypercalciuria and altered intestinal calcium absorption occurring independently of vitamin D in incomplete distal renal tubular acidosis. *Metab Clin Exp.* 1987;36:176–179.
36. Pak CY. Citrate and renal calculi: new insights and future directions. *Am J Kidney Dis.* 1991; 17:420–425.
37. Melnick I, Landes RR, Hoffman AA, Burch JF. Magnesium therapy for recurring calcium oxalate urinary calculi. *J Urol.* 1971;105:119–122.
38. Fetner CD, Barilla DE, Townsend J, Pak CY. Effects of magnesium oxide on the crystallization of calcium salts in urine in patients with recurrent nephrolithiasis. *J Urol.* 1978;120: 399–401.
39. Ogawa Y, Yamaguchi K, Morozumi M. Effects of magnesium salts in preventing experimental oxalate urolithiasis in rats. *J Urol.* 1990;144: 385–389.
40. Pak CY, Sakhaee K, Fuller C. Successful management of uric acid nephrolithiasis with potassium citrate. *Kidney Int.* 1986;30:422–428.
41. Zerwekh JE, Holt K, Pak CY. Natural urinary macromolecular inhibitors: attenuation of inhibitory activity by urate salts. *Kidney Int.* 1983;23:838–841.
42. Harvey JA, Pak CY. Gouty diathesis and sarcoidosis in patient with recurrent calcium nephrolithiasis. *J Urol.* 1988;139:1287–1289.
43. Morton WJ. Lesch-Nyhan syndrome. *Urology.* 1982;20:506–509.
44. Gigax JH, Leach JR. Uric acid calculi associated with ileostomy for ulcerative colitis. *J Urol.* 1971;105:777–779.
45. Singer A, Das S. Cystinuria: a review of the pathophysiology and management. *J Urol.* 1989;142:669–673.
46. Evans WP, Resnick MI, Boyce WH. Homozygous cystinuria—evaluation of 35 patients. *J Urol.* 1982;127:707–709.
47. Sakhaee K, Poindexter JR, Pak CY. The spectrum of metabolic abnormalities in patients with cystine nephrolithiasis. *J Urol.* 1989;141:819–821.
48. Griffith DP. Struvite stones. *Kidney Int.* 1978; 13:372–382.
49. Spirnak JP, Resnick MI. Anatrophic nephrolithotomy. *Urol Clin North Am.* 1983;10:665–675.
50. Preminger GM, Pak CY. Eventual attenuation of hypocalciuric response to hydrochlorothiazide in absorptive hypercalciuria. *J Urol.* 1987; 137:1104–1109.
51. Zerwekh JE, Pak CY. Selective effects of thiazide therapy on serum 1 alpha, 25-dihydroxyvitamin D and intestinal calcium absorption in renal and absorptive hypercalciurias. *Metab Clin Exp.* 1980;29:13–17.
52. Nicar MJ, Peterson R, Pak CY. Use of potassium citrate as potassium supplement during thiazide therapy of calcium nephrolithiasis. *J Urol.* 1984;131:430–433.
53. Pak CY. Should patients with single renal stone occurrence undergo diagnostic evaluation? *J Urol.* 1982;127:855–858.
54. Hosking DH, Erickson SB, Van Den Berg CJ, et al. The stone clinic effect in patients with idiopathic calcium urolithiasis. *J Urol.* 1983; 130:1115–1118.
55. Preminger GM, Peterson R, Peters PC, Pak CY. The current role of medical treatment of nephrolithiasis: the impact of improved techniques of stone removal. *J Urol.* 1985;134:6–10.
56. Yendt ER, Cohanim M. Absorptive hyperoxaluria: a new clinical entity—successful treatment with hydrochlorothiazide. *Clin Invest Med (Medecine Clinique et Experimentale).* 1986;9: 44–50.
57. Preminger GM. The metabolic evaluation of patients with recurrent nephrolithiasis: A review of comprehensive and simplified approaches. *J Urol.* 1989;141:760–763.
58. Uribarri J, Oh MS, Carroll HJ. The first kidney stone. *Ann Intern Med.* 1989;111:1006–1009.
59. Drach GW. Contribution to therapeutic decisions of ratios, absolute values and other measures of calcium, magnesium, urate or oxalate balance in stone formers. *J Urol.* 1976;116: 338–340.
60. Pak CY, Kaplan R, Bone H, et al. A simple test for the diagnosis of absorptive, resorptive and renal hypercalciurias. *N Engl J Med.* 1975;292: 497–500.
61. Pak CY, Fetner C, Townsend J, et al. Evaluation of calcium urolithiasis in ambulatory patients: comparison of results with those of inpatient evaluation. *Am J Med.* 1978;64:979–987.
62. Preminger GM, Peterson R, Pak CYC. Differentiation of unclassified hypercalciuria utilizing a sodium cellulose phosphate trial. In: Walker

VR, Sutton AL, Cameron ECB, et al., eds. *Nephrolithiasis.* New York: Plenum Press; 1989:325–340.

63. Pak CY, Skurla C, Harvey J. Graphic display of urinary risk factors for renal stone formation. *J Urol.* 1985;134:867–870.
64. Lycklama A, Nijeholt GA, Tan HK, Papapoulos SE. Metabolic evaluation in stone patients in relation to extracorporeal shock wave lithotripsy treatment. *J Urol.* 1991;146:1478–1481.
65. McCormack M, Dessureault J, Guitard M. The urine specific gravity dipstick: a useful tool to increase fluid intake in stone forming patients. *J Urol.* 1991;146:1475–1477.
66. Ackermann D. Prophylaxis in idiopathic calcium urolithiasis. *Urol Res.* 1990;18 Suppl 1: S37–S40.
67. Pak CY, Peters P, Hurt G, et al. Is selective therapy of recurrent nephrolithiasis possible? *Am J Med.* 1981;71:615–622.
68. Pak CY. Medical management of nephrolithiasis. *J Urol.* 1982;128:1157–1164.
69. Pak CY, Delea CS, Bartter FC. Successful treatment of recurrent nephrolithiasis (calcium stones) with cellulose phosphate. *N Engl J Med.* 1974;290:175–180.
70. Pak CY. Clinical pharmacology of sodium cellulose phosphate. *J Clin Pharmacol.* 1979;19: 451–457.
71. Pak CY. A cautious use of sodium cellulose phosphate in the management of calcium nephrolithiasis. *Invest Urol.* 1981;19:187–190.
72. Smith LH, Werness PG. Van Den Berg CJ, Wilson DM. Orthophosphate treatment in calcium urolithiasis. *Scand J Urol Nephrol.* (Suppl). 1980;53:253–263.
73. Thomas WC Jr. Use of phosphates in patients with calcareous renal calculi. *Kidney Int.* 1978; 13:390–396.
74. Pak CY. Effects of cellulose phosphate and sodium phosphate on formation product and activity product of brushite in urine. *Metab Clin Exp.* 1972;21:447–455.
75. Dudley FJ, Blackburn CR. Extraskeletal calcification complicating oral neutral-phosphate therapy. *Lancet.* 1970;2:628–630.
76. Pak CY, Peterson R, Sakhaee K, et al. Correction of hypocitraturia and prevention of stone formation by combined thiazide and potassium citrate therapy in thiazide-unresponsive hypercalciuric nephrolithiasis. *Am J Med.* 1985;79: 284–288.
77. Ettinger B, Oldroyd NO, Sorgel F. Triamterene nephrolithiasis. *JAMA.* 1980;244:2443–2445.
78. Carr MC, Prien EL Jr, Babayan RK. Triamterene nephrolithiasis: renewed attention is warranted. *J Urol.* 1990;144:1339–1340.
79. Leppla D, Browne R, Hill K, Pak CY. Effect of amiloride with or without hydrochlorothiazide on urinary calcium and saturation of calcium salts. *J Clin Endocrinol Metab.* 1983;57:920–924.
80. Pak CY, Tolentino R, Stewart A, Galosy RA. Enhancement of renal excretion of uric acid during long-term thiazide therapy. *Invest Urol.* 1978;16:191–193.
81. Pathroff RA, van Heerden JA, Segura JW. Urinary calculi and primary hyperparathyroidism: simultaneous surgical treatment. *J Urol.* 1987; 137:1221–1222.
82. Bone HG, Zerwekh JE, Haussler MR, Pak CY. Effect of parathyroidectomy on serum 1 alpha,25-dihydroxyvitamin D and intestinal calcium absorption in primary hyperparathyroidism. *J Clin Endocrinol Metab.* 1979;48:877–879.
83. Jabbour N, Corvilain J, Fuss M, et al. The natural history of renal stone disease after parathyroidectomy for primary hyperparathyroidism. *Surg Gynecol Obstet.* 1991;172:25–28.
84. Holdaway IM, Evans MC, Frengley PA, Ibbertson HK. Investigation and treatment of renal calculi associated with hypercalciuria. *J Endocrinol Invest.* 1982;5:361–365.
85. Coe FL. Uric acid and calcium oxalate nephrolithiasis. *Kidney Int.* 1983;24:392–403.
86. Pak CY, Barilla DE, Holt K, et al. Effect of oral purine load and allopurinol on the crystallization of calcium salts in urine of patients with hyperuricosuric calcium urolithiasis. *Am J Med.* 1978;65:593–599.
87. Pak CY, Holt K, Zerwekh JE. Attenuation by monosodium urate of the inhibitory effect of glycosaminoglycans on calcium oxalate nucleation. *Invest Urol.* 1979;17:138–140.
88. Pak CY, Peterson R. Successful treatment of hyperuricosuric calcium oxalate nephrolithiasis with potassium citrate. *Arch Intern Med.* 1986; 146:863–867.
89. Dobbins JW. Nephrolithiasis and intestinal disease. *J Clin Gastroenterol.* 1985;7:21–24.
90. Pak CY, Fuller C, Sakhaee K, et al. Long-term treatment of calcium nephrolithiasis with potassium citrate. *J Urol.* 1985;134:11–19.
91. Harvey JA, Zobitz MM, Pak CY. Calcium citrate: reduced propensity for the crystallization of calcium oxalate in urine resulting from induced hypercalciuria of calcium supplementation. *J Clin Endocrinol Metab.* 1985;61:1223–1225.
92. Preminger GM, Sakhaee K, Skurla C, Pak CY. Prevention of recurrent calcium stone formation with potassium citrate therapy in patients with distal renal tubular acidosis. *J Urol.* 1985;134: 20–23.
93. Pak CY, Fuller C: Idiopathic hypocitraturic calcium-oxalate nephrolithiasis successfully treated with potassium citrate. *Ann Intern Med.* 1986;104:33–37.
94. Koenig K, Padalino P, Alexandrides G, Pak CY. Bioavailability of potassium and magne-

sium, and citraturic response from potassium-magnesium citrate. *J Urol.* 1991;145:330–334.

95. Pak CY, Koenig K, Khan R, et al. Physicochemical action of potassium-magnesium citrate in nephrolithiasis. *J Bone Min Res.* 1992; 7:281–285.
96. Sakhaee K, Alpern R, Jacobson HR, Pak CY. Contrasting effects of various potassium salts on renal citrate excretion. *J Clin Endocrinol Metab.* 1991;72:396–400.
97. Sakhaee K, Nicar M, Hill K, Pak CY. Contrasting effects of potassium citrate and sodium citrate therapies on urinary chemistries and crystallization of stone-forming salts. *Kidney Int.* 1983;24:348–352.
98. Preminger GM, Sakhaee K, Pak CY. Alkali action on the urinary crystallization of calcium salts: contrasting responses to sodium citrate and potassium citrate. *J Urol.* 1988;139:240–242.
99. Rodman JS. Prophylaxis of uric acid stones with alternate day doses of alkaline potassium salts. *J Urol.* 1991;145:97–99.
100. Crawhall JC. Cystinuria—an experience in management over 18 years. *Min Electrolyte Metab.* 1987;13:286–293.
101. Pak CY, Fuller C, Sakhaee K, Zerwekh JE, Adams BV. Management of cystine nephrolithiasis with alpha-mercaptopropionylglycine. *J Urol.* 1986;136:1003–1008.
102. Sload JA, Izzo JL. Captopril reduces urinary cystine excretion in cystinuria. *Arch Intern Med.* 1987;147:1409–1412.
103. Streem SB, Hall P. Effect of captopril on urinary cystine excretion in homozygous cystinuria. *J Urol.* 1989;142:1522–1524.
104. Griffith DP, Khonsari F, Skurnick JH, James KE. A randomized trial of acetohydroxamic acid for treatment and prevention of infection-induced urinary stones in spinal cord injury patients. *J Urol.* 1988;140:318–324.
105. Williams JJ, Rodman JS, Peterson CM. A randomized double-blind study of acetohydroxamic acid in struvite nephrolithiasis. *N Engl J Med.* 1984;311:760–764.
106. Preminger GM, Harvey JA, Pak CY. Comparative efficacy of ''specific'' potassium citrate therapy versus conservative management in nephrolithiasis of mild to moderate severity. *J Urol.* 1985;134:658–661.

# 15

# Options in Stone Management

*Brian A. Feagins and Glenn M. Preminger*

Approximately 10% to 20% of all kidney stones may cause the patient enough problems to require surgical removal. Recent improvements in urologic equipment, fluoroscopic technology, and interventional radiologic techniques have given the patient and the urologist many choices of methods to remove kidney stones. When open renal and ureteral surgery are the means by which all new procedures are judged, it appears that percutaneous nephrostolithotomy, ureterorenoscopy, and extracorporeal shock wave lithotripsy offer the patient comparable success rates with significantly diminished morbidity and lowered costs.

As a consequence of the dramatic increase in the number of technologies available to the practicing urologist, a dilemma has been created concerning the application of these new modalities in the treatment of stone disease. There are several controversies in stone management which make it quite difficult to formulate absolute treatment guidelines. This chapter attempts to present many of the philosophies regarding surgical stone management. In an attempt to simplify this task, the text is divided into treatment philosophies for renal and ureteral calculi with discussion germane to the various options in each category.

## TECHNIQUES AVAILABLE FOR SURGICAL STONE MANAGEMENT

### Extracorporeal Shock-Wave Lithotripsy

Since the first patient with a renal calculus was successfully treated with extracorporeal shock-wave lithotripsy in 1980, rapid acceptance and widespread use have championed this form of stone therapy as the treatment of choice for the majority of patients with renal and ureteral calculi. Worldwide clinical studies have documented the efficacy of extracorporeal shock-wave lithotripsy.[1–3]

Shock waves are high-energy amplitudes of pressure generated in the air or water by an abrupt release of energy in a small space. They propagate according to the physical laws of acoustics and are transmitted through media with low attenuation. However, when a shock wave encounters a boundary between substances of differing acoustic impedance (density), compressive stresses are generated that may overcome the tensile strength of that object. Shock waves travel through water and the soft tissues of the body with low attenuation because these materials have similar densities. However, when kidney stones of any

**TABLE 1. Second-Generation Lithotripters**

| Manufacturer | Shock-Wave Generation | Patient Focusing Apparatus | Coupling | Localization |
|---|---|---|---|---|
| Diasonics | Piezoelectric | Spherical | Membrane | Fluoroscopy/Ultrasound |
| Direx | Spark gap | Ellipsoid | Membrane | Fluoroscopy/Ultrasound* |
| Dornier HM-4 | Spark gap | Ellipsoid | Membrane | Biplane fluoroscopy |
| EDAP | Piezoelectric | Spherical | Membrane | Ultrasound |
| Medstone | Spark gap | Ellipsoid | Membrane | Plain x-ray |
| Northgate | Spark gap | Ellipsoid | Membrane | Ultrasound |
| Siemens | Electromagnetic | Acoustic lens | Membrane | Biplane fluoroscopy |
| Technomed | Spark gap | Ellipsoid | Pool | Ultrasound |
| Wolf | Piezoelectric | Spherical | Pool | Ultrasound |

* This unit does not come with its own localization system; requires existing ultrasound or fluoroscopy equipment.

composition are contacted by a shock wave of sufficient energy, a compression wave is induced along the front face of the stone. As a result, the anterior surface begins to crumble. As the shock wave crosses the posterior surface of the stone, part of the energy is reflected, creating tensile stress and fragmentation along the posterior surface. Repeated shock waves eventually reduce the stone to small fragments (ideally 2 mm or less in diameter) which may be passed spontaneously.

Extensive clinical testing has determined that the compression–tensile wave phenomenon results in implosion rather than explosion of the fragments and that the total kinetic energy of all fragments can be minimized by using a large number of relatively low-energy shock waves rather than fewer shocks of higher energy. This finding explains the low incidence of adjacent tissue injury following successful stone fragmentation with high-energy shock waves.

Although the basic principles of shock-wave lithotripsy remain unchanged, a myriad of technologic advances and modifications in the currently available lithotripters have significantly expanded the clinical applications of lithotripsy.

**Instrumentation for Extracorporeal Shock-Wave Lithotripsy.** All lithotripters share four main features: an energy source, a focusing device, a coupling medium, and a stone-localization system. The original Dornier HM-3 design utilizes a spark-plug energy generator with an elliptical reflector for focusing the shock waves. A water bath transmits the shock waves to the patient, with stone localization provided by biplanar fluoroscopy. Modifications of the four basic components of this first-generation lithotripter have provided a class of second-generation lithotripters—ten of which are currently either available commercially or undergoing clinical trials (Table 1). This section on new instrumentation reviews the features and principal differences between the second-generation lithotripters with regard to shock-wave generation, focusing, patient coupling, and stone localization.

***Shock-wave generation.*** The two basic types of energy sources for generating shock waves are point sources and extended sources. The electrohydraulic devices (Dornier, Direx, Medstone, Northgate, and Technomed) utilize point sources for energy generation, whereas extended sources are incorporated in the piezoelectric (Diasonics, EDAP, and Wolf) and the electromagnetic (Siemens) devices.

The electrohydraulic shock-wave generator is located at the base of a water bath and produces shock waves using an electric spark-gap of 15,000 to 25,000 V of one microsecond duration (Fig 1). This high-voltage spark discharge produces the rapid evaporation of water which generates a shock wave by expanding the surrounding fluid ($F_1$). This electrohydraulic generator

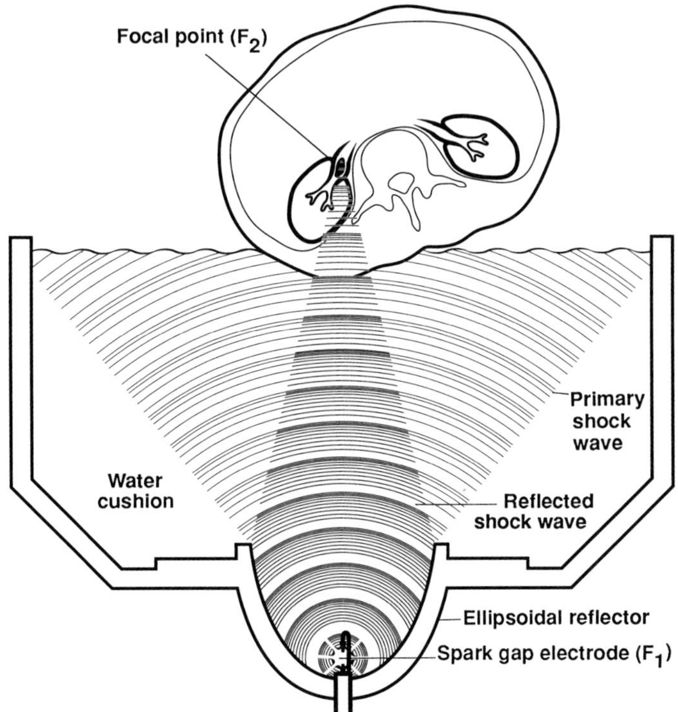


**Fig 1.** During spark-gap shock-wave generation, $F_1$ is the origin of the primary shock wave; $F_2$ is the concentration of reflected shock waves at a focal point such as a kidney stone.

is located within an ellipsoidal reflector that concentrates the reflected shock waves at the second focal point ($F_2$).

Multiple, repeated electrohydraulic shock waves from a first-generation machine produce pain at the skin level and within the focal region, thus requiring general or regional anesthesia during lithotripsy. ''Anesthesia-free'' second-generation electrohydraulic lithotripters have been developed by widening the aperture of the ellipse and decreasing the overall energy intensity of the shock-wave generator. However, some form of analgesia, sedation, or local anesthesia is usually required with the majority of second-generation electrohydraulic lithotripters (Table 2).

Piezoelectric shock waves are generated by the sudden expansion of ceramic elements excited by a high-frequency, high-voltage energy pulse. The motion of the piezoceramic elements generates an ultrasonic wave which in turn produces a shock wave directed to the focal point. The shock wave is then propagated through either a water-filled bag (as with EDAP and Diasonics machines) or basin (as with the Wolf machine). The spherical focusing mechanism of the piezoelectric lithotripters provides a wide region of shock-wave entry at the skin's surface and a very small focal region ($4 \times 8$ mm in the Wolf lithotripter). The combination of a wide aperture focusing sphere, a larger skin entry zone, a small focal region, and lower peak pressures generated by the piezoelectric machines has provided a truly anesthesia-free form of lithotripsy (Fig 2).[4,5]

In the electromagnetic (Siemens) device, shock waves are generated when an electrical impulse moves a metallic membrane that is housed within a ''shock tube.'' The resulting shock wave, produced in the water-filled shock-tube cylinder, is focused by

**TABLE 2. Anesthesia Requirements vs Lithotripter Efficiency**

| | Dornier HM-3 | Dornier HM-4 | Technomed Sonolith | Siemens Lithostar | EDAP LT-01 | Wolf Piezolith |
|---|---|---|---|---|---|---|
| Aperture | 156 mm | 170 mm | 205 mm | 120 mm | N/A | 300 mm |
| Focal size | 12 × 50 mm | 10 × 40 mm | N/A | 11 × 90 mm | N/A | 4×8 mm |
| Max. pressures | 500 Bar | N/A | 780 Bar | 440 Bar | 1050 Bar | 1140 Bar |
| Anesthesia | General | 75% Sedation | Sedation/general | Sedation local/tens | Sedation | None |
| Average # shock waves | 1200 | 2100 | 3600 | 3200 | N/A | 3600 |
| Secondary treatments | 16 | 22 | 13 | 18 | 32 | 29 |

N/A = not available

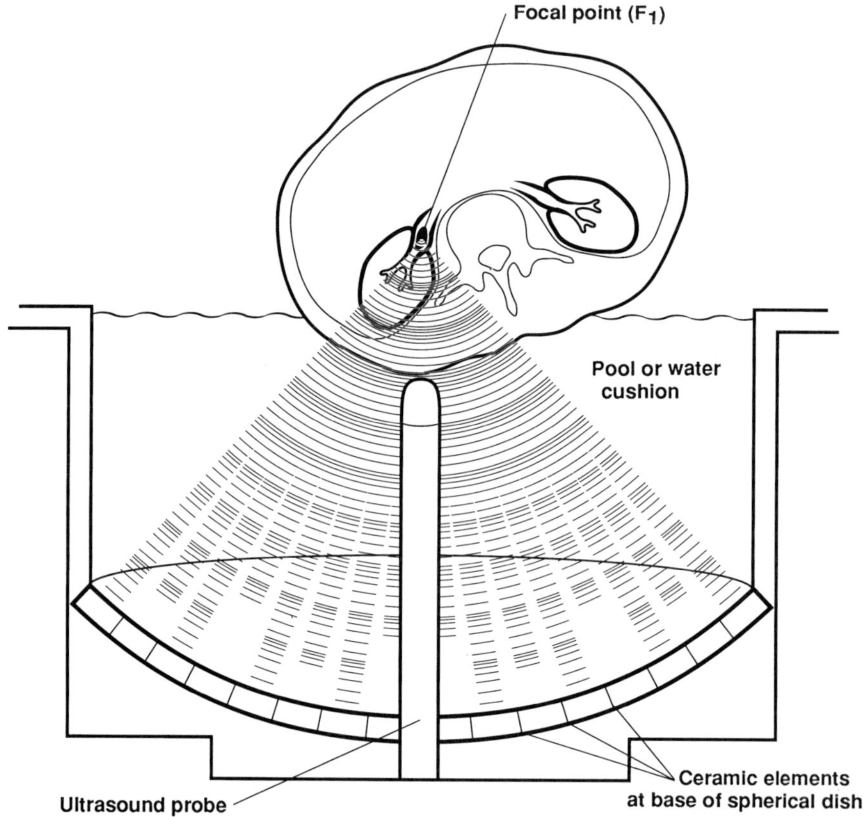


**Fig 2.** Piezoelectric shock-wave generation provides a wide point of shock-wave energy at the focal point ($F_1$).

an acoustic lens and coupled to the body surface with a water cushion (Fig 3). Some form of sedation and/or local anesthesia is usually required during treatment using this electromagnetic lithotripter due to the smaller aperture and moderate peak pressures generated. Recent studies have demonstrated that a transcutaneous electric

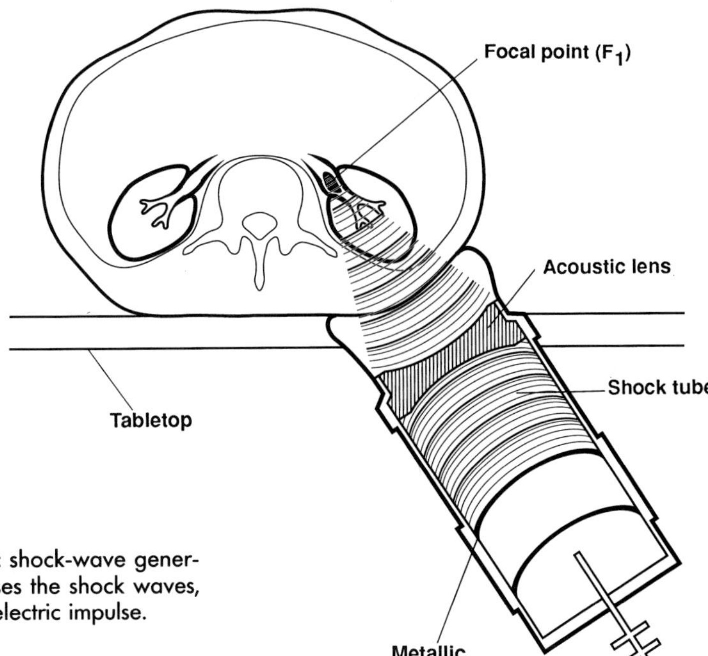


**Fig 3.** With electromagnetic shock-wave generation, an acoustic lens focuses the shock waves, which are produced by an electric impulse.

nerve stimulator (TENS) will provide adequate analgesia during lithotripsy with the Siemens machine.[6]

***Shock-wave focusing.*** Once shock waves are generated, they must be focused on the target calculus. The method of focusing is dictated by the type of shock-wave generation. Machines that utilize point sources, such as the electrohydraulic lithotripters (Fig 1), generate shock waves that travel in an expanding circular pattern and require ellipsoidal reflectors to focus the shock waves at the second focal point ($F_2$). The array of piezoceramic elements is positioned on a spherical disc that allows focusing at a very small focal region ($F_1$), whereas the vibrating metal membranes of the electromechanical lithotripter produce an acoustical wave that requires a lens for focusing the shock wave at $F_1$.

***Coupling of the shock wave.*** The coupling media currently utilized by the different lithotripters range from a 1000 L water bath to an enclosed water cushion. The water bath requires unique positioning of the patient in the tub so that the calculus is at the second focal point. Recent modifications in the patient gantry system used with the first-generation Dornier HM-3 lithotripter have allowed the treatment of children as well as patients with distal ureteral calculi. Second-generation machines have adopted designs for coupling that minimize the space requirements as well as the physiologic and functional disadvantages of a large water bath. Current models use either an enclosed water cushion, a small exposed pool of water, or a totally contained shock tube. The water-filled cushions and shock tubes contain the shock-wave source, conditioned water, and a coupling membrane to allow simplified positioning and "dry" lithotripsy. However, the direct water-skin interface utilized by two units (Technomed and Wolf) is believed by some to offer improved shock-wave coupling.

***Stone localization.*** Stone localization during lithotripsy is accomplished using either fluoroscopy or ultrasonography. Fluoroscopy provides the urologist with a familiar modality for effective renal and ureteral stone localization. Moreover, fluoroscopy facilitates the use of contrast

**TABLE 3. Third-Generation Lithotripters**

| Manufacturer | Shock-Wave Generation | Focusing | Patient Coupling Apparatus | In-Line Localization* |
|---|---|---|---|---|
| Dornier HM-5 | Spark gap | Ellipsoid | Membrane | Fluoroscopy |
| Siemens Lithostar plus | Electromagnetic | Acoustic lens | Membrane | 2 Fluoro-tubes |
| Storz Modulith SL 20 | Electromagnetic | Parabolic reflector | Membrane | Ultrasound |
| Wolf Piezolith 2500 | Piezoelectric | Spherical | Membrane | Ultrasound & fluoroscopy |

* Describes which of the localization systems is "in-line" with the shock-wave generator.

material to delineate the anatomy of the collecting system. However, fluoroscopy requires more space than ultrasonography, carries the inherent risk of delivering ionizing radiation to both the patient and medical staff, and is not useful in localizing radiolucent calculi.

Ultrasonography is becoming an increasingly important modality for the urologist. Sonography-based lithotripters offer the advantages of stone localization with continuous monitoring and effective identification of radiolucent stones, without the drawback of radiation exposure.[7] Additionally, ultrasound has been documented to be effective in localizing stone fragments as small as 2–3 mm, and is as good or better than routine KUB (kidney, ureter, and bladder plain radiographs of the abdomen) to assess patients for residual stone fragments following lithotripsy.[8] The ultrasound-based machines also have the important capability of gallstone localization for use in biliary lithotripsy (multi-purpose lithotripters: Direx, EDAP, Technomed, Wolf). The major disadvantages of ultrasound stone localization include the learning curve associated with basic mastery of the use of ultrasonic techniques by the urologist and the difficulty in localizing ureteral stones. Efforts are currently in progress to develop echogenic ureteral stents to aid in ultrasonic localization of ureteral calculi.[9]

**Third-Generation Lithotripters.** Currently, there are a number of third-generation lithotripters undergoing clinical trials; these devices attempt to incorporate many of the characteristics of an "ideal lithotripter." The basic design of the third-generation machines includes dual imaging capabilities, as well as variable shock-wave power. These machines include: Dornier MFL 5000 (HM-5), Siemens Lithostar Plus, Storz, Modulith SL20, and Wolf Piezolith 2500 (Table 3).

***Dual Imaging.*** Dual imaging capabilities entail having both fluoroscopic and sonographic localization systems available in the same machine. Such a design has the advantage of allowing the use of fluoroscopy for imaging stones within the kidney, as well as the ureter, and of sonography for the identification of radiolucent or biliary tract calculi. Moreover, sonographic capabilities allow one to initially target a stone using fluoroscopy and then switch over to ultrasound to avoid delivering an excessive amount of ionizing radiation. The inclusion of fluoroscopy capabilities may also lessen the learning curve for many urologists who are unfamiliar with sonographic stone localization procedures.

It is of interest that, while the Dornier, Siemens, and Storz machines have all added ultrasound capabilities to provide dual imaging, none of these systems provides "in-line" imaging for both the fluoroscopic and sonographic localization devices. For example, with the Dornier and Siemens machines, one can utilize sonography to target a radiolucent or biliary tract calculus, yet the patient must be moved "blindly" to the fluoroscopy unit which is in line with the shock-wave generator. Alternatively, one can utilize the fluoroscopic localization system with the Storz machine, yet only the ultrasound is in line with the shock-wave generator.

The Wolf Piezolith 2500 is the only third-generation device at this time that has both the fluoroscopy and sonography in line with the piezoelectric shock-wave generator. This permits rapid changes from fluoroscopic to sonographic stone localization, without moving the patient off the treatment dish.

***Variable Power.*** All four of the aforementioned third-generation devices have variable power shock-wave generators which allow the operator to apply the appropriate amount of shock-wave energy for a particular stone. One can turn down the generator power to provide significantly reduced anesthesia/analgesia requirements with the Dornier, Siemens, and Storz machines, and to provide anesthesia/analgesia-free lithotripsy with the Wolf device. Moreover, the shock-wave intensity can be increased using all four machines to allow adequate fragmentation of extremely hard or large calculi. However, when using these lithotripters in the "high-power mode," various forms of anesthesia/analgesia are necessary.

So, in fact, we still have not developed the "ultimate shock wave" that provides anesthesia-free lithotripsy with maximum efficiency. Yet, by varying the shock-wave energy, one can administer a highly efficient shock wave, using anesthesia/analgesia when high shock-wave pressures are indicated, or using significantly decreased shock-wave energy to provide minimal anesthesia lithotripsy.

While much of the industry has pushed for anesthesia-free capabilities over the past few years, many physicians have perhaps not been as aware and/or have ignored the potential deleterious effect that may result from excessive administration of the higher-powered electrohydraulic shock waves. Now, although variable-powered lithotripters that utilize electrohydraulic, electromagnetic, and piezoelectric energy sources are available, the physician must continue to closely monitor the total amount of energy delivered to a particular kidney to limit the incidence of significant renal injury.

### Percutaneous Nephrostolithotomy

The development of percutaneous endoscopic manipulation of stones in the renal collecting system is without precedent in the history of urologic surgery. Within one decade, the technique evolved from an adventure undertaken by only a few physicians to a routine procedure performed by thousands of urologists worldwide—only to be forced into the background by an even more revolutionary procedure for stone treatment, namely extracorporeal shock-wave lithotripsy.

**Techniques in Percutaneous Stone Manipulation.** Initially, a percutaneous nephrostomy tract must be established to gain access to the intrarenal collecting system. At our institution, this procedure is performed by a uroradiology team. The urologist is usually present during the access procedure to give suggestions concerning the optimal positioning of the nephrostomy tract. The access tract should enter the kidney through a posterior calyx; entry is usually facilitated by positioning the patient at a 30° angle on the fluoroscopy table. In most cases, the lower or middle pole calyces may be accessed below the 12th rib, but occasionally a supracostal approach is necessary to optimally reach the targeted stone.[10] One should anticipate possible cephalad renal movement during nephrostomy access placement, as this may alter the proposed approach.[11]

The nephrostomy tract is then formed by dilating the skin, fascia, muscles, and renal tissues over the guide wire. Nephrostomy tract dilatation can be performed using graduated plastic dilators (such as an Amplatz dilator) or a balloon catheter. After the nephrostomy tract has been dilated up to a 30 F (10 mm diameter) size, a hollow plastic sheath is placed in the renal pelvis. A variety of endoscopic instruments may then be passed directly into the renal collecting system to perform various manipulations.

Endoscopy is begun by performing rigid or flexible nephroscopy. Although specially designed nephroscopes with a 30° side-arm viewing system are available, a traditional panendoscope of 24 F is equally well suited for rigid nephroscopy, and allows visualization of, and manipulation inside, the renal collecting system. Once the renal pelvis and those calyces that are accessible to a rigid nephroscope have been visualized and the surgeon is familiar with the intrarenal anatomy, flexible nephroscopy can be performed to inspect individual calyces which may not be within the reach of the rigid instrument. With the help of these flexible instruments, the entire collecting system can be visualized by taking advantage of the tip deflection and rotating the instrument inside the kidney.

The diameter of the working sheath is usually 32 F, which equals about 1 cm. Therefore, stones up to this size can be extracted intact through the sheath. For the fragmentation of stones inside the renal collecting system (and the ureter) which are too large to be extracted (> 1 cm), three modalities of "power lithotripsy" are available: ultrasonic lithotripsy (UL), electrohydraulic lithotripsy (EHL), and laser lithotripsy.

***Ultrasonic Lithotripsy.*** The use of ultrasonic energy to fragment kidney stones was first described in 1979 by Alken.[12] Commercially available units consist of a power generator and an ultrasound transducer and probe (together forming the "sonotrode"). A piezoceramic element in the handle of the sonotrode is stimulated to resonate; this converts electrical energy into ultrasound waves (with a frequency of 23,000 to 27,000 Hz) which then are transmitted along the hollow metal probe, creating a vibrating action at its tip. When the vibrating tip is brought in contact with the surface of a stone, the calculus can be disintegrated. The probe must be rigid, since sound waves cannot be transmitted without energy loss along flexible probes. The probes are available in 10 F and 12 F sizes, and are passed through the straight working channel of a rigid (24 or 26 F diameter) nephroscope with a 30° or 90° offset lens. Suction tubing can be connected to the end of the sonotrode probe, thus converting the unit into a "vacuum cleaner" to remove stone fragments. Normal saline at body temperature should be used as irrigant.

UL should be the procedure of choice for fragmentation of large renal stones. However, some uric acid, calcium oxalate monohydrate, or cystine stones may not break up easily, necessitating the use of EHL. Besides the risk for perforation and extravasation of irrigant, UL is associated with noise levels of around 90 db at a distance of several inches from the transducer. Ear plugs are therefore recommended during lengthy UL sessions. Depending on the location of the stones, fragments are retained in 3% to 35% of all cases treated with ultrasonic lithotripsy. This cannot be considered a failure in many cases, because the UL is oftentimes performed with the goal of debulking of large stones to be followed by extracorporeal shock-wave lithotripsy as a planned two-stage procedure.

***Electrohydraulic Lithotripsy.*** The principles of EHL were described and developed by a Russian engineer in 1950. This technology has been used extensively for the destruction of bladder stones and in 1975, reports were published on its use for the fragmentation of kidney stones.[13] The EHL unit consists of a probe, a power generator, and a foot pedal. The probe consists of a central metal core and two layers of insulation with another metal layer between them. Probes are flexible and are available in 5, 7, and 9 F sizes to be used through either rigid or flexible nephroscopes.

Commercially available EHL units are manufactured with power up to 120 V. The electrical discharge is transmitted to the probe, where it generates a spark at the tip. The intense heat production in the immediate area surrounding the tip results in a cavitation bubble that produces a shock wave which radiates spherically in all directions. Collapse of the bubble causes a second shock wave. These shock waves, repeated at a frequency of 50–100 per second, result in destruction of the stone.

EHL will effectively fragment all kinds of urinary calculi, including the very hard cystine, uric acid, and calcium oxalate monohydrate stones. Since the probes are small and flexible, they can be passed through flexible nephroscopes and ureteroscopes to fragment stones in calyces that are unaccessible to UL, which must be performed through a rigid instrument. The primary disadvantage of EHL is the lack of an efficient method for removing the stone fragments. All particles must either be washed out during intraoperative irrigation or grasped with forceps. It is therefore advantageous to fragment the stone into the smallest number of particles allowing extraction with grasping devices (usually those sized $< 1.0$ cm). There is no virtue in transforming a large stone into hundreds of small particles or even sand-like material, because a significant amount of time will be required to remove the debris.

Overall, EHL should be used in the kidney as a technique of second choice for routine stone fragmentation, but may be the procedure of choice in the ureter. Its main application should be for very hard stones or stones not within reach of the rigid nephroscope/UL probe.

***Laser Lithotripsy.*** Laser lithotripsy is the newest modality available for stone fragmentation. The 250 μm quartz fiber of the pulsed-dye laser may easily be passed through the smallest flexible nephroscope for treatment of renal calculi. Although the indications for use of laser lithotripsy to disintegrate renal calculi are similar to those given for EHL, the major application of laser lithotripsy is to perform intraureteral fragmentation of stones and therefore will be discussed in the section on ureteroscopy.

## Ureteroscopy

The advent of ureterorenoscopy has dramatically altered the management of patients with symptomatic ureteral calculi. Rigid ureteroscopy has been used in conjunction with ultrasonic and electrohydraulic lithotripsy and pulsed-dye laser probes to successfully fragment ureteral calculi.[14,15] While improvements in fiberoptics and irrigation systems have fostered the use of smaller semi-rigid ureteroscopes (6.9 to 8.5 F), it was the introduction of flexible, deflectable ureterorenoscopes that made access to the upper ureter and intrarenal collecting system a safer and less tedious procedure.[14–16]

The extremely small working channel of the semi-rigid and flexible instruments, the sizes of which range from 2.4 to 4.0 F, limits the size and usefulness of instruments that can be passed through these ureterorenoscopes and used for stone removal. Indeed, for larger stones in the proximal ureter, the 3.0 F basket or grasping forceps are often inadequate to accomplish successful stone extraction. This limitation of the available instrumentation has prompted the use of intracorporeal lithotripsy for the management of larger upper ureteral and intrarenal calculi.

Currently the two most commonly employed methods for intracorporeal lithotripsy of ureteral stones via the flexible or semi-rigid ureterorenoscope are EHL and the pulsed dye laser. Ultrasonic lithotripsy is occasionally used for lower ureteral calculi, but its use has been supplanted to a large extent by EHL and laser lithotripsy. Although the choice of intracorporeal fragmentation is frequently based on the location and composition of the stone to be treated, the experience of the clinician and availability of equipment more often dictate this decision.

***Electrohydraulic Lithotripsy.*** The first experience with electrohydraulic lithotripsy in the ureter entailed use of a 6 F EHL probe which was fluoroscopically guided to the obstructing calculus.[17] The most common cause of failure in early experience was secondary to the operator's inability to pass the probe to the level of the stone. Additional early ureteral experience with EHL described the use of a 9 F probe which provided excellent fragmentation of the stone; however, ureteral extravasation was observed in 40% of the patients following the lithotripsy procedure.[18] This high complication rate was believed to be mainly due to the large probe size. The use of a smaller, 5 F EHL probe through the rigid ureteroscope was hindered by decreased stone visualization, as the probe occupied the majority of the working channel of the rigid ureteroscope.[19] The development of a smaller, 3 F EHL probe for use with a flexible ureteroscope was reported in 1988.[20] Recently, a 1.9 F EHL probe has been developed which is quite successful in fragmenting ureteral and intrarenal stones. An additional benefit of these small caliber probes is the possibility of improved visualization through the flexible ureteroscope, as a larger portion of the working channel is available for irrigation.[21]

***Laser Lithotripsy.*** As noted before, laser lithotripsy is also utilized for the management of ureteral calculi. The significant advances in laser fibers and power-generation systems have made laser lithotripsy, in many practitioners' hands, the treatment of choice for ureteral stones.[22] The pulsed-dye laser delivers short, 1 μsec, pulsations at 5–10 Hz that are produced by a tunable dye laser using coumarin R as the dye. This produces laser light in the 504 nm (green) range. The 504 nm wave length produced by the dye laser is selectively absorbed by the stone and not the surrounding ureteral wall.

As the energy is delivered in short pulses, minimal heat is generated, protecting the ureter.[22–24] Initial experience has yielded fragmentation rates from 64% to 95%.[25–27] Failures have been related to equipment malfunction (4% to 19%) or, more often, to stone composition. Moreover, use of EHL and/or basketing has been necessary as an adjunctive measure to laser lithotripsy in some cases of successful stone removal.[28] Use of the pulsed-dye laser in the ureter in all series appears to be safe, as no significant intraoperative or postoperative complications have been reported.

Continued developments in laser technology have yielded larger diameter laser fibers which are able to fragment hard calculi more effectively. Newer 300 μm and 320 μm laser fibers are superior to the 200 μm fibers in the fragmentation of calcium oxalate monohydrate and cystine stones,[29] and fragmentation rates of greater than 90% have been obtained with these new fibers. As the field continues to advance, new materials such as alexandrite are being tested as sources for new laser lithotripsy units.[30] Currently, cost is the most prohibitive aspect of laser lithotripsy, as most laser units command an initial investment of approximately $200,000 and have equally expensive yearly labor contracts.

## Open Lithotomy

As percutaneous nephrolithotomy, extracorporeal shock-wave lithotripsy, and ureteroscopy are now widely embraced as preferred treatments for the majority of patients with renal and ureteral calculi, the indications for open lithotomy have decreased dramatically. Currently, with use of the available technology, only 1% to 5% of stones will require open surgery for removal. Of 893 procedures to remove stones performed since the introduction of extracorporeal lithotripsy at their institution, Assimos et al found that 4.1% of cases required open lithotomy for renal calculi.[31] The most common indication for open lithotomy was failure of extracorporeal lithotripsy or percutaneous nephrolithotomy.

Morbidly obese patients often require open lithotomy, as their body habitus precludes fluoroscopic or sonographic localization or effective treatment of renal calculi (the shock waves become attenuated in the excess tissue). Also, a large amount of adipose tissue in the flank may prevent placement of an Amplatz sheath into the renal pelvis during percutaneous nephrostolithotomy. Percutaneous nephrostolithotomy often requires an extended operative period; patients with multiple medical problems or diminished cardiac reserve may benefit from a shorter open procedure. Stones found in a collecting system with distal obstruction may require open lithotomy and concomitant pyeloplasty. In addition, obstructed or scarred calyceal infundibula may be repaired with calyorrhaphy or calycoplasty after removal of the stone.[28] Coagulum pyelolithotomy may be helpful in patients with many small stones scattered throughout multiple calyces. This procedure may also be of benefit to clear small residual calculi in patients who have undergone anatrophic nephrolithotomy.[28,32]

For branched renal calculi, surgical procedures beyond simple open pyelolithotomy may be necessary for stone removal. Pyelonephrolithotomy may be used for isolated, lower-pole branched calculi in a small pelvis or in a system with stenotic infundibula. Anatrophic nephrolithotomy is based on the blood supply to the kidney using the relatively avascular plane of Brodel's line for the lateral renal parenchymal incision prior to entering the collecting system. This approach permits wide exposure of the renal pelvis and allows en bloc removal of the branched calculi leaving minimal amounts of residual calculi.[33] Patients with complex stones or evidence of parenchymal loss may benefit from either partial or complete nephrectomy for stone disease.[31]

## MANAGEMENT OF RENAL CALCULI

Several possibilities exist for the treatment of renal calculi. Extracorporeal shock wave lithotripsy, percutaneous nephrolithotripsy, ureterorenoscopy, and open lithotomy all provide the means to effectively remove renal calculi in given clinical situations. Other issues germane to any discussion of the treatment of renal calculi are the size of the stone being treated, stone composition (in particular, cystine or calcium oxalate monohydrate), location of the stone within the kidney, and renal anatomy.

### Small Calculi

Although multiple treatment options exist for small renal calculi, extracorporeal shock-wave lithotripsy has repeatedly been shown to be extremely effective for smaller stones. As a result, percutaneous nephrostolithotomy has been relegated to playing a less significant role in the management of small renal calculi. However, several indications still exist for percutaneous stone removal. Failure of either of these modalities to completely remove the renal stone burden may necessitate open lithotomy, or in some cases, flexible ureterorenoscopy.

The first generation Dornier HM-3 lithotripter represents the "gold standard" for efficacy of stone fragmentation, to which other second-generation lithotripters must be compared. As the shock-wave pressure (power), and focal region of the second-generation machines have been reduced, so have the requirements for anesthesia or analgesia. However, the price paid for anesthesia-free lithotripsy is a reduction in efficiency of stone fragmentation. For stones less than 1.5 cm in maximum dimension, the Dornier HM-3 lithotripter averages 1200 shocks per treatment, yielding a stone-free rate of approximately 85%, and a retreatment rate of 16%.[34,35] For stones less than 2 cm, an 81% stone-free rate can be expected. However, as one alters the configuration of the shock wave by widening the aperture of the ellipsoid (eg, when using the modified Dornier HM-3 and HM-4 machines), the average number of required shock waves increases to 2100 and the stone-free rate ranges from 56% to 82%, while the retreatment rate has been reported to increase from 22% to 37%.[36–39]

Similarly, there is a compromise in efficiency with the piezoelectric lithotripters. Clinical studies using piezoelectric lithotripsy (Wolf Piezolith 2300, EDAP LT.01) have reported an 84% to 90% stone-free rate at 3 months for patients with stones less than 1.5 cm in diameter. However, upwards of 30% of these patients may require a secondary treatment. Moreover, the average number of shock waves increases to approximately 3500 shocks per treatment.[5,7,40–44] The requirement for repeat treatments with the piezoelectric machines is somewhat offset by the fact that each treatment is performed as an "office" procedure, and does not require anesthesia, analgesia, or significant recovery time.

Electromagnetic lithotripsy is usually performed with intravenous or oral sedation; local anesthesia at the skin entry site may or may not be used. Some centers have found that a transcutaneous nerve stimulator unit provides adequate analgesia in 90% of treated patients. The mean number of shock waves per treatment is approximately 3600, and this type of lithotripsy is associated with a stone-free rate of 66% and a retreatment rate of 11%.[6]

Currently, many variable-power, third-generation lithotripters are in clinical use (Dornier HM-5, Sonolith 2000, and Wolf Piezolith 2500). Using the lower power setting, these machines have an approximate stone-free rate of 70%, and a retreatment rate of 14% to 25%.[45–51] Therefore, in order to achieve anesthesia-free status, the number of secondary treatments will probably increase and, therefore, the efficiency will be diminished.

Though extracorporeal lithotripsy represents the gold standard for treatment of renal calculi of less than 2 cm, some stones are recalcitrant to this mode of treatment. In these cases, percutaneous nephrostolithotomy would be the treatment of second choice. Stone-free rates of greater than 90% to 95% can be expected with renal calculi less than 2 cm in size. Morbidly obese patients often require percutaneous stone removal, as stone imaging and the effectiveness of the shock waves are hampered by the excess tissue. Hard stones, composed of cystine or calcium oxalate monohydrate, are relative indications for performing percutaneous nephrostolithotomy. Although extracorporeal shock-wave lithotripsy and percutaneous nephrostolithotomy occasionally fail, open lithotomy is only rarely necessary for the management of patients with small renal calculi.

## Large Calculi

Though the management of most patients with large renal calculi is similar to that of patients with smaller renal calculi, the clinician will find a larger population of patients that require some modality other than extracorporeal shock-wave lithotripsy for stone removal. Because fragmentation efficiency decreases with increasing stone size, percutaneous nephrostolithotomy may be, in certain cases, the treatment of choice. As with smaller stones, open lithotomy is required only for those stones resistant to previous treatment attempts.

As the stone volume increases, the efficacy of all lithotripters diminishes significantly. For example, for a stone burden of greater than 3 cm in a dilated collecting system, only 30% of the patients will be rendered stone free with Dornier HM-3 monotherapy.[52] While the stone-free rate for patients with large calculi will increase to approximately 70% for those with normal collecting system anatomy, many clinicians prefer the use of percutaneous nephrolithotripsy as the initial form of therapy for large renal calculi. Studies have found the combination of percutaneous nephrolithotripsy and extracorporeal shock-wave lithotripsy to be more effective than extracorporeal shock-wave lithotripsy alone. With this type of combination therapy, stone-free rates approaching 85% to 90% have been reported for those with large renal calculi.[3,53–56]

Previous studies have shown that the critical stone burden in considering extracorporeal lithotripsy monotherapy is a stone diameter of 2 cm.[57] In stones larger than 2 cm, the number of patients requiring ancillary procedures after extracorporeal shock-wave lithotripsy rises from 11% to 27%, and the incidence of significant residual fragments from 3% to 10% (up to 57% for stones greater than 3 cm in diameter). For stones larger than 2.5 cm, previous studies have shown an 83% stone-free rate after percutaneous nephrostolithotomy, with a 17% auxiliary procedure rate. Approximately 77% of all stones larger than 3 cm require additional treatment. Therefore, for complete and incomplete staghorn calculi, as well as for stones larger than 3 cm in diameter, percutaneous nephrostolithotomy should be the initial procedure, since it will occasionally be the only one required. The use of percutaneous nephrostolithotomy for stones between 2 and 3 cm depends on the preference of the physician. Percutaneous nephrostolithotomy is indicated if there is obstruction of the urinary tract between the stone location and the ureterovesical junction (eg, infundibular stenosis, primary or secondary ureteropelvic junction obstruction, ureteral stricture, or ureterovesical junction obstruction). Although the total hospital cost was slightly higher for patients undergoing percutaneous management of larger renal calculi, the convalescent period was significantly shorter than that observed in patients undergoing open lithotomy.[58]

Again, open lithotomy is not the principal therapeutic choice for large renal calculi, but must always be considered in patients with existing renal anomalies or previous failed treatment with either extracorporeal lithotripsy or percutaneous nephrostolithotomy.

## Staghorn Calculi

One of the current controversies in stone management is the treatment of staghorn calculi. Treatment philosophies vary, from single-modality treatment of all staghorn calculi with extracorporeal lithotripsy, to combined treatment with percutaneous nephrolithotomy and extracorporeal shock-wave lithotripsy, to open lithotomy. The differences in opinion are based on the inferior results obtained with the treatment of renal calculi by extracorporeal shock wave lithotripsy and the increased patient morbidity caused by the other modalities.

Initially, staghorn calculi were treated solely with open lithotomy with reasonable success rates. But with the advent of percutaneous nephrolithotomy in the early 1980s, new avenues were opened for treatment of this troublesome stone. Though one could expect anatrophic nephrolithotomy to render a patient free of stones in approximately 65% to 90% of cases, there was a high complication rate (up to 50%) and significant time is needed for convalescence.[59] Complete success in removal of staghorn calculi by percutaneous nephrolithotomy is achieved in 62% to 95% of patients, with a 20% to 57% complication rate.[59–61] Most authors employ a single treatment session but sometimes require multiple tracts to completely access a branched calculus percutaneously. Often, clinicians prefer to stage the percutaneous procedure, and ask the patients to return for a second percutaneous nephrolithotomy.[52]

As extracorporeal lithotripsy became widely available for the treatment of renal calculi, attempts to treat staghorn calculi with this modality were reported in the literature. Initially, the reports were dismal, as most patients underwent only a single treatment and follow-up was quite short. With multiple treatments, prolonged follow-up, and ureteral stenting, stone-free rates at 3–6 months have been reported to range from 36% to 72%, with complication rates similar to those associated with percutaneous nephrostolithotomy (12% to 64%).[62–67]

Recently, many clinicians have suggested the combined use of percutaneous nephrostolithotomy and extracorporeal lithotripsy for treatment of staghorn calculi. The initial treatment session debulks the stone through a percutaneous tract using ultrasonic and/or electrohydraulic lithotripsy (Table 4). If retained renal calculi are noted on postprocedure radiographs, extracorporeal lithotripsy—with or without internal ureteral stenting—is then used to fragment the remaining stone burden. Also, flexible nephroscopy may be used as a final procedure to remove additional fragments. Success rates of 80% to 95% have been reported with this combined approach.[68–70] Kahnowski et al studied combination therapy with extracorporeal lithotripsy and percutaneous nephrostolithotomy and found that percutaneous nephrostolithotomy was

**TABLE 4. Management of Staghorn Calculi**

| | Stone-Free Rate (%) | Complications (%) | Hospital Stay (Days) |
|---|---|---|---|
| Shock-wave lithotripsy | 31–67 | 28–50 | 10 |
| Percutaneous nephrolithotomy | 74–68 | 19–40 | 5–10 |
| Combined | 60–92 | 14–34 | 15 |
| Open surgery | 80–91 | 48–50 | 7–10 |

the only procedure required to render the patient stone free in 14 of 44 patients with complete staghorn calculi. Moreover, the incidence of urosepsis was reduced, and the nephrostomy tract allowed irrigation to be performed to wash out fragments and to allow postoperative chemolysis.[71] In a direct comparison between extracorporeal lithotripsy and percutaneous nephrostolithotomy, Winfield et al demonstrated that the number of re-hospitalizations after extracorporeal lithotripsy monotherapy was as high as 48% while it was only 6% to 13% following primary percutaneous nephrostolithotomy therapy. Placement of a nephrostomy tube was necessary in more than 40% of patients after extracorporeal lithotripsy. In this study, the stone-free rate after extracorporeal lithotripsy monotherapy was only 39% at 8 months. In contrast, only 14% of patients treated with percutaneous nephrostolithotomy alone had residual calculi.[72]

A few alternative methods have been explored to treat staghorn calculi. Aso and associates have used ureterorenoscopy and EHL to treat patients with partial and complete staghorn calculi. They report that 88.2% were successfully treated with this method, but also reported markedly increased operative time.[73] Ureteroscopy with ultrasonic stone fragmentation has also been used to debulk staghorn calculi prior to extracorporeal lithotripsy.[74]

As mentioned, controversy over the most appropriate treatment modality for staghorn calculi exists, as no modality seems to be clearly superior. Based on these reports, initial debulking with percutaneous nephrostolithotomy followed by extracorporeal shock-wave lithotripsy, if necessary, appears to be the procedure of choice for removal of complete and incomplete staghorn calculi. But for incomplete staghorn calculi, initial treatment could consist of either percutaneous nephrostolithotomy alone or extracorporeal shock-wave lithotripsy with internal ureteral stenting, especially if the lithotripter to be used is a high-power, spark-gap generator or a variable-power, third-generation machine. Residual calculi can be treated by repeat extracorporeal lithotripsy or staged percutaneous nephrostolithotomy using a flexible nephroscope in the established tract. For complete staghorn calculi, the combination of percutaneous nephrostolithotomy and extracorporeal lithotripsy is most efficacious.

Open pyelolithotomy or anatrophic nephrolithotomy may be considered for patients with extremely dilated collecting systems. Also, staghorn calculi with multiple calyceal extensions may best be managed with anatrophic nephrolithotomy, as multiple secondary percutaneous procedures may be required to clear all affected calyces. As previously mentioned, anatomic abnormalities associated with staghorn calculi may be surgically corrected at the time of stone removal. Moreover, those patients with calyceal or ureteropelvic junction obstruction may require adjunctive postprocedure measures and are at increased risk for complications during extracorporeal shock-wave lithotripsy or percutaneous nephrostolithotomy for treatment of staghorn calculi.

## Calyceal Diverticular Stones

Treatment of calculi in calyceal diverticula has long been a source of controversy. Some researchers question the clinical significance of these stones and their ability to cause symptoms of such severity as to mandate intervention. Experience with extracorporeal shock-wave lithotripsy as monotherapy is varied, with stone-free rates ranging from 20% to 56%. Though the stone-free rate for treatment of calyceal diverticular stones is routinely poor, 75% of patients in one series have reported an improvement in, or resolution of, their symptoms despite a 25% stone-free rate.[75] Recently, the success rates of extracorporeal lithotripsy, extracorporeal lithotripsy combined with percutaneous nephrostolithotomy, and percutaneous nephrostolithotomy alone were compared for the treatment of calyceal diverticular stones.[76] In the group treated with extracorporeal shock-wave lithotripsy alone, the stone-free rate was only 4% and the symptom-free rate was equally unimpressive (36%). In patients treated with percutaneous nephrostolithotomy alone or in combination with extracorporeal shock-wave lithotripsy, the stone-free rate was 92%, with 100% of the patients rendered symptom free. Therefore, percutaneous nephrostolithotomy may be the procedure of choice; small, residual calculi may require secondary treatment with extracorporeal shock-wave lithotripsy. Alternatively, with the noninvasive nature of extracorporeal shock-wave lithotripsy, the physician and patient may opt to use this modality as initial treatment for calyceal diverticular calculi, despite its apparent shortcomings.

## Lower-Pole Renal Calculi

As the results of the initial clinical studies using extracorporeal shock-wave lithotripsy were reported, it was clear that treatment of lower-pole renal calculi by extracorporeal shock-wave lithotripsy was associated with a lower stone-free rate when compared with results obtained with calculi located in other parts of the kidney. In 1986, the United States Cooperative Study of Extracorporeal Shock Wave Lithotripsy found, by stratifying stone-free rate by original location of calyceal stones, that the lower-pole calculi stone-free rate was 71.1% as compared with 83.8% for stones located in the renal pelvis. Of interest, only 64.1% of stones originally in the superior calyx, and 75.7% of middle calyx stones, were completely cleared at 3 months in this series. Also, 44.3% of all residual stone fragments were found in the lower-pole calyx.[77] A more obvious difference in the stone-free rate of dependent calyceal stones was noted in a later series, in which 58% of lower-pole calyces were rendered stone free by extracorporeal shock-wave lithotripsy versus 84%, 78%, and 76%, respectively, in the renal pelvis, upper-pole calyx, and middle calyx.[74]

One study has compared percutaneous stone extraction and extracorporeal shock-wave lithotripsy treatment of solitary lower-pole calculi. Of the patients treated with percutaneous nephrostolithotomy, 85% were stone free at 13 months, compared with 59% of those treated with extracorporeal lithotripsy. However, the hospital stay and recovery time were greater in the percutaneous nephrolithotomy group, as were the complication and retreatment/auxiliary procedure rates. Extracorporeal lithotripsy was therefore recommended as the treatment of choice for lower-pole calculi. In an attempt to overcome this apparent anatomical disadvantage, some centers employ positional techniques to improve clearance of lower-pole calyceal stone debris following extracorporeal shock-wave lithotripsy.[78]

## Horseshoe Kidney

Stones form in approximately 20% of patients with a horseshoe kidney. The ureters arise high in the renal pelvis and pass anteriorly. It is believed that this configuration leads to the common finding of hydronephrosis in patients with horseshoe kidneys, with resultant urinary stasis, infection, and subsequent stone formation. Approximately 50% of patients with stones in horseshoe kidneys treated with extracorporeal lithotripsy monotherapy will become stone free.[79] The antero-medial and inferior position of the horseshoe kidney makes stone localization with ultrasound, and often with fluoroscopy difficult, if not impossible, in some cases. Also, the dilated collecting system of the horseshoe kidney may prevent fragment passage after extracorporeal lithotripsy. A recent study reported treatment of 15 patients with calculi in horseshoe kidneys with percutaneous nephrostolithotomy.[80] Approximately 78% of these patients were stone free at follow-up; this figure improved to 88.8% when extracorporeal lithotripsy was used to treat residual fragments. Caution should be used by the inexperienced radiologist or urologist when treating horseshoe kidneys, as anomalous vessels may complicate development of a percutaneous nephrostomy tract.

## Solitary Kidney

Treatment of stones in a solitary kidney provides a significant challenge for the urologist. Prior to the introduction of percutaneous nephrostolithotomy and extracorporeal lithotripsy, retrospective studies failed to reveal any changes in renal function after anatrophic nephrolithotomy of a solitary kidney.[81,82] Experience with percutaneous nephrostolithotomy in solitary kidneys has been found to be safe and efficacious.[83] Treatment of renal calculi by extracorporeal lithotripsy also was shown to have minimal to no deleterious effect on renal function and was not associated with an increased incidence of complications.[84]

Recently, a long-term comparison of renal function in patients with solitary kidneys and/or moderate renal insufficiency after treatment of renal calculi by percutaneous nephrostolithotomy or extracorporeal lithotripsy was reported.[85] In patients with a solitary kidney and creatinine levels lower than 2 mg/dL, 13% of those undergoing percutaneous stone removal and 29% of those who underwent extracorporeal shock-wave lithotripsy showed at least a 25% deterioration of renal function approximately 4 years following the procedure. In patients with a solitary kidney, or two kidneys with creatinine levels from 2–3 mg/dL, no patients experienced renal deterioration. In contrast, of patients with creatinine levels greater than 3 mg/dL and either two kidneys or a solitary kidney, 80% who underwent extracorporeal lithotripsy showed a decrease in renal function compared to none of those who underwent percutaneous nephrostolithotomy. The investigators concluded that extracorporeal lithotripsy may be contraindicated in patients with a solitary kidney or in patients with two kidneys and creatinine levels greater than 3 mg/dL.

While it appears that most modalities available for stone removal are safe and effective in a solitary kidney, treatment philosophies for patients with stones in a solitary kidney should, for the most part, be based on those used in patients with paired kidneys.

## MANAGEMENT OF URETERAL CALCULI

Concomitant to the development of the technologies associated with extracorporeal lithotripsy has been the remarkable advance in modalities for treatment of ureteral calculi. The development of the rigid, and later, the semi-rigid and flexible fiberoptic ureteroscopes has made the entire ureter and renal pelvis accessible for treatment of ureteral and renal stones. Advances in the fiberoptic lens systems in more recent ureteroscopes have decreased the size of the instrument, allowing the ureter to be traversed without prior dilation. Additionally, intracorporeal stone fragmentation has improved with recent developments in electrohydraulic lithotripsy and laser lithotripsy. While most proximal ureteral stones are currently treated by extracorporeal shock-wave lithotripsy, ureterorenoscopy continues to be used by many physicians to treat mid- and distal-ureteral stones. Moreover, ureteroscopic and/or percutaneous access is often useful for the management of patients with ureteral calculi in whom shock-wave lithotripsy was ineffective.

### Proximal Ureteral Calculi

The options for treatment of proximal ureteral calculi are numerous. Proximal ureteral stones are easily localized and treated with the fluoroscopic and ultrasound imaging systems used with various first- and second-generation lithotripters. Stones in the proximal ureter may be easily approached by percutaneous antegrade techniques. With flexible ureteroscopy, the upper ureter is routinely accessible, and treatment of proximal stones with various modalities has been quite successful.

A large number of centers are using in situ extracorporeal shock-wave lithotripsy monotherapy to treat proximal ureteral stones. First- and second-generation lithotripters which employ fluoroscopy to localize ureteral stones may be used to achieve stone-free rates of between 61% and 100% when treating patients with upper ureteral stones.[25,86,87] Proximal ureteral calculi may also be pushed into the renal pelvis to facilitate extracorporeal visualization, targeting, and fragmentation (the so-called "push-bang" technique). Extracorporeal shock-wave lithotripsy of proximal ureteral stones can occasionally be tedious with second-generation units in which ultrasound is used for localization, but fragmentation rates of up to 90% can be expected. Placement of a ureteral stent appears to aid in the fragmentation and visualization of the stone. Recently, a brightly echogenic stent has been developed which may provide additional aid to the urologist using ultrasound to localize ureteral calculi.[9] The renal coil of this stent provides a sonographic landmark which may then be traced through the ureteropelvic junction to the level of the stone.

Proximal ureteral calculi may be approached endoscopically with the flexible ureteroscope and fragmented with either EHL or laser lithotripsy. Initial success with EHL was overshadowed by a relatively high complication rate (up to 40%).[18] With rigid ureteroscopy, 75% and 22% fragmentation rates, respectively, were reported for intracorporeal EHL of mid- and proximal ureteral calculi. Recent studies are more encouraging, and stone-free rates approach 95% using either a 3 F or 1.9 F EHL with flexible ureteroscopy; this success is associated with insignificant complication rates.[20,21,88] Laser lithotripsy of proximal ureteral calculi has proven to be highly efficacious, and is, to some investigators, treatment of choice. Several authors have reported achieving fragmentation rates ranging from 60% to 88%.[26,27,89,90] Cystine and calcium oxalate monohydrate calculi were often poorly fragmented with the early laser prototypes, but fragmentation rates have improved with the use of larger, higher-power laser fibers as well as the new Alexandrite lasers.

The percutaneous antegrade approach to proximal ureteral calculi is also a viable treatment option. In one series, 35 of 37 proximal ureteral calculi and 20 of 20 mid-ureteral calculi were successfully removed intact by flexible nephroscopy, fragmented with either EHL or ultrasonic lithotripsy, or basketed under fluoroscopic guidance.[91]

## Mid-Ureteral Calculi

Treatment of calculi in the mid-ureter has become significantly less troublesome with advent of the ureteroscope and associated instrumentation used for in situ fragmentation. Extracorporeal lithotripsy is now being used extensively for mid-ureteral stone fragmentation, although early studies reported decreased stone-free rates for patients with such calculi.[92,93] With treatment performed in the prone position, one series reported a 94% stone-free rate with treatment using the HM-3 lithotripter.[94] This positional change decreases the attenuation of shock waves that is normally encountered with traditional shock-wave entry through the patient's back. Again, incorporating the prone position, 100% of patients were stone free at 3 months after treatment with the second-generation Siemens Lithostar lithotripter.[95] Because of the presence of the bony pelvis and sacrum, as well as the lack of easily identified sonographic landmarks, extracorporeal shock-wave lithotripsy of mid-ureteral calculi using second-generation ultrasound-guided lithotripters has presented significant difficulty. Despite this, some series have shown stone-free rates in excess of 75% for in situ treatment of mid-ureteral stones using ultrasound-guided lithotripters.[96] As with proximal ureteral stones, mid-ureteral calculi may be pushed into the renal pelvis for "routine" extracorporeal shock-wave lithotripsy.

If a general anesthetic is required to perform extracorporeal shock-wave lithotripsy, ureteroscopy may be considered for stone removal. Mid-ureteral stones are easily accessible using both rigid and flexible ureteroscopy. New, small-diameter, semirigid fiberoptic ureteroscopes obviate the need for dilatation while providing excellent optics, enabling the urologist to treat ureteral calculi in a minimally invasive fashion, and in select cases, under sedation only. In most series, stones in the mid-ureter treated with ureteroscopy are removed in 80% to 95% of cases with either EHL, laser, or ultrasonic lithotripsy, with or without basketing. If extracorporeal shock-wave lithotripsy is available, it may be reasonable to make an initial attempt to fragment the mid-ureteral stone in situ or proceed with either the "push-bang" technique or with a stent past the stone. Failures may then be approached by using repeat extracorporeal lithotripsy or ureteroscopy. If the available lithotripter utilizes ultrasound for stone localization, or if extracorporeal shock-wave lithotripsy is not available, it seems prudent to make the initial attempt at stone removal with the ureteroscope, using either EHL or laser to fragment the stone, as stone-free rates with these techniques are equivalent or superior to those of extracorporeal shock-wave lithotripsy alone.

### Distal Ureteral Stones

For many clinicians, ureteroscopy is the preferred treatment for distal ureteral calculi, though extracorporeal shock-wave lithotripsy is used as treatment of choice at some centers. Recently, several investigators have touted the use of extracorporeal shock-wave lithotripsy for the treatment of distal and prevesicular stones, with the patient in a prone or modified sitting position. One study demonstrated an 87% stone-free rate after one treatment using the HM-3 lithotripter on patients positioned in the prone position.[97] Similar results have been noted in other series using the Dornier HM-3 lithotripter for in situ treatment of distal ureteral stones.[98,99]

Treatment of distal ureteral stones with rigid ureteroscopy has proven to be reliable and safe, and requires less technical expertise than when used in patients with more proximal calculi. Lower ureteral stones can be removed by ureteroscopy in approximately 90% to 99% of cases.[100–103] Although controversy exists as to which intraureteral fragmentation method is superior, it is clear that ultrasonic lithotripsy, EHL, or laser lithotripsy will be effective treatment for at least 90% of distal ureteral stones. Therefore, the means of intracorporeal fragmentation should be based primarily on the clinician's familiarity with the method chosen and the available equipment.

In summary, some investigators feel the treatment of distal ureteral stones may best be managed initially with endoscopic techniques. As excellent results have been obtained with in situ treatment of distal ureteral stones by extracorporeal shock-wave lithotripsy, this may become the treatment of choice for some clinicians. Of course, failure of both treatment options may require the use of antegrade percutaneous management or open ureterolithotomy.

## MEDICAL MANAGEMENT OF NEPHROLITHIASIS

The dramatic success of innovative surgical techniques for the removal of renal and ureteral calculi using percutaneous nephrostolithotomy, ureteroscopy, and extracorporeal shock-wave lithotripsy has prompted some physicians to disparage the need for medical evaluation and treatment of nephrolithiasis. Although these facilitative techniques have greatly reduced the pain and postoperative morbidity associated with conventional open surgical procedures, they are costly and may be attended by certain hazards and complications. Moreover, emerging evidence indicates that the recurrent formation of renal stones may be prevented by a variety of medical treatments designed to correct underlying metabolic derangements or disturbances in urinary biochemistry.[104] A remission rate of greater than 80% can be obtained in patients undergoing selective medical therapy for nephrolithiasis. In patients with mild to moderately severe stone disease, virtually total control can be achieved, as evidenced by remission rates of greater than 95%.[105]

The need for repeat stone removal may be dramatically reduced by a prophylactic medical program. Therefore, it is essential that an integrated approach to stone management be undertaken that encompasses both the actual removal of symptomatic calculi as well as the ability to investigate and medically treat patients to prevent recurrence of renal stones. It is only with this combined approach that one may be able to arrest recurrent nephrolithiasis.[104,105]

## REFERENCES


1. Chaussy C, Schmiedt E. Shock wave treatment for stones in the upper urinary tract. *Urol Clin North Am.* 1982;10(4):743–750.
2. Chaussy C, Schmiedt E, Jocham D, et al. First clinical experience with extracorporeally induced destruction of kidney stones by shock waves. *J Urol.* 1982;127:417–420.
3. Brown RD, Preminger GM. Changing surgical aspects in urinary stone disease. In: Resnick MI, ed. *Surgery Clinics of North America.* Philadelphia: WB Saunders Company; 1988:1085–1104.
4. Chuong CJ, Zhong P, Preminger GM. Pressure measurement in a Wolf Piezolith 2200 lithotripter. In: Lingeman JE, Newman DM, eds. *Shock Wave Lithotripsy: State of the Art.* New York: Plenum Press; 1988:395–398.
5. Preminger GM, Ewing JH. Piezoelectric lithotripsy: initial experience with the Wolf 2200. In: Lingeman JE, Newman DM, eds. *Shock Wave Lithotripsy: State of the Art.* New York: Plenum Press; 1988:281–284.
6. McClennan BL, Clayman RV. Lithostar: results of electromagnetic acoustic shock wave lithotripsy in over 250 patients. In: *Proc 5th Symp on Shock Wave Lithotripsy*; 1989.
7. Preminger GM. Sonographic, piezoelectric lithotripsy: more bang for your buck. *J Endourol.* 1989;3:321–327.
8. Abernathy BA, Wilson WT, Morris JS, Miller GL, Preminger GM. Evaluation of residual stone fragments following lithotripsy-sonography versus KUB. *J Urol.* 1989;141:176A.
9. Wilson WT, Feagins BA, Preminger GM. Development of an echogenic stent to aid in sonographic stent localization. *J Urol.* 1990; 143:260A.
10. Segura JW, Patterson DE, Leroy AJ, et al. Percutaneous removal of kidney stones: review of 1,000 cases. *J Urol.* 1985;134:1077–1081.
11. Preminger GM, Schultz S, Clayman RV, Curry TS, Redman HC, Peters PC. Cephalad renal movement during percutaneous nephrostolithotomy. *J Urol.* 1987;137:623–625.
12. Alken P. Percutaneous ultrasonic destruction of renal calculi. *Urol Clin North Am.* 1982; 9(1):145–151.
13. Raney AM, Handler J. Electrohydraulic nephrolithotripsy. *Urology.* 1975;6:439–442.
14. Preminger GM, Roehrborn CG. Special applications of flexible deflectable ureterorenoscopy. *Semin Urol.* 1989;7:16–24.
15. Beck EM, Vaughn ED, Sosa RE. Pulsed dye laser in the treatment of ureteral calculi. *Semin Urol.* 1989;7:25–29.
16. Huffman JL. Experience with the 8.5 F compact rigid ureteroscope. *Semin Urol.* 1989; 7:3–6.
17. Reuter HJ, Kern E. Electronic lithotripsy of ureteral calculi. *J Urol.* 1973;110:181–183.
18. Raney AM. Electrohydraulic ureterolithotripsy: preliminary report. *Urology.* 1978; 12:284–285.
19. Green DF, Lytton B. Early experience with direct vision electrohydraulic lithotripsy of ureteral calculi. *J Urol.* 1985;133:767–770.
20. Begun FP, Jacobs SC, Lawson RK. Use of a prototype 3 F electrohydraulic electrode with ureteroscopy for treatment of ureteral calculous disease. *J Urol.* 1988;139:1188–1191.
21. Feagins BA, Wilson WT, Preminger GM. Intracorporeal electrohydraulic lithotripsy with flexible ureterorenoscopy. *J Endourol.* 1990; 4:347–351.
22. Dretler SP. Laser photofragmentation of ureteral calculi: analysis of 75 cases. *J Endourol.* 1987;1:9–14.
23. Coptcoat MJ, Ison KT, Watson G, Wickham JEA. Lasertripsy for ureteral stones: 100 clinical cases. *J Endourol.* 1987;1:119–122.
24. Dretler SP, Watson G, Parhish L, Murray S. Laser fragmentation of ureteral calculi: initial experience. *J Urol.* 1987;137:386–389.
25. Morgentaler A, Bridge SS, Dretler SP. Management of the impacted ureteral calculus. *J Urol.* 1990;143:263–266.
26. Higashihara E, Horie S, Takeuchi T, et al. Laser ureterolithotripsy with combined rigid and flexible ureterorenoscopy. *J Urol.* 1990; 143:273–274.
27. Hoffman R, Hartung R. Use of pulsed Nd:YAG laser in the ureter. *Urol Clin North Am.* 1988;15:369–375.
28. Resnick MI, Pak CYC, eds. *Urolithiasis: a Medical and Surgical Reference.* Philadelphia: WB Saunders Co; 1990:225–227.
29. Dretler SP, Bhatta KM. Clinical results of high power (140 mJ) large fiber (320 μm) pulsed dye laser lithotripsy. *J Endourol.* 1990;4:S84.
30. Mattioli S, Cremona M, Benaim G, Metzen J. Pulsed dye and Alexandrite laser: in vitro and in vivo experimental results. *J Endourol.* 1990;4:S131.
31. Assimos DG, Boyce WH, Hamson CH, McCullough DL, Kroovand RL, Sweat KR. Role of open stone surgery since extracorporeal shock wave lithotripsy. *J Urol.* 1989;142:263–267.
32. Patel JJ. The coagulum pyelolithotomy. *Br J Surg.* 1973;60:230–236.
33. Blandy JP, Singh M. The case for a more aggressive approach to staghorn stones. *J Urol.* 1976;115:505–506.
34. Graff J, Diederichs W, Schulze H. Long-term follow up in 1003 extracorporeal shock wave lithotripsy patients. *J Urol.* 1988;140:479–483.

35. Lingeman JE, Newman DM, Mertz JHO, et al. Extracorporeal shock wave lithotripsy: the Methodist Hospital experience. *J Urol.* 1986;135:1134–1137.

36. Graff J, Schmidt A, Pastor J, et al. New generator for low pressure lithotripsy with the Dornier HM-3: preliminary experience of two centers. *J Urol.* 1988;139:904–907.

37. Jocham D, Liedl B, Schuster C, et al. New techniques and developments in extracorporeal lithotripsy: Dornier HM4 and MPL 9000. *Urol Res.* 1988;16:255A.

38. Rassweiler J, Gumpinger R, Mayer R, et al. Extracorporeal piezoelectric lithotripsy using the Wolf lithotripter versus low energy lithotripsy with the modified Dornier HM-3: a cooperative study. *World J Urol.* 1987;5:218–222.

39. Wilbert DM, Bichler K-H, Strohmaier WL, Fluchter SH. Initial experience with the second generation lithotripter Dornier HM4. *Urol Res.* 1988;16:262A.

40. Marberger M, Turk C, Steinkogler K. Painless piezoelectric extracorporeal lithotripsy. *J Urol.* 1988;139:695–699.

41. Philip T, Kellett MJ, Whitfield HN, Wickham JEA. Painless lithotripsy: experience with 100 patients. *Lancet.* 1988;2:41–43.

42. Vallancien G, Aviles J, Munoz R, et al. Piezoelectric extracorporeal lithotripsy by ultrashort waves with the EDAP LT01 device. *J Urol.* 1988;139:689–694.

43. Zwergel U, Neisius D, Zwergel T, Ziegler M. Results and clinical management of extracorporeal piezoelectric lithotripsy (EPL) in 1321 consecutive treatments. *World J Urol.* 1987; 5:213–219.

44. Rassweiler J, Westhauser A, Bub P, Eisenberger F. Second-generation lithotripters: a comparative study. *J Endourol.* 1988;2:193–204.

45. Jocham D, Liedl B, Schuster C, et al. New techniques and developments in extracorporeal lithotripsy: Dornier HM4 and MPL 9000. *Urol Res.* 1988;16:255A.

46. Turk C, Steinkogler I, Krings F, Marberger M. First experience with a lithotripter with in-line ultrasonic and flouroscopic stone localization. *J Endourol.* 1990;4:S90.

47. Neisius D, Zwergel TH, Jung P, Ziegler M. Extracorporeal piezoelectric lithotripsy (EPL) with the new Piezolith 2500—first clinical experiences. *J Endourol.* 1990;4:S92.

48. Haupt G, Benkert S, Graff J, Senge T. Results of more than 1500 EDWL treatments with the MFL 5000. *J Endourol.* 1990;4:S151.

49. Schlick R, Rodenbeck D, Gonnermann O, Jonas U. Experience in ESWL using the Modulith LS20: cost reduction by multifunctionality. *J Endourol.* 1990;4:S89.

50. Rassweiler J, Kohrmann KU, Wess O, Alken P. Modulith SL20: its clinical establishment. *J Endourol.* 1990;4:S90.

51. Seibold J, Rassweiler J, Schmidt A, Eisenberger F. Advanced technology in extracorporeal shock wave lithotripsy: the Dornier MPL 9000 versus the upgraded Dornier HM3. *J Endourol.* 1988;2:173–176.

52. Winfield HN, Clayman RV, Chaussy CG, Weyman PJ, Fuchs GJ, Lupu AN. Monotherapy of staghorn renal calculi: comparative study between percutaneous nephrolithotomy and extracorporeal shock wave lithotripsy. *J Urol.* 1988;139:895–899.

53. Chang CR, Webb DR, Payne SR, Wichhara JE. Comparison of treatment of renal calculi: by open surgery, percutaneous nephrolithotomy and extracorporeal shock wave lithotripsy. *Br Med J.* 1986;292:879–882.

54. Eisenberger F, Fuchs G, Miller K. Extracorporeal shock wave lithotripsy and endourology: an ideal combination for the treatment of kidney stones. *World J Urol.* 1985;3:41.

55. Kahnoski RJ, Lingeman JE, Lowry TA, Steele RE, Mosbaugh PG. Combined percutaneous and extracorporeal shock wave lithotripsy for staghorn calculi: an alternative to anatrophic nephrolithotomy. *J Urol.* 1986;135:679–681.

56. Schultz H, Hertu L, Graff J, Funke PJ, Serge T. Combined treatment of branched calculi by percutaneous nephrostolithotomy and extracorporeal shock wave lithotripsy. *J Urol.* 1986; 135:1138–1141.

57. Lingeman JE, Coury TA, Newman DM, et al. Comparison of results and morbidity of percutaneous nephrostolithotomy and extracorporeal shock wave lithotripsy. *J Urol.* 1987; 138:485–490.

58. Preminger GM, Clayman RV, Hardeman SW, Franklin J, Curry T, Peters PC. Percutaneous nephrostolithotomy versus open surgery for renal calculi: a comparative study. *JAMA* 1985; 254:1054–1058.

59. Rodrigues Netto N Jr, Lemos GC, Plama PC, Fiuza JL. Staghorn calculi: percutaneous versus anatrophic nephrolithotomy. *Eur Urol.* 1988; 15:9–12.

60. Mays N, Challah S, Patel S, et al. Clinical comparison of extracorporeal shock wave lithotripsy and percutaneous nephrolithotomy in treating renal calculi. *Br Med J.* 1988; 297:253–258.

61. Lee WJ, Snyder JA, Smith AD. Staghorn calculi: endourologic management in 120 patients. *Radiology.* 1987;65:85–88.

62. Vanden Bossche M, Simon J, Schulman CC. Shock wave monotherapy of staghorn calculi. *Eur Urol.* 1990;17:1–6.

63. Constantinides C, Recker F, Jaeger P, Hauri D. Extracorporeal shock wave lithotripsy as

monotherapy of staghorn renal calculi: 3 years experience. *J Urol.* 1989;142:1415–1418.

64. Gleeson MJ, Griffith DP. Extracorporeal lithotripsy monotherapy for large renal calculi. *Br J Urol.* 1989;64:329–332.

65. Karlsen S, Gjolberg T. Branched renal calculi treated by percutaneous nephrolithotomy and extracorporeal shock waves. *Scand J Urol Nephrol.* 1989;23:201–205.

66. Schulze H, Hertle L, Kutta A, Graff J, Senge T. Critical evaluation of treatment of staghorn calculi by percutaneous nephrolithotomy and extracorporeal shock wave lithotripsy. *J Urol.* 1989;141:822–825.

67. Tanda H, Kato S, Ohnishi S, Nakajima H, Mori K. Clinical experiences of renal and ureteral stones by extracorporeal shock wave lithotripsy (extracorporeal lithotripsy). IV: 3-year clinical experience of cases treated with extracorporeal lithotripsy. *Hinyokika Kiyo.* 1988;34:770–776.

68. Ferriere JM, Gaston R, Piechaud T, Brucher P, Le Guillou M. Current strategy in the treatment of urinary calculi since the introduction of the EDAP lithotripter. *Ann Urol.* 1988; 22:169–173.

69. Frick J, Kohle R, Kunit G. Experience with extracorporeal shock wave lithotripsy in children. *Eur Urol.* 1988;14:181–183.

70. Di Silverio F, Gallucci M, Alpi G. Staghorn calculi of the kidney: classification and therapy. *Br J Urol.* 1990;65:449–452.

71. Kahnowski RJ, Lineman JE, Coury TA, Steele RE, Mosbaugh PG. Combined percutaneous and extracorporeal shock wave lithotripsy for staghorn calculi: an alternative to anatrophic nephrolithotomy. *J Urol.* 1986;135:679–681.

72. Winfield HN, Clayman RV, Chaussy CG, Weryman PJ, Fuchs GJ, Lupu AN. Monotherapy of staghorn renal calculi: a comparative study between percutaneous nephrolithotomy and extracorporeal shock wave lithotripsy. *J Urol.* 1988;139:895–899.

73. Aso Y, Ohta N, Nakano M, Ohtawara Y, Tajima A, Kawabe K. Treatment of staghorn calculi by fiberoptic transurethral nephrolithotripsy. *J Urol.* 1990;144:17–19.

74. Valente R, Marini F, Signori G. Combined therapy of staghorn calculi with ureteroscopy and extracorporeal shock wave lithotripsy. Experience with 10 cases. *Eur Urol.* 1988; 14:349–352.

75. Ritchie AWS, Parr NJ, Moussa SA, Tolley DA. Lithotripsy in calyceal diverticula? *Br J Urol.* 1990;66:6–8.

76. Lingeman JE, Jones JA, Steidle CP. ESWL versus percutaneous management of calyceal diverticula. *J Endourol.* 1990;4:S140.

77. Drach GW, Dretler S, Fair W, et al. Report of the U.S. cooperative study of extracorporeal shock wave lithotripsy. *J Urol.* 1986;135:1127–1133.

78. Brownlee N, Foster M, Griffith DP, Carlton CE. Controlled inversion therapy: an adjunct to the elimination of gravity dependent fragments following extracorporeal shock wave lithotripsy. *J Urol.* 1990;143:1096–1098.

79. Smith JE, VanArsdalen KN, Hanno PM, Pollack HM. Extracorporeal shock wave lithotripsy treatment of calculi in horseshoe kidneys. *J Urol.* 1990;142:683–686.

80. Jones DJ, Wickham JEA, Kellett MJ. Percutaneous nephrolithotomy for calculi in horseshoe kidneys. *J Urol.* 1991;145:481–483.

81. Perry NM, Wickham JE, Whitfield HN. Hypothermic nephrolithotomy in solitary kidneys. *Br J Urol.* 1980;52:415–418.

82. Stubbs AJ, Resnick MI, Boyce WH. Anatrophic nephrolithotomy in the solitary kidney. *J Urol.* 1978;119:457–460.

83. Streem SB, Zelch MG, Risius B, Geisinger MA. Percutaneous extraction of renal calculi in patients with solitary kidneys. *Urology.* 1986;27:247–252.

84. Cohen ES, Schmidt JD. Extracorporeal shock wave lithotripsy for stones in solitary kidney. *Urology.* 1990;36:52.

85. Chandhoke DS, Albala DM, Clayman RV. Long-term comparison of renal function in patients with solitary kidneys and/or moderate renal insufficiency undergoing ESWL or percutaneous nephrolithotomy. *J Urol.* 1991; 145:323A.

86. Dretler SP, Keating MA, Riley J. An algorithm for the management of ureteral calculi. *J Urol.* 1986;136:1190–1193.

87. Ikemoto S, Sugimoto T, Yamamoto K, Kishimoto T, Maekawa M. Comparison of transurethral ureteroscopy and extracorporeal shock wave lithotripsy for treatment of ureteral calculi. *Eur Urol.* 1988;14:178–180.

88. Sanseverino R, Canton F, Salas M, Martin X, Gelet A, Dubernard JM. Treatment of upper ureteral stones. *Eur Urol.* 1988;14:111–114.

89. Denstedt JD, Clayman RV. Electrohydraulic lithotripsy of renal and ureteral calculi. *J Urol.* 1990;143:13–17.

90. Dretler SP. An evaluation of ureteral laser lithotripsy: 225 consecutive patients. *J Urol.* 1990;143:267–272.

91. Kahn RI. Endourological treatment of ureteral calculi: *J Urol.* 1986;135:239–243.

92. Mazone DJ, Chiang B. Extracorporeal shock wave lithotripsy of stones in the upper, middle, and lower ureter. *J Endourol.* 1988;2:107–111.

93. Tiselius HG, Pettersson B, Anderson A. Extracorporeal shock wave lithotripsy of stones in the mid ureter. *J Urol.* 1989;141:280–282.

94. Coptcoat MJ, Ison KT, Watson G, Wickham JE. Lasertripsy for ureteric stones in 120 cases: lessons learned. *Br J Urol.* 1988;61:487–489.

95. Rodrigues Netto N, Casterta Lemos G, Claro JFA. In situ extracorporeal shock wave litho-

tripsy for ureteral calculi. *J Urol.* 1990; 144:253.

96. Tung KH, Tan EC, Foo KT. In situ extracorporeal shock wave lithotripsy for upper ureteral stones using the EDAP LT-01 lithotripter. *J Urol.* 1990;143:481–482.
97. Jenkins AD, Gillenwater JY. Extracorporeal shock wave lithotripsy in the prone position: treatment of stones in the distal ureter or anomalous kidney. *J Urol.* 1988;139:911–915.
98. Becht E, Moll V, Neisius D, Ziegler M. Treatment of prevesical ureteral calculi by extracorporeal shock wave lithotripsy. *J Urol.* 1988;139:916–918.
99. Keele LL, McNamara TC, Dorey FO, Milster RE. De novo extracorporeal shock wave lithotripsy for lower ureteral calculi: treatment of choice. *J Endourol.* 1990;4:71–78.
100. Politis G, Griffith DP. Ureteroscopy in management of ureteral calculi. *Urology.* 1987; 30:39–42.
101. Blute ML, Segura JW, Patterson DE. Ureteroscopy. *J Urol.* 1988;139:510–512.
102. Daniels GF, Garrett JE, Carter MF. Ureteroscopic results and complications: experience with 130 cases. *J Urol.* 1988;139:710–713.
103. Lingeman JE, Sonda LP, Kahnoski RJ, et al. Ureteral stone management: emerging concepts. *J Urol.* 1986;135:1172–1174.
104. Preminger GM, Peterson R, Peters PC, et al. The current role of medical treatment of nephrolithiasis: the impact of improved techniques of stone removal. *J Urol.* 1985;134:6–10.
105. Preminger GM, Harvey JP, Pak CYC. Comparative efficacy of ''specific'' potassium citrate therapy versus conservative management in nephrolithiasis of mild-moderate severity. *J Urol.* 1985;134:658–661.

# 16

# Endourology: Noncalculus Indications

*Raju Thomas*

## INTRODUCTION

Over the past decade endourology has given urologists the ability to peer into the confines of the entire urinary tract. Thus, with an array of rigid and flexible endoscopes the entire length of the urothelium from the external urethral meatus to the far reaches of the distant renal calyces are within reach of diagnostic and therapeutic armamentaria. Endourology specializes in closed controlled manipulation of the urinary tract.

Approaches to the urinary tract are possible both in a retrograde fashion using the cystoscopes or ureteroscopes for retrograde diagnostics and therapeutics within the urethra, bladder, and ureter. Access to the urinary tract is also possible in an antegrade fashion via the percutaneous approach.

This chapter will briefly discuss the instrumentation, rationale, and techniques of the percutaneous approach to the urinary tract for noncalculus-related problems as outlined in Table 1. The advantages of an endourologic approach to these problems are as follows:

1. A less invasive mode of diagnosis and therapy
2. Quicker recovery
3. Quicker return to normal activity
4. Overall cost containment

**TABLE 1. Noncalculus Conditions of the Urinary Tract Amenable to Percutaneous Treatment**

| |
|---|
| **Obstruction to the Urinary Tract (see Fig 1)** |
| Intrarenal obstruction (infundibular stenosis, calyceal diverticulum) |
| Ureteropelvic junction (UPJ) obstruction |
| Ureteral strictures |
| **Nonobstructive Lesions** |
| Lesions in the renal collecting system (malignancy, blood clots, sloughed renal papillae, radiolucent calculi, etc.) |
| Renal cysts, solid tumors |
| Abscesses |
| Foreign body extraction |

## ANATOMIC RATIONALE FOR PERCUTANEOUS APPROACH

The principle for percutaneous access to the kidney is dependent on the segmental blood supply of the renal artery.[1] Thus, if one can approach the kidney in a posterolateral aspect (Fig. 2), it is evident that we are treading through a relatively avascular plane. The percutaneous puncture should be directed through a renal pyramid into a dorsal calyx. Puncturing the infundibulum should be avoided since this may cause bleeding from segmental and interlobar vessels. Direct puncture into the renal pel-

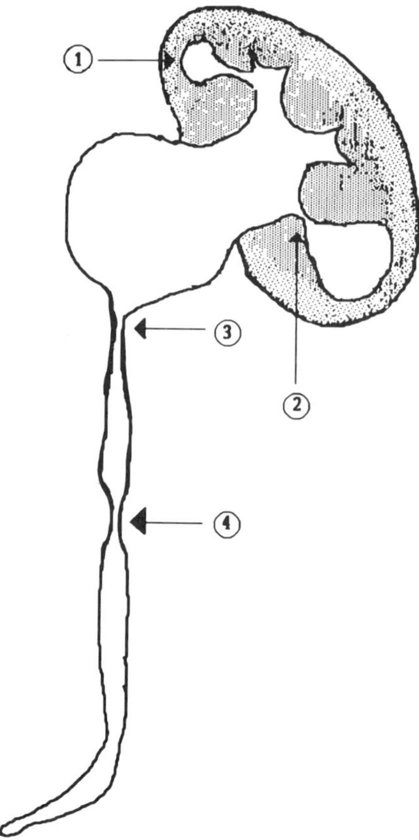


Fig 1. Sketch showing common obstructive lesions in the urinary tract. 1, calyceal diverticulum; 2, infundibular stenosis; 3, ureteropelvic junction obstruction; 4, ureteral stricture.

vis deprives one of the stabilizing effect of traversing through renal parenchyma. In most clinical situations, advance planning and accurate entry into an appropriate area of the renal collecting system is essential. This principle has fostered the basis of percutaneous access to the kidney. The technique and instrumentation used for access to the kidney is described in Chapter 17 of this Volume. But a wide array of needles, guidewires, and dilators are available for this purpose.[2,3] The imaging modality is either ultrasound- or fluoroscopy-guided.[4] Choice is dependent on availability, experience of user, size of patient, bony malformation in patient, relative position of kidney, etc. Once the tract from the skin to the predetermined location of the kidney

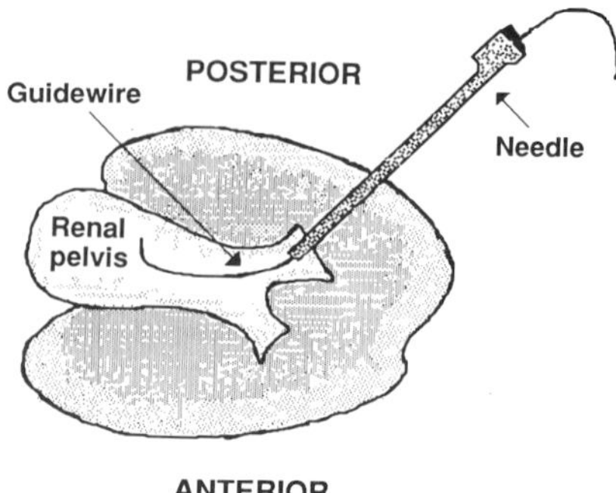


Fig 2. Posterolateral approach to kidney for percutaneous procedures (transverse view).

has been established, the interior of the kidney is visualized with the appropriate rigid or flexible nephroscopes. The interior of the kidney is then surveyed and the urologist focuses on the job at hand, which is either to diagnose and treat the obstruction (Fig 3) or to diagnose and/or treat neoplasia (Fig 4).

Fig 3. Obstruction to right kidney secondary to ureteropelvic junction obstruction (arrow).

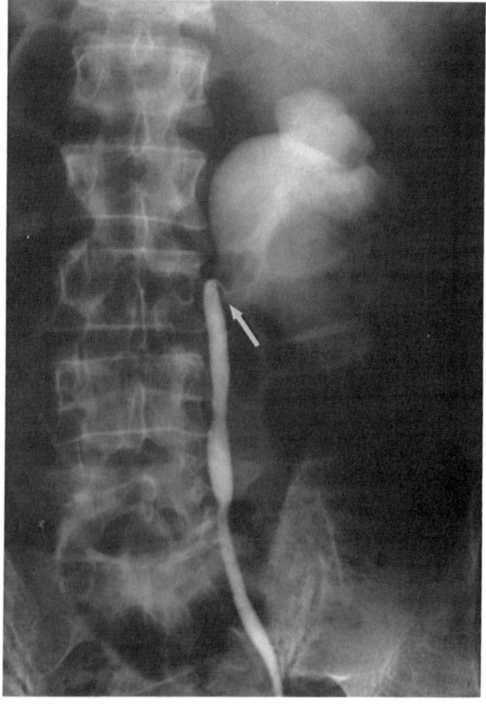

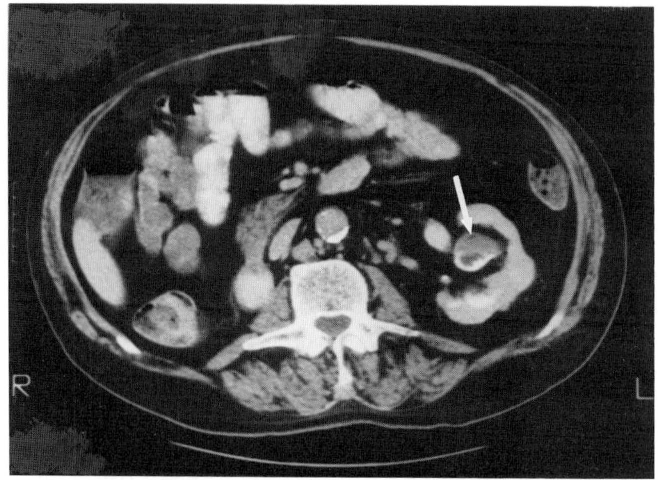


**Fig 4.** CT scan shows tumor of left renal pelvis (arrow).

## MANAGEMENT OF OBSTRUCTION IN THE URINARY TRACT

### Intrarenal Obstruction

Intrarenal obstructions are lesions causing obstruction at the calyceal and infundibular level of the kidney prior to drainage of urine into the renal pelvis.

**Calyceal Diverticulum.** Calyceal diverticulum is a cystic cavity situated peripheral to a calyx to which it is connected by a narrow opening (Fig 1). It is lined with transitional epithelium and may be congenital or acquired. The acquired causes include inflammatory processes, obstruction (secondary to infection or calculus), achalasia, or trauma. Such a diverticulum may be asymptomatic and incidentally diagnosed. It may be symptomatic secondary to obstruction, calculi, or infection. Traditionally, these lesions were treated by partial or segmental nephrectomy or nephrotomy with calyceal diverticulectomy. However, this obstructive lesion can now be managed percutaneously. Recent reports suggested percutaneous management in patients with calculi in such diverticuli. The percutaneous approach is the same as for the percutaneous approach to renal calculi[5–10] (see Chapter 17). However, one has to have a direct approach into the diverticulum. Guidewire is coiled within the diverticulum and judicious dilatation of this tract is accomplished under fluoroscopy. Dilatation equipment is the same as for any percutaneous procedure. Caution should be exercised during dilatation so as not to dislodge the guidewire. Once access to the kidney is obtained with a nephroscope, the calculi are removed. If an opening to the calyceal diverticulum is identified, this is cannulated with a guidewire and this tract is incised or dilated. Following incision/dilatation the neck of the infundibulum is stented for 6 to 8 weeks. The technique and instrumentation are similar to those used for managing ureteropelvic junction obstruction described below. Alternatively, the transitional cell lining of the diverticulum could be cauterized to obliterate the diverticulum and thus prevent its recurrence. A resectoscope (used for transurethral surgery) or Nd:YAG (neodymium:yttrium-aluminum-garnet) laser may be used for this procedure.

**Infundibular Stenosis.** Infundibular stenosis is caused by a narrowing of the infundibulum draining the calyx into the renal pelvis. This causes hydrocalycosis. These obstructing lesions can also be incised endourologically, replacing open surgical intervention in many patients.[11,12] The

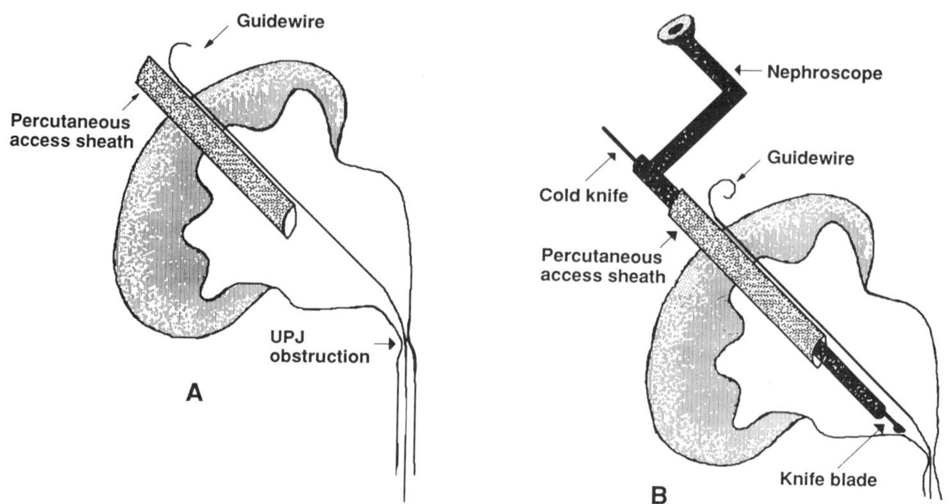


**Fig 5. A,** percutaneous sheath obtains access to right kidney; **B,** nephroscope visualizes ureteropelvic junction (UPJ) obstruction and is then incised.

technique used is essentially the same as for calyceal diverticulum. Access is obtained into the affected calyx. The affected infundibulum is traversed with a guidewire and the infundibulum is incised or dilated and then stented for approximately 6 weeks.

## Ureteropelvic Junction Obstruction

Ureteropelvic junction (UPJ) obstruction (Fig 3) is traditionally managed with open surgical intervention. Recently two approaches have been described to correct these obstructive lesions endourologically.

**Antegrade Percutaneous Endopyelotomy.** Antegrade percutaneous endopyelotomy is a technique used to incise the UPJ obstruction endoscopically. There are two approaches to the UPJ: antegrade percutaneous approach[13–15] and retrograde ureteroscopic approach. The antegrade technique is as follows: The percutaneous access to the kidney is usually obtained through one of the calyces in the upper half of the kidney. This gives a relatively straight access to the UPJ. If an approach is made through the inferior calyx, then it will be difficult to torque the instruments to gain access to the UPJ. A guidewire should be traversing the UPJ. This provides anatomic continuity between the ureter and the renal pelvis. After an appropriate approach has been obtained to the UPJ it is essential to ensure that the guidewire is still present across the UPJ. Once this is determined, the UPJ is incised laterally/posterolaterally using either the cold knife or electrocautery blade. If the electrocautery is used, the guidewire should be insulated with an open-ended catheter to prevent any propagation of the electrocautery current (Fig 5A, B).

The UPJ area is usually incised until fat is seen. This is based on the classic work described by Davis in 1943. The UPJ area is then balloon-dilated, if necessary, and stented as appropriate. Recent advances in stent technology have greatly improved the efficacy of such procedures since less reactive stent materials such as silicone are readily available.

The stenting of the UPJ area is accomplished by stents that either are passed percutaneously or can be self-contained as an

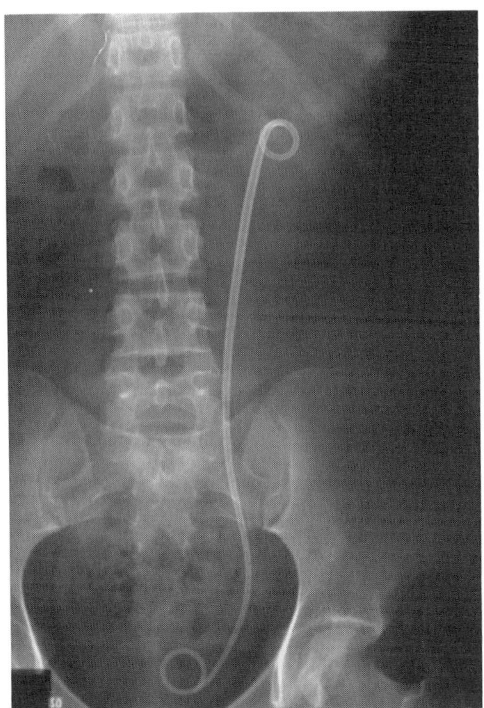

Fig 6. An indwelling endopyelotomy stent.

indwelling stent (Fig 6). The stent is usually left indwelling for approximately 6 to 8 weeks. Follow-up to evaluate the success of such procedures is by repeating radiographic or functional studies on the kidney. These include intravenous pyelograms (IVP), quantitative renal scans, ultrasound, and so forth. The percutaneous approach is preferred for treatment of patients with UPJ obstruction *and associated calculi* (Fig 7). Obstruction at the UPJ will not permit stone fragments from passing through if extracorporeal shock wave lithotripsy is performed.

**Retrograde Ureteroscopic Endopyelotomy.** This approach utilizes the ureteroscope to approach the UPJ in a retrograde fashion without need for developing a percutaneous tract.[16–21] In preparation for the retrograde approach, a 5 or 6 French size indwelling stent is placed to drain the kidney. This passively dilates the ureter and greatly facilitates subsequent ureteroscopy. Following this, an 11.5 French size insulated

Fig 7. **A,** calculi in left kidney seen on IVP; **B,** associated ureteropelvic junction obstruction (arrow).

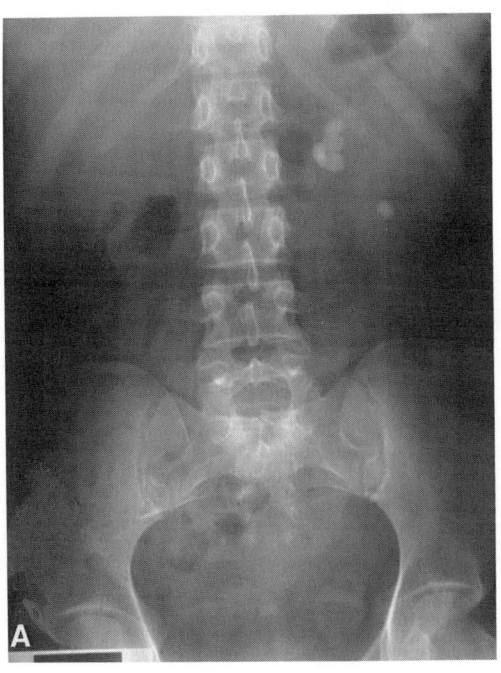


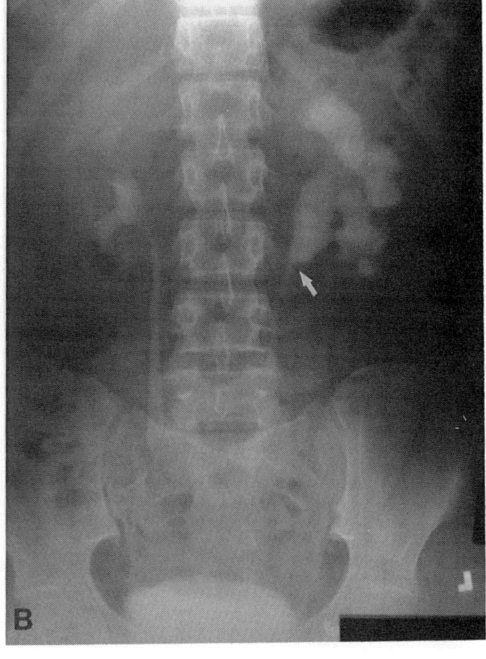

ureteroresectoscope is introduced in a retrograde fashion through the bladder and into the ureter. This ureteroscope is passed up to the UPJ. The UPJ is incised in the lateral/posterolateral aspect of the UPJ. Once again the incision is made with the cold knife or electrocautery current (Fig 8). The integrity of the UPJ is always maintained by the preplaced guidewire. The UPJ area is then balloon-dilated and stented with an indwelling ureteral endopyelotomy stent (Fig 6). This stent tapers from 14 French size in the UPJ area to 7 French size within the bladder. The stent is removed cystoscopically with grasping forceps after being in place for approximately 6 to 8 weeks.

**Summary.** Thus, a clear understanding of the renal anatomy, refinements in percutaneous instrumentation, paraphernalia, and techniques have given the urologist precise access to the kidney. This in turn has greatly increased the indications for percutaneous renal surgery. Thus, lesions mentioned above, which were traditionally managed with invasive open surgical techniques, can now be treated in a less invasive manner. This has been significantly aided by better understanding of stenting techniques and availability of better stenting materials.

Fig 8. Rigid ureteroscope with electrocautery attachment (arrow).

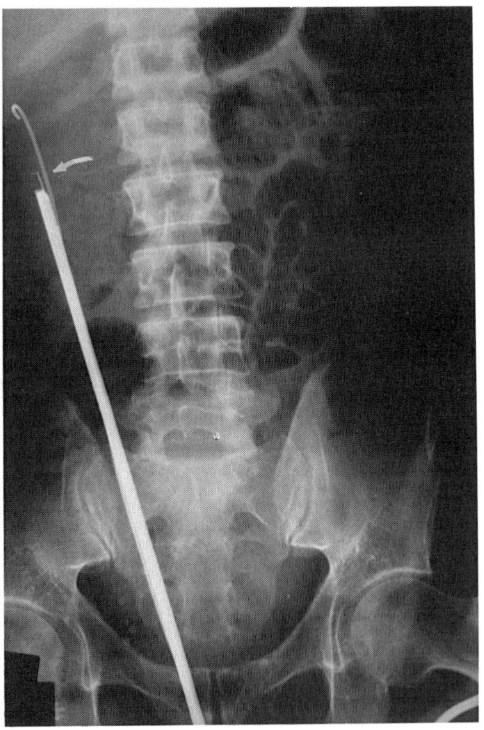

## Management of Ureteral Strictures

Ureteral strictures are narrowing within the lumen of the ureter and could be due to intrinsic or extrinsic causes. Intrinsic causes are congenital or secondary to inflammatory, iatrogenic, or traumatic processes.

The diagnosis is made with a variety of imaging techniques such as IVP, retrograde pyelograms, computerized tomography (CT) scannings (for extrinsic lesions), and endoscopic means.

Traditionally, ureteral strictures have been managed by the open surgical approach whereby the area of stricture is explored and after ensuring that there is no associated extrinsic pathology, the area of stricture is excised and the two free ends of the ureter are then anastomosed. The ureter is traditionally stented at this point to promote healing and to decrease any leakage of urine through the anastomosed area. The more recent endoscopic approach uses the same instrumentation as described for the endopyelotomy. With the retrograde ureteroscopic approach, one should have a guidewire traversing the strictured area,[22] and, depending on its location, the stricture is usually incised with a cold knife or the electrocautery knife[23,24] (Fig 8). The same precautions are taken as described above with the endopyelotomy procedure. The strictures in the upper ureter are usually incised laterally whereas strictures in the lower ureter are incised medially to respect the pattern of arterial blood supply to the ureter. The incised area is then stented for a period of approximately 6 to 8 weeks. The strictures in the upper ureter just distal to the UPJ can also be approached in a percutaneous antegrade fashion but the recent refinements in ureteroscopic instrumentation has greatly enhanced the ability to incise strictures along the entire length of the ureter. This permits treatment in a contained retrograde fashion without the need for any invasive percutaneous approaches.

The success in treating such strictures is dependent on both the etiology and the length of the strictures. Ideally, these strictures are suited to traumatic or iatrogenic causes up to a length of approximately 1.5 cm. Strictures that have been related to radiation inflammation or exceeding 1.5 cm have a lower success rate when managed endoscopically.

## MANAGEMENT OF NONOBSTRUCTIVE LESIONS

### Endourologic Approach to Urologic Malignancies

Traditionally, the diagnosis of upper urinary tract lesions has been through imaging modalities. Lesions within the urethra and bladder were diagnosed by direct vision through the cystoscope. Lesions in the ureter and within the kidney were diagnosed by a variety of imaging methods such as IVP, retrograde pyelogram, ultrasound, CT scan, brush biopsies, cytology, etc. Once these lesions were diagnosed, further diagnostic and therapeutic alternatives were limited to an open surgical approach. With the advances in fiberoptics and endoscopes one is able to approach these lesions endoscopically. This approach is used for diagnostic and even, in select cases, for therapeutic purposes. The "filling defects" or lesions *within the ureter* are diagnosed usually in a retrograde fashion using rigid or flexible ureteroscopes[25–27] (Fig 9). Thus after a guidewire has been introduced into the ureter the urologist is able to pass the ureteroscope to visualize lesions and biopsy these. Once the diagnosis is confirmed the therapeutic options are weighed. More recently, in patients who have low-grade malignancies, these lesions in the ureter can

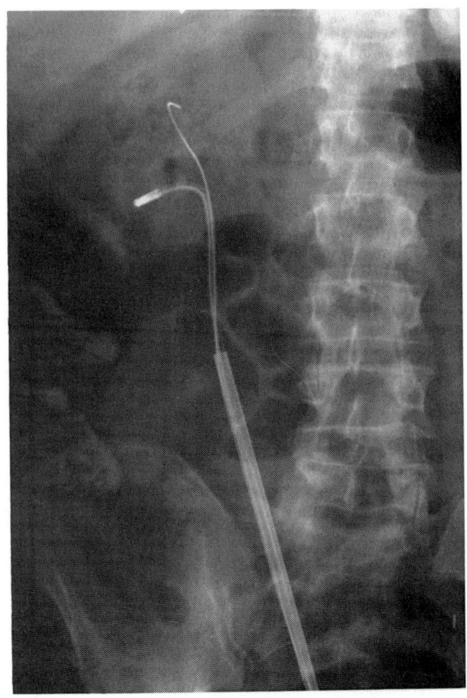

**Fig 9.** Flexible ureterorenoscope passed through rigid introduction sheath into renal calyces.

be treated endourologically. A variety of options such as (1) use of the ureteral resectoscope (to resect and coagulate lesions), (2) the Nd:YAG laser, etc., can be used for these purposes. These options are available to patients who have a low-volume, low-grade urothelial malignancy. Higher grade lesions and patients with more bulky lesions are usually managed via the open surgical approach.

Lesions *within the kidney* carry a differential diagnosis of urothelial malignancy, blood clots, sloughed renal papillae, radiolucent calculi, and the like. The definitive diagnosis is confirmed by various imaging modalities and by direct vision with the fiberoptic, usually flexible ureterorenoscopes. These ureteroscopes are passed in a retrograde fashion into the renal pelvis for diagnostic purposes.[25,26] Once the diagnosis is made the therapeutic approach can be outlined. For limited and low-grade malignancies, one can approach this in a

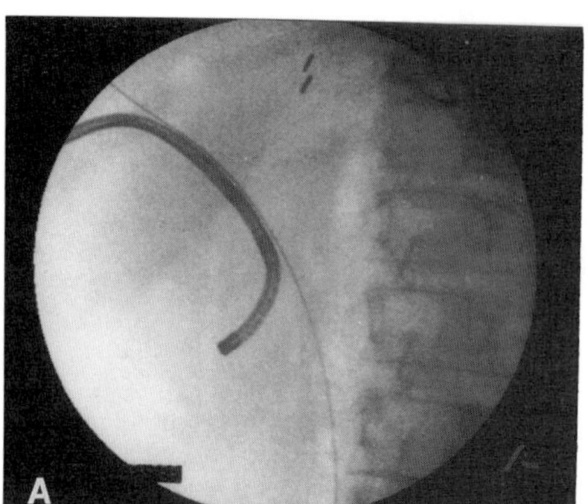


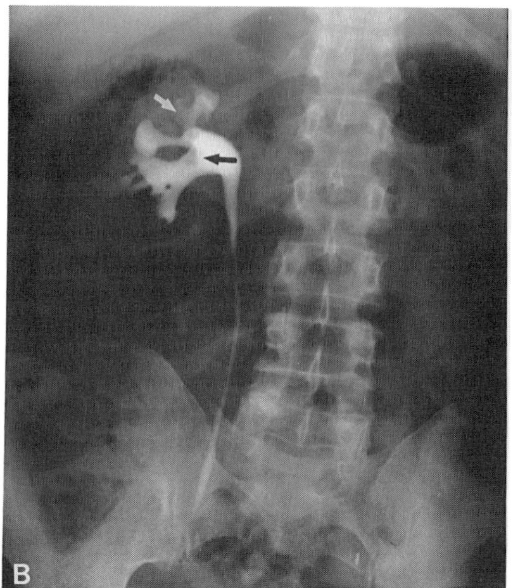


**Fig 10. A,** flexible nephroscope in place for percutaneous treatment of tumor in right renal pelvis seen in **B** (arrows).

retrograde fashion using the 200-μm Nd:YAG laser fiber through the ureteroscope to fulgurate these lesions. However, if these lesions are relatively bulky, then a percutaneous approach is recommended (Fig 10).

Lesions in the kidney are usually approached in an antegrade percutaneous fashion.[28–30] The approach was described earlier in the chapter; however, once the tract to the kidney has been established the lesion is then diagnosed and treated with a variety of options. These include use of resectoscope or Nd:YAG laser as described above. One has to be very cognizant of not spilling any tumor cells outside the confines

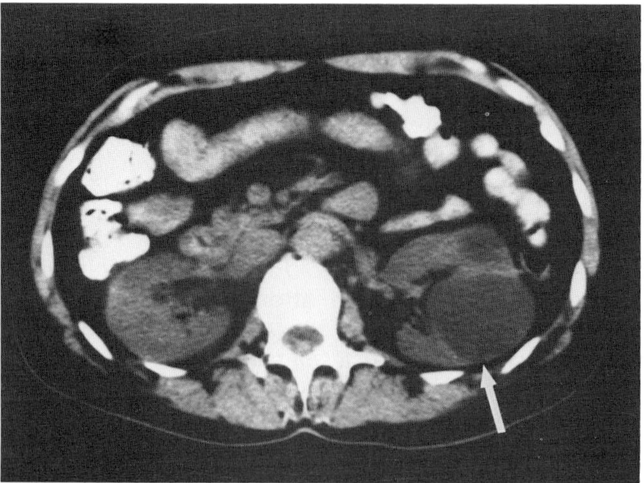

**Fig 11.** Simple renal cyst (arrow) seen on CT scan.

of the kidney. Such diligent approaches have been used in several series to treat patients in need of nephron sparing and have thus prevented imminent dialysis.

The kidneys are subsequently drained with a percutaneous nephrostomy tube and careful monitoring of these patients is done periodically. These surveillance cystoscopies and ureterorenoscopies are usually done every 3 months to ensure that there has been no recurrence of these ureteral malignancies. This endoscopic approach is usually restricted to patients who are in need of nephron-sparing surgery. These are patients with a history of having such a lesion in a solitary kidney or who have overall compromised renal function and in whom nephron sparing is preferable to dialysis-dependent survival.

## Renal Cysts

Renal cysts are the commonest space-occupying lesions in the kidney and are smooth-walled, spherical, and nonechogenic. Simple benign cysts are frequent "incidental" findings on intravenous pyelograms, sonograms, and CT scans (Fig 11). Simple cysts are rarely malignant. However, cysts with septations or multilocular cysts may be suspicious for malignancy. Cysts may be punctured for *diagnostic purposes* if patients have associated hematuria, irregular cyst wall, echoes on ultrasound, or suspicious CT evaluation (fluid density higher than serous fluid). Once these cysts are punctured with a needle, the fluid is analyzed (cytology, lactate dehydrogenase level, and fat content). These cysts are then injected with 60% contrast and multipositional views are obtained to rule out intrinsic lesions within the cyst. Cysts may also be punctured for *therapeutic purposes* if causing obstruction to the kidney or with associated pain.[31] After puncturing the cyst and obtaining diagnostic information (as described above), the cyst is injected with sclerosing agents such as 95% ethanol. Approximately 20% of original cyst volume is drained and replaced with 95% ethanol. The entire cyst volume is evacuated after 30 to 45 minutes (Fig 12).

Recently, the techniques of percutaneous renal surgery have been extended to treat select patients with symptomatic renal cysts[32–34] (obstruction to renal unit and/or associated pain). The renal cysts are punctured directly with an 18-gauge needle. Guidewires are introduced into the cyst. The tract from the skin to the cyst is dilated in a routine fashion. Once the dilator sheath (28 French size) is in position, the renal cyst is inspected with a nephroscope. The lining of the cyst is cauterized with a resectoscope loop or fulgurated with an Nd:YAG laser. The treated cyst is drained with a catheter for 1 to 2 days and then removed. Follow-up IVP, ultrasound, or CT scan should confirm obliteration and nonrecurrence of the cyst (Fig 12C).

## Solid Tumors

Solid tumors are usually diagnosed with available diagnostics such as ultrasound, CT scan, angiogram, MRI, etc. Rarely, ubiquitous lesions may need a needle biopsy of the lesions.[35] In such instances, CT or ultrasound-guided biopsy with a Biopty Gun™ or Tru-Cut needle is done for diagnosis.

The percutaneous approach to solid renal masses that are suspicious for malignancy is not recommended.[36] However, if the clinical picture is suggestive of an inflammatory lesion and a renal abscess is diagnosed, this can be managed with simple percutaneous drainage using a needle for initial access and subsequent placement of an 8 or 10 French nephrostomy-type drainage catheter. Occasionally, two catheters are placed within the abscess cavity. One of these is used for irrigation with antibiotic solution and the other is used to drain the cavity. Once again, percutaneous endoscopy of such cavities is not recommended.

## Foreign Body Extraction

Foreign bodies such as sheared-off ends of guidewires, bullets, and so forth can be

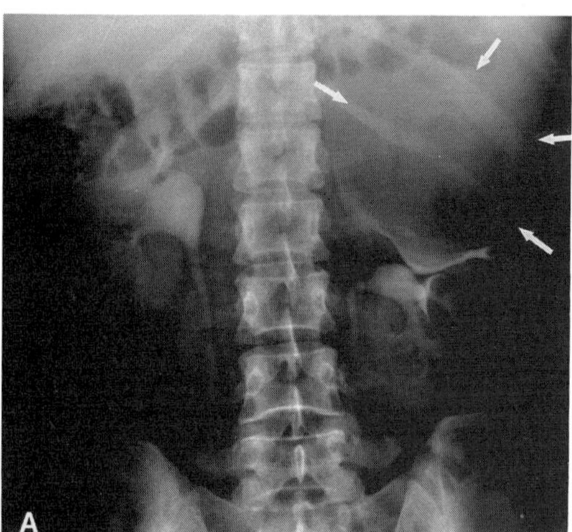

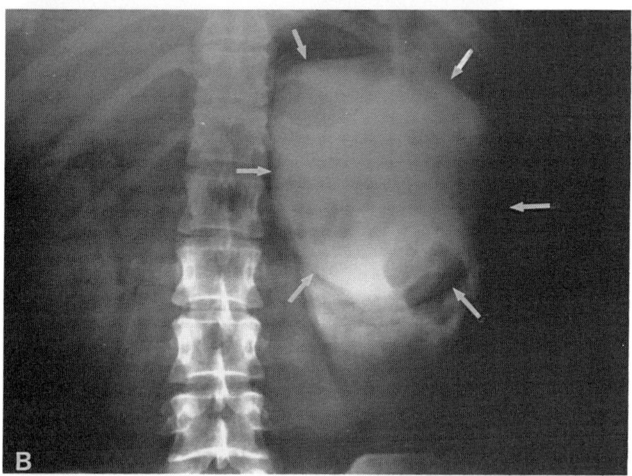

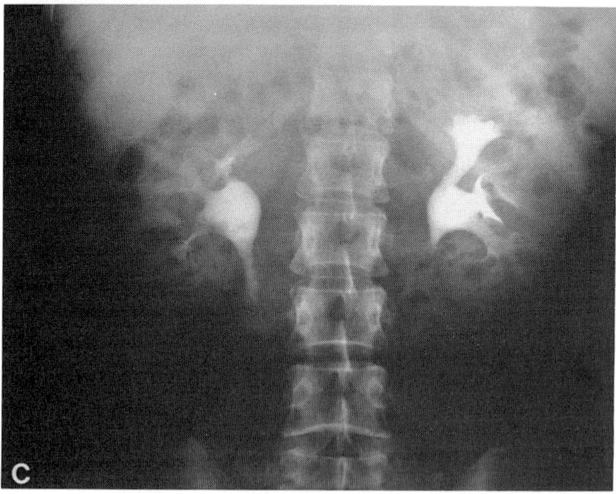

**Fig 12. A,** large cyst in upper pole of left kidney; **B,** contrast and ethanol injected into cyst; **C,** IVP a year later shows no recurrence of cyst.

removed from the renal parenchyma or collecting system using percutaneous renal surgery techniques described. Thomas et al described removal of an intrarenal bullet.[37]

## SUMMARY

The requirements for performing such complex closed controlled manipulation of the urinary tract are possession of a firm grasp of the anatomy and the wide array of instruments available, and knowledge of principles of stent placement and stent technology. It is evident that with the advent and rapid advances in fiberoptics and endoscope technology one can have a relatively rapid and easy access to the entire urinary tract. This combined with familiarity with the instrumentation, experience in performing percutaneous renal surgery, and improvement in imaging modalities has greatly enhanced the urologists' ability to diagnose and perform complex procedures within the urinary tract in a relatively noninvasive fashion. This has decreased the overall morbidity that the patient has to go through and has enabled patients to return to normal activity at a quicker pace.

## REFERENCES


1. Kaye KW, Goldberg ME. Applied anatomy of the kidney and ureter. *Urol Clin North Am.* 1982;9:3.
2. Smith A, Moldwin R, Karlin G. Percutaneous ureterostomy. *J Urol.* 1987;138:286.
3. Lange PH. Diagnostic and therapeutic urologic instrumentation. In: Wash PC, ed. *Campbell's Urology*, 5th ed. Philadelphia: WB Saunders; 1986.
4. Thüroff JW, Alken P. Ultrasound for renal puncture and fluoroscopy for tract dilatation and catheter placement: a combined approach. *Endourology.* 1987;2:1.
5. Goodwin WE, Casey WC, Woolf W. Percutaneous trocar (needle) nephrostomy in hydronephrosis. *JAMA.* 1955;157:891.
6. Bartley O, Chidekel N, Redberg C. Percutaneous drainage of the renal pelvis for uremia due to obstructed urinary outflow. *Acta Chir Scand.* 1965;129:443.
7. Clayman RV, Castaneda-Zuniga WR, Hunter DW, Miller RP, Lange PH, Amplatz L. Rapid balloon dilatation of the nephrostomy tract for nephrostolithotomy. *Radiology.* 1983;147:884.
8. Fowler JE Jr, Meares EM Jr, Goldin AR. Percutaneous nephrostomy: techniques, indications, and results. *Urology.* 1975;6:428.
9. Lang EK, Price ET. Redefinitions of indications for percutaneous nephrostomy. *Radiology.* 1983;147:419.
10. Smith AD, Badlani GH. Special use of retrograde percutaneous nephrostomy in endourology. *J Endourol.* 1987;1:23.
11. Clayman RV, Hunter D, Surya V, Castaneda-Zuniga W, Amplatz D, Lange PH. Percutaneous intrarenal electrosurgery. *J Urol.* 1984;131:864.
12. Eshgi M, Tuong W, Fernandez R, Addonizio JC. Percutaneous (endo) infundibulotomy. *J Endourol.* 1987;1:107.
13. Badlani G, Eshghi M, Smith AD. Percutaneous surgery for ureteropelvic junction obstruction (endopyelotomy): technique and early results. *J Urol.* 1986;135:26.
14. Badlani G, Karlin G, Smith A. Complications of endopyelotomy: analysis in series of 64 patients. *J Urol.* 1988;140:473.
15. Brannen GE, Bush WH, Lewis GP. Endopyelotomy for primary repair of ureteropelvic junction obstruction. *J Urol.* 1988;139:29.
16. Clayman RV, Basler J, Kavoussi L, Picus D. Ureterorenoscopic endopyelotomy. *J Urol.* 1990;144:246.
17. Thomas R. Ureteroscopic Retrograde Endopyelotomy. Video: Urology Times, Vol. 5, Program 1, 1992.
18. Thomas R, Cherry R. Ureteroscopic retrograde endopyelotomy for management of ureteropelvic junction obstruction. *J Urol.* 1991;145:414A.
19. Pérez-Castro E, Martinez-Piñeiro JA. Ureteral and renal endoscopy: a new approach. *Eur Urol.* 1982;8:117.
20. Thomas R. Rigid ureteroscopy: pitfalls and remedies. *Urology.* 1988;32:328–334.
21. Lyon ES, Huffman JL, Bagley DH. Ureteroscopy and ureteropyeloscopy. *Urology.* 1984; 23(5 Spec. No.):29.
22. Thomas R. Catheterizing a tortuous ureter. *J Urol.* 1988;140:778.
23. Thomas R. Endoureterotomy: Endoscopic Management of Ureteral Strictures. AUA Video Digest, Vol. 1, No. 4, 1989.
24. Netto NR, Ferreira U, Lemos G, Claro J. Endourological management of ureteral strictures. *J Urol.* 1990;144:631.
25. Bagley DH, Huffman JL, Lyon ES. Flexible ureteropyeloscopy: diagnosis and treatment in the upper urinary tract. *J Urol.* 1987;138:280.
26. Huffman JL, Bagley DH, Lyon ES, Morse MJ, Herr HW, Whitmore WF. Endoscopic diagnosis and treatment of upper-tract urothelial tumors: a preliminary report. *Cancer.* 1985;55:1422.
27. Kavoussi L, Clayman R, Basler J. Flexible, actively deflectable fiberoptic ureteronephroscopy. *J Urol.* 1989;142:249.

28. Tasca A, Zattoni F. The case for a percutaneous approach to transitional cell carcinoma of the renal pelvis. *J Urol.* 1990;143:902.

29. Smith AD, Orihuela E, Crowley AR. Percutaneous management of renal pelvis tumors: a treatment option in selected cases. *J Urol.* 1987;137:852.

30. Ziegelbaum M, Novick AC, Streem SB, Montie JE, Pontes JE, Straffon RA. Conservative surgery for transitional cell carcinoma of the renal pelvis. *J Urol.* 1987;138:1146.

31. Raskin MM, Poole DO, Roen SA, Viamonte M. Percutaneous management of renal cysts: results of a four year study. *Radiology.* 1975;115:551.

32. Hulbert JC, Hunter D, Young A, Castaneda-Zuniga W. Percutaneous intrarenal marsupialization of a perirenal cystic collection: endocystolysis. *J Urol.* 1988;139:1039.

33. Lang EK. Coexistence of cyst and tumor in the same kidney. *Radiology.* 1971;101:7.

34. Lang EK. Diagnosis and management of renal cysts. In: Lang EK, ed. *Percutaneous and Interventional Urology and Radiology.* New York: Springer-Verlag; 1986.

35. Wein AJ, Ring EJ, Freiman DB, Oleaga JA, Carpiniello VL, Banner MP, Pollack HM. Application of thin needle aspiration biopsy in urology. *J Urol.* 1979;121:626.

36. Gibbons RP, Bush WH Jr, Burnett LL. Needle tract seeding following aspiration of renal cell carcinoma. *J Urol.* 1977;118:865.

37. Thomas R, Suarez GM. Percutaneous removal of intra-renal bullet. *J Urol.* 1988;140:806.

# 17

# Urodynamics and Evaluation of the Incontinent Patient

*Richard F. Labasky*

In the broadest definition, urinary incontinence is the involuntary loss of urine. To the individual patient, the magnitude of the problems caused by the incontinence may range from mild to severe, and may affect a few or all aspects of quality of life, including social, employment, and recreational activities. Even more significantly, incontinence may be an initial symptom indicating a more serious or life-threatening disease, most commonly a disease of the neurologic or genitourinary systems. Incontinence is particularly prevalent (15% to 30%) among those older than 60 years; the prevalence increases to up to 50% of residents of nursing homes.[1,2] Indeed, urinary incontinence is a significant factor leading to placement of patients in nursing homes. Clearly, the psychosocial effects of incontinence on individuals can be immense.[1,2]

Incontinence is also a significant problem on a national scale, as it affects more than 10 million people at a cost that exceeds 10 billion dollars per year in the United States alone. Unfortunately, many "management" strategies are narrow-mindedly directed toward dealing with incontinence by using pads or diapers rather than by actually resolving the problem.[1,2]

The urologist must use a clear, straightforward approach to the evaluation and classification of incontinence to be able to offer an intelligent and appropriate choice of therapies to the patient. The data gathered with such an approach also provide the basic information necessary to effectively manage the possible presence of lower urinary tract dysfunction with a neurologic etiology. The approach discussed in this chapter is based on the patient history, physical examination, and basic diagnostic tests. Detailed neurophysiologic tests of the lower urinary tract—urodynamic evaluations—are occasionally performed in certain cases of general incontinence, and are often performed in cases of neurologic dysfunction, thus allowing a urodynamic diagnosis and classification of the incontinence.

## BASIC EVALUATION AND CLASSIFICATION

The evaluation for incontinence must be thorough and detailed enough to allow classification and diagnosis of the type of incontinence present and to allow the initiation of appropriate treatment. In addition to these primary goals, the evaluation also should facilitate the selection and use of further diagnostic tests, while minimizing unnecessary testing. The significance of the problem should be explained to the patient.

**TABLE 1. Steps in the Evaluation of Incontinence**

- History
- Physical examination
- Basic tests
  - —Urinalysis
  - —Culture & sensitivity
  - —Cytology
  - —Post-void residual
  - —Radiography (some situations)
- Endoscopy
- Urodynamics (See Table 4)

The patient may want information regarding noninvasive treatment or surgery, or may simply desire reassurance that the cause of the incontinence is probably benign. One of the simplest and most functional methods of describing the incontinence is based on symptomatology delineated by the patient's chief complaint and history and reinforced by the physical examination and basic diagnostic tests (Table 1). Within this system, five basic types of incontinence can be described: continuous, overflow, transient, stress, and urge (Table 2). One of these incontinence types will usually be present as the patient's chief complaint.

## The Patient History

The patient history should establish the type of incontinence that prevails. Questions should be designed to differentiate symptoms based on the following.

*Continuous incontinence* is urinary leakage occurring day and night in an unrelenting fashion; this type of incontinence is not associated with any specific activity or sensation in the bladder.

*Overflow incontinence* results from an inability to empty the bladder adequately. The patient may report some degree of voiding ability but also reports a slow leak that begins soon after voiding. The leakage may be enhanced by stress maneuvers.

*Transient incontinence* is characterized by a relatively acute and recent onset, and is usually due to a specific cause such as those summarized in Table 3.[2] Evaluation should reveal the inciting event, and should suggest a resolution to the problem.

*Stress incontinence* occurs in association with any maneuver that raises intraabdominal pressure such as standing up, coughing, laughing, sneezing, lifting, running, jumping, exercising, or sexual activity.

*Urge incontinence* is leakage associated

**TABLE 2. Symptomatic Classification of Incontinence**

| Type | Cause |
|---|---|
| Continuous | • Fistula<br>• Ectopic ureter<br>• Totally incompetent urethra (Type III stress incontinence) |
| Overflow | • Obstruction<br>—Anatomic—benign prostatic hyperplasia, stricture, tumor<br>—Neurologic—Detrusor-sphincter dyssynergia (multiple sclerosis, Parkinson's disease, spinal cord injury)<br>• Bladder decompensation<br>—Neurologic (including diabetes)<br>—Obstructive |
| Transient | • See Table 3 |
| Stress | • Type I, II, III (see also continuous incontinence) |
| Urge | • Infection<br>• Inflammation<br>• Neurologic disease<br>• Bladder tumor<br>• Foreign body<br>• Stone<br>• Obstruction<br>• Idiopathic causes |

**TABLE 3. Causes of Transient Incontinence ("Diappers" Mnemonic)**

| |
|---|
| D—Delerium |
| I—Infection, inflammation |
| A—Atrophy of the vaginal wall |
| P—Pharmaceutical agents |
| P—Psychologic/psychiatric |
| E—Endocrine (diabetes, hypercalcemia) |
| R—Restricted mobility |
| S—Stool impaction |

From Resnick.[2]

with a sudden onset of the need to urinate. Such urgency and incontinence may occur randomly, or may be triggered quite predictably by specific factors such as running water, washing dishes, attempting to get a key in the front door of the house, a sudden exposure to cold, or a sudden change in position.

After establishing the character of the patient's chief complaint, it is necessary to complete the details of the history to better establish the type of incontinence. The key categories of the history are discussed below.[2–6]

### Urinary Symptoms

***Onset, Duration, Suspected Cause, Course.*** Questions directed to the patient should establish when and how the incontinence began and the circumstances under which it occurs. If possible, determine what triggers the incontinence and what the patient is feeling in the bladder and urethra at those moments—the times of day incontinent episodes usually occur and how they relate to the most recent voidings, medications, or fluid intake. Also note any changes in activity, position, sensation, or environment that occur prior to the incontinence. Supine leakage usually does not denote simple stress incontinence, but is more likely to indicate continuous or another form of incontinence; a report of uncontrollable leak after a stress maneuver may indicate a stress-induced involuntary bladder contraction (detrusor instability) (see section on urodynamics testing). Determine the *severity* of incontinent episodes: does the patient need to change clothes? what is the number and type of pads or other devices used and how wet do they become? has the patient changed his or her daily routine or lifestyle in response to incontinence? Discover any *prior treatments* for incontinence, such as medications or catheters (either indwelling or intermittent self-catheterization); also note the duration, success or failure, and side effects of any therapy. If a medication did not cause at least mild side effects, the doses may have been inadequate to cure the incontinence.

***Irritative Urinary Symptoms.*** Irritative symptoms in patients with incontinence include nocturia, and urgency and frequency of voiding. Determine the presence of these symptoms and their relation to the incontinence and each other.[6,7] Irritative symptoms are often quite specific for urge incontinence, but are also present in about 30% of patients with stress incontinence.[8,9] When present, nocturia may be caused by insomnia rather than occurring as a result of being awakened because of a need to void. The patient may void more frequently to lessen incontinence rather than because of a sensation of the need to void. Finally, note the site and character of any dysuria or pain associated with urine storage or emptying which may indicate infection, inflammation, or sensory abnormalities of the bladder.

***Obstructive Urinary Symptoms.*** Patients with obstructive urinary problems may experience intermittent, slow, or dribbly urination; hesitancy, straining, or a feeling of incomplete emptying may also occur during voiding. Obstructive urinary symptoms are common to patients with urge, stress, and overflow incontinence.

In addition, the history should assess *bladder sensation:* the patient's ability to appreciate degree of filling, emptying, or even to notice the leakage; *infections:* the frequency, types, onset, treatments, and responses; *hematuria:* which may indicate the presence of infection, stones, or tumor; and the patient's *fluid intake:* volume and distribution throughout the day and whether intake is due to habit or thirst; consider the possibility of psychogenic water intoxication or response to polyuria from diabetes. Ask the patient to record urinary voiding and fluid intake in an *input/output log* for a week or so and to make a parallel listing of the times and amounts of incontinence. The input/output log can help to establish actual, functional bladder capacity.

**Nonurinary Symptoms.** Nonurinary symptoms provide information to further categorize the nature of the incontinence based on problems within other systems in the same anatomic region or regions served by the same branches of the sacral nerve (S2,3,4). The patient history should assess neurologic, gastrointestinal, and gynecologic symptoms.

Determine any *neurologic* symptoms that involve the perineum and lower extremities, noting paresthesias, numbness, weakness, pain. Also evaluate the patient's sexual capacity, noting impotence and the ability to have orgasm or to ejaculate. Has the patient ever had specific neurologic diseases such as cerebrovascular accidents, multiple sclerosis, Parkinson's disease, tumors, radiation treatment or trauma, disc disease, myelomeningocele, dementia? If so, determine the status/progression of the disease. Lower urinary tract dysfunction is a complaint in 10% of patients in the initial presentation of multiple sclerosis.[10,11]

*Gastrointestinal* symptoms to note include diarrhea, constipation, fecal soiling, or incontinence. Specify any treatments used for these conditions. *Gynecologic* symptoms include pelvic prolapse and dyspareunia; the physician should also discuss the patient's menstrual history.

**Medical History.** The medical history may help to determine the etiology of incontinence. Note the presence of the following signs and symptoms that may be related to incontinence:

- Renal: nonoliguric renal failure with high urine outputs
- Pulmonary: chronic cough associated with bronchitis, chronic obstructive pulmonary disease, tobacco use
- Cardiovascular: edema, venous insufficiency, medications resulting in large-volume diuresis
- Endocrinologic: diabetes causing polyuria or sensory or autonomic neuropathy
- Cancer: local or metastatic effects, including nervous system involvement
- Psychologic/psychiatric: the use of psychotropic drugs; somatization; attention-getting ploys
- Obstetric: urinary and obstetric problems ante- and postpartum; number of pregnancies, vaginal deliveries, Cesarean sections
- Gynecologic: menstrual history, ovarian/hormonal status, relationship of the incontinence to the menstrual cycle
- Radiation therapy: radiation to bladder, urethral, or pelvic areas

**Childhood/Adolescent History.** The childhood and adolescent histories are important if there is a history of prior surgery, infection, or incontinence; consider ectopic ureters, unresolved incontinence.[4]

**Surgical History.** The surgical history should assess:

- Genitourinary: urethral dilations, urethrotomies, bladder neck suspensions, bladder or urethral disease or surgery, stone disease, tumors
- Vaginal: cystocele, enterocele, rectocele, or anterior/posterior repairs or plications
- Pelvic: urologic, gynecologic, or general surgical, radical or not.
- General abdominal: vascular, bowel, or retroperitoneal surgery
- Neurologic: especially surgery to back or peripheral nerves

**Medications.** Almost every class of drugs can have some effect on the lower urinary tract. Practically speaking, it is more effective to simply remember the major and commonly used classes of drugs that have significant impact on lower urinary tract function: $\alpha$- and $\beta$-adrenergic agonists and blockers; cholinergics and anticholinergics; calcium channel blockers; diuretics; antidepressants; and antihistamines.

## The Physical Examination

The physical examination fulfills two main functions: it provides information which allows exclusion of anatomic or neurologic causes for incontinence and it may allow visualization of the cause of the incontinence, such as when incontinence is caused by a fistula, or stress.[2,3,5,6,12]

**Basic Examination.** Carefully check the abdomen, flank, and back for scars of prior surgery or trauma, a palpable bladder or tumor mass, hernias, or pain. Defects over the spine such as dimpling, patches of hair, or tenderness may indicate subtle spinal-cord abnormalities such as spina bifida occulta.

The vagina should be visualized with a single half of a standard speculum (Fig 1), placed to push the rectum away from the anterior vaginal wall, and then the bladder/urethra away from the posterior wall. The vagina should be examined at rest and during straining with the speculum to determine urethral mobility/descent, and the presence of cystocele, enterocele, rectocele, urethral caruncle, or prolapse. Assess the vaginal capacity, and note vaginal wall atrophy, fistulas, periurethral masses/diverticula, and the general condition of the cervix.[13] The bimanual examination should detect any masses or tenderness along the urethra, vaginal wall, bladder, uterus, or adnexa; repeating the examination with the patient standing with one foot on a footstool helps the physician to fully evaluate the extent of any vaginal wall or uterine prolapse.

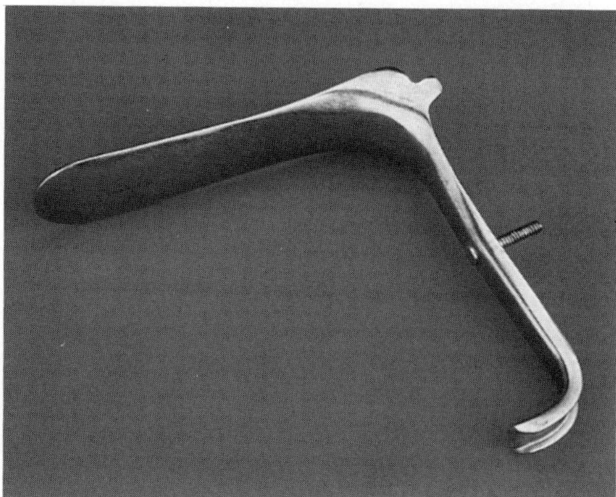

**Fig 1.** The lower half of a standard speculum is an excellent instrument with which to examine the vaginal vault.

As part of the detailed vaginal/genital and pelvic examination, it is important to have the patient strain or cough with a full or partially full bladder to elicit incontinence. Leakage associated with straining, in conjunction with a slight descent of the bladder neck and proximal urethra away from the pubic symphysis, indicates Type I stress urinary incontinence; in resting positions, the urethra is relatively normal and well supported. In patients with Type II stress incontinence, the urethral resting position shows poor support; with straining the urethra descends further (>2 cm) and leakage occurs.[14] Although often used, the Marshall and Q-tip tests do not provide unique diagnostic information beyond that provided by simple observation of the mobility and support of the bladder neck/urethra during vaginal examination.[15]

Incontinence may occur during a stress maneuver without any motion of the urethra. If such leakage is considered continuous and extreme by the patient—particularly when it occurs in those with a history of prior surgery or neurological injury—then Type III stress urinary incontinence, or an incompetent urethra, may be present.[14] In patients who complain of stress incontinence, yet in whom leakage cannot be demonstrated on physical or radiologic examination, the incontinence is called Type 0; more detailed evaluation is usually necessary in such cases.[14]

Examination of male genitalia should determine the presence of masses, tenderness, or discharge at the meatus or along the urethra. Also note any rectal masses and the status of the prostate.

The neurologic examination should discover the sensation in areas served by sacral roots 2, 3 and 4 (the perianal and perineal areas). Note changes of lower-extremity sensation in distributions consistent with disc disease or stocking/glove abnormality consistent with diabetic or alcoholic neuropathies. Also assess lower extremity reflexes and muscle tone/development; anal sphincter tone, voluntary contraction, and bulbocavernosus reflex (BCR) (elicited by squeezing the glans or clitoris gently, and feeling the contraction of the anal sphincter to test the sacral reflex arc; BCR can be absent in about 5% of normal men and 20% of normal women)[16]; any obvious hemiparesis or tremors; and the presence of abnormal mental status, gait, strength, balance, or speech patterns.

### Basic Diagnostic Tests

After the history and physical examination have been completed, basic tests can be of great value.[3,5] These include urinalysis to detect infection, hematuria, glucosuria or occult renal disease, urine culture and sensitivity to confirm suspected infection, and urine cytology to rule out bladder tumor in patients with hematuria or severe urgency/frequency. Urine cytology can be especially useful in patients with a history of tobacco use or industrial dye exposure. A further test is the measurement of postvoid residual urine: if less than 50 cc remains after voiding, urethral overactivity (obstruction) or bladder underactivity (acontractility) may be virtually eliminated as possible causes of incontinence. This test is especially important in patients older than 50 years, those with diabetes or neurologic disease, and those currently receiving anticholinergic or psychotropic drugs or who have undergone prior pelvic or vaginal surgeries.

**Radiography.** Intravenous pyelograms (IVP) or voiding cystourethrograms (VCUG) provide no unique information in the initial evaluation of incontinence unless continuous incontinence or a large cystocele is present. In patients with continuous incontinence, IVP and VCUG help make the diagnosis, and in patients with cystocele such tests grade the cystocele and help rule out ureteral obstruction.[13] However, an open bladder neck as visualized on a VCUG may be a normal variant, or the result of a bladder contraction which was not detected by the examiner. In patients with obstruction, the VCUG may help pinpoint the site of obstruction, if it is not already evident.

**Nonurinary Leakage.** It may be necessary to establish that the leakage about which the patient complains is truly urine. This would be particularly true in women, who may mistake vaginal discharge for urinary incontinence. Likewise, it may be important to get a better idea of the true location of urinary leakage. Oral medications like phenazopyridine hydrochloride stain the urine a distinct yellow-orange. A vaginal tampon stained at the apical end is indicative of a probable vesico- or ureterovaginal fistula. Staining at the end of the tampon resting near the urethral meatus may indicate either incontinence or a urethral fistula. Staining of the perineal pad alone is probably the result of simple incontinence. Dampness of tampon or pad without any staining indicates a nonurinary vaginal discharge.

### Summary

With the information provided by a basic but thorough history, physical examination, and basic tests, the urologist should know the type of incontinence—continuous, overflow, transient, stress, or urge, or perhaps a combination of two types—with an accuracy of at least 80%.[5] Based on this information, further evaluation will be necessary for those suspected of having overflow or continuous incontinence (Table 2). The information will also allow the reversal of causative factors and the relatively speedy resolution of transient incontinence (Table 3). For patients in whom simple stress or urge incontinence alone are suspected, therapy can be initiated. However, no irreversible or invasive therapy should be initiated until the cause of the incontinence is clearly demonstrated by either repeating the basic tests already discussed, or by using more invasive and detailed evaluations such as endoscopy or urodynamics tests.

## ENDOSCOPY

Cystourethroscopy can provide useful information about the bladder and urethra.[17] The bladder should be inspected for evidence of trabeculation, which may be associated with high-pressure storage or voiding characteristics. Foreign bodies, stones, bladder-wall inflammation, or tumor may not have been suspected as causes of the incontinence, although urinalysis or cytology is likely to be abnormal in most of these conditions. The absence or abnormal location of a ureteral orifice on cystourethroscopy may indicate an ectopic ureter, and inflammatory sites on the bladder wall in patients who have undergone prior surgery may confirm the site of a fistula.

Urethroscopy can be quite valuable. In women, urethroscopy is best performed with a female urethroscope with a 0°- or 5°-angle lens. This instrument has a blunt, nonfenestrated end rather than the beaked end of the standard cystourethroscope (Fig 2). The blunt end permits adequate distension of the urethra by fluid at the point of visualization, but does not distort the urethra during examination as the beaked cystoscope might.

Urethroscopy may be used to assess several aspects of the female urethra: mucosa and coaptation of the wall, mobility and descent with straining, length, and the presence of stricture, diverticula, or fistulas. The mucosa is best examined at the distal third of the urethra, where the mucosa should seal because of the healthy fullness of the submucosal vascular component of the urethra. With the water flow on at a height of about 50 cm, the mucosa will open. Failure to appropriately open and collapse may indicate atrophy from estrogen depletion or fibrosis from prior trauma, surgery, or infection which may be severe enough to cause Type III stress urinary incontinence (see below). At the mid-urethra, the water infusion will not necessarily separate the mucosal folds when urethral pressure is normal. This section of the urethral mucosa will open just prior to a detrusor contraction that might be induced by the examination.

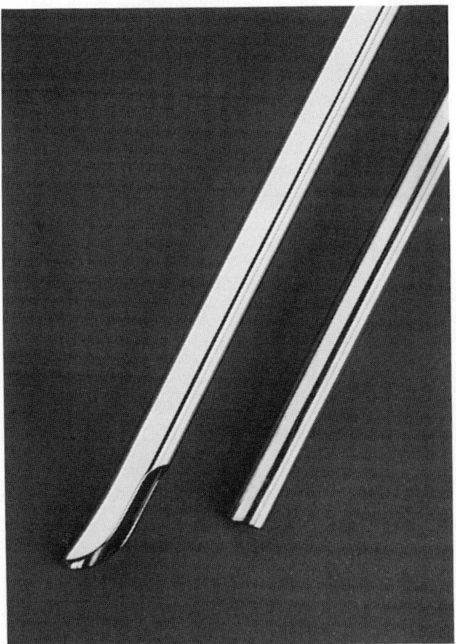

**Fig 2.** The female urethroscope (right) has a blunt end, which facilitates evaluation of the female urethra; the beaked end of the standard cystoscope sheath (left) is not as useful for evaluation of the female urethra.

The bladder neck will be closed at rest in a normal woman, but the bladder neck and proximal urethra may open with straining activity. While mobility (descent) and poor support of the proximal urethra and bladder neck may be obvious from the vaginal examination, they are clearly demonstrated by urethroscopy during straining. If leakage occurs with descent and straining, simple stress incontinence is the diagnosis. In general, a sudden, strong cough will show even the mildest amount of bladder neck incompetence; more gradual increases in straining pressure allow easier assessment of hypermobility and more severe incompetence at the bladder neck.

A tight stricture should be very evident on endoscopy. More subtle strictures can be detected by sounding the urethra using Bougie-a-boulés. A urethral caliber of less than 18 F in the adult woman is considered abnormal, but is significant only if there are associated symptoms of obstruction.[18]

Periurethral glands open into the urethral lumen which may be inflamed, or may be the sites of communication with urethral diverticula. In patients with diverticula, massaging the urethra over the endoscope will often force pus into the lumen and will allow identification of the site of communication between the diverticula and the urethral lumen. Fistulas may be suspected from the patient history; endoscopy may provide confirmation. Although possible during endoscopy, measurement of urethral length is rarely useful unless the urethra has been partially destroyed and the remaining length may affect the choice of a reconstructive procedure.

The endoscope may also be used to examine the vagina, a step most useful in patients with vesicovaginal or ureterovaginal fistulas.

Urethroscopy can be performed in men using a blunt-ended scope or the traditional fenestrated scope. The areas of prime concern are the bladder neck and prostatic urethra, the membranous urethra, and the bulbous/penile urethra. The status of the mucosa is significant in all areas, but is rarely indicative of pathology contributing or related to incontinence, with the exception of fistulas or diverticula, which might cause abnormal drainage patterns.

An open bladder neck may be indicative of urethral incompetence due to neurologic or traumatic injury (such as may occur after prostatectomy). The membranous urethra may be scarred or patulous and thus incompetent. In the most severe cases of incontinence, it is possible to look into the bladder during endoscopy from the region distal to the membranous urethra. When the membranous urethra is incompetent but the bladder neck remains closed at rest, incontinence is likely to occur only with significant stress maneuvers or with involuntary bladder contractions.

Evidence of marked urethral obstruction in the form of stricture is easy to diagnose. However, the diagnosis of prostatic obstruction is not reliable in patients with incontinence.

Other than fistula or diverticula, there are essentially no abnormalities in the bulbous and penile urethra which would in any way contribute to incontinence.

Endoscopy is not necessary for every patient with incontinence. It is of greatest value in patients who have undergone prior urethral or bladder surgery, especially surgery for incontinence; those who have a suspected urethral stricture or diverticulum; those with continuous incontinence; patients with urgency incontinence in whom basic therapy has failed; and in those for whom surgical intervention is planned.

## URODYNAMICS TESTING

While the basic history, physical examination, and simple tests allow diagnosis and guide treatment for the majority of patients with incontinence, it is sometimes necessary to perform urodynamic evaluations—a range of sophisticated and specific neurophysiologic tests of the lower urinary tract—to identify the lower urinary tract abnormality causing the incontinence and document its severity and prognosis. The instances in which urodynamics testing is often necessary to provide objective information about the lower urinary tract are summarized in Table 4.

**TABLE 4. General Indications for Urodynamic Evaluations for Incontinence**

- Failed medical or surgical therapies
- Known or potential neurologic causes
- Lower urinary tract alterations due to medications, disease, surgery, trauma
- Complex or combined types and causes of incontinence
- Contradictory, confusing, or noncontributory history or physical examination
- Total incontinence

Urodynamics tests provide objective information about the three elements of the lower urinary tract—the bladder, the urethra, and the sensation—allowing their functions to be classified as normal, overactive, or underactive. The six types of urodynamic tests used to obtain these data are: uroflowmetry, cystometry, voiding cystometry (pressure/flow study), electromyography, urethral-pressure profilometry, and videourodynamics (combinations of these tests conducted under fluoroscopic observation) (Table 5). The terminology that should be used to describe the urodynamic procedures and data have been compiled by the International Continence Society (ICS).[19–21] Each test will be discussed primarily in the context of the evaluation of incontinence.

**TABLE 5. Urodynamics Tests and the Data Provided**

| Test | Filling/Voiding | Bladder | Urethra | Sensation |
|---|---|---|---|---|
| Uroflowmetry | −/+ | I | I | I |
| Cystometry | +/− | D | I | D |
| Pressure/flow | −/+ | D | I | I |
| Urethral pressure | +/+ | — | D | — |
| Electromyography | +/+ | — | I | — |
| Videourodynamics | +/+ | * | * | * |

D = Direct measurement; I = Indirect measurement; * = Depends upon specific tests performed with fluoroscopy.

When conducting urodynamic tests, it is essential that the results be applied while considering the particular patient's clinical situation. To be considered significant, the tests should replicate accurately the patient's symptoms; if they do not, the tests must be repeated until they do. Conversely, if the tests produce findings unrelated to the patient's complaints the results are probably artifacts; clinically unrelated and irrelevant; or fortuitous and possibly related, yet clinically unexplainable at that point. To ensure the best results with urodynamic evaluations, the physician should observe or conduct the test personally, and should be very familiar with the details of the testing procedures and equipment as well as with the proper interpretation of the data provided.

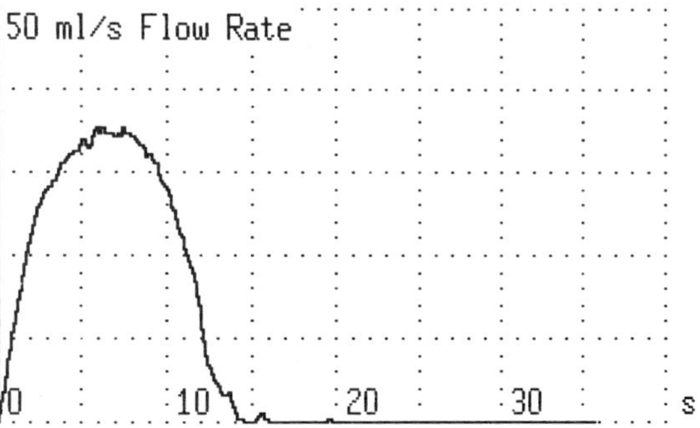


**Results of UROFLOWMETRY**

| | | | |
|---|---|---|---|
| Voiding Time | T100 | 16 | s |
| Flow Time | TQ | 15 | s |
| Time to max Flow | TQmax | 6 | s |
| Max Flow Rate | Qmax | 35.3 | ml/s |
| Average Flow Rate | Qave | 22.5 | ml/s |
| Voided Volume | Vcomp | 330 | ml |

**Fig 3.** A normal flow curve with normal maximum and mean flow rates and voided volumes; note the curve is relatively symmetrical about the midpoint of the flow.

## Uroflowmetry

Uroflowmetry provides an indirect measurement of the combined bladder, urethral, and sensory function during voiding. Obtaining a uroflow test requires only that the patient empty the bladder into a collection device that is capable of recording the rate of urinary flow. Most uroflow machines are electronic and have the capability of graphically depicting the curve of urinary flow rate vs time as shown in Figure 3. The figure includes the significant data points of the flow curve: the maximum and average flow rates and the voiding time. The shape of the flow curve, which is related to the flow rate magnitude as well as the voiding time, can vary from the normal shape with different lower urinary tract problems (Figs 4, 5).[19,22,23]

Normal values of maximum flow, average flow, voided volumes, and voiding time vary with patient age, sex, and the amount of urine within the bladder at the time of voiding, and may even vary from one test to another in the same patient. A number of tables and nomograms have been constructed to help determine whether the data from a specific uroflow test are normal for that patient, but general guidelines are that maximum flow rates less than 10 mL are clearly abnormal, greater than

15 mL are probably normal, and between 10 mL and 15 mL are equivocal.[22,24–35]

A normal uroflowmetry implies normal lower urinary tract function while voiding. Exceptions can occur when a patient empties well with a single Valsalva maneuver, or when a patient is actually obstructed, which necessitates a very high detrusor pressure to produce the normal flow curve. A low flow rate, correcting for the variables noted above, results from either detrusor underactivity (absent or low-pressure detrusor contractions) or urethral overactivity (obstruction). In some cases, a patient cannot void because of anxiety surrounding the testing situation; this is not unusual, especially in women. These conditions will be discussed more thoroughly in the section covering simultaneous cystometry/uroflowmetry.[22,23,26]

Very high maximum flow rates (>40 mL/sec) usually occur in patients with detrusor instability who can generate high detrusor pressures just prior to voiding.

While uroflowmetry can be useful as an indirect indicator of lower urinary tract function, it is minimally useful in the evaluation of the patient with incontinence, except to show that flow rate is low in the patient with retention and overflow incontinence. The issues surrounding this are summarized well by Aagaard and Bruskewitz.[37]

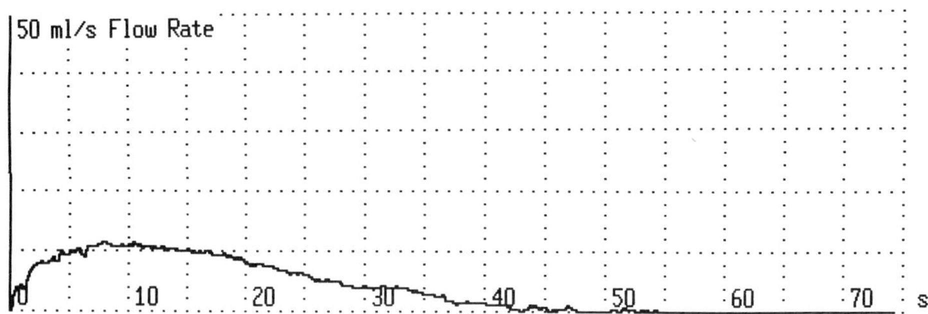


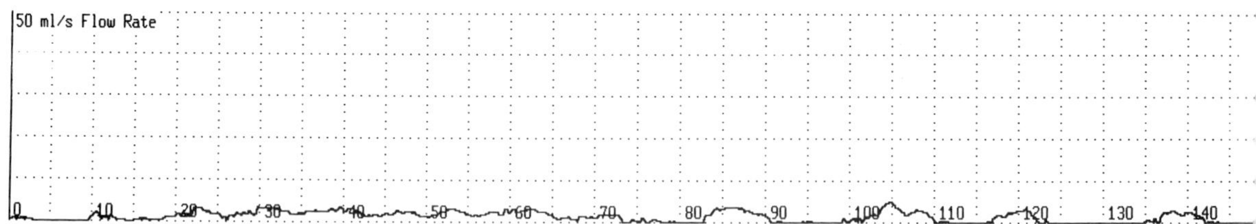

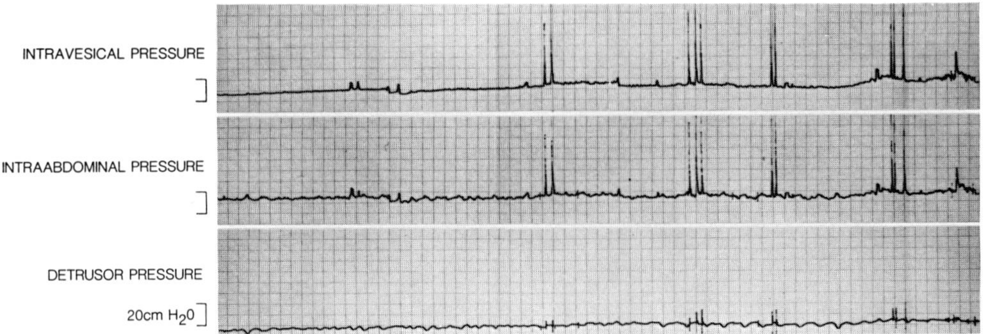


**Fig 6.** Normal cystometrogram; detrusor pressures remain relatively constant during bladder filling to capacity.

## Cystometry

The cystometrogram (CMG) provides data on the lower urinary tract during bladder filling and storage. Thus, cystometry is the most useful urodynamic test in the evaluation of urinary incontinence. A CMG provides direct information about the bladder and sensation, and indirect data about the urethra. This test is performed by filling the bladder with a fluid, either liquid or gas, and directly recording the pressure within the bladder (intravesical pressure) throughout the filling process. In most situations, intraabdominal pressure also is measured, usually with a rectal catheter. True detrusor pressure can then be calculated as the intravesical pressure minus intraabdominal pressure. As the bladder is filled and the measurements are made, the patient's sensation during the filling process is recorded and direct observations are made about the continence status.

Several variables must be considered when conducting a filling CMG: bladder access; catheter and transducer types; fluid type, usually either water or $CO_2$; fill rate; patient position; provocation maneuvers such as coughing, straining, or standing; fluid temperature; and the type of recording equipment. While the details affecting each of these considerations are too many to be discussed in this chapter, a number of references cover these questions thoroughly.[6,20,21,38]

**Bladder Function.** A CMG measures bladder function by capacity and storage pressure. The normal bladder capacity during a CMG will vary with the patient's age and sex. Generally, however, a bladder capacity of about 400 to 700 mL is normal for an adult man; the capacity is usually about 100 mL less in women. For the child, formulas such as "volume in ounces equals patient age in years plus 2," give reasonable approximations.[39] To be considered truly normal, the bladder capacity must be reached under normal bladder pressures, in the absence of involuntary contractions, and with little to no leakage.

Normally, the pressure within the bladder rises little during filling (Fig 6), and the detrusor does not contract despite provocation by the fluid, its fill rate or temperature, or patient activity. If the detrusor is overactive and does contract, phasic pressure increases may occur that cannot be suppressed despite a sense of urgency or a need to empty the bladder (Fig 7), and leakage (incontinence) might occur. Such contractions are abnormal; they are termed detrusor hyperreflexia (DH) when there is a known causative neurologic abnormality, and detrusor instability (DI) if there is no known causative neurologic abnormality. In the ICS definition, such involuntary contractions must displace greater than 15 cm of water to be considered significant. Practically, however, if such contractions replicate the patient's symptoms (including incontinence) they are clinically and uro-

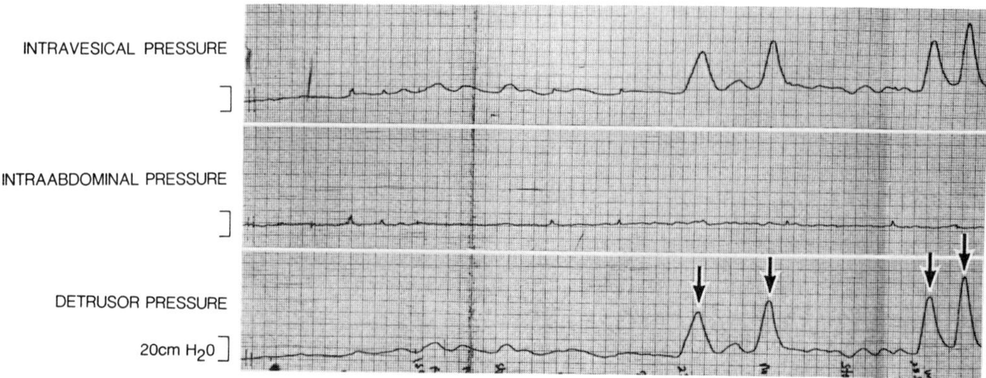


**Fig 7.** Detrusor instability or hyperreflexia; the cystometrogram shows a phasic increase of true detrusor pressure caused by involuntary bladder contractions which the patient cannot suppress (arrows).

dynamically significant, and indicate urge incontinence.[8,9,19,40]

Abnormal increases in bladder pressure can also occur steadily during the filling process, rather than in the phasic form of involuntary contractions. Such steady pressure increases are termed abnormal compliance, and denote the inability of the bladder to appropriately accommodate increased volume without a pressure increase (Fig 8). While compliance is defined as change in volume divided by change in pressure, there is no single numerical value defining abnormal compliance. However, since the adult bladder should be able to hold 400 to 600 mL with a pressure rise of less than 15 cm of water over this range of filling, any volume/pressure ratio less than this generally is considered to indicate low compliance. Though fluid or urine leakage can occur with the steady pressure increases of low compliance, there is no specific symptomatology correlated to incontinence of this type, as urge, overflow, continuous, or stress incontinence could all describe the clinical situation.

It is important to note the detrusor pressure at which leakage occurs (the leak-point pressure) in patients with low compliance or DI/DH. The leak-point pressure is especially important in the presence of neurologic disease, when urethral resistance often is fixed and the leak-point pressure defines the urethral resistance characteris-

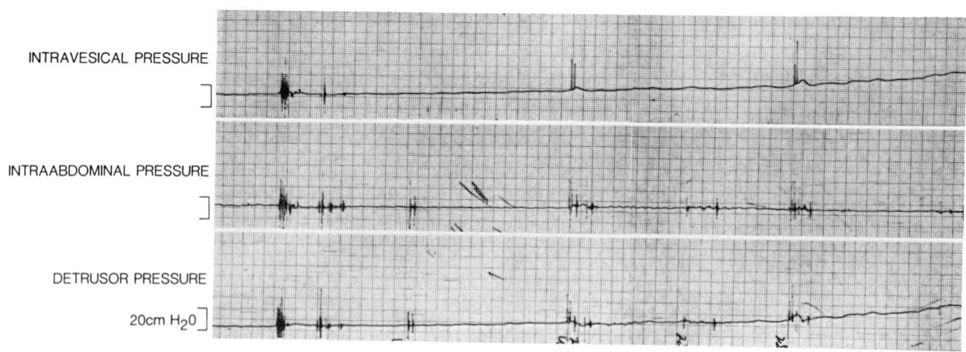


**Fig 8.** Low bladder compliance; the cystometrogram shows a gradual, steady increase in the true detrusor pressure to abnormally high levels. The bladder volume at the end of the tracing was 300 mL.

tics quite well. Leak-point pressures play a key role in determining the status of the upper urinary tracts of patients with bladder dysfunction and high storage pressures. A pressure of 40 cm of water has been accepted as a critical point, above which upper urinary tract damage and changes are almost certain to occur.[41–45]

**Urethral Function.** Urethral function (competence) during filling—ability to maintain continence—is assessed indirectly during the CMG by observing whether leakage occurs and, if it does, the detrusor pressure at that moment. Except for the leak-point pressure, no other objective data are obtained; any other conclusions about urethral competence are general, descriptive impressions about the competence of the urethra.

In any type of incontinence due solely to an underactive (incompetent) urethra, there must be no increase in detrusor pressure associated with urinary leakage. If DI/DH is present, the assumed urethral incompetence may simply reflect an inability to override the detrusor contraction and stop the normal urethral relaxation that occurs when the detrusor contracts. When the detrusor shows low compliance, the leak-point pressure is a discrete indicator of urethral competence. However, there is no "normal" leak point, since the situation usually arises only in the patient with neurologic disease.

A patient may demonstrate incontinence during the filling CMG when stress maneuvers such as coughing, straining, crouching, heel bouncing, and hopping are performed. If such leakage is observed, yet true detrusor-pressure does not rise, the diagnosis of genuine stress urinary incontinence (GSUI) is confirmed, and urethral incompetence (Type I, II, or III GSUI) is considered to be the cause (Fig 9).[19] Type III GSUI may be confirmed by a CMG with simultaneous fluoroscopy demonstrating an open, or relatively open, bladder neck/

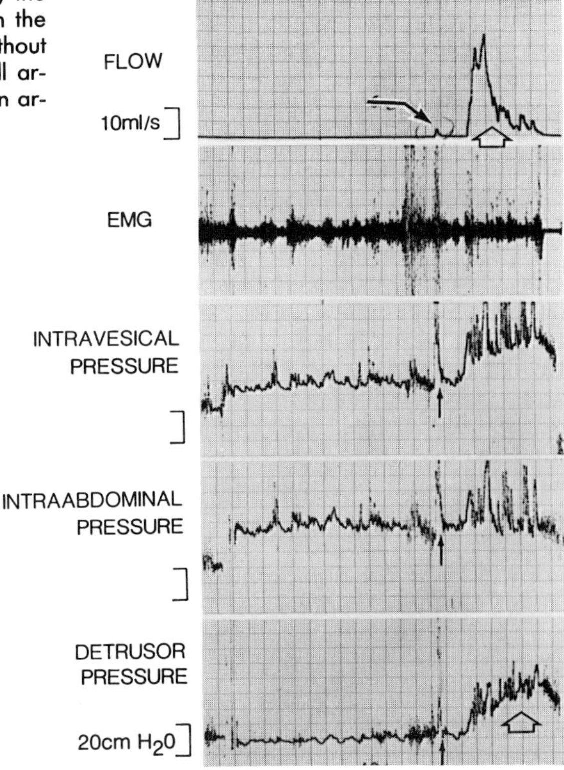


**Fig 9.** Genuine stress urinary incontinence; the cystometrogram shows the loss of urine on the uroflow (arrow) associated with a cough without an increase in true detrusor pressure (small arrows). The patient then voids normally (open arrow).

proximal urethra in the absence of detrusor activity (see section on videourodynamics). With urodynamic stress incontinence, the patient will usually report a consistent symptom complex.

In an uncommon form of urethral incompetence, incontinence during a CMG also can occur without detrusor pressure change, stress activity, a Type III urethra, or even patient awareness, as a result of intermittent, spontaneous drops in urethral closure pressure; this condition is known as urethral instability. DI may follow the urethral relaxation, creating a mixed problem. The patient's symptoms may indicate stress or urge incontinence, or may be nonspecific and unclear. Urethral pressure measurements and sphincter electromyography are necessary to confirm this diagnosis.[46,47]

Occasionally, a stress maneuver during a CMG generates a nearly immediate involuntary bladder contraction. Any leakage that results is associated not with the stress maneuver itself, but with the detrusor-pressure increase associated with the involuntary contraction; this is called stress-induced detrusor instability. Clinically, the patient may complain of symptoms indicating either stress or urge incontinence or both.

**Sensation.** Sensation during the CMG is evaluated by noting what the patient feels during the test. Normally, a patient has a "first desire" to void at a volume of about 100–200 mL, a "normal desire" to void beginning at volumes above 300 mL and ranging to near capacity, and "strong desire" at capacity. Increased, or overactive, sensation levels reduce these volumes and decreased, or underactive, sensation levels increase them. *Urgency* is the desire to void with a fear of impending leakage or pain; it is abnormal. Any indication of pain during CMG is also abnormal. An overactive sensation level without evident cause is termed sensory instability.

With two possible exceptions, sensation abnormalities rarely cause incontinence. A patient with overflow incontinence may have reduced or absent sensation, while a patient with increased sensation may have incontinence because discomfort prevents further holding; this patient may complain of urge incontinence.

Combinations of detrusor, urethral, and sensory abnormalities as revealed by the CMG are common, especially in patients with genuine stress urinary incontinence and DI.[9,40] Thus, it is important to investigate these possibilities adequately before the CMG is considered complete. Finally, it must be emphasized that correlation with the patient's clinical situation is vital, especially before invasive therapy is attempted.

Since all components of the lower urinary tract—bladder, urethra, and sensation—are assessed during the filling CMG, it represents the most valuable urodynamic test used in the evaluation of urinary incontinence. Valid concerns exist regarding the true usefulness of the CMG in evaluating patients with incontinence. However, when used in patients with the characteristics noted in Table 4, the CMG provides data that can be complementary to and supportive of the information provided in the basic evaluation, or when basic evaluation techniques are clearly inadequate.[5,37,48–57]

### Simultaneous Cystometry/Uroflowmetry (Pressure/Flow Study)

Simultaneous measurement of detrusor pressure (with a pressure-measurement catheter in the bladder) and the urine flow rate (with a flowmeter while voiding) constitutes simultaneous cystometry/uroflowmetry. This pressure/flow study provides direct data about bladder function during voiding as well as indirect information about urethral and sensory activity (Fig 10).[19]

Normal voiding pressures at maximum flow rates for men and women under 45 years old are approximately 60 to 75 cm and 50 to 60 cm of water, respectively, with respective corresponding normal maximum flow rates of about 20 mL/sec and 25 mL/sec.[6] Obstruction implies higher pressures with the same or lower flows, or the same pressures with lower flows. It has also been defined by sustained voiding

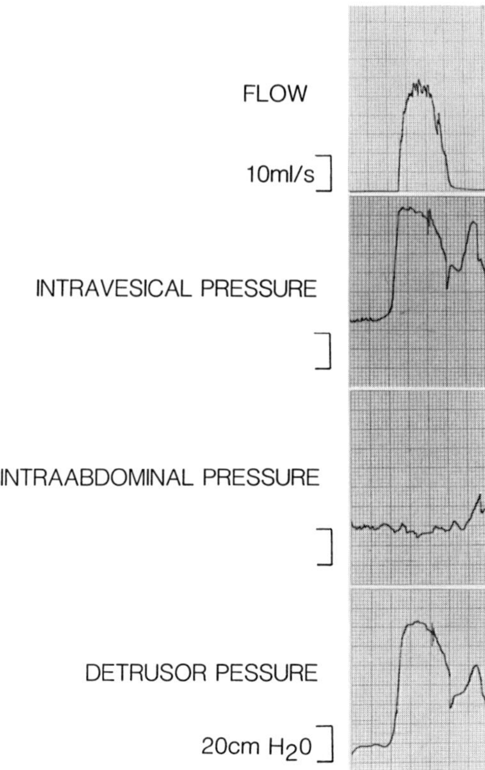


**Fig 10.** Normal pressure/flow study; the patient is voiding with a normal appearance to the flow curve, and an appropriate increase in detrusor pressure. The pressure rise after voiding is an after contraction, a normal variant.

pressures of greater than 30 cm (men) or 20 cm of water (women) with maximum flow rates below 12 mL/sec.[18,58,59] Attempts to create mathematical formulas to describe the pressure/flow relation, or urethral resistance, have been described. One formula is: R (Resistance) = $P/Q^2$, where Q = maximum flow rate and P = detrusor pressure corresponding to Q. Obstruction is then estimated as $R > 0.5$ for men and $> 0.2$ for women. Unfortunately, such crude approximations have not been consistently useful.[23,36,60]

Normal ranges of detrusor voiding pressures should be applied to a specific patient only if the patient has signs or symptoms of abnormal voiding function. Many normal women void without any increase occurring in bladder pressure. In addition, some patients cannot relax enough in the testing situation to generate a detrusor contraction and provide a pressure/flow study; this is not uncommon, especially among women or children and should not necessarily be considered indicative of an abnormality. Also, flow values in the pressure/flow study should be interpreted with the caveats pointed out in the prior section on uroflowmetry. Normal pressure and flow values mean that the pressure/flow relationship is normal.[19,36,60]

During voiding, the detrusor can be underactive absolutely—this type of detrusor never contracts, either voluntarily or involuntarily. In this case the detrusor is called areflexic when the cause of the absent contractility is neurologic, and acontractile for any other reason. A relatively underactive detrusor generates a low-pressure, short-duration contraction that is inadequate to empty the bladder. In this type of patient, the pressure/flow data will show low flow with absent or low detrusor contraction pressure (Fig 11).[19,22,23,36]

While voiding, the urethra should relax totally to minimize resistance, optimize flow, and minimize the work of the detrusor in emptying the bladder completely. Failure to relax and open adequately means the urethra is overactive (obstructive), whatever the cause. Such obstruction will be accompanied by a low flow rate with a normal or high detrusor pressure (Fig 12). While the detrusor can generate extremely high pressures during voiding, this apparent detrusor overactivity is actually secondary to the obstructive urethra.[18,22,23,36,58–63]

Normal voiding, obstruction, and acontractility are clearly defined by the pressure/flow relationship; however, there are many equivocal cases. Also, while the pressure/flow study can be useful in assessing the detrusor and urethra during voiding, the value of this test in the assessment of incontinence is quite limited. It can provide information to confirm that obstruction or an acontractile/areflexic bladder are contributing factors in overflow incontinence or in DI associated with obstruction (as in the man with benign prostatic hyperplasia [BPH]). Beyond such specific instances, it

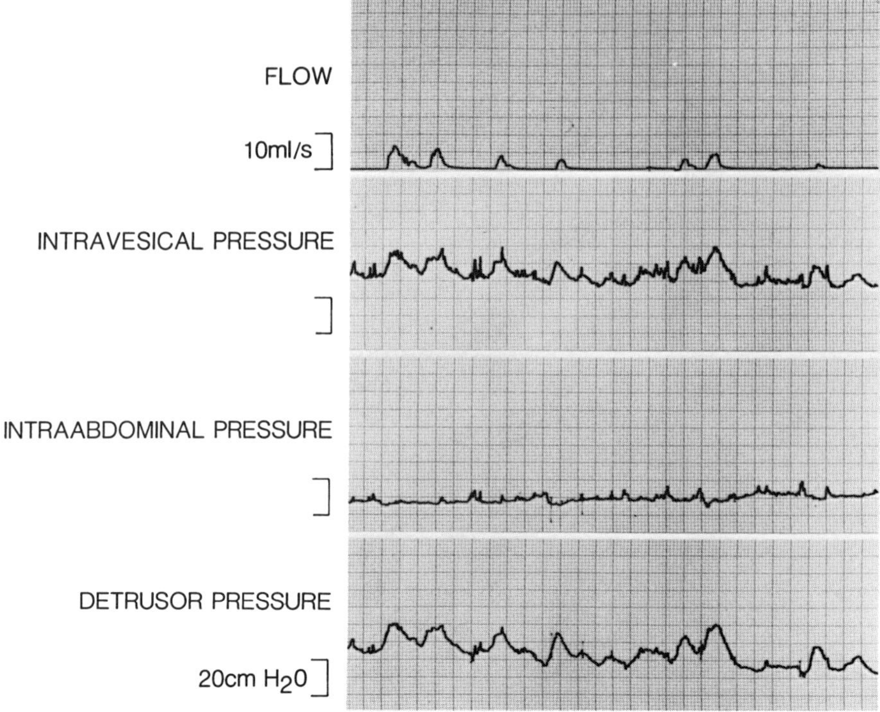


**Fig 11.** Fluctuating bladder underactivity (relative detrusor acontractility) on a pressure/flow study with low detrusor pressure and low intermittent flow.

is not an essential and rarely is a useful part of an assessment of incontinence.

## Electromyography

Electromyography (EMG) is the evaluation of electrical potentials generated by muscle depolarization. EMG of the periurethral sphincter muscles allows an indirect but valuable assessment of urethral function. A perianal EMG gives a reasonably accurate approximation of periurethral activity. However, the EMG provides no data on bladder function, and assesses sensory function only insofar as the patient may feel the application of the EMG electrodes.[19]

The EMG can be obtained using surface or needle electrodes. The former are adequate for most purposes; the latter are necessary for more detailed, precise assessments in patients with neurologic disease processes. EMG data is provided adequately for urodynamic evaluations in audio and strip chart form and is sometimes augmented with an oscilloscope for patients with neurologic disease.[19–21,64–68]

Besides use as an adjunct to the other urodynamic tests, the EMG can be used to assess sphincter function in voluntary contraction of the sphincter (full interference or recruitment pattern), and the BCR. In detailed neurologic evaluations, the EMG can be used to evaluate individual motor unit potentials, nerve conduction velocities, and evoked potentials thus providing the data needed to make a specific neurologic diagnosis.[19–21,64,65,69]

The normal EMG signal should increase gradually in intensity (recruitment) during bladder filling in response to the normal slight detrusor pressure increases. When voiding is initiated, the EMG signal should essentially disappear, heralding a decrease in urethral resistance which is followed by the initiation of voiding. The EMG signal should increase in intensity in response to an involuntary bladder contraction as the

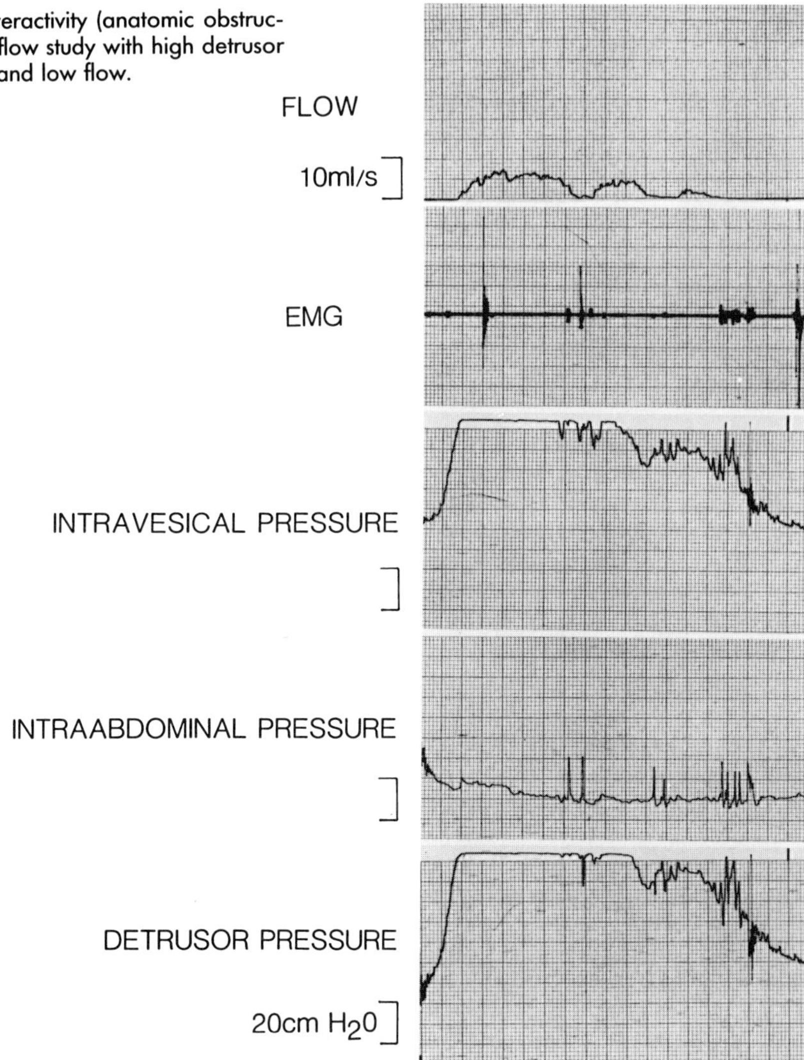


**Fig 12.** Urethral overactivity (anatomic obstruction) on a pressure/flow study with high detrusor pressure (off-scale) and low flow.

patient attempts to prevent incontinence by increasing urethral closure pressure; this is normal (Fig 13). In a patient with neurologic disease, who is unable to sense or voluntarily suppress a contraction, this same phenomenon is pathologic and is termed detrusor-sphincter dyssynergia (DSD). Like a high leak-point pressure, DSD can have adverse effects on the upper urinary tract.[41,42] A DSD pattern obtained during voluntary voiding from a patient without neurologic pathology is dysfunctional voiding, a learned, reversible pattern.[19,64,66,68,69,70–76]

The EMG is a useful adjunct to other tests in the assessment of incontinence, as it gives an indirect measure of the urethral response to the detrusor as well as of the level of urethral competence during the filling process.

## Urethral Pressure Measurements

Direct information on urethral function is gathered with the urethral pressure profile (UPP), a compilation of direct measurements of intraurethral pressures along the urethral length.[19,46] The measurements are

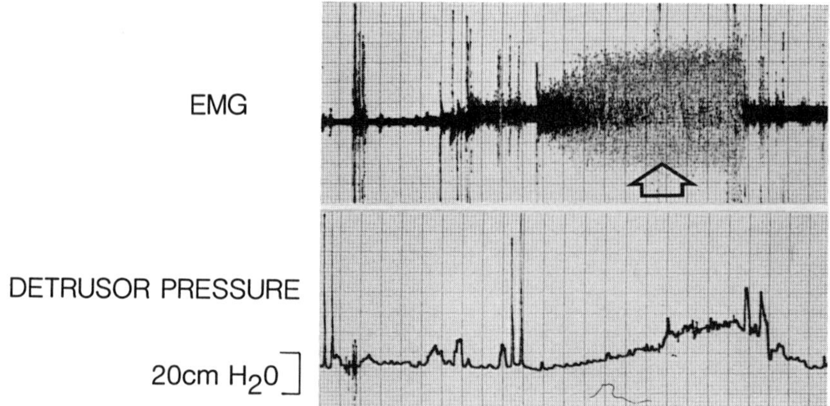


Fig 13. Detrusor instability with appropriate urethral sphincter EMG guarding (arrow). An identical pattern is seen in a patient with detrusor sphincter dyssynergia.

obtained using a variety of pressure measurement catheter systems. In a storage UPP, pressures are measured during the filling or storage process while the patient remains at rest (a resting UPP) or performs stress maneuvers (a stress UPP). Each type of UPP provides data about urethral closure pressures. A voiding UPP assesses urethral closure or opening pressures during voiding. The UPP provides no data on bladder or sensory function.

Conceptually, the UPP would seem to provide the most specific and ideal information to describe the urethral closure and relaxation capabilities. Unfortunately, the variety of tests performed and techniques used have resulted in data with overlaps between normal and abnormal patients which prevents the use of UPP in most clinical situations, including the use to make a definitive diagnosis of incontinence.[37,46] Thus, it is primarily a research tool.

## Videourodynamics

In some cases in the evaluation of urinary incontinence, it is necessary to know the anatomic appearance of the bladder neck/urethra while gathering other urodynamic data. An ideal way to obtain this information is by performing urodynamic tests under fluoroscopic observation, a process known as videourodynamics (VUD). The data of the various urodynamic tests are displayed simultaneously with the fluoroscopy picture of the bladder and urethra, allowing the most complete view possible of lower urinary tract function.

VUD is particularly valuable in the diagnosis of two conditions: the totally incompetent urethra (Type III GSUI) which should always be considered in a patient with prior urethral/bladder neck surgery or neurologic injury; and the location of urethral obstruction not discernable clinically, especially in cases of detrusor/bladder neck dyssynergia. A bladder neck and urethra which are incompetent and open at rest, or nearly so, on fluoroscopy, combined with urinary leakage and no detrusor pressure change confirms the diagnosis of Type III GSUI (Fig 14). The zone or point of urethral narrowing or closure as visualized by fluoroscopy in conjunction with other urodynamic data during voiding confirms the site and cause of obstruction. VUD allows accurate conclusions to be drawn about detrusor and urethral function that could not have been reached from separate examination by urodynamic testing and fluoroscopy. Confirmation of these complex diagnoses has a tremendous impact on the selection and ultimate success of therapy.[14]

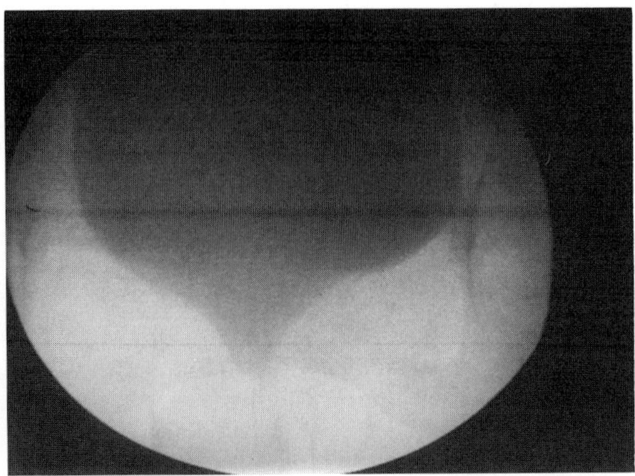
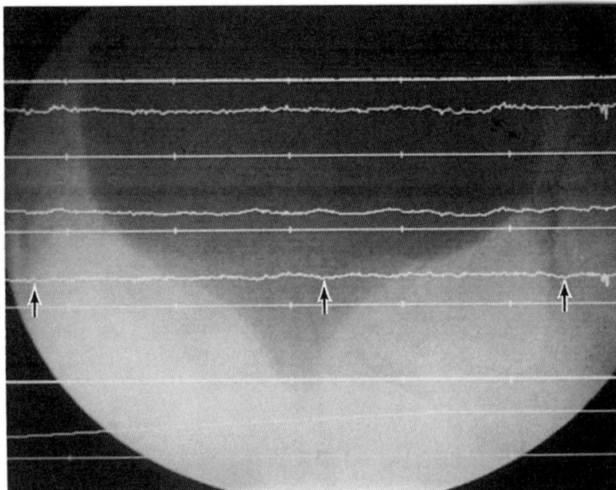

**Fig 14.** Videourodynamics; the left side of the figure shows a standing cystogram in the anterior/posterior view with an open bladder neck. The right side shows the corresponding stable detrusor pressures (arrows) with the same cystogram; in this case with the bladder neck open, leakage, and no increase in detrusor pressure the diagnosis is Type III stress urinary incontinence.

## Urodynamic Testing in Children

The full range of urodynamic evaluations can be performed in children. These tests are most useful when neurologic dysfunction must be ruled out; incontinence is progressive, or diurnal and nocturnal; pain or straining to void is present; or when the clinical situation needs further clarification.[77] The greater the numbers and invasiveness of the tests, the more difficult it may be to complete them successfully in a child who is likely to be anxious, frightened, and perhaps crying. Careful preparation of the patient and family can usually ensure successful placement of the necessary monitoring equipment and completion of the test. Interpretation of the test must consider the fact that the child may not respond as an adult would to all aspects of the evaluation. Repeating the study is often necessary, and the child usually tolerates this well if the early portions of the test and monitoring placement have gone smoothly. Sedation is rarely necessary to perform the evaluations, and there is essentially no indication for urodynamic evaluation under anesthesia.[74]

## Urinary Loss Measurement

The ICS has outlined a procedure for quantification of urinary loss.[19] This procedure requires about one hour and covers a full range of straining maneuvers with a bladder filled by hydrating the patient generously. Its primary use is in documenting the degree of a patient's incontinence and in research.

## Bedside Urodynamics

A simple, "poor man's" version of urodynamic tests, which can supplement the basic history and physical examination, is called "bedside" or "eyeball" urodynamics. This simple test has been found to be quite reliable as a screening tool to detect gross abnormalities contributing to incontinence.[3,5,56] The patient is placed in the supine or lithotomy position, a catheter placed in the bladder, and a catheter-tip syringe attached to the end of the catheter. The bladder is slowly filled with room temperature saline or water in fixed increments of about 50 mL. The volumes at which the various sensations of filling occur are noted. In addition, the rate at which the syringe empties is observed as is any reversal of the process that may indicate an involuntary bladder contraction. If bladder filling occurs relatively slowly, it can be concluded that the bladder capacity is either quite small or that the bladder has a low compliance. When capacity is reached, the catheter is removed and the patient is asked to perform a number of stress maneuvers to provoke incontinence. The patient can then void, and, because the volume infused is known, the amount of residual urine can be checked quite accurately if the bladder was emptied prior to the test.

## THE URODYNAMIC CLASSIFICATION OF INCONTINENCE

In the first part of this chapter, emphasis was placed on the importance of a thorough history and careful, directed physical examination to provide the basis for initial therapy or urodynamic evaluation for incontinence. The findings from urodynamics testing provide a urodynamic diagnosis, allowing an accurate classification of the patient's lower urinary tract dysfunction. Such a urodynamic classification can then guide therapy more precisely than when the therapy is guided by the history and physical examination alone.

Table 6 presents a classification scheme of lower urinary tract dysfunction based on urodynamic evaluation.[19] The system makes it possible to classify the urodynamic cause of any lower urinary tract dysfunction, including incontinence, and thus permit the selection of the most appropriate therapeutic options. As pointed out earlier, however, to be valid and useful the urodynamic evaluation must replicate as thoroughly as possible the patient's complaints so that the final urodynamic diagnosis correlates as closely as possible with the patient's signs and symptoms.

The urodynamic classification of lower urinary tract dysfunction shown in Table 6 divides the lower urinary tract into its three main components: the bladder, urethra, and sensation. The three components may have

**TABLE 6. Urodynamic Classification of Lower Urinary Tract Dysfunction†**

| Component | Activity | Dysfunction | Most Common Causes |
|---|---|---|---|
| Bladder | *Overactivity | Detrusor instability | Idiopathic<br>Infection<br>Foreign body<br>Obstruction |
| | | Detrusor hyperreflexia | Neurologic |
| | | Low compliance | Neurologic injury<br>Obstruction<br>Fibrosis |
| | **Underactivity (Absolute or relative) | Acontractility | Myogenic<br>Medications |
| | | Areflexia | Neurologic |
| Urethra | **Overactivity | Anatomic/Mechanical | BPH<br>Stricture<br>Bladder neck contracture |
| | | Dyssynergia | Neurologic |
| | *Underactivity | Total | Injury |
| | | Anatomic | Poor support |
| Sensation | Overactivity | | Infection<br>Tumor<br>Foreign body<br>Interstitial cystitis |
| | Underactivity | | Neurologic, psychogenic |

† Combinations of dysfunction are possible, eg, overactivity during filling but underactivity with voiding. The most common causes of incontinence are bladder overactivity and urethral underactivity.

* Applies to the period of bladder filling/storage.

** Applies to the period of bladder voiding.

From Abrams et al.[19]

a urodynamic description of normal, overactive, or underactive. Ranges of normal for each of the three lower urinary tract components have been discussed in the preceding sections. An overactive detrusor or underactive urethra during bladder filling are the most important abnormalities related to incontinence.

### Detrusor Function and Incontinence

Detrusor function becomes overactive when the detrusor is in a high-pressure state due to low bladder compliance or to detrusor instability/hyperreflexia. Low bladder compliance occurs commonly in a variety of neuropathic diseases such as spina bifida, spinal cord injury, and pelvic surgery. It may also result from bladder wall fibrosis due to longstanding catheter use or extensive infection, radiation, urethral obstruction, or bladder surgery; in addition many cases are idiopathic.[43] DH results from neurologic injury or dysfunction, while DI can be associated with stress incontinence, infection, inflammation, foreign bodies, stones, cancer, urethral obstruction, urinary retention, and high fluid output states such as diabetes or high fluid intake.[9] Many cases of DI are idiopathic.[40]

An absolutely underactive detrusor during voiding describes a low-pressure bladder state in which the bladder is either acontractile or areflexic. Causes of an acontractile bladder include myogenic decompensation (as after longstanding obstruction), medications, and psychogenic or idiopathic causes. An areflexic bladder results from neurologic injury or disease. A detrusor may also be relatively underactive; such a detrusor generates voiding contractions, but these contractions are of extremely low pressure and short duration and are thus ineffective in emptying efficiently, even in the face of appropriately low urethral resistance during voiding. The relatively underactive detrusor during voiding has no clear, quantitative ICS definition.[19,23,36,60]

The most common cause for incontinence resulting from abnormal detrusor function is overactivity—high-pressure storage from low compliance or DH/DI. In these instances the bladder pressure rises enough to overcome the closure resistance of the urethra and leakage occurs. In rarer instances, incontinence may occur with an underactive bladder with relatively low storage pressures; in these cases the volume present within the bladder is sufficient to open the urethra and bladder neck and cause overflow incontinence.

### Urethral Function and Incontinence

As with the detrusor, abnormal urethral function can be overactive or underactive. When overactive, the urethra is obstructive. Obstruction can be anatomic/mechanical at any point along the urethra, from the bladder neck to the urethral meatus. Such obstructions can be relatively static, taking the form of bladder neck contractures, urethral strictures, tumors, stones, or BPH.

A dynamic type of overactive urethral function, known as dyssynergia, results in an inappropriate level of striated or smooth muscle sphincteric activity in the presence of a detrusor contraction. Striated muscle dyssynergia—classic DSD—occurs with significant neurologic injuries and diseases between the conus medullaris and pons, especially spinal cord injury and multiple sclerosis.[19,70,71,75,76] A similar EMG and detrusor pressure pattern is found in dysfunctional voiders who have no neurologic dysfunction but instead have a "learned" incoordination of bladder and urethra; patients with the non-neurogenic neurogenic bladder provide excellent examples (see following section).[72–74] As there is no neurologic deficit, this type of dysfunction is not a true dyssynergia, though the overactivity is certainly dynamic.

Smooth muscle dyssynergia is a less well-understood phenomenon. It can occur in patients with neurologic dysfunction such as spinal cord injury above T-6. Detrusor/bladder neck dyssynergia, another variation of dysfunctional voiding, occurs in men and occasionally in women. These patients do not have neurologic disease or notable EMG abnormality, but rather have inadequate opening of the proximal urethra and bladder neck while voiding, and as a result have complaints of obstruction similar to those in an older man with BPH.[18,58,59,61–63]

The underactive urethra is incompetent—ie, it is incapable of performing its normal function of maintaining continence. Such a deficit results from anatomic abnormalities, and may produce genuine stress urinary incontinence of all types. The causes of Types I and II GSUI are not completely understood, but age, parity, and tissue atrophy contribute to changes in the normal anatomy. Total urethral incompetence is present in patients with Type III stress urinary incontinence. It results from direct injury to the urethra through surgery, dilations, or accidental trauma, or through neurologic injury in which the appropriate neurological input to the urethra—autonomic, somatic, or both—is no longer present.[14]

Incontinence associated with urethral dysfunction occurs most often as a result of underactivity. However, incontinence can occur with an overactive urethra; overactivity is usually concurrent with DH or DI due to obstruction with BPH, or to DSD.

### Sensory Function and Incontinence

Underactive sensory function is usually the result of specific neurologic lesions such as spinal cord injury, or more general problems such as diabetes mellitus or syphilis. Psychologic abnormalities may yield a urodynamic diagnosis of an underactive sensory mechanism in unusual circumstances.

An overactive sensory mechanism is usually caused by direct injury or insult to the bladder or urethra by such processes as infections, neoplasms, neurologic disease, foreign bodies, inflammatory processes, and interstitial cystitis. Psychologic abnormalities may also produce an overactive sensory perception. Sensory instability has an idiopathic cause and shows sensory overactivity.

Underactive sensory dysfunction can lead to overflow incontinence. Overactive sensation levels cause incontinence because of the inability to hold urine as a result of the associated discomfort.

## NEUROPATHIC BLADDER, INCONTINENCE, AND THE URODYNAMIC EVALUATION

Incontinence is one of the ways that neurologic injury or disease can manifest in the lower urinary tract. The urodynamic evaluation is often essential in delineating the cause of such incontinence as well as in guiding therapy and monitoring the therapeutic success.

In considering neurologic lower urinary tract dysfunction, whether incontinence is present or not, the most significant point to remember is that detrusor overactivity—high-pressure detrusor dysfunction from low compliance or DH, especially with DSD—can cause significant bladder dysfunction, and ultimately renal damage. Perhaps the greatest source of confusion, resulting in the neglect of the importance of high-pressure bladder dysfunction, is that lower spinal cord lesions are often areflexic and therefore assumed to have no long-term clinical significance. This assumption is clearly erroneous, however, as although a bladder may not demonstrate phasic pressure change to empty, the pressure can still change because of low compliance; it is this low compliance that can be so devastating to the kidneys. Likewise, the presence of high-pressure DH with DSD can have serious adverse effects upon the upper urinary tract. The significance of high bladder pressure is characterized best by the leak point pressure introduced in the section covering urodynamic evaluations.[41–45]

From the clinical standpoint, incontinence does not mean that there is a urethral "pop-off valve" guaranteeing that the upper urinary tract is going to be normal. At high leak-point pressures the risk to the kidneys is significant, and increasing the competence of the urethra to produce continence would only worsen the problem. In a patient with true urethral incompetence, simply increasing the urethral closure capability may trade one problem for another, as it is possible that the new urethral competence will allow the true high-pressure potential of the bladder to manifest. In this situation, the urodynamic evaluation must be conducted by occluding the bladder outlet to allow filling. This technique helps predict the effects of restoring urethral competence, thus preventing complications or anticipating them appropriately.

## Central Nervous System Disease

There are several major types of injury or disease affecting the central nervous system which can have a dramatic effect on the lower urinary tract, and which are thus of significance to the urologist: cerebrovascular accidents, Parkinson's disease, spinal cord injury, myelomeningocele, and multiple sclerosis. Each process involves neurologic abnormalities at different points in the central nervous system, so the effects upon the lower urinary tract differ.

**Cerebrovascular Accidents.** Initially after a cerebrovascular accident, a patient often develops urinary retention. Over several months, the lower urinary tract settles into an unpredictable, possibly dysfunctional, pattern, from which it later does not vary much. The most frequent abnormality is an overactive bladder (DH) with a normally active (competent) urethra, and normal sensation. If the DH exceeds the urethral competence, incontinence will result. An EMG in association with hyperreflexia will appear to indicate DSD; DSD is not present, however, as the increased EMG activity reflects the patient's voluntary attempt to close the urethra to suppress the contraction and not leak. Voiding function is essentially unchanged from the status before the accident.

A variation of this dysfunction is that the bladder, urethral, and sensory functions are as described above, but dementia has reduced the capability to appropriately perceive and respond to stimuli. This finding will usually be evident from the history, and urodynamic evaluation will only provide confirmation rather than add unique data.

Many patients who suffer a cerebrovascular accident will have other common types of lower urinary tract dysfunction present even before the accident, such as outlet obstruction from BPH, or simple stress incontinence. In such cases, the urodynamic evaluation must be tailored carefully to account for these possibilities, allowing the clinician to reach the proper diagnosis.

**Parkinson's Disease.** Up to 75% of patients with Parkinson's disease develop lower urinary tract dysfunction, which may include incontinence. Detrusor overactivity (DH) is present in up to 90% of such patients with dysfunction. Many patients have an underactive detrusor during voiding (poorly sustained detrusor contractions), and, in parallel with the remainder of the skeletal muscle system, a relative rigidity and dyskinesia in the urethral sphincter (urethral over- and underactivity). Sensation is normal.[78,79]

A careful urodynamic evaluation is quite valuable in the presence of combined abnormal bladder and urethral function, especially in men who may also have a bladder outlet obstruction from BPH. If the urodynamic evaluation with the pressure/flow study shows obstruction which may contribute to some of the involuntary bladder contractions, the wisdom of relief of the obstruction is not clear unless the characteristics of the sphincter are taken into account. The major complication of inappropriate transurethral resection of the prostate (TURP) in a male with Parkinson's disease is incontinence. Up to 83% of patients who have inadequate voluntary sphincter control or dyskinesia, as revealed by urodynamic evaluation with pressure/flow studies and EMG, will have incontinence after prostatectomy as compared with only 4% of patients who have proper voluntary sphincter control.[80] Obviously, a properly performed urodynamic evaluation is vital to the proper management of the patient with Parkinson's disease.

**Spinal Cord Lesions.** Spinal cord injury at any level can lead to bladder, urethral, or sensory dysfunction. While some generalizations can be made about the dysfunctions relative to level of injury, these assumptions should always be confirmed by urodynamic evaluation since treatment based upon wrong assumptions can be very damaging.[43,70,74]

With a complete cord lesion the sensory component is eliminated. With an incomplete lesion the degree of sensory underactivity can be variable.

For injuries above the sacral reflex arc, that is, above the conus medullaris, the bladder usually displays a high-pressure dysfunction (DH and sometimes low compliance), though low-pressure dysfunction (detrusor areflexia) can also occur. For injuries involving the sacral reflex arc at any point, a low-pressure dysfunction has usually been the assumed abnormality. However, high-pressure dysfunction abnormalities are common, especially those involving low bladder compliance. This type of abnormality can be devastating in patients in whom a relatively benign condition is assumed to exist, but in whom a life-threatening lower urinary tract dysfunction is actually present.

After spinal cord injury, urethral function is usually fixed. With an injury above the sacral reflex arc, the urethra is usually overactive (detrusor sphincter dyssynergia). The smooth portion of the sphincter functions normally, unless the injury is above T6, in which case it is possible that smooth sphincter dyssynergia can also be present. For injuries at the level of the conus medullaris and below, the smooth and striated sphincters are usually competent but maintain a fixed, non-relaxing tone.

Leak-point pressure and DSD are significant with spinal cord injuries, as they demonstrate the balance between bladder storage pressures and urethral competence. High urethral competence may lead to continence, but also to renal compromise if the bladder storage pressures are high.[41–45]

**Myelomeningocele.** Patients with myelomeningocele or myelodysplasia can exhibit the same abnormalities that may be present in patients with spinal cord injury. The variety and nature of the defects requires that a urodynamic evaluation be performed to specify the sensory, urethral, and bladder abnormalities present, including those contributing to incontinence. The evaluation is essential to establish the leak-point pressure.

**Multiple Sclerosis.** Lower urinary tract dysfunction is a presenting symptom in as many as 10% of patients with multiple sclerosis (MS). With disease progression, up to 80% of patients will have some type of lower urinary tract dysfunction.[10,11,81]

Sensory function is usually normal. The bladder dysfunction is caused by high pressure (DH) in up to 90% of patients. Low-pressure dysfunction (areflexia) also exists, but may change into DH at a later point of the disease process.[82–85]

Urethral function is usually intact, though overactivity (DSD) is reported in up to 65% of patients with detrusor hyperreflexia.[82–85] Care must be taken during the urodynamic evaluation to confirm that the diagnosis of DSD is accurate, since many patients will feel the involuntary contraction of hyperreflexia, and attempt to suppress this in a normal fashion.

The urodynamic evaluation is essential in patients with MS to clearly delineate the type of problem, to optimize care, and to clarify which patients are at high risk for damage of the upper urinary tracts because of sustained high bladder pressures.[10,11,81] Empiric treatment is successful in fewer than half of MS patients, while treatment guided by urodynamic evaluation is correct in more than 80% of such patients. For example, in MS patients with obstructive voiding symptoms, about 70% will have detrusor areflexia rather than true urethral overactivity and obstruction. Also, only about 60% of patients with urgency, frequency, and urge incontinence actually prove to have detrusor overactivity (hyperreflexia); the remainder may have obstruction or sensory overactivity.[10,11] Some patients will have an incompetent sphincter due to urethral instability, and thus are incontinent due to urethral dysfunction rather than bladder dysfunction.

## PERIPHERAL NERVOUS SYSTEM DISEASE

A number of diseases can cause a range of lower urinary tract dysfunction by affecting the peripheral nervous system. Among the most common diseases in this category are diabetes mellitus, syphilis, pernicious anemia, disc disease, and radical pelvic surgery.

### Diabetes Mellitus, Syphilis, Pernicious Anemia

Diabetes mellitus affects the lower urinary tract by causing abnormalities to autonomic and peripheral nerves. The primary dysfunction is one of sensory underactivity. It is believed that a slow process occurs in which the bladder is progressively allowed to fill beyond its normal capacity, eventually compromising the detrusor's capacity to appropriately contract, and making it underactive (acontractile). Urethral function is usually unaffected. During a voiding study, the bladder does not generate adequate detrusor contraction and the flow rate is low and increases only with abdominal straining. When present, incontinence is of the overflow type. Syphilis and pernicious anemia cause a similar syndrome.[74,86–89]

### Disc Disease

Prolapsed discs can affect lower urinary tract function. Sensation is usually normal, and the detrusor usually has low-pressure dysfunction (areflexia) resulting in urinary retention; however, high-pressure dysfunction from low compliance or hyperreflexia can also occur. Urethral function is usually normal but may show some evidence of denervation. The EMG is of particular value in these cases when precise needle techniques are used.[69,88]

### Radical Pelvic Surgery

Lower urinary tract dysfunction can occur after any surgery in the pelvis which may injure the pelvic nerves or the plexuses serving the bladder and urethra. Radical hysterectomy and abdomino-perineal resection are the two surgical procedures that pose the greatest threats to normal lower urinary tract function. The urodynamic evaluation is essential to confirm the diagnosis of the dysfunction present and to guide therapy.

Sensation is normal to underactive. Bladder dysfunction is usually of the overactive type; voluntary voiding is sometimes absent. Urethral dysfunction can be mixed, depending on the location and severity of nerve injury. If the sympathetic nerves are injured then the smooth sphincter is incompetent; the striated sphincter is usually overactive—competent but commonly fixed, and unable to relax appropriately.[74,91–93]

### Imperforate Anus, Sacral Agenesis

The child with an imperforate anus develops lower urinary tract dysfunction that is related to the level of the original defect, the associated corrective surgeries, and the presence of commonly associated vertebral defects. With sacral agenesis, the neurologic and lower urinary tract changes associated with the bony defect can range from subtle to severe. A urodynamic evaluation is necessary in these situations to specify the lower urinary tract dysfunction present as accurate prediction is impossible.[74,94]

## DYSFUNCTIONAL VOIDING (NON-NEUROGENIC/ NEUROGENIC BLADDER)

The non-neurogenic/neurogenic bladder, sometimes called the Hinman Syndrome, is a voiding dysfunction most often present in children.[72–74] It occurs as a consequence of a dysfunctional voiding pattern characterized by an overactive urethra, and produces an EMG signal increase during the voiding process. It is a learned behavior, and thus can be unlearned, correcting the urodynamic abnormality and resolving the associated symptoms, including incontinence.

Sensation is normal. Detrusor abnormalities can include overactivity (detrusor instability and low compliance). In some patients in whom the process has been longstanding, the detrusor may be underactive (acontractile) due to myogenic decompensation. The urethral function is usually overactive, and displays an obstructive pattern similar to DSD; however, it is separable from true dyssynergia by careful examination of the EMG/detrusor pressure patterns and the absence of objective neurologic abnormality, hence the name.[72–74]

## SUMMARY

The appropriate and successful evaluation of incontinence requires a thorough, systematic approach built on the history, physical examination, and basic tests, to yield a symptomatic classification of incontinence. Urodynamic tests are used in specific instances, including when the core evaluation does not yield an adequate or accurate diagnosis. Urodynamic tests allow urodynamic classification of the lower urinary tract dysfunction causing the incontinence, a step which is particularly valuable in patients with incontinence of complex etiology such as that associated with neurologic incontinence and lower urinary tract dysfunction.

## REFERENCES

1. Rowe JW, et al. Urinary incontinence in adults. *JAMA*. 1989;261:2685–2690.
2. Resnick NM. Urinary incontinence in the elderly. *Hosp Pract*. 1986;21:80C–80Z.
3. Bavendam TG. Geriatric female incontinence. *Probl Urol*. 1991;5:42–71.
4. Bruskewitz R. Female incontinence: signs and symptoms. In: Raz S, ed. *Female Urology*. Philadelphia: WB Saunders Co; 1983:chap 4.
5. DeBeau CE, Resnick NM. Evaluation of the causes and severity of geriatric incontinence. *Urol Clin North Am*. 1991;18:243–256.
6. Abrams P, Feneley R, Torrens M. *Urodynamics*. New York: Springer-Verlag, Berlin Heidelberg; 1983.
7. Burgio KL, Engel BT, Locher JL. Normative patterns of diurnal urination across 6 age decades. *J Urol*. 1991;145:728–731.
8. McGuire EJ, Savastano JA. Stress incontinence and detrusor instability/urge incontinence. *Neurourol Urodyn*. 1985;4:313–316.
9. McGuire E. Bladder instability and stress incontinence. *Neurourol Urodyn*. 1988;7:563–568.
10. Blaivas JG, Bhimani G, Labib KB. Vesicourethral dysfunction in multiple sclerosis. *J Urol*. 1979;122:342–347.
11. Blaivas JG. Management of bladder dysfunction in multiple sclerosis. *Neurology*. 1980;30:12–18.
12. Snyder JA, Lipsitz DU. Evaluation of female urinary incontinence. *Urol Clin North Am*. 1991;18:197–209.
13. Snyder JA, Westmacott R. Treatment of mild, moderate, and severe cystoceles. *Probl Urol*. 1991;5:85–93.
14. Blaivas JG, Olsson CA. Stress incontinence: classification and surgical approach. *J Urol*. 1988;139:727–731.
15. Walters MD, Shields LE. The diagnostic value of history, physical examination, and the Q-tip cotton swab test in women with urinary incontinence. *Am J Obstet Gynecol*. 1988;159:145–149.
16. Blaivas JG, Zayed AAH, Labib KB. The bulbocavernosus reflex in urology: a prospective study of 299 patients. *J Urol*. 1981;126:197–199.
17. O'Donnell P. Water endoscopy. In: Raz S, ed. *Female Urology*. Philadelphia: WB Saunders Co; 1983:51–68.
18. Axelrod SL, Blaivas JG. Bladder neck obstruction in women. *J Urol*. 1987;137:179–181.
19. Abrams P, Blaivas JG, Stanton SL, Andersen JT. Standardization of terminology of lower urinary tract function. *Neurourol Urodyn*. 1988;7:403–427.
20. Labasky RF. Urodynamics. In: Smith JA, ed. *High-Tech Urology*. Philadelphia: WB Saunders Co. In press.
21. O'Donnell PD. Pitfalls of urodynamic testing. *Urol Clin North Am*. 1991;18:257–269.
22. Siroky MG. Interpretation of urinary flow rates. *Urol Clin North Am*. 1990;17:537–542.
23. Blaivas JG. Multichannel urodynamic studies in men with benign prostatic hyperplasia. *Urol Clin North Am*. 1990;17:543–552.
24. Siroky MG, Olsson CA, Krane RJ. The flow rate nomogram, I: development. *J Urol*. 1979; 122:665–668.
25. Siroky MB, Olsson CA, Krane RJ. The flow rate nomogram, II: clinical correlation. *J Urol*. 1980;123:208–210.
26. Toguri AG, Uchida T, Bee DE. Pediatric uroflow rate nomograms. *J Urol*. 1982;127:727–731.
27. Toguri AG, Bee DE, Uchida T. Normal pediatric uroflow rates in nonclinical setting. *J Urol*. 1982;127:732–735.
28. Drach GW, Ignatoff J, Layton T. Peak urinary flow rate: observations in female subjects and comparison to male subjects. *J Urol*. 1979; 122:215–219.
29. Drach GW, Layton T, Bottaccini MR. A method of adjustment of male peak urinary flow rate for varying age and volume voided. *J Urol*. 1982;128:960–962.

30. Drach GW, Steinbronn DV. Clinical evaluation of patients with prostatic obstruction: correlation of flow rates with voided, residual or total bladder volume. *J Urol.* 1986;135:737–740.

31. Gierup J. Micturition studies in infants and children: normal urinary flow. *Scand J Urol Nephrol.* 1970;4:191–208.

32. Gierup J. Micturition studies in infants and children: intravesical pressure, urinary flow and urethral resistance in boys without infravesical obstruction. *Scand J Urol Nephrol.* 1970;4:217–230.

33. Gierup J, Ericsson NO. Micturition studies in infants and children: urodynamics in boys with disorders of the lower urinary tract. *Scand J Urol Nephrol.* 1971;5:1–16.

34. Hjalmas K. Micturition in infants and children with normal lower urinary tract. *Scand J Urol Nephrol.* 1976;37(suppl):1–106.

35. Haylen BT, Ashby D, Sutherest JR, Frazer MI, West CR. Maximum and average urine flow rates in normal male and female populations—the Liverpool nomograms. *Br J Urol.* 1989;64:30–38.

36. Chancellor MB, Blaivas JG, Kaplan SA, Axelrod S. Bladder outlet obstruction versus impaired detrusor contractility: the role of uroflow. *J Urol.* 1991;145:810–812.

37. Aagaard J, Bruskewitz R. Are urodynamic studies useful in the evaluation of female incontinence? *Probl Urol.* 1991;5:11–22.

38. Jorgensen L, Lose G, Andersen JT. Cystometry: $H_2O$ or $CO_2$ filling medium? A literature survey of the influence of the filling medium on the qualitative and quantitative cystometric parameters. *Neurourol Urodyn.* 1988;7:343–350.

39. Berger RM, Maizels M, Moran GC, Conway JJ, Firlit CF. Bladder capacity (ounces) equals age (years) plus 2 predicts normal bladder capacity and aids in diagnosis of abnormal voiding patterns. *J Urol.* 1983;129:347–349.

40. Coolsaet BLRA, Elhilali MM. Detrusor overactivity. *Neurourol Urodyn.* 1988;7:541–561.

41. Bauer SB, Hallett M, Khoshbin S, et al. Predictive value of urodynamic evaluation in newborns with myelodysplasia. *JAMA.* 1984; 252:650.

42. Galloway NTM, Mekras JA, Helms M, Webster GD. An objective score to predict upper tract deterioration in myelodysplasia. *J Urol.* 1991;145:535–537.

43. Labasky RF, Leach GE. Spinal cord injury and sacral arc denervation in the female. *Probl Urol.* 1991;5:155–170.

44. McGuire EJ, Woodside JR, Borden TA, Weiss RM. Prognostic value of urodynamic testing in myelodysplastic patients. *J Urol.* 1981;126:205–209.

45. Hackler RH, Hall MK, Zampieri TA. Bladder hypocompliance in the spinal cord injury population. *J Urol.* 1989;141:1390–1393.

46. Constantinou CE. Urethrometry: considerations of static, dynamic, and stability characteristics of the female urethra. *Neurourol Urodyn.* 1988;7:521–539.

47. Tapp AJS, Cardozo LD, Versi E, Studd JWW. The prevalence of variation of resting urethral pressure in women and its association with lower urinary tract function. *Br J Urol.* 1988;61:314–317.

48. McGuire EJ, Lytton B, Kohorn EI, Pepe V. The value of urodynamic testing in stress urinary incontinence. *J Urol.* 1980;124:256–258.

49. Jarvis GJ, Hall S, Stamp S, Millar DR, Johnson A. An assessment of urodynamic examination in incontinent women. *Br J Obstet Gynaecol.* 1980;87:893–896.

50. Cadogan M, Awad S, Field C, Acker K, Middleton S. A comparison of the cough and standing urethral pressure profile in the diagnosis of stress incontinence. *Neurourol Urodyn.* 1988; 7:327–341.

51. Cardozo LD, Stanton SL. Genuine stress incontinence and detrusor instability—a review of 200 patients. *Br J Obstet Gynecol.* 1980;87:184–190.

52. Castleden CM, Duffin HM, Asher MJ. Clinical and urodynamic studies in 100 elderly incontinent patients. *Br J Urol.* 1981;282:1103–1105.

53. Farrar DJ, Whiteside CG, Osborne JL, Turner-Warwick RT. A urodynamic analysis of micturition symptoms in the female. *Surg Gynecol Obstet.* 1975;141:875–881.

54. Friis E, Hjortrup A, Nielsen JER, Sanders S, Walter S. Urinary incontinence and genital prolapse: a prospective blind study of the value of urodynamic evaluation. *J Urol.* 1982;128:764–765.

55. Ouslander J, Staskin D, Raz S, Su HL, Hepps K. Clinical versus urodynamic diagnosis in an incontinent geriatric female population. *J Urol.* 1987;137:68–71.

56. Ouslander J, Leach G, Abelson S, et al. Simple versus multichannel cystometry in the evaluation of bladder function in an incontinent geriatric population. *J Urol.* 1988;140:1482–1486.

57. Sand PK, Hill RC, Ostergard DR. Incontinence history as a predictor of detrusor instability. *Obstet Gynecol.* 1988;71:257–260.

58. Norlen LJ, Blaivas JG. Unsuspected proximal urethral obstruction in young and middle-aged men. *J Urol.* 1986;135:972–976.

59. Webster GD, Lockhart JL, Older RA. The evaluation of bladder neck dysfunction. *J Urol.* 1980;123:196–198.

60. Schafer W. Principles and clinical application of advanced urodynamic analysis of voiding function. *Urol Clin North Am.* 1990;17:553–566.

61. Sheldon LA, Blaivas JG. Bladder neck obstruction in women. *J Urol.* 1987;137:179–181.

62. Mayo ME. Primary bladder neck obstruction in men: variation in detrusor response. *J Urol.* 1982;128:957–959.
63. Siroky MB, Goldstein L, Krane RJ. Functional voiding disorders in men. *J Urol.* 1981;126:200–204.
64. Dibenedetto M, Yalla SV. Electrodiagnosis of striated urethral sphincter dysfunction. *J Urol.* 1979;122:361–365.
65. Blaivas JG. Electromyography: other uses. In: Barrett DM, Wein AJ, eds. *Controversies in Neuro-Urology.* New York: Churchill Livingtone; 1984:chap 3C.
66. Barrett DM. Electromyography: the practical approach. In: Barrett DM, Wein AJ, eds. *Controversies in Neuro-Urology.* New York: Churchill Livingtone; 1984:chap 3A.
67. Siroky MG. Electromyography: needle. In: Barrett DM, Wein AJ, eds. *Controversies in Neuro-Urology.* New York: Churchill Livingtone; 1984:chap 3B.
68. Blaivas JG. A critical appraisal of specific diagnostic techniques. In: Krane RJ, Siroky MB, eds. *Clinical Neuro-Urology.* Boston: Little, Brown and Company; 1979:chap 5.
69. Siroky MB, Sax DS, Krane RJ. Sacral signal tracing: the electrophysiology of the bulbocavernosus reflex. *J Urol.* 1979; 122:661–664.
70. Blaivas JG. The neurophysiology of micturition: a clinical study of 550 patients. *J Urol.* 1982; 127:958–963.
71. Wein A, Barrett DM. Etiologic possibilities for increased pelvic floor electromyography activity during cystometry. *J Urol.* 1982;127:949–953.
72. Hinman F Jr. Nonneurogenic neurogenic bladder (the Hinman syndrome)—15 years later. *J Urol.* 1986;136:769–777.
73. Rudy DC, Woodside JR. Non-neurogenic neurogenic bladder: the relationship between intravesical pressure and the external sphincter electromyogram. *Neurourol Urodyn.* 1991; 10:169–176.
74. Barrett DM, Wein AJ. Voiding dysfunction: diagnosis, classification, and management. In: Gillenwater JY, Grayhack JT, Howards SS, Duckett JW, eds. *Adult and Pediatric Urology.* Chicago: Year Book Medical Publishers Inc; 1987:chap 28.
75. Blaivas JG, Sinha HP, Zayed AAH, Labib KB. Detrusor-external sphincter dyssynergia. *J Urol.* 1981;125:542–544.
76. Blaivas JG, Sinha HP, Zayed AAH, Labib KB. Detrusor-external sphincter dyssynergia: a detailed electromyographic study. *J Urol.* 1981;125:545–548.
77. Koff SA. Evaluation and management of voiding disorders in children. *Urol Clin North Am.* 1988;15:769–775.
78. Berger Y, Blaivas JG, DeLaRocha ER, Salinas JM. Urodynamic findings in Parkinson's disease. *J Urol.* 1987;138:836–838.
79. Pavlakis AJ, Siroky MG, Goldstein I, Krane RJ. Neurologic findings in Parkinson's disease. *J Urol.* 1983;129:80–83.
80. Staskin DS, Vardi Y, Siroky MB. Post-prostatectomy continence in the parkinsonian patient: the significance of poor voluntary sphincter control. *J Urol.* 1988;140:117–118.
81. McGuire EJ, Savastano JA. Urodynamic findings and long-term outcome management of patients with multiple sclerosis-induced lower urinary tract dysfunction. *J Urol.* 1984;132:713–715.
82. Wheeler JS Jr, Siroky MB, Pavlakis J, Goldstein I, Krane RJ. The changing neurologic pattern of multiple sclerosis. *J Urol.* 1983;130:1123–1126.
83. Schoenberg HW, Gutrich J, Banno J. Urodynamic patterns in multiple sclerosis. *J Urol.* 1979;122:648–650.
84. Philp T, Read DJ, Higson RH. The urodynamic characteristics of multiple sclerosis. *Br J Urol.* 1981;53:672–675.
85. Awad SA, Gajewski JB, Sogbein SK, Murray TJ, Field CA. Relationship between neurological and urological status in patients with multiple sclerosis. *J Urol.* 1984;132:499–502.
86. Wheeler JS Jr, Culkin DJ, O'Hara RJ, Canning JR. Bladder dysfunction and neurosyphilis. *J Urol.* 1986;136:903–905.
87. Frimodt-Moller C. Diabetes cystopathy, I: a clinical study on the frequency of bladder dysfunction in diabetes. *Danish Med Bull.* 1976;23:267–278.
88. Frimodt-Moller C. Diabetes cystopathy, II: relationship to some late diabetic manifestations. *Danish Med Bull.* 1976;23:279–294.
89. Kaplan SA, Blaivas JG. Diabetic cystopathy. *J Diabetic Complications.* 1988;2:133–139.
90. Sandri SD, Fanciullacci F, Politi P, Zanollo A. Urinary disorders in intervertebral disc prolapse. *Neurourol Urodyn.* 1987;6:11–19.
91. Blaivas JG, Barbalias GA. Characteristics of neural injury after abdominoperineal resection. *J Urol.* 1983;129:84–87.
92. Kadar N. Permanent retention following radical hysterectomy. *Neurourol Urodyn.* 1989;8:11–16.
93. Woodside JR, McGuire EJ. Detrusor hypertonicity as a late complication of a Wertheim hysterectomy. *J Urol.* 1982;127:1143–1145.
94. Koff SA, Deridder PA. Patterns of neurogenic bladder dysfunction in sacral agenesis. *J Urol.* 1977;118:87–89.

# 18

# Management of Urinary Incontinence

*Larry T. Sirls, K. Ganabathi, Philippe E. Zimmern, and Gary E. Leach*

## INTRODUCTION

It is estimated that incontinence-related health care costs exceed $10 billion per year in the U.S. Over 60% of the money spent is for *disposable* products such as diapers or laundry costs.[1] An estimated 10–12 million Americans have urinary incontinence, and one survey suggested that less than 10% of incontinent patients seek professional help. Of those seeking help, more than 50% reported no useful assistance from the consultation.[2] Heightened public awareness and education, coupled with effective management of presenting patients, can both satisfy an underserved population and save the health care system valuable resources. Nearly all patients who present to the urologist for help with incontinence can be greatly improved or cured. Of course, this is dependent on the etiology of the leakage and patient motivation and compliance to recommended therapies. This latter issue, patient motivation and compliance, cannot be emphasized enough and is a prominent factor in formulating the ultimate treatment plan. Each patient must be assessed physiologically and socially, often incorporating family support potential with self-care issues, eg, can and will the patient perform self-catheterization if required? Of great import is a clear understanding at the onset of treatment by the patient of what to expect during therapy. It is imperative that even in the busiest practice the urologist take the time to explain in detail the results of pretherapy evaluation, the management and its possible complications, as well as possible associated requirements such as self-catheterization. The majority of patients who present for evaluation and treatment have chosen to attack this problem and will comply when educated and guided.

History and physical examination (including a focused neurologic exam) are critical in initial assessment and characterization of the type of incontinence. Past surgical history such as failed bladder neck suspension or prior prostatectomy (open or transurethral) is obtained. In addition to documented neurologic history, the presence of neurologic symptoms should be taken seriously, as a number of patients with as of yet undiagnosed neurologic disease may present first to the urologist with voiding dysfunction.[3] Associated patterns including the timing of incontinence (day, night, total) and presence or absence of physical activity (stress, movement, spontaneous) are obtained. Other pertinent history such as stones, bladder malignancy, and cystitis are obtained. From this information one can *preliminarily* classify the type of incontinence and determine what further radiologic or urodynamic evalua-

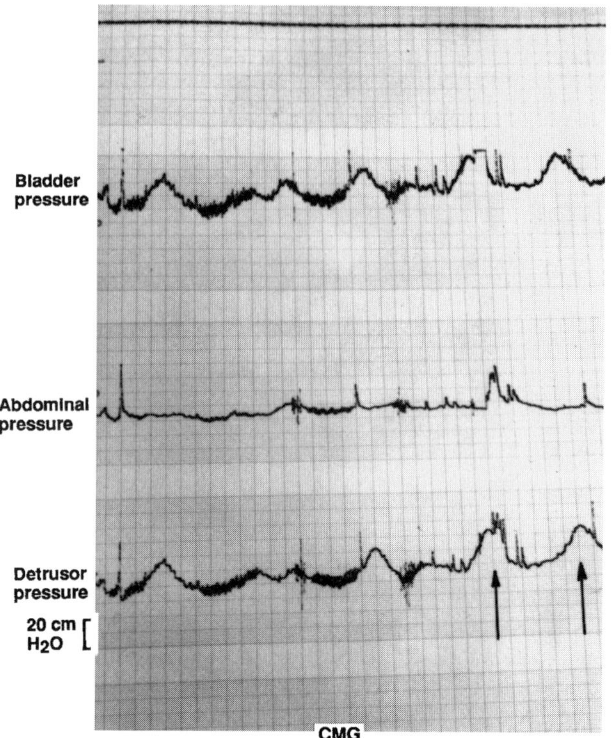


**Fig 1.** Urodynamic tracing demonstrating uninhibited bladder contraction typical of either detrusor hyperreflexia or detrusor instability. The arrows mark two of the many uninhibited contractions.

tion is needed. Caution should be exercised when definitively classifying a type of incontinence based on clinical evaluation alone as it will be misleading in nearly 50% of cases.[4,5]

## NOMENCLATURE

Any involuntary loss of urine by the patient is defined as incontinence. Further terms used to characterize urinary incontinence are descriptive and based on the symptoms relayed by the patient. *Total incontinence* is when the patient is wet at all times, day and night, regardless of stress or positional change. *Urge incontinence* is when the patient has the urge to urinate but cannot control urination until a socially acceptable situation presents itself. There are two types of urge incontinence: motor urgency and sensory urgency. Motor urgency is present when the patient has the urge to urinate that is accompanied by a urodynamically documented involuntary bladder contraction. Although involuntary bladder contraction was previously defined urodynamically as an uninhibited detrusor contraction of greater than 15 cm $H_2O$, many agree that lower amplitude uninhibited detrusor contractions associated with the sense of urgency are clinically relevant. Motor urgency from uninhibited detrusor contractions (Fig 1) is termed *detrusor instability* in the patient without known neurologic history or findings and *detrusor hyperreflexia* in the patient with documented neurologic disease. Sensory urgency is when the patient feels a strong urge to urinate but there is no demonstrable detrusor contraction on cystometrogram (CMG). In the authors' experience, sensory urgency rarely causes incontinence (but may cause severe frequency) and should alert the investigator to another potential etiology such as stone, cystitis, bladder tumor, and so on.

*Stress incontinence* is suggested by the loss of urine with activities that produce increases in abdominal pressure such as laughing, coughing, or sneezing, or with positional changes that occur at normal bladder pressures (not associated with a bladder contraction or elevated detrusor pressures). *Overflow incontinence* reflects a bladder that is full to capacity and cannot accommodate more volume, so that further urine production results in frequent, obligatory low-volume urine loss across the outlet. *Functional incontinence* implies a situational incontinence that is not related to the bladder or outlet per se, but instead reflects the patient's immobility or mental incapacitation. A simple example would be an arthritic patient who cannot make it to the toilet and subsequently wets. *Mixed incontinence* is the combination of stress and urge incontinence and is common in both men and women. Critical to proper management is identification and quantification of these separate components and their respective contribution to symptomatology. Examples of mixed incontinence are men after prostatectomy, where one study demonstrated that more than 50% had bladder dysfunction (poor compliance and/or instability) contributing to incontinence,[6] and women with genuine stress incontinence, where up to 60% have symptoms of urgency and urge incontinence suggestive of detrusor instability.

## OVERFLOW INCONTINENCE

Overflow incontinence is the involuntary loss of urine associated with a decompensated bladder that cannot accommodate more volume. It is simply a case of the bladder pressure being greater than outlet resistance with further urine production resulting in an obligatory loss of urine across the outlet. The common denominator is a bladder than cannot empty adequately. Although the condition can be idiopathic, it most commonly is a result of prolonged outlet obstruction or neurogenic bladder dysfunction. The detrusor muscle may be decompensated (myogenic), or may be underactive and unable to sustain a contraction (Fig 2). The detrusor that is acontractile from known neurologic disease is termed *areflexic.*

The patient with overflow incontinence from myogenic decompensation or neurogenic dysfunction needs initial manage-

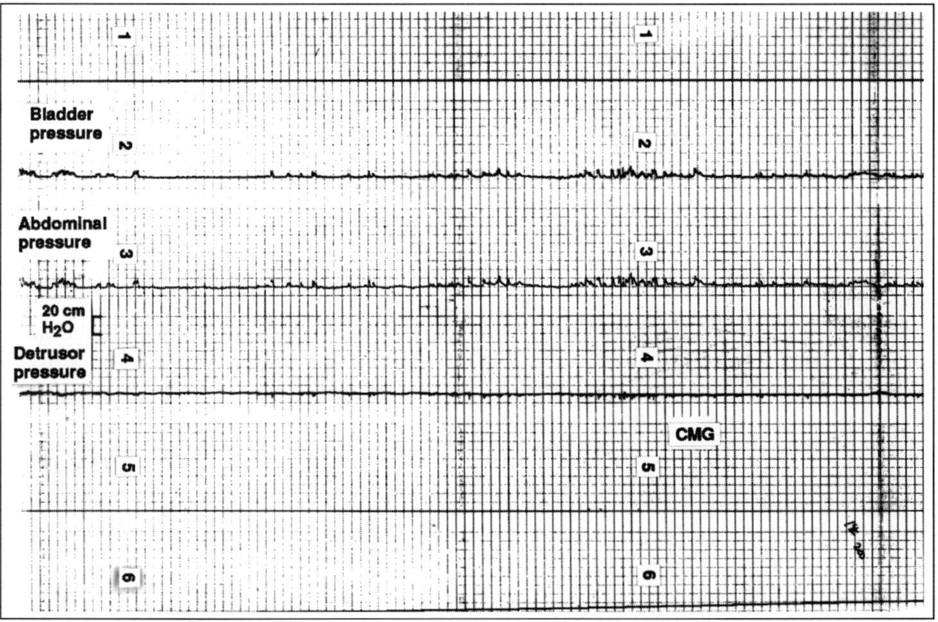


**Fig 2.** Urodynamic tracing of high-capacity, low-pressure bladder, characteristic of an acontractile or myogenically decompensated bladder. Note the absence of detrusor activity, or significant pressure change, up to 800 cm$^3$ volume.

ment with bladder drainage, preferably by clean intermittent catheterization (CIC). It is usually recommended that patients catheterize frequently enough to keep bladder volumes at less than or equal to normal capacity to allow bladder "recompensation." However, a recent study of 1702 patients suggests that catheterization frequency is not an indicator of bladder recovery.[7] These patients had varying etiologies of urinary retention; all were managed with CIC. Although only 13% had spontaneous return of voiding, there was a high percentage of patients with neurologic lesions. Renal function must be assessed acutely in the patient with urinary retention and then monitored for postobstructive diuresis. The authors use renal ultrasound and serum creatinine as initial evaluation of the upper tracts. These baseline studies can be used as a measure of therapeutic success if the upper tracts were adversely affected at presentation.

Patients who do not recover bladder function should remain on CIC and should not be managed with an indwelling urethral catheter. Chronic options for managing those who cannot catheterize (often high spinal cord lesions) or be catheterized include sphincterotomy with an external appliance, suprapubic catheter, or urinary diversion (though these are less desirable). Sphincterotomy may not result in complete bladder emptying; these patients often have continued high postvoid residual urine volumes.[8]

**Treatment of Outflow Obstruction.** Bladder outlet obstruction may be either anatomic or functional. Functional obstruction occurs in men and women, and includes incomplete external (striated) sphincter relaxation (nonneurogenic neurogenic bladder), true vesicosphincter dyssynergia (always of neurologic origin), or psychogenic retention. Management of nonneurogenic neurogenic dysfunction must be individualized but includes bladder retraining, biofeedback, and pharmacotherapy, targeted at reducing outflow resistance, usually with striated muscle relaxants such as diazepam. In severe cases (with upper tract dilation) iatrogenic pharmacologic retention using anticholinergics and CIC may be indicated. Similarly, vesicosphincter dyssynergia from a complete suprasacral neurologic lesion is most effectively managed with pharmacologic retention and CIC. Patients with cervical cord injuries and limited use of their upper extremities may not be able to catheterize or be catheterized, and their management again becomes individualized. Keeping the lower urinary tract free of foreign bodies (indwelling catheters) is the goal and options include sphincterotomy, insertion of urethral stent across the external sphincter, or a procedure such as the incontinent ileal vesical conduit. Retaining the natural continence mechanism of the outflow tract is preferable whenever possible. Psychogenic retention often results from a severe traumatic event, is usually temporary, and frequently resolves with management of the psychiatric disorder. Occasionally, myogenic decompensation may result and CIC may be required.

**Treatment of Outflow Obstruction in Men.** The most common cause of anatomic outflow obstruction in men is prostatic obstruction, either benign or malignant (Fig 3). When patients present in urinary retention with an acontractile bladder, return of bladder function should be documented before considering prostatectomy. Though transurethral prostatectomy remains the mainstay of therapy, other therapeutic modalities such as transurethral incision of the prostate (TUIP) and insertion of prostatic stents have received much attention. More technologically advanced procedures such as hyperthermia and transurethral laser ablation of the prostate are on the horizon. Pharmacologic options such as $\alpha$-blockade therapy (terazosin, prazosin) and hormonal antagonist including 5$\alpha$-reductase inhibitors (Proscar), antiandrogens (Flutamide), and luteinizing hormone–releasing hormone agonists may also be considered. It is the authors' view that without documented return of detrusor function there is no reason to submit a patient to the risk of anesthesia and surgery to relieve outlet obstruction since it may not result in spontaneous voiding. Other anatomic obstructions such as urethral stricture and bladder

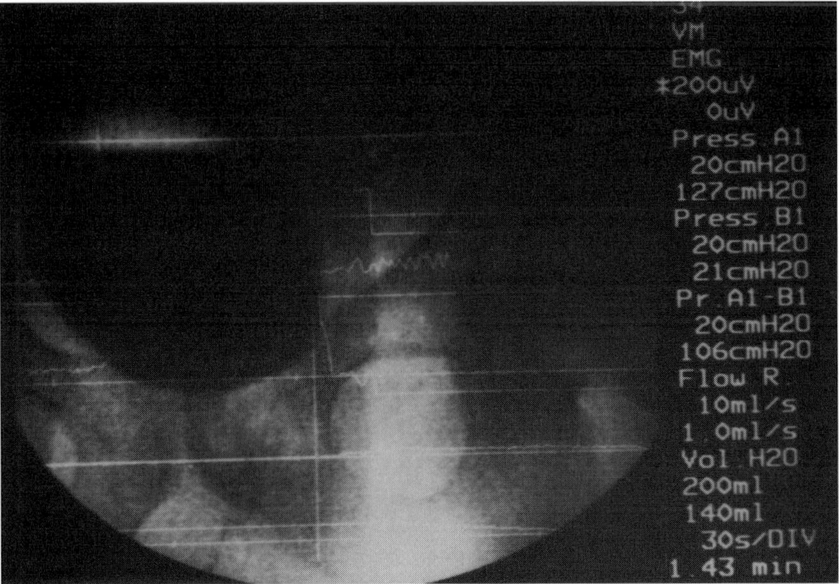


**Fig 3.** A video urodynamic study demonstrating bladder outlet obstruction. Note the bladder neck fails to open, the detrusor pressure is elevated at 106 cm $H_2O$, and the low uroflow rate of 1 $cm^3$/sec.

neck contracture are managed with incision under direct vision.

**Treatment of Outflow Obstruction in Women.** Obstruction of the lower urinary tract in women is rare. The most common cause is iatrogenic, ie, from previous surgical correction of stress urinary incontinence.[9] Technical advances and modifications of transvaginal needle suspension procedures allow elevation and stabilization of the bladder neck and proximal urethra to the retropubic position, yielding excellent surgical results without obstruction.[10] However, some of the procedures originally described, such as that by Marshall in 1949,[11] carried increased risk secondary to potential outlet obstruction. The mechanism of obstruction after a Marshall–Marchetti–Krantz (MMK) procedure was based on periurethral suture placement that could cause urethral angulation or result in periurethral scarring and fibrosis. The incidence of obstruction after MMK has been reported as 5.5%–11%.[12,13] Endoscopic suspension of the bladder neck (Stamey) has been shown urodynamically to cause obstruction by a similar mechanism, proximal urethral angulation, which sometimes requires removal of one or both suspension sutures.[14] Any bladder neck suspension procedure can cause outlet obstruction if the suspension sutures are placed periurethrally or if excessive tension is used to elevate the bladder neck and proximal urethra. Attention to anatomic detail during transvaginal suspension may allow long-term correction of incontinence without iatrogenic outlet obstruction.

Iatrogenic bladder outlet obstruction in the female clinically manifests as incomplete emptying, urinary retention, or detrusor instability with urgency and frequency. Once obstruction is documented (urodynamically), the optimal management is surgical urethrolysis. Zimmern and Raz[15] performed transvaginal urethrolysis followed by modified Pereyra bladder neck suspension on 13 patients with documented outflow obstruction after MMK, 12 of whom went on to void with a normal flow pattern and low postvoid residuals. McGuire[16] had success with urethrolysis alone in reducing voiding pressures of patients with iatrogenic obstruction and reports no recurrence of stress urinary incontinence (SUI). The authors feel the risk of recurrent SUI is sufficient after complete urethrolysis so that concurrent bladder neck suspension is warranted. Complete mobilization of the urethra and anterior vaginal wall is necessary to relieve the outlet obstruction while exercising care to avoid bladder or ureteral injury and periurethral suture placement. It is important to exclude type III stress incontinence prior to reoperation for iatrogenic outlet obstruction. In the rare woman who refuses urethrolysis, CIC with oral anticholinergics (to minimize the urgency symptoms) may be indicated.

Primary bladder neck obstruction is exceedingly rare in women. One report failed to identify a single case in almost 6000 women[17] while another demonstrated only four cases of 2500 women studied.[18] The etiology is unknown and the diagnosis is most accurately made using video urodynamics. Treatment is either medical (using an $\alpha$-antagonist such as terazosin) or surgical with transurethral incision or resection of the bladder neck or Y-V plasty.[19] Though the efficacy of transurethral management is documented, the risk of incontinence or fistula argues against this as first-line therapy.

Other less common causes of outlet obstruction in women include large cystocele that causes angulation of the proximal urethra. In addition, extrinsic compression of the bladder neck and proximal urethra by a pelvic mass may occur (rarely). Careful bimanual exam is essential and may suggest the presence of uterine leiomyoma, ovarian tumor, or urethral or vaginal wall mass such as diverticulum or carcinoma. The large cystocele can be managed transvaginally with formal repair and modified Pereyra bladder neck suspension (four-corner bladder neck suspension[20] for the moderate cystocele), whereas management of a pelvic mass is directed at the primary pathology.

## FUNCTIONAL INCONTINENCE

Factors other than lower urinary tract function may contribute to the development of incontinence. This is more evident in the elderly, as the prevalence of concurrent disease processes increases with age. Factors influencing continence include the presence of neurologic disease (stroke, Parkinson's, senile dementia), immobility (arthritis), and motivation (depression). Diurnal variation in urine production as seen with congestive heart failure (mobilization of peripheral edema when supine) and diuretic use, as well as the polyuria seen with poorly controlled diabetes may be major variables in multifactorial incontinence. Occasionally significant improvement results from simple recommendations like bedside commode, timing of diuretic use, or encouraging better management of peripheral edema or diabetes mellitus.

## URGE INCONTINENCE

Urge incontinence (UI) is the sudden desire to void with the inability to voluntarily control voiding until one reaches the toilet. There are two types of underlying bladder pathology: detrusor hyperactivity *(motor urgency),* identified by urgency with documented uninhibited detrusor contractions on filling cystometry, and detrusor hypersensitivity *(sensory urgency),* characterized by the urge to void on filling cystometry without an associated detrusor contraction. Another cause of UI is poor bladder *compliance,* in which the detrusor cannot accommodate increasing volumes of urine at a normal, low pressure. Poor compliance may result from chronic inflammatory conditions such as an indwelling urethral catheter, neurogenic lesions such as sacral arc denervation, fibrosis secondary to radiation therapy, and defunctionalized bladders left in situ after urinary diversion. Loss of compliance results in higher storage pressure that may overcome outlet resistance to cause incontinence and result in hydronephrosis. McGuire et al.[21] showed that myelomeningocele patients who do not leak, or "pop off," at detrusor pressures less than 40 cm $H_2O$ are at risk for damaging their upper tracts (Fig 4). The *duration* of elevated intravesical pressure may be more prognostic of upper tract deterioration in other patient populations.[22]

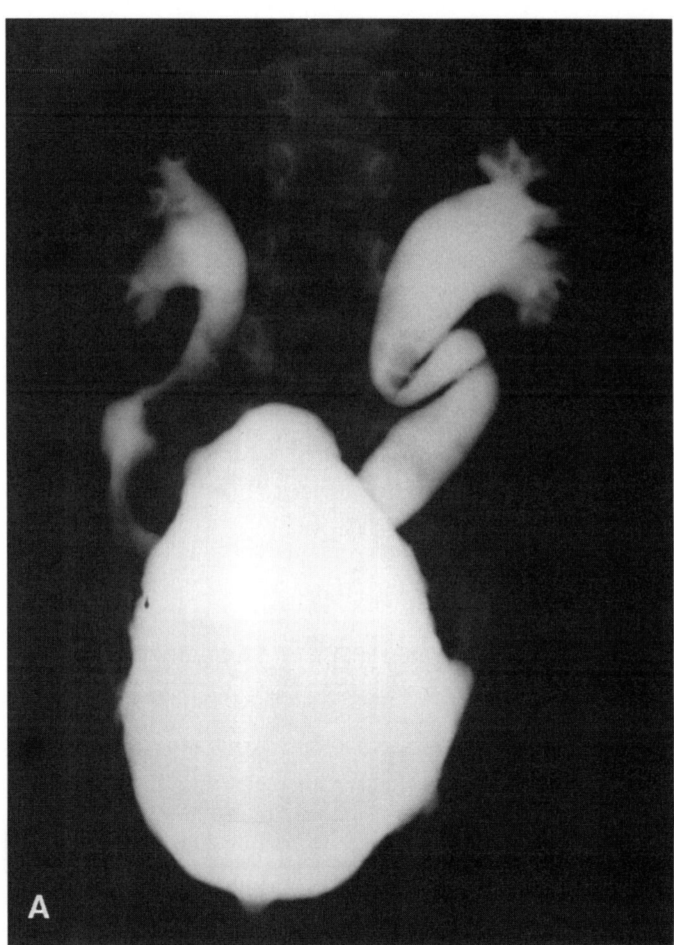


Fig 4. A: Cystogram in a myelomeningocele patient with a typical high-pressure "Christmas tree" bladder. Note the bilateral vesicoureteral reflux. B: Urodynamic tracing of same patient demonstrating elevated leak point pressure of 60 cm $H_2O$.

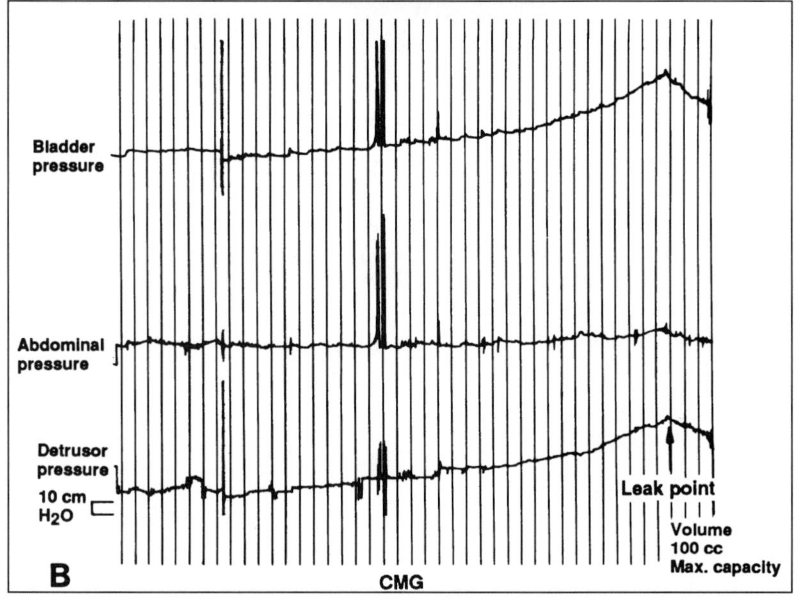

Patients with elevated leak point pressures require interval evaluation of the upper tracts including ultrasound and serum creatinine.

### Management

Management of UI can be difficult and may require management of coexisting pathology. UI may exist with, or be a result of, another process. Identification of UI with genuine stress incontinence (mixed incontinence) is important for therapeutic purposes and cannot be reliably differentiated on the basis of history alone. Urodynamic evaluation including slow-fill cystometry and pressure flow study to rule out obstruction (particularly in males and females after bladder neck suspension) is used routinely by the authors for diagnostic purposes. This urodynamic information, in conjunction with the voiding history, helps quantitate the relative contribution of each component (instability from obstruction, pure instability, or mixed incontinence) to the overall clinical picture. The authors' treatment approach, whether pharmacologic or surgical, is influenced by both symptomatology and findings on physical and urodynamic evaluation. For example, if a multiparous female with urethral hypermobility and documented genuine SUI has concurrent UI, then correction of the SUI with a routine bladder neck suspension may cure the UI in 59%–85% of cases.[23,24] However, if history suggests or evaluation reveals significant detrusor instability with a minor component of genuine SUI, pharmacologic and/or behavioral management of the detrusor instability may be indicated as first-line therapy. Patients must be assessed individually and often will require more than one form of treatment.

## NONOPERATIVE MANAGEMENT OF URINARY INCONTINENCE

Noninvasive management of urinary incontinence is usually indicated as first-line therapy. Some exceptions occur such as female patients with severe incontinence secondary to intrinsic urethral dysfunction (type III incontinence), female patients with associated pathology that will require surgical correction (such as a large cystocele, vaginal vault prolapse, or uterine descensus), and male patients with severe postprostatectomy stress incontinence (without associated bladder dysfunction). Most treatments discussed in the next sections may be applied to both male and female SUI and UI. Usually, the patient with documented severe SUI, requiring 10 heavy pads per day, will not be satisfactorily improved with pharmacotherapy, behavioral modification, or biofeedback alone. However, nonoperative therapies, even when not first-line therapy, are often useful adjuncts for successful postoperative management if surgery is ultimately required.

### Catheterization and External Devices

Bladder catheterization is utilized in different patient populations with urinary incontinence, often inappropriately. Patient subgroups requiring some form of urine collection include many in nursing homes, the mentally impaired, the immobile, and patients with total incontinence, usually from overflow. Catheterization options include internal (clean intermittent, indwelling urethral or suprapubic) or external devices such as condom catheters. Catheter-free status is the object of any therapeutic program; however, there are situations where catheters are the most realistic alternative. Indwelling urethral catheters have little role in the outpatient management of urinary incontinence. Most patients can perform CIC or have family or other support mechanisms to perform CIC for them. Clean intermittent catheterization[25] is easily learned and can be applied to patients of all ages. Although 40%–80% will have evidence of bacteriuria, symptomatic infections are seen in less than 2%.[26,27] Sterile technique in intermittent catheterization adds complexity and cost without significant benefit.

The complications of indwelling urethral catheters increase with duration of catheterization and include infection (urethritis, cystitis, pyelonephritis, and sepsis), stones, and urethral erosion. When a chronic indwelling catheter is required, the suprapubic approach is preferred because the incidence of significant bacteriuria is less than with indwelling urethral catheters and local complications such as urethritis and erosion are avoided.

External devices include condom catheters, penile clamps, female collection devices, and female occluding devices. Condom catheters may cause skin irritation and erosion, and external female devices are difficult to use. Penile clamps can cause skin erosion, urethral injury, or contribute to deterioration of the upper tracts and should therefore be avoided. An example of a female occlusive device is a small triangular foam pad, with a layer of hydrophilic adhesive, that is placed in the vestibule creating a seal over the urethral meatus. Though 80% of patients using this device reported significant improvement in their incontinence,[28] further clinical evaluation is needed.

Absorbent pads and undergarments may provide comfort and convenience when used temporarily. Unfortunately, for many these garments constitute the principal method of management and account for tremendous associated expense.

### Behavioral Modification and Biofeedback

Behavioral modification involves changes in the daily urination routine including timed voiding, avoidance of known stimulants of urination like caffeine, and restriction of total fluid intake. The authors recommend limiting fluid intake to 1000–1200 $cm^3$/d unless contraindicated for medical reasons such as a history of urinary stones, infection, or diabetes with polyuria. Fluid restriction may be quite effective for many patients, particularly those with minimal to moderate symptoms. Alterations in the daily ritual of urination may be charted (ie, Urolog) and the charts used as feedback that may support or change management decisions, and be used to reinforce clinical improvement. Many ''bladder training'' programs exist that include habit training, timed voiding, and scheduled ''retraining.'' Combining fluid restriction (to reduce total urine output) with a timed voiding program (to frequently empty the bladder) can minimize the bladder's filling to the volume that ''triggers'' an uninhibited contraction in the case of urge incontinence or being so full as to promote urine loss with stress maneuvers. These programs are most effective in patients with storage dysfunction (ie, sensory or detrusor instability) without a neurologic lesion. HIP[2] has published a 6-week bladder retraining program used at our institution for patients with UI. Fantl et al.[29] demonstrated a 75% improvement and a 12% cure in a prospective controlled trial of bladder training in elderly women (timed voiding, volitional inhibition, and charting), for urge and stress incontinence. The number of incontinent episodes, amount of fluid loss, and associated daytime and nighttime frequency were decreased. These authors recommended routine use of bladder training in selected elderly women with urge and stress incontinence, possibly precluding formal urodynamic evaluation in those responding to the bladder training program. These behavioral modification techniques play an important role in the management of less severe stress and urge incontinence.

The use of feedback stimuli of an auditory or visual nature has been successfully used to assist in voluntary control of such physiologic responses as blood pressure, heart rate, body temperature, and bowel motility. Biofeedback for urge incontinence depends on the patient's ability to recognize, and then suppress, the uninhibited contraction while voluntarily contracting the sphincter (to prevent the incontinent episode until the bladder contraction is suppressed). An effective biofeedback program is labor-intensive and quite dependent on a motivated patient. By observing filling cystometry real-time readings, the patient learns to identify bladder sensations as related to uninhibited detrusor contractions and subsequently attempts to control them (patients who cannot sense the uninhibited detrusor contractions have little chance of improvement with this type of program). Cardozo et al.[30] reported 40% cure and an additional 20% improved using

CMG feedback for idiopathic detrusor instability. Unfortunately, many of these studies suffer from variable design and response definitions and short follow-up. The use of biofeedback for genuine stress incontinence is discussed under "Pelvic Floor Exercises."

### Pelvic Floor Exercises

Treatment of urge incontinence with pelvic floor contraction relies on the patient's ability to suppress the bladder contraction once recognized, ie, contract the voluntary sphincter which may suppress or shut off the detrusor contraction by a reflex neurologic mechanism similar to, but reciprocal to, Bradley's loop #3. It is logical that a patient with a sustained high-amplitude detrusor contraction may not be able to control the detrusor contraction with contraction of the "voluntary" sphincter. However, in patients with severe urgency, a combination of fluid restriction, timed voiding, and pharmacologic agents that increase the uninhibited detrusor contraction "triggering" volume and decrease the strength of the contraction may provide the patient enough time to make it to the toilet.

Augmenting urethral closure by voluntary contraction of pelvic floor muscles can be a useful adjunct in both men and women with stress incontinence. The fast-twitch muscle fibers of the external or striated sphincter are not functionally adapted to maintain passive continence but are instead designed to augment closure pressure in time of sudden increases in abdominal pressure. Repetitive voluntary contractions of the pelvic and perineal muscles are designed to improve the resting tone and strengthen the reflex muscle contraction during provocative stress maneuvers. Kegel[31] described the use of a pneumatic perineometer placed in the vagina and connected to an external pressure gauge that supplied visual feedback to patients of the strength of the pelvic floor contraction. Other devices such as weighted vaginal cones and more sophisticated computer-aided feedback systems have been described. Basic exercises without the aid of complex feedback or expensive devices may be used routinely. Patient motivation is critical to any biofeedback program. There is no evidence that the more complex forms of biofeedback are more effective than simple feedback in a well-motivated patient. The authors have an instructional audiocassette tape available for patients who are candidates and are sufficiently motivated.[2] Success rates of 70%–80% are reported with biofeedback-assisted exercises vs. 50%–60% with verbal instruction alone.[32] However, relapse rates are high and long-term follow-up data sparse.

### Pharmacologic Therapy

The pharmacology of the anticholinergic and antispasmodic agents makes them applicable to patients with incontinence from uninhibited detrusor contractions but has no role in patients with genuine stress incontinence alone. However, drugs that augment outlet resistance such as the tricyclic antidepressant imipramine, the estrogens, and the $\alpha$-agonists may be used in patients with genuine stress incontinence. Clinically, these agents are most useful in patients with less severe incontinence and are generally used in combination with behavioral modification programs such as fluid restriction and timed voiding.

Integral to the successful management of UI is pharmacologic depression of the uninhibited detrusor contraction. The goal of therapy is to prevent or delay the uninhibited detrusor contraction in the storage phase of filling yet maintain complete emptying with micturition. This can be difficult, particularly in men with some component of outlet obstruction or in women with elevated postvoid residual volumes. These patients risk urinary retention with anticholinergics or antispasmodics and must be approached cautiously (or start pharmacologic therapy in conjunction with intermittent catheterization to monitor postvoid residual urine volume).

**Oral Agents.** ***Anticholinergics.*** Atropine and atropine-like agents inhibit the acetocholine neurohumoral effector mechanism for detrusor contraction thus depressing true involuntary bladder contractions of any etiology. The volume at which the first unstable detrusor contraction (UDC) is triggered is increased, the strength of the contraction is decreased, and total bladder capacity is increased. An important clinical caveat is that the interval between first urge and bladder contraction is not increased (the patient's "warning time" between the symptomatic urge and need to void is unchanged). Accordingly, a useful adjunct with anticholinergics is a behavioral modification program such as timed voiding or a toileting regimen to encourage bladder emptying before the volume stimulating urge and UI is reached. Propantheline bromide (Pro-Banthine) is the most commonly used antimuscarinic anticholinergic; the usual adult dosage is listed in Table 1.

Methantheline (Banthine), another oral agent differing from propantheline by an increased ratio of ganglionic blockade (which theoretically should further decrease UDCs), offers no increased clinical efficacy. Anticholinergic side effects, listed in Table 1, are often problematic and may limit patient compliance. A thorough discussion of the expected side effects with management advice such as oral lozenges for dry mouth and artificial saliva in severe cases is useful.

***Musculotropic Relaxants.*** The musculotropic relaxing agents are direct-acting smooth muscle relaxants but also have demonstrated anticholinergic activity and local anesthetic properties. Oxybutynin

**TABLE 1. Commonly Used Pharmacologic Agents in the Management of Urinary Incontinence**

| Class | Dosage[a] | Side Effects |
|---|---|---|
| Anticholinergics | | |
| Propantheline bromide (Pro-Banthine, others) | 15–30 mg po QID | Dry mouth, constipation, tachycardia, blurred vision (near objects)<br>Caution: bladder outlet obstruction |
| Methantheline (Banthine) | 50–100 mg po QID | Contraindicated: narrow-angle glaucoma, bowel obstruction |
| Musculotropics | | |
| Oxybutynin (Ditropan) | 5 mg po TID | Similar to the anticholinergics |
| Dicyclomine HCl (Bentyl) | 20–30 mg po TID | |
| Flavoxate HCl (Urispas) | 100–200 mg po TID, QID | |
| Tricylic Antidepressants | | |
| Imipramine (Tofranil) | 15–25 mg po TID | Systemic anticholinergic effects<br>CNS: sedation, confusion (elderly), tremor<br>Cardiovascular: postural hypotension, conduction disturbances (myocardial depression)<br>Other: increased LFT, obstructive jaundice, agranulocytosis<br>Do not withdraw abruptly |
| Estrogen | | |
| Vaginal cream (Dinesterol, Premarin, others) | ⅓ applicator 3 times weekly | May be contraindicated in women with history of breast or uterine carcinoma |
| Agonists | | |
| Ephedrine | 25–50 mg po QID | Hypertension, anxiety, insomnia, headache, palpitations, cardiac dysrhythmias |
| Pseudoephedrine (Sudafed, others) | 30–60 mg po QID | |
| Phenylpropanolamine HCl (Entex LA, others) | 25, 50, and 75 mg po BID | |

[a] Drug dosages may change. Please refer to the *PDR* for current dosage recommendations.

chloride (Ditropan) is the most commonly used agent for management of urgency and UI. Ditropan has been shown to decrease detrusor hyperreflexia in patients with neurogenic bladder dysfunction,[33] specifically in patients with multiple sclerosis.[34] Others have found little advantage of Ditropan over propantheline in the management of women with detrusor instability.[35] Other musculotropic agents with less potent anticholinergic activity include dicyclomine hydrochloride (Bentyl) and flavoxate hydrochloride (Urispas). These agents are clinically less effective but may have a role in the elderly population who cannot tolerate the side effects of the stronger anticholinergic agents. Side effects of the musculotropics are primarily anticholinergic and are listed with the usual adult dosage in Table 1.

***Tricyclic Antidepressants.*** The tricyclic antidepressants, particularly imipramine (Tofranil), are clinically useful to facilitate urine storage. Imipramine has been shown to decrease bladder contractility and increase outlet resistance at the bladder neck and proximal urethra. The mechanisms include both central and peripheral anticholinergic effects, inhibited reuptake of norepinephrine at the presynaptic nerve ending, and a direct inhibitory effect on bladder smooth muscle (neither anticholinergic nor adrenergic, possibly related to calcium influx). The augmented outlet resistance theoretically results from enhanced local α-adrenergic stimulation as a result of blocked norepinephrine reuptake into presynaptic nerve endings. Because of differing mechanisms of action, the clinical response to tricyclic antidepressants may be synergistic to those of anticholinergics and musculotropic agents; however, the anticholinergic side effects are often additive. Clinical judgment must be exercised in the use of tricyclic antidepressants. They are contraindicated in patients on monoamine oxidase inhibitors and should be used cautiously in the elderly with cardiac disease due to the risk of myocardial depression and conduction disturbances. Patients started on imipramine should be informed about the potential side effects (Table 1), and when discontinued should be tapered, not abruptly withdrawn (particularly in children).

***Estrogens and Alpha Agonists.*** The effects of estrogen on the urethra and bladder neck, particularly in postmenopausal women, are well recognized though the mechanisms of action are not entirely understood. Urethral outlet resistance is increased by suggested proliferation of submucosal vascular plexus, enhanced "mucosal seal,"[36] and augmented response to endogenous adrenergic stimulation either by increased α-receptor population or enhanced receptor function. Clinically, phenylpropanolamine and estriol were found to be individually effective in patients with SUI, but their effects were additive when combined.[37] α-Agonists such as phenylpropanolamine alone may be effective for genuine stress incontinence by enhancing proximal urethral outlet resistance. However, patients should be counseled that clinical relapse can be expected when the medicine is discontinued. Though estrogens are useful clinically in managing detrusor instability, particularly in elderly women with atrophic vaginitis, the mechanism is unclear.

***Other Oral Medications.*** Calcium channel blockers can diminish bladder contractility by uncoupling the calcium influx required for the excitation–contraction mechanism. Clinical use for motor urgency has been limited by the hemodynamic side effects experienced at doses required to inhibit detrusor contractility. Terodiline has been used extensively in Europe with promising results in treating detrusor instability and hyperreflexia but has been associated with cardiac arrhythmias and withdrawn from the market.[38] Verapamil (Isoptin) has been used as an adjunct in the management of urge incontinence, usually in combination therapy but few clinical data exist. Calcium channel blockers are contraindicated in patients with cardiac depression such as congestive heart failure, rhythm conduction disorders, or in patients on β-blockers. β-Adrenergic agonists theoretically should decrease uninhibited detrusor contractions by β-receptor–mediated relaxation of the bladder body, where β-receptors predominate. Terbutaline has shown some clinical effect in patients with urgency and urge incontinence.[39]

**Intravesical Agents.** Intravesical application of various agents including anesthetics (lidocaine) and oxybutynin (Ditropan) have been used for management of bladder dysfunction resistant to other forms of therapy. A 5-mg tablet of oxybutynin is dissolved in 20 $cm^3$ normal saline and instilled into the bladder by self-catheterization two to three times a day. The pharmacokinetics of topical use suggest the mechanism of action as enhanced systemic absorption vs. oral use, with more consistent bioavailability manifest as lower peak and higher trough serum levels, perhaps explaining the fewer systemic anticholinergic side effects.[40] Another possible mechanism accounting for fewer systemic side effects with intravesical Ditropan is that the absorbed oxybutynin is not initially metabolized by the liver as is oral Ditropan with gastrointestinal absorption. A hepatic metabolite of Ditropan not produced with intravesical administration may be responsible for the majority of the systemic side effects experienced. In the authors' experience, intravesical Ditropan has eliminated, or significantly improved, irritative voiding symptoms in 18 of 33 (55%) patients with DI, DH, or poor compliance who failed oral pharmacologic therapy.

Recent reports have suggested the use of intravesical atropine for urge incontinence in spinal cord injury patients.[41] Increases in cystometric capacity, volume triggering uninhibited contraction, and decrease in maximum detrusor pressure were statistically significant. Although no side effects were observed, further clinical experience is needed in different patient populations.

## Other Noninvasive Therapies

Electrical stimulation is used clinically to improve urinary continence by enhancing the activity of the compromised urethral closure mechanism (strengthening the sphincter) and/or by inhibiting the involuntary detrusor contractions. Management of urge incontinence does not depend on direct inhibition of detrusor function by the stimulated neuron but instead utilizes activated spinal inhibitory systems that prevent involuntary urine leakage during defecation and coitus (ie, detrusor inhibition occurs through reflex activity with afferent stimulation such as anal dilation or gentle mechanical stimulation of the genital region). Detrusor overactivity resulting from lack of central inhibition may respond to inhibitory signals from these and other system afferents. Clinically, electrodes can be placed in the anus and vagina or over the peroneal or posterior tibial nerve (S3 afferent) as described by McGuire et al.[42] Technical variables such as stimulation frequency, intensity, and pulse configuration are crucial in achieving maximal inhibition without patient discomfort. Though chronic stimulation has been used, short-term therapy is equally effective.[43] Short-term therapy may improve patient compliance and be more accountable for treatment success. Recently, statistically significant reductions in the frequency of urination and episodes of urgency in patients with idiopathic detrusor instability have been reported using a TENS unit over the S3 dermatome.[44] Success rates (with vaginal or anal stimulation) of 67% have been reported in incontinence secondary to detrusor overactivity[45] whereas somewhat less favorable results are seen with sphincteric insufficiency (53%).[43] Direct neurostimulation may be used to modulate voiding dysfunction and involves electrode stimulation of the sacral nerve roots or pudendal nerve. Typically, a single electrode is placed on a trial basis and if the patient experiences symptomatic improvement then chronic implantation is considered. Schmidt[46] reports greater than 50% improvement in patients with urge incontinence refractory to other therapies over a 6-year period.

Acupuncture has received recent attention in the management of patients with motor and sensory instability.[47] Though symptomatic improvement was noted, urodynamic confirmation was lacking. Potential mechanisms of action include depression of afferent impulses from the bladder or increases in the cerebrospinal fluid endogenous opiate levels.

## SURGICAL MANAGEMENT OF URINARY INCONTINENCE

### Stress Urinary Incontinence: Surgical Therapy in Men

Critical to accurate classification of SUI is urodynamic documentation of incontinence with cough or other provocative maneuvers with concurrent *normal detrusor pressure* (compliance) and the *absence of involuntary detrusor contractions.* The most common presentation of male urinary incontinence follows sphincteric damage during prostatectomy, occurring in less than 1% for transurethral resection and in 5%–10% of radical prostatectomy patients. Other etiologies include sphincteric disruption after pelvic trauma and theoretically with lesions that result in denervation of the proximal urethra secondary to myelomeningocele, thoracolumbar cord injury, or radical pelvic surgery. Genuine SUI is associated with sphincteric incompetence and treatment is directed at augmenting sphincter function or artificially increasing outlet resistance. Leach and Yun[6] demonstrated that 34% of men with postprostatectomy incontinence after detailed urodynamics had mixed incontinence, ie, bladder dysfunction (overactivity and/or poor compliance) coexisting with sphincter insufficiency. Initial management in men with a component of bladder dysfunction should be directed at controlling the overactive bladder with pharmacotherapy (Fig 5). This therapy was effective in achieving ''social continence'' (two pads per day or less) in 39% of the treatment group. Proper diagnostic evaluation of the male with incontinence is critical and must include urodynamics to assess the possibility of sphincteric insufficiency and exclude bladder dysfunction. Surgical procedures (such as artificial sphincter and periurethral injection) that create outlet obstruction in the face of high-pressure bladder dysfunction may result in continued or exacerbated high detrusor pressures and deterioration of the upper tracts, particularly in children.[48]

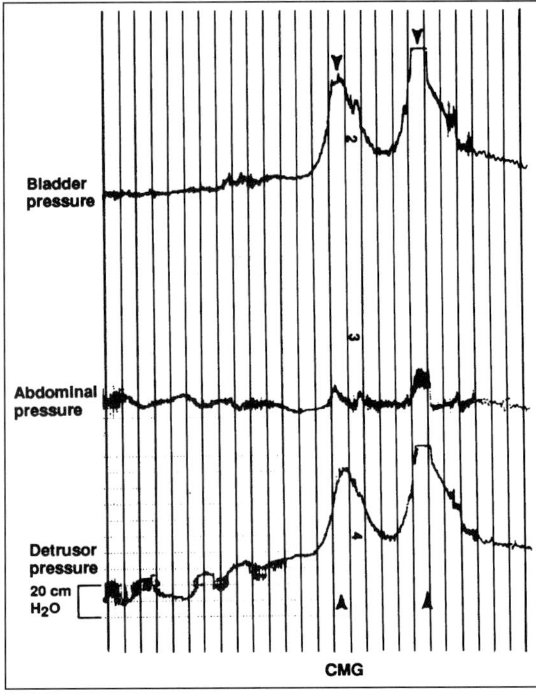


**Fig 5.** Detrusor instability and poor compliance before pharmacologic therapy in a patient with postprostatectomy incontinence.

### Periurethral Injection

Periurethral injection of polytetrafluorourethane (Polytef), collagen, and fat provide enhanced proximal periurethral bulk and mechanically increase urethral outlet resistance. In the absence of bladder dysfunction this minimally invasive therapy is conceptually appealing for management of SUI.

**Teflon.** Polytetrafluorourethane has been used for male SUI although concerns exist regarding the documented migration of Teflon particles to lymph nodes, lung, and brain.[49] Though the impact of such migration is unknown, it has not been shown to be clinically significant. Polytef is a thick paste requiring a high-pressure gun–like device for injection. The paste is injected transurethrally near the proximal membranous urethra under direct endoscopic visualization (others use a transperineal approach with cystoscopic monitoring). The surgeon can observe the material layering

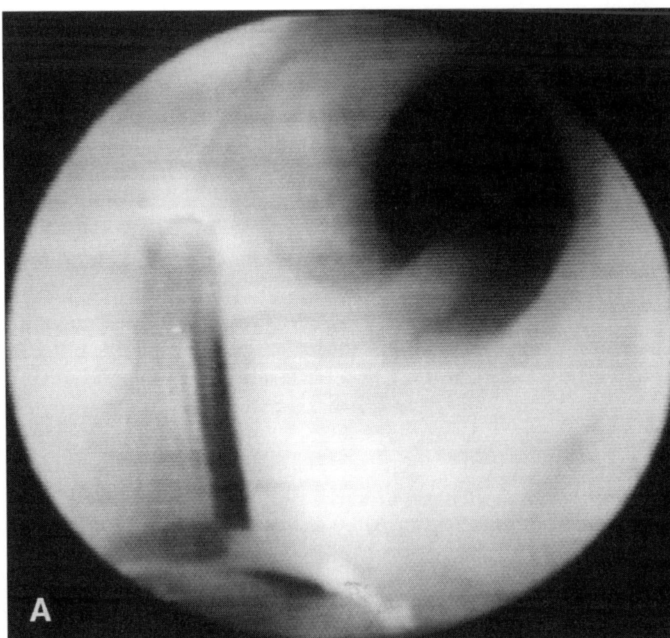


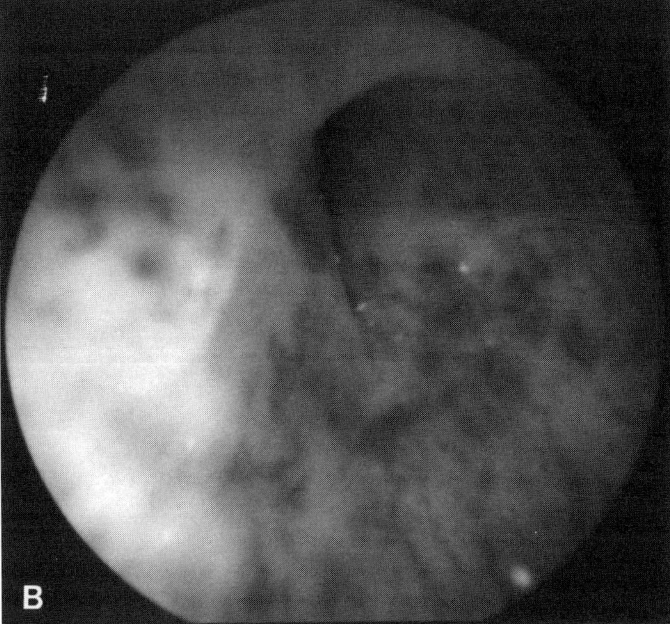


**Fig 6. A:** Cystoscopic view of proximal urethral lumen (demonstrating transurethral needle placement) before periurethral injection in a male. **B:** After injection, note the visual occlusion of the urethral lumen.

beneath the mucosa gradually occluding the proximal urethral lumen (Fig 6). A clinical caveat is to avoid multiple urethral puncture sites or mucosal splitting or the material will extrude into the urethral lumen. It is this potential ''leakage'' of material from the needle puncture site that prompts some surgeons to use the transperineal access avoiding urethral mucosal puncture. The technique is minimally invasive and can be performed under local anesthesia on an outpatient basis. The pioneering work of Politano[50] on incontinent men after transurethral prostatectomy revealed a success rate of 75% (average 1.8 injections per patient) with follow-up of 6 months to 16 years. As with other injectable periurethral substances, more than one injection is usually required to achieve continence. Patients after radical prostatectomy, radiation, and with neurogenic bladder have not had similar success rates with most series reporting durable response of 30%–50%.[51] Complications include transient urinary retention.

**Collagen.** Gax collagen (Contigen), a gluteraldehyde crosslinked natural substance derived from bovine skin, is currently used as a treatment for both male and female SUI. The Gax collagen is thought to be replaced by natural collagen via a "remodeling process" after 4–6 months. Cystoscopically controlled injections are placed at multiple positions just proximal to the membranous urethra until the lumen is visually coapted. The multicenter study of 115 men, 77 with greater than 2-year follow-up, reported only 8 men who were not dry or clinically improved. Leak point pressures increased over baseline by 61 cm $H_2O$ in the 2-year success group after 2.2 treatments using an average of 21 $cm^3$ collagen per patient.[52] Side effects include possible allergic reaction, which has prompted the recommendation of routine dermal skin testing prior to treatment. Appell[53] reported no hypersensitivity reactions in 239 patients but 3 patients had a positive skin test precluding collagen use. For periurethral injection, the potential cost advantages of an outpatient procedure usually under local anesthesia must be weighed against the cost of the collagen itself and the potential need for reinjection if the response is limited. Long-term results are needed to further assess the efficacy and potential cost implications of collagen injection.

**Fat.** Blaivas and Santarosa[54] used autologous fat harvested by liposuction for periurethral bulk enhancement in five men with postprostatectomy incontinence. Only one patient had a sustained response, which was "moderate." Nonetheless, periurethral injection of autologous fat avoids some of the issues concerning the other injectable materials such as cost, allergic response, and migration.

### Artificial Urinary Sphincter

Management of sphincteric incompetence using implanted artificial prosthetic devices has been employed for 40 years. Initial attempts were directed at urethral compression by strategically placed acrylic or silicone blocks. Critical to the concept of implantable circumferential urethral occluding devices is that excessive occlusion pressure results in vascular compromise, atrophy, or urethral erosion while insufficient pressure allows persistent incontinence. Scott et al.[55] in 1973 introduced the prototype for the modern artificial urinary sphincter (AUS) whose components included an inflatable cuff, reservoir for fluid, and pump with one-way valve for inflating and deflating the periurethral cuff. This early device was not mechanically reliable and the rate of urethral erosion was unacceptably high. Currently the most commonly used device is the AMS 800 GU sphincter introduced in 1983. The main advantages are a control assembly that contains a deflation pump with a deactivation button that allows transcutaneous deactivation (by scrotal manipulation), a procedure previously requiring reoperation. Criteria for patient eligibility are strict and include genuine stress incontinence for more than a year (refractory to pharmacologic therapy), sterile urine, absence of bladder outlet obstruction, and the manual dexterity to operate the AUS pump. The authors prefer a perineal approach for cuff placement around the proximal bulbar urethra (Fig 7); others use a retropubic approach for cuff placement at the bladder neck. A second incision is made in the inguinal region, the reservoir placed in the preperitoneal space, and the pump placed in the scrotum through a subcutaneous tunnel. The system is filled with *isotonic* (to prevent osmotic fluid shifts) 12.5% Hypaque for future radiographic identification. Achieving appropriate cuff pressure

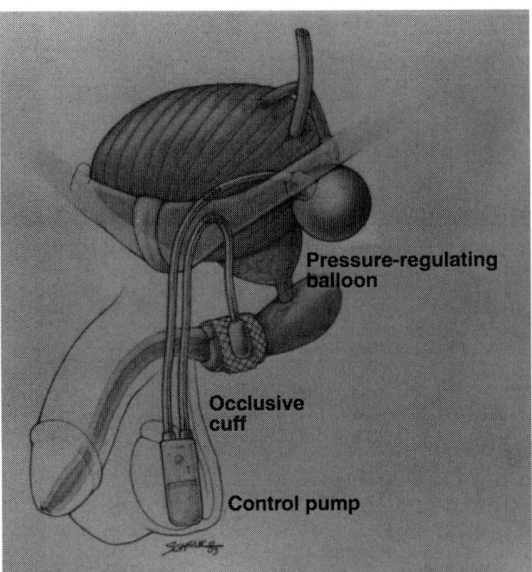


**Fig 7.** Artificial urinary sphincter, with cuff placement around the bulbar urethra.

for effective urethral compression without urethral compromise is critical. Various reservoirs are available with pressures ranging from 51–60 cm $H_2O$ to 81–90 $H_2O$. The lowest pressure required to allow continence is preferred; the authors routinely use the 51–60 cm $H_2O$ reservoir. Intraoperative perfusion sphincterometry as described by Leach and Raz[56] is a simple technique that allows intraoperative determination of occluding pressure and confirms proper device function. In the authors' experience, 13 of 55 men required operative revision of the artificial urinary sphincter, 6 of whom had urethral atrophy, 4 mechanical failure, 1 persistent perineal pain, and 2 unsatisfactory scrotal reservoir placement. No urethral erosion or prosthetic infections occurred. Serious complications of erosion, infection, and device malfunction in up to 15% of patients at 3 years have been reported. Urethral atrophy is the most common cause of recurrent incontinence; however, device malfunction, cuff erosion, and bladder dysfunction must be excluded. Many patients with iatrogenic outlet obstruction (ie, neurogenic bladder) induced by the AUS are at risk for detrusor changes that result in high pressures. In this population interval evaluation of the upper tracts is recommended.

## Stress Urinary Incontinence: Surgical Therapy in Women

Continence in the female depends on a complex balance of many factors including an anatomically well-supported urethra, intact urethral innervation, hormonally influenced mucosal coaptation, and reflex pelvic floor contraction at the time of cough or strain. Any of these factors may be individually compromised yet continence remains because of the cumulative effect of the others. This balance may explain why not all of the women with loss of anatomic support have incontinence and why, for example, the multiparous female with urethral hypermobility who is continent develops incontinence after menopause and loss of hormonal influence. The authors employ the classification of SUI presented in Table 2. SUI can be conceptually divided into two distinct groups: those with loss of anatomic support, ie, hypermobility (type I or II) and those with intrinsic urethral dysfunction (type III). Risk factors for type III incontinence include prior suspension surgery, radiation therapy for pelvic malignancy, pelvic trauma, and sacral arc denervation. Type III may reflect a spectrum of severe incontinence manifest by an open bladder neck and proximal urethra (VCUG) at rest, and a well-supported ure-

**TABLE 2. Commonly Used Classification of Female Stress Urinary Incontinence**

| | |
|---|---|
| Type O | History of incontinence but cannot be demonstrated by physician |
| Type I | Incontinence with proximal urethral or bladder neck hypermobility |
| Type II | Incontinence with demonstrable proximal urethral and bladder neck hypermobility and cystocele |
| Type IIA | Cystocele descending 2–5 cm below inferior aspect of pubic symphysis on cystogram, AP straining view |
| Type IIB | Cystocele descending >5 cm below inferior aspect of pubic symphysis on cystogram, AP straining view |
| Type III | Incontinence secondary to intrinsic urethral dysfunction |

thra, often scarred and fixed in the retropubic position. More recently, low active leak point pressures (less than 20 cm $H_2O$) are being used as criteria for type III incontinence. Leak point pressure measurement involves urodynamic observation of the change in abdominal pressure (generated by the patient's straining or coughing) required to cause urine leak.

Anatomic incontinence (types I and II) may be treated with a variety of therapies depending on the severity of incontinence, presence of associated cystocele or other pelvic pathology, and, importantly, the patient's motivation and compliance. Thorough explanations of the therapies available, anticipated duration of treatment, and reasonably expected outcomes must be discussed once the diagnosis is confirmed. Patients should know that behavioral modification and pharmacotherapy, while possibly effective, must be continued indefinitely or relapse is likely. Intraoperative and postoperative complications of bladder neck suspension surgery are discussed in detail by Kelly et al.[23]

### Anatomic Stress Urinary Incontinence: Types I and II—Suprapubic Approaches

**Marshall–Marchetti–Krantz (MMK).** Marshall et al.,[11] in 1949, pioneered the fixation of the proximal urethra and bladder neck to the pubic bone for restoring continence. As originally described, number 1 chromic sutures placed through the vaginal wall incorporating a partial thickness of the urethral wall were secured to the periosteum of the symphysis pubis. Additional sutures were placed through the anterior bladder wall and fixed to the rectus muscle for further anterior elevation. Though this technique allows for support of the proximal urethra and bladder neck, periurethral suture placement increased the likelihood of urethral obstruction. Subsequently, in 1957, the position of suture placement was modified to decrease the risk of periurethral placement and urethral obstruction[57] (Fig 8). Complications of MMK include osteitis pubis (1%–10%), prolonged urinary retention (10%), and postoperative instability (secondary to obstruction). Reported success rates are 57%–98% (Spencer et al.[12] reported a long-term success rate of 57% in 54 women with mean follow-up of 68.2 months after MMK urethropexy (Table 3).

Burch[58] modified the MMK procedure in 1961 by fixing the suspension sutures laterally to Cooper's ligament (ileopectineal line), an advantage in the ability to repair mild to moderate associated cystoceles (Fig 9). The technique involves retropubic exposure of the bladder neck, proximal urethra, and Cooper's ligament through a low midline or Pfannenstiel incision. Exposure of the lateral vaginal wall is facilitated by placing a finger or preferably a sponge stick in the vagina. A 0 polydiaxanone (PDS, or nonabsorbable suture) "figure 8" is placed full thickness through the vaginal wall at the level of the midurethra and bladder neck. The suture is then placed through Cooper's ligament at a point allowing stabilization. Further sutures may be placed proximally to reduce concurrent cystocele with caution to avoid ureteral injury. Most advocate cystoscopy to assess urethral support, rule out urethral and bladder injury, and confirm bilateral ureteral efflux. Others suggest open cystotomy with suture placement under direct vision to avoid ureteral injury. Reported success rates are 80%–100%.[59] The authors prefer the Burch colposuspension when an abdominal approach is required to manage concurrent pelvic pathology such as ovarian or uterine lesions or during augmentation cystoplasty.

### Transvaginal Approaches

**Modified Pereyra Bladder Neck Suspension (MPBNS).** Pereyra, in 1959, described vaginal suture placement with needle transfer to the suprapubic position for elevation of the bladder neck and proximal urethra.[60] Many modifications have been described including the use of polypropylene sutures for suspension (instead of wire as originally described) and routine use of cystoscopy to confirm the absence of urethral or bladder perforation, assess elevation of the proximal urethra and bladder neck, and document bilateral ureteral efflux. The au-

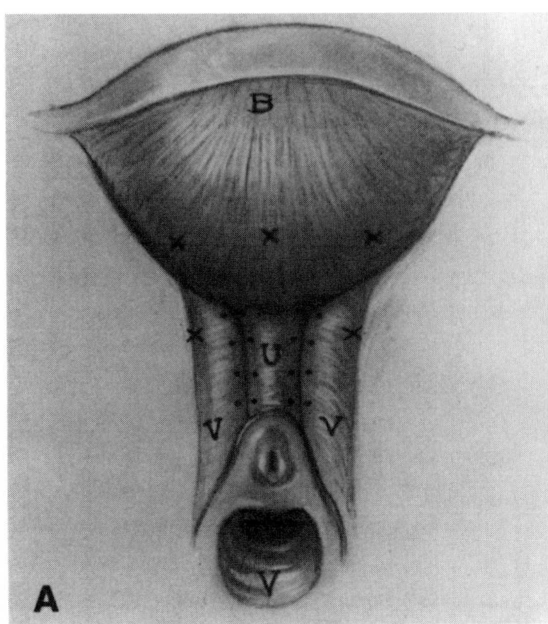


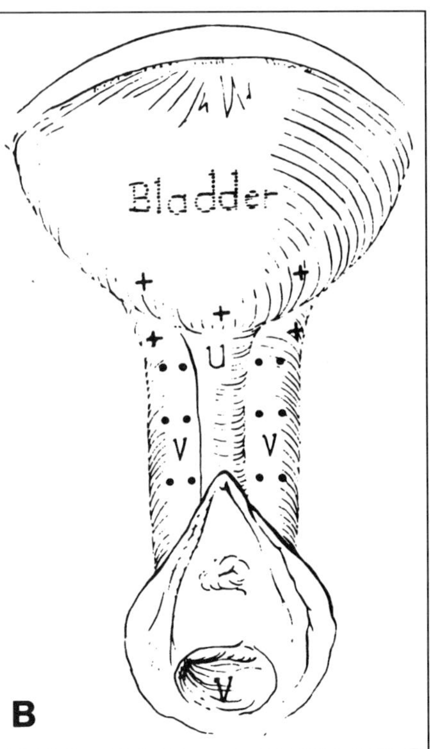


**Fig 8. A:** Location of MMK suture placement as originally described in 1949. The periurethral location increased the risk of outlet obstruction. (From Marshall VF, et al.,[11] by permission of *Surgery, Gynecology & Obstetrics.*) **B:** After modification in 1957, the suspension sutures were placed lateral to the urethra in the anterior vaginal wall. (From Marchetti AA, et al.,[57] with permission.)

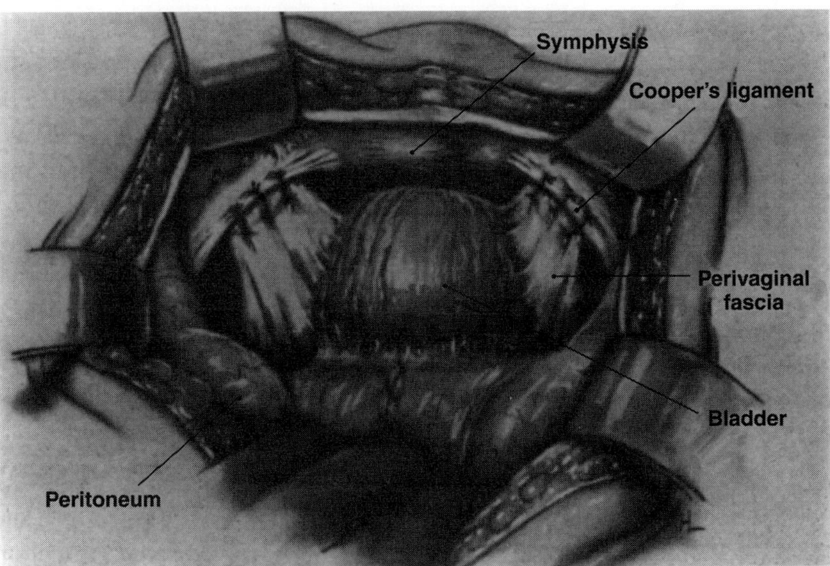


**Fig 9.** Diagram of suture placement in Burch suspension. Note the additional cephalad sutures for reducing a mild to moderate cystocele, as well as the fixation to Cooper's ligament laterally.

thors' technique (Fig 10) employs lateral anterior wall incisions at the bladder neck (the inverted ''U'' depicted in the diagram is no longer used) with sharp dissection along the ''shining white'' relatively avascular plane of the endopelvic fascia laterally to the undersurface of the pubic bone. Early digital confirmation of bone location avoids dissection lateral toward the levators or superficially into the labia. Brisk bleeding implies the wrong plane of dissection. After the bone is cleaned *the bladder is drained* and the endopelvic fascia is sharply penetrated. The retropubic space

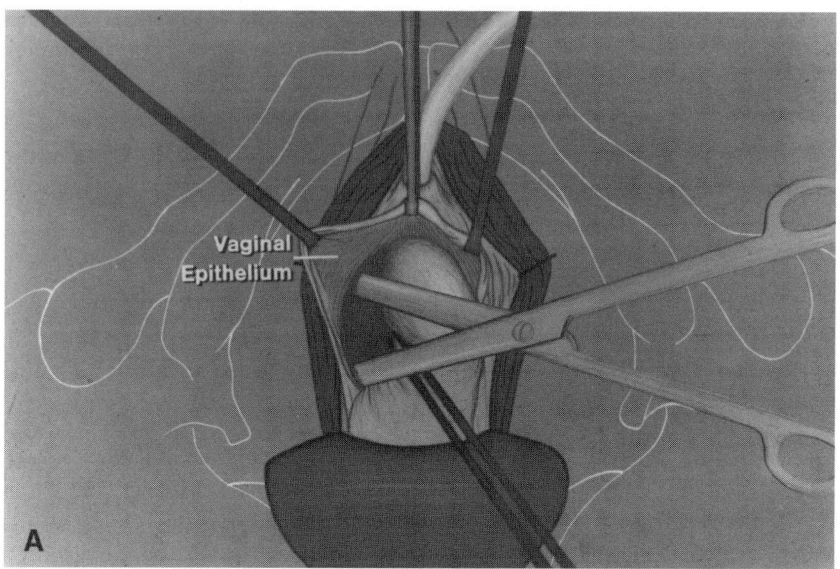


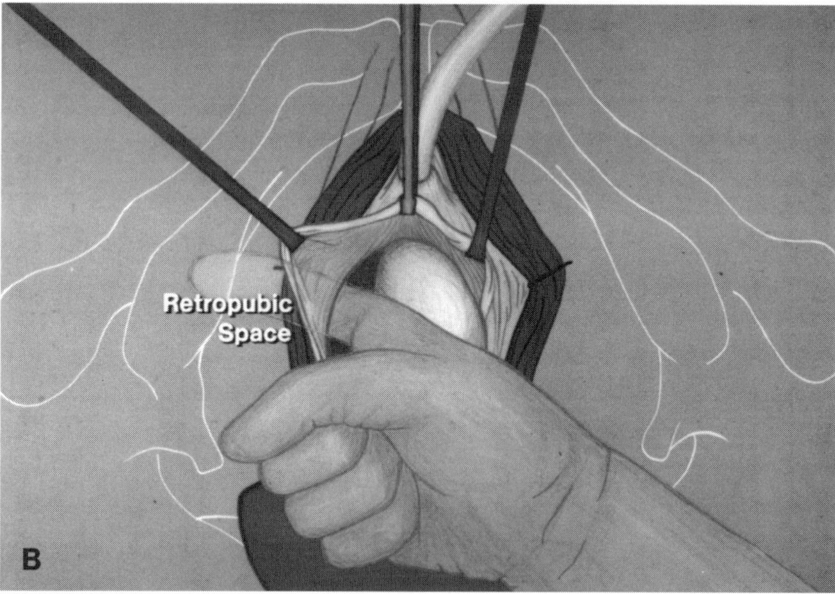


**Fig 10.** Technique of modified Pereyra bladder neck suspension (MPBNS). **A:** The inverted "U" anterior vaginal wall incision exposes the shiny white pubocervical fascia. Sharp dissection lateral to the bladder neck perforating the endopelvic fascia. [From *Urol Clin North Am.* (1991;18:327), with permission.] **B:** Blunt finger dissection of the retropubic space anteriorly to the fascia.

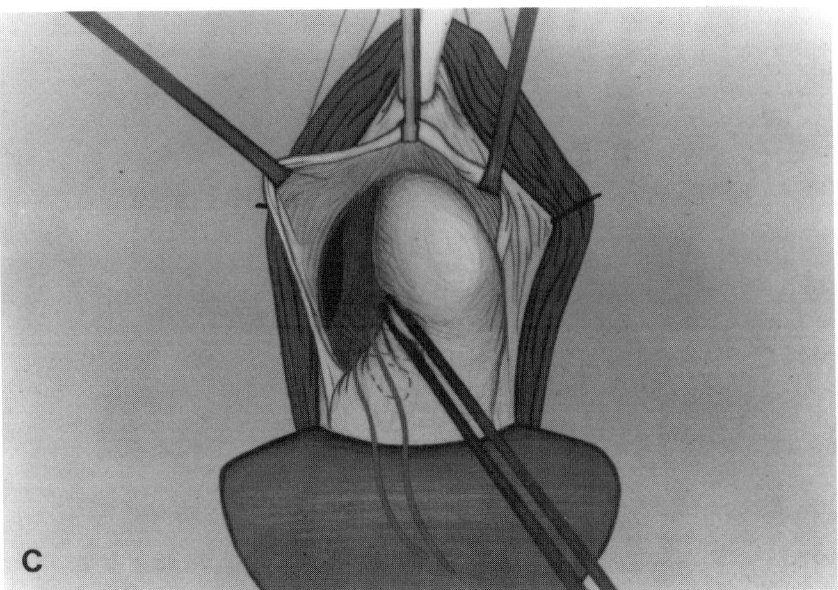


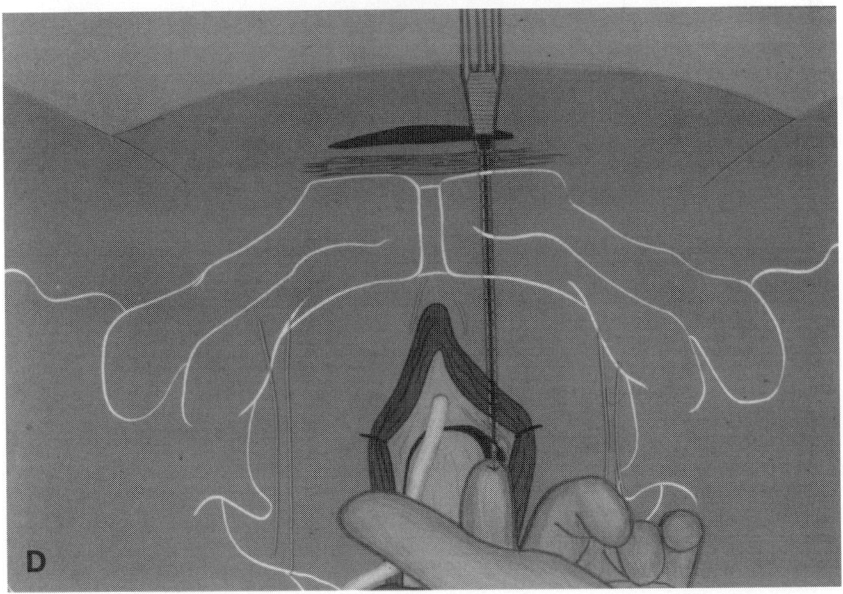


**Fig 10. C:** Helical #1 polypropylene suture placement through the anterior vaginal wall, at the level of the bladder neck. **D:** Passage of the Pereyra needle with *finger guidance* from the suprapubic incision through the retropubic space out of the vaginal incision.

lateral to the bladder is developed bluntly with finger dissection anteriorly toward the undersurface of the rectus muscle and inferiorly to the ischial tuberosity to assure complete mobilization of the anterior vaginal wall. Number 1 polypropylene sutures are placed in a helical fashion including the full thickness of the anterior vaginal wall, excluding the epithelium, at the level of the bladder neck (localized by feeling the Foley balloon). It is critical at this point to avoid periurethral suture placement to minimize the risk of outlet obstruction. The insertion of the rectus fascia and pubic

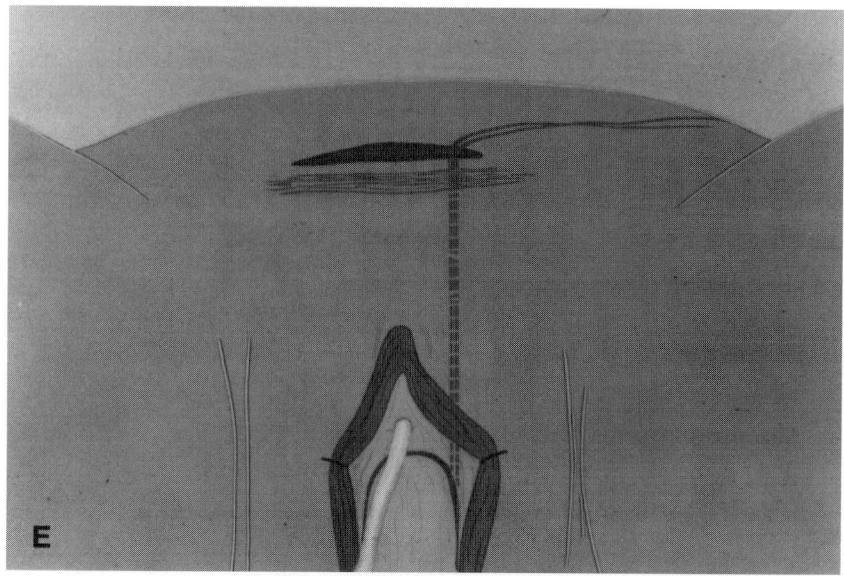


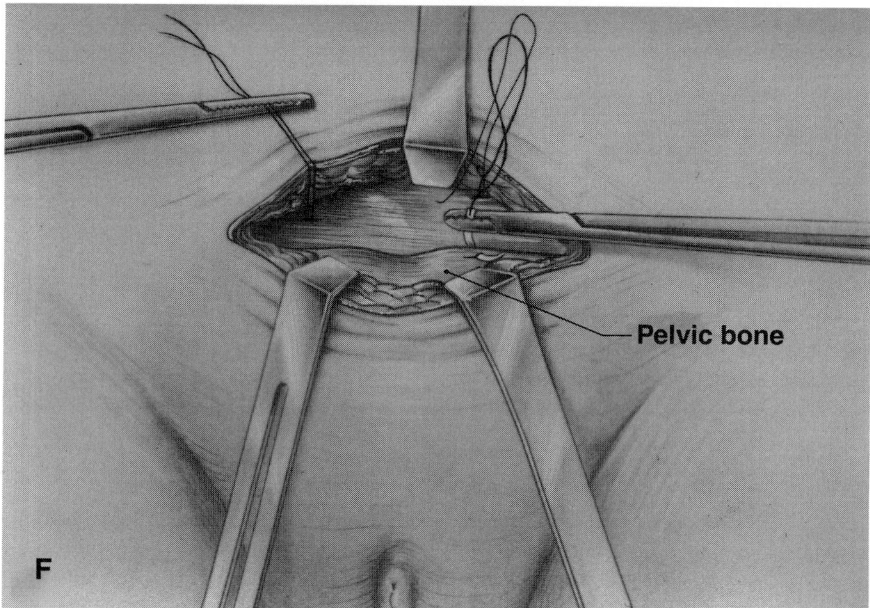


**Fig 10. E:** Transfer of the suspension suture through the retropubic space to the suprapubic position. **F:** Anchoring the suspension suture to the pubic tubercle bilaterally.

symphysis is exposed via a 3- to 4-cm suprapubic incision. A finger is placed vaginally through the perforation of the endopelvic fascia and the Pereyra needle passed under *direct finger guidance,* after the bladder is drained, through the retropubic space and delivered into the vagina. The polypropylene suture on each side is threaded into the eye of the Pereyra needle and transferred to the suprapubic position. Following cystoscopy, the anterior vaginal incisions are closed with absorbable suture (after the suspension sutures are tied the anterior vaginal wall is difficult to reach).

A variety of procedures have been described to secure the suprapubic suspension sutures. The authors favor bone fixation as it provides an excellent anchoring site, reduces the chance of nerve entrapment, thus minimizing the incidence of postoperative pubic pain.[61] When using anterior abdominal wall fascial fixation care should be taken in suture placement as sensory branches of the ilioinguinal nerve or genital branches of the genitofemoral nerve are at risk of injury if the sutures are placed too laterally. An important technical point is that the tension applied to the suspension sutures should only *stabilize* the proximal urethra and bladder neck. Excessive suture tension is avoided lest early failure from suture "pull-through" from the vaginal anchoring tissue or prolonged postoperative urinary retention results. The vaginal pack and Foley catheter are removed on the first postoperative day and the patient begins self-catheterization if residual urine levels are high. Postoperative management is greatly facilitated by *preoperative* teaching of intermittent catheterization. Similarly, in those unable to perform preoperative self-catheterization a temporary suprapubic tube is placed at the time of bladder neck suspension with a modified Lowsley tractor.

Success rates for MPBNS are 51%–96% (Table 3), though few objective studies are available that examine long-term results.[59] A study from the authors' institution in conjunction with the University of Wisconsin reported on 114 women with median follow-up of 42 months. Fifty-one percent were cured of their stress incontinence, 76% were "significantly improved," and 43% still required padding for stress incontinence. Importantly, 23% of patients noted recurrence of their incontinence more than 2 years after the suspension. Thus, success rates of suspension procedures should be viewed cautiously until long-term follow-up data are available.

**TABLE 3. Reported Success Rates of Bladder Neck Suspension Procedures**

| Procedure | Reported Success Rates (%) Overall | Long-Term Follow-up (>3 yr) |
|---|---|---|
| MMK | 60–98 | 57–72 |
| Burch | 80–100 | 89 |
| MPBNS | 51–96 | 76 |
| Stamey | 57–91 | 61 |

MMK, Marshall–Marchetti–Krantz; MPBNS, modified Pereyra bladder neck suspension. Adapted from Kelly MJ, Leach GE,[59], with permission.

**Stamey Needle Suspension.** Technical differences of the Stamey procedure from other transvaginal suspension procedures include the use of a Dacron "bolster" to buttress the anterior vaginal wall suture. Mobilization of the retropubic space is not performed and the transferring needle is passed blindly through the retropubic space without finger control. Reported success rates are 57%–91% (Table 3). Spencer et al., using a strict definition of cure (freedom from stress urinary incontinence), reported a cure rate of 61% in 41 women with a mean follow-up of 46.1 months.[12] Of concern is the potential for bolster erosion into the urethra as well as outflow obstruction from periurethral suture placement and excessive suspension suture tension. Outflow obstruction from periurethral suture placement may occur with the Stamey needle suspension procedure and may reflect the mechanism of continence after the Stamey procedure.[14,62]

## Type III Incontinence

Intrinsic urethral dysfunction resulting from denervation, prior periurethral surgery, trauma, or radiation therapy requires external compression to increase outflow resistance for restoration of continence (Fig 11). Treatment options include periurethral injection for "bulk enhancement" (Teflon, collagen, fat), artificial sphincter, or pubovaginal sling. Patients with type III incontinence may have periurethral scarring with a urethra "fixed" in the retropubic space from scarring or urethral hypermobility. Restoration of a hypermobile or poorly supported type III urethra to the retropubic position will not achieve continence as the primary deficit is not one of anatomic support but of intrinsic urethral damage.

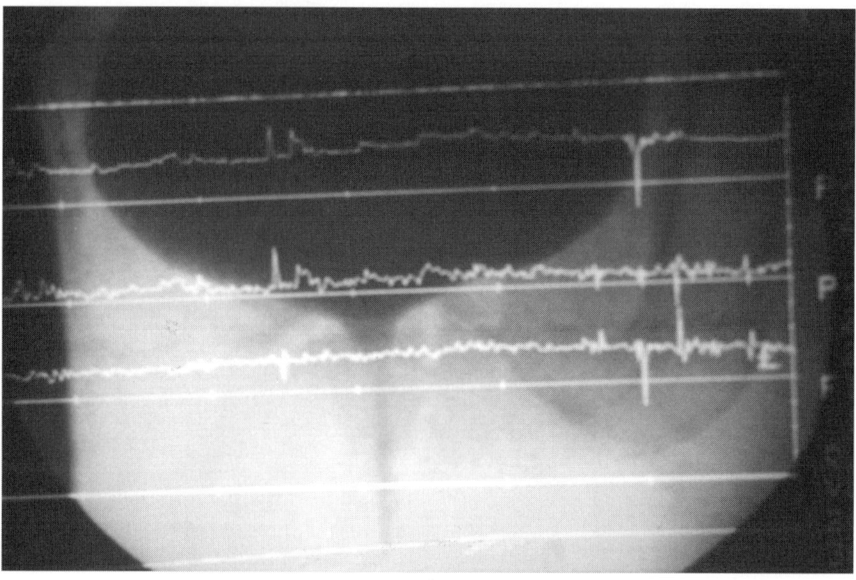

**Fig 11.** Video urodynamic study of a well-supported urethra with an open bladder neck at rest. There loss of contrast with low-pressure Valsalva (<20 cm $H_2O$), indicating type III stress incontinence.

**Pubovaginal Sling.** Many varieties of the sling procedure have been proposed to create a hammock effect beneath the damaged urethra including anterior rectus fascia, fascia lata of the thigh (Fig 12), dermis (skin), vaginal wall, dura mater, and synthetic ma-

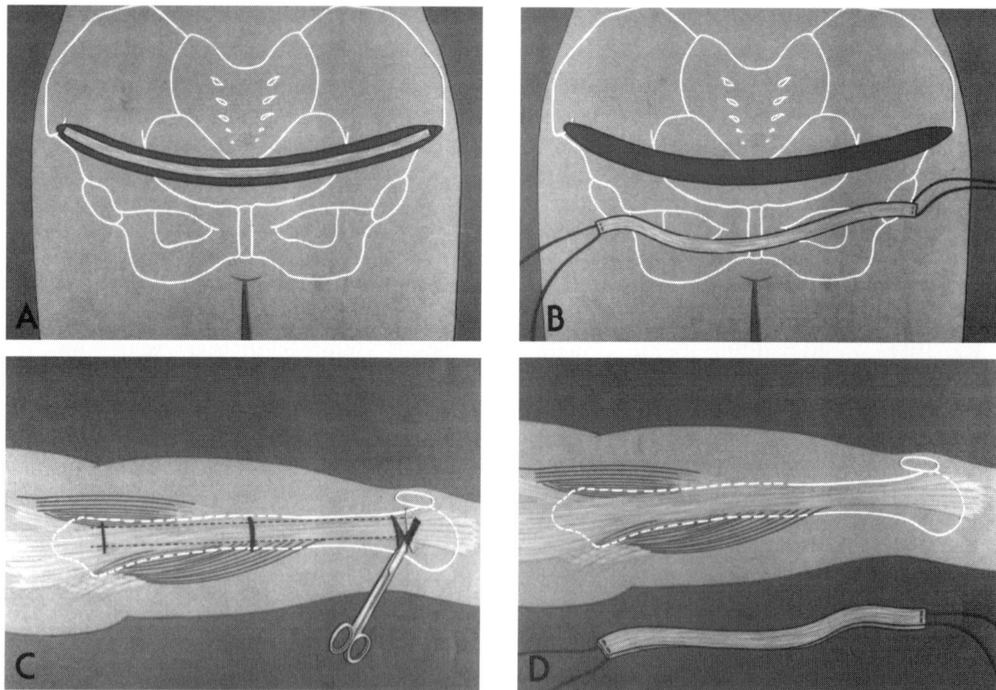


**Fig 12. A, B:** Representation of abdominal fascia harvest for pubovaginal sling. Number 1 nylon is used to secure the fascial strip to the pubic tubercle. **C, D:** Fascia harvest from the lateral thigh (fascia lata).

terial. The authors have used fascia lata almost exclusively in the last 1.5 years with the advantage of reliable strength, ease of harvest, and limited postoperative abdominal pain. The rectus fascia may be scarred and attenuated from prior suprapubic incisions or radiation often encountered in a type III patient population. The technique employed is similar to that described by McGuire and Lytton[63] (Fig 13). Important considerations are complete mobilization of the urethra and bladder neck from the dense periurethral scarring usually present after multiple prior surgeries. The retro-

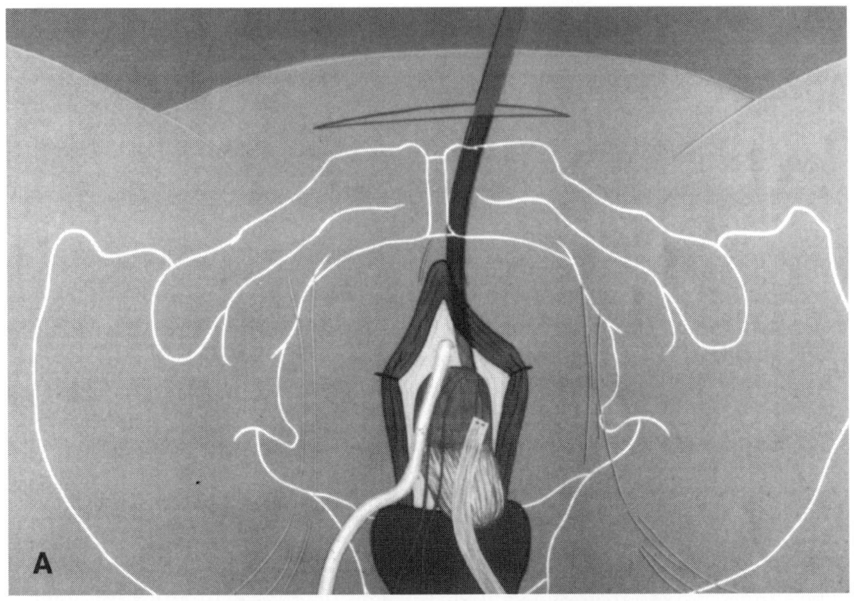


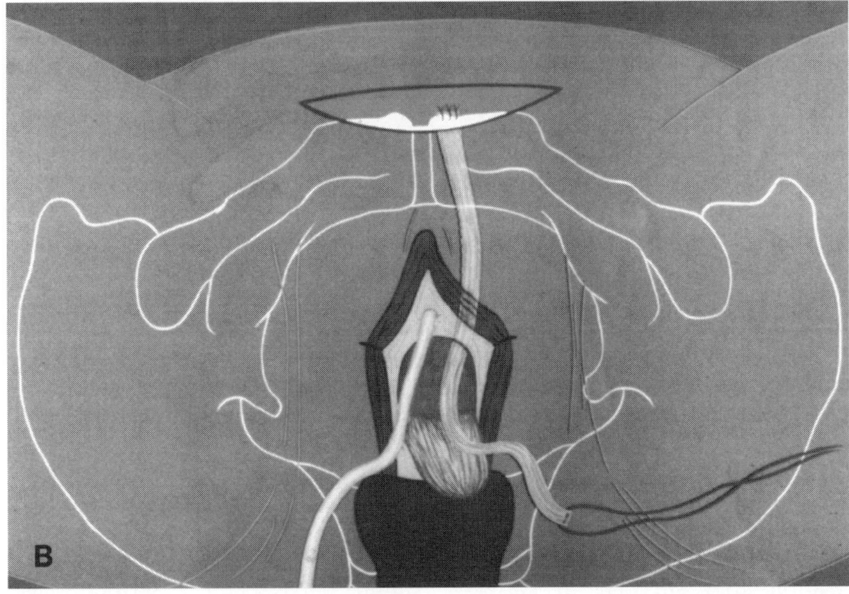


**Fig 13.** Technique of pubovaginal sling. The retropubic space is entered and developed in a fashion similar to steps A and B in Fig 10. **A:** Fascia transfer through retropubic space using a large, blunt-curved clamp. **B:** The fascial strip is secured to the pubic tubercle.

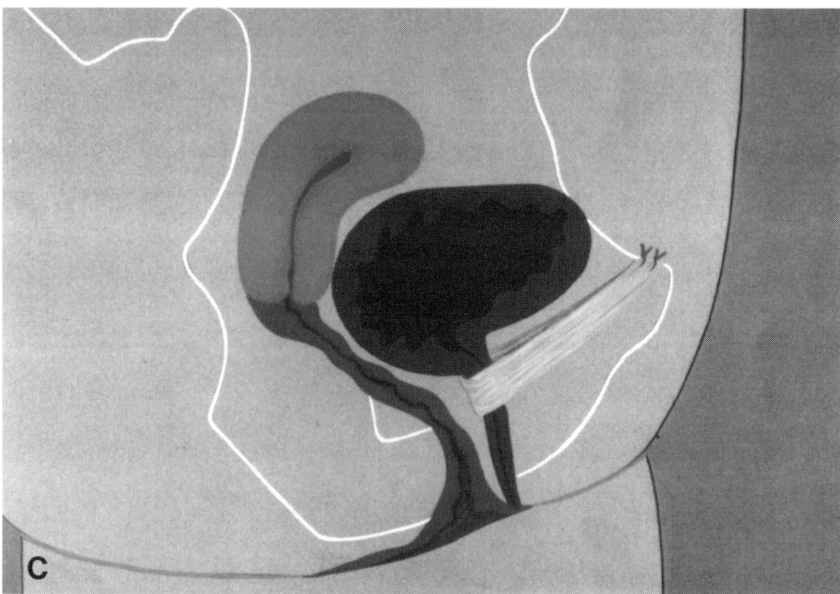


**Fig 13. C:** After carefully adjusting the tension, the fascial strip is positioned beneath the proximal urethra creating a "hammock" effect.

pubic space is carefully entered and dissected sharply as the bladder is often adherent to the pubic bone and may be inadvertently entered with blunt finger dissection. The sling is passed from the vagina through the lateral endopelvic perforation and retropubic space to the suprapubic incision. Sling tension is adjusted while endoscopically observing the urethra. The authors apply just enough tension to the fascia to see minimal impression on the floor of the urethra and are careful not to cause compression of the urethra. Excessive tension may result in urethral obstruction, prolonged urinary retention, and possibly troublesome postoperative detrusor instability. Fixation techniques vary. The authors prefer the pubic tubercle to minimize the chance of nerve entrapment and provide a strong anchor as discussed previously. The McGuire et al. series[64] reported an 81% success rate with 8 of 15 failures secondary to detrusor dysfunction (instability or low compliance). Though almost all patients require temporary self-catheterization after surgery, in patients with normal bladder function the pubovaginal sling causes permanent urinary retention in less than 5%. In patients with neurogenic bladder (myelomeningocele or spinal cord injury) the goal after pubovaginal sling is complete retention with postoperative CIC.

The vaginal wall sling involves using a rectangular piece of attached vaginal wall supported by four-corner nonabsorbable sutures and passed to a suprapubic position similar to MPBNS.[65] Vaginal inclusion cysts have not been a problem[66] but long-term follow-up is not available.

**Artificial Urinary Sphincter.** Indications for an AUS in the management of type III SUI are the same as for a pubovaginal sling with some additional caveats (a patient who refuses CIC is not a candidate for pubovaginal sling). In addition to normal urodynamic parameters such as bladder compliance, adequate capacity, and no instability, the patient must be motivated and have the manual dexterity to operate the pump. AUS has no role in the management of type I or II SUI.

Transabdominal and transvaginal techniques have been described.[67] Reported success rates are 66%–91% with follow-up ranging from 3 months to 6 years.[68,69] Complications include mechanical failure requiring reoperation in up to 21%, infection, urethral atrophy, and cuff erosion into the urethra or vagina. The authors prefer procedures that restore continence in women without the use of a prosthetic device particularly in patients with compromised periurethral tissue such as after prior periurethral surgery or radiation therapy.

**Periurethral Injection.** Periurethral injection of bulk-enhancing materials to increase outflow resistance is a conceptually attractive therapy for type III SUI. Periurethral injection is not indicated for type I and II "anatomic" SUI as the urethral closure mechanism is not compromised. Advantages to periurethral injection include technical simplicity, local anesthesia, and outpatient procedure.

***Collagen.*** Application is by periurethral needle penetration next to the urethral meatus (Fig 14). The needle is guided to a submucosal position at the proximal urethra under cystoscopic control. Although transurethral injection has been described, the authors prefer periurethral injection to decrease the chance of extrusion of the injected substance into the urethral lumen. With injection, one can observe the material layering submucosally gradually occluding the urethral lumen. Multiple quadrants are injected until visual occlusion of the proximal and midurethra occurs. The multicenter study group on GAX collagen[70] reported an 80% success at 2 years (average 1.7 injections and 16 $cm^3$). In those maintaining continence for more than 2 years, the mean rise in leak point pressure was 41 cm $H_2O$. Because of possible hypersensitivity reaction routine skin testing is recommended.

***Teflon.*** The technique of polytetrafluorourethane (Polytef) injection is similar to collagen although a high-pressure gun-like instrument is required to inject the thick paste. In the authors' experience, although all women have initial symptomatic improvement, the durable results (24-month follow-up) of periurethral Teflon in women with type III SUI suggest that 60% have some symptomatic improvement but only

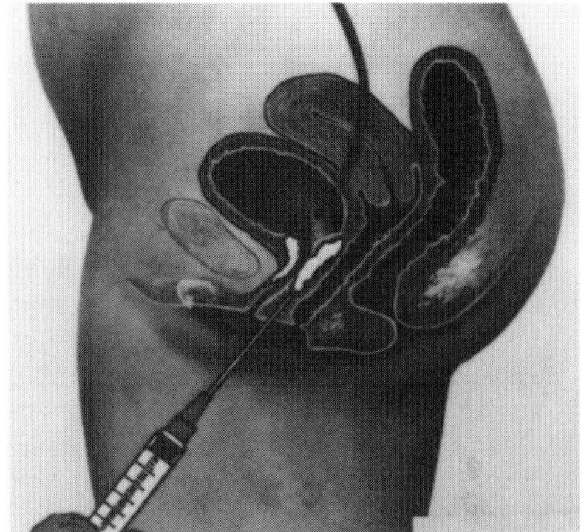

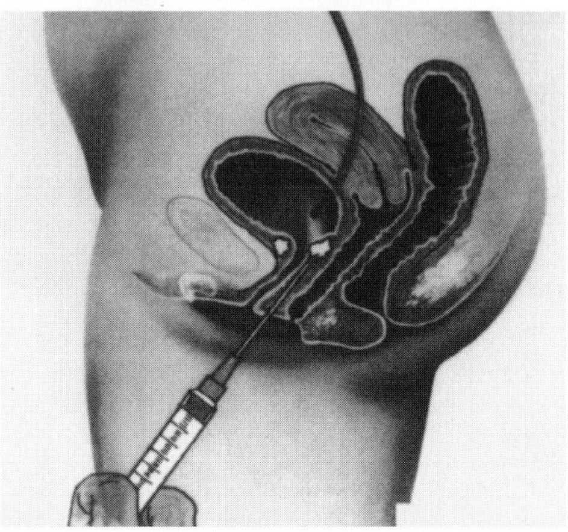

**Fig 14.** Sagittal view of periurethral injection in the female. Note the deposition of material (that may represent collagen, Teflon, or fat) in proximal urethra and midurethra.

10% are totally continent. Multiple injections are required (1.5–1.8) and those failing injection therapy may still be salvaged with pubovaginal sling. As with men, concerns regarding particle migration limit the application on this substance to older women (>60 years). FDA approval for use in women has not yet been granted.

***Other Periurethral Substances.*** In the report by Blaivas and Santarosa[54] in which liposuction harvested autologous fat for periurethral injection, 60% of women were improved (40% cured and 20% improved) after a mean of three injections with a follow-up of 6 months (range 3–10 months).

All of the failures had hypermobility in addition to urethral dysfunction. In those without hypermobility, 88% improved. The cost advantage of this outpatient procedure performed under local anesthesia as well as the autologous nature of the fat (circumventing the migration and allergic concerns with the other injectables) makes this procedure attractive. Although MRI studies have demonstrated persistence of the injected fat for 3 months,[71] resorption may result in recurrence of the incontinence and long-term results are pending at this time.

### Surgical Treatment of Urge Incontinence

**Denervation Procedures.** Denervation procedures are of historical interest and are rarely indicated. Denervation implies functional destruction of the nerve supply to an organ. This cannot be done effectively to the bladder because the peripheral ganglia are so close to the muscle; therefore, these procedures result at best in partial denervation or "decentralization." The decentralized bladder may become acutely areflexic but in the long term poor compliance usually develops. The high intravesical pressure from poor compliance may manifest as incontinence, urgency and frequency, or hydronephrosis.

Reported methods of denervation include peripheral approaches such as transvaginal subtrigonal dissection of detrusor afferents (Ingleman–Sundberg procedure), subtrigonal phenol injection, and open suprapubic procedures such as detrusor myotomy (multiple incisions through the detrusor muscle to the mucosa), cystocystoplasty (supratrigonal bladder transection with immediate reattachment), and cystolysis (division of superior neurovascular pedicle and superior aspect of inferior neurovascular pedicle as in cystectomy without removing the bladder). The long-term efficacy of peripheral "denervation" procedures has not been demonstrated and clinically these procedures have not achieved widespread acceptance.

The Ingleman–Sundberg procedure was reported to be effective in 72% of patients with follow-up of at least one year.[72] However, the authors feel that transvaginal partial denervation should only be used as a last resort in those who improve with a trial transvaginal subtrigonal injection of marcaine after failing all other conservative therapies.

Central attempts of denervation stem from the anatomic description of S3 as the major motor root to the bladder.[73] Selective ablation has been attempted by direct transection (selective dorsal rhizotomy, presacral neurectomy) or destruction (injection of phenol or alcohol into the root). Lack of selectivity has resulted in inadvertent loss of motor or sensory function at sites other than the detrusor (ie, impotence, fecal incontinence). Though the expected clinical areflexic bladder may be observed acutely, in the long term poor compliance often results secondarily to decentralization. Potential complications of subtrigonal phenol injection including ureteral necrosis and vesico vaginal fistula make this procedure prohibitively risky.

**Augmentation Cystoplasty.** The use of an intestinal segment to enlarge the small contracted bladder is not a new one; Mikulicz[74] used ileum in 1898 for enterocystoplasty. Augmentation cystoplasty has emerged as the definitive form of management of patients with severe, refractory hyperreflexia/instability and/or poor compliance only since the widespread acceptance of intermittent catheterization.[75] Though in-depth discussion of augmentation cystoplasty is beyond the scope of this chapter, some basic principles must be reviewed. The goal of the augmented bladder is to create a pain-free, adequate capacity reservoir that stores urine at low pressure. However, patients must accept permanent urinary retention as a trade-off for eliminating urinary incontinence. The use of detubularized bowel to prevent high pressures from intestinal contractions was recognized by Goodwin et al.[76] Detubularized bowel configured into a spherical shape will hold more volume than a cylinder (nondetubularized) and with a contraction will generate less pressure.[77] Properly detubularized, any segment of bowel can be an effective low-pressure reservoir, although jejunum should not be used because of fluid and electrolyte considerations. Different segments of bowel used in augmentation include ileum, ileocecum, colon, and stomach and the many configurations of intestinal segments have been reviewed and described.[78] Whether supratrigonal cystectomy is necessary for successful augmentation is controversial. Historically, contracted bladders from chronic tuberculosis were resected. Subsequent work suggested that contracted bladders left intact forced urine upward into the augmented portion rendering the bowel segment a functional diverticulum.[79,80] Others contest this and have shown satisfactory results in those patients whose bladders were not resected.[81] The authors do not routinely resect the detrusor prior to augmentation. Concurrent management of the incompetent outlet (which may coexist with high-pressure bladder dysfunction), particularly with neurologic disease like myelomeningocele and sacral arc denervation, includes sling and artificial sphincter, and is discussed elsewhere.[82] An absolute contraindication to augmentation is a history of bladder cancer and those unwilling to perform intermittent catheterization. Relative contraindications are a medically unstable patient and significantly impaired renal function.

A review of major series of augmentation cystoplasty[83] demonstrates success rates of 80%–90%, with the exception being patients after radiation therapy for pelvic malignancy where poor wound healing reduces favorable results to about 50%.

### Management of Mixed Incontinence

An example of mixed incontinence is postprostatectomy incontinence. Leach and Yun[6] reviewed 107 incontinent men postprostatectomy (71 after radical prostatectomy, 26 transurethral, and 10 open prostatectomy) with in-depth urodynamics and found that only 37% had incontinence as a result of sphincteric incompetence alone. Thirty-four percent had combined sphincteric incompetence and bladder dysfunction (uninhibited detrusor contractions and/or poor compliance) while 20% had bladder dysfunction alone as the sole cause of their incontinence. Overall, 39% of their treatment group became socially continent using medical management (behavioral and pharmacotherapy) alone. Clearly, effective management of bladder dysfunction in this patient population is critical for successful treatment of clinical symptomatology. Recently, Perez and Webster[84] reported that in men with postprostatectomy incontinence, poorly controlled bladder dysfunction *does not* increase the risk of upper tract deterioration after AUS placement in the patients' hands, although these high-risk patients had more postoperative incontinence than those with no bladder dysfunction. Until this experience is confirmed by other investigators, the authors continue to emphasize the importance of adequate low-pressure bladder storage before an AUS is inserted.

Preoperative urgency symptoms may be found in up to 60% of women with SUI with CMG-documented instability in 15%–30%.[24,85] The relative severity and contribution of the SUI and UI must be assessed symptomatically and confirmed urodynamically for effective treatment planning. When stress symptoms predominate and evaluation confirms type II SUI, anatomic correction of the hypermobility may resolve the urge symptoms. McGuire and Savastano[86] reported 85% of patients with instability (ie, with urgency symptoms or proven detrusor instability) respond to a bladder neck suspension (BNS) without need for subsequent use of pharmacotherapy to control urge symptoms. Kelly and Leach[59] found resolution of urgency complaints in 59% of patients after BNS. De novo detrusor instability from outlet obstruction may complicate the clinical picture after BNS and require the addition of pharmacotherapy.

It is controversial whether the urgency symptoms or proven detrusor instability before BNS adversely influences the outcome of surgery. Some authors suggest postoperative urgency symptoms and detrusor instability are highly related to recurrent stress leakage and subjective failure rates.[87,88] In the presence of preoperative instability, the authors routinely counsel patients that symptomatic urgency may persist and additional medical management of the instability may be necessary after BNS.

Another common clinical scenario is the woman presenting with predominant urge and urge incontinence who is found on urodynamic evaluation to have detrusor instability with type II SUI. These patients receive management of the symptomatically dominant urge component with behavioral programs and pharmacotherapy after which further assessment is made to evaluate the severity of any pertinent SUI.

## SUMMARY

The key to effective management of urinary incontinence is proper evaluation and diagnosis of the underlying pathophysiology. A thorough understanding of the expected outcomes of therapy provides the groundwork for treatment. Management of urinary incontinence should proceed logically, incorporating initial nonoperative therapies followed by surgical procedures when indicated. Clear understanding of the benefits and limitations of various therapies for urinary incontinence will equip the urologist to effectively treat a currently underserved patient population.

## REFERENCES

1. Hu T. Impact of urinary incontinence on health care costs. *J Am Geriat Soc.* 1990;38:292.
2. Help for Incontinent People (HIP), P.O. Box 544, Union, SC 29397.
3. Dula E, Leach GE. The role of the urologist in the diagnosis of multiple sclerosis. *Urology.* 1989;7:124.
4. Katz GP, Blaivas JG. A diagnostic dilemma: when urodynamic findings differ from the clinical impression. *J Urol.* 1983;129:1170.
5. Wise BG, Cutner A, Cardozo LD, et al. Do detailed symptom questionnaires negate the need for urodynamic investigation? *Neurourol Urodyn.* 1992;11:353.
6. Leach GE, Yun S. Post prostatectomy incontinence. 1. The urodynamic findings in 107 men. *Neurourol Urodyn.* 1992;11:91–97.
7. Braendjord LW, Bakke A, Klenmark B. Incidence of improvement of bladder emptying in 1702 patients on clean intermittent catheterization. *Neurourol Urodyn.* 1992;11:411(A).
8. Light JK, Beric A, Wise PG. Predictive criteria for failed sphincterotomy in spinal cord injury patients. *J Urol.* 1987;138:1201.
9. Bass JS, Leach GE. Bladder outlet obstruction in women. *Prob Urol.* 1991;5:141.
10. Leach GE, Yip C, Donovan BJ. Mechanism of continence after modified Pereyra bladder neck suspension. *Urology.* 1987;29:328.
11. Marshall VF, Marchetti AA, Krantz KE. The correction of stress incontinence by simple vesicourethral suspension. *Surg Gynecol Obstet.* 1949;88:509.
12. Spencer JR, O'Connor VJ, Schaeffer AJ. A comparison of endoscopic suspension of the vesical neck with suprapubic vesicourethropexy for treatment of stress urinary incontinence. *J Urol.* 1987;137:411.
13. McDuffie RW, Litin RB, Blundon KE. Urethrovesical suspension (Marshall–Marchetti–Krantz): experience with 204 cases. *Am J Surg.* 1981;141:297.
14. Constantinou CE, Govan DE, Stamey TA. Modification of urethral resistance, and detrusor stability by endoscopic bladder neck suspension. In: *Proceedings of the Third Joint Meeting of the International Continence Society and the Urodynamic Society.* Boston: 1986;236.
15. Zimmern PE, Hadkey HR, Leach GE, Raz S. Female urethra obstruction after Marshall–Marchetti–Krantz operation. *J Urol.* 1987;138:517.
16. McGuire EJ, Letson W, Wang S. Transvaginal urethrolysis after obstructing urethral suspension procedures. *J Urol.* 1989;142:1037–1039.
17. Massey JA, Abrams PH. Obstructed voiding in the female. *Br J Urol.* 1988;61:36.
18. Farrar DJ, Osborne JL, Stephenson TP, et al. A urodynamic view of bladder outflow obstruction in the female: factors influencing the results of treatment. *Br J Urol.* 1976;47:815.
19. Diokno AC, Hollander JB, Bennett CJ. Bladder neck obstruction in women: a real entity. *J Urol.* 1987;132:294.
20. Raz S, Kutke C, Golumb J. Four-corner bladder and urethral suspension for moderate cystocele. *J Urol.* 1989;142:712.
21. McGuire EJ, Woodside JR, Borden TA, et al. Prognostic value of urodynamic testing in myelodysplastic patients. *J Urol.* 1981;26:205.
22. Staskin DR. Hydroureteronephrosis after spinal cord injury. *Urol Clin North Am.* 1991;18:309.
23. Kelly MJ, Zimmern PE, Leach GE. Complications of bladder neck suspension procedures. *Urol Clin North Am.* 1991;18:339.
24. McGuire EJ, Lytton B, Kohorn EI, Pepe V. The value of urodynamic testing in stress urinary incontinence. *J Urol.* 1980;124:256.
25. Lapides J, Diokno AC, Silber SJ, Lowe BS. Clean intermittent self-catheterization in the treatment of urinary tract disease. *Trans Am Assoc Genitourin Surg.* 1971;63:92.

26. Rink RC, et al. Intermittent catheterization and the artificial urinary sphincter: compatible techniques in children with neurogenic bladder dysfunction. *J Urol.* 1985;133:352.
27. Bennett CJ, Diokno AC. Clean intermittent catheterization in the management of the neurogenic bladder in children. *J Urol.* 1984;132:526.
28. Newman AK, Smith DA, Harris T, Diokno A. An external female barrier device in the management of urinary incontinence. *Neurourol Urodyn.* 1992;11:368(A).
29. Fantl JA, Wyman JF, McClish DK, Harkins SW, et al. Efficacy of bladder training in older women with urinary incontinence. *JAMA.* 1991;65:609.
30. Cardozo LD, Abrams PD, Stanton SL. Idiopathic bladder instability treated by biofeedback. *Br J Urol.* 1978;50:427.
31. Kegel AH. Stress incontinence of urine in women. Physiologic treatment. *J Int Coll Surg.* 1956;25:487.
32. Burgio KL, Robinson JC, Engel BT. Comparison of bladder sphincter feedback and Kegel exercises. Bethesda, MD: Gerontology Research Center National Institute on Aging; 1985.
33. Thompson I, Lauvetz R. Oxybutynin in bladder spasm, neurogenic bladder and enuresis. *Urology.* 1976;8:452.
34. Gajewski JB, Awad JA. Oxybutynin versus propantheline in patients with multiple sclerosis and detrusor hyperreflexia. *J Urol.* 1986;135:966.
35. Holmes DM, Monty FJ, Stanton SL. Oxybutynin versus propantheline in the management of detrusor instability: a patient regulated variable dose trial. *Br J Obstet Gynaecol.* 1989; 96:607.
36. Raz S, Ziegler M, Caine M. The role of female hormones in stress incontinence. *Proceedings of the 16th Congress of Société Internationale d'Urologie.* Vol 1. Paris: Doin; 1973;397.
37. Biesland HO, Fossberg E, Moer A, et al. Urethral sphincteric insufficiency in postmenopausal females: treatment with phenylpropanolamine and estriol separately and in combination. *Urol Int.* 1984;39:211.
38. Connolly MJ, Astridge PS, White EG, et al. Torsades de pointes ventricular tachycardia and terodiline. *Lancet.* 1991;338:344.
39. Lindholm P, Lose G. Terbutaline (Bricanyl) in the treatment of female urge incontinence. *Urol Int.* 1986;41:158.
40. Madersbacher H, Knoll M, Kiss G. Intravesical application of oxybutynin: mode of action in controlling detrusor hyperreflexia. Proceedings of the 21st annual meeting of the International Continence Society. *Neurourol Urodyn.* 1991; 10:375.
41. Glickman S, Tsokos N, Glass J, Bywater HJ, et al. Intravesical atropine suppression of detrusor hyperreflexia. Proceedings of the 22nd annual meeting of the International Continence Society. *Neurourol Urodyn.* 1992;11:330.
42. McGuire EJ, Zhang S, Horwinski ER. Treatment of motor and sensory detrusor instability by electrical stimulation. *J Urol.* 1983;129:78–79.
43. Pelvnik S, Janez J, Vodusek DB. Electrical stimulation. In: Krane RJ, Siroky MB, eds. *Clinical Neuro-Urology.* 2nd ed. Boston: Little, Brown; 1991;559.
44. Webb RJ, Powell PH. Transcutaneous electrical nerve stimulation in patients with idiopathic detrusor instability. Proceedings of the 22nd annual meeting of the International Continence Society. *Neurourol Urodyn.* 1992;11:327.
45. Pelvnik S, Janez J, Yrtacnik P. Short-term electrical stimulation: home treatment for minor incontinence. *W J Urol.* 1986;4:24.
46. Schmidt RA. Experience with neurostimulation in urology. In Webster GD, ed. *Prob Urol.* 1989; 3:135.
47. Philip T, Shah PJR, Worth PHL. Acupuncture in the treatment of bladder instability. *Br J Urol.* 1988;61:490.
48. Perlmutter AD. Urinary tract reconstruction and the abnormal bladder. *Urol Clin North Am.* 1980; 7:379.
49. Malizia AA, Reiman JM, Meyers RP, et al. Migration and granulomatous reaction after periurethral injection of Polytef (Teflon). *JAMA.* 1984; 251:3277.
50. Politano VA. Periurethral Teflon injection for urinary incontinence. *Urol Clin North Am.* 1978; 5:415.
51. Kaufman M, Lockhart JL, Silverstein MJ, Politano VA. Transurethral polytetrafluoroethylene injection for postprostatectomy incontinence. *J Urol.* 1984;132:459.
52. Appell RA, McGuire EJ, DeRidder PA, et al. Updated multicenter study on the use of GAX-Collagen for male urinary incontinence due to outflow incompetence. *J Urol.* 1992; 147:399A.
53. Appell RA. Injectables for urethral incompetence. *W J Urol.* 1990;8:208.
54. Blaivas JG, Santarosa RP. Periurethral fat injection for sphincteric incompetence. *Neurourol Urodyn.* 1992;11:403(A).
55. Scott FB, Bradley WE, Timm GW, Kothari D. Treatment of incontinence secondary to myelodysplasia by an implantable prosthetic urinary sphincter. *South Med J.* 1973;66:987.
56. Leach GE, Raz S. Perfusion sphincterometry; a method of intraoperative evaluation of artificial urinary sphincter function. *Urology.* 1983;21: 312.
57. Marchetti AA, Marshall VF, Shultis LD. Simple vesicourethral suspension. *Am J Obstet Gynecol.* 1957;74:57.
58. Burch JC. Urethrovaginal fixation to Cooper's ligament for correction of stress urinary incontinence, cystocele and prolapse. *Am J Obstet Gynecol.* 1961;81:281.

59. Kelly MJ, Leach GE. Long term results of bladder neck suspension procedures. *Prob Urol.* 1991;5:94.
60. Pereyra AJ. A simplified surgical procedure for the correction of stress incontinence in women. *W J Surg Obstet Gynecol.* 1959;67:223.
61. Leach GE. Bone fixation technique for transvaginal needle suspension. *Urology.* 1988;31:388.
62. Mundy AR. A trial comparing the Stamey bladder neck suspension with colposuspension for the treatment of stress urinary incontinence. *Br J Urol.* 1983;55:687.
63. McGuire E, Lytton B. Pubovaginal sling procedure for stress incontinence. *J Urol.* 1978;119: 82.
64. McGuire EJ, Bennett C, Konnak J, et al. Experience with pubovaginal slings for urinary incontinence at the University of Michigan. *J Urol.* 1987;138:525.
65. Raz S, Sigel A, Short J, Snyder J. Vaginal wall sling. *J Urol.* 1989;141:43.
66. Phillips TH, Zeidman EJ, Thompson IM. Fate of buried vaginal epithelium. *J Urol.* 1992;148: 1941.
67. Hadley HR. The artificial urinary sphincter in the female. *Prob Urol.* 1991;5:123.
68. Scott FB, Fishman IJ, Shabshig R. The impact of the artificial urinary sphincter in the neurogenic bladder on the upper urinary tracts. *J Urol.* 1986;136:636.
69. Diokno AC, Hollander JB, Alderson TP. Artificial urinary sphincter for recurrent female incontinence: indications and results. *J Urol.* 1987; 138:778.
70. Appell RA, McGuire EJ, DeRidder PA, Bennett AH, Webster GD, Bennett JK, Badlani GH. Updated multicenter study on the use of GAX-Collagen for female type III stress urinary incontinence. *J Urol.* 1992;147:279A.
71. Palma PCR, Netto NR, Vidal BC, Campinas SSL. Magnetic resonance imaging of urethra after periurethral injection for urinary stress incontinence. *J Urol.* 1992;147:652A.
72. Wan J, McGuire EJ, Wang S. Ingleman–Sundberg bladder denervation for detrusor instability. *J Urol.* 1991;145:358(A).
73. Heimburger RF, Freeman LW, Wilde NJ. Sacral nerve innervation of the human bladder. *J Neurosurg.* 1948;5:154.
74. Mikulicz J. Zur operation der augeborenen blasenspalte. *Zentralbl Chir.* 1898;26:641.
75. Linder AL, Leach GE, Raz S. Augmentation cystoplasty in the treatment of neurogenic bladder dysfunction. *J Urol.* 1983;129:491.
76. Goodwin WE, Winter CC, Barker WF. ''Cup patch'' technique of ileocystoplasty for bladder enlargement or partial substitution. *Surg Gynecol Obstet.* 1959;108:240.
77. Hinman F. Selection of intestinal segments for bladder substitution: physical and physiologic characteristics. *J Urol.* 1988;139:519.
78. Benson MC, Olsson CA. Urinary diversion. In: Walsh PC, Retik AB, Stamey TA, Vaughn ED, eds. *Campbells Urology.* 6th ed. Philadelphia: WB Saunders; 1992:2654.
79. Gittes RF. Bladder augmentation procedures. In: Libertino JA, Zinman L, eds. *Reconstructive Urologic Surgery: Pediatric and Adult.* Baltimore: Williams and Wilkins; 1977: 216.
80. Zinman L, Libertino JA. Technique of augmentation cystoplasty. *Surg Clin North Am.* 1979;6: 137.
81. Smith RB, Van Cangh P, Skinner DG, et al. Augmentation enterocystoplasty: a critical review. *J Urol.* 1977;118;35.
82. Bauer SB. Urologic management of the myelodysplastic child. *Prob Urol.* 1989;3:86.
83. Webster GD, Coldwasser B, Kreder KJ. Management of the contracted bladder. In: Krane RJ, Siroky MB, eds. *Clinical Neuro-Urology.* 2nd ed. Boston: Little, Brown; 1991:593.
84. Perez LM, Webster GD. Successful outcome of artificial urinary sphincters in men with post-prostatectomy urinary incontinence despite adverse implantation features. *J Urol.* 1992;148: 1166.
85. Kelly MJ, Nielson K, Roskamp D, et al. Symptom analysis of patients undergoing modified Pereyra bladder neck suspension for stress urinary incontinence. *Urology.* 1991;37:213.
86. McGuire EJ, Savastano JA. Stress incontinence and detrusor instability/urge incontinence. *Neurourol Urodyn.* 1985;4;313.
87. Webster GD, Sihelnik SA, Stone AR. Female urinary incontinence: the incidence, identification and characteristics of detrusor instability. *Neurourol Urodyn.* 1984;3:235.
88. Lockhart JL, Tirado A, Morillo G, Politano VA. Vesicourethral dysfunction following cystourethropexy. *J Urol.* 1982;128:943.

# 19

# Interstitial Cystitis and Female Urethral Syndrome

*Philip Hanno*

## INTRODUCTION

The two most common and least understood entities that are encompassed by the term *painful bladder* are the urethral syndrome and interstitial cystitis (IC). The painful bladder disease complex includes a large group of urologic patients with pain in the bladder, irritative voiding symptoms (urgency, frequency, nocturia, dysuria), and sterile urine. There are painful bladder diseases with a well-known etiology and pathogenesis. These include radiation cystitis, cyclophosphamide cystitis, carcinoma in situ, malacoplakia, and systemic diseases affecting the bladder.[1] Cystitis and/or urethritis caused by organisms in low "insignificant" colony counts or by organisms such as *Chlamydia,* that are not routinely cultured for are common infectious processes causing symptoms that used to be ascribed to urethral syndrome.[2] The differential diagnosis of pelvic pain also includes endometriosis in females and epididymitis, prostatodynia, and nonbacterial prostatitis in males.[3] In fact, symptoms attributed to prostatodynia in males are remarkably reminiscent of urethral syndrome in females.[4]

While the etiology of both the urethral syndrome and interstitial cystitis remains in doubt, there is reason to believe that they may be varying manifestations of a single spectrum of disease, with the more self-limited forms and those with less in the way of clinical findings categorized as urethral syndrome. As current methods of investigation continue to shed light on this group of problems, we will likely see a continuation in the trend to diminish the use of the very nonspecific diagnosis of urethral syndrome.

## URETHRAL SYNDROME

As recently as May 1985, *Urologic Clinics of North America* covering "female urology" had a chapter on the urethral syndrome[3] and only an isolated page on IC.[5] In the last few years the tables have turned, and an enormous funding effort and body of literature on IC has evolved,[6,7] with little being written or researched regarding the urethral syndrome.

The term *urethral syndrome* was first mentioned in a clinicopathological study of the female urethra in 1949 by Powell and Powell.[8] Four years earlier the distinguished American physician Richard Cabot was quoted as having stated that "any pain within two feet of the female urethra for which one cannot find an adequate explanation should be suspected of coming from the female urethra.[9] The urethral syndrome can be defined as a symptoms complex consisting of urinary frequency, urgency, dysuria, and suprapubic discomfort without any objective findings of urologic pathology. Typically, these symptoms occur in women; however, there is no reason to assume that a similar entity does not occur in the male.[10]

The diagnosis is one of exclusion. Urinalysis, cultures, cytologic studies, and cystoscopy—including cystoscopic examination under anesthesia if a diagnosis of IC is entertained—are all unremarkable. Nocturia is unusual.[11]

Theories as to the etiology of urethral syndrome are varied. Hormonal imbalances, reactions to ingested or environmental chemicals, and allergic conditions have been proposed with little supporting evidence and are not widely accepted.[12] Many authors have supported the idea of urethral stenosis and reported good results with urethral dilatation.[13–16] However, diagnostic criteria are inconsistent, histologic studies claiming to document periurethral fibrosis are not reproducible, and a truly stenotic urethra in these patients is probably very rare.[17,18]

Neurogenic and psychogenic causes of urethral syndrome have been explored, but the case for either of these is highly controversial.[10] If the condition is strictly defined as occurring with sterile urine and negative urine cytology, evidence for an anatomic, infectious, inflammatory, or neurogenic cause is weak.[12] One can then speculate that it might be psychogenic[19] or that it may fall into the spectrum represented in its extreme by IC. One must remember that in few if any papers written about urethral syndrome were patients clinically evaluated to exclude IC as it is now defined.

While infection often causes symptoms of the urethral syndrome, by definition bacterial urethritis, if diagnosed, would not be urethral syndrome. Stamm et al reported that many patients with urethral syndrome have pyuria, and a significant proportion of these patients actually have a chlamydial urethritis that can be treated successfully with appropriate antibiotics.[2] Wilkins et al[20] proposed an infectious theory of urethral syndrome and IC, but their finding of fastidious organisms (*Gardnerella vaginalis* and *Lactobacillus sp*) in urine specimens or bladder biopsies in a group of 20 patients with painful bladder disease was not compared to a control group. In a carefully controlled clinical and microbiological study of the urethral syndrome, Gillespie was unable to find any difference in the incidence of positive cultures with fastidious organisms in disease and control groups, and concluded that the urethral syndrome is not caused by bacterial or chlamydial infection.[21] Certainly one can justify a trial of antibiotics, especially in patients with pyuria, even in the absence of positive cultures in symptomatic patients.

The same diagnostic techniques used in the evaluation of IC and detailed in the following section are useful in diagnosing the urethral syndrome. Indeed, as both are essentially diagnoses of exclusion, one must be sure that specific disease entities (nicely detailed in the National Institutes of Health [NIH] "research definition" of interstitial cystitis below) are indeed not responsible for the symptom complex. While urine and urethral cultures are critical, urodynamics and cystoscopy under anesthesia with bladder distention can be postponed until symptoms have persisted for 6 to 9 months, as many patients will experience spontaneous and long-lived remission of their symptoms. Urine cytology and imaging studies to rule out other conditions can also be withheld assuming the symptoms resolve in a matter of weeks.

A course of antibiotics would seem to be the mainstay of treatment, even in the absence of positive cultures. Doxycycline, erythromycin, and flagyl have been recommended to treat the fastidious organisms and anaerobes potentially missed on routine culture.[12] When antibiotics fail, numerous other treatments have been recommended including endoscopic and open surgical procedures designed to treat urethral stenosis, local fulgeration, or scarification of the urethra, and virtually the entire gamut of treatments used for interstitial cystitis and mentioned in the following section. The physician's time and reassurance may be the best medicine.

## INTERSTITIAL CYSTITIS

Possibly one of the most challenging diseases in the urologic spectrum, IC has only recently been recognized as the major health problem that it is.[22] The exponential growth in clinical and basic research is largely due to the efforts of patient groups who demanded that more attention be paid to this problem.[23] Unfortunately, IC can only be diagnosed with cystoscopic examination under anesthesia, perhaps explaining why many cases are often overlooked even by urologists.

### Definition

Interstitial cystitis remains essentially a diagnosis of exclusion. With little certain about its etiology and little distinctive about its pathology, groups of basic scientists and clinicians working through the NIH have arbitrarily proposed a set of characteristics that have come to define the disease.[24] While originally meant to be criteria for entry into NIH-funded research projects on IC, for lack of anything better they seem to have evolved into the de facto definition. Clearly, there are many patients with the syndrome who fall outside of these guidelines. The NIH diagnostic criteria for interstitial cystitis are as follows:

Criteria required for *inclusion* as diagnostic of IC:

A. One of the following two cystoscopic findings must be present:
   1. Glomerulations.
   2. A classic Hunner's ulcer—a discreet bladder ulceration typically noted at the time of bladder distention and present in a distinct minority of patients. An examination for glomerulations should be undertaken after distention of the bladder with the subject under anesthesia and the fluid inflow pressure at 80 to 100 cm $H_2O$ for 1 to 2 minutes. The bladder may be distended up to two times before evaluation. The glomerulations must be diffuse—present in at least three quadrants of the bladder—and there must be at least 10 glomerulations per quadrant. The glomerulations must not lie along the path of the cystoscope (to eliminate artifacts due to instrumentation contact).

B. One of the following two subjective symptoms must be present:
   1. Pain associated with the bladder.
   2. Urinary urgency.

Criteria required for *exclusion* as diagnostic of IC:

1. A bladder capacity of >350 mL on cystometry carried out in conscious subjects using either a gas or liquid medium.
2. Absence of an intense urge to void in patients whose bladder has been filled to 100 mL gas or 150 mL water during cystometry at a fill rate of 30 to 100 mL/min.
3. Demonstration of phasic involuntary bladder contractions on cystometry using the fill rate described above.
4. Duration of symptoms of <9 months.
5. Absence of nocturia.
6. Occurrence of symptoms that are relieved by antimicrobials, urinary antiseptics, anticholinergics, or antispasmodics.
7. Frequency of urination during waking hours of less than eight times per day.
8. Diagnosis of bacterial cystitis or prostatitis within a 3-month period.
9. Presence of bladder or lower ureteral calculi.
10. A finding of active genital herpes.
11. Occurrence of uterine, cervical, vaginal, or urethral cancer.
12. A finding of urethral diverticulum.
13. Presence of cyclophosphamide (or any type of chemical) cystitis.
14. Occurrence of tuberculous cystitis.
15. Demonstration of radiation cystitis.
16. Presence of benign or malignant bladder tumors.
17. A finding of vaginitis.
18. Age <18 years.

Certain of the exclusion criteria serve mainly to make one wary of a diagnosis of IC but should by no means be used for categorical exclusion of such a diagnosis. However, because of the ambiguity involved, these patients should probably be eliminated from research studies or separately categorized; thus, the above definition is best considered a "research definition" of IC. In particular, exclusion criteria 4–6, 8, 9, 11, 12, 17, and 18 are only relative. Specific pathologic findings represent a glaring omission from the criteria, as there is a lack of consensus as to which pathologic findings, if any, are required for a tissue diagnosis of IC.[25]

As part of the painful bladder complex, IC is one of a group of diseases manifested by bladder pain, irritative voiding symptoms (urgency, frequency, nocturia, dysuria), and negative urine cultures. Diseases of known etiology include radiation cystitis, cyclophosphamide cystitis, cystitis caused by microorganisms that are not detected by routine culture methodologies, malacoplakia, and systemic diseases affecting the bladder. The Danish have characterized the painful bladder of unknown etiology into four subgroups: IC, detrusor myopathy, chronic unspecific cystitis, and eosinophilic cystitis.[1]

There appear to be three groups of patients who show symptoms without an obvious cause.[26] One group develops lower tract symptoms that resolve before any formal evaluation can be instituted. These appear to be patients we would diagnose as suffering from the urethral syndrome. A second group of patients has the symptom complex long enough to be referred to a urologist who elects to perform an evaluation including cystoscopy under anesthesia with hydrodistention of the bladder and biopsy. Those patients with glomerulations are considered to have IC. Those without these "typical findings of IC" are in a twilight zone, but are generally treated as if they have IC. The specificity of the finding of bladder glomerulations and the percentage of the normal population that would be found to have glomerulation if the bladder were distended under anesthesia to 80 cm of water pressure are unclear. The number of patients with urethral syndrome that would have findings of IC if they were evaluated with bladder distention under anesthesia is also unknown.

## Epidemiology

The sole resource of IC incidence and prevalence data until 1990 was Oravisto's regional population-based study.[27] Studies of the metropolitan area of Helsinki, Finland, showed a prevalence of the disease in women of 18.1/100,000. The joint prevalence of both sexes was 10.6/100,000, and the annual incidence of new female cases was 1.2/100,000. Severe cases accounted for 10% of the total. Ten percent of cases were in men. The disease onset was commonly subacute rather than insidious, and full development of the classical symptom complex occurred in a short time. Generally the disease did not progress continuously, but reached its final stage rapidly and then stabilized at that level. Subsequent major deterioration was the exception rather than the rule.

Many of the above findings were confirmed in a recent major population-based study in the United States.[22] Among a wealth of interesting data, the study revealed the following:

1. The prevalence of diagnosed IC in the United States approximates 43,500 cases—double the incidence found by Oravisto in Finland.
2. Late deterioration in symptoms is unusual (as per Oravisto).
3. Up to 50% of patients experience spontaneous remissions with a duration ranging from 1 to 80 months (mean 8 months).
4. Patients with interstitial cystitis are 10 to 12 times more likely than controls to report childhood bladder problems.
5. Patients with IC are twice as likely as controls to report a history of urinary tract infection; however, over half of all IC patients report less than one such infection per year before the onset of IC.
6. The time from symptom onset to diagnosis varied from 24 months for patients most recently diagnosed to 51 months for members of the Interstitial Cystitis Association, a patient advocacy group.
7. Women who were diagnosed by the

sampled urologists as actually having IC represented only 20% of the cases presenting with symptoms that were suggestive of this disease. The remaining cases were women who had been classified by a urologist as having painful bladder syndrome and sterile urine but had not been diagnosed. Based on these data, *one can extrapolate a possibility of almost half a million patients with this disease in the United States alone*.

8. Household size, marital status, number of male sexual partners, and educational status did not seem to significantly differ between those patients diagnosed as having IC and the general adult female population.
9. Using well-developed quality-of-life indicators, which employed responses to subjective statements, IC females scored lower on nine such tests, compared with an identical set of tests given to a sample of U.S. females with chronic renal failure undergoing dialysis.

## Etiology

While there is no lack of theories, the etiology of IC remains obscure. This is not necessarily surprising in a disease as difficult to objectively categorize as this one. Today the general opinion is that the etiology is multifactorial and that we may be dealing with a syndrome rather than a specific disease.[28]

Numerous studies have failed to find evidence of causative bacterial, fungal, and viral infection.[29–35] The vast majority of patients have received treatment with antibiotics during the years of symptoms prior to diagnosis and by definition the symptoms are unresponsive. While some still propose an infectious etiology,[36] with the possible exception of some type of slow-growing virus or unknown organism, this theory of etiology has almost been abandoned. The finding that *Helicobacter pylori* (formerly *Campylobacter pylori*) infection has been linked to chronic atrophic gastritis[37,38] has sparked renewed interest in the possibility that a bacterial infection, not demonstrated by standard urine culture techniques, may play a role in IC. This theory is tantalizing, as the disease often presents acutely, and patients may remember the week or even the day that symptoms began.

Potential etiologies of IC tend to fall into and out of favor, and one of the most popular now concerns a possible deficiency in the bladder glycosaminoglycan layer (GAG) lining the luminal surface as a possible initiating event. Parsons and Hurst[39] proposed that a defective transitional epithelium may lead to molecular leaks of normal urine constituents into the bladder wall, setting up the symptom complex. He showed experimentally that one can damage the GAG layer with protamine sulfate with resultant back-diffusion of urea through the bladder lumen, and that this urea loss can be prevented with a bladder instillation of exogenous GAG (heparin).[40] By placing a solution of concentrated urea into the bladder of IC patients and measuring absorption versus controls, Parsons was able to confirm his theory in patients with interstitial cystitis.[41]

Fowler et al[42] studied 14 IC patients and 10 normal controls for the presence of intraurothelial Tamm–Horsfall protein. He found the protein in ten of the former group and only one control. Pathologic controls (bladder cancer, inflammation) did not have intraurethelial Tamm–Horsfall protein. Neal et al[43] reported anti–Tamm–Horsfall protein serum antibody titers to be significantly elevated in IC patients.

However, ultrastructural, biochemical, and functional studies of bladder GAG have failed to support this theory.[33,44–46] One wonders if it is a GAG abnormality that symptoms tend to respond so well to treatments that damage GAG, including transurethral resection and laser of ulcerated areas, bladder distention, silver nitrate administration, and chlorpactin administration. Speculation about what might initiate a GAG abnormality is absent, and the possibility that if such an abnormality exists it might be secondary to a primary unknown insult certainly is not unreasonable. Nevertheless, some patients do respond to treatment with GAG (see below), and at least some cases of IC may be related to GAG abnormality.

Another intuitively enticing possibility is that the urine of IC patients is itself carrying a pathologic substance accounting for the disorder. Lynes et al[47] were unable to find a urinary myotropic substance unique to interstitial cystitis patients. Parsons and Stein[48] found IC urine to result in higher cell death of cultured transitional cells than normal urine, suggesting a toxic compound in the urine of some IC patients. The Temple University research group[49] was able to induce glomerulations in rabbit bladder following repeated intravesical exposure to the urine of IC patients. However, a follow-up study[50] did not demonstrate increased rabbit urothelial permeability after exposure to either the high or low molecular weight fractions of IC urine. While an intriguing theory, the toxic urine etiology remains to be proven.

Many studies have noted the presence of a mast cell infiltrate in the bladder wall in a subset of IC patients suggesting a potential pathogenic role of the mast cell.[51] The bladder mast cell contains many granules, each one of which can secrete many vasoactive and nociceptive molecules. A number of conditions such as extreme cold, drugs, neuropeptides, stress, trauma, and toxins can trigger the mast cell to secrete some of its contents. In turn, these chemicals can sensitize sensory neurons, which can further activate mast cells by releasing neurotransmitters or neuropeptides. Additionally, the mast cell can directly cause vasodilatation and bladder mucosal damage while attracting inflammatory cells, thus causing many of the problems observed in IC.[52] It has been demonstrated in vitro that in the presence of urothelial damage, urine can penetrate subepithelially and induce degranulation of mast cells with release of mediators.[53] Aldenborg and Fall[54] are proponents of the theory that mast cell activation may be central to IC and that some of the symptoms and findings, such as frequency, pain, and mucosal edema, may be related to the release of preformed or secondarily generated mast cell mediators. Proliferation of autonomic nerve fibers has been reported to occur within the bladder wall in IC,[55] and it is tempting to speculate that the autonomic nervous system might in some way control mast cell function in IC, as postulated in the colon in ulcerative colitis.[56]

The question becomes, why have antihistamines been largely ineffective in treatment?[52] Although the evidence suggests that it may be related to the pathogenesis of the symptoms of IC in some patients,[54] and, indeed, treatments such as amitriptyline and the experimental agent nalmefene have pharmacologic activity that is partly based on mast cell stabilization,[57] the presence of mast cells is not necessary for a diagnosis of IC, nor can detrusor mastocytosis be considered a marker for the disease. In a study of 115 patients with IC, Holm-Bentzen et al[58] could not correlate the severity of symptoms with the number of mast cells. We and others have found mast cell infiltration in the bladder to be a nonspecific finding, associated with not only IC but also other bladder pathology.[25,56] With mast cell counts being elevated primarily in patients with the ulcerative form of IC,[59] the question as to whether these cells play a primary or a secondary role in pathogenesis is unknown, but they currently have no place in diagnosis.

For many years the autoimmune character of IC has been commented on.[60] However, the lack of pathologic findings, the variable and usually poor response to immunosuppressants and anti-inflammatory agents, and the usual immediate relief upon diversion of the urine stream speak against an autoimmune etiology.[12] While the immune mechanism may have at least a partial role in the pathophysiology of IC,[61] many studies continue to shed doubt on this as a significant causative factor.[62–64]

Finally, new research into etiology may focus on the knowledge that the sensory nervous system can generate some of the manifestations of inflammation.[65] Polymodal nociceptor activation generates axon reflexes in the terminal arborizations of primary afferent neurons. These reflexes cause the C fibers to release neuropeptides that initiate inflammatory changes. Neuropeptides can exert direct effects on vascular smooth muscle and endothelium to increase flow and permeability. Histamines released from mast cells may also participate in neurogenic inflammation. In a disease manifested primarily by sensory abnormalities, this possibility that the sensory nervous system itself might be the underlying culprit is worth exploring.

Abelli et al demonstrated in the rat urethra that mechanical irritation alone can cause neuropeptide release from peripheral capsaicin-sensitive primary afferent neurons resulting in neurogenic inflammation.[66] Hohenfellner et al suggest that IC is associated with increased sympathetic outflow into the bladder and altered metabolism of vasoactive intestinal polypeptide and neuropeptide Y.[67] Ongoing immunohistochemical studies on the neuropeptides and muscarinic receptors of the bladder in IC and non-IC populations promise to reveal important data regarding the pathogenesis of IC.[68]

## Diagnosis

The diagnosis of IC is best based on the techniques necessary to elicit the criteria established at the conferences held by the National Institute of Arthritis, Diabetes, Digestive and Kidney Diseases.[24] Essentially, this requires a thorough history, appropriate cultures to document the sterility of the urinary tract, a urodynamic evaluation, and cystoscopy carried out in subjects under anesthesia with hydrodistention of the bladder and bladder biopsy. Cystometry in conscious IC patients generally demonstrates normal function, the exception being decreased bladder capacity and hypersensitivity, perhaps exaggerated due to gas. Very small volumes are required to initiate discomfort. Patients with discrete involuntary bladder contractions often respond to anticholinergic medication and do not tend to respond to standard therapy for IC,[69] and thus should not be given this diagnosis.

Biopsy and cytology are essential to rule out carcinoma in situ and other pathologic conditions. It should not be surprising that in a disease so difficult to diagnose definitively, pathognomonic findings on biopsy material are essentially unknown, and not for lack of trying. While one can easily differentiate ulcerative from nonulcerative disease by both cystoscopic and light microscopic changes, there is nothing pathognomonic about the histologic changes specific for IC. Despite the same severe symptoms in both groups, patients with nonulcer disease have relatively unaltered mucosa with a sparse inflammatory response in some cases.[59] The finding of mast cells in the mucosa and/or detrusor is extremely nonspecific, and the histologic light and scanning electron microscopic findings have failed to reveal surface characteristics specific for IC, or the presence of specific immunoreactive cells.[70–72]

Benson's somewhat facetious comment, "We may be doing our patients a disservice by diagnosing 'interstitial cystitis.' I would much prefer to say, 'I believe you have symptoms, I don't know what's wrong with you, but I'll do my best to make you symptomatically better,' may have more truth than we would like to admit."[73]

## Treatment

The ultimate goal of therapy of any disease process is to neutralize the factor or factors responsible for the disease. As long as causative factors are unknown, treatments will be based on empiricism. Although the symptoms of IC can be controlled with one of a variety of treatments in the overwhelming majority of patients, there is little evidence that treatment accomplishes anything more than influencing the symptomatic expression of the disease rather than curing the condition.

Hydraulic distention is generally the initial therapeutic modality used in the treatment of IC, as it is an initial part of the diagnostic process. Approximately 30% of patients experience some symptomatic relief following distention,[12] although we have been impressed that an almost equal number experience some exacerbation of their symptoms. Both effects seem to be short-lived. There are no standard methods for distention. Simple bladder filling at cystoscopy gives relief to some patients. Dunn and associates[74] reported that 16 of 25 patients remained free of symptoms at a mean of 14 months after they had undergone distention for up to 3 hours while under anesthesia during which their bladder pressure was increased to the level of the systolic blood pressure; 2 patients suffered bladder rupture. At initial cystoscopy, we distend the bladder for 1 minute at 80 cm water pressure, empty it, refill it to establish the diagnosis, and let it remain distended for another 7 minutes. In our recent experience with 130 patients, we obtained excellent results in 13% of patients with bladder capacities >600 $cm^3$ and 28% of patients with bladder capacities <600 $cm^3$. Only one subject in the former group showed a response that lasted for >3 months, and none of the patients in the latter group showed a 9-month response. The average response lasted less than 3 months.[75]

Intravesical lavage with one of a variety of preparations remains the standard therapy for IC against which other treatments may be measured.[72] Pool and Rives[76] reported on 74 patients treated with intravesical silver nitrate. Excellent to good results were obtained in 89% of patients, with an average duration of response of 7.6 months. Burford and Burford[77] also reported good results after using silver nitrate in conjunction with bladder fulguration. O'Conor[78] introduced the use of intravesical chlorpactin (WWCS-90) in the treatment of IC. Messing and Stamey[79] reported a 72% success rate and a duration of response of 6 months.

One of the principal treatments for IC is the intravesical instillation of dimethylsulfoxide (DMSO), a product of the wood pulp industry and a derivative of lignum. Its pharmacologic properties include membrane penetration, enhanced drug absorption, anti-inflammatory and analgesic effects, collagen dissolution, muscle relaxation, and mast cell histamine release. Stewart[80] popularized the use of this agent in treating IC. For theoretical reasons we administer the 50 $cm^3$ DMSO (Rimso 50) with 5000 units of heparin, 10 mg triamcinolone acetonide (Kenalog), and 44 mEq bicarbonate. Treatments are weekly for 6 weeks. We recently reported on 73 patients treated and followed for 2 years.[75] The response rate was 60%, with two thirds of those responding reporting excellent relief of symptoms. The average duration of response to a 6-week course was 10 months. In all, 25% of our patients are currently on monthly maintenance. Our results are comparable to those of Perez-Marrero et al,[81] who reported a 53% response rate versus an 18% response to placebo.

Just to illustrate that almost any treatment for IC seems to be effective at first glance, Khanna and Loose[82] recently reported dramatic improvement in three patients treated with intravesical doxorubicin, calling it possibly the "breakthrough drug for interstitial cystitis." No follow-up studies have been reported. Parsons and Koprowski[83] reported on the success of bladder retraining in IC patients in order to increase voiding intervals. This seems to be most successful in patients where pain is not a major manifestation of symptomatology. In this author's experience, while many patients can control their frequency if motivated, the extreme discomfort and pain engendered makes the tradeoff far from worthwhile.

The tricyclic antidepressant amitriptyline has many actions that are theoretically beneficial to patients with IC.[57] It is the most potent tricyclic antidepressant in terms of blocking H1 histaminergic receptors, stabilizes mast cells in vitro, and has actions that might tend to stimulate predominantly β-adrenergic receptors in the bladder body smooth musculature, an action that would further facilitate urinary storage by decreasing the excitability of smooth muscle in that area. It has analgesic actions that are not clearly understood and sedative properties that can be potentially beneficial to IC sufferers. In a dosage gradually increasing to 75 mg hs over 3 weeks, responses have been over 50% with little tachyphylaxis.[75,84]

Experimental oral medications showing promise include sodium pentosanpolysulfate (elmiron), a synthetic GAG partially excreted in the urine,[85] and nalmifene, an opiate antagonist thought to prevent mast cell degeneration.[86] Both have shown some efficacy in initial trials. Elmiron has been studied in four placebo-controlled trials in this country and abroad. Parsons and Mulholland initially reported on 62 patients.[87] In terms of patient subjective symptoms of pain, urgency, frequency, and nocturia, the drug was significantly better than placebo in all categories. Of the patients on sodium pentosanpolysulfate, 45% experienced at least a 50% reduction in pain compared to 18% on placebo. Average voided volumes increased 17.3 mL, significant statistically but of questionable clinical significance. The average number of voids per day was unchanged. Holm-Bentzen et al[88] studied 115 patients in a similar trial and found no differences between before and after trial values in the elmiron and placebo groups with regard to symptoms, urodynamic parameters, cystoscopic appearance of the bladder, and mast cell counts. Two recent multicenter U.S. studies[85] (one awaiting publication) have shown some symptomatic improvement in less than one third of patients (about double the placebo improvement rate) with no improvement in objective parameters other than the extra tablespoon in average voided volumes. Nevertheless, the drug seems to be quite safe and bereft of significant side effects. Nalmifene is currently undergoing initial double-blind placebo-controlled testing. As with all drug trials, one must heed the caution that statistical significance does not always translate clinically. A difference, to be a difference, must make a difference.

Small, uncontrolled series have reported efficacy with the old antihistamine hydroxyzine[89] and the calcium channel antagonist nifedipine.[90] The latter drug is known to inhibit smooth muscle contraction and cell-mediated immunity.

The rare patient with a discreet Hunner's ulcer can be treated with transurethral resection, fulguration, or laser irradiation.[91,92] Transcutaneous electrical nerve stimulation is effective in some patients.[93] Long-term results of subtrigonal phenolization have been dismal,[94] and this therapy should be abandoned.

It is certainly worthwhile to exhaust all reasonable conservative measures before proceeding to surgical therapy in a disease such as IC, which is chronic, not life threatening, and subject to spontaneous remission of symptomatology. Augmentation cystoplasty with supratrigonal cystectomy can be considered in patients with a small-capacity bladder measured under anesthesia.[95] Patients with large-capacity bladders and intractable symptoms may best be treated with diversion, with or without cystectomy.[96] In fact, for patients "at the end of their rope" we recommend urinary diversion rather than substitution cystoplasty, as good results with the latter procedure are anything but assured,[97,98] and a need for clean intermittent catheterization in about 25% of women after cystoplasty turns what would still be considered a success for other disease processes into a failure, as intermittent catheterization is excruciating for an IC patient. Anecdotal reports of pain developing in continent diversions performed in IC patients make some cautious about this form of diversion until more long-term data become available.[99]

## REFERENCES


1. Holm-Bentzen M. Pathology, pathophysiology, and pathogenesis of painful bladder disease. *Urol Res.* 1989;17:203–209.
2. Stamm WE, Wagner KF, Amsel R, et al. Causes of the acute urethral syndrome in women. *N Engl J Med.* 1980;303:409.
3. Schmidt RA. Pelvic pain. *Problems Urol.* 1989;3:270–281.
4. Fowler J. *Urinary Tract Infection and Inflammation.* Chicago: Yearbook Medical Publishers; 1989:291–322.
5. Parsons CL. Urinary tract infections in the female patient. *Urol Clin North Am.* 1985;12:359.
6. Striker GE. Urology program: data on research support. *Semin Urol.* 1991;9:73.
7. Hanno PM, Staskin DR, Krane RJ, Wein AJ (eds). *Interstitial Cystitis.* London: Springer-Verlag; 1990.
8. Powell NB, Powell EB. The female urethra: a clinico-pathological study. *J. Urol.* 1949; 61:557–570.
9. Charlton CAC. Historical review: confusions in definition. In: George NJR, Gosling JA, eds. *Sensory Disorders of the Bladder and Urethra.* Berlin: Springer-Verlag; 1986:81–83.
10. Bodner DR. The urethral syndrome. *Urol Clin North Am.* 1988;15:699–704.
11. Scotti RJ. The urethral syndrome and urethral infections. *Infect Surg.* 1989;8:102–181.

12. Messing EM. Interstitial cystitis and related syndromes. In: Walsh PC, Retik AB, Stamey TA, Vaughan ED, eds. *Campbell's Urology*. 6th ed. Philadelphia: WB Saunders; 1992:982–1004.
13. McCannel DA, Haile RW. Urethral narrowing and its treatment. *Intl Urol Nephrol*. 1982; 14:407–414.
14. Davis DM. Vesical orifice obstruction in women and its treatment by resection. *J Urol*. 1955;73:112–116.
15. Richardson FH. External urethroplasty in women: technique and clinical evaluation. *J Urol*. 1969;101:719–723.
16. Roberts M, Smith P. Non-malignant obstruction of the female urethra. *Br J Urol*. 1968;40:694.
17. Splatt AJ, Weedon D. The urethral syndrome: morphological studies. *Br J Urol*. 1981;52:263.
18. Mabry EW, Carson CC, Older RA. Evaluation of women with chronic voiding discomfort. *Urology*. 1981;18:244.
19. Carson CC, Osborne D, Segura JW. Psychogenic characteristics of patients with female urethral syndrome. *J Clin Psychol*. 1979;35:312.
20. Wilkins EGL, Payne SR, Pead PJ, Moss ST, Maskell RM. Interstitial cystitis and urethral syndrome: a possible answer. *Br J Urol*. 1989;64:39–44.
21. Gillespie WA, Henderson EP, Linton KB, Smith JB. Microbiology of the urethral (frequency and dysuria) syndrome. *Br J Urol*. 1989;64:270–274.
22. Held PJ, Hanno PM, Wein AJ, Pauly MV, Cahn MA. Epidemiology of interstitial cystitis. In: Hanno PM, Staskin DR, Krane RJ, Wein AJ, eds. *Interstitial Cystitis*. London: Springer-Verlag; 1990:29–48.
23. Ratner V, Slade D. The interstitial cystitis association: patients working for a cure. *Semin Urol*. 1991;9:72.
24. Nyberg LM. Advances in the diagnosis and management of interstitial cystitis. In: Rous S, ed. *Urology Annual*. Norwalk, CT: Appleton & Lange; 1991:181–191.
25. Hanno PM, Levin RM, Monson FC, et al. Diagnosis of interstitial cystitis. *J Urol*. 1990;141:846–848.
26. Hanno PM. Interstitial cystitis: unresolved issues. In: McGuire E, Lytton B, eds. *Advances in Urology*. vol 3. Chicago: Yearbook Medical Publishers; 1990:237–242.
27. Oravisto KJ. Epidemiology of interstitial cystitis. *Ann Chir Gynaecol Fenn*. 1975;64:57–58.
28. Holm-Bentzen M, Nordling J, Hald T. Etiology: etiologic and pathogenetic theories in interstitial cystitis. In: Hanno PM, Staskin DR, Krane RJ, Wein AJ, eds. *Interstitial Cystitis*. London: Springer-Verlag; 1990:63–77.
29. Smith BH, Dehner LP. Chronic ulcerating interstitial cystitis (Hunner's ulcer). *Arch Pathol*. 1972;93:76–81.
30. Hanish KA, Pool TL. Interstitial and hemorrhagic cystitis: viral, bacterial, fungal studies. *J Urol*. 1970;104:705–706.
31. Hedelin HH, Mardh P, Brorson J, et al. Mycoplasma hominis and interstitial cystitis. *Sexually Transm Dis*. 1983;10(4):327–330.
32. Fall M, Johansson S, Vahlne A. A clinicopathological and virological study of interstitial cystitis. *J Urol*. 1985;113:771–773.
33. Collan Y, Alfthan O, Kivilaakso E, Oravisto KJ. Electronic microscopic and histological findings in IC. *Eur Urol*. 1976;2:242–245.
34. Siegel SW, Guz B, Suit P. Silver staining of mucosal biopsy specimens in chronic IC. *J Urol*. 1989;141:267A.
35. Lynes WL, Sellers RG, Shortliffe LMD. The evidence for occult bacterial infections as a cause for IC. *J Urol*. 1989;141:268A.
36. Wilkins EGL, Payne SR, Pead PJ, Moss ST, Maskell RM. Interstitial cystitis and the urethral syndrome: a possible answer. *Br J Urol*. 1989;64:39–44.
37. Marshall BJ, Warren JR. Unidentified curved bacilli in the stomach of patients with gastritis. *Lancet*. 1984;1:1311–1315.
38. Parsonnet J, Friedman GD, Vandersteen DP, Chang Y, et al. Helicobacter pylori infection and the risk of gastric carcinoma. *N Engl J Med*. 1991;325:1127–1136.
39. Parsons CL, Hurst RE. Decreased urinary uronic acid levels in individuals with IC. *J Urol*. 1990;143:690–693.
40. Lilly JD, Parsons CL. Bladder surface GAG is a human epithelial permeability barrier. *Surg Gynecol Obstet*. 1990;171:493–496.
41. Parsons CL, Lilly JD, Stein P. Epithelial dysfunction in nonbacterial cystitis (interstitial cystitis). *J Urol*. 1991;145:732–735.
42. Fowler JE, Lynes WL, Lau JLT, Ghosh L, Mounzer A. IC is associated with intraurothelial Tamm–Horsfall protein. *J Urol*. 1988; 140:1385–1389.
43. Neal DE, Dilworth JP, Kaack MB. Tamm–Horsfall autoantibodies in interstitial cystitis. *J Urol*. 1991;145:37–39.
44. Dixon JS, Holm-Bentzen M, Gilpin CJ, et al. Electron microscopic investigation of the bladder urothelium in IC. *J Urol*. 1986;135:621–625.
45. Johansson SL. Light microscopic findings in bladders of patients with IC. In: Hanno PM, Staskin DR, Krane RJ, Wein AJ, eds. *Interstitial Cystitis*. London:Springer-Verlag; 1990:83–90.
46. Ruggieri MR, Steinhardt GF, Hanno PM. Antiadherence of IC bladder extracts. *Semin Urol*. 1991;9:136–142.
47. Lynes WL, Shortliffe LD, Stamey TA. Urinary myotropic substances in interstitial cystitis. *J Urol*. 1990;143:373A.
48. Parsons CL, Stein P. Role of toxic urine in interstitial cystitis. *J Urol*. 1990;143:373A.

49. Balagani RK, Hanno PM, Ma M, et al. Induction of glomerulations in rabbit bladder after exposure to IC urine. *J Urol.* 1991;145:258A.

50. Perzin AD, Hanno PM, Ruggieri MR. Effect of protamine and IC urine on dye penetration across urothelium. *J Urol.* 1991;145:259A.

51. Sant GR. Diagnosis of IC: a clinical, endoscopic, and pathologic approach. In: Hanno PM, Staskin DR, Krane RJ, Wein AJ, eds. *Interstitial Cystitis.* London: Springer-Verlag; 1990:107–114.

52. Theoharides TC, Sant GR. Bladder mast cell activation in interstitial cystitis. *Semin Urol.* 1991;9:74–87.

53. Ugaily-Thulesius L, Thulesius O. The effects of urine on mast cells and smooth muscle of human ureter. *Urol Res.* 1988;16:441–447.

54. Aldenborg F, Fall M, Enerback L. Mast cells and interstitial cystitis. In: Hanno PM, Staskin DR, Krane RJ, Wein AJ, eds. *Interstitial Cystitis.* London: Springer-Verlag; 1990:95–106.

55. Christmas TJ, Rode J, Bottazzo GF, et al. Nerve fibre proliferation in interstitial cystitis. *Virchows Arch A.* 1990;416:447–451.

56. Christmas TJ, Rode J. Characteristics of mast cells in normal bladder, bacterial cystitis and IC. *Br J Urol.* 1991;68:473–478.

57. Hanno PM, Buehler J, Wein AJ. Use of amitriptyline in the treatment of interstitial cystitis. *J Urol.* 1989;141:846–848.

58. Holm-Bentzen M, Jacobsen F, Nerstrom B. Painful bladder disease: pathoanatomical differences in 115 patients. *J Urol.* 1987;137:500–502.

59. Johansson SL, Fall M. Clinical features and spectrum of light microscopic changes in IC. *J Urol.* 1990;143:1118–1124.

60. Hanno PM, Wein AJ. Interstitial cystitis. *American Urological Association Update Series,* vol 6, lessons 9 and 10.

61. Harrington DS, Fall M, Johansson SL. IC: bladder mucosa lymphocyte immunophenotyping and blood cytometry. *J Urol.* 1990;144:868–871.

62. Zhou ZZ, Monson FC, Hanno PM, et al. Immunohistochemical analysis of the urinary bladder in IC and non-IC. *J Urol.* 1990;143:278A.

63. MacDermott JP, Miller CH, Levy N, Stone AR. Cellular immunity in interstitial cystitis. *J Urol.* 1991;145:274–278.

64. Anderson JB, MacIver AG, Bradbrook RA, Gingell C. Immunological factors in the aetiology of interstitial cystitis. *J Urol.* 1990;143:279A.

65. Forman JC. Peptides and neurogenic inflammation. *Br Med Bull.* 1987;43:386–400.

66. Abelli L, Conte B, Somma V, et al. Mechanical irritation induces neurogenic inflammation in the rat urethra. *J Urol.* 1991;146:1624–1626.

67. Hohenfellner M, Nunes L, Schmidt RA, et al. IC: increased sympathetic innervation and related neuropeptide synthesis. *J Urol.* 1992; 147:587–591.

68. Shickley TJ, Luthin GR, Ruggieri MR. Immunohistochemical examination of neuropeptides in IC bladders. *J Urol.* 1992;147:462A.

69. Perez-Marrero R, Emerson L, Juma S. Urodynamic studies in interstitial cystitis. *Urology.* 1987;29:27–30.

70. Lynes WL, Flynn SD, Shortliffe LD, Stamey TA. The histology of interstitial cystitis. *Am J Surg Pathol.* 1990;14:969–976.

71. Anderstrom CRK, Fall M, Johansson SL. Scanning electron microscopic findings in interstitial cystitis. *Br J Urol.* 1989;63:270–275.

72. Hanno PM, Wein AJ. Intravesical therapy of interstitial cystitis. In: Hanno PM, Staskin DR, Krane RJ, Wein AJ, eds. *Interstitial Cystitis.* London: Springer-Verlag; 1990:147–151.

73. Benson G. Interstitial cystitis. In: Hanno PM, Staskin DR, Krane RJ, Wein AJ, eds. *Interstitial Cystitis.* London: Springer-Verlag; 1990:131.

74. Dunn M, Ramsden PD, Roberts JBM. Interstitial cystitis treated by prolonged bladder distention. *Br J Urol.* 1977;49:641–654.

75. Hanno PM, Wein AJ. Conservative therapy of interstitial cystitis. *Semin Urol.* 1991;9:143–147.

76. Pool TL, Rives HF. Interstitial cystitis: treatment with silver nitrate. *J Urol.* 1944;51:520–525.

77. Burford EH, Burford CE. Hunner ulcer of the bladder: a report of 187 cases. *J Urol.* 1958;79:952–955.

78. O'Conor VJ. Chlorpactin WCS90 in the treatment of interstitial cystitis (abstract). *Q Bull Northwest Univ Med School.* 1955;29:392.

79. Messing EM, Stamey TA. Interstitial cystitis, early diagnosis, pathology, and treatment. *Urology.* 1978;12:381–392.

80. Stewart BH, Persky L, Kiser WS. The use of dimethylsulfoxide in the treatment of interstitial cystitis. *J Urol.* 1967;98:671–672.

81. Perez-Marrero R, Emerson LE, Feltis JT. A controlled study of dimethylsulfoxide in interstitial cystitis. *J Urol.* 1988;140:36–39.

82. Khanna OP, Loose JH. Interstitial cystitis treated with intravesical doxorubicin. *Urology.* 1990; 36:139–142.

83. Parsons CL, Koprowski PF. IC: successful management by increasing urinary voiding intervals. *Urology.* 1991;37:207–212.

84. Kirkemo AK, Miles BJ, Peters JM. Use of amitriptyline in interstitial cystitis. *J Urol.* 1990; 143:279A.

85. Mulholland SG, Hanno PM, Parsons CL, et al. Pentosanpolysulfate sodium for therapy of interstitial cystitis. *Urology.* 1990;35:552–558.

86. Stone NN, Sherman F. Pilot study of the opiate antagonist nalmefene in patient with IC. *J Urol.* 1990;143:280A.

87. Parsons CL, Mulholland SG. Successful therapy of interstitial cystitis with pentosanpolysulfate. *J Urol.* 1987;138:513–517.

88. Holm-Bentzen M, Jacobsen F, Nerstrom B, et al. A prospective trial of elmiron in the treatment of IC. *J Urol.* 1987;138:503–507.

89. Theoharides TC, Sant GR. Hydroxyzine for the treatment of interstitial cystitis. *J Urol.* 1992; 147:461A.

90. Fleischmann JD, Huntley HN, Shingleton WB, Wentworth DB. Clinical and immunological response to nifedipine for treatment of IC. *J Urol.* 1991;146:1235–1239.

91. Fall M. Reappraisal of transurethral resection in classic IC. In: Hanno PM, Staskin DR, Krane RJ, Wein AJ, eds. *Interstitial Cystitis.* London: Springer-Verlag; 1990:175–182.

92. Shanberg AM, Malloy TR. Treatment of interstitial cystitis with the neodymium YAG laser. In: Hanno PM, Staskin DR, Krane RJ, Wein AJ, eds. *Interstitial Cystitis.* London: Springer-Verlag; 1990:183–188.

93. Fall M. Use of transcutaneous electrical nerve stimulation in IC. In: Hanno PM, Staskin DR, Krane RJ, Wein AJ, eds. *Interstitial Cystitis.* London: Springer-Verlag; 1990:169–173.

94. McInerney PD, Vanner TF, Matenhelia S, Stephenson TP. Assessment of the long-term results of subtrigonal phenolisation. *Br J Urol.* 1991;67:586–587.

95. Webster GD, Maggio MI. The management of chronic interstitial cystitis by substitution cystoplasty. *J Urol.* 1989;141:287–291.

96. Eigner EB, Freiha FS. The fate of the remaining bladder following supravesical diversion. *J Urol.* 1990;144:31–33.

97. Kisman OK, Lycklama AAB, Nijeholt A, vanKrieken JHJM. Mast cell infiltration in intestine used for bladder augmentation in IC. *J Urol.* 1991;146:1113–1114.

98. Nurse DE, Parry JRW, Mundy AR. Problems in the surgical treatment of interstitial cystitis. *Br J Urol.* 1991;68:153–154.

99. Baskin LS, Tanagho EA. Pelvic pain without pelvic organs. *J Urol.* 1992;147:683–686.

# 20

# Erectile Dysfunction

*Ronald W. Lewis*

## INTRODUCTION

Impotence or male erectile dysfunction is the inability to achieve or maintain an erection of adequate rigidity for sexual intercourse. This condition can be primary, ie, never having had this ability, or secondary. The loss of rigidity can be total or partial. Occasional or intermittent problems suggest a psychologic etiology. This disorder is not to be confused with lack of ejaculation or orgasm, and often the patient who presents with "impotence" may, in fact, on first questioning identify his true problem, such as premature ejaculation. Erectile dysfunction is a common problem, particularly in the aging male; the largest number of patients who present with this complaint are in the sixth and seventh decades of life. Not so long ago many physicians tried to convince their patients to accept the inevitable and consider their affliction an unsolvable problem, or, if the patients were younger than 50 years of age, send them for psychologic counseling or try empiric testosterone injections. Now as the average age of the population is shifting to older and the life span is increasing with better general health in these later years, this type of approach is less than optimal. It is currently felt that most of the causes of impotency are organic or physical, almost always with psychologic overtones, as opposed to primarily psychologic or emotional. Well over 15 million American men suffer from this disorder, and these patients should expect this disorder to be treated with the same degree of expertise and compassion as with any other functional loss.

## BASIC ANATOMY AND PHYSIOLOGY

Erection is a psychosomatic-dependent event, an integration of several mutually occurring actions in several different systems (vascular, endocrine, and neurologic). Erection can begin with sexual thoughts, visual stimuli that arouse an individual that can vary from one to the next, or other sensory stimulation such as touch. In the physically intact male, mental aversion or disease can override the local sensory stimulation of the genital organs to reflexogenically produce an erection. Similarly, in patients with complete upper level spinal cord injury, reflexogenic erections can occur although often not sustained or spontaneous as desired. More is known about the lower reflexogenic neural pathways than the psychogenic ones. Sensory stimuli elicited in the glans, penile, and other perineal and inguinal areas are eventually carried by the dorsal penile and other sensory nerves to the sacral spinal cord via the pudendal nerve. The efferent limb originates in the parasympathetic center in the sacral cord, which contributes fibers to the pelvic nerve that enters the cavernosal tissue as the cavernous nerves. Careful attention to preserving these nerve tracts has gained importance in radical pelvic cancer surgery in the potent patient. In the brain, several regions modulate the psychogenic component of erection, including the thalamic nucleii, the rhinenencephalon, and the limbic structures, with integration of these various areas occurring perhaps in the medial preoptic anterior hypothalamic

**Fig 1.** Diagram of the sympathetic, parasympathetic, and somatic efferent pathways to the penis. Sympathetic pathways emerge from the thoracolumbar T11 to L2 segments of the cord and pass via the white rami to the sympathetic chain ganglia and then via the lumbar splanchnic nerves to the prevertebral ganglia in the inferior mesenteric and superior hypogastric plexuses, from which fibers travel in the hypogastric nerves to the pelvic plexus. Sympathetic preganglionic fibers also descend in the sympathetic chain to the sacral ganglia from which postganglionic fibers pass in gray rami to the sacral nerves, at which point they join the pelvis or pudendal nerves. Sacral parasympathetic preganglionic axons arise in the S2 to S4 segments of the spinal cord and travel to the pelvic plexus via the pelvic nerve. Ganglion cells in the pelvic plexus send axons into the cavernous nerve, which lies in close proximity to the prostate gland on its posterior surface en route to the penis. Branches of the pudendal nerve innervate the external sphincter and the bulbocavernous (BC) and ischiocavernous (IC) muscles, as well as providing sensory fibers to the dorsal nerve of the penis. The pudendal nerve arises in the S2 to S4 segment of the spinal cord. [From de Groat WC, Steers WD. Neuroanatomy and neurophysiology of penile erection. In: Tanagho EA, Lue TF, McClure RD, eds, *Contemporary Management of Impotence and Infertility* (Baltimore: Williams and Wilkins; 1989:5), with permission.]

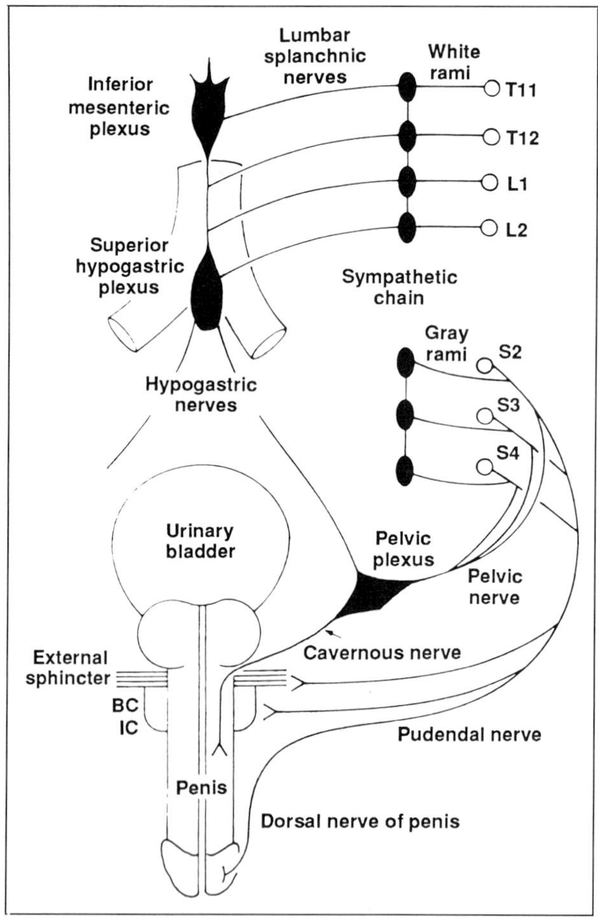

area.[1,2] A classic article dealing with the neuroanatomy and neurophysiology of erection is that prepared by de Groat and Steers.[3] As stressed by these authors, the following three sets of peripheral nerves have a role in erectile function: thoracolumbar sympathetic, sacral parasympathetic, and sacral somatic (Fig 1). The pelvic plexus (occasionally referred to as the inferior hypogastric plexus in humans) found in the pelvic fascia on either side of the lower genitourinary tract and the rectum is a very important site for the integration of autonomic input to the penis via the cavernous nerves. Physiologic studies and the presence of cholinergic nerves in the cavernous tissue implicate the parasympathetic nervous system as the primary effector of penile erection. Pharmacologic data indicate that acetylcholine is unlikely the intracavernous transmitter primarily responsible for human penile erection. Noncholinergic-nonadrenergic (NANC) neurotransmitters play a significant role in penile erection. Also the most important neurotransmitter in initiation of penile erection may be nitric oxide, which may be the endothelium-derived relaxing factor.[4] The sympathetic nervous system has an important role in the mediation of penile detumescence and flaccidity via the neurotransmitter norepinephrine, but the sympathetic nervous system may also have a role in penile tumescence.

The arterial blood supply to the cavernous tissue is primarily the deep penile or cavernous artery (Fig 2), which is usually a terminal branch of the common penile artery. The internal pudendal artery, which usually arises from the anterior division of the hypogastric or internal iliac artery, is usually the source for the penile arteries. However, accessory internal pudendal arteries arising from the obturator or other pelvic arteries are not uncommon. Also, the dorsal penile artery can supply the cavernous tissue with multiple branches along the shaft of the penis as a normal variant. There also can be rich anastomotic networks of vessels between the arteries of the

**Fig 2.** Diagram of the terminal branches of the internal pudendal artery. It first gives a branch to the urethral bulb. Occasionally, this branch continues as the urethral artery or the urethral artery is a separate branch. The two most terminal branches are the deep penile artery (or the cavernosal artery) and the dorsal penile artery.

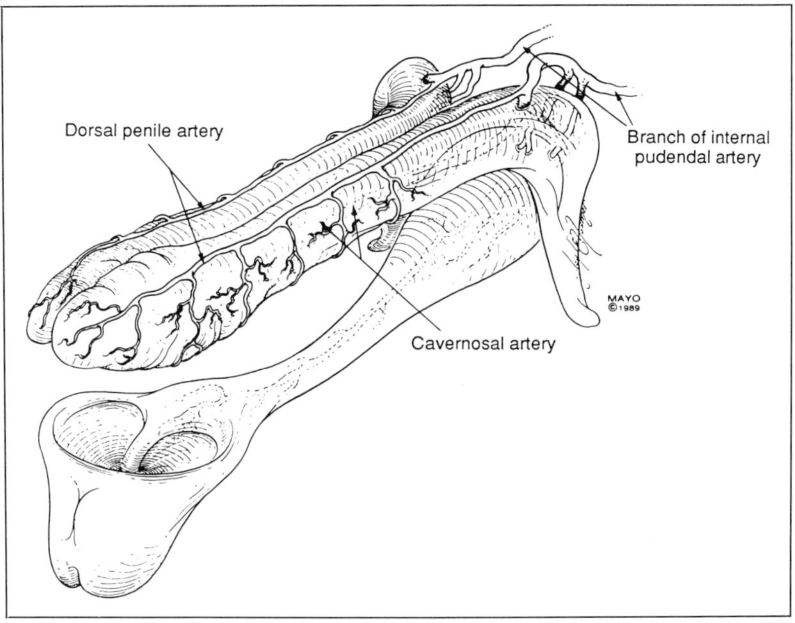

pelvic area, and one side may also supply both corporeal spaces as a normal variant. At any rate, the sinus tissue is supplied by a usually slightly eccentric central vessel (medial to center toward the midseptum of the cavernous bodies), which branches to form the helicine arteries, which supply the sinus spaces. The sinus spaces drain into a system of venules that coalesce on the outer surface of the cavernous tissue just beneath the tunica albuginea of the corpus cavernosum. These venules form a number of veins transversing the tunica albuginea called emissary veins, which usually drain into the circumflex veins on the outer surface of the tunica albuginea. The circumflex veins in turn drain into the deep dorsal vein of the penis in the dorsal midline of the penile shaft between the dorsal arteries lying usually just laterally adjacent, all beneath Buck's fascia. Occasionally, the deep dorsal vein consists of more than one trunk on the most distal shaft of the penis, and occasionally the deep dorsal vein re-

**Fig 3.** Diagrammatic representation of the three major vein divisions draining the penis. The superficial dorsal vein can communicate with the intermediate veins, and it drains into the external pudendal vein and to the saphenous vein eventually. This is called the superficial system. The intermediate system is the deep dorsal vein, which receives the circumflex veins along the shaft of the penis and direct emissary veins from the corpora cavernosa. It terminates in the infrapubic region by joining the retropubic venous plexus (the pelvic preprostatic plexus) or the internal pudendal vein. There can be communications in the retropubic venous plexus between the internal pudendal vein and the preprostatic veins. The crural veins and the cavernosal veins are the deep system and originate from the penis in the infrapubic region. Cavernosal veins can drain into the deep dorsal vein complex or the retropubic venous plexus. The crural veins usually drain into the internal pudendal veins or can also drain into the retropubic venous plexus.

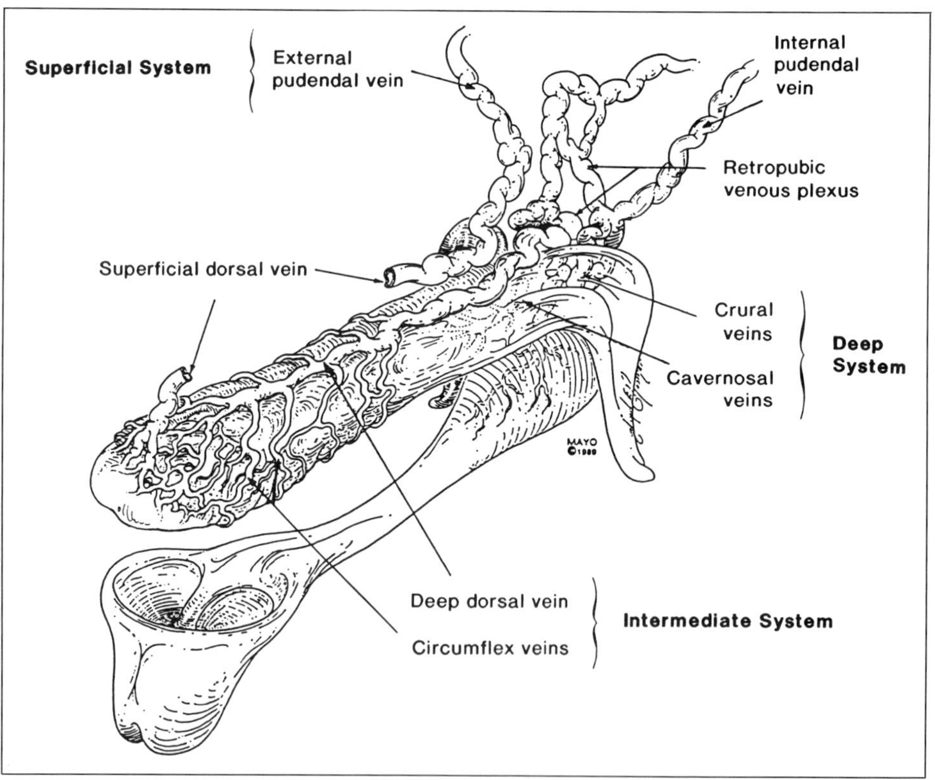

ceives direct emissary veins from the cavernous tissue in the dorsal midline. The deep dorsal vein near the glans penis also is initially constituted by numerous trunks from the glans and many of the circumflex vessels anastomosis with small tributaries from the spongiosum. The deep dorsal vein in the infrapubic region (where it can also receive tributaries from the prepubic fat) usually consists of one trunk that drains into the pelvic preprostatic venous plexus or the internal pudendal veins. This system of the deep dorsal vein is referred to as the intermediate venous system. The superficial venous system, which lies superficial to Buck's fascia and primarily drains the penile skin, can also have anastomotic connections to the deep dorsal vein. This superficial system drains into the femoral vein via the saphenous and the external pudendal veins. The deep penile drainage system consists of the cavernosal and/or crural veins that drain the deeper cavernous tissue. The cavernosal veins are really extensions of emissary veins from the infrapubic cavernous tissue that drain directly into the pelvic plexus or the deep dorsal vein in the deep infrapubic area. The crural veins are direct emissary veins from the antero- to posterolateral surface of the crura of the cavernous tissue that usually drains into the internal pudendal veins or the pelvic plexus. What should be emphasized are the rich anastomosis and the number of venous channels capable of draining the cavernous spaces (Fig 3).

Functionally, in the flaccid state, there is a high-resistance, low-flow arterial state in the cavernous tissue, primarily regulated by the contracted smooth muscles surrounding the cavernous spaces. Intracavernous pressure in this flaccid state is usually resting venous pressure. With the initiation of erection, relaxation of the sinus and arterial smooth muscle occurs and a low-resistance system is produced with blood flow increasing six to ten times that of the flaccid state. At full tumescence, the intracavernous pressure rises to approximately 50 mm Hg. As the sinus spaces expand, the subtunical venules are collapsed beneath the tunica albuginea. The emissary veins are also further collapsed by the expanding tunica albuginea, so that venous efflux is markedly decreased and intracavernous pressure rises to 80 to 100 mm Hg, the pressure necessary for rigidity. Maintenance of rigidity is influenced by tactile sensory stimulation mediated by a spinal reflex system. Ischiocavernosus muscle contraction probably causes intracavernosal pressure to rise higher than the 100 mm Hg but is not necessary for rigidity and is probably intermittent (see Table 1).

**TABLE 1. Phases of Human Penile Erection**

| Phase | |
|---|---|
| Flaccid | Minimal blood flow<br>Intracavernous pressure low (5–20 mm Hg) |
| Latent or filling | Blood flow highest (6–10 times that of flaccid phase) |
| Tumescence | Penis expands and elongates<br>Intracavernous pressure approximately 50 mm Hg |
| Full erection | Good rigidity of penis<br>Intracavernous pressure approximately 90–100 mm Hg |
| Rigid (or skeletal muscle) erection | Highest intracavernous pressure due to constriction of ischiocavernosus muscles (>100 mm Hg)<br>Short duration because of striated muscle fatigue |
| Detumescence | Consists of two subphases: early rapid detumescence (to 50 mm Hg) followed by slow decrease to flaccid phase pressure |

Data from Batra AK, Lue TF. The physiology of penile erection. In: Lewis RW, Barrett DM, eds. *Problems in Urology: The Impotent Man.* vol 5 (Philadelphia: JB Lippincott; 1991:489–495).

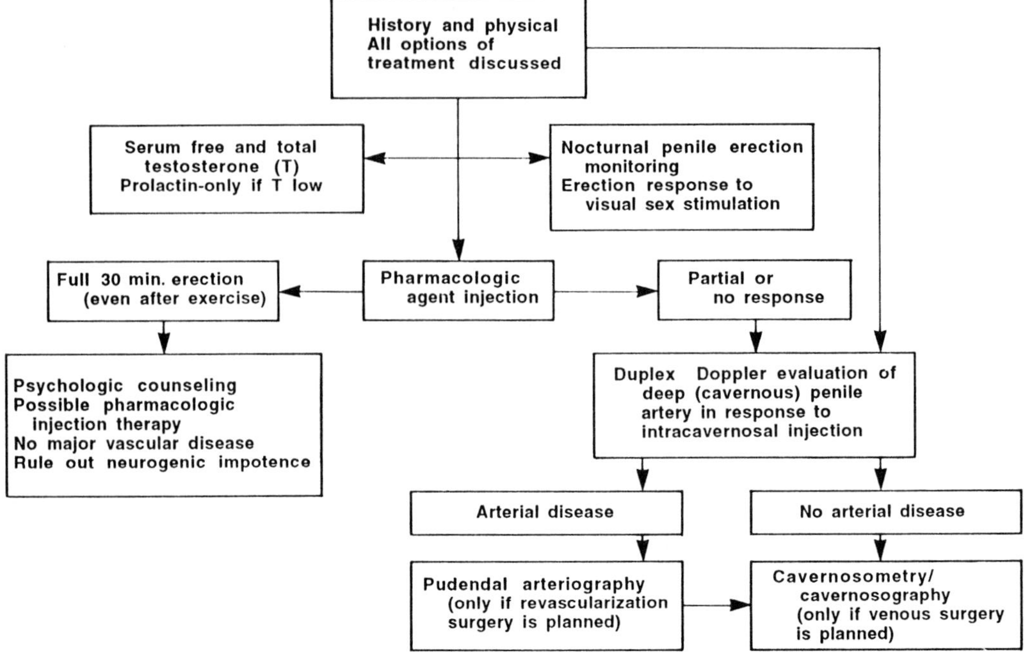


**Fig 4.** A flow sheet for the evaluation of impotency that is used at the Mayo Clinic.

## EVALUATION OF ERECTILE DYSFUNCTION (Fig 4)

### History and Physical

It cannot be stressed enough that the single most important step in the evaluation of the impotent patient is the initial history and physical. Important elements to stress are listed in Tables 2 and 3. Symptoms and signs of endocrine disorders of the pituitary, adrenal, or thyroid glands can be determined at this initial evaluation, and laboratory tests can be ordered in a more cost-effective and appropriate manner. A family history of diabetes mellitus alerts the examiner to consider further screening for this disorder, particularly in the individual who has not had much routine health screening. Medication history and use of tobacco in any form are to be particularly stressed because this has implications not only for eti-

**TABLE 2. Evaluation of Impotency: History**

- Genitourinary disease or surgery
- Vascular, neurologic, spinal, or inguinal surgery
- Medications
- Smoking, drug abuse or use
- Neurologic disease
- Marital and sexual history
- Systemic debilitating disease
- Genital, pelvic, or spinal trauma
- Symptoms of vascular or endocrine disease
- Nocturnal, early morning, nonintercourse erections

**TABLE 3. Evaluation of Impotency: Physical Exam**

- Secondary sex characteristics
  - Gynecomastia
- Genitalia
- Neurological
  - Perineal and penis sensation
  - Bulbocavernosus reflex
- Pulses
  - Femoral
  - Distal extremities
  - Penile

ology but also for choice of treatment. History of trauma or surgery to the penis, pelvis, or perineum should be carefully ascertained. Other signs and symptoms of vascular disease clearly suggest a possible vascular etiology for the erectile dysfunction. Neurogenic impotence is certainly best suspected by obtaining a positive neurologic disease history. Mental depression in man is commonly seen at the same time of life in which impotence occurs, and a causal relationship may be first suggested by this initial encounter with the patient. The physical examination should concentrate on the genitalia, peripheral pulses in the lower extremities, a sensory evaluation of the penis and perineum, and a thorough rectal evaluation for evaluation of the prostate and presence of a bulbocavernosus reflex.

At some of the larger or academic centers, a clinical psychologist or psychiatrist or other trained sex therapist is part of the evaluation team.[5] This individual usually evaluates the patient at the first visit. This may also be associated with some sort of self-administrated mental status or sexual inventory questionnaire, although there has been much debate in the literature about the value of individual types of these evaluations.[6] Even in the most simple office setting, however, some effort should be made to determine the mental status of the erectile dysfunction patient, preferably at the first visit.

It is at this first visit that also the goals of treatment for that individual patient must be established. Lue was the first to discuss this concept.[7] This goal establishment determines the remainder of the evaluation for the patient (see Table 4). For instance, if the patient is a 70-year-old with total erectile dysfunction who desires to try a vacuum constriction device, then there is really no need for further evaluation. It is important that the patient be presented with a rational and unbiased description of the alternatives available for the modern day treatment of impotence. Today many patients are well informed about alternatives, but many misconceptions about the potential complications and realistic expectations of the various alternatives exist.

**TABLE 4. Choice of Therapy for Impotence**

- Patient's and partner's goals
- Age and medical condition of patient
- Careful systematic diagnostic approach
- An unbiased presentation to the patient of all options available to treat the particular erectile dysfunction problems

Finally, at the first visit or certainly before major therapeutic decisions are made, there is great value to the patient and his sex partner to have that partner involved in the evaluation process. This person can often provide information that will amplify or clarify the patient's history. More importantly, goal-directed therapy is best accomplished when both individuals involved in sexual intercourse are well and evenly informed of the techniques of their particular therapeutic choice.[8]

## Laboratory Tests

Laboratory test ordering can be pragmatic. If the patient has not had any routine medical evaluation, then a complete blood count, serum chemical screen, and urinalysis are in order. A glycosylated hemoglobin as opposed to a fasting blood sugar is preferred in almost all individuals, but particularly in those with a strong family history of diabetes mellitus, those with signs or symptoms suggesting the disease, and those patients who are known diabetics to assess their current control status. A free and total serum testosterone is obtained in almost all patients but in particular in those who have partial erectile dysfunction or intermittent erectile problems. An initial serum prolactin is usually not obtained, except in the face of a definite history of suppressed libido or symptoms of visual blurring or intense headaches. If the serum testosterone is decreased, prolactin should always be ordered to rule out a prolactin-secreting pituitary tumor. Serum luteinizing hormone and follicle-stimulating hormone levels can be obtained in the face of low testosterone levels to determine if the hypogonadism is hyper- or hypogonadotropic. The treatment, however, in the partially impotent man is the same in either of these cases and that is parenteral testosterone, if elected in the patient who can be followed with rectal examinations. Urethral and/or prostatic cultures can be obtained in the patient who has suggestion of infection as a possible factor affecting his potency, but this is not usually necessary or cost-effective in every patient. Other hormonal tests such as thyroid and adrenal ones are only performed in patients with signs or symptoms of endocrine disease. A serum lipid panel should also be obtained in any patient found to have arteriogenic impotency who has not had routine medical evaluations or also as a later laboratory test in any young patients who are being considered as possible candidates for arterial surgery.

Many experts in this field would recommend nocturnal tumescence testing (NPT) as one of the first evaluation steps.[9,10] This evaluation is certainly necessary when psychogenic impotence is suggested by the history (ie, excellent erections with partners other than the wife or symptoms of depression), when secondary gain is suggested such as workmen's compensation or insurance claims cases, when a major sleep disorder is suspected from the history (such as extreme daytime sleepiness), or when the patient shows an excellent response to injection agents but gives a definite history of total erectile dysfunction. If performed, measurement of number of events, length of time of erection, and rigidity are necessary components for a test to have any accuracy. Testing methods that cannot provide these data are gross screening tests at best. A formal sleep lab test is the optimal evaluation since it is the only one that provides sleep disorder data as well as NPT data, but the cost of such a study makes it almost prohibitive as a routine evaluation. Only one patient take-home unit provides the necessary components for evaluation of NPT.[11]

Other sophisticated neurologic testing such as biothesiometry, bulbocavernosus reflex latency, and penile nerve evoked potentials may increase the accuracy of diagnosing sensory deficits but decreased tactile sensation in the penis or perineum on physical evaluation or a history of an inability to sustain erections and a sense of a decreased feeling of contact with sexual intercourse can also be determined during the initial patient visit.[2] In addition, checking for increased rectal sphincter tone on the examining finger at the time of squeezing the glans penis (the bulbocavernosus reflex) also measures the same spinal arc as the other more sophisticated tests, not with the same degree of accuracy but certainly in a more cost-effective manner. There are no tests that are currently proved to measure autonomic nerve defect. Sarica and Karacan suggested that by measuring a bladder neck stimulation (through a special catheter) to rectal sphincter contraction latency time, an afferent arc of the autonomic nervous system is measured, but this has not been verified.[12] In addition, measurement of nerve potentials by special needle electrodes has been introduced as a possible direct measurement of cavernous tissue nervous activity.[13,14] A good history will detect most disease or surgery that will affect the nerves responsible for erection, and these patients will almost always, in the face of this being the single etiology for the impotency, have a supersensitivity to small doses of injection of smooth muscle relaxing and vasoactive agents intracavernously.

## Pharmacologic Agent Injection

Often it is convenient and a great source of information at the first office visit to perform an injection of an intracavernous agent to determine the ability of these agents to produce an erection.[15] This can also serve as a test to see if this may be a therapeutic choice for that particular individual. Agents popularly used are papaverine alone (usually at doses of 15 to 60 mg), a mixture of papaverine and phentolamine (15 to 30 mg/0.5–1 mg), prostaglandin E1 (PGE-1) (5 to 20 μg), or, as preferred at the Mayo Clinic, a mixture of all three of the agents papaverine, phentolamine, and PGE-1 (4.4 mg/0.15 mg/1.5 μg, respectively). The latter choice can be given in a 0.25-mL dose. Because of the synergism obtained with the agent combination, a much lower dose of each of the individual agents is possible. The development of a full rigid erection by 10 minutes that is fully sustained for 30 minutes is indicative of no major vascular disease, ie, normal arterial inflow and the presence of an intact veno-occlusive mechanism. Lue suggested that if no spontaneous erection is achieved by 10 minutes, manual stimulation should be added by the patient to see if an adequate erection can be obtained.[7] A good response to this office test can serve as a dose-determining session for the patient wishing to use this method as a therapy. The patients tested should be carefully assessed for priapism before leaving the physician's office since this tends to occur in the initial office test 5% to 10% of the time regardless of the agents used. The preference at the Mayo Clinic is to wait for 2 hours before pharmacologic reversal, but the erection will also be reversed if it is particularly painful for the patient. For reversal, a 19-gauge needle is placed in one of the corpora at the lateral base, 20 to 30 mL of blood is aspirated, and the patient is observed for 10 minutes. If the erection reoccurs, another 20 to 30 mL of blood is aspirated and 200 μg of phenylephrine flushed into the corpora through the tubing attached to the butterfly needle. (The phenylephrine is kept refrigerated in a 500 μg/mL stock solution.)

A patient's failure to achieve a full erection cannot be taken as definite evidence of vascular disease. In the nervous patient who has showered the area with norepinephrine with a sympathetic response or in some patients with psychologic impotency, a similar type of pattern of no response may occur. Additional definitive testing must be performed to determine vascular abnormalities. A slow erectile response taking 30 minutes or longer to produce any erection suggests arterial disease, and a rapid full erection by 10 minutes that quickly dissipates over the next 10 minutes suggests deficient veno-occlusion. For the patient who has selected intracavernous therapy at this first office visit and in whom a poor response is obtained, this should not be disqualifying for this particular therapy. Further injection on a return office visit or arranging an injection so that the patient may try sexual intercourse with his partner in a private, more congenial setting is the next step.

## Duplex Doppler Evaluation

For the patient who desires to know the exact etiology of his impotency, and actually preferred as a very important assessment of the vascular status of the erectile mechanism, the performance of a color duplex Doppler test is the next step in the diagnosis of erectile dysfunction after the initial history and physical session.[16] Lue was the first to describe the use of duplex Doppler as a more accurate way to diagnose arterial disease in 1985.[17] We and others have expanded this evaluation to include the use of color imaging to more easily and quickly identify the cavernous artery and to use the end-diastolic velocity of flow in the artery to evaluate the veno-occlusive mechanism. These imaging units, although expensive, are available in most major hospitals for evaluation of carotid and other peripheral vessels, and these programs can easily be adapted to perform the evaluation of the cavernous arteries. (See Figs 5 to 7 and Table 5 for some of the information from the standards of interpretation used at the Mayo Clinic regarding this study.) If

**Fig 5.** The color duplex Doppler probe is scanned over the corpora through a ventral approach.

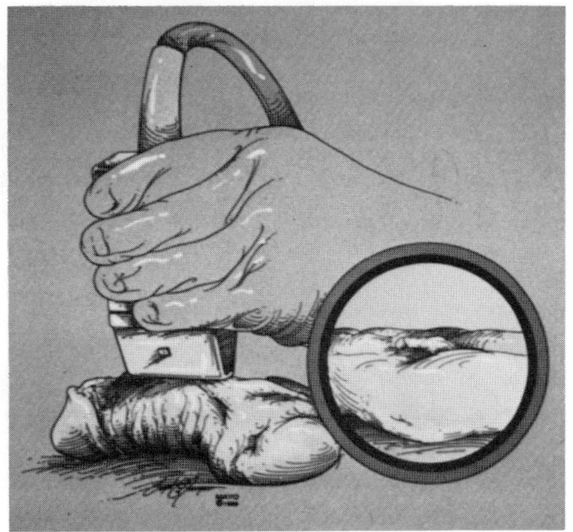

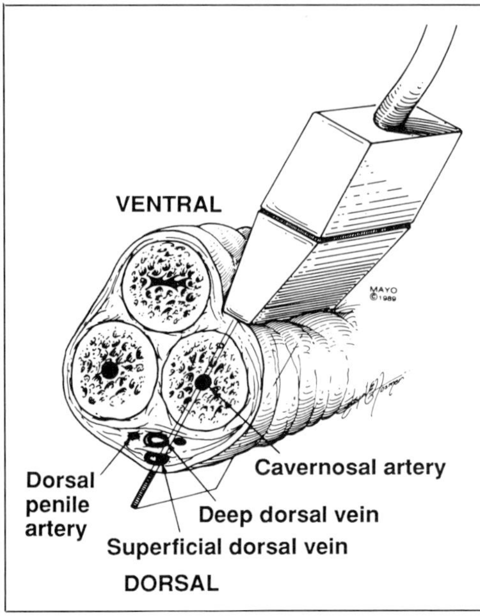


**Fig 6.** The duplex Doppler probe allows for accurate assessment of the cavernosal artery and can be easily detected in the ventral approach.

the patient has normal peak systolic velocity of flow (>30 cm/s) in both arteries and has a 30-minute lasting good firm erection, then there is no significant vascular disease. Again, however, it should be stressed that some patients with mild to moderate arterial disease can still respond to injection therapy; therefore for the patient motivated for this type of therapy, further trials of injection should be made. Patients with normal bilateral arterial peak systolic velocities with poor erections from the injected agents and who have end-diastolic velocities of flow ≥3 to 5 cm/s usually have veno-occlusive disease. If interested in surgery for this disorder, after informing them of the 40% to 50% success rate for this operation, then the more definitive diagnostic tests, cavernosometry and cavernosography, should be the next evaluation. Similarly, for patients who are found to have significant arterial disease and are acceptable candidates for revascularization surgery, the next diagnostic test is pelvic and internal pudendal arteriography.

**Fig 7.** An example of an image obtained from color duplex Doppler. (A color representation would show that the cavernosal artery demonstrates forward flow in a brilliant red, which is appreciated in the middle of the upper cavernosal ultrasound image.) A computer-generated arterial wave form is also presented at real time from which a peak systolic arterial velocity and an end-diastolic artery velocity are computed.

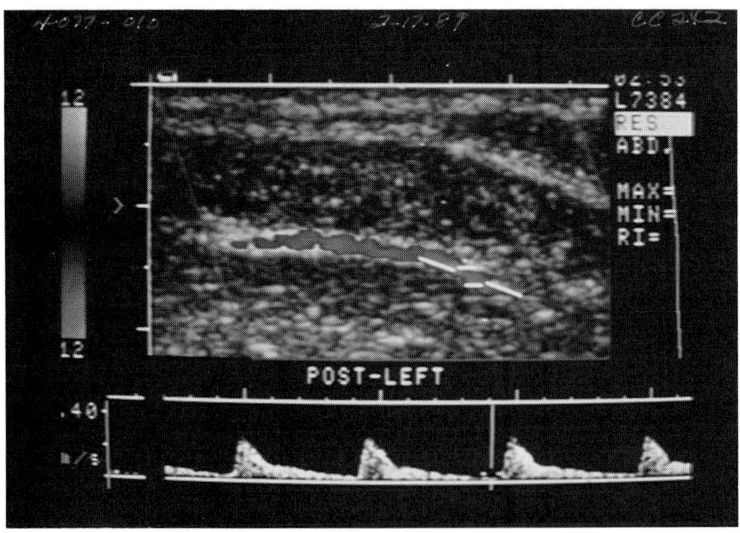

| TABLE 5. Duplex and Color Doppler Imaging Vasculogenic Impotence |
|---|
| • Specific evaluation of deep penile arteries<br>• Conventional duplex Doppler spectral analysis and color Doppler imaging<br>• Qualified/designated ultrasound technician(s)<br>• Studies performed prior to and after intracorporeal injection of a smooth muscle relaxing agent<br>• Parameters<br>Echotexture of corpora cavernosa is performed to detect plaque fibrosis or other abnormalities<br>Cavernosal artery diameter is difficult to measure preagent injection but should increase to a diameter of 0.7 mm afterward<br>Cavernosal artery peak systolic velocity (PSV) should increase to >30 cm/s to be considered normal (25–30 cm/s is indeterminate) (multiple measurements are required to optimize detection of maximum PSV, suggested time is 5, 10, 15, and 20 minutes)<br>Cavernosal artery end-diastolic velocity, if ≥3–5 cm/s venous leak is suggested to be followed by definitive diagnostic tests, which are cavernosometry and cavernosography (reversal of flow at diastole is indicative of good veno-occlusive function)<br>Abnormally high cavernosal artery peak systolic velocity may suggest vascular spasm or poststenotic dilatation flow<br>Deep dorsal vein velocity is not indicative of venous leak<br>Systolic flow reversal suggest variation of vascular anatomy, proximal arterial disease prior to insertion into the cavernous tissue, or arterial sinusoidal fistula<br>A clinical response to the pharmacologic agent is also made at the time of the testing |

| TABLE 6. Diagnosis of Venogenic Impotence |
|---|
| • Cavernosometry or pharmacocavernosography/infusion by pump maintenance flow rate<br>• Gravity pharmacocavernosometry<br>• Pharmacocavernosography<br>• Evaluation of pressure decay from steady state (ie, second phase of dynamic infusion cavernosometry and cavernosography [DICC] |

## Invasive Testing for Evaluation of Vascular Disease

The more invasive tests for the evaluation of vascular disease mentioned above should be reserved for those patients who, after being presented with the expected results from vascular surgery, wish to select this type of therapy over the other options.[18] (See Tables 6 to 11 and Figs 8 to 12 for

| TABLE 7. Technique of Cavernosometry/Cavernosography |
|---|
| • Two 19-gauge needles placed into each corpus cavernosum (obliquely, toward patient's head), without anesthesia, laterally along shaft of penis under sterile conditions<br>• One needle connected for pressure measurement via a transducer connected to a physiologic recorder or monitor<br>• Other needle connected to an infusion roller pump for infusion of heparinized saline solution (1000 U/1000 mL)—prewarmed to body temperature<br>• Record baseline pressure<br>• Infuse fluid at 50 mL/min increments until full erection occurs (90–100 mm Hg), then decreased flow to obtain flow rate needed to maintain erection (do not infuse above 300 mL/min)<br>• Inject pharmacologic agent (usually 45 mg of papaverine and 2.5 mg of phentolamine) through needle<br>• Record baseline pressure 10 minutes later<br>• Repeat flow study obtaining flow rate to maintain erection (do not infuse above 150 mL/min)<br>• Inject 30% diatrozoate or iothalomate meglumine (60 mL full strength or 120 mL 50% dilution with saline) at same rate as last maintenance flow rate and obtain cinefluoroscopic images, or spot static x-ray images (AP and oblique) for cavernosography |

**TABLE 8. Infusion Pump Cavernosometry**

Consider positive (indicative of venous leak or poor veno-occlusion) if:

- Maintenance flow without pharmacologic agents is >100 mL/min (75–100 indeterminate)
- Maintenance flow rate after pharmacologic agents is >50 mL/min (30–50 indeterminate)

**TABLE 9. Diagnosis for Arteriogenic Impotence**

- Penile blood pressure indices and/or pulse wave analysis probably not accurate by a simple Doppler
- Color duplex Doppler ultrasonography of central deep penile artery in response to pharmacologic agent
- Gradient between cavernosal arteries systolic occlusion pressure and brachial artery (third phase of DICC)
- Pudendal arteriography

**TABLE 10. Pelvic Arteriography**

- Vasculogenic impotence is suggested by deep penile artery screening studies or by history (ie, pelvic trauma)
- Only candidates for revascularization should be studied
- Femoral percutaneous approach
- Includes pelvic flush study, bilateral hypogastric arteries, and selective internal pudendal arteriography
- Nonionic contrast material
- Simultaneous intracavernosal pharmacologic injection is necessary
- Magnification views or subtraction studies may aid in visualization of these small arteries
- Intra-arterial vasodilators used
- Left anterior oblique for left artery study and right anterior oblique for right artery study

**TABLE 11. Arteriographic Signs of Significant Vascular Disease**

- Delay in filling of cavernosal arteries compared to other penile vessels
- Abrupt termination of arteries, particularly in the perineal segment of the penile artery
- Late collateral filling
- Retrograde filling of the cavernous artery from the dorsal artery
- Nicking, beading, or narrowing of the deep penile or cavernous artery and tributaries

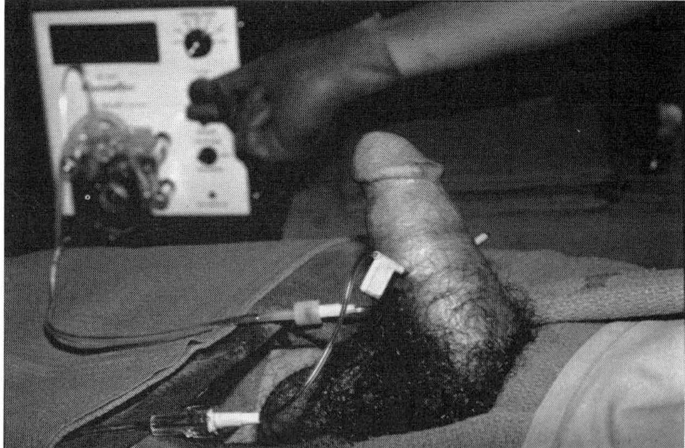

**Fig 8.** Infusion pump cavernosometry. Two 19-gauge needles have been placed into the corpora on the lateral surface of the penis. One is connected to an infusion pump that has an adjustable constant digital readout of flow, and the other is connected to a pressure manometer (not shown).

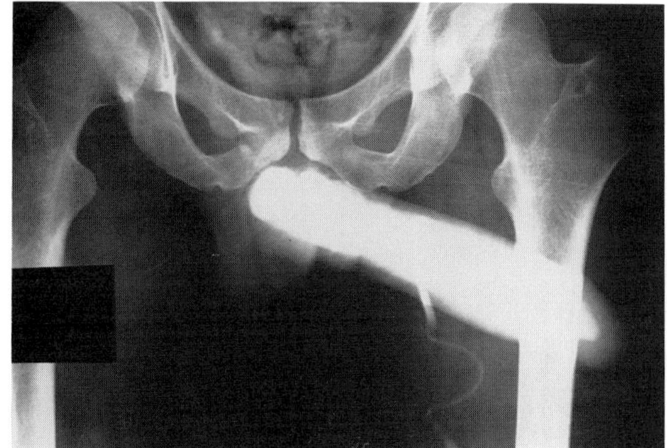

**Fig 9.** Example of a patient who has an intact veno-occlusive function as indicated by no significant leak at the time of infusion of contrast into the corpora.

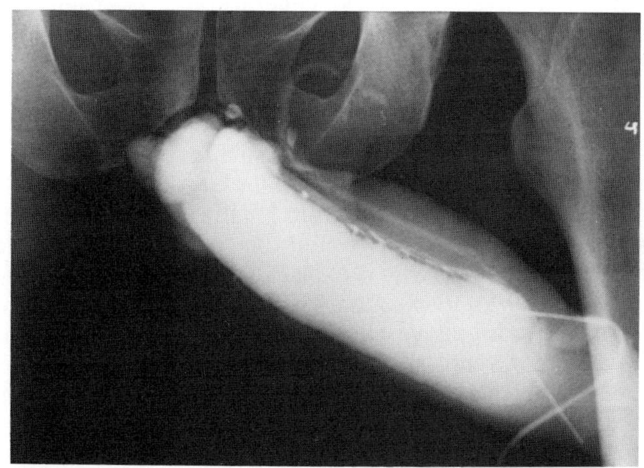

**Fig 10.** A cavernosogram in a patient with a significant venous leak. A large deep dorsal vein being filled by direct emissary and circumflex vessels is clearly seen. Communications to a superficial penile vein that drains into the left external pudendal system are also seen. This superficial vein subsequently drains into the saphenous vein (not shown on this figure).

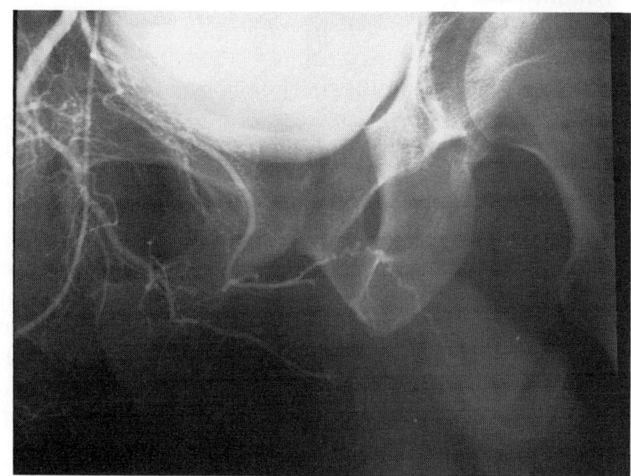

**Fig 11.** An abrupt termination of the deep dorsal artery on the patient's arteriography. The penile vessels are supplied by an aberrant internal pudendal artery, and there is an abrupt termination of the deep penile artery (the cavernosal artery) in the perineum. There is a continuation of the dorsal artery of the penis that is seen to lie along the shaft of the penis. This is the common type of pattern that is seen in perineal trauma.

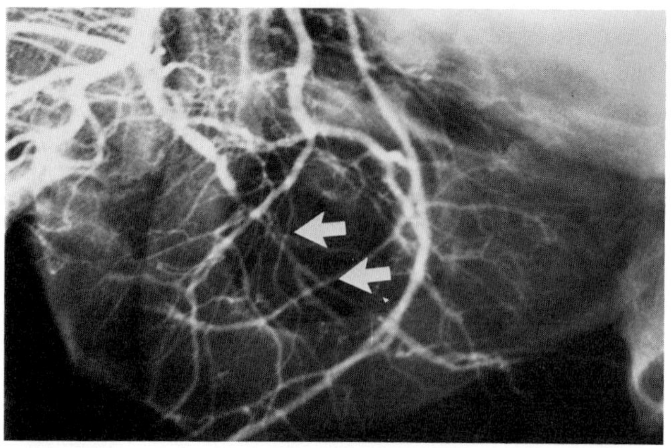

**Fig 12.** Arteriogram showing the common pattern found in focal arteriosclerosis in a patient with erectile dysfunction of an arteriogenic nature. The internal pudendal artery is seen to be diseased (as indicated by the large white arrows in the projection over the obturator foramen in the oblique positioning of the patient) in its course through Alcock's canal.

specifics of cavernosometry, cavernosography, and arteriography.) The more preferable test for diagnosis of veno-occlusive dysfunction is infusion pump pharmacocavernosometry and pharmacocavernosography.[19,20] Both a functional test, such as color duplex Doppler evaluation of the cavernous arteries, and an anatomic localization test, arteriography should be performed in the patient who is to be evaluated for arterial revascularization. The patient who has arteriography should also have evaluation for veno-occlusive dysfunction before the planned arterial surgery because venous dissection and ligation can be accomplished at the same surgery.

Dynamic infusion cavernosometry and cavernosography (DICC) is a four-phase evaluation of the vascular system responsible for erection that has been described by Goldstein and his associates.[21] The measurement of the systolic arterial occlusion pressure seems to be an excellent alternative for diagnosis of arterial disease to the color duplex Doppler evaluation, but the pressure decay measurement from a steady-state value is not specific for veno-occlusive disorders.[20]

## MANAGEMENT OF ERECTILE DYSFUNCTION

As mentioned in the evaluation section, the patient with erectile dysfunction, and preferably his partner, must be carefully counseled as to the therapeutic choices available for the management of the disorder. Often more than one of the subsequently discussed management options can be used together. Although each will be described separately, it does not mean that only one of these options should be used for the management of any one individual's impotence. For example, the patient may use intracavernous injection therapy and a vacuum device as combination therapy. Once the patient's goal of therapy is chosen, then further workup and intervention must go hand in hand.

Often improving management in a poorly controlled insulin-dependent diabetic can reverse a partial erectile failure in that patient. Changing one type of antihypertensive medicine to another that is least likely to cause erectile dysfunction will improve the erectile ability for a given patient. Similar adjustments in some of the psychotropic medications may produce similar results. Successful treatment of other endocrine disorders, such as hypothyroidism, may result in reversal of an associated erectile failure. Management of a sleep disorder by a physician who is a specialist in this field will often reverse an associated sexual disorder. Patients with minor or even moderate vascular disorders who use tobacco should be encouraged to stop and certainly to stop before any vascular surgery is planned.

Behavioral therapy or psychotherapy has an obvious role in the management of erectile dysfunction that is mostly due to a psychogenic disorder. Clearly, treatment of depression in the male who is also impotent often reverses the impotency. This psychological management should be performed by a psychiatrist or other mental health worker with credentials in sexual therapy.

## Testosterone Therapy

Partial erectile failure in patients consistently found to have low serum testosterone will often respond to testosterone therapy. This treatment should be given in a parenteral form on an every 2–3 week basis with proper evaluation and follow-up of the prostate for cancer and benign prostatic hyperplasia. In the presence of low serum testosterone, serum prolactin should be obtained since parenteral therapy with testosterone in the presence of a prolactin-secreting tumor will not successfully reverse the associated impotence and the usual associated decreased libido. Surgical ablation of the pituitary tumor or medical treatment with bromocriptine would be necessary, but also testosterone parenteral therapy might have to be added to reverse the impotence even though the elevated serum prolactin is successfully managed.

## Vacuum Devices

Regardless of etiology, almost every impotent patient should be presented with the therapeutic option of vacuum devices quite early in the evaluation. The use of this device is contraindicated in the patient who has a disorder likely to be associated with priapism, such as sickle cell trait, has a blood dyscrasia prone to affect the clotting mechanism, or has significant capillary fragility. Available devices are numerous and any one of the prescription-requiring devices seems to be adequate with only minor differences among the various choices. This type of therapy is probably the most cost-effective and satisfaction compares favorably with other therapeutic options. Nadig, one of the pioneers in this field, has reviewed this subject very well.[22]

## Pharmacologic Injection Therapy

A very popular type of therapy today is pharmacologic injection therapy.[15,23] The agents most commonly used are papaverine, alone or with phentolamine, prostaglandin E-1 (PGE-1), or various two- or three-drug combinations of these agents. At the Mayo Clinic, the most commonly prescribed injectable is a triple agent containing papaverine, phentolamine, and PGE-1 (4.4 mg, 0.15 mg, and 1.5 μg, respectively, in a dose of 0.25 mL). The synergy of action of the three agents allows for a marked reduction in the dose of each of the individual agents. It is imperative that the patient be tested in the clinic in order to be able to select the proper minimal dose necessary for the individual patient and also to instruct the patient in the proper sterile injection technique. The injection site is the lateral corpora cavernosa on either side of the penis from just below the glans to the base of the penis. It is recommended to the patient that injections be performed no more than twice weekly and to vary the injection site. The initial first test dose should be minimal for those with neurologic disease or those in whom injury to the nerves is suspected since these patients are usually quite sensitive to the agents and are more prone to have prolonged erections or priapism. This type of therapy has high success in those patients who have had radical pelvic surgery for cancer. Priapism occurs in approximately 5% to 10% of patients at first testing, less commonly with PGE-1 alone. After deciding a safe dose, priapism with home use is usually about 1% regardless of the agent used. The patient who is using home self-injection therapy should be carefully instructed to seek priapism treatment as an emergency should a resulting erection last more than 3 hours or become a painful prolonged erection. Significant fibrosis is rare, particularly in patients using the agents no more than twice weekly and varying the injection sites. Infection has rarely been reported. The dropout rate for patients who elect this type of therapy is approximately 30% to 35%. Although none of these agents are approved for this indication by the U.S. Food and Drug Administration, the therapy has become a much accepted and widely practiced choice for the impotent male.[24] Alternate agents other than those discussed above have been described, but they have not become popular in the United States and have not gained wide acceptance.[15]

## Penile Prostheses

Penile prosthetic devices have evolved over the last 15 years and many improvements have resulted in types that are more dependable regarding mechanical wear or breakdown (Fig 13). This therapy should be considered irreversible although some patients have had successful use of the vacuum devices after removal of the prosthetic. Basically, there are two major types of devices: semirigid and inflatable. The semirigid devices currently available are Silastic rods with some type of metallic core or interlocking plastic components centered by a metallic cable covered with a synthetic covering. The inflatable devices are either self-contained inflatable, two-piece systems with a single-combination scrotal pump and reservoir, or three-piece systems with a separate scrotal pump and postrectus muscle reservoir. The latter devices offer the best flaccidity, rigidity, and girth, particularly suitable for those patients who elect this type of therapy who also have a significant curvature of the penis due to Peyronie's disease. Several current papers deal with the advantages of each of the more popular and available prostheses.[25–29] Basically, the semirigid devices have less tendency for mechanical wear and are surgically easier to place, but flaccidity, concealability, and girth are not optimal. In addition, erosion is more common with the semirigid devices. Two-piece inflatable penile devices are particularly useful for patients in whom there may be difficulty placing an abdominal reservoir. They are also slightly easier to surgically place but

**Fig 13.** Penile prosthetic devices consist of semi-rigid devices, self-contained inflatable, or 2- and 3-piece inflatable prosthetic devices.

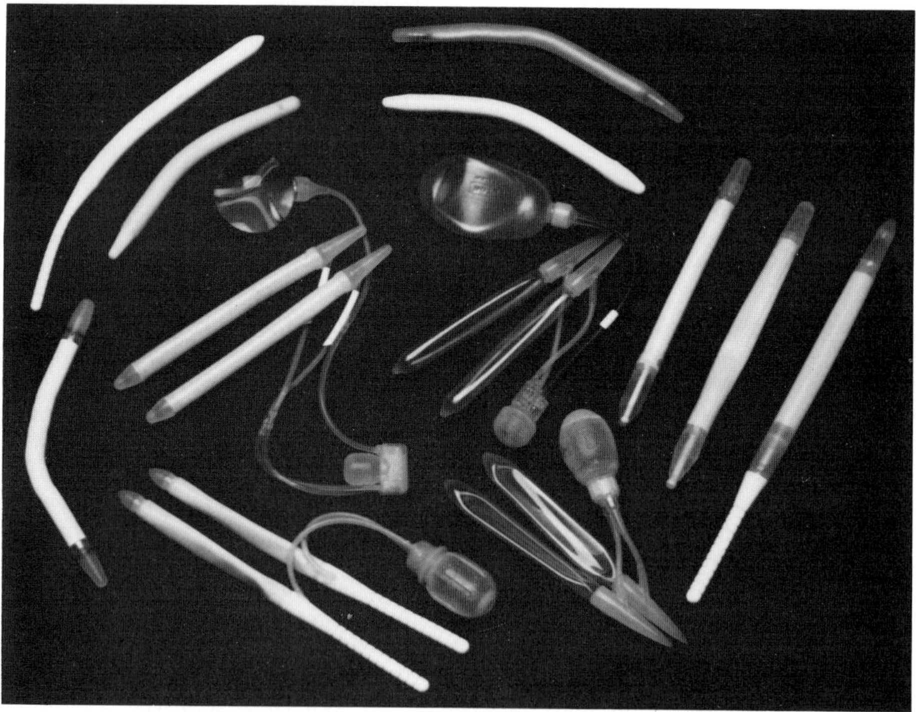

produce approximately 80% to 85% of the girth change or rigidity of the three-piece devices and less flaccidity in the deflated state. Both of the major three-piece devices are now available connectorless in the tubing from the pump to the cylinders, and one has an expandable length feature in the cylinders. Silastic material is the main component of the penile prostheses except for one company whose two- and three-piece inflatable devices have the cylinders and other parts of the device made of a plastic polymer, which is very wear-resistant. The surgical approach for placement of the penile prosthesis depends on the type of device selected. Semirigid devices and self-contained inflatable devices are usually placed through circumcision-like incisions or penile-scrotal incisions. Inflatable devices are usually placed via infrapubic or penile-scrotal incisions. The patient who selects the penile prosthesis should understand that reoperation may be necessary, particularly if the device is present over 5 to 10 years. Mechanical failure of the devices has accounted for approximately 50% of the reason for reoperation at the Mayo Clinic. Table 12 lists the 1397 reasons for reoperation in 1358 cases in 555 patients who had reoperation for penile implant at the Mayo Clinic. Infection occurs in approximately 1% to 9% of patients who have placement of penile prostheses and when occurring usually require total implant removal.[30] Recently some have suggested salvage maneuvers, but this must be done cautiously and currently probably only at large prosthetic centers.[31] (See Table 13 for guidelines for salvage therapy.) Overall patient and partner satisfaction for the penile prosthesis is high, 90% to 95%. However, informed consent regarding infection, mechanical failure possibility, and the rare intolerable pain must be given to each patient accepting this modality of treatment.

**TABLE 12. Reoperation for Penile Prosthesis**

| Reason | No. (%) |
|---|---|
| • Mechanical failure or device malfunction | 770 (56.7) |
| • Infection | |
| Without erosion | 99 (7.3) |
| With erosion | 57 (4.2) |
| • Unknown fluid loss | 104 (7.7) |
| • Patient dissatisfaction or pain | 86 (6.0) |
| • Poor position | 85 (5.0) |
| • Staged procedure | 56 (4.1) |
| • Hematoma or seroma | 28 (2.0) |
| • Encapsulation | 21 (1.5) |
| • Could not be determined | 91 (6.7) |

## Vascular Surgery

Vascular surgery for male erectile dysfunction is only indicated for highly selected patients.[32,33] Patients who have sustained major pelvic trauma and have identified arterial lesions are an example of the type of patient who might be encouraged to have arterial revascularization. Generalized arteriosclerosis, high serum lipids, lack of specific focal lesions affecting the internal pudendal arteries or any of its terminal penile branches, the presence of insulin-dependent diabetes, the inability of the patient to refrain from the use of

**TABLE 13. Salvage Techniques for Penile Prosthesis**

- Options
  - New components to same space (drains are always used) or a new site
  - Retention of some components of the device
  - Perineal urethrostomy diversion with immediate repair of urethral perforation
  - Early replacement after local and systemic antibiotics over 3 weeks
- Tubular fenestrated drains (irrigation with antibiotics)
  - Old infected sites
  - Same site with immediate replacement
  - Corpora spaces without devices to decrease future fibrosis
  - 1–5 drains may be used in a patient
  - Majority are irrigated around the clock with 2–7 ml every 4–8 hours for 5–7 days
- Dabs antibiotic solution for irrigation consist of:
  - 50 mg of neomycin, 80 mg gentamicin, 100 mg polymyxin — 1000 ml isotonic saline
- Long course of postoperative oral antibiotics

tobacco in any form, and an age over 60 years are all contraindications for penile revascularization. Basically, after demonstrating specific focal arterial lesions on pelvic arteriography and testing the patient with intracavernous agents to see if this would be an alternative therapy, the young patient with arterial disease is offered the option of revascularization with the prognosis of success to reverse the impotence of approximately 60% to 70%, including conversion to successful injection therapy. The surgery of penile revascularization consists of using the inferior epigastric artery or saphenous vein bypass from the femoral artery to a receptor vessel, which can be the dorsal penile artery, an isolated deep dorsal vein, or a combination of the two (Fig 14, Table 14). Postoperative persantine (50 mg 3 times a day for 6 months) and aspirin (2.5 grains/d for the remainder of the patient's sex life) is recommended after revascularization surgery. Glanular hyperemia is seen in approximately 5% of those patients who have deep dorsal vein arterialization and great care should be taken to ensure that tributaries from the glans penis and from the corpus spongiosum are ligated as the receptable dorsal vein is prepared.

**Fig 14.** Diagrammatic representation of the current steps in penile revascularization. **A,** a midline incision is recommended so that either inferior epigastric artery can be reached without a separate incision; **B,** inferior epigastric vessel bundle is dissected away from the inferior margin of the rectus muscle by retracting the muscle laterally from the midline. The branches are ligated with fine silk or small clips, and both the artery and the vein are taken together; **C,** the inferior epigastric artery can be microscopically connected end-to-side (as shown) or end-to-end in the dorsal artery; **D,** similar microvascular surgery can be performed by arterializing an isolated segment of deep dorsal vein.

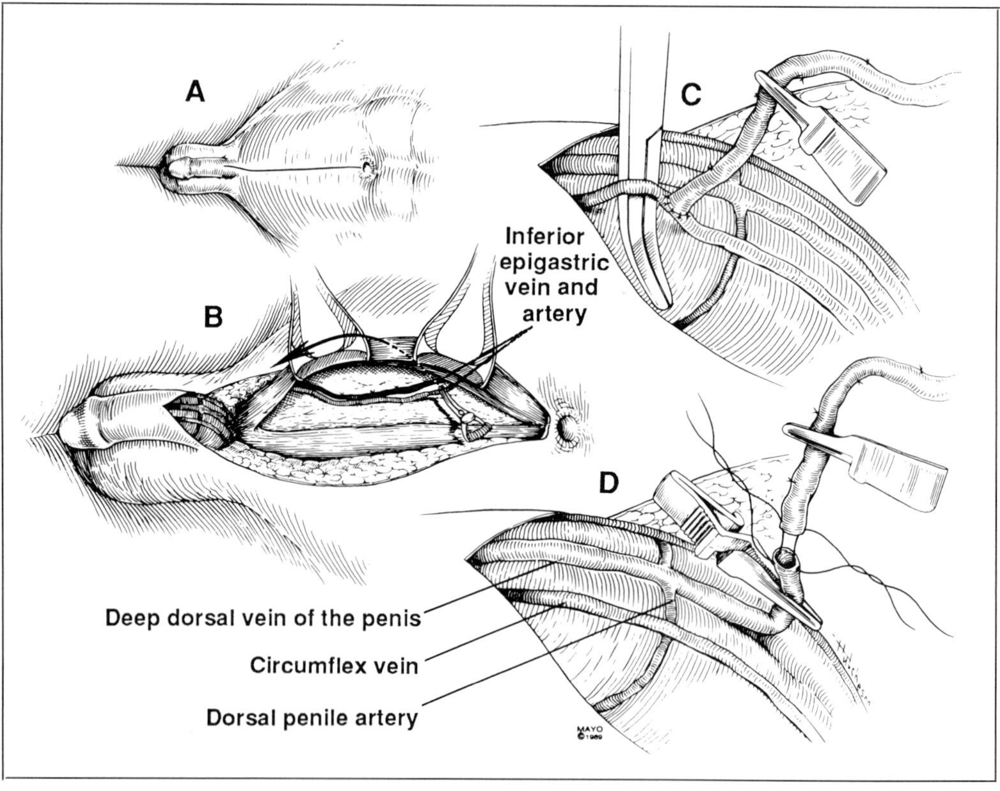

**TABLE 14. Current Major Penile Revascularization Procedures**

- Use of inferior epigastric artery or saphenous vein bypass from femoral vein as input source
- Microvascular surgery
- Modification of Michal procedure—distal or proximal end to end to dorsal artery—end to side to dorsal artery
- Arterialization (modification of Virag procedure) of isolated segment of deep dorsal vein
- Direct anastomosis to deep penile cavernous artery

## Venous Surgery

Deep penile vein dissection is indicated in an even more select type of patient[19,34–36] (Table 15). Because veno-occlusion is often faulty secondary to poor arterial inflow or poor engorgement of the cavernous tissue due to sinus smooth muscle disease for which there is no current specific diagnostic test, it is rare to find the patient who is a candidate for venous surgery. Some have advocated deep dorsal vein arterialization for patients with veno-occlusion, but this is not widely accepted. There are rare individuals who have congenital or developmental abnormal venous channels that are not properly occluded with normal arterial infow or sinus tissue relaxation. Basically every effort is made to rule out concomitant arterial disease in individuals found to have veno-occlusive dysfunction. Then a prognosis of cure of only 50% to 60% is presented to these patients (Table 16). They should not be able to get an erection with an intracavernous agent and should not use tobacco. Surgery should eliminate all possible effluxing veins visualized on pharmacocavernosography and should not be ligation of the deep dorsal vein only.

**TABLE 15. Criteria of Venous Surgery for Veno-Occlusive Disorder**

- Compatible history and physical
- No or poor response to pharmacologic agents intracavernously
- Normal arteries by color duplex Doppler evaluation
- Positive leak on cavernosometry/cavernosography

**Technique of Penile Vein Dissection and Ligation.** The procedure begins with the standard anterior scrotal peripenile incision (Fig 15A). Penile edema is less likely to occur with this incision. The penile shaft is then inverted into the peripenile incision (Fig 15B, C). The entire penile shaft can be approached by this inversion, and the infrapubic region can be easily reached through it. As the penile skin is stripped away from the penile shaft, there is often a connection between the deep penile veins and the superficial penile veins. The junction between these two systems can be identified and ligated during this step (Fig 15D).

Figure 15E shows the next two important steps. A 19-gauge needle is placed into one of the corpora, usually on the side of the incision. After the injection of a pharmacologic agent, indigo carmine is injected to demonstrate effluxing veins. (In addition, as shown in Fig 15H, this same line can be used for controlled infusion cavernosometry.) Fixation of the butterfly wing by the chromic suture allows for less chance of dislodgement during the procedure. The infrapubic suspensory ligament is then sharply dissected. Please note that care should be taken in this area because often superficial draining veins from the pubis can join the more superficial of the penile veins. The figure shows a deeper incision of the suspensory ligament. The less defined superficial fundiform ligaments have already been cut. The suspensory ligament will be reapproximated with silk ligature at the end of the procedure.

A large silk suture is then placed around the deep dorsal vein in the infrapubic region. Figure 15F shows the vein fully exposed with the artery to its left margin. Buck's fascia has been removed in the illustration to show the orientation of the arteries and vein. Sometimes, the deep dorsal vein consists of more than one trunk along the shaft of the penis, but usually in the infrapubic region these coalesce to form one large draining vein. This vein also has

**TABLE 16. Results of Surgery for Veno-Occlusive Sexual Dysfunction**

| Study (Years of Study) | No. Patients | Excellent | Improved | Immed. Success/ Later Failure | Failures | Average Follow-up (Months) |
|---|---|---|---|---|---|---|
| Lewis—Tulane Series (1981–1987)[38] | 49 | 12 (24%) | 12 (24%) | 8 (16%) | 17 (35%) | 15 |
| Wespes et al (1982–1986)[39] | 67[a] | 31 (46%) | 16 (24%) | | 20 (30%) | 24 |
| Austoni et al (1987)[40] | 234 | 129 (55%) | | 21 (9%) | 84 (36%) | 9 |
| Lue (1986–1988)[41] | 68[b] | 36 (53%) | 17 (25%) | 4 (6%) | 11 (16%) | Unknown |
| Bondil et al (1981–1988)[42] | 60 | 25 (42%)[c] | | | 35 (58%) | 22 |
| Lunglmayr et al (1984–1986)[43] | 29 | 9 (31%)[c] | | 10 (34.5%) | 10 (34.5%) | to 24 |
| Weidner et al (1984–1988)[44] | 51 | 28 (55%) | | 8 (16%)[d] | 15 (29%)[d] | 20 |
| Treiber and Gilbert (1985–1987)[45] | 115 | 28 (24%) | 39 (34%) | | 48 (42%) | 12.9 |
| Lewis—Mayo Series[46] | | | | | | |
| (1987–1988) | 28 | 7 (25%) | 4 (14%) | 8 (29%) | 9 (32%) | 36 |
| (1988–1989) | 32 | 9 (28%) | 13 (41%) | 5 (15.5%) | 5 (15.5%) | 18 |
| Knoll et al (1987–1989)[47] | 41 | 22 (54%) | Unknown | Unknown | 19 (46%) | 18 |
| Kropman et al (1987–1989)[48] | 20 | 6 (30%) | 4 (20%) | 8 (40%) | 2 (10%) | 15 |
| Rossman et al (1985–1988)[49] | 16 | 2 (12.5%) | 2 (12.5%) | 10 (62.5%) | 2 (12.5%) | Unknown |
| Claes and Baert (1987–1989)[50] | 72 | 30 (41.7%) | 23 (31.9%) | | 19 (26.4%) | >12 |

[a] Sixty-seven patient questionnaire responses to 105 letters sent.
[b] Four not reported because too soon after surgery or no follow-up.
[c] Series reported as excellent or improved as a group, not in each individual category.
[d] Fourteen of 23 are now able to get pharmacologic agent injection erection.

to be eliminated in order to approach the deeper cavernosal veins that sometimes join directly to this vein as a common trunk in the infrapubic region or sometimes drain directly into the pudendal plexus or the internal pudendal veins.

The deep dorsal vein is then carefully dissected along the shaft of the penis to the region of the glans where several trunks can be seen to coalesce and begin the deep dorsal vein (Fig 15G). Circumflex and direct emissary veins that drain into this deep dorsal vein are identified as this vein is dissected, divided between clamps, or divided between ligatures. It is extremely important to stay in the midline because of the close proximity of the dorsal arteries and penile nerve bundles that lie lateral to this vein on either side. The dissection is taken to approximately 1 to 2 cm from the glans edge since the nerves tend to fan out over the veins in this area. Any ligatures used on the penile shaft are absorbable.

Controlled cavernosometry is performed after the penile vein dissection and ligation (Fig 15H) to compare with preoperative cavernosometry data. This is accomplished after another 30 mg of papaverine has been injected into the corpora. Ten minutes later this controlled cavernosometry is obtained. If adequate venous dissection has been performed, maintenance flow rate is usually well below 5 to 10 mL/min.

Some have advocated percutaneous oc-

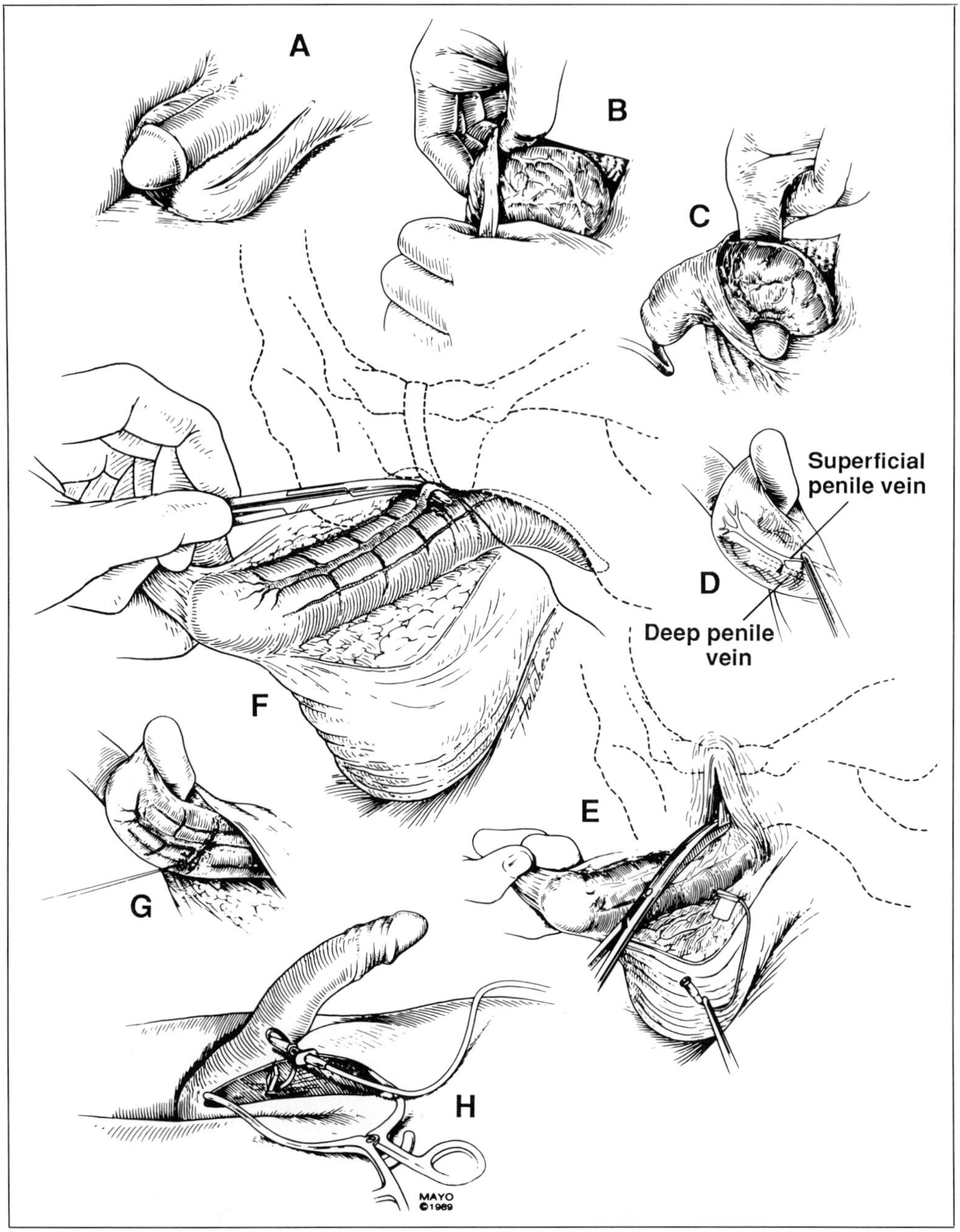

**Fig 15.** Penile vein dissection and ligation. **A,** the standard anterior scrotal peripenile incision; **B, C,** the inversion of the penile shaft into the peripenile incision; **D,** the penile skin is stripped away from the penile shaft; **E,** a 19-gauge needle is placed into one of the corpora; this step also shows a sharp dissection of the infrapubic suspensory ligament—note the deeper incision; **F,** placement of a large silk suture around the deep dorsal vein in the infrapubic region; **G,** careful dissection of the deep dorsal vein along the shaft of the penis. [From *Semin Urol* (1990;8:119), with permission of the Mayo Foundation.]

clusion as an alternative to surgery although supportive data are scant.[37] Alternative therapy such as spongiosolysis and crural compression have also been described but are advised by others and ourselves as secondary procedures only.[34,45]

## SUMMARY

The diagnosis and treatment of male erectile dysfunction has become quite complex and variable. As more information becomes available regarding the physiology of erection and the pathophysiology of impotence, these therapeutic options may become clearer and other options of treatment with a greater precision of prediction of success may become available. However, the basic precept of goal-directed therapy for the patient burdened with this disorder and his sexual companion will remain a basic tenet.

## REFERENCES


1. Krane RJ, Goldstein I, de Tejada IS. Impotence. *N Engl J Med.* 1989;321:1648–1659.
2. Padma-Nathan H, Gerstenberg TC. Neurogenic erectile dysfunction—diagnosis and management. In: Lewis RW, Barrett DM, eds. *Problems in Urology: The Impotent Man.* vol 5. Philadelphia: JB Lippincott; 1991:527–540.
3. de Groat WC, Steers WD. Neuroanatomy and neurophysiology of penile erection. In: Tanagho EA, Lue TF, McClure RD, eds. *Contemporary Management of Impotence and Infertility.* Baltimore: Williams and Wilkins; 1988:3–27.
4. Rajfer JB, Aronson WJ, Bush PA, Dorey FJ, Ignarro LJ. Nitric oxide as a mediator of relaxation of the corpus cavernosum in response to nonadrenergic non-cholinergic neurotransmission. *N Engl J Med.* 1992;326:90–94.
5. Williams DE. Impotence: psychologic contributions to etiology and management. In: Lewis RW, Barrett DM, eds. *Problems in Urology: The Impotent Man.* vol 5. Philadelphia: JB Lippincott; 1991:510–518.
6. Segraves RT, Schoenberg HW, Segraves KAB: Evaluation of the etiology of erectile failure. In: Segraves RT, Schoenberg HW, eds. *Diagnosis and Treatment of Erectile Disturbances: A Guide for Clinicians.* New York: Plenum Press; 1985:165–195.
7. Lue TF. Impotence: a patient's goal-directed approach to treatment. *World J Urol.* 1990;8:67–74.
8. Leiblum SR, Rosen RC. Couples therapy for erectile disorders: conceptual and clinical consideration. *J Sex Med Ther.* 1991;17:147–159.
9. Karacan J. Clinical value of nocturnal REM erections in the differential diagnosis of sexual impotence. *Med Aspects Hum Sex.* 1970;4:27–34.
10. Thon WF. Monitoring of penile tumescence and rigidity. In: Jonas U, Thon WF, Stief CG, eds. *Erectile Dysfunction.* New York: Springer-Verlag; 1991;171–177.
11. Kessler WD. Nocturnal penile tumescence. *Urol Clin North Am.* 1988;15:81–86.
12. Sarica Y, Karacan I. Bulbocavernosus reflex to somatic and distal nerve stimulation in normal subjects and in diabetics with erectile dysfunction. *J Urol.* 1987;138:55–58.
13. Wagner G, Gerstenberg T, Levin RJ. Electrical activity of corpus cavernosum during flaccidity and erection of the human penis: a new diagnostic method? *J Urol.* 1989;142:723–725.
14. Stief CG, Djamilian M, Schaebstaup F, Truss MC, Schlick RW, Abicht JH, Allhoff EP, Jonas U. Single potential analysis of cavernous electric activity: a possible diagnosis of autonomic impotence? *World J Urol.* 1990;8:75–79.
15. Lewis RW. Pharmacologic erection. In: Lewis RW, Barrett DM, eds. *Problems in Urology: The Impotent Man.* vol 5. Philadelphia: JB Lippincott; 1991;541–558.
16. Hattery RR, King BF, Lewis RW, James EM, McKusick MA. Vasculogenic impotence: duplex and color Doppler imaging. *Radiol Clin North Am.* 1991;29:629–645.
17. Lue TF, Hricak H, Marich KW, et al. Vasculogenic impotence evaluated by high-resolution ultrasonography and pulsed Doppler spectrum analysis. *Radiology.* 1985;155:777–781.
18. Lewis RW, Parulkar BG, Johnson CM, Miller WE. Radiology of impotence. In: Lytton B, Catalona WJ, Lipschultz LI, McGuire EJ, eds. *Advances in Urology.* Chicago: Year Book Medical Publishers; 1990;159–189.
19. Lewis RW, Venogenic impotence: diagnosis, management, and results. In: Lewis RW, Barrett DM, eds. *Problems in Urology: The Impotent Man.* vol 5. Philadelphia: JB Lippincott; 1991;567–576.
20. Meuleman EJH, Wijkstra H, Doesburg WH, Debruyne FMJ. Comparison of the diagnostic value of pump and gravity cavernosometry and evaluation of the cavernous veno-occlusive mechanism. *J Urol.* 1991;146:1266–1270.
21. Goldstein I. Vasculogenic impotence: its diagnosis and treatment. In: deVere W, ed. *Problems in Urology: Sexual Dysfunction,* vol 1. Philadelphia: JB Lippincott; 1987:547–563.
22. Nadig PW. Vacuum devices for erectile dysfunction. In: Lewis RW, Barrett DM, eds. *Problems in Urology: The Impotent Man.* vol 5. Philadelphia: JB Lippincott; 1991;559–565.

23. Jünemann KP, Alken P. Pharmacotherapy of erectile dysfunction: a review. *Int J Impotence Res.* 1989;1:71–93.
24. Vasoactive intracavernous pharmacotherapy for therapy: papaverine and phentolamine (diagnostic and therapeutic technology assessment—DATTA). *JAMA.* 1990;264:752–754.
25. Knoll LD, Furlow WL, Motley RC. Clinical experience implanting an inflatable penile prosthesis with controlled-expansion cylinder. *Urology.* 1990;36:502–504.
26. Jonas U. Long-term results with a Jonas-Eska silicone-silver penile prosthesis: a critical evaluation. *Urologe[A].* 1991;30:277–281.
27. Fein RL. The GFS Mark II inflatable penile prosthesis. *J Urol.* 1992;147:66–68.
28. Steinkohl WB, Leach GE. Mechanical complications associated with Mentor inflatable penile prostheses. *Urology.* 1991;38:32–34.
29. Woodworth BE, Carson CC, Webster GD. Inflatable penile prosthesis: effect of device modification on functional longevity. *Urology.* 1991;38:533–536.
30. Carson CC. Infections in genitourinary prostheses. *Urol Clin North Am.* 1989;16:139–147.
31. Furlow WL, Goldwasser B. Salvage of the eroded inflatable penile prosthesis: a new concept. *J Urol.* 1987;138:312–314.
32. Sohn M, Sikora R, Bohndorf K, Deutz FJ. Selective microsurgery in arteriogenic erectile failure. *World J Urol.* 1990;8:104–110.
33. Lewis RW. Vascular surgery in the management of erectile dysfunction. In: Rous SN, ed. *Urology Annual:* Norwalk, CT: Appleton & Lange; 1990:1–25.
34. Lewis RW. Venous ligation surgery for venous leakage. *Int J Impotent Res.* 1990;2:1–19.
35. Lewis RW, Fallen MJ. Diagnosis of management of venogenic impotence. *AUA Update Series.* 1991; Vol X (Lesson 31):242–247.
36. Wespes E. Penile venous surgery for cavernovenous impotence. *World J Urol.* 1990;8:97–100.
37. Courtheoux P, Maiza D, Henriet JP, Vaislic CD, Everard C, Theron J. Erectile dysfunction caused by venous leakage: treatment with attachable balloons and coils. *Radiology.* 1986;161:807–809.
38. Lewis RW. Venous surgery for impotence. *Urol Clin North Am.* 1988;15:115–121.
39. Wespes E, Delcour C, Prejzerowicz L, Struyven J, Schulman CC. Long-term follow-up of patients operated for venous leakage. In: Proceedings of Sixth Biennial International Symposium for Corpora Cavernosum Revascularization and Third Biennial World Meeting on Impotence. Boston: International Society of Impotence Research (ISIR). 1988:193.
40. Austoni E, Belloroforte C, Mantovani F. Improved results with intracavernous vasoactive drug infusion following new surgical techniques for vasculogenic impotence. *World J Urol.* 1987;5:182–189.
41. Lue TF. Penile venous surgery. *Urol Clin North Am.* 1989;16:607–611.
42. Bondil P, Schauvliege T, Nguyen Qui JL. Venocavernous leakage: considerations in 60 operated cases. In: Proceedings of Sixth Biennial Corpora Cavernosum Revascularization and Third Biennial World Meeting on Impotence. Boston: International Society of Impotence Research (ISIR). 1988:189.
43. Lunglmayr G, Nachtigall M, Gindl K. Long-term results of deep dorsal penile vein transaction in venous impotence. *Eur Urol.* 1988;15:209–212.
44. Weidner W, Weiske WH, Rudnick J. Deep dorsal vein dissection for treatment of venous leakage review of the results after a four-year period. *Urologe[A].* 1989;28:217–222.
45. Treiber V, Gilbert P. Venous surgery in erectile dysfunction: a critical report of 116 patients. *Urology.* 1989;34:22–27.
46. Lewis RW. Venous ligation for venogenic impotence. In: Whitehead ED, Nagler HM, eds. *Management of Impotence and Infertility.* Philadelphia: JB Lippincott; 1992, submitted for publication.
47. Knoll LD, Furlow WL, Benson RC. Penile venous surgery for the management of cavernosal venous leakage. *Int J Impotence Res.* 1990;2:21–27.
48. Kropman RF, Nijeholt AABL, Giespers AGM, Swarten IJK. Results of deep penile vein resection in impotence caused by venous leakage. *Int J Impotence Res.* 1990;2:29–34.
49. Rossman B, Mieza M, Melman A. Penile vein ligation for corporeal incompetence: an evaluation of short-term and long-term results. *J Urol.* 1990;144:679–682.
50. Claes H, Baert L. Cavernosometry and penile vein resection in corporeal incompetence: an evaluation of short-term and long-term results. *J Impotence Res.* 1991;3:129–137.

# 21

# Renal and Ureteral Trauma

*Michel A. Pontari and E. James Seidmon*

## RENAL INJURY

Trauma to the kidney is the most common urologic injury in both children and adults.[1,2] Approximately 1 of every 3000 hospital admissions is for renal trauma,[3] and 3% of all trauma patients admitted have renal injuries.[4] Renal injuries are reported in about 10% of all abdominal trauma.[5] The risk to either kidney is equal. Males more commonly sustain renal injuries, with a male-to-female ratio of 3:1, and 4:1 in children.[6]

Anatomically, the kidney is relatively well protected by virtue of its retroperitoneal location, the ribs, vertebral bodies, and anterior viscera. Children are at greater risk for renal injuries than adults because as compared with adults the kidneys are greater in size relative to the rest of the body, there is less renal fat and less development of the flank and abdominal muscles, and there is the presence of fetal lobulations that can separate and disrupt more easily than adult parenchyma. The kidney is the most commonly injured organ in blunt abdominal trauma in the pediatric population.[7]

At least 75% of all renal injuries are due to blunt trauma.[8,9] The remainder are from penetrating trauma,[3,10,11] which can result from external injury such as a gunshot wound or stabbing, or increasingly iatrogenic injuries from procedures involving the kidney such as percutaneous renal biopsy, percutaneous nephrostomy, ureterorenoscopy, and ureteral catheterization. Table 1 lists the etiology of renal injuries at our institution over the past 5 years.

**TABLE 1. Etiology of Renal Injuries**

| Type | % |
|---|---|
| Automobile | 45 |
| Fall | 20 |
| Direct blow | 16 |
| Sports | 10 |
| Gunshot | 6 |
| Stab | 3 |

The kidneys are infrequently the only organ injured by a penetrating injury. The liver, small intestine, colon, and stomach are the most commonly involved organs when the kidney is injured. High-velocity bullets, defined as a muzzle velocity greater than 2500 ft/sec will produce more tissue damage, as the amount of kinetic energy of the bullet is equal to $\frac{1}{2} mv^2$, where $m$ is the mass of the bullet and $v$ the velocity.[12] High-velocity missiles pass through tissue neatly, but create a cavity 30–40 times their size because of the exertion of high pressure on adjacent tissues; these pressures may reach thousands of pounds per square inch.[13] The ''blast effect'' describes the damage that can be done to an organ by the energy of the bullet even in the absence of direct contact. Whereas in the past high-velocity weapons were limited to military use, more civilian high-velocity weapon injuries are being seen. Stab wounds anterior to the anterior axillary line will often involve intraabdominal organs as well, whereas lesions posterior to this less commonly have associated injuries.[14]

Pedicle injuries can be seen following blunt or penetrating trauma. Following blunt trauma, total or partial avulson of the renal artery and vein may occur, as well as segmental injuries to these structures. If the renal artery is stretched without avulsion as in a deceleration injury, a tear may occur in the intima, which is less elastic than the media and adventitia, leading to renal artery thrombosis.[15] With penetrating wounds, the left renal vein is at higher risk than the right side because it is longer and crosses the midline.

The extent of renal injury is variable. Minor injuries include contusions and superficial parenchymal lacerations. Major injuries include deeper parenchymal lacerations, renal fragmentations, or pedical injuries. Table 2 lists one classification, after Federle.[16] Overall, contusions account for 85% of renal injuries, 10%–13% are major lacerations, 4% are fragmented or shattered kidneys, and less than 3% are pedicle or ureteropelvic junction (UPJ) disruptions.[17–19] Children sustain more severe injuries than adults from blunt trauma, with up to 17% of such injuries being significant renal lacerations and 4% pedicle injuries, as compared to 10% and 0.3%, respectively, in adults.[20]

The presentation of renal trauma is variable. Patients with gunshot wounds to the torso and abdomen that involve the kidney often present in hemorrhagic shock from multisystem injury, as can patients with severe blunt renal injuries. In stable patients with suspected renal injuries, the physical exam may reveal ecchymosis in the flank area (Gray–Turner sign) or ecchymosis of the periumbilical area (Cullen's sign), indicative of retroperitoneal hemorrhage. A retroperitoneal bleed can also manifest as nausea, vomiting, ileus and abdominal distension, often without distinct abdominal pain. Physical exam can reveal abdominal rigidity, indicative of bowel injury. The size of the entrance site of a stab wound has little correlation with the extent of injury and depth of penetration. Stab wounds can also present in hemorrhagic shock.

**TABLE 2. Blunt Renal Injuries**

| Category | Injury |
|---|---|
| I | Contusions, intrarenal hematomas, sequential infarctions, subcapsular hematoma |
| II | Large subcapsular hematoma, corticomedullary laceration, complete renal laceration (parenchymal lacerations communicating with the renal collecting system), renal fracture |
| III | Shattered kidneys, renal pedicle damage (occlusion/avulsion) |
| IV | Disruption of the ureteropelvic junction (occlusion/avulsion) |

Hematuria is not a constant sign in renal injuries, and the degree of hematuria does not correlate with the severity of injury. Approximately 70% of penetrating injuries will present with gross hematuria. Pedicle injures are not always associated with hematuria.[21–23] Any patient with a penetrating injury and more than 5 RBC per high power field (HPF) should undergo an imaging study to assess the kidneys. Additionally, patients with no hematuria, but in whom there is suspicion of a renal injury based on the path of a bullet or stab wound, should also undergo radiologic evaluation. In a review of 1146 consecutive patients with renal injuries, 1007 from blunt trauma and 139 penetrating, Mee et al.[24] found that patients with microscopic hematuria who did not present in shock (systolic blood pressure $< 90$ mm Hg) were unlikely to have a significant renal injury. They suggested that patients with gross hematuria or those having hypotension should be radiologically evaluated if stable. Other authors have reached the same conclusions.[25,26] This policy is not advocated in children, however, as children are able to maintain a normal blood pressure despite significant blood loss.[27] Clinically, hypotension is not as good an indicator of significant renal injury in the pediatric population as gross hematuria and a low hematocrit.[6]

Patients presenting in hemorrhagic shock will not have the time for a full radiologic workup prior to proceeding to open exploration. In these patients a limited intravenous pyelogram, either in the trauma area or on the operating room table, should be performed.[28] A dose of 100–150 ml of 50%–60% contrast is recommended.[29] This dose is somewhat larger than the standard intravenous pyelogram (IVP) dose, but compensates for decreased renal perfusion and the dilution effect of parenteral fluids. The status of the contralateral kidney may dictate therapy on the involved side. For patients who are stable on admission, the older literature suggests proceeding with an IVP, but currently our study of choice is a CT scan with intravenous and oral contrast. The CT is a more sensitive test for evaluating parenchymal lacerations and urinary extravasation than IVP and is helpful in determining the presence of nonviable segments of tissue, hematoma size, and the status of associated injuries.[30–32] Herschorn et al.[25] found that of seven patients who had a normal IVP after blunt trauma, four had an abnormal CT scan. For kidneys that are nonfunctioning or hypoperfused on IVP or CT, an angiogram is obtained to rule out vascular injury. A chest film should be obtained in the emergency room to rule out a hemothorax and/or pneumothorax.

Retrograde pyelography has little use in renal parenchymal trauma and is only used rarely in cases of suspected UPJ disruption when the diagnosis is in question. Renal scans have been used in blunt trauma to demonstrate areas of poor perfusion or extravasation.[33] Ultrasonography with Doppler has a limited role in assessing renal trauma and can be used to evaluate a penetrating injury for a pedicle injury or a fistula.

Renal injuries from blunt renal trauma infrequently require surgical exploration. Small hematomas and even larger ones without hemodynamic instability can be managed by observation (Fig 1). In a large series, McAninch et al. reported that 2.4% of blunt renal trauma required exploration.[34] Absolute indications for renal exploration, for both penetrating and blunt renal trauma, include uncontrolled hemorrhage and an expanding or pulsatile hematoma, whereas relative indications for exploration include extensive urinary extravasation, large segments of nonviable tissue, and vascular injury.[34] These findings may be encountered at the time of open exploration in a patient taken to the operating room by the trauma team for hemodynamic instability, or they may be found on preoperative imaging studies. Small amounts of urinary extravasation most often resolve

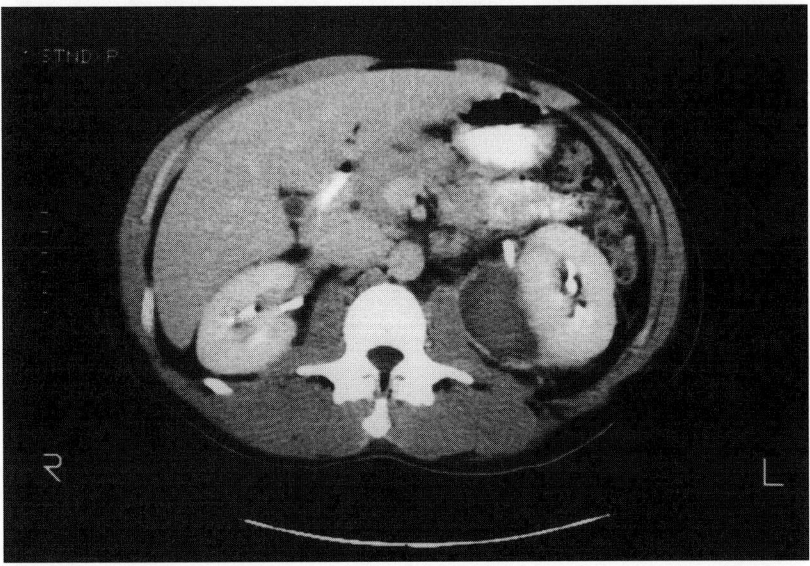


**Fig 1.** CT scan with contrast shows left renal subcapsular hematoma from blunt trauma motor vehicle accident. The patient was managed conservatively.

spontaneously. Even larger amounts of extravasation may subside, but this must be weighed against the risks of urinoma and abscess formation. An increasing number of patients with penetrating renal trauma are being managed nonoperatively. For gunshot wounds, this decision must include consideration of the type of weapon if known, for as the muzzle velocity of the weapon used increases, the chance of injury from the blast effect also increases.

For stab wounds, there is no such blast effect, and when the entrance site is posterior to the anterior axillary line, the incidence of associated abdominal injury is low. Up to 90% of patients with stab wounds in this area have been successfully managed nonoperatively.[14] For stab wounds managed expectantly that develop delayed bleeding or signs of an arteriovenous fistula, angiography can be both diagnostic and therapeutic with the use of embolization.[35] We have used angioembolization as well in cases of blunt trauma with isolated branch renal injuries (Fig 2).

The management of nonfunctioning renal fragments that result from trauma remains under debate. Petersen[36] had success with observation in such situations. Of 15 patients observed, only 2 (15%) developed a complication, ie, hypertension in one child that responded to partial nephrectomy, and delayed hematuria in an adult that was treated with angioembolization. The other 11 have been followed for 5–10 years with no sequelae. Husmann and Morris[37] reported an 85% complication rate in patients observed with devascularized renal fragments after blunt trauma, including perinephric abscesses, infected urinomas, and delayed hemorrhage. Interestingly, 75% of those who developed a perinephric abscess had an associated pancreatic laceration or colon injury. Thus observation of devascularized segments is an option, but may have a higher complication rate in the face of concomitant pancreatic or colonic injury.

For the exploration of renal injuries, the preferred approach is a midline transperitoneal incision.[38] This allows for assessment of other abdominal viscera as well as quick access to the renal vessels if necessary. Repair of major vascular, liver, spleen, or bowel injuries should precede renal exploration unless the renal bleeding is causing hemodynamic instability. Some feel that vascular control should be ob-

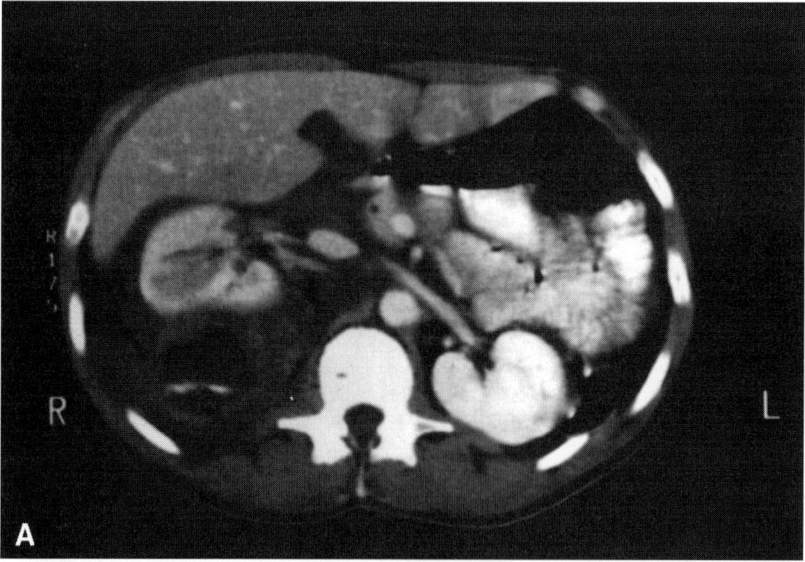


**Fig 2A.** CT scan with contrast after motor vehicle accident shows large right perirenal and retroperitoneal hematoma, with urinary extravasation. After initial period of observation, the patient became hemodynamically unstable.

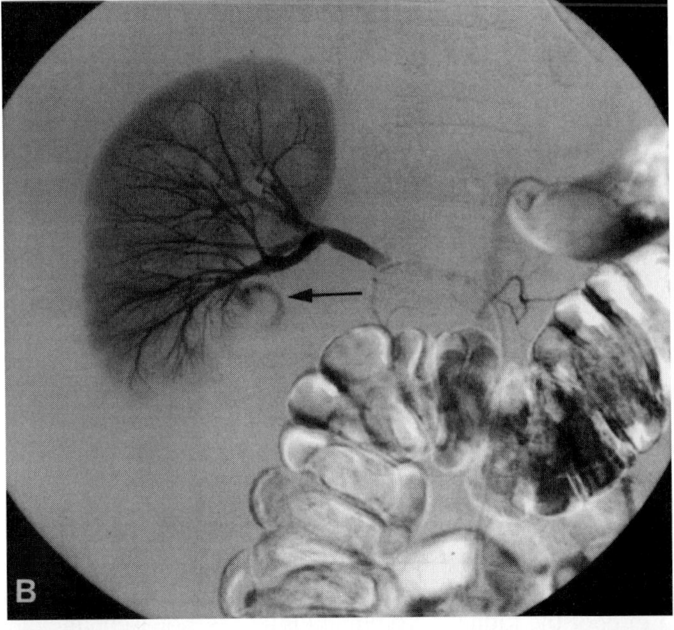


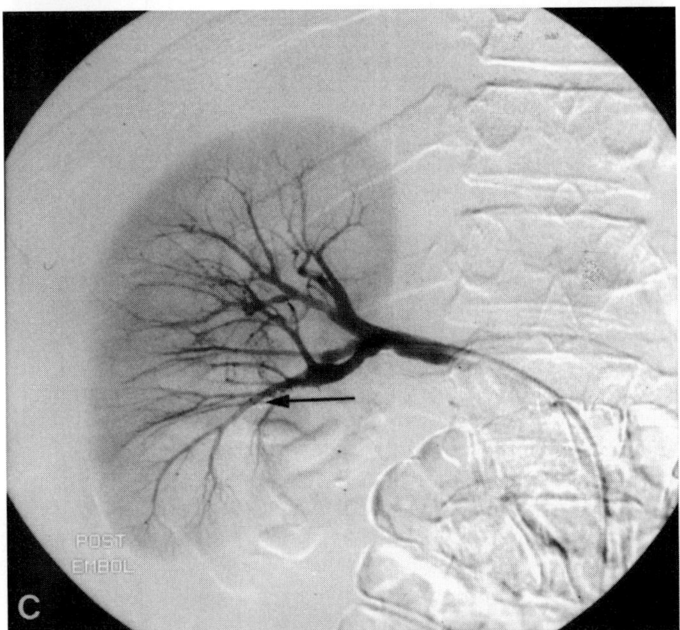


**Fig 2B,C. B:** An arteriogram was performed and showed hemorrhage from lower pole renal vessel *(arrow)*. **C:** Vessel was successfully embolized with coils *(arrow)*.

tained prior to exploring any renal injury. Some centers now obtain vascular control first only if there is a wound and hematoma overlying the renal vessels suggesting a vascular injury.[39] For an isolated hematoma away from the pedicle, exploration can proceed by entering Gerota's fascia laterally and obtaining rapid manual control of any bleeding that occurs.[40]

When vascular control is necessary, the small bowel is reflected to expose the retroperitoneum. An incision is made over the aorta just above the inferior mesenteric artery. If a large hematoma prevents identification of the aorta, the incision should be made just medial to the inferior mesenteric vein.[41] Once onto the aorta, dissection proceeds up to the level of the left renal vein. At this level, the renal artery and vein on each side can be identified and vessel loops placed around the vessels ipsilateral to the injury. The vessels are not clamped unless bleeding is excessive. The kidney is then approached by incising the line of Toldt and reflecting the colon to expose Gerota's fascia and the hematoma.

Total renal exposure is carried out. If bleeding necessitates clamping of the vessels for more than 30 min, iced slush should be used to cool the kidney. Nonviable tissue is debrided, and as much viable tissue, ie, any tissue that bleeds when cut, is preserved.[41] For a devitalized polar lesion, a heminephrectomy may be necessary. Bleeding is controlled by suture ligation and figure of eight 4-0 chromic sutures. Rents in the collecting system are closed with running 4-0 chromic suture. The integrity of the collecting system can be assessed by injecting indigo carmine via a fine-gauge needle into the collecting system while compressing the ureter distally with the fingers. Renal defects are ideally covered by the renal capsule.[34] If this is not available, omentum can be sutured to the wound margin, or absorbable gelatin sponges can be used to bolster and cover the repair. Absorbable mesh can be placed around the kidney if a large repair in the midportion of the kidney has been performed and the ends of the kidney cannot be approximated without tension or after amputation of the lateral aspect of the kidney.[42] Lacerations of the renal artery or vein are repaired with a 5-0 interrupted vascular suture. Extensive injury to a segmental vessel may require ligation. Closed suction drains are placed around the repair and systemic antibiotics are given.

A nephrectomy is performed if there is irreparable damage to the vessels or the collecting system, if a congenital lesion such as a UPJ obstruction is present, or if the patient is hemodynamically unstable.[40] Sagalowsky et al.[43] reported a nephrectomy rate of 26% for patients with renal trauma undergoing renal exploration. With emphasis on early vascular control and attempt at renorrhaphy, the San Francisco group reported an 11% rate of nephrectomy for renal exploration after trauma.[34] Delayed exploration after a major renal injury more often results in total nephrectomy than renorrhapy.[28,38,44,45] For pedicle injuries Carroll et al.[23] recommend attempts to repair/revascularize injuries to the main artery and/or vein in cases of bilateral vascular injury or in case of a solitary kidney. In other patients with a unilateral vascular injury and a normal contralateral kidney, repair is recommended only if the injury is incomplete, amenable to repair, and the kidney is not ischemic. In cases of complete arterial thrombosis or injury with renal ischemia and/or extensive associated other injuries, the patient often is best served by a nephrectomy. After 12 hr of ischemia, the chance for salvage is slim.[46] If recognition is delayed, a nephrectomy is performed only if the patient is being explored for other injuries. If left alone, the kidney will atrophy.[41]

Postoperatively, the patient ambulates once the urine has cleared of gross blood. The blood pressure is monitored, and at 6 weeks to 3 months a follow-up IVP is obtained to evaluate the reconstruction. After any renal injury and repair, or during observation of a renal injury, patients are at risk for developing delayed bleeding, abscess formation, urinary extravasation, fistula formation, and hypertension. Delayed bleeding may represent the formation of an arteriovenous fistula, especially in stab wounds. An arteriogram in this setting can both be diagnostic and allow for therapeutic embolization of the bleeding site. Low-grade fever and continued pain in the area of injury should prompt a CT scan to look for a urinoma or abscess; if present, percutaneous drainage can be carried out. Hypertension may be transient and subside over a few months. If persistent, it usually responds to medical therapy.

## URETERAL INJURY

Injuries to the ureter and renal pelvis account for up to 1% of genitourinary (GU) injuries from external trauma.[47] Most ureteral injuries come from penetrating trauma, and of these, the majority are from gunshot wounds with far fewer the result of stab wounds.[48] The incidence of ureteral injuries with gunshot wounds to the abdomen ranges from 2.5% to 5% in recent series.[49] Ten to fifteen percent of ureteral injuries from external trauma are attributable to blunt injuries, and most of these are confined to the UPJ area.[50,51] Trauma patients with ureteral injuries tend to be severely injured. Presti et al.[47] noted that 53% of their patients with ureteral trauma presented in shock, as defined by a systolic BP <90 mm Hg. However, with improved trauma evacuation and stabilization methods, more patients are surviving serious injuries and as a result the number of recognized ureteral injuries from both penetrating and blunt trauma is increasing.[52]

Penetrating injuries can involve the upper, mid-, or distal ureter, with more injuries seen involving the upper or midureter.[53,54] Patients who sustain penetrating ureteral injuries almost always have associated intraabdominal injuries. The small bowel is most commonly involved, followed by the colon, liver, vascular structures, stomach, bladder, and kidney.[51] Middle ureteral injuries especially are often associated with vascular injuries.[49]

On the initial evaluation, the urinalysis may not show hematuria in 23%–42% of cases.[49,55] Urinary extravasation and obstruction on the IVP indicate injury, but the IVP is nondiagnostic in up to two thirds of cases in which it is performed.[52] Hypovolemia and hypotension will contribute to a poor study. Also, many patients do not get a complete study due to their clinical instability. Such limited studies can be useful to document renal function in an injured kidney and the presence of a functioning contralateral kidney but appears to have its limitations with regard to the diagnosis of ureteral injury.[47] Most penetrating ureteral injuries will be discovered at the time of the trauma. Retrograde pyelography has little role in the acute setting but can be useful in making the diagnosis in the few delayed cases. The role of the CT scan in penetrating ureteral trauma is limited but can be helpful in some situations. Campbell et al.[52] found that the CT finding that helps to delineate proximal ureteral injury from renal parenchymal injury is medial perirenal extravasation of contrast, but that only one of three scans they obtained was helpful or diagnostic.

Many patients will be too unstable at presentation to undergo any radiologic evaluation to rule out a ureteral injury. In these patients, indigo carmine should be given intravenously in the operating room at the time of exploration. If the patient is hypotensive or if there is ipsilateral renal injury that may limit function, the dye can be directly injected into the renal pelvis with a 25-gauge needle to assess the ureteral integrity.[47] Direct inspection of the collection system should be performed as well, looking for a urinoma or retroperitoneal hematoma, which may suggest a ureteral injury. An injury to the intramural or distal ureter must be considered when the bladder is injured.

The ureter injured from a gunshot may actually be more severely damaged than it appears. The energy associated with the bullet can produce injury even if the bullet does not come into direct contact with the ureter.[12] The blast effect can produce damage to the intima of the small vessels in the ureteral wall, leading to extravasation of blood into the ureteral lumen causing hematuria and into the ureteral wall causing bruising.[56] More severe damage can lead to thrombosis of small vessels, ischemia of the ureter, delayed necrosis, and urine leakage.[57] Cass[56] reported on 12 patients explored for ureteral injuries from civilian gunshot wounds. The patients had hematuria with a normal IVP. Two had obvious contusion at exploration and underwent repair or diversion. There was no apparent injury in the other 10; on long-term follow-up, however, two of these patients (20%) developed urinary fistulas through the abdominal wound 2–6 days after the injury, and both eventually died from complications of urosepsis. Rohner observed delayed ureteral fistulas in three of seven ureteral injuries from gunshot wounds in Vietnam.[57] In the past, high-velocity bullet injuries to the ureter were mainly limited to military combat, but more are being seen now in civilian life.

Blunt trauma is an uncommon cause of ureteral injury. The ureter is usually protected from blunt trauma by the vertebral column and overlying abdominal contents. When it does occur, it is usually in children and usually at the UPJ, rarely affecting the lower two thirds of the ureter.[58] A common scenario is in the setting of a pedestrian hit by a car. The right ureter is involved in two thirds of cases.[59] Proposed mechanisms for ureteral injury with blunt trauma include sudden cephalad movement of the kidney associated with downward traction on the ureter, a direct blow to the second or third lumbar vertebra, or compression of the kidney and renal pelvis against the twelfth rib or transverse process, associated with lateral flexion.[52,60] The generally accepted mechanism of injury is from sudden acceleration–deceleration, with acute hyperextension of the lumbar spine causing traction on the ureter.[60,61] It was previously thought that only children were flexible enough to survive a severe hyperextension injury, but more adults are being seen with blunt ureteral injuries.[52] The same mechanism can produce a renal pedicle injury, as seen in four of nine patients with ureteral injuries from blunt trauma in one series.[62]

Recognition of blunt ureteral injuries is usually delayed, and it is suspected in the setting of a flank mass, fever, pain, or a draining external urinary fistula after the injury. Only 40% of such injuries are discovered within 24 hr of the time of the trauma.[59] Severe cases can result in delayed ureteral rupture and intraabdominal abscess formation.[58] Rising serum creatinine may be from urinary ascites from a missed injury, with peritoneal absorption of creatinine.[58] Hematuria often is not present in the admission urinalysis,[60] or if present can be transient.[63] A high index of suspicion is helpful in making the diagnosis.

The radiologic diagnosis of ureteral injury in the setting of blunt trauma is made on IVP. However, it may be difficult to distinguish ureteral disruption caused by extravasation from a renal calyx. As with penetrating trauma, hypotension and hypovolemia can impair the study. IVP findings that are diagnostic of ureteral rupture are good excretion of contrast; undamaged calyces; contrast extravasation at the pelviureteric level; nonvisualization of the ureter in delayed films; and ectasia of the renal pelvis and calyces.[64] Deviation and dilation of the ureter also are suggestive of the diagnosis.[52] CT scan has been used as well in blunt trauma (Fig 3). In children with ureteral disruptions, fluid collections can be seen in the anterior pararenal space and psoas muscle, and the extravasation of contrast may not necessarily be limited to just the medial aspect of the ureter or renal pelvis.[65] A plain film of the abdomen after a CT scan is helpful in the search for extravasation of contrast and nonvisualization of the ureter.

### Surgical Injury

A common source of ureteral trauma is iatrogenic injury from surgical procedures. These include procedures performed by urologists, gynecologists, and general surgeons. Ureteral injury has even been described after percutaneous lumbar disk nucleotomy.[66] The injury can take many forms including direct injury from ligation, transection, crush, excision of part of the ureter, and indirect injury by extensive adventitial dissection or stripping leading to ischemia and necrosis with sloughing. Ureteral injury complicates 0.5%–2.5% of all pelvic operations, and the risk of ureteral injury increases with anatomic deviation, such as with pelvic inflammatory disease, endometriosis, tumors, previous radiation therapy (RT), and redo surgery.[67]

From 1.5% to 2.5% of gynecologic procedures are complicated by ureteral injury, including 10%–30% of radical hysterectomies, 1% of abdominal hysterectomies, 0.05%–0.3% of vaginal hysterectomies, and 0.1% of cesarean sections.[68,69] Of injuries in gynecological procedures, 75% occur during routine hysterectomy for benign conditions, usually described by the

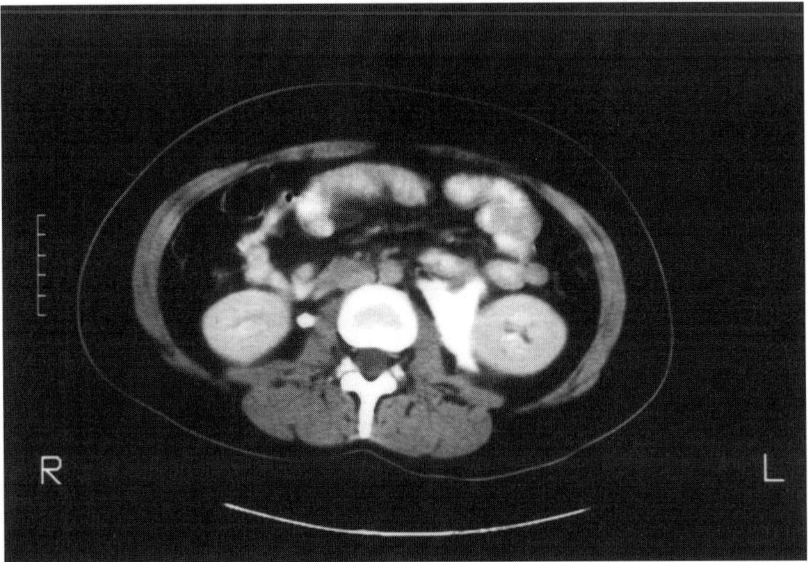


**Fig 3.** CT scan with contrast shows traumatic UPJ disruption after motor vehicle accident. Note medial extravastion of contrast material.

surgeon as uncomplicated.[70] The most common sites of injury in gynecologic surgery are at the level of infundibulopelvic ligament where the ureter courses under the uterine artery, and at the pelvic brim where the ureter lies in close approximation to the ovarian vessels.[71]

Colon and rectal surgery can be complicated by ureteral injury. The incidence of ureteral injury with abdominoperineal resection is 3.7%, and the left ureter is more often injured due to its proximity to the sigmoid.[72] With complicated colonic cases, retroperitoneal cases, and any redo pelvic surgery, the ureter is often injured at the level of the inferior mesenteric artery (IMA) ligation.[71] Ureteral injuries also occur in vascular surgery. Ureteral injuries are most likely in the setting of aortic aneurysm repair associated with perianeurysmal fibrosis, redo vascular reconstruction, extensive retroperitoneal dissection, and hemorrhage.[73,74] At the time of surgery, entrapment of the ureter in perianeurysmal fibrosis is reported in 5%–23% of aortic aneurysms.[75] A graft placed anterior to the ureter can cause compression leading to obstruction, as well as an increased risk of ureteral fistula.[76,77] Ureteral injury is also reported with inferior vena cava (IVC) ligation for the treatment of recurrent pulmonary emboli.[76]

Urologists are not immune from causing iatrogenic ureteral injury. Open ureterolithotomy can cause local damage at the site of the procedure and prolonged wound drainage in up to 17% of cases.[78] Bladder neck suspension procedures can produce angulation of the distal ureter. Increasingly, ureteroscopy is a cause of iatrogenic ureteral injury. Huffman[79] reviewed 15 series reporting on 1696 ureteroscopic procedures. There was a 9% rate of complications, including 1.6% that required surgical intervention. A common injury with these procedures is perforation, caused by either a guidewire, the ureteroscope, a lithotripsy probe, or a biopsy forceps. Ureteral manipulation can also lead to stricture formation, whether or not a frank perforation has occurred, and is often at the site of a stone.[80] Strictures are more common in the ureter below the pelvic brim.[81] Stricture formation can follow initial balloon dilation, mucosal tears, extravasation, or thermal injury with intraureteral lithotripsy, either with electrohydraulic lithotripsy (EHL), ultrasound, or laser.[82–84] The largest increase in temperature is with EHL, and therefore this method of stone dissolution presents the biggest risk to the ureter.[79] Among the most serious of complications is ureteral avulsion, usually from trying to extract a calculus that is too large for the diameter of the ureter to pass. Another major complication of ureteroscopy is the creation of a false passage in the submucosa with a guidewire or the ureteroscope, which can cause extensive ureteral ischemia and injury especially if large amounts of irrigation fluid are forced into the submucosal space.

It is less common to have injuries with ureteroscopy in diagnostic cases than in cases where stone manipulation or extraction occurs.[85] More injuries occur as stone size exceeds 8 mm and with multiple stones.[86] More injuries occur in the proximal ureter because the wall is thinner and there is less muscular support.[79] Fewer injuries occur as instruments get smaller, and even fewer occur with the use of flexible scopes. Many of the earlier series used ureteroscopes up to 11.5 Fr for rigid scopes,[81] larger than many of the semirigid scopes, which are as small as 6 Fr, used today. As with open procedures, previous pelvic operations may cause the course of the ureter to deviate from normal and lead to a higher risk of injury. Pelvic radiation may decrease the ureteral blood supply, and small injuries in patients who have received pelvic radiation may heal poorly. Another source of ureteral injury is laparoscopic surgery. This technique is a standard method of performing gynecologic procedures and is becoming increasingly used by the urologist. Grainger et al.[87] reviewed 13 reported cases of ureteral injury during gynecologic laparoscopy. These occurred during laparoscopic sterilization in four cases, treatment of endometriosis in four, lysis of adhesions in three, uterine sacral ligament transection in one, and trocar placement in one. The injury was clinically apparent within 48–72 hr in all cases. All injuries except those of the trocar involved electrocautery, both unipolar and bipolar. The most common area of injury was near the uterine-sacral ligaments. The ureter can usually be easily seen through the posterior peritoneum in the upper pelvis, and it is less easily identified in the distal portion near these ligaments. The incidence of ureteral injury from laparoscopic pelvic lymph node dissection performed by urologists was reported at 0.5% in a large series compiled from several centers and consisted of two transections, one identified intraoperatively and one discovered in the postoperative period.[88]

Fewer than one third of iatrogenic ureteral injuries are recognized at the time of injury.[71] Of 27 iatrogenic injuries in one series, only 4 were immediately recognized intraoperatively, and the other 23 presented at 10–34 days postoperatively.[68] Delayed ureteral injuries can manifest as fever, flank pain, ileus, abdominal distension, ureterovaginal fistula, ureterocutaneous fistula, urinoma, and abscess. The workup for suspected ureteral injuries in the postoperative period begins with an IVP. Retrograde ureteropyelography may be needed to localize the site of injury, and anterior pyelography can be helpful as well in localization.

### Repair of Ureteral Injuries

The type of repair needed for ureteral injuries depends on the site of injury, the amount of ureter involved, the mechanism of injury, and the general condition of the patient. The standard method of repair for all but lower ureteral injuries is ureteroureterostomy.[55] One of the principles of ureteral repair includes debridement of nonviable tissue. This is important with gunshot wounds and especially with high-velocity bullets. Although only a small part of the ureter may appear to be involved by the bullet, much more of the ureter may be devitalized.[49] Debridement is recommended until bleeding, viable tissue is seen. It is important, however, to avoid skeletonizing the ureter, which could compromise the blood supply. If the ureter is contused, a segmental resection, debridement, and ureteroureterostomy are performed. A tension-free, spatulated anastomosis with good mucosal apposition, and wrap of omentum or coverage with fat is used. A nephropexy can be used to avoid tension on the anastomosis. Some have recommended a watertight anastomosis to prevent stricture.[53] However, Petersen and Pitts[55] showed that even among patients who had urine leaks, none had subsequent ureteral obstruction or stricture on postoperative evaluation.

Partial transections can be closed primarily if from a stab wound and there is no blast effect. All repairs are stented and drained. Campbell et al.[52] report a 92% success rate with primary ureteral repair. Ureteral primary repair is undertaken regardless of associated injuries, such as contamination from bowel trauma.[55] In all cases, control of infection is important and antibiotics should be given. For lesser injuries, consider stenting. Since a ureter that looks nearly normal or slightly bruised from a gunshot may progress to necrosis and extravasation,[62] consider stenting any ureter in proximity to the path of a bullet, especially a high-velocity round.

Lower ureteral injuries can be managed with a ureteroneocystostomy, usually with a psoas hitch. A tunneled anastomosis is not essential in view of the questionable significance of adult urinary reflux.[55] Contraindications to the psoas hitch include a small, thickened bladder, scarring from prior procedures that prohibits mobilization, and prior pelvic radiation.[89] As for all ureteral surgery, bladder outlet obstruction must be corrected or temporized to ensure adequate drainage. A suprapubic tube and ureteral stents are used. Defects of up to 5–6 cm can be correct with the reimplant and psoas hitch.[90]

For longer ureteral defects, a Boari flap can bridge the distance. If both ureters have been injured, bilateral Boari flaps can be created.[91] Using this technique, defects can be bridged that extend up not only above the pelvic brim but to the lower pole of the kidney.[92,93] The Boari flap is not recommended for patients who have had much prior renal or pelvic surgery predisposing to retroperitoneal fibrosis and adhesions. Konigsberg et al.[94] reported a satisfactory result in 15 of 21 patients reconstructed with a Boari flap. Poor results were seen with patients who had previous pelvic radiation and in whom the flap was not pexed to the psoas muscle. Flynn et al.[95] reported on 41 patients treated in this manner for iatrogenic ureteral injuries and reported no cases of postoperative obstruction or failure. Benson et al.[96] in his series noted that one third of his patients had urinary tract infections (UTIs), which may have been due to colonization from previous procedures and stents, and 50% had reflux.

Other measures may be needed for extensive ureteral loss or damage. An ileal interposition can be used. The use of a simultaneous psoas hitch can shorten the bowel segment required to bridge the ureteral defect.[97] One complication from interposing bowel is hyperchloremic metabolic acidosis. This usually compensates with a normal contralateral side, however, and shortening the segment helps avoid this.[96] Boxer et al.[98] reported a series of 89 patients who received an ileal ureter. Of these, 24 required the ureter for ureteral injury. The success rate in this subgroup was 85%, and 81% overall. They identified a subset of patients who did poorly; 45% of those with a preoperative creatinine of 2 mg/dl or greater had progressive renal failure postoperatively. Thus, an elevated creatinine above 2 mg/dl should be a relative contraindication to this procedure. Benson et al.[96] used no antireflux procedure and all of their patients had normal upper tracts, as the bowel peristalsis is thought to dampen transmitted pressures. Of their patients, 60% had at least one UTI, and several patients had multiple infections. This procedure is a good choice for patients with adhesions and fibrosis in the operative area. Another part of the bowel that can be employed is the appendix, which can be used to repair defects in the right ureter.[99] In females the fallopian tube can also be used, but the tube does not have peristaltic movement and therefore if used will gradually dilate causing hydronephrosis of the proximal ureter and renal pelvis.[99,100]

Another option to compensate for extensive ureteral loss is renal autotransplantation. A renal autotransplant requires minimal hilar inflammation, vascular experience on the part of the operating surgeon, a preoperative angiogram of both the renal and pelvic vasculature, and is contraindicated in the face of severe pelvic atherosclerosis.[96,101] Long-term results can be excellent, with Bodie et al. reporting 20 of 23 patients postautotransplant with creatinine improved or stable from preoperative at 1.5–14 years of follow-up.[101]

A less desirable option for treating extensive ureteral injuries is a transureteroureterostomy (TUU). This often requires the anastomosis of the least vascularized midureter, and can potentially jeopardize the contralateral ureter and kidney.[55] Hodges et al. reported a 92% success rate for 100 patients undergoing TUU,[102] but others have not had such success, even in the best of settings.[103] This procedure is contraindicated in the face of distal obstruction of the recipient ureter, retroperitoneal fibrosis, and transitional cell carcinoma of the donor kidney.[104]

In some cases, a nephrectomy may be necessary. Attempts at sparing the kidney should be attempted, and before nephrectomy, determination of the status of the contralateral renal unit is essential. There is a higher rate of nephrectomy for treatment of injuries with a delayed diagnosis. McGinty and Mendez[105] reported a 32% incidence of nephrectomy in cases of delayed recognition compared with 4.5% when the injury was recognized immediately.

Ureteral repairs should be performed over a stent, either a double J, a ureteral catheter, or a pediatric feeding tube. This applies for primary ureteroureterostomy as well as reimplants with psoas hitch and/or Boari flap. Franco et al.[106] noted a 90% complication rate for proximal ureteral injuries repaired without stents compared to 30% with the use of a stent, and complication rates of 13% and 20%, respectively, in the midureter. Steers et al.[107] noted persistent drainage in two of three ureteral repairs performed without stents, as compared to no complications in 11 repairs in which this group used ureteral stents.

The use of a (percutaneous) nephrostomy for proximal diversion in ureteral repair in penetrating trauma is individualized, and may be most helpful in proximal ureteral injuries, in the face of associated bowel or pancreatic injuries, or with a vascular prosthesis in place.[106] Percutaneously placed ureteral stents can also be used as an adjunct for complications of ureteral repair. Toporoff et al.[108] used a percutaneous antegrade ureteral stent in the treatment of six patients with ureteral anastomosis dehiscence, or late recognized injuries that led to full-thickness disruptions; five had perfect healing, and one healed with a stricture that necessitated reanastomosis. If drainage from a ureteral fistula persists despite nephrostomy drainage, reflux must be ruled out as the cause.[77]

The treatment of a ureteral disruption following blunt trauma is a primary repair. As the disruption usually occurs at the UPJ, the repair usually consists of a dismembered pyeloplasty. A ureterocalicostomy is also an option. In a majority of patients with ureteral injuries from blunt trauma, there is a delay in diagnosing the injury. This may make the subsequent repair technically more difficult due to inflammation, and fixation of the renal pelvis and distal aspect of the ureter, which may be retracted. Downward displacement of the kidney and fixation posteriorly to the psoas can help bring the two ends together and reduce tension on the anastomosis. Some patients have been treated with an autotransplant, or ileum interposition.[109] If the repair is too difficult or if the patient's condition is tenuous, a nephrectomy may have to be performed.[52] Another alternative is the placement of a temporary percutaneous nephrostomy, especially if other injuries need attention.[62] This can allow the patient to stabilize and be more prepared to withstand a long and difficult repair. Palmer and Drago[59] reported good results with six repairs in five of their patients (one bilateral). In a review of the literature, 29 patients were repaired by dismembered pyeloplasty, with good results in all but five, only three of whom required nephrectomy. No apparent adverse effect on outcome was associated with a delay in diagnosis. Campbell et al.[52] reported worse results in three patients with delayed diagnosis of a blunt ureteral injury; two underwent a nephrectomy, and the third had a prolonged urinary leak at the anastomosis site.

The treatment of iatrogenic ureteral injuries depends on the type of injury, the type of procedure being performed, and whether the injury was recognized at the time it occurred or the diagnosis was reached sometime postoperatively.

For ureters that have been clamped or ligated for short periods, removal of the clamp or deligation should suffice.[110] Depending on the condition of the ureter after this maneuver, a stent may be used if a delayed deterioration of the ureter is a concern. If the ureter has been extensively damaged, resection of the involved ureter is performed followed by a primary reanastomosis, or reimplant if the injury involves the distal ureter. For a complete transection, a primary repair is performed, or a reimplant for a distal injury. If the patient is unstable, consider a cutaneous ureterostomy.[110]

The treatment of an iatrogenic ureteral injury discovered sometime after the procedure is variable and can be handled in several different ways. The presentation can be fever, flank pain, ureterovaginal or ureterocutaneous fistula, ileus, and/or hematuria. The first diagnostic procedure of choice in a suspected ureteral injury is an IVP. In the setting of an IVP diagnostic for a ureteral injury, which includes hydroureteronephrosis, nonvisualization of the ipsilateral collecting system, or pooling of contrast in the vagina, a retrograde pyelogram can be helpful to delineate the exact level of the injury. At the time of a retrograde, an attempt can be made to pass a ureteral catheter or stent retrograde. This maneuver is extremely helpful if successful, but can rarely be achieved. Dowling et al.[68] reported that in 20 attempts at retrograde stenting of an iatrogenic ureteral injury, his group was successful only once (5%).

Should the attempt at retrograde stenting be unsuccessful, the choice becomes one of placing a percutaneous nephrostomy for the purpose of primary therapy in some cases, passing a stent antegrade, or temporizing for a delayed open repair. In some select cases of ureteral ligation, placing a percutaneous nephrostomy may be all that is required. Harshman et al.[111] reported three cases of ureteral obstruction from suture entrapment that resolved with temporary drainage by percutaneous nephrostomy alone. Dowling et al.[68] reported similar success in six of seven patients with ligation of the ureter. Chromic suture loses its tensile strength in 3 weeks and is reabsorbed in about 8 weeks,[112] so that a conservative trial of 8 weeks of percutaneous nephrostomy drainage is justified if it is suspected that the ureter is ligated with chromic suture. Obstruction that persists beyond this point is unlikely to resolve without other intervention. Other advantages of percutaneous nephrostomy is that with a tube in place, an antegrade study can be performed to help localize the injury, and the diversion will decrease the morbidity of the wetness from a continuously draining urinary fistula.[113] An indwelling tube is not without risks, however. Up to two thirds of patients in some series with ureteral injuries temporized by indwelling percutaneous nephrostomy tubes required tube change or had pyelonephritis requiring hospitalization and antibiotics.[68]

The passage of a stent antegrade may help greatly to speed healing of the ureteral injury. This maneuver is usually more successful than the passage of a stent retrograde. Lang[114] was able to pass a stent antegrade in 11 of 13 patients with ureteral injury, from either iatrogenic or external violence. Ureteral fistulas seem to respond best to stenting alone, with resolution in 83%–100% of cases reported after 4–14 weeks of stenting.[115,116] Fistulas treated with percutaneous drainage alone without stenting are far less likely to resolve.[68] A stent placed antegrade can also be very useful for intraoperative localization if an open repair is needed (Fig 4).

If a retrograde ureteral catheter cannot be placed, an alternative to percutaneous nephrostomy is an immediate open repair. Even if an open repair in the acute setting is chosen, the percutaneous nephrostomy can be a useful adjunct as a means to pass a stent antegrade to the site of injury and make intraoperative location of the ureter easier. The issue of timing of repair after an iatrogenic ureteral injury is debatable. Blandy et al.[91] point out that the traditional view that iatrogenic injuries after a gynecologic operation must not be repaired un-

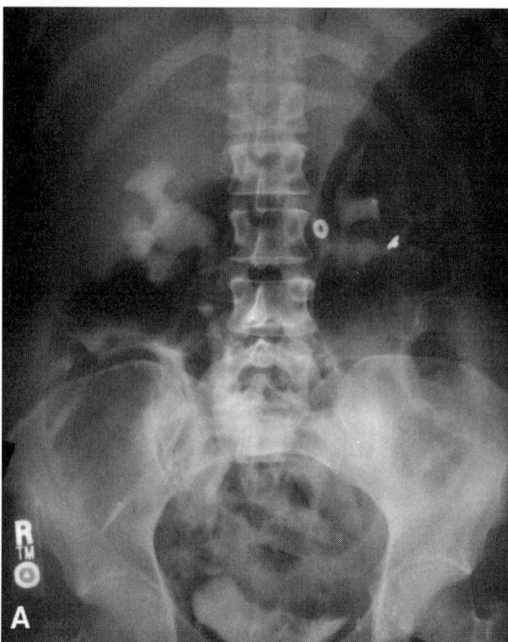


**Fig 4A.** IVP in patient status post (s/p) an abdominal hysterectomy with right flank pain and fever. Right ureter is obstructed just proximal to the ureterovesical junction.

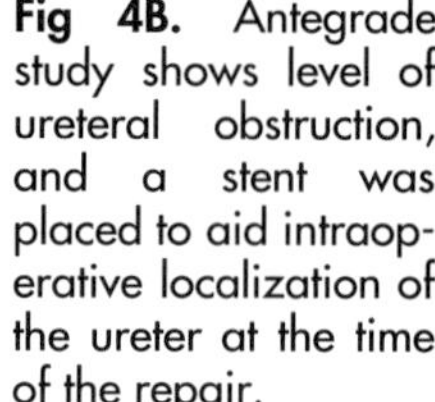
**Fig 4B.** Antegrade study shows level of ureteral obstruction, and a stent was placed to aid intraoperative localization of the ureter at the time of the repair.

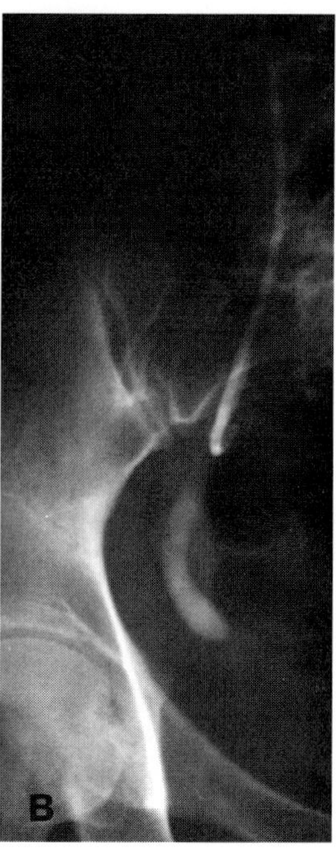


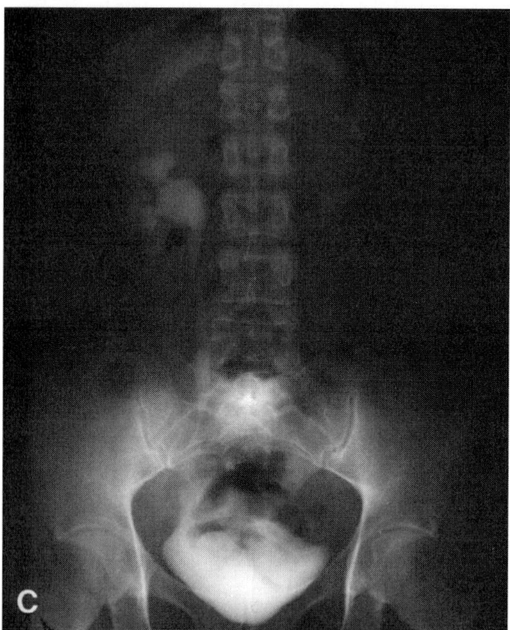


**Fig 4C.** IVP 4 weeks s/p ureteroneocystostomy with psoas hitch shows continuity of ureter down to the bladder.

til several months have passed is largely unsupported in the literature by results showing that this approach produces results superior to those for immediate repair. The obvious advantage of immediate repair is a marked decrease in patient morbidity as compared to spending several months with an indwelling diversion or, worse, with leaking from a ureteral fistula.

There is a large body of literature to support the repair of ureteral injuries soon after they are discovered in the postoperative setting. In the acute setting with intraoperative recognition of the injury, the only reason to delay a repair is if the patient is hemodynamically unstable. Hoch et al.[117] reported successful early repair in 16 of 19 patients with iatrogenic ureteral injuries not discovered at the time of operation. This included primary ureteral repairs, reimplants, Boari flaps, and primary closure of lacerations. All but four of these were repaired within 3½ weeks of recognition. Blandy et al.[91] reported no complications following early repair of 28 iatrogenic ureteral injuries that presented postoperatively as a ureterovaginal fistula or obstruction. Tarkington et al.[71] reported the successful repair of iatrogenic ureteral injuries in 12 patients within 3 weeks of their primary gynecologic procedure. All 12 injuries were treated with a tunneled reimplant and psoas hitch, with renal mobilization performed if needed. This group advocates prolonged stenting of the repair for at least 21 days because the blood supply to the lower part of the ureter is usually compromised by the original injury. Flynn et al.[95] suggest that delay in repair renders dissections more difficult secondary to the formation of dense fibrous tissue in the retroperitoneum.

Ureteral injury can result in stricture formation. For strictures of the upper ureter and ureteropelvic junction after a failed pyeloplasty, an endopyelotomy can be successful in up to 86% of cases.[118] For failures of endopyelotomy to salvage an open UPJ, a ureterocalycostomy is the procedure of choice, as it is difficult to redo the UPJ repair due to scar, fibrosis, and diminished blood supply. Overall success with percutaneous or retrograde balloon dilation is 47%–63%, with distal ureteral strictures responding much more favorably than upper or midureteral strictures.[119] Endoscopic dilation is most successful for strictures <1 cm in length.[120] For strictures at the UVJ, a ureteral meatotomy and stenting is recommended as the initial procedure, performed with a wire placed antegrade as a guide. Failure of conservative management will require an open procedure.

The management of ureteral injuries at the time of vascular surgery involving the placement of a vascular graft is evolving. In the past, some have recommended nephrectomy due to the risk of ureteral anastomotic leak leading to graft infection.[74,121] However, more recent reports advocate repair of the injury and salvage of the renal unit.[73] Primary repair is reasonable when the transected margins are viable, urine is uninfected, and contralateral kidney is normal. The repair is stented to separate the anastomosis from the vascular repair. An effective way to do this is to wrap the repair in omentum.[104,122] Live animal experiments by Finney and Rinker[123] have shown that omentum as a sleeve results in rapid sealing of the anastomosis, minimizing leakage of urine. Using this technique, Spirnak et al.[122] reported on primary repair of seven patients with ureteral injuries sustained during placement or revision of a vascular graft. Significantly, no patient had a graft infection as a complication, even when the diagnosis was delayed and significant urinary extravasation had occurred, such as in two of three patients who eventually required nephrectomy for persistent extravasation. Some have recommended using a proximal nephrostomy as well in conjunction with the repair.[76] If these conditions for immediate repair cannot be met but salvage of the kidney is desired, ligation of the ureter and placement of a percutaneous nephrostomy can temporize the situation and permit a later repair.[73] For ureteral compression by a graft placed anterior to it, an alternative to dividing the ureter is to divide the graft and reanastomose posterior to the ureter.[76]

Most ureteral injuries from ureteroscopy, including small ureteral perforations, can be managed conservatively with the passage of a stent. If a stent will not pass, a percutaneous nephrostomy with antegrade stenting should be considered. It is not recommended to place a nephrostomy alone as this can create a dry ureter and lead to total occlusion.[124] For a documented perforation, the stent is left for 6 weeks and a contrast study is performed prior to its removal to confirm that the injury has healed.[79] In the setting of a documented perforation, antibiotics should be given. Exceptions to this are ureteral avulsion, ureteral necrosis, and large perforations. These injuries will require an open repair. The procedure required will depend on the site of injury.

Recommended treatment for ureteral injuries with delayed recognition after laparoscopy is stenting, either antegrade percutaneous or retrograde. For injuries discovered at the time of surgery, immediate repair is indicated. This can be done by converting to an open procedure or, as has been reported, by repairing the damage laparoscopically.[125,126] For laparoscopic repair, a stent is placed cystoscopically and the ureter repaired over the stent.

## REFERENCES


1. Hessel SJ, Smith EH. Renal trauma: a comprehensive review and radiological assessment. *CRC Crit Rev Radiol Nucl Med.* 1974;5:251–293.
2. McAninch JW. Renal injuries. In Gillenwater JY, Grayhack JT, Howards SS, Duckett JW, eds. *Adult and Pediatric Urology.* 2nd ed. St. Louis: Mosby Year Book; 1991:475–490.
3. Mertz JH, Wishard WN Jr, Nourse MH. Injury of the kidney in children. *JAMA.* 1963;183:730.
4. Krieger, JN, Algood CB, Mason JT, et al. Urological trauma in the pacific northwest. *J Urol.* 1984;132:70.
5. Bretan PN Jr, McAninch JW, Federle MP, et al. Computerized tomographic staging of renal trauma. *J Urol.* 1986;136:561.
6. Quinlan DM, Gearhart JP. Blunt renal trauma in childhood. Features indicating severe injury. *Br J Urol.* 1990;66:526.
7. Morse TS. Renal injuries. *Pediatr Clin North Am.* 1990;22:379.
8. Mendez R. Renal trauma. *J Urol.* 1977;118:698.
9. Banowsky LH, Wolfel DA, Lackner LH. Considerations in the diagnosis and management of renal trauma. *J Trauma.* 1970;10:587.
10. Scott R Jr, Carlton CE Jr, Goldman M. Penetrating injuries of the kidney. *J Urol.* 1969;101:247.
11. Tynberg TLH, Hoch WH, Perksy L, et al. The management of renal injuries coincident with penetrating wounds of the abdomen. *J Trauma.* 1973;13:502.
12. Stutzman RE. Ballistics and the management of ureteral injuries from high velocity missiles. *J Urol.* 1977;118:947.
13. O'Connell KJ, Clark M, Lewis RH, Christenson PJ. Comparison of low- and high-velocity ballistic trauma to genitourinary organs. *J Trauma.* 1988;28(Suppl):S139.
14. Bernath AS, Schutte H, Fernandez RRD, Addonizio JC. Stab wounds of the kidney: conservative management in flank penetration. *J Urol.* 1983;129:468.
15. Fey R, Brosman S, Lindstrom R, et al. Renal artery thrombosis: a successful revascularization by autotransplantation. *J Urol.* 1974;111:572.
16. Federle M. Evaluation of renal trauma. In: Pollock HM, ed. *Clinical Urography.* Philadelphia: WB Saunders; 1990:1472–1494.
17. Waterhouse K, Gross M. Trauma to the genitourinary tract: a 5-year experience with 251 cases. *J Urol.* 1969;101:241.
18. Glenn JF, Harvard BM. The injured kidney. *JAMA.* 1960;173:1189.
19. McDougal WS, Persky L. *Traumatic Injuries of the Genitourinary System.* Baltimore: Williams and Wilkins; 1981.
20. Monstrey SJM, Vander Werken C, Debruyne FMJ, Goris RJA. Rational guidelines in renal trauma assessment. *Urology.* 1988;31:469.
21. Hai MA, Pontes JE, Pierce JM Jr. Surgical management of major renal trauma: a review of 102 cases treated by conservative surgery. *J Urol.* 1977;118:7.
22. Cass AS, Luxenberg M. Unilateral non-visualization on excretory urography after external trauma. *J Urol.* 1984;132:225.
23. Carroll PR, McAninch JW, Klosterman P, Greenblatt M. Renovascular trauma: risk assessment, surgical management, and outcome. *J Trauma.* 1990;30:547.
24. Mee SI, McAninch JW, Robinson AL, et al. Radiographic assessment of renal trauma: a 10-year prospective study of patient selection. *J Urol.* 1989;141:1095.
25. Herschorn S, Radomski SB, Shoskes DA, et al. Evaluation and treatment of blunt renal trauma. *J Urol.* 1991;146:274.
26. Hardeman, SW, Hussman DA, Chinn HKW, Peters PC. Blunt urinary tract trauma: identifying those patients who require radiological diagnostic studies. *J Urol.* 1987;138:99.
27. Jevitch MJ, Montero GG. Injuries to the renal vessels by blunt trauma in children. *J Urol.* 1969;102:493.
28. Cass AS, Bubrick M, Luxenberg M, et al. Renal trauma found during laparotomy for intra-abdominal injury. *J Trauma.* 1985;25:997.
29. Pollock HM, Wein AJ. Imaging of renal trauma. *Radiology.* 1989;172:297.
30. Petersen NE, Schulze KA. Selective diagnostic urography for trauma. *J Urol.* 1987;137:449.
31. Fanney DR, Casillas J, Murphy JB. CT in the diagnosis of renal trauma. *Radiographics.* 1990;10:29.
32. McAninch JW, Federle MD. Evaluation of renal injuries with computerized tomography. *J Urol.* 1982;128:456.
33. Flax S, McLorie G, Churchill BM, Gilday DL. A comparative study of intravenous urograms and radionuclide renal scans in diagnosis of renal trauma. *Urology.* 1989;34:62.
34. McAninch JW, Carroll PR, Klosterman PW, et al. Renal reconstruction after injury. *J Urol.* 1991;145:932.
35. Eastham JA, Wilson TG, Larsen DW, Ahlering TE. Angiographic embolization of renal stab wounds. *J Urol.* 1992;148:268.
36. Petersen NE: Fate of functionless post-traumatic renal segment. *Urology.* 1986;27:237.
37. Husmann DA, Morris JS. Attempted nonoperative management of blunt renal lacerations extending through the corticomedullary junction: the short-term and long-term sequelae. *J Urol.* 1990;143:682.
38. McAninch JW, Carroll PR. Renal trauma: kidney preservation through improved vascular

control—a refined approach. *J Trauma.* 1982; 22:285.

39. Atala A, Miller FB, Richardson JD, et al. Preliminary vascular control for renal trauma. *Surg Gynecol Obstet.* 1991;172:386.
40. Corriere JN, McAndrew JD, Benson GS. Intraoperative decision-making in renal trauma surgery. *J Trauma.* 1991;31:1390.
41. McAninch JW, Carroll PR. Renal exploration after trauma: indications and reconstructive techniques. *Urol Clin North Am.* 1989;16:203.
42. White RA, Ramos SM, Delany HM. Renorrhapy using knitted polyglycolic acid mesh. *J Trauma.* 1987;27:689.
43. Sagalowsky AI, McConnell JD, Peters PC. Renal trauma requiring surgery: an analysis of 185 cases. *J Trauma.* 1983;23:128.
44. Morgensen P, Agger P, Ostergaard AH. A conservative approach to the management of blunt renal trauma. *Br J Urol.* 1980;52:338.
45. Osias MB, Hale SD, Lytton B. The management of renal injuries. *J Trauma.* 1976;16:954.
46. Cass AS, Luxenberg M. Conservative or immediate surgical management of blunt renal injuries. *J Urol.* 1983;130:11.
47. Presti JC, Carroll PR, McAninch JW. Ureteral and renal pelvic injuries from external trauma: diagnosis and management. *J Trauma.* 1989; 29:370.
48. Guerriero WG. Ureteral injury. *Urol Clin North Am.* 1989;16:237.
49. Rober PE, Smith JB, Pierce JM Jr. Gunshot injuries of the ureter. *J Trauma.* 1990;30:83.
50. Carlton CE, Scott R, Guthrie AG. The initial management of ureteral injuries: a report of 78 cases. *J Urol.* 1971;105:335.
51. Bright TC, Peters PC. Ureteral injuries due to external violence: 10 years experience with 59 cases. *J Trauma.* 1977;17:616.
52. Campbell EW, Filderman, PS, Jacobs SC. Ureteral injury due to blunt and penetrating trauma. *Urology.* 1992;40:216.
53. Holden S, Hicks CC, O'Brien DP III, et al. Gunshot wounds of the ureter: a 15-year review of 63 consecutive cases. *J Urol.* 1976;116:562.
54. Fisher S, Young DA, Malin JM Jr, Pierce JM Jr. Ureteral gunshot wounds. *J Urol.* 1972;108: 238.
55. Petersen NE, Pitts JC III. Penetrating injuries of the ureter. *J Urol.* 1981;126:587.
56. Cass AS. Ureteral contusion with gunshot wounds. *J Trauma.* 1984;24:59.
57. Rohner TJ. Delayed ureteral fistula from high velocity missiles: report of 3 cases. *J Urol.* 1971;105:63.
58. Wilkinson S, Loughhead MG, Holmes AB, Brothers L. Delayed intraperitoneal ureteric rupture following blunt abdominal trauma: case report. *J Trauma.* 1989;29:1292.
59. Palmer JM, Drago JR. Ureteral avulsion from nonpenetrating trauma. *J Urol.* 1981;125:108.
60. Beamud-Gomez A, Martinez-Verduch M, Estornell-Moragues F, et al. Rupture of the ureteropelvic junction by nonpenetrating trauma. *J Pediatr Surg.* 1986;21:702.
61. Ainsworth T, Weems WL, Merrell WH. Bilateral ureteral injury due to non-penetrating external trauma. *J Urol.* 1966;96:439.
62. Cass AS. Blunt renal pelvic and ureteral injury in multiple-injured patients. *Urology.* 1983;22: 268.
63. Wallijn E, DeSy W, Fonteyne E. Blunt ureteral trauma with perineal urine fistulization: review of the literature. *J Urol.* 1975;114:942.
64. Beckly DE, Waters EA. Avulsion of the pelviureteric junction—a rare consequence of nonpenetrating trauma. *Br J Radiol.* 1972;45:423.
65. Siegel MJ, Balfe DM. Blunt renal and ureteral trauma in childhood: CT patterns of fluid collections. *AJR.* 1989;152:1043.
66. Flam TA, Spitzenpfeil E, Zerbib M, et al. Complete ureteral transection associated with percutaneous lumbar disk nucleotomy. *J Urol.* 1992;148:1249.
67. Neuman M, Eidelman A, Langer R, et al. Iatrogenic injuries to the ureter during gynecologic and obstetric operations. *Surg Gynecol Obstet.* 1991;173:268.
68. Dowling RA, Corriere JN, Sandler CM. Iatrogenic ureteral injury. *J Urol.* 1986;135:912.
69. Brubaker LT, Wilbanks, GD. Urinary tract injuries in pelvic surgery. *Surg Clin North Am.* 1991;71:963.
70. Symmonds RE. Ureteral injuries associated with gynecologic injury: prevention and management. *Clin Obstet Gynecol.* 1976;19:623.
71. Tarkington, MA, Dejter SW Jr, Bresette JR. Early surgical management of extensive gynecologic ureteral injuries. *Surg Gynecol Obstet.* 1991;173:17.
72. Andersson A, Bergdahl L. Urologic complications following abdominoperineal resection of the rectum. *Arch Surg.* 1976;111:969.
73. Adams JR Jr., Mata JA, Culkin DJ, Venable DD. Ureteral injury in abdominal vascular reconstructive surgery. *Urology.* 1992;39:79.
74. Bright TC, Peters PC. Ureteral injuries secondary to operative procedures. *Urology.* 1977;9: 22.
75. Sethia B, Darke SG. Abdominal aortic aneurysm with retroperitoneal fibrosis and ureteric entrapment. *Br J Surg.* 1983;70:434.
76. Schapira HE, Li R, Gribetz M, et al. Ureteral injuries during vascular surgery. *J Urol.* 1981; 125:293.
77. St Lezin MA, Stoller ML. Surgical ureteral injuries. *Urology.* 1991;38:497.
78. Furlow WL, Buchiere JJ. The surgical fate of ureteral calculi: review of Mayo Clinic experience. *J Urol.* 1976;116:559.
79. Huffman JL. Ureteroscopic injuries to the upper urinary tract. *Urol Clin North Am.* 1989;16:249.

80. Shultz A, Kristensen, JK, Bilde T, Eldrup J. Ureteroscopy: results and complications. *J Urol.* 1987;137:865.
81. Kramolowsky EV. Ureteral perforation during ureterorenoscopy: treatment and management. *J Urol.* 1987;138:36.
82. Huffman JL, Bagley DH, Lyons ES, et al. Transurethral removal of large ureteral and renal pelvic calculi using ureteroscopic ultrasonic lithotripsy. *J Urol.* 1983;130:31.
83. Dretler SP, Watson G, Parrish JA. Pulsed dye laser fragmentation of ureteral calculi: initial clinical experience. *J Urol.* 1987;137:386.
84. Green DF, Lytton B. Early experience with electrohydraulic lithotripsy of ureteral calculi using direct vision ureteroscopy. *J Urol.* 1985; 133:767.
85. Daniels GF Jr, Garnett JE, Carter MF. Ureteroscopic results and complications: experience with 130 cases. *J Urol.* 1988;139:710.
86. Carter SC, Cox R, Wickham JEA. Complications associated with ureteroscopy. *Br J Urol.* 1986;58:625.
87. Grainger DA, Soderstrom RM, Schiff SF, et al. Ureteral injuries at laparoscopy: insights into diagnosis, management, and prevention. *Obstet Gynecol.* 1990;75:839.
88. Kavoussi LR, Sosa E, Chandhoke P, et al. Complications of laparoscopic lymph node dissection. *J Urol.* 1993;149:322.
89. Ehrlich RM, Melman A, Skinner DG. The use of vesico-psoas hitch in urologic surgery. *J Urol.* 1978;119:322.
90. Kishev SV. Psoas-bladder hitch procedure: our experience with repair of the injured ureter in men. *J Urol.* 1975;113:772.
91. Blandy JP, Badenoch DF, Fowler CG, et al. Early repair of iatrogenic injury to the ureter or bladder after gynecological surgery. *J Urol.* 1991;146:761.
92. Thompson IM, Ross G. Long-term results of bladder flap repair of ureteral injuries. *J Urol.* 1974;111:483.
93. Olsson CA, Norlen LJ. Combined Boari bladder flap-psoas hitch procedure in ureteral replacement. *Scand J Urol Nephrol.* 1986;20:279.
94. Konigsberg H, Blunt KJ, Muecke EC. Use of Boari flap in lower ureteral injuries. *Urology.* 1975;5:751.
95. Flynn JT, Tiptaft RC, Woodhouse CRJ, et al. The early and aggressive repair of iatrogenic ureteric injuries. *Br J Urol.* 1979;51:454.
96. Benson MC, Ring KS, Olsson CA. Ureteral reconstruction and bypass: experience with ileal interposition, the Boari flap-psoas hitch and renal autotransplantation. *J Urol.* 1990;143:20.
97. Olsson CA. Ileal ureter and renal autotransplantation. *Urol Clin North Am.* 1983;10:685.
98. Boxer RJ, Fritzsche R, Skinner DG, et al. Replacement of the ureter by small intestine: clinical application and the results of the ileal ureter in 89 patients. *J Urol.* 1979;121:728.
99. Komatz Y, Itoh H. A case of ureteral injury repaired with appendix. *J Urol.* 1990;144:132.
100. Schein CJ, Sanders AR, Hurwitt ES. Experimental reconstruction of ureters: substitution with autogenous pedicled fallopian tube grafts. *Arch Surg.* 1956;73:47.
101. Bodie B, Novick AC, Rose M, Straffon R. Long-term results with renal autotransplantation for ureteral replacement. *J Urol.* 1986;136: 1187.
102. Hodges CV, Barry JM, Fuchs EF, et al. Transureteroureterostomy: 25 year experience with 100 patients. *J Urol.* 1980;123:834.
103. Sandoz IL, Paul DP, MacFarlane CA. Complications with transureteroureterostomy. *J Urol.* 1977;117:39.
104. Zinman LM, Libertino JA, Roth RA. Management of operative ureteral injury. *Urology.* 1978;12:290.
105. McGinty DM, Mendez R. Traumatic ureteral injuries with delayed recognition. *Urology.* 1977;10:115.
106. Franco I, Eshgi M, Schutte H, et al. Value of proximal diversion and ureteral stenting in management of penetrating ureteral trauma. *Urology.* 1988;32:99.
107. Steers WD, Corriere JN, Benson GS, Boileau MA. The use of indwelling ureteral stents in managing ureteral injuries due to external violence. *J Trauma.* 1985;25:1001.
108. Toporoff B, Sclafani S, Scalea T, et al. Percutaneous antegrade ureteral stenting as an adjunct for treatment of complicated ureteral injuries. *J Trauma.* 1992;32:534.
109. Seiler RK, Filmer RB, Reitelman C. Traumatic disruption of the ureteropelvic junction managed by ilieal interposition. *J Urol.* 1991;146: 392.
110. Spence HM, Boone T. Surgical injuries to the ureter. *JAMA.* 1961;176:1070.
111. Harshman MW, Pollack HM, Banner MP, Wein AJ. Conservative management of ureteral obstruction secondary to suture entrapment. *J Urol.* 1982;127:121.
112. Clark DE. Surgical suture materials. *Contemp Surg.* 1980;17:33.
113. Persky L, Hampel N, Kedia K. Percutaneous nephrostomy and ureteral injury. *J Urol.* 1981; 125:298.
114. Lang EK. Antegrade ureteral stenting for dehiscence, strictures, and fistulae. *AJR.* 1984; 143:795.
115. Lang EK, Lanaso JA, Garrett J, et al. The management of urinary fistulas with percutaneous ureteral stent catheters. *J Urol.* 1979;122:736.
116. Chang R, Marshall FF, Mitchell S. Percutaneous management of benign ureteral strictures and fistulas. *J Urol.* 1987;137:1126.

117. Hoch WH, Kursh ED, Persky L. Early, aggressive management of introperative ureteral injuries. *J Urol.* 1975;114:530.
118. Smith AD. Management of iatrogenic ureteral strictures after urological procedures. *J Urol.* 1988;140:1372.
119. Silverstein JI, Libby C, Smith AD. Management of ureteroscopic ureteral injuries. *Urol Clin North Am.* 1988;15:515.
120. Kramolowsky EV, Tucker RD, Nelson CMK. Management of benign ureteral strictures: open surgical repair or endoscopic dilation? *J Urol.* 1989;141:285.
121. Fry DE, Milholen L, Harbrecht PJ. Iatrogenic ureteral injury. *Arch Surg.* 1983;118:454.
122. Spirnak JP, Hampel N, Resnick MI. Ureteral injuries complicating vascular surgery: is repair indicated? *J Urol.* 1989;141:13.
123. Finney HR, Rinker JR. Live omentum as a substitute for the fatty periureteral sheath: an experimental study. *J Urol.* 1969;102:414.
124. Chang C, Marshall FF. Management of ureteroscopic injuries. *J Urol.* 1987;137:1132.
125. Gomel V, James C. Intraoperative management of ureteral injury during operative laparoscopy. *Fertil Steril.* 1991;55:416.
126. Nezhat C, Nezhat F. Laparoscopic repair of ureter resected during operative laparoscopy. *Obstet Gynecol.* 1992;80:5.

# 22

# Trauma to the Lower Urinary Tract and Genitalia

*Robert E. Steckler and Robert A. Riehle, Jr.*

Certainly, there is no task in surgery more challenging than the initial evaluation of the trauma victim in the emergency room. Although rapid, effective management of ventilatory and circulatory compromise is now commonplace, a delay in the identification and treatment of genitourinary injuries is still more frequent than is desirable. Prompt evaluation of the lower urinary tract during resuscitation will allow effective management of the injury in the acute state. Immediate recognition and treatment will significantly decrease unnecessary morbidity and late urologic complications.

## BLADDER INJURY

The bladder, located within the pelvic cavity, is protected by the bony pelvis and cushioned by perivesical fat, the sigmoid colon, and the levator muscle sling. It is an extraperitoneal structure, except for the dome and the posterior surface superior to the trigone and the ureteral hiatus. This superior portion, covered by the visceral peritoneum, protrudes into the peritoneal cavity during filling and lacks the support of surrounding tissues. It is susceptible both to direct (penetrating or nonpenetrating) injury and to hydraulic rupture resulting from pelvic or perineal impact. Although the empty bladder is rarely injured, when filled the bladder rises out of its protected intrapelvic position and is much more susceptible to trauma. This is especially likely in women during late pregnancy and in children whose bladders have not descended into the bony pelvis. In addition, a filled bladder has a thin and stretched detrusor layer; the higher the intraluminal pressure, the less force required to rupture it.

Trauma to the urinary bladder may result from (a) blunt impact to the lower abdomen or pelvis (as seen with motor vehicle or pedestrian accidents), crush injuries occurring in mining or building demolition, skiing, horseback riding, fights, contact sports, or falls; (b) penetrating injuries such as gunshot, knife, and projectile wounds; or (c) intraoperative injury to the bladder during surgical procedures involving adjacent organs. These injuries can all cause bladder contusion, intraperitoneal and extraperitoneal bladder rupture, or a combination of these conditions. The type of injury sustained can usually be predicted from the mode of injury and findings on initial physical and radiologic examination of the patient, including whether pelvic fracture (which is frequently associated) is present.[1] In addition, bladder rupture in the setting of apparently insignificant trauma may suggest underlying bladder pathology.

The spectrum of bladder injuries encountered depends on the individual trauma center's patient base and referral patterns. During the 5-year period from 1971 to 1976, at Detroit General Hospital there were 79 patients treated for ruptures of the bladder; 63 of these ruptures (61 gunshot wounds, 2 knife wounds) were from penetrating trauma.[2] In contrast, however, Brosman and Faye reported that 80% of 90 bladder injuries at Harbor General/UCLA Medical Center were caused by blunt trauma, presumably mostly from vehicular accidents.[3] In addition, they reported a high number of associated pelvic fractures.

Patients with bladder trauma may present with localized or generalized lower abdominal pain, hematuria, or urinary retention. They may have associated pelvic and acetabular fractures, as well as perineal and suprapubic hematomas. Abdominal distension usually signifies a reflex ileus or massive intraabdominal hemorrhage, but urinary ascites, especially in children, can cause a similar distension.[4] Rarely, particularly when delayed rupture occurs, patients may display the signs or symptoms of appendicitis or diverticulitis, without evidence of traumatic injury.

If the patient does not have gross hematuria, bladder injury may be missed; suspicion should automatically be aroused by the nature of the injury and by the abovementioned subtle signs and symptoms. It is important to inquire about the nature of the force that caused the injury. Often, the patient will describe a direct blow to the abdomen during sports, a fight, or even sexual intercourse. If he is inebriated, even the history of a fall or stumble with impact to an overdistended bladder could suggest the mode of injury. However, since many of these patients are unconscious and unable to relate pertinent information, an inability to void or the ability to void only a small amount of bloody urine may alert the physician to the presence of a bladder injury.

## Diagnosis

Recently, large trauma centers have begun to use computerized tomography (CT) as the primary means of radiologic evaluation for hemodynamically stable patients.[5–7] Simultaneous CT assessment of the chest, abdomen, and pelvis in search of soft tissue, organ, and skeletal injury is efficient and accurate, especially for injuries to the upper urinary tract. In addition, within the bony pelvis, visualization of pelvic fracture lines, hematomas, and bladder displacement provides important information. However, CT is not a substitute for urethrography and cystography in the evaluation of the lower urinary tract. Unless staff are available to operate the CT scanner 24 hours a day, the routine performance of excretory urograms is necessary—as is the case in most community hospitals caring for trauma patients (Fig 1).

For years, urologists have advised that retrograde urethrography be performed before the passage of a urethral catheter in the severely traumatized patient. Unfortunately, this advice is rarely heeded, and the consulting urologist often arrives to find the Foley catheter already in place or a pile of used catheters, none of which could be passed into the bladder, on the trauma stretcher. Although urine output is rarely of any significance during the first 15 minutes of resuscitation, the ritual passage of the Foley catheter seems to occupy anxious hands while minds decide on priorities and actions.

Retrograde urethrography should be the initial urographic investigative procedure performed on every patient with perineal, pelvic, or lower abdominal trauma. In order to reduce the morbidity and mortality in these high-risk patients, prompt diagnosis of lower urinary tract trauma requires a high index of suspicion. The incidence of concomitant lower urinary tract injuries in patients with pelvic fractures has been reported to range from a low of 7.5% to a high of 25%,[8] and probably most reliably approaches the 13.5% reported by Palmer et al.[9] Furthermore, the frequent association of bladder and urethral injury (a 10% to 29% incidence of bladder rupture has been observed in cases of rupture of the posterior urethra),[10] mandates performance of retrograde urethrography and cystography prior to catheter passage. Correspondingly, bladder and urethral trauma are usu-

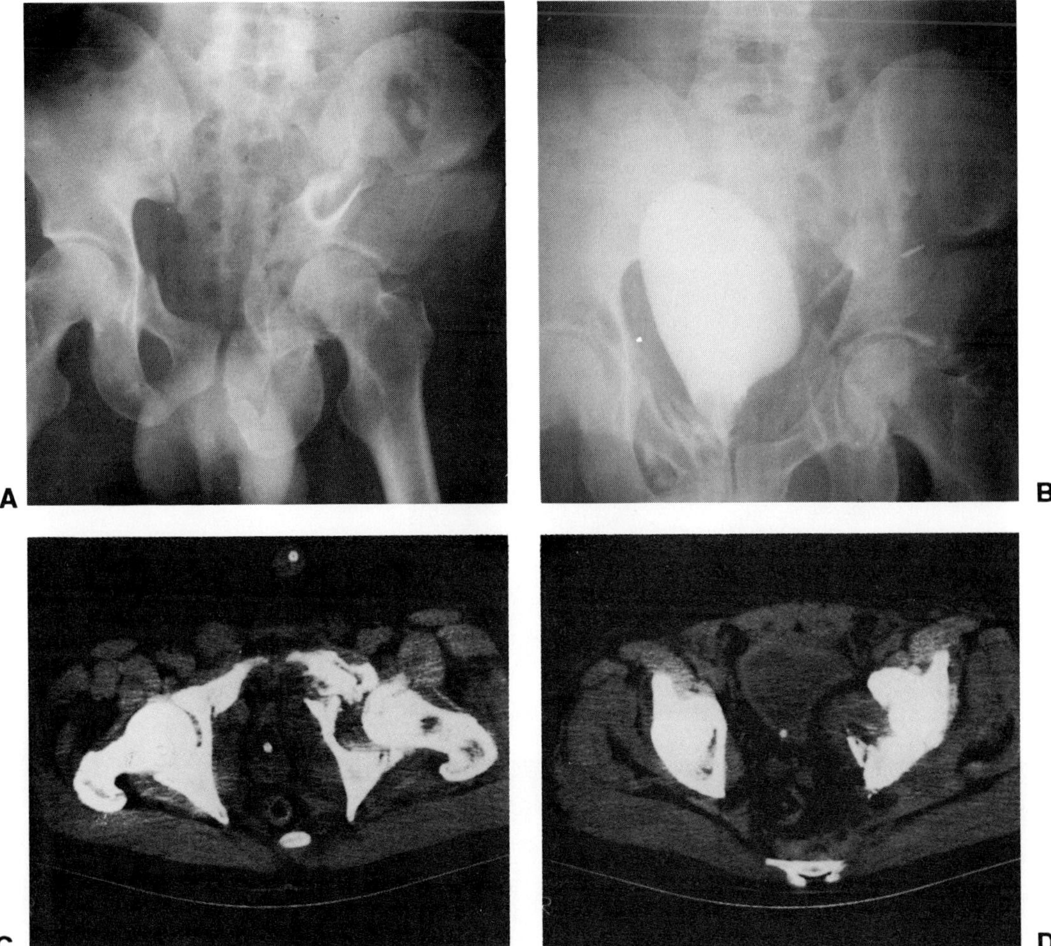

**Fig 1.** This 40-year-old man hit by a truck had multiple transverse processes fractures, unstable pelvic fracture, and left femur fracture. Resuscitation required transfusion of 11 units of whole blood. Note displacement of acetabular fragments into perivesical space. A, B, cystogram reveals perivesical hematoma; C, CT reveals acetabular fracture; D, additional view demonstrates bladder displaced by pelvic hematoma.

ally associated with significant injuries elsewhere in the majority of patients. Cass[8] found associated injuries in 390 (94%) of 417 patients with bladder trauma. The most commonly associated injury was fracture of the pelvis, which was found in 83% of the patients with bladder trauma. Not surprisingly, the mortality rate in patients with bladder ruptures is high, and has been variously reported to range from 12%[11] to 44%.[10]

Retrograde urethrography is performed by slowly injecting 20 to 30 mL of water-soluble contrast material using a piston syringe, with the patient in a slightly oblique position. In men, the penis should be stretched over the medial aspect of the flexed thigh and the glans held firmly around the penetrating syringe.

When the urethra is demonstrated to be intact, the catheter may be placed and cystography should be performed using the technique described by Cass and Ireland.[12] Initially, 250 mL of a 30% solution of sodium meglumine diatrizoate (Renografin) is placed by gravity drainage into the bladder, and anteroposterior and oblique views are obtained (Fig 2). If there is no extrav-

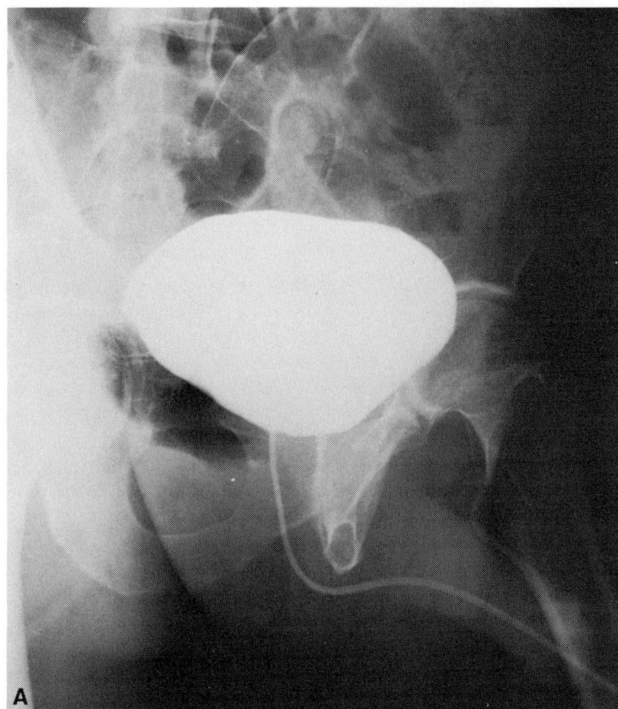


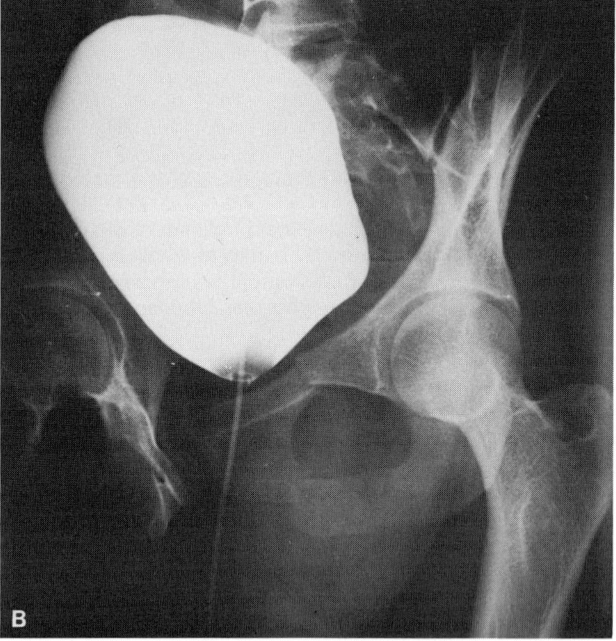


**Fig 2.** Cystograms: A, properly filled bladder in the oblique projection; B, anteroposterior view showing pelvic hematoma with elevated but intact bladder secondary to pubic arch fracture sustained in an automobile accident.

asation, an additional 150 mL is instilled, again by gravity or under slight pressure, if necessary, and additional views are taken. The contrast material is then allowed to drain from the bladder, and after gentle normal saline irrigation, additional post-drainage films are obtained to detect extravasation. At this point, some examiners prefer to place the patient in a modified Trendelenburg position.

Pitfalls with cystography include the following: If the bladder is not adequately distended and multiple views including oblique and post-drainage exposures are not taken, subtle extravasation of dye may not be noted. Occasionally, an associated intramural hematoma from penetrating trauma or a perivesicular hematoma (seen with pelvic fractures) may produce tamponade at the point of rupture and not allow extravasation. In penetrating injury, bladder lacerations tend to seal themselves with hematoma dissection in the wall of the bladder. Intraperitoneal ruptures will seal off after deflation of the bladder, and herniated loops of small intestine may plug mucosal defects.[13] Cass and Ireland reported false-negative cystograms in three patients from a series of 19 extraperitoneal bladder ruptures.[12] Only 250 mL of contrast was instilled in two of these patients, and in the third, a post-washout film had not been obtained. Diagnoses were made at laparotomy (two) and autopsy (one). Similarly, Carroll and McAninch studied 51 cases of traumatic bladder rupture and found that, with adequate bladder distension and drainage films, the diagnostic accuracy of cystography should approach 100%. Alternatively, if adequate distension is not achieved and drainage films are omitted, the accuracy of the cystogram falls to 79%.[14]

The cystogram obtained at infusion intravenous pyelography (IVP) is not an adequate examination of the bladder. The frequently recommended quantitative irrigation of the bladder to assure the integrity of the wall is mentioned here only to be condemned. Bladder lacerations can capriciously seal and unseal, and this test has no place in the diagnosis of acute bladder injury.

After lower-tract evaluation, an IVP or CT is commonly performed to evaluate the function and status of the upper tracts, although this is not universally practiced if the mechanism of injury does not suggest an upper tract injury.

## Treatment

**Bladder Contusion.** Assuming that the upper tracts are normal, hematuria accompanying edema and irregularity of the bladder contour on the cystogram (without extravasation) suggest bladder contusion. Bladder contusions are caused by direct impact to the distended bladder or by impact from the bony spicules or fragments of the fractured pelvis. Contusions rarely need to be confirmed cystoscopically, and these cases should be treated conservatively with bladder drainage if hematuria and clots cause significant symptoms or retention.

Of note are reports of cystoscopically confirmed contusions associated with jogging or marathon running.[15] The cause is presumably repetitive impact of the bladder posterior wall against the firmly fixed trigone. It should be emphasized that without cystoscopic evidence of contusion, hematuria associated with this minimally traumatic exercise is unusual and must be investigated, especially in middle-aged and older joggers, as it may herald previously undiagnosed upper or lower urinary-tract pathology.

Contusions usually resolve without sequelae; however, with lysis of bladder wall hematomas and necrosis of surrounding tissue, delayed rupture may occur. This mechanism probably explains many of the idiopathic bladder ruptures reported sporadically in the literature.[16] Spontaneous rupture without either preceding urologic endoscopy, self-instrumentation, or minor unnoticed trauma remains rare unless there is a preexisting pathologic bladder condition such as tumor, radiation injury, or virulent necrotizing infection.

**Extraperitoneal Rupture.** Extraperitoneal rupture, documented most often by the cystogram series, is usually associated with pelvic fractures. Of course, penetrating injuries to the perineum, groin, or lower abdomen may yield a similar clinical picture. The lacerations most often are observed on the dome or the anterolateral surface of the bladder near the bladder neck, and were previously believed to occur secondary to penetration of the bladder wall by bony fragments of the pubic rami. More recent evidence, however, suggests that the most common mechanism is the bursting or shearing injury that is similarly responsible for the intraperitoneal ruptures.[17,18] Blood and urine extravasate into the pelvic soft tissues, causing a classic hourglass or half-moon bladder deformity as revealed by the cystogram (Fig 3). Occasionally, acetabular blowout fractures send bony missiles into the bladder, and displaced femoral

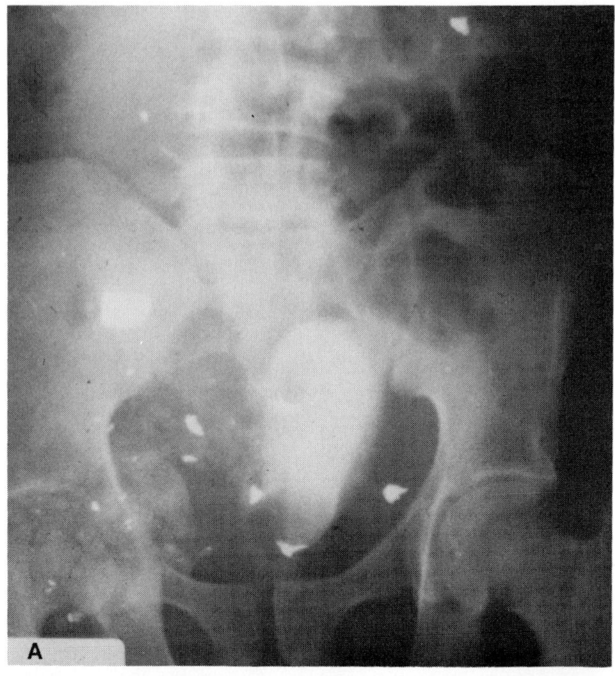

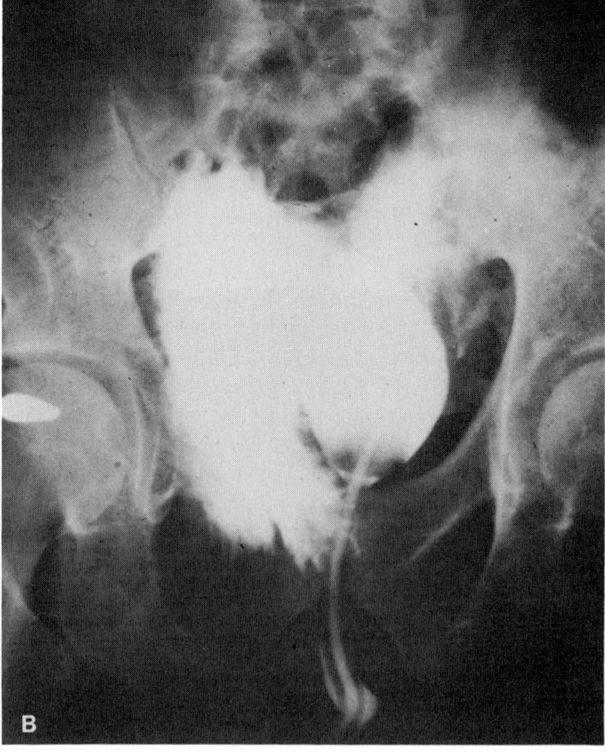

**Fig 3.** Cystograms: A, bilateral pelvic hematomas compress the bladder into a gourd or hour-glass deformity; B, gross extraperitoneal extravasation of contrast after a penetrating gunshot wound.

head penetration of the bladder has been reported.

If the extraperitoneal leak is minimal, urethral catheterization and urinary diversion for a period of 7 to 10 days is usually sufficient treatment,[11,17,19] since 88% of patients will heal in 10 days.[11,17] Corriere and Sandler managed 41 of 62 patients who had extraperitoneal ruptures with catheter drainage only—using a Foley catheter in 32, percutaneous cystotomy in 4, and an open cystotomy in 5—with a 12% complication rate limited to persistent extravasation at 10 days; all symptoms resolved after prolonged catheterization.[17] An additional 14 patients underwent bladder closure and cystotomy tube placement (although the reasons for this course of action were not stated); seven died before intervention.

For moderate extravasation accompanied by pelvic hematoma or pelvic fracture requiring external fixation, cystotomy diversion is a more appropriate therapeutic option. Exploration of pelvic hematomas to locate bladder lacerations is often a time-consuming, bloody, and fruitless procedure, and, as such, should be avoided. Closure of a large bladder defect can be achieved transvesically through an anterior cystotomy by simple two-layer muscle and mucosal approximation; urinary diversion should be achieved by cystotomy drainage. In contrast to Corriere and Sandler,[11,17] Carroll and McAninch recommend surgical repair and suprapubic drainage of all extraperitoneal ruptures, arguing that an open bladder laceration managed with an indwelling urethral catheter could lead to possible infection of a retroperitoneal hematoma. In addition, since a high percentage of these patients require laparotomy for associated injuries anyway, Carroll and McAninch argue, the bladder rupture should be managed at that time, thereby avoiding the potential problems associated with prolonged urethral catheterization.[18]

**Intraperitoneal Rupture.** Bladder perforations (and intraabdominal leakage of urine) should certainly be suspected when penetrating injury to the lower abdomen occurs (Fig 4). However, blunt suprapubic impact to a filled bladder may cause a classic rupture at the dome, where surrounding soft-tissue cushioning is absent.[8,18] There may be associated pelvic injury, but the mechanism of rupture is transmission of force across fluid under pressure rather than bony spicule penetration. The patient is more acutely ill than patients with other types of injury and has lower abdominal pain that

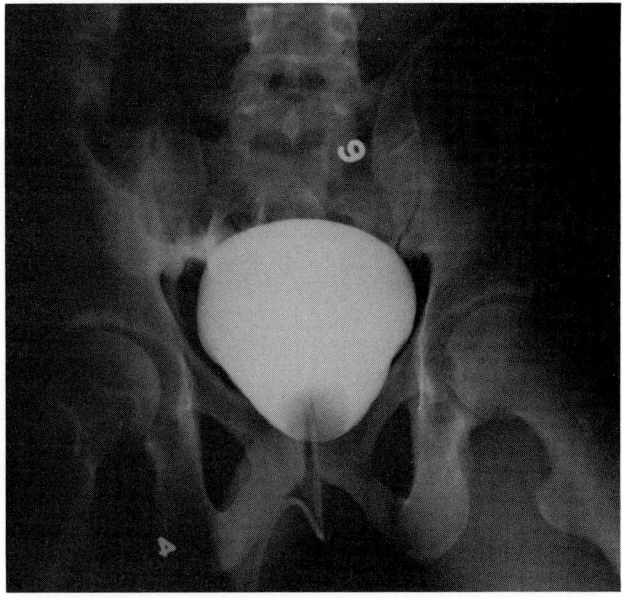


**Fig 4.** A gunshot wound of the lower abdomen (marker 6 on entrance, 4 on exit) produced intraperitoneal bladder perforation; note dye tracking along right colon gutter intraabdominally.

is often indistinguishable from that associated with pelvic fracture. Voiding may be impossible despite an intact urethra because of intense detrusor spasms, or the urine output may have leaked into the abdominal cavity. Note that blood urea nitrogen (BUN) and creatinine levels are not good indicators of urinary reabsorption by the peritoneum.

These injuries need immediate exploration and repair. Exploration is performed through a vertical lower-abdominal incision, which allows simultaneous evaluation of other intraabdominal organs. The peritoneal surface of the bladder should be carefully examined, and after the point of rupture is located, the bladder should be closed from the peritoneal side. Sutures of 2–0 chromic catgut are used for approximation of the detrusor; a second layer of peritoneal running sutures, 2–0 chromic, is used to reinforce this closure.

The bladder may then be entered through a vertical anterior cystotomy to allow inspection of the ureteral orifices. All devitalized bladder tissue must be debrided. If there is any suggestion of penetrating injury, indigo carmine may be given intravenously, or stents may be passed, to identify disruption either within the bladder wall or extravesical disruption. When present, this injury may be dealt with at the time of bladder repair. The mucosal edge of the laceration should then be closed, using a running 3–0 plain catgut suture, and the bladder drained using suprapubic cystotomy in the male and a large (22- or 24-F) urethral catheter in the female. Furthermore, no attempt should be made to explore the pelvic hematoma because of the risk of inducing uncontrolled hemorrhage or pelvic infection.

Suprapubic cystotomy drainage in the male decreases the potential for development of urethritis or epididymitis during the recommended 7- to 10-day period of urinary diversion. If the injured area is adequately debrided and closed in multiple layers, postoperative hematuria should not be a problem and normal healing of the well-vascularized bladder will occur. A cystogram is recommended prior to removal of the suprapubic catheter, but rarely shows persistent leakage.

During laparotomy, the rectum and anterior surface of the sigmoid colon should also be inspected; if an injury is found here, a diverting colostomy or repair of bowel laceration should be performed.

It should be reemphasized that the accepted principles of care of the ruptured bladder are (a) debridement, (b) multiple-layer closure with absorbable suture material, (c) drainage of the perivesical space, (d) urinary diversion, and (e) avoidance of dissection into the pelvic hematoma.

**Combined Injuries.** Combined intra- and extraperitoneal bladder ruptures are in general uncommon, but have been reported to have an incidence as high as 12% by Carroll and McAninch.[18] Such combined injuries are usually associated with severe pelvic trauma. The challenge is to identify both aspects of this injury simultaneously and to repair them promptly[20] as described above. The initial retrograde urethrogram, performed prior to cystography, will aid in the diagnosis of an associated urethral injury.[21]

The pediatric bladder resides within the abdomen, and thus the vesical neck is susceptible to blunt anterior abdominal trauma. Vesicourethral and vesicovaginal ruptures, both anterior and posterior to the bladder neck, have occurred, and the traumatic laceration of the vesicovaginal septum in the young female can lead to a traumatic vesicovaginal fistula. Since the bladder neck is a region of primary continence control, especially in females, Merchant recommends primary surgical repair under direct vision with reconstruction of the vesicourethral area.[22] Vaginal injuries may be simultaneously repaired, resulting in improved continence and normal vaginal maturation.

**Operative Injury to the Bladder.** The operative procedures in which the bladder is most commonly injured include cystoscopy and transurethral resections, caesarean section, laparoscopy,[23] dilatation and curettage, hysterectomy (vaginal or transabdominal), repair of sliding hernias involving the bladder, and occasionally, extirpative operations on the rectum and sigmoid colon. The challenge in these cases is to recognize that injury has occurred, so that adequate repair can be performed immediately. Failure to recognize such a condition may lead to serious increase in morbidity.

With the increasing rate of cesarean section deliveries, the urologist will see a small but significant number of bladder lacerations incurred during delivery. Since the classic cesarean vertical incision has been replaced by the Pfannenstiel incision, less uterine bleeding and fewer uterine ruptures during labor have occurred; however, an increased rate of bladder injuries has been incurred while separating the bladder from the lower uterine cervical segment.[24] In some gravid patients, the anatomical transition between the lower uterus and the cervix is indistinct, and the bladder does not separate well from the upper vagina. If the bladder is not mobilized adequately, laceration can occur. Serious complications, such as vesicovaginal and vesicouterine fistulae, can be avoided with prompt attention to primary repair.

During vaginal hysterectomy, the bladder injury is usually in the trigonal area just superior to the interureteric ridge. The bladder should be inspected by means of suprapubic cystotomy, the integrity of the ureteral orifices noted, and primary repair performed. Closure of the bladder from the perineum combines difficulty in achieving sufficient exposure with uncertainty as to ureteral injury, and is therefore not recommended.

## URETHRAL INJURY

The male urethra, extending from the bladder neck to the glandular meatus, is susceptible to trauma at several points along its path (Fig 5).

The posterior urethra can be subdivided into three portions: the prostatic urethra; the supradiaphragmatic urethra, stretching from the prostatic apex to the superior limit of the urogenital diaphragm; and the intradiaphragmatic portion, known as the membranous urethra. The urogenital diaphragm lies between the inferior ischial rami and is made up of an inferior fascia and a superior fascia, which together enclose the deep transverse muscle of the perineum, the bulbourethral glands, and branches of the pudendal artery. The urogenital diaphragm, quite prominent in the male, contains the membranous urethra; this fixed point is often the site of urethral rupture. The male continence mechanism lies just proximal to the superior fascia, and the autonomic nerves involved in sexual potency travel along the membranous urethra. Thus, injuries in this area may cause incontinence and impotence as well as subsequent stricture.

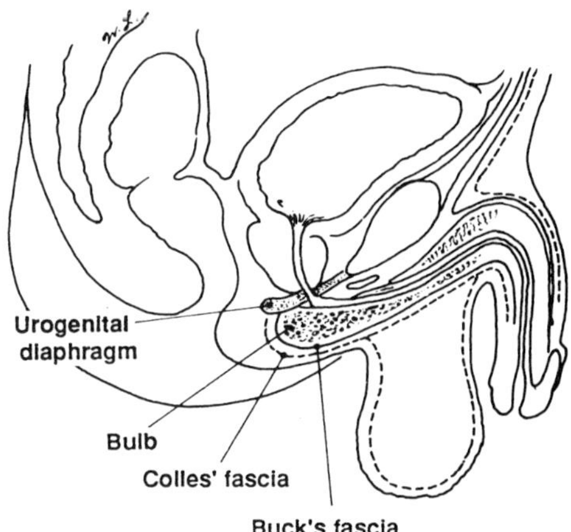

**Fig 5.** Anatomy of the male urethra.

The anterior urethra, that portion distal to the urogenital diaphragm, is encircled by the corpus spongiosum and is held against the corporal bodies by Buck's fascia. The proximal portion, the bulbar urethra, is covered inferiorly by the bulbocavernosus muscle. The distal pendulous urethra is mobile, cushioned by the soft tissues of the penis as well as the fibrous Buck's fascia, and less prone to blunt injury. If an anterior urethral injury ruptures Buck's fascia, the hematoma and possible urinary extravasation can spread under the superficial layers of the scrotum and extend onto the abdominal wall beneath Scarpa's and Colles' fasciae (Fig 6).

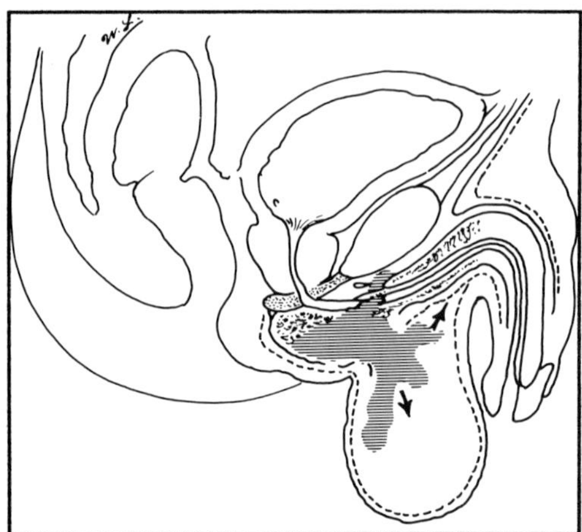

**Fig 6.** Diagram depicting the path of urine and blood extravasation when Buck's fascia is ruptured.

Posterior urethral injuries occur in 3.5% to 25% of patients sustaining pelvic fractures.[9,25,26] From 1971 to 1976 at the Detroit General Hospital, there were 26 urethral injuries (15 anterior and 11 posterior) out of 311 reported genitourinary injuries.[2] Most of the anterior urethral injuries were penetrating, while blunt trauma—with associated pelvic fracture—was the most frequent cause of posterior urethral rupture. In general, however, straddle injuries are the most common disruptive lesions of the anterior urethra.[27]

Patients with anterior urethral disruption present with urethral hemorrhage of varying amounts; they may manifest either meatal spotting or profuse urethral bleeding. Since the injury is below the genitourinary diaphragm, continence is maintained and the urine is clear. There are associated soft-tissue injuries to the penis, and perineal or scrotal discoloration secondary to extravasation along the above-described planes may be the necessary clue for diagnosis.

Straddle injury to the bulbar urethra occurs when a man falls astride a hard object such as the bar of a bike, a fence crossbar, or a ladder rung.[28] The bulbar urethra is crushed against the symphysis pubis, causing contusion or partial (or, rarely, complete) rupture of the urethra. Injury usually occurs about 2 cm to 3 cm distal to the inferior leaf of the urogenital diaphragm, and there may be considerable bleeding through the urethra. The hallmark of this injury is bleeding from the urethra with clear urine during voiding. There is frequently a perineal hematoma if Buck's fascia is violated, and, more rarely, there may be an associated fracture of the pubic arch.

The pendulous urethra is rarely injured by blunt trauma when the penis is flaccid. However, with erection, acute angulation during sexual gymnastics may cause a tear in the tunica albuginea and subsequent penile hematoma, in which the urethral integrity must be suspect.

Penetrating injuries to the pendulous and bulbar portions of the urethra have been caused by gunshot wounds, knife wounds, fans, zippers, vacuum sweepers, and bites. The absence of cutaneous entrance or exit wounds should suggest the possibility of self-induced injuries secondary to the attempted passage of foreign bodies such as pencils, hat pins, or files up the urethra.

Posterior urethral disruption is most often accompanied by an unstable pelvic fracture. Although only 30% of pelvic fractures are complicated and unstable, patients with severe injuries sustaining soft tissue loss (from open fractures), associated abdominal and rectal injuries, and possible iliac vessel tears requiring multiple transfusions, may have posterior urethral injuries.[29] Beyond the mechanism of injury, which alone should raise suspicion for urethral trauma, clinically, one may find a distended bladder or high-riding and nonpalpable prostate on rectal examination. MAST trousers or orthopedic external fixation devices may make such an examination impossible. Furthermore, as stated earlier, concomitant bladder ruptures[20,21] will be found in 10% to 29% of the patients with posterior urethral injuries.[10]

## Diagnosis

As discussed previously, proper radiologic evaluation of urethral trauma mandates retrograde urethrography before any diagnostic or therapeutic passage of a catheter.[30] The urethrogram will demonstrate

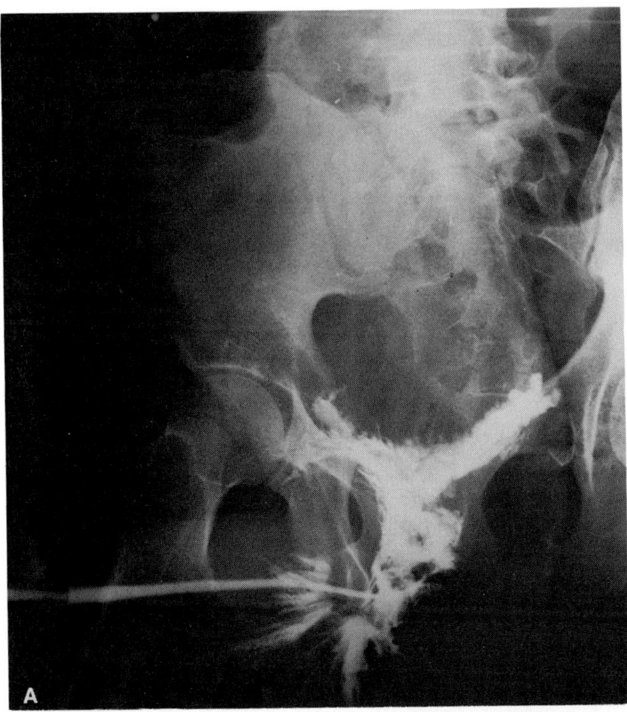


**Fig 7.** A, retrograde urethrogram showing gross extravasation from the posterior urethra (membranous and prostatic) after butterfly pelvic fracture sustained in an automobile accident; B, radiograph showing fracture.

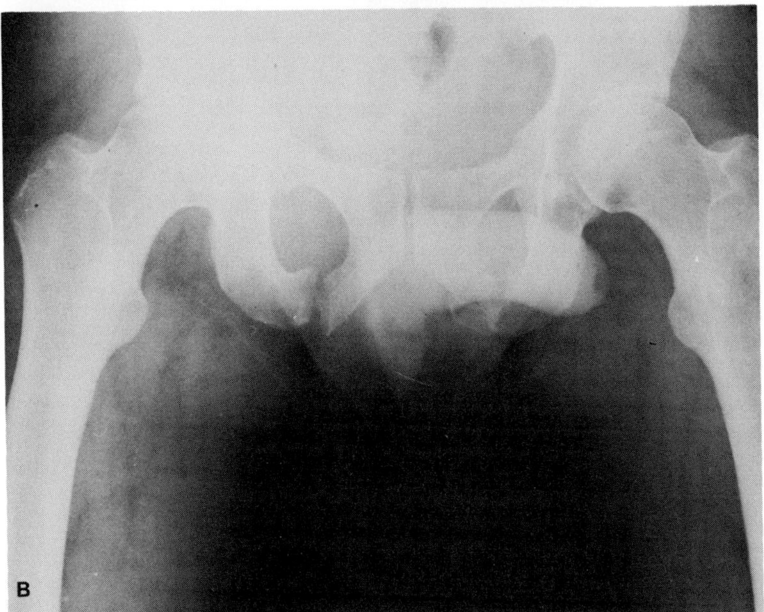


urethral rupture, with accompanying extravasation, as well as passage of contrast material into the bladder, the presence of which precludes complete urethral disruption (Figs 7, 8). The technique used has been previously described. It need only be added that gently performed urethrography will provide the information desired without the undesirable reflux of contrast into blood vessels that injection under pressure often produces. A patient is rarely too ill for this procedure, and evidence of scle-

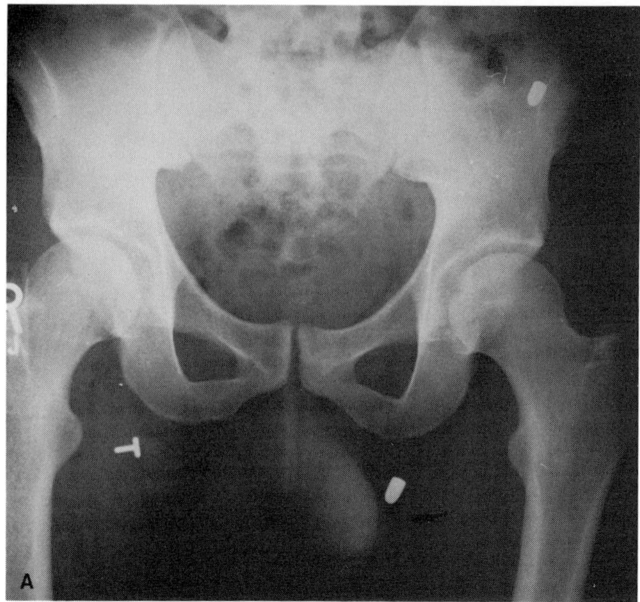


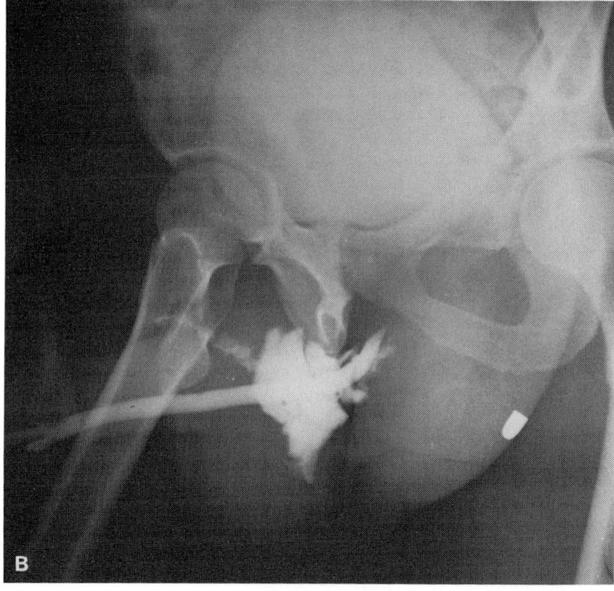


**Fig 8.** A, gunshot wound penetrating bulbar urethra (marker T at groin entrance wound) with swelling of perineum and scrotum; B, retrograde urethrogram showing partial urethral disruption with dye tracking retrograde along bullet's path. The patient was treated by suprapubic cystotomy.

rosis or fibrosis of periurethral tissue produced by extravasated water-soluble contrast is less than anecdotal.

Urethrography should be performed before the passage of a catheter.[31] Mitchell has warned that many urethral disruptions are partial, in which stretched but bridging strands of mucosa and urethra remain intact.[32] With the resolution of the pelvic hematoma, the partial disruption often realigns, occasionally without secondary stricture formation. Blind passage of a urethral catheter by inexperienced hands can convert a partial disruption to a full one and should, as a rule, be avoided. However, Blandy's group in London reportedly passed a small urethral catheter routinely in trauma patients without causing damage to the urethra.[33]

If the urologist called to evaluate a lower-abdominal trauma patient finds that a catheter has already been inserted, it should not be removed. Urethrography should be performed by passing a small-gauge (16 F or 18 F) intravenous catheter into the urethral meatus alongside the urethral catheter; an injection through this catheter will demonstrate any rupture of the urethra. If extravasation is demonstrated, the patient must be managed as discussed below.

### Treatment

**Anterior Urethra Injury.** Despite accumulating experience, controversy continues to flare between advocates of primary repair and those who prefer primary treatment with urinary diversion and later urethral reconstruction, if necessary. At Detroit General Hospital, of 19 patients with trauma to the anterior urethra (14 gunshot wounds, 2 shotgun blasts, 2 blunt injuries, and 1 dog bite), 16 were treated with suprapubic cystotomy combined with local debridement as necessary; three had urethral catheter diversions.[34] Of those treated with suprapubic cystotomy alone, 15 needed no further treatment, suggesting that most partial urethral injuries heal satisfactorily without primary repair.

The management of straddle injuries is currently less controversial than in the recent past. Accumulating experience has revealed that a significant percentage of these injuries will heal with urinary diversion alone, using suprapubic cystotomy.[27,35] Follow-up voiding cystourethrography can be performed after 10 to 14 days. The cystotomy tube may be removed once the injury has healed. Dixon and McAninch recommend the use of uroflowmetry at 3-month intervals and a voiding cystourethrogram at 3 and 12 months[35] for follow-up of the injured urethra. Secondary strictures, which are in general short (<0.5 cm), can often be managed by internal urethrotomy at the first or second occurrence; however those rare recurrences are best treated by urethroplasty with excision and a spatulated end-to-end anastomosis.[27,35]

Although some authors have reportedly employed primary reapproximation over a catheter, the periurethral hematoma, urethral edema with infection and necrosis secondary to blast effect, and the rate of subsequent urethrocutaneous fistula formation make this approach undesirable.[36] A small laceration or knife wound may be handled by this primary approach, but this situation is unusual.

If the traumatic urethral injury is extensive, with loss of several centimeters of urethra, the use of exteriorization urethroplasty allows wound healing and urethral regeneration and obviates the need for a later first-stage urethroplasty. If the bulbar urethra is involved, perineal urethrostomy allows removal of the cystostomy tube as well as continued drainage of the surrounding devitalized tissue.

Complications reported with all types of treatment of anterior urethral trauma include stricture, urinary tract infection, and urethritis secondary to indwelling catheters and stents. Most secondary strictures are short and, when mature, can easily be managed by direct-vision internal urethrotomy[37] as stated above.

**Posterior Urethral Injury.** More controversy surrounds primary management of the patient with a disrupted posterior urethra. This injury is frequently associated with the crushed pelvis of vehicular, industrial, or mining accidents.

The posterior urethra is fixed to the inferior aspect of the inferior pubic rami by the urogenital diaphragm and the puboprostatic ligaments. The urethra itself is stretched and torn when these ligamentous structures are stressed in the following injuries[1]: the diametric or Malgaigne fracture causing cephalad displacement of the hemipelvis; the bilateral fracture of the superior and inferior pubic rami, with posteroinferior displacement and retrocession of the urogenital diaphragm; diastasis of the symphysis pubis with rupture of puboprostatic ligaments and the urogenital diaphragm; and direct transection of the prostatic urethra by bony spicules from

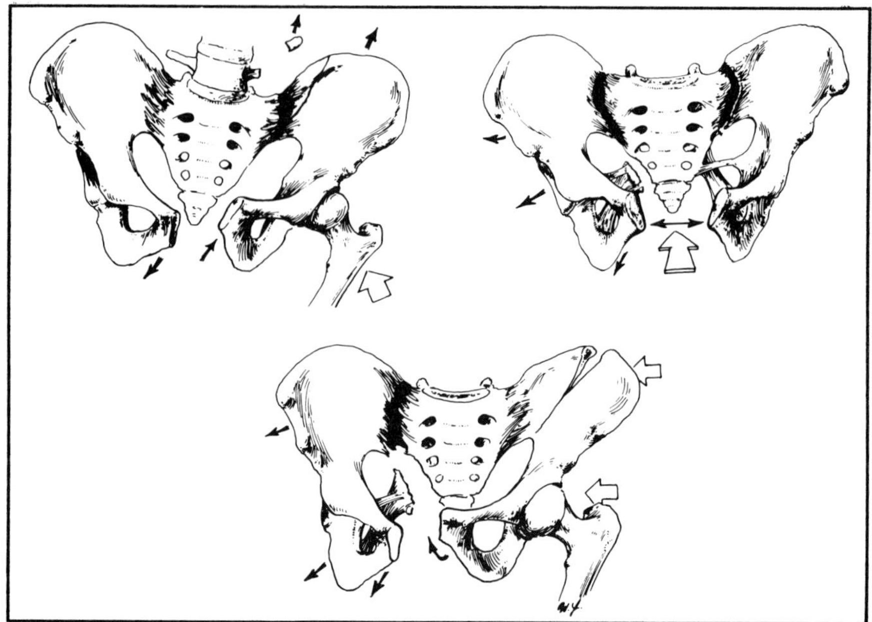

**Fig 9.** Diagrammatic representation of injury forces causing pelvic fractures. [From Pierce JM, Riehle RA, Lower genitourinary tract trauma, in Resnick M [ed], *Current Trends in Urology,* Vol 1 (Baltimore: Williams & Wilkins; 1981), with permission.]

fractures of the pubis close to the midline (Figs 9, 10). Once disruption has occurred, the bladder and prostate may float freely up and out of the pelvis (Fig 11).

However, if the puboprostatic ligaments and urethra are only partially severed, displacement may be minimal. The amount of urinary extravasation from the bladder depends on the competence of the bladder neck, which often reacts to injury with spasm.

In the past, management of patients with posterior urethral dismemberment localized just above the urogenital diaphragm involved exploration of the pelvis, with reestablishment of urethral continuity over a rubber catheter acting as a stent.[38] These indwelling catheters were usually left in place for 6 weeks. Currently, however, disagreement centers around the efficacy of primary reapproximation versus primary suprapubic cystotomy diversion combined with delayed urethroplasty.

The primary objectives during the initial treatment of any posterior urethral injury are to limit the extent and degree of future stricture formation, to avoid compounding the initial injury, and to minimize the risks of incontinence and impotence.[39] Despite the clear objectives, considerable controversy surrounds the means to that end. Primary suprapubic cystotomy combined with delayed urethroplasty yields an impotence rate of 10% and incontinence rates ranging from 1% to 3%.[35] Comparable results using primary realignment and urinary diversion have recently been reported.[40]

Those who advocate exploration and drainage with primary approximation report that a dense stricture or a segment of urethral obliteration is certain unless the proximal and distal portions of the urethra are approximated over a stent.[41–46] After primary repair, any resulting stricture is less complex and more easily repaired. DeWeerd recommends the use of interlocking sounds and traction to the bladder neck by means of a Foley catheter to reposition the prostate in the pelvis.[47] In this series, fewer than 50% of patients developed strictures; most of these were treated by dilatation or internal urethrotomy. Only

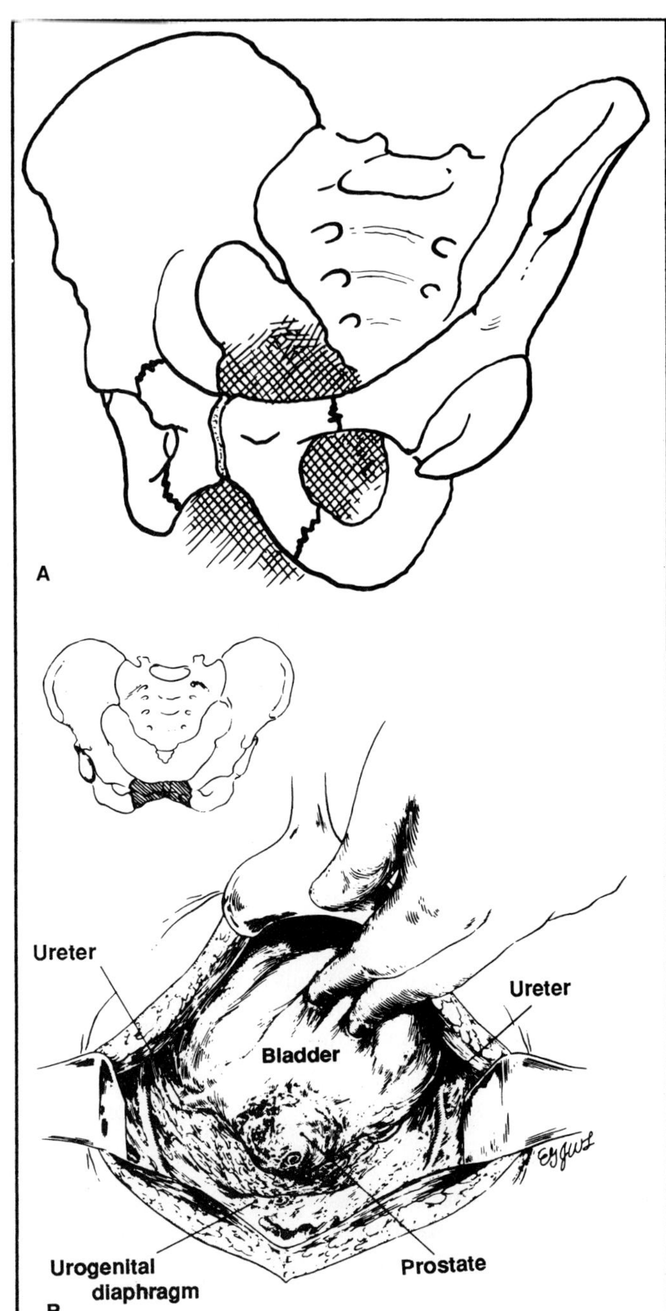


**Fig 10.** A, bilateral pubic arch fracture is often accompanied by posterior displacement of the fragment; B, the supradiaphragmatic portion of the posterior urethra avulsed from the urogenital diaphragm; note that spasm at the bladder neck often maintains urinary continence. [From Pierce JM, Riehle RA, Lower genitourinary tract trauma, in Resnick M [ed], *Current Trends in Urology,* Vol 1 (Baltimore: Williams & Wilkins; 1981), with permission.]

2 of 22 patients needed surgery for secondary stricture. Less impressive are Cass' results with primary realignment: 62% of the patients studied by Cass developed strictures, one half of whom needed further surgery.[45] Devine and associates emphasize the necessity to divide the puboprostatic ligaments (if they are still intact) to facilitate the descent of the prostate without tension or the need for traction.[46]

If there is gross distraction between the urethra and the prostate caused by pelvic

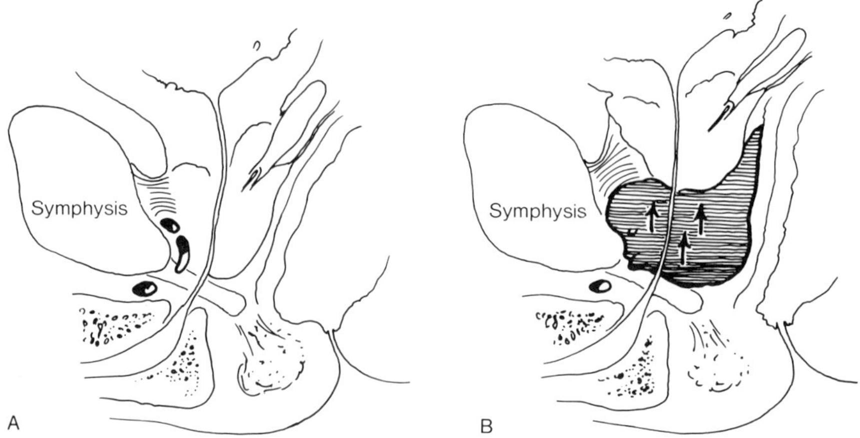


**Fig 11.** A, normal sagittal posterior urethral anatomy; B, pelvic hematoma often accompanies a stretched or torn posterior urethra.

hematoma or pelvic fragments, Turner-Warwick prefers bladder-neck traction over an anatomically restored, suture-free urethra stented by a fenestrated urethral catheter. This type of catheter allows better drainage of urethral exudates, and perineal traction decreases the incidence of later development of complex posterior urethral strictures.[48]

These reports make no mention of blood loss, the presence of partial tears, or the inherent risk of opening pelvic hematomas. Exploration of the traumatized pelvis may cause excessive hemorrhage, facilitate pelvic abscess formation, or produce greater degrees of fibrosis due to increased extravasation.

Several points should be made regarding primary exploration and realignment:

- Interlocking sounds often traumatize the bulbar and membranous urethra. Traumatic attempts at reestablishing urethral continuity at the time of injury may only result in the creation of false passages in the membranous urethra and bladder neck, thus compounding the severity of the injury. Scar formation along the posterior urethra may increase stricture length and make subsequent urethroplasty more difficult. In addition, proper postoperative bladder-neck function is essential for full continence in these patients, and an inelastic bladder outlet may compromise the functional results of a quite adequate anatomical repair.
- Posterior urethral disruptions are often partial tears; determination of this is very difficult during the operation.[47,49]
- Exposure of the pelvic hematoma often causes increased hemorrhage, and control of lacerated veins can be quite difficult once the hematoma is evacuated.

After consideration of the patient's condition, blood loss, and accompanying injuries, an effective, conservative approach for posterior urethral injury is simply the placement of a cystostomy tube for urinary diversion. As a result, the complications of iatrogenic impotence and incontinence secondary to dissection in the periprostatic area during pelvic exploration are avoided.

If an attempt at antegrade catheter passage is made, only a soft latex catheter should be used. If a Foley catheter can be successfully negotiated through the pendulous urethra, it may be pulled retrograde into the bladder and left indwelling as a stent for 4 to 6 weeks.

Traction by means of a urethral catheter to approximate the proximal and distal portions of the urethra should be avoided. This sometimes produces irreversible ischemic damage to the vesical neck continence

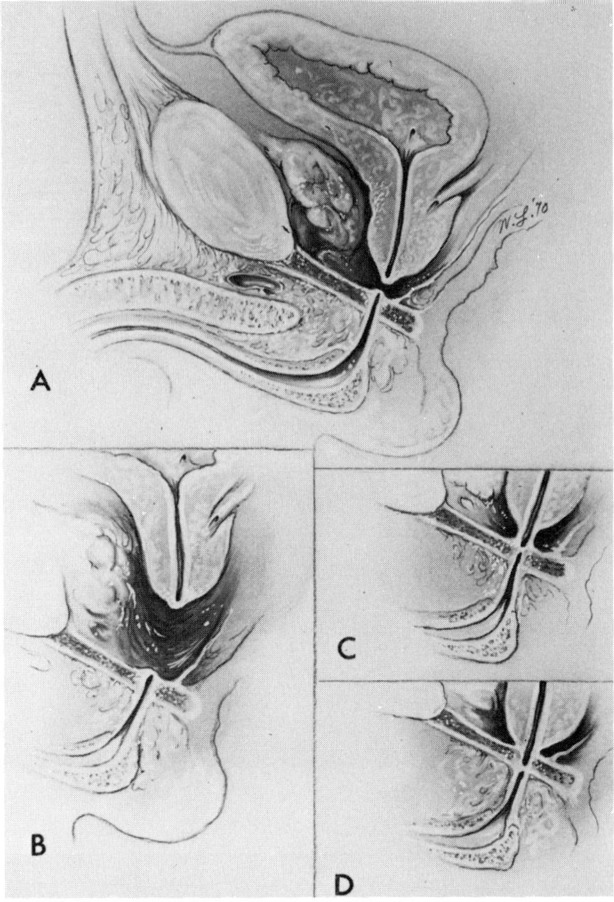


**Fig 12.** Types of posterior urethral disruption and resulting obliteration of urethra. The situation in (B) may resolve to that in (A) with time and resorption of pelvic hematoma. C, D, short, though dense, membranous strictures.

mechanism—the primary mechanism controlling urination following repair of posterior urethral injury.

After the pelvic hematoma and edema have resolved, the proximal prostatic urethra settles surprisingly close to the urogenital diaphragm; if the tear sustained was only partial, continuity may be preserved. Most secondary strictures can be handled by direct-vision urethrotomy. If fibrous obliteration of the urethra or impassable stricture develops, an elective surgical approach for repair can be planned (Figs 12, 13).

However, in this situation, the timing of urethroplasty is critical. The minimum duration of suprapubic cystotomy drainage following injury is 3 months.[35,50] If, after 3 months, the measured length of obliteration on the x-ray film is more than 1 cm, repair may be postponed. Often, resolution and absorption of pelvic hematoma are not complete until as long as 18 months after injury.[48,51]

## Surgical Options and Techniques

The traditional options for delayed reconstruction of the obliterated or disrupted posterior urethra are perineal or transpubic approaches for direct urethral anastomoses, tube grafts, or multistaged scrotal inlay urethroplasty. Recently, however, endoscopic internal urethrotomy has been advocated to reestablish urethral continuity while maintaining continence and potency.[52–54] However, reported experience with this approach remains small. Lieberman reported 4 male patients, with posterior urethral strictures measuring 2.0 to 3.5 cm in length, who underwent cystoscopic internal urethrotomy guided by si-

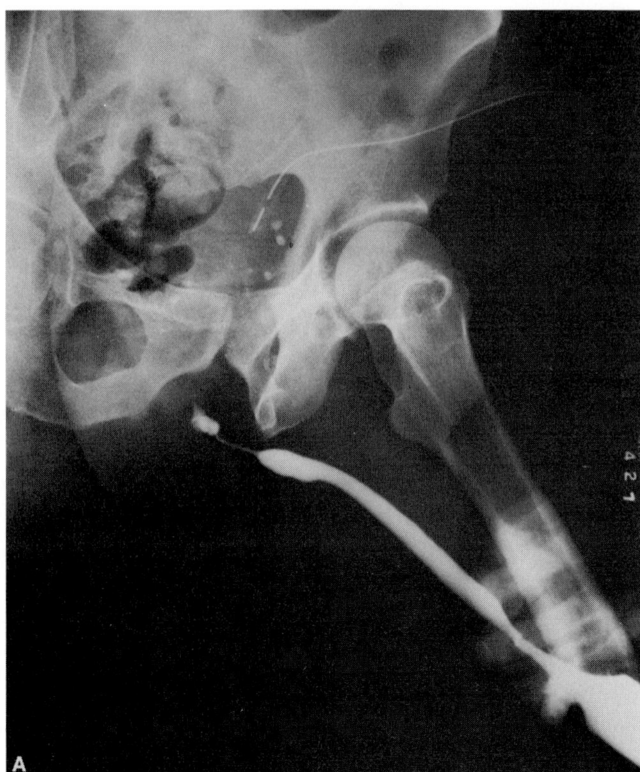

**Fig 13.** A, retrograde urethrogram showing lengthy posttraumatic bulbar stricture; B, voiding cystourethrogram with evidence of obstruction.

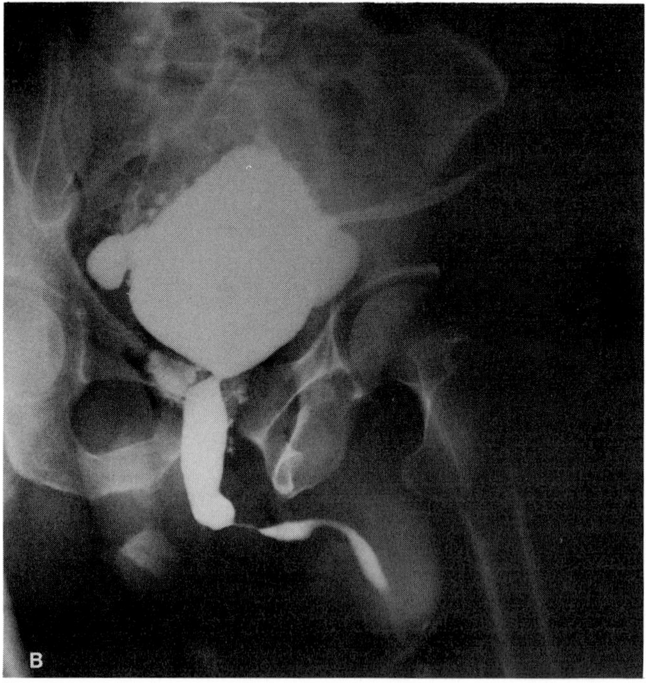

multaneous bladder endoscopy.[52] Urethrotomy was performed 4 to 12 months after injury. Only one patient required repeat urethrotomy during the follow-up period of 9 months, and potency status was not altered from that observed immediately following injury. Antegrade dilation and catheterization of the posterior urethra via cystotomy tract endoscopy allows a combined approach if bulbar or urethral false passages must be bypassed.[53]

Marshall has extended follow-up of patients treated with these endoscopic techniques even further, and reports 7 patients who are voiding at least 1 year after the last procedure.[54] The patients were initially evaluated 3 to 6 months after their injury and suprapubic diversion. If physical examination, radiographic studies, and endoscopy were consistent with urethral obliterations of less than 3.0 cm in length, the patient was deemed a candidate for endoscopic reconstruction. The patients underwent endoscopy from above and below, and a trocar was passed through the scar under fluoroscopic guidance through which a guidewire was passed. A van Andel balloon catheter was then used to dilate the tract. It was then possible to remove excessive scar using a pediatric resectoscope. The procedure is terminated after injection of the scar with triamcinolone and passage of a 22 F or 24 F Foley catheter. All patients required at least one additional urethrotomy; however, all have remained continent, but potency is absent or impaired in four. Long-term follow-up of patients handled in this way is yet to be reported, and, of course, proper patient selection is crucial to this technique's success.

Surgically, the most satisfactory approach to the uncomplicated posterior traumatic membranous stricture is a perineal one-stage end-to-end urethral anastomosis. Full-thickness free-tube grafts have been successful, but seem better suited for use in more anterior urethral strictures.[55]

Preoperative cystoscopic and radiologic evaluations of the strictured area should be made. Note that simultaneous voiding cystourethrography and retrograde urethrography often exaggerate the length of urethral obliteration, because the prostatic urethra may not be visualized. The most accurate means to assess stricture length is by the simultaneous passage of suprapubic and urethral sounds (Figs 14, 15); recently, magnetic resonance imaging has been re-

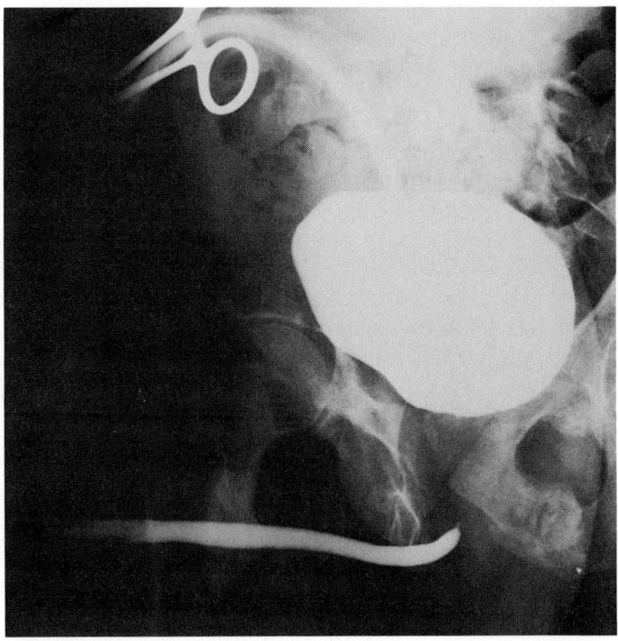

**Fig 14.** Simultaneous retrograde urethrography and voiding cystourethrography.

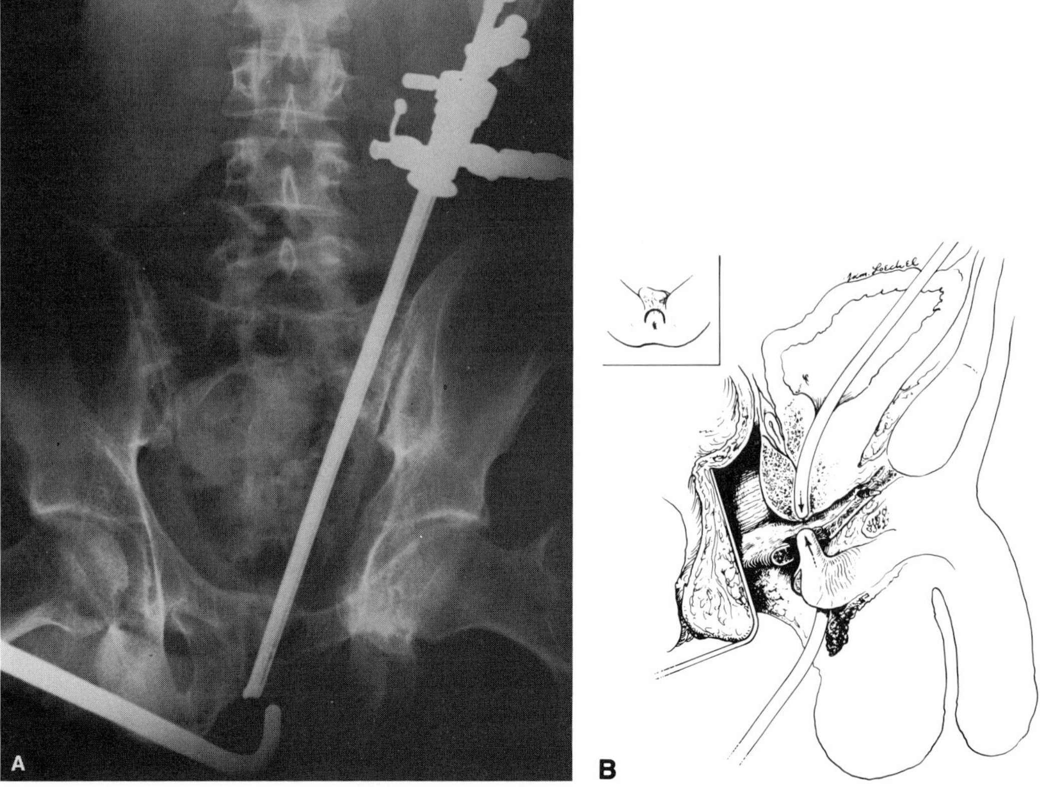


**Fig 15.** A, combined antegrade and retrograde instrumentation can illustrate the length of the obliterated posterior urethral segment more precisely, as depicted diagrammatically in B.

ported to better define the length and position of posterior urethral strictures.[56] In most patients, the separation is less than 1 cm 6 months after injury. Longer strictures or obliterations are the result of interposed bony fragments, extensive hematoma fibrosis, previous early attempts at surgery, or extreme pelvic distortion. In the last case, pelvimetry can be helpful in assessing the pelvic outlet. A narrowed outlet or ossified, obliterated pubic arches may necessitate a combined anterior-posterior approach with pubectomy. On the other hand, Turner-Warwick stresses the importance of simultaneous voiding cystourethrography and retrograde urethrography to define any fistulae or false passages; however, he emphasizes that radiographic demonstration of prostatobulbar strictures is inadequate to determine the surgical approach and that the nature of repair needed can only be determined at exploration.[50]

The anterior urethra should be inspected cystoscopically to identify any nontraumatic simultaneous strictures. While under anesthesia, the patient should be placed in extreme lithotomy position to assess the degree of hip mobility allowed by the healed bony pelvis.

**Technique for Transperineal Repair (Single-Stage).** For single-stage transperineal repair, the patient is placed in exaggerated lithotomy position and a midline perineal incision is made.[57,58] In the face of a previously failed urethroplasty or numerous draining sinuses, the surgeon may elect a perineal scrotal flap incision (Fig 16). This allows the first-stage exteriorization type of urethroplasty, if urethral scarring or ante-

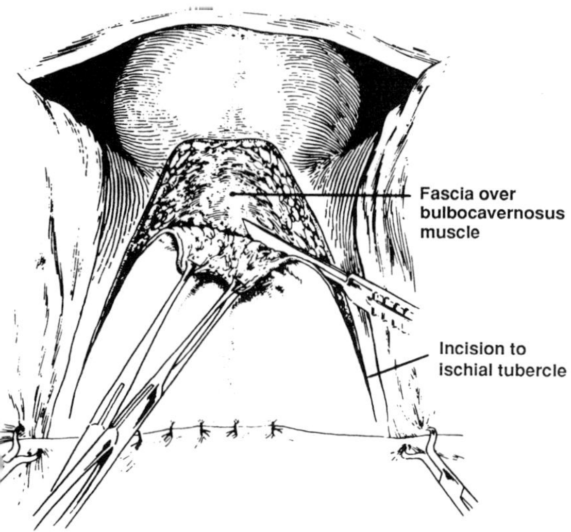


**Fig 16.** A perineal Leadbetter flap incision, as an alternative to the usual midline incision for transperineal repair of an interrupted posterior urethra. [From Pierce[57].]

rior urethral inelasticity contraindicates the one-stage procedure. The bulbocavernosus muscles are divided, the bulb and infradiaphragmatic portions of the urethra are mobilized down to the diaphragm, and the urogenital diaphragm is incised vertically in the midline (posterior or anterior to the membranous urethra). The placement of this incision should preserve autonomic fibers as they traverse the diaphragm. The membranous and supradiaphragmatic urethra are dissected until the strictured area is encountered, and then the membranous urethra is divided distally, freeing the bulb (Fig 17). A half-circle sound is passed into the cystotomy tract through the posterior prostatic urethra and then pushed gently toward the perineum, until the tip can be palpated through the fibrous obliteration. The fibrous tissue is incised, until the sound penetrates the perineum, identifying the apex of the proximal prostatic urethra. Notably, the apical prostatic segment is often

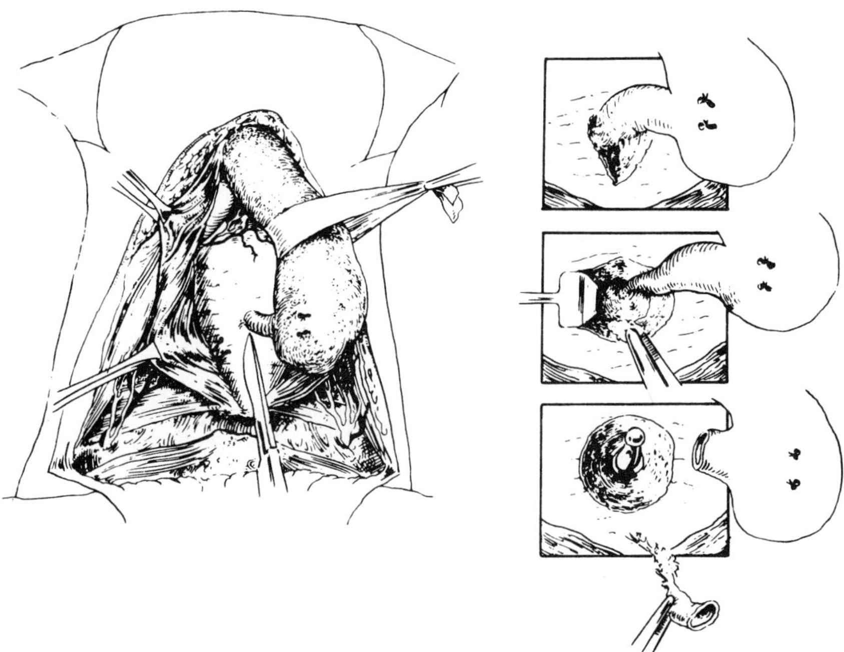

**Fig 17.** In transperineal repair of an interrupted posterior urethra, a 1-cm vertical incision in the urogenital diaphragm anterior or posterior to the urethra is usually sufficient. Use of malleable suction tube facilitates visualization. Views A–C show dissection of strictured urethra through the membranous diaphragm and excision of fibrotic segment. Proximal and distal urethra are ready for anastomosis. [From Pierce[57].]

also obliterated from the injury in children and this portion must be excised or bypassed as well. Complete excision of all paraurethral and retropubic fibrosis and scar is recommended to achieve a complication-free anastomosis.[50,56] The proximal prostatic urethra should easily accept a 36 F sound.

Urethral margins are debrided to give fresh clean bleeding edges, and the pendulous urethra can be dissected extensively to gain needed length for a tension-free repair. A spatulated end-to-end anastomosis is then performed over an 18 F Foley catheter using six to eight 4–0 to 6–0 chromic or PGA sutures (Fig 18). The placement of the proximal sutures is facilitated by the use of Turner-Warwick posterior urethral needles and a curved tonsillar suction tube passed through the bladder into the prostatic urethra. The urethral bulb is attached to the inferior aspect of the urogenital diaphragm using interrupted chromic sutures to seal the repair. Turner-Warwick recommends the use of a pedicled omental graft to obliterate any significant perianastomotic dead space; however, this is only feasible in a combined abdominoperineal approach.[50] A perineal Penrose drain should be placed lateral to the incision, which is closed with subcuticular absorbable sutures (eg, Dexon).

The urethral catheter may be removed after 3 weeks, and if no extravasation is evident on retrograde urethrography, the patient is allowed to void and the cystotomy is removed. Patients are evaluated postoperatively by visual inspection of urinary stream. Flow rate and urodynamic evaluation are undertaken only if problems with control or anastomotic stricture occur. Retrograde urethrography is not performed, except in the immediate postoperative period. Others recommend uroflowmetry every 3 months for the first year, accompanied by a voiding cystourethrogram and retrograde urethrography at 3 and 12 months.[35] If anastomotic stricture occurs, it can be easily managed by dilatation or, rarely, internal urethrotomy.

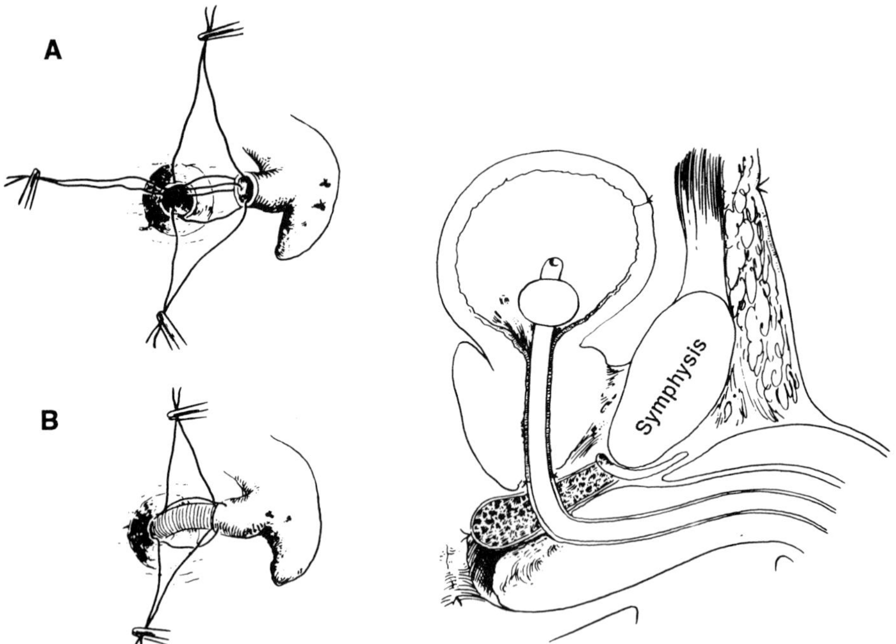


**Fig 18.** Primary end-to-end anastomosis in transperineal repair of an interrupted posterior urethra. Four quadrant chromic sutures are placed and then tied under direct vision (A, B). The urethral catheter is left indwelling for 3 wks (right).

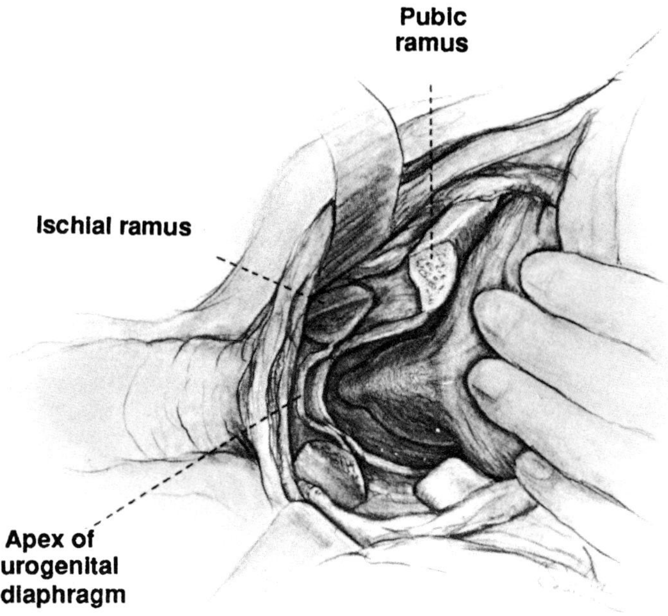


**Fig 19.** The much-improved access to the posterior urethra following pubectomy is shown.

**Technique for Transpubic Repair (Single-Stage).** A pubectomy is recommended to improve exposure of the prostatomembranous urethra, thereby allowing excision of all fistulae and scar tissue, with the end result of a tension-free prostatobulbar anastomosis.[56] The transpubic approach may also be used in cases of severe pelvic distortion and in children with a small perineum who require a combined abdominal and perineal approach. Pubectomy is performed as described by Pierce,[57] Waterhouse and colleagues,[51,59] McAninch,[56] and others[60–62] (Fig 19).

The anterior surface of the symphysis is exposed and the suspensory ligament of the penis divided. The dissection is carried anteriorly and posteriorly under the inferior arch, the puboprostatic ligaments are sharply divided, and the dorsal vein complex is tied off and divided. After a right-angle clamp is used to punch through the remaining tissue, a Gigli's wire saw can be used to resect the wedge of symphysis pubis. A bone chisel used subperiosteally can achieve the same exposure. Care must be taken to divide both the superior and inferior (arcuate) pubic ligaments, to allow the symphysis to spring apart. The bulbar urethra is then dissected free. Additional bulbar length can be obtained by dividing the intracrural septum, thereby allowing the urethra to be passed more anteriorly toward the prostate. Prostatobulbar anastomosis can then be performed. However, care must be taken to create a sufficiently large oval window through the prostatic anterior lobe and to permit a wide-open (> 30 F) anastomosis to prevent secondary stricture formation.

After pubectomy, bed rest is generally maintained for 4 to 5 days (however, McAninch recommends ambulation on the first postoperative day),[56] followed by increased periods of ambulation. The postoperative management is otherwise as described above for the perineal repair. In general, gait disturbances and pelvic instability have not been observed.

In summary, increasingly refined techniques for the management of posterior urethral stricture have been developed over recent decades. Effective use of antibiotics, the availability of less-irritating silastic catheters, and better understanding of the natural history of the traumatized urethra have eliminated the infected perineum with weeping fistulae previously encountered in these patients. Now, staged urethroplasties using scrotal inlay and perineal full-thickness flaps are rarely indicated, and endoscopic urethrotomy and one-stage perineal urethroplasty have significantly decreased the number of operations needed for restoration of urethral continuity.[63] Secondary or repeat direct-vision internal urethrotomy has replaced repetitive dilatations and numerous office visits. But the persistently increasing rate of traumatic injuries with significantly lower mortality figures assures that the urologist must keep a "bag full of tricks" to successfully meet the challenge of posterior urethral repair.[64]

## EXTERNAL GENITAL INJURY

Although mobile and supple, the penis, scrotum, and testes can be injured by a variety of mechanisms, and subsequent hemorrhage along the previously described anatomical planes can obscure the initial or simultaneous injuries. The primary objective of therapy for genital trauma is preservation of function, and because the genitalia have such a rich vasculature, one should guard against overzealous debridement since marginally viable tissue will often heal nicely.[65]

### Penis

The corpora cavernosa are invested bilaterally by the fibrous tunica albuginea; a laceration of the tunica or rupture caused by acute angulation of the erect penis during intercourse can be accompanied by a massive penile hematoma deep to Buck's fascia. Penile edema and distortion usually ensue, and, if Buck's fascia has been violated, extravasation of blood can extend into the perineum, down to the medial portions of the thighs, or onto the anterior abdominal wall. Usually, the urethra itself is intact, unless the initial injury was self-inflicted by inserting an object into the urethra. However, retrograde urethrography should be performed to insure urethral integrity. If a urethral defect is demonstrated, the principles of primary urinary diversion and observation should be employed, since these injuries are usually small tears with normal urethral margins. Rarely, urethral disruption and inability to pass a catheter may mandate exploration, according to Gross.[66] If the urethrogram is negative, an indwelling catheter is not necessary, unless edema or hematoma cause temporary urethral obstruction.

To control hemorrhage and prevent contracture deformities of the penis with healing, penetrating penile corporal injuries should be explored and debrided, and any corporal tears should be closed using a permanent suture. Exploration can be performed using a circumcision skin incision followed by telescoping the penile skin to the base of the penis. Alternatively, a longitudinal shaft incision can be made directly over a localized hematoma for drainage and visualization of corporal injury. Finally, penile exploration can be performed via an inguinoscrotal or infrapubic incision, as is recommended for venous ligation surgery for impotence. If there is a large defect in the corpora tunica accompanied by profuse hemorrhage, this area can be packed with iodoform gauze to provide adequate hemostasis. If there is a skin defect, the use of petroleum gauze or Xeroform dressing allows granulation and reepithelialization. Later, skin grafts can be used for coverage.[36]

Penile fractures should be suspected when a hematoma overlying a palpable corporal defect is observed with curvature away from the side of the fracture.[65] Retrograde urethrography should be performed if a urethral injury is remotely suspected; however, some centers routinely use urethrography, since it is not unusual for the fracture to involve the spongiosum.[67]

Certainly, many urologists have advocated that the penile hematoma resulting from intercourse angulation of the erect penis can be treated conservatively by local elevation and ice, although tunica fibrosis and subsequent Peyronie's disease or flail penis may result. Devine considers these sequelae unacceptable, and he recommends immediate exploration, with evacuation of hematoma and repair of the torn tunica with 4–0 or 5–0 nylon sutures (eg, Prolene)[68]; however, nonabsorbable sutures are less likely to cause patient discomfort and are recommended by Bertini and Corriere.[65]

Penile amputations, although usually self-inflicted, can also occur after machinery crush injuries. Hemostasis, debridement, and cystotomy diversion are the principles of primary management. These can later be followed by partial penectomy after the injury has demarcated. Primary penile anastomosis using microsurgical technique has been reported.[65,67]

Penile degloving injuries are managed by immediate local care and later grafting.[69] Initially, biologic or petroleum dressings can be used, and at a later date, split-thickness skin grafts can be applied to cover the penile shaft. If the scrotum is preserved, the surgeon may elect to bury the penis in the scrotum, using the Allen-Spence technique of urethroplasty. The second stage releases a penis covered with scrotal skin.

## Scrotum

Scrotal injuries, in the absence of associated testicular injury, can be handled by local care, debridement, and closure. Scrotal ultrasound may be helpful in distinguishing between an isolated scrotal contusion/hematoma and testicular injury. The rugated skin and good blood supply make rapid healing the rule. If the majority of the scrotal skin is avulsed, or debrided secondary to necrosis from Fournier's gangrene, the testes can be covered with a biologic dressing while reepithelialization occurs. Regrowth of scrotal skin across a granulating surface is slow, but effective, and skin grafting is rarely necessary.

## Testes

Testicular injuries, both blunt and penetrating, are relatively rare, occurring usually with straddle injuries, kicks and blows to the groin, or bites. Many occur during sports activities. In such injury, the testis is entrapped or impinged against the pubic symphysis or thigh, and rupture may occur (Fig 20). The resulting scrotal mass usually enlarges rapidly and becomes quite tender, making examination other than inspection difficult. Rarely, the testes may be displaced from the scrotum into the inguinal canal.[70,71]

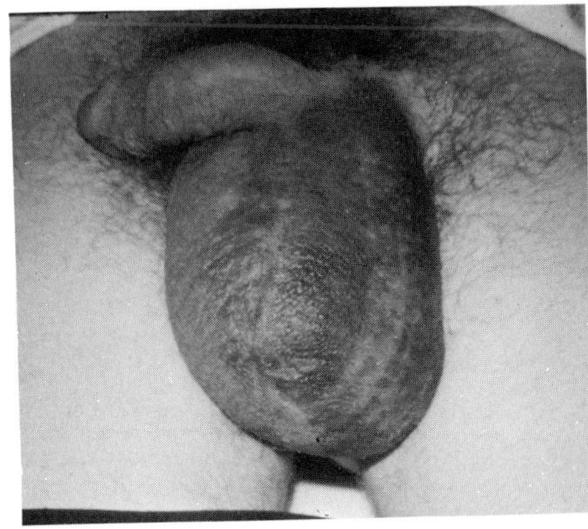

**Fig 20.** Left scrotal hematoma after automobile impact to pedestrian's right hip.

Traumatic intrascrotal lesions must be differentiated from underlying epididymitis or tumor that has been traumatized because of the testis size or prominence. This usually can be done by careful history taking, urinalysis, and sonography.

The treatment objective here is preservation of hormonal function and spermatogenesis, while minimizing the often prolonged convalescent period. Although conservative management of nonpenetrating testicular trauma has often been advocated, this frequently leads to delayed diagnosis of testis rupture, pressure atrophy of the testis secondary to hematocele, and subsequent decreased testicular function.

Ultrasonography of the scrotum and its contents can detect testicular rupture and distinguish it from traumatic hydrocele, and epididymal or cremasteric hematoma. Fractures are nearly always associated with hematoceles, and extravasated seminiferous tubules may also be visualized.[67] Therefore, ultrasonography can also identify the rare rupture unaccompanied by a traumatic hematocele.[72,73]

Testicular salvage rates vary, depending on delay before exploration. In 15 cases of testicular rupture secondary to blunt scrotal trauma in Texas, orchiectomy was performed in 80% of the cases.[74] Yet, while exploring all cases of blunt testicular trauma, Cass reported an incidence of rupture of 48%, and early exploration resulted in an orchiectomy rate of only 8% and was associated with decreased hospital stay, disability, and convalescence.[75]

An expanding scrotal mass, a tense hydrocele, or a suspected testis rupture should be explored immediately to preserve function and prevent prolonged convalescence.[76,77] The hematocele should be drained, and the tunica albuginea closed over the remaining testicular tissue. If the defect in the tunica is large, a piece of tunica vaginalis can be used as a graft.

## REFERENCES

1. Pokorny M, Pontes JE, Pierce JM. Urologic injuries associated with pelvic trauma. *J Urol.* 1979;121:455.
2. Pontes JE. Urologic injuries. *Surg Clin North Am.* 1977;57:77.
3. Brosman S, Faye R. Diagnosis and management of bladder trauma. *J Urol.* 1973;13:687.
4. Redman JF, Siebert J, Arnold W. Urinary ascites in children owing to extravasation of urine from the bladder. *J Urol.* 1979;122:409.
5. Ertuk E, Sheinfeld J, DiMarco P, et al. Renal Trauma: evaluation by computerized tomography. *J Urol.* 1985;133:946.
6. Nicholaisen G, McAninch J, Marshall G, et al. Renal Trauma: reevaluation of indications for radiographic assessment. *J Urol.* 1985;133:183.
7. Kane NM, Francis IR, Ellis JH. The value of CT in the detection of bladder and posterior urethral injuries. *AJR.* 1989;153:1243.
8. Cass AS. The multiple injured patient with bladder trauma. *J Trauma.* 1984;24:731.
9. Palmer JK, Benson GS, Corriere JN Jr. Diagnosis and initial management of urologic injuries associated with 200 consecutive pelvic fractures. *J Urol.* 1983;130:712.
10. Cass AS. Diagnostic studies in bladder rupture: indications and techniques. *Urol Clin North Am.* 1989;16:267.
11. Corriere JN Jr, Sandler CM. Management of the ruptured bladder: seven years experience with 111 cases. *J Trauma.* 1986;26:830.
12. Cass A, Ireland G. Bladder trauma associated with pelvic fractures in severely injured patients. *J Trauma.* 1973;13:205.
13. Nowak A, Ziebriski J. Difficulties in bladder rupture diagnostics. *Eur Urol.* 1977;3:351.
14. Carroll PR, McAninch JW. Major bladder trauma: the accuracy of cystography. *J Urol.* 1983;130:887.
15. Blacklock N. Bladder trauma in the long distance runner: 10,000 meter hematuria. *Br J Urol.* 1977;49:129.
16. Turnbull A, Smart C, Jenkins J. Delayed rupture of the bladder. *Br J Urol.* 1978;50:162.
17. Corriere JN, Sandler CM. Mechanisms of injury, patterns of extravasation and management of extraperitoneal bladder rupture due to blunt trauma. *J Urol.* 1988;139:43.
18. Carroll PR, McAninch JW. Major bladder trauma: mechanisms of injury and a unified method of diagnosis and repair. *J Urol.* 1984;132:254.
19. Cass A, Johnson C, Khan A, et al. Nonoperative management of bladder rupture from external trauma. *Urology.* 1983;22:27.
20. Cass AS, Gleich P, Smith C. Simultaneous bladder and prostatomembranous urethral rupture from external trauma. *J Urol.* 1984;132:907.
21. Belis J, Recht K, Milam D. Simultaneous traumatic bladder perforation and disruption of the prostatomembranous urethra. *J Urol.* 1979; 122:412.
22. Merchant WC III, Gibbons MD, Gonzales ET Jr. Trauma to the bladder neck, trigone and vagina in children. *J Urol.* 1984;131:747.
23. Hamburg R, Sega T. Perforation of urinary bladder by laparoscope. *Am J Obstet Gynecol.* 1978;130:597.
24. Faricy P, Augspurger R, Kaufman J. Bladder injuries associated with cesarean section. *J Urol.* 1978;120:762.
25. Devine PC, Devine CJ. Posterior urethral injuries associated with pelvic fractures. *Urology.* 1982;20:467.
26. Fallon B, Wendt JC, Hawtrey CE. Urological injury and assessment in patients with fractured pelvis. *J Urol.* 1984;131:712.
27. Pierce JM. Disruptions of the anterior urethra. *Urol Clin North Am.* 1989;16:329.
28. Persky L. Childhood urethral trauma. *Urology.* 1978;11:608.
29. Mucha P Jr, Farnell MB. Analysis of pelvic fracture management. *J Trauma.* 1984;24:379.
30. Colapinto V, McCallum R. Injury to the male posterior urethra in fractured pelvis: a new classification. *J Urol.* 1977;118:575.
31. Mitchell JT. Trauma to the urinary tract. *N Engl J Med.* 1973;288:90.

32. Mitchell JT. Injuries to the urethra. *Br J Urol.* 1968;40:649.

33. Glass R, Flynn J, King J, Blandy J. Urethral injury and fractured pelvis. *Br J Urol.* 1978;50:578.

34. Pontes JE, Pierce JM. Anterior urethral injuries: four years of experience at the Detroit General Hospital. *J Urol.* 1978;120:563.

35. Dixon CM, McAninch JW. Minimizing consequences of urethral trauma. *Contemp Urol.* 1990;2:25.

36. Salvatierra O, Ridgon W, Norris D, et al. Vietnam experience with 252 urologic war injuries. *J Urol.* 1969;101:615.

37. Walther P, Parsons C, Schmidt J. Direct vision internal urethrotomy in the management of urethral stricture. *J Urol.* 1980;123:497.

38. Pierce JM. Management of dismemberment of prostatic membranous urethra and ensuing stricture disease. *J Urol.* 1972;107:259.

39. Fowler JW, Watson G, Smith MF, MacFarlane JR. Diagnosis and treatment of posterior urethral injury. *Br J Urol.* 1986;58:167.

40. Gelbard MK, Heyman AM, Weintraub P. A technique for immediate realignment and catheterization of the disrupted prostatomembranous urethra. *J Urol.* 1989;142:52.

41. Waterhouse K, Gross M. Trauma to the genitourinary tract: a 5-year experience with 251 cases. *J Urol.* 1969;101:241.

42. Moorehouse D, Velitsky P, MacKinnon K. Rupture of the posterior urethra. *J Urol.* 1972; 107:255.

43. Myers R, DeWeerd J. Incidence of stricture following primary realignment of the disrupted proximal urethra. *J Urol.* 1972;107:265.

44. Moorehouse D, MacKinnon J. Urologic injuries associated with pelvic fractures. *J Trauma.* 1969;9:479.

45. Cass AS, Godek CJ. Urethral injury due to external trauma. *Urology.* 1978;11:607.

46. Devine CJ, Jordan GH, Devine PC. Primary realignment of the disrupted prostatomembranous urethra. *Urol Clin North Am.* 1989;16:291.

47. DeWeerd JH. Immediate realignment of posterior urethral injury. *Urol Clin North Am.* 1977;4:75.

48. Turner-Warwick R. Complex traumatic posterior urethral stricture. *J Urol.* 1977;118:564.

49. Glassberg K, Tolete-Velcek F, Ashley R, Waterhouse K. Partial tear of prostato-membranous urethra in children. *Urology.* 1979;13:500.

50. Turner-Warwick R. Prevention of complications resulting from pelvic fracture urethral injuries and from their surgical management. *Urol Clin North Am.* 1989;16:335.

51. Waterhouse K, Laungani C. The surgical repair of membranous urethral strictures: experience with 105 consecutive cases. *J Urol.* 1980; 123:500.

52. Lieberman SF, Barry JM. Retreat from transpubic urethroplasty for obliterated membranous urethral strictures. *J Urol.* 1982;128:379.

53. Lee WJ, Greenbaum R, Susi R, et al. Percutaneous antegrade urethral catheterization of the traumatized urethra. *Radiology.* 1984;151:250.

54. Marshall FF. Endoscopic reconstruction of traumatic urethral transections. *Urol Clin North Am.* 1989;16:313.

55. Devine P, Wendelken J, Devine C. Free full thickness skin graft urethroplasty: current technique. *J Urol.* 1979;121:282.

56. McAninch JW. Pubectomy in repair of membranous urethral stricture. *Urol Clin North Am.* 1989;16:297.

57. Pierce JM. Posterior urethral stricture repair. *J Urol.* 1979;121:739.

58. Webster GD, Selli C. Management of traumatic posterior urethral stricture by one stage perineal repair. *Surg Gynecol Obstet.* 1983;156:620.

59. Waterhouse K, Abrams J, Gruber H, et al. The transpubic approach to the lower urinary tract. *J Urol.* 1973;109:486.

60. Khan A, Furlow A. Transpubic urethroplasty. *J Urol.* 1976;116:447.

61. Brock W, Kaplan G. Use of the transpubic approach for urethroplasty in children. *J Urol.* 1981;125:496.

62. Patil UB, Ackerman NB, Waterhouse K. The transpubic approach in the management of problems of the lower genitourinary and intestinal tracts. *Surg Gynecol Obstet.* 1982;155:97.

63. Olsson C, Krane R. The controversy of single versus multi-staged urethroplasty. *J Urol.* 1978;120:414.

64. Pierce JM. Urethroplasty. *J Urol.* 1981;125:508.

65. Bertini JE, Corriere JN. The etiology and management of genital injuries. *J Trauma.* 1988; 28:1278.

66. Gross M, Arnold T, Peters P. Fracture of the penis with associated laceration of the urethra. *J Urol.* 1977;117:725.

67. Jordan GH, Gilbert DA. Male genital trauma. *Clin Plast Surg.* 1988;15:431.

68. Devine CJ. Surgery of the penis and urethra. In: Harrison, Walsh P, Gittes R and Perlmutter A (eds.). *Campbell's Urology.* 4th ed. Philadelphia: WB Saunders; 1979:2405.

69. Grewal S, Dalal S, Singh S, et al. Traumatic degloving of penis. *Br J Urol.* 1982;54:296.

70. Edson M, Meck J. Bilateral testicular dislocation with unilateral rupture. *J Urol.* 1979;122:419.

71. Cos L, Rabinowitz R. Trauma-induced testicular torsion in children. *J Trauma.* 1982;22:244.

72. Anderson KA, McAninch JW, Jeffrey RB, et al. Ultrasonography for the diagnosis and staging of blunt scrotal trauma. *J Urol.* 1983;130:933.

73. Jeffrey RB, Laing FC, Hricak H, et al. Sonography of testicular trauma. *AJR.* 1983; 141:993.

74. McConnell JD, Peters PC, Lewis SE, et al. Testicular rupture in blunt scrotal trauma: review of 15 cases with recent application of testicular scanning. *J Urol.* 1982;128:309.

75. Cass AS. Testicular trauma. *J Urol.* 1983; 129:299.

76. Gross M. Rupture of the testicle: the importance of early surgical treatment. *J Urol.* 1969; 101:196.

77. Warden S, Schellhammer P. Bilateral testicular rupture: report of a case with an unusual presentation. *J Urol.* 1978;120:257.

# 23

# Treatment of Urethral Stricture Disease

*Gerald H. Jordan*

## URETHRAL ANATOMY

### Anatomic Divisions

To understand the treatment of urethral stricture disease, an appreciation of urethral anatomy is important. The urethra begins at its point of intersection with the bladder trigone. It is divided into a posterior and an anterior division in men. The posterior urethra is arbitrarily defined as that portion proximal to Müller's tubercle, which in the adult corresponds to the location of the verumontanum (Fig 1). These divisions are based on the embryologic anlage. The anterior urethra thus corresponds only to that portion of the urethra that in men begins as a flat strip and then undergoes a process of ventral fusion during fetal development. Using this definition, women have only the posterior portion of the urethra.

This anatomic anterior-posterior division of the urethra is not, however, cogent to influence surgical decision making. However, a division of the urethra into five components is useful in determining the surgical approach to lesions in the male urethra:

1. Prostatic urethra, or the portion of the urethra proximal to the verumontanum and surrounded by the prostatic glandular tissue
2. Membranous urethra, or the portion of the urethra that penetrates beneath the triangular ligament and is surrounded distally by the external urethral rhabdosphincter
3. Bulbous urethra, or the portion of the urethra that is invested by the corpus spongiosum and covered by the midline fusion of the ischiocavernosus musculature
4. Penile or pendulous urethra, or the portion invested by the corpus spongiosum but distal to the fused ischiocavernosus muscles
5. Fossa navicularis, or the portion of the urethra that is surrounded by the erectile tissue of the glans penis and terminates at the junction of the urethral epithelium with the glanular epithelium (Fig 2)

The female urethra is the equivalent only to the prostatic urethra.[1]

An important concept in urethral anatomy is that of the genitourinary diaphragm. The genitourinary diaphragm per se does not exist as a true anatomic entity. The prostate gland is fixed to the pubic symphysis by the puboprostatic ligaments, and the membranous urethra is therefore commonly depicted as that portion which penetrates the genitourinary diaphragm. However, the genitourinary diaphragm is actually only the plane between the de-

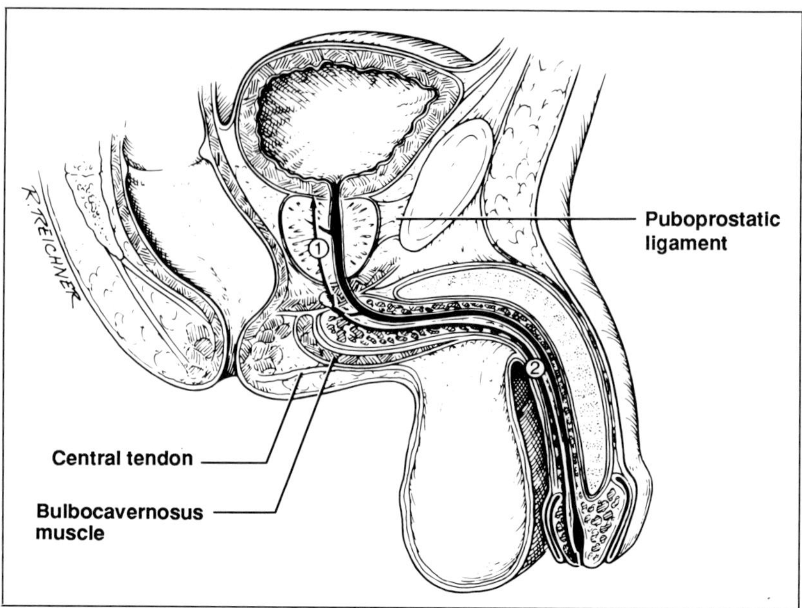


**Fig 1.** Cross-sectional diagram of the pelvis showing the anatomical divisions of the urethra. 1, posterior; 2, anterior. [From Jordan GH, Schellhammer PF. Urethral surgery and stricture disease. In: Droller MJ, ed. *Surgical Management of Urologic Disease: An Anatomic Approach* (St. Louis: Mosby; 1992: 815–832), with permission.]

**Fig 2.** Cross-sectional diagram of the pelvis showing the anatomic divisions of the urethra. 1, prostatic urethra; 2, membranous urethra; 3, bulbous urethra; 4, pendulous portion of the penile urethra; 5, fossa navicualris. (Permission as in Fig 1.)

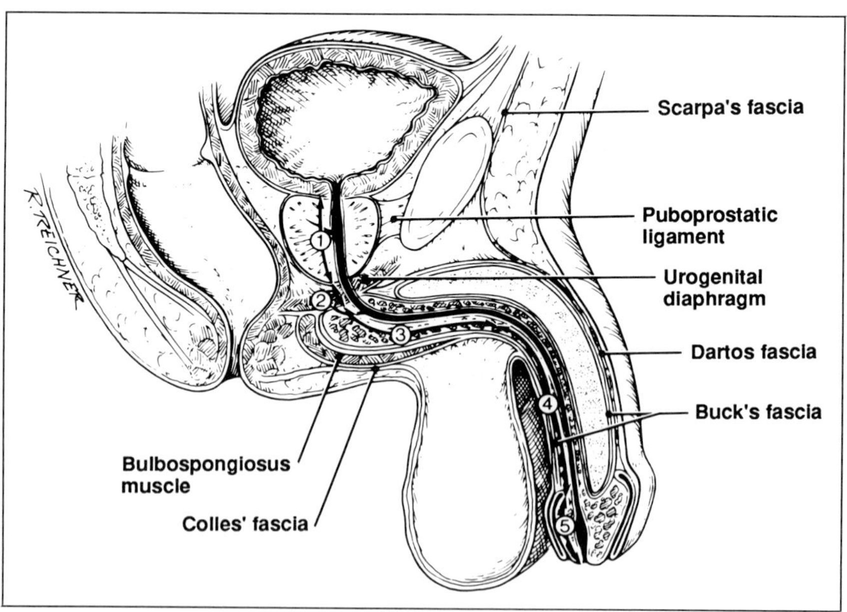

cussation of the corpora cavernosa, posterior to the triangular ligament anterior to the transverse perinei muscles. The membranous urethra is not bound in a true diaphragm. Indeed, the concept of a true diaphragm surrounding the urethra is probably derived from the observation made during bulbomembranous or membranoprostatic urethral reconstruction in trauma patients. The observed diaphragm is hence actually a scar.[2]

## Vasculature

The urethral vasculature is well defined. The deep structures of the male penis are, for the most part, totally dependent on branches of the internal pudendal arteries. The pudendal arteries are distal branches of the hypogastric arteries that then perforate to the perineum via Alcock's canal. The pudendal artery branches in the perineum to form the artery to the scrotum and then to continue as the common penile artery. The common penile artery branches to form the artery to the corpus spongiosum (artery of the bulb), the deep artery of the corpus cavernosum (the cavernosal artery), the circumflex arteries of the crus of the corpus cavernosum, and the dorsal arteries of the penis. Small vascular connections also exist in the "urethral groove," which link the corpora cavernosa with the corpus spongiosum (Fig 3).

In the female, the pudendal artery gives off several superficial branches to the perineum and then extends as the perineal artery. The artery then branches giving off the posterior labial artery (analogous to the scrotal artery). There is vasculature equiv-

**Fig 3.** The blood supply of the corporal bodies originates from the internal pudendal artery, which is a branch of the hypogastric artery. The internal pudendal artery branches into the dorsal artery of the penis and the cavernosal artery. Branches of these supply the external and internal portions of the cavernosal body. Additional branches of the internal pudendal artery form the lateral arteries of the urethra, which feed the penile portions of the urethra distal to the bulbar artery. An early branch of the pudendal artery is the bulbar artery, which supplies the bulbar part of the urethra. As the artery then passes over the dorsum of the corporal bodies, it gives rise to a number of circumflex and cavernosal arteries, which supply the various external and internal portions of the corporal bodies. The terminal portion of the dorsal artery supplies the spongy tissue component of the glans penis. (Permission as in Fig 1.)

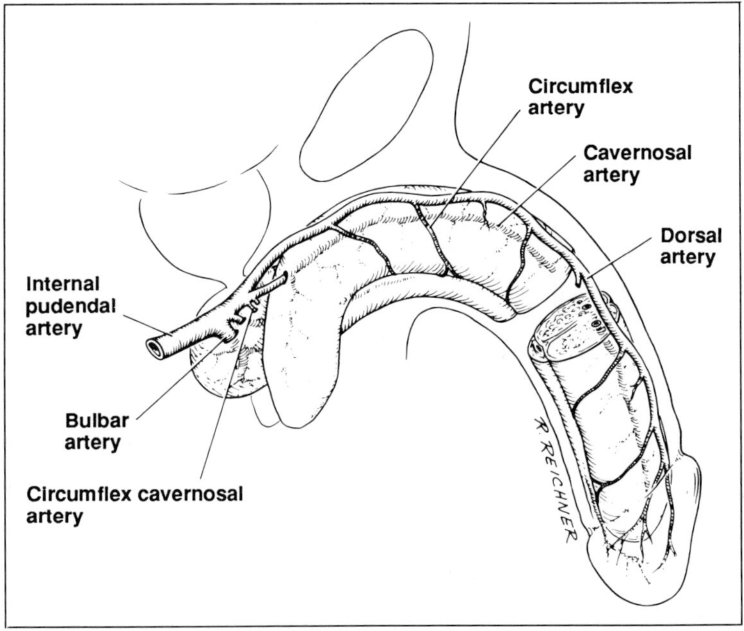

alent to the common penile vasculature that goes into the clitoris; however, from the standpoint of significance as related to surgery, there is none. There is a "urethral strip" that extends from the female urethral meatus to become contiguous with the glans clitoridis. This structure is analogous to the corpus spongiosum.

In the male, the venous drainage of the penis consists of the following:

1. The superficial dorsal venous system, exiting in the dartos layer and communicating with the femoral and superficial iliac arteries
2. The deep dorsal venous system passing over the dorsum of the penis within Buck's fascia and eventually piercing the "genitourinary diaphragm" to join the periprostatic plexus
3. The crural vessels, leaving the corpora cavernosa at the crus of the corpora and draining into the periprostatic plexus
4. The cavernosal venous system, leaving the corpora proximal to the crus and joining the dorsal vein of the penis and periprostatic plexus (Fig 4)

In about 60% of individuals, there is communication between the superficial veins and the deep dorsal vein of the penis. The clitoris has similar venous drainage. The female urethral venous and lymphatic drainage for the most part is identical to the venous drainage of the prostate.[3–5]

The genital skin has a dual blood supply in both males and females. The fasciocutaneous system is an extension of and represents the terminal arborization of the external pudendal artery, a medial branch of the femoral artery. In both males and females, the scrotum and labia majora have

**Fig 4.** Venous drainage of the penis and corporal bodies. Distally a plexus arising from the glans penis feeds into the deep dorsal vein, which runs the length of the corporal body. It takes into it venous drainage via the circumferential veins, and ultimately leads into the plexus of Santorini, which lies superolateral to the prostate. Crural veins and some of the medial cavernosal veins also feed into the plexus. The periurethral vein, running the length of the urethra on its lateral aspects, communicates with the circumferential veins and thereby also feeds into Santorini's plexus. The superficial dorsal vein of the penis drains the more superficial structures of the penis. Lateral cavernosal veins and some of the medial cavernosal veins drain the internal aspects of the corporal bodies and drain into the hypogastric plexuses and internal iliac veins. (Permission as in Fig 1.)

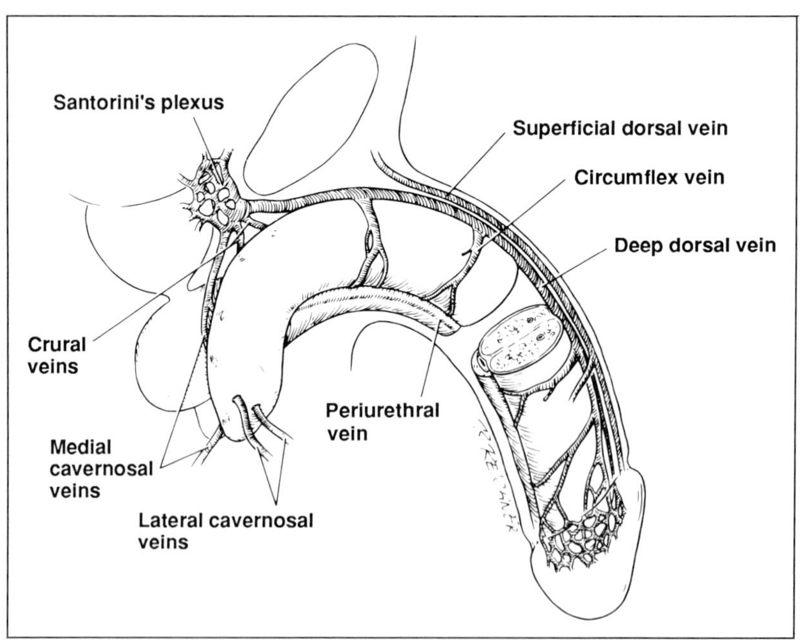

areas of the fasciocutaneous blood supply that are the distal ramifications of both the internal pudendal and external pudendal arterial systems. Additionally, in the genital skin, the subdermal plexus of vessels is extremely well defined and developed. This vasculature has been well documented in studies of the fasciocutaneous vascular supply of the genital skin. Practical studies during urethral reconstructive surgery show the genital skin to reliably survive on the basis of these vessels after skin islands have been elevated and transposed on the fasciocutaneous system. The skin that remains thus survives essentially on a random, but very predictable, blood supply.[6–8]

## CLASSIFICATION OF STRICTURES

A true urethral stricture is a scar, the natural result of tissue injury and/or destruction. Scars contract in all axes. Then when a scar is oriented as a circle, as is the case in the urethra, contracture decreases the circumference of that circle, compromising its lumen.[9,10]

A classification of anterior urethral stricture disease was proposed by Drs Charles and Patrick Devine in 1983 (Fig 5). According to this classification, urethral strictures are categorized by precise anatomic definitions—including length and location of the stricture, and an estimate of the depth and density of spongiofibrosis.[11] These measurements are made from the appearance of the stricture at urethroscopy, by using contrast studies, and by imaging via either B-scan ultrasound using high-megahertz transducers or high-megahertz real-time ultrasonography.[12]

In addition to the more common anterior urethral strictures, there are also less common posterior urethral strictures. The term *posterior urethral stricture* is used in reference to portions of the urethra proximal to the bulbous urethra. Strictly speaking, the only posterior urethral strictures are the rare strictures of the female urethra, prostatic urethra, bladder neck contractures, and the above-mentioned bulbomembranous/prostatomembranous strictures. Strictly speaking, membranous urethral strictures are a misnomer. These strictures inevitably follow urethral distraction injuries and should be referred to as urethral distraction defects. The stricture of the sphincter-active portion of the urethra, which usually occurs in patients following

**Fig 5.** Classification of urethral stricture disease according to the anatomy of the stricture. Classification as described by Devine. [From Jordan GH: Management of anterior urethral stricture disease. In: Webster GD, ed. *Problems in Urology.* Vol 1, No 2 (Philadelphia: JB Lippincott; 1987:199–225), with permission.]

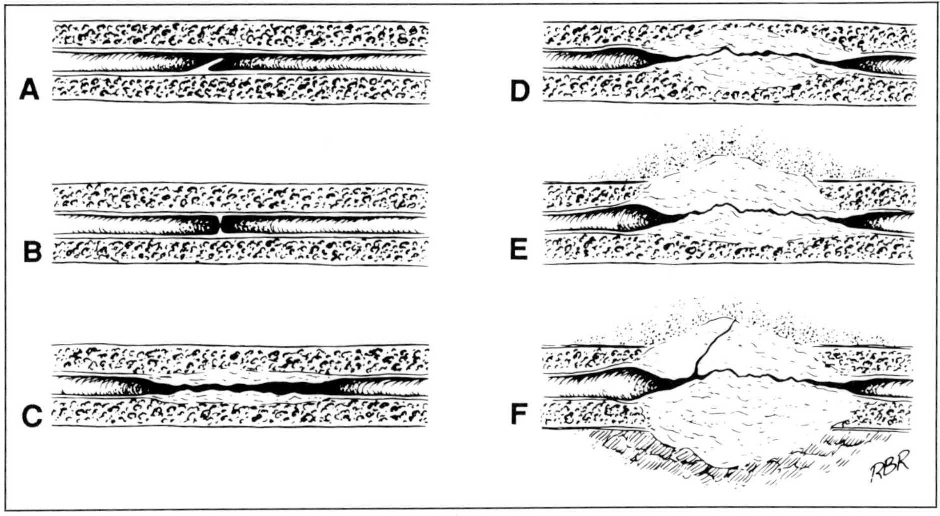

instrumentation and especially transurethral resection of the prostate (TURP), and because of the circumstances (ie, incompetence of the bladder neck sphincter), is a totally unique situation and will be addressed as such.

## APPROACH TO TREATMENT

### Reconstructive Ladder

One approach to the treatment of stricture disease is known as the reconstructive ladder. This approach is based on treatment beginning with the simplest procedure and progressing to the more complex procedures, as simple ones fail. Applying this concept to the treatment of urethral stricture disease, all strictures would be treated with dilation, followed by internal urethrotomy, and then full-thickness skin graft urethroplasty. This concept has become outdated, however, due to literature support of diminished success rates in urethroplasty after multiple dilations, as well as marked progress in modern tissue transfer techniques.[10]

### Anatomic Approach

A more recent protocol for the treatment of urethral stricture disease, known as the anatomic approach, matches a particular tissue transfer technique to the anatomy of the specific stricture disease determined at the time of diagnosis. Application of this protocol requires that the techniques of tissue transfer be individualized for each patient (Fig 6). The anatomic approach to treatment of urethral stricture disease has been proven to offer patients a statistically better chance of cure from a single one-stage procedure—achieving a 90% to 93% success rate.[10,13,14]

**Fig 6.** Flow chart of the approach to anterior urethral stricture disease as dictated by the anatomy (classification of stricture; Fig 5) of the stricture. FTSG = full-thickness skin graft. (Permission as in Fig 5.)

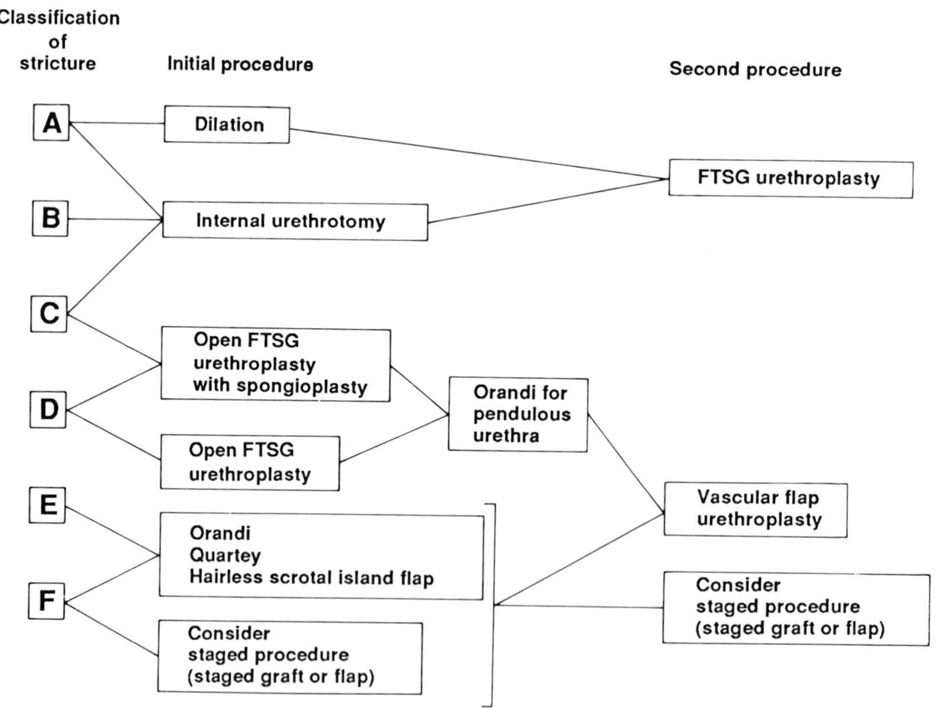

## DIAGNOSIS OF URETHRAL STRICTURE

### Symptoms

Most urethral stricture patients present with an insidious onset of voiding symptoms, prostatitis, and/or epididymitis. Some patients will present with urinary retention secondary to anterior urethral stricture disease. On close inquiry, however, many if not all of these patients have tolerated severe voiding symptoms for a significant time period prior to their presentation in retention. Evaluation of patients with these symptoms often leads to the diagnosis of urethral stricture.

### Anatomy of the Stricture

The precise anatomy of the urethral stricture must be determined prior to formulation of a treatment plan. The location and true length of the urethral stricture disease can be established only by evaluation with both voiding and retrograde urethrography. Although ultrasound study can precisely show the length of urethral stricture disease and perhaps give some illusion concerning "subclinical fibrosis," the exact location of the stricture is not as obvious on ultrasound as on urethrography.

The depth of spongiofibrosis in a stricture, used in classification and treatment plans, can be alluded to by ultrasound study. With experience, the appearance of a urethral stricture on urethroscopy can also give the surgeon insight regarding the depth and density of stricture fibrosis. In addition, palpatory examination of the corpus spongiosum through the penile skin, scrotum, or perineum gives much insight concerning the depth of spongiofibrosis.

### Imaging

Retrograde urethrography should always be performed with the instillation of contrast suitable for intravenous administration. In many patients, if retrograde urethrography is performed prior to having the patient void, sufficient contrast can be refluxed proximally through the sphincter mechanism to sufficiently opacify the bladder urine. One can then have the patient void and obtain a voiding urethrogram without the need for catheterization to instill the contrast.

### Preparation for Surgery

Should one be contemplating reconstruction in the immediate time frame, great care must be taken to not dilate the stricture during urethroscopy. It is imperative that the stricture be stable, and "at its worst" at the time of open reconstruction. Should instrumentation of a stricture be required, then reconstruction should be delayed for a period of 3 to 4 months, to allow the scarring process to stabilize and the stricture to maximally contract.

The vast majority of strictures that are currently encountered are the result of trauma. Inflammatory strictures, particularly those associated with gonococcal urethritis, are fortunately not seen with any marked frequency. There is a category of inflammatory stricture disease, however, that is seen quite frequently and that is the stricture associated with balanitis xerotica obliterans.

The author's experience has shown the stricture disease of balanitis xerotica obliterans to be the result of high-pressure voiding. Many patients, if not all, present with isolated urethral meatal stenosis. They void through a normal urethra to encounter severe obstruction at the distalmost aspect of the urethra. In time, this causes dilation of the glands of Littre with intravasation of urine into those glands (Fig 7). It appears in many patients that either subclinical infection then develops in those dilated glands of Littre or sufficient inflammation develops in the glands to cause deep spongiofibrosis. The stricture disease associated with balanitis xerotica obliterans tends to be associated with deep if not panspongiosal spongiofibrosis. There is some evidence to suggest that early reconstruction of the meatal stenosis associated with early balanitis xerotica obliterans may arrest and prevent the consequences of panurethral

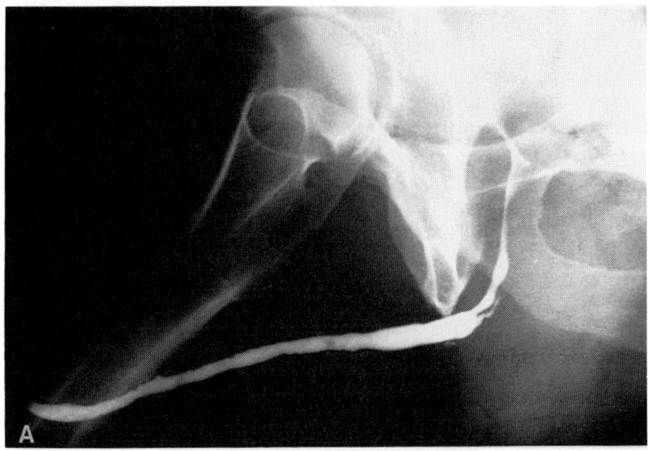


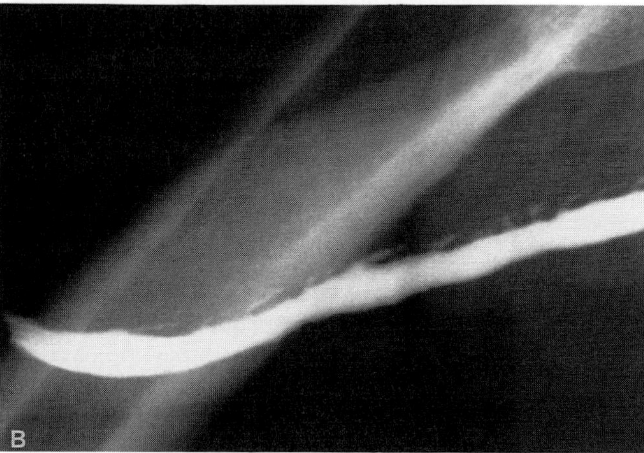


**Fig 7. A,** retrograde urethrogram in a patient with the changes of balanitis xerotica obliterans on the glans and panurethral stricture disease. It should be noted that this patient has had essentially no prior urethral instrumentation; **B,** close-up of the midportion of the retrograde urethrogram showing the dilated glans of Littre with extravasation of contrast into the dilated glans.

stricture disease that is frequently associated with balanitis xerotica obliterans.[15]

A patient suspected of urethral injury due to trauma must undergo immediate evaluation. Many of these patients will present with blood at the meatus. In others, however, the injury must be suspected to be found. Posterior urethral stricture injuries, which go unrecognized following pelvic trauma, can evolve to serious complications with difficult-to-manage consequences. There is a misconception that diversion "prevents" the development of urethral stricture following posterior urethral trauma. Clearly, the development of a stricture associated with posterior urethral trauma is determined at the time of impact. Diversion serves to limit the sequela.

In some centers, there is enthusiasm for placement of an aligning urethral catheter following posterior urethral trauma. In the author's experience, this practice is worthwhile and in many patients, while not completely preventing the development of stricture, it leads to the development of a stricture that often is managed by very conservative techniques. In the vast majority of adults, posterior urethral trauma leads to urethral distraction defects confined to the urethra below the prostate but proximal to the departure of the urethra from the bulbospongiosum. Classically, the injury occurs at the juncture of the membranous urethra and the bulbous urethra, where the bulbous urethra departs the bulbospongiosum. However, the injury can also occur at the juncture of the membranous urethra with the apical prostatic urethra or at any point midway on the membranous urethra. In children, however, because the prepubescent prostate does not protect the child's posterior urethra to the same extent as in adults, disruption of the urethra can extend to the prostatic urethra and can lead to extension of the stricture process proximally.

In patients suspected of anterior urethral stricture disease, retrograde urethrogram will define the watertight integrity or lack thereof of the urethra. Again, contrast suitable for intravenous administration should be utilized for these studies. Immediate management then can be accomplished via diverting urethral catheter or suprapubic catheter.

The posterior urethra is more difficult to visualize than the anterior urethra. Because of the association of pelvic fracture with intra-abdominal injury, any patient suspected of urethral injury should undergo some form of excretory imaging of the kidneys. The bladder is often visualized on this study. It should be kept in mind, however, that the cystogram phase of an intravenous pyelogram (IVP) is not sufficient to totally rule out bladder injury. A CT scan seems to be more sensitive to the detection of bladder injury, but again does not totally define the watertight competence of the bladder. The diagnosis of the posterior distraction injury itself is then made with retrograde urethrography. With a posterior urethral distraction injury, a large pelvic hematoma often displaces the bladder and prostate cephalad into the pelvis, giving it the "pie-in-the-sky" radiographic appearance. In that contrast is hyperosmolar, in suspected trauma, retrograde urethrography should be accomplished with small volumes of contrast and, if possible, under fluoroscopic control. This limits the extravasation of the hyperosmolar contrast material and also avoids the total obscuration of the pelvis with contrast should other studies need to be done in the immediate trauma course. Suitable diversion can then be accomplished. The author does not favor the use of percutaneous techniques for catheter placement in the case of pelvic trauma associated with bladder and/or urethral injury.

## TREATMENT MODALITIES

### Dilation

Medical reports indicate that the Egyptian and Hindu medical practitioners used dilation as early as the 6th century BC as a treatment for what we now know to be urethral stricture disease.[16] Dilation as a management modality persists. Dilation is seldom curative. However, for strictures that represent superficial scars or folds in the mucosa, dilation can be a curative modality.

In current times, it is not uncommon for dilation to be accomplished by the urologist placing as many sounds as may be fit through the stricture without having to "push too hard." In many cases dilation is forced until there is bleeding. It should be recognized that if bleeding is caused by dilation, then there has been tissue disruption. Tearing of the strictured area leads to further scarring and increase in the length and density of the stricture. For dilation to be effective, it must be a gradual process of stretching, carried out in a manner that will not lead to further trauma to the urethra.

If at first treatment the urethra will not accept an 18 French sound for initial dilation, a guidewire with followers should be used. The tips of the smaller Van Buren sounds are sharp and easily penetrate the urethra causing false passage. With the development of the guidewire system with followers, filiforms with followers are used less and less. With the ready availability of flexible endoscopes now, guidewires can be passed under direct vision through the "true" lumen of the stricture. The followers are then advanced over the guidewire.

Filiforms may be straight, or have a Coude or spiral tip. The latter instruments are easier to pass, especially when the urethra has been filled with lubricating jelly. If the stricture is short and soft, a small follower should pass easily. Larger followers can then be passed in sequence until one meets mild resistance. At this point, a catheter can be placed if indicated. Sequential dilation is then done via soft dilation in which the catheter is changed at 2- to 3-day intervals and sequentially enlarged until an adequate lumen is reestablished. Optionally, patients can be returned to the office and sequentially dilated with sounds at 2- to 3-day intervals. The dilation should be advanced 2–4 French at a setting until the desired lumen is achieved. In most patients an interval of redilation will be established and in the rare patient cured by dilation, eventually the need for subsequent dilation will define itself as nonexistent. Optionally, patients can be placed on home self-dilation protocols using dilators, catheters, sounds, or balloon dilators.

If dilation is accomplished gently as described above, the chances of successful management will be increased, both from the standpoint of successful scar management and from the standpoint of patient compliance. The patient will be more likely to return for further treatments if the experience has not been painful. If the density of stricture makes it impossible to pass dilating instruments, a suprapubic tube is inserted and further treatment planned. In some patients, with suprapubic diversion there will be remarkable improvement in the stricture probably because of diminishment of the inflammatory response attendant to all strictures. Many strictures that are "impassable" after several days to weeks of diversion are easily dilated or managed with internal urethrotomy.[10]

## Internal Urethrotomy

A second procedure that is used for patients not considered to be candidates for open reconstruction is internal urethrotomy. The principle of internal urethrotomy is that of an incision causing disruption of the urethral stricture and allowing the underlying soft elastic tissue to expand the urethra. For internal urethrotomy to be effective, the incision must extend through the depth of the spongiofibrosis. With diversion and stenting during the period of urethral regeneration, the diameter of the urethra is increased.

Studies have shown that in some cases all elements of the urethra can regenerate. However, it takes 4 to 6 weeks for 50% of the circumference of the urethra to regenerate, implying that catheterization would be required for this length of time for internal urethrotomy to be successful. In fact, studies have shown that internal urethrotomy can be effective with shorter lengths of catheterization, suggesting either that urethral regeneration proceeds at a faster rate than the laboratory studies indicate, or that diversion and stenting are not required for the entire time required for complete urethral regeneration. A third explanation for these reports of effective results from internal urethrotomy with short-length posturethrotomy diversion is that internal urethrotomy is most effective in strictures with only superficial spongiofibrosis. Hence, the defect to be reepithelialized is smaller. To effectively widen the lumen of the urethra in strictures of this type, there is a relatively small gap for regeneration to span after incision. In applying the protocol outlined under the anatomic approach section of this chapter, internal urethrotomy has been shown to be most successful when used in patients with superficial stricture such as mucosal fold configurations or strictures of an iris configuration (Devine classification types A and B). The author has found that the length of catheterization and diversion necessary for a successful procedure is 5 to 7 days in these types of cases.

Internal urethrotomy can be accomplished blindly with instruments such as the Otis urethrotome. In general, however, visual internal urethrotomy has supplanted blind internal urethrotomy. Urethrotomy is accomplished with a sharp "cold" urethrotome used as a unit instrument, with the blade extended through the area of stricture, and the entire instrument then rocked as the stricture band is incised. The incision, as already mentioned, must be carried through the entire depth of spongiofibrosis. Effective internal urethrotomy usually does not result in inordinate bleeding; however, if a small artery is divided, delicate Bugby electrode catheterization can be used.

Although the urethra is often presumed to run down the center of the corpus spongiosum, it actually is eccentrically placed toward the dorsal aspect of the corpus spongiosum. It departs the bulb of the corpus spongiosum well prior to the attachment of the bulbospongiosum to the perineal body.

It is customary practice to perform internal urethrotomy at the "12 o'clock" position. In the area of the bulbous urethra, there is little of the spongy erectile tissue between the urethral lumen and the triangular ligament or the tunica albuginea of the corpora cavernosa. The author prefers two incisions at the 10 and 2 o'clock positions or three incisions with the third cut at 6 o'clock. Care must be taken with the cuts at the 10 and 2 o'clock positions as deep cuts through the spongy erectile tissue of the corpora cavernosa can possibly precipitate focal veno-occlusive dysfunction. In the area of the pendulous urethra, even further caution must be exercised. Even incisions at 12 o'clock can, if extended deeply, enter the cavernosal interior with focal veno-occlusive phenomena as the result. The literature supports an increased incidence of erectile dysfunction occurring after internal urethrotomies for strictures of the pendulous urethra.

If the first attempt at internal urethrotomy does not succeed, one should critically reassess the situation. If x-rays and cystoscopy show improvement, the process may be repeated. However, two or three times should be the limit, and continued improvement should be noted after each procedure. When the epithelium and spongy tissue of the urethra have been severely damaged by the disease or trauma that caused the stricture or as a result of treatment, they will not regenerate to bridge the defect, and an open surgical procedure will be necessary.

In all situations of internal urethrotomy, the surgeon fights a race between wound contracture, an integral part of healing by secondary intention, and reepithelialization. If reepithelialization wins while the lumen is still adequate, then a successful result is achieved. If, however, wound contracture proceeds to the point that the lumen is again constricted, then failure is the result. Strictures at the level of the suspensory ligament of the penis that occur after urethral instrumentation (eg, TURP, or complication of an indwelling catheter) often involve the full thickness of the corpus spongiosum and usually do not respond to internal urethrotomy. Such a stricture is usually short. A single attempt at management with internal urethrotomy is warranted. However, these strictures are readily managed via excision of the stricture with primary anastomosis.[10]

## Internal Urethrotomy with Dilation

Because of the aforementioned race between contracture and epithelialization, contracture can often be delayed by a combination of internal urethrotomy followed by home dilation. This modality is especially effective for select patients who are not thought to be candidates for open reconstruction but who are not optimally suitable for curative internal urethrotomy either. In these cases, internal urethrotomy can be performed such that the urethra accepts an 18 to 20 French catheter following internal urethrotomy. The catheter is left in place to allow for onset of healing of the urethra. The length of this catheterization is subject to some controversy; however, the author usually prefers leaving catheters in place in these cases for 10 to 14 days, and in rare cases for up to 21 days. The catheter should be a soft silicone silastic catheter. When it is removed, the patient is provided with a 20 to 22 French red Robinson catheter and instructed to pass the catheter through the area of stricture three times daily. After a period of 2 to 3 months, the interval is tapered such that many patients only require self-obturation once or twice a week. In these patients, however, if self-obturation is discontinued, with assurity the stricture will eventually recur and require another definitive procedure.[17]

### Dilation and/or Internal Urethrotomy with Implantable Urethral Stent

Another option now currently available to help with the fight between wound contracture and epithelialization is the implantable urethral stent.[18] The stent has been widely used in Europe with mixed reviews. Clinical trials are currently underway in the United States and Canada. In Europe, the most commonly employed implantable urethral stent is the Wallstent/UroLume device (American Medical Systems, Minnetonka, Minnesota). This device is a stainless steel alloy that is totally noncorrosive and was originally designed for use intravascularly. Prior to implantation, the urethra is dilated to 28 to 30 French. Dilation can be done acutely or can be done via soft techniques during a period of a week to 10 days prior to implantation. The implantation is then accomplished under direct vision using a specially designed implantation instrument. Protocols in this country for anterior urethral stricture disease limit the use of the stent to the bulbous urethra and require a short segment of normal urethra distal to the external sphincter. The stent cannot extend beyond the penoscrotal junction. Bulbous strictures of approximately 5 cm in length are considered appropriate for entry into the study protocols.

The stents exert gentle pressure, keeping the lumen of the urethra expanded, ostensibly resisting the forces of wound contracture. The stent then becomes totally incorporated into the wall of the urethra and is reepithelialized. Experience has shown poor results in the use of the stent with strictures associated with very deep spongiofibrosis or full-thickness spongiofibrosis. This thus limits, if not contraindicates, the use of the implantable stents for posterior urethral distraction defects. Likewise, strictures that have been previously managed with multiple internal urethrotomies, laser, multiple dilation, etc., often are associated with very deep scarring. In these cases, the scar grows through the latticework of the stent. The scar can be resected, and the interval of resection of the scar is often much less than the previously required intervals of dilation or internal urethrotomy. The stent therefore may find a place as a management modality in some patients.

The author feels that the implantable stents will clearly find a place in the management of urethral stricture disease; however, they do not represent a panacea. They will never replace open urethral reconstruction.[17]

In Israel, a different concept of implantable urethral stent is employed. These stents are tightly coiled, thus limiting, if not preventing, the ingrowth of tissue into the stent latticework. These stents are designed to be removed; they are left in place until the stricture process/scar process has stabilized following internal urethrotomy. Epithelialization occurs around the stent. When the stricture is stable, then the stent is removed. These stents exist in a number of configurations and have been used for prostatic urethral stenotic processes as well as posterior urethral stricture disease.[19]

### Tissue Transfer Techniques

In 1914, Hamilton Russell described a technique that represented the first of the modern approaches to urethral reconstruction.[20] In this procedure, a stricture (scar) was excised, one wall of the remaining normal urethra was then reapproximated, and the remaining wall was left to heal by secondary intent. His approach was limited by lack of knowledge in two areas. First, it was not appreciated that the urethral vascularity (vasculature of the corpus spongiosum) was based on both proximal vessels (artery to the bulb and circumflex cavernosal arteries) and distal vessels (the dorsal arteries of the penis as they arborize in the glans and distal spongiosum). In many cases, Hamilton Russell might have been able to perform primary circumferential anastomosis. Second, concepts of tissue transfer were still in their infancy. Thus, in those cases in which a larger urethrotomy defect existed, failure by Hamilton Russell's technique is now a success by the inlay of transfer tissue into the urethrotomy defect. These techniques are grouped under the name of *substitution ure-*

*thral reconstruction*. As the name implies, a substance other than urethra is substituted into the urethrotomy defect, thus expanding the lumen of the urethra. These procedures will be covered in detail later in this chapter.

## GENERAL PRINCIPLES OF URETHRAL SURGERY

### Positioning and Incisions

Today's anatomic approach to the treatment of urethral stricture disease deals with open stricture excision and reconstruction of the urethra. Surgical access to the urethra can be gained via a number of approaches. The pendulous portion of the penile urethra can be reached via a circumcising degloving incision or via ventral longitudinal incisions. A common technique used to reconstruct distal anterior urethral strictures involves the use of penile or preputial fascial flaps to support a skin island. In these situations, placement of the incision is determined by the location of the planned flap. The subscrotal penile urethra can either be reached through a ventral penile or perineal incision, or directly by incising the scrotal raphe and intrahemiscrotal septum. The bulbous, membranous, and apical prostatic portions of the urethra are easily approached via a perineal incision in most patients. In the perineum, the author prefers an incision that is lambda in shape. However, a number of authors prefer a straight midline perineal incision (Fig 8).

Perineal surgery requires that the patient be placed in exaggerated lithotomy position. The exaggerated lithotomy position is associated with some morbidity. However, a recent review by the author of over 200 cases placed in exaggerated lithotomy position shows the morbidity associated with

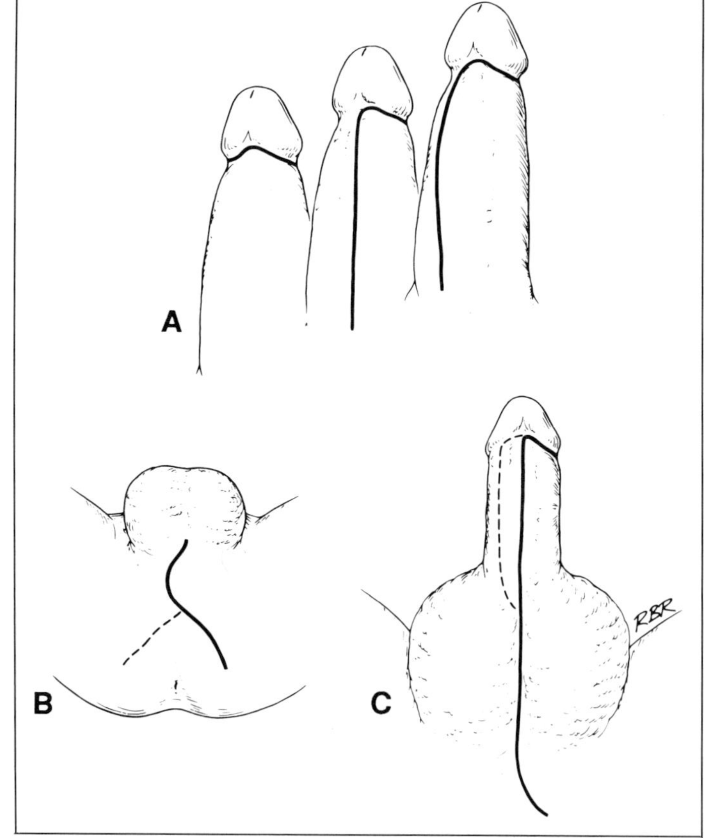


**Fig 8.** Incisions useful for access in urethral surgery. **A,** incisions useful for penile or pendulous urethral surgery; **B,** incision preferred for the perineal approach to the urethra; **C,** incision useful for panurethral reconstruction. [From Jordan GH. Management of anterior urethral stricture disease. In: Webster G, ed. *Problems in Urology* (Philadelphia: JB Lippincott; 1987:200), with permission.]

positioning to be minimal and more than acceptable. A number of key steps are necessary, however, to avoid complications of positioning. It is imperative that the feet and legs be well secured and suspended with the patient in position. The new boot-style stirrups work well. Great care must be taken, however, to avoid pressure on the posterior calves or the area of the anterior peroneal nerve. Additionally, it is imperative that the patient be placed in lithotomy by the elevation of the hips as opposed to "cranking" the patient into position by rotating the stirrups. The stirrups serve to suspend the legs only, the exaggerated lithotomy position being achieved by elevation of the buttocks. A number of tables are now available with elevating buttocks plates for placing the patient in exaggerated lithotomy. Likewise prior to shave-prepping the patient, it is imperative that the areas of nonhirsute skin be accurately identified and marked. This should be accomplished even in cases in which excision of the stricture with primary anastomosis is contemplated. It is not uncommon, after opening the urethra, to encounter subclinical fibrosis that would preclude the use of an excisional procedure and require the use of a substitution-type procedure. With the patient properly prepared and in the exaggerated lithotomy position, the perineal incision can be marked. The lambda incision is oriented with its apex in the midline of the scrotum and the tips of the posterior limbs extending just medial to the ischial tuberosities. It is essential to place the incisions medial to the ischial tuberosities. Placing the incisions over the ischial tuberosities creates a great deal of sitting pain for the patient in the postoperative course. Opening the skin reveals the Colles fascia (Fig 9). As the fascia is opened, the aponeurosis of the ischiocavernosus muscles (bulbospongiosus muscles) is seen in the midline. Dissecting distally reveals the edge of the muscles with the uninvested corpus spongiosum located beneath the scrotum. With a combination of sharp and blunt dissection, the muscles can be freed from the corpus spongiosum and divided in the midline (Fig 10). Dissection is carried back to the insertion of the muscles intto the perineal body, which

**Fig 9.** Dissection of the bulbous urethra. Central tendon is divided, revealing the midline fusion of the ischiocavernosus muscles with the "bare" corpus spongiosum visible beneath the scrotum.

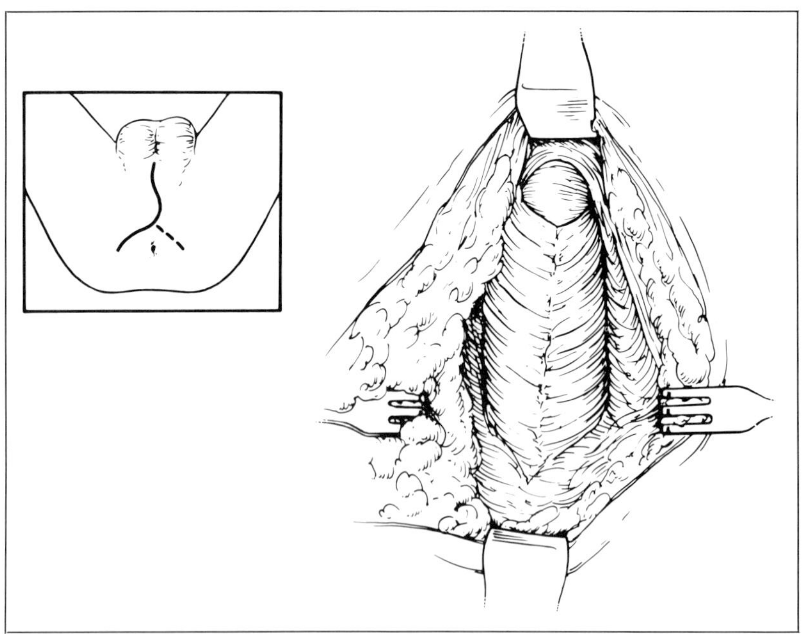

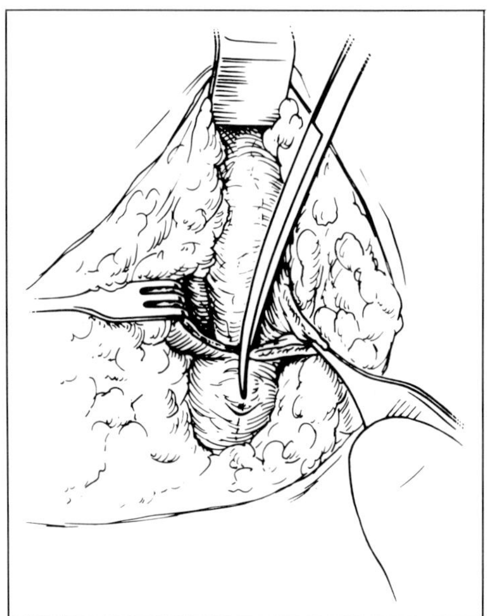

**Fig 10.** The ischiocavernosus musculature is divided in the midline and detached from the corpus spongiosum and bulbospongiosum.

allows exposure of the entire length of the bulbospongiosum. The bulbospongiosus muscles are relatively loosely attached to the bulbospongiosum, and the bulb is easily freed by a combination of sharp and dull dissection. It is not necessary in all cases to completely dissect the muscle from the bulbospongiosum, nor is it necessary to detach the muscles from both sides of the bulbospongiosum.

The urethra, as already mentioned, lies eccentrically placed in the corpus spongiosum. The urethra tends to be closer to the cavernosal aspect of the corpus spongiosum. Hence, mobilizing the urethra on the lateral aspect limits bleeding from the corpus spongiosum as well as improving the exposure of the urethra and urethrotomy defect. In some cases, a dorsal urethrotomy is preferred.

## Mobilization of the Corpus Spongiosum

The corpus spongiosum can be dissected completely free from its attachments to the muscles, triangular ligament, and perineal body, but except for excision of stricture with primary reanastomosis, urethroplasty in the bulb rarely requires such complete mobilization (Fig 11).

It is of essential importance that the vascular supply to the urethral tissues not be interrupted as a result of the surgical procedure. The dual blood supply to the male corpus spongiosum and, hence, the urethra proximally enters the corpus spongiosum via the arteries to the bulb and the circumflex cavernosal arteries. The vasculature of the distal anterior urethra is provided by the dorsal arteries of the penis via the communicators to the glans penis. In most cases, the male urethra can be expected to survive mobilization on either end as a result of this dual vascularity.

If the artery to the bulb is interrupted, the corpus spongiosum can serve as a vascular channel between the dorsal arteries of the penis and the proximal portion of the anterior urethra. However, if there is coexisting anterior urethral stricture disease, the proximal portion of the anterior

**Fig 11.** Corpus spongiosum is dissected from the adjacent muscular attachments and detached from the corpora cavernosa.

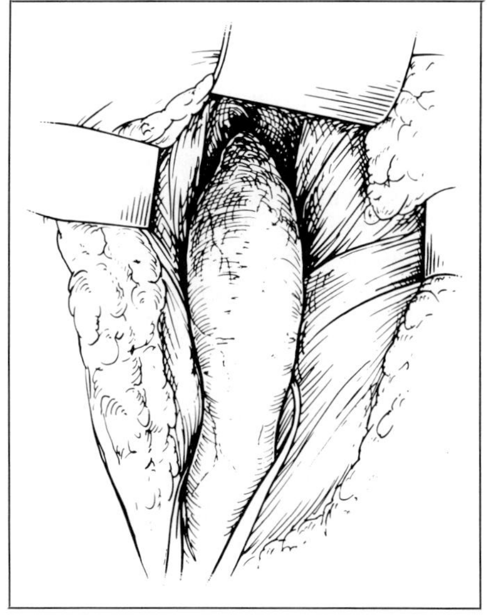

urethra may not reliably survive when widely mobilized in that the spongiofibrosis in the corpus spongiosum associated with concomitant urethral stricture disease may not provide sufficient vascularity to the proximally mobilized urethral segment. Likewise, if the distal corpus spongiosum is detached from the glans penis, the converse will be true. In this case, the coexisting anterior urethral stricture disease would prevent the vascularity provided by the artery to the bulb from reaching the distal mobilized corpus spongiosum and distal anterior urethra.[1]

Caution is warranted in the case of the patient with a history of hypospadias and reconstruction with proximal urethral stricture disease. During the excision of chordee, the bifid corpus spongiosum is often detached from the glans penis. When the patient exhibits proximal urethral stricture disease later, one must be careful in mobilizing the proximal anterior urethra.

Severe pelvic trauma can also compromise urethral mobilization. Since all of the distal urethral blood supply represents the branches of the pudendal arteries, disruption of those arteries makes mobilization of the corpus spongiosum risky. In general, the pudendal arteries are not disrupted; however, the proximal common penile arteries just distal to Alcock's canal or the dorsal arteries of the penis can be disrupted by trauma. If such a patient then has proximal urethral stricture disease possibly associated with pelvic fracture, it may not be possible to mobilize the anterior urethra reliably without risking ischemic damage to the mobilized segment. In fact, most series from centers performing large numbers of posterior urethral reconstructions would support the fact that failures arise not from technical problems with the anastomosis but rather from ischemic problems of the mobilized anterior urethra. Additionally, in the case of severe pelvic trauma, it is not unusual to encounter the patient who has had surgical ligation of the hypogastric arteries or embolization of the hypogastric or pudendals in the acute trauma phase. Arteriography is indicated in all cases in which there is evidence of interruption of the pudendal or dorsal vasculature of the penis. Additionally, patients presenting with numbness of the glans penis after trauma or after failed urethral reconstruction must be suspected as these findings may indicate concomitant vascular injury due to the close proximity of the common penile vessels to the nerves of the glans penis. Should these studies demonstrate bilateral pudendal or dorsal common penile arterial damage, it is advisable to resort to a method of urethral reconstruction that involves tissue transfer as opposed to one that depends on excision of the stricture with wide mobilization and primary anastomosis. Alternatively, in posterior urethral stricture disease, some of the offshoots of the "cut-for-light" procedure or endoscopic realignment procedures could serve as an option.[21,22]

## Diversion

After excision of stricture with primary anastomosis or after reconstruction via tissue transfer, the repair is stented and diversion is maintained until the urethra has healed sufficiently to be watertight. The author prefers the use of stenting catheters with suprapubic diversion. Thin-walled silicone catheters are used for stenting of repairs with standard latex or silicone Foley catheters used instead for suprapubic diversion. In proximal repairs, the Foley catheter is passed through the area of reconstruction into the bladder and used as a stent. For distal repairs, a 14 French thin-walled silicone tube is placed such that it extends several centimeters proximal to the repair but does not extend through the external urethral sphincter. These tubes are secured with prolene sutures at the urethral meatus. In general, the small-caliber urethral catheters used for stenting are not adequate for diversion, and larger catheters that would be needed for adequate diversion risk the consequences of trauma to the repair. In the vast majority of patients, for urinary diversion, a Foley catheter is easily placed in the dome of the bladder using the Hurwitz suprapubic cystostomy placement trocar. Use of these Foley catheters is associated with fewer bladder spasms than with other forms of percutaneous diversion and Foley catheters also provide better drainage.

Diversion is maintained for varying periods of times following reconstruction, depending on the type of reconstruction employed. Should grafts be used, diversion is generally maintained for a period of about 28 days postoperatively. For flap repairs, diversion is maintained for 14 to 21 days. For repairs employing excision of stricture with primary reanastomosis, diversion again is maintained for 14 to 21 days. At the end of the selected diversion interval, the patient is returned to the office where his stenting catheter is removed. Using the suprapubic cystostomy catheter, contrast is instilled and a voiding urethrogram is performed. If that shows no evidence of extravasation and adequate healing of the inlay suture line, then the suprapubic catheter is plugged. The patient leaves the office voiding per urethra. Urine cultures are obtained at that time. The suprapubic catheter is left in place for a period of 5 to 7 days. During that time the patient voids per urethra. He is maintained on suppressive antibiotics. Should no problems arise at the end of that time frame, the suprapubic catheter is removed and the patient is treated with culture-specific antibiotics for the almost inevitable bladder colonization. Treatment of colonization generally requires between 7 and 10 days. The patient is returned to the office at 2 to 3 weeks following extubation for a urine culture, which should be sterile.[10]

Because of the field effect associated with monopolar cautery, in general all cautery associated with dissection of the urethra is accomplished via bipolar electrocautery forceps. It is imperative during mobilization of the fascial flaps and skin islands that cautery be accomplished with bipolar forceps. The field effect transmitted via the dartos fascia and inherent plexus could adversely affect the vascularity to the skin island. Due to the size of the vessels in the fascial plexus, in general the bipolar is set to minimal settings. These settings will adequately coagulate the small vessels of the dartos fascial plexuses. In general, all urethral reconstructive surgery is accomplished under magnification. In the adult, 2½ power loupe magnification suffices. In the child, 3½ power loupe magnification may be helpful.

### Excision with Primary Anastomosis

In the author's opinion, the optimal anterior urethral stricture reconstruction is accomplished by total excision of the area of stricture with primary anastomosis of normal urethra to normal urethra (Fig 12). In the pendulous urethra, the ability to mobilize the urethra to close the defect following the excision of a stricture is limited as the spatulation required for the primary anastomosis after excision of a 1.5-cm stricture approaches or exceeds the limits of mobilization. Excessive mobilization of the pendulous portion of the urethra distal to the suspensory ligament of the penis risks the creation of chordee. In the very proximal bulbous or membranous urethra, however, longer defects can be easily spanned and a primary reanastomosis accomplished.

In a primary anastomosis, the stricture is excised and the urethra mobilized such that the normal ends can overlap 1 to 1.5 cm. To accomplish this, the urethra has to be extensively mobilized by freeing it from its attachments to the corpora cavernosa and the triangular ligament. The attachment of the bulbospongiosum from the perineal body can also facilitate mobilization proximally. Care must be taken, however, to not interrupt the proximal blood supply. After primary anastomosis is complete, the urethra must be reattached to the corpora cavernosa. Spatulating incisions are placed in apposing aspects of the urethral ends. The proximal anterior urethra is spatulated on the dorsal aspect, thus limiting the incision into the spongioerectile tissue of the corpus spongiosum. Distally, where the urethra lies more centrally placed, the spatulating incision can be made on the ventral aspect. The ends are brought together by placing initial sutures of PDS in the adventia of the corpus spongiosum on the dorsal aspect. These sutures do not penetrate the lumen; the knots are tied outside. The urethral epithelium is then reapproximated in watertight fashion using inter-

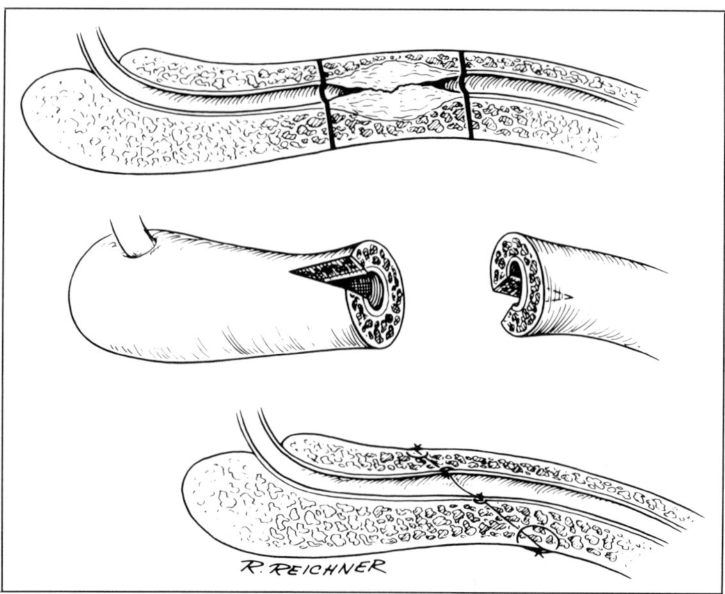


**Fig 12.** Technique of excision of an area of narrow-caliber/short-length stricture of the anterior urethra with a two-layer spatulated reanastomosis of the urethra. (Permission as in Fig 1.)

rupted chromic or small PDS sutures. Watertightness is tested by instilling saline. The remaining lateral and ventral adventia of the corpus spongiosum is then reapproximated with further epithelial chromic sutures and extraepithelial PDS sutures.

When a stricture in the urethra proximal to the pendulous portion is too long for a primary anastomosis, excision of the stricture and mobilization of the urethra may still be useful if the dorsal wall of the urethra can be brought together. This thus leaves a ventral urethrotomy defect that can be repaired by one of the substitution urethral reconstruction techniques described later in this chapter. However, in the pendulous portion of the penile urethra, if the patient is still having good straight erections, the involved urethra would not be excised. Instead, after opening the stricture, the open segment of the urethra would be incorporated into a repair as a dorsal strip, leaving it as a ''trellis'' to help prevent contraction of the newly formed substitution urethral onlay.

## Full-Thickness Skin Graft Urethral Reconstruction

Full-thickness skin graft urethral reconstruction is one of the most versatile of open urethral reconstructive procedures. The operation, developed and popularized in the author's institution, has been applied to all types of urethral strictures.[23,24] However, as the anatomic protocol would indicate, the best results are obtained in patients who have relatively superficial spongiofibrosis. Likewise, the best results are obtained in the bulbous urethra, where the overlying ischiocavernosus musculature provides an optimal graft host bed. Full-thickness skin grafts, used as indicated in the algorithm (Fig 6), provide good results in 90% to 93% of patients. Patients with longstanding stricture disease who have had multiple dilations and/or internal urethrotomies or prior attempts at open urethral reconstruction have not been shown to be good candidates for skin grafts, as they will have deep spongiofibrosis or adjacent scarring following these procedures. For the most part, full-thickness skin grafts are now used for bulbous urethral strictures that have not been subjected to multiple prior procedures. Should the stricture extend into the pendulous portion of the urethra, a graft can be used proximally in the bulb with a flap (to be discussed later) in the distal portion that is not covered by the bulbospongiosus muscles.

**Graft Take Process.** Grafts are excised from their blood supply and must acquire new vascularity from the host bed to which they are transferred. This process, termed graft take, occurs over a period of approximately 96 hours and takes place in two stages known as imbibition and inosculation, respectively. Initially, the graft survives through imbibition, or the process of imbibing tissue fluid from its surroundings. Inosculation follows, as new vessels grow as buds from vessels in the bed to penetrate and anastomose with the vessels on the deep aspect of the graft. There are requirements for successful graft take as follows:

1. *The host bed must be well vascularized.* Scar tissue, excessive cauterization, seroma, hematoma, purulent collections, and infection all interfere with vascularity and result in graft failure.
2. *Imbibition must be effective.* The graft must be capable of absorbing tissue fluid furnished by the vascular bed. Grafts that are allowed to dry during harvesting and onlay will form a more or less impermeable surface, thus limiting imbibition.
3. *Inosculation must be rapid and effective.* This is accomplished by immobilization of the graft on the host bed. In the urethra, catheters or stents serve poorly as bolsters. Immobilization is achieved via the use of quilting sutures.

**Graft Sites.** Due to its minimal contraction, the preputial skin is the full-thickness skin best suited for urethral reconstruction. There are a few other areas of hairless or nearly hairless skin suitable for use as a full-thickness graft for urethral reconstruction. Full-thickness skin grafts taken from sites other than the penis can contract by 15% to 25%, a factor that must be allowed for when the graft is designed. Split-thickness grafts in unsupported tissue may contract as much as 100% and should therefore be used only for urethral reconstruction in specialized applications (see below).[25]

Bladder epithelium is used for urethral reconstruction on occasion. Bladder epithelium is prone to desiccation and special care must be taken to keep it moist during the harvesting and onlay procedure. Bladder epithelial grafts are reliable and at maturation are truly nonhirsute. The grafts tend to maintain good compliance. Some claim that bladder epithelial grafts are prone to diverticular formation. It is the author's feeling, however, that during harvesting inadequate tailoring leads to diverticular formation. It is imperative during the tailoring phases of harvesting that the graft be maximally distended, thus preventing the harvesting of a redundant graft onlay. It is presumed that bladder epithelial grafts contract in the same ratio as preputial or penile full-thickness skin grafts and that contraction is generally less than 5%.[25]

In pediatric patients, buccal mucosa has been used as a full-thickness graft unit of transfer. This donor site has not been used for open urethral reconstruction in adults. These buccal mucosal grafts appear, in early small series, to be very reliable, nonhirsute, and essentially noncontractile.[26]

**Graft Technique.** Exposure of the bulbous urethra is gained through a perineal incision, as described earlier in the section on general principles of urethral surgery. The urethra is situated eccentrically in the corpus spongiosum of the bulb, thus lying closer to its deep surface. In cases with minimal spongiofibrosis, an incision of the bulb and the urethra can be made through the ventral aspect, allowing the spongy tissue to be spread out. The graft is then inlaid to the urethral epithelium, with the spongy tissue and corpus spongiosum closed over the graft (spongioplasty). In cases with marked spongiofibrosis, spongioplasty is not practical. Especially in the case of full-

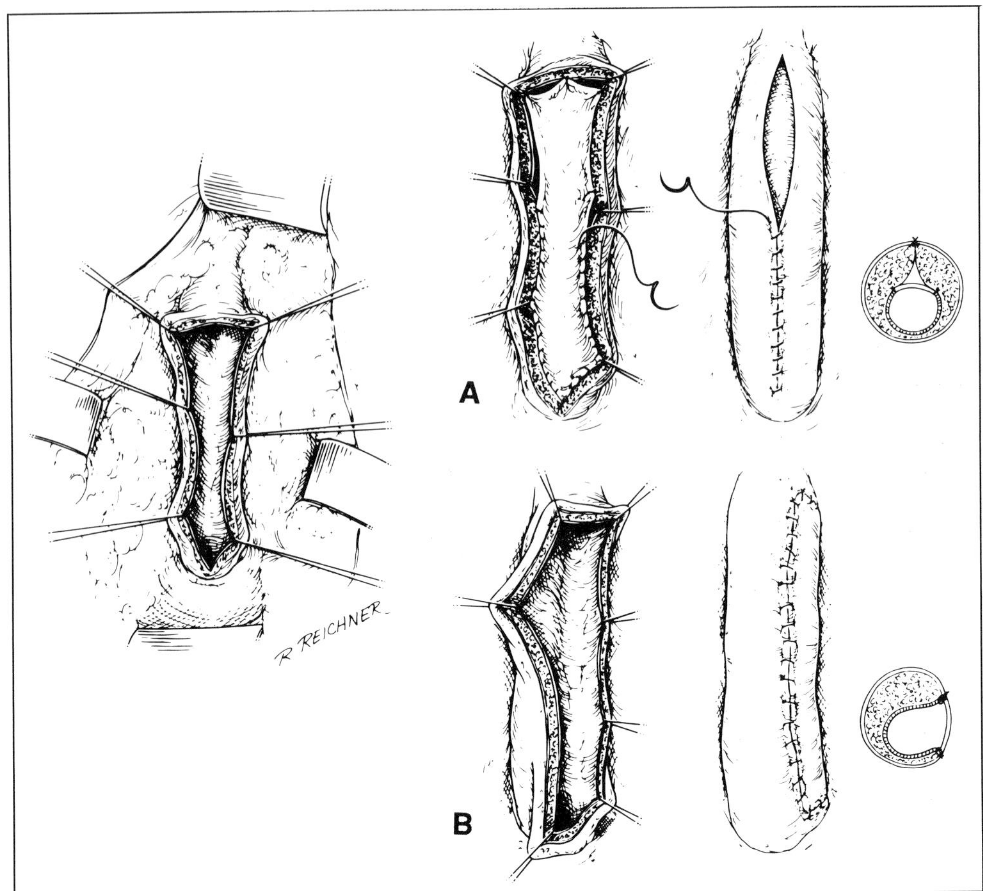


**Fig 13.** Urethrotomies with grafting. Closure is in accordance with the location of the urethrotomy incision. **A,** midline ventral incision, the graft sutured to the mucosa, and spongioplasty performed; **B,** urethra opened on the lateral aspect, graft sutured in place. [From Jordan GH, Devine CJ Jr. *Difficult Problems in Urologic Surgery.* (Chicago: Year Book; 1989), with permission.]

thickness skin graft patch onlay urethral reconstruction, a lateral urethrotomy is useful (Fig 13). A full-thickness skin graft is harvested, with all of the underlying adipose or fibrovascular tissue removed from the dermal aspect of the graft. This ''defatting'' ensures good apposition of the subdermal plexus vessels to the graft host bed recipient vessels, allowing for quick onset of inosculation. The graft is measured and tailored to fit the defect, with allowance made for contracture depending on the donor site. The graft is sutured into the urethrotomy with its epithelial surface toward the lumen. This is accomplished by placing tacking sutures of small PDS or chromic to secure the graft to the defect. These knots are, in general, tied toward the urethral lumen. A subepithelial running PDS suture, which is placed in an extraepithelial fashion, creates a watertight inlay. A stenting catheter is placed through the repair with a suprapubic diversion accomplished as already mentioned.

In the case of graft or reconstruction, optimal hemostasis is essential. Again, this is accomplished using bipolar electrocautery forceps. With hemostasis assured, the bulbocavernosus muscles are carefully quilted to the graft as they are reapproxi-

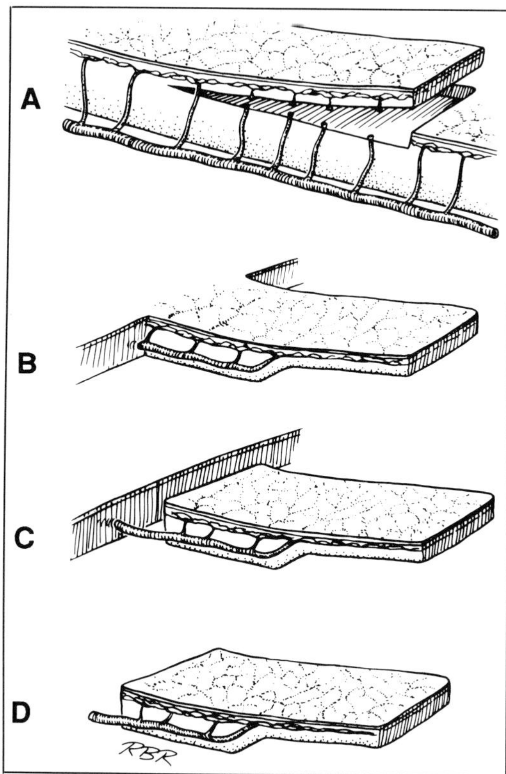


**Fig 14.** **A,** random peninsula flap; **B,** axial peninsula flap; **C,** axial island flap; **D,** free microvascular transfer ("free") flap. [From Jordan GH, McCraw JB. *Tissue Transfer Techniques in Genitourinary Reconstructive Surgery,* Part 2 (AUA Update Series, Vol 7, Lesson 10, 1988:74), with permission.]

mated in the midline. Fusion of these muscles in the midline is accomplished with individual sutures. The quilting process optimizes graft host bed apposition, and the individual sutures fusing the muscles in the midline allow for collections that could form beneath the muscles to escape and reach a suction drain placed superficial to the closed muscle but deep to the Colles fascia.

## Flap Procedures for Anterior Urethral Stricture Reconstruction

Utilizing skin flaps involves transferring a composite of skin and underlying tissue while maintaining or reestablishing the blood supply. Flaps do not take but rather survive. If a flap survives, it does not contract. If a flap does not survive, the tissue is completely lost, as it will not reliably take as a graft. Flaps used for urethroplasty should be axial flaps, planned with an identifiable vascular pedicle entering at the base of the flap and elevated with it (Fig 14). The mainstay of flap urethral reconstruction procedures are semantically correctly termed *skin islands* on fascial pedicles. They are elevated with a cutaneous paddle divided from the base, but vascular continuity is maintained. Common usage terms these "island flaps" (Fig 15). On the penis, the pedicle of these flaps is a fascial flap that can be aggressively mobilized in some cases to allow the skin paddle to be moved to any segment of the urethra.[25]

For anterior urethral strictures of the pendulous urethra, a longitudinal ventral penile skin island is useful. The pedicle of these longitudinal ventral skin islands needs not be widely mobilized as it is used most commonly to repair strictures contiguous with the location of the flap. In some cases of panurethral stricture disease, a longitudinal skin island may be useful for the distal portion of the repair combined with a full-thickness skin graft or hairless scrotal island flap for the proximal segment. A combination of distal flap and proximal graft capitalizes on the vascular bed provided by

**Fig 15.** The concept of skin islands or paddles. **A,** fascial flap with a skin island (paddle); **B,** muscle flap with a skin island (paddle). [From Glenn JF, ed. *Urologic Surgery.* 4th ed. (Philadelphia: JB Lippincott; 1991:1085), with permission.]

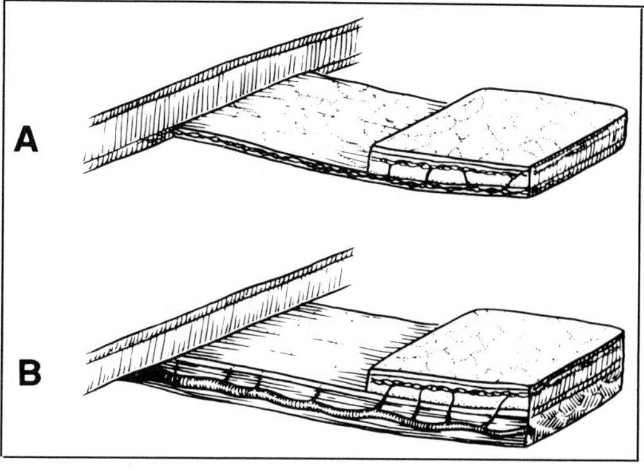

the musculature overlying the more proximal urethra while providing good vascularized tissue for the distal urethra. The author prefers to use flaps for the complete repair if nonhirsute genital skin is available.

**Orandi Flap Procedure.** Orandi originally described the concept of a longitudinal skin island based on a fasciocutaneous pedicle.[27,28] Subsequently, the author has modified significant details of the technique to allow for easier inlay of the flap (Fig 16). An incision is made in the ventral penile skin lateral to the midline and carried sharply through the dartos fascia and Buck's fascia to expose the underlying tunica of the corpora cavernosa and the adventia of the corpus spongiosum. By dissecting medially beneath Buck's fascia, the fascial flap is elevated in the plane superficial to these structures. Proceeding past the midline, the tunica of the contralateral corpus cavernosum is exposed.

A lateral incision is then made into the side of the urethra ipsilateral to the pedicle of the flap. A sound is introduced into the

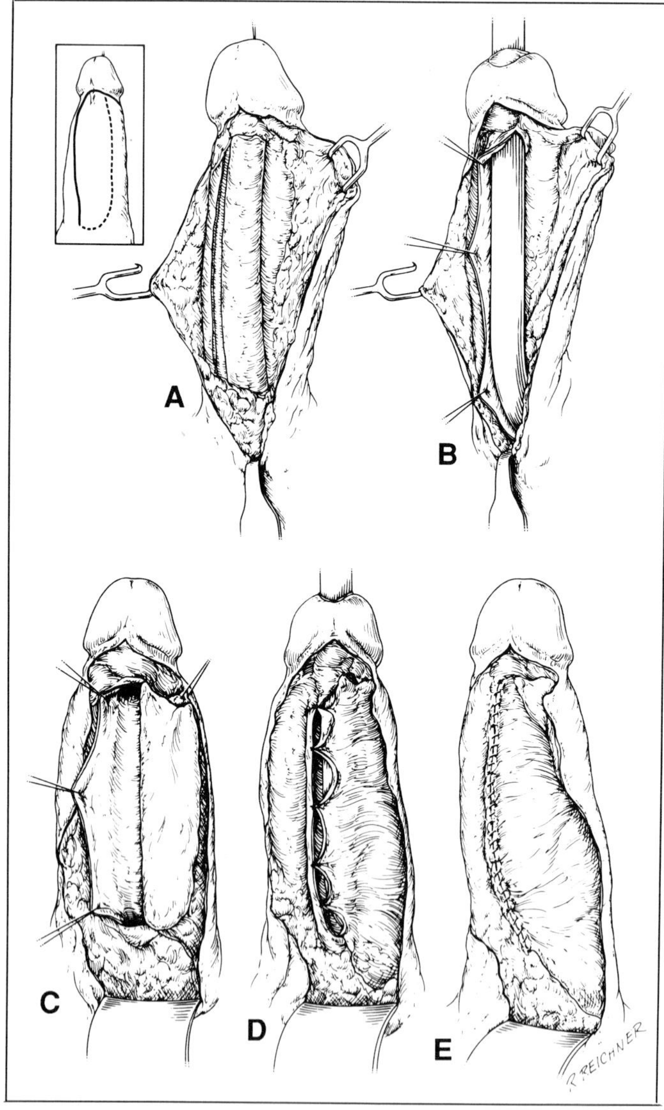


**Fig 16.** The Orandi urethroplasty. **A,** flap is developed in the layer immediately beneath Buck's fascia; **B,** urethrotomy is performed on the lateral aspect of the urethra contralateral to the original incision in the penile skin; **C,** flap is sutured into position with a running submucosal suture; **D,** flap is then inverted into the urethrotomy defect with tacking sutures; **E,** submucosal suture line is then completed. (Permission as in Fig 5.)

urethra to define the distal extent of the stricture and the lateral urethrotomy incision continued proximally from there. The normal urethra is open 1 to 1.5 cm proximal and distal to the stricture. If the meatus is involved in the stricture, the urethrotomy will extend to the tip of the penis, mobilizing the glans tissue bilaterally, thus leaving a dorsal strip of urethra in the midline. The size of the flap necessary to reconstruct the urethra is carefully measured and designed as a longitudinal skin island based on the lateral fascial vascular pedicle. The island is carefully tailored limiting the opportunity for redundancy of the inlay.

Smaller stent tubes are used for flap reconstruction as compared to graft reconstruction. Rather, in flap reconstruction they serve as supports for the flap during the immediate postoperative period and limit the formation of synechiae at the suture lines. As mentioned, hemostasis is accomplished using bipolar electrocautery forceps.

Electrocautery forceps limit the electrical field effects to the tissue just between the tips of the instrument. This is particularly important with flap procedures as it avoids the effect of the current on the tiny vessels of the fascial pedicle.

The incision is closed in layers with absorbable suture. In most cases, the skin is reapproximated with interrupted suture of chromic gut or small PGA. In some cases chromic is preferred for closure of the preputial and penile skin as the skin does not contain sufficient moisture to rapidly dissolve polyglycolic acid or related sutures, thus causing them to linger and in some cases become inflamed. Occasionally it is beneficial to reapproximate the skin with small PGA or nylon sutures even though they may have to be removed later. They support the healing wound longer than chromic sutures. The longitudinal ventral skin island can be aggressively mobilized for more proximal strictures should that donor site provide the only available nonhirsute genital skin.

For a stricture in the pendulous or mid-proximal penile urethra, a dorsal transverse skin island as described for hypospadias repair by Duckett may be elevated and used as a patch inlay.[6] The dorsal position of the vascular pedicle of this flap in some individuals limits its mobility and the flap is therefore difficult to mobilize for very proximal strictures. However, if that donor site represents the only available area of redundant nonhirsute genital skin, then the islands can, in most patients, be mobilized to reach the distal membranous urethra.

A dorsal transverse preputial island flap procedure is initiated with a ventral skin midline incision over the stricture, extending it to, but not into, Buck's fascia, where it overlies the corpus spongiosum. The urethra is exposed and the urethrotomy is performed. If better exposure is required, the skin incision can be extended into the anterior aspect of the scrotum through the raphe. In most cases, the skin of the penis is mobilized in the plane immediately superficial to the outer lamina of Buck's fascia. The dissection is carried proximally, lifting the skin of the penis and the full thickness of the dartos fascia with it. Dissection must be done with care, preserving the vessels in the dartos fascia and staying superficial to Buck's fascia to avoid the dorsal vessels and nerves.

The urethrotomy defect is measured, and a skin paddle of proper size is created transversely on the dorsal surface of the penile/preputial skin. If the patient has been circumcised, the island is created just proximal to the circumcision scar. Incisions are made to outline the skin paddle and the remaining proximal skin is elevated to mobilize the vascular pedicle. Care must also be taken to preserve the superficial vessels in the skin as it is elevated from the dartos fascia, as these vessels provide random vascularity to the remaining penile skin.

After proper elevation of the pedicle, the island flap can be transposed to the ventral surface of the penis or beneath the scrotum to the exposed perineal portions of the urethra. First the edge of the inlay that will be beneath the pedicle is sewn in a watertight fashion. Then the remainder of the inlay is completed in the same fashion and the skin is closed.

**Quartey Flap Procedure.** In most cases of proximal anterior urethral strictures, a ventral skin island as first described by Quartey has proven to be useful. Quartey positioned his skin island in circumferential orientation with the island extending from the raphe laterally.[7,8] The positioning of the island has been modified depending on the length and location of the flap. Using a perineal incision, the stricture is opened with a laterally placed incision, so that the skin paddle of the flap will fit easily into the urethrotomy without distortion or tension. In some cases an area of short-segment, narrow-caliber stricture is excised; the flap can then be fit into a dorsal spatulating urethrotomy defect.

The inlay consists of a ventral penile skin island elevated on the ventral dartos fascia. Elevation of a skin paddle from the midline of the ventrum of the penis allows the vascular pedicle to be elevated from the ventrolateral aspect of the penis. This makes the fascial pedicle wider and limits the amount of remaining penile skin that must survive on random blood supply. The incision is deepened through Buck's fascia. As the skin paddle of the flap is mobilized,

**Fig 17.** The Quartey (ventral longitudinal/transverse preputial island) flap. **A,** flap is elevated in the layer immediately beneath Buck's fascia; **B,** flap is passed beneath the scrotum to the perineal incision where urethrotomy has been performed through the stricture; **C,** flap is sutured in place with a running subepithelially placed suture; **D,** flap in place showing the pedicle extending up beneath the scrotum. (Permission as in Fig 5.)

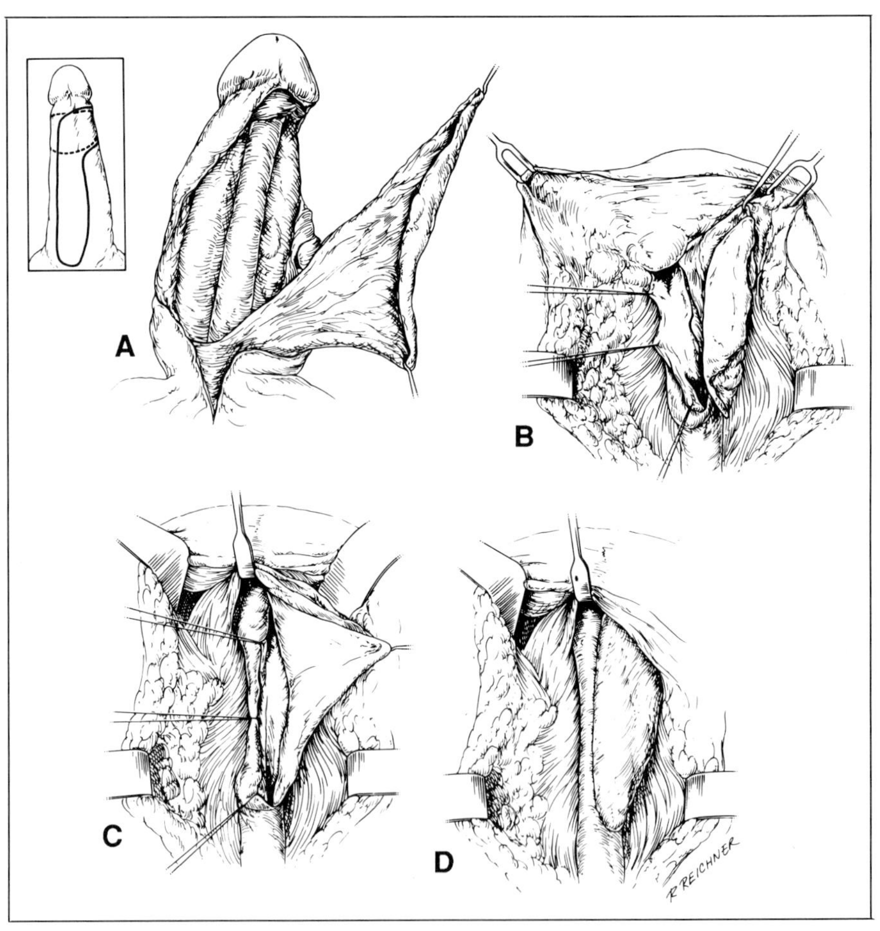

the tunica of the corporal bodies is denuded. The pedicle can then be easily mobilized proximally beneath the scrotal skin allowing the flap to be inverted and transposed beneath the scrotum to the most proximal portions of the anterior urethra. For longer strictures, the island flap is designed with its longitudinal portion running the length of the penis, swinging laterally to the left or right as it approaches the frenulum and coronal margin (Fig 17). The longest flap that the author has developed in this fashion measured 3 × 13 cm and was closed primarily with no problems with its vascularity. In some cases, depending on the redundancy of the skin, the skin island is oriented circumferentially and encompasses the entire circumference of the distal penile skin. Quite long islands can be elevated in that fashion as well.[29] The choice of skin island orientation depends on the relationship of the length, location, and shape of the urethrotomy defect coupled with the site of redundancy of the nonhirsute penile skin (Fig 18).

After completing the suture line, watertightness is tested as described under general principles. If the repair is proximal enough that the stent would bridge the sphincter of the urethra, a small silicone silastic Foley catheter is placed through the reconstruction into the bladder. However, it is emphasized that these catheters cannot be relied on for drainage and suprapubic diversion is placed.

**The Hairless Scrotal Island Flap Procedure.** A hairless scrotal skin island also has good applicability in select patients with proximal urethral strictures (Fig 19). Compared to the extensive mobilization required when the ventral island flap prior to above was applied to the bulbous urethra, in a patient who has a large enough area of nonhirsute scrotal skin, creation of a flap mobilizing this hairless island requires less dissection and still allows reconstruction of the urethra with vascularized tissue. The scrotal island flap is a fascial-based flap with a skin island. The hairless island should truly have no hair. Histologic studies of these islands in cadavers show that the hair follicles are readily visualized. Truly nonhirsute areas do exist on the scrotum of some males. If a few hair follicles are noted, they can be destroyed by placing a small needle down the hair follicle and applying low-power monopolar cautery. Extensive ablation with the cautery, however, is not recommended in the acute phase. Rather extensive scrotal nonhirsute islands can be developed with epilation, but the epilation should be done in a staged fashion.

Genital skin flaps do not contract unless there is ischemia upon elevation of the flap. Genital skin flaps that are created from scrotal skin have remarkable distensibility. The skin is quite elastic, and the dartos layer of the scrotum has a pronounced musculature component that tends to contract the skin. It is essential that these islands be measured with the scrotal skin fully stretched. When not properly tailored, these flaps are prone to diverticulum formation. Recent review of in excess of 40 patients reconstructed with scrotal hairless skin islands show the flaps to be remarkably dependable. This is felt to be due to the dual vascularity with the artery to the scrotum, a branch of the common penile artery extending onto the scrotum posteriorly and the distal branches of the external pudendal artery, branching from the femoral artery, coming onto the scrotum in a superolateral fashion.

Since the vessels in the dartos fascia extend onto the scrotum from the lateral direction, the fascial pedicle must be developed laterally and not be based on the midline. Although some flaps can be based on scrotal midline vessels, the presence of these vessels is not dependable and these vessels must be demonstrable prior to basing the flap on that pedicle. A pedicle developed from the scrotal raphe is not reliable and may not support the skin island. As in the previously described flap procedures, the deep edge of the flap is secured to the edge of either a lateral or dorsal urethrotomy with a running subepithelial suture. The flap is then inverted into the defect and the closure accomplished in watertight fashion as described in the section on general principles.[30]

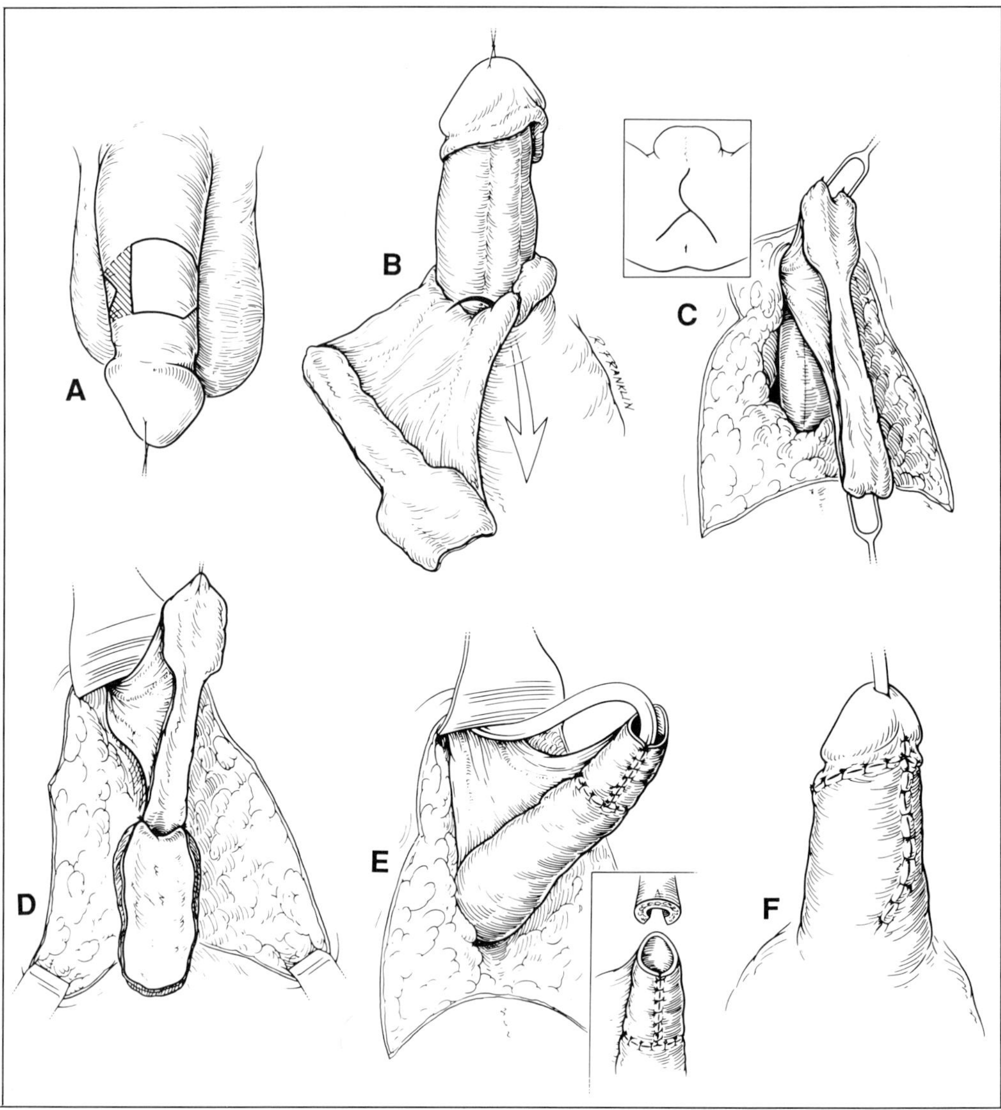


**Fig 18.** A distal circumferential skin island based on the dartos fascia. **A,** skin island is carefully tailored and marked on the foreskin; **B,** skin island is elevated on the dartos fascia and inverted beneath the scrotum; **C** (inset), perineal incision with the skin island transposed into the area of the perineum; **D,** spatulated corpus spongiosum. Note that the corpus spongiosum has been spatulated on the dorsal aspect. The skin island inlay is begun with the inlay accomplished at the spatulation into the membranous urethra; **E,** inlay is complete with the distal portion of the flap tubed (see inset). The tubed portion of the flap is anastomosed via widely spatulated technique into the proximal portion of the distal anterior urethra; **F,** skin closure on the penis with a stenting urethral catheter in place.

## Strictures of the Fossa Navicularis

An entirely different challenge is presented by strictures of the fossa navicularis and urethral meatus. Strictures of other portions of the anterior urethra require careful attention for good functional results; however, strictures of the fossa and meatus require both good functional and good cosmetic results. The anatomy of the fossa

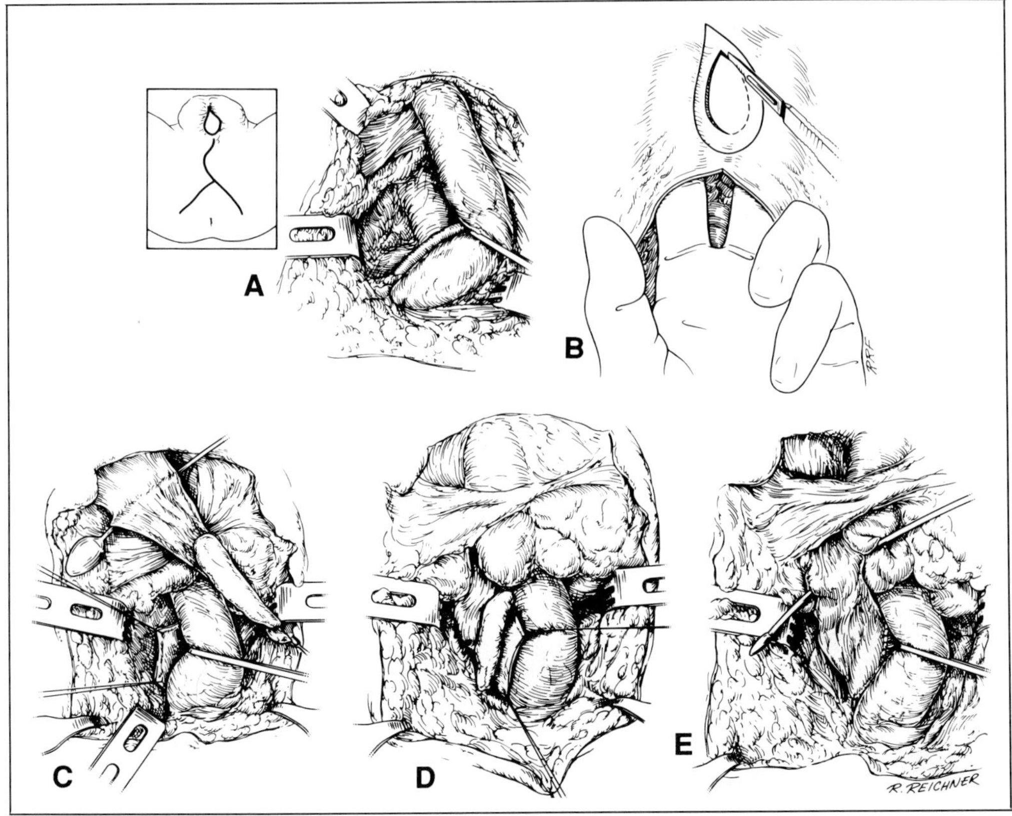


**Fig 19.** Hairless scrotal island flap. **A,** dissection of the bulbomembranous portion of the urethra; **B,** it is essential in tailoring and developing the skin island that the scrotal skin be distended to its limits. This will avoid the creation of a redundant skin island; **C,** flap is elevated on the dorsolateral pedicle with a lateral urethrotomy created on the lateral aspect of the bulbomembranous portion of the urethra; **D, E,** flap is sutured into the urethrotomy defect. Note the probe beneath the vascular pedicle.

navicularis stricture with accompanying balanitis xerotica obliterans (BXO) or the stricture in that area following transurethral resection is a completely different entity than the meatal stenosis seen in children, a sequela of ammoniacal meatitis/balanitis. In true meatal stenosis, the stenotic entity consists of a diaphragm, which is in essence a fusion of the meatus following irritation of the tip of the glans in the infant or young child in diapers. Hence the entity is readily managed with meatotomy. Some centers prefer a dorsal Y-V flap procedure. A simple ventral meatotomy in the vast majority of children is curative. The dorsal Y-V flap technique trades the relative redundancy of tissue of the dorsal glans for the paucity of tissue of the stenotic meatus or distal fossa. A V flap is elevated from the tissues of the dorsal glans. An incision is created through the area of stenosis. The V flap is then advanced into the incision, widening the area of stenosis.

**Fossa Reconstruction Procedures.** Devine described a graft procedure for reconstruction of fossa strictures that he termed "resurfacing of the fossa navicularis." This procedure has been used with good functional and cosmetic success in a small number of patients. The procedure, however, is not useful in the patient with balanitis xerotica obliterans, as the BXO process seems capable of involving the graft (Fig

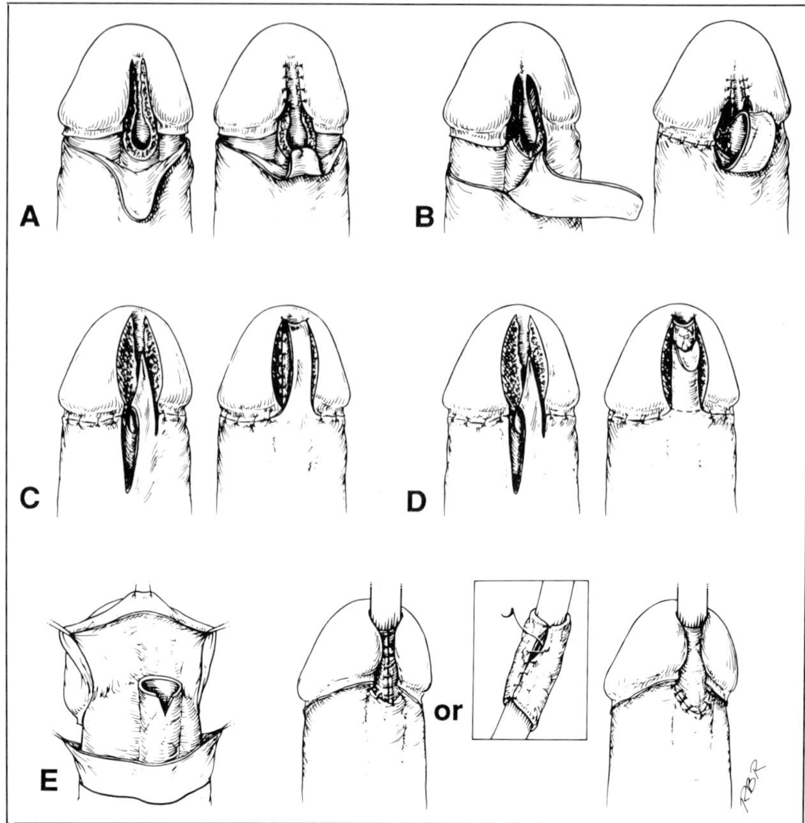


**Fig 20.** Collage of the techniques of fossa reconstruction: **A,** Blandy; **B,** Cohney; **C,** Brannen; **D,** DeSy; **E,** Devine. (Permission as in Fig 5.)

20). Cohney in 1963 and Blandy in 1967 described flap procedures based on the V-Y principle for reconstruction of the fossa navicularis. The cosmetic results of both techniques were criticized due to the postoperative deformity of the glans and the retrusive nature of the meatus. Brannen described a modification of the Blandy procedure, which was designed to place the meatus further toward the tip of the glans. This procedure involved the elevation of a peninsula flap based on the ventral dartos fascial blood supply that was then aggressively advanced into the meatotomy defect. The longer flap was designed to allow the meatus to be placed further distally. In reality, because of the degree of advancement required, most patients were left with a retrusive meatus and functional results were little better than those of Cohney's and Blandy's original flaps.

In 1984 DeSy presented a modification of the Brannen procedure in which a longitudinally oriented skin island is mobilized on the ventral dartos fascia. The skin island is advanced and inverted into the meatotomy defect. The description of the procedure implies that the island is mobilized on a relatively thin dartos pedicle. The dartos pedicle is advanced and the ventral glans is fused over the fascial strip. DeSy recently reported a series of approximately 30 patients with excellent functional and cosmetic results. His procedure does, however, require rather lengthy advancement of the midline dartos fascia.[31]

The author in 1987 described a procedure for reconstruction of the fossa navicularis that consisted of a transverse ventral penile skin island elevated on a broad dartos fascial pedicle.[32] The island is transposed and inverted into the meatotomy defect (Fig 21). The broad dartos pedicle allows vigorous mobilization of the ventral fascial pedicle but in so doing also requires more aggressive dissection of the lateral glans flaps in order to assure a tension-free ventral fusion of the glans. Application of this procedure requires confinement of the stricture to the fossa navicularis. However, this procedure has been successfully used for strictures as long as 5 cm.

All patients must be evaluated with retrograde and voiding contrast medium studies as well as urethroscopy. In most patients urethroscopy can be performed using a small pediatric rigid cystopanendoscope. In those in which preoperative urethroscopy cannot be performed, yet contrast studies indicate that the stenotic process is confined to the fossa, endoscopy is done immediately on performance of the urethrotomy through the area of stenosis, thus assuring that the more proximal urethra is uninvolved with stricture. To date, the author has reconstructed 15 patients. In 14 patients follow-up has exceeded 1 year. One patient has been followed for 6 months following reconstruction. Median follow-up is greater than 3 years. There have been no recurrences and no fistulas in that series of patients.[33]

Occasionally a patient will present with distal anterior urethral stricture disease that is not confined to the fossa navicularis yet is confined to the pendulous portion of the anterior urethra. In these patients, a longitudinal skin island, as was previously described in this chapter, can be elevated on a lateral dartos fascial pedicle. However, in these cases, in order to allow for advancement of the skin island into the meatus, more vigorous mobilization of the lateral dartos fascia is required. By orienting

**Fig 21.** Reconstruction of the fossa navicularis using a ventral transverse island flap. Urethrotomy is performed well into urethra of normal caliber. Then small, partial-circumferential incision is created. Note outline of flap. Flap is transposed and inverted into urethrotomy defect. Flap tips are sutured with chromic catgut and lateral edges of flap are sutured with 5–0 or 6–0 polydioxanone sutures. Suturing of flap is complete. Note wide mesentery extending proximally. Glans flaps have been elevated. Note tip of exposed corporal body. [From *J Urol* (1987;138:102), with permission.]

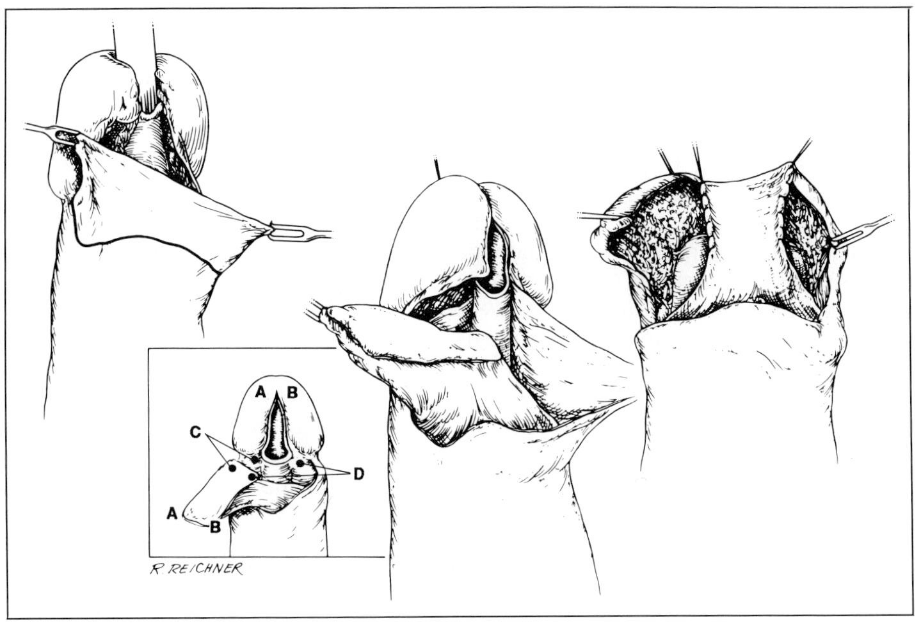

the skin island in a longitudinal orientation, however, longer defects can be reconstructed.

Occasionally a patient will present with stenosis of the fossa navicularis but will have redundancy of skin on the dorsum of the penis. In these cases, a transverse skin island can be elevated from the redundant dorsal skin. In these cases, the deep dissection is accomplished in the layer immediately superficial to the outer lamina of Buck's fascia. The island is then transposed to the ventrum of the penis and applied as an onlay much in the fashion as it would be in hypospadias.

All of the aforementioned procedures can be accomplished in the patient who has been circumcised. Care must be taken to orient the skin islands proximal to the circumcising incision. Depending on the method of circumcision, the preputial skin distal to the circumcising incision may not be predictably vascularized by the proximal dartos fascia. It is essential, in those procedures requiring fusion of the glans ventrally, that the glans be fused in a tension-free fashion around the neomeatus and neofossa navicularis.

### Post-TURP: Strictures of the Sphincter-Active Portion of the Urethra

Strictures of the membranous urethra in the area of the external urethral sphincter are technically highly reconstructible. However, in many cases the strictures arise in a patient following TURP. Hence, open reconstruction risks incontinence. Additionally, the open reconstruction makes subsequent management of the incontinence by the implantation of an artificial urethral sphincter a tenuous situation. In these cases, there is a higher incidence of sphincter cuff erosion.

These strictures are, however, very manageable with dilation. The author prefers to use balloon dilations in these cases. The dilations predictably have to be repeated but usually only at intervals of 6 months to a year. These dilations can generally be accomplished in the office and the patient's continence is usually quite acceptable.

### Complex Strictures

Classically, multistage urethral reconstruction begins with marsupialization of the urethra followed by staged tubularization of the adjacent scrotal or perineal skin. Many of these procedures have invariably placed hair-bearing skin in the urethra and the results were fraught with complications such as diverticula, hair bezoar, fistula formation, and urethral calculus. Modern tissue transfer techniques have replaced these procedures with excellent results. However, there still is a place for multistaged procedures, although the nature of those procedures is entirely different from that just described. Schreiter and Noll describe an alternative procedure for the multioperated complex patient,[34] and that procedure has been termed the mesh graft urethroplasty. They report excellent results in over 100 patients. Other centers in Germany likewise report large series. The author has had good experience with this procedure and the majority of patients do well in all series.

The mesh graft urethral reconstruction first involves either complete excision of the strictured urethra or subtotal excision leaving only a small dorsal strip of urethral epithelium (Fig 22). The dartos fascia is mobilized to cover the ventral tunica albuginea of the penis and in the perineum. A split-thickness graft is harvested from a relatively nonhirsute area. That graft is harvested approximately 15/0.0001 in. It is then meshed on a carrier that creates a 1.5:1 ratio. The mesh graft is then placed as an open-faced graft. The graft is placed in an unexpanded fashion. A meticulous bolster dressing is then placed. That bolster consists of Xeroform gauze padded with Dacron batting and secured in place with tie-over sutures. A stenting catheter is left in the proximal urethrostomy, and if there is a patent distal urethra, then a distal urethrostomy is likewise created.

The patient is kept on broad-spectrum antibiotics and at bedrest for a period of 5 to 7 days. At that time the bolster is removed and the patient is ambulated and taught to care for his graft with standard wound care.

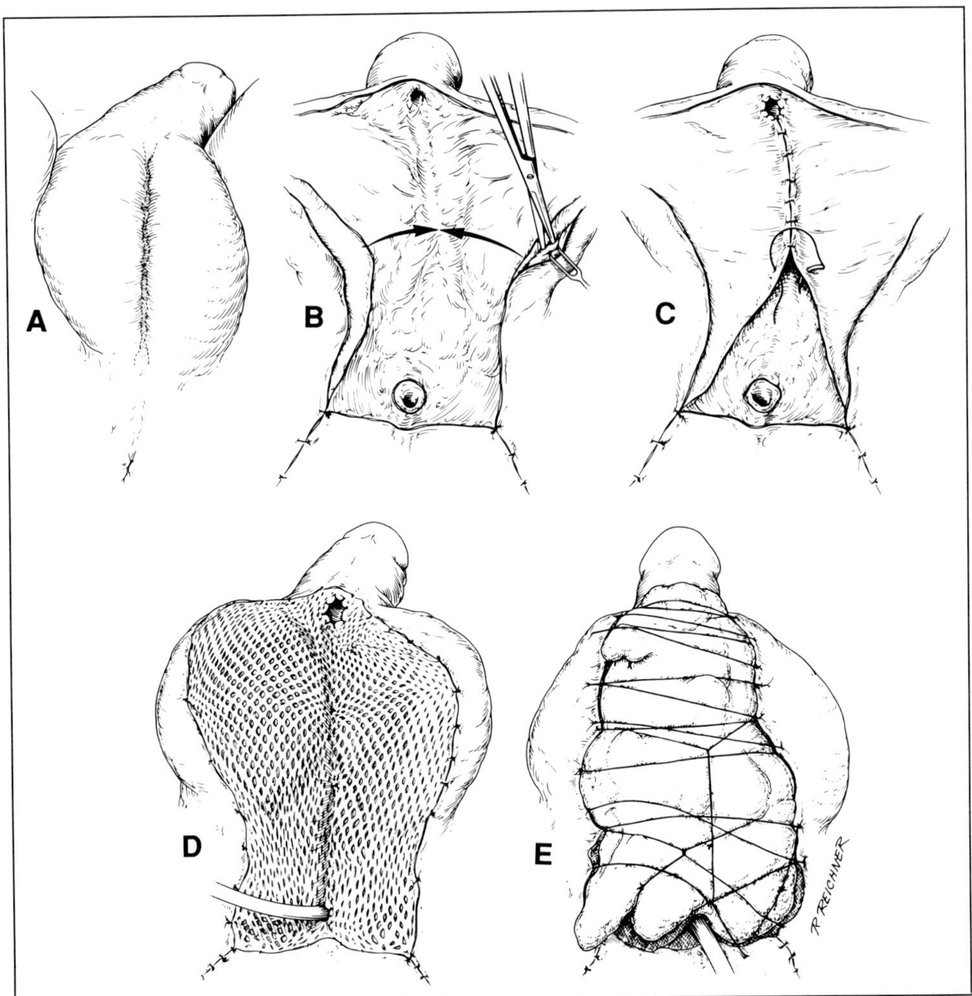


**Fig 22.** Mesh graft urethroplasty—stage 1, placement of the graft. **A,** the condition of the patient with a proximal stenotic urethrostomy and a distal urethrostomy. Note that patient had only the pendulous portion of the anterior urethra; **B,** incision with transposition of the adjacent dartos fascia to the midline; **C,** transposition is completed with the dartos fascia bed in place for placement of the graft; **D,** inlay of a mesh split-thickness skin graft cut approximately 0.0016 in. thick with a mesh ratio of 1.5 to 1; **E,** bolster in place. [From Devine CJ, Jordan GH. *Strictures of the Anterior Urethra,* Part 2 (AUA Update Series, Vol 9, Lesson 26, 1990:205), with permission.]

The patient is then followed and is returned to the operating room in 6 months to a year depending on maturity of the graft (Fig 23). In some patients, preputial skin can be meshed. Maturation of those grafts seems to occur in accelerated fashion and some patients can be returned to the operating room as quickly as 4 to 6 months after graft placement. The new nonhirsute epithelial surface is smooth and elastic. At the second stage, in essence a Thiersch–Duplay tubularization is accomplished. The strip is not undermined but dissected laterally. Due to the mobilization of the dartos fascia in the initial procedure, the tube can be closed without difficulty, with the wound then closed in layers over that. In general, the author does not excise the

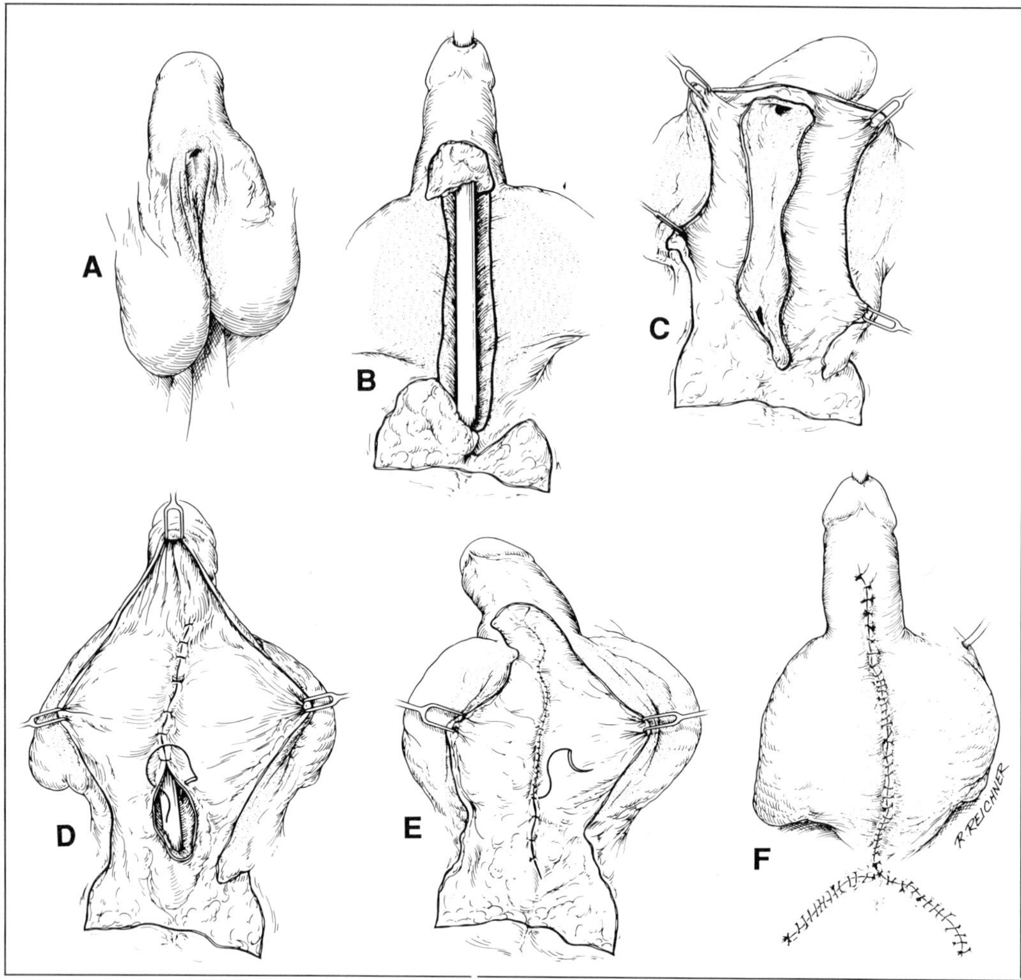


**Fig 23.** Mesh graft urethroplasty, stage 2. **A,** condition of the patient after maturity of the graft at 6 months; **B,** midline strip is created with a spatulation of the strip into the proximal urethrostomy and distal urethrostomy; **C,** closure of strip is begun; **D,** epithelium is opposed with a chromic absorbable suture with the knots toward the lumen; **E,** several layers of extraepithelial absorbable monofilament suture are placed to reinforce tube closure; **F,** closure of the perineum and scrotal incision. (Permission as in Fig 22.)

extra graft material but rather leaves it in place should subsequent procedures be required. To date, subsequent procedures have only been required in one patient. The appearance of the extra graft material on the genitalia is cosmetically acceptable.

## Posterior Strictures

**Pelvic Trauma and Acute Management of Urethral Distraction Injuries.** Discussion of the management of posterior urethral strictures must begin with a discussion of urethral trauma as associated with pelvic fractures. Acute treatment of the fractured pelvis with urethral injury must take into account the patient's total condition as well as the experience of the urologist involved. If nothing further is done, all of these patients require suprapubic diversion. There again is the misconception that the suprapubic diversion may obviate stricture formation. Indeed, the suprapubic diversion merely prevents the adverse sequela that would arise if the patient were not diverted. The author favors placement of a suprapubic diversion and at the same setting an attempt at placement of a primary aligning catheter. With the ready availability of flexible endoscopes, in more cases than not aligning catheters can be placed. Obviously, the patient's total condition must allow for the added time required to endoscope the patient and attempt placement of an aligning catheter. The author does not favor percutaneous methods of suprapubic catheter placement in the trauma patient. In patients in whom an aligning catheter has been placed, a number have healed with virtual hairline scars at the area of the distraction defect. In patients not so fortunate, delayed excision and primary repair can be accomplished. There is enthusiasm for the cut-for-light procedures or the endoscopic realignment procedures. In the author's experience and that of the vast majority of centers performing these procedures, the posterior stricture becomes manageable but not cured. These patients inevitably require interval dilation. The author does not favor these endoscopic alignment procedures in the vast majority of patients. Certainly in certain patients in whom orthopedic injuries would prevent approach to the proximal urethra or general health needs would preclude extensive reconstruction, endoscopic alignment with management of the stricture from that point may be desirable.[35]

**Preoperative Evaluation.** In patients who have been diverted and in whom a distraction defect develops, attempts at reconstruction should be accomplished at 4 to 6 months following the trauma. The author favors an interval of 6 months. During that time frame, urethral instrumentation should be avoided. As the time for reconstruction arrives, the patient is then evaluated with contrast studies and endoscopy. Simultaneous retrograde urethrogram and cystogram often nicely outline the posterior urethra and accurately define the length of the distraction defect. However, it is not unusual to not be able to visualize the posterior urethra. In adults, the posterior urethra is inevitably uninvolved in the trauma and essentially normal anatomically and in length. Occasionally, by asking the patient to try and relax to void while contrast is in the bladder, a bladder spasm will fill the posterior urethra. Using the flexible endoscope, the anterior urethra to the site of total obstruction is examined. Again, in most patients the entire anterior urethra is normal. The scope is then introduced through the suprapubic sinus and the bladder neck appearance noted. In patients in whom the bladder neck is closed on contrast studies and in whom the endoscopic appearance is that of a normally closed bladder neck, postoperative continence is almost guaranteed. The flexible endoscope can be passed down the posterior urethra very nicely defining its length and confirming the lack of involvement of the traumatic process in that area.

In virtually all patients who have suffered posterior urethral distraction injuries, reconstruction can be accomplished by excising the area of fibrosis and defect and performing a spatulated anastomosis of the bulbous urethra to the apical prostatic urethra. This does require mobilization of the corpus spongiosum and in some patients rather extensive mobilization out to the area of the penoscrotal junction. The proximal corpus spongiosum, hence, is converted to a flap. For it to survive, the distal blood supply must be intact. That blood supply consists of the aborization of the termination of the dorsal arteries of the penis in the glans, which then flow in retrograde fashion into the corpus spongiosum.

In many patients in whom there has been profound pelvic bleeding, we are finding that embolization has been performed in the acute trauma phases. All of these patients must be suspect. Additionally, lateral compression fractures and blowout fractures of the pubis often disrupt the pudendal arteries and/or common penile arteries. The vascularity to the corpus spongiosum in these patients must likewise be suspect.

The author has noted an association between numbness of the glans and common penile artery injury. Any patient with numbness of the glans beginning following the trauma must be suspected of having inadequate vascularity to the corpus spongiosum. The elevation of the corpus spongiosum requires sacrifice of the arteries to the bulb and the circumflex cavernosals.

At this center, these patients are all subjected to evaluation with pudendal/penile angiography. This procedure very adequately confirms the presence of the blood supply to the distal aspects of the penis or defines the lack of such blood supply. In patients in whom the distal blood supply to the penis is found to be inadequate, then the stricture must be addressed by one of the methods of tissue transfer already described for anterior urethral reconstruction. The literature supports the fact that the vast majority of failures of posterior urethral reconstruction are not technical failures at the anastomosis but rather represent ischemia of the mobilized corpus spongiosum. These patients generally are left with relatively long anterior urethral stricture defects.[21,22]

**Operative Technique Perineal Approach.** At the author's institution, virtually all patients are approached in the exaggerated lithotomy position. The urethra is exposed as already described in the general principles section of this chapter (Fig 24). The corpus spongiosum is then detached from the corpora cavernosa to the level of the scrotum and then further as required. The bulbospongiosum is detached from the perineal bodies and the proximal blood supply is cauterized and divided. Eventually, proximally the urethra remains detached

**Fig 24.** Dissection of the bulbous urethra. **A,** central tendon is divided revealing the midline fusion of the ischiocavernosus muscles with the "bare" corpus spongiosum visible beneath the scrotum; **B, C,** muscles are divided in the midline; **D,** muscles have been divided all the way to the insertion of the perineal body; **E,** corpus spongiosum is dissected from the adjacent muscular attachments. (Permission as in Fig 5.)

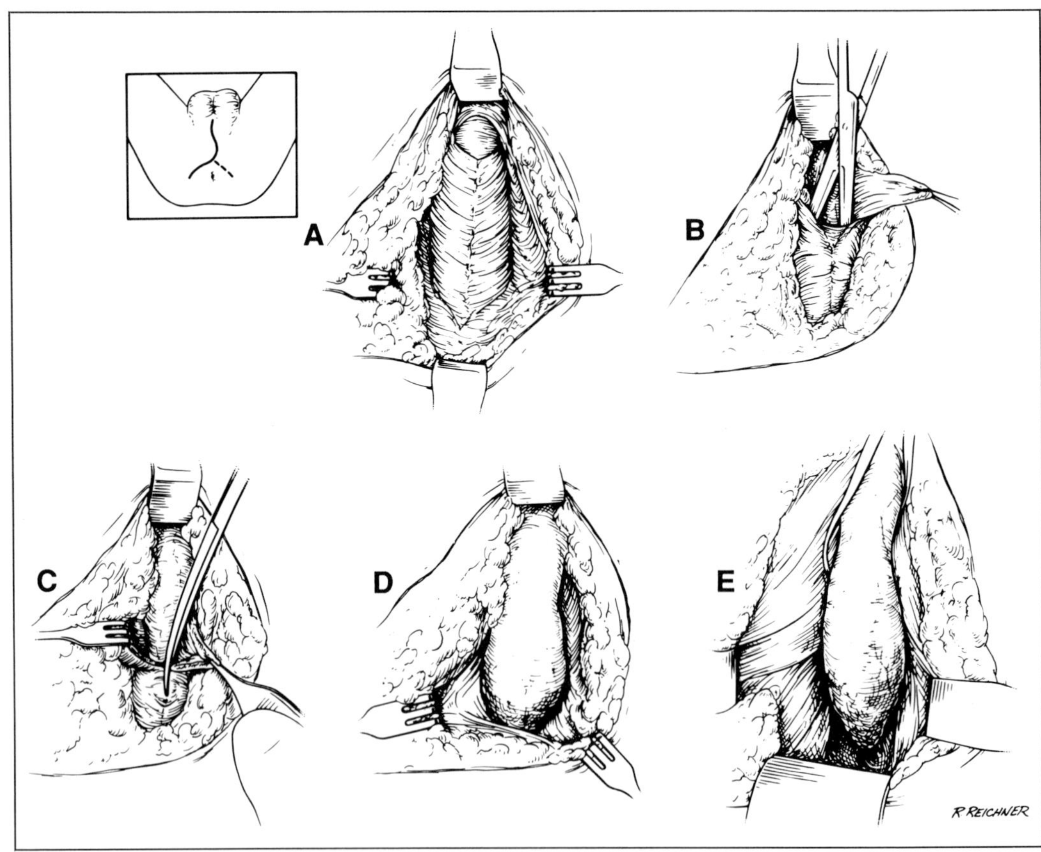

only to the distraction defect, which is then divided.

The triangular ligament is then divided and the intracrural space developed. The dorsal vein is encountered in most patients and is ligated and divided (Fig 25).

A modified Gelpi retractor is then placed to retract the corpora laterally. Using periosteal elevators, the space beneath the pubis is dissected and the prostatic attachments detached there. The fibrosis in the area of the distraction defect is entirely excised. A Hey–Grooves staff is placed in the suprapubic sinus and advanced down through the bladder neck. The distalmost limits of the posterior urethra are palpated. The fibrosis is totally excised prior to the opening of the distal urethra. When the sound is concealed only by the remaining epithelial layer, then an incision into the apex of the posterior urethra is made. A stitch is withdrawn back through the path of the sound and endoscopy is then performed, which should confirm the presence of a normal-appearing verumontanum, prostatic lobes, and bladder neck. When it is confirmed that the urethrotomy has been created at the distalmost limits of the posterior urethra, then spatulation of that urethra is accomplished such that a 32 French bougie-à-boule can be passed without difficulty. The bulbous urethra is then likewise prepared and spatulated. It is imperative that the normal epithelial tissues of the prostatic urethra evert from the wound. The success of this procedure demands a hairline epithelial-to-epithelial apposition. If that is achieved, patients will, following reconstruction, have virtually undetectable evidence of ever having had trauma or reconstructive surgery for the trauma.

The anastomotic sutures are initially placed in the proximal urethra. They are then placed in their respective positions in the proximal anterior urethra. Prior to seating the anastomosis, a stenting soft silicone silastic catheter is passed through the reconstruction. The anastomosis is then seated with the surgeon and his assistant, tying opposite sutures simultaneously, thus keeping the anastomosis tied under equal tension and widely splayed. The wound is then closed in layers as already described. Because of the dead space created, suction drains are placed.

It is emphasized that the corpus spongiosum should not be detached out on the pendulous portion of the penis. Mobilization there will inevitably create ventral chordee. In the older patient, the creation

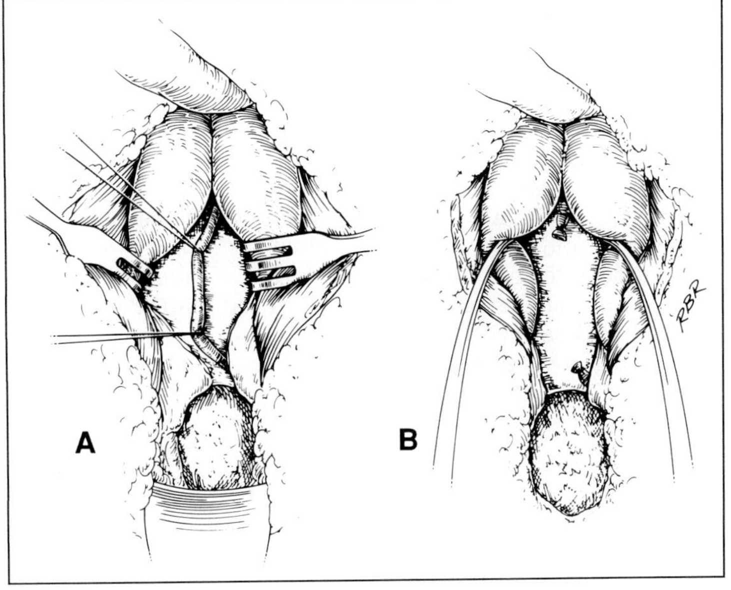


**Fig 25. A,** division of the triangular ligament with dissection between the corpora cavernosa demonstrating the exposed dorsal vein of the penis; **B,** division of the triangular ligament with dissection of the intracorporal space with the dorsal veins ligated. (Permission as in Fig 5.)

of chordee may be inconsequential. There is no question that the results of the procedures of scar excision and primary reanastomosis are far superior to any procedures of tissue transfer for posterior urethral reconstruction. The use of full-thickness skin grafts in posterior urethral reconstruction is not advocated. The scarring does not support graft take. Even "importation of blood supply" by heroic measures such as elevating gracilis flaps and so forth has been shown to give far less than optimal results.

**Operative Technique Transpubic Approach.** In some centers, there is considerable enthusiasm for transpubic reconstruction of the posterior urethra. The author has found little advantage to that approach. The transpubic approach is clearly attached with more morbidity than perineal reconstruction. It is emphasized that infrapubectomy, if not total pubectomy, is possible and easily accomplished via the perineal approach. In the anterior transpubic approach, there is far more risk of injury to the dorsal penile neurovascular bundles. In the anterior transpubic approach, it is essential that the pubis be dissected subperichondrially or subperiosteally in order to avoid damage to the dorsal nerves and arteries of the penis.

A clear disadvantage of the perineal approach is the inability to address the bladder neck. In reality, few patients require lysis of the bladder neck or bladder neck reconstruction. In those who do, a combined perineal abdominal approach can be used. In a recent review of 60 patients with posterior strictures that were reconstructed by the author, only two patients required intervention at the level of the bladder neck. One patient at the time of trauma had a bladder neck laceration from having a section of his pubis pushed into the bladder. A second patient had undergone a failed attempt at endoscopic realignment. The alignment was unfortunately performed between the proximal bulbous urethra and the bladder directly through the dorsal aspect of the bladder neck. In both, successful bladder neck reconstruction was performed simultaneously with perineal reconstruction of the posterior urethra.

**Distraction Defects Requiring Tissue Transfer.** The flap procedures that have already been described for anterior urethral reconstruction can be successfully applied to the patient with a posterior urethral distraction defect.

Even in the patient who has been aggressively circumcised, there should be adequate nonhirsute penile or preputial skin to perform the reconstruction. If there is difficulty with closing the penis, then the penis can be closed and reconstructed with split-thickness skin grafts.

**Postoperative Management.** The author keeps the patients at bedrest for a short time following reconstruction. The drains are removed as drainage allows. As the patients are ambulated, they are discharged from the hospital with their diverting suprapubic cystostomy tube for gravity drainage and their stenting urethral catheter to a catheter plug. A voiding trial with contrast is performed in most patients on the 21st postoperative day. With good healing confirmed, the suprapubic tube is plugged to be removed in 5 to 7 days. Colonization of the bladder is treated with culture-specific antibiotics once the patient is tube-free.

## SUMMARY

The combination of understanding of the nature of urethral stricture disease combined with the evolution of modern tissue transfer techniques has allowed the reconstructive surgeon to deal with urethral stricture disease assuredly. A cure is possible in the vast majority of patients. Even patients with the most complex situations, by use of aggressive techniques of transfer, can be completely cured. There will be some patients in whom reconstruction of the urethra is not possible. These patients, however, now can be dealt with by techniques that allow catheterizable access to the bladder through abdominal continent stomas. The issue of continent catheterizable bladder augmentation clearly has a place in the treatment of severely complicated urethral stricture patients.

## REFERENCES


1. Jordan GH, Schellhammer PF. Urethral surgery and stricture disease. In: Droller MJ, ed. *Surgical Management of Urologic Disease: An Anatomic Approach.* St. Louis: Mosby; 1992:815–832.
2. Turner-Warwick R. A persona view of the management of traumatic posterior urethral stricture. *Urol Clin North Am.* 1977;4:111.
3. Jukiewenski S, Vaysse PH, Moscovici J, et al. A study of the arterial blood supply to the penis. *Anat Clin.* 1982;4:101.
4. Kodos AB. The vascular supply of the penis. *Arkh Anat Embriol.* 1967;43:525.
5. Lich R Jr, Howerton LW, Amir M. *Campbell's Urology.* 4th ed. Philadelphia: WB Saunders; 1978.
6. Duckett JW. The island flap technique for hypospadias repair. *Urol Clin North Am.* 1981;8:503.
7. Quartey JKM. One-stage penile/preputial cutaneous island flap urethroplasty for urethral stricture: a preliminary report. *J Urol.* 1983;129:284.
8. Quartey JK, Accra G. One stage penile/preputial island flap urethroplasty for urethral strictures. Abstract #123, American Urological Association, Seventy-ninth Annual Meeting, May 6–10, 1984, New Orleans.
9. Singh M, Blandy J. The pathology of urethral stricture. *J Urol.* 1976;115:693.
10. Jordan GH. Management of anterior urethral stricture disease. In: Webster GD, ed. *Problems in Urology.* vol 1, no 2. Philadelphia: JB Lippincott; 1987:199–225.
11. Devine CJ Jr, Devine PC, Felderman TP, et al. Classification and standardization of urethral strictures. Abstract #325, American Urological Association, Seventy-eighth Annual Meeting, April 17–21, 1983, Las Vegas.
12. McAninch JW, Laing FC, Jeffrey RB. Sonourethrography in evaluation of urethral strictures. Abstract #427, American Urological Association, Eighty-first Annual Meeting, May 18–22, 1986, New York. *J Urol.* 135:210A.
13. Webster GD, Koefoot RB, Sihelnik SA. Urethroplasty management in 200 cases of urethral stricture: a rationale for procedure selection. *J Urol.* 1985;134:892.
14. Webster GD, Robertson CN. The vascularized skin island urethroplasty: its role and results in urethral stricture management. *J Urol.* 1985;1333:31.
15. Schellhammer PF, Jordan GH, Schlossberg SM. Tumors of the Penis. In: Walsh PC, Retik AB, Stamey TA, Vaughan ED, eds. *Campbell's Urology.* 6th ed. vol 2. Philadelphia: WB Saunders; 1992:1264–1298.
16. Attwater HL. The history of urethral stricture. *Br J Urol.* 1943;15:39.
17. Jordan GH. Management of anterior urethral stricture disease. In: Webster GD, Kirby R, King LR, Goldwasser B, eds. *Reconstructive Urology.* Oxford: Blackwell Scientific (in press).
18. Milroy EJ, Chapple C, Eldin A, Wallsten H. A new treatment for urethral strictures: a permanently implanted urethral stent. *J Urol.* 1989;141:1120–1122.
19. Yachia D, Beyar M. The use of three types of self-expanding and self-retaining temporary coil stents in the treatment of recurrent strictures in various parts of the urethra. Abstract 628. *J Urol.* 1992;147:369A.
20. Russell RH. The treatment of urethral stricture by excision. *Br J Surg.* 1914;2:375.
21. Jordan GH. Wide mobilization of the urethra: a cause for caution? Abstract 677. *J Urol.* 1988;139:332A.
22. Jordan GH, Secrest CL. Arteriography in select patients with posterior urethral distraction injuries. Abstract 308. *J Urol.* 1992;147:289A.
23. Presman D, Greenfield D. Reconstruction of the perineal urethra with a free full-thickness skin graft from the prepuce. *J Urol.* 1953;69:677.
24. Devine P, Fallon B, Devine C. Free full-thickness skin graft urethroplasty. *J Urol.* 1976;226:444.
25. Jordan GH. Principles of plastic surgery. In: Droller MJ, ed. *Surgical Management of Urologic Disease: An Anatomic Approach.* St. Louis: Mosby, 1992:1218–1237.
26. Dessanti A, Rigamonti W, Merulla V, Falchetti D, Caccia G. Autologous buccal mucosa graft for hypospadias repair: an initial report. *J Urol.* 1992;147:1081–1084.
27. McAninch JW, Laing FC, Jeffrey RB. Sonourethrography in evaluation of urethral strictures. Abstract #427, American Urological Association. Eighty-first Annual Meeting, May 18–22, 1986, New York.
28. Orandi A. One stage urethroplasty: 4-year follow-up. *J Urol.* 1972;207:977.
29. Jordan GH, Schlossberg SM. Genital skin islands based on dartos fascial pedicles. *Contemporary Urology* (in press).
30. Jordan GH, Secrest CL, Devine PC, Devine CJ Jr. Urethroplasty using scrotal skin islands based on the dartos fascia: A long-term followup (in preparation).
31. Jordan GH. Reconstruction of the meatus/fossa navicularis using flap techniques. In: Schreiter F. ed. *Plastic Reconstructive Surgery in Urology.* Stuttgart: Theime Verlag (in preparation).
32. Jordan GH. Reconstruction of the fossa navicularis. *J Urol.* 1987;138:102–104.

33. Jordan GH, Secrest CL. Fossa navicularis reconstruction: series with long-term followup (in preparation).
34. Schreiter F, Noll F. Meshgraft urethroplasty using split thickness skin graft of foreskin. *J Urol.* 1989;142:1223.
35. Jordan GH, Devine PC. Immediate management of external urethral injury. In: Cass AS, ed. *Genitourinary Trauma.* Boston: Blackwell Scientific; 1988:197–207.

# 24

# Benign Lesions of the Prostate and Vesical Neck and Their Surgical Management

*Stephen N. Rous*

Probably there is no single part of the male anatomy that is the cause of more rumors, misconceptions, apprehension, and distress than the prostate gland. The functions of this gland, along with the seminal vesicles, are to produce the fluid that serves as the vehicle in which the spermatozoa are conveyed to the outside and to furnish the latter with nutrient matter. The average man, unfortunately, fancies that his prostate gland is the seat of his sexual power and prowess and is intimately connected to his male ego; therefore he believes that any malfunction of this gland will lead to impotence, sterility, prostatic cancer, enlargement of the prostate, and a host of other conditions which are in no way connected with this gland. There is, moreover, probably no other organ in the body more prone to psychoneurotic manifestations, both real and imaginary.

## EMBRYOLOGY

During the twelfth week of embryonic life, the prostate gland develops from outgrowths of the prostatic urethra. Sprouts of urethral epithelium, which herald the appearance of the prostate, penetrate surrounding mesenchymal tissue and form five distinct groups of tubules. Two lateral groups originate from furrows on either side of Müller's hillock, the site of the future verumontanum. A middle group arises from the floor of the urethra proximal to the openings of the wolffian ducts; a posterior group appears distal to Müller's hillock. Anteriorly, a small group arises from the roof of the prostatic urethra. During the fourth month of fetal life these outgrowths develop into five groups of glands. They represent primitive lobes of the prostate. By the time of birth, the tubules have become enveloped in fibromuscular stroma, and the gland is surrounded by a capsule.[1]

Prior to the appearance of the prostate, the lower ends of the wolffian ducts migrate distally to open into the urethra at the site of the future verumontanum. The proximal part, extending from the vesical trigone to the verumontanum, originates from the terminal portion of the excretory ducts which are mesodermic. The distal segment, extending from the openings of the wolffian ducts to the membranous urethra, arises from an entodermal fundament, the pars pelvina of the urogenital sinus. Although the reason is obscure, these separate origins seem to account for the fact that benign hyperplasia almost universally develops from the region of the proximal urethra (the periurethral glands), whereas carcinoma originates from structures arising from the distal segment (the true prostate, chiefly the posterior lobe).[2]

## ANATOMY

The prostate gland is a musculoglandular organ that surrounds the prostatic urethra and may be likened to a very small apple with the core removed. The lumen formed by so removing the "core" is thus actually the prostatic urethra. The prostate is encased in a fibrous capsule (the true capsule), which may be likened to the skin of the apple. In size and shape the adult prostate gland resembles a horse chestnut, with an average weight of 20 g. The base of the gland is applied to the neck of the urinary bladder, with which it is contiguous. The apex of the gland abuts the superior leaf of the urogenital diaphragm. Posteriorly, the prostate lies against the anterior wall of the rectum, from which it is separated by a thin layer of rectovesical fascia; this fascia was first described by Denonvilliers and bears his name. It is formed by a fusion of the anterior and the posterior layers of pelvic peritoneum. The midanterior surface of the gland is attached to the undersurface of the pubis by two puboprostatic ligaments.

Many of the problems associated with prostatic surgery arise from the location of the gland. Since it lies deep within the bony pelvis, operative approach is a considerable problem. If approached by the suprapubic route, the bladder must be incised. Retropubically, there is an extensive vascular network. Perineally, there is danger of injury to the rectum and to the nerves that control urination and erection. In all approaches the proximity of the external urinary sphincter and the lower ends of the ureters create a hazard (Fig 1). In most operations the internal urinary sphincter is ablated. Sole dependence is thereby placed on the external sphincter.

The inferior vesical arteries, which are branches of the internal iliacs, provide the main blood supply (Fig 2). At the base of the prostate, these vessels branch into two groups of arteries; the urethral group enters the prostate at the vesicoprostatic junction to supply the vesical neck and the periurethral portion of the gland (Fig 3); the second group, the capsular arteries, enters the gland laterally and supplies the peripheral portion of the prostate and the distal portion of the prostatic urethra. In addition, the apex of the gland receives twigs from the internal pudendal artery.[3]

Veins from the prostate communicate freely with each other and with veins from the penis, bladder, and seminal vesicles (Fig 4). An anterior venous plexus (of Santorini) lies within the anatomic capsule of the prostate. The deep veins of this sinus are the ones most frequently perforated during transurethral prostatectomy. Veins from lateral venous plexuses coalesce to form the inferior vesical veins, which drain into the internal iliacs. The lateral venous plexuses may give rise to serious hemorrhage during total prostatectomy unless they are ligated early in the operation. In addition to free anastomoses with each other, the anterior and the lateral plexuses communicate with the hemorrhoidal and vesical plexuses and thence with the portal system.

The prostate is rich in lymphatics. Each glandular acinus is surrounded by a network of fine lymph vessels, and these unite into larger channels that lead to the periphery of the gland. They empty into lymph nodes lying alongside the external and the internal iliac arteries (Fig 5). In addition to following blood vessels, many lymphatics pursue the course of the ureters and the vasa deferentia.

The prostate is innervated by the autonomic nervous system, which supplies the smooth musculature; nerve impulses are relayed through the superior hypogastric, aortic, and pelvic plexuses.

In addition to the "classic" prostatic anatomy just described, more recent work on the structure of the prostate suggests that the prostate can be divided into several glandular and nonglandular components, all of which are encased in a common capsule.[6–10] The nonglandular components consist of the sphincters, fibromuscular stroma, and the prostatic capsule itself, and much of this tissue is concentrated in the anteromedial portion of the prostate.

Four distinct glandular portions of the

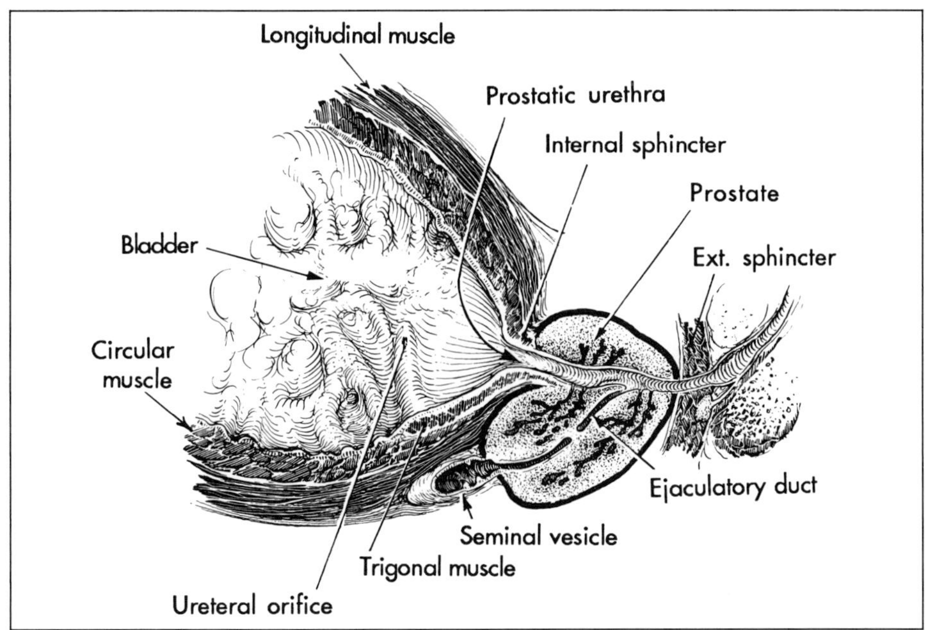


**Fig 1.** Normal prostate. Relationship to structures of urinary and genital tracts.*

**Fig 2.** Arterial supply of prostate.

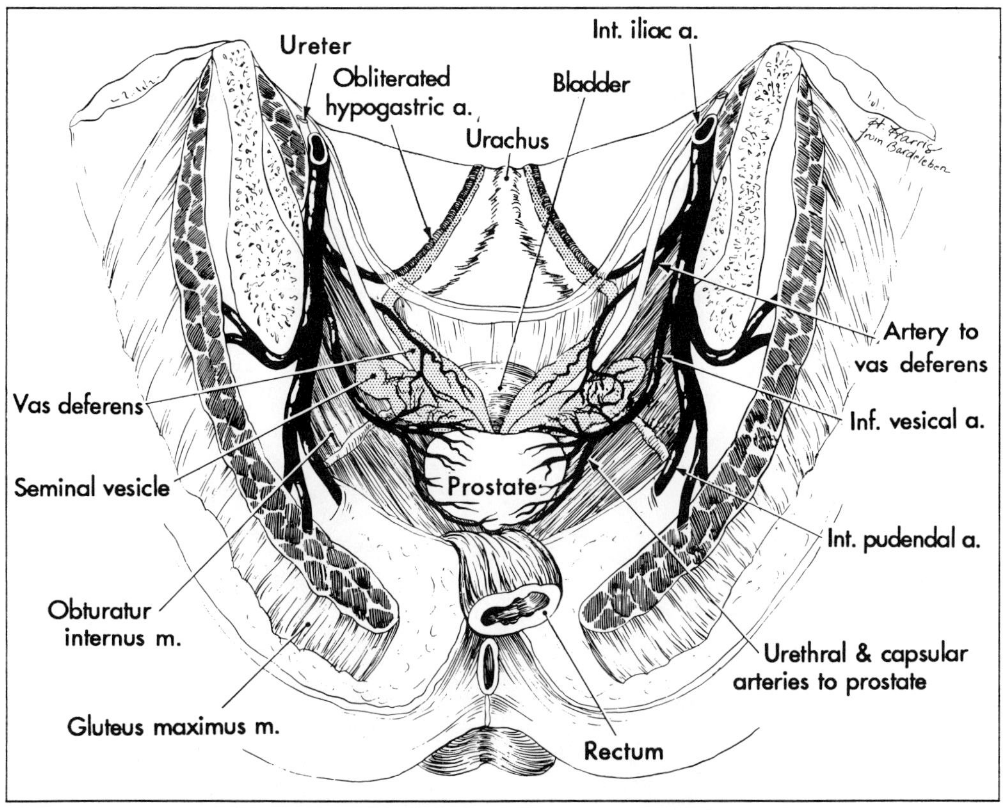


*Except for Figs 52, 65, and 66, the illustrations used in this chapter are reproduced from HM Weyrauch's *Surgery of the Prostate*, with permission of the publisher, WB Saunders, Philadelphia.

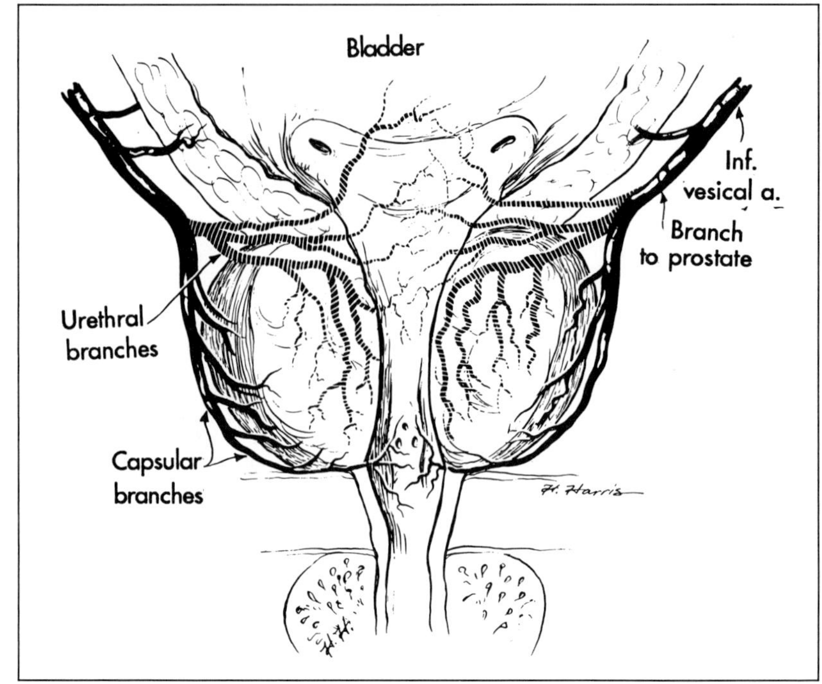


**Fig 3.** Branching of prostatic artery. Urethral and capsular distribution. (After Flocks.)

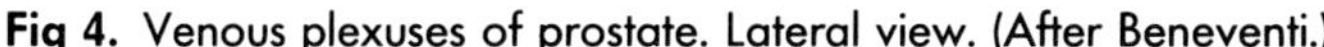

**Fig 4.** Venous plexuses of prostate. Lateral view. (After Beneventi.)

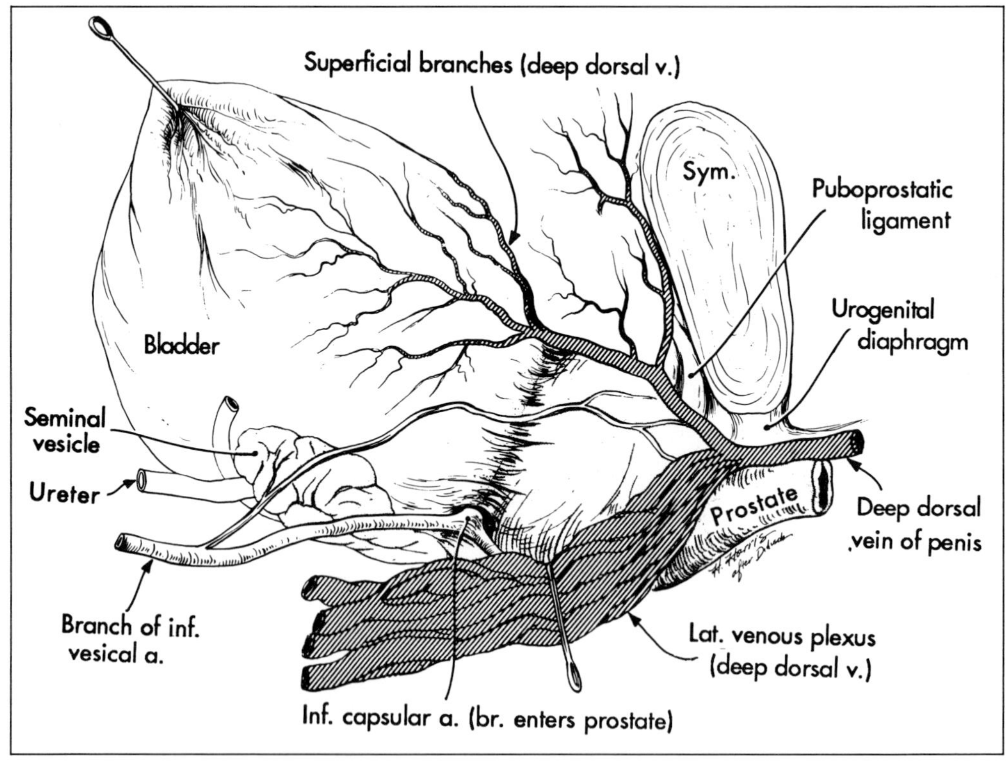

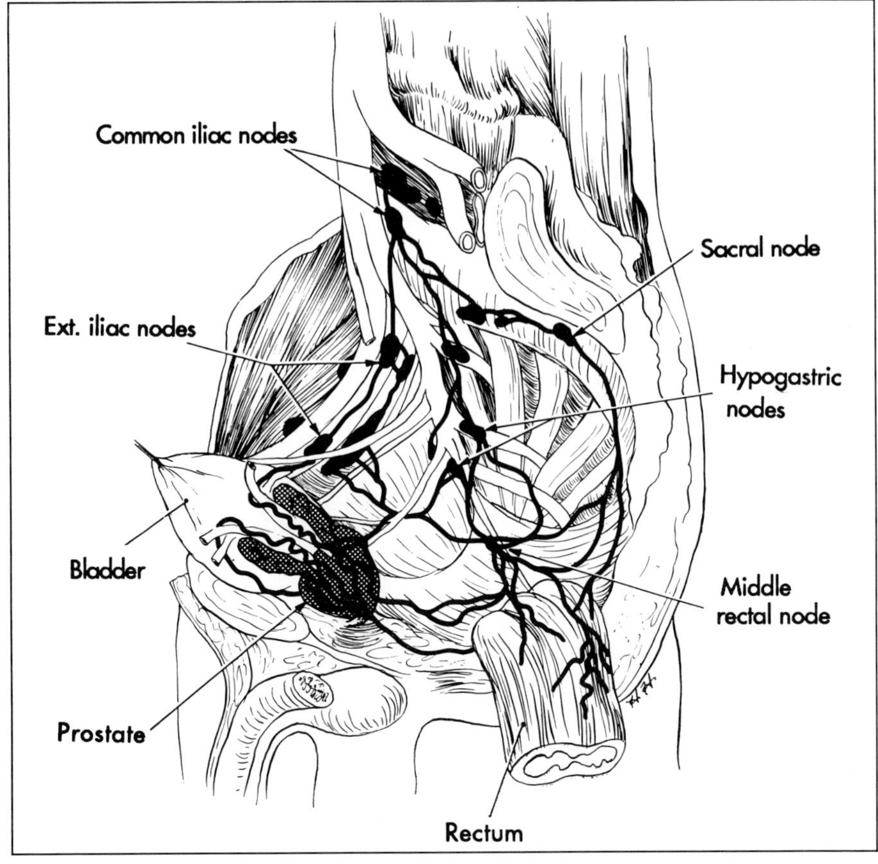


**Fig 5.** Lymphatic drainage of prostate.

prostate can be identified, and it is perhaps easiest to visualize these considering the urethra itself as a landmark that is divided into proximal and distal segments. The ducts of the great majority of the glandular prostate as well as the ejaculatory ducts empty into the distal urethral segment.

The peripheral zone, the largest of the four glandular zones, comprises about 70% of the prostatic mass. It is this peripheral zone that is the site of origin of most prostatic carcinomas. The central zone comprises about one fourth of the total prostate gland and forms much of the base of the prostate. The most proximal portion of the prostatic urethra is related to the transition zone and to the periurethral gland region, which is much smaller than the transition zone itself. The transition zone and the periurethral zone together are the sites of origin of benign prostatic hyperplasia, and this condition is predominantly one of transition zone enlargement, which manifests itself as lateral lobe hyperplasia.

## PHYSIOLOGY

The sole function of the prostate is external secretion. The gland manufactures and stores fluids that convey sperm during copulation. Prostatic and seminal vesicle secretions constitute 95% of the volume (2 to 4 mL) of spermatic fluid. These secretions provide a vehicle for conveying sperm and furnish the latter with extracellular foodstuffs, supplementing their intracellular nutritional reserve.[4,5]

High concentrations of fructose, calcium, citric acid, and phosphorylcholine, as well as enzymes, are found in prostatic and seminal vesicle secretions. Acid prosphatase and prostate specific antigen (PSA) are found in the prostate, and their serum level is of clinical significance. Elevated serum levels are almost always diagnostic of disseminated cancer of the prostate. Liquefaction of seminal fluid results from a proteolytic prostatic enzyme.

## SURGICAL PATHOLOGY

Because of the prostate's anatomic location, most diseases produce urinary obstruction either by compressing the posterior urethra or by occluding the vesical neck; either or both of these entities are often referred to simply as bladder outlet obstruction. Intelligent management depends upon a knowledge of the type and pathogenesis of the causative lesion.

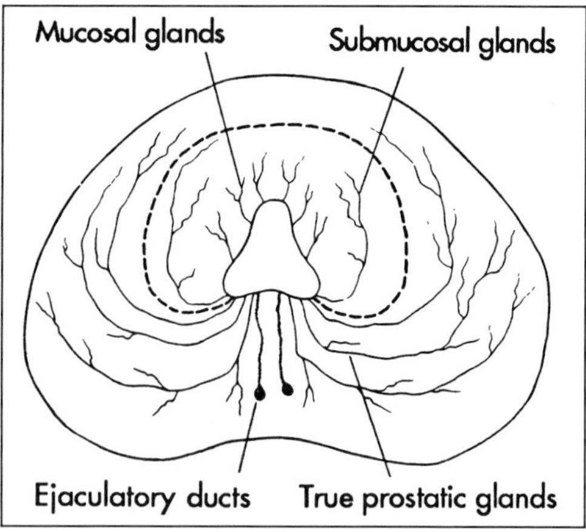


**Fig 6.** Origin of benign prostatic hyperplasia. Periurethral glands within dotted line. True prostatic glands (**outside dotted line** ) become compressed with development of hyperplasia. Cross-section of prostate. (After Young, 1926.)

### Benign Prostatic Hyperplasia

This is the most common cause of bladder outlet obstruction. Its incidence, as indicated by Randall's study of 1,215 necropsy cases, is greater than 50% in men over the age of 50 years; its occurrence rises to 75% in men past the eighth decade.[11]

The precise etiology of benign prostatic hyperplasia remains unknown, although it is felt to be related to the action of dihydrotestosterone on the cells of the prostatic acini.[12]

Of numerous terms used to designate benign prostatic hyperplasia, the only accurate one is *periurethral adenoma*. The site of enlargement is the periurethral glands and not the true prostatic glands (Fig 6). The process is one of hyperplasia, which consists of an increase in the number of cells rather than hypertrophy of the tissues.

In hyperplasia, areas of fibrous and muscular tissue develop from the acini and the stroma of the mucosal and submucosal glands. With progressive enlargement, the true prostate is displaced peripherally. It is gradually compressed into a narrow, fibroglandular structure. Between the hyperplasia and the compressed prostatic tissue, a well-defined cleavage plane is marked by a layer of fibrous tissue known as the "surgical capsule." On cross section the false encapsulation of the hyperplastic tissue is easily visible and can readily be separated by enucleation. This characteristic is invaluable to the surgeon and influences the surgical technique of open adenectomy (conservative prostatectomy).

Benign hyperplasia is classified according to the point of origin of the lobes of hyperplastic tissue. Middle-lobe hyperplasia arises from the posterior vesical neck and grows in a direction away from the examining digital rectal finger. It is, therefore, due to this intravesical location, not possible to detect a middle-lobe hyperplasia upon rectal examination. By its "ball-value" action, this type of enlargement may result in severe urinary obstruction and retention.

On the other hand, when hyperplasia develops in the lateral lobes, massive enlargements well situated for rectal palpation may result in little urinary obstruction. This is because passageways that permit the escape of urine are formed around the lobes (Fig 7A). It is also because greater enlargement of the lateral lobes toward the periphery of the gland (the lobes therefore being palpable) does not always mean great enlargement of the lateral lobes inwardly to obstruct the prostatic urethra. By providing passageways, lateral lobe enlargements may compensate for a median lobe

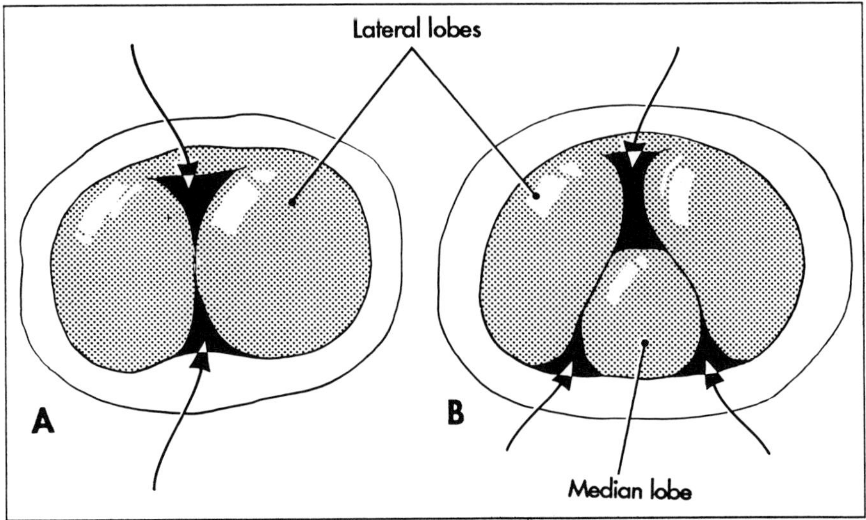


**Fig 7.** Hyperplastic lobes may allow passageway for urine. **A:** Simple bilateral lobe hyperplasia. **B:** Bilateral lobe hyperplasia accommodates for middle lobe enlargement.

(Fig 7B). Thus, the degree of obstruction is not proportional to the magnitude of obstructing tissue nor to the severity of the symptoms.

Posterior commissural hyperplasia is frequently confused with middle-lobe hyperplasia. Instead of lying in a submucosal position, this hyperplasia arises from glandular acini located more deeply, below the floor of the urethra. The hyperplastic tissue is separated from the urethra by the heavy musculature of the trigone. This must be kept in mind during surgery for benign hyperplasia to ensure that hyperplastic tissue is not left intact beneath the vesical neck.

Although the glandular tissue of the anterior commissure usually undergoes prepubertal atrophy, it occasionally persists. Such an anterior lobe lies in the roof of the prostatic urethra. If careful inspection is not directed anteriorly during transurethral prostatectomy, this type of hyperplasia may escape detection and perpetuate the obstructive symptoms.

In rare instances a small group of glandular acini gives rise to subtrigonal lobe hyperplasia in the midportion of the trigone.

Prostatic hyperplasia frequently presents as a multilobed enlargement involving more than one group of glands. Combinations of lateral lobes with a middle lobe or with posterior commissural hyperplasia comprise the most common multilobe types.

## Median Bar

Of the benign causes of vesical neck obstruction, median bar ranks next to benign prostatic hyperplasia in frequency of occurrence. Usually appearing before the patient reaches the age of 45, the lesion constitutes an elevation of the posterior vesical neck. It is composed mainly of fibrous tissue; however, glandular and muscular elements may participate. The lesion is often secondary to infection of the posterior urethra and vesical neck. It is not associated with any form of prostatic enlargement.

Cystoscopically, a median bar appears as an abrupt elevation of the posterior aspect of the vesical neck. It is to be differentiated from contracture of the vesical neck, usually a congenital or an iatrogenic lesion, in which fibrous tissue involves the entire periphery of the internal sphincter. A major cause of persistent prostatic infection is some form of obstruction, such as benign hyperplasia or median bar, which must be removed to attain a cure.

### Tuberculosis of the Prostate

Whereas primary tuberculosis of the prostate is a pathologic rarity, secondary tuberculosis is a frequent clinical problem. Spread, in the latter type, is either from the kidney via the urinary tract or from the epididymis by way of the vas and the ejaculatory ducts. With the availability of effective chemotherapy, the need for surgery in tuberculous prostatitis has been practically eliminated.

### Prostatic Calculi

From a surgical standpoint, prostatic calculi are of threefold significance: (1) they may lead to a mistaken diagnosis of carcinoma,[13] (2) they frequently occur in association with benign hyperplasia and carcinoma of the prostate and should be completely removed at the time of prostatectomy, and (3) they may cause urinary obstruction and require surgical removal.

When calculi are associated with benign hyperplasia they tend to develop around the periphery of the adenomatous process, either in the surgical capsule or superficially in the compressed cortex. Investigative work seems to suggest that corpora amylacea, thought to be the result of normal aging processes, may be the precursors of pathologic concretions (prostatic calculi).[14]

### Traumatic Lesions

Because of its protected position deep within the bony pelvis, the prostate is rarely injured by external trauma, although a shearing of the prostatic urethra just distal to the veru may occur with pelvic fractures and/or straddle injuries. Surgery on or in the vicinity of the prostate and improper urethral instrumentation are the usual causes of injury to the gland.

Injuries may result in (1) urinary extravasation, (2) hemorrhage, (3) secondary infection, (4) urinary obstruction from disruption of the prostatic urethra, (5) stricture formation, and (6) urinary incontinence from damage to the internal and external sphincters.

### Congenital Anomalies

Congenital anomalies of surgical interest include hypertrophy of the verumontanum, valves of the posterior urethra, contracture of the vesical neck, and cysts of the prostate. All are rare.

## PROSTATIC AND/OR VESICAL NECK OBSTRUCTION

### Diagnosis

As is perhaps evident from the discussion of the surgical pathology of bladder outlet obstruction, voiding is simplistically a function of two parameters: contractions of the detrusor muscle on the one side and urethral resistance anyplace from the bladder neck to the meatus on the other side.[15] The urethral resistance area of primary interest is the prostatic urethra including the bladder neck.

As the benign prostatic hyperplasia (periurethral adenoma) develops, there is increased resistance to the flow of urine. The detrusor muscle is the same as muscle anywhere else in the body, and when it must work against an increased resistance it will undergo a work hypertrophy. The bladder trigone, because it is different embryologically from the rest of the bladder (it is of mesodermal origin while the rest of the bladder is of endodermal origin), happens to be the first part of the bladder to undergo this work hypertrophy and also happens to be the most sensitive part of the bladder. Since it additionally is the most dependent portion of the bladder, small amounts of urine, by coming in contact with the trigone, are detected by the hypertrophied trigone which is extremely sensitive to stimuli; this is perceived by the patient as a desire to void.[16]

### Symptoms

It is this hypertrophied and sensitive (irritable) bladder trigone that is responsible for the most frequent early symptom of bladder outlet obstruction: nocturia (being awakened during the night to void). The nocturia occurs because the urine formed during sleep irritates the hypertrophied and irritable trigone and produces a voiding urge that is sufficient to waken an individual. One may ask why this trigonal hypertrophy that produces a nocturia does not produce a daytime frequency as well, since in theory both should be present. When most individuals are busy working during the day, they are usually not aware of early voiding urges, which tend to be overlooked in favor of the usual daytime occupation. At night, with no diversions except sleep, the voiding urge produced by the hypertrophied trigone is readily perceived, bringing about a state of wakefulness and a desire to void. In fact, as the disease process progresses and the trigonal hypertrophy and irritability become greater, daytime frequency does become a reality, bringing with it a desire to void when much smaller amounts of urine than usual are in the bladder.

The pathologic process of prostatic enlargement (periurethral adenomatous enlargement) is an inexorable one and progresses steadily, whether it be slowly or rapidly. As it progresses, the patient will often notice a weakening of his urinary stream; the best way to elicit this symptom from the patient is to inquire about the strength of his urinary stream when he is voiding into a standup type urinal such as is commonly seen in public restrooms. The patient must be asked whether his stream goes straight out and hits the back of the urinal or whether it arches in a downward trajectory and hits for the first time at or near the bottom of the urinal. Another sign of increasing weakness of the urinary stream may be the observation of the patient or his wife that the floor is frequently wet in front of the toilet bowl at home. The patient, being used to a stronger stream, still stands a little farther back from the urinal than his weakened stream will now allow, and the floor frequently gets wet.

During this period, which may last from many months to a few years, the bladder musculature progressively undergoes a work hypertrophy secondary to the increased resistance to the flow of urine presented by the gradually enlarging prostatic obstruction (periurethral adenomatous obstruction). This hypertrophy of the bladder musculature is uneven and irregular, since the bladder wall itself is not uniform; it is composed of three interdigitating muscle layers. When viewed cystoscopically, the bladder wall hypertrophy or trabeculation sometimes gives the appearance of a piece of Swiss cheese, with prominent bands of muscle interspersed among thinned out areas of bladder wall (cellules) that eventually may "blow out" and become diverticulae if the obstructive process is allowed to continue indefinitely. As the bladder outlet obstruction progresses, the bladder trabeculation, with or without diverticulae formation, usually becomes more severe.

As long as the bladder is able to empty itself following voiding, the bladder is said to be compensated; during this period of time the patient's symptoms are usually limited to those already noted, ie, nocturia, frequency, and weakness of the urinary stream. Obviously, however, the bladder musculature cannot hypertrophy without limit in its efforts to empty itself against an increased resistance, and as the prostatic obstruction becomes more progressive the bladder is no longer able to empty itself during voiding. At this point, the bladder is considered to be decompensated, and a residual urine will remain in the bladder following voiding. When such bladder decompensation occurs, a whole new set of symptoms will sooner or later develop. The patient will probably not perceive any of these symptoms while the residual urine is very low (less than an ounce); however, the buildup of residual urine is an inevitable phenomenon, and as the amount of urine increases the patient will notice such things as intermittency (a cessation of the urinary stream before voiding has been completed, followed within seconds by a continuation of the stream). This phenomenon of intermittency occurs because, following the initial detrusor contraction, a significant amount of urine still remains in the bladder; therefore, following the refractory period for the bladder smooth musculature, a second and weaker contraction occurs, bringing about the resumption of the urinary stream. Terminal dribbling may occur for these same reasons: the patient thinks he has finished voiding, closes his trousers, and then wets himself with another half-ounce or ounce of urine that appears because of this secondary bladder contraction.

As the residual urine builds up, it is clear that there will be a short postvoiding time interval before the patient feels the desire to void again. This is because urine normally forms in the kidneys and runs into the bladder at about a rate of 1 $cm^3$ per minute. If a patient normally has a voiding urge when there is 6 to 8 ounces of urine present in the bladder, and if that individual normally leaves 4 to 6 ounces behind following voiding, it will not take very long before the additional urine necessary to produce a voiding urge has come from the kidneys into the bladder. Perhaps most important, however, in the bladder that has become decompensated and that carries residual urine is the inevitable onset of infection. Bacteria that may normally be present in the distal urethra and ordinarily are nonpathogenic to a normal bladder sooner or later produce acute bladder infection when allowed to grow in the perfect culture medium that residual urine provides. The onset of such acute cystitis dramatically increases the patient's frequency, producing an urgency (the desire to void immediately) and a marked discomfort on urinating (dysuria), as well as foul-smelling urine. The latter is due to the release of large amounts of ammonia that is produced by the presence of urea-splitting organisms such as *Proteus,* if that is the etiologic organism. In fact, many clinicians believe that almost any urinary tract pathogen can split urea and thereby release ammonia if it is present in a large enough quantity. The symptoms of acute cystitis can be relieved by appropriate antimicrobial therapy, but the return of these symptoms again and again is inevitable until the bladder outlet obstruction is relieved and residual urine no longer exists. A complication of acute cystitis may be the sudden and unexpected onset of gram-negative sepsis, should the infected bladder urine gain a portal of entry into the bloodstream through one of the bladder vessels.

The symptomatology of bladder outlet obstruction that has just been described depicts the commonest findings that the physician will encounter in taking a history when he is trying to determine if his patient is suffering from this condition. However, there may be as many as 10% to 15% of individuals with severe bladder outlet obstruction in whom these symptoms will not be apparent in the course of interviewing the patient. The aptly named condition of "silent prostatism" applies to those few individuals who are honestly quite unaware of any change whatever in their voiding pattern. The complete absence of these symptoms as far as the patient is concerned may be because they have been so very slow and insidious in onset, over a long period of time, that he is truly unaware of any change in his voiding pattern; it is also possible that in view of the close correlation in the minds of many men between their voiding function and their sexual function, some individuals subconsciously deny that anything could be "wrong" with their voiding pattern. Regardless of the reason, the fact remains that a number of patients will not give a "classic" history for bladder outlet obstruction. Such individuals characteristically present one day in the hospital emergency room or the physician's office in acute urinary retention, and it is incumbent on the examining physician to initiate a diagnostic workup for bladder outlet obstruction, even though the patient does not give a history compatible with such a diagnosis. Finally, a small number of patients who may either have had the classic symptomatology of bladder outlet obstruction or may have had "silent prostatism" present with the seeming paradox of urinary incontinence. When a man over the age of 40 presents with such incontinence, the first thought the examining physician should have is that this may be an overflow or a paradoxic incontinence based upon bladder outlet obstruction and a high residual urine with a resulting leakage of "overflow" urine that just cannot be accommodated in the bladder. Whether an individual develops an acute urinary retention or an overflow incontinence is probably a function of the obstructive pattern of his prostatic lobes within the prostatic urethra and whether or not an open channel exists for overflow urine.

Certain individuals with bladder outlet obstruction, regardless of their history and presenting findings, may additionally have signs and symptoms that are secondary to uremia; these may range from loss of appetite, malaise, nausea, vomiting, headache, and lethargy, to convulsions, coma, and even death. While the findings associated with uremia are not often seen as the presenting symptoms of bladder outlet obstruction, this condition does occur often enough that a brief discussion of its etiology is indicated. Uremia results from a residual urine that causes significant back pressure upon the ureters and the collecting system of the kidneys and that is sufficiently high to therefore diminish the glomerular filtration rate and lead to an elevation of the blood urea nitrogen and the creatinine levels. Recognition of this possibility is incumbent upon the examining physician in those individuals whose symptoms suggest uremia.

## Physical Examination

A complete physical examination, which ideally should be carried out, is often not done by the practicing urologist because of time constraints and because his patient has usually been referred by an internist or a generalist who presumably has already carried out a complete exam. In any case, it is the author's firm conviction that if the patient ultimately comes to surgery, a thorough preoperative physical examination should be carried out, preferably by a competent internist.

The urologic portion of the physical examination is mandatory; it might begin with an abdominal examination to detect enlarged kidneys. The kidneys are not normally palpable, and in cases in which one can readily feel the lower pole of either kidney, strong consideration must be given to the diagnosis of an enlarged kidney, a kidney in an unusually thin individual, or an unusually mobile kidney. In addition, lower abdominal palpation and percussion is indicated to look for a distended bladder or for suprapubic tenderness that might result from infection in the bladder. Particular attention must be paid to an examination of the external genitalia; in uncircumcised men this should include retraction of the foreskin to permit a careful examination of the glans. Palpation along the course of the urethra is indicated to detect any scarring or fibrosis that may accompany urethral stricture. The testes should be carefully palpated to be certain that a testicular tumor does not exist, and the cord and the inguinal canals should also be palpated for abnormalities. Finally, and possibly most important in the diagnosis of bladder outlet obstruction, digital rectal examination of the prostate must be carried out. It is important in the course of this examination to sweep the examining finger around in a 360° arc to make sure that a palpable rectal carcinoma is not overlooked because of its posterior or its lateral location. The sphincter tone should also be noted, and once the finger is inserted well up into the rectum, the glans penis should be briskly squeezed so as to elicit the normal bulbocavernosus reflex. When this reflex is normal, squeezing the glans penis will produce a sharp contraction of the anal sphincter on the examining finger, thereby signifying an intact sacral reflex arc. The absence of this bulbocavernosus reflex may indicate abnormal bladder innervation and perhaps a neurogenic bladder. Even though the pudendal nerve innervates the anal sphincter and the pelvic nerve innervates the bladder, the two nerves travel in close anatomic proximity; a defect in the pudendal innervation is usually accompanied by a defect in pelvic nerve innervation. A neurogenic bladder may often be suspected when a patulous anal sphincter is noted upon initial insertion of the examining finger; nonetheless, the bulbocavernosus reflex should always be tested whenever a rectal examination is done.

Palpation of the prostate gland itself, while necessary to a complete urologic examination, may or may not be diagnostic in determining bladder outlet obstruction. Some types of obstruction, such as median lobe or median bar enlargement, absolutely cannot be detected on rectal examination since they are inward encroachments upon the lumen of the prostatic urethra and do not grow outward toward the periphery of the gland. Additionally, rectal palpation of enlarged lateral lobes is not an unfailing sign that the lateral lobes are also enlarged intraurethrally and are producing symptoms of outlet obstruction.

In lateral lobe hyperplasia, rectal palpation will usually disclose a more or less symmetric enlargement of both lateral lobes, with an elastic consistency and a smooth surface. The median sulcus, which is present in early lateral lobe enlargement, is usually obliterated as the hyperplastic process progresses (Fig 8). The posterior lobe of the prostate gland does not participate in the process of benign bladder outlet obstruction. It is significant in that it is the site of origin of the majority of prostatic cancers, most of which are palpable.

## Laboratory Tests

Routine urinalysis and culture should be performed on a midstream clean catch specimen, with the foreskin retracted and the glans penis thoroughly scrubbed in uncircumcised individuals. Such examination of the urine should include the physical, chemical, and microscopic components of the urine and should preferably be done by the urologist. Culture of the urine may be warranted if there has been any history of urinary tract infection, if the patient's symptomatology would suggest an infection, or if an infection needs to be ruled out. Moreover, the presence of more than a very few white cells per high power field should also call for a urine culture. The urine specimen should be collected prior to rectal examination to avoid contamination of the urine with prostatic secretions.

Renal function tests are helpful and are often necessary to determine the presence and degree of renal impairment. The phenolsulfonphthalein (PSP) test is a simple test that measures renal tubular excretory function; it is most conveniently done while the patient is still in the waiting room. This is a very rough screening test for tubular function, and many factors can produce falsely depressed values. Normally, 25% to 50% of the intravenously injected dye is excreted

**Fig 8.** Rectal findings in benign hyperplasia of prostate.

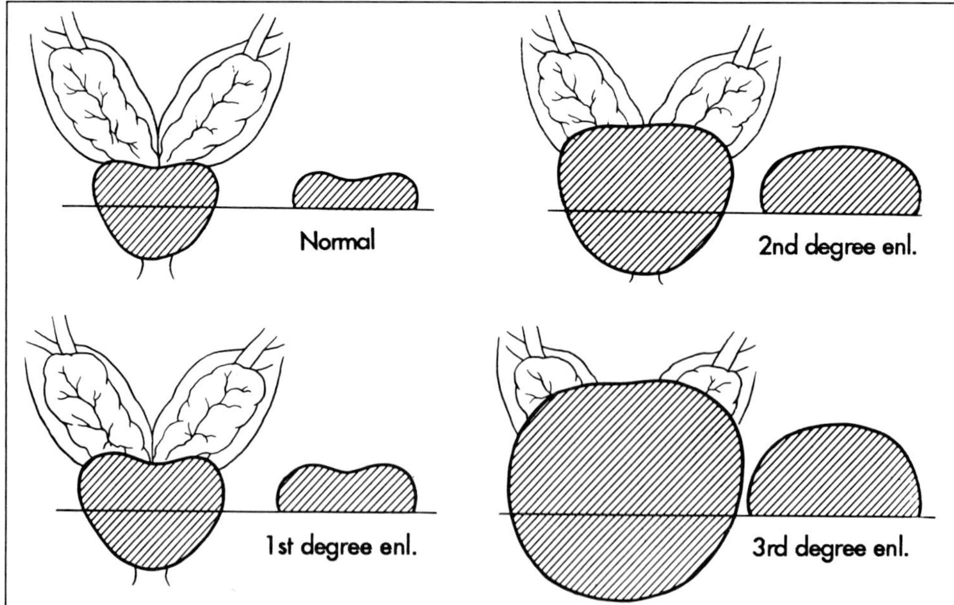

in the urine in 15 minutes if renal tubular function is normal and if there is no significant retention of urine in the bladder after voiding. Many individuals cannot, however, urinate on demand, and this is one of the failings of the test. Other commonly performed tests of renal function are blood urea nitrogen and serum creatinine levels, although these must usually be done in a professional laboratory and not in the urologist's office.

## Roentgenologic Studies

Excretory urography is frequently indicated in cases of bladder outlet obstruction to determine the status of the upper urinary tract prior to any contemplated surgery. In advanced cases of bladder outlet obstruction, unilateral or bilateral hydroureteronephrosis may be present and catheter drainage prior to surgery may be advantageous in these individuals. In addition, excretory urography with voiding antegrade cystourethrography can detect unexpected urethral strictures that might alter the planned surgical approach. On the excretory cystograms, intravesical protrusion of median or lateral lobes will produce a filling defect in the base of the bladder and thereby provide additional information on the exact status of the bladder outlet obstruction. Bladder wall changes such as hypertrophy and trabeculation may also be seen in the excretory cystogram. The postvoiding film supplies information concerning the amount of residual urine without the disadvantages of catheterization; it may also permit visualization of a bladder diverticulum that was not noticed on the regular cystogram. Finally, the bladder and the prostatic regions may be inspected on the preliminary film [kidney, ureter, and bladder (KUB)] for the presence of bladder and/or prostatic stones.

Although some have recently advocated omitting the excretory urogram in patients about to undergo prostatic surgery, I feel that it still has a place in the preoperative assessment of the patient's urinary tract. It is often a major factor in deciding whether or not prostatic surgery is indicated, and it is very helpful to have a baseline excretory urogram for reference should a patient be found to have hydroureteronephrosis or nonfunction of a kidney following surgery. Also, the potential of finding significant genitourinary tract pathology unrelated to the prostatic enlargement would seem to add to the wisdom of preliminary urograms.

It must be pointed out, however, that excretory urography is not without risk of both morbidity and even mortality (death rates as high as 1 in 20 000 have been reported).[15] In patients with microscopic or gross hematuria, an excretory urogram is essential for the evaluation of the upper urinary tract. However, for those patients with benign prostatic hyperplasia (BPH) who do not have microscopic or gross hematuria, the upper urinary tracts can very adequately be evaluated by means of renal nuclear imaging and renal ultrasound.

**Prostatic Ultrasound and CT Scans.** Although very ingenious rectal probes have been developed to measure the size of the prostate by ultrasound, I feel that such diagnostic modalities do not add significantly to the knowledge that may be gained from the excretory urogram, cystoscopy, and the digital rectal examination, particularly when the rectal examination is done at the same time as cystoscopy, thereby allowing the examiner to estimate the bulk of prostatic tissue between the cystoscope and the examining finger.[17] Similarly, although CT scans of the pelvis can delineate the prostate quite graphically, they do not really have a place in establishing the diagnosis of bladder outlet obstruction.

**Urodynamic Studies.** Another very helpful parameter in determining the presence and the degree of bladder outlet obstruction is the peak voiding rate. Although sophisticated studies using costly urodynamic equipment can be helpful in measuring such things as intravesical pressure and intraurethral pressure, I feel that the most helpful and valid measurement in the patient with bladder outlet obstructon is the peak voiding flow rate. Although this measurement can be made in a most sophisticated manner using costly devices, it may be determined just as well by means of a stop watch and a measuring container, with the patient allowing the peak volume middle portion of his voiding stream to go into the container while the examiner holds a stop watch (during this peak voiding period). Flow rates are age-related, but in general rates of 20 mL/second or greater are normal, and a diagnosis of bladder outlet obstruction may very safely be made (in the absence of a urethral stricture or a neurogenic bladder) when the flow rate is 10 mL/second or less. Such measurements should be undertaken only when the bladder is full and when the patient has a strong voiding urge.

## Cystourethroscopy

Endoscopic visualization of the urethra and the bladder will contribute vital confirmatory information concerning the existence (or absence) of bladder outlet obstruction, as well as the specific type of obstruction if present (Fig 9). This information is most important in determining the need for operation, as well as in selecting the most advantageous surgical procedure. The introduction into the bladder of a cystourethroscope carries with it the potential hazard of infection, particularly in patients carrying a residual urine; it is therefore wise to delay cystourethroscopy in those individuals in whom a significant residual urine is suspected or documented until the patient is hospitalized. Endoscopic examination following hospitalization can be done as a final diagnostic step a day or so before surgery or it can preferably be carried out immediately prior to surgery under the same anesthetic when it is strongly felt that surgical intervention will be necessary. When cystoscopy is done under an anesthetic, it greatly facilitates a digital rectal examination simultaneous with cystoscopy, and this "bimanual" approach allows for more accurate prognostications on the size of the prostate gland than either cystoscopy alone or digital rectal examination alone.

**Fig 9.** Cystourethroscopy. Small trilobed benign hyperplasia. First-degree enlargement. Small median and small intraurethral lateral lobe enlargement.

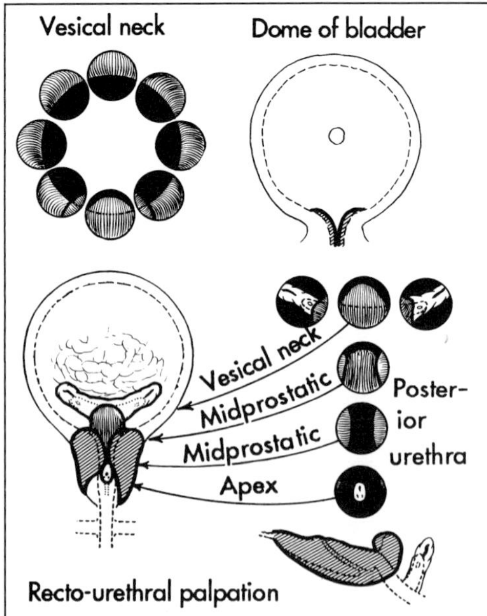


## Treatment

### Nonsurgical*

**Surgical.** Surgical measures remain the preferred method for removing benign obstructions of the prostate and vesical neck. I generally place the indications for surgery into subjective and objective categories. The first, subjective, consists of the patient's symptoms as reported by the patient; if there are *no* objective indications for surgery, I will generally let the patient determine if and when he wants to have surgery.[16] However, if the patient has objective indications for surgery, with or without any subjective indications, then I will usually recommend surgery. The greater (in number or in severity) the objective symptoms, the greater the urgency for surgery.

*Subjective* symptoms are:

1. Nocturia
2. Frequency
3. Weak urinary stream
4. Intermittency
5. Hesitancy
6. Terminal dribbling

*Nonsurgical techniques will be discussed in Chapter 00.

The *objective* findings warranting surgery are[18]:

1. Evidence of bladder outlet obstruction such as residual urine (should probably be well over 100 $cm^3$ before it becomes the sole indication for surgery)
2. Bladder trabeculation
3. Back pressure on kidneys producing decreased renal function and/or
4. Dilation of kidneys and ureters and recurrent urinary tract infection

Other indications for surgery include acute urinary retention and overflow incontinence. A final, and very uncommon, indication for surgery is hemorrhage from dilated blood vessels related to the BPH.

The patient's general condition is assessed during the preliminary examination, preferably by a competent internist. Any coexisting disease is recognized and is treated before operation.

Intercurrent urologic conditions may influence the proper time for prostatectomy. When there is neoplasm of the urinary bladder, this should usually be treated first. Operation on a large bladder neoplasm at the same time as prostatectomy may lead to implantation of neoplastic cells in the prostatic fossa; operation on a small bladder tumor may properly be done at the same time as the prostate surgery. If the preoperative excretory urograms reveal a space-consuming lesion of the kidney suggestive of malignancy, the kidney should be further investigated and possibly explored prior to prostatectomy.

Concurrent infection should be treated by appropriate antimicrobial agents. Chronic urinary infection is, however, difficult or impossible to eradicate prior to removing an obstruction.

The need for preliminary catheter drainage is determined by the degree of impairment of renal function caused by back pressure. A prime indication for preliminary drainage is decreased renal function in the presence of hydroureter and hydronephrosis. However, if initial blood urea nitrogen and creatinine levels indicate minimal or no reduction in renal function, preliminary catheter drainage is not usually necessary prior to surgery.

If preliminary catheter drainage is indicated, it should continue until the patient's creatinine and blood urea nitrogen (BUN) levels have "bottomed out"; that is, catheter drainage should continue until maximal improvement in renal function has been obtained, at which time prostatic surgery may be carried out with far less risk to the patient than would have been the case had surgery been undertaken before the renal function had reached its maximum status. Preliminary catheter drainage may also prove beneficial in the presence of acute infection and to control hemorrhage from massive prostatic hyperplasia. When preoperative urinary drainage is indicated, an indwelling urethral catheter is preferable; suprapubic cystostomy becomes necessary when a patient cannot tolerate a urethral catheter or when a severe urethral stricture precludes its insertion.

Prophylactic bilateral vasectomy (Fig 10) has reduced the incidence of postprostatectomy epididymitis from 25% to less than 1%. In my experience, however, uncomplicated epididymitis occurs so infrequently as to suggest that there is just no need to do routine vasectomies prior to transurethral resection (TUR). However, in the patients with infected urine, a history of epididymitis, or in those who have had preliminary catheter drainage, prophylactic vasectomy may be beneficial.

## SELECTION OF OPERATION

Selection of the operation best suited to the individual patient is fundamental to a successful result. In some cases, circumstances permit only one satisfactory operation; in others, two or more options are available. Sometimes a surgeon's deficiencies in one procedure will indicate the choice of another. The transurethral, perineal, suprapubic, and retropubic approaches are in common usage today. Each has its advantages and its disadvantages.[19]

There is a prevalent misconception that transurethral prostatectomy is less hazardous than open prostatectomy. This is true only when the circumstances are propitious, ie, when the caliber of the urethra is adequate and the amount of tissue to be

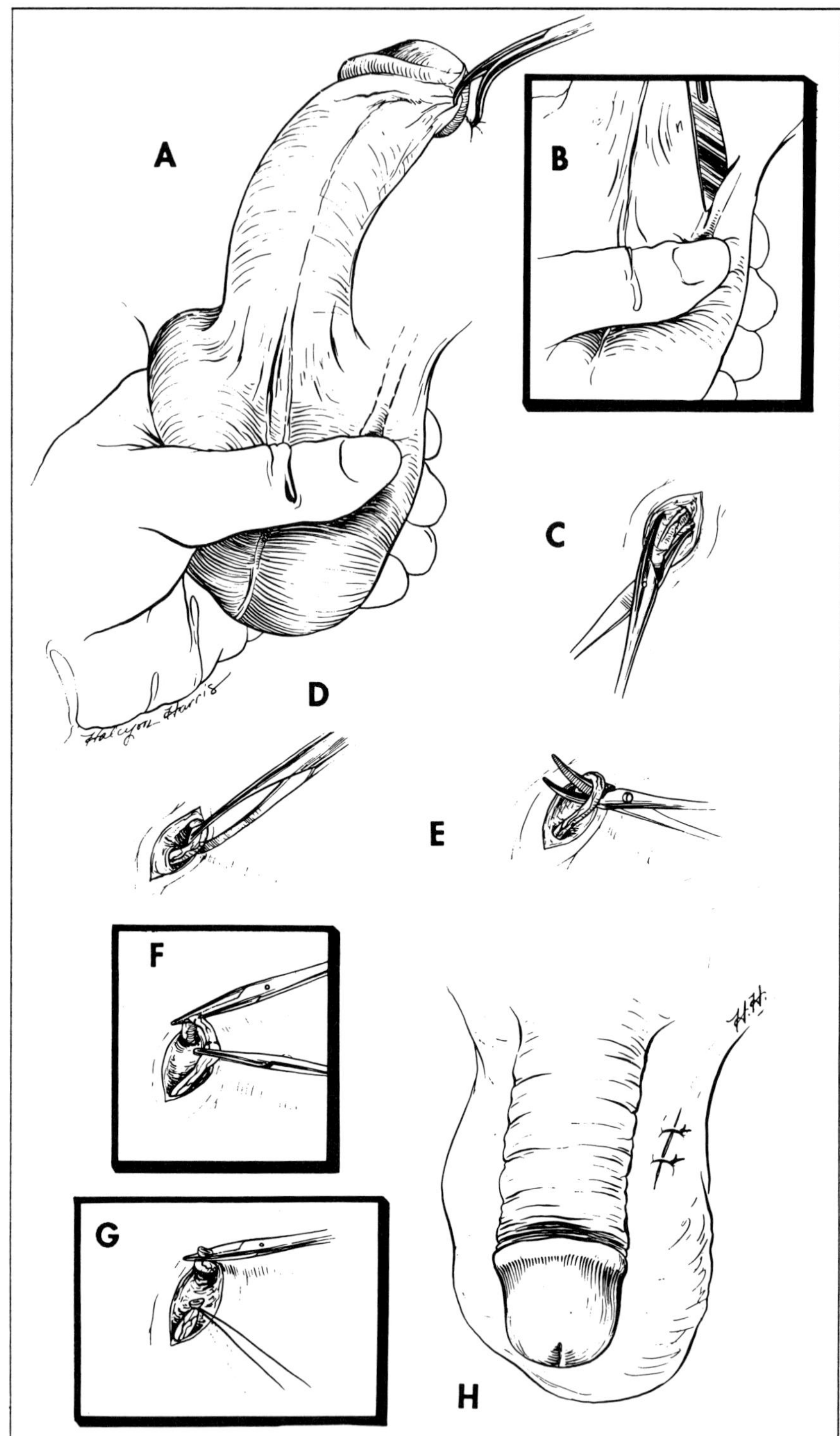


**Fig 10.** Prophylactic vasectomy. **A:** Penis retracted from operative field; left vas secured in upper part of scrotum by fingers of left hand. **B:** Incision 1 cm long made over, and in line with, vas. **C:** Overlying tissues spread apart with small curved clamp. **D:** Vas grasped with Allis forceps. **E:** Vas separated with sharp-tipped clamp. **F:** One-centimeter segment of vas isolated between mosquito clamps. **G:** Segment excised; ends tied with fine cotton. Cotton causes less cellular reaction than catgut. **H:** Scrotal skin closed with No 00 plain catgut. Identical procedure is executed on right side.

removed is not massive. On the contrary, in massive benign hyperplasia, transurethral prostatectomy may be more hazardous than open operation.

Basic to the application of the general principles of prostatic surgery is consideration of the characteristics of the pathologic process: What is the type of lesion? Is it fibrous, muscular, glandular, or composed of other tissue? What is its size, shape, and location? Is it intraurethral, intravesical, or limited to the vesical neck?

Benign hyperplasia of the prostate is unique in that its pathologic characteristics render it suitable for any type of prostatectomy. Its surgical capsule facilitates enucleation by open prostatectomy, yet in small to moderate enlargements, transurethral prostatectomy is ideally performed. Other indications permitting, an adenoma weighing 50 g or less is probably best removed by the transurethral route.

Median bar and contracture of the vesical neck are ideal lesions for transurethral resection. However, in tenacious fibrotic processes, such as recurrences following electroresection, retropubic excision with Y-V closure may be preferable.

Prostatic calculi, when small, can be removed by any route. If calculi are large and there is complicating infection, total perineal or retropubic prostatectomy is the method of choice. It is necessary to keep in mind that, regardless of approach, it is essential that *all* calculi be removed. If any calculi remain in the prostatic cortex and fail to slough, they act as foreign bodies and cause persistent infection and continuing symptoms.

Traumatic lesions of the prostatic urethra are sometimes treated by direct perineal approach at the time of injury. The retropubic approach may also be effective, but recent urologic thinking would suggest that a viable and thoroughly accepted alternative approach is simply to place a cystostomy tube and definitively repair the prostatic urethra approximately 6 months after the original injury.

For contracture of the vesical neck in children, the retropubic or suprapubic approach is usually preferable, although transurethral excision is appropriate in selected cases. Despite the fact that a 14 Fr resectoscope can be readily introduced into the bladder, vision is limited and the cutting loop is so shallow it may prove impossible to remove adequate tissue. This problem is greatly obviated, however, with the newer pediatric resectoscopes. There is the additional danger following transurethral surgery of the bladder neck in children of urethrorectal fistula in boys and urethrovaginal fistula in girls; these conditions may develop following slough of delicate tissues that have inadvertently been damaged by electrosurgical currents. On the other hand, congenital valves of the posterior urethra are best suited to transurethral excision or fulguration.[20,21] Cysts of the prostate and vesical neck in the adult are best removed transurethrally; müllerian duct cysts are best removed by the perineal route.

Obesity complicates all open operations and lends positive support to selection of the transurethral route. Suprapubic prostatectomy usually presents less difficulty than the retropubic route in obese patients.

When there is severe complicating urinary and/or prostatic infection transurethral prostatectomy may be less desirable than open operation, since the latter operation permits more adequate postoperative drainage. Of the open operations, perineal prostatectomy has the advantage of affording dependent drainage.

The caliber and the condition of the urethra also influence the choice. Open prostatectomy is advisable when the urethra is of very small caliber, scarred, or infected. However, perineal urethrostomy or internal urethrotomy may enhance endoscopic resection.

Factors that limit positioning of the patient preclude certain approaches. It is impossible to perform perineal prostatectomy if the patient's hip joints cannot be flexed. The execution of transurethral prostatectomy is compromised as well if there is limitation of hip movement. A narrow bony pelvis renders both the perineal and the retropubic approaches more difficult.

Previous operations on the prostate merit attention. If there has been previous prostatectomy and there are a few remaining fragments of obstructive tissue or fibrous bands, transurethral resection is the method of choice. After a previous transurethral prostatectomy the retropubic approach may offer difficulty in control of bleeding. The prostate itself may have been reduced to such tissue-paper thinness as to preclude satisfactory closure of the capsule. If the perineum is extensively scarred from an anorectal operation, perineal operation should be avoided. On the other hand, after proctectomy, perineal prostatectomy may be ideally performed since there is no danger of injury to the rectum.

Large vesical calculi are most easily removed at the time of open prostatectomy, but litholapaxy in skilled hands is quite efficient when the calculi are less than 2.5 cm in size.

## ANESTHESIA IN PROSTATIC SURGERY

Most patients who undergo prostatectomy (more accurately referred to as adenomectomy) are in the older age group. Selection of the proper anesthetic and its skillful administration is of special importance. All other things being equal, spinal anesthesia is preferred. It combines analgesia and relaxation ideally without postoperative respiratory problems, items that are often difficult to obtain with a general anesthetic. In certain cases, eg, in severe cardiovascular disease, epidural anesthesia is the method of choice. General anesthesia is best for the hypotensive patient since spinal anesthesia often causes further lowering of the blood pressure.

## GENERAL PRINCIPLES OF PROSTATIC SURGERY

Progress in prostatectomy (adenomectomy) depends upon measures designed to prevent the numerous complications which may attend this operation. General rules, broad in scope and germane to all surgical approaches, for performing successful prostatectomy include the following:

1. Attain adequate exposure.
2. Avoid damage to vital structures.
3. Remove all obstructive tissue.
4. Control bleeding.
5. Assure proper treatment of the vesical neck.
6. Execute precise closure and make adequate provision for postoperative drainage.
7. Utilize proper suture material.
8. Maintain asepsis.
9. Replace blood loss and maintain satisfactory fluid balance.
10. Avoid all technical errors.

As in all types of surgery, exposure is one of the keystones to success. Ideal exposure depends upon adequate anesthesia, proper positioning of the patient, and knowledge by the surgeon of anatomic structures and pathologic variations.

Damage to vital structures is imminent during almost every step of every type of prostatectomy. The surgeon must devote special care to preserve the external urinary sphincter. Danger of tearing or excising the sphincter or its nerve supply is greatest during perineal exposure of the prostate. During transurethral prostatectomy there is danger that the external sphincter may be ruptured by inexpert introduction of the resectoscope or divided during resection of tissue. In any type of open prostatectomy, the sphincter may be avulsed by rough enucleation of benign hyperplasia. For this reason, the urethra must be divided at the apex of the adenoma with scissors or scalpel in preference to tearing or twisting it free.

Injury to the rectum is most common in perineal prostatectomy. However, the rectum may be damaged during any type of prostatectomy if the prostatic capsule is perforated.

Although damage to the anterior urethra is more likely during transurethral prostatectomy, it may be injured by the inexpert passage of catheters or sounds during any approach.

The lower ends of the ureters may be injured during transurethral resection or they may be included in a suture inexpertly applied to the vesical neck in any open prostatectomy.

With adequate exposure, complete removal of obstructive tissue presents little difficulty. During enculeation of benign hyperplasia, close adherence to the natural surgical cleavage plane facilitates complete removal of the adenoma. Before closure the surgeon must make a careful examination to be certain that all adenomatous tissue has been removed and that no fragments or calculi remain in the bladder. Adequate removal of tissue during transurethral prostatectomy depends upon careful inspection with the resectoscope lens, aided by rectourethral palpation with the resectoscope in the urethra.

Advances in surgical technique have aided the development of effective methods for the control of bleeding. By attaining adequate exposure, keeping the field dry, and replacing serious blood loss by transfusion, leisurely attention can be given to hemostasis. Spot coagulation is employed for smaller blood vessels; large vessels are secured by free sutures or by suture ligatures. Angulated needle holders facilitate placing sutures in difficult locations.

Hemorrhage must be controlled at the operating table. The surgeon must never return the patient to bed in hopes that bleeding will cease after watchful waiting. Frequently, as the blood pressure rises after operation, bleeding becomes more profuse. Prior to closure the physician must evacuate all blood clots from the prostatic fossa and bladder. Clots which remain act as foreign bodies. In attempting to expel them the bladder contracts, spasms are induced, and fresh bleeding is excited.

In all approaches the surgeon must direct attention to the patency of the vesical neck. Unless provision is made for a wide-open orifice, whether by resection or wedge excision, postoperative contracture may ensue. During open operation one must ascertain the size of the vesical neck by inserting a finger in the opening. When there is resistance, a wedge is excised posteriorly. Postoperative stenosis of the vesical neck is most frequent in fibrous lesions and following retropubic and transurethral prostatectomy.

Following open operation, accurate approximation of tissue layers accelerates healing. Precise closure of the prostatic capsule decreases the likelihood of urinary seepage and formation of fistulas. Provision must be made for urinary drainage. This minimizes bleeding, clot formation, and bladder distention. A urethral catheter is preferable to one placed suprapubically. The drain is placed in the periprostatic tissue spaces (of Retzius). There is always the possibility of urinary leakage and secondary infection. Failure to obtain precise tissue approximation and to ensure adequate drainage may lead to periprostatic cellulitis, abscess, osteitis pubis, and urinary and rectal fistulas.

Since some degree of infection is almost inevitable after prostatic operations, there is no justification for the use of nonabsorbable suture material (with the exception of skin sutures). For ligatures and for closure of the vesical neck, No 00 or No 0 plain catgut is the material of choice. Chromic catgut may provide the nidus for incrustation and delay healing because of the prolonged time required for absorption. The surgeon must use as little suture material as is consistent with the arrest of bleeding and precise closure of tissue layers. This avoids "burying" large amounts of catgut, a practice which deters healing and contributes to secondary infection.

In former years little stress was placed on asepsis in prostatic surgery. It has become abundantly evident, however, that asepsis diminishes appreciably the dangers of the operation. The desirability of operation in a clean field has led to a policy of limiting preoperative catheter drainage to those patients in whom it is overwhelmingly indicated and delaying cystoscopy, if possible, until the time of operation.

The surgeon must exercise meticulous care to avoid technical errors. It is always simpler to keep out of than to get out of difficulty. The surgeon must be constantly alert to recognize immediately any operative complication. Prompt allocation of appropriate corrective measures minimizes whatever danger exists.

### Antimicrobial Usage in Prostatic Surgery

I feel rather strongly that there is no valid indication for prophylactic antimicrobial usage in the vast majority of patients undergoing prostatic surgery.[22] Specifically, antimicrobials need not be used for the patient at minimal risk with sterile urine preoperatively who does not require an indwelling catheter prior to surgery. This statement applies to all forms of prostatic surgery, but it is particularly germane for the patient undergoing transurethral surgery, since this surgical approach is by far the most common one used in the United States for the relief of bladder outlet obstruction due to benign conditions. On the other hand, the patient who has advanced carcinoma, the diabetic, the patient on steroids, and other such poor-risk patients obviously do not fall under the category of "at-minimal-risk" patients, and for these prophylactic antimicrobial therapy is undoubtedly proper. A specimen of urine should always be obtained at the time of surgery when the resectoscope or cystoscope is introduced into the bladder so that the appropriate antimicrobial may be used if and when the patient develops bacteriuria in the postoperative period.

## TYPES OF OPERATIONS

### Conservative Perineal Prostatectomy

Perineal prostatectomy is the oldest of the four modern approaches to the prostate. Earliest attempts grew from the ancient operation of perineal lithotomy for removal of vesical calculi (Ammonius Lithotomus, 460 to 367 BC). After approximately 2000 years of primitive attempts, it was left to the brilliance and enterprise of Dr. Hugh Hampton Young to become the "father of perineal prostatectomy." The operation that he devised in 1903 is the fundamental operation performed today.[23]

Conservative perineal prostatectomy has a few theoretic advantages: the perineum affords the most direct surgical approach to the prostate, and this approach is through a relatively avascular field; the incision itself provides for a physiologically dependent drainage of the operative wound; it is specifically indicated for repair of trauma to the prostatic and the bulbous urethra; and it also affords the best exposure for drainage of prostatic abscesses. There are few or no practical advantages to this approach, however.

The perineal approach is contraindicated in patients with ankylosis of the hips where the extreme lithotomy position would be impossible. If a patient has had extensive rectal surgery, the scarring would probably prohibit adequate perineal dissection.

This operation never gained widespread acceptance, most likely because of occasional complications such as sexual impotence and urinary incontinence. In the experience of many surgeons, these complications have been more frequent than in other conventional approaches. In most clinics the approach is used only for radical prostatectomy for carcinoma; in a few clinics the operation is still utilized for benign prostatic hyperplasia.

**Position of the Patient.** The patient is placed on a perineal board in the extreme lithotomy position. This is accomplished by flexing the thighs sharply on the abdomen; the position is maintained by fixing the legs to pivots on either side of the operating table. Any standard operating table can be made suitable for perineal prostatectomy by the addition of leg supports.

In the extreme lithotomy position, almost the entire weight of the body rests upon the shoulders. If the shoulders are not adequately cushioned against the shoulder guards, pressure on the brachial plexus may lead to nerve palsy. Foam rubber is well suited for this purpose. Likewise, the pivots are cushioned to prevent pressure on the legs. The sacrum is elevated by the use of sandbags on a perineal elevator. In proper position the perineum projects beyond the end of the operating table and is parallel to the floor of the operating room.

**Procedure.** Place the Young seminal vesicle tractor into the bulbous urethra (Fig 11A). By introducing the tractor at the beginning of the operation, it can be conveniently passed into the bladder at any moment the dissection warrants. Do not advance the tractor into the bladder until after the rectum has been freed, since passage of a rigid instrument into the bladder forces the pros-

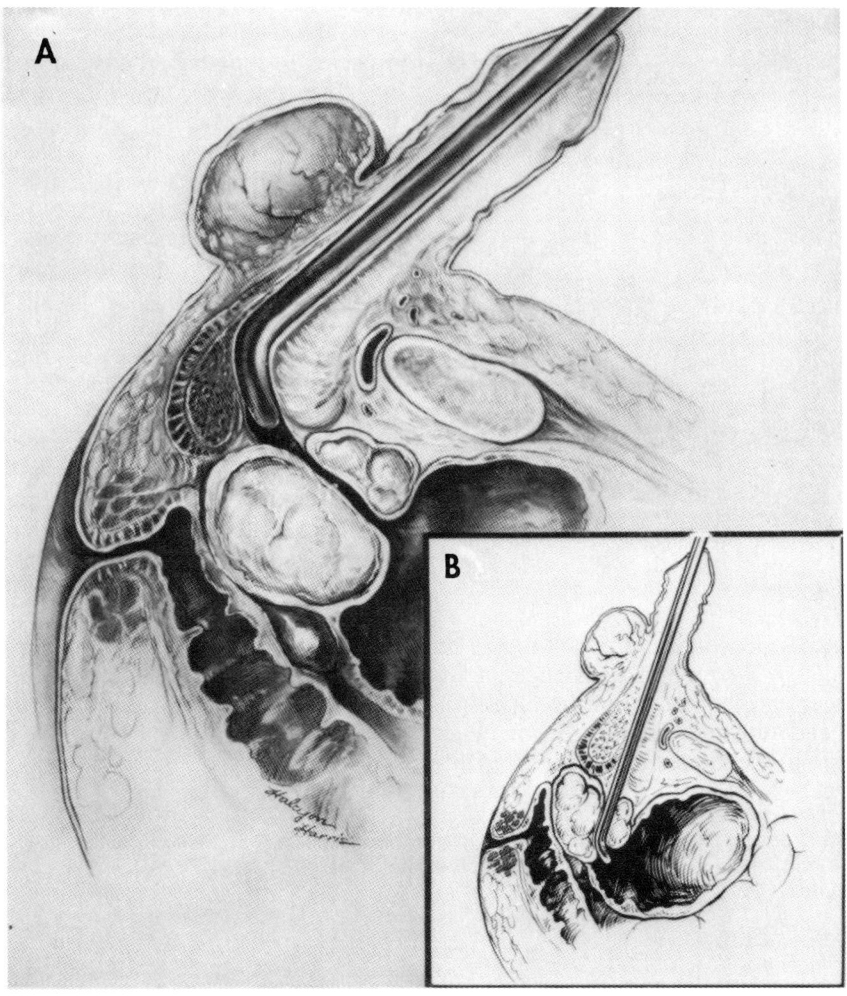


**Fig 11.** Perineal prostatectomy. Introducing seminal vesicle tractors. **A:** Instrument placed into bulbous urethra. **B:** There is danger of inserting tractor into bladder before dissection. Note precarious position of rectum.

tate toward the perineum. If this is done before the central tendon is divided, the rectum will be tented up over the prostate (Fig 11B), thus increasing the danger of perforation. Make an inverted U skin incision with the center 3 cm above the anal margin (Fig 12). Curve the edges backward within the ischial tuberosities, to the level of the anus. By carrying the incision well posteriorly, the rectum is released. This permits the perineum to be pushed inward and facilitates access to the prostate. If the incision is placed too high, two difficulties are encountered: there is danger that the bulb of the urethra will be cut, and the surgeon is forced to work down into a deep hole to reach the prostate. The incision is curved within, not over, the ischial tuberosities to avoid postoperative pain from pressure of the scar on these bony prominences. In making the incision, leave the subcutaneous fat attached to the skin. This removes it from the operative field and ensures a well-nourished flap.

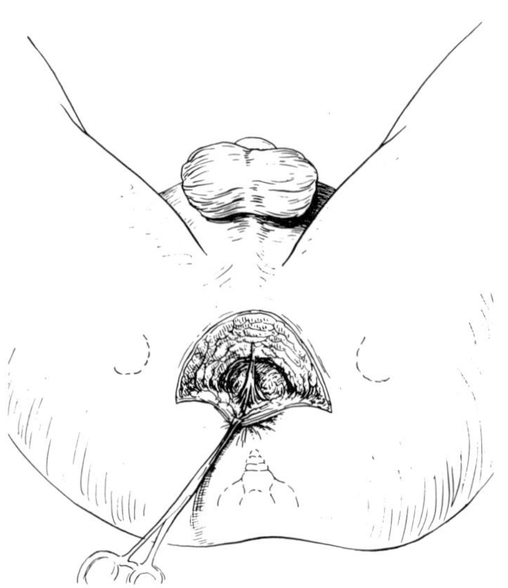

**Fig 12.** Perineal prostatectomy. Inverted U incision.

Next, develop the ischiorectal fossae on either side of the rectum. Introduce the index finger and the handle of a scalpel in a lateral and upward direction from either extremity of the incision. If this proves difficult, cut more deeply with the scalpel to divide the superficial perineal fascia. Be sure to keep the dissection close to the rectum and behind the transverse perineal muscles. If the perineum is entered in front of these muscles, one comes down upon the anterior surface of the triangular ligament and further dissection damages the external urinary sphincter. While keeping close to the rectum, be sure not to damage this structure. If there is any question concerning its location, do not hesitate to place a finger in the rectum and locate it by bimanual palpation through the operative wound. A perineal sheet assures asepsis during this maneuver without the necessity of changing gloves.

When the ischiorectal fossae are well developed, divide the central tendon. Tent up this structure by applying traction to the skin flap with an Allis forceps, placing it under tension. Incise the tissue transversely to separate the rectum from the bulb of the urethra (Fig 13A). An alternative method is to divide the central tendon over an index finger, gently insinuated over the rectum from one ischiorectal fossa to the other (Fig 13B).

Bring the prostate into the operative

**Fig 13.** Perineal prostatectomy. Dividing central tendon. **A:** With tension on skin flap. **B:** Over finger insinuated from one ischiorectal fossa to the other.

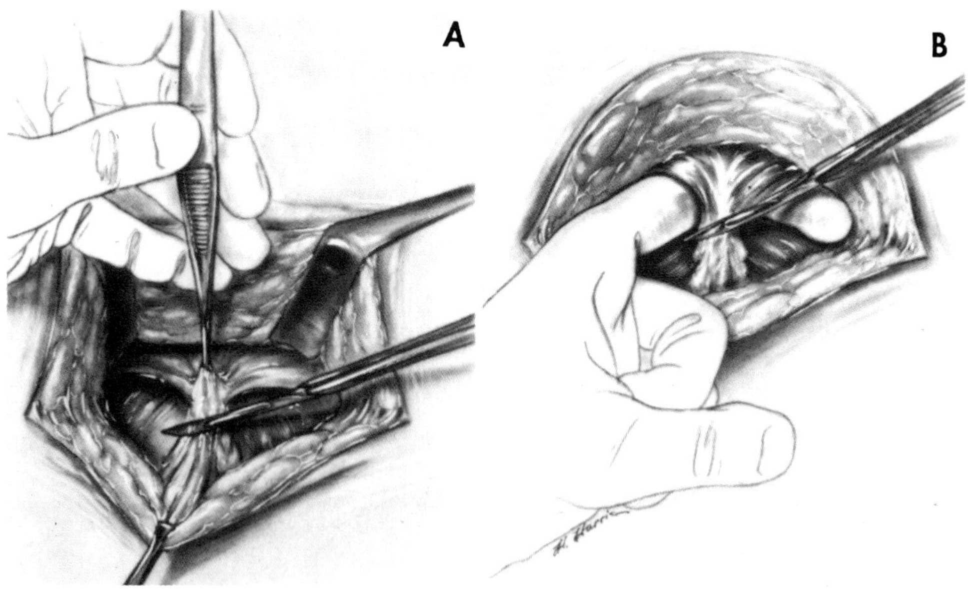

wound by advancing the seminal vesicle tractor into the bladder, opening the blades, fixing them with the set screw, finally shifting the instrument upward in the direction of the abdomen (Fig 14). The symphysis acts as a fulcrum, forcing the prostate toward the perineum.

Covering the entire posterior surface of the prostate are the two layers of Denonvilliers' fascia. Tented over the posterior surface is the rectum. Above is the rectourethralis muscle. Incise this muscle transversely (Fig 15) in the plane between the two layers of Denonvilliers' fascia. The glistening white surface of the prostatic capsule, which Young terms the "pearly gates," indicates the proper place. The handle of the scapel is a convenient aid (Fig 16).

An alternative method is to incise the posterior layer of Denonvilliers' fascia over one lateral aspect of the prostate and progress medially to free the rectum. Do not hesitate to put a finger in the rectum if there is confusion regarding the landmarks at this stage or at any stage of the dissection.

Do not attempt to incise Denonvilliers' fascia too close to the membranous urethra. Here both layers are firmly attached to the apex of the prostate and there is danger of injuring the sphincter. To complete exposure of the prostate, maintain the tissue planes as they are developed, using gauze over an index finger. If, once separated,

**Fig 14.** Perineal prostatectomy. Forcing prostate into perineal wound. Seminal vesicle tractor displaced toward abdomen; symphysis acts as a fulcrum.

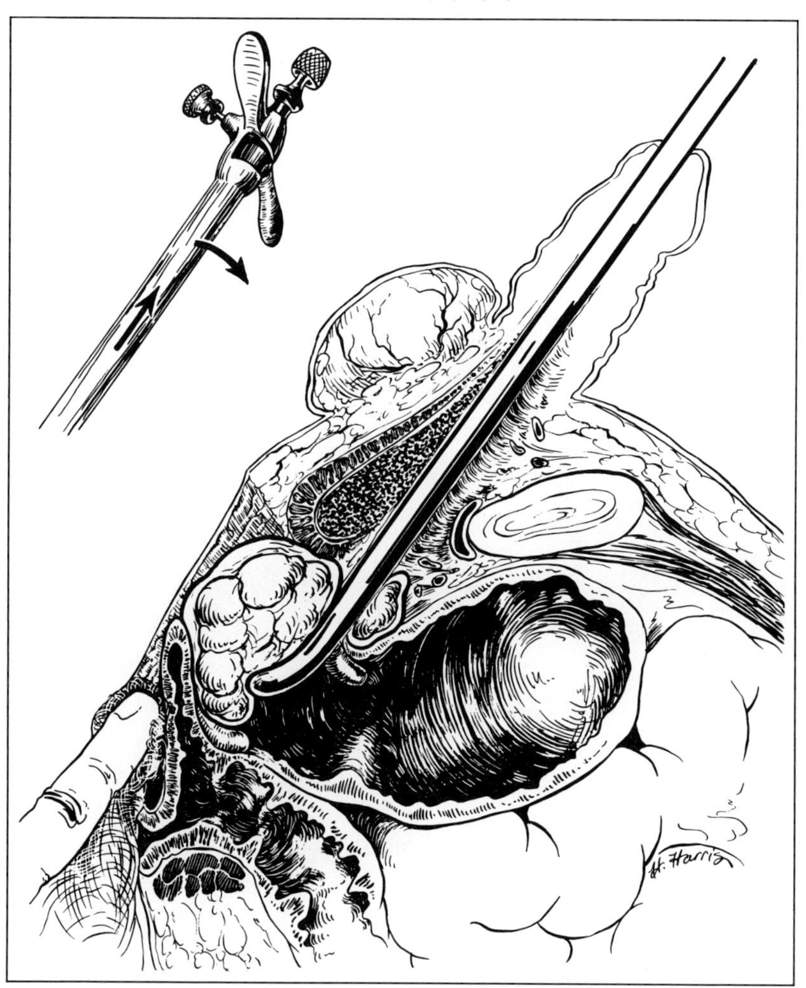

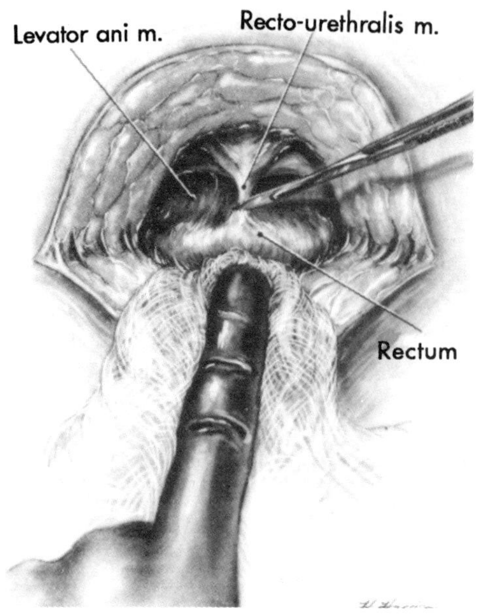


**Fig 15.** Perineal prostatectomy. Dividing rectourethralis muscle.

the tissues are permitted to fall together after the correct plane has been entered, it may be necessary to start the deep perineal dissection all over again. To expose the prostate completely, free the rectum so that the gland is exposed from the apex above, to both sides laterally, and to the seminal vesicles posteriorly. When there is massive hyperplasia, divide a few of the inner fibers of the levator ani muscles transversely on either side to permit delivery of the adenoma.

With the prostate exposed, protect the rectum with a gauze sponge and hold it out of the field with a posterior perineal retractor of proper depth (Fig 17).

To enucleate the adenoma, make an inverted U incision through the posterior aspect of the prostate. Place the transverse part of the incision between the apex and the verumontanum. The latter structure occupies a soft area that can be felt by palpation against the seminal vesicle retractor. Deepen the incision into the prostatic urethra, identified by the seminal vesicle tractor. The verumontanum and the ejaculatory ducts are contained in the reflected flap (Fig 18). At this state the surgical capsule is identified between the adenoma and the true prostate. Develop this cleavage plane with the joker (Fig 19, left) or the blunt ends of the curved scissors (Fig 19, right). Using scissors, sharply divide the portion of prostatic urethra bearing the verumontanum from the posterior commissural area of the

**Fig 16.** Perineal prostatectomy. Exposing prostate. Opening plane between two layers of Denonvilliers' fascia.

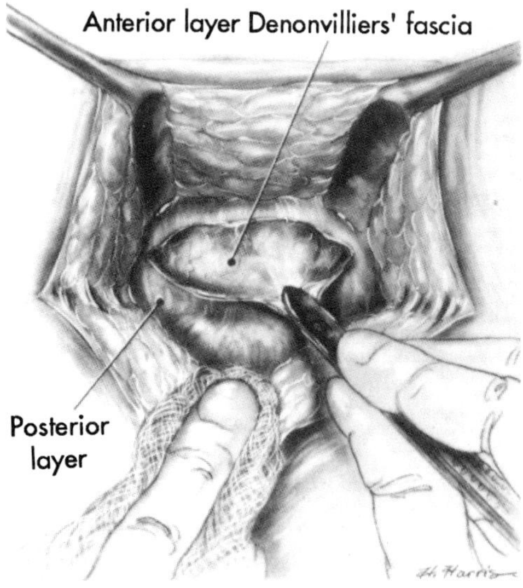


**Fig 17.** Perineal prostatectomy. Prostate exposed. Dotted line marks the line of incision for enucleation.

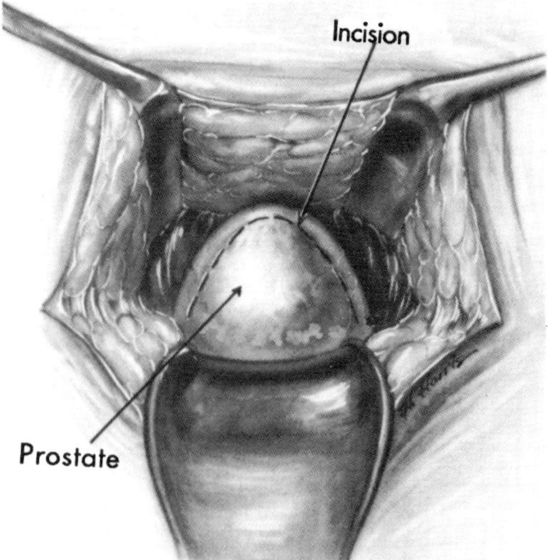

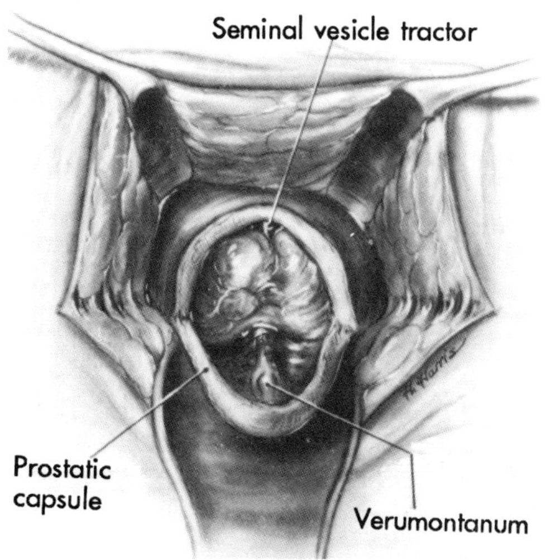


**Fig 18.** Perineal prostatectomy. Posterior flap reflected. Verumontanum exposed.

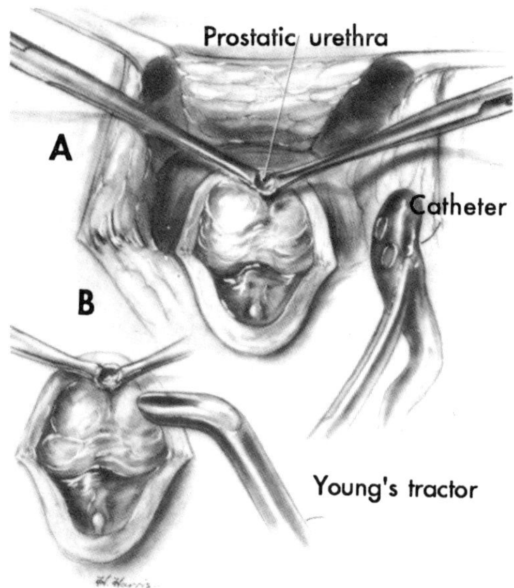


**Fig 20.** Perineal prostatectomy. Preparation for delivery of adenoma. **A:** Catheter is introduced to evacuate the fluid in the bladder. **B:** Inserting Young's prostatic retractor.

hyperplasia. Delay further enucleation until the seminal vesicle tractor has been replaced with a prostatic tractor. With the prostate under tension there is danger of starting false tissue planes and tearing the prostate.

After defining the posterior aspect of the adenoma, remove the seminal vesicle tractor and insert Young's short perineal tractor. Hold the urethra open with the Allis forceps and remove the fluid from the bladder with a urethral catheter (Fig 20A) be-

**Fig 19.** Perineal prostatectomy. Developing plane for enucleation. **Left:** With a joker. **Right:** With curved scissors.

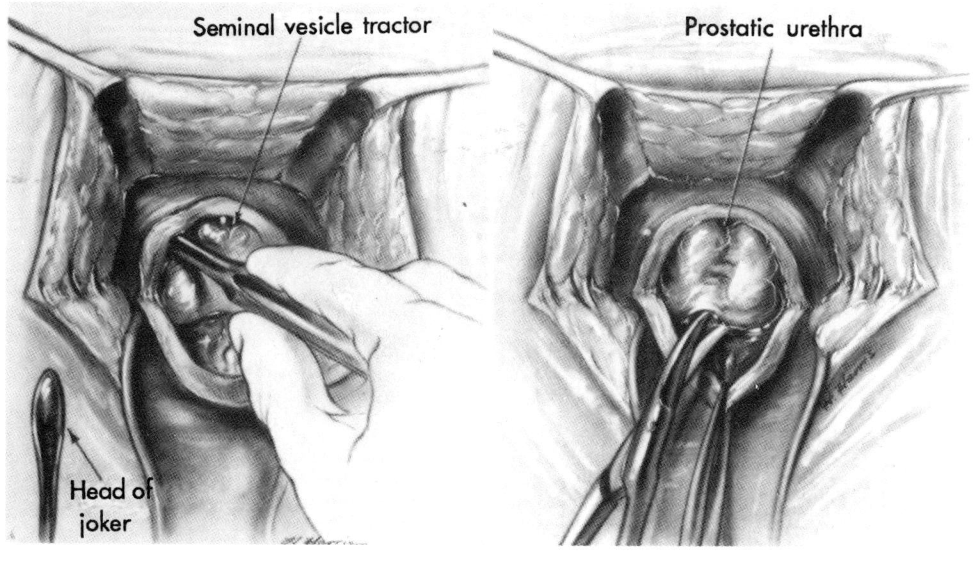

fore introducing the Young tractor into the bladder (Fig 20B). Finally, open the blades and fix them in position with the set screw. At this point remove all retractors and clamps from the wound to prevent injury to the rectum during enucleation. Complete division of the urethra in situ to avoid damage to the external sphincter (Fig 21). With the apex free, work around the circumference of the surgical capsule with an index finger. Leave the attachment at the vesical neck until last. Deliver the adenoma with prostatic lobe forceps or thyroid clamps. In massive hyperplasia it is advisable to deliver one lobe at a time, though still removing all the hyperplastic tissue in one piece. This avoids tearing the capsule.

Strip backward the cone of the vesical neck as it comes into view. Develop a cylinder of mucosa at the point where the bladder mucosa joins the musoca of the posterior urethra. Incise the cone transversely (Fig 22) and apply Allis forceps to the vesical neck (Fig 23).

Be certain to remove all adenoma, including any median or subtrigonal lobe. If a large median lobe is present it may be necessary to dilate the vesical neck to permit its delivery.

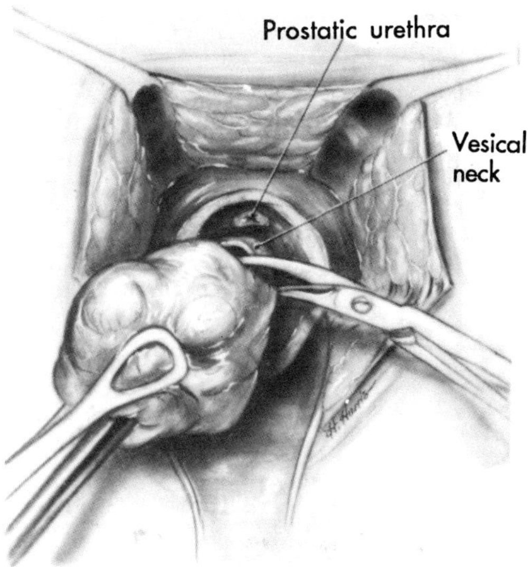


Fig 22. Perineal prostatectomy. Dividing mucosa of vesical neck.

Secure bleeding vessels as they appear during the enucleation. Identify additional bleeders by drawing up the vesical neck

Fig 21. Perineal prostatectomy. Dividing distal urethra.

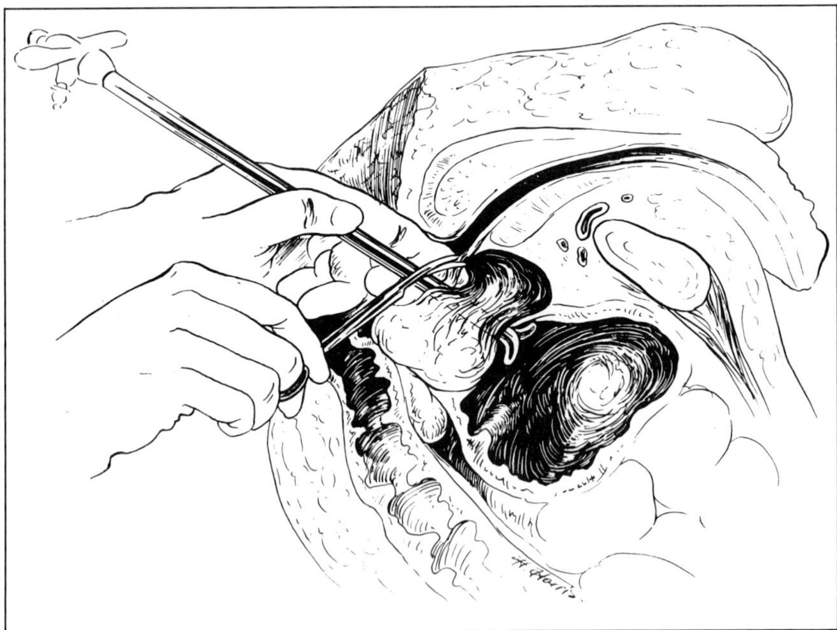

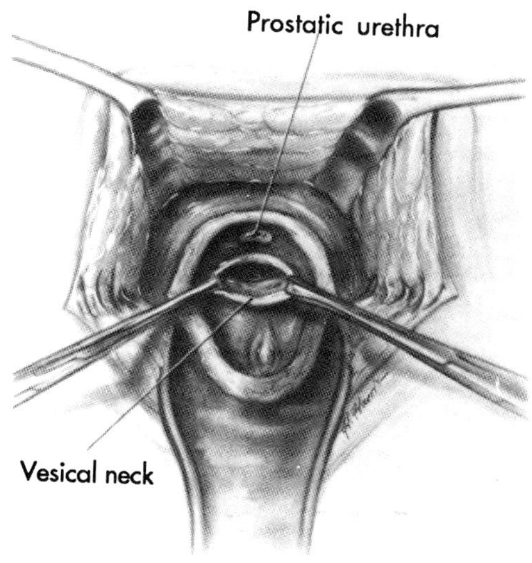


**Fig 23.** Perineal prostatectomy. Enucleation complete. Allis forceps identify vesical neck.

with Allis clamps. Secure them with mattress sutures of No 0 plain catgut (Fig 24). Make a plastic closure of the vesical neck by joining the divided mucosa of the bladder to the prostatic fossa. For this purpose introduce interrupted sutures around the circumference of the bladder neck. These

**Fig 24.** Perineal prostatectomy. Placing anchor sutures at inferior quadrants of vesical neck. **Inset:** Avoid danger to the adjacent ureter.

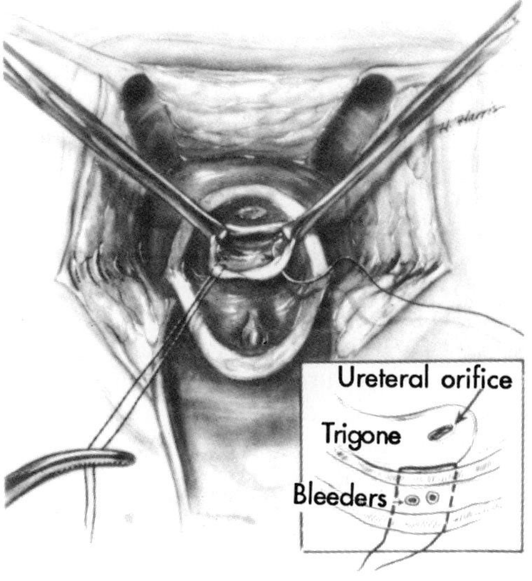


sutures arrest bleeding along the free margin and prevent separation of the vesical neck. Make a final inspection of the prostatic fossa to make certain hemostasis has been secured.

Introduce a 24 F 30-mL Foley bag catheter through the urethra into the bladder (Fig 25). Irrigate the bladder to remove any blood clots before closing the prostatic incision. Inflate the Foley bag (Fig 26). Close the posterior flap with a running No 0 chromic catgut suture (Fig. 27). Do not perforate the bag or include the catheter in the suture. Place a mattress suture of No 0 plain cutgut between the urogenital diaphragm and the apex of the prostate to reinforce the external sphincter.

Inspect the rectum to make sure it has not been injured. Close the perineum by interposing the medial portions of the levator ani muscles between the prostatic capsule and the rectum with interrupted sutures of No 0 plain catgut. Place a few additional sutures of the same material in the subcutaneous tissues. Place a Penrose drain down to the prostatic capsule. Close the skin with skin clips or with interrupted sutures (Fig 28).

## Suprapubic Prostatectomy

Similar to the perineal approach, suprapubic prostatectomy was an outgrowth of cystolithotomy and has progressed from a blind to a visual procedure. Blind perineal prostatectomy has been abandoned. Blind suprapubic prostatectomy, however, is still practiced.

The transvesical suprapubic approach was initiated by Pierre Franco who in 1556 removed a bladder stone by means of cystotomy. In 1834, Amusset performed the first primitive suprapubic prostatectomy. It was not until 1896 that Freyer developed the method of blind suprapubic prostatectomy; to this day it is called the Freyer operation.

Credit for originating open (visual) suprapubic prostatectomy goes to Thompson Walker in 1909. Performing the operation under vision, bleeding was controlled by suture ligatures of the vesical neck.

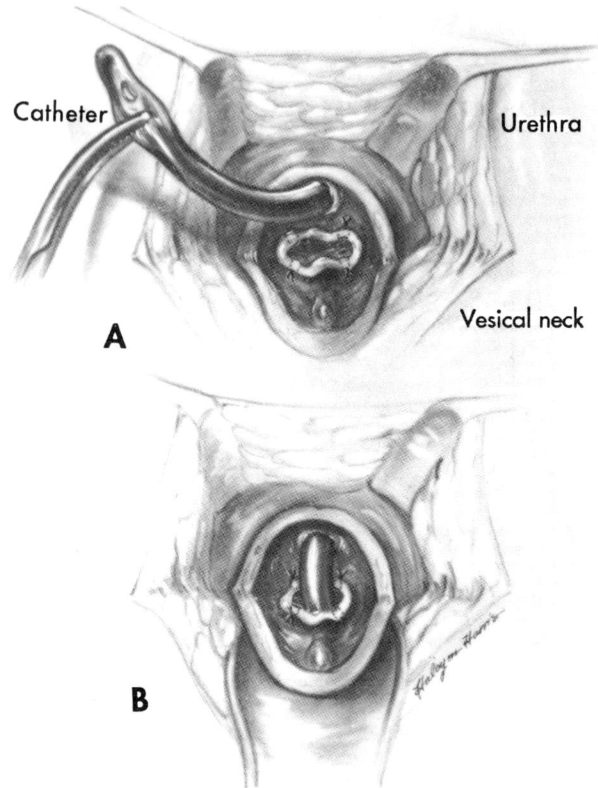


**Fig 25.** Perineal prostatectomy. Introducing urethral catheter. **A:** Catheter appears in prostatic fossa. **B:** End placed into bladder.

**Fig 26.** Perineal prostatectomy. Bag secures catheter in bladder.

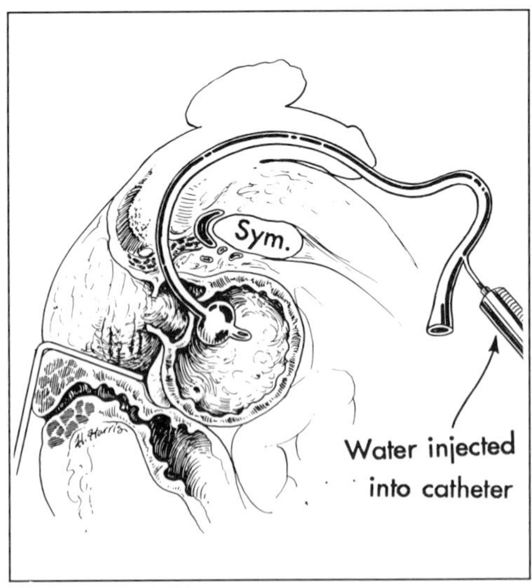


**Blind Suprapubic Prostatectomy.** The prime advantage of this procedure is that it is relatively easy to do and a minimum of special equipment is needed. It can also be done without benefit of excellent relaxation or exposure. However, its use is limited to benign prostatic hyperplasia. The primary disadvantage of the technique is the difficulty in controlling bleeding since the points of bleeding are not visualized. There are few, if any, specific indications for this type of procedure except perhaps the absence of surgical assistance and a paucity of specialized urologic instruments. The procedure is contraindicated in carcinoma of the prostate.

Place the patient in the dorsal decubitus or low lithotomy position. Place well-bolstered shoulder guards to permit a subsequent shift to Trendelenburg position.

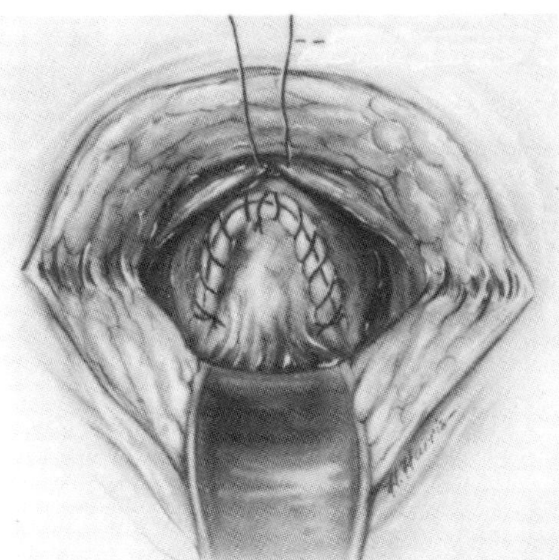


**Fig 27.** Perineal prostatectomy. Closing prostatic capsule. U flap reconstructed. Reinforcing suture to urogenital diaphragm.

Insert a urethral catheter into the bladder and distend the bladder with water to approximately 300 mL. Retain the fluid by tying an open 4 × 4-inch sponge around the penis, by applying a penis clamp, or by clamping the catheter and leaving it in place (Fig 29).

After distending the bladder, prepare the operative field and drape the patient. With the patient in the dorsal decubitus position, strap the right leg to the operating table. Leave the left leg free to permit insertion of a finger in the rectum during enucleation. Use of the low lithotomy position permits cystocopy with one draping and facilitates placing a finger in the rectum.

The only urologic instruments needed are prostatic lobe forceps, a hemostatic bag or gauze pack for control of hemorrhage, and a cystostomy tube.

Make a low midline abdominal incision starting 3 cm above the symphysis pubis and extend it upward a distance of 4 to 6 cm (Fig 30A). Deepen the incision to the rectus sheath and incise this structure in the midline between the recti muscles. Divide the fascia to both extremities of the incision but do not divide the pyramidalis muscle. Separate the recti muscles from the midline with the tips of the index fingers (Fig 30B).

Expose the dome of the bladder by stripping back the peritoneum with the index finger covered with gauze (Fig 30C). Do not open the space of Retzius or the lateral recesses of the bladder. It is neither necessary nor desirable to open these tissue spaces in this operation. Dissect the peritoneum from the vault of the bladder so it will not be incised when the bladder is opened. If the peritoneal attachment extends down to the symphysis pubis, make a few superficial strokes with the scalpel to free it. Do not confuse the single layer of perivesical fascia with the peritoneum. This thin layer is closely applied to the detrusor. The bladder wall is easily recognized by the interlacing bundles and closely attached blood vessels (Fig 30C). If the peritoneal cavity is inadvertently entered, repair the rent.

Select the site for cystotomy high in the vault of the bladder. A low incision leads to the danger of tearing into the prostatic capsule during enucleation and compromises placing the cystostomy tube.

Place stay sutures of heavy silk in the bladder wall above and below the cystotomy site and make preparation for suction. Plunge the tip of the scalpel into the cavity of the bladder (Fig 31A) and apply Allis forceps to the edges of the incision. Widen the incision laterally with scissors until there is room to introduce three fingers for enucleation and delivery of the adenoma (Fig 31B). Secure bleeding vessels in the wall of the bladder.

In this method of suprapubic prostatectomy, satisfactory inspection of the bladder cannot be made. Reliance is placed on previous cystoscopy and upon palpation to determine whether calculi may be hidden in a deep bas-fond.

Before starting enucleation of the benign adenoma, place the patient in the Trendelenburg position and remove all clamps and retractors from the wound.

To gain access to the surgical capsule, insert an index finger through the vesical neck into the prostatic urethra. Break through the urethra anteriorly at the distal

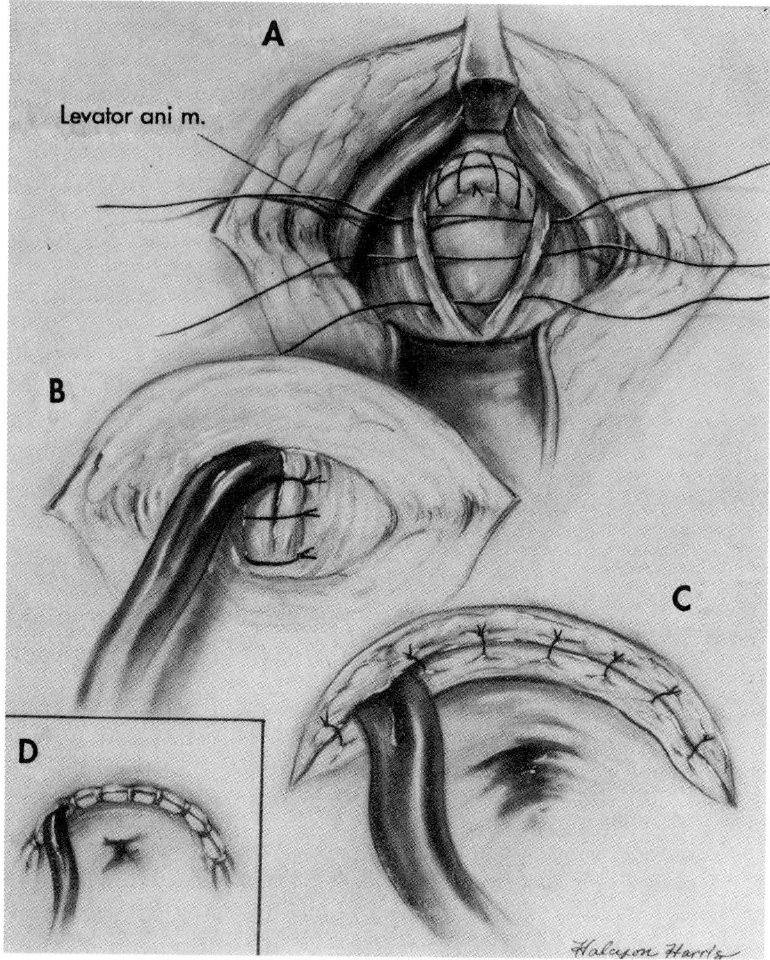


**Fig 28.** Perineal prostatectomy. Closure of incision. **A:** Levator ani muscles interposed between prostatic capsule and rectum. **B:** Space left for Penrose drain. **C:** Closure of subcutaneous tissues. **D:** Skin closed with skin clips.

extent of the adenoma at the apex of the prostate. In the blind operation, if the enucleation is started at the vesical neck and the adenoma is freed before breaking through the urethra at the prostatic apex, traction of the adenoma may avulse the membranous urethra from the external sphincter and lead to urinary incontinence. Another advantage in deferring until last the separation of the adenoma from the vesical neck is that opening the main blood supply to the adenoma is delayed and bleeding is minimized.

Once the mucosa has broken and separation of the adenoma discloses that the plane of the surgical capsule has been reached, do not penetrate deeper (Fig 32). In this area there is danger of lacerating the deep branches of the anterior venous plexus, an accident that causes profuse venous bleeding.

If the patient is obese or if the pelvis is deep, do not hesitate to insert a finger into the rectum to elevate the prostate (Fig 33A).

After breaking through the mucosa anteriorly, sweep the tip of the enucleating finger laterally and develop the plane of the surgical capsule. Sever the urethral mucosa at the apical extent of the hyperplasia (Fig

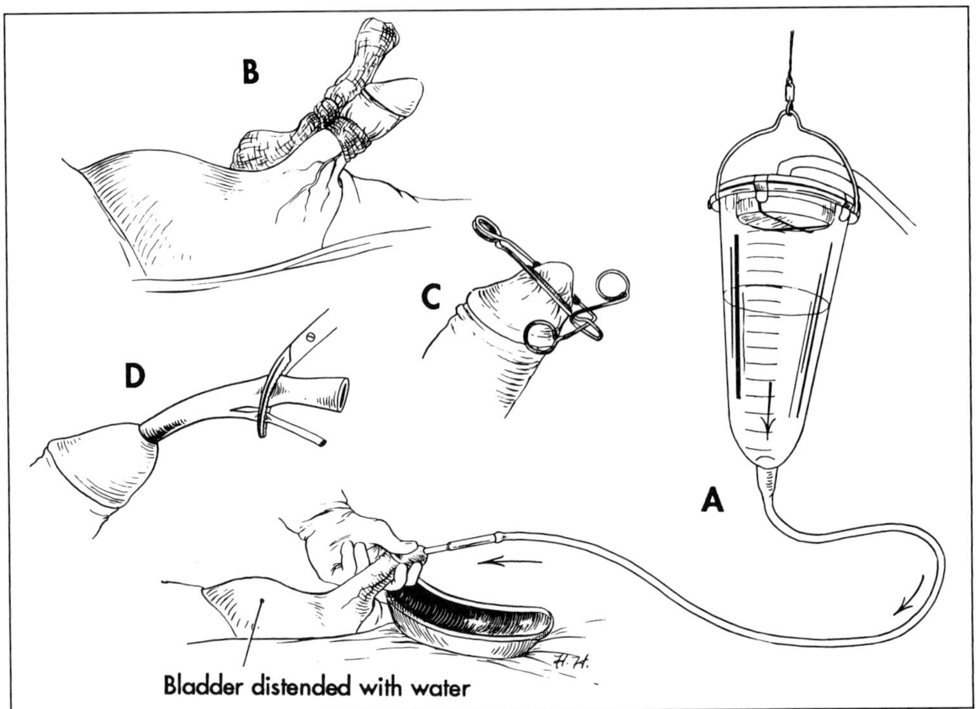


**Fig 29.** Suprapubic prostatectomy. Distention of bladder. **A:** Distending bladder with water. **B:** Constricting urethra with a sponge. **C:** Constricting urethra with penile clamp. **D:** Retaining fluid in bladder with Foley catheter.

33B). The urethra is more easily divided at this time than after the adenoma has been freed, when forceful maneuvers to pinch or twist off an intact urethra may damage the external sphincter.

Having defined the surgical capsule, continue the enucleation with the flat surface of one or more fingers using a circular sweeping motion. Closely hug the adenoma to lessen danger of perforation of the true capsule. In some cases the true capsule is extremely thin.

In small adenomas, one index finger suffices for enucleation. In massive hyperplasias, two or even three fingers are required to sweep around the adenoma. Free one lateral lobe and then free the remaining lateral lobe. Finally, progress posteriorly to enucleate the posterior commissure and the middle lobe. En masse enucleation is desirable to avoid leaving nodules of adenoma behind. Retained fragments hinder contraction of the capsule, lead to continued bleeding, and predispose to infection.

Once the proper plane has been developed in one region, it is usually easy to continue the enucleation around the entire periphery of the adenoma. However, in the presence of fibrosis, development of the cleavage plane may require bizarre angulation of the elbow to bring pressure to bear in critical areas.

Do not exert undue force when resistance is met. If a point of adherence is met, continued force may perforate the true capsule. Withdraw the enucleating finger and free the adherent area from a different approach within the surgical capsule. When an adenoma is separated over most of its circumference, adherent areas separate more easily. If the urethra remains attached after the adenoma has been freed from the capsule, separate the mucosa by pinching it off between the tips of two fingers or by

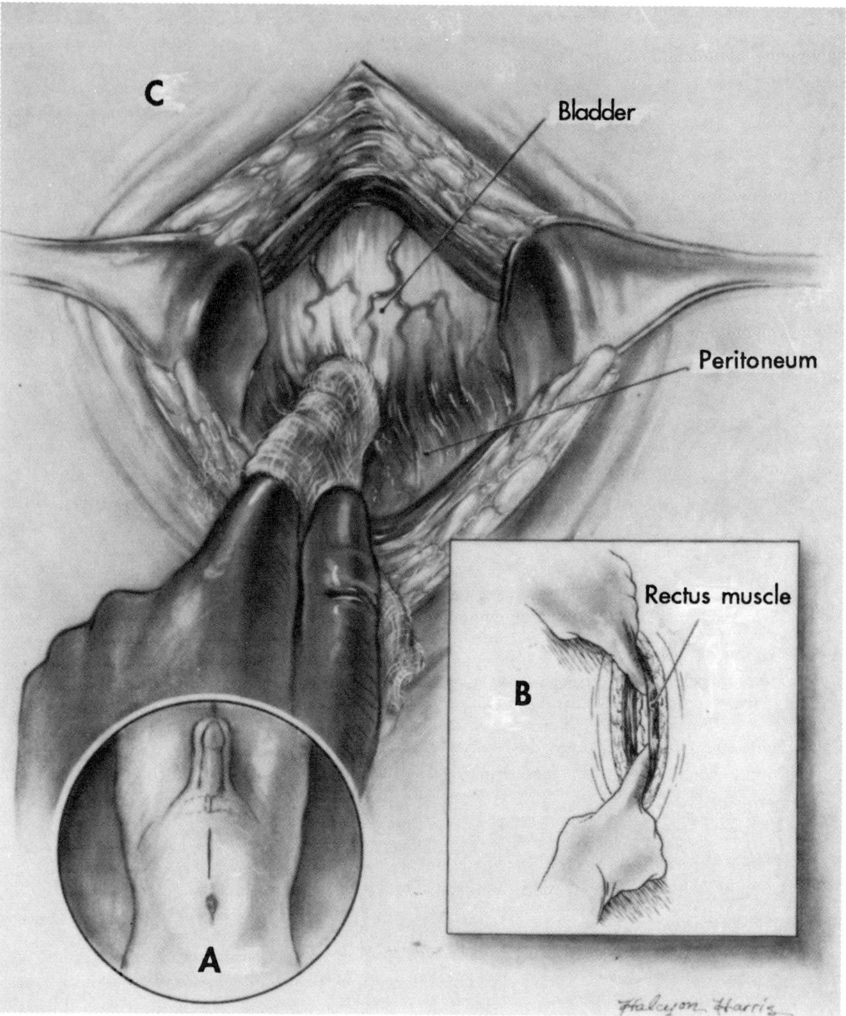


**Fig 30.** Suprapubic prostatectomy. Exposure of bladder. **A:** Low midline skin incision. **B:** Separating the recti muscles. **C:** Dome of bladder exposed by stripping back peritoneum.

one finger pressing the adenoma against the wall of the prostatic fossa. If the attempt is made to deliver the adenoma before the urethra is completely severed, the external sphincter may be ruptured (Fig 34).

When the adenoma is completely freed, grasp and remove it with the fingers or with a lobe forceps (Fig 35). In massive hyperplasia it may be necessary to deliver the adenoma through the bladder incision one lobe at a time or with the lobe forceps. A forceps occupies less space than the fingers.

When the bladder neck is small, it is sometimes difficult to extract the adenoma from the prostatic fossa. Resolve this difficulty by using the fingers to dilate the bladder neck; then deliver the adenoma with a slender uterine tenaculum. An adenoma can sometimes be "popped" through the vesical neck by pressure from a finger in the rectum.

Examine the tissue to make sure all lobes have been removed. As a final check, palpate the prostatic fossa to make sure that no remnants remain.

Following blind suprapubic prostatectomy, use of a hemostatic bag is the usual method to control bleeding. One of three

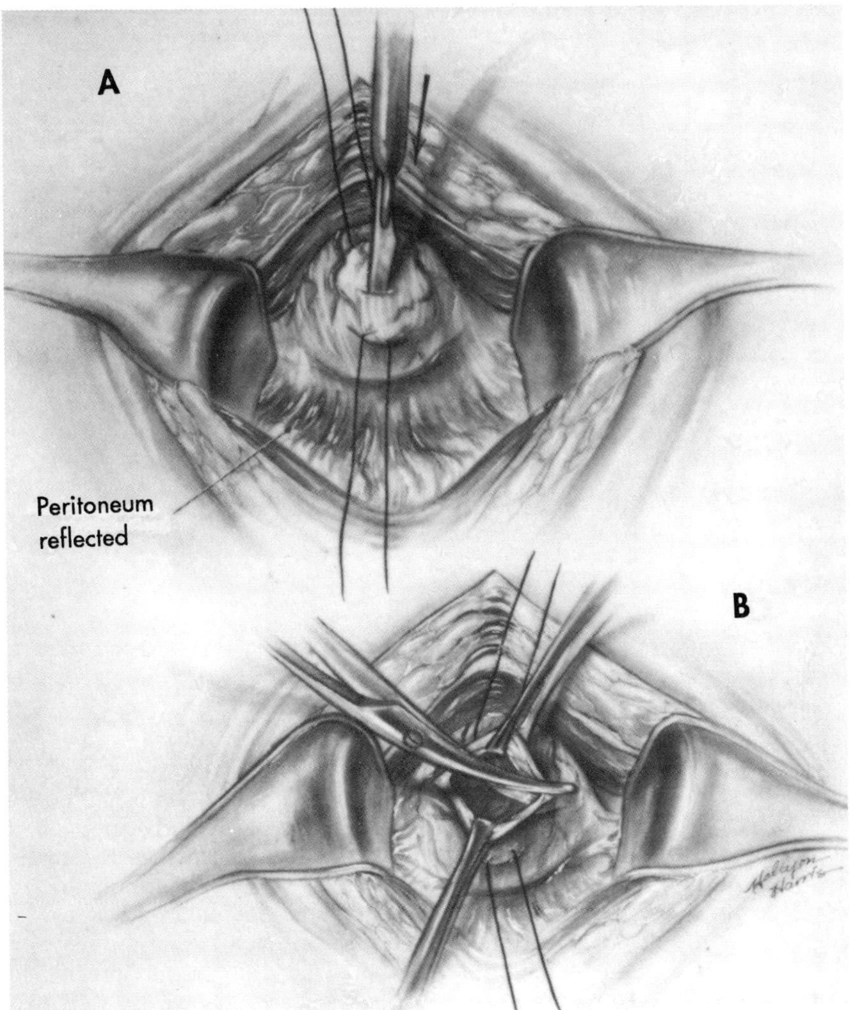


**Fig 31.** Suprapubic prostatectomy. Incising bladder. **A:** Silk stay sutures mark site for opening. **B:** Opening enlarged with scissors.

types of bag may be selected: (1) a bag catheter inserted and removed transurethrally (eg, the Foley), (2) a bag inserted and removed suprapubically (eg, the Pilcher or the Hagner), or (3) a combination in which a suprapubic bag is locked to a urethral catheter (eg, the Brake).

Prior to introducing any type of bag, pack the prostatic fossa with a 2-inch gauze pack for 5 minutes or longer (Fig 36). This minimizes bleeding by permitting the capsule to contract. During this time select the appropriate bag for the conditions found in the individual patient. Remove all blood clots from the fossa and the bladder while an assistant distends the bag. As the bag is drawn against the vesical neck, palpate the vesical neck to be certain that edges of mucosa are directed toward the prostatic fossa. Introduce sufficient fluid to keep the bag within the vesical neck when traction is applied. In adjusting the bag, apply sufficient traction to arrest bleeding into the bladder. Urethral bleeding around the catheter may be ignored. While closing the wound, continue traction until the device to maintain traction is applied.

After blind suprapubic prostatectomy it

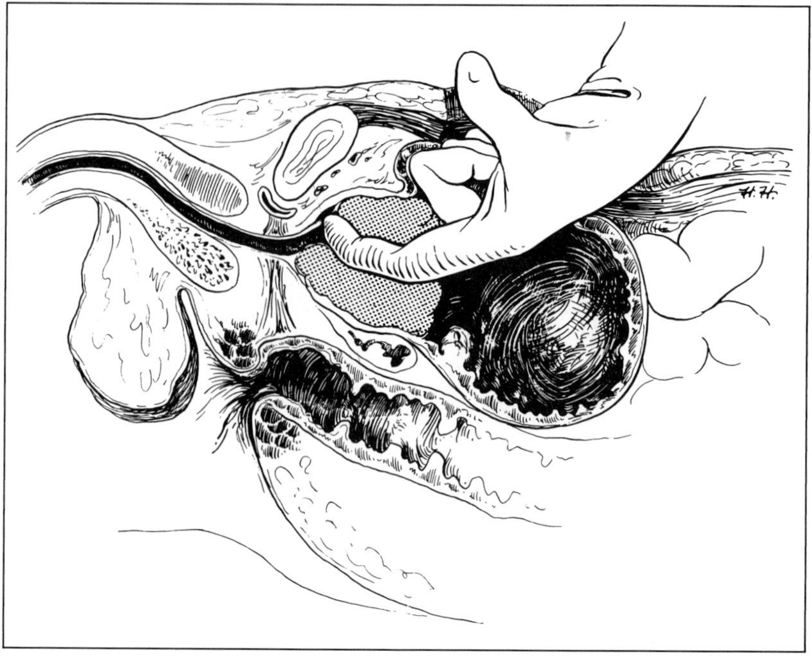

**Fig 32.** Suprapubic prostatectomy. Start of enucleation. Breaking through urethra anteriorly with tip of index finger.

is advisable to provide for cystostomy drainage. A No 28 Fr Malecot catheter is a convenient size. Adjust the catheter so that its cuff is just within the dome of the bladder. With interrupted sutures of No 0 chromic catgut, close the bladder wall around the catheter down to, but not including, the mucosa (Fig 37A).

In closing the abdominal wound, suspend the dome of the bladder to the abdominal wall with two sutures of the bladder closure. This obliterates dead space and facilitates exposure should secondary operation become necessary. Place a drain next to the cystostomy tube and bring the rectus fascia together with interrupted sutures of No 0 chromic catgut. When the patient is obese or if tissues are poor, use retention sutures as well. Finally, close the subcutaneous tissues and the skin (Fig 37B).

**Open Suprapubic Prostatectomy.** This operation is indicated for benign prostatic hyperplasia and may also be applied to excision of bars and vesical neck contractures. It is particularly applicable to massive adenomas and has the same general advantages as blind suprapubic prostatectomy. Its particular advantage over the blind approach is that the bladder neck is visualized; this permits precise control of bleeding and the plastic treatment of the vesical neck. The procedure is contraindicated in carcinoma of the prostate.

The preparation and position of the patient are similar to those in the blind operation. With regard to anesthesia, muscular relaxation is essential. Special prostatic instruments are required.

Make the abdominal incision longer than in the blind operation. Start it at the upper margin of the symphysis pubis and extend it upward to the vicinity of the umbilicus (Fig 38A). The more obese the patient, the longer is the incision required. Expose the dome of the bladder over an area sufficiently wide to permit a transverse incision at least 6 cm long (Fig 38B). Make the incision into the bladder according to the technique described for the blind op-

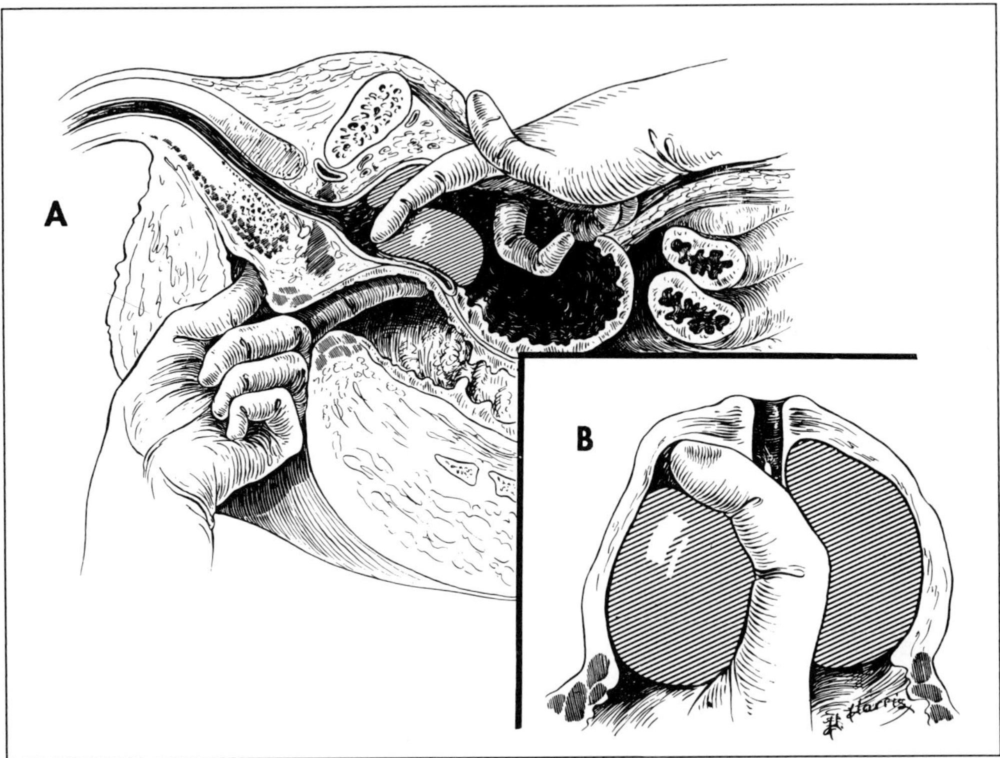


**Fig 33.** Suprapubic prostatectomy. Enucleation of adenoma. **A:** Finger in rectum to elevate prostate. **B:** Severing urethra and developing cleavage plane around apex.

**Fig 34.** Suprapubic prostatectomy. Danger of avulsing urethra from external sphincter. Traction applied to adenoma before urethra is freed.

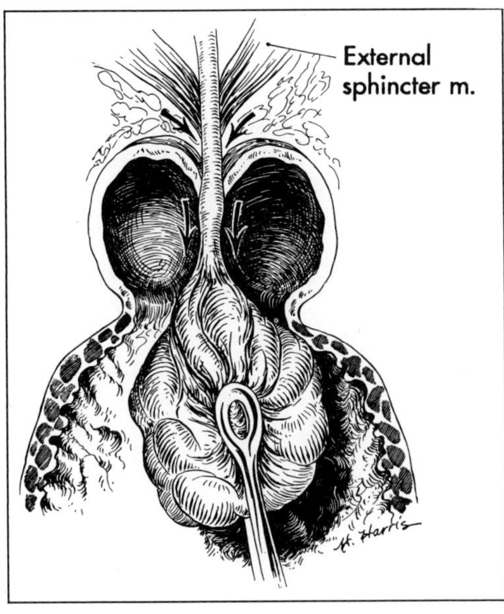


eration, and expose the interior by introducing a three-bladed self-retaining retractor (Fig 39).

Inspect and palpate the bladder and the vesical neck to assess the obstructive lesion.

Preliminary to enucleation of an adenoma, raise a cuff of mucous membrane at the vesical neck with an electrocautery knife (Fig 39A). Preserve as much of this layer as possible for plastic closure. With the curved scissors, raise the cuff of mucosa to avoid tearing it during enucleation (Fig 39B).

Remove the self-retaining retractor and perform the enucleation as in the blind procedure. If there is difficulty in separating adherent areas or in severing the urethra at the apex of the prostate, use the tips of long curved scissors, guided by the finger. Once the adenoma has been freed and the urethra has been severed, apply a prostatic lobe forceps or a uterine tenaculum to aid in the

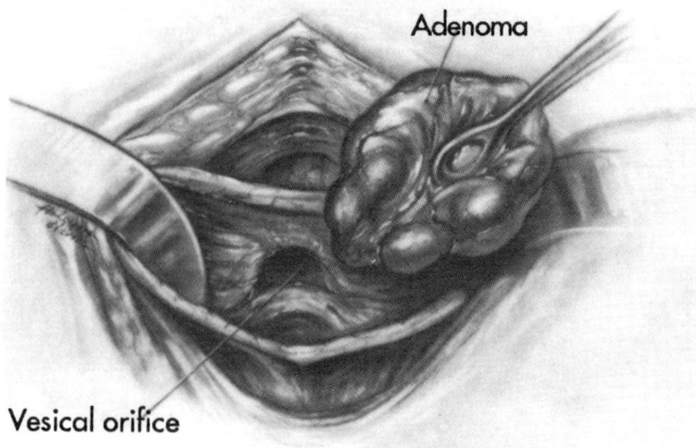


**Fig 35.** Suprapubic prostatectomy. Removing adenoma with lobe forceps.

final separation of the adenoma from the vesical neck.

Reinsert the self-retaining bladder retractor while keeping the field dry with suction and inspect the prostatic fossa. Excise any remaining fragments of tissue with long curved scissors and secure bleeding vessels that can be identified.

Pack the fossa with 2-inch gauze and retain the pack with the tip of a Deaver retractor. Leave the posterior lip of the vesical neck free to receive hemostatic sutures (Fig 40). Employ figure-of-eight sutures of No 0 plain catgut at the quadrants of the vesical neck. Avoid the ureteral orifices. If the pelvis is deep, use a long, angulated

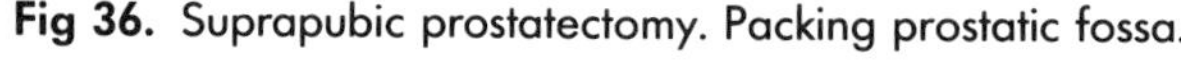
**Fig 36.** Suprapubic prostatectomy. Packing prostatic fossa.

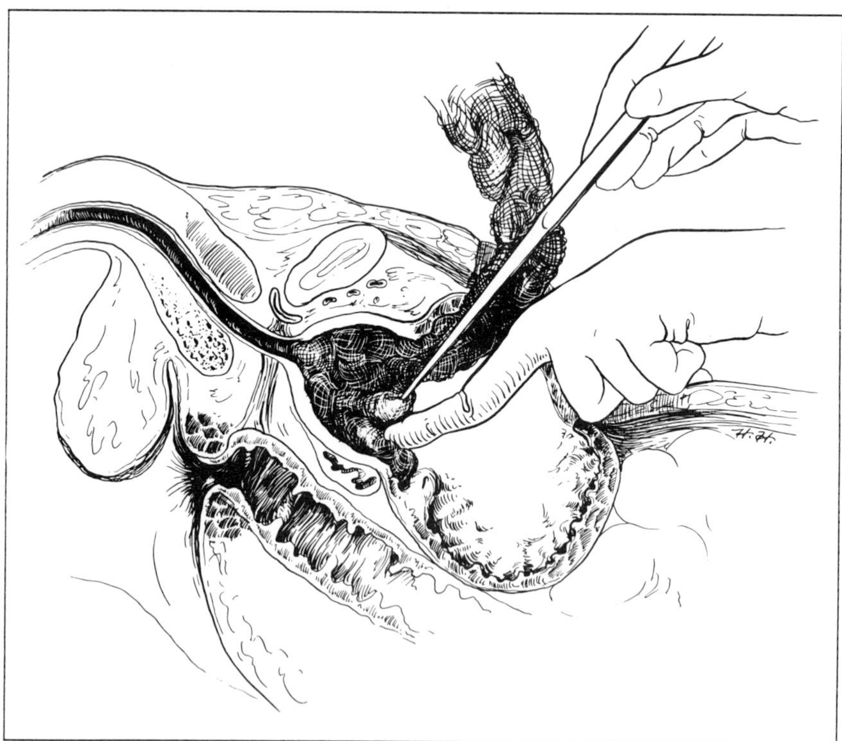

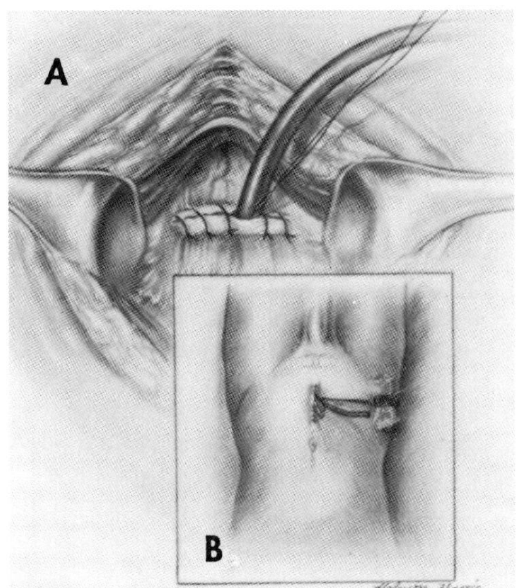


Fig 37. Suprapubic prostatectomy. Closure with Foley bag catheter. **A:** Musculature united around Malecot catheter. **B:** Malecot catheter, long safety suture, and cigarette drains led out abdominal wall.

needle holder to place these sutures. Traction on the first suture will bring up the vesical neck; this facilitates completing the plastic closure.

If the vesical neck is small or fibrotic, excise a wedge of tissue from the posterior aspect. When bleeding continues, search out and ligate or fulgurate the vessel. The hemostatic sutures around the vesical neck usually reduce the size of the orifice so that a 30-$cm^3$ bag catheter is adequate.

A modification of the open suprapubic prostatectomy involves the placing, for hemostatic purposes, of deep interrupted No 0 or No 00 plain catgut sutures at the vesical neck starting posteriorly. These sutures are taken approximately 1 cm lateral to the edge of the bladder neck and extend an equal depth into the fossa. These sutures may then either be tied directly over a No 24 Fr Foley catheter, or they may be brought out suprapubically and tied snugly over a button, the No 24 Fr Foley catheter having been inserted before the bladder was closed. In either of these modifications, the snug sutures around the bladder greatly minimize postoperative bleeding, and there does not appear to be any resulting postoperative vesical neck contracture or prostatic urethral stricture resulting.

**Suprapubic Resection of Vesical Neck.** This method is also applicable to resection of fibrous lesions of the vesical neck. Place an Allis forceps in the central portion of the posterior vesical neck and draw it upward. With curved scissors or with cervical biopsy forceps, excise a wedge of tissue through the entire depth of the fibrous ledge (Fig 41). Control bleeding with suture of No. 0 plain catgut. Close the bladder without cystostomy drainage.

## Conservative Retropubic Prostatectomy

The retropubic approach is the most recently developed[24,25] of the four presently used approaches to the prostate. As with the open suprapubic approach, this operation is indicated when a massive adenoma is present. It is also indicated, as is the suprapubic technique, in patients in whom ankylosis of the hips precludes the lithotomy position. It is contraindicated in the presence of carcinoma of the prostate.

The advantages of the retropubic approach are that it permits ideal exposure of the prostatic bed and vesical neck and greatly facilitates precise control of bleeding and the plastic treatment of the bladder neck. Also advantageous is the absence of the necessity to use a postoperative suprapubic catheter, as in the suprapubic approach. Disadvantages are that special equipment is needed and that the exposure can be very difficult in obese persons or in those with a narrow or deep pelvis. The incidence of osteitis pubis is reportedly higher with this approach than with any other. Postoperative bleeding is minimal; nevertheless, the approach is through an extremely vascular field, which renders control of bleeding difficult in an occasional case. Also, there is wide opening of poorly drained tissue spaces, which may predispose to infection.

Von Stockum first utilized this approach in 1909, and Terrence Millen established

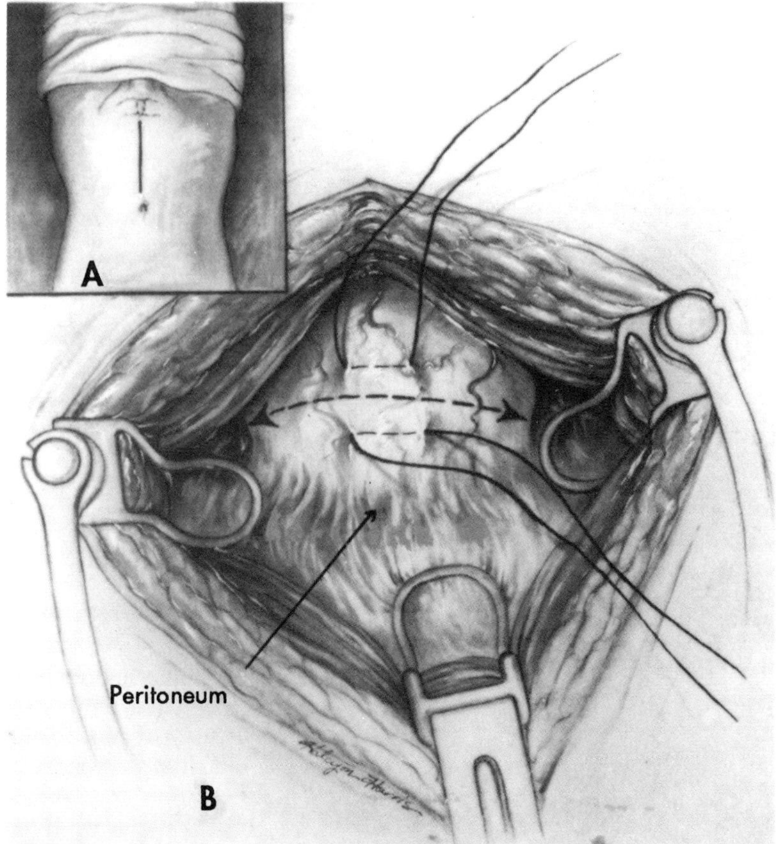


**Fig 38.** Open suprapubic prostatectomy. Method of exposure. **A:** Long low-midline abdominal incision. **B:** Line of wide transverse incision in dome of bladder.

the procedure on a firm surgical foundation in 1945.

The operation may be performed in the conventional decubitus or the low lithotomy position. I prefer the latter position because it affords simultaneous access to the urethra (for cystoscopy), scrotum (for vasectomy), retropubic region, and rectum. In both positions elevation of the hips, as with a sandbag, facilitates access to the retropubic region.

Prepare the operative field and drain the bladder with a catheter. Urine in the bladder compromises exposure of the prostate. If cystoscopy has not been carried out previously, make the examination at this point.

Retropubic prostatectomy requires special instruments. These include long-handled curved clamps, Allis forceps, and tissue forceps, as well as the special instruments shown in Fig 42.

Make a low midline abdominal incision starting at the symphysis pubis. Extend it to the region of the umbilicus (Fig 43A). Deepen the incision through the rectus fascia and separate the recti muscles in the midline. Divide the pyramidalis muscles and carry the incision down to the symphysis pubis to gain all possible exposure of the retropubic space. In obese patients this may bring the skin incision to the base of the penis.

Develop the retropubic space by using the gauze-covered index finger to gently draw the extravesical fat and transversalis fascia upwards to the vesical neck. Insert

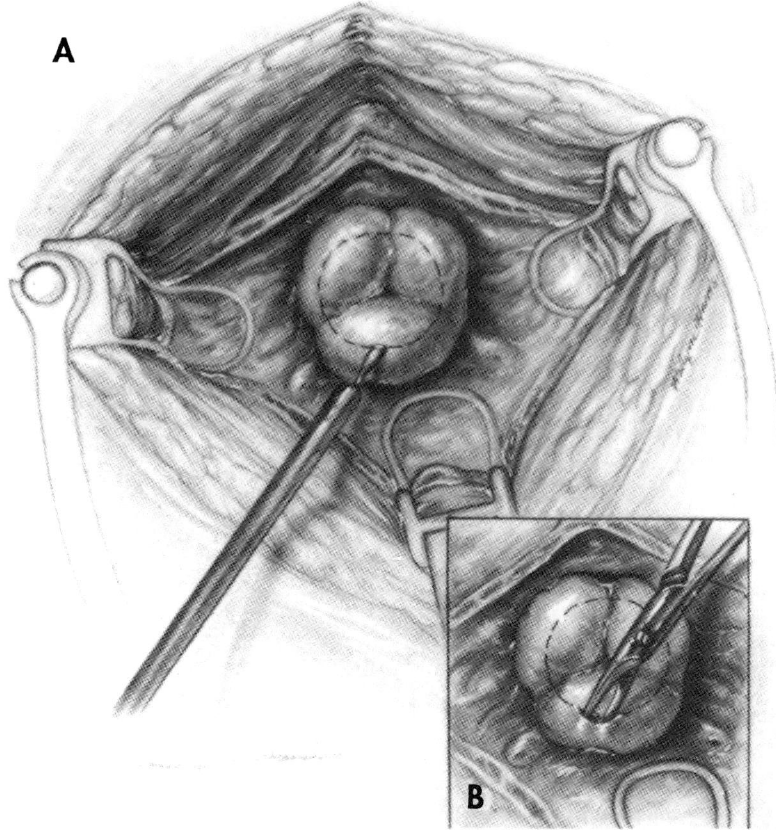


**Fig 39.** Open suprapubic prostatectomy. Exposure of bladder maintained with Jacobson retractor. **A:** Incision with coagulation current for plastic treatment of vesical neck. **B:** Freeing cuff of mucosa with curved scissors.

a self-retaining retractor to spread the recti muscles apart. Fix the middle blade to depress the bladder upward.

Inspect the retropubic space to locate vessels outside the prostatic capsule. Clamp, divide, and coagulate them at this time. Gently divest the anterior aspect of the prostate of any adherent fat. Use a cherry sponge or Kittner dissector to tease the fat to either side or upward (Fig 43B).

Palpate the extent of the prostatic hyperplasia and observe the location of the anterior capsular veins. The vesical neck is identified as a ridge where the firm glandular texture of the prostate gives way to the softer tissues of the bladder musculature.

It is not necessary to remove the self-retaining retractor during enucleation, although some surgeons prefer to do so. In contrast to suprapubic prostatectomy, the enucleation can be effected with minimal use of fingers inside the prostatic capsule. If the prostate is deeply located, elevate it by pressure exerted through the rectum. In the low lithotomy position this is accomplished by the second assistant who stands between the patient's legs. Make the capsular incision in a transverse direction 1 cm below the vesical neck. Stay sutures may be placed above and below the site selected (Fig 44A). Start the incision over the midportion of one lateral lobe and extend it across the midline to the midpoint of the opposite lateral lobe. This permits access to the entire periphery of the adenoma. Bleeding may be brisk, so keep suction available. Deepen the incision to the sur-

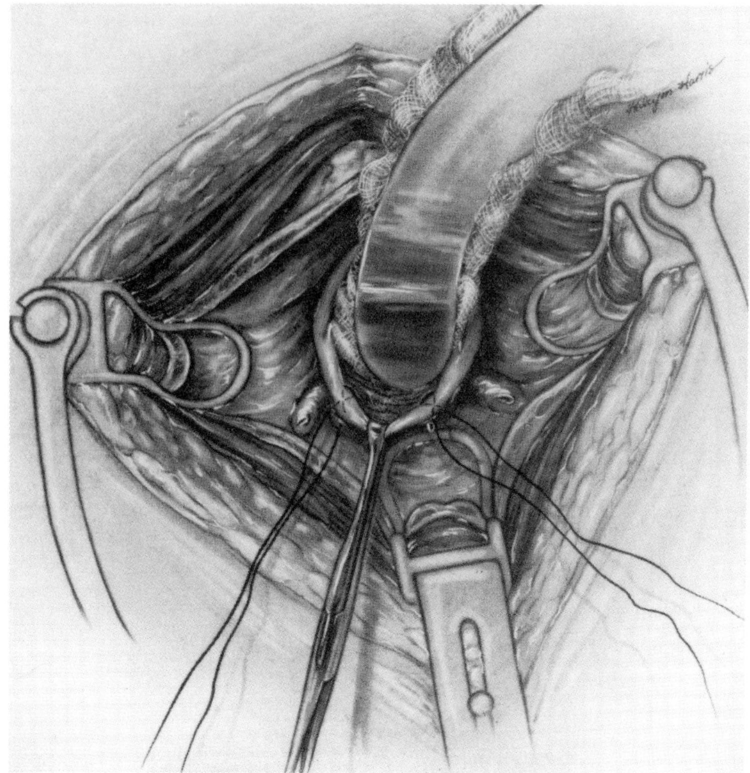

**Fig 40.** Open suprapubic prostatectomy. Placing sutures in vesical neck. Prostatic fossa packed with gauze to minimize bleeding.

gical capsule, recognized by the white texture of the adenoma and felt by the ''give'' of the scalpel as it penetrates the capsule. Grasp the capsular vessels with straight hemostats as they are seen to bleed, and electrocoagulate them.

Start the enucleation by undermining the distal flap of the capsule, inserting and opening the blades of long-curve scissors (Fig 44B). As the line of cleavage is developed, substitute the tip of an index finger to free the adenoma from the lateral aspects of the prostatic fossa, but avoid tearing the capsule. If a wider capsular opening is required, use a scissors. When the adenoma has been freed over its anterior and lateral aspects, grasp it with a uterine tenaculum to tent up and identify the prostatic urethra as it emerges from the apical extent of the adenoma. Divide the urethra with curved scissors. Avoid any traction which might injure the external sphincter. The verumontanum and ejaculatory ducts are preserved by dividing the urethra close to the adenoma (Fig 44C).

After mobilizing the apex of the adenoma, apply gentle traction and deliver it through the capsular incision (Fig 45A). Sweep an index finger around the periphery of the adenoma, thereby freeing it from the capsule, and withdraw the adenoma from the depths of the fossa. The adenoma now remains attached only at the vesical neck (Fig 45B). If the lateral lobes are extremely large, one lobe may be delivered at a time; this step does not preclude en masse enucleation.

Separate the adenoma from the circular fibers of the internal sphincter. Be sure to include any median lobe or posterior commissural hyperplasia in the dissection. Divide the mucosa of the vesical neck throughout its circumference as it is separated (Fig 46A). Clamp and ligate any

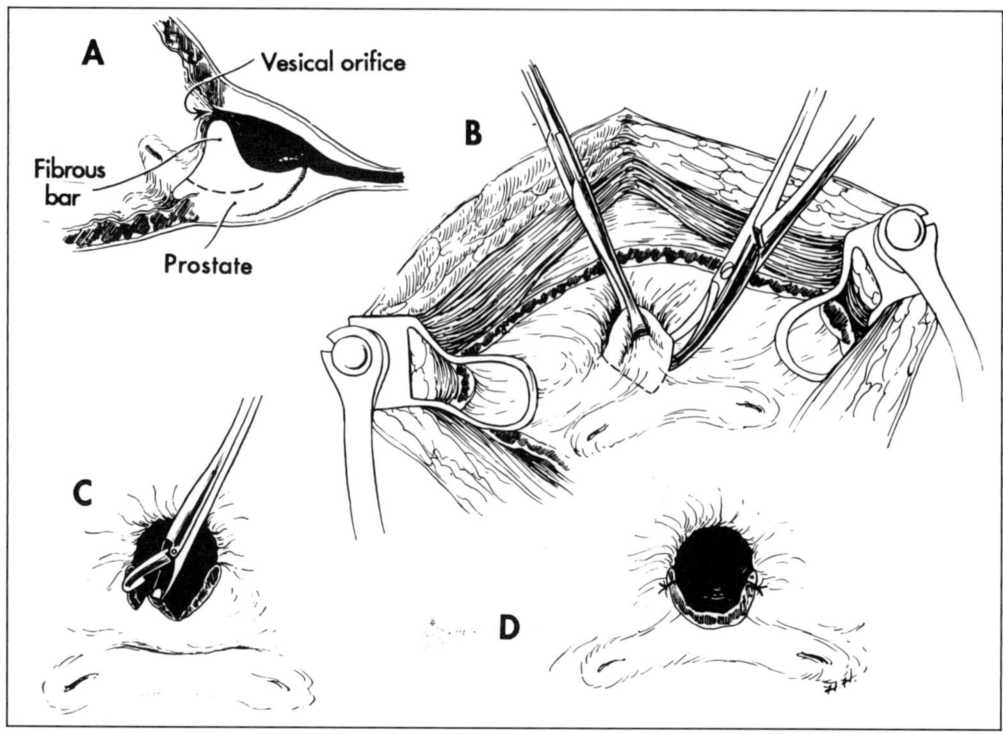


Fig 41. Suprapubic resection of vesical neck. Excision of fibrous median bar. **A:** Depth of resection indicated. Excising bar with scissors (**B**) and with cervical biopsy forceps (**C**). **D:** Sutures to control bleeding.

vessels which come into view. Inspect the widely exposed prostatic fossa for adherent nodules of adenoma or tags of tissue (Fig 46B).

Pack the prostatic fossa with 2-inch gauze. Keep the pack out of the field with a Deaver retractor (Fig 47) while the bladder is explored, a wedge is resected from the vesical neck, and hemostatic sutures are introduced. Wedge resection of the vesical neck is extremely important in this operation. It prevents postoperative stenosis.

Inspect the removed tissue and palpate the interior of the bladder to be certain no nodules have separated and fallen off. If indicated for any reason, do not hesitate to make a cystotomy opening.

Grasp the posterior lip of the vesical neck in the midline and excise a generous wedge of tissue (Fig 48). Keep the line of incision at least 1 cm distant from the urteral orifices. Cervical biopsy forceps may be used to deepen the wedge and to grip the edges. Control bleeding and secure the divided mucosa with interrupted sutures of No 0 plain catgut. In excising the wedge of tissue, some surgeons preserve a flap of mucosa to suture over the divided posterior vesical lip (Fig 49).

Place mattress sutures of No 0 plain catgut in the inferior quadrants of the vesical neck to secure the main prostatic blood vessels. Complete the closure of the vesical neck by taking additional interrupted sutures around the entire circumference of the neck. This provides hemostasis and prevents retraction of the mucosa (Fig 50A).

After plastic treatment of the vesical neck, remove the gauze pack, inspect the fossa, and electrocoagulate any bleeding points. When hemostasis is secure, introduce a No 24 Fr, 30-$cm^3$ Foley catheter through the urethra and advance it far into the bladder cavity (Fig 50B) so that it will not slip out during closure of the capsule. Do not inflate the bag at this time. There

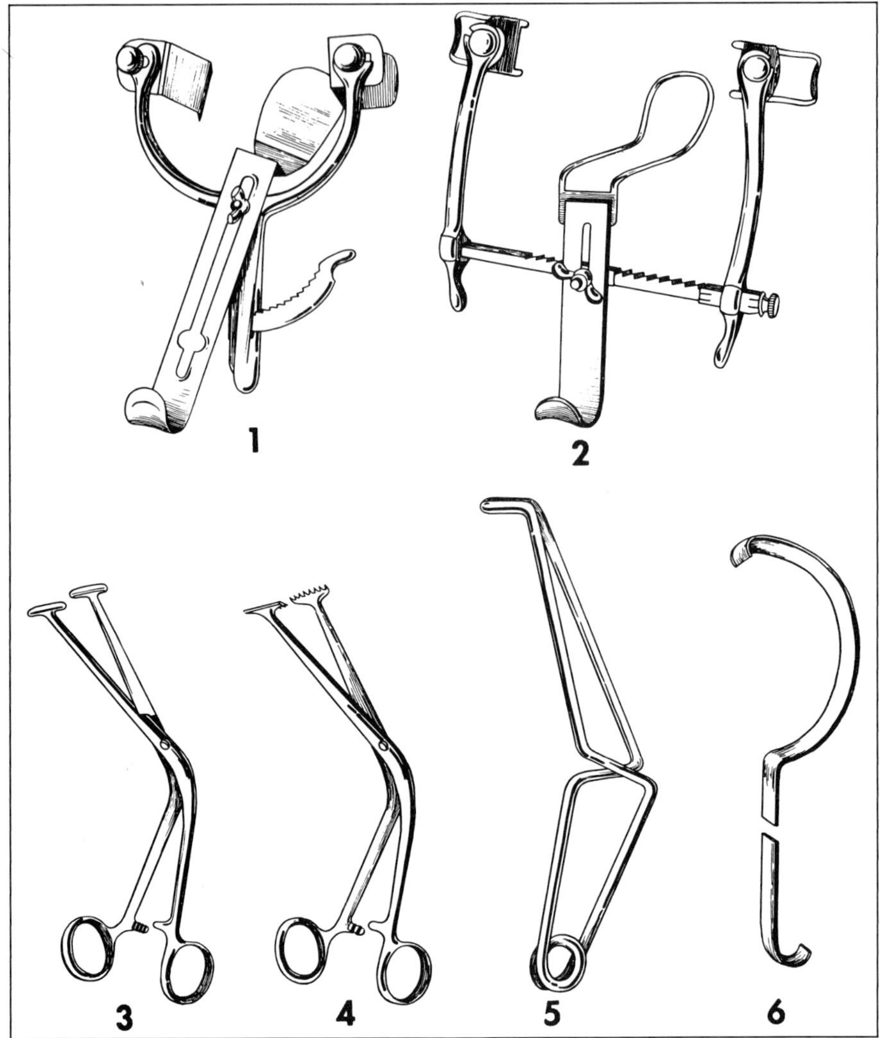


**Fig 42.** Retropubic prostatectomy. Special instruments for operation. **1:** Millin retractor. **2:** Jacobson retractor. **3:** Millin capsule forceps. **4:** Millin volsellum. **5:** Millin bladder neck spreader. **6:** Nelson retractor.

is danger of perforating it during closure of the capsule. Irrigate the bladder to flush out all blood clots.

Close the incision in the capsule with a continuous suture of No 0 chromic catgut starting with two sutures, each one lateral to either extremity of the incision. Tie the two in the middle. This technique minimizes danger of leakage at the vulnerable extremities of the incision. Do not pierce the urethral catheter with a suture. Secure a watertight capsular closure. Then inflate the catheter with approximately 20 mL of water, draw it to the vesical neck, and again irrigate the bladder.

Irrigate the wound with normal saline. Place two cigarette drains down to the capsular incision. Approximate the recti muscles with a few interrupted sutures of No 0 plain catgut. Close the rectus fascia with interrupted sutures of No 0 chromic catgut. Bring together the subcutaneous tissues with No 00 plain catgut. Close the skin with silk, cotton, or skin clips.

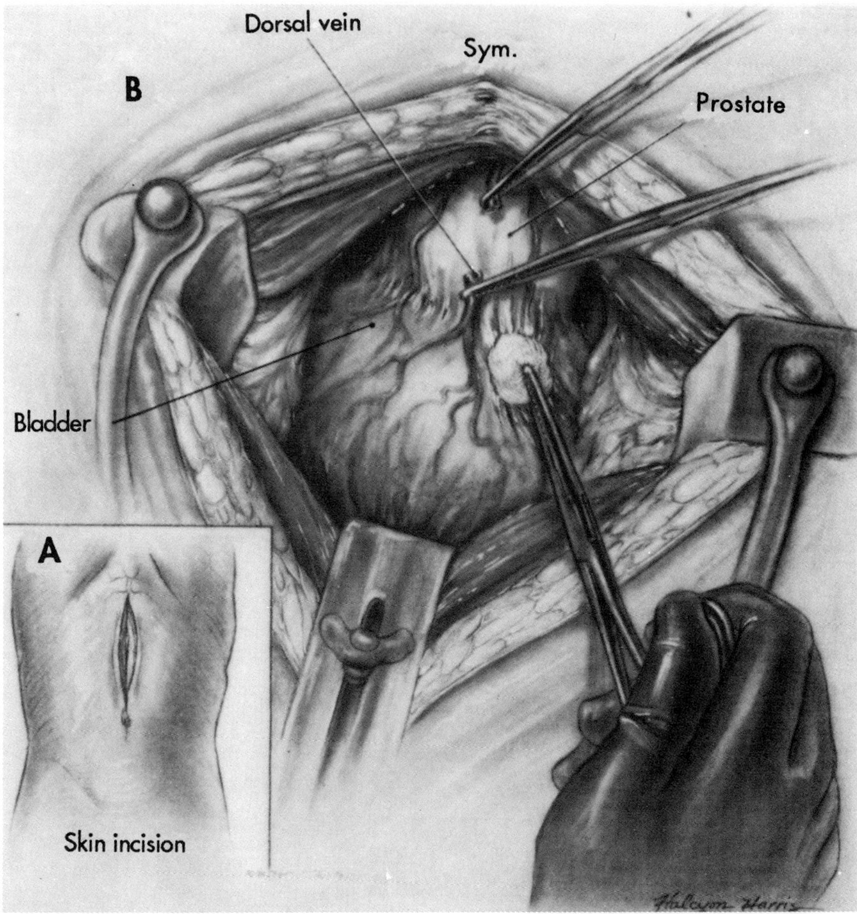


**Fig 43.** Retropubic prostatectomy. Exposure of prostate. **A:** Abdominal incision. **B:** Dissecting superficial fat from anterior aspect of prostate; dividing superficial vein.

## Y-V Plasty

This procedure has been used in the surgical treatment of fibrotic obstructions to the vesical neck in both children and adults.

Make a low midline abdominal incision as for a retropubic prostatectomy, and expose the anterior aspect of the vesical neck and adjacent proximal portion of the prostate.

Inflate the bladder through a urethral catheter with about 200 $cm^3$ of a sterile solution. Place a stay suture of No 0 chromic catgut in the midline of the prostatic capsule just proximal to the puboprostatic ligaments. Use a curved blade and make the limbs of the Y incision over the lower aspect of the bladder just above the vesical-prostatic junction. Stay within an area approximately 2 cm on either side of the midline of the bladder to avoid large blood vessels. Continue the incision through the roof of the prostatic urethra and overlying capsule so as to make the stem of the Y incision (Fig 51A). Secure bleeding points and fulgurate.

Elevate the V flap of bladder wall that has just been made. This provides ideal exposure of the bladder trigone, posterior vesical lip, and prostatic urethra. Excise a deep wedge from the posterior vesical neck as in conservative retropubic prostatectomy. Make sure hemostasis is secure and insert a No 24 Fr, 30-$cm^3$ Foley catheter into the bladder, but do not inflate the bag until the Y incision has been closed. Close

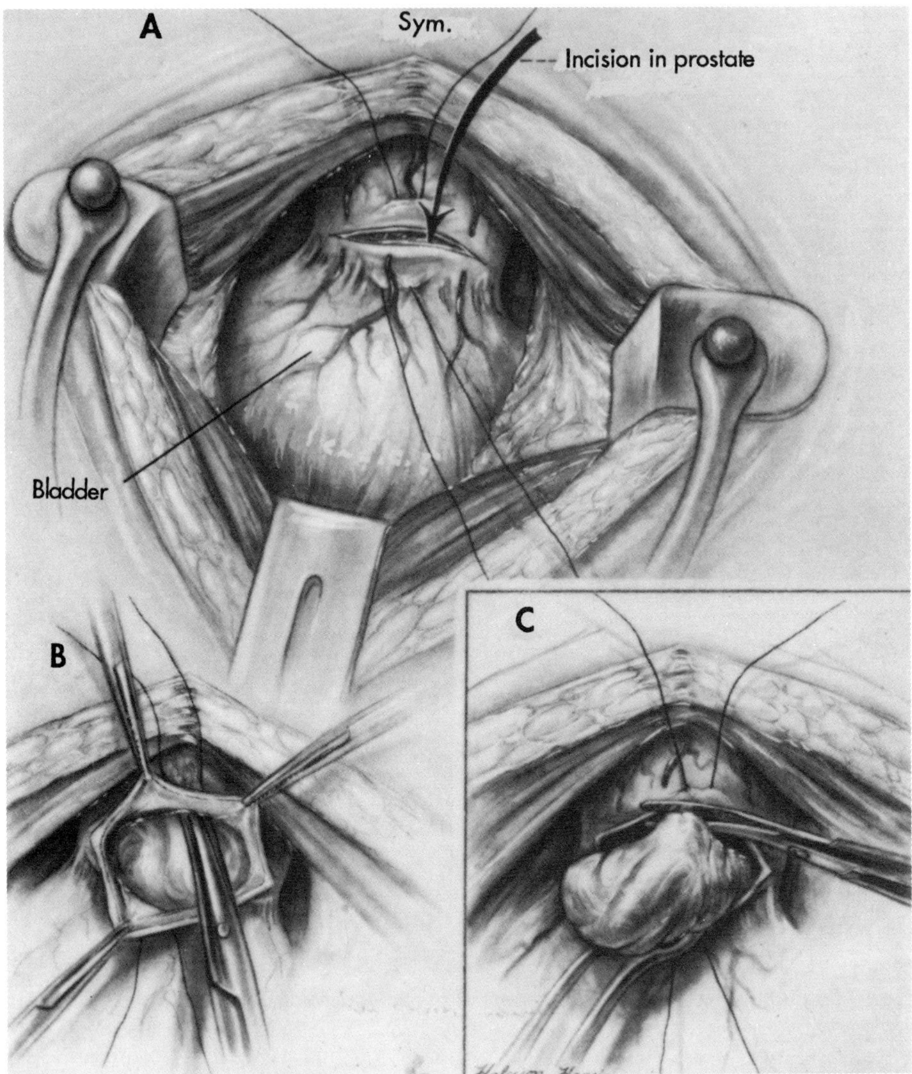


**Fig 44.** Retropubic prostatectomy. Enucleation of adenoma. **A:** Transverse incision 1 cm below vesical neck. **B:** Start of enucleation by undermining distal flap. **C:** Adenoma elevated with uterine tenaculum; division of urethra at apex.

the incision with a running suture using the previously placed stay suture for this purpose (Fig 51A). By bringing this wedge of bladder wall down to the lower angle of the incision, a tongue of vesical neck musculature is interposed anteriorly at the vesical neck, which is thereby enlarged. Leave cigarette drains in the space of Retzius, and close the abdominal incision as previously described.

## Transurethral Prostatectomy

Transurethral prostatectomy has gained widespread acceptance only in the United States, and it is, by any criterion, one of the most difficult of all operations to master.

The modern era of this surgical procedure really dates back only as far as the mid 1930s, when tremendous improve-

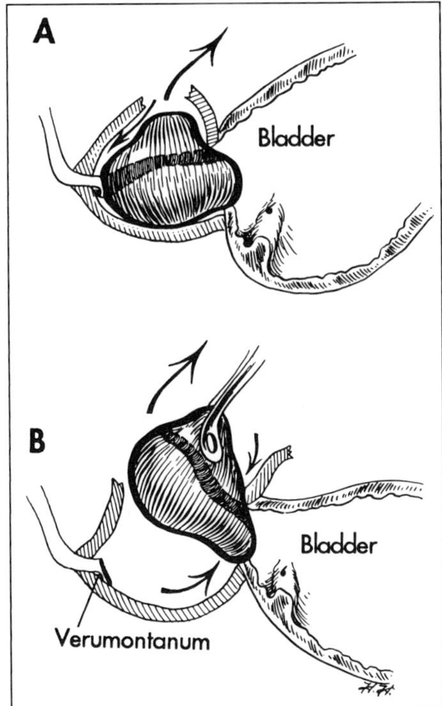


**Fig 45.** Retropubic prostatectomy. Method of enucleation. **A:** Adenoma mobilized by dividing urethra. **B:** Adenoma delivered, separating it from apex to base.

ments were effected both in the widely used electroresection and the lesser known "cold punch" techniques.

The procedure is indicated for small and moderate adenomas and for median bar and vesical neck contractures, as well as for cysts of the prostate and for tags from past prostatectomy surgery. It is also indicated in carcinoma of the prostate not amenable to total prostatectomy and in the poor-risk patient who nevertheless requires surgery.[26] It is most difficult to do in massive adenomas (over 100 g) and, for the average urologist, in adenomas over 50 g. It is not indicated in cases in which the urethra is unusually narrow, although the use of internal or perineal urethrotomy may obviate this somewhat. It is similarly contraindicated in patients with hip ankylosis precluding the lithotomy position.

The principal advantages of the transurethral approach are that the patient is usually hospitalized half the number of days required in "open" operation and the morbidity is much less. Disadvantages are that the procedure is technically much more difficult than any of the open procedures, and special equipment is required. The risks of great blood loss and of urinary incontinence are very real, as are the risks of postoperative bladder neck contracture or urethral stricture.

The transurethral approach is probably the procedure of choice for the skilled urologist who is competent with any approach. Massive adenoma (over 100 g) is the chief indication for the choice of an open operation rather than a transurethral approach.

With either type of resectoscope an irrigation system is required that will ensure a continuous supply of fluid during the operation. Many irrigation systems are satisfactory; even a Valentine flask reservoir refilled with fluid as needed is perfectly functional, although the vast majority of urologists prefer to use the commercially available bags or plastic bottles that contain an isotonic irrigating solution. These bags or bottles usually are of 3-L size, and the number of times that bag replacement is necessary during the course of a transurethral surgical procedure will depend upon the duration of the operation.

There are some urologists who prefer to use water (and not an isotonic solution) for irrigation throughout the operative procedure. I feel that this is potentially dangerous if large amounts of it are absorbed into the circulation during prolonged procedures or when many venous sinuses are opened. This water absorption leads to intravascular hemolysis and very often to subsequent oliguria and anuria due to acute tubular necrosis. With increasing frequency, therefore, urologists are now tending to use the isotonic irrigating solutions, although many feel that they cannot see as well when using these solutions as they can with water. It is probably not dangerous to use water for a very small and relatively bloodless resection. Where the gland is larger and the bleeding brisk, isotonic solutions should be mandatory.

Recent clinical and investigational ex-

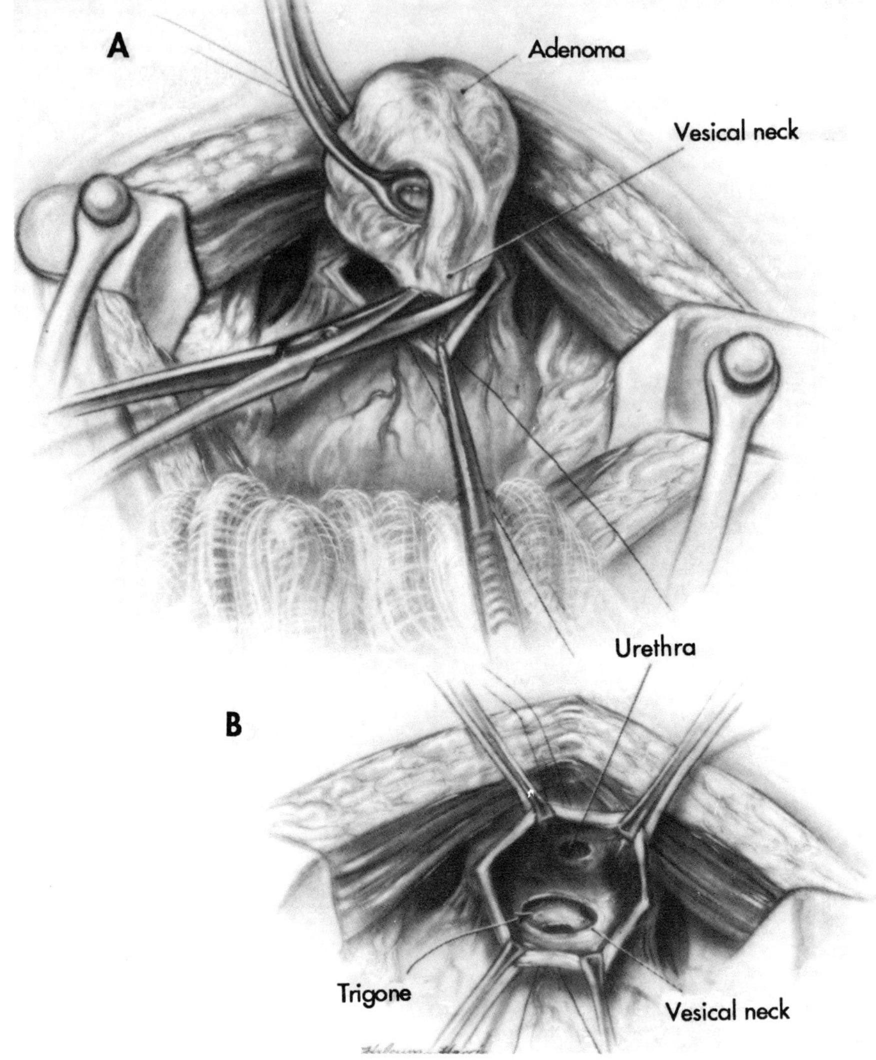


**Fig 46.** Retropubic prostatectomy. Completing enucleation. **A:** Final division at vesical neck. **B:** Prostatic fossa after enucleation.

perience indicates, however, that even the isotonic irrigating solutions are not a panacea for all potential problems that can occur as a result of fluid absorption into the circulation.[27] When isotonic irrigating solutions are used, the risk of intravascular hemolysis is virtually nonexistent and this certainly provides a reason to use these agents rather than sterile water for irrigation. However, the two most frequently used isotonic irrigating solutions (mannitol and glycine) do indeed present problems of their own.

With either, for example, a dilutional hyponatremia can occur depending on the volume of irrigating fluid that is absorbed into the circulation. Equally important are the more recently described side effects of these isotonic irrigating solutions, such as hyperkalemia and hyperammonemia. The irrigants containing glycine produce hyperkalemia and usually a prickling or a burning skin sensation as well as a slight nausea. The severity of these symptoms correlates with the elevated blood ammonia level and increases significantly after gly-

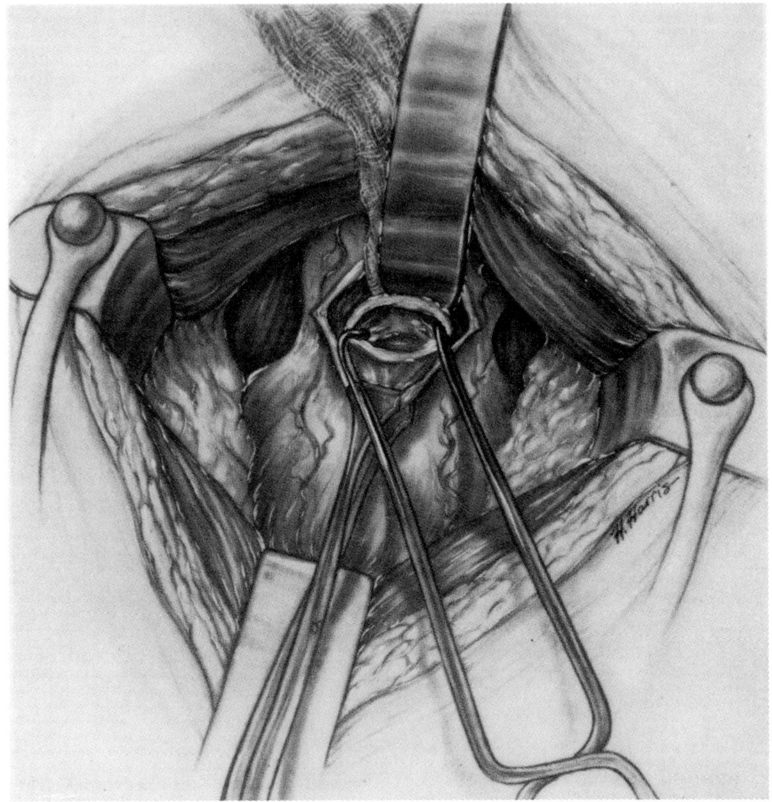

**Fig 47.** Retropubic prostatectomy. Preparation for plastic treatment of vesical neck. Prostatic fossa packed with gauze. Bladder neck held open with Millin spreader.

cine infusion but not following mannitol infusion. Infusion of mannitol results in pronounced but transient increase in blood volume and a hyponatremia that is more prolonged than that which occurs with glycine infusion. The experimental use of 1% ethanol, combined with either the mannitol or the glycine, provides an interesting and noninvasive method of monitoring absorption of either of these irrigant solutions by measuring the amount of ethanol in the expired breath. It is important to note that, notwithstanding the problems that can occur when either mannitol or glycine are used for irrigation during the TUR, either of these agents poses far less of a threat to a patient than does distilled water with its attendant risk of intravascular hemolysis and renal shutdown.

In addition to the "cold-punch" resectoscope, there are basically two types of electroresectoscopes: the two-hand model, such as the Stern–McCarthy, and a spring modification of this instrument, such as the Nesbit. The latter allows the surgeon a free hand to apply rectal counterpressure during a resection. The "cold-punch" resectoscope, as it is most commonly used, is a two-hand instrument, necessitating the presence of an assistant who can supply the rectal counterpressure during resection.

Low spinal anesthesia is ideal for transurethral prostatectomy. Relaxation is excellent, and the patient is able to complain if the bladder becomes overdistended or if extravasation occurs.

Calibrate the urethra with Otis bulbs Nos 26 Fr, 28 Fr, and 30 Fr. If any of these do not easily pass the meatus and the fossa navicularis, do a meatotomy to No 32 Fr

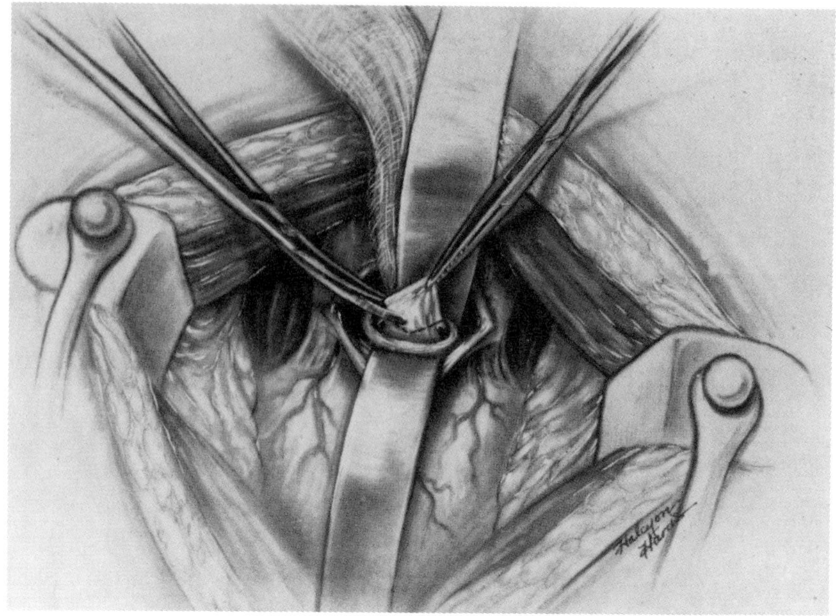

**Fig 48.** Retropubic prostatectomy. Excising wedge from posterior vesical lip.

**Fig 49.** Retropubic prostatectomy. Mucosal flap method of wedge excision. **A:** Mucosal flap raised over site selected for wedge excision. **B:** Wedge excised. **C:** Mucosal flap sutured over denuded surface, prostatic vessels being secured with mattress sutures.

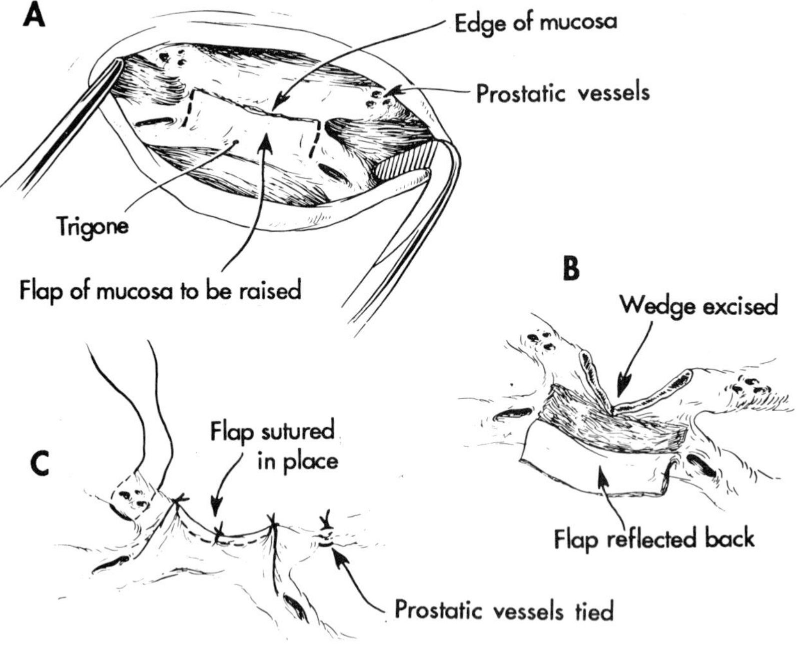

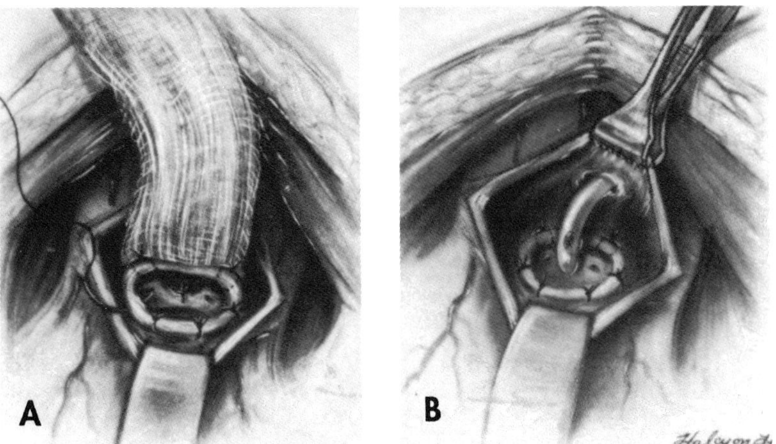


**Fig 50.** Retropubic prostatectomy. Completion of plastic closure. **A:** Sutures placed around vesical neck. **B:** Introducing Foley catheter into bladder.

**Fig 51.** Retropubic excision of vesical neck. Application of Y-V incision. **A:** Y started over lower aspect of bladder and continued into prostatic urethra. **B:** Bladder musculature interposed at vesical neck in closure.

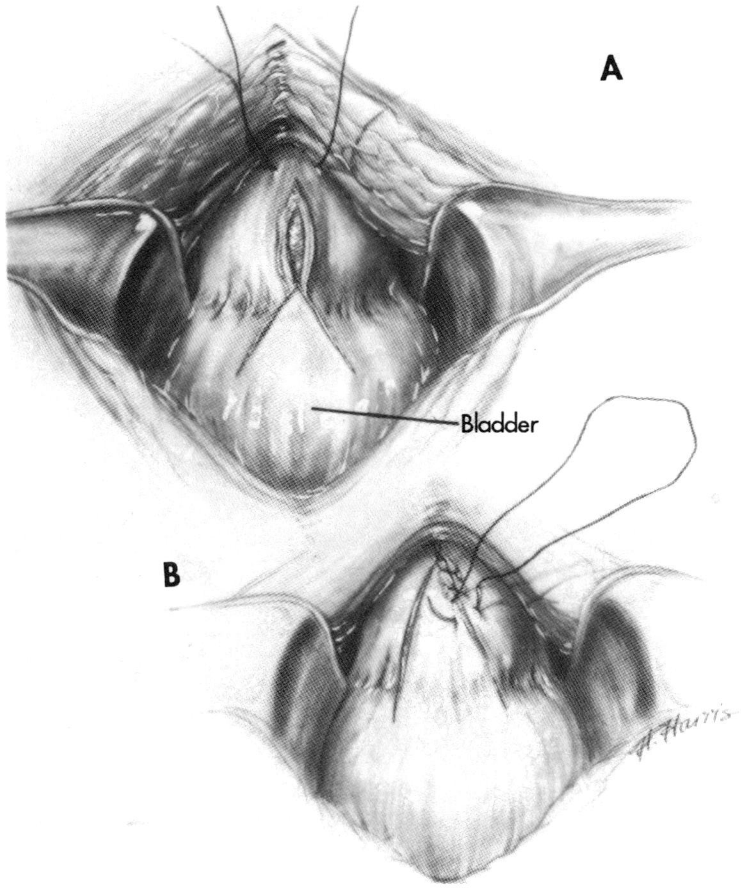

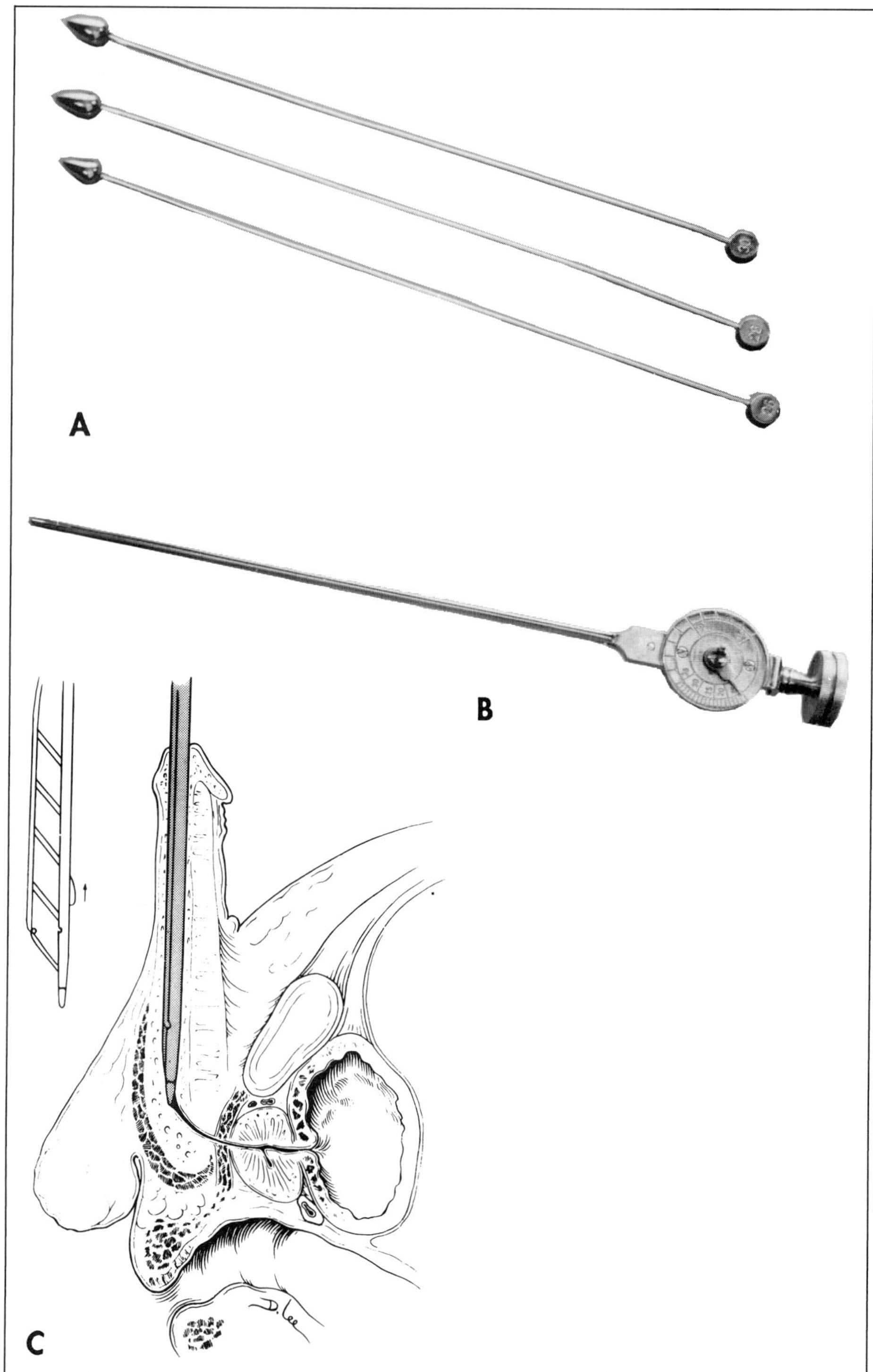


**Fig 52. A:** Otis bulbs, 26 Fr, 28 Fr, 30 Fr, used to calibrate the urethra from the bulb all the way distally to the meatus. **B:** An Otis urethrotome that is used to cut narrowed portions of the urethra as needed. The blade has been removed, and the groove on the front surface of the urethrotome (in which the blade normally rests) can clearly be seen. The numbered dial at the larger end of the urethrotome is calibrated in French units and shows the size to which the urethrotome has been opened prior to incising the urethra. **C:** The urethrotome is in place within the urethra after the patient has been anesthetized. The urethrotome has been opened so that the urethra can be incised to the size noted on the dial in the front of the urethrotome.

using an Otis urethrotome. The meatus can be cut at either the 12 o'clock or the 6 o'clock position. Next pass each Otis bulb in turn down as far as the bulb of the urethra, and if any resistance at all is felt to any of these bulbs, do an internal urethrotomy to No 35 Fr with the Otis urethrotome (Fig 52). This should be done in the 12 o'clock position. One of the very real complications of transurethral resection of the prostate is stricture of the urethra or of the meatus. This results from moving the resectoscope about vigorously in a urethra that is not large enough to accommodate it easily. By doing the meatotomy and/or the internal urethrotomy, the postsurgical incidence of stricture can be decreased to approximately 1%.[28] (Some surgeons prefer to do a perineal urethrostomy instead of an internal urethrotomy, and this is clearly an acceptable alternative.)

Introduce the resectoscope into the well-lubricated urethra and carefully inspect the interior of the bladder and the prostatic urethra. Plan the methodical execution of the operation. If cystoscopy has not previously been performed, this should be done because the fore-oblique lens of the resectoscope does not give an adequate view of the interior of the bladder. Note carefully the type of prostatic enlargement (Fig 53). Particularly note the position of the obstructive tissue with relation to the ureteral orifices and the trigone. Intravesical extension of prostatic tissue may obscure the trigone and the ureteral orifices and the danger of resecting a ureteral orifice is a very real one. A similarly real danger, in these cases of intravesical extension of prostatic tissue, may be that of resecting too deeply and perforating the bladder. Moreover, in a median bar, for example, anteriorly and laterally there is only a narrow rim of tissue separating the urethra from the internal sphincter. In such instances, removal of one loopful of tissue penetrates the muscular fibers of the vesical neck and an additional bit may cause perforation (Fig 54A). In benign prostatic hyperplasia, however, adenomatous tissue assures a wider margin of safety (Fig 54B). Also note very carefully the region of the apical tissue

**Fig 53.** Transurethral prostatectomy. Inspection of operative field. Trilobed benign hyperplasia.

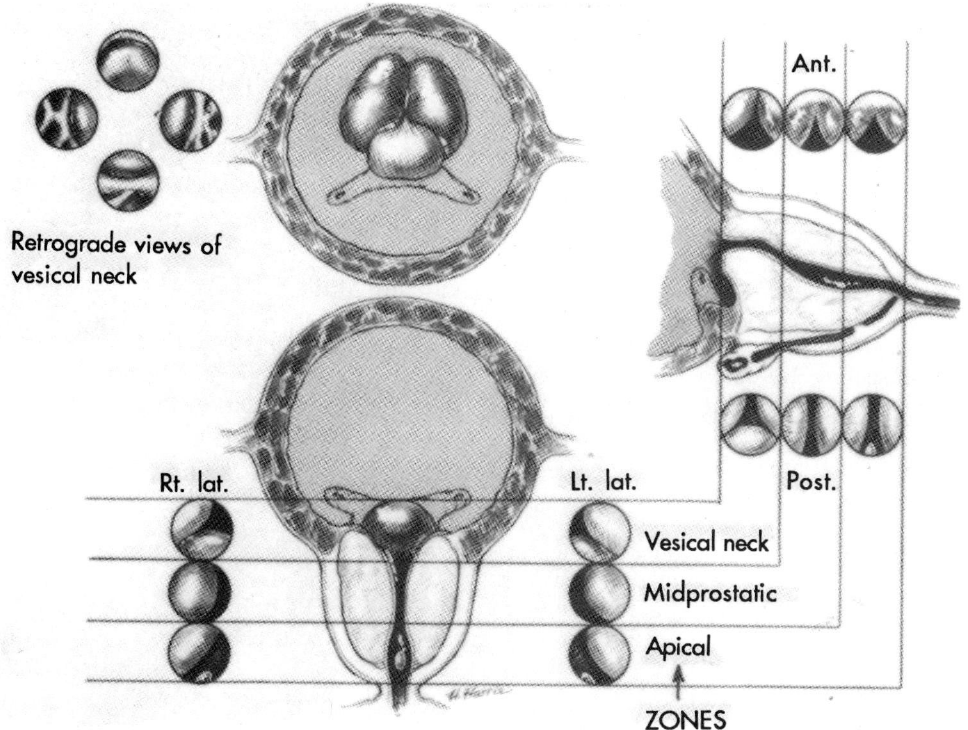

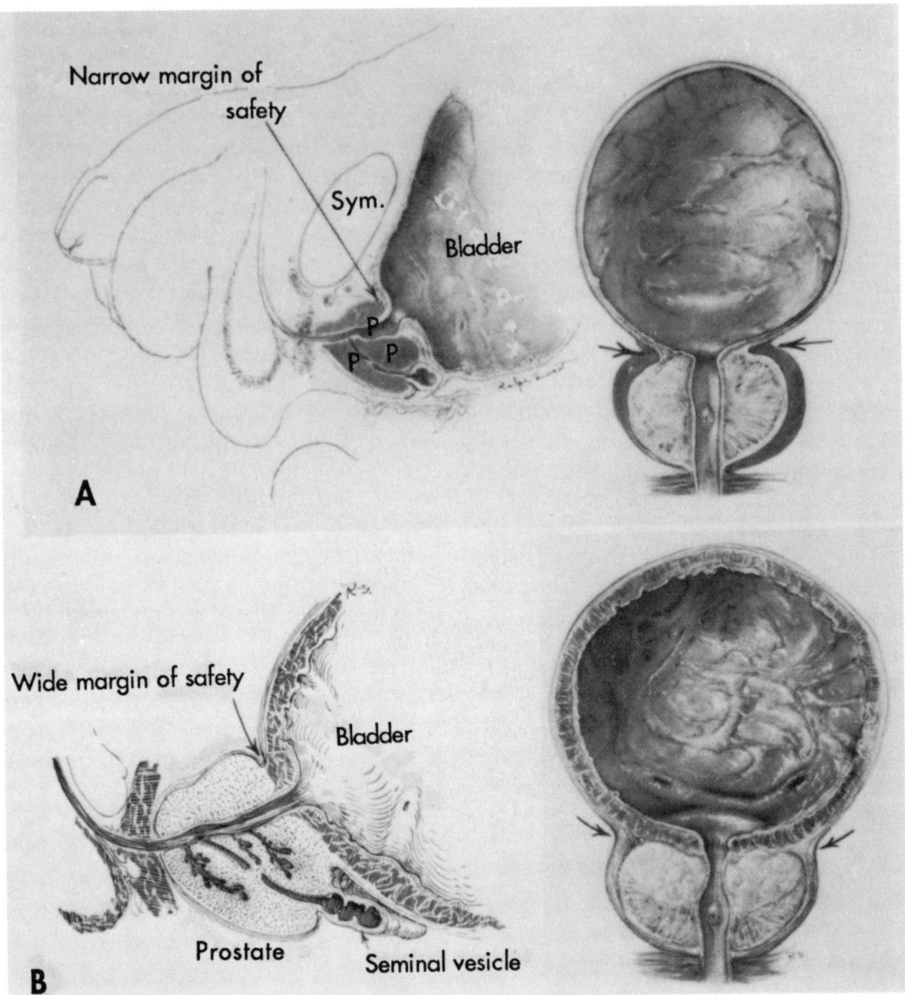


**Fig 54.** Transurethral prostatectomy. Margins of safety at vesical neck. **A:** Median bar with narrow rim of tissue anteriorly and laterally. **B:** Benign hyperplasia and hypertrophy of the detrusor afford a wider margin of safety.

and the verumontanum and realize that just distal to the verumontanum is the easily damaged external sphincter.

In resecting tissue the prevailing principle is to take bites as long as and as deep as conditions permit. Routine cuts are made toward the surgeon when the electroresectoscope is used (Fig 55).

The ability to identify cut tissue is a fundamental requirement of transurethral prostatectomy. Only by recognizing such cut tissue can the surgeon completely remove the obstruction yet avoid perforation. The tissue structures encountered during transurethral resection are illustrated in Fig 56. The easiest tissue to identify is the musculature of the vesical neck; this is seen as circular fibers (Fig 56, 1). Benign adenoma looks dull and fuzzy without a regular pattern (Fig 56, 2). The false prostatic capsule may be very difficult and even impossible to identify as one progresses from adenoma to prostatic cortex. When enough false capsule is exposed, one can see a pattern that aids in identification (Fig 56, 3). True prostatic tissue has more of a pattern than does adenoma, but it is difficult to distinguish from adenoma. The true anatomic capsule of the prostate has a readily identifiable pattern of fibrous tissue (Fig 56, 4). A near perforation is shown in Fig 56, 5, and a true perforation is shown in Fig 56,

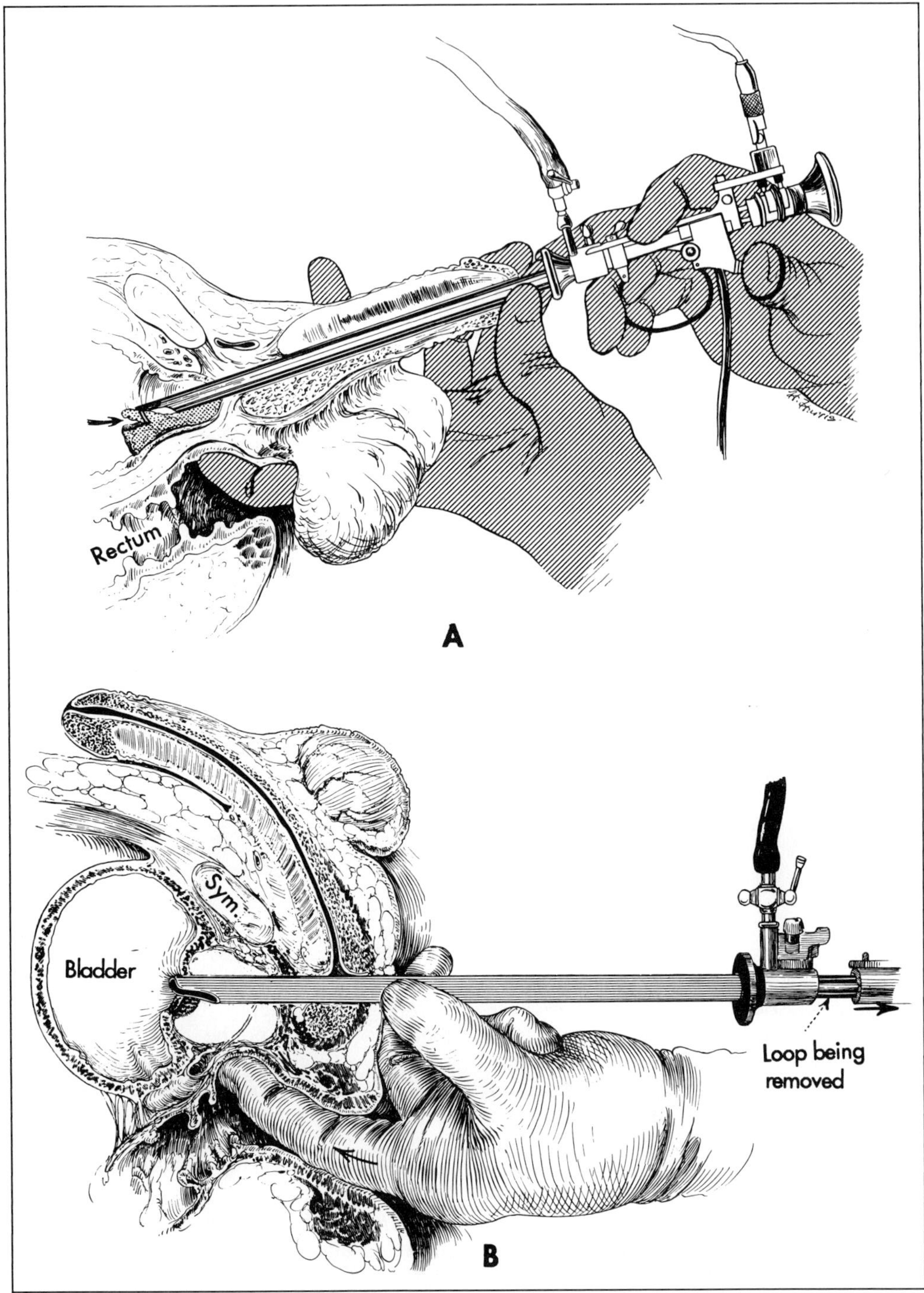


**Fig 55.** Transurethral prostatectomy. Cutting aided by rectal elevation of prostate. Iglesias resectoscope. **A:** Usual technique. **B:** Resecting through perineal urethrotomy.

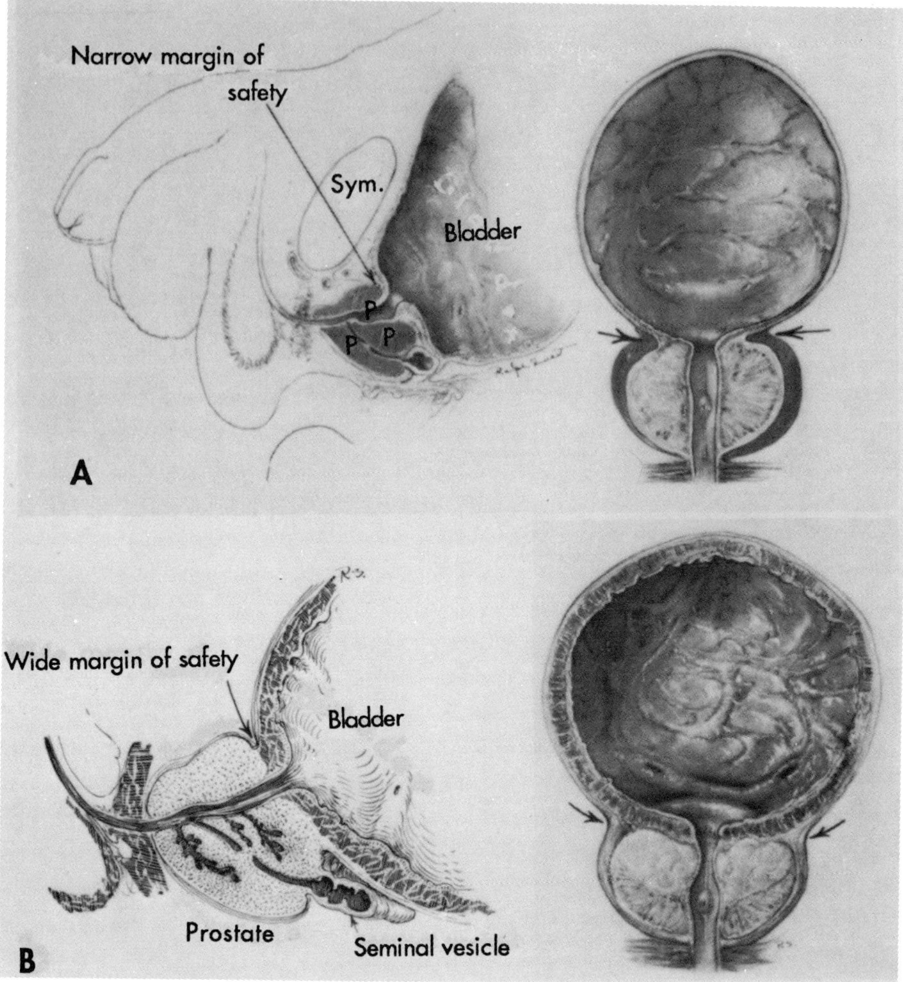


**Fig 56.** Transurethral prostatectomy. Identification of tissue.

6. Characteristically, entry to a venous sinus is indicated by a gush of blood from the opening (Fig 56, 7). Other structures which may be encountered during resection are the ejaculatory ducts and the calculi in prostatic ducts (Fig 56, 8). The fibers of the external sphincter are illustrated in Fig 56, 9, and prostatic carcinoma with a tendency toward circular whorls is shown in Fig 56, 10. Since the most delaying factor in transurethral prostatectomy is the control of bleeding, care should be taken to meet the problem systematically. The objectives are to prevent excessive loss of blood and to maintain a clear operative field. Bleeding is arrested by the application of the fulgurating electrode to the bleeding point; ideally, this should be done as soon as bleeding is noticed, unless the surgeon intends to resect more deeply in that same area, in which case the fulguration of the bleeding vessel can await the termination of resection in that area. Widespread and indiscriminate coagulation must be avoided since necrotic tissue provides a nidus for infection and gives rise to delayed slough and secondary hemorrhage.

Arterial spurters send out jets of blood that are so forceful as to sometimes obscure a ''head-on'' view. Locate this type of bleeder by a sideways approach along the wall of the prostatic fossa. A careful search

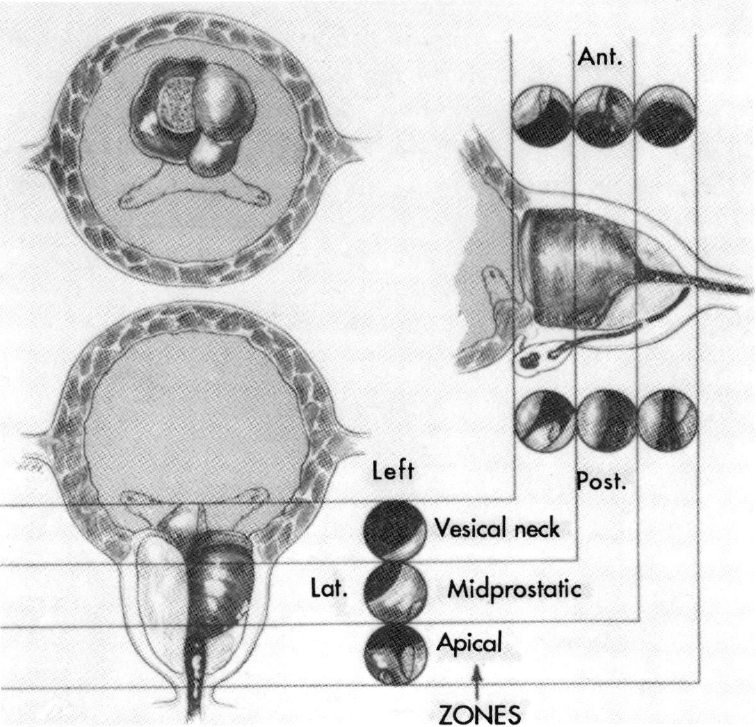


**Fig 57.** Transurethral prostatectomy for benign hyperplasia. First stage complete; vesical neck and midprostatic tissue on left removed.

of all sides of the fossa may reveal the error of mistaking the "splash" of a spurter against the opposite wall for the bleeding artery. Bleeding from veins is easier to locate since it ceases with a slight rise in intravesical pressure. Locate the source by first distending the bladder and then searching the field carefully while water flows out of the instrument. When the intravesical pressure falls to a level such that venous bleeding ensues, the vessel is easily identified. The objective on endoscopic transurethral prostatectomy (adenomectomy) is to remove all tissue encroaching upon the vesical neck and the posterior urethra and, ideally, all tissue down to the surgical capsule. Before removal of the resectoscope, the water draining out of the bladder should be clear or, at most, very faintly pink tinged, with the patient's blood pressure at its normal level. It should be pointed out that in the event the patient becomes hypotensive toward the end of surgery, the return irrigation may be clear, but heavy bleeding may start in the recovery room after the patient's blood pressure has returned to normal. Attempts should be made to have the patient's blood pressure at its resting level prior to the completion of surgery.

Successful transurethral surgery depends on the development of a methodical operative technique; the techniques are based upon the sequence in which segments of tissues are removed.

1. Lateral and trilobar benign hyperplasia is treated in four stages: (1) excision of all vesical neck and adjacent midprostatic tissue on the left (Fig 57); (2) excision of all vesical neck and adjacent midprostatic on the right; (3) excision of remaining midprostatic and apical tissue on the left (Fig 58); and (4) excision of remaining midprostatic and apical tissue on the right (Fig 59).
2. Isolated middle lobe hyperplasia requires an individual approach. Start the

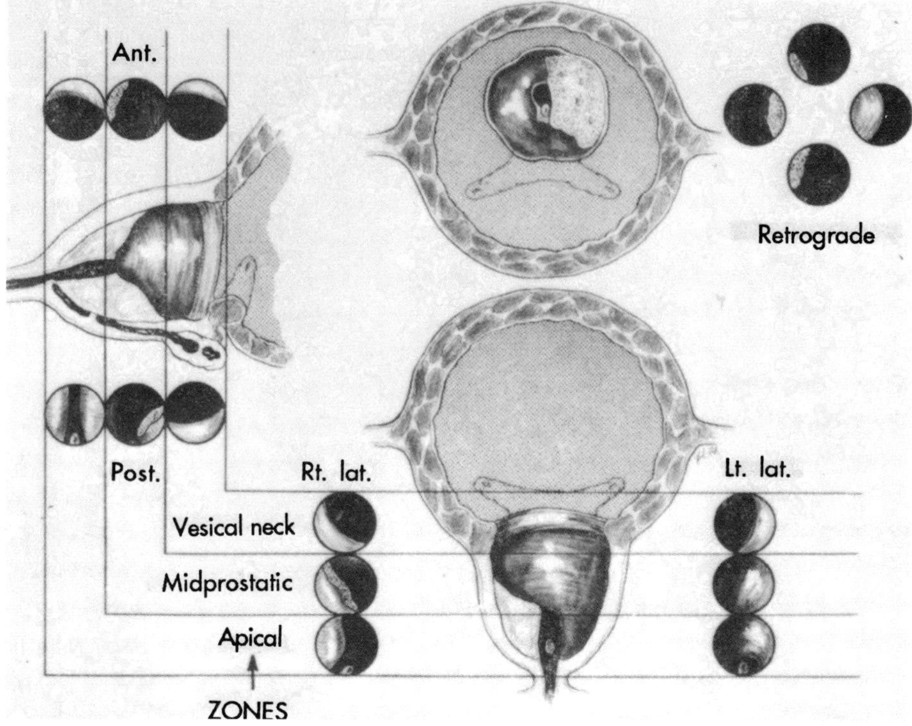


**Fig 58.** Transurethral prostatectomy for benign hyperplasia. Third stage complete. All of tissue on left has been excised at two levels.

morcellation of the lobe at the summit, leveling it by horizontal cuts. If the resection is started at the base of the isolated middle lobe, it is easy to pedunculate it, after which a large piece of prostatic tissue may fall loose into the bladder, and its recovery and removal can be extremely difficult. In resecting the isolated middle lobe, take care not to perforate the vesical neck and the underlying trigone (Fig 60).

3. To uncover posterior commissural hyperplasia, it is necessary first to excise the overlying musculature of the vesical neck. Performing this with the finger in the rectum helps in judging the depth of the enlargement.
4. To excise anterior lobe hyperplasia, start the line of resection at the vesical neck in either lateral sulcus (at the 10 o'clock or the 2 o'clock position). Expose the circular fibers of the vesical neck with one or two bites and fragment the remainder of the lobe. Progress systematically across the midline to the opposite sulcus.

   In carcinoma of the prostate the procedure is, in general, the same as that for benign prostatic hyperplasia, and the chief difficulty is knowing how deep to go. Since the normal anatomic guideposts may no longer be visible, considerable judgement must be used. In general, the aim is to remove enough tissue to permit urination without incontinence; therefore, there is no need to resect all the way down to the surgical capsule.
6. When a fibrotic lesion of the vesical neck is confined to the vesical lip, as in fibrous median bar, it is well to leave the anterior aspect of the vesical neck intact to deter future fibrous ring formation (Fig 61).

Following the operative procedure, evacuate all the excised fragments of tissue that have gone into the bladder. Many of

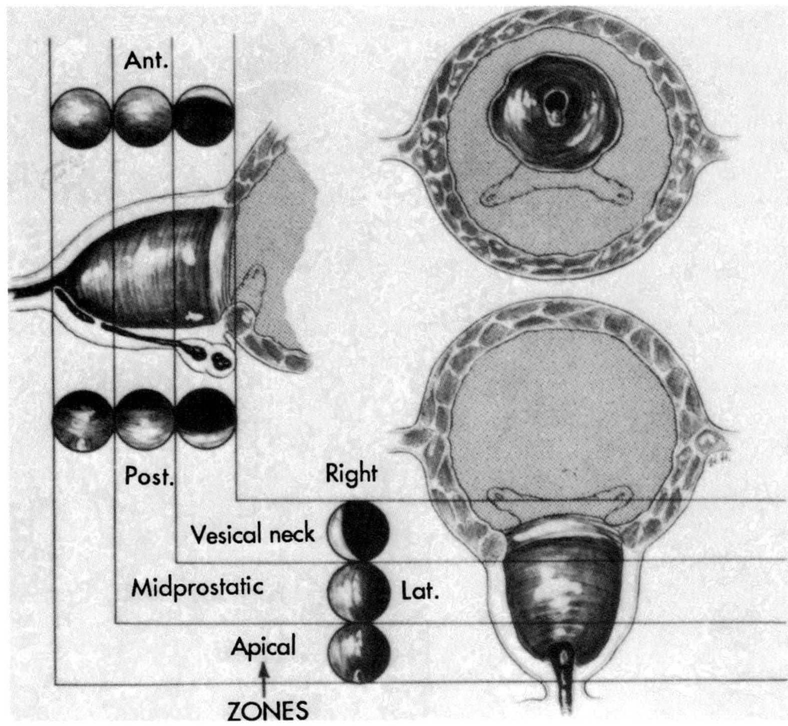


**Fig 59.** Transurethral prostatectomy for benign hyperplasia. Complete resection.

**Fig 60.** Transurethral prostatectomy for benign hyperplasia. Resecting middle lobe. **A:** Cuts are made horizontal at summit, in an upward direction at base to avoid perforation. **B:** Lifting up lowest segment with cold loop to prevent damage to trigone.

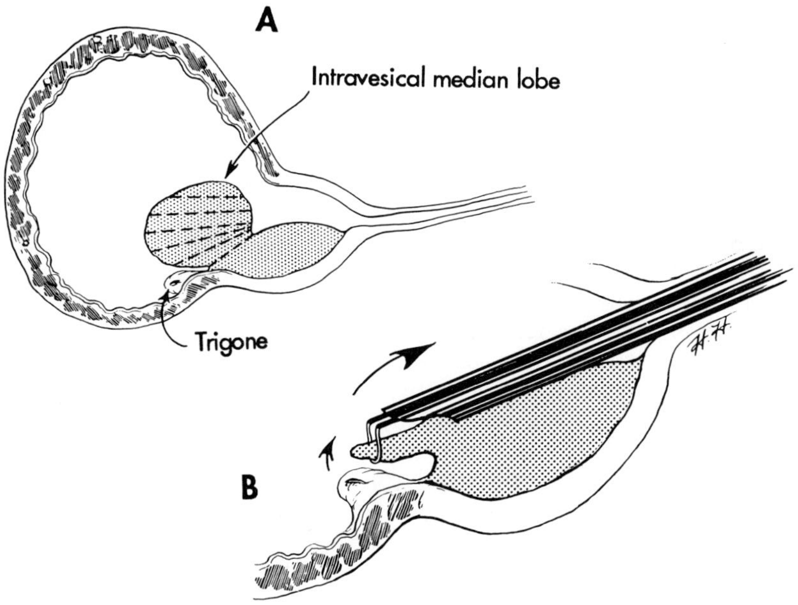

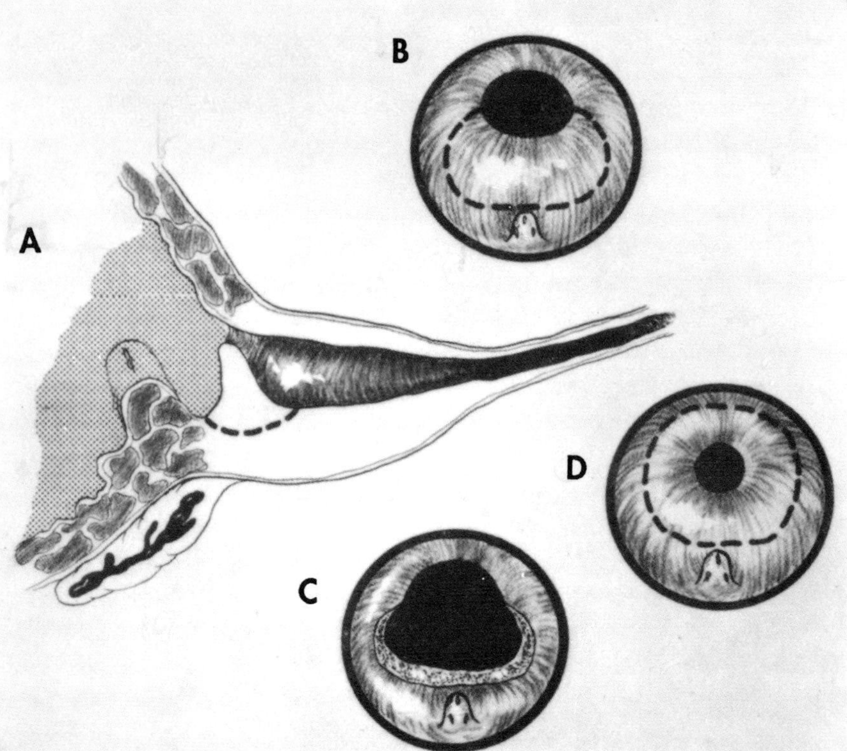


**Fig 61.** Transurethral prostatectomy. Excision of fibrotic lesion of vesical neck. **A:** Median bar, depth of resection indicated by dotted line. **B:** Cystoscopic view, line of resection. **C:** Resection completed. **D:** Line of resection in contracture of vesical neck.

these can be removed easily by employing the resectoscope sheath alone (Fig 62). The difficult-to-remove fragments can be delivered with an Ellik or a McCarthy evacuator (Fig 63).

Within the last several years, "continuous-flow" resectoscopes have found considerable favor with some urologists who find that the time saved during the course of a prostatic resection is considerable and who also prefer not having to remove great amounts of prostatic tissue with one of the evacuators following the surgical procedure. The continuous-flow resectoscope allows for the continuous removal of all but the larger chips of tissue, along with the irrigating fluid. These continuous-flow instruments have not achieved widespread usage because of various technical difficulties to which they are sometimes prone, and many experienced urologists have returned to the more conventional type of resectoscope after a brief stint with the continuous-flow resectoscope.

After final inspection of the operative field, insert the urethral catheter, usually a No 24 Fr with a 30-$cm^3$ bag. Some urologists prefer to use a two-way Foley catheter so that the bladder can be continuously irrigated. The urethra should be well lubricated, and if any resistance is met, the catheter should be inserted over a metal stylet.

## Transurethral Prostatectomy Using the Cold Punch

The fundamental principles of resection and hemostasis with a punch instrument are the same as with the electrotome, although basic differences between the instruments exist (Fig 64).

The prime advantage of the cold-punch instrument for prostatic resection is that a

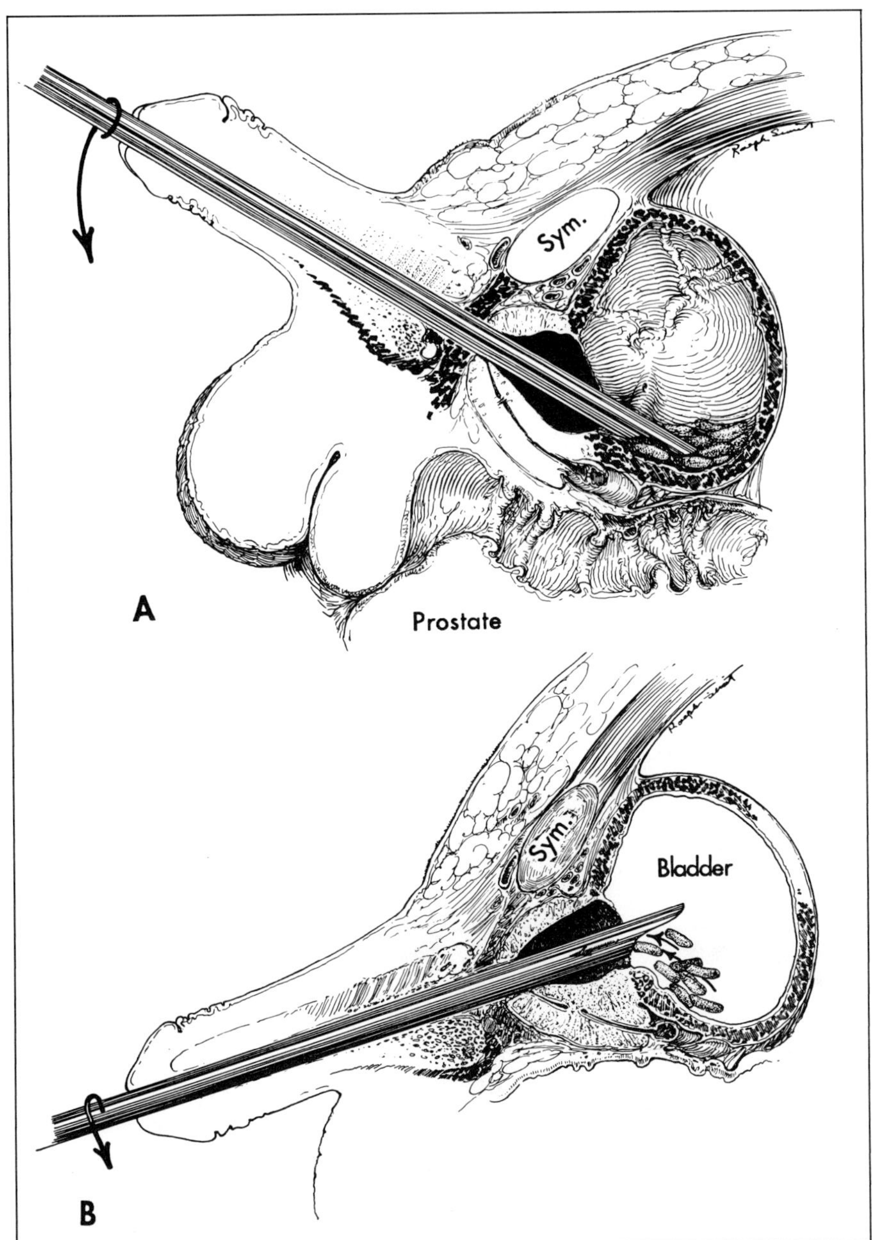


**Fig 62.** Transurethral prostatectomy. Removal of fragments. Routine method of aiding their passage through the sheath during the progress of the operation. **A:** Inner end of sheath placed over fragments in base of bladder. **B:** As fluid flows out of bladder, outer end of sheath is lowered; fragments are carried out by gush of outflowing current.

tubular knife blade instead of an electrical cutting current is used to excise tissue; this largely eliminates the destruction of tissue adjacent to that which is being resected by the thermal effect of electrosurgical currents. Additionally, the absence of any thermal effect transmitted through the resectoscope sheath may minimize the incidence of postoperative urethral stricture. Another major advantage of the cold-punch

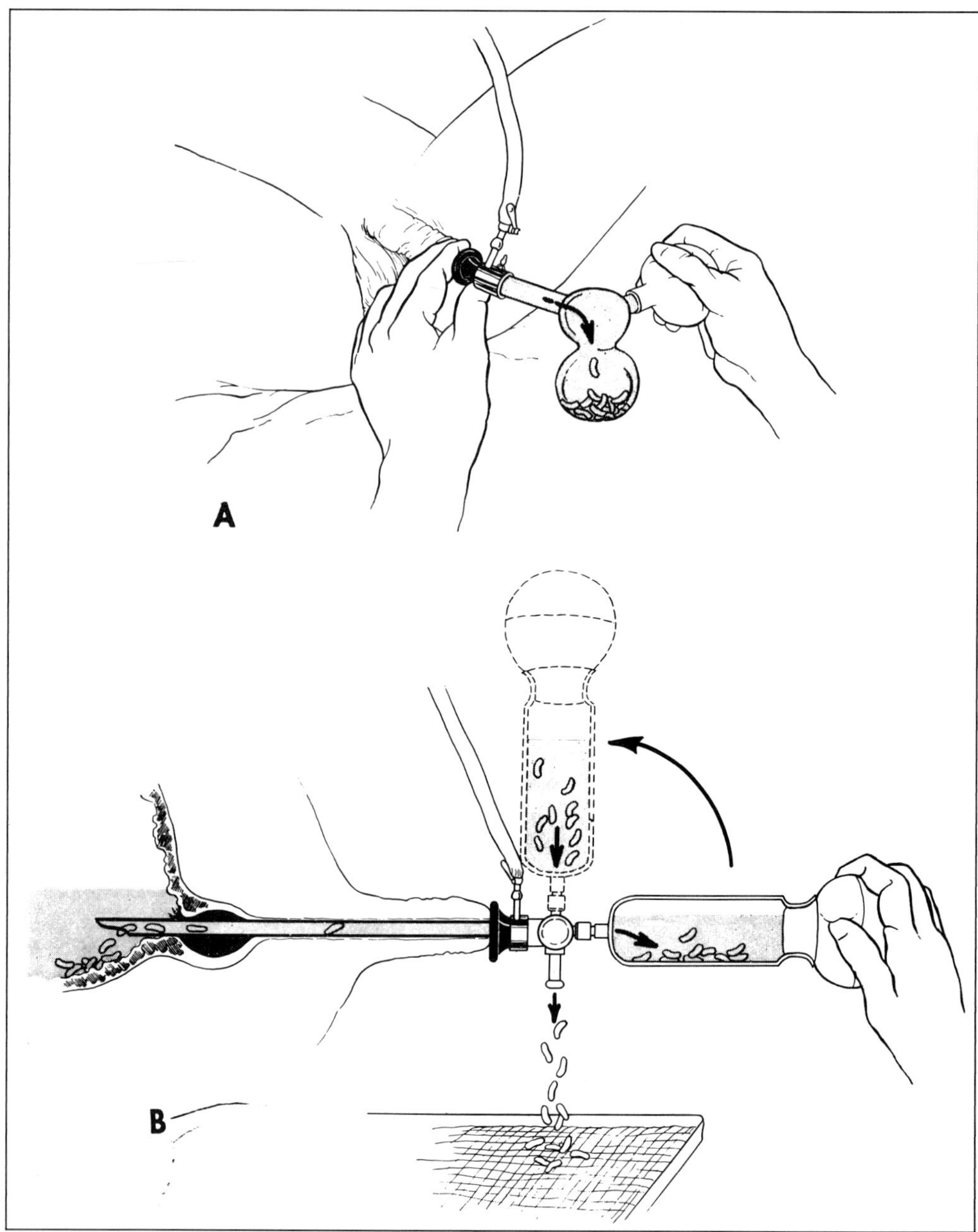


**Fig 63.** Transurethral prostatectomy. Removal of fragments. Use of bladder evacuator. **A:** Ellik. **B:** McCarthy.

instrument is that, because it is basically just a hollow steel tube, greater amounts of irrigating solution under a higher head of pressure can pass through it than through the electrotome. This means that bleeding, even very brisk bleeding, is not as likely to obscure the resectionist's vision with this instrument as compared with the electro-resectoscope.

Control of bleeding is with point electrofulguration, and it is therefore possible to fulgurate only the bleeding vessel itself

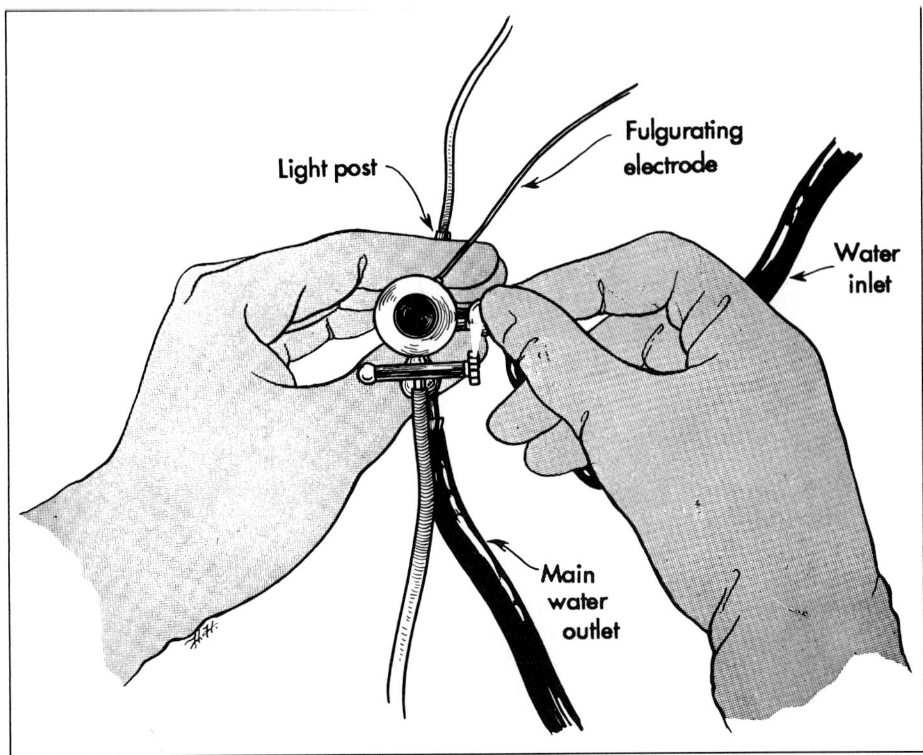


**Fig 64.** Transurethral prostatectomy. Punch operation. Method of holding instrument.

and not any of the tissue around it, as might occur when the electrotome is used. The cold-punch resectoscope is fitted with a closed system for continuous bladder irrigation and evacuation. This allows for removal of the resected chips of prostatic tissue as well as the used irrigation fluid that is in the bladder and thereby avoids the time-wasting and messy maneuvers necessary when the electrotome operating element must be removed from its sheath for the purpose of periodic bladder emptying. The cold-punch resectoscope that was the standard instrument of its kind for many years was the one perfected by Thompson. Within the past few years,

**Fig 65.** The Frohmuller resectoscope seen in profile with the eyepiece on the left, the water and the resected tissue outflow valve on the bottom, the fulgurating electrode and the light contact on the top, and the cutting fenestrum (closed) on the far right.

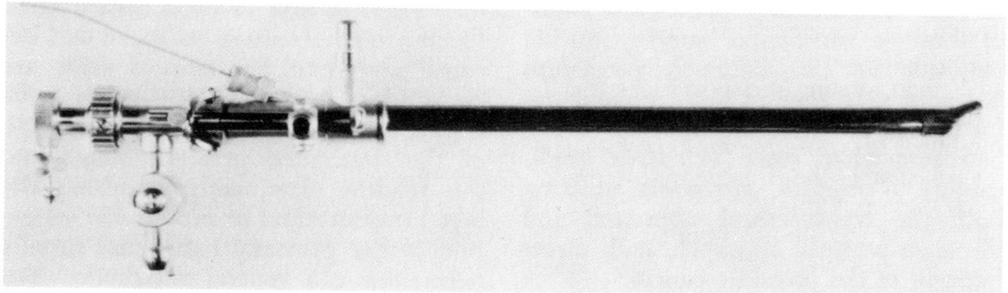

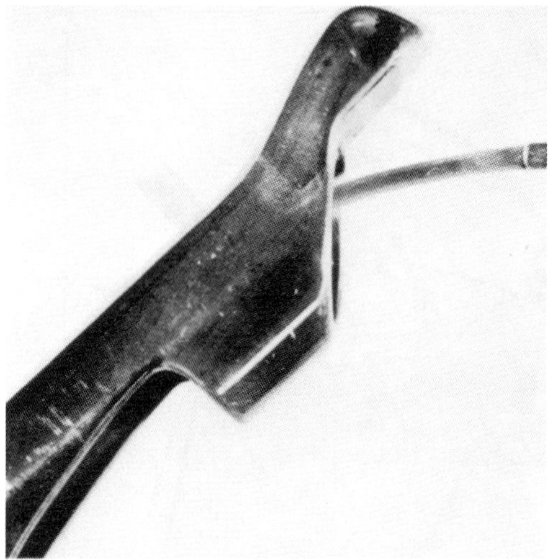

**Fig 66.** A close-up and slightly oblique view of the cutting fenestrum seen in the open position. A tubular knife blade comes across the fenestum and resects adenomatous tissue that has been engaged in the fenestrum. Note also the fulgurating electrode in an extended position for fulgurating purposes. It is ordinarily retracted into the sheath when not being used.

Frohmüller has modified the Thompson resectoscope with a fiber-optic light system and a somewhat greater mechanical advantage incorporated in a superiorly manufactured product, and it is now most likely the standard instrument of its kind in use. It is a two-hand model, and the cutting of prostatic tissue is carried out by means of "punching" the tubular knife blade against the tissue to be resected (Figs 65 and 66).

Transurethral prostatic resection with the cold-punch instrument has never achieved widespread use because it is undoubtedly a more difficult instrument to master than the electrotome and also because some urologists feel that they do not have adequate vision because of a lack of magnification and because they are "looking down a tube" at the tissue to be resected rather than looking through a lens that is directly adjacent to the operative site. The cold-punch resectoscope works on the same visual system as the Braasch cystoscope in which there is virtually no magnification, and most urologists not familiar with the use of this instrument are not comfortable with it.

The cold-punch resectoscope is an excellent instrument for the purpose for which it was designed, but it is doubtful if one could truly objectively say whether it is better than the electrotome. In the final analysis, it takes many years to become a master with either type of resectoscope, and the individual urologist will generally prefer the instrument with which he has had the most experience.

## POSTOPERATIVE COURSE AND COMPLICATIONS

### Hemorrhage

Probably the most frightening and distressing immediate postoperative complication is that of hemorrhage from the prostatic fossa. This complication can occur with any of the methods used for prostatectomy, although with all of the open techniques except the blind suprapubic approach, it is usually possible to suture ligate the areas from which major bleeding is likely to occur. Regardless, there are numerous smaller capsular and urethral branches of the inferior vesical artery that open into the prostatic fossa and that may not be controlled by suture ligatures. These vessels usually constrict and retract in the postoperative period but they may, on occasion, be the source of frightening and even life-threatening hemorrhage. In the case of transurethral surgery, where no suture ligation is possible, bleeding can indeed be a formidable postoperative problem. Corrective measures that may be used in the hopes of controlling the hemorrhage involve the use of the urethral catheter placed on traction with the bag at the vesical neck or even, at times, pulled down into the prostatic fossa for its tamponade effect. Cystostomy with packing of the prostatic fossa is sometimes also necessary. In rare cases, surgical ligation of both hypogastric arteries may become a necessity, and this will usually control the hemorrhage. In such cases of uncontrollable hemorrhage, one must give serious consideration to the possibility that disseminated intravascular coagulopathy (DIC) secondary to the prostatic carcinoma might be the principal cause of the bleeding. This is an uncommon occurrence (less than 1% of all TURs) and is usually associated with widespread prostatic carcinoma. Fibrinolysis may occur secondary to the DIC and it may also very uncommonly be primary. When acute DIC exists there is bleeding and oozing of blood from many sites (oral cavity, IV puncture sites) in addition to the prostatic fossa. If DIC is suspected clinically, the following will usually be found: prolonged prothrombin time, prolonged partial thromboplastin time, prolonged thrombin time, low platelet count, and elevated fibrin split products. The clot lysis time, often done, is not of very much value. DIC is treated with replacement of clotting factors and platelets using cryoprecipitate and fresh frozen plasma. Heparin may at times also be indicated. If primary fibrinolysis is suspected, fibrin split products will be elevated, circulating free plasmin will be present, and the platelet count will be normal. Epsilon aminocaproic acid (Amicar) is used to treat primary fibrinolysis and secondary fibrinolysis (to the DIC) as well.

### Intravascular Hemolysis and Water Intoxication

This is not a problem with any of the open forms of prostatectomy; however, it may be a major problem with the transurethral approach. Large amounts of irrigating fluid are often used during the course of a transurethral resection, and it is inevitable that venous sinuses will be opened during such surgery. Obviously, a certain quantity of irrigating solution is going to be absorbed through these venous sinuses into the general circulation; the larger the gland being resected, the longer the resection will take, the more venous sinuses are opened, and, therefore, the more irrigating fluid will be absorbed into the circulation. The problem of intravascular hemolysis becomes a severe one when distilled water is used for the irrigating fluid instead of an isotonic solution such as Cytal. Some urologists prefer to use distilled water as the irrigating solution for the resection because they feel that vision through the resectoscope when one of the isotonic solutions is used is not nearly as clear as when distilled water is used. Other urologists feel that they do such a quick resection with a minimum of bleeding that it is not necessary to worry about absorption and therefore not necessary to use isotonic solution. Regardless, when distilled water is used for the irrigating solution, a significant number of patients may develop intravascular hemolysis because the tonicity of their red blood cells is greater than the tonicity of the surrounding fluid, which becomes hypotonic from the absorption of large amounts of the distilled water. This intravascular hemolysis can be detected by running a hemoglobin determination on the patient's serum postoperatively and finding it vastly elevated over the 50 to 100 mg/100 mL that is the normal serum hemoglobin level. Intravascular hemolysis may lead postoperatively to renal shutdown secondary to renal tubular necrosis. It is indeed a complication greatly to be feared.

Simple water intoxication, on the other hand, occurs when large amounts of isotonic solution used for the irrigation during the resection are absorbed into the circulation producing a dilutional hyponatremia. This condition may be suspected, usually several hours after surgery, by unusual lethargy and lassitude on the part of the patient and a check of the blood sodium level will reveal it to be less than 120 mg/100 mL. This condition may be readily corrected, if it is recognized, by the infusion of hypertonic saline.

### Vesical Neck Contracture

This complication, in which the vesical neck contracts to a small aperture with resulting difficulty in urination, may theoretically result from any form of prostatectomy but is most often seen as a complication of transurethral resection. It occurs when the resection is carried out circumferentially around the vesical neck and where normal bladder mucosa and submucosa (and not prostatic adenoma) is resected. The contracture most likely will not occur if this circumferential resection involves no more than one half or two thirds of the circumference of the vesical neck; it is a very distinct possibility if the resectionist resects over a 360° angle and resects normal bladder tissue. This condition usually develops within 6 weeks postoperatively, and it may be suspected when the patient complains of great difficulty in voiding and a weak stream. Diagnosis is made by retrograde urethrogram, in which the characteristic "toothpaste" sign is noted; this sign results from the appearance of squiggly lines of contrast medium entering the bladder after passing through the narrowed vesical neck and looks not unlike the appearance of toothpaste leaving a tube that has been vigorously squeezed. Treatment of this condition is by incising the vesical neck in the 5 o'clock and in the 7 o'clock positions, and it results in a "falling apart" of the vesical neck contracture. If the contracture is large enough to allow the Colling's knife to pass through it, incision of the vesical neck is relatively simple. If the contracture is too small to allow passage of the knife blade, it may be dilated with filiforms (passed through the panendoscope) and followers until the Colling's knife can be passed through it. If the vesical neck contracture recurs following the incisions, the procedure may be repeated. Recurring contracture beyond this point is probably best treated with the "open" Y-V plasty procedure.

## Urethral Stricture

This very unpleasant complication can occur with any form of prostate surgery but, again, it is far more prevalent with transurethral surgery. The etiology is the manipulation of a resectoscope sheath within a urethra that is not large enough to accommodate the sheath without producing considerable friction and trauma to the mucosa during the course of the resection. Prevention of urethral stricture is usually successful if an adequate urethral caliber is ensured by internal urethrotomy, when indicated, prior to resection. Alternatively, performing the transurethral resection prostate through a perineal urethrostomy will obviously obviate manipulating a resectoscope in a urethra that is too small for the calibre of the sheath. This is another means of preventing a posttransurethral resection prostate stricture. Once the urethral stricture has developed, usually 3 to 6 weeks following surgery, treatment varies, depending on the extent of the stricture. An occasional urethral dilatation may be satisfactory, or the individual may require internal urethrotomy with indwelling silastic catheter for 6 weeks in an effort to prevent recurrence of the stricture. In extreme cases, plastic surgical procedures on the urethra may be necessary. This condition may be suspected when the individual complains of voiding difficulty postoperatively, and its presence may be confirmed by a retrograde urethrogram and by the inability to pass a No 20 Fr or larger Van Buren sound into the bladder. Urethral strictures usually become symptomatic when they are No 18 Fr or smaller.

## Residual Prostatic Tissue

Failure to remove all of the obstructing tissue may actually result in more severe symptoms of bladder outlet obstruction than the patient had preoperatively if the residual tissue is located in such a manner as to encumber the outflow of urine. If the patient has difficulty voiding, with a slow and weak stream within the first week or so after the catheter has been removed, the problem is probably residual prostate tissue (unless the patient has an unsuspected neurogenic bladder). Residual prostate tissue may therefore be differentiated from urethral stricture and vesical neck contracture, all of which will produce similar symptoms, by the relatively early onset following surgery. Definitive diagnosis may be made by cystoscopic examination, and treatment is directed towards removing the residual prostatic tissue.

## Persistent Pyuria or Bacteriuria

Pyuria is perfectly normal for 3 or 4 months following prostatic surgery, during which time the prostatic fossa is undergoing a process of reepithelialization. It is therefore of great importance that the referring physician realize such pyuria to be a normal postoperative condition, because in my experience it is not at all unusual for referring physicians to become extremely concerned over such pyuria, usually to the point of placing the patient on antimicrobial therapy. Bacteriuria, however, is *not* a normal postoperative occurrence, and it should be treated with appropriate antibiotic therapy (based upon culture and sensitivity studies) whenever it occurs. Persistent or recurrent bacteriuria should lead to a complete reinvestigation of the patient's urinary tract in an effort to turn up conditions that may or may not have been overlooked. Such conditions include renal calculi, bladder diverticula, chronic infection in the prostate, residual or necrotic prostatic tissue in the prostatic fossa, and so forth. Therapy can then be directed to any underlying problem that may be revealed. As indicated earlier in this chapter, I do *not* feel that prophylactic antimicrobial therapy is indicated for the patient undergoing prostatic surgery, but it most assuredly should be employed promptly and properly in the patient developing bacteriuria in the postoperative period.

## Epididymitis

Acute epididymitis is a complication of any form of prostatic surgery and results from bacteria from infected urine going down the ejaculatory duct, into the vas, and then into the epididymis. The incidence of epididymitis is far greater after transurethral surgery as the volumes of irrigating fluid that are used can facilitate the forcing of bacteria into the ejaculatory duct and thence to the epididymis. Some have estimated the incidence of post transurethral resection epididymitis as high as 10% to 15%, but this is really most often a problem in individuals who have had a history of epididymitis, a history of infection in the bladder, or indwelling catheter (with its inevitable infection) during the preoperative course. In these individuals, prophylactic bilateral vasectomy is indicated immediately prior to the surgery. Even though the incidence of epididymitis is not as high with one of the open forms of prostatectomy, prophylactic vasectomy is frequently carried out during these operations also. Epididymitis, if it is going to occur, will usually have its onset between 2 and 6 weeks following surgery, and a sudden temperature spike or intrascrotal pain will usually be the warning signs that this condition is present. Treatment is symptomatic and is usually quite successful.

## Incontinence

Incontinence may follow any of the forms of prostate surgery if sufficient damage occurs to the smooth or the striated musculature of the posterior urethra and it probably occurs, to a greater or lesser degree of severity, about 1% of the time. It is no longer felt that incontinence occurs exclusively as a result of damage to the external sphincter although, undoubtedly, damage to a large part of this sphincter is a major factor in the production of incontinence.

This incontinence is manifested by a leakage of urine following removal of the catheter. It must be pointed out, however, that leakage of urine covers a broad spectrum that can range anywhere from total urinary incontinence to a mild degree of stress incontinence. It is rather commonplace to have a certain amount of involuntary urine leakage the first few hours to the first few days following removal of the catheter. Before one can say that a true problem exists, the patient should be unable to have adequate urinary control for a minimum of 6 to 9 months and preferably for a year following surgery. As already noted, this incontinence may be mild and may only be present with stress such as sneezing or walking fast, or it may be a total incontinence with inability to hold any urine at all. Not to be overlooked in the differential diagnosis of postoperative incontinence is the overflow incontinence that may occur secondary to residual or recurrent prostatic adenoma, vesical neck contracture, or urethral stricture. Diagnosis of the various stages of incontinence is usually self-evident, but therapy can frequently be most vexing and difficult. Alpha-adrenergic stimulating agents such as ephedrine sulfate, 25 to 50 mg qid by mouth, may be most helpful and should be tried unless there is a specific contraindication to this medication. If the incontinence appears to be of an urgency type, anticholinergic agents such as propantheline bromide (Probanthine), 15 to 30 mg qid, may also be helpful. Also, Ditropan, 5 mg tid, has been extremely helpful in selected patients. Cystoscopic evaluation should be carried out to determine the extent, if any, of the posterior urethral damage.

Historically there have been many operative procedures devised for the correction of postprostatectomy (whether TUR or one of the "open" procedures) incontinence, and none have been entirely satisfactory for all patients. At present, the best device available is probably the AMS (American Medical Systems) 800 Artificial Sphincter, and it offers a short-term (2 years) success rate of around 80%.[29] Unfortunately, the very nature of these sphincters is such that many tend to separate from the underlying urethra with the passage of time, thereby leading again to varying degrees of incontinence.

The periurethral injection of bovine collagen has met with considerable patient success in the research and experimental setting, and it may well be the best approach to the difficult problem of urinary incontinence at a future time.

### Hernias and Benign Prostatic Hyperplasia

I feel strongly that any man over 50 who has a direct inguinal hernia of short duration (1 to 2 years) should be evaluated for bladder outlet obstruction *before* the hernia is repaired. In my opinion, one of the major causes of direct inguinal hernia, and *recurrent* direct inguinal hernia, is overlooked bladder outlet obstruction in which straining to void—whether consciously or otherwise—leads to the hernia.

Patients with these hernias, regardless of the urologic history they give, should be evaluated—at the very least—with a peak voiding flow rate. If outlet obstruction is found, it should be repaired at the same time the hernia is repaired.[30]

### Overall Results and Mortality

The vast majority of patients having surgery for BPH (in the United States better than 90% of these operations are via the transurethral route) do extremely well. Indeed, in my opinion, there is probably no other major surgical procedure done in the same age group with a better benefit/risk ratio.

The mortality following TURP is extremely low, and this low figure borders on the phenomenal when the advanced age of patients undergoing the surgery is considered. In the most recent and extensive review done of over 3300 TURs in 13 different centers, the mortality rate was 0.2%.[31] A similar study in 1974 showed a mortality rate of 1.3%,[32] and a study done in 1962 showed a mortality rate of 2.5%.[33] The precipitous drop in the reported mortality rate over the past 30 years reflects better surgical techniques, better antibiotics, and better general medical care of the hospitalized patient.

## ALTERNATIVE INVASIVE PROCEDURES FOR THE TREATMENT OF BENIGN PROSTATIC HYPERPLASIA

### Balloon Dilatation of the Prostate

Balloon dilatation of the prostate had a great flurry of activity in the urologic community in the late 1980s[34] but by the early 1990s most had come to the conclusion that its clinical applicability was very limited. With this procedure, which can be done on a very cost-effective outpatient basis, a balloon catheter is inserted through the urethra and into the bladder. It is positioned so that the distensible balloon portion of the catheter is within the prostatic urethra (Fig 67). This positioning of the catheter can be done under fluoroscopic control with the patient sedated and with a local anesthetic inserted into the urethra. Alternatively, the balloon can be properly positioned within the prostatic urethra by palpating a "button" on the dilating balloon catheter using a finger in the patient's rectum. Once the

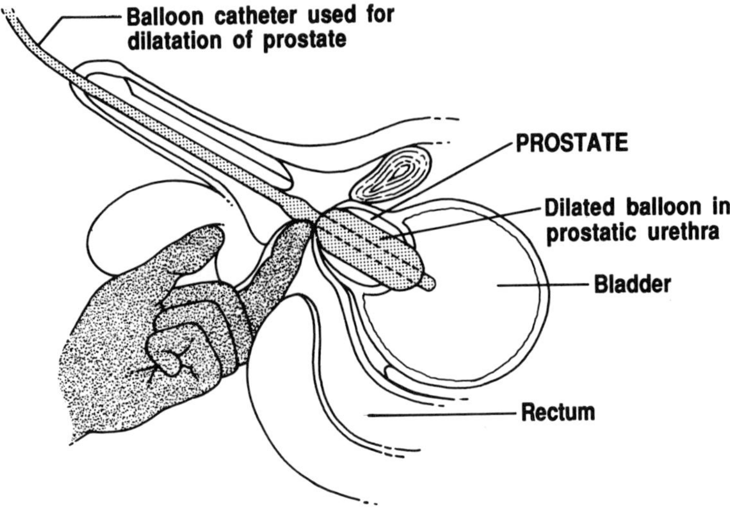


**Fig 67.** Balloon dilatation of the prostate. Note the inflated balloon within the prostatic urethra and bladder neck. The illustration shows the balloon being properly positioned by the examiner's finger in the patient's rectum where it is palpating a "button" on the dilating catheter thereby ensuring the correct position of the catheter.

catheter has been properly positioned the balloon is dilated to a diameter of between 2 and 3 cm and this inflation with its great resulting pressure is maintained on the prostate for about 10 minutes after which the balloon is deflated and withdrawn. A regular catheter is then inserted into the bladder and left in place for a few days because there is invariably a modest amount of bleeding following this procedure.

Although several thousand patients have had this procedure done in the past several years, the long-term results are not particularly satisfactory and neither are the objective measurements of improvement in the voiding pattern. Between half and three quarters of the patients in whom the procedure is done believe they have considerable relief of their symptoms but the duration of this improvement seems to be no longer than a year or two in most cases. Also, objective measurements of improvements such as voiding flow rate and residual urine usually are not commensurate with the patient's subjective impression of improvement. It is generally agreed among urologists that balloon dilatation should be limited to those patients with a relatively small prostate gland and only minimal enlargement of the median lobe, and it is also generally recognized that any improvement noted will be a transient one.

One of the major justifications offered for the use of balloon dilatation is that it presumably does not result in retrograde ejaculation. However, in fact, retrograde ejaculation does occasionally occur following this procedure and even incontinence has occurred following this procedure. While a place may well remain now and in the future for balloon dilatation in the treatment of benign prostatic hyperplasia, it is probably fair to say that the initial enthusiasm for this technique has passed.

## Hyperthermia of the Prostate

It has long been known that heat can congeal tissue, which then presumably shrinks and retracts as healing occurs. The problem with delivering heat to the prostate has historically been one of not injuring the urethra when the transurethral method of delivering heat has been employed and not injuring the rectum when a transrectal method of heating the prostate has been employed. Numerous hyperthermia devices have had experimental use in the past few years using either the transurethral or the transrectal approach, and most of these devices have required up to 10 or 12 separate 1-hour sessions to achieve any degree of clinical shrinkage of the prostate.

Although many companies are experimenting with heat-generating microwave machines, one such machine (the Prostatron, Fig 68) has had extensive clinical trials in France and in England in the late 1980s as well as in the U.S. since the early part of 1991.[35,36] The heat generated by this machine is conducted through a probe that is placed within the prostatic urethra under local anesthetic. The machine has been engineered so that a cooling fluid is applied to the lining of the prostatic urethra and this actually limits the degree to which the urethra is heated to something under 45°C while the deeper portions of the prostate gland are heated to approximately 55°C. This lower temperature does not result in any significant changes in the tissues of the prostatic urethra but the higher temperature serves to congeal the deeper portions of the prostate gland, which results in shrinkage of this tissue within a few weeks. Because the heat within the prostatic urethra is not sufficient to damage the delicate mucosa in this area, the problems of bladder neck contracture and retrograde ejaculation are not seen. The heat with this particular machine is applied one time only for a period of 30–60 minutes and it is done entirely on an outpatient basis. The Prostatron is extremely costly and will run in the neighborhood of nearly $1 million if and when it ultimately receives FDA approval for general use. Presently, other companies are rapidly trying to develop a machine quite similar to Prostatron that presumably will be less costly.

One of the centers in the U.S. that has been conducting clinical trials on Prostatron, as of early 1993, has been able to follow 150 patients who have had this treatment for BPH for a full year and the initially promising results have indeed stood up. At the end of this 1-year follow-up period about half of the patients treated with Prostatron had a definite and statistically significant improvement in their maximum voiding flow rates and there was a reported success rate of 77% taking both subjective and objective symptoms and findings into account. Overall, 84% of the patients who were followed for this 1-year period re-

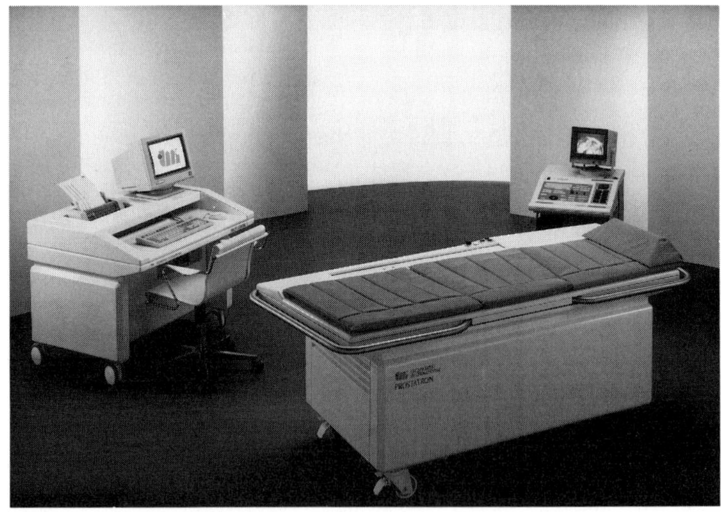

**Fig 68.** The Prostatron transurethral thermal therapy machine. On the left is the operator's console with computer, keyboard, and printer, and all the necessary software to operate the device. In the center is the patient treatment module in which is housed all the necessary equipment to perform the treatment. On the right is an ultrasound machine that is used to localize the treatment catheter.

ported that they were satisfied with the results of their treatment.

These figures are certainly no better and they may indeed not be quite as good as the "gold standard," which is the TURP. One must bear in mind, however, that the Prostatron operation is done on an outpatient basis with local anesthesia only and, therefore, there is virtually no morbidity and no mortality. If the long-term follow-up for the next several years results in the same favorable improvement in symptoms and in objective findings as did the 1-year follow-up period it is certainly likely that the Prostatron will become the new gold standard for relief of bladder outlet obstruction in selected patients. Presently, although still an investigational instrument that is not on the open market, the Prostatron should be considered a viable alternative to pharmacologic therapy for BPH and, in very selected patients, to a transurethral prostatic resection.

## Laser Surgery

As of 1993 laser surgery on the prostate is considered to be investigational by the FDA. This does not mean that its use is forbidden but it does mean that, in general, reimbursement for surgical procedures done with the laser may well not be forthcoming. However, at the very end of 1992, the FDA Office of Device Evaluation did note that the use of side-firing laser catheters for the treatment of outlet obstruction due to BPH is not considered investigational provided that the urologist makes the determination that performing a laser prostatectomy is therapeutically appropriate. Whether or not reimbursement will actually be forthcoming until lasers are totally removed from the category of investigational equipment will probably vary from case to case and region to region. The FDA has taken the tack that there have not been enough clinical trials using the laser for BPH to take it out of the investigational category but its use per se is not forbidden in the treatment of diseases of the prostate.

In any case, lasers have been used in urology at least since the 1970s for the treatment of urethral strictures and, more recently, cutaneous lesions of the external genitalia. With the great impetus of the last few years to find alternative methods of treating BPH, lasers of various types have been used for this purpose. All of these have been Nd:YAG lasers. One particular kind that has been used investigationally in well over 100 patients is the transurethral ultrasound-guided laser-induced prostatectomy (TULIP); this procedure is done by imaging the entire prostate gland by means of ultrasound while blindly moving the laser window longitudinally along the length of the urethra from the bladder neck to the apex of the prostate and doing this circumferentially. Results have been good and, in the hands of those who have done most of these investigational procedures, patient satisfaction has been high, operative morbidity has been rare, and there has been a statistically significant improvement in symptoms score and in peak flow rate.[37] With this procedure, as with other laser ablations of the prostate gland, patients are in the hospital for one night postoperatively as a rule and they are often discharged with a small suprapubic tube in place because the edema in the prostatic urethra and the discomfort in that area combine to make voiding difficult for a period of time postoperatively.

More recently, a side-firing laser was developed using a quartz crystal to deflect the laser beam at right angles to the laser catheter and the entire catheter is passed through a cystoscope so that the transurethral resection, using the laser, can be done under direct vision. The light from the Nd:YAG laser is directed from the fiber to the prostatic tissue at an 80° angle and the initially visualized zone of coagulation expands in time to a larger zone of sloughing. The procedure is done using a 20 or 22 Fr cystoscope and a standard cystoscopic bridge is used for introduction of the laser fiber. The laser energy is directed in four radial positions at the 2, 4, 8, and 10 o'clock positions and the fiber is dragged in each of these positions from the bladder neck to the level of the verumontanum. The power setting usually is in the region of 30 W but some researchers have suggested that a setting in the region of 10 or 15 W, dragged more slowly from the bladder neck to the verumontanum, produces a greater area of tissue destruction. The goal is to coagulate a sufficient depth of tissue so that after sloughing occurs a cavity is produced. There is no attempt made to coagulate and vaporize a volume of prostatic tissue similar to that which would be resected during a conventional TURP. Following the operative procedure a catheter is placed in the urethra where it may remain for several days and up to 2 or 3 weeks depending on the size of the prostate preoperatively. Additionally, some urologic surgeons choose to insert a small suprapubic catheter which then enables earlier removal of the urethral catheter so as to permit a voiding trial with measurement of residual urine. It usually takes 1 to 2 months following laser surgery of the prostate for the prostatic urethra to be reepithelialized and for it to achieve its maximum interior dimension.

Those surgeons who have had experience with this side-firing laser fiber that is introduced through the cystoscope are uniformly enthusiastic about the results achieved and about the future of this type of prostate surgery. Clearly, prudence and caution would dictate a "wait-and-see" approach regarding the complications, efficacy, and long-term results of laser ablation of the prostate but at the time of this writing it appears that it may indeed offer a viable alternative to the TURP for patients with a prostate that is small to moderate in size (less than 40 or 50 g) and in whom the median lobe is not particularly large.

### Transurethral Incision of the Prostate

Originally advocated in the early 1970s, the transurethral incision of the prostate (TUIP) did not catch on with most urologists until very recently. It has undergone a renaissance of interest because of the great push for alternative methods to relieve the symptoms of patients with BPH.[38] It is generally agreed that this procedure is only indicated in patients in whom the estimated amount of tissue to be removed is 30 g or less, and in the hands of those surgeons

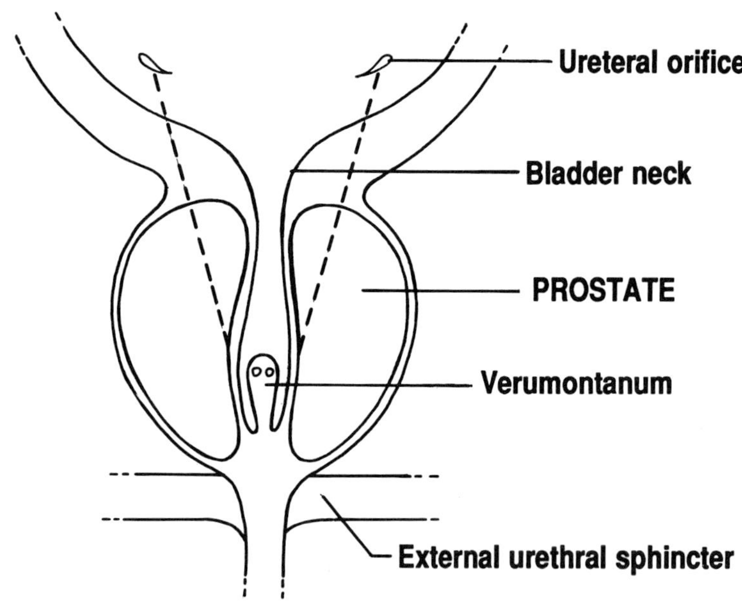


**Fig 69.** Transurethral incision of the prostate. Dotted lines indicate the two positions (5 o'clock and 7 o'clock) in which deep cuts are made beginning just below the ureteral orifices in the bladder and extending outward to a point just inside the verumontanum. These incisions go all the way through the prostate gland as far as the surgical capsule of the prostate.

advocating this procedure, the duration of hospitalization, operating time, blood loss, and overall morbidity are considerally less than with TURP and the results are as good as with TURP. In this procedure two incisions are made, one at the 5 o'clock and one at the 7 o'clock position, and these begin at the bladder neck and extend deeply into the fat surrounding the bladder but not through the prostatic capsule, and these incisions extend distally all the way to the verumontanum (Fig 69). No tissue is removed with this procedure and it is therefore necessary to determine as best as possible by means of digital rectal exam, prostate-specific antigen level, and prostatic ultrasound whether or not prostate cancer exists prior to doing this procedure. These same precautions to rule out the presence of prostate cancer are necessary before laser prostatectomy as well. The incisions from the bladder neck to the verumontanum, it should be noted, are usually made with a Collins knife. Advocates of this procedure point out that the incidence of bladder neck contracture, urethral stricture, and retrograde ejaculation are extremely low as compared with conventional TURP. In most cases, the patient is able to leave the hospital the day after surgery with his catheter removed.

### Intraurethral Stents

The driving force to find alternatives to the conventional TURP have led urologists and biomedical engineers to try the use of intraurethral stents.[37] These are placed within the prostatic urethra, distal to the bladder neck but proximal to the external urethral sphincter, and they expand circumferentially after they are placed to increase the lumen of the prostatic urethra over its original size. Insertion of these stents is rapid and there is no need for an indwelling catheter after placement. Patients are usually able to go home later that day or the next day. The stents must become covered with epithelium or else they tend to become encrusted and also tend to migrate and cause considerable discomfort. There are presently two types of stents in use in clinical investigation trials (as of 1993 urethral stents are not approved for general usage). One of these is a tubular device made of titanium that is rigid and nonflexible and requires balloon dilatation in order to expand it within the prostatic urethra. Once fully expanded, the stent provides an outward radial force which tends to keep open the prostatic urethra. The other device undergoing investigational trials is a prosthesis that is made of a woven, tubular mesh of a nonmagnetic alloy, is self-expanding, and, after placement in its contracted state within the prostatic urethra (under direct vision), expands considerably to keep the prostatic urethra well open.

When properly placed, there is apparently little difficulty with infection, migration, erosion, incontinence, or potency and it is possible to remove the stent at any time without traumatizing the external sphincter or the urethra. It is likely that these intraurethral stents will achieve their maximum benefit in those patients felt to be too ill to undergo any form of prostatic surgery or who just do not want any kind of surgery. The irritative symptoms complained of by many people with these stents will in all likelihood preclude their widespread use except as just noted.

## REFERENCES


1. Arey RB. *Developmental Anatomy: A Textbook and Laboratory Manual of Embryology*. 5th ed. Philadelphia: WB Saunders; 1949.
2. Lowsley OS. The development of the human prostate gland. *Am J Anat*. 1912;13:299.
3. Flocks RH. The arterial distribution within the prostate gland: its role in transurethral prostatic resection. *J Urol*. 1937;37:524.
4. Huggins C. The physiology of the prostate gland. *Physiol Rev*. 1945;25:281.
5. Huggins C, Clark PJ. Quantitative studies of prostatic secretions: II. The effect on castration and of estrogen injection on the normal and on the hyperplastic glands of dogs. *J Exp Med*. 1940;72:747.
6. McNeal JE. Normal histology of the prostate. *Am J Surg Pathol*. 1988;12:619–633.
7. McNeal JE: The prostate gland: morphology and pathobiology. In: Stamey TA, ed. *1983 Monographs in Urology*. Princeton, NJ: Custom Publishing Services; 1983: 3–33.
8. Stamey TA, McNeal JE, Freiha FS, Redwine EA. Morphometric and clinical studies on 68

consecutive radical prostatectomies. *J Urol.* 1988;139:1235.

9. Kabalin JN, McNeal JE, Price HM, Freiha FS, Stamey TA. Unsuspected adenocarcinoma of the prostate in patients undergoing cystoprostatectomy for other causes: incidents, histology and morphometric observations. *J Urol.* 1989; 141:1091.
10. McNeal JE. The prostate gland: morphology and pathobiology. In: Stamey TA, ed. *1988 Monographs in Urology*. Princeton, NJ: Custom Publishing Services; 1988;9:36–63.
11. Randall A. *Surgical Pathology of Prostatic Obstruction*. Baltimore: Williams & Wilkins; 1931.
12. Walsh PC. Benign prostatic hyperplasia. In: Walsh PC, Gittes R, Perlmutter AT, Stamey TA, eds: *Campbells Urology*. 5th ed. Philadelphia: WB Saunders; 1986;2:1248–1265.
13. Crystal DS, Emmett JL: The incidence of coincident prostatic calculi, prostatic hyperplasia and carcinoma of the prostate gland. *JAMA*. 1944;124:646.
14. Spector M, Magura CE, Lilga JC. Prostatic calculi. In: Smith LH, Robertson WG, Finlayson B, eds. *Urolithiasis*. New York: Plenum Press; 1981.
15. Rous SN. *Urology: A Core Textbook*. Norwalk, Conn: Appleton & Lange; 1985.
16. Rous SN. *The Prostate Book*. New York: WW Norton; 1993.
17. Resnick MI. Transrectal ultrasonography of the prostate. In: Rous SN, ed. *Urology Annual*. Norwalk, Conn: Appleton & Lange; 1988; 2:59–78.
18. Weyrauch HM. *Surgery of the Prostate*. Philadelphia: WB Saunders, 1959.
19. Higbee DR. Benign prostatic obstruction: a comparison of results following suprapubic, transurethral and perineal operative procedures. *J Urol.* 1946;56:83.
20. Presman D. Congenital valves of the posterior urethra. *J Urol.* 1961;86:602.
21. Waterhouse K, Hamm FC. The importance of urethral valves as a cause of vesical neck obstruction in children. *J Urol.* 1962;87:404.
22. Holl WH, Rous SN. Is antibiotic prophylaxis worthwhile in patients with transurethral resection of prostate? *Urol.* 1982;19:43.
23. Young HH, Davis DM. *Young's Practice of Urology*. Philadelphia: WB Saunders; 1926.
24. Millin T: Retropubic prostatectomy: new extravesical technique: report on 20 cases. *Lancet.* 1945;2:693.
25. Millin T. *Retropubic Urinary Surgery*, Edinburgh: Churchill-Livingstone; 1947.
26. Greene, LF, Thompson GJ. Transurethral prostatic resection in patients with advanced renal insufficiency. *J Urol.* 1945;54:166.
27. Hahn RG, Stalberg HP, Gustafsson SA. Intravenous infusion of irrigating fluids containing glycine or mannitol with and without ethanol. *J Urol.* 1989;142:1102.
28. Emmett JL, Rous SN, Greene LF, et al. Preliminary internal urethrotomy in 1,036 cases to prevent urethral stricture following transurethral resection: caliber of normal adult male urethra. *J Urol.* 1963;89:829.
29. Marks J, Light K. Management of urinary incontinence after prostatectomy with the artificial urinary sphincter. *J Urol.* 1989;142:302.
30. Brugh R, Rous SN. The incidence of bladder outlet obstruction in male inguinal hernia patients over 50 years of age. *Urology.* 1977;10:550.
31. Mebust WK, Hotigrewe HL, Cockett ATK, Peters PC. Transurethral prostatectomy: immediate and postoperative complications: a cooperative study of thirteen participating institutions evaluating 3385 patients. *J Urol.* 1989;141:243.
32. Melchior J, Valk WL, Foret JD, Mebust WK. Transurethral prostatectomy: a computerized analysis of 2223 consecutive cases. *J Urol.* 1974;112:64.
33. Hotigrewe JL, Valk WL. Factors influencing the mortality and morbidity of transurethral prostatectomy: a study of 2015 cases. *J Urol.* 1962; 87:45.
34. Klein LA, Lerming B. Balloon dilatation for prostatic obstruction. Long-term follow-up. *Urology.* 1989;33:198.
35. Blute ML, Tomera KM, Hellerstein DK, et al. Transurethral microwave thermotherapy for Prostatron: early Mayo Foundation experience. *Mayo Clin Proc.* 1992;67:417.
36. Blute ML, Lewis RW. The use of hypothermia in benign prostatic hyperplasia. In: Rous SN, ed. *Urology Annual, Vol. 7*. New York: Norton; 1993;171.
37. Khoury S. Future directions in the management of benign prostatic hyperplasia. *Br J Urol.* 1992;70 (Suppl 1):27–32.
38. Riehmann M, Bruskewitz R. Transurethral invasion of the prostate and bladder neck. *J Androl.* 1991;12:415.

# 25

# Nonsurgical Management of Benign Prostatic Hyperplasia

*Robert E. Vlach, Jr. and Reginald C. Bruskewitz*

Transurethral resection of the prostate (TURP) has become the preferred treatment for benign prostatic hyperplasia (BPH) over the last 50 years. Improvements in surgical instrumentation and perioperative care, as well as the low mortality, have contributed to this trend. The decade of the 1980s has seen an upsurge toward alternative therapies for BPH (Table 1).

TURP achieved prominence due to its safety and effectiveness. In 1962, Holtgrewe and Valk reported a mortality of 2.5% and a morbidity of 18%, mostly due to coronary artery disease and infections, respectively.[1] Melchoir et al noted 1.3% mortality in 1974.[2] A mortality of 0.2% and morbidity of 18% was recently reported in a multi-institutional study of 3385 patients.[3] In addition, TURP is highly effective in relieving bladder outlet obstruction. Lepor and Rigaud found an improvement of 108% in urinary flow rates, 87% in obstructive symptom scores, and 67% in irritative symptom scores.[4]

**TABLE 1. Therapeutic Options for BPH**

- Prostatectomy
  - —Open
  - —TURP
- Prostatic incision (TUIP)
- Bilateral orchiectomy (Historical)
- Pharmacologic
  - —α-Blocker
  - —Antiandrogens
- Balloon dilation
- Hyperthermia
- Prostatic stents

Why has the trend toward alternative therapies for BPH occurred, if TURP is so effective?

Several epidemiologic studies have shed some light on the prevalence of BPH; 77% of older men exhibit some sign or symptom of BPH and approximately 29% of all males will undergo prostatectomy, according to the Boston Normative Aging Study.[5] In 1985, 350,000 TURPs were performed[6] at an average cost of $12,070 per procedure.[7] Thus, the high surgical rate and the cost of TURP have made it a major public health issue.

Berry et al reported the results of combined data from ten studies, and has shed further light on the growth rate and prevalence of BPH.[8] Eight percent of men aged 31 to 45 were found to have pathologic evidence of BPH, as opposed to 50% of those in their sixth decade of life. Between the ages of 10 and 20, the prostate undergoes its greatest growth. Thereafter, a

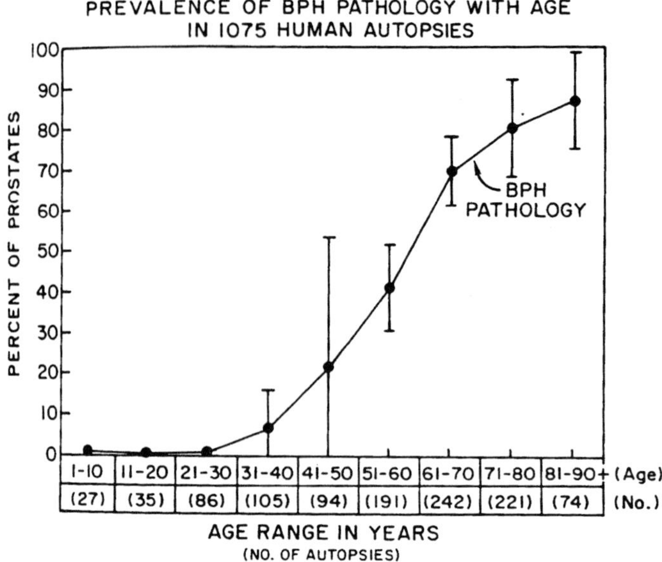


**Fig 1.** Age-associated increase in human male subjects (%) with pathologic evidence of BPH at autopsy determined during 10-year intervals from five studies. Mean ± standard error is shown. Number below age range indicates number of samples used to calculate each point and represents combined data from studies in Table 2. [From Berry.[8]]

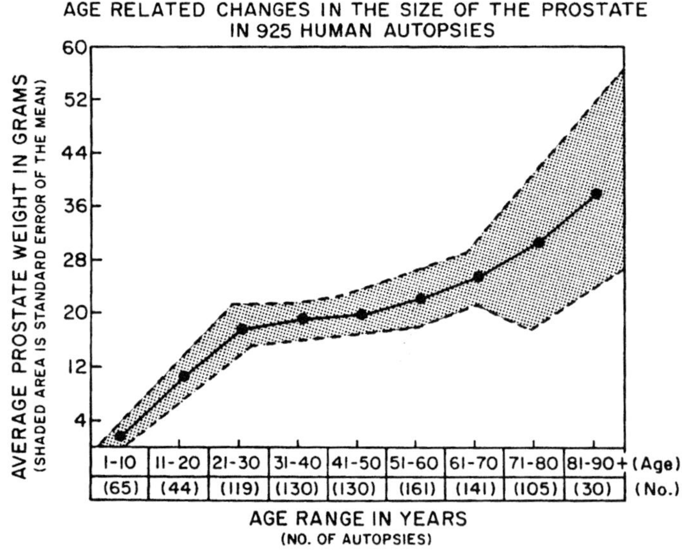


**Fig 2.** Age-related increase in average weight of human male prostate. Average prostatic weights (mean ± standard error) are presented for 10-year intervals. Prostates were obtained at autopsy after 925 samples collected from studies in Table 3. [From Berry.[8]]

much slower growth rate occurs (Figs 1, 2). A substantial degree of growth occurs in less than 5% of men later in life. BPH is associated with continued, although slow, increases in prostatic size and weight after age 30. From this data, the investigators concluded that the onset of BPH occurs before age 30 and most do not exhibit an extreme degree of growth. The data presented by Berry et al and the Normative Aging Study imply that BPH is probably a normal part of the aging process, is very prevalent, and leads to clinical symptoms in the majority of men. Hence, if TURP were the only effective treatment and was liberally utilized, then our health care delivery system most certainly would be taxed.

Other epidemiologic studies have called to question the safety and effectiveness of TURP and open prostatectomy. Wide variations in the prostatectomy rate were noted within small areas of similar medical demographics.[9] These variations were greater than expected due to differences in access to care or BPH prevalence.

Recent investigators also dispute the efficacy and safety of TURP as reported by Mebust et al.[3] Wennberg et al reported a higher mortality rate and a 20% prostatic and urethral reoperation rate after a period of 8 years.[10] It also has been suggested that improvements in voiding symptoms and quality of life after prostatectomy are only significant in patients with severe symptoms or acute retention.[11]

Given the differing views about the safety and efficacy of TURP and the wide variations in the prostatectomy rates, there appears to be significant uncertainty about the indications for prostatectomy and about which patients are likely to benefit from this procedure.[12] Also, there is a distinct lack of large-scale, randomized trials that would best answer these questions about the surgical management of BPH.

It appears that these epidemiologic studies have fueled the search for alternative therapies for BPH over the last decade. However, since the inception of therapy for BPH, alternative treatments have been sought.

## PATHOGENESIS OF BPH

The role of the testes in the development of BPH was noted over 100 years ago. In the 1890s, two investigators reported the use of castration in the treatment of BPH. White[13] and Cabot,[14] reporting on 111 and 61 patients, respectively, documented "improvement" in more than 80% of those treated with castration for symptomatic BPH. There were no objective measurements of response, and no attempts to distinguish BPH from prostatic carcinoma. The development of effective resection techniques and instrumentation—as well as subsequent conflicting reports of castration's efficacy—led to the decline of castration as treatment for BPH.

The presence of functioning testes and aging appear to be essential for the development of BPH. This is supported by the observations of Scott, who found BPH rarely occurred when castration is performed before the age of 30.[15] McNeil has reported that the pathogenesis of BPH results from the reawakening of the embryonic potential of the stoma to induce epithelial budding.[16] The specific biochemical factor that initiates growth of the prostate remains unknown. The leading candidates include an androgen, specifically dihydrotestosterone, which may play a synergistic role with an estrogen, probably estradiol.[17] Estrogens have been found to increase the level of androgen receptors in the dog prostate.[18,19]

The testes produce testosterone, and then dihydrotestosterone, via the action of 5α-reductase.[17] Estrogens are also directly produced by the testes. In addition, testosterone is converted to estradiol peripherally via a process called aromatization. Both dihydrotestosterone and estradiol must be considered as potential targets for preventing or reversing BPH. This hormonal milieu, as recently depicted graphically by Geller (Fig 3),[20] must be kept in mind when reviewing the antiandrogen approaches to BPH management.

Some questions remain unanswered regarding BPH and hormonal therapy. What is the proper timing of antiandrogen therapy: before or after BPH symptoms develop? Are all the symptoms of BPH due to prostatic growth or are other mechanisms operative? Jones and Schoenberg have found that the uninhibited bladder contractions commonly found in men with BPH are also present in approximately 11% of

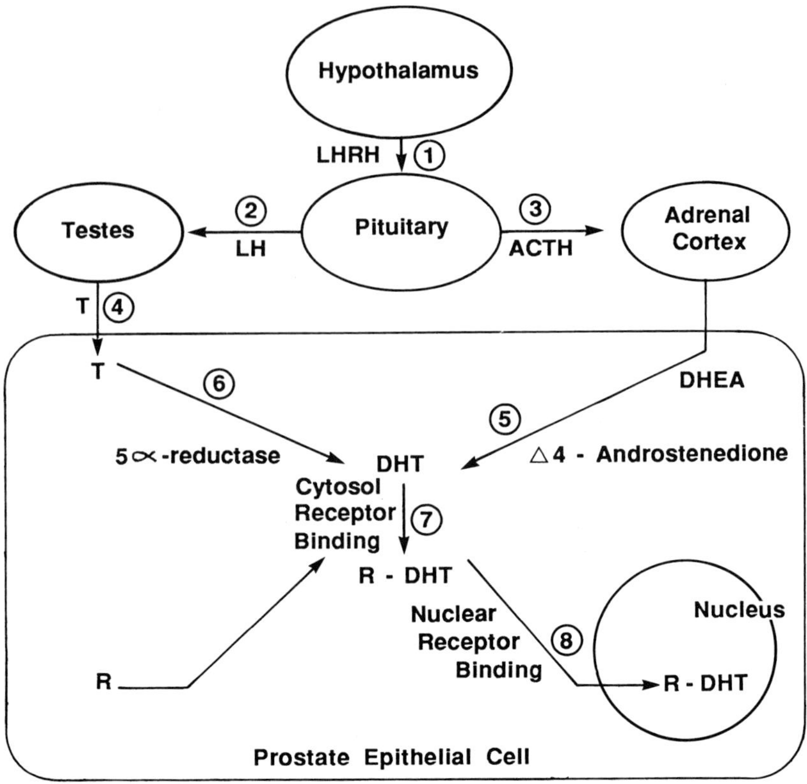


**Fig 3.** Multiple factors contributing to androgen-mediated action. Pathway for synthesis of DHT is shown; primary loci at which various androgen withdrawal therapies block androgen action are indicated by numbers as follows: 4, surgical castration; 2, 3, 4, 6, 7 medical castration with progestational antiandrogens; 7, androgen blockade with pure antiandrogens; 1, medical castration with gonadotropin-releasing hormone (GnRH) agonist androgen blockade with 5α-reductase inhibitors; 5, 6, no therapy is known to block step 5. LHRH = luteinizing hormone-releasing hormone; LH = luteinizing hormone; ACTH = adrenocorticotropic hormone; T = testosterone; DHEA = dehydroepiandrosterone; R = androgen receptors; R·DHT = androgen receptor-steroid complex. [From Geller.[20]]

older women.[21] This study suggests that some age-related changes in bladder function are independent of prostatic growth. Also, the role of the prostatic smooth muscle in prostatism suggests other mechanisms play a role in the development of BPH.

## ANTIANDROGENS

Nonsurgical castration has been attempted by a number of different approaches. These include using luteinizing hormone-releasing hormone (LHRH) analogs, flutamide, 5α-reductase inhibitors, cyproterone acetate, megestrol acetate, and candicidin.

### LHRH Analogs

The LHRH analogs block testicular androgen production by inhibiting pituitary gonadotropin release. This effect occurs via desensitization of the LHRH receptor complex in the pituitary gland. These effects lead to decreases in luteinizing hormone, follicle-stimulating hormone, testosterone, dihydrotestosterone, and estradiol levels (Fig 4).[22] Three months of therapy with a long-acting LHRH analog resulted in a 90%

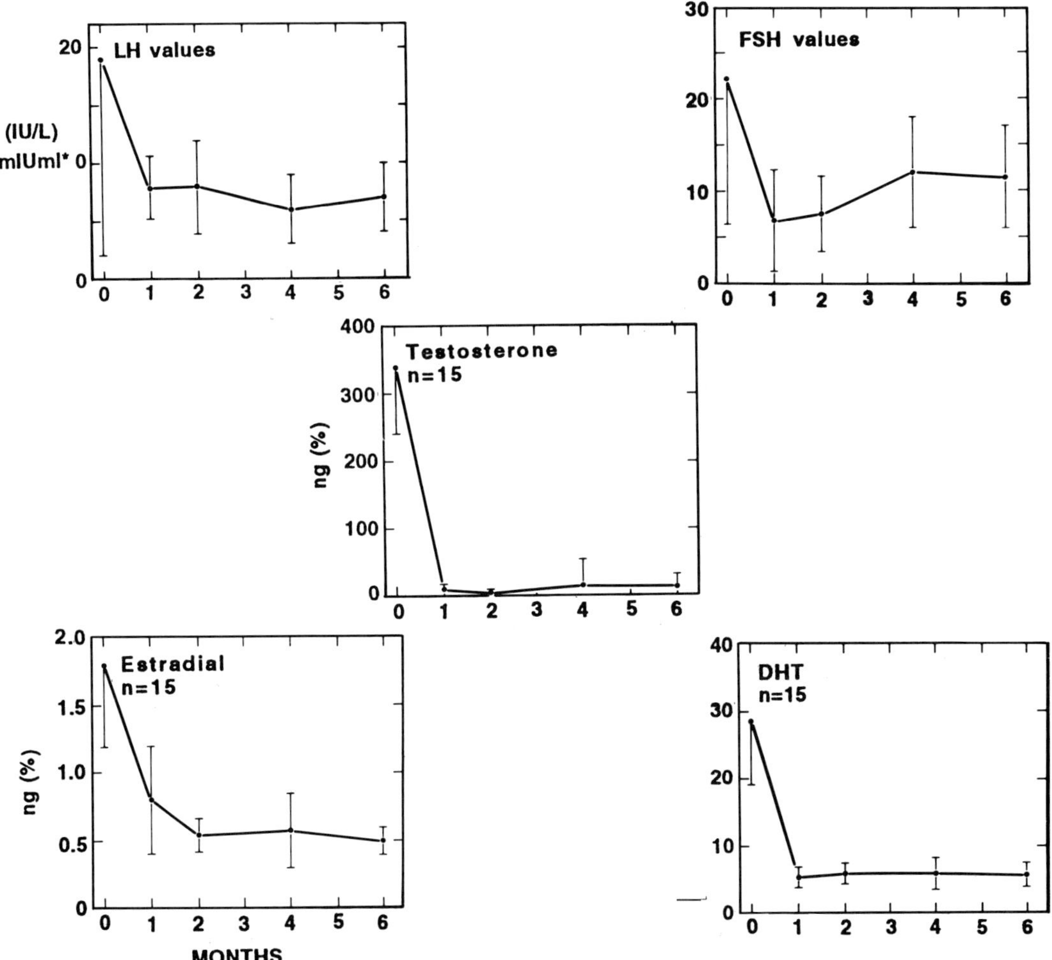


**Fig 4.** Mean (± standard deviation) of serum LH, FSH, T, DHT, and E concentrations in 15 men with BPH receiving leuprolide therapy. [From Gabrilove.[22]]

reduction in prostatic dihydrotestosterone and a 75% reduction in prostatic testosterone.[23,24] There also appears to be a decrease in 5α-reductase activity concomitant with a decrease in nuclear androgen receptor levels.[23] Thus, LHRH analogs affect prostatic growth by decreasing androgen levels and the tissue responsiveness to androgens.

Peters and Walsh reported their results of a non-controlled trial treating nine BPH patients with nafarelin acetate (400 μg daily administered subcutaneously) for 6 months.[25] Testosterone levels fell to castrate levels within 1 month of initiation of therapy and returned to normal levels within 2 months after cessation of therapy. Six of nine patients experienced improvement in symptoms, and three of nine reported overall clinical improvement. The prostate size regressed, as determined by prostate sonography, an average of approximately 24%. This regression reached a plateau at 4 months and prostate sizes returned to normal by 6 months after cessation of treatment. Morphometric analysis of biopsy specimens demonstrated a 40% reduction of epithelial volume due to epithelial atrophy which reversed after therapy. Three of the nine patients exhibited substantial improvements in peak urine flow, but no change in posttreatment, postvoid residual urine was noted. The peak flow and obstruction symptom changes correlated with the prostatic size change. Patients noted reversible impotence, hot flashes, fatigue, and weight gain.

Gabrilove et al demonstrated the effects of treating 15 men with BPH with leuprolide (1 mg daily given subcutaneously) for a minimum of 4 months.[22] This study lacked objective uroflowmetry data, but the average total symptom score dropped from 4.7 (out of 8) to 1.8. The prostate size, measured by transrectal ultrasonography, decreased by an average of 40% after 4 months and 46% after 6 months. All 15 men experienced impotency, hot flashes, and decreased libido during treatment. Schroeder and associates demonstrated an average reduction of 31% in prostatic size in four patients who underwent orchiectomy and one who underwent LHRH analog therapy.[26] Again, these studies demonstrate the ability of LHRH analog therapy to effect prostatic shrinkage.

Other investigators have reached different conclusions regarding the possible benefits of medical castration. Matzkin and colleagues recently reported testing 20 patients with a monthly injection of depot LHRH analog.[27] After 6 months of therapy, the prostatic volume decreased an average of 63%, which did not correlate with objective clinical improvement. Approximately 30% of the patients attained normalization of urinary flow rates, and 40% reported overall clinical improvement. Keane et al studied 20 patients receiving the LHRH analog buserelin (1.6 mg daily given in four divided doses administered intranasally).[28] These researchers noted no significant improvement in urinary flow rates or residual volume, despite maintaining castrate levels of dihydrotestosterone. Additionally, biopsies showed no evidence for epithelial cell height reduction. Another study comparing buserelin (12 mg daily given in three divided doses administered intranasally) with the antiandrogen cyproterone acetate (100 mg bid) reported that with both agents only minimal urodynamic changes occurred despite a 29% reduction in prostate volume after 12 weeks.[29] In addition, impotency was experienced by all men. These studies indicate that although LHRH analog therapy does exhibit a clinical effect (decreasing prostatic volume and reducing hormone levels to castrate levels), it is not practical for the great majority of men.

## Flutamide

Because impotency results from LHRH analog treatment, an approach at medical castration that spares potency would be preferable. Flutamide, an orally active nonsteroidal antiandrogen, is converted by hydroxylation to a competitive inhibitor of the cytoplasmic androgen receptor (Fig 5).[30,31] Side effects include tender gynecomastia and diarrhea.

Two groups have investigated the use of flutamide in the treatment of BPH. In 1975, Caine and coworkers evaluated 30 patients in a double-blind, placebo-controlled study lasting 12 weeks; patients received 300 mg flutamide daily.[32] A significant increase in urinary flow rate was noted and prostatic biopsies demonstrated no significant changes after 12 weeks. Seven of 15 patients developed nipple pain and gynecomastia, thought to be secondary to unopposed estrogen action in the breast. Testosterone levels markedly increased, while dihydrotestosterone levels decreased. Patients receiving 750 mg of flutamide per day were studied by Stone recently in a multicenter, randomized, double-blind study.[31] At the time of reporting, only 12 of 84 patients had been studied for 6 months, and 58 had been followed for 12 weeks or more. Peak urinary flow rate values increased 12% in the placebo group and 30% in the flutamide group after 12 weeks. A 30% reduction in symptoms occurred in both groups. At 24 weeks, an average 41% decrease in prostatic volume was noted by ultrasonography in patients treated with flutamide. Eleven percent of patients in the flutamide group experienced severe tender gynecomastia or diarrhea. However, this study is not yet completed, and it may take longer than 12 weeks to see the full effects of flutamide therapy.

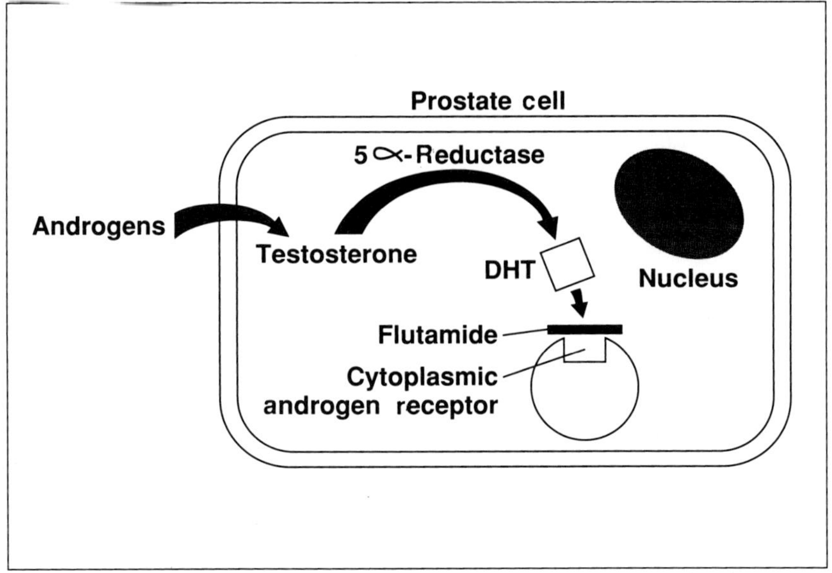


**Fig 5.** Method of action of the antiandrogen flutamide.

## 5α-Reductase Inhibitor

As seen in Figures 3 and 5, testosterone is converted to dihydrotestosterone by the enzyme 5α-reductase. An inherited form of male pseudohemaphroditism has been found to occur secondary to defective or deficient production of 5α-reductase.[33,34] These patients exhibit nonpalpable testes despite aging, while retaining potency and the ability to ejaculate. 5α-reductase blockade results in regression of BPH or, theoretically, in prevention of BPH development if administered early enough.

A potent, reversible inhibitor of 5α-reductase (MK-906, finasteride, Proscar) is currently being tested in a large, prospective, multicenter, placebo-controlled study. Finasteride induces castrate levels of prostatic dihydrotestosterone without affecting plasma testosterone levels or the androgen cytoplasmic receptor.[35,36] Preliminary results indicate that 6 months of therapy with finasteride results in approximately a 30% reduction in prostatic size, and roughly one third of patients demonstrated improvement in symptomatology and urinary flow rates.[37] No significant side effects have been noted. The final determination of the efficacy of 5α-reductase inhibitor therapy for BPH awaits the results of the large clinical trial.

## Cyproterone Acetate

Cyproterone acetate, a synthetic antiandrogen with progestational activity, inhibits the androgen receptor as well as pituitary gonadotropin release. In an uncontrolled study, Scott and Wade used cyproterone acetate in 13 patients with BPH for up to 15 months.[38] Nine patients experienced urinary flow rate improvement, while 11 exhibited improved symptomatology. Prostatic needle biopsy revealed a decrease in epithelial cell height in eight of the 11 patients evaluated. Impotency developed in four of 13 men. In a previously discussed study, Bosch and associates used either cyproterone acetate or buserelin and found an approximately 30% decrease in prostatic volume.[29] Clinical improvement was deemed to be minimal, however.

## Megestrol Acetate

Megestrol acetate, a progestational hormone, also inhibits gonadotropin release and blocks androgen receptors. Geller et al performed a double-blind, placebo-controlled study of 61 patients for a period of 20 weeks.[39] Peak urinary flow rates did not differ between the two groups, but 78% of megestrol-treated patients compared with 57% of the placebo-treated group experienced subjective improvement. In addition, 70% of the megestrol-treated patients reported loss of libido. This study again illustrates the tendency to have spontaneous symptomatic or uroflowmetry improvement in placebo-treated patients. Similarly, Donkervoort et al found minimal objective improvement in megestrol-treated patients.[40] The sexual side effects have generally limited therapeutic use of steroidal antiandrogens for patients with BPH.

### Conclusions About Antiandrogen Therapy

Most elderly men with prostatism have primarily stromal cell rather than epithelial cell enlargement. A 5:1 stromal-to-epithelial ratio usually occurs in men with BPH. Antiandrogen treatments appear to reduce the epithelial component of BPH, as witnessed by Higgins et al, who studied histologic sections of prostates from three castrated patients.[41] Generally, there appears to be a 25% to 35% reduction in prostate volume with antiandrogen therapy.

About one third to one half of patients treated with antiandrogens experience beneficial effects on clinical and urodynamic indices when compared to TURP. Whether this is sufficient from a clinical standpoint remains to be seen. Also, it may be difficult to shrink the prostate and relieve symptoms once BPH is established. Antiandrogen therapy may need to be instituted prior to the development of BPH, at a relatively young age. If this conclusion is correct, it raises largely unanswered questions about treating BPH at a younger age: Treat every male? Protect pregnant females from semen containing the drug to prevent teratogenic effects on a male fetus? Risk heretofore recognized ill effects of counteracting testicular steroids over a long period of time? Treat for the life of the patient?

## ANTI-STEROIDAL THERAPY

Because the prostatic epithelial component is rich in cholesterol, drugs that inhibit cholesterol metabolism may be used to shrink the prostate. Candicidin, an antifungal agent, is one such drug. Sixty-two patients received candicidin (300 mg/day) over a 6-month period in a study by Abrams.[42] No significant difference was found in the symptom score, urinary flow rates, and overall improvements between the candicidin- and placebo-treated groups. Again, a significant placebo effect was demonstrated.

## SMOOTH MUSCLE RELAXANTS

In 1986, Caine postulated that benign prostatic enlargement causes obstruction to urinary flow by both static and dynamic factors.[43] The hyperplastic stromal and epithelial tissue constitutes the static component, while the dynamic component is related to the tone of the prostatic smooth muscle. The human prostate is surrounded by a dense capsule containing abundant smooth muscle fibers and, in addition, contains numerous smooth muscle fibers within the stroma. The variable tone of this smooth muscle is thought to account for the day-to-day variations in symptoms characteristic of BPH. Hence, pharmacologic agents that relax smooth muscle might represent an effective therapeutic approach for men with BPH.

The receptors within the prostate, prostatic capsule, and bladder neck have recently been characterized. These smooth muscle fibers appear to be innervated by $\alpha_1$-adrenergic nerve fibers.[43,44] The role of the $\alpha_2$-adrenergic receptors is unclear. The $\alpha_2$-adrenoreceptors, both pre- and postjunctional, may modulate norepinephrine release via presynaptic receptors (with the postsynaptic receptors located on prostatic epithelium or vascular smooth muscle).[45] Muscarinic cholinergic receptors are located within prostatic adenomas and are thought to modulate prostatic secretions.[46,47] $\alpha_1$-adrenoreceptors are abundant in the bladder base and prostate, and are found in fewer numbers in the bladder body and urethra.[48]

A number of clinical effects have been associated with α-blocker therapy. α-blockade has been shown to reduce residual urine (although this may be due to improved detrusor function), increase urinary flow rates, and reduce urethral pressure.[49] A reduction in uninhibited bladder contractions with α-blocker therapy has been postulated to occur as a result of a direct effect on the obstructed detrusor. Chronic obstruction might produce a change from the normal β-receptors of the detrusor (relaxation) to α-receptors (contraction).[50,51]

### Phenoxybenzamine

This noncompetitive $\alpha_1$- and $\alpha_2$-blocker was the first studied in men with BPH. In one of the earliest placebo-controlled studies, Caine et al administered phenoxybenzamine 10 mg twice daily to 49 patients for 15 days.[49] Although no quantitative symptom score analyses were performed, overall symptom improvement was reported. The peak urinary flow rate improved by 1.2 mL/sec in the placebo group as compared with 6.2 mL/sec in the phenoxybenzamine-treated group. A sedative effect that might have contributed to the reduction in nocturia was noted. Subsequent trials have reported 50% to 80% improvement in various parameters in patients treated with phenoxybenzamine.[52,53]

However, other investigators have reached different conclusions. Abrams et al conducted a double-blind placebo study of 41 patients with BPH.[54] Peak flow rates improved from 6.5 mL/sec to 7.1 mL/sec in patients who received placebo vs a change from 7.2 mL/sec to 10.3 mL/sec in phenoxybenzamine-treated patients. This study did not show as much benefit as the Caine study. Two studies have found no benefit from using phenoxybenzamine at a dose of 10 mg/day.[55,56] A lack of side effects suggests this dose of phenoxybenzamine may be insufficient for adequate α-blockade.

Side effects with phenoxybenzamine are noted to occur in approximately 30% of patients,[53] and include palpitations, tachycardia, tiredness, dizziness, impaired ejaculation, nasal congestion, dryness, and difficulty with visual accommodation. Ten percent of patients are unable to tolerate this therapy. Phenoxybenzamine also has been associated with intestinal malignancy in rats. Because of these significant side effects—thought to be due to nonspecific α-blockade—trials of selective α-blockers have been instituted.

### Prazosin

Prazosin, a selective α-blocker, has recently been tested for the treatment of symptomatic BPH. Hedlund et al reported the results of a double-blind, crossover study.[57] These investigators noted significant improvement in peak urinary flow rates, and reduced residual volumes, without significant irritative symptomatic improvement. A significant placebo effect was also noted. Fifty-five patients were treated with prazosin (2 mg bid) during a placebo-controlled study in 1987.[58] The drug was titrated in a stepwise fashion to reduce orthostasis. A significant increase was noted in the peak urinary flow rate: 4.8 mL/sec in prazosin-treated patients vs 0.5 mL/sec in placebo-treated patients. Similar results were seen by Martorana and associates.[59]

Due to its lack of $\alpha_2$-blockade, prazosin produces fewer side effects than phenoxybenzamine and selective blockade may also explain its lesser effectiveness in ameliorating irritative symptoms. When using prazosin, one must consider the first-dose phenomenon of orthostatic hypertension that has been reported to occur. Doses of 2 to 6 mg daily are generally used, with an initial dose of 0.5 mg at bedtime.

### Long-Acting Selective $\alpha_1$-Blockers

Because phenoxybenzamine and prazosin are relatively short-acting agents, trials of longer-acting selective $\alpha_1$-blockers have been instituted. The α-adrenoceptor properties of the three long-acting, selective $\alpha_1$-blockers, terazosin, doxazosin, and YM-12617, have recently been characterized.[60–62]

Three clinical trials have reported using terazosin for treatment of symptomatic BPH. Dunzendorfer performed a single-blinded dose titration study in 15 men using terazosin in doses of up to 10 mg daily.[63] He noted 62% and 31% improvement in the obstructive and irritative symptom scores, respectively, without significant side effects. The peak urinary flow rate increased from 5.9 mL/sec to 7.7 mL/sec. A randomized, placebo-withdrawal study using a maximum dose of 10 mg daily was reported by Fabricius et al.[64] These researchers noted an improvement of 68% in obstructive symptom scores and 54% in peak urinary flow rates. Recently, a terazosin dose-titration study in 45 normotensive patients was reported by Lepor and coworkers.[65] Complete urodynamic evaluation and symptom scores were recorded using doses of up to 5 mg per day. The peak urinary flow rate improved by 42% and obstructive and irritative symptoms scores decreased by 63% and 35%, respectively. No change in blood pressure was noted. Sixty-seven percent of the patients indicated their voiding symptoms were markedly improved while receiving terazosin. Five of 45 patients did not complete the study because of experiencing severe adverse reactions, including erectile dysfunction (7%), tiredness (7%), lightheadedness (4%), palpitations (4%), nasal congestion (2%), and asymptomatic hypotension (2%). A large-scale, randomized, placebo-controlled study evaluating terazosin at dosages of 2, 5, and 10 mg is now completed and is undergoing statistical analysis.

Doxazosin and YM-12617 are also currently under study. Kawabe et al recently reported their work with YM-12617.[66] In this placebo-controlled, dose-titration study, a significant increase in urinary peak flow rate was not found, although approximately 80% of patients who received doses of 0.2 mg and 0.4 mg daily noted some improvement (as compared with 56% of patients in the placebo group).

### α-Blocker Therapy: Assessment and Indications

Most of the above studies have been of short duration, and many are not placebo-controlled or blinded. The older studies tend not to include symptom analysis or quality-of-life assessments. Most studies have used small numbers of patients and there may well be selection bias. Side effects do occur and cannot be minimized in the older patient population. However, α-blockers appear to be associated with a modest improvement in peak urinary flow rates, and obstructive symptoms tend to improve more than irritative symptoms. A large placebo effect is often present in all studies of men with BPH.

Indications for α-blocker therapy include prostatism without chronic urinary retention, urinary tract infection, or chronic renal insufficiency. Acute postoperative urinary retention may be prevented or treated with α-blockers as described by Goodman et al.[67] The use of such agents should probably be limited in those with cerebrovascular disease, cardiovascular disease, or who experience persistent side effects.

### Prostatic Balloon Dilation

Over the last 5 years, prostatic balloon dilation has been actively pursued as an alternative to prostatectomy. The origin of prostatic urethral dilation dates back to the mid-1800s, when investigators such as Mercier designed metal dilators.[68] In 1956, Deisting reported the results of treating 324 patients with a moveable transurethral metal dilator to disrupt the anterior and posterior prostatic commissures (Fig 6).[69] Although he did not publish objective measurements, he reported success rates of 95%, 83%, 74%, and 48% at 0, 3, 5, and 8 years postdilation, respectively. Other investigators during this period confirmed the efficacy of this procedure.

The enthusiasm for prostatic urethral dilation abated secondary to the results of two studies and improvements in endoscopic resection instruments. Kollberg published results showing that only 22% of 55 cases so treated showed favorable results at 1 to 2 years.[70] Then, Aalkjaer reported results of 296 patients receiving treatment with prostatic dilation or TURP.[71] Seven-year follow-up was available; in the TURP treatment group, 18 out of 110 patients required reoperation within 7 years, a value comparable to currently reported rates.[3] Of the 186 patients in the group treated with

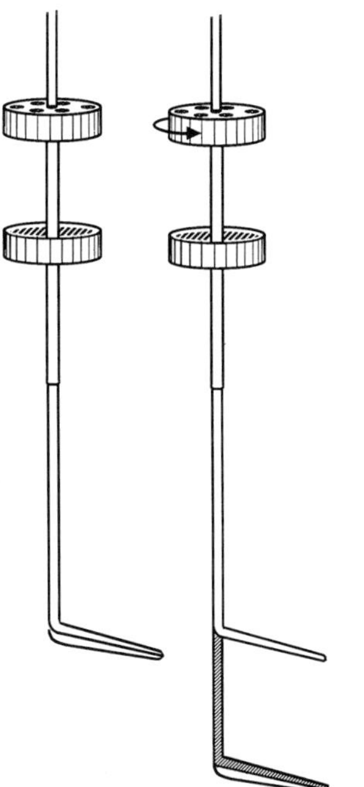

**Fig 6.** The Deisting prostatic dilator consists of a 24F shaft with two dilator branches and two handwheels. One handwheel serves as a handle for the instrument and the other for operation of the dilatation mechanism. [From Reddy PK, *Urol Clin North Am* (1988;15:529), with permission.]

dilation, 14% required immediate TURP—predominately to treat acute retention—and 38% required re-dilation—half within 9 months of the original procedure. Interestingly, Aalkjaer was the Chief of Urology at Diesting's institution and subsequently reported on some of Diesting's patients. These reports helped decrease enthusiasm for Diesting's technique.

Enthusiasm for prostatic balloon dilation was rekindled in the 1980s with experimental work on dogs and cadavers. Burhenne et al dilated 10 cadavers (and himself) using a 24 F balloon and a hand-held syringe.[72] Five of 7 cadavers exhibited a 30% to 100% increase in prostatic urethral diameter by urethrogram. Five of 6 dogs dilated by Quinn and associates exhibited widening of the prostatic urethra lasting 8 to 23 weeks.[73] The authors emphasized that the human prostate is predominately stromal with a strong capsule, as opposed to the dog prostate which is predominately epithelial with a weak capsule. Hence, the dog model may not be that useful. Castaneda et al determined that dilation to 60 F for at least 10 minutes was required for long-term results in dogs.[74]

The mechanism of action of prostatic balloon dilation is uncertain. The predominant mechanism might be disruption of the prostatic commissures as postulated by Castaneda et al.[75] Other postulated mechanisms include: gland compression and dehydration to enlarge the urethral lumen, stretch the elastic capsule, lessen smooth muscle tone by pressure provocation, or disrupt the α-adrenergic receptor.[76] Intraprostatic hemorrhages have been noted, but no other serious side effects have been reported.[73]

Three major techniques for prostatic balloon dilation have been employed. These include digital, fluoroscopic, and endoscopic positioning of balloons. Dowd and Smith recently reported results from 50 patients treated with digitally positioned balloons inflated to 90 F at 4 atms pressure for 15 minutes (Fig 7).[76] Forty-two percent of the patients had complete urinary retention and 62% had failed treatment with α-blockers. Follow-up ranged from 1 to 41 months; 72% of patients had excellent or acceptable results. Placement of a chronic catheter or TURP was required in 28% of the patients. Secondary treatment with dilators was not beneficial, and the response to the treatment was known within the first 2 weeks after treatment. Complications were minor and included hematuria and a urethral stricture.

A prospective, uncontrolled study of 73 subjects with moderate to severe prostatism was recently reported by Wasserman and colleagues.[77] They used 75 F fluoroscopically positioned balloons inflated to 3 to 5 atms for 10 minutes (Fig 8). Ninety-six percent of patients were successfully dilated, and follow-up averaged 16.2 months. Symptoms scores improved in 66% (38% if median lobe enlargement was present). Fifty-four percent of the patients exhibited an improvement in their peak urinary flow rate. Symptom score changes were significant through 24 months, while peak urinary flow improvements were

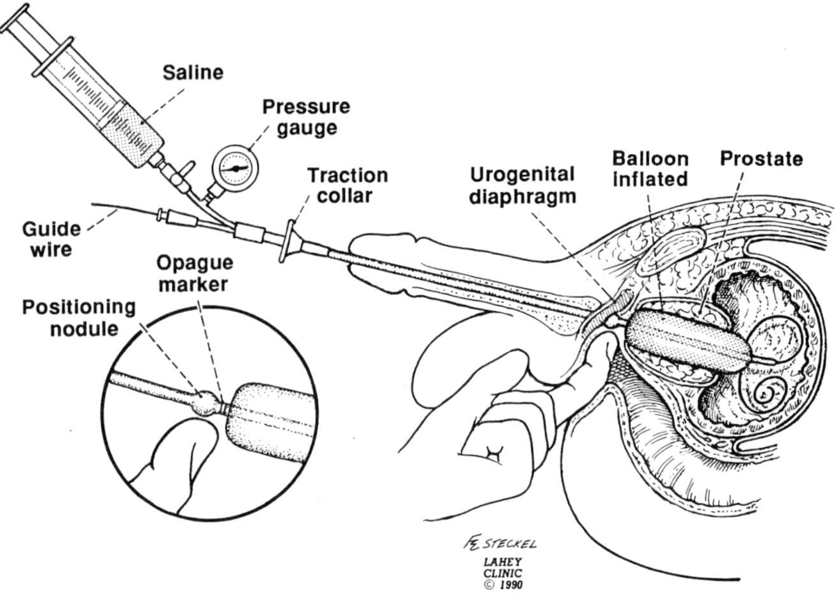


**Fig 7.** Technique of balloon dilation of the prostate. [From Dowd JB, Smith JJ, Prostatic balloon dilatation in 115 unequivocally obstructed patients, *J Endourol* (1991;5(2)99–104), with permission.]

maintained through 12 months. Sixty-eight percent of the nonresponders were identified during the first 6 months and 28% of these men responded to a second dilation. Only 28% of those with urinary retention showed clinical improvement. No complications were reported.

Goldenberg et al described the use of the endoscopic method in a Phase I study of 42 patients with BPH and bladder neck hyperplasia.[78] A 75 F, 3 atm balloon was inflated for 10 minutes (Fig 9). These investigators noted at 6-month follow-up that 46% of the patients demonstrated at least a 25% improvement in symptom score and peak flow rate. Additionally, 21% of the men experienced a greater than 50% improvement in symptom score without any change in peak flow rates. The durability of the symptom score and flow rate improvements were noted through 6 months. Complications included mild hematuria, pain, and transient urinary retention.

Further clinical trials are needed to determine the efficacy of balloon dilation as compared with placebo. The debate over optimal method, balloon length and shape, pressure, and diameter awaits further study. Apparent relative contraindications include a noncompliant bladder, active urinary tract infection, long or large glands, middle lobe hypertrophy, chronic obstruction with bladder atony, stones, and recurring urethral stricture disease.

## PROSTATIC HYPERTHERMIA

Prostatic hyperthermia was first used to treat carcinoma of the prostate, based on the observation that cancer cells were more sensitive to hyperthermia than normal cells. Subsequently, transrectal and transurethral hyperthermia have been investigated in the treatment of men with BPH.

Initial investigations focused on transrectal hyperthermia in dogs. Mendecki et al developed a coaxial microwave device that, when inserted rectally, produced prostatic urethral temperatures of 43.0°C to 43.5°C without rectal injury.[79] This device was ensheathed in a water-cooled jacket. Dose-response curves in normal dog prostates were generated by Leib and associates in 1986.[80] They found heating at 42.5°C for 90 minutes was harmless.

Phase I clinical studies of transrectal prostatic hyperthermia have recently been performed. Servadio et al treated a diverse

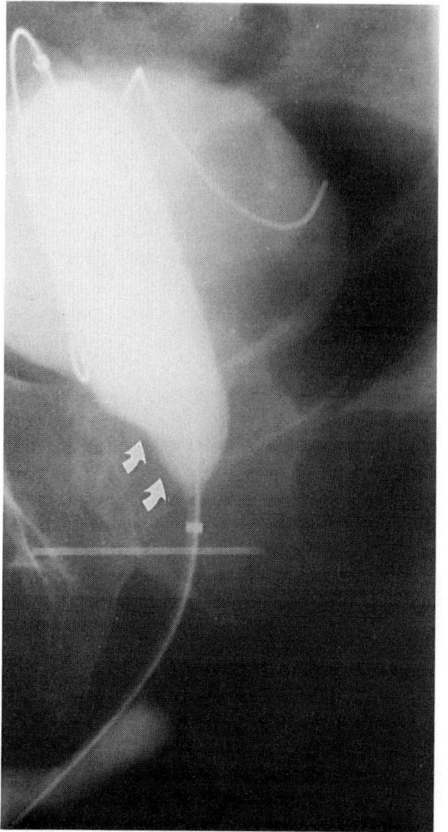


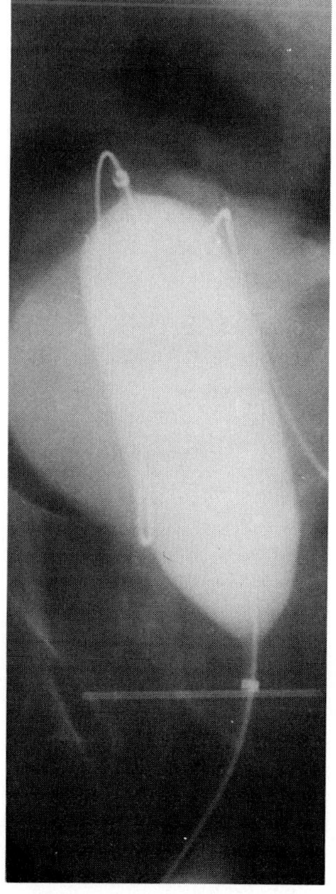


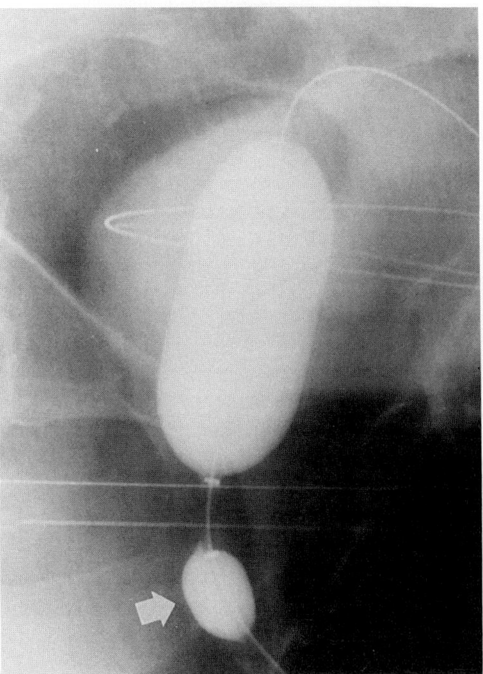


**Fig 8.** A, deformity of the balloon (arrows) indicates incomplete compression of prostatic tissue at 2.5 atm; B, further inflation to 4 atm achieves fully effective dilatation; C, superior and inferior margins of external sphincter are indicated by metal markers on drape. Fixation balloon is inflated with contrast in proximal bulbous urethra (arrow) immediately below the external sphincter, preventing upward migration of distended dilating balloon. [From Wasserman et al.[77]]

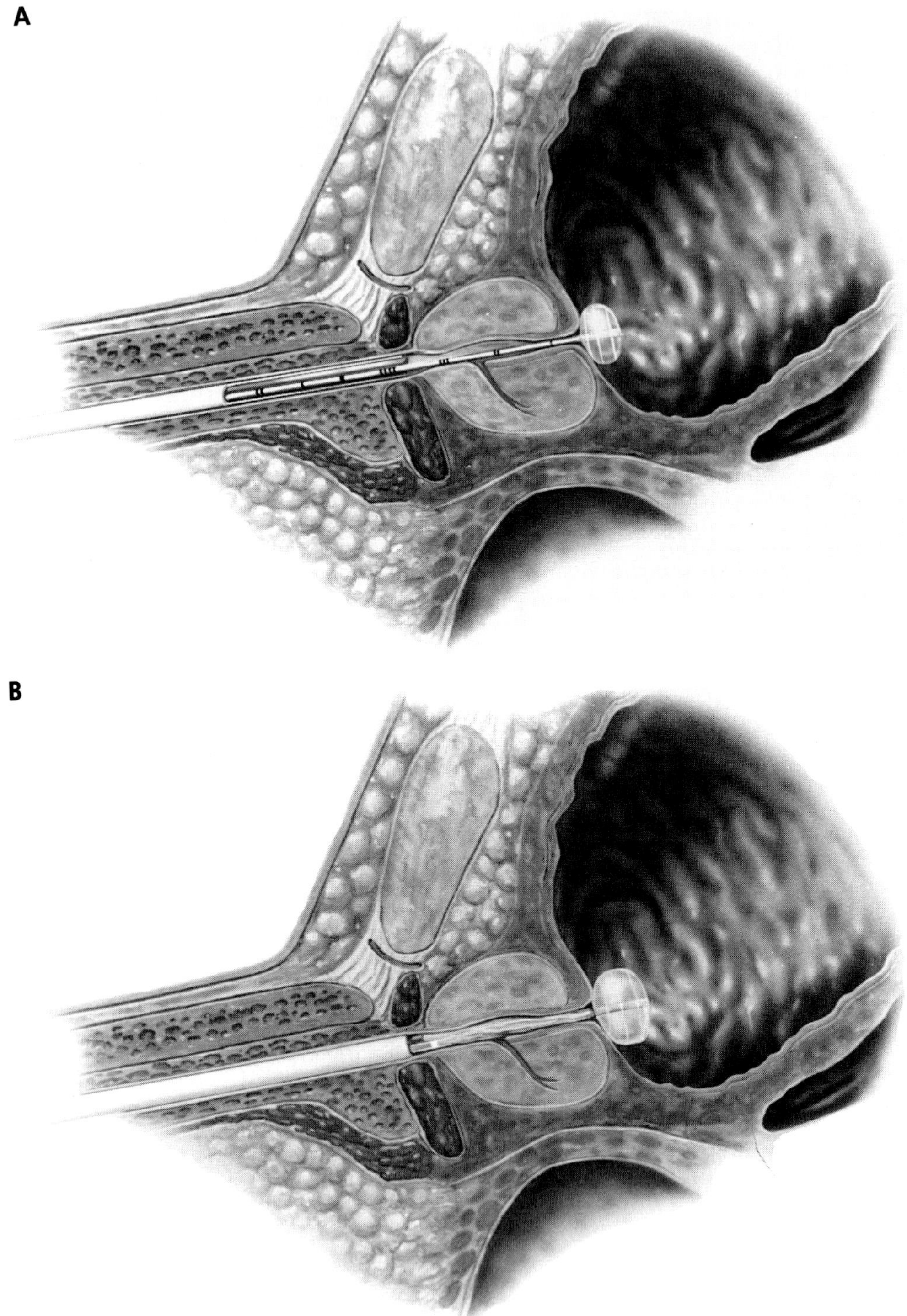


**Fig 9.** A, urethral calibration catheter positioned in prostatic urethra with inflated balloon against bladder neck. Anatomical length of urethra is determined with centimeter markings on catheter shaft; B, dilation balloon in prostatic urethra with Foley balloon pulled back against bladder neck and

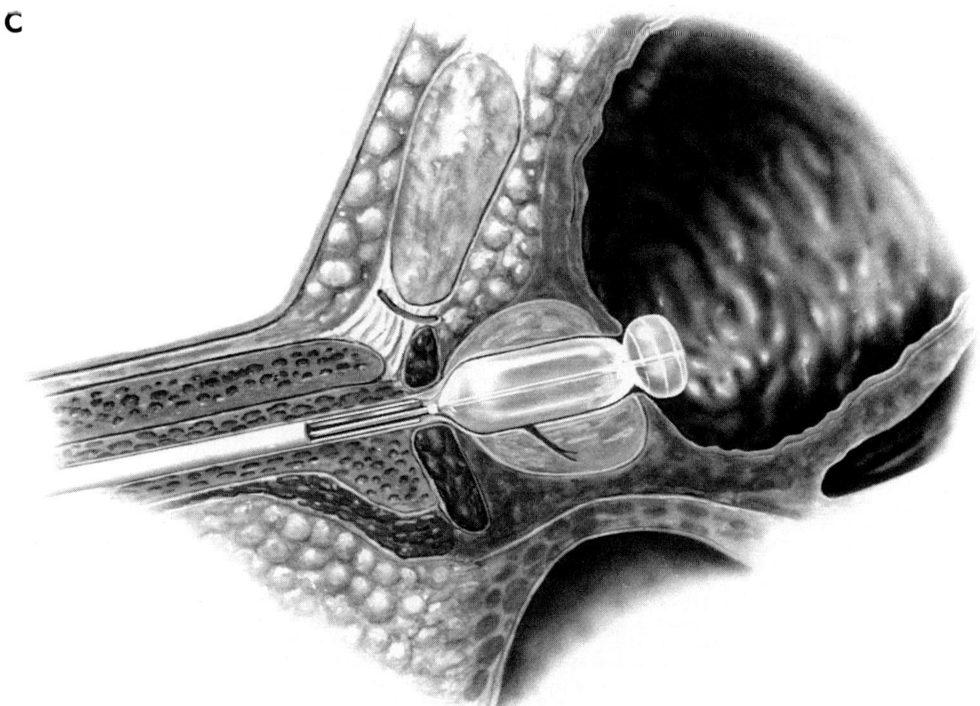


uninflated dilation balloon appropriately positioned in prostatic fossa; C, dilation balloon is inflated in prostatic urethra. Sheath has been positioned just beyond and proximal balloon marker at external sphincter. [From Goldenberg et al.[78]]

group of patients, including untreated controls, advanced prostatic carcinoma patients, poor-risk BPH patients, and chronic nonbacterial prostatitis patients.[81] Six to 10 treatments per patient at weekly intervals resulted in improved voiding ability in 15 of 23 catheter-dependent patients and improved average symptoms scores from 3.3 to 6.4. Two patients, one with a history of chronic bacterial prostatitis and one with previous surgery, developed prostatorectal fistulas which healed spontaneously. Five of six poor-risk, catheter-dependent patients no longer needed the catheter after 5 to 10 outpatient hyperthermia treatments in a study by Lindner et al.[82] Seventy percent of 20 catheter-dependent patients treated with 7 to 18 treatments once or twice weekly have voiding ability after up to 51 months of follow-up in a study by Yerushalmi.[83] Additionally, 47 severely symptomatic patients were treated with hyperthermia; improvement was noted in 81% of the patients studied.

More recent reports of the use of transrectal hyperthermia are less optimistic. Saranga and colleagues reported 28% improvement in both subjective and objective parameters in a group of 83 patients with severe symptomatology.[84] Additionally, 61% of 31 patients with acute urinary retention were able to dispense with catheter use. Lindner et al reported a 40% 1-year catheter-free rate in 72 patients treated for urinary retention.[85] However, the best results were obtained in patients who also received cyproterone acetate. A 7.1% success rate was reported by Strohmaier et al in 30 patients with symptomatic BPH.[86]

Transrectal prostatic hyperthermia is generally well tolerated, and is associated with an overall complication rate of 6.6%.[87] Prostatic volume and prostate-specific antigen levels do not appear to change.[86,88] Weekly outpatient treatments at 916 mHz with heating to 42.5°C represent the therapeutic norm. Several disadvantages exist, including difficulty in maintaining proper position and orientation, and the distance of the irradiation source from the targeted hyperplastic tissues. The development of transurethral hyperthermia catheters was pursued to overcome these problems.

Transurethral prostatic hyperthermia utilizes a microwave antenna wrapped around a Foley catheter. Sapozink et al presented their experience in treating 21 patients with this approach (Fig 10).[89] In this study, 75% of the prostatic loci were heated to 43°C. Patients were noted to have an increased urine flow rate (11–15.9 mL/sec), decreased postvoid residual urine (177–91 mL), and decreased urinary frequency. Three patients required TURP after a median follow-up period of 12.5 months. Mild toxicity included bladder spasms (26% of patients), hematuria (23%), and dysuria (9%). Substantial objective and subjective improvement was noted in 80% of 15 patients treated recently by Baert and associates.[90] Three patients were considered to be treatment failures and required prostatectomy. Chronic bladder atony, middle lobe hypertrophy, and asymptomatic lateral lobes were thought to be factors contributing to failure. The mechanism of action, based on pathologic examination, appeared to be periurethral scarring leading to urethral dilation.

Future clinical trials will further delineate the role of prostatic hyperthermia in the treatment of men with BPH. Transurethral delivery methods might prove to be most efficacious. Hyperthermia has little associated morbidity and can be performed under local anesthesia; however, the need for multiple treatments reduces its attractiveness.

## PROSTATIC STENTS

Recently, prostatic stents have been used to treat patients with BPH who are unfit for or refuse surgery. Some of the stents are modified versions of those used in the treatment of intraarterial occlusive disease. Recent urologic applications include treat-

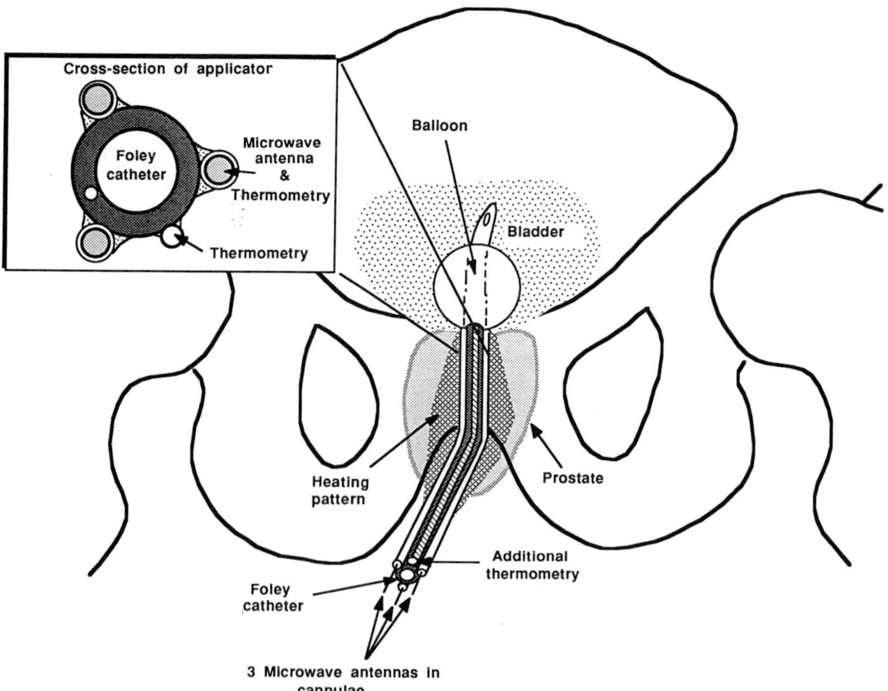


**Fig 10.** Transurethral prostatic hyperthermia utilizes a microwave antenna wrapped around a Foley catheter. Inset shows cross-section of applicator. [From Sapozink et al.[89]]

ment of urethral strictures, dyssynergic external urinary sphincters, and prostatic and bladder neck obstructions.

Ideally, stents should be easy to place, should remain in proper position, and should have a long, durable lifespan. In addition, they should be resistant to encrustation and infection. Currently, stents come in two forms: temporary and permanent.

## Temporary Stents

The first reports of clinical trials utilizing prostatic stents dates back to 1980. In 1989, Nordling et al published their results with the "Prostakath," an intraprostatic steel spiral with gold plating to prevent encrustation (Fig 11).[91] These investigators successfully placed the spiral under local anesthesia in 41 of 45 patients with acute or chronic urinary retention. The patients were considered to be poor surgical candidates, with a history of stroke, dementia, or cardiovascular disease. Stents were successfully placed via ultrasonic guidance in 33 patients and by endoscopy in six. Significant problems in maintaining proper stent position were noted. Eight stents were removed secondary to urinary retention or incontinence, and six patients required endoscopic repositioning of the stents. Of 33 patients who achieved voiding ability and underwent uroflowmetry, the mean peak flow rate was 13.6 mL/sec. Overall, 28 of 41 patients had a satisfactory outcome. No severe complications were noted, but irritative symptoms were reported in two patients, urge incontinence in one, and local discomfort with pressure on the perineum was noted in two patients.

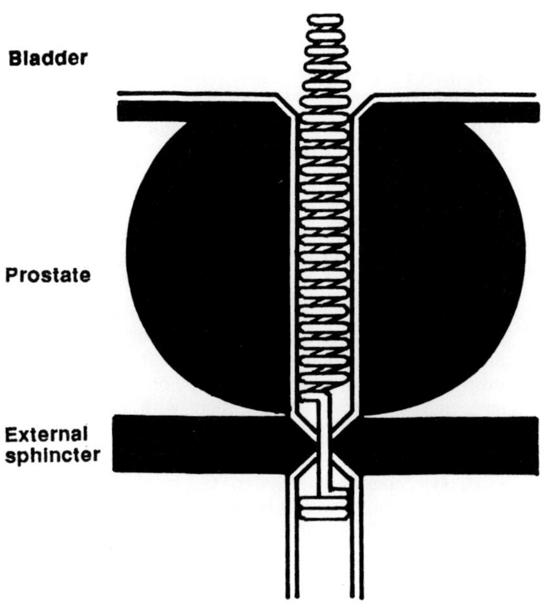


**Fig 11.** Spiral in situ. [From Nordling et al.[91]]

Vincente et al evaluated use of a similar stent in 22 patients with urinary retention and anesthetic contraindications.[92] A bulbar urethral perforation was noted in one patient, and stent immigration occurred in four patients (iatrogenically in two). Follow-up at 12 months revealed a 93% proper positioning rate and 74% normal voiding rate. Sixty-seven percent of the patients experienced peak urinary flow rates between 6 mL/sec and 14 mL/sec. Negative urine cultures were noted in 60% of those studied. Four patients reported irritative voiding symptoms and two had incontinence.

A polyurethane, double-ended malecot intraprostatic urethral stent has been described by Nissenkorn.[93] Eight of 10 patients with urinary retention achieved voiding ability and were continent after 2 to 7 weeks of follow-up. The main complaint in these patients was urinary frequency. Nissenkorn believes that this is a reasonable short- or median-term alternative to use of an indwelling catheter.

## Permanent Prostatic Stents

A permanent, stainless-steel stent that becomes completely epithelialized by 4 to 6 months was described by Williams et al in 1989.[94] Nine patients with urinary retention who were felt to be unfit for surgery voided with peak flow rates of 12 mL/sec to 22 mL/sec.

It thus seems that these stents work reasonably well for a short period in those unfit for surgery. The stents can be successfully placed using local anesthesia. Epithelialized stents should theoretically decrease infection and encrustation risks, but the inability to remove these stents may be a significant problem. Long-term follow-up is needed to determine the therapeutic role of stents for patients with moderate BPH.

## CONCLUSIONS

The last decade has seen an upsurge of interest in developing nonsurgical alternatives for management of BPH. Relatively few of these new therapies have been evaluated in randomized trials comparing them to observation or prostatectomy, and we must resist pressure to use these newer modalities without caution until safety and efficacy have been proven. This is especially true since the surgical treatment of BPH and observation work so well.

## REFERENCES

1. Holtgrewe HL, Valk WL. Factors influencing the mortality and morbidity of transurethral prostatectomy: a study of 2,015 cases. *J Urol.* 1962;87:45.
2. Melchoir J, Valk WL, Fout JD, Mebust WK. Transurethral prostatectomy: a computerized analysis of 2223 consecutive cases. *J Urol.* 1974;112:64.
3. Mebust WK, Holtgrewe HL, Cockett ATK, et al. Transurethral prostatectomy: immediate and postoperative complications. A cooperative study of thirteen participating institutions evaluating 3,385 patients. *J Urol.* 1989;141:243.
4. Lepor H, Rigaud G. The efficacy of transurethral resection of the prostate in men with moderate symptoms of prostatism. *J Urol.* 1990;143:533.
5. Glynn RJ, Campion EW, Bouchard GR, Silbert JE. The development of benign prostatic hyperplasia among volunteers in the normative aging study. *Am J Epidemiol.* 1985;121:78.
6. Holtgrewe HL, Mebust WK, Dowd JB, et al. Transurethral prostatectomy: practice aspects of the dominant operation in American urology. *J Urol.* 1989;141:248.
7. *Metropolitan Life Insurance Company: Statistical Bulletin.* 1989;70(3):20.
8. Berry SJ, Coffey DS, Walsh PC, Ewing LL. The development of human benign prostatic hyperplasia with age. *J Urol.* 1984;132:474.
9. Wennberg J, Gittelsohn A. Variations in medical cases among small areas. *Sci Am.* 1982;246:120.
10. Wennberg J, Roos N, Sola L, et al. Use of claims data systems to evaluate health care outcomes: mortality and reoperation following prostatectomy. *JAMA.* 1987;257:933.
11. Fowler FJ Jr, Wennberg JE, Timothy RP, et al. Symptom status and quality of life following prostatectomy. *JAMA.* 1988;259:3018.
12. Graverson PH, Gasser T, Wasson J, et al. Uncertainty about prostatectomy. *J Urol.* 1989; 141:475.
13. White JW. The results of double castration in hypertrophy of the prostate. *Ann Surg.* 1895;21:1.
14. Cabot AT. The question of castration for enlarged prostate. *Ann Surg.* 1896;24:265.
15. Scott WW. What makes prostates grow? *J Urol.* 1953;70:477.
16. McNeil JE. Origin and evolution of benign prostatic enlargement. *Invest Urol.* 1978;15:340.
17. Walsh PC. Benign prostatic hyperplasia. In: Walsh PC, Gittes RF, Perlmutter AD, Stamey TA, eds. *Campbell's Urology.* 5th ed. Philadelphia: WB Saunders; 1986;2:1248–1265.
18. Coffey DS, Berry SJ, Ewing LL. An overview of current concepts in the study of benign prostatic hyperplasia. In: Rodgers CH, et al, eds. *Benign Prostatic Hyperplasia.* Bethesda: National Institutes of Health; 1987;2:1.
19. Wilson JD. The pathogenesis of benign prostatic hyperplasia. *Am J Med.* 1980;68:745.
20. Geller J. Overview of benign prostatic hypertrophy. *Urology.* 1989;34(suppl):57.
21. Jones KW, Schoenberg HW. Comparison of the incidence of bladder hyperreflexia in patients with benign prostatic hypertrophy and age-matched female controls. *J Urol.* 1985;133:425.
22. Gabrilove JL, Levine AC, Kirschenbaum A, et al. Effect of long acting gonadotropin releasing hormone analog (leuprolide) therapy on prostatic size and symptoms in 15 men with benign prostatic hypertrophy. *J Clin Endocrinol Metab.* 1989;69:629.
23. Forti G, Salerno R, Moneti G, et al. Three months treatment with a long-acting gonadotropin-releasing hormone agonist of patients with benign prostatic hyperplasia: effects on tissue androgen concentrations, 5α-reductase activity and androgen receptor content. *J Clin Endocrinol Metab.* 1989;68:461.
24. Salerno R, Moneti G, Forti G, et al. Simultaneous determination of testosterone, dihydrotes-

tosterone, and 5α-androstan 3α, 17β-diol by isotopic dilation mass spectrometry in plasma and prostatic tissue of patients affected by benign prostatic hyperplasia: effects of a 3-month treatment with a GnRH analog. *J Androl.* 1988; 9:234.

25. Peters CA, Walsh PC. The effect of nafarelin acetate, a luteinizing hormone/releasing hormone agonist, on benign prostatic hyperplasia. *N Engl J Med.* 1987;317:599.
26. Schroeder FH, Westerhof M, Bosch RJLH, et al. Benign prostatic hypertrophy treated by castration or the LH-RH analog burselin: a report on six cases. *Eur Urol.* 1986;12:318.
27. Matzkin H, Chan J, Lewysohn O, et al. Treatment of benign prostatic hypertrophy by a long-acting gonadotropin-releasing hormone analog: one-year experience. *J Urol.* 1991;145:309.
28. Keane PF, Timong AG, Kiely E, et al. The response of the benign hypertrophied prostate to treatment with an LHRH analog. *Br J Urol.* 1988;62:163.
29. Bosch RJLH, Griffiths DJ, Blom JHM, et al. Treatment of benign prostatic hyperplasia by androgen deprivation: effects on prostate size and urodynamic parameters. *J Urol.* 1989;141:68.
30. Surfin G, Coffey DS. Mechanism of action of a new nonsteroidal antiandrogen: flutamide. *Invest Urol.* 1975;13:429.
31. Stone N. Flutamide in the treatment of benign prostatic hypertrophy. *Urology.* 1989;34 (suppl):64.
32. Caine M, Perlberg S, Gordon R. The treatment of benign prostatic hypertrophy with flutamide (SCH 13521): a placebo-controlled study. *J Urol.* 1975;114:564.
33. Walsh PC, Madden JD, Hanod MJ, et al. Familial incomplete male pseudohermaphroditism, type 2: decreased dihydrotestosterone formation in pseudovaginal perineoscrotal hypospadias. *N Engl J Med.* 1984;291:944.
34. Imperato-McGinley J, Guerrero L, Gautier T, et al. Steroid 5α-reductase deficiency in man: an inherited form of male pseudohermaphroditism. *Science.* 1974;186:1213.
35. McConnell JD, Wilson JD, George FW, et al. An inhibitor of 5α-reductase, MK-906, suppresses dihydrotestosterone in men with benign prostatic hyperplasia. *J Urol.* 1989;141:299A. Abstract.
36. Liang T, Hess CE, Cheung AH, et al. 4-Azasteroid 5α-reductase inhibitors without affinity for the androgen receptor. *J Biol Chem.* 1984; 259:734.
37. McConnell JD. Androgen ablation and blockade in the treatment of benign prostatic hyperplasia. *Urol Clin North Am.* 1990;17(3):661.
38. Scott WW, Wade JC. Medical treatment of benign nodular hyperplasia with cyproterone acetate. *J Urol.* 1969;101:81.
39. Geller J, Nelson CG, Albert JD, et al. Effect of megestrol acetate on uroflow rates in patients with benign prostatic hypertrophy: a double-blind study. *Urology.* 1979;5:467.
40. Donkervoort T, Sterling AM, Van Ness J, et al. Megestrol acetate in treatment of benign prostatic hyperplasia. *Urology.* 1975;6:580.
41. Huggins C, Stevens RA. The effect of castration on benign prostatic hypertrophy of the prostate in men. *J Urol.* 1940;43:705.
42. Abrams PH. A double-blind trial of the effects of candicidin in patients with benign prostatic hypertrophy. *Br J Urol.* 1977;49:67.
43. Caine M. The present role of alpha-adrenergic blockers in the treatment of benign prostatic hypertrophy. *J Urol.* 1986;136:1.
44. Lepor H, Gup DI, Bauman M, et al. Laboratory assessment of terazosin and alpha-1 blockade in prostatic hyperplasia. *Urology.* 1988;32 (suppl):21.
45. Lepor H. Alpha adrenergic antagonists for the treatment of symptomatic BPH. *Int J Clin Pharmacol Ther Tox.* 1989;27:151.
46. Lepor H, Kuhar MJ. Characterization and localization of muscarinic cholinergic receptors in human prostatic tissue. *J Urol.* 1984;132:397.
47. Smith ER, Ilievski V, Hadiclan Z. The stimulation of canine prostatic secretion by pilocarpine. *J Pharmacol Exper Ther.* 1966;151:59.
48. Shapiro E, Lepor H. $Alpha_1$ adrenergic receptors in canine lower genitourinary tissues: insight into development and function. *J Urol.* 1987;138:1.
49. Caine M, Perlberg S, Meretyk S. A placebo-controlled double-blind study of the effect of phenoxybenzamine in benign prostatic obstruction. *Br J Urol.* 1978;50:551.
50. Perlberg S, Caine M. Adrenergic response of bladder muscle in prostatic obstruction: its relation to detrusor instability. *Urology.* 1982; 20:524.
51. Restorick JM, Mundy AR. The density of cholinergic and alpha and beta adrenergic receptors in the normal and hyperreflexic human detrusor. *Br J Urol.* 1989;63:32.
52. Boreham PF, Braithwait P, Milewski P, et al. Alpha-adrenergic blockers in prostatism. *Br J Surg.* 1977;64:756.
53. Caine M, Perlberg S, Shapiro A. Phenoxybenzamine for benign prostatic obstruction: review of 200 cases. *Urology.* 1981;17:542.
54. Abrams PH, Shah PJR, Stone R, et al. Bladder outflow obstruction treated with phenoxybenzamine. *Br J Urol.* 1982;54:527.
55. Brooks ME, Sidi AA, Hanani Y, et al. Ineffectiveness of phenoxybenzamine in treatment of benign prostatic hypertrophy: a controlled study. *Urology.* 1983;21:474.
56. Ferrie BG, Paterson PJ. Phenoxybenzamine in prostatic hypertrophy: a double-blind study. *Br J Urol.* 1987;59:63.
57. Hedlund H, Anderson K-E, Ek A. Effects of prazosin in patients with benign prostatic obstruction. *J Urol.* 1983;130:275.

58. Kirby RS, Coppinger SWC, Corcoran MD, et al. Prazosin in the treatment of prostatic obstruction. A placebo controlled study. *Br J Urol.* 1987;60:136.
59. Martorana G, Giberti C, Damonte P, et al. The effect of prazosin in benign prostatic hypertrophy: a placebo-controlled study. *IRCS Med Sci.* 1984;12:11.
60. Lepor H, Baumann M, Shapiro E. The alpha adrenergic binding properties of terazosin in the human prostate adenoma and canine brain. *J Urol.* 1988;140:664.
61. Lepor H, Baumann M, Shapiro E. The binding and function properties of doxazosin in the human prostate adenoma and canine brain. *Prostate.* 1990;16:29.
62. Lepor H, Baumann M, Shapiro E. The sterospecificity of LY 253 352 for $\alpha_1$-adrenoceptor binding sites in the brain and prostate. *Br J Pharmacol.* 1988;95:139.
63. Dunzendorfer MV. Clinical experience with symptomatic management of BPH with terazosin. *Urology* 1988;32(suppl):27.
64. Fabricius PG, Weizert P, Dunzendorfer U, et al. A randomized, double-blind, placebo-controlled trial on the efficacy of once a day terasozin in prostate hyperplasia. *Prostate.* 1990;3:85.
65. Lepor H, Knapp-Maloney G, Sunshine H. A dose titration study evaluating terazosin, a selective, once-a-day $\alpha_1$-blocker for the treatment of symptomatic benign prostatic hyperplasia. *J Urol.* 1990;144:1393.
66. Kawabe K, Ueno A, Takimoto Y, et al. Use of $\alpha_1$-blocker, YM617, in the treatment of benign prostatic hypertrophy. *J Urol.* 1990;144:908.
67. Goldman G, Leviav A, Mazor H, et al. Alpha-adrenergic blocker for posthernioplasty urinary retention. *Arch Surg.* 1988;123:35.
68. Mercier F. Recherches sur les valvules des col de la vessie. Paris, 1850 (as cited in Hinman F Jr, ed. *Benign Prostatic Hypertrophy.* New York: Springer-Verlag; 1983:chap 5.
69. Deisting W. Transurethral dilation of the prostate: a new method in the treatment of prostatic hypertrophy. *Urol Int.* 1956;2:158.
70. Kollberg S. *Erfarenhetes av transurethral prostatadilatation enlight Deisting.* Stockholm: Foredrag vid Med riksstamma; 1959.
71. Aalkjaer V. Transurethral resection: prostatectomy vs. dilatation treatment in hypertrophy of the prostate. II. A comparison of late results. *Urol Int.* 1965;20:17.
72. Burhenne HJ, Chisholm RJ, Quenville NF. Prostatic hyperplasia. Radiologic intervention. *Radiology.* 1984;152:655.
73. Quinn SF, Dyer R, Smothers R, et al. Balloon dilatation of the prostatic urethra. *Radiology.* 1985;157:57.
74. Castaneda F, Lund G, Larson BW, et al. Prostatic urethra: experimental dilatation in dogs. *Radiology.* 1987;163:645.
75. Castaneda F, Isorna S, Hulbert JC, et al. The importance of separation of prostatic lobes in relief of prostatic obstruction by balloon catheter urethroplasty: studies in dogs and humans. *AJR.* 1989;153:1301.
76. Dowd JB, Smith JJ. Balloon dilatation of the prostate. *Urol Clin North Am.* 1990;17:671.
77. Wasserman NF, Reddy PK, Zhang G, et al. Experimental treatment of benign prostatic hyperplasia with transurethral balloon dilation of the prostate: preliminary study in 73 humans. *Radiology.* 1990;177:485.
78. Goldenberg SL, Perez-Marrero RA, Lou LM, et al. Endoscopic balloon dilation of the prostate: early experience. *J Urol.* 1990;144:83.
79. Mendecki J, Friedenthal E, Botstein C, et al. Microwave applicators for localized hyperthermia treatment of cancer of the prostate. *Int J Radiat Oncol Biol Phys.* 1980;6:1583.
80. Leib Z, Rothem A, Lev A, et al. Histopathological observations in the canine prostate treated by local microwave hyperthermia. *Prostate.* 1986;8:93.
81. Servadio C, Lieb L, Lev A. Diseases of the prostate treated by local microwave hyperthermia. *Urology.* 1987;30:97.
82. Lindner A, Golomb J, Siegel Y, et al. Local hyperthermia of the prostate gland for the treatment of benign prostatic hypertrophy and urinary retention. A preliminary report. *Br J Urol.* 1987;60:567.
83. Yerushalmi A. Localized, noninvasive microwave hyperthermia for the treatment of prostatic tumors: the first five years. *Cancer Res.* 1988;107:141.
84. Saranga R, Matzkin H, Braf Z. Local microwave hyperthermia in the treatment of benign prostatic hypertrophy. *Br J Urol.* 1990;65:349.
85. Lindner A, Braf Z, Lev A, et al. Local hyperthermia of the prostate gland for the treatment of benign prostate hypertrophy and urinary retention. *Br J Urol.* 1990;65:201.
86. Strohmaier WL, Bichler KH, Fluchter SH, et al. Local microwave hyperthermia of benign prostatic hyperplasia. *J Urol.* 1990;144:913.
87. Lindner A, Siegel YI, Saranga R, et al. Complications in hyperthermia treatment of benign prostatic hyperplasia. *J Urol.* 1990;144:1390.
88. Lindner A, Siegel YI, Korcyak D. Serum prostate specific antigen levels during hyperthermia treatment of benign prostatic hyperplasia. *J Urol.* 1990;144:1388.
89. Sapozink MD, Boyd SD, Astrahon MA, et al. Transurethral hyperthermia for benign prostatic hyperthermia. Preliminary clinical results. *J Urol.* 1990;143:944.
90. Baert L, Ameye F, Willemen P, et al. Transurethral microwave hyperthermia for benign prostatic hyperplasia: preliminary clinical and pathological results. *J Urol.* 1990;144:1383.
91. Nordling J, Holm HH, Klarskov P, et al. The

intraprostatic spiral: a new device for insertion with the patient under local anesthesia and with ultrasonic guidance with 3 months of follow-up. *J Urol.* 1989;142:756.

92. Vincente J, Salvador J, Chechile G. Spiral urethral prosthesis as an alternative to surgery in high risk patients with benign prostatic hyperplasia: prospective study. *J Urol.* 1989; 142:1504.

93. Nissenkorn I. Experience with a new self-retaining intraurethral catheter in patients with urinary retention: a preliminary report. *J Urol.* 1989;142:92.

94. Williams G, Jager R, McLoughlin J, et al. Use of stents for treating obstruction of urinary outflow in patients unfit for surgery. *Br Med J.* 1989;298:1429.

# 26

# Molecular Biology of Urologic Cancer: Principles and Practice

*William C. DeWolf and Michael A. O'Donnell*

## INTRODUCTION

Cancer will be the overall leading cause of death by the year 2000.[1] Although this fact is more reflective of a decreasing mortality from heart disease than an increase in cancer mortality,[2] it underscores the importance and obligation of the scientific and medical community to improve treatment and cure of this disorder. The process of investigation of how to eliminate cancer begins with an exact understanding of cell proliferation and those factors that regulate cell behavior in response to its environment. Major progress was made in our understanding of cell biology in the 1970s with advances in knowledge of immunology, but the real change occurred in the 1980s with the explosion of information resulting from the application of new techniques in biochemistry and molecular genetics. This chapter will define the terms and then dissect the process of malignant transformation into its component parts such that a better understanding may eventually lead to cure and prevention.

### What Is Cancer?

All normal vertebrate cells have a limited capacity to proliferate, a phenomenon that has come to be known as the Hayflick limit or replicative senescence.[3] In human fibroblasts this limit occurs after 50–80 population doublings after which the cells remain in a viable but nondividing senescent state. In contrast, most cancer cells have escaped from the controls limiting their proliferative capacity and are essentially immortal. This is especially brought out by the interesting paradox that the frequency of tumor incidence in humans and rodents is correlated with the fractional life span in a similar manner, even though the life spans of these two species differ by an order of magnitude.[4] The molecular basis for this difference remains obscure.

To gain a foothold on where to begin to understand malignant transformation, three basic principles appear from the last half decade of cancer research. The first is that most, if not all, cancer cells contain genetic damage that appears to lie at the heart of tumorigenesis. This was originally stated by Boveri in 1914 with his somatic mutation theory.[5] Recent advances in the molecular biology of cancer with the discovery of oncogenes and suppressor genes have provided definitive evidence.[6] The second basic principle of carcinogenesis is that more than one genetic mistake must occur for cancer to develop. In a sense, cancer is a multistage (multifactor) phenomenon in which cancers arise by stepwise evolution involving progressive genetic changes, cell proliferation, and clonal expansion. Indeed, statistical analysis of the frequency of cancer incidence with age in humans indicates that possibly five or six steps are required for the genesis of a diagnosable tumor.[4] In most cases it is still unclear as to what specific genetic errors must occur or how they occur. Nonetheless, the multievent requirement for carcinogenesis is well established in both animal models and human tumors. In the 1940s several investigators began to present evidence that carcinogenesis could occur through multiple steps. These reports, which culminated in a publication by Berenblum and Shubik in 1947, define the models referred to as *initiation* and *promotion.*[7] This "staged" terminology is based on the observations that neoplasia, as with many disease conditions, is preceded by a latent period from the time of the first administration of a carcinogenic agent to the development of physically visible neoplastic lesions. Initiation, then, reflects a permanent and irreversible change in the DNA of the cell, while promotion generally refers to reversible changes that enhance malignancy.

The third basic principle of carcinogenesis is based on the well-known observation that DNA replication is not 100% faithful; that is to say, cell division provides an opportunity, although small, for a mistake to be made with any gene including those responsible for cancer development. DNA damage and replication errors that go unrepaired become part of the genome in subsequent cell progeny. Thus cell replication contributes to carcinogenesis by providing opportunities for somatic mutations to occur that may perpetuate themselves because of defective repair mechanisms.

With these principles in mind, this chapter will explain and unravel the various control mechanisms that are a part of cellular homeostasis and then determine how these mechanisms, when defective, lead to malignancy. The next section will define some of the important tools and concepts, including terminology, that are important. The third section will look at the molecular basis for alteration of growth control. The fourth section will analyze the very unique and special property of malignant cells to metastasize. The fifth section will include important component parts of immunobiology and malignancy especially emphasizing immunotherapy and its potential in clinical urology. Finally, the future will be addressed looking at new directions and the novel approaches to cancer treatment including programmed cell death (apoptosis), gene therapy, and terminal differentiation therapy (retinoids) as a possible treatment to halt malignancy.

## A PRIMER OF MOLECULAR GENETICS: THE BASICS

DNA is the molecule of life; it acts as the brain of all cells. The structure of DNA dictates the structure of proteins that subsequently go on to provide the ordering signals for cell homeostasis including growth control. The entire system contains many checks and balances with positive and negative growth regulators. A basic understanding of how DNA functions therefore is necessary for a complete understanding and an appreciation of what might malfunction when growth control is lost. In general, the elucidation of DNA structure has allowed us to apply many of the laws of chemistry and physics to questions of biology and disease. DNA represents the sole biochemical basis for information *storage* and *transfer;* it also provides signals for *regulation.* In fact, the regulatory capability is so strong that it can be translated into diverse bodily functions such as regulation of circadian rhythm,[8,9] and sexual behavior.[10]

### DNA Structure and Organization

How can DNA successfully hold such a position of power and influence? Surprisingly, one of the reasons lies in its elegantly simple structure. Its messages are clear and there is rarely a mistake; or if there is a mistake, it usually can be fixed. In a way, DNA resembles proteins in the sense that it is constructed of many building blocks with a repeating fundamental structure and the blocks are linked end-to-end. In the case of proteins, the building blocks are amino acids and in the case of DNA they are nucleotides. Nucleotides consist of three components: a phosphate group, a sugar group (eg, ribose), and a base that is either a purine [adenine (A) or guanine (G)] or a pyrimidine [thymine (T) or cytosine (C)]. In RNA, thymine is replaced by uracil (Fig 1A). Amazingly, the protein "alphabet" consists of 20 amino acids while the DNA "alphabet" consists of only 4 bases (A, T, G, or C). The triphosphate of the nucleotide is a high-energy compound that can react with polymerases to form a polymer, ie, RNA or DNA. These acidic polymers of polynucleotides are termed *nucleic acids*. The DNA molecule is then made up of two chains of polynucleotides with the sugar phosphate backbones on the outside of the DNA molecule and the purine and pyrimidine bases on the inside as Watson and Crick originally described[11] (Fig 1B). Importantly, the bases are oriented in such a way that they hydro-

Hydrogen bond
THYMINE (Pyrimidine)
ADENINE (Purine)
Deoxyribose
CYTOSINE (Pyrimidine)
GUANINE (Purine)
URACIL
A

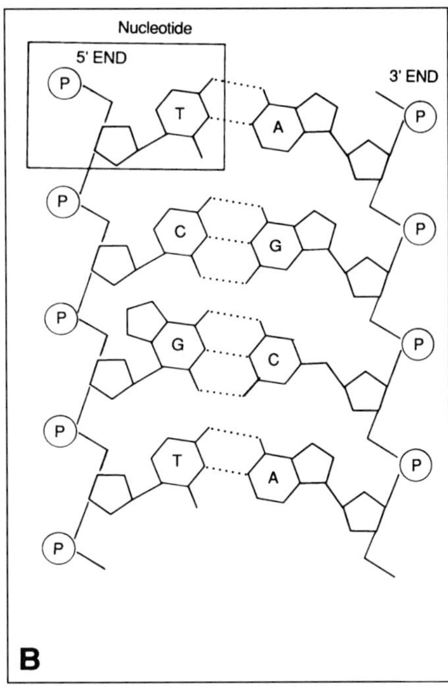


5' END
3' END
Transcription
C

**Fig 1A–C.** The structure of DNA. **A:** The alphabet consists of four bases: the purines adenine (A) and guanine (G) and the pyrimidines thymine (T) and cytosine (C). Uracil (U) is substituted for thymine in the case of RNA. The combination of a base and sugar (deoxyribose) is referred to as a nucleoside. **B** and **C:** The combination of a sugar phosphate group and a base constitutes a nucleotide. The double helix is made from two polynucleotide chains each of which consists of a series of 5′- to 3′-sugar phosphate links that form a backbone from which the bases protrude. The double helix maintains a constant width because purines always face pyrimidines in complementary A-T and G-C base pairs, respectively.

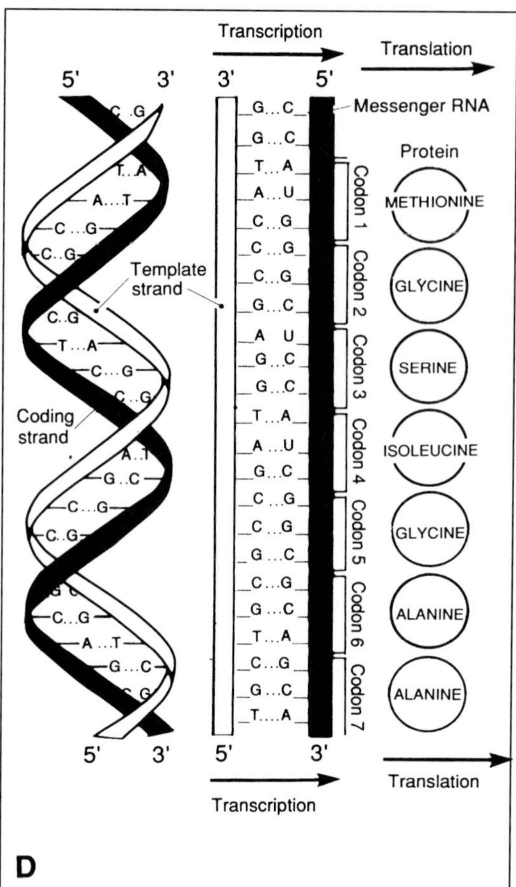


**Fig 1. D:** During transcription the coding strand conveys its message through the template strand to make mRNA that is eventually translated into polypeptides by ribosomes. The relationship between DNA sequence and corresponding protein is called the genetic code, which is read in triplets or codons.

gen-bond to bases on the opposing chain, ie, a purine on one chain is always hydrogen-bonded to a pyrimidine on the other chain. The bonding is extremely specific such that adenine (A) can only pair with thymine (T) whereas guanine (G) can only pair with cytosine (C) (Fig 1A). The hydrogen bonding will also allow the two chains to temporarily split like a "nature's velcro." This occurs, for example, in the process of transcription when the two chains temporarily separate. If the sequence of one chain is known, the other can be deduced and the opposing sequences are referred to as *complementary* (Fig 1D). Despite the relative weakness of the hydrogen bonds holding the base pairs together, each DNA molecule contains so many base pairs that the complementary chains never spontaneously separate under physiologic conditions. Experimentally, however, if DNA is exposed to near-boiling temperatures or to extremes of pH ($<3$ or $>10$), the base pairs quickly fall apart and the double helix separates into its complementary strands—a process called *denaturation* (Table 1). This will be referred to in later sections. Perhaps more important is the fact that denaturation is reversible such that at cooler temperatures at near-neutral pH, complementary single strands recombine to form native double helices. This annealing process is called *renaturation* and forms the basis for southern and northern blotting as will be described later in this section. Because three hydrogen bonds link guanine to cytosine while only two link adenine to thymine, there is some interchain variability with respect to how "sticky" the two strands really are.

This simplicity of structure allows for several other interesting properties aside from renaturation. For example, base pairing forms not only between bases on opposing strands but also between bases on single strands that have nearby inverted repetitive sequences that allow the formation of hydrogen-bonded hairpin loops called *palindromes* (Fig 2). These loops are then able to act as "guideposts" to interact with DNA-binding proteins which are important in regulating DNA activity. Regulator protein binding to DNA can be affected by other epigenetic changes in the DNA structure (ie, changes that do not involve the actual architectural structures of DNA). For example, cytosine residues can exist in a modified form in which a methyl group is attached to the 5′ carbon atom of the pyrimidine ring to make 5-methyl cytosine (Fig 3). Such methyl groups do not affect the way their respective molecules can hydrogen-bond (ie, the base pairs formed by the 5-methyl cytosine with guanine are equivalent in strength to those formed by cytosine). In eukaryotic DNA, cytosine

**TABLE 1. Glossary of Terms**

*Allele:* An alternative form of a gene. For example, the sickle mutation is one of the β-globin gene alleles. Alleles can also be recognized that differ from one another only at the gene sequence level, ie, they do not produce an altered gene product.
*Blotting:* The process of using a radioactive single-stranded DNA or RNA molecule (a probe) to detect a complementary polynucleotide sequence that is bound (or blotted) to a solid support, usually a sheet of nitrocellulose paper. Usually, blotting is used to identify DNA restriction endonuclease fragments or specific mRNAs from a complex mixture of molecules that have been separated on the basis of their length by electrophoresis in a semisolid gel (agarose).
*cDNA:* Complementary DNA copied from an mRNA molecule.
*Denaturation:* A process whereby the two strands of DNA molecule are separated by interrupting the hydrogen bonds that (weakly) hold the two strands of DNA together. The process is reversible (renaturation or annealing) and occurs when pH is lowered (from alkaline) or temperature is lowered.
*Exon:* A gene sequence that corresponds to part of the mature mRNA (sometimes also called a *coding sequence*).
*Fragment:* The DNA cleavage product of a restriction endonuclease. A specific length (fragment) of DNA between two cleavage sites.
*Genomic clone:* A selected host cell with a vector containing a fragment of genomic DNA from a different organism.
*Genomic DNA:* All DNA sequences of an organism.
*Host cell:* A cell (usually a bacterium) in which a vector can be propagated.
*Hybridize* (verb): To anneal two complementary single-stranded polynucleotides, either DNA or RNA, to one another.
*Intron (Intervening sequence):* A sequence that is spliced out of a primary RNA gene transcript to form mature mRNA.
*Library:* A complete set of genomic clones from an organism (genomic library) or of cDNA clones from one cell type (cDNA library).
*Plasmid:* A small, circular, extrachromosomal DNA molecule capable of reproducing independently in a host cell.
*Polymorphism:* Different forms of the same gene maintained in a population.
*Probe:* A piece of DNA of varying length that is homologous to a specific DNA sequence within a genome; hybridization of the probe to DNA (or RNA) preparations allows for localization of the sequence.
*Restriction enzyme:* A restriction endonuclease, one of a class of enzymes that digests DNA at specific sites.
*Reverse transcriptase:* The RNA-dependent DNA polymerase enzyme that catalyzes the synthesis of a DNA strand on an RNA template. The resultant single strand of DNA is complementary to its RNA template and is called cDNA.
*Vector:* The genetically simple carrier element, usually a plasmid, bacteriophage, or animal virus, into whose genome a foreign segment of DNA has been inserted. There are two major types of vectors used in human genetics (although more are available). *Plasmid*—an element consisting only of a double-stranded circular DNA genome that is capable of replicating in the cytoplasm of a bacterial host. It is usually genetically simple (it has few genes) and can be used as an acceptor (vector) for foreign DNA. Since it is replicated independently of its host's chromosome and usually is present as several copies per host cell, and since it can be introduced into its host as naked DNA (transformation), it is a useful vector system. It is especially useful for secondary cloning operations. *Viral*—an animal virus used as a DNA cloning vehicle. The major advantage of viral vectors is that they can be used to infect animal cells and carry cloned genes into a living cell where their function can be assayed.

residues that contain methyl groups are always located next to guanine residues on the same chain, ie, CpG (p is the phosphodiester bond between adjacent nucleotides). The importance of methylation is that it seems to hinder regulatory protein binding to DNA in the sense that highly methylated DNA is usually genetically silent.

As one can imagine, the structure of DNA with its relatively simple construction allows it to be pliable and durable (Fig 1). Externally there are two outer grooves, a major (larger one) and a minor (smaller one), that are important because regulatory proteins fit into these grooves. The bases are perpendicular to the axis of symmetry and there are 10 base pairs per turn; the diameter of the double helix is 20 Å (the diameter of a hydrogen molecule is 1 Å and the diameter of a human red blood cell is $8 \times 10^4$ Å). This type of construction ren-

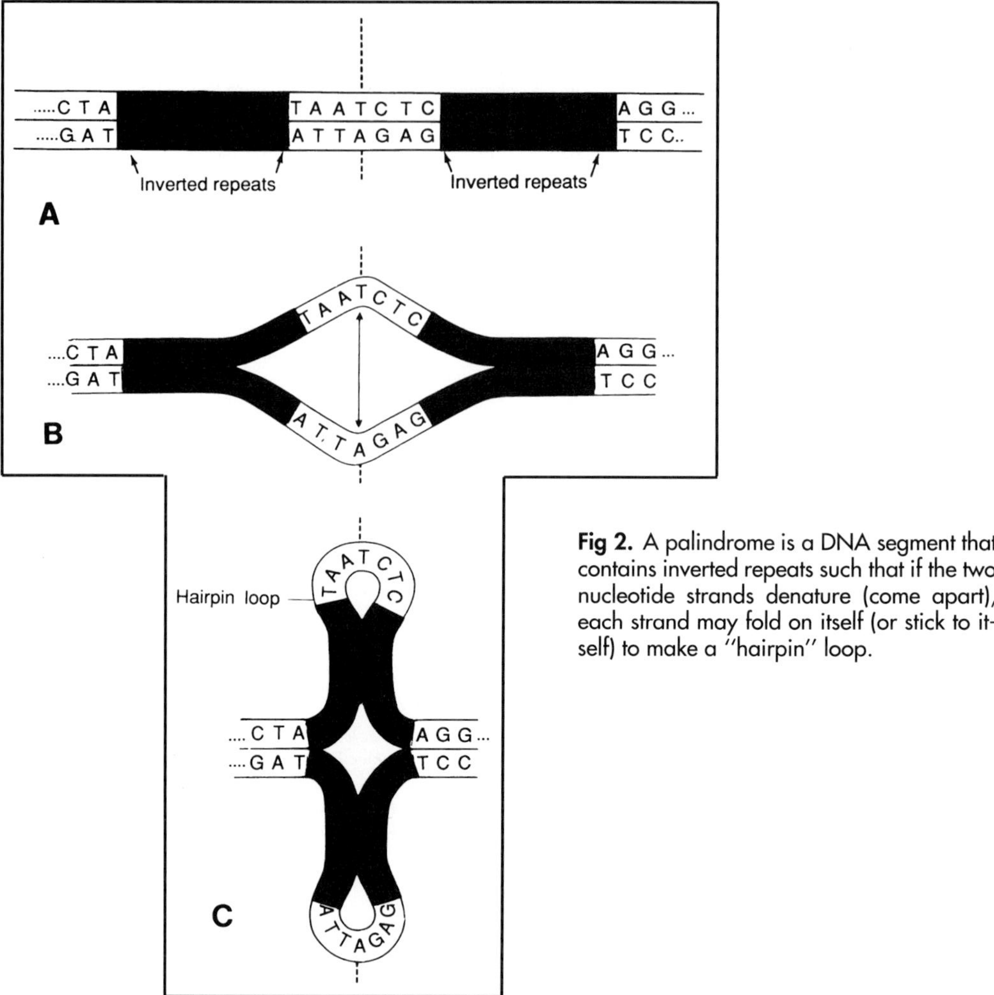


**Fig 2.** A palindrome is a DNA segment that contains inverted repeats such that if the two nucleotide strands denature (come apart), each strand may fold on itself (or stick to itself) to make a "hairpin" loop.

ders the DNA molecule extremely resistant to all types of denaturing substances such as phenol and chloroform, sizable temperature shifts, and pH changes that are not too extensive.

As noted above, DNA is a long, thin molecule; in fact, each chromosome consists of a single molecule of DNA on the average of 2 m long. All of the DNA within a diploid cell contains 6 billion ($6 \times 10^9$) base pairs to make the DNA content of each cell, which is called the *genome.* The genome is the same within each cell of an organism; cells from different tissues of the

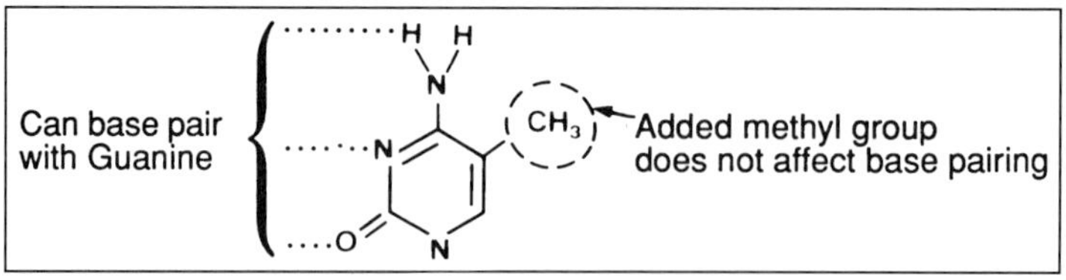

Can base pair with Guanine

Added methyl group does not affect base pairing

**Fig 3.** 5-Methylcytosine.

body are genetically distinguished from one another not by their DNA (which is the same) but by which parts of the genome are active, ie, which genes are operational. This notion of tissue-specific differential gene expression is currently challenging the best genetic laboratories in the world with respect to a proper mechanistic explanation. The actual amount of information represented by number of bases per nucleus, however, is almost beyond imagination. If the genome were compared to a book, then there would be $6 \times 10^9$ letters (A, T, G, C, or bases) in the book; assuming 2000 letters per page, there would be 3 million pages or 3000 volumes of 1000 pages each. With this information, the real challenge then is how does 2 m of DNA get packaged into a 10-μm ($10^{-5}$-m nucleus)? And, the mechanism by which this is done must allow replication into 46 daughter chromosomes without tangling. The key to packaging is the *histone* proteins (Fig 4.) The double helix is wound twice around a spool of eight histone molecules to form nucleosomes, which are the fundamental repeating units of chromatin. Six of these nucleosomes form a solinoid to form a 30-μm-diameter fiber that forms the *chromatin thread.*[12,13] These fibers then undergo a series of coordinated loops attached to the nuclear matrix (which is like an internal nuclear skeleton) such that the packaging ratio or the fold condensation of the length of packaged DNA is $10^5$. Judging from this information it is easy to imagine how this ''tight'' DNA packaging may have an important regulatory effect on how genetic material is transcribed. Not only must the active genes be ''exposed'' for processing, but also transcriptional regulatory proteins and the transcriptional apparatus (see below) must be able to access the DNA for transcription to occur. For example, it is easy to see how DNA in its ''resting state'' actually represses transcription: consider that one side of the double helix is occluded because it faces the core histones (see Fig 4). The solinoid will thereby render large segments of DNA invisible to DNA-binding proteins (which regulate transcription). In a sense, this may

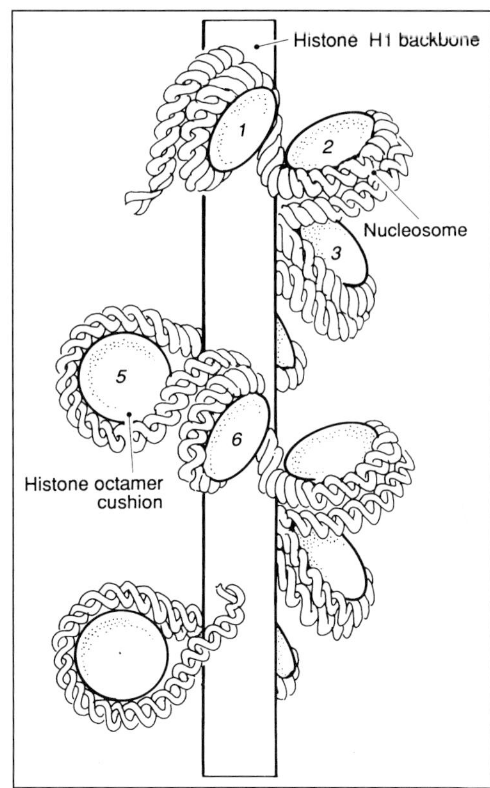


**Fig 4.** The chromatin thread is actually a solenoid with a string of nucleosomes coiled helically with a pitch of six nucleosomes per turn in an axial fashion. Each nucleosome has an octameric protein core and is cylindrical in shape. DNA runs continuously from nucleosome to nucleosome.

be advantageous in reducing the amount of DNA that a eukaryotic transcription factor has to search in order to find its binding site.[14] Moreover, each transcription complex that does form may, by disrupting the fiber, act as a highly visible signpost to RNA polymerase (the enzyme that binds to DNA to begin transcription).[15] Whatever the answer to these issues, it is apparent that alterations in histone sequence, nucleosome structure, and folding of chromatin fiber influence both activation and repression of genes through alteration of accessibility of DNA to both transcriptional factors and RNA polymerase, and progression of RNA polymerase along the chromatin fiber (for review, see Ref. 16).

Another simplistic feature of DNA that adds to its "strength" is that *its structure is independent of its sequence.* In other words, the sequence of nucleotides from which DNA is constructed is important not to determine the general structure of DNA but rather to code for the sequence of amino acids that constitutes the corresponding polypeptide. The relationship between the sequence of DNA and the sequence of the corresponding protein is the *genetic code* (Fig 1D). A *gene* includes a series of triplets (three nucleotides that encode an amino acid) or *codons* that are read in a series from a starting point at one end to a termination point at another, always in a 5′- to 3′-direction (direction in the polynucleotide chain as indicated by carbon atoms on the deoxyribose ring; see Fig 1C). Surprisingly, most DNA, estimated at 90%, does not code for proteins but acts as "filler." In fact, it is usually found that genes themselves contain interrupting noncoding sequences that do not code for protein. The reason for this circumstance of nature is not known. The coding portions of genes are called *exons* and the noncoding interrupting portions of genes are called *introns.* It is required that the noncoding portion of mRNA (ie, the message from DNA) be excised from the coding portion of mRNA. Although some of the noncoding portion has use for certain regulatory activities,[17,18] most of it has been considered genetic rubbish and has baffled geneticists with regard to its evolutionary value or even where in evolution this modification occurred.[19]

## Transcription

DNA basically has two jobs: the first is to self-replicate, which is required to make a new cell, and the second is to transcribe its code into RNA, which is then shipped to the cytoplasm where it directs the production of protein (called *translation*). Transcription, then, is the process or mechanism whereby DNA information is copied into RNA language. The only difference in DNA and RNA structure is that uracil (U) replaces thymine (T) (Fig 1D).

The enzymes that copy DNA are called *polymerases.* Logically those that make more DNA from DNA are called DNA polymerases and those that make RNA from DNA are called RNA polymerases. All eukaryotic cells (cells containing a nucleus; organisms without a nucleus are called prokaryotic) contain three distinct types of RNA polymerase. Each is responsible for making a different kind of RNA. For example, RNA polymerase I (Pol I) synthesizes ribosomal RNA; Pol II transcribes protein-coding genes; and Pol III is responsible for the synthesis of small RNA species such as transfer RNA (tRNA) and ribosomal (5S) RNA. It is not known exactly why the job of RNA synthesis is divided between three enzymes but the roles of the RNAs clearly differ as to the sites of synthesis. In general, Pol I and Pol III act to produce RNA that will act as the machinery to be used in translating the Pol II product (mRNA) into protein. Current work has now established that RNA polymerases require accessory proteins to acquire specificity. For example, in the case of Pol II, several general transcription factors have been identified (Fig 5), some of which recognize specific DNA sequences to help "set" the transcriptional apparatus (see below).[20,21]

This information leads one to consider one of the most fundamental questions of

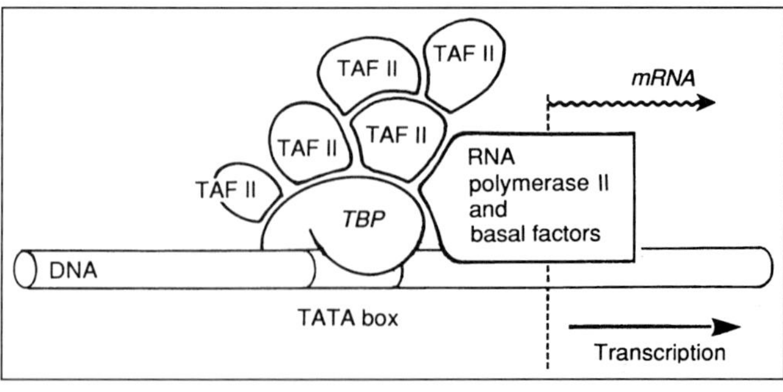


**Fig 5.** Transcriptional apparatus for polymerase II. Distinct multiprotein complexes with a common subunit, the TATA-binding protein (TBP), participate in specific promoter recognition by Pol II. Several other "TBP-associated factors" (TAFs) are required.

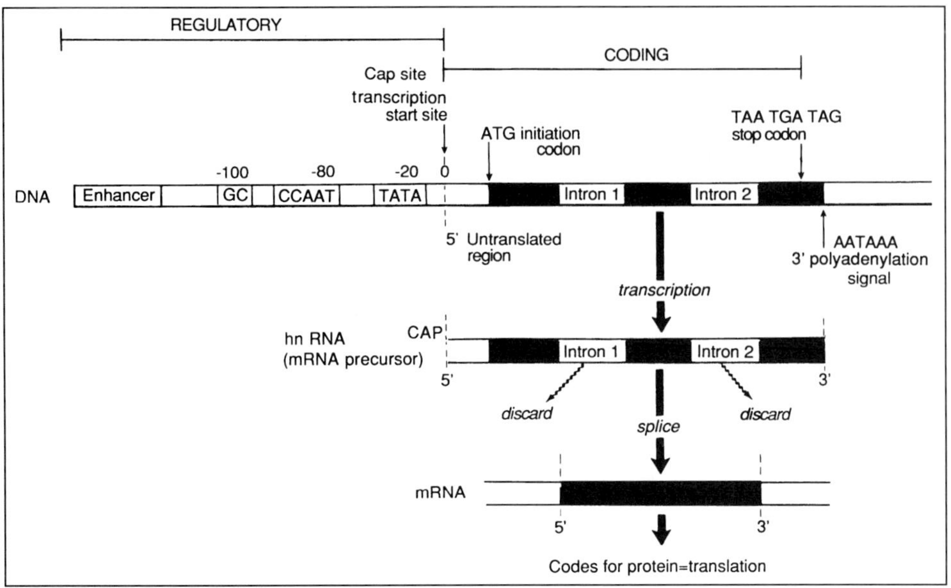


**Fig 6.** Structural landmarks in the transcription of mRNA from DNA.

molecular genetics and perhaps in all of biology: if all cells in the body contain the same genetic content, how does the cell know which gene to turn on? The exact answer is not clear but enough is known to offer a good perspective. In the nucleus, free Pol II molecules collide randomly with the DNA chromosome sticking only weakly to most DNA. However, the polymerase binds very tightly when it collides with a specific DNA sequence, called a *promoter,* that contains the start site for RNA synthesis and signals where RNA synthesis should begin (Fig 6). Two principal DNA promoter elements located upstream (5′) of the gene are commonly used for transcription. The first is an AT-rich region located approximately 28 base pairs (bp) 5′ from the gene start site. This region contains a consensus sequence (a conserved sequence found in all DNA samples) of TATAAA or ATAAA, which is commonly known as the *TATA box* (Figs 5 and 6). This sequence can serve as a recognition site for binding of proteins that control the transcription of DNA. In fact, the first step during formation of a transcription-competent complex on a TATA-containing promoter is the association of a protein called a TATA-binding protein, or TBP, with the TATA sequence.[22] Binding of TBP provides the site through which Pol II and the rest of the general transcription factors can sequentially associate to form a transcriptionally competent complex (Fig 5). Some promoters, however, do not have TATA sequences to direct transcription initiation. These genes have a second type of sequence called the *initiator* (Inr) element, which encompasses the transcription start site. The multiprotein complex that directs transcription from this start site is not completely understood but also involves participation from the TBP.

Other regulatory sequence elements are located further upstream and can enhance or repress initiation of transcription. Examples include the CCAAT consensus (CAAT box) and the GGGCC consensus, which were among the first regulatory sequences identified (Fig 6). These have been called *promoter-proximal sequences* because of their proximal position to the gene. These elements are conserved in several but not all known promoters, where they are often located close to 80 bp 5′ to the gene. However, they can function at distances that vary considerably from the gene start point. It is possible that hundreds as of yet unidentified proteins exist within the cell that interact with these sequences to regulate transcription.

Aside from promoters, there exists a second class or type of DNA sequences that are associated with gene activation and these are called *enhancers*. Like promoters, these sequences bind specific proteins that positively or negatively regulate transcription. The difference, however, is that they can be positioned in unusual ways relative to the gene, ie, they can be in reverse orientation or they can be located at great distances from the gene (approximately 40 kb) either upstream or downstream from the gene. They can even be located within the gene, usually within introns located between coding sequences of a gene. It is thought that enhancer elements form loops in DNA to exert their effects.

**DNA-Binding Proteins.** The initiation of transcription, then, involves a Pol II recognition of a specific promoter-enhancer region near the start site for transcription of a gene followed by the generation of mRNA. The exact question of specificity, that is, *which* gene to activate in a cell, is the part that continues to be unclear. The role of sequence-specific *DNA-binding proteins* is the key. This information should hold the secret to selective activation of promoters.[23–25] A few clues exist as to the nature of these regulatory proteins. For example, DNA-binding proteins, in general, exhibit a limited number of structural designs. These are termed helix-turn-helix proteins, zinc finger proteins, leucine zipper proteins, and helix-loop-helix proteins (Fig 7).

1. The *helix-turn-helix* proteins all bind as dimers. They are principally found associated with *homeotic genes* that regulate spacial development and embryogenesis. Helix 3 (Fig 7A) is the "recognition sequence" that makes the major contacts with DNA. Helices 1 and 2 lie on top of helix 3 and are able to make contact with other proteins.
2. The *zinc finger* protein motif was discovered as part of the first well-characterized eukaryotic positive-acting regulatory protein, ie, transcription factor IIIA ($TF_{IIIA}$), which is required for RNA polymerase III transcription of the 5S RNA genes. The basic molecule consists of two cysteine residues (C) and two histidine residues (H) coordinated around a zinc molecule. In the structural model of this protein, the helix on the right (Fig 7B) is believed to contact the major groove of the DNA molecule.[26]
3. The *leucine zipper* protein family act as dimers of two subunits (Fig 7C). At the carboxyl terminus of each subunit there is a stretch of about 35 amino acids containing 4–5 leucine residues separated from each other by 6 amino acids.[27] The leucines are located on one side of the protein helix and the leucines on two such helices interdigitate leading to dimerization. The "zipper" is immediately preceded by a region rich in positively charged amino acids and it is thought that the dimerization arranges the basic regions of the subunits in a configuration that allows specific interaction with a DNA recognition sequence. It is this type of bond that is responsible for joining different proteins as heterodimers that then bind DNA as regulators. An example includes the *fos-jun* protooncogene heterodimer, which together acts as a powerful regulatory complex.[28] The finding that leucine zippers are responsible for specific heterodimer formation provides a conceptual framework for understanding combinatorial models for gene regulation. In this case, dimerization, which is becoming a unifying property of sequence-specific DNA-binding proteins, physically allows DNA-binding proteins to bind to their targets at far more dilute concentrations than monomers. The complexity involved in achieving a highly specific pattern of gene activation required for growth and development of eukaryotic organisms is staggering; this specificity may be achieved, at least in part, by novel protein–protein interactions made possible by dimerization of regulatory proteins.

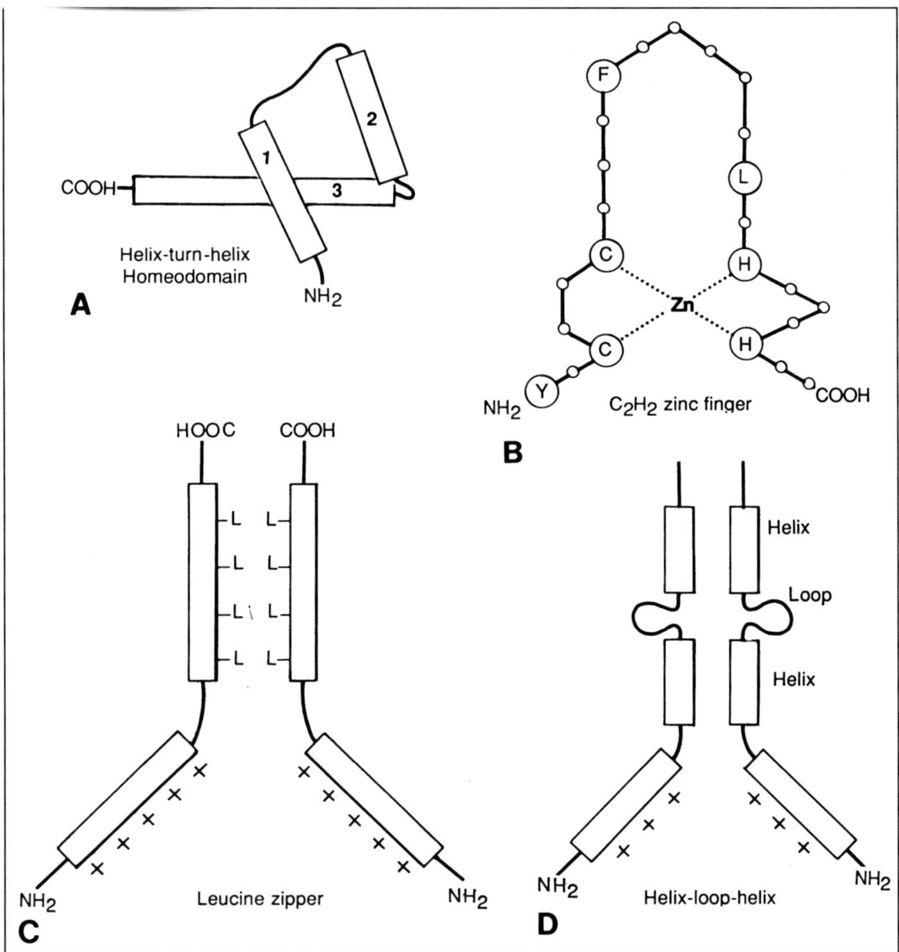


**Fig 7.** DNA binding motifs. **A:** Helix-turn-helix motif found in several prokaryotic regulatory proteins and the homeotic protein of eukaryotes. Helix 3 is the "recognition helix" that contacts the DNA. **B:** Zinc finger motif. The helix *(right)* is believed to contact the major groove of the DNA molecule. **C:** The leucine zipper motif is formed as a dimer of two subunits. Amino terminal to the interdigitating leucines is a region rich in positively charged amino acids believed to contact DNA. **D:** Helix-loop-helix protein motif contains two helices linked by a loop of unknown structure that allows protein dimer formation.

4. *Helix-loop-helix* proteins comprise the fourth transcription factor family. These proteins are similar to the leucine zipper family in that they bind DNA as dimers—either heterodimers or homodimers—and they have a positively charged domain that recognizes the DNA site. They also contain two helices linked by a loop of unknown structure (Fig 7D). In this family are several proteins with important roles in the control of cell growth and division. Among them is the protein encoded by the *c-myc* protooncogene.

A common feature to most of these proteins is that DNA binding and transcriptional activation reside within discrete domains and thus consist of independently functioning modules. Experimentally, the activation domain of one factor can be joined to the DNA-binding domain of the other and the resulting hybrid is fully active in cells. However, as previously noted, the exact mechanism of action of transcription factors and how they interact with Pol II (and its associated transcription factors to make the transcription apparatus) is not exactly clear. It is thought they can do one of two things: either help RNA polymerase bind to the promoter or accelerate the rate at which bound RNA polymerase initiates transcription. It is important to remember that chromosomal DNA is tightly packed into higher order nucleoprotein structures; it is possible that transcription factors may act to free DNA from nucleosomes so that the promoter is accessible to the large transcription complex. In this process it is possible that transcription factors bind to enhancers (at distant sites) and to the transcription complex, which then efficiently "loops out" intervening DNA (Fig 8).

After initiation of RNA transcription the RNA polymerase proceeds by opening up a local region of the DNA double helix with the aid of such enzymes as helicases, gyrases, and topoisomerases to expose nucleotides on a short stretch of DNA on each strand. One of the two exposed DNA strands acts as a template for complementary base pairing with incoming ribonucleoside triphosphate monomers, two of which are joined together by the polymerase to begin an RNA chain. The RNA polymerase molecule then moves stepwise along the DNA, unwinding the DNA helix just ahead to expose a new region of template for complementary base pairing. In this way, the growing RNA chain is extended by one nucleotide at a time in a 5′- to 3′-direction. The rate of progression is on the order of 1 μm/min, which means that the RNA chain grows at a rate of 50 nucleotides/sec; or that it takes RNA polymerase no more than two hundredths of a second to try various nucleoside triphosphates for fit, find the right one, substitute one bond for another, move on through the next base pair in the DNA double helix, and get ready for another round of the same kind. Although this may seem fast, consider the fact that transcription of some large genes, such as the giant dystrophin gene, would take up to 11 hr to complete. Overall this rate of transcription has strategic implications during embryogenesis where cell division is often measured in minutes, thus eliminating some genes from ever getting transcribed.

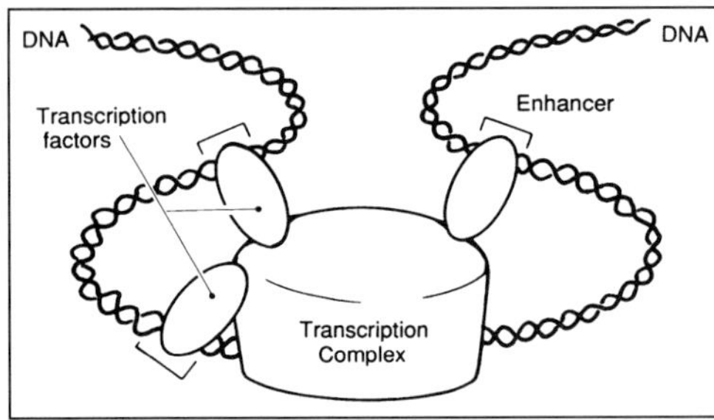


**Fig 8.** A conceptual illustration of how transcriptional factors can bind to DNA recognition sites distant from a gene (enhancer) and then, by simultaneously binding to the transcriptional complex, loop out large pieces of DNA. This may help "unwind" DNA to help in the transcriptional process.

Interestingly, mRNA transcripts begin and end in a uniform way. For example, most sequences begin with an AUG that codes for methionine; usually this sequence is followed by a purine-rich sequence (ie, AGGA) that may help to position the starting AUG opposite the ribosomal cavity containing the initiating amino acid tRNA complex (see below). All mRNA is ordered such that the first codons encode the amino terminal amino acids and finish with the carboxyl terminal amino acid. One or several amino terminal amino acids that were encoded by the initiating AUG and associated sequences are frequently cleaved away by proteolytic (protein-degrading) enzymes to produce functional polypeptide products that have different amino terminal amino acids from those of the primary translation products.

Within about 1 sec after initiation of transcription, before the RNA is more than 30 nucleotides long, a chemically protective cap is added to the nucleotide at the beginning of the chain (the 5′ end). The cap, which consists of a methylated guanosine (a nucleotide incorporating the base guanine), is linked to the first nucleotide by a triphosphate bridge.

After the cap is attached, the polymerase continues to add nucleotides to the 3′ end of the chain until the enzyme encounters a second special sequence in DNA, the *termination signal* in the form of the sequence AAUAAA (poly A) located 10–30 nucleotides upstream from the actual site of cleavage. Usually the RNA polymerase overshoots the actual end of the gene, and as the poly A sequence is transcribed (in addition to other less well-understood events), cleavage occurs and a poly A polymerase enzyme adds 100–200 residues of adenylic acid (as poly A) to the 3′ end of the RNA chain to complete the primary RNA transcript. Meanwhile the Pol II polymerase fruitlessly continues transcribing for hundreds or thousands of nucleotides until termination occurs at one end of several later sites. The extra ''mRNA'' is quickly degraded presumably because it lacks the methylated guanosine cap that is on the functional mRNA. The function of the poly A tail is not known for certain but it may play a role in the export of mature mRNA from the nucleus. It also may stabilize mRNA by retarding degradation in the cytoplasm. In general, transcription is usually unidirectional—a one-sided process in which only one side of the two DNA strands is transcribed.

To make a mature mRNA to be exported to the cytoplasm for translation into protein, the primary transcript, called pre-mRNA, must be processed to remove the introns and join the coding sequences into a contiguous mRNA molecule (Fig 6). This process is appropriately called *splicing* and is extremely important because if an exon is missed, or if a splice occurs even one nucleotide away from the correct location, the correct protein will not be translated from the resulting mRNA because a base pair will either be added or subtracted from the reading frame (DNA coding sequence). When that happens a mutation has occurred. For example, when a base pair is added or subtracted, the codon reading frame is ''offset'' (remember that every third base pair forms a codon that codes for an amino acid). If the start site is moved over by 1 bp, then a ''frame shift'' mutation occurs. The splicing process takes place in splicosomes, which are large ribonucleoprotein particles akin to ribosomes. Although the exact mechanism is not completely clear, it is understood that splicing is a two-step process. First, the 5′ splice site is cut freeing the upstream exon and generating a lariat molecule containing the intron still joined to the downstream exon. In the second step, the 3′ splice site is cut and the exons are joined, freeing the intron as a lariat.[29] Many factors are involved in this process, both small nuclear ribonucleoproteins (sn RNPs) and several protein components.

The process of transcription is not reversible under normal circumstances. Once mRNA molecules are made they serve as templates that order the amino acids within the peptide chains of proteins during the process of *translation*—so named because the nucleotide language of nucleic acids is translated into amino acid language of proteins. *This scheme—that information flows from DNA to RNA to protein—has become known as the central dogma of molecular biology.* In general, the only exception to this rule involves retroviruses whose genomes consist of single-stranded RNA molecules. During infection, RNA is converted to single-stranded DNA and then to double-stranded DNA by a process called *reverse transcription.* This process is commonly employed in experiments in which DNA probes are made from mRNA transcripts using the *reverse transcriptase* enzyme.

## Mutations

If during the process of DNA replication a ''mistake'' is made resulting in a change in the coding sequence of a gene, then a *mutation* occurs. The occurrence of mutations is important because they are responsible for inherited diseases and other diseases such as cancer, and they are the source of phenotypic variation on which natural selection acts. The processes by which mutation produces variability and natural selection favors any resulting advantageous variants are the driving forces in evolution.

There is a wide variety of terminology to describe mutations. For example, *transition* refers to a base substitution by a base of the same class, eg, a purine by a purine

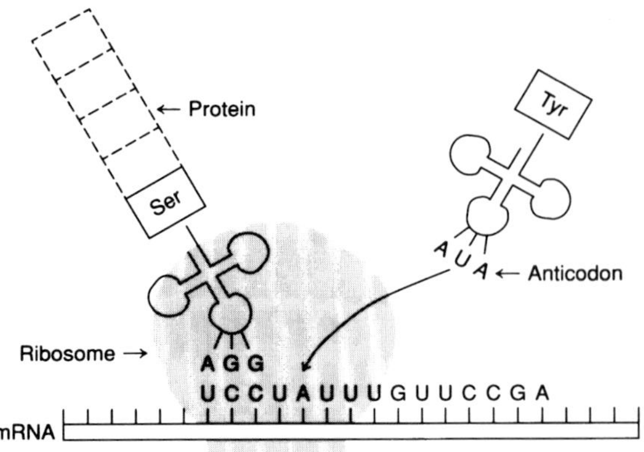


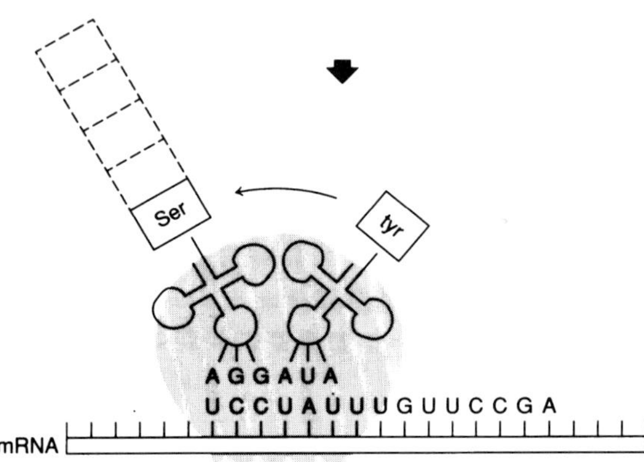


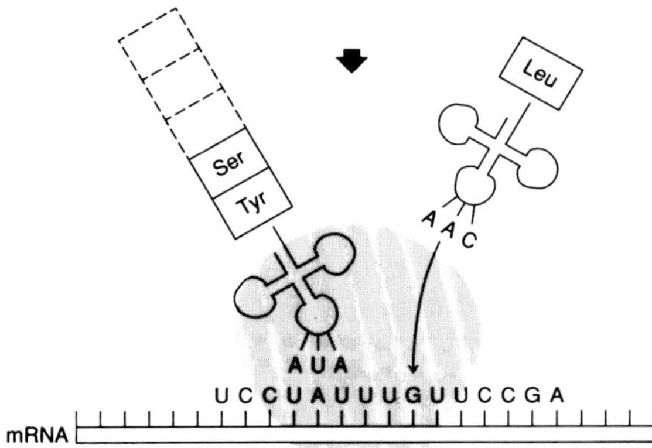


**Fig 9.** Translation is the synthesis of protein on a messenger RNA (mRNA) template. Each nucleotide triplet, or codon, on the mRNA chain encodes a specific amino acid. Each molecule of transfer RNA (tRNA) in turn binds only the amino acid corresponding to a particular codon. A tRNA recognizes a codon by means of a complementary nucleotide sequence called an anticodon. Here the addition of one amino acid to a protein chain is shown. An incoming tRNA molecule carrying the amino acid tyrosine binds to the codon exposed at a binding site on a ribosome. The lysine forms a peptide bond with the serine, the last amino acid in the peptide chain. As the ribosome advances onto the codon, exposing the binding site to the next incoming tRNA, the serine tRNA is released. [From Walsh PC, et al, eds. *Campbell's Urology*, 6th ed (Philadelphia: WB Saunders Co. 1992), with permission.]

or pyrimidine by pyrimidine. Conversely, *transversion* refers to a base substitution by another class base, eg, a purine by a pyrimidine. A *nonsense mutation* refers to a point mutation that converts a codon to a stop codon and therefore results in a premature termination of the polypeptide chain. Similarly, a *missense mutation* occurs when a mutation alters the codon so that an incorrect amino acid is produced. Often this has little effect on the function of the protein unless it is in a critical portion of the protein. Finally, *deletions* and *insertions* usually have drastic effects on proteins because they alter the triplet groupings in which the bases are read.

## Translation

In the process of translation, mRNA molecules serve as templates that order the amino acids within the polypeptide chain. "Translation" is an appropriate name because the nucleotide language of nucleic acids is translated into the amino acid language of proteins. In simplistic terms, the mRNA is read within the ribosome, a structure that is composed principally of RNA. Each amino acid is attached to a special kind of RNA called transfer RNA (tRNA), which serves as a reading device through base pairing (Fig 9). Each tRNA recognizes and binds to a single one of the 20 different amino acids found in proteins. At the opposite end of the tRNA molecule is a loop containing the anticodon, which is a nucleotide triplet that is complementary to a specific mRNA codon. The tRNA molecules carrying an amino acid are brought in contact with an mRNA molecule on the surface of a ribosome. As the ribosome moves along the mRNA one codon at a time, tRNAs with the appropriate anticodons are selectively bound to the mRNA and the amino acids they carry are linked to a growing polypeptide chain. The sequence of codons on the mRNA dictates the amino acid sequence. The process of translation is complex, involving perhaps 100 components, and is not yet completely understood.

## Special Strategies in Molecular Genetics

**Southern and Northern Blotting.** Two of the most commonly used methodologies in a molecular biology laboratory are southern and northern blotting developed by E. M. Southern of the University of Edinburgh.[30] The procedures are used to determine the presence of specific base pair sequences in samples of DNA (southern blotting) or RNA (northern blotting) as defined by a probe that contains complementary sequences to those that are sought. (See Table 1 for a review of terms.)

The ability of the DNA double helix to separate and reform during replication, for example, without disrupting covalent bonds (only hydrogen bonds are disrupted; see Fig 1) is an important physical property called *denaturation* (Table 1). In southern blotting, as will be described, DNA strands are separated and then join complementary sequences on the probe. The double strand is broken simply by disrupting the noncovalent forces that stabilize the double helix through the use of heat, exposure to high salt, or high pH. As expected, *renaturation* is the ability of the two separate complementary strands to be reformed into a double helix. It would therefore be expected that the success of an artificially made segment of single-stranded DNA (the probe) to renature to a piece of single stranded genomic DNA (DNA from the native genome) would depend on how well matched the complementary sequences are between the genomic DNA (in southern blotting) or RNA (in northern blotting) and the probe.

The renaturation process (probe annealing to genomic DNA strands—southern—or RNA strands—northern) occurs in two stages. First, DNA single strands in solution encounter one another by chance. If the sequences are complementary, the two strands base-pair to generate a short double-helical region. Then additional base pairing occurs along the molecule by a zipper-like effect through hydrogen bonding, ie, the "velcro effect," to form a long double-helix molecule. The renaturation of the DNA helix forms the basis for one of the most important phenomena in DNA technology known as *hybridization.* Hybridization refers to the tendency of any two complementary single-stranded nucleic acid sequences, whether from DNA or RNA, to anneal with each other to form a duplex structure. In other words, the ability of two nucleic acid preparations to hybridize constitutes a precise test for their complementary sequences.

Molecular biological investigations are able to exploit this property of DNA in studies designed to locate particular regions of DNA within the human genome. The strength of interaction between the strands of nucleic acid and the probe is important to understand and is dependent on numerous factors such as temperature, ionic strength of the reaction, molar percentage of G-C base pairs in the probe, probe length, percentage of noncomplementary bases between the probe and the target (percent mismatch), and percent formamide (a duplex-destabilizing agent) in the solution. Increasing the ionic strength, probe length, and G-C content increases duplex stability. Increasing temperature, percent formamide, and percent mismatch decreases duplex stability. The *stringency* of a hybridization reaction refers to the degree to which the reaction conditions favor duplex dissociation; high-stringency conditions include high temperature as well as low salt or high formamide concentrations. Duplexes formed when the two strands have a high degree of base homology withstand a higher stringency wash than do duplexes of a lesser homology.

*Restriction enzymes* are an important tool and are used in almost every experiment of molecular genetics. These are extremely important enzymes, isolated from bacteria, that cut DNA at specific sequences, usually specified by either four or six base sequences. Enzymes that bind to only four bases cut many more times in a given DNA molecule than the ones that have to recognize a specific group of six. A six-base restriction sequence may not even exist once in a given viral DNA molecule. For example, the GAATTC recognition sequence from the *Escherichia coli* *Eco*RI enzyme is not present in phage T7 DNA, which is 40,000 bp long. Currently there are over 250 restriction endonucleases known with over 100 different cut sites.

In order to analyze and identify the fragments that result from digestion of genomic DNA with restriction enzymes, the resultant fragments must be separated from one another. This is easily accomplished by using agarose gel electrophoresis. (Fig 10), which is the first step in performing a southern blot. The mixture of DNA fragments following digestion with a designated *restriction endonuclease* is loaded at one end of a horizontally placed agarose gel that is submerged within an electrophoresis tank; an electric current is then passed through the gel. The fragments move through the gel at a rate proportional to their length, ie, the smaller fragments move quickly and the larger fragments move slowly. Staining the gels with dyes that bind to DNA generates a series of bands, each corresponding to a restriction fragment (or a cut piece of DNA) whose base pair length can be estimated by calibrating the gel using DNA molecules with known base pair lengths. It therefore follows that different restriction enzymes give different restriction patterns for the same digested DNA molecule.

A southern blot is performed to determine the presence of a genomic nucleotide sequence or an alteration of a sequence within a DNA digest. To perform a southern blot, genomic DNA is cut with one or several restriction enzymes and the resultant fragments are separated by size on an agarose gel (Fig 10). Because double-stranded DNA does not undergo hybridization, the DNA, while still in the agarose gel, is denatured by alkaline treatment to yield single-stranded fragments. The gel is then overlaid with a sheet of nylon or nitrocellulose filter and a flow of buffer is drawn up through the gel toward the nitrocellulose filter. This causes the DNA fragments to be carried out of the gel onto the filter where they bind. This is necessary not only to form a replica of the DNA that was on the gel but also to provide a "scaffolding" to permanently hold apart the complementary DNA strands which, if in a solution (other than alkaline), would tend to renature. It is important that the two strands remain apart so that a labeled probe specific for the gene (or nucleotide sequence under study) can be hybridized to the single-stranded DNA on the nitrocellulose paper (or nylon membrane). The probe can be a purified RNA, a cloned DNA that has been made single-stranded, or a short synthetic oligonucleotide. The labeled probe will hybridize to the specific molecules containing a complementary sequence; thus each complementary sequence gives rise to a labeled band at a position determined by the size of the DNA fragment.

This technique can also be performed with RNA immobilized on the nitrocellulose paper, eg, to determine whether a certain mRNA is being produced by a specific cell type. In this case, the RNA is mixed with formaldehyde or a similar agent to prevent hydrogen bonding between base pairs and to ensure that RNA is in unfolded linear form. In accordance with laboratory jargon, the procedure is then known as *northern blotting.* (When proteins are fixed to nitrocellulose and probed with antibodies, the procedure is called *western blotting.*) These procedures form some of the backbone of molecular genetics.

**Gene Cloning and the Polymerase Chain Reaction—PCR.** DNA cloning traditionally refers to a process whereby a fragment of DNA is reproduced essentially with unlimited quantities by using the "growth machinery" of either a bacterium or virus. Therefore, in theory what is done is fairly simple: a piece of DNA that is to be amplified is obtained either by laboratory synthesis, reverse-transcribing mRNA into a

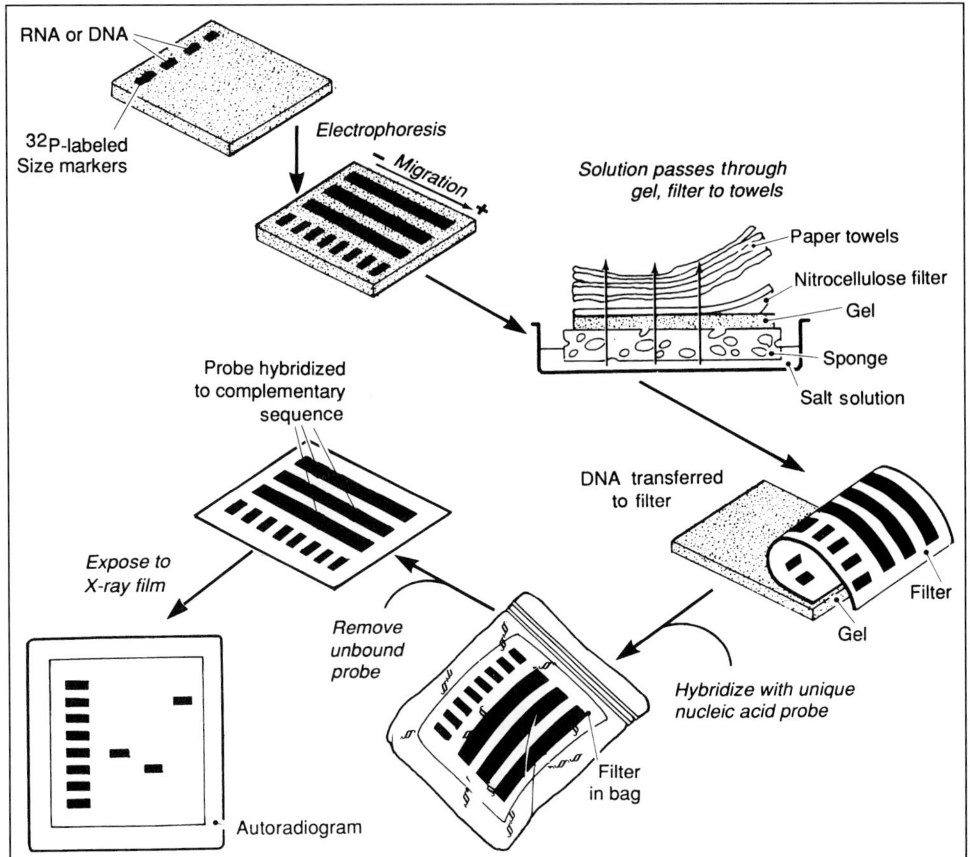


**Fig 10.** Southern and northern blotting (analyzing DNA and RNA by gel electrophoresis and blotting). DNA cleaved with restriction enzymes (or RNA isolated from cells) is applied to an agarose gel and electrophoretically separated by size. The single-stranded nucleic acids in the gel are then transferred to a nitrocellulose filter to make a precise replica of the gel. When transferring DNA, the nitrocellulose acts to "fix" the single strands of DNA such that they will not reanneal, thereby making them accessible to probes. The transfer is usually done by placing the gel atop a sponge sitting in a tray of buffer. The nitrocellulose filter is laid over the gel and covered with a stack of paper towels that acts as a wick pulling buffer up through the sponge, gel, and filter. DNA (or RNA) fragments from the gel are carried up onto the filter where they are fixed by heating. The filter is then hybridized with a radiolabeled probe. Hybridization thereby specifically tags the sequence of interest even though it may constitute a very minute fraction of nucleic acid on the filter. Unbound probe is washed off and the filter exposed to x-ray films where the position of the DNA fragment (or RNA fragment) that is complementary to the probe appears as a band on the film. The procedure is termed southern blotting when DNA is transferred to nitrocellulose, northern blotting when RNA is transferred, and western blotting when protein is transferred from an SDS-polyacrylamide gel. In western blotting the protein of interest is identified using an antibody that specifically recognizes it.

DNA copy or cDNA, or by digesting nuclear DNA with restriction endonucleases. The selected piece of DNA is then replicated in a foreign cell by putting the DNA into certain genetic carriers, ie, plasmids or viruses, which nature has endowed with the ability to move from one place within the genome to another or from one kind of cell to another (Fig 11). In a sense, these factors can carry "hitchhiking" genes. A number of techniques are available for introducing the new DNA into recipient cells, a process called *transfection.* It can be microinjected, helped across the plasma membrane by

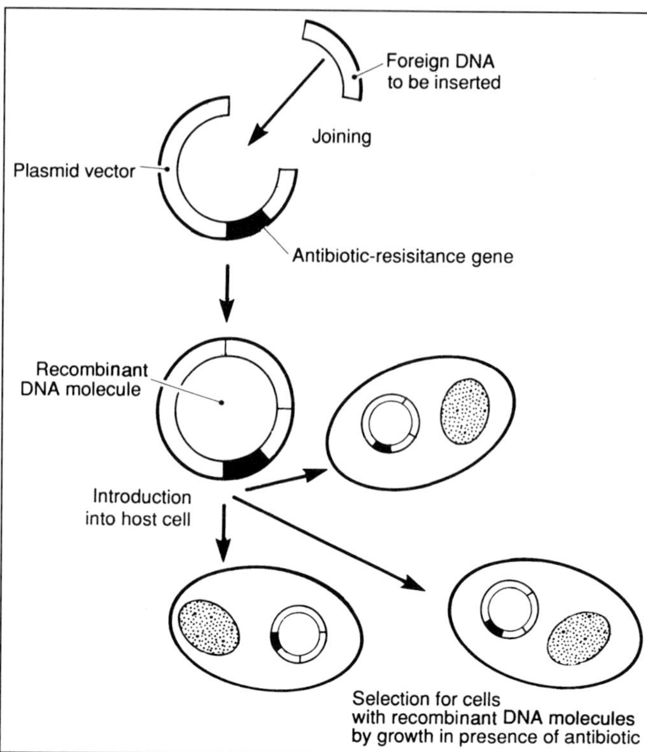


**Fig 11.** Cloning of DNA in a plasmid.

certain chemical treatments such as calcium chloride, enclosed within small membranous sacs or artificial phospholipid vesicles (liposomes) that fuse to the plasma membrane, or brought into the cell by electrical current. When applicable, the method of choice is to attach the DNA to the DNA of a vector, usually a plasmid, which is a self-replicating circular extrachromosomal DNA molecule, or some viral particle that happens to be naturally endowed with the appropriate means for introducing its DNA content into selected cells. This technique has the additional advantage that the vectors used often carry genetic markers such as resistance to certain antibiotics that allow recognition and isolation of the transferred cells very easily (Fig 11).

The tools for attaching the DNA to its vector are all borrowed from nature. They include restriction enzymes for cutting the DNAs at specific sites; nonspecific terminal deoxynucleotidyltransferases for fitting the vector and its passenger with sticky ends (poly-dG on one and poly-dC on the other); and DNA polymerase to fill in the gaps and DNA ligase to do the final stitching. The passenger DNA may be a simple piece of native DNA, a more complex mixture of such pieces, or the contents of a complete genome fragmented by a restriction enzyme. Bacteria are the obvious recipients for all cloning and manufacturing elements in view of their rapid generation rate, ease of culture and selection, and large number of possible vectors. Interestingly, some of the initial objections to genetic engineering arose largely from the fear that some bacteria, unwittingly transformed into highly pathogenic species, might escape into the environment. This risk appeared particularly hazardous because the most widely used bacterium is *E. coli,* which is, of course, a natural inhabitant of the human digestive tract. These fears, however, have not proven to be the case and no serious accidents have occurred.

**Polymerase Chain Reaction.** The polymerase chain reaction (PCR) is a rapid procedure for in vitro enzymatic amplification of a specific segment of DNA.[31] In a sense, the procedure has made it possible to artificially clone specific DNA sequences rapidly without the need of a living cell like all other cloning procedures. Furthermore, the starting DNA "mixture" does not need to be homogeneously pure and can even be fragmented. It is possible to amplify DNA sequences from as short as 50 bp to over 2000 bp in length, more than a millionfold in only a few hours. Moreover, the ability to propagate specific DNA (for subsequent analysis) from amounts too minute for standard amplification (eg, cloning) gives the method such extraordinary power and sensitivity that the DNA from fixed pathologic specimens, buccal cells from mouthwashes, human hairs, single lymphoid or sperm cells, or ancient mummies can now be amplified.

The theoretical basis for PCR is described in three steps and is illustrated in Fig 12. The first step of the cycle is the *heat denaturation* of the native double-stranded DNA, which breaks the hydrogen bonds holding the two strands thus liberating single strands of DNA (which can hybridize to other DNA with complementary sequences). In the second step, two short DNA primers are annealed to complementary sequences on opposite strands of the target DNA. These primers are chosen to encompass the desired DNA. Importantly, they define the two ends of the stretch of DNA to be amplified.

The final step is the actual synthesis of a complementary second strand of DNA. The primers are designed and annealed such that their 3′ ends are facing each other so that synthesis by DNA polymerase (which catalyzes growth of new strands in a 5′- to 3′-direction) extends across the segment of DNA between them. A new single strand of DNA is synthesized for each annealed primer. Each new strand consists of the primer and its 5′ end trailed by a string of linked nucleotides complementary to those of the corresponding template.

An essential feature of the PCR is that all previously synthesized products act as templates for new primer—extension reactions (eg, DNA synthesis)—in each ensuing cycle. The result of this aptly named chain reaction is the geometric amplification of new DNA products. Since the primers form the kernels of all new DNA strands, each of the two different primers as well as the four deoxyribonucleoside triphosphates (the building blocks of the

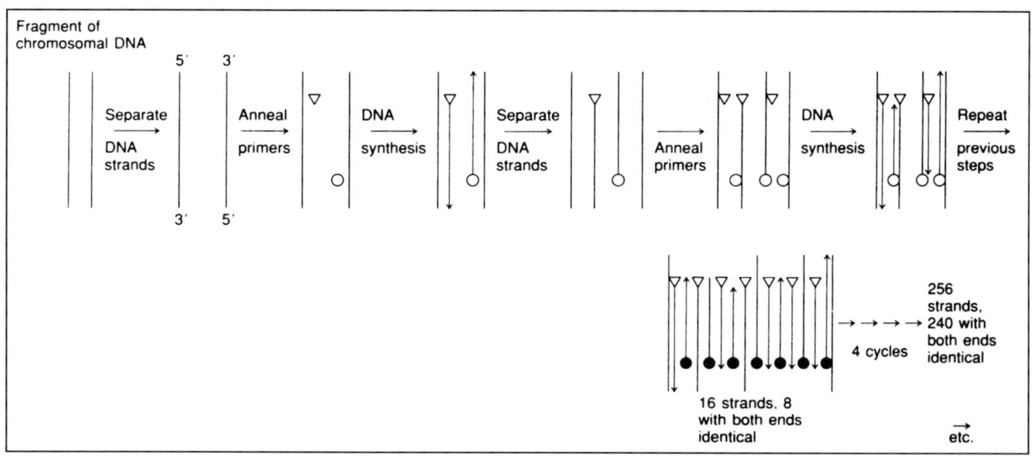


**Fig 12.** The polymerase chain reaction for amplifying specific DNA sequences in vitro. DNA that is isolated from cells is heated to separate the complementary strands. These strands are then annealed with oligonucleotide primers, which "outline" the region to be amplified, generally 50–2000 bp in length. DNA synthesis is then catalyzed by DNA polymerase, which copies the DNA between the sequences corresponding to the two oligonucleotides. After multiple cycles, a large amount of double-stranded DNA fragments of a specific length is formed. [From Walsh PC, et al, eds. *Campbell's Urology,* 6th ed (Philadelphia: WB Saunders Co. 1992), with permission.]

DNA molecule) must initially be present in massive amounts relative to the quantity of target (substrate) DNA. The exquisite *specificity* of the annealing reaction (second step) and the *geometric amplification* of the PCR products (third step) together give the methods its extraordinary sensitivity. Each cycle of replication is temperature-controlled, ie, the temperature is raised so that all double-stranded DNAs are converted to single-stranded DNAs (thus aborting any ongoing polymerizations); the temperature is then lowered to allow the steps of annealing and extension. Typically, 30 full cycles are completed.

The PCR has the ability to synthesize defined fragments of DNA in unlimited amounts and shares this property with standard gene cloning. The advantage of gene cloning is that it does not require the synthesis of primers that are needed by the PCR, and it therefore remains the method of choice for many experiments, particularly those in which the sequence of the target DNA is unknown. On the other hand, PCR surpasses standard cloning in its simplicity, speed, and ability to amplify vanishingly small amounts of impure starting material.

With an understanding of the principles of PCR, it can be seen that the methodology is potentially useful in any situation that requires examination of DNA. In its most commonly applied form, the PCR is best suited to help answer the often raised question, does a given sequence of DNA exist in a given clinical specimen? This approach has numerous clinical applications and in many cases can provide answers that often can be difficult or impossible to obtain. For example, the PCR is useful in determining the sex of human embryos associated with in vitro fertilization, the prenatal diagnosis of genetic disorders, and the detection of human immunodeficiency virus (HIV) in people whose sera cannot be determined to be HIV-positive by conventional means, such as infants born to HIV-infected mothers and seronegative people at high risk for AIDS.

## Genetic Analysis

Extraordinary progress has been made in understanding the structure and function of human genes with respect to certain disease states. Most of our understanding has related to disorders associated with a defect in a single gene. There are two basic strategies used to find a gene, characterize its defect, and therefore define the genetic disease (Table 2). The first and most straightforward protocol for genetic analysis assumes that either the abnormal or normal gene product (a protein) is known. With that prerequisite, amino acid sequence analysis can be performed on part of the protein. From that, an oligonucleotide can be synthetically made that is then equivalent to a cDNA molecule. This can then be used to probe a cDNA library from various tissues or chromosomes with resultant identification of the cDNA (or mRNA), the tissue of origin, or the chromosome of origin, according to the experiment done.

This type of approach can also be used when an antibody is available to the protein in question; it can be used to precipitate protein–mRNA complexes. After conversion of mRNA to cDNA, an identical approach to that outlined above can be used to isolate the gene. Once the gene is identified, specific abnormalities such as deletions, insertions, rearrangements, or point

**TABLE 2. Genetic Analysis and "Reverse" Genetic Analysis**

| From Gene to Protein | From Protein to Gene |
|---|---|
| Isolate mRNA; make cDNA | Isolate protein |
| Sequence cDNA | Partial amino acid sequence |
| Deduce amino acid sequence from cDNA sequence | Make oligonucleotides that correspond to amino acid sequence |
| Make peptides specified by sequence; inject into animals to produce antibodies | Use labeled oligonucleotides to select cDNA clone from cDNA library |
| Isolate pure protein by affinity to antibody | Sequence selected gene |

mutations can be sought in the diseased patient to account for the abnormal protein production (or lack of protein production).

### In-Situ Hybridization

cDNA probes can also be used for in-situ hybridization experiments for the purpose of chromosomal localization of the gene or tissue localization of the mRNA. In such cases, nucleic acid probes are used in much the same way as labeled antibodies to locate specific nucleic acid sequences in situ. A $^{32}$P-labeled cDNA probe can be hybridized to chromosomes that have been exposed briefly to very high pH to disrupt their DNA base pairs. The chromosomal regions that bind the radioactive molecule during the hybridization step are visualized by autoradiography. In-situ hybridization methods that reveal the distribution of specific RNA molecules in cells within tissues have also been developed. In this case, the tissues are not exposed to high pH; thus, the chromosomal DNA remains double-stranded and cannot bind the probe. Instead, the tissue is gently fixed so that its RNA is retained in an exposed form that will hybridize when the tissue is incubated with the cDNA probe.

In general, the advantages of in-situ hybridization are localization of the cellular source of mRNA in complex tissues; increased specificity over conventional techniques when the probe is directed at untranslated portions of the gene; and elimination of the need for processing frozen tissue. No freezing that may cause artifact is necessary. Tissues are fixed, which eliminates the "risk" associated with clinical specimens.

### Antisense RNA Strategy

One of the principal goals of genetic engineering is to selectively turn off specific genes or genetic function in cells. This will be important, for example, in cells producing an abnormal or deleterious gene product or in experiments designed to determine the function of a protein by observing the cell or organism after production of the protein in question has been turned off. One of the more creative strategies that is not new but has recently become more widely used because of recent advances in technology is that of the use of antisense RNA.[32] The idea is to introduce into cells an RNA or single-stranded DNA molecule that is complementary to the mRNA of the target gene. The *antisense* molecule then can base-pair (or hybridize) with mRNA so as to extinguish its signal and prevent translation of the mRNA into protein. Several strategies have been used to introduce antisense nucleic acids into cells. In the earliest experiments, antisense RNA was synthesized in vitro using bacteriophage RNA polymerase and then microinjected into cells. Injection of antisense RNA for the gene encoding actin, a major constituent of the cytoskeleton that maintains cell shape, causes the cytoskeleton to disintegrate and the cells to change their shape. More recently, however, expression vectors have been designed to produce high levels of antisense RNA in transfected cells (Fig 13). In this case, cells are transfected with a plasmid that carries a portion of the target gene downstream (or 3′) from a strong promoter. The key, however, is that the orientation of the target gene in the plasmid is opposite in orientation to the target gene (the template strand and coding strand are reversed), so that the RNA transcribed from the plasmid is *complementary* in sequence to the mRNA transcribed from the corresponding cellular gene. If the complementary (antisense) RNA is present in large excess, it base-pairs to virtually all mRNA to form a double-strand RNA that cannot be translated into protein and is thought to be rapidly destroyed. The effect is that the protein product of the target gene is not produced. Particularly dramatic results have been achieved with antisense constructs for oncogenes. In several instances, antisense oncogene constructs have reverted the growth properties of tumor cells to near normal or slowed their growth.

### Transfection: Transferring DNA and Genes Into Cells

The ability to transfer genes (or any DNA for that matter) into cells, especially

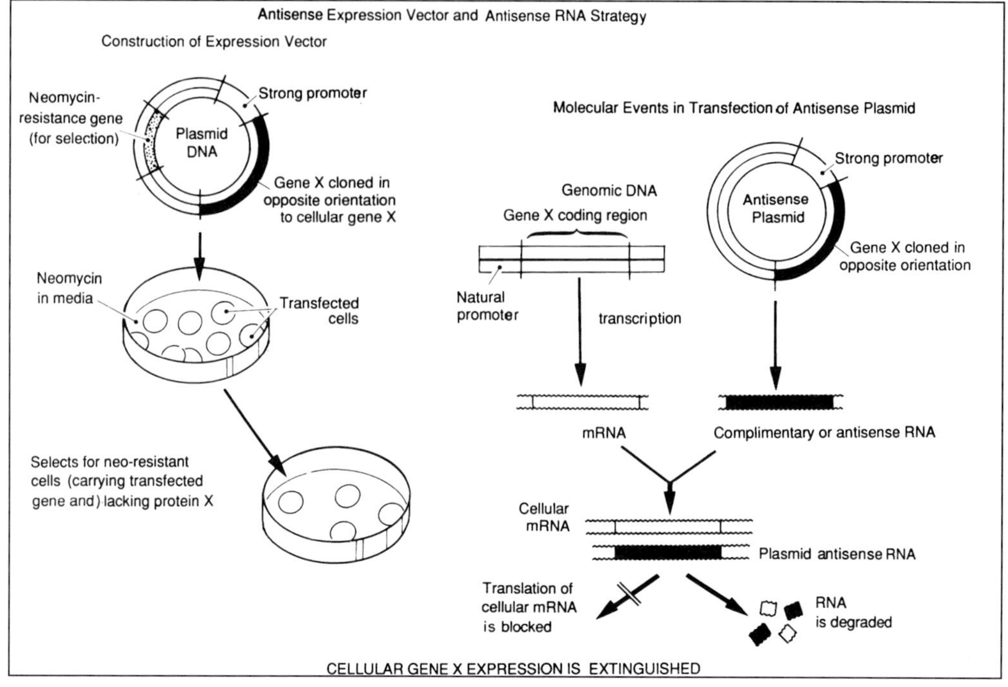


**Fig 13.** Use of antisense RNA to extinguish cellular gene expression. Cells are transfected with a plasmid that carries a portion of the target gene (gene x) downstream of a strong promoter. Since the orientation of the target gene in the plasmid is backward (ie, the coding strand and template strand are reversed—see Fig 1), the RNA transcribed from the plasmid is complementary in sequence to the mRNA transcribed from the corresponding cellular gene. If the antisense RNA is present in large excess, it base-pairs to virtually all mRNA to form a double-stranded RNA that cannot be translated into protein and is thought to be rapidly destroyed.

mammalian cells, is a complex process that has extreme importance. For such to occur it is necessary to isolate the gene in question by cloning, manipulate the sequence of the gene in vitro, and return the altered gene to cells to determine how it functions.

The earliest gene transfer experiments were done with DNA tumor viruses. This was a natural because tumor viruses infect mammalian cells, insert their genetic material into host DNA, and "hijack" the cellular biosynthetic machinery to manufacture more virus. Basically, DNA was isolated from purified viruses and introduced into cultures of uninfected cells that eventually produced infectious virus. This DNA-mediated transfer of infectious virus was termed *transfection* to distinguish it from *infection,* the natural route of entry for viruses.

To make this work properly, special techniques were required to get the DNA into cells; throughout evolution cells have developed several natural barriers against invading DNA. Conceptually, the simplest form of transfection is *microinjection* in which DNA is injected directly into the nucleus of cells through painstakingly constructed fine-glass needles. This is an efficient way to get the job done on a per-cell basis but, unfortunately, only a few hundred cells can be injected in a single experiment.[33]

The earliest method for the large-scale introduction of DNA into cells was to incubate the DNA with an inert carbohydrate polymer (dextran) to which a positively charged chemical group (DEAE or diethylaminoethyl) has been coupled. The DNA sticks to the DEAE-dextran via its negatively charged phosphate groups. The large DNA-containing particles stick to the surfaces of the cells which then take them in by *endocytosis,* which is a normal consequence of membrane turnover. Some of the DNA evades destruction in the cytoplasm and then enters the nucleus where it is transcribed to RNA like any other gene in the cell. A simpler method that was more reliable supplanted the DEAE-dextran method and is in use today. The technique, called the calcium phosphate coprecipitation technique, is based on the initial finding that cells efficiently take up DNA in the form of a precipitate with calcium phosphate. This discovery arose from previous work showing that divalent cations such as calcium and magnesium promoted the uptake of DNA into bacteria. It was this technique that led the way to our advanced understanding of the genes (oncogenes) underlying cancer.

Interestingly, some cells such as lymphocytes are resistant to the calcium phosphate coprecipitation method to introduce DNA past the cell membrane. In such cases other, newer methods are available. One example is *electroporation* in which cells are placed in a solution containing DNA and subjected to a brief electrical pulse that causes holes to open transiently in the host cell membrane. DNA passes through the holes and enters the cytoplasm. In another method called *lipofection,* DNA is encapsulated into artificial lipid vesicles, or *liposomes,* which resemble spheres of synthetic membrane filled with DNA. They fuse spontaneously with cell membranes, delivering their contents directly into the cytoplasm.

## Selectable Markers

Another important technical requirement for experimental transfection is that a system must be used to identify or isolate cells that have been successfully transfected because only a small minority of cells undergoing this experimental manipulation actually achieve a stable transfected state. To meet this goal, *biological markers* have been developed. In bacteria these are commonly drug resistance genes. In other words, a drug resistance gene (eg, neomycin resistance) is tagged onto the transfected gene of interest so that after transfection, by whatever technique, the resultant bacterial population can be placed in the drug (such as neomycin) and all bacteria that did *not* take up the transfected gene construct will be killed by the neomycin leaving only cells that are stably transfected (Fig 13). Other genes besides neomycin resistance have been used. For example, the thymidine kinase gene will allow selective growth of cells transfected with this gene (along with the experimental gene of interest) when the transfected cells are grown in selective HAT (hypoxanthine, aminopterine, thymidine) medium. Thymidine kinase is an enzyme that catalyzes a step in the synthesis of thymidine triphosphate, one of the four precursor nucleotides for DNA synthesis. Mammalian cells possess two distinct routes for synthesizing DNA triphosphates for DNA synthesis. Mammalian cells can make them from scratch or they can salvage free purine and pyrimidine bases. Aminopterine blocks two steps in the biosynthesis of purines and one in the biosynthesis of thymidine. If cells are provided with hypoxanthine and thymidine they can survive aminopterine treatment by using the salvage pathways with thymidine kinase. This selection can also be used for *hprt,* the gene that encodes the key salvage enzyme (hypoxanthine phosphoribosyltransferase—HPRT) for purines.

## Viral Vectors

Although the above-noted methodologies are unique and provide a means to transfect cells with genes or DNA segments, the fraction of cells taking up the DNA may be quite low. To increase the efficiency of transfection, viruses have been used. As noted previously, this is a natural move because viral growth depends on the ability of the viral genome to get into cells, and several natural viral mechanisms have been developed in nature to do just that. When the goal is to introduce a gene into a cell in a stable fashion, the most commonly used vector is a *retrovirus.* Retroviruses are RNA viruses that are able to convert their RNA into DNA by the enzyme reverse transcriptase when they enter a cell. Viral DNA is efficiently integrated into the host genome where it permanently resides and is called a *provirus* after integration. The integrated provirus steadily produces viral RNA from a strong promoter at the end of the viral genome within a sequence called a *long terminal repeat* (LTR). Retroviruses therefore make attractive vectors because they permanently express a foreign gene in cells. Retroviruses are commonly used to study the effects of foreign genes on cells. For example, oncogenes and tumor suppressor genes are commonly studied by placing them in retrovirus vectors and subsequently transfecting cells. Cells that have been transfected can be marked; for example, if the retrovirus construct carries the *E. coli* Lac Z gene, encoding β-galactosidase, descendents of the infected cells can be easily identified in tissue samples by treating them with x-gal, a molecule that is turned blue by β-galactosidase. Because of their obvious versatility, retroviruses have become the vector of choice in gene therapy.

Retroviruses do have drawbacks, however. For example, they can only integrate into cells that are dividing (therefore leaving out cells such as mature neurons). It is also possible for retroviruses to cause cancer, perhaps through activation of a quiescent oncogene or inactivation of a suppressor gene. The likelihood of this happening seems to be low if the viral vectors are prevented from reproducing. This is accomplished with a clever strategy (Fig 14). Retroviral RNA is made by replacing the three major genes [*gag, pol,* and *env,* which specify proteins of the viral core, the enzyme reverse transcriptase (allowing the production of viral DNA from RNA, respectively), and constituents of the coat of the virus] with the therapeutic gene. This altered retrovirus with no instruction for making viral proteins produces no progency by itself. This modified virus is inserted into a packaging cell containing a packaging provirus that produces all of the proteins required for packaging of viral RNA into the infectious virus particles but is unable to package its own RNA. The viral DNA directs the synthesis of viral RNA but, lacking viral "housekeeping" genes, cannot give rise to proteins needed to package RNA into particles for delivery to other cells. The missing proteins are supplied by a "helper" provirus from which the ψ region has been deleted. ψ is critical to the inclusion of RNA in viral particles. Without it, no virus-carrying helper RNA can form. The particles that escape the cell then carry therapeutic RNA and no viral genes. They can enter other cells and splice the therapeutic gene into cellular DNA, but they cannot reproduce.

### Gene Transfer

The two main problems associated with gene transfer methodologies are that when DNA is taken up by cells it is frequently lost and that in those rare instances (based on odds per cell) that DNA integrates stably into the host genome the integration occurs at random. This means that for gene therapy experiments, there may be wide fluctuations in the expression levels of the transfer gene and perhaps in the pattern of its regulation. In some cases the foreign gene integrates in the vicinity of a highly expressed cellular gene and comes under the influence of a gene's regulatory apparatus, or the integrated gene may unintentionally disrupt the proper function of the "bystander" gene. It should also be remembered that this methodology only brings information into cells. Unfortunately, it does not provide for the removal of genes. Sometimes the study of the function of introduced genes can be complicated by the presence of the normal counterpart of the gene in recipient cells. The problem at hand, therefore, is *gene targeting,* which is one of the most actively studied areas in research dealing with gene therapy. Currently, when foreign genes recombine in the host genome, it occurs by *heterologous recombination,* ie, by gene recombination with an unrelated sequence. In some cases, however, a gene can recombine precisely into the identical sequence in the genome by *homologous recombination.* This process is frequently observed in bacteria and yeast but unfortunately is exceedingly rare in mammalian cells, occur-

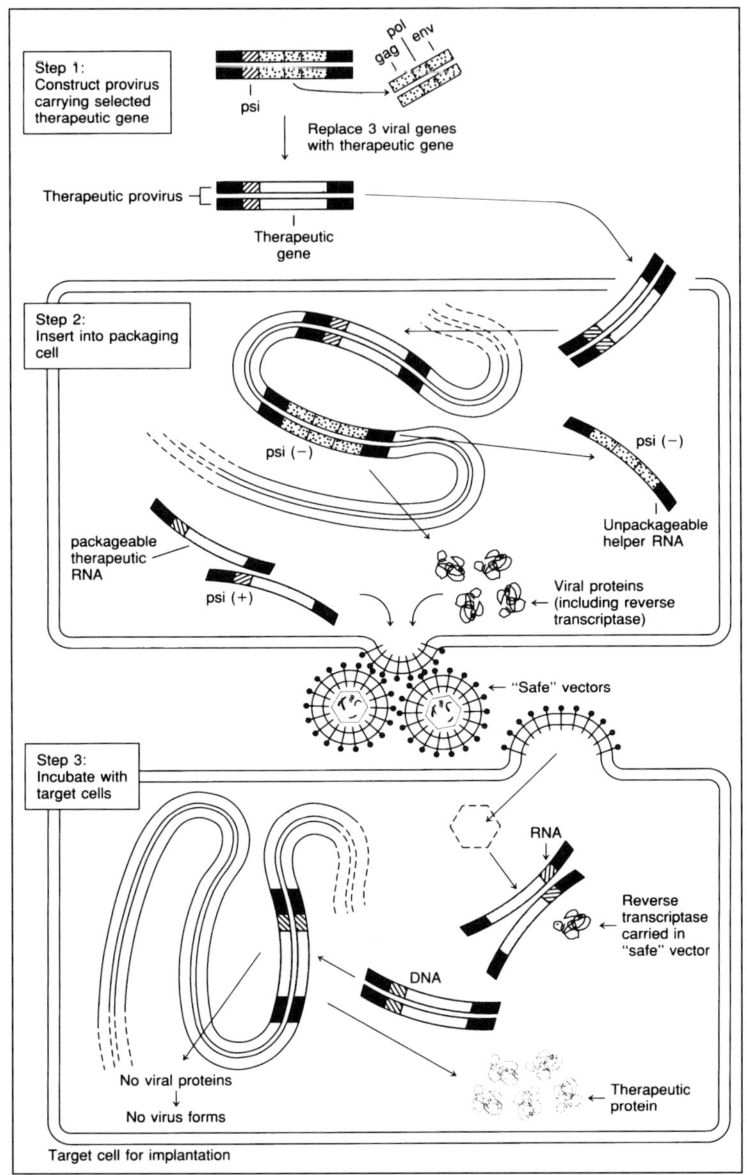


**Fig 14.** Gene therapy may use retroviral vectors to deliver therapeutic genes. In such case, viruses are made in which viral genes encoding the proteins of the viral core (gag), the enzyme reverse transcriptase (pol), and the constituents of the coat (env) (all of which are necessary for proper packaging of RNA into particles for delivery to other cells) are removed and therapeutic gene substituted. The virus is then inserted into a packaging cell. Here the defective "therapeutic virus" is helped to replicate and repackage with the aid of a "helper" virus that "lends" the missing viral protein products to the therapeutic virus. The helper virus, however, is also defective because the ψ region is deleted (necessary for inclusion of RNA into viral particles). This prevents the helper virus from leaving the cell. The particles that escape the cell, then, carry therapeutic RNA and no viral genes. They can enter other cells and splice the therapeutic gene into the cellular DNA, but they cannot reproduce. [From Walsh PC, et al, eds. *Campbell's Urology,* 6th ed (Philadelphia: WB Saunders Co. 1992), with permission.]

ring 1 per 1000 heterologous insertions. In the future it may become possible to perform *gene transplacement* by which an endogenous gene is precisely replaced with an engineered derivative.

## Introduction of Genes into Animals: Transgenes

In the previous section, methodology was discussed directed at the introduction of genetic material into individual cells in tissue culture. The next order of complexity is the study of introduced genes into animals, usually mice. An animal that gains new permanent genetic information from the addition of new foreign DNA is described as *transgenic.* A transgenic animal then carries in its genome gene sequences inserted by laboratory techniques. Transgenic animals provide the opportunity to identify genetic elements that determine tissue-specific gene expression to broaden understanding of human disease conditions including developmental defects and cancer.

There are various ways to construct the transgenic models, but the most common practice is to microinject cloned DNA into one of the two pronuclei (either the male or female haploid nucleus contributed by the parents) of a fertilized mouse egg before they fuse (Fig 15).[34] A few hundred copies of the foreign DNA in about 2 pL of solution are microinjected directly into one of the pronuclei. The injected embryos are then transferred to the oviduct of a foster mother and, upon subsequent implantation in the uterus, may develop to term. Of the survivors, the number that have foreign DNA integrated into their chromosomes is usually 10%–30%. The introduced DNA appears to integrate randomly without preference for a particular chromosomal location, usually a tandom array of many copies at a single locus. Again, mice that carry the foreign gene are referred to as transgenic and the foreign DNA is termed a *transgene.*

Transgenic therapy is still not available clinically because of incomplete understanding of gene targeting (replacing the old gene) as well as regulation of function. For example, in the progeny of injected mice, expression of the donor gene can be quite variable. The level of expression does not always correlate with the number of genes that were integrated.

The transgenic model has become an important investigative tool for urologic sci-

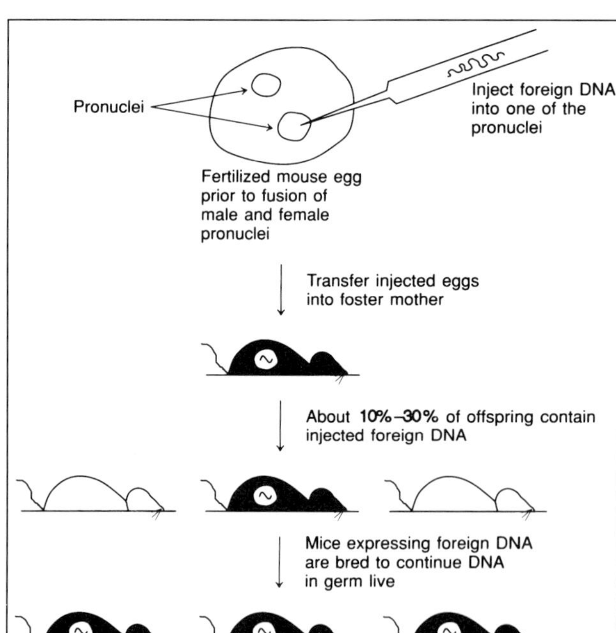


**Fig 15.** Introduction of foreign DNA into a mouse and establishment of a homozygous transgenic mouse strain. [From Walsh PC, et al, eds. *Campbell's Urology,* 6th ed (Philadelphia: WB Saunders Co. 1992), with permission.]

ence. Perhaps the best example is the transgenic model of benign prostatic hyperplasia (BPH), which provides the first solid evidence for genetic disruption as one of the causative factors in the genesis of BPH.[35] This approach is radically different from conventional historical studies of BPH. In this transgenic model, the promoter/enhancer for the mouse mammary tumor virus (MMTV) was "fused" to the *int-2* protooncogene and the DNA microinjected into the male pronucleus of a zygote. Following microinjection, the eggs were washed and transferred to the oviducts of pseudopregnant mice. The transgene also contained the SV-40 promoter/enhancer, which acted as a "marker" so that expression of the transgene *int-2* RNA (in contrast to constituent *int-2* RNA) could be identified by using SV-40 promoter probes. The rationale for performing the original experiments was that *int* genes appear to be common targets for proviral integration during MMTV-mediated mammary carcinogenesis and are transcriptionally activated in virally induced neoplasms. The founder mice passed the transgene in Mendelian fashion, and the transgene was expressed mainly in breast, prostate, and salivary glands. All males were sterile. Pathologic evaluation of the prostate in transgenic males exhibiting prostate-specific transgene expression showed enlarged prostates that revealed hyperplasia by microscopic examination. Interestingly, there was no stromal hyperplasia or presence of nodules. Malignancy did not develop in any of the animals. Although this model does not precisely describe BPH, it provides an important first step in realizing our thoughts to making BPH a disorder of growth factors in addition to an androgen-related disorder.

The transgene model has provided new insights into other urology-related diseases. For example, transgenic rats have been developed bearing an extra gene for renin.[36] As expected, hypertension develops in the animals; oddly enough, however, concentrations of renin in the plasma and kidney are low. In fact, the model has certain similarities with human essential hypertension; ie, blood pressure increases as the animal matures and concentrations of renin in the plasma are normal or low. The distribution of blood pressure and renin levels was not normal in the transgenic animals (as it is in the human population), suggesting a new model for low-renin hypertension. Finally, another model has been developed in which a mutant transgenic mouse (mpv 17) expresses a recessive lethal trait for focal segmental glomerulosclerosis.[37] In homozygous adults, nephrotic syndrome and chronic renal failure develop. The strain was originally generated by introduction of a replication-defective retrovirus into the germ line.

## MOLECULAR BASIS FOR CANCER

### A Disease of Cellular Dysregulation

The abilities to grow without restriction, invade locally, and spread distantly are typical characteristics of the cancer cell. However, during embryonic development most normal cells display these same features. The notable difference between cancer and embryonic development is not one of fundamental cellular properties but rather one of growth control. In this sense, cancer can be thought of as primarily a disease of cellular dysregulation. How these controls become dysfunctional forms the molecular basis for understanding carcinogenesis.

### The Signal Transduction Pathway

Cells interact with their environment on the basis of both external stimuli and genetically determined preprogrammed responses (Fig 16). External information is transmitted into the interior of cells through *signal transduction* pathways that ultimately result in the production of specific proteins that regulate cell behavior.[38] These external signals may be in the form of relatively nonspecific environmental factors such as physical stress or nutrient availability, or they may be much more specific. Thus, distinct pathways exist to allow communication between cellular neighbors via cell contact, between more distant neighbors via short-acting *paracrine* growth factors, and between cells in distant organs via

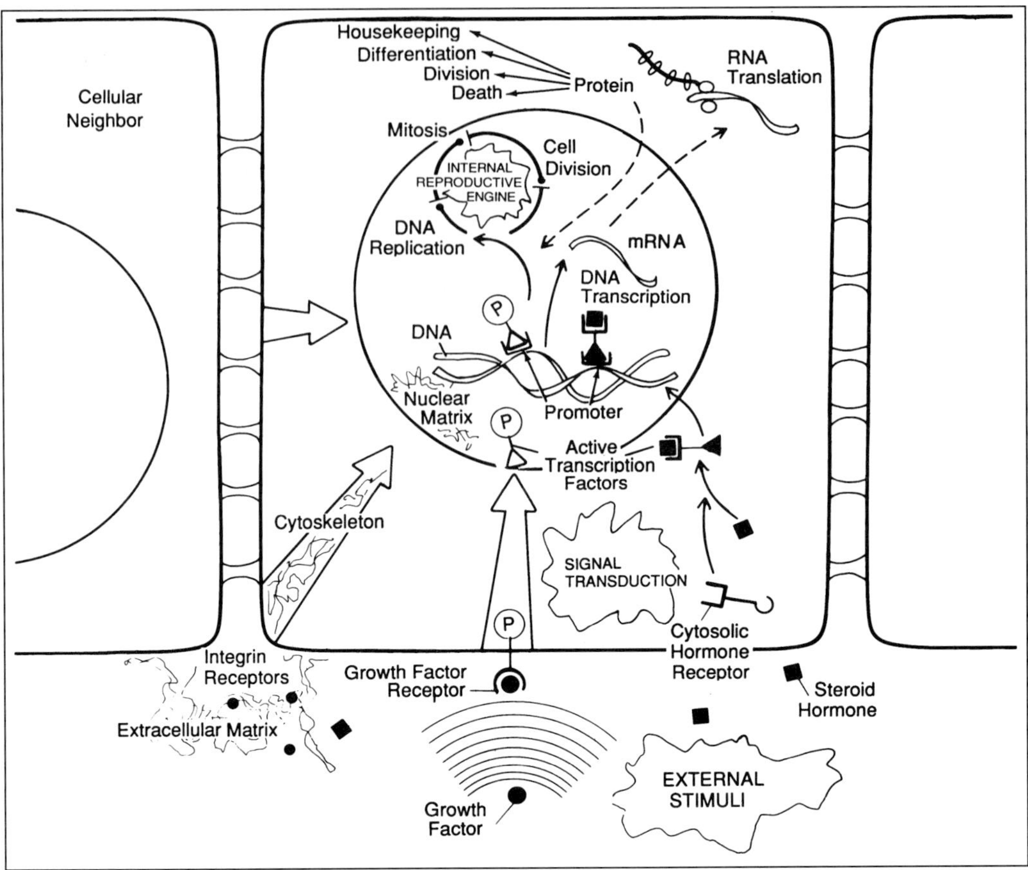


**Fig 16.** External stimuli elicit specific responses from the cell by changing gene expression patterns. Signals are transmitted to the cell nucleus via specialized signal transduction pathways that result in the activation of DNA-binding proteins known as transcription factors. These in turn initiate the transcription of messenger RNA leading to specific protein production. Ultimately it is the synthesis of these proteins that drives the cell to undertake specialized functions including differentiation, cell division, and even programmed cell death.

long-range *endocrine* type growth factors. Direct interactions also exist between the cell interior and the external scaffolding *(extracellular matrix)* either through soluble mediators or via cytoskeletal elements.[39] Coordinated responses are produced by the convergence and interaction of pathways at multiple levels much like the integrated circuits of a computer chip.

The pathway of signal transduction can be simple or complex. In the case of steroid hormone receptors, binding of the signal (eg, androgen) to the appropriate receptor is accompanied by direct transport of the complex into the nucleus where it binds to a specialized promoter region on DNA to initiate gene transcription into messenger RNA. In most cases, however, the signal is processed through a cascade of intermediaries that amplify the signal and eventually translate it into direct-acting DNA-binding proteins known as *transcription factors* (Fig 17).[40] This cascade effect is usually accomplished through enzymes that modify proteins by either adding phosphate groups *(kinases)* or removing phosphate groups *(phosphatases).* Widespread propagation of responses throughout the cell may be orchestrated through small and rapidly diffusible molecules known as *second messengers.* Examples of such messengers include cyclic AMP and GMP, diacylglycerol (DAG), inositol triphosphate (ITP or IP3), and intracellular calcium.

While this indirect method for cell signaling may appear cumbersome, it allows the cell to exercise a great deal of control. Operating like a squelch on a radio, background noise from interfering signals can be prevented from eliciting unproductive responses. At the same time, true signals exceeding certain threshold limits can be greatly amplified to achieve rapid and dynamic responses. Mechanisms also exist to permit ''cross-talk'' between different signal pathways, so that antagonistic responses are intercepted at an early stage before the cell has invested a great deal of precious energy and raw material (Table 3).[41] This exquisite system of regulation is disrupted in cancer by either inappropriate signal amplification *(oncogenes)* or by the loss of mechanisms responsible for dampening out inappropriate responses (*tumor suppressor genes* or *antioncogenes*).

## Oncogenes and Tumor Suppressor Genes

Oncogenes were first discovered by genetic analysis of nucleotide sequences isolated from certain animal RNA tumor viruses. Specific genetic sequences termed viral oncogenes (v-*onc*) were found that conferred on these viruses the ability to transform normal cells into cancer cells. More importantly and quite unexpectedly, these viral oncogenes were found to correspond with a high degree of similarity to DNA sequences found in normal cells. These cellular oncogenes or *protooncogenes* (c-*onc*), as they began to be called, were remarkably preserved across species boundaries as diverse as man and yeast. Clearly they had not evolved for the purpose of causing cancer but rather had persevered because they served a vital function in normal cellular physiology. However, while tumor viruses may have acquired these sequences as a result of random DNA capture during infection, they have persisted in viruses because they conferred a distinct growth advantage. The inappropriate activity of these oncogenes deregulates cellular physiology, allowing more activated raw materials to be available for viral replication.

Over 40 such protooncogenes have now been identified.[42] While many were originally found through the study of tumor viruses, more have been identified recently through their ability to transform cells in tissue culture. The classic cell line used in these *gene transfection* experiments has been the immortalized but nontumorigenic mouse fibroblast cell line NIH 3T3. Indeed, the ability of a gene when functionally overexpressed to cause cancer is the hallmark of an oncogene.

Structural analysis of oncogenes has revealed that they fall into distinct functional categories stretching along the entire signal transduction pathway (Fig 17).[43] Some, such as c-*sis,* code for growth factors, which if expressed by the same cell containing the appropriate receptor allows for a positive feedback *autocrine loop.* Others such as c-*erb* B/*neu* code for growth factor receptors that possess the ability to phosphorylate the tyrosine residues of several other kinases, changing their enzymatic potential. The *ras* family represents an important class of protooncogenes responsible for generating a kinase signal cascade. These special GTP-binding proteins are found on the inner surface of the cell membrane and couple signals from growth factor receptors to intermediate compounds that eventually reach the cell nucleus. Other intermediaries of signal transduction include cytoplasmic tyrosine kinases (en-

**TABLE 3. Motifs in Cellular Growth Regulation**

| |
|---|
| Growth factors |
| Growth factor inhibitors |
| Differentiation factors |
| GTP exchange proteins |
| GTPase activating proteins |
| Kinases — via ± feedback loops |
| Phosphatases — via ± feedback loops |
| Subunit activation requirements |
| Nuclear transport mechanisms |
| Transcription factors |
| DNA methylation and demethylation |
| Regulators of mRNA stability, splicing, and transport |
| Regulators of protein synthesis and degradation |

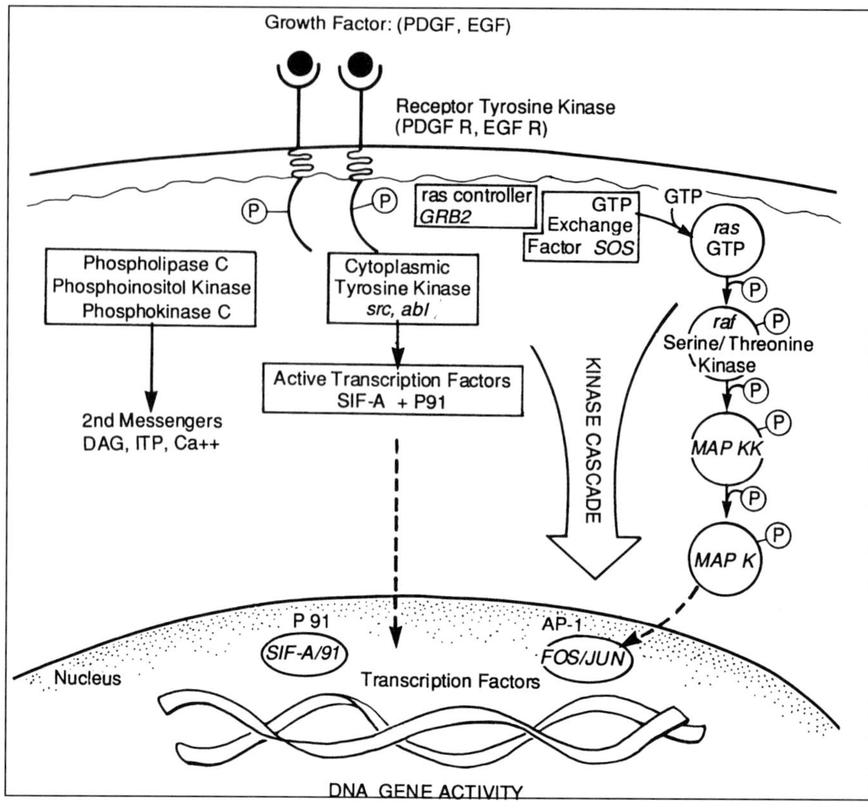


**Fig 17.** The receptor tyrosine kinase pathway is currently the best-understood signal transduction pathway. Binding of growth factor to the receptor is accompanied by receptor aggregation and activation of tyrosine kinase activity. Phosphorylation of specific proteins, many of which are themselves kinases, produces a cascade effect resulting in the production of second-messenger molecules and culminating in the activation of nuclear transcription factors.

coded for by c-*src* and c-*abl*) or serine/threonine kinases (c-*mos* and c-*raf*). Transcription factors may also act as protooncogenes. The protein products of the c-*myc*, c-*fos*, and c-*jun* genes bind directly to DNA after appropriate subunit pairing to initiate the transcription of messenger RNA. A relatively new player to the field, *mdm-2*, encodes a cytosolic membrane protein that works as an oncogene in a more indirect manner by sequestering the p53 protein, a known tumor suppressor gene product.[44]

Because of the pivotal roles these protooncogene proteins play in normal cellular homeostasis, it is not surprising that aberrations in their structure or production may have profound effects on cellular behavior. In general, oncogenes achieve their deleterious effect through mechanisms that are either qualitative (gene mutations) or quantitative (overexpression of normal genes). The prototype example of the qualitative mechanism is provided by the *ras* oncogene, first described in bladder cancer.[45] A simple point mutation in the *ras* gene at either amino acid position 12, 59, or 61 results in the production of a GTP-binding protein that is permanently trapped in the on position. The best example of a quantitative mechanism for oncogene activation is furnished by c-*myc* and a related gene N-*myc*. The N-*myc* gene is physically amplified (several additional copies of the normal gene) in very aggressive forms of neuroblastoma. In other cases, such as in Burkitt's lymphoma, the c-*myc* gene is physically translocated from chromosome 8 to chromosome 14, downstream from a very active immunoglobulin promoter region. Both situations result in a large increase in messenger RNA synthesis (and thus protein) derived from this gene.

While actual DNA abberations of *ras* and *myc* can be detected in several forms of human cancer, the vast majority of cancers display more subtle oncogene aberrations. Usually this is in the form of increased expression of the oncogene protein product without an actual change in the DNA blueprint. This may be due either to message overexpression (usually via overactive transcription factors) or to decreased message or protein degradation. The latter situation occurs in the case of bladder cancer where an overexpression of the epidermal growth factor receptor is commonly found.[46] However, because other factors such as the cellular proliferation rate can also affect protein expression, one is often faced with a ''chicken-and-the-egg'' paradox. Thus, the simple demonstration of increased oncogene expression is not sufficient to prove cancer causation. Indeed, this scenario makes the search for etiologic oncogenes in clinical cancers very difficult.

Largely through the inability to explain clinical carcinogenesis simply through the upregulation of positively acting oncogenes, it was soon realized that another mechanism of cellular dysregulation existed involving the removal of negatively acting cellular signals. It was through this type of analysis that *antioncogenes* or *tumor suppresor genes* were discovered.[47]

The existence of aberrations in negative regulatory signals leading to cancer was first deduced from epidemiologic data concerning the frequency of the rare heritable childhood tumors retinoblastoma and Wilms' tumor. Based on the discrepancies in frequency found between sporadic and heritable forms of these diseases, Knudson in 1971 deduced that two hits must be occurring, one in each of two alleles or copies of the same gene.[48] In the hereditable form, one mutant allele was transmitted genetically while the other was acquired as a result of a somatic mutation. The sporadic form, by contrast, required two somatic events. In fulfillment of this prediction, genes responsible for retinoblastoma and Wilms' tumor have been identified, cloned, and partially characterized. The retinoblastoma (RB) protein has been found to play a pivotal role in regulating cell cycle–specific DNA transcription[49] and has been implicated in both bladder cancer and prostate cancer.[50,51] The Wilms' tumor protein (WT1) represses DNA transcription at a specific stage of embryogenesis in the developing kidney possibly allowing a default program to be initiated.[52] Loss of WT1 is responsible for most but not all cases of this childhood cancer indicating there are likely other downstream events controlled by different genes that result in the same phenotypic cancer type.[53]

Since the original identification of the retinoblastoma and Wilms' tumor genes, several more tumor suppressor genes have been isolated and cloned. Many have been identified using the technique of *restriction fragment length polymorphism* (RFLP) in which losses in one of the alleles of a gene are identified as a band loss on a southern blot. By using DNA probes that span a chromosome of interest, deletions of the *APC* (adenoma polyposis coli) and *DCC* (deleted in colon carcinoma) genes were discovered to play a vital role in familial polyposis and colon carcinoma, respectively.[54] The *DCC* gene encodes a cell membrane protein thought to supply a negative proliferative signal. The function of the *APC* gene is unknown. The gene lost in von Recklinghausen's neurofibromatosis, *NF-1,* has been implicated in keeping *ras* in its inactive off state.[55] A tumor suppressor gene on the short arm of chromosome 3 (3p21) lost in over 80% of renal cell carcinomas was recently identified.[56] Evidence for other loci encoding putative tumor suppressor genes have also recently been found on chromosomes 9p, 9q, and 11p in bladder cancer[57] and on chromosomes 8p and 16q in prostate cancer.[58] The search for specific genes involved in these cancers is currently underway. Perhaps the most important and widespread example of a tumor suppressor gene in human cancer, however, is the *p53* gene.[59]

Located on the short arm of chromosome 17, position 13 (17p13), *p53* was first identified in family pedigrees of the Li-

Fraumeni syndrome, a disease marked by multiple familial cancers. This gene was subsequently found to be lost or mutated in over 50% of all human cancers including many high-stage bladder cancers and prostate cancers. Like RB and WT1, p53 is a nuclear protein involved in regulating a gamut of cellular genes through its ability to directly bind with DNA. Unlike the other tumor suppressor gene products, however, the p53 protein loses functional activity even when mutated at one of its two DNA alleles. This is because functional p53 exists as a homotetramer composed of four identical subunits. Mutation of even one single component is enough to significantly quench the activity of the entire complex (so-called *dominant-negative* effect).[60] Tumors with mutant *p53* usually show increased expression of the protein product when stained immunohistochemically as this complex is also more resistant to protein degradation. Mutations in *p53* are associated with a worsened prognosis for both bladder cancer and prostate cancer.[61,62] Recently p53 was implicated to have a major role in both apoptosis and DNA repair.[63]

Not surprisingly, certain tumor viruses have been found to take advantage of these same tumor suppressor gene mechanisms for their own benefit. Three types of DNA viruses—adenovirus, parvovirus, and papillomavirus—depend on the host cell to supply them with raw materials for DNA synthesis. This material is only available during a specific stage of the cell cycle. By deregulating the cell cycle these viruses create a situation more favorable for their own replication. They are able to do this by producing specific viral products that inactivate both the RB protein and the p53 protein, essentially unlocking the cell to divide while preventing the cell from undergoing abortive apoptotic cell death. In the case of the SV-40 virus, the large T antigen binds and sequesters both p53 and RB. By contrast, both adenovirus and papillomavirus employ two separate proteins to accomplish the same functional result. The adenovirus E1a protein binds RB while E1b binds p53. Likewise the papilloma protein E7 binds RB while its companion E6 binds p53. Binding of E6 in turn targets p53 for rapid degradation.[64] Thus, these viruses mimic the same cellular changes found in cancer cells genetically deficient of either RB or p53 proteins and are, in fact, commonly used in the laboratory to immortalize normal cells in tissue culture.

A comparison between oncogenes and tumor suppressor genes reveals several important differences. Oncogenes exert their effects through activation/alteration of cellular protooncogenes while tumor suppressor genes, in order to cause cancer, require the deletion or inactivation of a normally expressed gene. Oncogenes are not transmitted in the germ line while tumor suppressor genes can be, resulting in sporadic forms of the former and both sporadic and hereditary forms of the latter. Finally, oncogenes act in a dominant fashion; only one bad copy of the gene is needed to cause the deleterious effects. Tumor suppressor genes (with the exception of *p53* and *Erb* A, which are dominant-negative) are recessive; both copies of the gene must be inactivated before an untoward effect is manifested.

### Multiple Disruptions of Oncogenes and Tumor Suppressor Genes

It is very difficult to prove either clinically or experimentally that a single genetic event is sufficient to cause cancer. Experimentally, in the minimal case, at least two oncogenes (such as *ras* and *myc*) or one oncogene and one tumor suppressor gene (such as *ras* and *p53*) are required in transfection experiments to produce tumors. The situation in clinical cancer is even more complex. Indeed, it would appear from a statistical analysis of cancer incidence vs. age that at least five events or hits are necessary before the average cell becomes cancerous.[65] Multiple-hit scenarios have been partially worked out in the case of both colon cancer and bladder cancer (Fig 18).[66,67] In the case of clinically significant prostate cancer, the number of hits has been estimated to be as high as 12.[68]

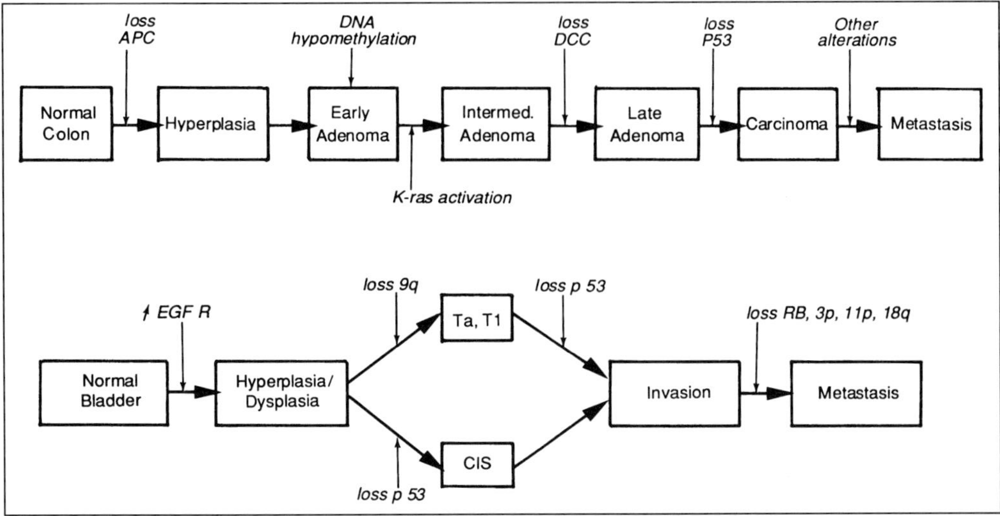


**Fig 18.** A model of the multistep process of carcinogenesis for colon and bladder cancer. In colon cancer the genetic alterations occur in a preferred order but many cases show deviations from this scheme. Invasive bladder cancer appears to evolve via one of two routes characterized by early (CIS) or late (Ta, T1) acquisition of *p53* mutations.

## Genetic Instability

The reason why so many aberrations are necessary to produce cancer may be due to several factors including counteracting homeostatic forces, redundancy in function for critical cellular components, and the ability of cells to undergo cell death when significantly damaged. However, if the chance of a genetic event occurring in a given gene is estimated at one in a million, five events would require $10^{30}$ divisions. Yet the average number of cell divisions occurring during a human lifetime is $10^{16}$. If cancer were purely a statistical event, it would affect less than one in a trillion, not the one-in-four prevalence observed today. Thus, early genetic events must predispose the cell to subsequent genetic events leading to the so-called *mutator phenotype*.[69] Such genetic instability could then allow for a process of *clonal evolution* whereby specific clones of cells are selected because of a growth advantage over their neighbors. The key to understanding how this genetic instability becomes manifest requires an investigation into the proliferative cell cycle pathway itself.

## Internal Mechanisms for Cell Proliferation: Analysis of the Cell Cycle

Each eukaryotic cell from yeast to man is governed by a complex regulatory program that dictates the life cycle of the cell from birth through replication to eventual death. As in the case of the signal transduction pathway, many of these processes and even the actual enzymes responsible for these processes have been highly conserved across species and across millennia. Cancer represents loss of control of these internal processes whereby cells develop an unlimited propensity for proliferation (immortality) coupled with an insensitivity to internal feedback signals responsible for preventing and perpetuating DNA damage (loss of fidelity).[70] While a complete understanding of the mechanics of the cell cycle is not yet available, nonetheless significant inroads have been made with regard to how cancer unbalances this vital program.

Most cells in the human body are in a relatively quiescent state performing specialized tasks but failing to proliferate. Certain cells are able to exit out of this so-

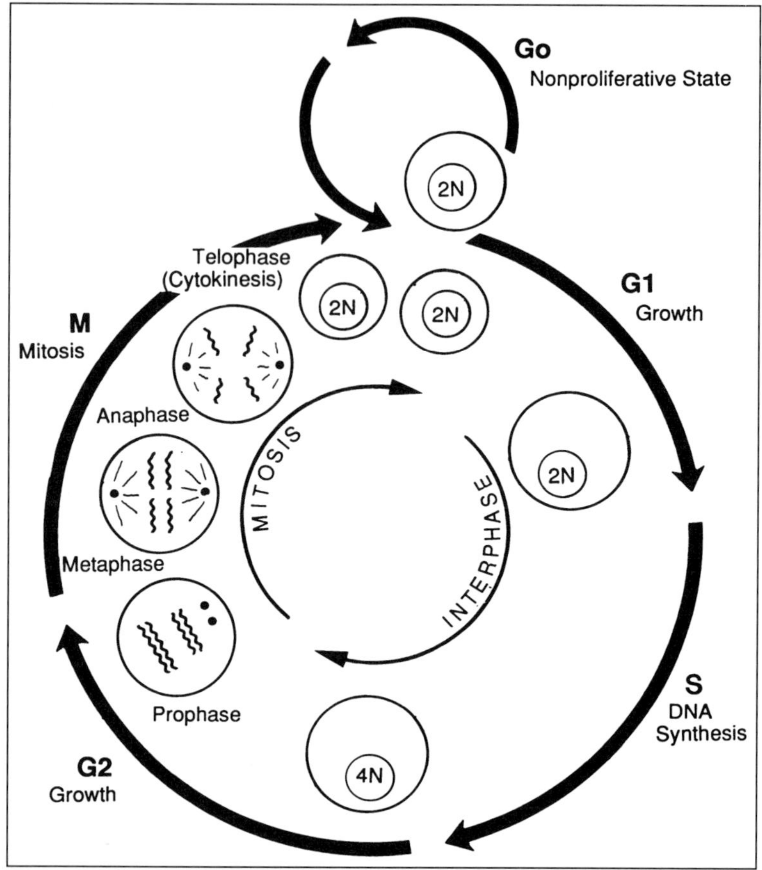


**Fig 19.** Replicating cells pass through four distinct growth phases: the G1 (gap 1) phase during which the cell grows accumulating nutrients and proteins, the S (synthesis) phase during which DNA is replicated, the G2 (gap 2) phase during which DNA repair occurs, and the M (mitosis) phase culminating in chromosomal separation and actual cellular division (cytokinesis). Cycling cells may exit into the G0 resting phase upon completion of the cell cycle and reenter it upon appropriate stimulation.

called G0 resting phase into the G1 phase of the proliferative cell cycle upon exposure to external growth factors. However, progress through the remainder of the replicative cell cycle is relatively independent of external growth factors and relies on internal programs and feedback controls to accomplish eventual cell replication. A depiction of the stages of the cell cycle is given in Fig 19.

The driving force behind progress through the cell cycle are *cell division kinases* (cdk's), proteins whose enzymatic activities vary with the stage of the cell cycle. A paradigm of cell cycle control is illustrated (Fig 20) for fission yeast where a single cdk known as cdc-2 or p34 appears to be the key player.[71] Similar to the mechanism used in signal transduction pathways to exert enzymatic control, the cdc-2 kinase activity is dependent on appropriate phosphorylation and dephosphorylation. In addition, cdk's must combine with other proteins known as *cyclins* to become enzymatically active. Cyclins were so designated because they are periodically synthesized and degraded during the cell cycle forming an internal biological clock for the cell. Another significant feature of this system is that this periodic fluctuation of cdk

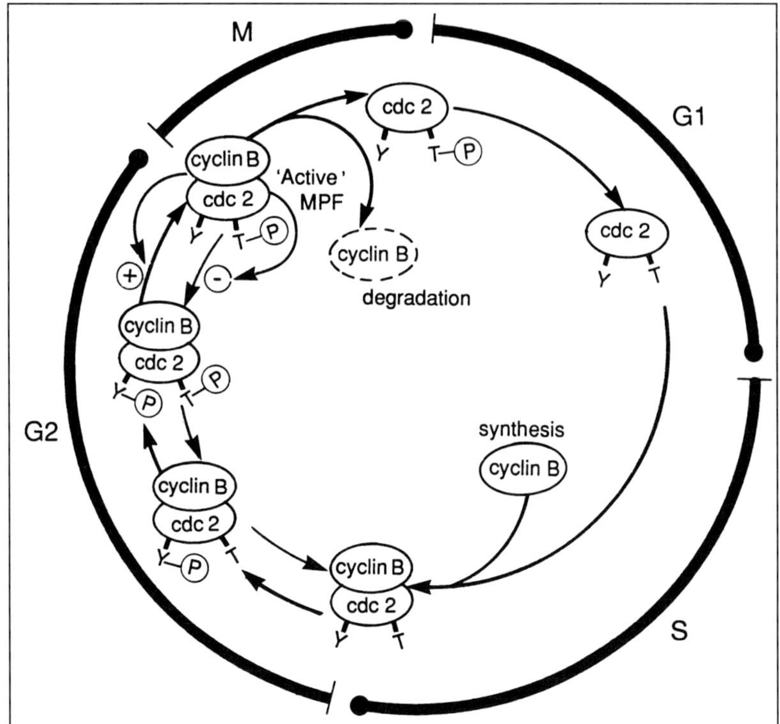


**Fig 20.** A paradigm of eukaryotic cell cycle control is found in budding yeast. Entry into mitosis is triggered by the association of the cell division kinase cdc-2 with cyclin B followed by its activation through phosphorylation. This creates active maturation-promoting factor (MPF), an enzymatic moiety responsible for triggering several downstream mitotic events including nuclear membrane breakdown and chromosomal separation. Exit from mitosis requires the destruction of MPF achieved via cyclin B degradation. The cdc-2 is not consumed during this process and is recycled into the next round of cell replication.

activity forms a self-sustaining cellular engine that modulates cell proliferation.

A similar though more complex system exists in mammalian cells to drive cells through the cell cycle. Six different cdk's (cdk 1–6; cdc-2 = cdk1) and five cyclin families (A–E) have now been identified in humans.[72] It would appear that different cdk–cyclin combinations are operative in specific phases of the cell cycle (Fig 21).

Growth control is established through feedback mechanisms that regulate the passage through specific checkpoints in the cell cycle.[73] These feedback controls ensure that cells finish DNA replication, DNA repair, and chromosomal segregation before they divide. A specific point prior to DNA replication at the G1–S boundary forms one of the most crucial decision points in the cell cycle. Passage through this "restriction point" or "START" requires that the cell attain both a minimal cell size and have appropriate nutrients available. In mammalian cells, positive-acting signals from growth factors facilitate passage through this checkpoint. In some cases at least two complementary factors are required: a *competence factor* and a *progression factor*.[74] Epidermal growth factor, for instance, is competent to bring G0 cells into G1 but requires the additional action of another growth factor, insulin-like growth factor 1 (IGF-1), to progress through this restriction point. Commitment is not absolute, however, as TGF-β, a known growth-inhibiting and differentiation factor, can inhibit the onset of DNA synthesis even when added in the late

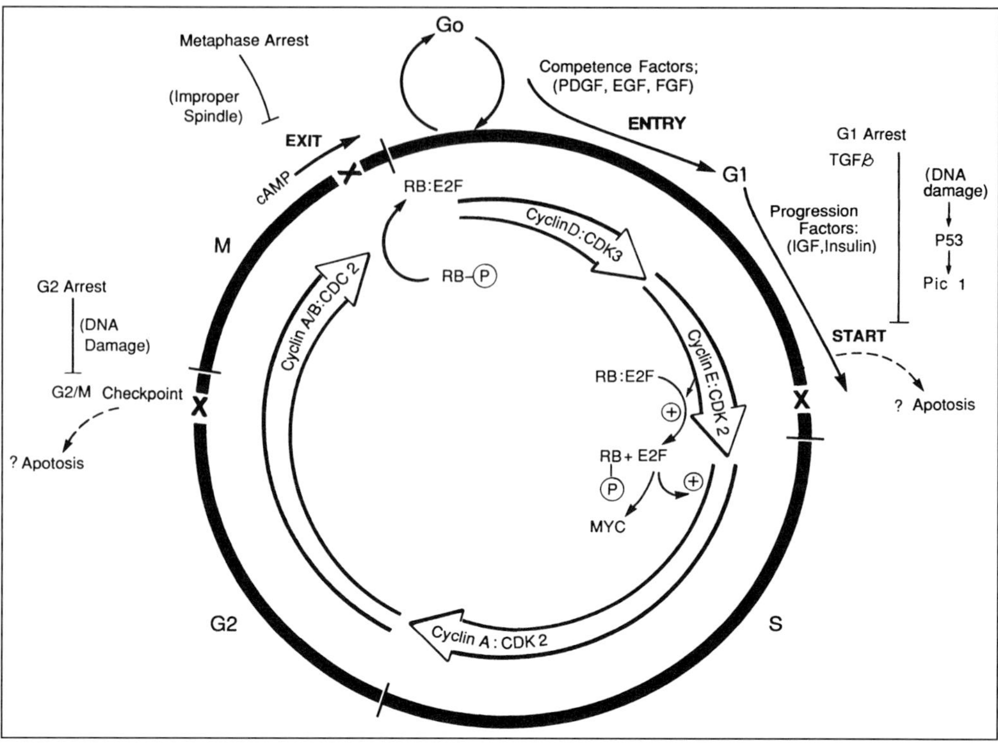


**Fig 21.** Entry into the cell cycle from G0 is achieved by the action of competence factors such as platelet-derived growth factor (PFGF) or epidermal growth factor (EGF), which operate through receptor tyrosine kinases. Progression through the major restriction point, START, however, requires additional progression factors such as insulin or insulin-like growth factor (IGF). Activation of both cyclin D–cdk3 and cyclin E–cdk 2 is required for progress through this restriction point. Negative growth factors such as TGFβ destabilize this complex and arrest cell growth in G1. DNA damage elicits the production of p53, which both by itself and through other downstream regulators such as *pic-1* acts as a brake in slowing down passage through START until DNA repair is complete. Failure to complete DNA repair may result in programmed cell death or apoptosis. The retinoblastoma protein RB also regulates progression through START by sequestering a necessary transcription factor E2F. RB is prompted to release E2F upon phosphorylation by cyclin E–cdk 2. The result of E2F release is the activation of the cyclin A–cdk2 complex as well as production of other transcription factors such as myc. Entry into mitosis likely requires the association of either cyclin A or B with cdc-2, not unlike the situation found in yeast. A checkpoint at the G2–M boundary exists to sense DNA damage incurred during DNA replication resulting in either G2 arrest or apoptosis. Chromosomal separation and exit from mitosis are likely subject to an additional checkpoint that monitors spindle assembly. Cyclic AMP accelerates passage through this point. Upon degradation of the cyclin B–cdc-2 complex, RB is dephosphorylated to allow it to resequester E2F in preparation for another round of cell division. The mechanisms responsible for exit into G0 are poorly understood.

G1 phase. The mechanisms by which this occurs is probably by destabilizing the cdk2–cyclin E complex, a critical step in passage through START.[75]

Both the retinoblastoma protein and p53 appear to play significant roles in mediating passage through this first checkpoint. The RB protein is known to complex an important transcription factor called E2F.[49] Upon phosphorylation of RB by one of the cdk–cyclin complexes (possibly cdk2–cyclin E), free E2F is released to accelerate transcription of DNA synthesis enzymes. E2F also appears to play a role in assembly of the next crucial cdk complex, cdk2–cyclin A. Loss of functional RB protein by either gene deletion or mutation, inappropriate protein phosphorylation, or viral protein sequestration would be expected to uncouple this normally tightly regulated process resulting in premature passage through this checkpoint.

The G1/S transition checkpoint is the first point in the cell cycle where DNA damage is sensed and repaired. The p53 protein plays a significant role in this process.[76] Under normal circumstances DNA damage from ionizing radiation results in the upregulation of p53 protein expression. By an as yet poorly understood process, an increase in p53 is associated with cell cycle arrest in G1 until DNA repair is complete. Furthermore, it would also appear that p53 mediates apoptosis in the event of unsuccessful DNA repair.[77] Cells lacking wild-type p53 are unable to arrest in G1 and are hampered in initiating apoptosis. The result is potential perpetuation or accentuation of genetic damage in the following phase of DNA replication. Indeed, the incidence of gene amplification increases with loss of functional p53.[78]

Once DNA replication is complete there are at least two other critical checkpoints in the cell cycle that must normally be passed before cell division can occur. Unfortunately, little is known about the molecular mechanisms at work in these latter checkpoints. At the G2/M checkpoint, DNA damage and incomplete replication is assessed through an unknown mechanism. This protective feature ensures that the cell does not divide until DNA replication and DNA damage induced during replication is repaired. Patients with the disease ataxia telangiectasia lack this protective feature and are unable to arrest in either G1 or G2.[79] These patients exhibit a very high incidence of cancer. Agents that increase the intracellular concentration of cyclic AMP facilitate passage through this checkpoint.[80]

Exit from mitosis is regulated by degradation of cyclin B. Arrest during mitosis in the metaphase stage is accomplished in certain animal oocytes by maintaining high levels of active cdc2–cyclin B through interaction with the c-*mos* protein product.[81] Exit from mitosis is also prevented in yeast by a mechanism that senses improper spindle assembly.[82] While a mammalian counterpart has not yet been found, loss of such a mechanism could explain the high degree of aneuploidy and chromosomal breakage observed in many mammalian cancers.

Completion of mitosis is also accompanied by dephosphorylation of the RB protein to its active E2F-binding form. It is logical to expect that the phosphatase involved in this process would qualify as a tumor suppressor gene once identified.

One final note regarding the cell cycle concerns exit out of the cycle into G0. While all cells, including cancer cells, can exit into G0 under conditions of appropriate nutrient starvation, the molecular events orchestrating this pathway remain largely unexplored. It may well be that differentiation factors play an important role here.

## SUMMARY

Cancer arises out of a dysregulation of cellular processes involving both the signal transduction pathway and the cell cycle. Positively acting mitogenic signals supplied by growth factors or intermediates, enhanced as a result of qualitative or quantitative overexpression of oncogenes, drive cells into a proliferative state. In addition, loss of tumor suppressor genes responsible for the maintenance of fidelity of DNA replication allows cells to proceed through critical checkpoints in the cell cycle leading to progressive DNA damage in the form of deletions, chromosomal breaks, and aneuploidy. The cumulative result of the interaction between growth accelerators and loss of growth regulators is a genetically unstable cell capable of evolution into the autonomous and destructive disease we know as cancer.

## METASTASES

Clinically not all cancers are equal. That is to say, tumors can be divided into two major groups: benign and malignant. Benign tumors are noninvasive growths that do not spread to distant organs. Unless located at a functionally vital site (eg, the brain), they pose little threat to the patient and usually can be removed surgically. In contrast, malignant neoplasms are readily invasive, metastasize to other organs in the body, and eventually kill their host.[83] *The biochemical events that distinguish malignant from benign neoplasms remain unknown but are the target of intense investigation.*

The term *metastasis* was coined by Joseph Claude Recamier, a French physician, in his 1829 treatise *Recherches du Cancer.* He was the first to provide anatomic evidence that metastases are caused by cancer cells that enter the circulation and travel to distant sites in the body. Before this work, surgeons and anatomists believed that colonies of tumors "in more distant organs" arose independently.

The ability to metastasize, then, represents the principal life-threatening component of cancer. Only a fraction of parental tumor cells acquire this property, perhaps fewer than 1 in $10^4$. The earliest indication that cells in a single tumor may differ in their ability to metastasize came from studies that demonstrated that only a few of many clones derived from a single tumor are able to generate metastases when transplanted into another tumor-compatible animal such as a nude mouse.[84] These differences were not the result of adaptation to local organ environment by the clones but represented a subpopulation already existing within the parent tumor. The mechanisms by which tumor cells diversify and become heterogeneous are not fully understood. Most human tumors result from the proliferation of a single transformed cell. The cellular diversity observed within such tumors probably results from a continuous process of tumor progression and evolution resulting from genetic instability. When this variability is subjected to host selection pressures, new sublines emerge whose growth advantage is manifested by increased malignancy. In other words, the more metastatic a tumor cell population becomes, the higher its spontaneous mutation rate.[85]

This observation has led to the important principle that tumor metastasis is not merely the result of the high growth rate but rather the product of a complex series of events and changes in cell behavior. A metastasizing tumor cell must break loose from its parent tumor, invade the matrix between cells, and penetrate the membrane of a blood vessel. It must survive its passage in the bloodstream, when it is subject to immune surveillance and hence immune-mediated destruction, and emerge from the bloodstream in a favorable spot. After lodging in the surrounding tissue, it must induce the growth of new blood vessels to support the new tumor. Each of these steps undoubtedly is controlled by a different molecular system. A failure in any one of these systems would most likely render a tumor cell incapable of metastasizing (Fig 22).

Perhaps the most important characteristic required by a metastasizing cell is invasiveness. A metastatic cell must cross a basement membrane barrier at several points. Basement membranes, which consist of a complex of proteins including collagen IV, laminin, and fibronectin, underlie the epithelial cells from which the common cancers are derived. They also surround the

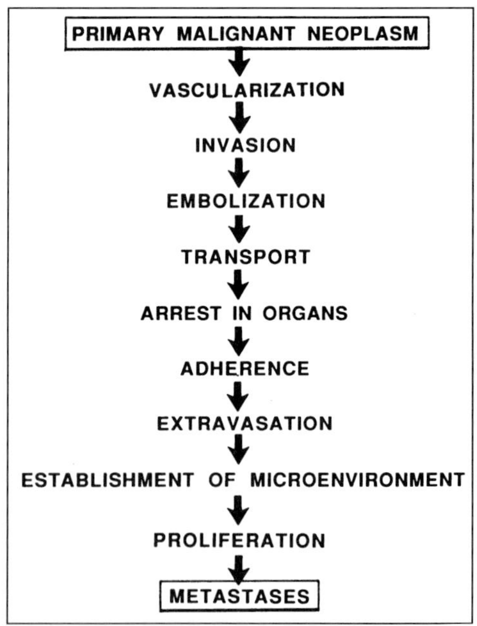


**Fig 22.** Formation of a cancer metastasis. The process is sequential and requires that cells survive a series of highly selective events.

smooth muscles of blood vessels. Tumor cells adapt by increased secretions of enzymes that facilitate cell movement through such barriers. Examples are lysosomal hydrolases, collagenases, and the serine protease plasminogen activator.

After invading a vessel, tumor cells grow locally at the site of penetration or detach to be carried off to distant sites. Animal studies reveal that the efferent venous blood from an organ containing 1 g of implanted tumor can carry several million released cancer cells over a 24-hr period.[86] Radiolabeled tumor studies, however, demonstrate that less than 1% of shed cancer cells survive passage through the circulation and less than 0.1% result in metastases.[87] Clearly the majority of tumor emboli do not survive to develop into new cancers. Two distinct mechanisms are probably responsible for their ultimate death. The first is nonspecific immune surveillance carried out by macrophages, natural killer cells, and neutrophils. However, even under optimal circumstances, the system cannot account for the rapid destruction of almost all circulating tumor cells. Instead, passive mechanical processes such as turbulence probably are responsible for most tumor cell deaths. Unlike blood cells, tumor cells are not sufficiently deformable to survive the high shear forces imposed on them by the microcirculation. It is apparent, however, that if a cell is indeed able to survive its journey to a distant organ it must then undergo a three-step process to implant. The first step is the adhesion of the tumor cell to the basement membrane. The adhesion is mediated by specific receptors on the tumor cell surface that recognize components of the basement membrane. The second step is activation of destructive enzymes that cleave or unravel basement membrane molecules immediately beneath the tumor cell. The third step is the protrusion of the tumor cell into the zone of lysis followed by migration of the entire tumor cell. It is interesting to note that the genetic mechanisms responsible for this process are not unique to tumor cells. For example, similar invasive behavior occurs during implantation of the placenta in the wall of the uterus and during formation of organs in the embryo. Likewise, circulating white blood cells must penetrate the walls of the vessels to reach a site of infection.

### Distribution of Metastasis

Is the distribution of metastasis random or selective? Familiar examples include the propensity of prostate cancer to metastasize to bone and renal cell cancer to metastasize to the adrenal. Experimental animal studies with radiolabeled tumor cells have demonstrated that tumor cells become arrested in the microenvironment of many organs but the arrested cells grow into metastases in only specific organs.[88]

In 1928, Ewing postulated that the location of metastasis was the result of mechanical factors such as circulatory anatomy and rate of blood flow.[89] Although this may account for regional metastasis, such as adrenal metastasis from renal cell carcinoma, it does not account for the distribution of more distant metastasis, such as contralateral adrenal metastases associated with renal cell carcinoma. A more likely explanation was set forth in the "seed-and-soil" hypothesis originally set forth by the British surgeon Stephen Paget in 1889.[90] He analyzed the metastasis pattern of breast carcinoma and concluded that the distribution was nonrandom and that certain types of cancers tended to metastasize preferentially to certain organs. He proposed that cancer cells, like plant seeds, may travel in all directions but can only grow if they fall on congenial soil. Experimental support for Paget's theory is derived from the evaluation of metastatic patterns in animals with ectopically implanted organs. Tumor cells with a predilection for lung metastases were injected into animals that harbored ectopically placed tissue fragments including lung. Metastases occurred in the ectopically grafted lung tissue as well as in the in situ lung; metastases to other grafted control organs did not occur. The phenomenon was not due to "homing" of the tumor cells since radiolabeled tumor cells within the animals were distributed evenly to all sites irrespective of whether they contained ectopic organs.[91]

The principle is that the sites of metastasis are not determined solely by the characteristics of the neoplastic cells but also by the microenvironment provided by the host tissue.

Finally, once tumors have found the proper ''soil'' they begin to grow, and their ability to continue to grow, at least after the first several days, is dependent on their ability to induce their own blood supply—a process called *angiogenesis.*

## Angiogenesis

Exponential growth of tumor cells requires the support of nutrient blood vessels. Angiogenesis is important to this end because it is the fundamental process by which new blood vessels are formed. In simple terms, tumor growth and metastasis are angiogenesis dependent.[92] The importance of angiogenesis is recognized by the fact that without organized vascularization, solid tumors are incapable of growing beyond 1–2 mm in diameter.[93]

Research directed at this process began with the idea of learning more about malignant transformation and understanding aspects of ''antiangiogenesis'' for use in therapeutics. With models developed that utilized naturally transparent structures such as the cornea of the eye, several interesting facts about normal angiogenesis became known. For example, it is possible for capillary channels to develop in a pure culture of endothelial cells that obviously do not contain blood and are otherwise empty. These and other experiments demonstrated that blood pressure and blood flow are not necessary for the formation of a capillary network. A second important observation was that, in general, endothelial cells form new capillaries only where there is a need for them, and their growth can be induced, for example, by local infections and damaged tissue.

It is now known that specific angiogenic molecules can initiate this process and that specific inhibitory molecules can stop it. These molecules with opposing functions appear to be continuously acting in concert to maintain a quiescent microvasculature in which endothelial cell turnover is normally measured in thousands of days. At the present time several angiogenic factors and inhibitors have been discovered, and while their properties can be listed (Table 4), the elucidation of their interaction with each other is only beginning to be uncovered.[94]

Currently, there are eight angiogenic polypeptides that have been completely purified, sequenced, and cloned and seem to have diverse properties. For example, angiogenin isolated from human colon cancer has ribonucleolytic properties. Vascular endothelial growth factor (VEGF), vascular permeability factor (VPF), and platelet-derived endothelial cell growth factor (PD-ECGF) act mainly as mitogens for vascular endothelial cells. Finally, fibroblastic growth factors (FGFs) are pleiotropic in that they stimulate the growth of endothelial cells, smooth muscle cells, fibroblasts, and certain epithelial cells.

Angiogenesis, especially as it relates to malignancy, is affected not only by the named angiogenic factors (and probably more) but also by factors that inhibit an-

**TABLE 4. Angiogenic Polypeptides[94]**

| | |
|---|---|
| bFGF and aFGF | Both bFGF and aFGF are mitogenic for a wide variety of cells types, stimulate endothelial cells to migrate and form tubes, and act as embryonic inducers. |
| VEGF/VPF | Proliferation activity is highly specific for vascular endothelial cells; increases vascular permeability; is structurally related to PDGF. |
| PD-ECGF | Stimulates endothelial cell DNA synthesis and chemotaxis; amplifies DNA synthesis activity of FGFs on endothelial cells. |
| TGFα | Transforms normal cells into malignant phenotype; binds EGF receptor. |
| Angiogenin | Stimulates endothelial cells to form diacylglycerol and secrete prostacyclin by activating phospholipase C and phospholipase $A_2$. |
| TGFβ | Enhances extracellular matrix production; chemotactic for monocytes. |
| TNFα | Induces production of bFGF in endothelial cells and enhances its secretion. Chemotactic for monocytes and activates macrophages. |

giogenesis. Undoubtedly the onset of angiogenic activity in tumors is determined by the balance of these factors. An example would be tumor cell proteases (eg, plasminogen activator) and inhibitors (plasminogen activator inhibitor). The balance between them precisely regulates the level of extracellular proteolysis and thus promotes or suppresses angiogenesis.[95]

After the angiogenic phenotype has been established through factors secreted either by the tumor cells or macrophages, a number of barriers in the microvasculature may have to be overcome. For example, resting endothelial cells are surrounded by specialized cells, pericytes, which help to maintain the endothelium in a quiescent, nonproliferating state. Pericytes in the microvasculature appear to inhibit endothelial proliferation. The contact between pericytes and endothelial cells leads to activation of latent TGF-β produced by both cells. It is not known how tumors overcome this barrier.

### Clinical Correlation

Angiogenesis research is currently applied to cancer treatment in two ways: diagnostic applications and inhibition of angiogenesis in neoplasia. Quantitation of oncogenesis in biopsy specimens of breast cancer provides an independent marker of future metastatic risk.[96] This same application may prove beneficial in differentiating invasive from noninvasive prostate cancer.[97] Likewise the excretion of acidic FGF in urine may prove to help in diagnosis and prognosis of transitional cell carcinoma.[98]

## IMMUNOBIOLOGY OF CANCER

### Immune Surveillance

The idea that the immune system's capability to recognize foreign invaders could be extended to include aberrant tumor cells was put forth as early as 1908 by Erlich. By the late 1950s Burnet and Thomas had formalized the idea of *immune surveillance* whereby a major function of the immune system was to recognize and destroy malignantly transformed cells before they grew into tumors.[99] Evidence that such a phenomenon was occurring included the rare but documented cases of spontaneous regression of tumors, particularly malignant melanomas and renal cell carcinomas, and the notable infiltration of several tumor types such as seminomas with inflammatory cells. This theory gradually fell into disrepute, however, with the recognition that conditions associated with immunodeficiency or immunosuppression were rarely responsible for the emergence of the common solid malignancies such as breast cancer, prostate cancer, lung cancer, and colon cancer. Nevertheless, the basic concept that the immune system could be harnessed as a vehicle by which cancer cells could be targeted has remained strong. Indeed, as the fundamental knowledge of the immune system has increased, immunotherapy has begun to be a viable clinical option in the treatment of cancer, and in some urologic cancers (bladder and renal) may even become the treatment of choice.

### Antigenic Features of Cancer Cells

The immune system possesses the fundamental ability to distinguish self from nonself. This property emerges out of the selective deletion of autoreactive clones during embryonic development as well as the active suppression of autoreactive responses that may have escaped developmental restriction.[100] The big question in immunotherapy of cancer is whether the immune system is capable of distinguishing self from altered self. Cancers resulting from treatment with a variety of chemical or physical carcinogens such as methylcholanthrene (a surface carcinogen) or ultraviolet radiation can clearly be recognized and rejected by immunocompetent animals. In many cases it has been unequivocally established that mutations in a single DNA base pair causing a change in one amino acid of a protein is sufficient to incite a protective immune response.[101] Likewise, the few human cancers associated with viral pathogens such as Burkitt's lymphoma and nasopharnygeal carcinoma (induced by the Epstein–Barr virus) or HTLV I–induced lymphoma can engender virus-specific antitumor responses.[102] In these cases it is the presence of specific foreign viral antigens on tumor cells that triggers immune rejection. For years it was feared that spontaneously arising tumors might not be sufficiently different from normal cells to allow immune recognition. However, now it is apparent that even these cancers possess recognizable alterations perceptible to the immune system.

Recent investigations have shown that the same biochemical and genetic alterations present in cancer cells can result in perceptible changes in cell antigenicity. For instance, mutant oncoproteins such as ras, p53, and RB can themselves be immunogenic.[103] As genetic instability appears to be frequent in cancer, it is likely too that amino acid alterations in other proteins might commonly occur. Another consequence of genetic dysregulation in cancer is the expression of previously unexpressed or actively repressed *oncofetal* proteins. Such is clearly the case with α-fetoprotein expression by certain malignant germ cell tumors.[104] Likewise, loss of more differentiated biochemical processes such as protein glycosylation appears to occur frequently in cancers. This may result, for instance, in the expression of previously cryptic antigens such as the Thompsen–Friedenreich antigen or the Lewis X antigen that occur in bladder cancer.[105] It is even possible that more subtle changes associated with malignant transformation such as the induction of stress proteins or alterations in membrane lipid constitution can be perceived by the immune system.[106] The big question is, why aren't these changes normally sufficient to incite a protective immune response?

The reason why cancer cells are not eliminated by an immune system theoretically capable of recognizing them is unknown. Many hypotheses have been ventured ranging from blocking antibodies to active cellular tumor suppressors.[107] While specific examples of each of these mechanisms can be found in select systems, evidence is emerging that immune unresponsiveness to cancer is the result of a failure of spontaneous tumors to be properly processed for immune recognition.[108]

### Basis for Immune Recognition

The immune system is composed of two general arms of defense: (1) an innate or natural defense system that possesses the ability to respond rapidly but somewhat nonspecifically to foreign pathogens and (2) a highly specific but more delayed defense system that remembers previous encounters with past foes.[109] The innate immune system includes the granular leukocytes (neutrophils, eosinophils, and mast cells), macrophages, and natural killer (NK) cells. The specific immune system includes B cells responsible for humoral antibody production and T cells that orchestrate specific cellular responses on the basis of membrane-bound receptors. Communication between and within each system is achieved through short-lived trafficking proteins produced by these cells termed *cytokines.*[110] Cytokines regulate cell migration, proliferation, and specific functional activation. In this way specific mechanisms are brought to bear on sites flagged by acute inflammation. In turn, specificity can be conferred to cells of the innate immune system by antibodies. Thus, binding of specific antibody can facilitate phagocytosis or complement dependent lysis. Direct binding of antibodies via Fc receptors to NK cells and macrophages can also allow directed cellular killing, a process referred to as *antibody-dependent cellular cytotoxicity* (ADCC). Chemotactic factors produced by reconnaissance cells of the specific immune system may also recruit less specific effector cells to the scene.

Generation of specific immunity requires a coordinated system of antigen presentation and recognition. With the exception of certain polyvalent antigens, professional *antigen-presenting cells* (APCs), which include macrophages, dendritic cells, and activated B cells, must process antigen before it can be recognized by T cells.[111] This processing results in the surface expression of small pieces of degraded proteins known as peptides bound to molecules known as *major histocompatibility complex* (MHC) antigens. Although originally defined by their ability to mediate tissue transplantation rejection, it

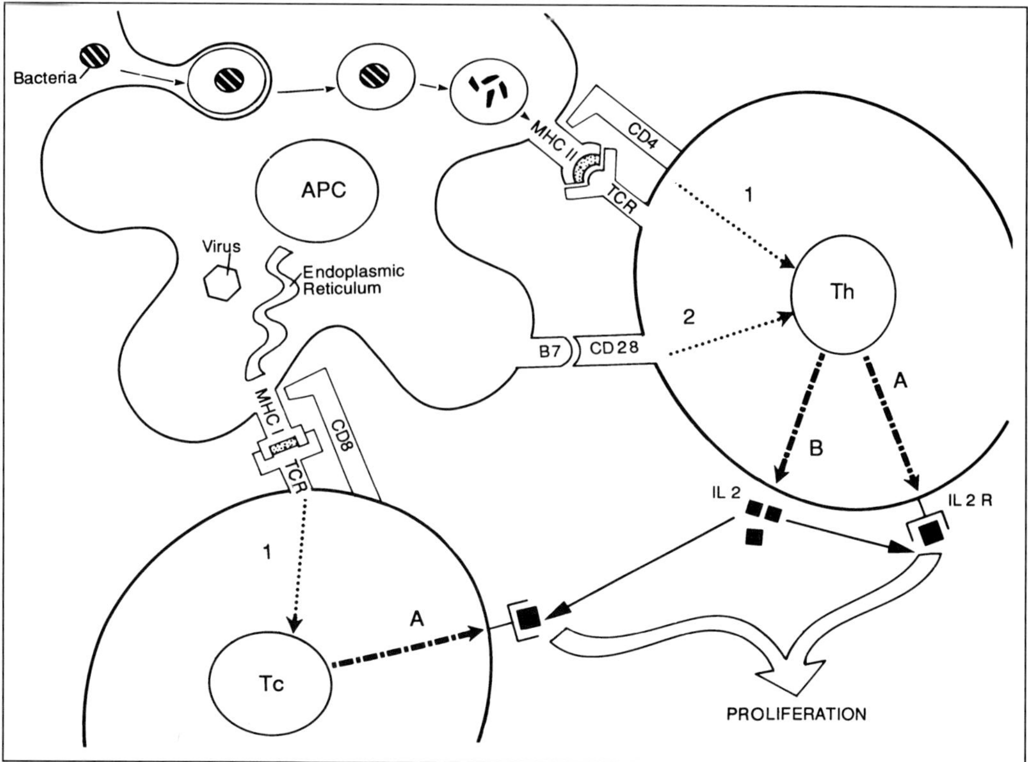


**Fig 23.** Antigen presenting cells (APCs) process exogenous antigen for presentation on their cell surface in the form of small peptides bound to class II major histocompatibility complex molecules (MHC II). Helper T cells (Th) bearing the appropriate T-cell receptors (TCR) recognize the peptide:MHC complex and stabilize it through the CD4 molecule. As a result of this interaction, a signal (1) is transduced to the cell nucleus leading to the production of high specificity interleukin-2 receptors (IL-2R). This also primes the Th cell for production of IL-2 upon receiving the second signal (2) delivered by a costimulatory molecule (in this case binding of B7 to CD28). If both signals are present, an autocrine feedback loop is established to drive the clonal proliferation of the Th cell. Failure to receive this second signal results in anergy or even programmed cell death of the Th cell. Cytotoxic T cells recognize endogenous antigens albeit in the context of a class I MHC and CD8 molecule. However, because they are somewhat less proficient at generating the second signal, the additional presence of IL-2-secreting helper cells is often necessary for their clonal expansion.

is now known that these MHC proteins play a vital role in the presentation of antigen to T cells.

Two general classes of MHCs exist with distinctive functionality. Class I MHC proteins typically express foreign peptides that have invaded a cell. For example, as viruses commandeer the normal intracellular protein synthesis machinery, virus peptides are presented at the cell surface on class I MHCs. Class II MHCs, on the other hand, present peptides derived from external sources such as bacterial pathogens (Fig 23). Only T cells expressing the CD4 antigen react with class II MHC peptides while T cells bearing the CD8 antigen react with class I MHC peptides. Classically, CD4 T cells have been known as *helper T cells* and CD8 T cells as *cytotoxic T lymphocytes* or CTLs, though it is now apparent that these strict functional divisions are not always kept.[112] Further subdivision of labor is present within each T-cell subset. CD4 T cells that provide T cell help are known as TH1 cells while those that primarily help B cells are known as TH2

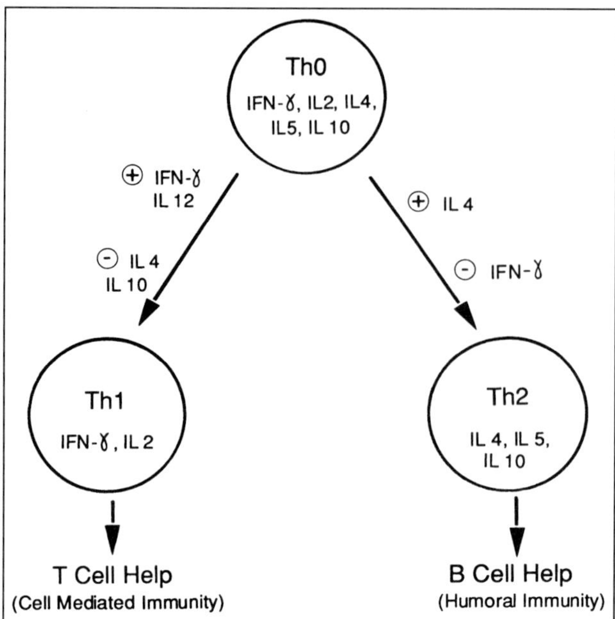


**Fig 24.** Upon short-term stimulation, T-helper 0 cells produce a wide range of cytokines. Under chronically stimulated conditions, however, Th0 cells differentiate along one of two pathways to provide for preferential T-cell help and cell-mediated immunity (Th1) or B-cell help and humoral immunity (Th2). The stimulus for divergence is not completely understood but in part depends on the activity of other cell types such as macrophages, which shunt either toward or away from TH1 differentiation by the production of IL-12 or IL-10, respectively. In addition, dominance of one T-helper response effectively switches off the other by the production of mutually antagonistic cytokines such as IL-4 and interferon-γ.

cells[113] (Fig 24). A similar subdivision among CD8 cells may distinguish CTLs from suppressor cells. T cells bearing neither CD4 nor CD8 surface antigens exist that possess a completely different T-cell receptor known as γδ (to differentiate from the αβ T cell receptor found on CD4/8 T cells). γδ T cells do not recognize antigens on either class I or class II MHCs.[114] The normal function of these γδ T cells is unknown but may play a role in the recognition and elimination of specific pathogens or even "stressed" or senescent cells.

As part of the closely knit system of mutual regulation and coordination between various components of the immune system, cytokine pathways exist to regulate the control of MHC expression and directionality of the immune response.[115] Thus, *interferons* and *tumor necrosis factor* (TNF) can upregulate MHC expression. Other cytokines such as *interleukin 4* and *interleukin 10* promote TH2 differentiation favoring humoral responses while *γ-interferon* and *interleukin 12* promote cell-mediated immunity through TH1 differentiation[116] (Fig 24).

The final level of complexity and control is achieved by the use of *costimulatory signals* provided by APCs to T cells.[117] Lack of such a signal effectively vetoes the generation of the classical T-cell immune response in spite of appropriate receptor to MHC–peptide binding. Thus, immune responses are achieved only when specific conditions are met: (1) antigen is processed by an APC; (2) antigenic peptide fragments are expressed in association with the appropriate MHC molecule; (3) a specific T-cell receptor engages the peptide–MHC complex; and (4) a costimulatory signal is issued by the APC to the T cell. Event 3 results in the expression of high-affinity interleukin 2 (IL-2) receptors on the T lymphocyte. Event 4 results in the production of IL-2, a mitogenic signal that feeds back in a positive autocrine manner to cause clonal T-cell proliferation thus promulgating the immune response (Fig 23). Absence of any of these four conditions effectively prevents T-cell activation. Absence of the costimulatory signal usually within the first 24 hr, in particular, results in T-cell *anergy* or a state of unresponsiveness.[118]

## Strategies in Cancer Immunotherapy

**Antibody-Targeted Therapy.** The recognition of the existence of *tumor-associated antigens* (TAAs) together with the development of technological procedures to manufacture *monoclonal antibodies* of defined specificity has permitted several cancer-targeting approaches using antibodies.[119] By linking moieties such as bacteria toxins, chemotherapeutic drugs, or even radioisotopes to monoclonal antibodies, the hope has been to develop a "magic bullet" for cancer. However, while antibody-directed tumor localization has been possible in some instances, therapeutic success has been limited by several problems. Penetration into large tumor masses is often poor although it may be improved using smaller antibody fragments that maintain specificity. Liver and spleen toxicity has occurred due to uptake of antibody complexes by the reticuloendothelial system. Normal cells expressing low levels of cross-reacting antigen are also a problem. Finally, the development of immune reactivity against the antibody (usually of mouse origin) has resulted in rapid clearance of the antibody. Recent advances in the development of human or humanized monoclonal antibodies with greater specificities may solve some of these problems.[120]

Variants of toxin targeting utilizing other localizing molecules besides antibodies are currently under investigation. One of the most promising approaches involves the use of growth factors that bind to cancer cells expressing increased amounts of growth factor receptors. Bladder cancer has been of particular interest because of its heightened expression of the epidermal growth factor (EGF) receptor and the ease of intravesical drug delivery. This permits high dosing with a significantly lower chance of systemic toxicity.[121]

**Tumor Vaccine Therapy.** With the exception of malignant melanoma, clinical attempts to generate systemic immunity by immunization with native or modified tumor products alone have been uniformly unsuccessful.[122] Indeed, in situ angiographic infarction of renal cell carcinoma was at one time advocated as a theoretical means to liberate stores of tumor antigens to provoke an immune response.[123] The reason these attempts failed is not altogether clear but probably relates to a failure to appropriately activate MHC-dependent antigen presentation to specific T cells via APCs.

**Bacterial Adjuvant Therapy (BCG).** It has long been appreciated that bacterial products are potent nonspecific stimulators of the immune system. Before immune mechanisms were well understood, tumors in the vicinity of local suppurative infections had been observed to regress.[124] This idea gradually led to testing of agents such as BCG (bacille Calmette Guérin) and *Corynebacteria* against a variety of cancers and the eventual demonstration of BCG's clinical efficacy in both melanoma and bladder cancer. Indeed, BCG immunotherapy is currently the most effective agent against superficial bladder cancer with complete response rates in the 60%–80% range.[125]

The mechanism by which BCG effects bladder tumor destruction remains unknown. Evidence exists suggesting a localized inflammatory response in the bladder that recruits and activates macrophages and both CD4 and CD8 T cells.[126] Cytokines such as Il-2, IL-6, TNF, and interferon-γ peak during the latter stages of treatment and are associated with prominent expression of MHC class II antigens on the urothelium.[127,128] However, since systemic immunity is not generated, it is unlikely that a classical cytotoxic T cell (CTL) response to tumor antigens is occurring. It remains to be seen whether tumor cells are killed by virtue of their altered state or simply because they are bystander victims in a hostile humoral and cellular environment.

**Adoptive Cellular Immunotherapy.** Based on the concept that the immune system is capable of mounting antitumor responses when properly stimulated, methods have been developed to harvest lymphocytes from cancer patients and activate and expand them in vitro. *Peripheral blood lymphocytes* (PBLs) activated in this manner by IL-2 results in the generation and proliferation of so-called *lymphokine-activated killer* (LAK) cells possessing markedly enhanced though somewhat nonspecific tumoricidal activity.[129] The actual cell type responsible for LAK activity is not completely understood but may represent a form of activated NK cell or T cell. Clinical trials with LAK cell therapy has resulted in dramatic responses and even cures in patients with widely metastatic renal cell carcinoma and melanoma.[130] Complete responses and actual cures, however, have disappointingly remained at the 10% level. This therapy has also been extremely toxic owing to the concomitant administration of large doses of IL-2 causing a generalized capillary leak syndrome. It has also failed to be effective in many other forms of genitourinary cancer including bladder and prostate cancer.[131]

As a means to improve on this therapy, it was hoped that lymphocytes isolated from tumors themselves, so-called *tumor-infiltrating lymphocytes* or TILs, might possess greater specificity and efficacy.[131] Unfortunately, no significant improvement over LAK cell therapy has yet been realized.[132]

**Cytokine Therapy.** The direct administration of powerful *biological response modifiers* such as IL-2, TNF, and interferons has achieved limited clinical success against certain cancers. Interferon-α, for instance, results in complete clinical remissions in over 90% of hairy cell leukemias.[133] Its efficacy as a single agent in renal cell carcinoma is approximately 15%[134] and as an intracavitary agent against refractory superficial bladder cancer, about 30%.[135] When combined with IL-2, roughly 30% of patients with renal cell carcinoma can achieve long-term remissions.[136] The mechanism of cytotoxicity is not clear but may involve the in vivo generation of LAK, NK, or CTL cells. TNF alone has met with much less clinical success but some limited activity has been observed against superficial bladder cancer.[137] New agents on the horizon include IL-12, a potent activator of both CTLs and NK cells that also possesses the capacity to facilitate TH1 cell-mediated responses.[138]

**Future Approaches.** With an increased understanding of the mechanism of T-cell activation coupled with the advent of gene transfer technology, it is likely that many new approaches to cancer immunotherapy will be investigated. The most promising approaches to date include the transfer of cytokine genes and genes encoding co-stimulatory signals into tumor cells.[139,140] Upon reintroduction of lethally irradiated transduced tumor cells, systemic memory against subsequent tumor challenge has been observed in several animal model systems. The eventual clinical impact of this technology is unknown but several phase I trials are currently underway.

## NEW DIRECTIONS: PRESENT AND FUTURE

### Programmed Cell Death

Cell death occurs normally during the planned development of both vertebrates and nonvertebrates and probably occurs as part of a controlled genetic process.[141] As a matter of fact, if cells don't die at the right times and in the right places, the developing brain, for example, can't form its myriad of precise connections between nerve cells.[142] Historically this is defined as *apoptosis.* Based on morphologic characteristics of cell disintegration in a variety of tissues, the concept of apoptosis was developed to describe the naturally occurring cell death that plays a complementary but opposite role to mitosis in regulation of animal cell populations.[143] In a sense, it was suggested that cells have a metabolic cascade that when activated will lead to removal of the cell. Initially apoptosis involves enzymatic degradation of genomic DNA into nucleosomic oligomers, which gives a typical "step-ladder" appearance after gel electrophoresis.[144] This DNA fragmentation is subsequently followed by irreversible morphologic changes such as chromatic condensation, nuclear disintegration, cell surface blebbing, and eventually cellular fragmentation into a cluster of membrane-bound apoptotic bodies.[145] In contrast to this energy-dependent process of programmed cell death is another type of cell death process termed *necrotic cell death,* which is energy-independent and induced by noxious stimuli to cells such as heat, freezing, exposure to detergents, and so forth. Therefore cell death that results from severe environmental perturbations and not from a process intrinsic to the cell should be considered distinctly different from apoptosis and only the latter type should be considered necrosis.

The regulation of programmed cell death is determined by several genes in invertebrates.[141] However, its regulation in vertebrates is poorly understood. The *Bcl-2* oncogene located on chromosome 18 has provided some useful information in this regard. Many types of lymphoid neoplasms exhibit characteristic chromosomal translocations that juxtapose the powerful transcriptional regulatory regions of the immunoglobulin or T-cell receptor loci and protooncogenes resulting in overexpression of the oncogene in question. In a high proportion of human follicular B-cell lymphomas, the *Bcl-2* oncogene is found next to the immunoglobulin heavy-chain locus on chromosome 19. The Bcl-2 oncoprotein is unique by virtue of the fact that it seems to act by promoting survival rather than by promoting proliferation. For example, introduction of the *Bcl-2* gene into the myeloid or pre-B cell lines that are IL-3–dependent does not change their dependence on IL-3 for growth; however, removal of IL-3 no longer induces the rapid apoptosis seen in nontransfected cells.[146] Instead, the cells stop growing but remain viable for long periods of time. Thus, *Bcl-2* seems to prevent programmed cell death. Although still early, some data indicate that the effects of *Bcl-2* can be modulated by both oncogenes and suppressor genes. This is somewhat intuitive because abnormalities of *Bcl-2* cannot make cancers on their own. For example, the oncoprotein myc, in addition to stimulating cell proliferation, can stimulate apoptosis as well. In a sense, the myc oncoprotein can give the cell two options: proliferate or die.[147] Which of these two actually happens depends on what other signals the cell receives; if the *Bcl-2* signal is given, the cell survives and proliferates. If not, apoptosis occurs. There is also evidence that some cancer suppressor genes may work through the induction of apoptosis (or lack thereof). For example, the p53 tumor suppressor protein seems to act like a "brake" on tumor growth. There is growing evidence that this may, in part, occur through apoptosis. Likewise, a mutation in the p53 gene may impair its ability to induce apoptosis.

The overall goal in achieving knowledge of mammalian apoptosis, especially relative to tissues with high rates of malignancy such as breast and prostate, is to eventually "harness" the control mechanisms such that apoptosis can be artificially induced early in the course of disease to cure the cancer and avoid metastasis. Significant work has already been done with prostate cancer. Experimental studies in animals have demonstrated that tumor regression following androgen ablation involved first an inhibition of cell proliferation, followed by an activation of programmed cell death as defined by typical biochemical and morphologic events.[148] Associated with this response was an enhanced expression of transforming growth factor-β, which is a potent inhibitor of cell proliferation and itself has been shown to induce apoptosis in other tissues.[149] *TRPM-2* is another gene that is "activated" in prostate in association with apoptosis following androgen ablation.[150] Although its function is not known, it has been demonstrated to be induced during programmed cell death in a large variety of other tissues.[151]

The evolutionary conservation of programmed cell death among different species as well as the ability of both normal and malignant cells to undergo programmed cell death via what appears to be a common process suggests a well-defined genetic program for this mode of cell death. Further study of its genetic control could lead to methodologies to "tap into" the system and induce cell death. For example, as previously noted, experiments have shown that overexpression of the *p53* gene in some tumor cells leads to apoptosis and eventual cell death. *p53* is loosely defined as a tumor suppressor gene and is known to stop growth in most transformed cells into which it has been introduced.[152,153] Furthermore, overexpression of *p53* causes cell cycle arrest near the G1–S boundary.[154] This rationale was exploited in an experiment in which the *p53* gene was placed under control of the metallothionein MT-1 promoter, which was then stably transfected into a human colon tumor–derived cell line E13.[155] When the transfected cells were treated with zinc chloride, which then induced the expression of *p53,* soft agar colony formation was inhibited, and established tumors in nude mice underwent regression. The most interesting part, however, was that regressing tumors showed histologic features of apoptosis and that it was induced both in vitro and in vivo. The apoptosis of cells in culture was quite rapid, being essentially complete after 4 days of *p53* induction. In contrast, established tumors in vivo took approximately 2 months to complete apoptosis.

Finally, research on apoptosis may shed light on one of the toughest problems in cancer therapy—the development of resistance to chemotherapeutic drugs. One of the best examples demonstrated that transfection of a pre–B-cell leukemia with a *Bcl-2*–containing retrovirus rendered it resistant to several chemotherapeutic agents.[156] It may therefore be necessary to derive drugs that can circumvent the block by *Bcl-2* as well as drugs that can activate apoptosis.

## Gene Therapy

Probably the most logical conclusion for much of genetic research is the hope of gene therapy, a concept based on the assumption that definitive treatment for genetic disease should be possible by directing treatment to the site of the defect itself within the genome.

There are two basic strategies for gene therapy: *gene replacement* and *gene augmentation.* Gene replacement is the most ideal of the two. In what is called homologous recombination, the healthy or therapeutic gene would replace the damaged copy exactly. This approach has the theoretical advantage of the introduced gene functioning correctly. In addition, there would be a reduced likelihood that random insertion will activate a quiescent oncogene or inactivate a cancer suppressor gene. This approach, however, is fraught with problems relating to control of the fate of the DNA introduced into cells. For every gene spliced into the correct place, more than 1000 may fit randomly into the genome.

The most reliable laboratory method for gene targeting requires the use of an embryo-derived stem cell (ES) as the recipient. A targeting vector containing the derived gene is introduced into ES cells by electroporation or microinjection (Fig 25). In a few cells, the targeting vector pairs with the cognate chromosomal DNA sequence and transfers the gene to the genome by homologous recombination. Screening or enrichment procedures (or both) are then used to identify the rare ES cell in which the targeted event has occurred. The appropriate cell is then cloned and maintained as a pure population. The altered ES cells are injected into the blastocele cavity of a preimplantation mouse embryo and the blastocyst is surgically

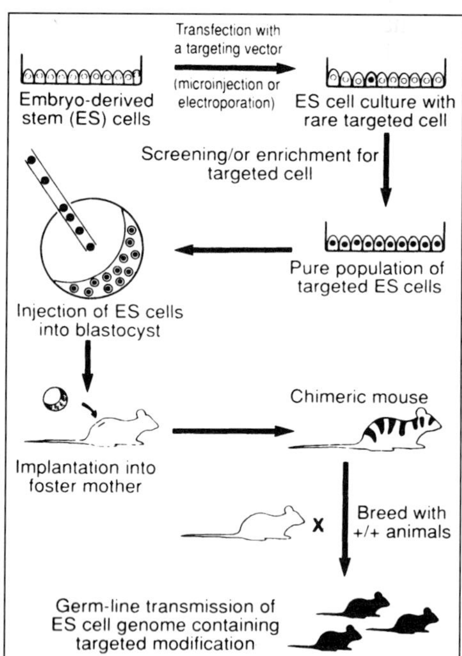


**Fig 25.** Generation of mouse germ line chimeras from embryo-derived stem (ES) cells containing a targeted gene disruption. (From Capecchi M, *Science.* 1989; 244: 1289, with permission.)

transferred into the uterus of a foster mother where development is allowed to progress to term. This process is similar to the technique described for generation of transgenic animals (Fig 15). The resulting animal is chimeric in that it is composed of cells derived from both the donor stem cells and the host blastocyst. In the particular example shown in Fig 25, the ESs are derived from a mouse homozygous for the black coat color allele and the recipient blastocyst derived from albino. The resulting chimeric mouse has both colors. Finally, interbreeding of heterozygous siblings yields animals homozygous for the desired mutation. This technology has already been used to create germ line chimeras containing targeted disruption in such genes as n-*myc,* $\beta_2$-microglobulin, *HPRT,* and *int-1.* Unfortunately, despite such achievements relatively little is known about the recombination mechanisms underlying gene targeting in mammalian cells. For example, it is not clear as to what the normal function might be of the machinery required for homologous recombination. One function must be DNA repair; in an evolutionary sense, the machinery might even participate in the generation, maintenance, and divergence of gene families and in the shuffling of exons between genes sharing stretches of homologous DNA sequences. An ideal strategy for disrupting or replacing a gene not expressed in ES cells has not yet emerged.

More established than gene replacement are several techniques of gene augmentation in which a healthy gene is added to the genome in addition to the missing or defective gene. This approach is especially helpful when a genetic derangement results in little or no production of a protein (each gene encodes a single protein); this approach, however, would not be good when a mutated or damaged gene yields overproduction of a protein or synthesis of a destructive substance (eg, sickle cell anemia). In that case, therapy would have to include delivery of both a healthy gene and one capable of inactivating the mutated version. At present, gene augmentation strategy requires removal of cells from patients followed by the introduction of the therapeutic gene into those cells and the reinfusion of the altered cells back into the patient.

Nontargeted delivery of genes into cells can be accomplished by chemical or physical means as previously mentioned. The delivery of nucleic acids into mammalian cells can be made more efficient than permitted by physical methods through the use of viral vectors capable of infecting virtually every cell in a target population.[157] The only problem with this technique, as noted above, is the lack of site specificity of integration. It is possible, then, for the virus vector to damage host cells by many mechanisms including insertion of the vector into an essential gene of the host cell, the activation of a silent protooncogene by introduction of viral promoter and enhancer sequences, the activation of latent viruses encoded by the genome, or the rescue of infectious virus from the defective vector by recombination with cellular sequences.

The most useful vector models for the efficient introduction of foreign genes into target mammalian cells have been derived from murine and avian retroviruses. The mechanisms of infection, replication, integration, and gene expression from these replication defective vectors are reviewed elsewhere.[158,159]

Although retrovirus vectors are capable of infecting a broad class of cell types, cell replication and DNA synthesis are required for provirus integration. This effectively restricts efficient use of retrovirus vectors to replicating cells. To be used clinically, retrovirus vectors would have to lead to efficient infection and stable gene expression.

Despite the technical success of gene targeting, several ''nuisance'' difficulties have come into focus. For example, promoter–enhancer combinations that worked well in transient expression or stable transformation experiments in cultured cells may work poorly or not at all in whole-animal experiments. In many gene therapy experiments, low levels of expression or complete shutdown over time may be encountered. One possible solution to this problem is to introduce genes into myoblasts ex vivo or into muscle in vivo as an alternative to hematopoietic cell or fibroblast gene therapy.[160]

The overall concept of gene therapy seems perfectly suited for the treatment of cancer. At the moment, the simplest genetic models involve neoplasia resulting from deficiencies of cancer suppressor genes. These cancers presumably arise from inactivation of both alleles of a wild-type (normal) gene. Therefore, the cancer phenotype might be suppressed or possibly reversed by restoring functional expression from a wild-type gene.

The loss of cancer suppressor genes has been described for several urologic cancers including kidney,[161-164] bladder,[165,166] prostate,[167] and testis.[163] As previously noted, these cancers arise in association with inactivation of both alleles of a wild-type (normal) gene. Therefore, the cancer phenotype might be suppressed or possibly reversed by restoring functional expression of the wild-type gene. In fact, this has already been done in an animal model of Wilms' tumor[168] as well as prostate cancer.[169]

### Immunotoxins

Immunotoxins are a special type of recombinant toxin in which toxin entry is mediated by antibody binding. The toxin must be modified so that its interactions with cellular receptors are diminished or abolished. For example, when *Pseudomonas* exotoxin (PE) (which acts by arresting the synthesis of proteins) is selected as the toxin, the antibody (to the target cell) is coupled to domain I of PE, which interferes with the binding of this region to the PE receptor. Likewise domain I may be entirely deleted with coupling of antibody to domain II. It is important to select a surface target, or epitope, that naturally enters cells by endocytosis such that the toxin, as part of the "toxic complex," will eventually kill the cell.

Many immunotoxins produce selective killing in cell culture but only a few are able to cause substantial or complete tumor regression in animals. However, regression of human carcinomas growing in immunodeficient mice has been achieved by treatment with monoclonal antibodies reacting with ovarian, colon, and breast cancers coupled to PE.[170] Immunotoxins that have been developed for human trials are of two types. The first involved the ex vivo addition of immunotoxins to harvested bone marrow to eliminate contaminating tumor cells before reinfusion in patients undergoing autologous bone marrow transplantation. A second type involves the parenteral administration of immunotoxins either regionally (such as peritoneal cavity) or systemically to patients with cancer. Most significant responses involve hematologic malignancies.[171] Antibodies used for preparation of immunotoxins to treat solid tumors have been found to react with important normal tissues (eg, normal tissue and bone marrow) and produce dose-limiting toxicity without significant clinical responses.

Before toxin therapy is seriously considered for use, a few problems must be successfully confronted. For example, it is well known that toxins are highly immunogenic and therefore neutralizing antibodies commonly develop about 10 days after exposure; likewise antibodies to diphtheria toxin (DT) already exist in most individuals who have received immunizations with diphtheria pertussis and tetanus (DPT). It may be necessary therefore for concomitant immunosuppression to be administered for long-term treatment.

In another approach, targeted introduction of a drug sensitivity gene specifically into tumor cells is designed to make them uniquely susceptible to pharmacologic treatment. One candidate of potential use is the herpes simplex virus 1 thymidine kinase (HSV1-TK) gene. This enzyme alone is not harmful to cells and in thymidine kinase–negative cells ($TK^-$) it can allow cell survival. The pathogenic effects of herpes simplex virus infection have led to the development of a nucleoside analog that selectively blocks viral spread as a consequence of its metabolism by the herpes simplex enzyme but not by the usual cellular counterpart. The analog, acyclovir (ACV), is converted by HSV1-TK to toxic nucleotide intermediates, which disrupts cellular DNA replication, thus leading to cell death. Furthermore, the toxicity is proportional to both the levels of HSV1-TK and ACV to which the cells are exposed. Because neither ACV nor HSV1-TK alone is harmful to cells, this approach could have widespread applicability in inducing selective cell death.[172]

**Antisense Strategy.** The potential for modulating the expression of oncogenes and other genes through the use of antisense oligonucleotides suggests another approach to the suppression of the cancer phenotype. The basic concept behind it is quite simple (as previously noted).[173] Antisense oligonucleotides (sequences that are complementary to the target) are made and thereby bind specifically with the targeted gene's RNA message, thereby inactivating it. The exact mechanisms of inactivation, however, are not known. For example, it is not clear as to which mRNA processing stage is interrupted (DNA before transcription, mRNA either before or after splicing, the process of splicing itself, ribosomal function, elongation of the polypeptide, or degradative processes that affect mRNA).

Although the mechanisms involved with inactivation of gene expression by antisense sequences are not thoroughly understood, it is probably necessary to deliver high concentrations of antisense information to compete either with efficient gene transcription or with the function of transcription factors. Eventually, however, therapy will be directed at correction of abnormal transcription elements that are responsible for deregulation. The obvious problems now are identification of those regulatory elements and, once identified, tissue-specific targeting. Despite potential technical difficulties and problems, this methodology has been used to inactivate plant enzymes, with resultant change in color.[174] In other experiments, antisense c-*raf*–transfected Scl-20B squamous cell carcinoma cell lines were found to be less tumorigenic and more radiosensitive in nude mice.[175]

No matter how efficient and stable the techniques of gene delivery and expression become, most potential clinical applications are likely to require faithful regulation of foreign gene expression. Qualitative or quantitative mistakes as well as inappropriate timing of transcriptional products will make disease correction difficult. There is still much to be learned about the many levels of transcriptional and translational regulation before medically relevant genetic complementation can become commonplace.

### Retinoids: Differentiation and Neoplasia

The coordination of the differentiation and proliferation processes is an essential feature of successful development and replenishment of tissues. However, it is not yet clear as to how the decline of one is causally related to the onset of the other or how this results in the decreased proliferation of differentiated cells. This issue is the focus of much attention since uncoupling of the normally interdependent processes of proliferation and differentiation is an obligatory step in the generation of the transformed phenotype and, hence, cancer. Simply put, the growth of cancer cells may be characterized by the blocking of normal differentiation. It is therefore not surprising that retinoic acid, a known inducer of differentiation, has been used in many experimental settings to alter the normal expression of the malignant phenotype.

The most striking example of the differentiation effects of retinoic acid is produced by the murine embryonal carcinoma cell model. The most studied is the F-9 cell system. These cells respond to retinoic acid by differentiating into primitive endoderm (Fig 26); eventually primitive endoderm progresses to become visceral endoderm. In the presence of retinoic acid and diburityl cyclic AMP, parietal endoderm is formed. The formation of visceral endoderm is characterized by an increase in the expression of α-fetoprotein. Differentiation toward parietal endoderm in the presence of cAMP is accompanied by a marked increase in the biosynthesis of laminin and type IV collagen.[176,177] From this work it is clear that retinoic acid has a profound effect on the ability of F-9 cells to form an extracellular matrix.

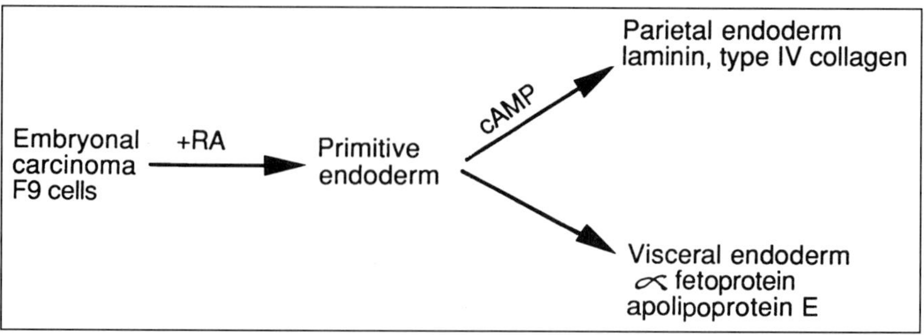


**Fig 26.** Schematic representation of differentiation pathways and products of F9 cells.

With this information, a logical direction of investigation was to determine the effects of retinoic acid on other tumors, and indeed positive inhibitory effects were noted both in vivo and in vitro.[178,179] In retrospect this was not surprising because about 70 years ago Wolbach and collaborators established that vitamin A deficiency causes squamous metaplasia and keratinization of most columnar epithelia of the body.[180] Because epithelial cancer is a major subset of malignancy, retinoids became of interest to cancer researchers because they afforded a way to control epithelial differentiation and possibly prevent alterations caused by exposure to chemical carcinogens. The concept of *chemoprevention* was formulated to indicate an approach distinct from chemotherapy.[181] Retinoic acid or similar compounds were thought to prevent epithelial tumorigenesis by directing cells to differentiate in their normal manner, thus preventing or reversing the squamous metaplastic phenotype normally considered (at least in the respiratory epithelium) an early lesion in the path toward tumor formation. Pioneering efforts showed that retinoids could in fact inhibit tumorigenesis in the skin and in the respiratory, buccal, stomach, and mammary epithelia of rodents.[178] Recently there have been optimistic reports on the prevention of second primary tumors in patients with squamous cell carcinoma of the head and neck[182] and skin cancer in xeroderma pigmentosum patients using 13-*cis*-retinoid acid.[183]

This approach may prove beneficial for some urologic-related disorders. For example, it was previously shown that a synthetic retinoid *N*-(4-hydroxyphenyl) retinamide or (4-HPR, fenretinide) can significantly reduce the development of bladder cancer as well as prostate cancer in mice[184] and rats.[185,186] Although the mechanism of action is not known, it is thought to be related to the inhibition of angiogenesis and endothelial cell motility and tubule formation.[186]

Insight into the mechanism of action may be gained by reviewing the use of retinoic acid and derivatives, such as trentoin (all-*trans*-retinoic acid). Interest in the drug increased in 1988 when investigators in Shanghai reported their experience with the drug in patients with acute promyelocytic leukemia.[187] They used trentoin because of difficulty in obtaining enough blood products to support standard chemotherapy. Complete responses were achieved in 23 of 24 patients, 8 of whom had originally failed to respond to chemotherapy. Likewise, trentoin was well tolerated and treatment was not complicated by disseminated intravascular coagulopathy that often occurs in this disease and is exacerbated by therapy. These figures have since been confirmed by others.[188] Of greater surprise, however, was that this disease is associated with a chromosomal translocation [t(15;17)(q22;q12–21)] and the breakpoint site occurs within the coding exons of the retinoic acid receptor α (RAR∝) on chromosome 17q 11.2. The t(15;17) translocation results in the fusion of the RAR∝ gene to a newly identified oncogene on chromosome 15, the PML gene. This new fusion gene encodes for a novel PML–RAR∝ fusion messenger RNA and protein. The fusion protein can be identified in leukemia cells in virtually all cases by PCR amplification.[189]

The relationship, if any, between the differentiation effects of retinoic acid on leukemia cells and the translocation of the RAR∝ gene remains to be characterized, but this latter phenomenon puts on a solid molecular footing previous expectations that retinoids are involved in neoplastic transformation. Although the biological consequences of the translocation of the RAR∝ gene and the new PML locus are not clear, the generation of new PML–RAR∝ transcripts may well influence differentiation and growth potential of the cells. Interestingly, a dominant-negative mutation has been discovered in the RAR∝ gene of an embryonal carcinoma cell that confers resistance to the differentiating action of retinoic acid.[190]

The complexity of retinoic acid and its effects on cells became even greater when it was discovered by two groups that the receptors for retinoids were similar to that of steroid and thyroid hormone receptor being localized to the nucleus. Retinoid receptors therefore belong to the steroid/thyroid hormone receptors superfamily.[191,192] These receptors act as transcriptional activators by binding as heterodimers to specific nucleotide sequences in the response elements of target genes. This is an important consideration because response elements for retinoic acid so far have been identified for rat growth hormone and phosphoenolpyruvate carboxy kinase, the mouse complement H and laminin B1, human and mouse RARβ, and the human osteocalcin and alcohol dehydrogenase genes. The retinoic acid response element for the rat growth hormone gene is also a thyroid hormone response element. The AP-1 binding site of the human osteocalcin promoter is both a vitamin D response element as well as a retinoic acid response element. From this information, it is easily appreciated that the retinoic acid "road map" is potentially complex and truly involves cellular homeostasis. "Differentiation therapy" is only at the beginning of its adolescence.

## REFERENCES

1. Henderson BE, Ross R, Pike M. Toward the primary prevention of cancer. *Science.* 1991; 254:1131.
2. Department of Health and Human Services (DHHS). Publication PHS 85-1232. Washington, DC: Public Health Service; 1984.
3. Hayflick L, Moorhead PS. The serial cultivation of human diploid cell strains. *Exp Cell Res.* 1961;25:585.
4. Peto R, Roe FJC, Lee PN, et al. Cancer and aging in mice and men. *Br J Cancer.* 1975;32: 411.
5. Boveri T. *Zur Tragee der Entstehung maligner Tumoren.* Jena: G Fisher; 1914.
6. Bishop JM. Molecular themes in oncogenesis. *Cell.* 1991;64:235.
7. Berenblum I, Shubik P. A new quantitative approach to the study of the stages of chemical carcinogenesis in the mouse's skin. *Br J Cancer.* 1947;1:384.
8. Takahashi JS. Circadian clock genes are ticking. *Science.* 1992;258:238.
9. Kornhauser J, Nelson D, Mayo K, Takahashi J. Regulation of jun-B messenger RNA and AP-1 activity by light and a circadian clock. *Science.* 1992;255:1581.
10. Hamer D, Hu S, Magnuson V, et al. A linkage between DNA markers on the X chromosome and male sexual orientation. *Science.* 1993;261: 321.
11. Watson JD, Crick FH. Molecular structure of nucleic acid: a structure for deoxyribose nucleic acid. *Nature.* 1953;171:737.
12. Richmond TJ, Finch JT, Rushton B, et al. Structure of the nucleosome particle at 7A resolution. *Nature.* 1984;311:532.
13. Arents G, Burlingame RW, Wang BW, et al. The nucleosomal core histone octomer at 3.1Å resolution: a tripartite protein assembly and a left handed superhelix. *Proc Natl Acad Sci USA.* 1991;88:10148.
14. Lin S-Y, Riggs AD. The general affinity of lac repressor for *E. coli* DNA: implications for gene regulation in prokaryotes and eukaryotes. *Cell.* 1975;4:107.
15. Wolffe AP, Brown DD. Developmental regulation of two 5S ribosomal RNA genes. *Science.* 1988;241:1626.
16. Wolffe AP. New insights into chromatin function in transcriptional control. *FASEB J.* 1992; 6:3354.
17. Augustin S, Moller MW, Schweyen RJ. Reverse self splicing group II intron RNAs in vitro. *Nature.* 1990;343:383.
18. Perlman P, Butnow R. Mobile introns and intron encoded proteins. *Science.* 1989;246:1106.
19. Roger A, Doolittle W. Why introns in pieces? *Nature.* 1993;364:289.

20. Weis L, Reinberg D. Transcription by RNA polymerase II: initiater-directed formation of transcription-competent complexes. *FASEB J.* 1992;6:330.
21. Gill G. Complexes with a common core. *Curr Biol.* 1992;2:565.
22. Carcamo J, Maldonado E, Ahn M, et al. A TATA-like sequence located downstream of the transcription initiation site is required for expression of an RNA polymerase II transcribed gene. *Genes Dev.* 1990;4:1611.
23. Levine M, Manley J. Transcriptional repression of eukaryotic promoters. *Cell.* 1989;59:405.
24. Peterson MG, Tanese N, Pugh B, Tigian R. Functional domains and upstream activation properties of cloned human TATA binding proteins. *Science.* 1990;248:1625.
25. Ptashne M. How gene activators work. *Sci Am.* 1989;260:40.
26. Rhodes D, Klug A. Zinc fingers. *Sci Am.* 1993; 268:56.
27. Vinson C, Sigler P, McKnight S. Scissors-grip model for DNA recognition by a family of leucine–zipper proteins. *Science.* 1989; 246:911.
28. Oshae E, Rutkowski R, Stafford W, Kim P. Preferential heterodimer formation by isolated leucine zippers from Fos and Jun. *Science.* 1989;245:646.
29. Maniatis T, Reed R. The role of small nuclear ribonucleoprotein particles in pre-mRNA splicing. *Nature.* 1987;325:673.
30. Southern EM. Detection of specific sequences among DNA fragments separated by gel electrophoresis. *J Mol Biol.* 1975;98:503.
31. Mullis K. The unusual origin of the polymerase chain reaction. *Sci Am.* 1990;262:56.
32. Singer M, Jones OW, Nirenberg M. The effect of secondary structure on the template activity of polyribonucleotides. *Proc Natl Acad Sci USA.* 1963;49:392.
33. Capecchi M. High efficiency transformation by direct microinjections of DNA into cultured mammalian cells. *Cell.* 1980;22:479.
34. Brinster PL, Chen H, Trumbauer M. Somatic expression of thymidine kinase in mice following injection of a fusion gene into eggs. *Cell.* 1981;27:223.
35. Muller WJ, Lee FS, Dickson C, et al. The int-2 gene product acts as an epithelial growth factor in transgenic mice. *EMBO J.* 1990;9:907.
36. Mullins JJ, Peters J, Ganten D. Fulminant hypertension in transgenic rats harboring the mouse Ren-2 gene. *Nature.* 1990;344:541.
37. Weiner H, Noda T, Gray D, et al. Transgenic mouse model of kidney disease: insertional inactivation of ubiquitously expressed gene leads to nephrotic syndrome. *Cell.* 1990;62:425.
38. Varmus H, Weinberg R. *Genes and Biology of Cancer.* New York: WH Freeman; 1993.
39. Lin CQ, Bissell MJ. Multi-faceted regulation of cell differentiation by extracellular matrix. *FASEB J.* 1993;7:737.
40. Egan SE, Weinberg RA. The pathway to signal achievement. *Nature.* 1993;365:781.
41. Marx J. Two major signal pathways linked. *Science.* 1992;262:988.
42. Bos TU. Oncogenes and cell growth. *Adv Exp Med Biol.* 1992;321:45.
43. Karin M. Signal transduction from cell surface to nucleus in development and disease. *FASEB J.* 1992;6:2581.
44. Leach FS, Tokino T, Meltzer P, et al. p53 mutation and MDM2 amplification in human soft tissue sarcomas. *Cancer Res.* 1993;53:2231.
45. Reddy EP, Reynolds RK, Santos E, Barbacid M. A point mutation is responsible for the acquisition of transforming properties by the T24 human bladder carcinoma oncogene. *Nature.* 1982;300:149.
46. Sidransky D, Messing E. Molecular genetics and biochemical mechanisms in bladder cancer. *Urol Clin North Am.* 1992;19:629.
47. Weinberg RA. Tumor suppressor genes. *Science.* 1991;254:1138.
48. Knudson A. Mutation and cancer: statistical study of retinoblastoma. *Proc Natl Acad Sci USA.* 1971;68:820.
49. Bandara LR, Adamczewski JP, Hunt T, La Thangue NB. Cyclin A and the retinoblastoma gene product complex with a common transcription factor. *Nature.* 1991;352:249.
50. Benedict WF. Altered RB expression is a prognostic clinical marker involved in human bladder tumorigenesis. *J Cell Biochem.* (Suppl) 1992;161:69.
51. Isaacs WB, Bova GS, Morton RA, Ewing CM. Genetic alterations and tumor suppression in prostate cancer. *Proc Annu Meet Am Assoc Cancer Res.* 1993;34:627.
52. Madden SL, Cook DM, Morris JR, et al. Transcriptional repression mediated by the WT1 Wilm's tumor gene product. *Science.* 1991;253: 1550.
53. Schwartz CE, Haber DA, Stanton VP, et al. Familial predisposition to Wilm's tumor does not segregate with the WT1 gene. *Genomics.* 1991; 10:927.
54. Yaremko ML, Wasylyshyn ML, Westbrook CA, Michelassi F. Oncogenes, suppressor genes, and allele losses in colon cancer. *Adv Surg.* 1993;26:323.
55. O'Connell P, Cawthon R, Xu GF, et al. The neurofibromatosis type 1 (NF1) gene: identification and partial characterization of a putative tumor suppressor gene. *J Dermatol.* 1992;19: 881.
56. Reiter RE, Zbar B, Linehan WM. Molecular genetic studies of renal cell carcinoma: potential biologic and clinical significance for genitourinary malignancy. In Walsh PC, Retik AB, Sta-

mey TA, Vaughan ED, eds. *Campbell's Urology,* 6th Ed., Update 7. Philadelphia: WB Saunders; 1993.

57. Olumi AF, Tsai YC, Nichols PW, et al. Allelic losses of chromosome 17p distinguishes high grade from low grade transitional cell carcinomas of the bladder. *Cancer Res.* 1990;50:7081.
58. Rinker-Schaeffer CW, Isaacs WB, Isaacs JT. Molecular and cellular markers for metastatic prostate cancer. *Cancer Metast Rev.* 1991;12:3.
59. Levine AJ, Momand J, Finlay CA. The p53 tumor suppressor gene. *Nature.* 1991;351:453.
60. Kern SE, Pietenpol JA, Thiagalingam S, et al. Oncogenic forms of p53 inhibit p53-regulated gene expression. *Science.* 1992;256:827.
61. Sarkis AS, Dalbagni G, Cordon-Cardo C, et al. Nuclear overexpression of p53 protein in transitional cell bladder carcinoma: a marker for disease progression. *JNCI.* 1993;85:53.
62. Navone NM, Troncoso P, Pisters LL, et al. p53 protein accumulation and gene mutation in the progression of human prostate carcinoma. *JNCI.* 1993;85:1657.
63. Kastan MB, Onyekwere O, Sidransky D, et al. Participation of p53 protein in the cellular response to DNA damage. *Cancer Res.* 1991;51: 6304.
64. Scheffner M, Werness BA, Huibregtse JM, et al. The E6 oncoprotein encoded by human papillomavirus types 16 and 18 promotes the degradation of p53. *Cell.* 1990;63:1129.
65. Cairns J. *Cancer: Science and Society.* New York: WH Freeman; 1978.
66. Frearon ER, Vogelstein B. A genetic model for colorectal tumorigenesis. *Cell.* 1990;61:759.
67. Dalbagni G, Presti J, Reuter V, et al. Genetic alterations in bladder cancer. *Lancet.* 1993;342: 469.
68. Carter HB, Piantadosi S, Isaacs JT. Clinical evidence for and implications of the multistep development of prostate cancer. *J Urol.* 1990;143: 742.
69. Loeb LA. Mutator phenotype may be required for multistage carcinogenesis. *Cancer Res.* 1991;51:3075.
70. Murray A, Hunt T. *The Cell Cycle.* New York: WH Freeman; 1993.
71. Tyson JJ. Modeling the cell division cycle: cdc2 and cyclin interactions. *Proc Natl Acad Sci USA.* 1991;88:7328.
72. Sherr CJ. Mammalian G1 cyclins. *Cell.* 1993; 73:1059.
73. Murray AW. Creative blocks, cell cycle checkpoints and feedback controls. *Nature.* 1992; 359:599.
74. Gadbois DM, Crissman HA, Tobey RA, Bradbury EM. Multiple kinase arrest points in the G1 phase of nontransformed mammalian cells are absent in transformed cells. *Proc Natl Acad Sci USA.* 1992;89:8626.
75. Koff A, Ohtsuki M, Polyak K, et al. Negative regulation of G1 progression in mammalian cells: inhibition of cyclin E–dependent kinase by TGFβ. *Science.* 1993;260:536.
76. Perry ME, Levine AJ. Tumor-suppressor p53 and the cell cycle. *Curr Opin Genet Dev.* 1993; 3:50.
77. Shaw P, Bovey R, Tardy S, et al. Introduction of apoptosis by wild-type p53 in a human colon tumor-derived cell line. *Proc Natl Acad Sci USA.* 1992;89:4495.
78. Livingstone LR, White A, Sprouse J, et al. Altered cell cycle arrest and gene amplification potential accompany loss of wild type p53. *Cell.* 1992;70:923.
79. Hartwell L. Defects in a cell cycle checkpoint may be responsible for the genomic instability of cancer cells. *Cell.* 1992;71:543.
80. Lau CC, Pardee AB. Mechanisms by which caffeine potentiates lethality of nitrogen mustard. *Proc Natl Acad Sci USA.* 1982;79:2942.
81. Sagata N, Watanabe N, Vande Woude G, Ikawa Y. The c-mos proto-oncogene product is a cystostatic factor responsible for meiotic arrest in vertebrate cells. *Nature.* 1989;342:512.
82. Li R, Murray AW. Feedback controls of mitosis in budding yeast. *Cell.* 1991;66:519.
83. Poste G, Fidler IJ. The pathogenesis of cancer metastasis. *Nature.* 1980;283:139.
84. Fidler IJ, Kripke ML. Metastases results from pre existing variant cells within a malignant tumor. *Science.* 1977;197:893.
85. Ciferge MA, Fidler IJ. Increasing metastatic potential is associated with increasing genetic instability of clones isolated from murine neoplasms. *Proc Natl Acad Sci USA.* 1981;78: 6949.
86. Butler TP, Gullino PM. Quantitation of cell shedding into efferent blood mammary adenocarcinoma. *Cancer Res.* 1975;351:512.
87. Fidler IJ. Metastasis: quantitative analysis of distribution and fate of tumor emboli labeled with $^{125}$I-5-iodo-2′-deoxyuridine. *JNCI.* 1970; 45:773.
88. Hart IR. "Seed and soil" revisited: mechanisms of site specific metastases. *Cancer Metast Rev.* 1982;1:5.
89. Ewing J. *Neoplastic Diseases,* 6th ed. Philadelphia: WB Saunders; 1928.
90. Paget S. The distribution of secondary growth in cancer of the breast. *Lancet.* 1889;1:571.
91. Hart IR, Fidler IJ. Role of organ selectivity determination of metastatic patterns of B16 melanoma. *Cancer Res.* 1981;41:1281.
92. Folkman J. What is the evidence that tumors are angiogenesis dependent? *JNCI.* 1990;82:4.
93. Folkman J, Cotran R. Relocation of vascular proliferation to tumor growth. *Int Rev Exp Pathol.* 1976;16:207.

94. Folkman J, Shing Y. Angiogenesis. *J Biol Chem.* 1992;267:10931.
95. Pepper MS, Ferrara N, Orci L, Mantesano R. *Biochem Biophys Res Commun.* 1991;181:902.
96. Weidner N, Semple JP, Welch WR, Folkman J. Tumor angiogenesis and metastasis: correlation in invasive breast carcinoma. *N Engl J Med.* 1991;324:1.
97. Brawer MK, Bigler SA, Deering RE. Quantitative morphometric analysis of the microcirculation in prostate cancer. *J Cell Biochem (Suppl).* 1992;16H:62.
98. Chopin DK, Caruelle JP, Colombel Poucy S, et al. Increased immunodetection of acidic fibroblast growth factor in bladder cancer detectable in urine. *J Urol.* 1993;150:1126.
99. Burnet FM. The concept of immunological surveillance. *Prog Exp Tumor Res.* 1970;13:1.
100. Abbas AK, Lichtman AH, Pober JS. *Cellular and Molecular Immunology.* Philadelphia: WB Saunders; 1991.
101. Prehn RT, Main MJ. Immunity to methylcholanthrene-induced sarcomas. *JNCI.* 1957;18: 769.
102. Purtilo DT. Defective immune surveillance in viral carcinogenesis. *Lab Invest.* 1984;51:373.
103. Urban JL, Schrieber H. Tumor antigens. *Annu Rev Immunol.* 1992;10:617.
104. Kloppel G, Caselitz J. Epithelial tumor markers: oncofetal antigens (carcinoembryotic antigen, alpha fetoprotein) and epithelial membrane antigen. *Curr Topics Pathol.* 1987;77:103.
105. Graham SD. Immunology of the bladder. *Urol Clin North Am.* 1992;19:541.
106. Young RA. Stress protein and immunology. *Annu Rev Immunol.* 1990;8:401.
107. Beverley P. Tumor immunology. In Roitt I, Brostoff J, Male D, eds. *Immunology.* St. Louis: Mosby; 1993.
108. Travers P. Immunological agnosia. *Nature.* 1993;363:117.
109. Janeway CA. How the immune system recognizes invaders. *Sci Am.* 1993;269:72.
110. Aggawal BB, Pocsik E. Cytokines; from clone to clinic. *Arch Biochem Biophys.* 1992;292:335.
111. Harding CV, Unanue ER. Cellular mechanisms of antigen processing and the function of class I and class II major histocompatability complex-encoded molecules. *Cell Reg.* 1990;1:499.
112. Kupfer A, Singer SJ. Cell biology of cytotoxic and helper T-cell functions. *Annu Rev Immunol.* 1989;7:309.
113. Romagni S. Human TH1 and TH2 subsets: doubt no more. *Immun Today.* 1991;12:256.
114. Doherty PC. The function of gamma delta T cells. *Br J Haematol.* 1992;81:3321.
115. Arai K, Lee F, Miyajima A, et al. Cytokines: coordinators of immune and inflammatory responses. *Annu Rev Biochem.* 1990;59:783.
116. Scott P. IL-12: initiation cytokine for cell-mediated immunity. *Science.* 1993;260:496.
117. Cohen J. New protein steals the show as ''costimulator'' of T cells. *Science.* 1993;262:844.
118. Gimmi CD, Freeman GJ, Gribben JG, et al. Human T-cell clonal anergy is induced by antigen presentation in the absence of B7 costimulation. *Proc Natl Acad Sci USA.* 1993;90:6586.
119. Hellstrom KE, Hellstrom I. In DeVita VT, Hellman S, Rosenberg SA, eds. *Cancer: Principles and Practice of Oncology.* Philadelphia: JB Lippincott; 1991.
120. Trail PA, Willner D, Lasch J, et al. Cure of xenografted human carcinomas by BR96-doxorubicin immunoconjugates. *Science.* 1993;261: 212.
121. Theuer CP, Fitzgerald DJ, Pastan I. A recombinant form of Pseudomonas exotoxin A containing transforming growth factor alpha near its carboxyl terminus for the treatment of bladder cancer. *J Urol.* 1993;149:1626.
122. Berd D, Maguire HC, McCue P, Mastrangelo MG. Treatment of metastatic melanoma with an autologous tumor-cell vaccine: clinical and immunologic results in 64 patients. *J Clin Oncol.* 1990;8:1858.
123. Gottesman JE, Crawford ED, Grossman HB, et al. Infarction-nephrectomy for metastatic renal disease carcinomas: Southwest Oncology Group Study. *Urology.* 1985;25:248.
124. Nauts HC, Fowler GA, Bogatka F. A review of the influence of bacterial infection and of bacterial products (Coley's toxins) on malignant tumors in man. *Acta Med Scand.* 1953;276:5.
125. Lamm DL. Long term results of intravesical therapy for superficial bladder cancer. *Urol Clin North Am.* 1992;19:573.
126. Ratliff TL, Ritchey JK, Yuan JJ, et al. T-cell subsets required for intravesical BCG immunotherapy for bladder cancer. *J Urol.* 1993;150: 1018.
127. Fleischmann JD, Toossi Z, Ellner JJ, et al. Urinary interleukins in patients receiving intravesical BCG therapy for superficial bladder cancer. *Cancer.* 1989;6:1447.
128. Stafanini FF, Bercovich E, Mazzeo V, et al. Class I and class II HLA antigen expression by transitional cell carcinoma of the bladder: correlation with T cell infiltration and BCG treatment. *J Urol.* 1989;141:1449.
129. Rosenberg SA, Lotze MT. Cancer status of interleukin-2 and interleukin-2-activated lymphocytes. *Annu Rev Immunol.* 1986;4:681.
130. Tartour E, Mathhiot C, Friedman WH. Current status of interleukin-2 therapy in cancer. *Biomed Pharmacother.* 1992;46:473.
131. Hermann GG, Geertsen PF, von der Maase H, et al. Recombinant interleukin-2 and lymphokine-activated killer cell treatment of advanced bladder cancer. *Cancer Res.* 1992;52:726.

132. Kedar E, Klein E. Cancer immunotherapy. Are the results discouraging? Can they be improved? *Adv Cancer Res.* 1992;59:245.

133. Vedantham S, Gamliel H, Golomb HM. Mechanisms of interferon action in hairy cell leukemia: a model of effective cancer biotherapy. *Cancer Res.* 1992;52:1056.

134. Buzaid AC, Roberstone A, Kisala C, Salmon SE. Phase II study of interferon alpha-2a, recombinant (Roferon-A) in metastatic renal cell carcinoma. *J Clin Oncol.* 1987;5:1083.

135. Horoszicz JS, Murphy GP. An assessment of the current use of human interferons in therapy of urologic cancers. *J Urol.* 1989;142:1173.

136. Figlin RA, Belldegrun A, Moldawer N, et al. Administration of recombinant human interleukin-2 and recombinant interferon alfa-2A: an active outpatient regimen in metastatic renal cell carcinoma. *J Clin Oncol.* 1992;10:414.

137. Ferri WA, Bahnson R, Hakala T, et al. Phase I trial of intravesical recombinant human tumor necrosis factor (rHuTNF) in patients with superficial transitional cell carcinoma or carcinoma in-situ of the urinary bladder. *Proc Am Soc Clin Oncol.* 1990;9:153.

138. Gately MK. Interleukin-12: a recently discovered cytokine with potential for enhancing cell-mediated immune responses to tumors. *Cancer Invest.* 1993;11:500.

139. Fathman CG. Stimulating the lymphocytes. *Curr Biol.* 1993;3:558.

140. Pardoll D. Immunotherapy with cytokine gene-transduced tumor cells: the next wave in gene therapy for cancer. *Curr Opin Oncol.* 1992;4:1124.

141. Ellis H, Horvitz HR. Genetic control of programmed cell death in the nematode. *C. elegans. Cell.* 1986;44:817.

142. Barinaga M. Death gives birth to the nervous system. *Science.* 1993;259:762.

143. Kerr JFR, Wyllie AH, Currie AR. A basic biologic phenomenon with wide ranging implications in tissue kinetics. *Br J Cancer.* 1972;26:239.

144. Wyllie AH. Glucocorticoid induces in thymocytes a nuclease-like activity associated with the chromatin condensation of apoptosis. *Nature.* 1980;284:555.

145. Wyllie AH, Kerr JFR, Currie AR. Cell death: the significance of apoptosis. *Int Rev Cytol.* 1986;68:251.

146. Vaux DI, Corey S, Adams JM. Bcl-2 gene promotes hematopoietic cell survival and cooperates with c-myc to immortalize pre B cells. *Nature.* 1988;335:440.

147. Marx J. Cell death studies yield cancer clues. *Science.* 1993;259:760.

148. Kyprianou N, English H, Isaacs J. Programmed cell death during regression of PC-82 human prostate cancer following androgen ablation. *Cancer Res.* 1990;50:3748.

149. Oberhammer FA, Pavelka M, Sharma S, et al. Induction of apoptosis in cultured hepatocytes and in regressing liver by transforming growth factor beta 1. *Proc Natl Acad Sci USA.* 1992;89:5408.

150. Montpetit ML, Lawless KR, Tenniswood M. Androgen repressed messages in the rat ventral prostate. *Prostate.* 1986;8:25.

151. Buttyan R, Olsson C, Pintar J, et al. Induction of the TRPM-2 gene in cells undergoing programmed cell death. *Mol Cell Biol.* 1989;9:3473.

152. Baker S, Markowitz S, Fearon E, et al. Suppression of human colorectal carcinoma cell growth by wild type p53. *Science.* 1990;249:912.

153. Chen P, Chen Y, Bookstein R, Lee W. Genetic mechanism of tumor suppression by the human p53 gene. *Science.* 1990;250:1576.

154. Michalovitz D, Halevy O, Oran M. Conditional inhibition of transformation and of cell proliferation by a temperature sensitive mutant of p53. *Cell.* 1990;62:671.

155. Shaw P, Bovey R, Tardy S, et al. Induction of apoptosis by wild type p53 in a human tumor-derived cell line. *Proc Natl Acad Sci USA.* 1992;89:4495.

156. Miyashita T, Reed J. Bcl-2 oncoprotein blocks chemotherapy-induced apoptosis in a human leukemia cell line. *Blood.* 1993;81:151.

157. Gluzman Y, Hughes S. *Viral Vectors.* Cold Spring Harbor, NY: Cold Spring Harbor Laboratory; 1988.

158. Shimotohno K, Temin HM. Formation of infectious progeny virus after insertion of herpes simplex thymidine kinase gene into DNA of an avian retrovirus. *Cell.* 1981;26:67.

159. Wei C, Gibson M, Spear PG, Scolnick EM. Construction and isolation of a transmissable retrovirus containing the src gene of Harvey sarcoma and the thymidine kinase gene of herpes simplex type 1. *J Virol.* 1981;39:935.

160. Dai Y, Roman M, Naviaux RK, Verma I. Gene therapy via primary myoblasts: long term expression of factor 1X protein following transplantation in vivo. *Proc Natl Acad Sci USA.* 1992;89:10892.

161. Koufos A, Hansen MF, Lamplin BC, et al. Loss of alleles at loci on chromosome 11 during genesis of Wilms' tumor. *Nature.* 1984;309:107.

162. Orkin SH, Goldman DG, Sallan S. Development of homozygosity for chromosome 11p markers in Wilms' tumor. *Nature.* 1984;309:172.

163. Rukstalis D, Bubley G, Donahue J, et al. Regional loss of chromosome 6 in 2 urologic malignancies. *Cancer Res.* 1989;49:5087.

164. Zbar B, Branch H, Talmadge C, Linehan M. Loss of alleles of loci on the short arm of chromosome 3 in bladder cancer. *Nature.* 1987;327:721.

165. Fearon E, Feinberg AP, Hamilton SH, Vogelstein B. Loss of genes on the arm of chromosome 11 in bladder cancer. *Nature.* 1985;318: 377.

166. Horowitz J, Park SH, Bogenmann E, et al. Frequent inactivation of the retinoblastoma antioncogene is restricted to a subset of human tumor cells. *Proc Natl Acad Sci USA.* 1990;87:2775.

167. Carter B, Ewing C, Ward S, et al. Allelic loss of chromosome 16q and 10q in human prostate cancer. *Proc Natl Acad Sci USA.* 1990;87:8751.

168. Weissman BE, Saxon PJ, Pasquale SR, et al. Introduction of a normal human chromosome 11 into a Wilms' tumor cell line controls its tumorogenic expression. *Science.* 1987;236: 175.

169. Bookstein R, Shew JY, Chen PL, et al. Suppression of tumorigenicity of human prostate cancer cells by replacing a mutated Rb gene. *Science.* 1990;247:712.

170. Pai LH, Batra JK, Fitzgerald DJ, et al. Antitumor activities of immunotoxins made of monoclonal antibody B3 and various forms of pseudomonas exotoxin. *Proc Natl Acad Sci USA.* 1991;88:3358.

171. Vitetta ES. Phase I immunotoxin trial in patients with B cell lymphoma. *Cancer Res.* 1991; 51:4052.

172. Burelli E, Heyman R, Hsi M, Evans R. Targeting of an inducible toxic phenotype in animal cells. *Proc Natl Acad Sci USA.* 1988;85:7572.

173. Weintraub H. Antisense RNA and DNA. *Sci Am.* 1990;262:40.

174. Van der Krol H, Lenting P, Veenstra J, et al. An antisense chalcone synthetase gene in transgenic plants inhibit flower pigmentation. *Nature.* 1988;333:866.

175. Kasid U, Pfeifer A, Brennan T, et al. Effect of antisense c-raf-1 on tumorigenicity and radiation sensitivity of a human squamous carcinoma. *Science.* 1989;243:1354.

176. Hogan BL, Taylor A, Adamson E. Cell interactions modulate embryonal carcinoma differentiation into parietal or visceral endoderm. *Nature.* 1981;291:235.

177. Marotti KR, Brown GD, Strickland S. Two stage hormonal control of type IV collagen mRNA levels during differentiation of F9 teratocarcinoma cells. *Dev Biol.* 1985;108:26.

178. Moon RC, McCormack DL, Mehta RG. Inhibition of carcinogenesis by retinoids. *Cancer Res.* 1983;43:24696.

179. Lotan R, Lotan D, Sacks PG. Inhibition of tumor cell growth by retinoids. *Meth Enzymol.* 1990;190:100.

180. Wolbach SB, Howe PR. Tissue changes following deprivation of fat soluble A vitamin. *J Exp Med.* 1925;42:753.

181. Sporn MB, Dunlop NM, Newlon DL, Smith JM. Prevention of chemical carcinogenesis by vit A and its synthetic analogs (retinoids). *Fed Proc.* 1976;35:1332.

182. Hong WK, Lippman SM, Itri LM, et al. Prevention of second primary tumors with isotretinoin in squamous cell carcinoma of the head and neck. *N Engl J Med.* 1990;323:795.

183. Kraemer KH, DiGiovanna JJ, Moshell AN, et al. Prevention of skin cancer in xeroderma pigmentosum with the use of oral isotretoin. *N Engl J Med.* 1988;318:1633.

184. Moon RC, McCormick DL, Becci PJ, et al. Influence of 15 retinoic acid amides on urinary bladder carcinogenesis in the mouse. *Carcinogenesis* (Lond). 1982;3:1469.

185. Pollard M, Luckert P, Sporn MB. Prevention of primary prostate cancer in Lobund–Wistar rats by N-(4-Hydroxphenyl) retinamide. *Cancer Res.* 1991;51:3610.

186. Pient KJ, Nguyen NM, Lehr JE. Treatment of prostate cancer in the rat with synthetic retinoid fenretinide. *Cancer Res.* 1993;53:224.

187. Huang M, Ye Y, Chen S, et al. Use of all-trans retinoic acid in the treatment of acute promyelocytic leukemia. *Blood.* 1988;72:567.

188. Warrell RP Jr, Frankel SR, Miller WH, et al. Differentiation therapy of acute promyelocytic leukemia with all-trans-retinoic acid. *N Engl J Med.* 1991;324:1385.

189. Castaigne S, Balitrand N, de The' H, et al. A PML retinoic acid alpha fusion transcript is constantly detected by RNA based polymerase chain reaction in acute promyelocytic leukemia. *Blood.* 1992;79:3110.

190. Pratt MA, Kralova J, McBurney M. A dominant negative mutation of the alpha retinoic acid receptor gene in a retinoic acid-nonresponsive embryonal carcinoma cell. *Mol Cell Biol.* 1990; 10:6445.

191. Petkovich M, Brand NJ, Krust H, Chambon P. A human retinoic acid receptor which belongs to the family of nuclear receptors. *Nature.* 1987;330:444.

192. Giguere V, Ong ES, Segui P, Evans RM. Identification of a receptor for the morphogen retinoic acid. *Nature.* 1987;330:624.

# 27

# Tumors of the Kidney

*Carla D. Chiapella and Barry S. Stein*

## INTRODUCTION

Renal cell carcinoma comprises 87%–90% of the primary malignant masses of the kidney. Seven to eight percent of renal tumors originate from the urothelium of the collecting system and will be discussed in another chapter. The remaining 2%–3% constitute sarcomas and adult Wilms' tumors.

Historically, many patients presented with advanced disease because symptoms occur late. The location of the kidney in the retroperitoneum allows for uninhibited growth of a renal mass to a large size before symptoms occur. Hematuria, whether microscopic or macroscopic, is one presenting symptom that is often ignored by the patient and/or physician. Thus, 25%–30% of patients with renal cell carcinoma (RCC) have distant metastasis at the time of diagnosis.

Familiar diagnostic techniques such as ultrasound and computed tomography (CT) have improved with newer models. A new imaging modality, magnetic resonance imagine (MRI), has emerged in recent years. These modalities have been used more frequently by primary care physicians for diagnosis and a coincident increase in incidental renal masses has emerged. The incidental tumor is more likely to be a low-stage lesion with a better survival outcome projected. Unfortunately, the death rate from renal cell carcinoma has not yet improved.

The estimated projection for renal tumors is 24,000 yearly, of which 15,000 will be in males and 9000 in females. Death due to upper tract disease (including tumors of the collecting system) is 10,000 yearly. Historically, survival improved with the advent of radical nephrectomy for parenchymal tumors and nephroureterectomy with a cuff of bladder for tumors of the collecting system. During 1960–1963, 5-year survival of tumors of the renal pelvis and kidney was 37% for whites and 38% for blacks. In the mid-1970s, the same statistics showed 50% survival for these same groups. In 1980–1985, the 5-year survival was slightly better for blacks, 55% compared to whites at 52%.[1,2]

## BENIGN RENAL TUMORS

### Renal Medullary Fibroma

Renal medullary fibromas are the most common benign tumors, found in 35% of autopsies.[3] There is no sex predilection and 50% are bilateral. They are usually 1 cm or less in size and cause no symptoms. They are more common with increasing age and are rare in children and young adults.

Symptomatic lesions are primarily found in females and present with flank pain and hematuria,[4] and are not associated with hypertension. Accurate diagnosis is rare because the lesions appear as a filling defect on excretory urogram and are hypovascular at angiography. A partial nephrectomy would be adequate treatment; however, in most patients, a radical nephrectomy is performed due to the difficulty in determining the appropriate diagnosis preoperatively.

On gross examination, the lesion is similar to a uterine fibroid. Typically, they are gray–tan, well-demarcated, round nodules originating in the renal medulla. No distinct capsule is present. Microscopically, they are composed of a mixoid to densely fibrous stroma with interwoven collagen bundles in a "brush stroke" pattern. There are scattered spindle cells and small groups of entrapped tubules. These tubules are considered to be indicative of the etiology of the tumor.

In the past, fibrous tissue found in the renal parenchyma, perinephric tissues, and the renal capsule were termed renal fibromas. Petersen[5] and Lerman et al.[6] recommend the more specific name of renomedullary interstitial cell tumor to exclude renal capsular tumors and fibroepithelial polyps of the renal pelvis.

## Angiomyolipoma

Angiomyolipoma (AML) is a rare benign tumor of the kidney, also known as renal hamartoma, and consists of three elements: fat, abnormal blood vessels, and smooth muscle. The term angiomyolipoma was coined by Morgan et al. in 1951.[7] The incidence of this tumor in the general population is uncertain. It must be differentiated from RCC and the very rare tumor, renal liposarcoma, as the management is different; however, the presentation may be similar.

There are two distinct clinical entities of AML. The first form is found in 80% of tuberous sclerosis (TS) patients. Inheritance in TS is thought to be autosomal dominant with incomplete penetrance.[8] The syndrome consists of mental retardation, epilepsy, adenoma sebaceum of the face, Shagreen patches in the lumbosacral region, brain gliosis, submucosal fibromas, and hamartomas of the retina, lungs, liver, pancreas, bone, and kidneys.[8–12] AML are commonly bilateral, multifocal, and asymptomatic in this population. Only 50% of patients with AML have tuberous sclerosis. In the second category, there is no evidence of tuberous sclerosis and the lesions are usually solitary and symptomatic. Females between 35 and 60 years of age are predominantly affected, with the mass most often described as on the left side.

The mass has a variety of presentations ranging from symptomatic to those with chronic vague symptoms of abdominal discomfort or flank pain. In extreme cases, acute sharp pain results from hemorrhage in or around the tumor. Abdominal mass, gross hematuria, fever, and lightheadedness are less common complaints. Hypertension may be present. Alternately, hypotension and shock combined with a decreasing serial hemoglobin represent acute bleeding from the angiomyolipoma. Asymptomatic lesions are incidentally discovered on abdominal CT scans and ultrasounds more frequently than in the past due to increasing use of these modalities. These lesions are sometimes associated with microscopic hematuria.

Prior to the advent of computed tomography, AML was difficult to differentiate from RCC. Excretory urography detects a solid mass in most patients but is not diagnostically specific. Ultrasonography has improved with new technology, and AML appears as an intensely echogenic mass on ultrasound. This is not as specific as CT in distinguishing AML from malignancy and a confirmatory CT is recommended. Blute et al. report that six of eight renal masses with fat attenuation consistent with AML were detected by CT.[12] Houndsfield (H) units are usually low, −10 to −80 due to the negative density of fat, and are considered pathognomonic for AML. Normal renal parenchyma (15–25 H) does not contain fat. RCC has areas of necrotic degeneration with attenuation values of 0 to −10 H, clearly separating AML from RCC. Fat has been reported in some cases of Wilms' tumor; however, identification of fat in a renal mass in an adult is most suggestive of AML.[13] Ninety-five percent of the time CT can differentiate AML from RCC.[14] Renal angiography shows hypervascularity and pathologic vessels including arteriovenous fistulas.[10] Angiography is not generally indicated for diagnosis; however, it is useful for infarction of smaller lesions as a form of treatment for active bleeding. MRI with T1- and T2-weighted images has the same degree of reliability in detecting fat as CT; but reliability is decreased in evaluating small lesions.[13] Considering cost facts, CT is preferred over MRI when angiomyolipoma is suspected.

Pathologically, the gross appearance depends on which of the three elements predominates and varies from yellow, in those with high fat content, to gray. The mass is not encapsulated and may be solid or cystic. Hemorrhage and necrosis are present in some tumors. Histologically, the tumors are composed of the three components in varying proportions: mature fat cells, smooth muscle, and abnormal vessels. The fat cells have large central vacuoles and small peripheral nuclei. The smooth muscle originates from the muscle layers of the vessels. The vessels resemble arteries but are neither arteries nor veins; however, they do function and contain red blood cells. The size of the vessels ranges from capillaries to larger vessels with thick, muscular walls but normal elastic tissue is absent. Slightly pleomorphic nuclei are seen in the muscular component but bizarre mitotic activity is not evident.[15] The presence of nuclear pleomorphism in combination with multifocality and extension into the perirenal tissue has resulted in misinterpretations of the lesions as metastatic or as liposarcoma in the past. There are multiple reports of concurrent lymph node involvement in nephrectomy specimens, and there is one report of splenic involvement.[16–20] It is significant that no reports of death attributable to metastatic AML are reported in the literature, although AML has been noted to extend into the inferior vena cava.[21] Local recurrence is probably due to inadequate resection. Whether multicentricity represents the congenital presence of precursor cells or "benign metastasis" such as those seen with endometriosis and leiomyoma is not known.[19]

Renal-conserving therapy is indicated in AML. At least 10% of patients with AML develop acute hemorrhage requiring intervention. Initial management consists of bed rest and serial hematocrits unless shock is present. In those requiring treatment, a CT scan or intravenous pyelogram (IVP) should be done prior to an operation to determine the functional status of the contralateral kidney and exclude the presence of a mass in the opposite kidney as well. Angioinfarction of the bleeding vessels has been successful, sparing valuable parenchyma.

Blute et al. encouraged conservative management by observation in the asymptomatic or minimally symptomatic small lesions.[12] They have followed 11 patients without tuberous sclerosis from 1 to 6 years with annual radiologic evaluation. All have stable renal function and none have demonstrated increasing size or change in appearance. In their patients with TS, three of four in their series required an operation because of pain and/or hemorrhage.

A review by Osterling and associates used symptoms and size to determine management.[22] They recommend following lesions that are asymptomatic with yearly CT or ultrasound for lesions under 4 cm and biannually for lesions greater than 4 cm. Symptomatic lesions were managed initially by observation if less than 4 cm, and by selective embolization or surgical intervention for those larger than 4 cm. In our institution, we attempt embolization of symptomatic or bleeding lesions initially unless shock is present. We wait 6 weeks after successful embolization for hemorrhage to allow for healing and distinction of tissue planes. A partial nephrectomy is undertaken at that time if necessary.

RCC associated with AML has been reported in patients with the majority also suffering the stigmata of tuberous sclerosis. Newly diagnosed tuberous sclerosis patients should have an initial renal evaluation and yearly screening ultrasounds if no lesions are found initially. If AML is found, an annual or biannual CT scan or ultrasound should be performed depending on the size of the lesion. AML with calcification should be considered highly suspicious for malignancy and a nephrectomy or partial nephrectomy is recommended.

Renal-sparing surgery is encouraged for AML with sampling of hilar lymph nodes due to multicentricity. Complete removal of all involved tissue is the key to prevention of local recurrence.

### Lipoma

Primary intrarenal lipomas are found in about 1% of all autopsies.[23] Lipomas of a size significant enough to cause symptoms are rare. The kidney itself does not normally contain fat. There are multiple theories to explain the origin of these tumors. They are thought to arise from embryonal nests of fat or alternatively from multiplication of perivascular and intertubular connecting tissues that undergo fatty metamorphosis.

Unilateral pain is the representing symptom ranging from a dull ache to sharp colic. Renal lipomas are most common in middle-aged women and become symptomatic as they grow larger. Perirenal lipomas are more common than intrarenal lipomas and often are huge and bilateral. There are no reported cases of malignant transformation, and they are not associated with tuberous sclerosis. Replacement lipomatosis secondary to degenerative changes within the parenchyma is a separate entity.

On pathologic examination, gross characteristics are similar to any lipoma, ie, lobules interposed with streaks of blood vessels. An intrarenal lipoma is completely surrounded by the renal capsule and its blood supply is derived from renal arterial branches.[24] The diagnosis of perirenal lipoma should be entertained if the renal capsule is found within or between the tumor and renal parenchyma. Microscopic examination shows uniform fat cells. The differential diagnosis includes angiomyolipoma and liposarcoma. Compared to liposarcoma, there is an absence of local invasion, hemorrhage, and necrosis. Radiographic diagnosis is best made by CT scan. Typical fat density is observed allowing preoperative consideration of lipoma as the diagnosis. Nephrectomy is usually undertaken as excision of the lipoma alone is seldom possible. Nephrectomy cures the pain that is usually the primary symptom.

### Leiomyoma

Symptomatic urinary leiomyomas are uncommon but may arise from any structure or organ containing smooth muscle. In 5% of autopsies small, frequently multiple, leiomyomas are found associated with the renal capsule. Leiomyomas of renal origin occur in three basic types: small, often multiple asymptomatic subcortical lesions; large, solitary neoplasms associated with vessels of the renal capsule; and, rarely, those arising within the renal pelvis.[25]

Clinically, significant renal leiomyomas are rare and usually present with a mass or pain in the flank area or abdomen. They infrequently present with hematuria.[26] The peak frequency is in the fourth or fifth decade, although they have been diagnosed in a newborn.[27] There is a predilection for women. There is no specific appearance on intravenous urogram and angiographically there is no evidence of neovascularity.

The gross appearance of the cut surface is ivory to tan color and has a whorled appearance. There is no evidence of hemorrhage or necrosis. Microscopic examination discloses bundles of smooth muscle with no mitotic figures and minimal nuclear pleomorphism. These tumors should be differentiated from leiomyosarcoma, angiomyolipoma, and congenital mesoblastic nephroma. Gross invasion of adjacent structures and lack of circumscription denote malignancy as does the presence of mitosis.

Leiomyoma should be suspected if an exophytic renal mass is seen that is well circumscribed on CT scan and appears at exploration to be attached to the kidney but separate from the parenchyma. Excision of the mass alone is the treatment of choice, but usually the diagnosis is made at nephrectomy.[28]

### Hemangioma

Renal hemangioma is an uncommon lesion that can occur at any age. The diagnosis has been made from a 4-day-old infant to a 72-year-old, but the peak incidence is between 30 and 40 years of age. Intermittent hematuria is the presenting symptom 95% of the time, some with colic secondary to passage of clots. Rarely, a large arteriovenous shunt in the kidney leads to signs of cardiomegaly and heart failure. There is an equal distribution between sexes, and there is no side predilection. Twelve percent are multiple but the hemangiomata are usually unilateral. They range in size from pinpoint to extremely large but the majority are 1–2 cm.[29]

The diagnosis should be suspected in a person less than 40 years old with gross hematuria. In the past, the correct diagnosis was made only after nephrectomy for suspected tumor; however, improved diagnostic techniques allow for accurate preoperative diagnosis. The lesion can be lateralized during cystoscopy by visualization of bloody efflux from a ureteral orifice. A dark red lesion may be seen on flexible ureteroscopy of the renal pelvis. Selective angiography is helpful for diagnosis, with arteriovenous shunting within the hemangioma visualized in 8 of 13 patients at angiography.[30,31] Campistol et al. diagnosed a renal hemangioma with sequestration of radionuclide red blood cells.[32]

Pathologic examination reveals a well-demarcated cluster of blood-filled vascular channels that may contain thrombus. The formations are generally venous but may be arterial or mixed arteriovenous. They are generally cavernous but may be capillary. Some hemangiomas that give rise to hematuria are very small, almost pinpoint, and they seldom exceed 1–2 cm in diameter. They are typically blood-filled tributaries in a disorganized tangle that appear to arise from the renal medulla or submucosa of the renal collecting systems. Cytologic features are of benign tumors arising from the endothelium allowing for differentiation from angiosarcoma.

If the correct preoperative diagnosis is made, a partial nephrectomy can be undertaken or a wait-and-see attitude can be taken as they are usually not life threatening. Invasive radiologic techniques allow some hemangioma to be selectively embolized. Laser therapy via endoscopy may be a viable alternative in some cases.

### Juxtaglomerular Cell Tumor

The juxtaglomerular cell tumor is an important benign tumor of the kidney because it secretes renin causing profound hypertension. It is an uncommon neoplasm first described by Robertson et al. in 1967,[33] while the term was coined by Kihara et al. in 1968,[34] and 20 cases have been documented in the literature. They usually present in a young adult or adolescent with diastolic hypertension and hypokalemia. The hyperreninemia causes secondary hyperaldosteronism followed by hypokalemia. The diagnosis should be suspected in a young person with elevated serum renin. Radiographically the lesion is difficult to detect because most are less than 2.5 cm although they have been reported as large as 8 cm. An excretory urogram may reveal a mass while CT scan shows contrast enhancement. Angiography usually shows abnormal vessels.[35] Renal vein renin determinations demonstrate lateralization.

On gross inspection, the mass is small, gray–yellow, with hemorrhagic areas. Histologically, it resembles a hemangiopericytoma with sheets of cells, abundant pink cytoplasm, and oval, slightly irregular nuclei. Renin-secreting granules are detected with Bowie's stain, and tumor extract contains a high concentration of renin. Electron microscopy reveals juxtaglomerular cells, which are closely compacted uniform cells. The cytoplasm contains pools of particulate glycogen and lipid vacules. Some cells contain neurosecretory granules of various shapes with hypertrophied Golgi apparatus characteristic of juxtaglomerular cell tumor. Juxtaglomerular cell tumors are always benign and should be distinguished from the larger, nonfunctional renal hemangiopericytoma that is considered malignant. A partial nephrectomy should be considered if the diagnosis is made preoperatively.[36] Recently, a case was reported with a concomitant elevated erythropoietin that normalized after removal of the tumor.[37] Elevated renin levels normalize after nephrectomy and those patients remaining hypertensive postoperatively had sustained arterial damage in a portion of the kidney not involved by the tumor.[38]

## QUESTIONABLY BENIGN RENAL TUMORS

### Adenoma

Renal cortical adenomas are the second most common ''benign'' lesions of the kidney after renal medullary fibroma.[39] They are rarely symptomatic and are not associated with paraneoplastic syndromes. They are uncommon in children and young adults but are common after age 40. Seven percent to twenty-three percent are reported in adult autopsy series with males predominating more than 2:1.[3] They are located peripherally beneath the renal capsule, are less than 3 cm in size, and have tubular or papillary histology. They are frequently multiple but are rarely metastatic.

There are no x-ray characteristics on intravenous urogram, renal ultrasonography, angiography, or CT that reliably distinguish adenoma from carcinoma. MRI has not shown promise in differentiating the two thus far. With improved equipment, adenomas are increasingly found incidentally on roentgenographic studies.

Controversy exists regarding the benign nature or potential malignancy of renal adenomas. Adenomas of less than 3 cm have been known to metastasize and renal carcinoma arising from renal adenoma has also been reported.[40,41] Nonetheless, small adenomas are still regarded as benign lesions, particularly by our pathology colleagues. Previously adenomas were reported in autopsy series and in kidneys removed for nonmalignant disease. A classic autopsy study by Bell shows metastasis from a 1.5-cm lesion and a progressively higher rate of metastasis as the lesions grow larger. In his original paper in 1938, he states that ''the small tumors (so-called adenomas) are early stages of the large growths, and no certain distinctions can be made between adenomas and carcinoma.''[42] In a 1950 text he appears to contradict his prior statement by classifying these lesions as benign cortical adenomas if less than 3 cm vs. renal adenocarcinomas if greater than 3 cm.[43] The latter nomenclature has been perpetuated in the literature. Murphy and Mostofi report 29 nephrectomy patients in whom they believe an RCC arose in a renal adenoma.[41] In a follow-up on these patients 5 years later, 11% (1 in 9) of those with a lesion less than 3 cm in diameter and 70% (14 in 20) of those with a lesion greater than 3 cm had clinical metastases.

Bell's unfortunate use of the term ''benign adenoma'' for lesions under 3 cm was popularized and perpetuated despite his own qualification that the distinction between adenoma and carcinoma is often arbitrary especially in the case of solid adenoma. Few patients with clinically evident metastases have been reported in the literature. It has been a commonly held premise that an arteriosclerotic kidney with multiple peripheral adenomas will follow a benign course. Whether these peripheral adenomas will undergo malignant transformation in the future is unresolved.

Certainly the onus is on the clinician, not the pathologist. A long-term controlled study with a surgical arm and an observation arm on patients with incidentally found adenomas is needed to settle the controversy. The study may not be ethical in light of the fact that even 1.5-cm lesions have metastasized. Also, it becomes the physician's responsibility to monitor the patient and ensure that the requisite radiologic examination is obtained every 6–12 months to rule out enlargement of the ''benign'' adenoma to the ''carcinoma'' range.

We believe surgery is the conservative route for clinically evident renal adenomas and surveillance is risky particularly in adults in their fourth, fifth, and sixth decades where the anesthesia risk is low. Radical nephrectomy remains the standard treatment; however, bilateral partial nephrectomy or wedge resection with excision of adjacent fat may be considered. Enucleation is not recommended due to the possibility of leaving active tumor behind in the remaining bed.

Gillenwater et al.[11] recommend nephron-sparing surgery in asymptomatic incidentally found adenomas because the prognosis of patients with RCC treated with subtotal nephrectomy in solitary kidneys or with bilateral lesions has been similar to those treated with radical nephrectomy (with a normal contralateral kidney). Partial nephrectomy is also considered by some when the contralateral kidney may be affected by another process, such as Lindau–von Hippel disease, diabetes, or calculus. The presence of the paraneoplastic syndrome or calcifications in the adenoma should dictate radical nephrectomy when a normal contralateral kidney is present.

Regarding the pathology of small adenomas, macroscopically the nodules are off-white to yellow and lie superficially beneath the capsule.[39] Some have a well-defined capsule but infiltration and perforation are possible.[44] Occasional calcification is observed, but hemorrhage and necrosis are rare. Microscopically, the adenomas are composed of small cuboidal cells with a large, dark-staining round nuclei arranged in a papillary, cyst papillary, or tubular pattern with rare mitosis.

We believe the adenoma has low malignant potential and lies in a spectrum from benign adenoma to frank carcinoma. Incidental adenomas are on the rise due to increasing usage of abdominal ultrasound and CT scans. We recommend treatment as if these are early carcinomas since the biologic potential of any given lesion cannot be reliably predicted. Life expectancy, anesthesia, and surgical risk should be considered in each individual case. Any symptoms associated with a cortical mass including hematuria, flank pain, or paraneoplastic syndrome should be considered -indications for surgery.

## Oncocytoma

Renal oncocytomas comprise 5%–7% of renal tumors. The term was introduced in 1932 by Jaffe[45] as a description for tumors of the salivary gland. It is composed of large polygonal cells possessing abundant cytoplasm called oncocytes. Other glandular organs with these tumors include the thyroid, parathyroid, and kidney. The first series of renal oncocytoma was reported in 1976 with 13 patients with renal proximal tubular adenomas with so-called oncocytic features.[46] Retrospective reviews of granular or dark cell tumors determined that many oncocytomas were classified as RCCs. Oncocytes are differentiated from granular cell adenocarcinoma because they contain abundant mitochondria but not other organelles in their cytoplasm. The two tumors follow different clinical courses and should be distinguished for this reason. While oncocytomas are clinically benign, granular cell adenocarcinoma is a more aggressive lesion. Retrospective reviews show a rising incidence whereas others have not observed clustering in recent years.[46–48] Local involvement of lymph nodes and renal veins has been reported but distant metastasis is rare.

Klein and Valensi documented characteristics of these tumors.[46] These include a large mass with well-differentiated borders usually found incidentally. Sixty-five percent are symptomatic and are found on autopsy or abdominal roentgenographic studies done for other reasons. The tumor usually follows a benign clinical course with a long recurrence-free interval. The risk of metastasis does not correlate with size as it does in RCC. These tumors may be multicentric and bilateral.

Commonly, the tumor is found in males with a peak incidence in the sixth to eighth decades, although they are reported from age 15–102 years. Thirty-five percent present with pain, hematuria, or a mass. Spontaneous hemorrhage or rupture into the perirenal adipose tissue is unusual as is a paraneoplastic syndrome. Radiologic examination does not reliably differentiate these tumors from RCC. Ultrasound and intravenous urography show a circumscribed solid mass. Reports of a characteristic angiographic pattern are one of its hallmarks. A spoke-wheel pattern of interlobar arteries or stellate pattern in the arterial phase without arteriovenous fistula or venous pooling is largely responsible for its identification as a specific clinical entity. These patterns occur in malignant tumors more frequently and thus are not pathognomonic of oncocytoma. CT also may demonstrate a spoke-wheel pattern with central necrosis but, once again, caution must be used.

On gross examination, a tan or mahogany red–brown color in a well-demarcated large solid tumor with a central fibrous scar is classic. They average around 7 cm with the largest reported being 26 cm. They are surrounded by a capsule in most cases and there is a characteristic absence of extensive hemorrhage, hypervascularity, or necrosis. Focal cystic changes, polycystic disease, and RCC may be located adjacent to an oncocytoma.

Large homogeneous eosinophilic cells, usually in nests, cords, or tubules of tumor cells in loose edematous stroma, are seen microscopically. Sheets of tumor cells or microcysts lined by oncocytic cells are less common. These cells are uniformly polygonal with round or oval hyperchromatic nuclei. Low-grade nuclear atypia or occasional cells with enlarged bizarre nuclei are seen. Nucleoli may be prominent or inconspicuous, but mitosis is rare.[49]

Electron microscopy demonstrates an ultrastructure with a profusion of mitochondria and a paucity of Golgi apparatus and rough endoplasmic reticulum. Microvilli are inconsistently present. This is in contrast to granular cell tumors with numerous mitochondria as well as Golgi apparatus and endoplasmic reticulum. The electron micrography picture is also similar to proximal convoluted tubule cells, indicating a common site of origin with RCC.

Lieber et al. described 90 cases of "pure" oncocytomas in a retrospective review.[47] They classified the tumors into grade I with similar regular cells, round smooth nuclei, and abundant eosinophilic cytoplasm. Grade II cells were more varied in size; configuration and the nuclei were larger and more irregular. They also allow abundant mitotic figures in their grade II classification. None of the grade I but four (14%) of the grade II tumor patients died of metastatic disease during an 18-month follow-up. They acknowledge that multiple areas of tumor were rarely sampled, so other elements of renal carcinoma or spindle cells cannot be entirely excluded. Also, most authors would classify only those tumors with rare mitosis as oncocytoma,[49,50] whereas tumors with multiple mitosis were included in this series. Barnes and Beckman identified 10 oncocytomas and 6 congeners; the latter had areas inconsistent with oncocytoma on gross and histologic section.[51] One of the six patients in the oncocytoma congeners group died, and they suggest there may have been inadequate sectioning of the tumor. Their recommendation is for total excision of oncocytomas for complete examination. They stress that needle aspiration or biopsy with frozen section could lead to misdiagnosis of the tumor. One needs to be aware that there are areas of oncocytic cells in RCC, and this could lead to an error in diagnosis.

Other large series on renal oncocytoma are retrospective reviews of pathologic material where the tumors were not carefully sectioned; therefore, a component of RCC cannot be excluded. No proven metastasis of grade I renal oncocytomas has occurred. Most reported metastases occur in grade II oncocytoma but are usually not biopsy- or autopsy-proven to be oncocytoma. One grade II renal oncocytoma metastasized to the lung 14 years after a nephrectomy and biopsy confirmed the histology to be oncocytoma.[52,53]

Flow cytometry on archival pathologic specimens demonstrates that the DNA histograms are the same as normal renal parenchyma.[54] Rainwater et al.'s[55] retrospective study shows a large percentage of DNA tetraploid and DNA aneuploid tumors. Histologic grade I and II tumors were evaluated in this study. When analyzed by grade, DNA polyploidy was found in 39% of grade I and 43% of grade II tumors. An aneuploid pattern was documented in 11% of grade I and 24% of grade II tumors. Conversely, Eble and Sledge[54] found no evidence of aneuploidy in the seven oncocytomas studied. The clinical use of flow cytometry to classify and predict the behavior of oncocytomas may not prove useful in the future even if grade II tumors are excluded since 50% of the unequivocal grade I oncocytomas have abnormal DNA ploidy.[55]

Recent analysis of renal tumors includes chromosomal analysis in an attempt to classify and predict the behavior of renal tumors, oncocytomas included. Thus far, chromosomal analysis has not shed light on the subject.

Six percent of these tumors penetrate the renal fat, 2% involve regional lymph nodes, 9% extend into the renal pelvis, and 3% extend into the renal vein or vena cava. One percent are bilateral or multifocal. Although renal oncocytoma rarely metastasizes and usually follows a benign course, it can be locally aggressive. We recommend a radical nephrectomy with adequate surgical margins as the treatment of choice. A small polar oncocytoma found incidentally could be considered for a partial nephrectomy. We do not recommend observation as these tumors may contain a focus of RCC that can be missed by biopsy alone.

## INTRODUCTION TO RENAL CELL CARCINOMA

Renal cell carcinoma represents 2%–3% of all adult malignancies, and is more common in males by a ratio of 2:1. In the past, these tumors presented most often in the fifth to seventh decades of life; however, with the advent of abdominal ultrasound and CT, RCCs are increasingly diagnosed in younger patients.

The etiology of RCC is unknown, but the cell of origin is considered the proximal tubular cell.[56] Variable reports on smoking implicate cigarettes whereas others suggest that pipe and cigar smoking carry a higher risk. Brownson[56] showed an elevated risk of RCC in truck drivers and a weaker association observed for mechanics. These reports are consistent with work in laboratory animals where kidney carcinoma has been associated with prolonged exposure to unleaded gasoline vapors[57] and components of petroleum byproducts such as dimethylnitrosamines. Further risk factors include exposure to cadmium, obesity, and living in an urban environment. There is a familial incidence in sporadic family trees.[58] There is an increased incidence of RCC in patients with Lindau–von Hippel disease, an autosomal dominant genetic disorder with variable penetrance.[59,60]

### Presentation

Renal cell carcinoma has been called the "internist tumor" because of its protean manifestations. The classic triad of symptoms—hematuria, flank pain, and a flank mass—occurs in only 10% of patients. Hematuria is the most common presenting sign, present in approximately 60% of patients. Microscopic hematuria may be found on routine physical examination or the patient may complain of gross hematuria which is usually painless. RCC is associated with pain in four instances: (1) spontaneous renal parenchymal hemorrhage; (2) invasion of surrounding structures; (3) clot colic associated with gross hematuria; and (4) distant metastatic disease to bone or brain. About 25%–30% of patients present with metastatic disease, many with the complaint of bone pain due to metastatic deposits.

Physical signs are few in RCC. Bimanual examination of the flank and upper quadrants of the abdomen may reveal a ballotable flank mass. New onset of symptomatic varicocele, one that does not recede in the recumbent position, is most common on the right due to renal vein or vena caval tumor thrombus. The recent onset of a varicocele in an older male is pathognomonic for renal mass but is only present in 2%–3%. Generalized weight loss and cachexia is present in up to one third of patients with RCC.

Hematuria can be associated with flank pain or suprapubic discomfort and clot retention. The patient may complain of persistent day and/or night sweats due to pyrexia. Release of endogenous pyrogens from the tumor are thought to cause the pyrexia and is present in 15% of the patients. Hypertension is common in the age group that develops RCC, but 10% of patients will have resolution of their hypertension after nephrectomy. The tumor may produce a renin-like substance, or mechanical effects of a large mass or an arteriovenous fistula may induce the juxtaglomerular apparatus to produce increased endogenous renin.

Laboratory findings are nonspecific and include gross or microscopic hematuria on urine analysis. Urine cytology is rarely helpful for diagnosis in RCC. More than half of the patients have an elevated erythrocyte sedimentation rate. Anemia is common and is usually the anemia of chronic disease (normocytic, normochromic) and, less frequently, hypochromic, microcytic variety due to blood loss. At the other end of the spectrum, erythrocytosis due to production of erythropoietin or a similar substance generated by the tumor is observed. Erythropoietin is presumed to be produced in response to localized hypoxia. Ectopic ACTH production and hyperprolactinemia have also been reported. Hypercalcemia is present in 3%–13% of patients and can be life threatening. A parathormone-like substance produced by the tumor is the cause of the elevated calcium in some whereas those with metastatic deposits in the bone may have release of calcium from osteolytic lesions.

Abnormalities of liver function occur in patients with RCC with and without hepatic metastasis.[61] The diagnosis of Stauffers' syndrome, ie, individuals without hepatic metastasis but with elevated liver enzymes, requires at least three of the following biochemical abnormalities: elevation of alkaline phosphatase or α-globulin, prolonged prothrombin time, hypoalbuminemia, hypergammaglobulinemia, or increased bilirubin and glutamyl transpeptidase. Half of these patients will have nontender hepatomegaly. The syndrome is not related to the prognosis and liver function parameters usually resolve with nephrectomy. Nonresolution of the syndrome after nephrectomy portends a poor prognosis with 90% of patients with abnormal liver function tests after nephrectomy ultimately demonstrating metastasis.[62] Only 26% of patients in whom the syndrome does not resolve will survive one year. Monitoring patients who had resolution of Stauffers' syndrome after nephrectomy with serial liver function studies is recommended as return of the hepatic dysfunction is associated with recurrent disease.[63]

The majority of patients with hypercalcemia have high-stage lesions but the morphologic cell type may vary. The source of the elevated calcium may be from osteolytic osseous metastasis of RCC or be the humoral hypercalcemia of malignancy. Albright first suggested a syndrome of pseudohyperparathyroidism, demonstrating hypercalcemia in the presence of malignancy without osseous metastasis. Tumors have been shown to express parathormone and a parathyroid hormone-like peptide. One must exclude primary hyperparathyroidism, particularly if the hypercalcemia persists after nephrectomy.[64]

Fever is associated with RCC in 20%–40% of patients. It may be the initial or sole manifestation of the tumor. The fever may be caused by tumor necrosis with release of pyrogens, secretion of pyrogens by the tumor cells, or prostaglandin release.[65] It does not correlate with tumor stage or degree of tumor necrosis, and is more common in the granular than clear cell pattern. It also occurs in female more often than in male patients. Tumor recurrence is associated with the reappearance of fever. Prostaglandin production has also been associated with pyrexia.

### Genetics

Renal cell carcinoma most commonly occurs sporadically and rarely in family lineage. The familial form may carry a defective gene as these tumors present at an earlier age, tending toward bilaterality and multifocality.[66] The best example is Lindau–von Hippel disease, which is autosomal dominant with incomplete penetrance.

The most common chromosomal change observed in RCC is deletions and translocations in the short arm of chromosome 3 (3p).[67] Sporadic RCC shows a high incidence of changes in chromosome 3 on cytogenetic studies.[68] Deletion of DNA sequences on chromosome 3p may play a role in tumor initiation or progression. Three of the family RCC lineages (without Lindau–von Hippel disease) gave a translocation of chromosome 3p to chromosomes 6, 8, or 11 consistent within each family.

### Flow Cytometry

Approximately 50% of RCCs contain aneuploid cells as measured by flow cytometry while the remainder have a normal diploid pattern.[69] In a study of 68 RCC patients, there was correlation between tumors with aneuploid DNA histograms and recurrent tumor. In tumors with diploid histograms, there was a 21% recurrence rate in contrast to 89% of those with aneuploid histograms.[70] Most of the diploid tumors were classified as grade I or II (out of four grades). The tumors that were low grade but aneuploid had an 87% rate of metastasis. Baisch et al. had similar findings where 8 of 17 aneuploid tumors and 1 of 14 diploid tumor patients died or relapsed although length of follow-up was short.[71]

Flow cytometry showing aneuploidy correlates well with progression to metastasis in the future in several studies.[70,71] High-grade tumors tend to have more aneuploid cells but ploidy does not strictly correlate with tumor grade. Ploidy may have prognostic implication and be used to determine which patient should have adjuvant therapy in the future. Ploidy combined with tumor grade has had a good correlation with prognosis. High grade combined with aneuploid flow cytometry portends a poor prognosis while low-grade tumors with a diploid pattern predicts a good prognosis.

## Imaging of Renal Masses

Renal imaging for renal masses is thoroughly covered in Chapter 20. The following is a summary of imaging studies for the evaluation of renal masses.

In the past, excretory urogram with tomography followed by angiography and venacavography were the only diagnostic tools available to the urologist. Surgical exploration and biopsy were necessary to determine the nature of a renal mass visualized with radiologic studies. New technologies have been developed in uroradiology and have changed the practice of urology. Advances have been made in nuclear medicine, ultrasonography, computerized tomography (CT), and magnetic resonance imaging (MRI). The imaging diagnosis of a simple cyst or angiomyolipoma may obviate the need for surgery. The solid mass with documented distant metastasis would preclude surgery for cure as well. Imaging techniques assist the urologic surgeon in planning the surgical approach to a solid mass.

Intravenous urogram (IVU) with tomography continues to be the initial study for hematuria, the most common reason for diagnostic studies (Fig 1). Irregularity of the

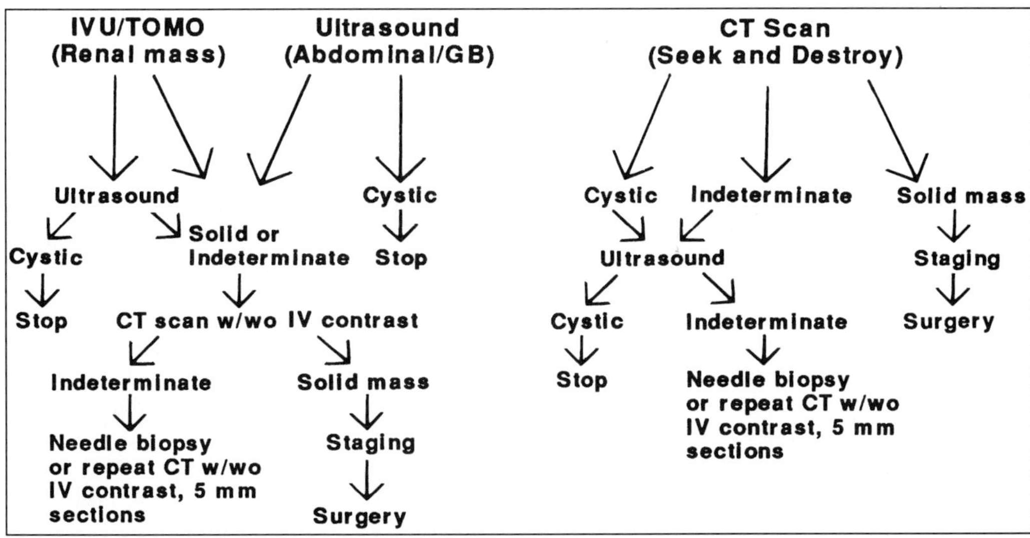


**Fig 1.** Algorithm for evaluation of a renal mass.

renal shadow may show an exophytic mass. The collecting system is also visualized on IVU and an intraluminal filling defect may represent a tumor in the collecting system. When a parenchymal mass is detected on IVU, it should be followed by a renal ultrasound. A simple cyst requires no further studies.[72,73] A solid or indeterminate mass requires a CT scan with and without intravenous contrast and with Houndsfield units on the mass. A solid mass on CT scan requires surgical exploration unless the presence of fat suggests an angiomyolipoma. Enlargement of the renal vein or vena cava should raise suspicions for tumor thrombus. An indeterminate mass on CT scan is usually followed by biopsy with CT or ultrasound guidance or, as an alternative to biopsy, a repeat renal CT with and without contrast, with 5-mm sections and bolus infusion to clarify the consistency of the mass.[74]

Venous tumor extension determination by CT is accurate only 78% of the time.[75] MRI is more accurate than CT and less invasive than venacavography. It has the added benefit of not requiring intravenous contrast.[76,77] Coronal and sagittal sections should be done when patients undergo MRI. Ultrasound for renal vein or venacaval thrombus is highly technician-dependent and therefore not recommended in most cases.

Angiography does not play as significant a role in the diagnosis of renal masses as it did in the past. Angiography is helpful in planning surgery where partial nephrectomy or autotransplantation after bench surgery is concerned. Bilateral tumors, a tumor in a solitary kidney, or a small tumor amenable to a partial nephrectomy all benefit from angiography to map the blood supply of the affected renal unit.

Most solid renal masses are considered surgical lesions. A history of fever and rigors may indicate a renal caruncle or abscess, and a focal mass may be a lobar nephronia. An abscess should be percutaneously or surgically drained and treated with appropriate intravenous antibiotics alone selected on the basis of urine culture. A renal mass in a lymphoma, leukemia, or cancer patient should undergo percutaneous biopsy, particularly if the mass persists after appropriate chemotherapy for the underlying disease.

## Staging

Staging procedures in RCC include a history, physical examination, laboratory tests, roentgenographic studies of the kidneys, and a chest PA and lateral. History may reveal bone pain or recent weight loss suggesting advanced disease. Physical exam may show a varicocele or caput medusa, leg edema, flank or abdominal mass. Laboratory tests do not correlate with stage but may direct the investigator. Elevated liver enzymes suggest metastatic disease to the liver or Stauffers' syndrome. Elevated alkaline phosphatase or hypercalcemia may result from bony metastasis and should be followed up with a bone scan. Routine bone scans without clinical or chemical indication are not warranted. Complete blood count will show anemia of chronic disease or erythrocytosis. Rarely, microcytic, hypochromic anemia is present due to blood loss. Baseline renal function is assessed with a blood urea nitrogen and creatinine.

Roentgenographic examinations include the chest to determine the presence of lung metastasis. An abnormal chest x-ray should be pursued with a chest CT to determine the number of suspicious lesions present and to direct a biopsy. An abdominal CT is helpful in staging RCC. Abdominal lymph nodes can be evaluated for enlargement; however, 50% of enlarged lymph nodes are due to inflammation and hyperplasia, not to metastasis. No patient should be denied a potentially curative operation based solely on enlarged abdominal lymph nodes. The liver and other organs should be studied for metastasis. The CT shows the extent of the tumor and vena cava or renal vein involvement. An MRI is suggested to document the extent of vena cava tumor extension if it is suspected. Venacavography is an alternative, albeit invasive, way to study venous involvement if MRI is not available. Ultrasonography is accurate for staging in only 70%.

Robson et al.[78] modified a staging classification based on works by Flocks and Kadesky.[79] This system is easy to use but

**TABLE 1. Staging Systems**

| Robson's | |
|---|---|
| Stage I | Tumor confined within the kidney |
| Stage II | Perirenal fat involvement confined within Gerota's fascia |
| Stage III | Local spread |
| | a. Involvement of renal vein or inferior vena cava |
| | b. Involvement of regional lymph nodes |
| | c. Vascular and lymphatic involvement |
| Stage IV | Extensive disease |
| | Adjacent organs other than adrenal |
| | Distant metastases |

| TNM | |
|---|---|
| *Tumor (T)* | |
| TX | Primary tumor cannot be assessed |
| TO | No evidence of primary |
| T1 | Small tumor, minimal renal deformity |
| T2 | Large tumor, with renal enlargement and/or deformity |
| T3 | Tumor extending into perinephric tissues |
| T4 | Tumor invading adjacent organ or abdominal wall |
| *Nodes (N)* | |
| NX | Nodal involvement cannot be assessed |
| N0 | No involvement of regional nodes |
| N1 | Involvement of single homolateral regional node |
| N2 | Involvement of contralateral, bilateral, or multiple nodes |
| N3 | Fixed nodes at surgical exploration |
| N4 | Involvement of juxtaregional nodes |
| *Metastases (M)* | |
| MX | Distant metastases cannot be assessed |
| M0 | No evidence of distant metastases |
| M1 | Distant metastases present |
| M$^1$a | Occult metastases |
| M$^1$b | Solitary in single organ |
| M$^1$c | Multiple in single organ |
| M$^1$d | Multiple in multiple sites |

does not correlate well with prognosis. The TNM system is the most accurate but it is lengthy and cumbersome to use. It has been applied to large retrospective studies but patients in each category remain few in number thus limiting its usefulness for predicting an individual patient's outcome (Table 1).

Radical nephrectomy for Robson stage I tumors have 5- and 10-year survivals of 65% and 56%, respectively. Stage II tumors involve the perinephric fat but are confined within Gerota's fascia. The 5-year survival is 45% and decreases to 20% in 10 years. Robson stage III includes local spread to the lymph nodes and/or major veins as well as vena cava. Prognosis in stage III tumors is not as clear as the other stages. Complete resection of a tumor with renal vein involvement (IIIa) may not adversely affect survival. On the other hand, vena caval involvement affects longevity in proportion to the extent of the tumor thrombus. Complete excision of infradiaphragmatic tumor thrombus (IIIa) portends a poorer prognosis. The fact that incompletely resected inferior vena cava thrombus, thrombus in the hepatic veins, or supradiaphragmatic thrombus are more difficult to resect completely is reflected in lower survival. Regional lymph node involvement (IIIb) is a dire prognostic indicator with only a 20% 5-year survival. Selective series have shown up to 35% 5-year survival with extensive lymph node dissection; however, patients in poor general condition are excluded in these reports.[80]

The Robson staging classification, although easy to use, does not correlate well with the outcome of the patients particularly with respect to stage III lesions. The limitation of this classification prompted the development of the TNM classification. This classification is also based on the pathologic specimen.[81] Urologic surgeons need to become facile with the TNM system as it is used by many tumor registries.

In the TNM system, patients with vena caval involvement (T3c) and no perinephric fat extension (T3a) are separated from those with both (T3ac). This system is somewhat awkward to use but will eventually result in more accurate survival curves. Nodal involvement by volume is a separate entity in this system. Direct extension to the adrenal gland is classified as T3a in the TNM system.[82]

## ADULT WILMS' TUMOR

Wilms' tumor or nephroblastoma is the most common renal tumor of childhood but is rarely found in the adult population, accounting for less than 1% of Wilms' tumors. It is difficult to evaluate because of the many synonyms, 53 in number, and errors in reporting tumor types.[83,84] It is found in young adults, average age of 40–50 years, with flank pain, sciatica, abdominal or flank mass, weight loss, and occasionally hematuria. There is no side or sex predilection. The prognosis in adults is generally not as good as in their pediatric counterparts stage for stage, and adults often present with more advanced tumors.[85,86] While death usually occurs in children within the first 2 years, many of the adult deaths occur as late as 6 years. It is possible that adults tend to have unfavorable histology, but this is not well documented. Byrd et al. report 31 adults with Wilms' tumor who received aggressive chemotherapy and found an overall survival of 24% at 3 years.[85] Survival in stages I and II was 48%, whereas those with distant metastases faced a dismal prognosis with only 11% survival.

Staging is according to the criteria of the National Wilms' Tumor Study Grouping System: group I, tumor limited to the kidney; group II, tumor extending beyond the kidney but resected completely and excised completely; group III, residual nonhematogenous tumor metastasis; group IV, hematogenous metastasis; and group V, bilateral Wilms' tumor (synchronous or metachronous).[87]

Wilms' tumor originates from the totipotential cells of the metanephric blastema that undergoes malignant transformation. Diagnosis requires documentation of three components: epithelial, stromal, and blastemal. Typically, there are varying proportions of epithelial components composed of tubules and glomerular structures in a background of spindle cell stromal components and densely cellular blastemal tissue.[88] Tumors are classified as epithelial, stromal, blastemal prominent or mixed. There can be no area of the tumor diagnostic for RCC. Unfavorable prognosis includes tumors with areas of anaplasia.

Preoperative staging is similar to RCC. There are no specific features to distinguish Wilms' tumor for RCC on radiologic studies. IVP shows subtle calcifications in 10%–30%, half being punctuate and the remainder curvilinear. Nonfunction may be present. Both tumors may be hypovascular or hypervascular on arteriogram but no arteriovenous fistulas will be present in Wilms' tumor.

Initial treatment includes radical nephrectomy or open biopsy if nephrectomy is not technically feasible. The contralateral kidney is infrequently biopsied as the diagnosis is not suspected preoperatively. Less than 1% of adult cases are bilateral, therefore, Roth et al.[86] believe biopsy of the contralateral kidney is not necessary for that reason. Biopsy should be undertaken only if a contralateral mass is present.

All patients should have adjuvant chemotherapy as adults have a poorer prognosis than children. This usually consists of actinomycin D for stage I disease with the addition of vincristine alone or with doxorubicin for higher stage disease. Radiation of the renal fossa should be considered in all stages. One can argue that children who present with stage I disease have an excellent prognosis without radiation. Radiation therapy is less toxic to adults than children and is recommended to optimize survivability. The lung is the most common site of metastasis followed by liver, bone, skin, bladder, sigmoid colon, orbit, brain, and spinal cord. Whole-lung radiation is very successful with pulmonary metastasis.

## SARCOMAS

Sarcomas represent 1%–2% of malignant tumors of the kidneys. The incidence increases with advancing age, with over 100 cases having been reported. The most common signs and symptoms are similar to those of RCC: flank pain, abdominal or flank mass, and hematuria. They do not have distinctive radiologic characteristics (with the exception of osteogenic sarcoma) making preoperative differentiation from RCC difficult. The majority are thought to arise from the renal capsule; however, they may also arise from the renal parenchyma. They are generally large, circumscribed, and may be encapsulated or nonencapsulated tumors that compress the renal cortex and sometimes invade the collecting system with rare venous invasion.

Treatment consists of radical nephrectomy. Prognosis is poor with surgery alone. Adjuvant therapy is recommended. Chemotherapy has shown some minor success with doxorubicin on a short-term basis. Radiation therapy has not proven beneficial. The long-term prognosis is unknown because so few sarcomas have been treated, but it appears to be no greater than a 10% 5-year survival.

## SECONDARY TUMORS OF THE KIDNEY

Lymphomas and leukemia are the most common secondary malignancies to affect the kidney. Clinical detection of metastatic tumors to the kidney is rare, although they are common on necropsy studies. Secondary tumors excluding lymphoma and leukemia have an incidence of 7%–11% in autopsy studies performed on patients who died of malignant disease.[89–91] Forty to fifty percent are bilateral.

One third of lymphoma patients dying of their disease have renal metastasis.[92] It is a rare primary site for lymphoma, and bilateral involvement with metastasis is high (75%). Non-Hodgkin's lymphoma affects the kidney more frequently than Hodgkin's disease. Morphologically, a nodular or diffuse distribution through the kidney is present.[93] Occasionally, a poorly demarcated solitary mass is observed, occurring late in the disease process.[94] Ten percent have hydronephrosis due to ureteral obstruction by lymphatous nodes but uremia is decidedly rare. Radiation and chemotherapy dramatically improve renal function secondary to lymphoma.

Leukemic infiltration of the kidney is rarely clinically evident but is present in two thirds of autopsies on patients who have died of leukemia. Lymphocytic leukemias involve the kidney more frequently than myelogenous leukemias. Histologically, leukemic cells infiltrate the interstitium in a patchy or diffuse pattern sparing the glomerulus. Hemorrhage is common. There is usually bilateral involvement of the renal units, but uremia is unusual.

Solid tumors most likely to metastasize to the kidney by primary site are melanomas and tumors of the adrenal gland, testes, and lung. With the exception of lung cancer, these are uncommon tumors. The most frequent metastatic tumors found on autopsy studies are those from the lung, breast, gastrointestinal sites, and melanomas. The age of presentation is in the fifth to seventh decades with the sexes affected equally. Clinical detection is rare despite high prevalence on necropsy. The diameter of metastasis documented by Bracken et al. on a large autopsy series was 29% less than 1 cm, 22% between 1 and 3 cm, 10% greater than 3 cm, and the remainder were not recorded by size.[89] There was no predilection for upper, middle, or lower poles and in several cases multiple ureteral satellites were present.

Albuminuria is present in virtually all urine specimens while only 31% had microscopic evidence of red blood cells in the spun sediment.[91] In regard to renal function, mild to moderate renal impairment is usually present but less than 5% of the patients die of uremia. There are no specific findings for renal metastasis on intravenous urogram or angiography. We recommend ultrasound or CT prior to and after intravenous contrast administration. The fact is that a large number of metastases have a small diameter, making detection difficult. Hydronephrosis may be present. Retrograde pyelograms are helpful if satellite lesions of the ureter are suspected but urine cytologies are not generally diagnostic. Suspicious lesions on ultrasound or CT scan should be fine needle–biopsied to show a metastatic lesion and exclude a primary kidney tumor such as RCC.

## REFERENCES


1. Silverberg E, Lubera JA. *Cancer Statistics.* 1989; 39(1):3.
2. Silverberg E, Boring CC, Squires. *Cancer Statistics.* 1990;40(1):9.
3. Culp DA, Loening SA, eds. *Genitourinary Oncology.* Bks. Demand; 1985.
4. Glover SD, Buck AC. Renal medullary fibroma: a case report. *J Urol.* 1981;127:758.
5. Petersen RO, ed. *Urologic Pathology.* Philadelphia: JB Lippincott; 1986.
6. Lerman RJ, Pitcock JA, Stephenson P, et al. Renomedullary interstitial cell tumor (formerly fibroma of renal medulla). *Hum Pathol.* 1972;3: 559.
7. Morgan GS, Staumfjord JV, Hall EJ. Angiomyolipoma of the kidney. *J Urol.* 1951;65:525.
8. Bissada NK, White HJ, Sun CN, et al. Tuberous sclerosis complex and renal angiomyolipoma. *Urology.* 1975;6(1):105.
9. Drago JR, Nesbitt JA, Leb R. Renal angiomyolipomas. *J Surg Oncol.* 1988;39:64.
10. Morgan GS, Staumfjord JV, Hall EF. Diagnosis and management of renal angiomyolipoma. *Urology.* 1985;25(5):461.
11. Gillenwater JY, Grayhack JT, Howard SS, Duckett JW. *Adult and Pediatric Urology.* Chicago: Year Book; 1987.
12. Blute ML, Malek RS, Segura JW. Angiomyolipoma clinical metamorphosis and concepts for management. *J Urol.* 1988;139(1):20.
13. Pollack HM (ed). *Clinical Urography.* Philadelphia: WB Saunders, 1990.
14. Stillwell TJ, Gomez MR, Kelalis PP. Renal lesions in tuberous sclerosis. *J Urol.* 1987;139(3): 477.
15. Pitts WR, Kazam E, Gray G, Vaughn ED. Ultrasonography, computerized transaxial tomography and pathology of angiomyolipoma of the kidney: solution to a diagnostic dilemma. *J Urol.* 1980;124(6):907.
16. Busch FM, Bark CJ, Clyde HR. Benign renal angiomyolipoma with regional lymph node involvement. *J Urol.* 1976;116(6):715.
17. Taylor RS, Joseph DB, Kohaut EC, et al. Renal angiomyolipoma associated with lymph node involvement and renal cell carcinoma in patients with tuberous sclerosis. *J Urol.* 1989;141(4):930.
18. Friis J, Hjortrup A. Extrarenal angiomyolipoma diagnosis and management. *J Urol.* 1982;127: 528.
19. Bloom DA, Scardino PT, Ehrlich RM, Waisman J. The significance of lymph nodal involvement in renal angiomyolipoma. *J Urol.* 1982;128(6): 1292.
20. Hulbert JL, Graf R. Involvement of the spleen by renal angiomyolipoma: metastasis or multicentricity? *J Urol.* 1983;130(2):328.
21. Arenson AM, Graham RT, Shaw P, et al. Angiomyolipoma of the kidney extending into the inferior vena cava: sonographic and CT findings. *AJR.* 1988;51:1159.
22. Osterling JE, Fishman EK, Goldman SM, Marshall FF. The management of renal angiomyolipoma. *J Urol.* 1986;35:1121.
23. Robertson TD, Hand JR. Primary intrarenal lipoma of surgical significance. *J Urol.* 1941;46: 458.
24. Dineen MK, Venable DD, Misra RP. Pure intrarenal lipoma—report of a case and review of the literature. *J Urol.* 1984;132(1):140.
25. Mohler JL, Casale AJ. Renal capsular leiomyoma. *J Urol.* 1987;138(4):853.
26. Belis JA, Post GJ, Rochman SC, Milam DF. Genitourinary leiomyomas. *Urology.* 1979; 13(4):424.
27. Fisher KS, vanBlerk PJP. Childhood leiomyoma of kidney. *Urology.* 1983;21(1):74.
28. Steiner M, Quinlan D, Goldman S, et al. Leiomyoma of the kidney: presentation of four new cases and the role of computerized tomography. *J Urol.* 1990;143:994.
29. Peterson NE, Thompson HT. Renal hemangioma. *J Urol.* 1971;105(1):27.
30. Andersen JB, Rasmussen T. Renal haemangioma diagnosed preoperatively by renal angiography. *ACTA Radiologica Diag.* 1964;2:201.
31. Ekelund L, Gothlin J. Renal hemaniomas: 13 cases diagnosed by angiography. *AJR.* 1975;125: 788.
32. Campistol JM, Agusti C, Tomas A, et al. Renal hemangioma and renal artery aneurysm in the Klippel–Trenauny syndrome. *J Urol.* 1988; 140(1):134.
33. Robertson PW, Klidjian A, Harding LK, Walters G. Hypertension due to a renin-secreting renal tumor. *Am J Med.* 1967;43:963.
34. Kihara I, Kitamura S, Hoshino T, et al. A hitherto unreported vascular tumor of the kidney: a proposal of "juxtaglomerular cell tumor." *ACTA Pathol Jap.* 1968;18:197.
35. Conn JW, Cohen EL, McDonald WJ, et al. The syndrome of hypertension, hyperreninemia, and secondary aldosteronism associated with renal juxtaglomerular cell tumor (primary reninism). *J Urol.* 1973;109(3):349.
36. Skinner DG, Lieskowvsky G, eds. *Diagnosis and Management of Genitourinary Cancer.* Philadelphia: WB Saunders; 1988.
37. Remynse LC, Begun FP, Jacobs SC, Lawson RK. Juxtaglomerular cell tumor with elevation of serum erythropoietin. *J Urol.* 1989;142(6): 1560.
38. Dennis RL, McDougal WS, Glick AD, MacDowell RC Jr. Juxtaglomerular cell tumor of the kidney. *J Urol.* 1985;134:334.
39. Xipell JM. The incidence of benign renal nodules (a clinicopathologic study). *J Urol.* 1971;106: 503.
40. Murphy GP, Mostofi FK. The significance of cy-

toplasmic granularity in the prognosis of renal cell carcinoma. *J Urol.* 1965;94:48.

41. Murphy GP, Mostofi FK. Histologic assessment and clinical prognosis of renal adenoma. *J Urol.* 1970;103:31.
42. Bell ET. A classification of renal tumors with observations on the frequency of the various types. *J Urol.* 1938;39:238.
43. Bell ET, ed. Tumors of the kidneys. In: *Renal Diseases.* Philadelphia: Lea and Febiger; 1950.
44. Pfannkuch F, Leistenschneider W, Nagel R. Problems of assessment in the surgery of renal adenomas. *J Urol.* 1981;125:95.
45. Jaffe RH. Adenolymphoma (oncocytoma) of parotid gland. *Am J Cancer.* 1932;16:1415.
46. Klein MJ, Valensi QJ. Proximal tubular adenomas of kidney with so-called oncocytic features. A clinicopathologic study of 13 cases of a rarely reported neoplasm. *Cancer.* 1976;38:906.
47. Lieber MM, Tomera KM, Farrow GM. Renal oncocytoma. *J Urol.* 1981;125(4):481.
48. Fairchild TN, Dail DH, Brannen GE. Renal oncocytoma—bilateral, multifocal. *Urology.* 1983; 22(4):355.
49. Peterson RO (ed.). *Urologic Pathology.* Philadelphia: JB Lippincott; 1986.
50. Psihramis KE, Althausen AF, Yoshio AA, et al. Chromosome anomalies suggestive of malignant transformation in bilateral renal oncocytoma. *J Urol.* 1986;136(4):892.
51. Barnes CA, Beckman EN. Renal oncocytoma and its congeners. *Am J Clin Pathol.* 1982;79(3): 312.
52. Lewi HJE, Alexander CA, Fleming S. Renal oncocytoma. *Br J Urol.* 1986;58:12.
53. Lewi H. Renal oncocytoma (letter). *Urology.* 1986;28(1):78.
54. Eble JN, Sledge G. Cellular deoxyribonucleic acid content of renal oncocytomas: flow cytometric analysis of paraffin-embedded tissues from light tumors. *J Urol.* 1986;136(2):522.
55. Rainwater LM, Farrow GM, Lieber MM. Flow cytometry of renal oncocytoma: common occurrence of deoxyribonucleic acid polyploidy and aneuploidy. *J Urol.* 1986;135(6):1167.
56. Brownson RC. A case-control study of renal cell carcinoma in relation to occupation, smoking, and alcohol consumption. *Arch Environ Health.* 1988;43(3):238.
57. MacFarland HN, Ulrich CE, Holdsworth CE, et al. A chronic inhalation study with unleaded gasoline vapor. *J Am Coll Toxicol.* 1984;3:231.
58. Doyal HH, Wilkinson GS. Epidemiology of renal cell cancer. *Semin Urol.* 1989;7(3):139.
59. Lynch HT, Walzak MP. Genetics in urologic cancer. *Urol Clin North Am.* 1980;7:815.
60. Kuhlman JK, Fishman EK, Marshall FF, Siegelman SS. CT diagnosis of unsuspected von Hippel–Lindau disease. *Urology.* 1987;30(5): 505.
61. Utz DC, Warren MM, Gregg JA, et al. Reversible hepatic dysfunction associated with hypernephroma. *Mayo Clin Proc.* 1970;45:161.
62. Suffin G, Chasan S, Golic A, Murphy GP. Paraneoplastic and serologic syndromes of renal adenocarcinoma. *Semin Urol.* 1989;7(3):158.
63. Case Records of the Massachusetts General Hospital. *N Engl J Med.* 1941;225:789.
64. Fahn HJ, Lee YH, Chen MT, et al. The incidence and prognostic significance of humoral hypercalcemia in renal cell carcinoma. *J Urol.* 1991; 145(2):248.
65. Gilman AG, Goodman LS, Gilman A. *The Pharmacological Basis of Therapeutics.* New York: Macmillan; 1975.
66. Malek RS, Omess PJ, Benson RC, Zincke H. Renal cell carcinoma in von Hippel–Lindau syndrome. *Am J Med.* 1987;82:236.
67. Daniel LN, Linehan WM. Genetics of renal cell carcinoma. *Semin Urol.* 1989;7(4):258.
68. Levinson KA, Johnson DE, Strong LC, et al. Familial renal cell carcinoma: hereditary or coincidental? *J Urol.* 1990;144:849.
69. Grignon DJ, Ayala AG, El-Naggar A, et al. Renal cell carcinoma: a clinicopathologic and DNA flow cytometric analysis of 103 cases. *Cancer.* 1989;64:2133.
70. Otto U, Baisch H, Huland H, Kloppel G. Tumor cell deoxyribonucleic acid content and prognosis in human renal cell carcinoma. *J Urol.* 1984;132: 237.
71. Baisch H, Otto U, Konig K, et al. DNA content of human kidney carcinoma cells in relation to histological grading. *Br J Cancer.* 1982;45:878.
72. Cronan JJ. Practical approach to renal masses, unpublished, 1989.
73. Kissane JM. The morphology of renal cystic disease. *Persp Nephrol Hypertension.* 1976;4:31.
74. Zeman RK, Cronan JJ, Rosenfield AT, et al. Renal cell carcinoma: dynamic thin-section CT assessment of vascular invasion and tumor vascularity. *Radiology.* 1988;167:393.
75. Johnson CD, Dunnick NR, Cohan RH, Illescas FF. Renal adenocarcinoma: CT staging of 100 tumors. *Am J Roentgenol.* 1987;148:59.
76. Goldfarb DA, Novick AC, Lorig R, et al. Magnetic resonance imaging for assessment of vena caval tumor thrombi: a comparative study with venacavography and computerized tomography scanning. *J Urol.* 1990;144(5):1100.
77. Horan JJ, Robertson CN, Choyke PL, et al. The detection of renal carcinoma extension into renal vein and inferior venacava: a prospective comparison of venacavography and magnetic resonance imaging. *J Urol.* 1989;142:943.
78. Robson C, Churchill BM, Anderson W. The results of radical nephrectomy for renal cell carcinoma. *J Urol.* 1969;101:297.
79. Flocks RH, Kadesky MC. Malignant neoplasms of the kidney: an analysis of 353 patients followed 5 years or more. *J Urol.* 1958;79:196.

80. Skinner DG, Lieskovsky G, eds. *Diagnosis and Management of Genitourinary Cancer.* Philadelphia: WB Saunders; 1988.
81. Bassil B, Dororetz D, Prout GR Jr. Validation of the tumor, nodes and metastasis classification of renal cell carcinoma. *J Urol.* 1985;134:450.
82. Hermanek P, Schrott KM. Evaluation of the new tumor, nodes and metastases classification of renal cell carcinoma. *J Urol.* 1990;144(2):238.
83. Gupta OP, Dube MK. Rare primary renal sarcoma. *Br J Urol.* 1971;43:546.
84. Godec CJ, Smith SJ, Belzer MB, Strom RL. Triple therapy for adult Wilms' tumor. *Urology.* 1987;30(2):147.
85. Byrd RL, Evans AE, D'Angio GJ. Adult Wilms' tumor: effect of combined therapy on survival. *J Urol.* 1982;127:648.
86. Roth DR, Wright J, Cawood CD, Pranke DW. Nephroblastoma in adults. *J Urol.* 1984;132:108.
87. D'Angio GJ, Evans A, Breslow N, et al. The treatment of Wilms' tumor: results of the second national Wilms' tumor study. *Cancer.* 1981;47:2302.
88. Petersen RO, ed. *Urologic Pathology.* Philadelphia: JB Lippincott; 1986.
89. Bracken RB, Chica G, Johnson DE, Luna M. Secondary renal neoplasms: an autopsy study. *South Med J.* 1979;27(7):806.
90. Roy JB, Walton KN. Secondary tumors of the kidney. *J Urol.* 1970;103:411–413.
91. Wagle DG, Moore RH, Murphy GP. Secondary carcinomas of the kidney. *J Urol.* 1975;114:30.
92. Pascal RR. Renal manifestations of extrarenal neoplasms. *Hum Pathol.* 1980;11(1):7.
93. Richmond J, Sherman RS, Diamond HD, et al. Renal lesions associated with malignant lymphomas. *Am J Med.* 1962;32:184.
94. Osborne BM, Brenner M, Weitzner S, Butler JJ. Malignant lymphoma presenting as a renal mass: four cases. *Am J Surg Pathol.* 1987;11(5):375.

# 28

# Management of Renal Carcinoma

*Jong Woo Choe, Edward W. Campbell, Jr., Michael J. Naslund, and Stephen C. Jacobs*

## INTRODUCTION

The cure of renal carcinoma is essentially by surgical means. Other treatment modalities, however, may play a role in the management of the disease. Renal carcinoma has been known as a cancer with considerable vagaries in its progression and these behavioral uncertainties need to be considered when weighing courses of patient treatment. In the 1990s urologists have the impression that surgical cure rates for renal cancer are improving. Much of this is due to the current early detection of the disease. Patients rarely present with the classic triad of flank mass, flank pain, and hematuria. The average patient now presents with a renal mass found incidentally on an imaging study or, at most, one of the three from the classic triad. With smaller tumors being found earlier, surgical cure rates should improve as the risk of nodal and distant metastases falls with smaller primary cancers.

Radiation therapy fills a very small niche in the management of renal carcinoma. We are now in the second decade of promises of advances in both chemotherapy and immunotherapy, and basically no substantial impact on renal cancer management has been made thus far. If patients with metastatic disease are living longer or more comfortably today, then the improvements in supportive care are primarily responsible.

## RESULTS OF RADICAL NEPHRECTOMY

Radical nephrectomy is the unilateral en bloc excision of the contents of Gerota's fascia. In the past, surgeons generally cut through cancer and did simple nephrectomies for large renal tumors that presented with flank mass, flank pain, and hematuria. A major problem with this approach was local recurrence. In the 1930s the first principles of an en bloc resection of renal cancer were espoused, but it was not until after World War II that Chute et al described a true radical nephrectomy.[1] Robson popularized the operation[2] and stressed the importance of an accompanying lymph node dissection. The survival data Robson presented were much better than the 1930s results. But, in fact, data on the additive value of current lymph node dissection do not support his survival statistics.[3]

Currently, radical nephrectomy for stage I renal carcinoma (see Table 1) produces a 56% to 82% 5-year survival and a 20% to 72% 10-year survival.[4–8] For stage II renal carcinoma the reported values are 93% to 100% 5-year survival and 0% to 67% 10-year survival. For stage III renal carcinoma, radical nephrectomy will pro-

**TABLE 1. Comparison of Conventional and TNM Staging Classification of Renal Cell Cancer**

| Robson Stage | T | N | M |
|---|---|---|---|
| I. Tumor combined by renal capsule | T1 (small tumor with minimal calyceal distortion)<br>T2 (large tumor with calyceal deformity) | | |
| II. Tumor extension to perirenal fat or ipsilateral adrenal but confirmed by Gerota's fascia | $T_{3a}$ | | |
| IIIa. Renal vein or inferior vena cava involvement | $T_{3b}$ (renal vein involvement)<br>$T_{3c}$ (renal vein and caval involvement below the diaphragm)<br>$T_{4b}$ (caval involvement above the diaphragm) | $N_0$ (nodes negative) | $M_0$ (lack of distant metastases) |
| IIIb. Lymphatic involvement | $T_{1-3}$ | $N_1$ (single homolateral regional node involved)<br>$N_2$ (multiple regional, contralateral, or bilateral nodes involved)<br>$N_3$ (fixed regional nodes)<br>$N_4$ (juxtaregional nodes involved) | |
| IIIc. Combination of IIIa and IIIb | $T_{3-4}$ | $N_{1-4}$ | |
| IVa. Spread to contiguous organs except ipsilateral adrenal | $T_{4a}$ | $N_{0-4}$ | |
| IVb. Distant metastases | $T_{1-4}$ | $N_{0-4}$ | $M_1$ |

duce an 8% to 51% 5-year survival and a 0% to 38% 10-year survival. For stage IV renal carcinoma, the long-term results of radical nephrectomy are poor: 0% to 13% 5-year survival and 0% to 7% 10-year survival. Obviously, favorable biologic characteristics of the cancer—not the nephrectomy—are responsible for the few survivors with stage IV renal cancer.

As the presenting renal carcinomas become smaller, the absolute necessity of the radical nature of the excision falls. For example, the ipsilateral adrenal gland can be spared unless directly invaded. Often partial nephrectomies are feasible if necessary with less risk of tumor spillage than in Robson's day.

## Technique of Radical Nephrectomy

The purpose of the radical nephrectomy incision is to best encompass the particular tumor and give the surgeon the clearest operative exposure, but still give the patient the least morbid skin and muscle incision. Figure 1 shows five incisions; each incisional exposure has its benefits and detractions.

The standard flank incision places the patient in a flank-up position, but jackknifed with kidney rest up and the table flexed. This position increases the risk for (1) a brachial plexus injury, (2) dependent lung hypoventilation, (3) diminished venous return due to the flexed position, par-

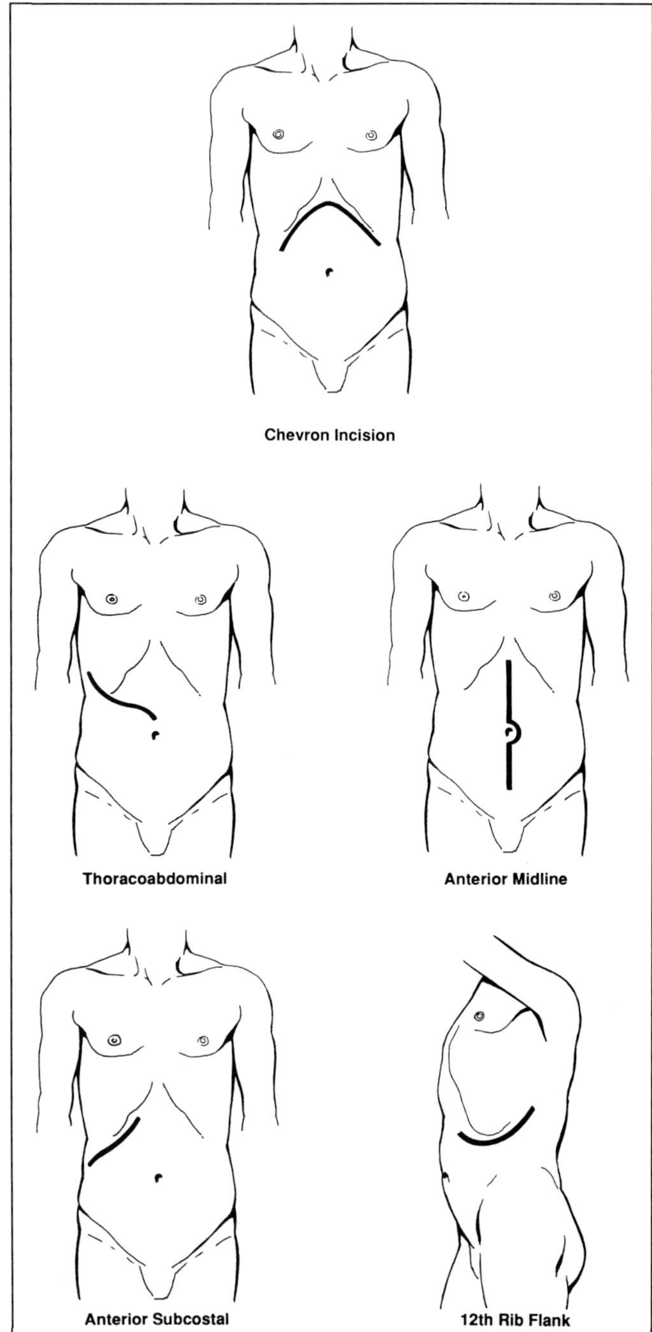


**Fig 1.** Incisions for radical nephrectomy.

ticularly in elderly or dehydrated patients, and (4) pneumothorax (small). The advantages of the standard flank incision are that (1) its extraperitoneal nature results in shorter postoperative ileus, (2) wound infections are extremely rare, and (3) there is very good exposure of all sides of the kidney (renal hilum least well seen).

The anterior subcostal approach produces slightly less incisional pain, but exposure of the kidney is more difficult. This approach gives a good view of renal vessels but poorer visualization of the posterior kidney and the upper pole. The anterior subcostal approach should not be used for large tumors.

The anterior midline approach is favored by most general surgeons. The incisional pain is probably the least, but this incision requires the most difficult retraction intraoperatively. The renal vessels can be well controlled and the exposure can be bilateral, but upper pole and posterior exposure is poor.

The chevron incision provides good exposure to the entire anterior abdomen, but requires cutting the rectus muscles, which can result in prolonged postoperative incisional pain. This incision also requires a transperitoneal approach.

The thoracoabdominal incision provides the best exposure of the kidney and the great vessels. The primary disadvantages of this incision are increased operative time during closure and the need for a postoperative chest tube.

The laparoscopic approach provides the best incision for postoperative patient comfort. However, currently the laparoscopic approach to nephrectomy is tedious, time consuming, and unproven in terms of its ability to avoid tumor spillage. To date, experience with laparoscopic nephrectomy has been with simple, not radical, nephrectomy.[9]

After the incisional exposure has been completed, the peritoneum is separated from Gerota's fascia by pulling the peritoneal contents medially. On the right side the ascending colon, the colonic mesentery, and the duodenum together bluntly separate from Gerota's fascia and expose the vena cava. On the left the descending colon and colonic mesentery similarly separate from Gerota's fascia to expose the renal vein at the level of the aorta. The extensive dilated veins will be inside Gerota's unless the renal carcinoma has perforated through Gerota's fascia. Ligation of the renal artery close to the aorta shrinks the tumor mass and diminishes subsequent blood loss (see Fig 2). Early ligation of the vessels also theoretically decreases intraoperative tumor shedding into the vascular system. The renal vein is ligated at the vena cava on the right or over the aorta on the left. On the right side, the short adrenal vein must be ligated at the vena cava. On the left side, the adrenal, gonadal, and lumbar veins enter the renal vein and are individually tied during dissection of the renal vein. Lumbar vessels may need to be ligated a second time as they exit Gerota's fascia posteriorly. After ligation of the renal vessels, Gerota's fascia and its contents are freed from surrounding structures; all nodal tissue anterior, posterior, and lateral to the great vessel is taken with the kidney. The perinephric fat and Gerota's fascia are pulled off the diaphragm superiorly and freed from the posterior body wall bluntly. The ureter is ligated distally and the gonadal vein is ligated again distally. The entire contents of Gerota's fascia are removed. Drains are generally not needed. The kidney can be bivalved on a side table and sent for frozen section diagnosis if there is concern that transitional cell carcinoma is present and that a distal ureterectomy is necessary.

## RESULTS OF LYMPHADENECTOMY

There is some debate as to whether a lymphadenectomy for renal carcinoma improves the prognosis. Approximately 25% of patients with renal carcinoma have positive lymph nodes. Of all patients who have metastases, only 15% have lymph node metastases alone.[10] This is the pool that might benefit from lymph node dissection. Several series document patients with very small amounts of lymph node metastases with as high as a 40% to 50% 5-year survival for those who have lymph node dissection.[6,11,12]

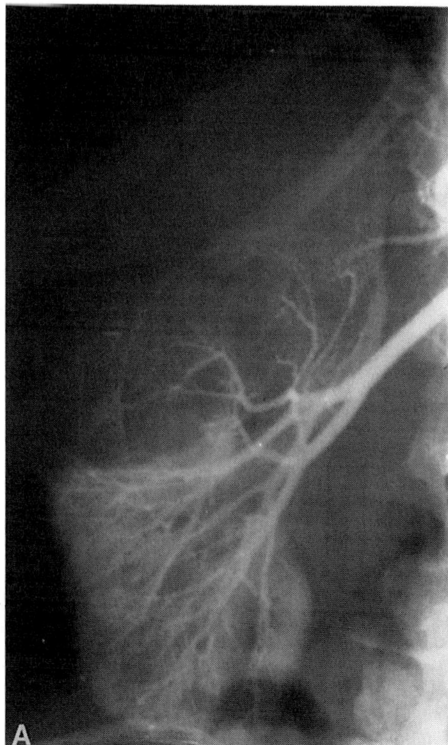


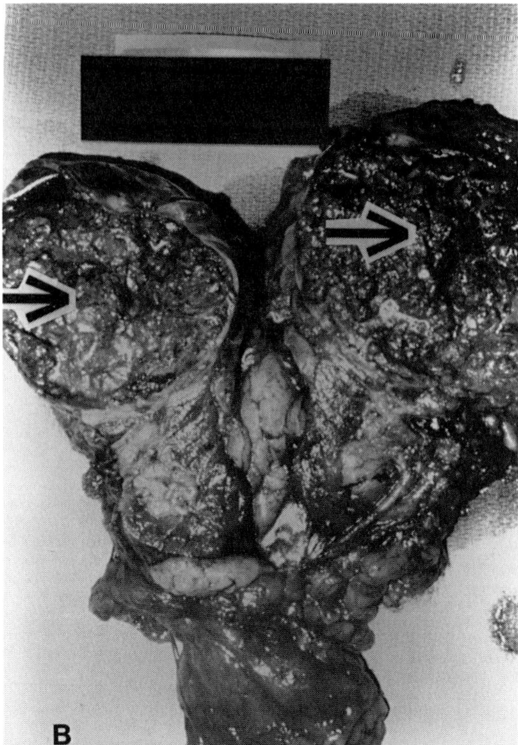


**Fig 2.** Hypovascular renal carcinoma. Some renal carcinomas are remarkably hypovascular at angiography, as opposed to the usual hypervascular appearance. **A** demonstrates a large right upper pole hypovascular mass; **B** shows the fresh bivalved nephrectomy specimen with a totally necrotic renal carcinoma (arrows). Instead of the usual golden yellow color, these tumors are a necrotic muddy brown. The prognosis for such patients who have necrosed their own tumors is probably better.

Complications of lymphadenectomy are few and the procedure does not add much operative time. Lymphocele formation is possible but quite rare, as is chylous ascites. Injury to the superior mesenteric artery is possible and dissection of the celiac ganglion leads to longer postoperative ileus.

### Technique of Lymphadenectomy

For a complete lymphadenectomy, all nodal tissue surrounding the great vessel on the tumor side is removed from the bifurcation of the aorta to the diaphragm. While the interaortocaval, anterior, lateral, and posterior nodal tissue is removed, usually the resection does not require sacrifice of all lumbar arteries and veins as in a testis tumor node dissection. Fat and lymph nodal tissue from under the crus of diaphragm is also extracted. The sympathetic chain usually is sacrificed on the tumor side and patients will complain mildly of a relative vasodilatation in the ipsilateral leg (or a cold contralateral foot). On the aorta anteriorly, dissection around the superior mesenteric artery and celiac trunk should be done with extreme care. On the vena cava anteriorly, the hepatic veins limit the resection. Drains are generally unnecessary.

## RESULTS WITH VENOUS INVASION

Approximately one third of renal carcinomas have involvement of the venous system. Most of these have venous invasion still within the kidney and less than 5% actually extend into the inferior vena cava. Less than 1% of venous invasion extends all the way into the atrium.[13–16] Survival in cases of venous invasion is primarily dependent on the presence or absence of metastases, either nodal or distant.[17,18] Certainly if all tumor cannot be removed, then the 5-year survival for these patients approaches 0%.

Preoperative delineation of the extent of the tumor thrombus dictates the approach. Venography is still probably the most accurate method for determining tumor thrombus extent, but from a practical standpoint, angiography is being replaced by computerized tomography (CT) and magnetic resonance imaging (MRI). MRI is sensitive in detecting and delineating caval extension. CT scanning is accurate in determining whether tumor is present but is not as useful at showing the extent of the thrombus.

In an unobstructed vena cava, the tumor thrombus grows in the same direction as the blood flow. However, if the vena cava is obstructed and blood flow is low, then the renal cancer may grow retrograde in the cava and out venous branches, including the lumbar, gonadal, and contralateral renal veins.

## Surgical Technique with Vena Caval Involvement

Surgical approaches to caval involvement depend on the tumor thrombus extent (Figs 3 and 4). Radiographic evaluation is extremely important in defining this extent. The thoracoabdominal approach is clearly best when handling all but the most minor of vena caval tumor thrombi. Tumor thrombi within the vena cava are conveniently divided into infrahepatic, intrahepatic, and supradiaphragmatic because the approach to each is distinctly different.

**Infrahepatic Thrombus.** Smaller tumors involving the infrahepatic vena cava are usually free-floating and do not invade the caval wall. First control of the vena cava above and below the tumor thrombus is obtained. A controlling loop is also passed around the contralateral renal vein for control. Early ligation of the renal artery will cause the tumor thrombus to shrink. A venacavotomy close to the entrance of the affected renal vein will allow the tumor thrombus to come out with the kidney. Repair of the vena cava with 5–0 prolene is done before use of release tourniquets. Because the vasculature is well controlled, there is little need for a cell saver in most cases.

**Intrahepatic Thrombus.** Intrahepatic caval extension of renal carcinoma is more likely to have caval wall invasion. For these cases, the diaphragm is opened. The triangular ligaments holding the liver are cut and the right liver is rotated medially to allow visualization of the retrohepatic cava. The hepatic veins are ligated and divided as they enter the anterior surface of the vena cava until a tourniquet can be placed around the vena cava above the tumor thrombus. Obviously, an absolute requirement is that some major hepatic venous drainage be spared. If the vena cava is clotted off, then the cava can be ligated and sectioned above the tumor. If the vena cava is open, then the patient must be tested intraoperatively to determine whether the cardiovascular system can adapt to the diminished venous return.

In cases of right renal carcinoma, the left renal venous return is not permanently compromised by a vena caval resection. Left renal venous return will adapt to return via adrenal, phrenic, lumbar, and gonadal venous routes. However, in cases of left renal carcinoma, vena caval resection cannot be done without providing venous drainage for the right renal vein. Right renal vein to portal vein bypass to protect the remaining right kidney is possible, but very difficult technically. Free-floating thrombus above the site of vascular control can be retrieved by extraction under back bleeding, often with a Foley catheter balloon above the tumor thrombus aiding the extraction. Clearly the potential for blood loss is higher in these intrahepatic cava cases and a cell saver can be very useful (Figs 5 and 6).

**Supradiaphragmatic Thrombus.** Most tumor thrombi involving the supradiaphragmatic cava and right atrium cannot be re-

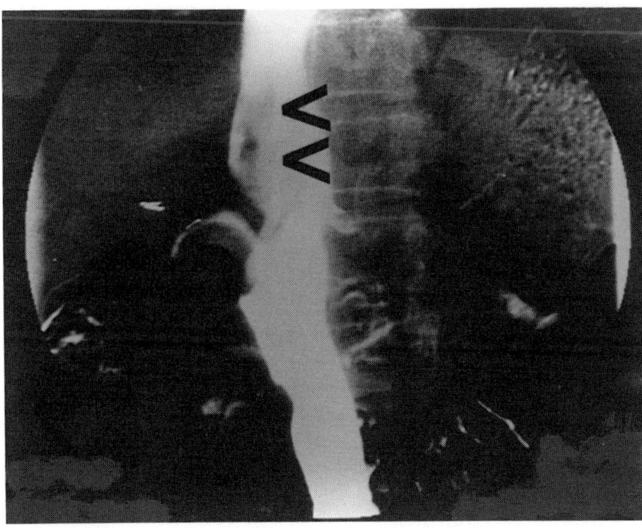

**Fig 3.** Vena caval thrombus. Digital angiography demonstrates a tumor thrombus (arrows) emanating from the right renal vein and floating freely in the vena cava.

trieved from below because the risk of tumor embolus during manipulation of the thrombus is substantial. Most surgeons now recommend hypothermic circulatory arrest under cardiopulmonary bypass. The patient is approached through a midline sternal and abdominal incision. The kidney and tumor are freed for radical nephrectomy with the exception that the renal vein is left untouched. The vena cava is controlled and the patient is put on bypass. The right atrium is opened and the tumor thrombus inspected from above. The cavotomy and section of the renal vein is performed and the tumor is extracted from below using a Foley catheter. Any tumor emboli are seen and retrieved using suction by the cardiac surgeon.

Resection of large caval tumor thrombi present significant operative risks to the patient. The intraoperative mortality from embolus alone is 4%, and postoperative mortality from bleeding, sepsis, or multiorgan failure ranges from 2% to 7%. The

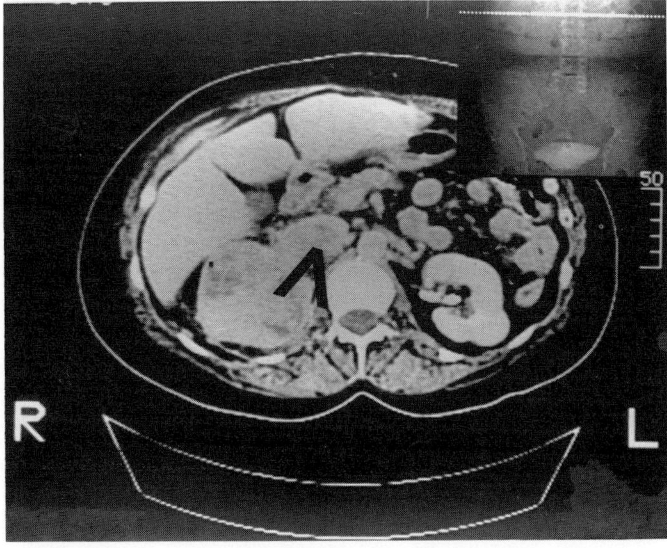


**Fig 4.** Venal caval involvement. Computed tomography demonstrates that the right renal carcinoma is extending into the vena cava (arrow).

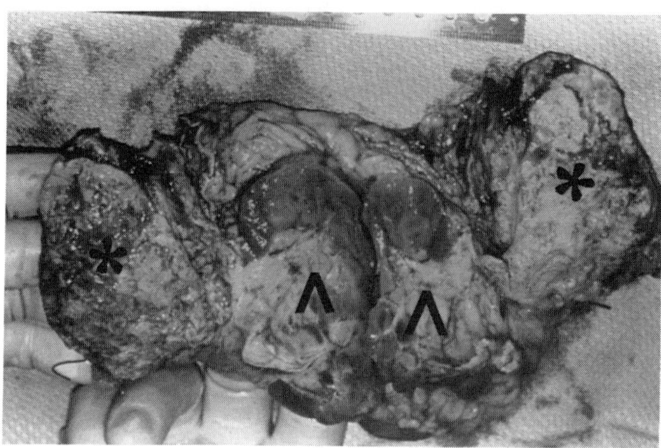

**Fig 5.** Vena caval resection. The fresh bivalved radical nephrectomy specimen demonstrates that the intrahepatic vena cava tumor mass (asterisk) may considerably exceed in size the primary renal cancer (arrows).

average experience may not be as successful as the reported series.[17–22] Furthermore, the morbidity from transient renal, cardiac, or respiratory failure is substantial. Long-term survival with supradiaphragmatic cases is in the 20% to 33% range.[19]

## MANAGEMENT OF RENAL CARCINOMA IN THE SOLITARY KIDNEY

For patients with a renal carcinoma in a solitary functioning kidney, the goal must be not only to cure the cancer but to maintain renal function and avoid dialysis. For patients with low-grade stage I renal carcinoma, the 5-year survival for renal sparring resection is the same as for radical nephrectomy.

Partial nephrectomy yields good tumor margins but takes away functioning renal parenchyma. The blood loss from a partial nephrectomy is generally greater than from a radical nephrectomy. Enucleation of the tumor as an alternative involves excising the tumor at a cleavage plane at the level of the tumor pseudocapsule.[23] Enucleation does not result in much blood loss. However, enucleation has a high positive margin rate and may result in the leaving of some cancer cells at the base of the tumor.[24,25] For patients with multicentric renal cancers within one kidney, enucleation is often the only alternative to nephrectomy and dialysis.

### Technique of Partial Nephrectomy

**Enucleation.** The renal artery and vein are controlled as for a radical nephrectomy, but vessel loops are used instead of ligatures. Gerota's fascia is opened and the perinephric fat is dissected off the normal kidney leaving it to cover the tumor only. The junction of the tumor and the normal renal parenchyma is exposed and the renal capsule is incised around the bulging tumor. A blunt instrument is used to tease the tumor off the renal parenchyma. In the base there will be a feeding vessel entering the tumor. This is cauterized or oversewn. The entire cavity is fulgurated in an attempt to minimize the viable tumor cells that might remain. The cavity can be left open or packed with vascularized fat. A postoperative drain is usually used (Fig 7).

**Partial Nephrectomy.** The same exposure is used for partial nephrectomy as for enucleation except the tumor/parenchymal junction is not directly visualized. The renal capsule is incised 1 cm away from the tumor. The renal capsule is elevated circumferentially away from the tumor for another 1 cm. The renal parenchyma is then cut 2 cm away from the tumor. In cases of small polar resections, compression of the renal parenchyma by the assistant's hand will control bleeding. Open renal parenchymal vessels are then suture-ligated with 3–0 chromic. The collecting system is closed to prevent hematuria. Mattress sutures of 2–0 chromic are used to compress capsule and bleeding parenchyma. The cut surface of the kidney is packed with fat or gelfoam and the surface drained.

**Hypothermic Ischemia.** Doing the partial nephrectomy under cold ischemia results in a much lower blood loss. However, older kidneys or atherosclerotic kidneys do not tolerate ischemia as well as younger or healthier kidneys. After exposure and control of the renal vessels, a rubber or plastic sheet is placed around the kidney to hold the ice slush. The kidney is anticoagulated by giving the patient heparin 5000 U IV and an osmotic diuresis is started with mannitol 12.5 g IV. Bulldog vascular clamps are used to occlude the renal vessels, and iced saline and slush are used to immediately cool the kidney to 4°C. The partial nephrectomy is then done in a bloodless field. Closure of the vessels, collecting system, and renal capsule is much easier under cold ischemia. After release of the vascular occlusion clamps, hemostasis is completed prior to drainage and closure (Fig 8).

**Bench Surgery and Autotransplantation.** Some partial renal resections are very difficult because the major renal vessels are involved in the cancer and they need to be reconstructed in order to salvage parenchyma. Midpolar or hilar cancers especially cause sufficient problems that they may have to be resected and then microvascular techniques used to repair or reconstruct the vasculature. Basically the radical nephrectomy is done in the manner of a donor nephrectomy. The kidney and Gerota's fascia are completely freed up so that only the renal artery and vein are left. Heparin 5000 U and mannitol 12.5 g are given IV and the renal vessels are clamped and sectioned. The tumor-bearing kidney is immediately cold-perfused with Euro-

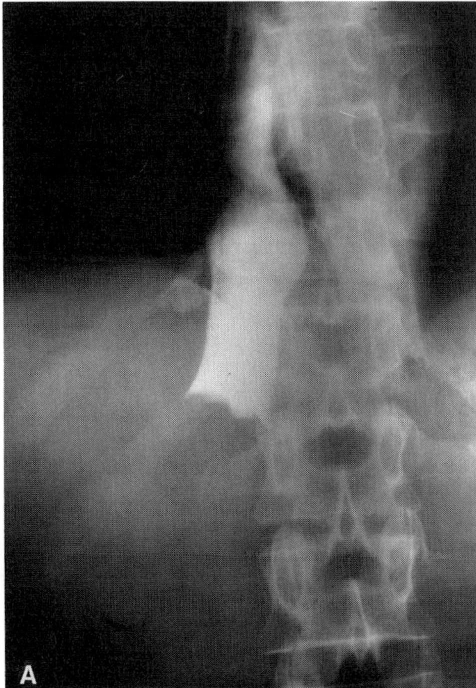


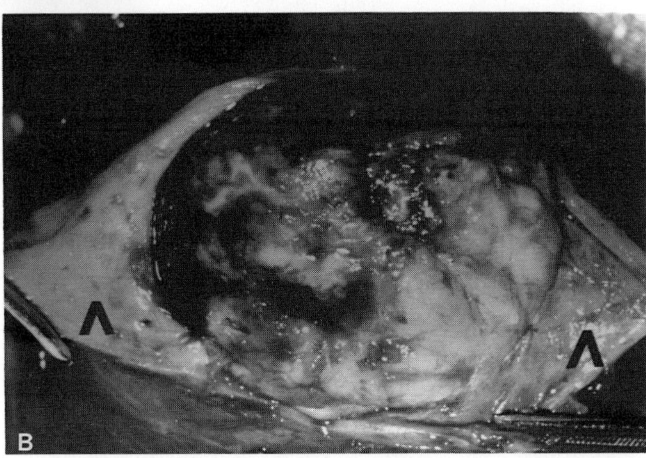


**Fig 6.** Vena caval invasion. **A** shows a superior vena cavagram demonstrating a renal carcinoma completely obstructing the inferior vena cava below the diaphragm; **B** shows the open vena cava (arrows) with a bulging tumor mass that invades the wall of the vena cava circumferentially.

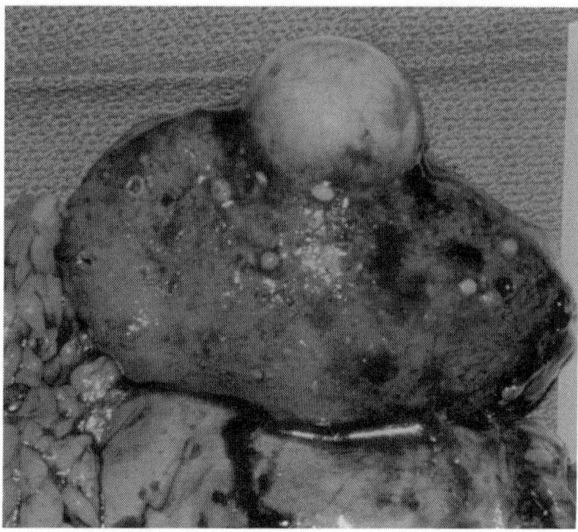

Fig 7. Enucleation of renal carcinoma. The surface-bulging round renal carcinoma growing by symmetric expansion rather than invasion is possibly suited to enucleation. This kidney shows additional small renal carcinomas indicative of a multicentric origin.

collin's solution that approaches intracellular electrolyte concentrations. The systemic heparin is reversed and an assistant closes the patient's incision.

Meanwhile on the bench under cold ischemia the tumor is exposed and resected. The renal arteries and veins are reconstructed using microvascular technique. The collecting system may also need extensive reconstruction. When the bench work is completed, a lower quadrant transplant incision is made and a recipient artery and vein are prepared. The kidney is transplanted back into the patient. The ureter can be left intact during the entire cold ischemic period, but this presents a risk because the ureteral blood supply can reperfuse and warm the kidney during the cold ischemia. Furthermore, leaving the ureter attached prevents the surgeon from sitting comfortably at a separate bench for

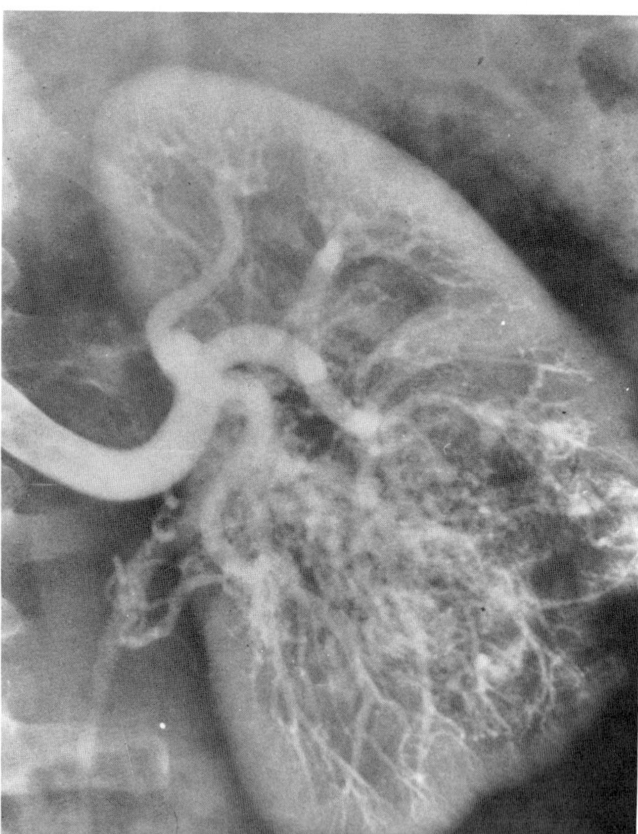

Fig 8. Partial nephrectomy under cold ischemia. The renal arteriogram shows a hypervascular tumor involving the left lower pole, which was amenable to resection in situ under cold ischemia. The cancer does not involve the main renal artery, main renal vein, or ureter, so that reconstruction is relatively easy and does not require bench work.

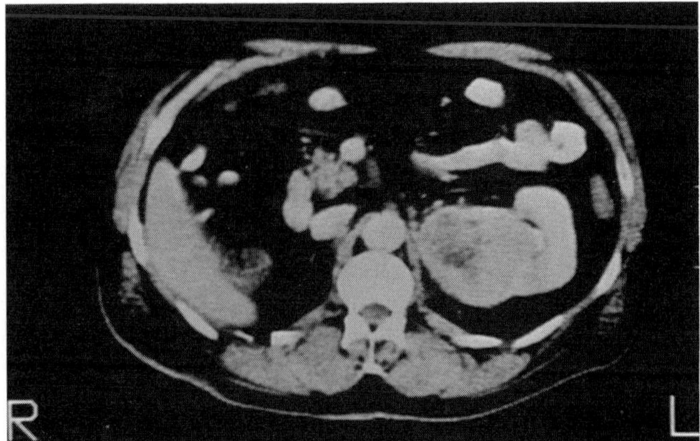


**Fig 9.** Partial nephrectomy on the bench. This solitary left kidney with a large hilar carcinoma required ex vivo resection under cold ischemia and autotransplantation. Despite the effort, the patient succumbed to metastatic renal carcinoma.

the microvascular repairs that might be required. Usually the ureter is reimplanted in the bladder.

Patients who undergo these bench resections are obviously carefully selected. Local recurrence rates have been reported at 11%.[26] Overall survival is approximately 69%, which approaches survival from radical nephrectomy[26,27] (Fig 9).

## MANAGEMENT OF BILATERAL RENAL CARCINOMA

Bilaterality in renal carcinoma does not imply a worse tumor prognosis. Although there is some controversy,[28,29] the current belief is that survival with synchronous bilateral renal carcinoma is dependent only on the grade and stage of the tumors.[30–32] Patients with a synchronous bilateral renal carcinoma do not do as well as the synchronous cancer group. Zincke and Swanson found that the 5-year survival rate for synchronous bilateral renal carcinoma (77.8%) was significantly higher than for a synchronous bilateral renal carcinoma (37.5%).[32] Topley et al found 5-year survival rates for patients with unilateral carcinoma in a solitary kidney or bilateral synchronous renal carcinoma of 71%, but a 5-year survival rate of only 38% in patients with bilateral asynchronous tumors.[33]

When faced with synchronous bilateral renal cell carcinoma, which side to operate on first is a major question. The size and extent of the tumors involved will dictate the procedures required. A large tumor involving the major portion of a kidney requires a radical nephrectomy. Polar or peripheral tumors are candidates for partial nephrectomy. There are two schools of thought on which side to do first. A radical nephrectomy on the more involved side first allows compensatory hypertrophy to occur in the lesser involved kidney prior to its partial nephrectomy. This compensatory hypertrophy hypothetically allows the surgeon to obtain a better tumor-free margin. Furthermore, solitary kidneys appear to be more resistant to acute tubular necrosis from operative ischemia. However, performing a partial nephrectomy on the lesser involved kidney first does allow the more involved kidney to maintain enough of the renal function load to keep the patient off of hemodialysis while the partial renal remnant recovers. After the recovery of renal function has been clearly demonstrated by radionuclide scanning, radical nephrectomy can be carried out.

### Bilateral Nephrectomy and Renal Transplantation

Because of the extent of the bilateral renal carcinomas, bilateral radical nephrectomy may be the only way to render the patient free of cancer. The surgery is followed by chronic dialysis and possibly renal transplantation at a later date. The disease-free interval demanded by transplant surgeons prior to renal allografting has

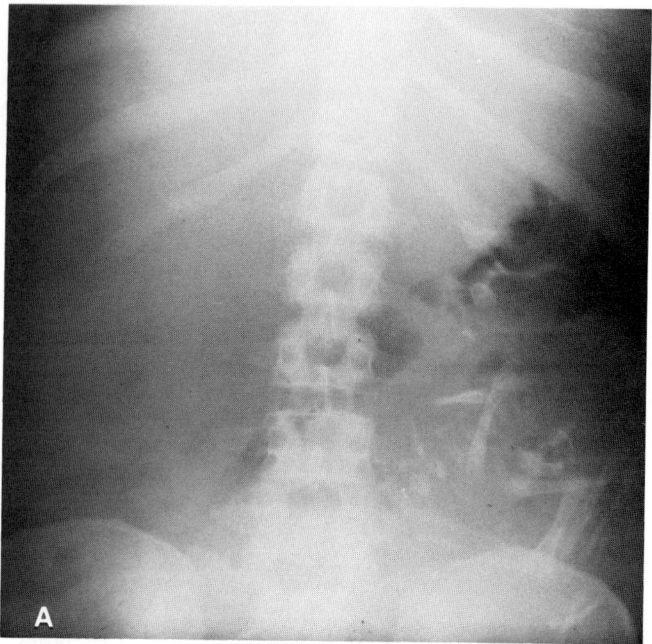


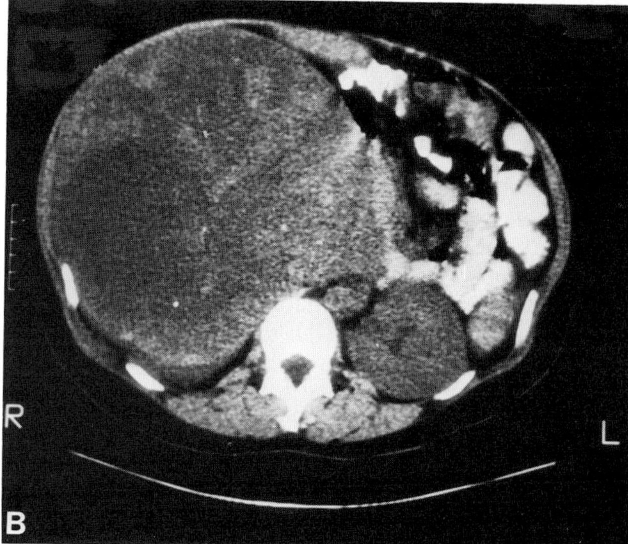


**Fig 10.** Renal carcinoma in pregnancy. **A** shows that the patient has a very large right abdominal mass pushing her 32-week fetus to the left; **B** delineates the actual size of the renal mass on the right. Caesarean section and radical nephrectomy were performed concomitantly. The tumor directly invaded the liver and required partial hepatectomy.

dropped from 5 years to about 18–24 months. Though the quality of life on hemodialysis for that time period is poor, the survival is excellent. The 5-year survival on hemodialysis is 40% to 50%, which is significantly higher than that of untreated renal cell carcinoma.

## MANAGEMENT OF RENAL CARCINOMA IN CONJUNCTION WITH OTHER SURGERY

Many incidental renal carcinomas are now detected in patients undergoing imaging studies for other surgical diseases.

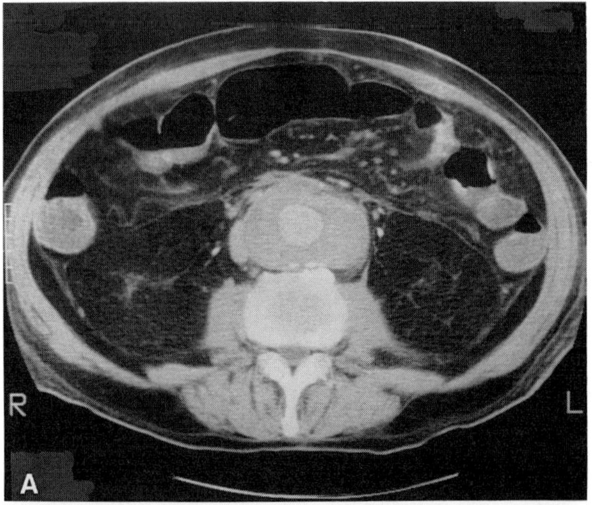


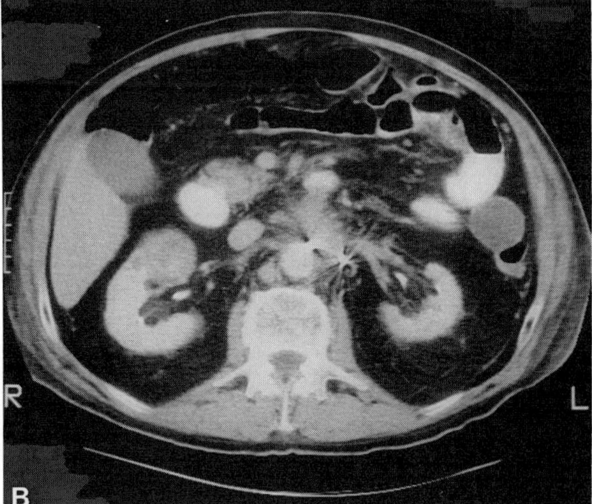


**Fig 11.** Aortic aneurysm and renal carcinoma. **A** demonstrates the patient's abdominal aortic aneurysm requiring replacement; **B** shows an anterior, midpolar right renal carcinoma and a small, poorly functioning left kidney. The patient underwent aortic replacement, followed 4 weeks later by a left anterior segmental renal resection.

The surgical requirements of the other disease may materially affect any plans for resection of the renal carcinoma.

Some elective surgical cases can clearly wait for the renal resection to be completed. For example, in cases of elective joint replacement or elective vascular grafting, the surgeons usually prefer the renal surgery to proceed first so that there is a diminished risk of graft infection later. However, in only semielective vascular or cardiac surgery, the additional renal reserve provided by the carcinomatous kidney may help patients through the postoperative period and the nephrectomy can follow several weeks later. Some concomitant surgical conditions should be relieved to prevent postoperative complications following the nephrectomy. These might include symptomatic cholelithiasis and gastrointestinal bleeding. Some surgical conditions can be attended to during the same anesthesia as the nephrectomy. Examples of these might be asymptomatic cholelithiasis and herniorrhaphy; also see Figures 10 and 11.

## DIRECT INVASION OF OTHER STRUCTURES

Renal carcinomas can become very large and invade adjacent organs in about 10% of patients. Usually, renal carcinomas that grow to a large size locally present with invasion of the tumor into the posterior abdominal wall, nerve routes, or paraspinous muscles. The tumor may involve the duodenum, ascending colon, liver, and head of the pancreas on the right. The tumor may invade the descending colon, spleen, and tail of the pancreas on the left. The mesentery and diaphragm may be invaded from either side. Invasion of these organs gives the patient an extremely poor prognosis. Total excision of the tumor and part of the involved adjacent organ is essential. Direct invasion of the ipsilateral adrenal gland occurs in 10% to 15% of patients, but the prognosis of patients with ipsilateral adrenal involvement is no different from that of stage II renal carcinoma.

In many cases, surgical intervention involving partial resection of the colon, tail of the pancreas, spleen, or liver may be feasible. However, most reports suggest that less than 5% of the patients with extension into adjacent viscera survive 5 years after surgery. Careful preoperative staging with CT scan or MRI to evaluate tumor involvement into adjacent organs is useful but may be misleading. For example, CT scan frequently overstates the possibility of direct liver invasion.

## MANAGEMENT OF LOCAL RECURRENCES

Local recurrence of renal carcinoma following radical nephrectomy may be in the renal fossa, the incision, or residual lymph nodes. In any of these situations, repeat resection can be palliative and in rare cases may provide some hope of salvage. For wound recurrences, an excision must be performed with wide margins, which can make wound closure quite difficult. Recurrences in the renal fossa require en bloc partial resection of the psoas and the overlying peritoneum and potentially its intraperitoneal structures. Residual periaortic or pericaval lymph nodes that develop metastatic renal carcinoma can be resected in the same manner as a testis tumor node dissection. In all of these situations, postoperative adjuvant external beam radiation therapy may aid in preventing a second local recurrence.

Local renal recurrence of a renal carcinoma following partial nephrectomy may follow an actual positive resection margin or may represent a second primary renal carcinoma. A second partial nephrectomy may be attempted, but will be difficult due to the extensive perinephric scarring seen following a partial nephrectomy. In most cases a nephrectomy will be required. In the transplanted or autotransplanted kidney there will be no perinephric fat and the tumor margins of resection will be necessarily thin (Fig 12).

## ANGIOINFARCTION OF RENAL CARCINOMA

Some very large tumors have been treated preoperatively by transcatheter embolization using a variety of absorbable or nonabsorbable materials. Although absorbable gelatin sponge and steel coils have been the most widely used embolic agents, cellulose, autologous blood clots, sodium tetradexysulfate, and ethanol have been used.[34–39] Theoretically, angiographic infarction of renal carcinoma followed by nephrectomy might induce a stimulation of postinfarction immune response.[34]

Preoperative renal arterial embolization may aid the surgeon by decreasing operative blood loss. In patients with unresectable tumors, embolization may be used as a palliative measure to decrease hematuria or alleviate intractable pain. The principal risk of angioinfarction is the inadvertent reflux of embolic particles or agents into adjacent normal organs. Angioinfarction causes significant side effects: severe abdominal pain, nausea, diarrhea, fever, paralytic ileus, hypertension, and potentially sepsis.

Transcatheter embolization can be a reasonable approach to the patient with a large, symptomatic, nonresectable primary renal cell carcinoma. Serial selective infarction of segmental renal arterial branches mini-

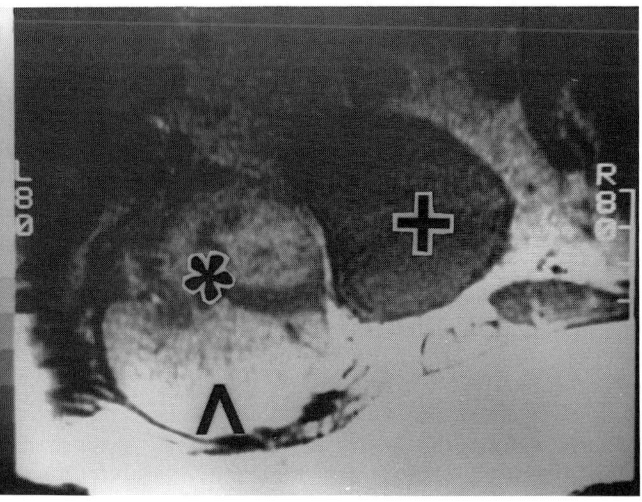


**Fig 12.** MRI of autotransplanted renal remnant. The patient with renal carcinoma in a solitary kidney underwent partial nephrectomy under ex vivo hypothermic ischemia and autotransplantation to the left iliac fossa. Follow-up MRI at 2 years demonstrates a local recurrence. The bladder (+) has the autotransplanted remnant pressing slightly on the left dome. The posterior half of the renal remnant (arrow) is uninvolved. The anterior half of the renal remnant (asterisk) is replaced by recurrent renal carcinoma necessitating a nephrectomy and hemodialysis.

mizes the postinfarction syndrome and risk of tumor rupture.

The embolization route has also been used to deliver therapeutic radiation therapy[40] or chemotherapy[41] to unresectable renal carcinomas in order to render them resectable. Though these methods have not been popularly employed, they do appear to relieve tumor symptoms and often allow resection of the renal cancer. For example, using radioactive seed embolization, Lang and deKernion[40] reported a 2-year survival rate of 59% and a 5-year survival rate of 30% in 22 patients with extensive localized renal cell carcinoma. Excellent tumor size reduction and symptom relief were seen.

## TREATMENT OF METASTATIC RENAL CARCINOMA

### Palliative Nephrectomy

As many as 30% of patients with renal carcinoma have metastatic disease at the time of presentation with lungs, bone, liver, and brain being the most common sites involved. While their survival is low (10% at 1 year), flank pain and hematuria are often major problems in patients with advanced or metastatic renal cell carcinoma. Palliative nephrectomy is most effective in patients with severe hemorrhage, severe pain, paraneoplastic syndromes, or symptomatic compression of adjacent organs. Although angiographic infarction is a reasonable alternative, palliative nephrectomy often results in a quicker resolution of the symptoms and a shorter, more comfortable hospitalization.

### Adjunctive Nephrectomy

Spontaneous regression of renal carcinoma metastases occurs extremely rarely (<0.4%).[42] Adjunctive nephrectomy is the removal of the primary renal carcinoma in patients with metastatic disease in order to increase their survival or cause regression of the metastatic lesions. Due to reports of spontaneous regression of metastasis after removal of the primary tumor and a lack of other effective therapeutic options, urologists may feel justified in performing adjunctive nephrectomy. Actually, there is no randomized prospective study that demonstrates that adjunctive nephrectomy provides any survival advantage over no surgery. Montie et al reported a <1% short-lived regression rate following adjunctive nephrectomy, but a 2% to 15% operative mortality rate.[43] Myers et al reported a 0% regression rate in a series of 533 adjunctive nephrectomies.[44] deKernion et al reported that the average survival of patients with distant metastases was 4 months and only 10% were alive at 1 year.[45] Survival of the patients undergoing adjunctive nephrectomy was the same. The addition of preoperative embolization by Gottesman and associates in 30 patients resulted in only one partial response.[46] These reports strongly suggest that there should be no support for routine adjunctive nephrectomy in patients with metastatic disease.

## Resection of Renal Carcinoma Metastases

**Solitary Metastases.** Adjunctive nephrectomy may be indicated in patients with solitary pulmonary, brain, or liver metastases. However, only 1.6% to 3.6% of patients with metastases to these organs have such solitary metastasis. Bone metastases are usually multiple, though occasionally a solitary metastasis to a long bone is seen. Nephrectomy and resection of a solitary pulmonary metastasis has yielded excellent reported 5-year survival results: 30% to 36.5%.[47–50] However, these patients were all carefully selected. A more typical experience might be the report of Dineen et al.[51] In their series of 29 patients with apparent solitary metastasis either at the time of presentation (11 patients) or later (18 patients), only 2 were long-term survivors following resection of the metastasis.

**Multiple Metastases.** Resection of multiple metastases from renal carcinoma is futile. However, some renal cancers display rather slow doubling times and resection of metastases for palliation may be undertaken. Because the resection of a metastasis is enucleative surgery without the necessity for wide margins, the morbidity of the resection is lower. Lesions that might be considered for palliative resection include symptomatic metastases to the brain. Metastases to long bones may be very disabling and internal fixation leads to both comfort and mobility with little morbidity except for intraoperative blood loss. For the pain in a non-weight-bearing bone, external beam radiation therapy generally offers better palliation than resection. Some local metastatic tumor masses may be palliated by resection if they are compressing a bronchus or the gastrointestinal tract (Figs 13 and 14).

## Radiation Therapy

Radiation therapy is a significant and important treatment technique in the palliative management of patients with bone metastases. However, there is very little role for radiation in the primary management of renal cancer. Werf-Messing[52] reported on a randomized prospective trial comparing nephrectomy alone with preoperative radiotherapy (3000 rads) followed by nephrectomy. She found no improvement in survival with preoperative radiotherapy. Cox et al[53] did demonstrate that preoperative radiation therapy may have a small impact on improving local control (regional lymph nodes and renal bed), but no impact on long-term survival. If tumor spill occurs, then external beam therapy may be

**Fig 13.** Renal carcinoma metastasis. The patient presented with a pathologic fracture of the humeral head (arrow). Treatment for this can be by internal fixation (if there is enough humeral head to hold the rod) or by rotational external beam radiation therapy.

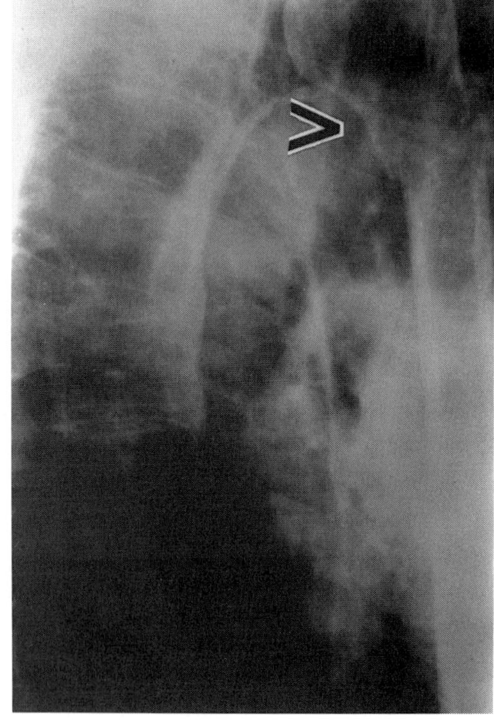

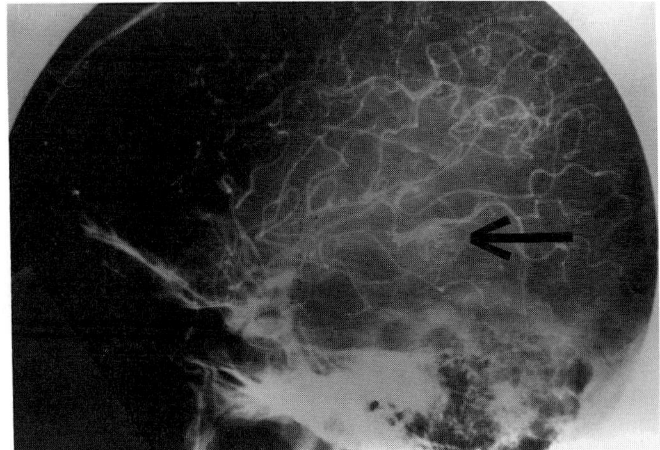

**Fig 14.** Cerebral angiography demonstrates the hypervascular renal carcinoma metastasis (arrow). The patient went on to survive 5 years by undergoing resections of brain (3), pulmonary (2), and nodal (1) metastases on five occasions. Palliation was excellent for 4 of the 5 years.

warranted to slightly diminish the risk of wound seeding. For recurrent metastatic lymph nodes, resection and postoperative radiotherapy seems by default to be the therapy of choice.

## Chemotherapy

Metastatic renal cell carcinoma is generally refractory to chemotherapeutic agents. Although more than 40 single-agent phase II trials have been reported, the results have been consistently disappointing.[54] Vinblastine has been the most effective agent, with partial response rates of 10% to 25%.[55,56] Trials with combination chemotherapy have also been ineffective.[57]

A positive palliative effect has been seen with lonidamine 350 mg/m$^2$ as an oral daily dose. This study showed one complete and one partial response in 19 patients. In addition, there was no tumor progression in 13 patients for a median duration of 100 days. The 5-year survival in these 19 patients was 37% with moderate toxicity.[58]

Promising results have been reported using continuous infusion chemotherapy. In a study of 42 patients, the continuous infusion of 5-floxuridine yielded three complete responses and three partial responses. In addition, 18 patients had no progression for a median of 7 months (range 3–73 months). The remaining 18 patients progressed.[59] In another report, one patient with metastases to the brain, lungs, mediastinum, and retroperitoneum from renal cell carcinoma received daily infusion of fluorodoxyuridine for 31 months with a complete response seen in all metastases except those in the brain.[60]

Trials with suramin[61] and Taxol[62] have been unsuccessful.

There is convincing evidence that the resistance of renal cell carcinoma to chemotherapeutic agents is due to the expression of a multidrug resistance (*MDR-I*) gene. This gene encodes a membrane-bound protein, P-170 glycoprotein, which acts as an efflux pump capable of extruding chemotherapeutic agents from cancer cells.[63] In a study by Mickisch et al, P-170 expression was found in 18 of 25 tumors that were highly resistant to chemotherapy and in no tumors that were sensitive to chemotherapy.[64] Another report by Goldstein et al found *MDR-I* gene expression in 38 of 46 human renal cell carcinoma specimens.[65] In addition, this study and others have demonstrated that the P-170 efflux mechanism can be inactivated in vitro by calcium antagonists such as verapamil, nifedipine, and diltiazem.[66]

## Hormonal Therapy

Medroxyprogesterone (Provera) is widely used to treat metastatic renal cell carcinoma. It has been used postoperatively in patients with positive lymph nodes and also in patients who are not surgical candidates. Bloom described a 16% objective response rate using Provera and androgens in metastatic renal cell carcinoma. Other series report a 7% to 25% response rate.[67] It has not been possible to predict which patients with advanced renal cell carcinoma will respond to Provera or other hormonal manipulations. A recent study by Stahl et al using high doses of tamoxifin (150 mg/m$^2$ orally for 6 months followed by 50 mg/m$^2$ until tumor progression) showed two complete responses and one partial response in 25 patients and the cessation of tumor progression in an additional 16 patients. The median duration of response was 150 days (range 28–355) and the 5-year survival was 35%.[58]

Although the response rate for medroxyprogesterone is poor, it is approximately equivalent to the response seen with chemotherapy. In addition, medroxyprogesterone is generally well tolerated by patients and is FDA-approved for the treatment of renal cell carcinoma.

## Immunotherapy

For the past 15 years immunotherapy has held forth the promise that the body's own immune system might regain its presumed lost surveillance and eradicate metastatic renal carcinoma. Unfortunately, to date, the clinical effectiveness of any immunotherapy regimen for significant responses in renal cancer is still minimal.

There are four basic approaches to immunotherapy that have been tried in patients with metastatic renal carcinoma:

1. Active nonspecific immunotherapy
2. Active specific immunotherapy
3. Adoptive transfer of immunocompetent cells
4. Cytokines

**Active Nonspecific Immunotherapy.** Initially, active nonspecific immunostimulation with BCG (bacillus Calmette-Guerin) was the most widely used approach. Minton et al[68] reported that 4 of 9 patients with metastatic renal cell carcinoma responded to BCG with a partial regression, primarily in pulmonary metastases. Morales and Eidinger[69] found that 5 of 8 patients similarly derived a short partial regression. Brosman[70] performed a prospective study on 22 patients using BCG as nonspecific immunostimulation and found only a slight increase in survival, not statistically significant. Essentially these studies demonstrated that active nonspecific immunostimulation with BCG yielded little survival advantage.

**Active Specific Immunotherapy.** Active specific immunotherapy is based on the premise that a specific T-cell response will be elicited by immunization of the patient with inactivated autologous tumor cells with adjuvants. The vaccine of autologous tumor cells may consist of cells homogenized into polymer particles, irradiated tumor cells with a bacterial adjuvant, or a single-cell suspension of autologous or allogeneic tumor cells complexed with a chemical adjuvant. Tykka and associates reported that 6 of 16 patients with pulmonary metastasis had complete response after receiving an intradermal injection of a soluble fraction of autologous tumor polymerized to ethylchlorformate.[71] The survival of the treated patients was improved, but data are difficult to interpret because of the heterogeneity of the treated patients and a bias in the selection of control patients. Prager and associates used a similar approach using irradiated autologous cells polymerized with dichlorodiphenyltrichloroethane injected percutaneously and they saw a slight increase in survival in 27 patients.[72] In a prospective study, Neidhart and associates used a vaccine consisting of a mixture of modified tumor antigens with tuberculin or phytohemagglutinin as adjuvant in the treatment of stage IV renal cell carcinoma. In the series of 30 patients, two complete responses and two partial responses were observed. The overall survival rate was equivalent in patients treated with or without immunotherapy.[73]

**Adoptive Transfer of Immunocompetent Cells.** In this modality, anticancer immunity is transferred to the patient by infusing lymphocytes known to react with the tumor. The source of the lymphocytes is the patient's peripheral blood or the fresh tumor tissue removed at surgery. The number of cells retrieved that are actually reactive to the tumor-associated antigens is very small and therefore must be expanded. This is done in vitro by a number of methods.

Interleukins are a class of cytokines that activate and regulate growth and/or differentiation of leukocytes. More than ten different interleukins are known at this time, but to date interleukin 2 (IL-2) is the major interleukin involved in clinical studies. IL-2 is derived from T-helper lymphocytes and induces proliferation of antigen-triggered cytotoxic T-lymphocytes, but does not stimulate nonlymphoid cells. Upon activation with IL-2, some peripheral lymphocytes acquire the ability to lyse tumor target cells, but not normal cells. This heterogeneous subpopulation of peripheral lymphocytes are called lymphocyte-activated killer cells or LAK cells. The IL-2 stimulation of the LAK cells may be in vitro, in vivo, or both.

Rosenberg and associates[74] from the National Cancer Institute (NCI) reported objective response rates in the range of 20% to 30% in a large series of patients with renal cell carcinoma who received IL-2 and LAK cells. Their report has been reproduced by a multicenter study group.[75] Patients given LAK cells and IL-2 were treated in an intensive care unit because of possible life-threatening side effects, due primarily to high-dose IL-2 therapy. The most common side effect of IL-2 therapy was fluid retention leading to hypertension. Other side effects of IL-2 are fever, chills, malaise, renal and hepatic dysfunction, respiratory distress, nausea, vomiting, diarrhea, and mental disturbance. Toxic side effects of IL-2 therapy have been found to be dose-dependent and reversible. Although side effects of the LAK cells themselves are less severe than the IL-2, 73% of the patients after LAK cell therapy developed severe anemia that required a blood transfusion. Other side effects include fever, chills, and decreased pulmonary function.

An improved approach for adoptive transfer of in vitro–activated lymphocytes was introduced by Beldegrun et al[76] from the same NCI laboratory. Instead of expanding human peripheral blood lymphocytes, tumor-infiltrating lymphocytes (TIL) from a human renal carcinoma were isolated and expanded. These cells already sensitized to the tumor in vivo and have been shown to possess 50 to 100 times more killer activity than LAK cells. In their series of 7 patients, Kradin and associates reported that 2 had objective tumor response after the therapy.[77] Since the side effects of TIL therapy are generally milder than those of LAK cell therapy, therapy could be given in the ward setting instead of an intensive care unit.

The bolus infusion of high doses of IL-2, as used by Rosenberg and coworkers,[74] was felt to be necessary to maintain the activity of the LAK cells infused. However, Thompson and associates demonstrated that continuous infusion of IL-2 and LAK cells demonstrated a better biological activity than bolus injections.[78] Furthermore, West et al[79] demonstrated that continuous infusion of IL-2 significantly reduces treatment-related toxicity. However, so far there is no randomized study to show that continuous infusion decreases toxicity. The future of this therapy in renal carcinoma is not only in augmentation of the tumoricidal effects but also in reduction of toxicity to allow widespread application in a general ward setting.

Osband et al[80] reported on a form of adoptive immunotherapy in which the lymphocytes are exposed to cytokines in vitro and reinfused without IL-2. An attempt is made to selectively inactivate suppressor T cells, which might actually hasten tumor growth.[81] The side effects are minimal, consisting primarily of fever, and the response rate is encouraging.

**Cytokines.** Cytokines alone may have direct antineoplastic action or may act indirectly through modulation of the immune system. To date there is little evidence that combinations work any better against renal carcinoma than single agents.

Interferons are a family of three different immunoregulatory glycoproteins termed alpha, beta, and gamma. The interferons are produced by cells in response to viral infection or other inducers. They have antiviral and antineoplastic activities that are mediated by direct tumor cytotoxicity or by indirect cytotoxicity through natural killer cell stimulation or both. Of the three interferons, alpha interferon appears to have more efficacy in renal carcinoma than beta or gamma interferon. In phase II clinical trials, deKernion et al[82] reported a 16.5% objective response rate after giving $3 \times 10^6$ U of natural human leukocyte alpha interferon 5 days a week for 6 weeks. Quesada et al[83] reported that 5 of 19 patients had a partial response with a mean duration of 4 months. Most of the responses were seen in pulmonary metastasis. Figlin and associates[84] used alpha interferon and vinblastine in a phase II clinical trial and found a 30% partial response rate. They concluded that the efficacy of a combination of alpha interferon and vinblastine was similar to that of alpha interferon alone.

These initial encouraging objective responses seen in metastatic renal cell carcinoma using interferons has led to a great number of additional studies using both natural and recombinant interferons. These studies have shown that response rates ranged from 5% to 27% with a median duration of response ranging from 3 to 16 months.[85] The various subtypes of alpha interferons do not differ significantly in overall response rates: 19% for human leukocyte interferons, 17% for partially purified lymphoblastoid interferon, and 14% for recombinant alpha interferons. The preliminary results of clinical trials using beta and gamma interferons indicate that these do not have any greater activity than alpha interferons.[86,87] In addition, a combination of alpha interferons and a variety of chemotherapeutic agents has not shown any clinical benefit in response or survival compared to alpha interferon alone, and toxicity appeared to be greater using combination therapy.[88]

Although optimal doses of alpha interferon have not been determined, the use of intermittent or high doses appears to give a better response. Two different randomized trials by Kirkwood and associates[89] and Quesada et al[90] demonstrated that higher doses ranging from $10 \times 10^6$ U to $20 \times 10^6$ U of alpha interferon provided better objective responses. They demonstrated that adverse effects of alpha interferons are proportional to dosage, but are reversible on termination of treatment. Some of the acute side effects of alpha interferon are seen in the first week of treatment and include fever, chills, tachycardia, myalgia, headache, arthralgia, and nasal congestion. Some of the chronic side effects are fatigue, weakness, and anorexia. Other common side effects are nausea, vomiting, diarrhea, elevation of liver enzymes, proteinuria, and myelosuppression.

An important aspect of failure of interferon therapy is a potential development of anti-interferon antibodies. In some series this has been seen in up to 44% of the patients receiving interferons.[91] Its clinical relevance is unclear, however. Reportedly the response to interferon has been shortened due to anti-interferon antibodies.[92]

Tumor necrosis factor (TNF) is a macrophage-derived protein that may be cytotoxic or cytostatic for human tumor cells in vitro, especially renal cell carcinoma. Two species are known: TNF-$\alpha$ and $\beta$. In vivo, TNF causes hemorrhagic necrosis from its effect on vascular endothelium and the coagulation cascade. In addition, peripheral blood leukocyte cytotoxicity is enhanced after infusion of TNF.

In phase II clinical trials, intravenous TNF resulted in two objective responses in 22 patients.[93] Because TNF has a half-life of only 20 to 30 minutes, sufficient serum levels may only be achieved through intravenous injection. Because TNF is an important mediator of endotoxic shock, the side effects of TNF are fever, hypertension, and water retention.[94] In order to improve the efficacy of TNF, Otto and associates[95] tried it in combination with alpha interferon and found a 43% objective response rate in 14 patients. Although TNF is promising in the treatment of advanced renal cell carcinoma, further prospective clinical trials are required to clarify the role of TNF in the host defense against tumors.

## REFERENCES

1. Chute R, Soutter L, Kerr WS Jr. The value of the thoracoabdominal incision in the removal of kidney tumors. *N Engl J Med.* 1949;241:951.

2. Robson CJ. Radical nephrectomy for renal cell carcinoma. *J Urol.* 1963;89:37.
3. Williams RD. Renal, perirenal and ureteral neoplasms. In: Gillenwater JY, ed. *Adult and Pediatric Urology*. Chicago: Year Book; 1987:527.
4. Robson CJ, Churchill BM, Anderson W. The results of radical nephrectomy for renal cell carcinoma. *J Urol.* 1969;101:297.
5. Wagle DG, Scal DR. Renal cell carcinoma: a review of 256 cases. *J Surg Oncol.* 1970;2:23.
6. Giuliani L, Giberti C, Martorana G, et al. Radical extensive surgery for renal cell carcinoma: long-term results and prognostic factors. *J Urol.* 1990;143:468.
7. Siminovitch JP, Montie JE, Straffon RA. Lymphadenectomy in renal adenocarcinoma. *J Urol.* 1982;127:1090.
8. Golimbu M, Joshi P, Sperber A, Tessler A, Al-Askari S, Morales P. Renal cell carcinoma: survival and prognostic factors. *Urology*. 1986;27:291.
9. Clayman RV, Kavoussi LR, et al. Laparoscopic nephrectomy: initial case report. *J Urol.* 1991;146:278.
10. Tsukamoto T, Kumamoto Y, Miyao N, et al. Regional lymph node metastasis in renal cell carcinoma: incidence, distribution and its relation to other pathological findings. *Eur Urol.* 1990;8:88.
11. Herrlinger A, Schrott KM, Sigel A, et al. Results of 381 transabdominal radical nephrectomies for renal cell carcinoma with partial and complete en-bloc lymph node dissection. *World J Urol.* 1984;2:113.
12. Pizzacaro G, Piva L, Salvioni R. Lymph node dissection in radical nephrectomy for renal cell carcinoma: is it necessary? *Eur Urol.* 1983;9:10.
13. McDonald JR, Priestley JT. Malignant tumors of the kidney: surgical and prognostic significance of tumor thrombosis of the renal vein. *Surg Gynecol Obstet.* 1943;77:295.
14. Riches EW, Griffiths IH, Thakray AD. New growths of the kidney and ureter. *Br J Urol.* 1951;23:297.
15. Waters WB, Richie JP. Aggressive surgical approach to renal cell carcinoma: review of 130 cases. *J Urol.* 1979;122:306.
16. Marshall VF, Middleton RG, Holswade GR, et al. Surgery for renal cell carcinoma in the vena cava. *J Urol.* 1970;103:414.
17. Libertino JA, Zinman L, Watkins E Jr. Long term results of a resection of a renal cell cancer with extension into inferior vena cava. *J Urol.* 1987;137:21.
18. Hatcher PA, Anderson EE. The management of renal cell carcinoma with renal vein and vena cava tumor thrombus. *Problems Urol.* 1990; 4:273–283.
19. Krane RJ, White R, Davis Z, et al. Removal of renal cell carcinoma extending into the right atrium using cardiopulmonary bypass, profound hypothermia and circulatory arrest. *J Urol.* 1984;131:945.
20. Kearney GP, Waters WB, Klein LA, et al. Results of inferior vena cava resection for renal cell carcinoma. *J Urol.* 1981;125:769.
21. Novick AC, Kaye MC, Cosgrove DM, et al. Experience with cardiopulmonary bypass and deep hypothermic circulatory arrest in the management of retroperitoneal tumors with large vena caval thrombi. *Ann Surg.* 1990;212:472.
22. Skinner DG, Pritchett TR, Lieskovsky G, et al. Vena caval involvement by renal cell carcinoma. *Ann Surg.* 1989;210:387.
23. Vermooten V. Indications for conservative surgery in certain renal tumors: a study based on the growth pattern of the clear cell carcinoma. *J Urol.* 1950;64:200.
24. Marshall FF, Taxy JB, Fishman EK, Chang R. The feasibility of surgical enucleation for renal cell carcinoma. *J Urol.* 1986;135:231.
25. Blackley SK, Ladaga L, Woolfitt RA, Schellhammer PF. Ex situ study of the effectiveness of enucleation in patients with renal cell carcinoma. *J Urol.* 1988;140:6.
26. Novick AC. Extracorporeal renal surgery and autotransplantation. In: Novick AC, Straffon RA, eds. *Vascular Problems in Urologic Surgery*. Philadelphia: WB Saunders; 1982:305.
27. Zincke H, Sen SE. Experience with extracorporeal surgery and autotransplantation for renal cell and transitional cell cancer of the kidney. *J Urol.* 1988;140:25.
28. Malek RS, Utz DC, Culp OS. Hypernephroma in the solitary kidney: experience with 20 cases and review of the literature. *J Urol.* 1976;116:553.
29. Marberger M, Pugh RCB, Auvert J, Bertermann H, Constantini A, Gammelgaard PA, Petterson S, Wickham JEA. Conservative surgery of renal carcinoma: the EIRSS experience. *Br J Urol.* 1981;53:528.
30. Jacobs SC, Berg SI, Lawson RK. Synchronous bilateral renal cell carcinoma: total surgical excision. *Cancer.* 1980;46:2341.
31. Smith RB, deKernion JB, Ehrlich RM, Skinner DG, Kaufman JJ. Bilateral renal cell carcinoma and renal cell carcinoma in the solitary kidney. *J Urol.* 1984;132:450.
32. Zincke H, Swanson SK. Bilateral renal cell carcinoma: influence of synchronous and asynchronous occurrence on patient survival. *J Urol.* 1982;128:913.
33. Topley M, Novick AC, Montie JE. Long-term results following partial nephrectomy for localized renal adenocarcinoma. *J Urol.* 1984; 131:1050.
34. Swanson DA, et al. Angioinfarction plus nephrectomy for metastatic renal cell carcinoma: an update. *J Urol.* 1983;130:449.

35. Kaisary AV, Williams G, Riddle PR. The role of preoperative embolization in renal cell carcinoma. *J Urol.* 1984;131:641.
36. Ekelund L, Mansson W, Olsson AM, Stigsson L. Palliative embolization of arterial renal tumor supply. Results in 10 cases. *Acta Rad Diag.* 1979;20:323.
37. Goldin AR, Barnes DR, Jacobsen I. Percutaneous infarction of renal tumors: comparison between gelatin sponge embolization and cyanoacrylate occlusion. *Urology.* 1978;11:197.
38. Wallace S, Gianturco C, Anderson JH, Goldstein HM, Davis LJ, Bree RL. Therapeutic vascular occlusion utilizing steel coil technique: clinical applications. *Am J Roentgenol.* 1976;127:381.
39. Goldstein HM, Medellin H, Beydoun MT, Wallace S, Ben-Menachem Y, Bracken RB, Johnson DE. Transcatheter embolization of renal cell carcinoma. *Am J Roentgenol.* 1975;123:557.
40. Lang EK, deKernion JB. Transcatheter embolization of advanced renal cell carcinoma with radioactive seeds. *J Urol.* 1981;126:581.
41. Kato T, Nemoto R, Mori H, et al. Transcatheter arterial chemoembolization of renal cell carcinoma with microencapsulated mitomycin C. *J Urol.* 1981;125:19.
42. Freed SZ, Halperin JP, Gordon M. Idiopathic regression of metastases from renal cell carcinoma. *J Urol.* 1977;118:538.
43. deKernion JB, Ramming JB, Smith RB. The natural history of metastatic renal cell carcinoma: a computer analysis. *J Urol.* 1978;120:148.
44. Montie JE, Stewart BH, Straffon RA, et al. The role of adjunctive nephrectomy in patients with metastatic renal cell carcinoma. *J Urol.* 1977; 117:272.
45. Myers GH, Gehrenbaker LG, Kellais PP. Prognostic significance of renal vein invasion by hypernephroma. *J Urol.* 1968;100:420.
46. Gottesman JE, Crawford ED, Grossman HB, et al. Infarction-nephrectomy for metastatic renal carcinoma: Southwest Oncology Group Study. *Urology.* 1985;25:248.
47. O'Dea MJ, Zincke H, Utz DC, Bernatz PE. The treatment of renal cell carcinoma with solitary metastasis. *J Urol.* 1978;120:540.
48. Tolia BM, Whitmore WF Jr. Solitary metastasis from renal cell carcinoma. *J Urol.* 1975; 114:836.
49. Middleton RG. Surgery for metastatic renal cell carcinoma. *J Urol.* 1967;97:973.
50. Skinner DG, Colvin RB, Vermillion CD, Pfister RC, Leadbetter WF. Diagnosis and management of renal cell carcinoma. A clinical and pathologic study of 309 cases. *Cancer.* 1971;28:1165.
51. Dineen MK, Pastore RD, Emrich LJ, Huben RP. Results of surgical treatment of renal cell carcinoma with solitary metastasis. *J Urol.* 1988; 140:277.
52. van der Werf-Messing B. Carcinoma of the kidney. *Cancer.* 1973;32:1056.
53. Cox CE, Lacy SS, Montgomery WG, Boyce WH. Renal adenocarcinoma: a 28-year review with emphasis on rationale and feasibility of preoperative radiotherapy. *J Urol.* 1970;104:51.
54. Yagoda A. Phase II cytotoxic chemotherapy trials in renal cell carcinoma: 1983–1988. *Prog Clin Biol Res.* 1990;350:227.
55. Hrushesky WJ, Murphy GP. Current status of the therapy of advanced renal carcinoma. *J Surg Oncol.* 1977;9:277.
56. Bodey GP. Current status of chemotherapy in metastatic renal carcinoma. In: Johnson DE, Samuels ML, eds. *Cancer of the Genitourinary Tract.* New York: Raven Press; 1979:67.
57. Lupera H, Theodore C, Ghosn N, Court B, Wibault P, Droz J. Phase II trial of combination chemotherapy with dacarbazine, cyclophosphamide, cisplatin, doxorubicin, and bindesine in advanced renal cell cancer. *Urology.* 1989;34:281.
58. Stahl M, Schmoll E, Becker H, Schlichter A, Hoffman L, Wagner H, Possinger K, Mullerm W, Kollerman N, Weidenhammer W. Lonidamine vs. high-dose tamoxifin in progressive advanced renal cell carcinoma: results from ongoing randomized phase II study. *Semin Oncol.* 1991;18:33.
59. Damascelli B, Marchiano A, Spreafico C, Lutman R, Salvetti M, Bonalumi MG, Mauri M, Garbagnati F, Del Nero A, Comeri G. Sarcadian continuous chemotherapy of renal cell carcinoma with an implantable programmable infusion pump. *Cancer.* 1990;66:237.
60. Damascelli B, Marchiano A, Frigerio LF, Salvetti M, Spreafico C, Garbagnati F, Zanoni F, Radice F. Flexibility and efficacy of automatic continuous fluorodeoxyuridine infusion in metastases from a renal cell carcinoma. *Cancer.* 1991;68:995.
61. LaRocca R, Stein C, Danosi R, Cooper M, Uhrich M, Myers C. A pilot study of suramin and the treatment of metastatic renal cell carcinoma. *Cancer.* 1991;67:1509.
62. Einzig A, Gorowski E, Sasloff J, Wiernik P. Phase II trial of taxol in patients with metastatic renal cell carcinoma. *Cancer Invest.* 1991;9:133.
63. Fojo AT, Shen DW, Mickley LA, et al. Intrinsic drug resistance in human kidney cancer is associated with expression of a human multi-drug resistance gene. *J Clin Oncol.* 1987;5:1922.
64. Mickisch G, Kossig J, Keilhauer G, Schlick E, Tachada R, Aiken P. Effects of calcium antagonists in multi-drug resistant primary human renal cell carcinomas. *Cancer Res.* 1990;50:3670.
65. Goldstein L, Galski H, Fojo A, et al. Expression of a multi-drug resistance gene in human tumors. *Proc Am Assoc Cancer Res.* 1988;29:298.
66. Mickisch G, Merlino G, Aiken P, Gottesman N, Pastan I. New potent verapamil derivatives that reverse multi-drug resistance in human renal carcinoma cells and in transgenic mice expressing the human MDR I gene. *J Urol.* 1991;146:447.

67. Bloom HG. Medroxyprogesterone acetate (Provera) in the treatment of metastatic renal cancer. *Br J Cancer.* 1971;25:250.
68. Minton JP, Pennline K, Nawrocki JG, Kibbey WE, Dodd MC. Immunotherapy of human kidney cancer. Abstract c-258. *Proc Am Assoc Cancer Res Am Soc Clin Oncol.* 1976;17:301.
69. Morales A, Eidinger D. Bacillus Calmette-Guerin in the treatment of adenocarcinoma of the kidney. *J Urol.* 1976;115:377.
70. Brosman S. Non-specific immunotherapy in GU cancer. In: 4th Chicago Symposium of Neoplastic Immunity. Chicago: Franklin Institute Press; 1977:97.
71. Tykka H, Oravisto KH, Lehtonen T, Sarna S, Tallberg T. Active specific immunotherapy of advanced renal cell carcinoma. *Eur Urol.* 1978;4:250.
72. Prager MD, Baechtel FS, Peters PC, Brown GL, Greene CL. Specific immunotherapy of human metastatic renal cell carcinoma. *Proc Am Assoc Cancer Res.* 1981;22:163.
73. Neidhart JA, Murphy SG, Hennick LA, Wise HA. Active specific immunotherapy of stage IV renal carcinoma with aggregated tumor antigen adjuvant. *Cancer.* 1980;46:1128.
74. Rosenberg SA, Lotze MT, Muul LM, et al. A progress report on the treatment of 157 patients with advanced cancer using lymphokine activated killer cells and interleukin-2 or high dose interleukin-2 alone. *N Engl J Med.* 1987; 316:889.
75. Fisher RI, Coltman CA, Doroshow JH, et al. Metastatic renal cancer treated with interleukin-2 and lymphokine activated killer cells. *Ann Intern Med.* 1988;108:518.
76. Beldegrun A, Muul LM, Rosenberg SA. Interleukin-2 expanded tumor filtrating lymphocytes in human renal cancer: isolation, characterization and anti-tumor activity. *Cancer Res.* 1988;48:206.
77. Kradin RL, Kurnick JT, Lazarus DS, Preffer FI, et al. Tumor-infiltrating lymphocytes and interleukin-2 in treatment of advanced cancer. *Lancet.* 1989;1:577.
78. Thompson JA, Lee DJ, Lindgren CG, Benz LA, Collins C, Shuman WP, Levitt P, Fefer A. Influence of interleukin 2 and lymphocyte activated killer cells. *Cancer Res.* 1989;49:235.
79. West WH, Taeur KW, Yanellie JTR, Marshall GD, Orr DW, Thurman GB, Oldham RK. Constant-infusion recombinant interleukin-2 in adoptive immunotherapy of renal cancer. *N Engl J Med.* 1987;316:898.
80. Osband ME, Lavin PT, Babayan RK, Graham S, Lamm DL, Parker B, Sawczuk I, Ross SD, Krane RJ. Autolymphocyte therapy for metastatic renal cell carcinoma significantly prolongs survival with good quality of life: clinical outcome from a randomized, controlled multi-site study. *Lancet.* 1990;335:994–998.
81. Sahasrabudhe DM, McCune CS, O'Donness RW, Henshaw EC. Inhibition of suppressor T lymphocytes (Ts) by cimetidine. *J Immunol.* 1987;138:2760.
82. deKernion J, Lindner A, Figlin R, Sarna G, Smith RB. The treatment of metastatic renal cell carcinoma with a leukocyte interferon. *J Urol.* 1983;130:1063.
83. Quesada JR, Swanson DA, Trindale A, et al. Renal cell carcinoma: Antitumor effects of leukocyte interferon. *Cancer Res.* 1983;43:940.
84. Figlin RA, deKernion JB, Mukamel E, Schnipper EF, et al. Recombinant leukocyte A interferon (rIFN alpha) antibody development in advanced renal cell carcinoma. *Proc Am Soc Clin Oncol.* 1988;5:222.
85. Muss HB. Interferon therapy for renal cell carcinoma. *Semin Oncol.* 1987;14:36.
86. Rinehart J, Young D, LaForge J, et al. Phase I/II trial of interferon b-serine in patients with renal cell carcinoma: immunological and biological effects. *Cancer Res.* 1987;47:2581.
87. Recombinant Human Interferon Gamma (S-6810) Research Group on Renal Cell Carcinoma: Phase II study of recombinant human interferon gamma on renal cell carcinoma. *Cancer.* 1987;60:929.
88. Spiegel RJ. Clinical overview of alpha interferon: studies and future directions. *Cancer.* 1987;59:626.
89. Kirkwood JM, Harris JE, Vera R, et al. Randomized trial of two doses of leukocyte interferon (IFNa) in metastatic renal cell carcinoma: American Cancer Society Collaborative Trial. *Cancer Res.* 1985;45:863.
90. Quesada JR, Rios A, Swanson DA, et al. Antitumor activity of recombinant-derived interferon alpha in metastatic renal cell carcinoma. *J Clin Oncol.* 1985;3:1522.
91. Itri LM, Campion M, Dennin RA, et al. Incidence and clinical significance of neutralizing antibodies in patients receiving recombinant interferon alpha-2a intramuscular injection. *Cancer.* 1987;59:668.
92. Steis RG, Smith JW, Urba WJ, et al. Resistance to recombinant interferon alpha-2a in hairy cell leukemia associated with neutralizing anti-interferon antibodies. *N Engl J Med.* 1988;318:1409.
93. Frei E III, Spriggs D. Tumor necrosis factor: still a promising agent. *J Clin Oncol.* 1989; 7:291.
94. Schirmer WJ, Schirmer JM, Fry DE. Recombinant human tumor necrosis factor produces hemodynamic changes characteristic of sepsis and endotoxemia. *Arch Surg.* 1982;124:445.
95. Otto U, Conrad S, Schneider AW, Kempeni J, Schlick E, Klosterhalfen H. Combined therapy with TNF-alpha and IFN-alpha 2a: a promising approach to treatment of metastatic renal cell carcinoma. *Proc Am Soc Clin Oncol.* 1990; 8:A573.

# 29

# Superficial Transitional Cell Carcinoma Stages Tis, Ta, T1: Bladder and Upper Urinary Tract

*Robert C. Flanigan*

## INTRODUCTION

The most common form of bladder cancer at its presentation is disease involving the epithelium and/or submucosa with no underlying muscular invasion, commonly known as superficial bladder cancer (stages Tis, Ta, and T1). In recent years, increasing information has suggested that these superficial tumors have a markedly different prognosis in terms of the potential for muscle invasion, metastases, and patient death determined by tumor grade and stage. Our knowledge of what ultimately determines tumor behavior, however, continues to remain limited. To date, it is not possible for us to predict in an individual patient which tumor will remain confined locally to the bladder and which tumor will subsequently metastasize and cause the patient's death. The purpose of this chapter is to review the current concepts of epidemiology, pathology, natural history, methods of diagnosis, staging, and approaches to treatment of superficial urothelial cancer, including those tumors that arise in the upper urinary tract as well as the urinary bladder.

## EPIDEMIOLOGY

### Incidence and Mortality Rates

Newly diagnosed bladder cancer will account for approximately 51,600 cases in the United States in 1992. Of these, 38,500 will involve males and 13,100 will involve females. Upper tract urothelial cancers are much less common, occurring in 5000 cases, 3750 in men and 1250 in women. Transitional cell carcinoma (TCC) of the urinary tract is three to four times more common among men than women, accounting for 10% of cancers among men and only 3% of cancers among women. Furthermore, TCC of the bladder occurs with approximately twice the incidence (cases per 100,000 person-years) among whites as compared to blacks (31.5 versus 16.2 when comparing white men to black men and 7.8 versus 5.0 when comparing white women to black women).[1] This apparent difference in incidence between white and black people in the United States may be explained by variables in diagnosis and reporting as suggested by recent studies that have shown that the increased risk in whites is limited to patients with noninvasive tumors, and that among patients with muscle-invasive tumors, whites were actually at a slightly reduced risk compared to blacks. Mortality rates from bladder cancer (deaths per 100,000 person-years) are similar for blacks and whites (white men 6.0, black men 4.2, white women 1.7, black women 2.5), also suggesting that the differences in incidence may reflect variable diagnosis and reporting.[1] Geographic distribution in the United States has been correlated with mortality rates from bladder cancer. Urban areas and in particular the northeastern United States, a location of chemical manufacturing, are associated with a higher risk of development of bladder cancer.[2,3]

## Risk Factors

**Occupational Exposure.** In 1895, Rehn reported that aniline dyes were acting as urothelial carcinogens involving workers involved in the manufacture of these dyes.[4] Subsequently, it was appreciated that the intermediates 2-naphthylamine and benzidine, rather than the aniline dyes themselves, were responsible for the increased incidence of bladder cancer.[5] Similar associations of aromatic amines (β-naphthylamine, 4-aminobiphenyl, 4-nitrobiphenyl) and the development of bladder cancer were subsequently reported.[6]

Epidemiologists now believe that occupational exposure may account for approximately one fourth to one third of all cases of bladder cancers seen in industrialized societies.[7,8] Long latency periods after exposure have been reported, some of which have appeared to approach 40 to 50 years after exposure. A quantitively greater exposure to carcinogen seems to shorten the latency period without significantly increasing the risk.[9]

In addition to the dye industry, several other industries have been found to be associated with an increased risk of bladder cancer, including the leather industry, metal machining, and the organic chemical industry.[10] Cancer risk is not limited to industrial exposure from nitrosamines. Azo dyes found in common sewage may be broken down by bacteria to aromatic amines.[11] Endogenous formation of aromatic amines in the intestines by bacterial synthesis from dietary sources (eg, nitrates and nitrites used as food preservatives) has been suggested, but recent studies suggest that endogenous metabolites do not significantly contribute to the formation of human bladder cancers.[12,13]

**Cigarette Smoking.** The association between cigarette smoking and bladder cancer was first noted in the 1950s.[14] These early studies and subsequent investigations have suggested roughly a fourfold excess risk for the development of bladder cancer among male smokers as compared to male nonsmokers. It is therefore postulated that approximately 30% to 40% of bladder cancers may be directly associated with cigarette smoking.[15] The length of time smoking occurs and the degree of inhalation have been correlated with an increased mortality from bladder cancer.[16] Ex-cigarette smokers have been shown to have a reduced incidence of bladder cancer as compared to current cigarette smokers.[17] The increased risk of bladder cancer associated with smoking is observed in both men and women.

Although the specific carcinogen present in cigarette smoke that may lead to the development of transitional cell carcinoma has not been identified, it is known that cigarette smoke does contain nitrosamines as well as 2-naphthylamine.[18] In addition, tryptophan metabolites also are present in increased concentration in the urine of cigarette smokers.[12,19]

**Analgesics.** The analgesic phenacetin, when consumed in large quantities (5 to 15 kg over a 10-year period), has been associated with an increased risk of TCC of the renal pelvis, particularly in women.[20] The overall increased risk of developing bladder cancer in this setting has been estimated to be 2.6–4 to 1.[21,22] A latency period of approximately 15 to 20 years has been reported for the development of upper tract tumors with a longer latency period associated with the development of bladder cancer.[23] The precise mechanism by which analgesic compounds induce transitional cell carcinoma is unclear, although phenacetin is an aniline derivative and is metabolized to orthohydroxyamines.[24,25]

**Chronic Infection or Irritation.** Chronic bladder irritation, especially when associated with urinary calculi, indwelling catheters, or bladder diverticulae, is associated with an increased risk for the development of squamous cell carcinoma of the bladder.[26] Spinal cord injury patients who are predisposed to infection, stone formation, obstruction, and chronic foreign body reactions may have a risk for the development of squamous cell cancer that is 16 to 20 times higher than normal.[27,28] Chronic infection with *Schistosoma haematobium* is also associated with a significantly higher incidence of squamous cell carcinoma of the bladder in countries bordering the Nile River where these infections are endemic.[29] In addition, patients with defunctionalized bladders who develop pyocystis may also be at an increased risk for the development of squamous cell carcinomas.[30]

**Cyclophosphamide (Cytoxan).** Several investigators have suggested that patients treated with cyclophosphamide have a ninefold increased risk of bladder carcinoma.[31,32] These carcinomas appeared to occur after a relatively short latency period of 6 to 13 years. The mechanism responsible for the formation of transitional cell carcinoma in this setting is the presence of the metabolite acrolein in the bladder. Carcinogeneses associated with this agent can be reduced by the use of uro-protective agents, eg, mesna,[33] during periods of chemotherapy.

**Other Etiologies.** Other associated factors include those shown in Table 1.

## PATHOLOGY

### Normal Bladder Urothelium

The normal bladder urothelium is composed of three to seven layers of transitional cells with large umbrella cells overlapping the cells of the intermediate cell layers which in turn rest on a basal cell layer (Fig 1). Characteristically the nuclei of the intermediate cells are oval-shaped and oriented with their long axis perpendicular to the basement membrane. Below the epithelium lies the lamina propria and submucosal layer. The submucosal layer contains the muscularis mucosa and multiple vascular spaces (Fig 2). Below the submucosal layer lies the detrusor muscle. Tumor involvement of the muscularis mucosa must be distinguished from involvement of

**TABLE 1. Other Etiologies of Bladder Cancer**

| Etiologic Factor | Relative Incidence of Cancer | Reference |
|---|---|---|
| Regional differences | 30%–50% higher in northern regions of U.S. as compared to southern regions | Cutler[34] |
| Age | Bladder cancer is uncommon in patients <50 years old and tends to be present with a more differentiated histology in younger patients | Benson[35] |
| Artificial sweeteners (Saccharine, cyclamates) | These compounds have been shown in large doses to induce bladder cancers in rodents; case-controlled epidemiologic studies reveal little significant evidence to suggest an association in humans | Risch[36] |
| Pelvic irradiation | Ionizing radiation for carcinoma of the cervix has been associated with a 2- to 4-fold increase in the development of TCC of bladder; careful epidemiologic studies have not clearly established this relationship | Duncan[37] |
| Heredity | May occur in familial clusters; genetic differences in hepatic arylamine acetyltransferase may play a role (slow acetylators more susceptible to bladder tumors than fast acetylators) | Fraumeni[38]<br>McCullough[39]<br>Kadlubar[40] |

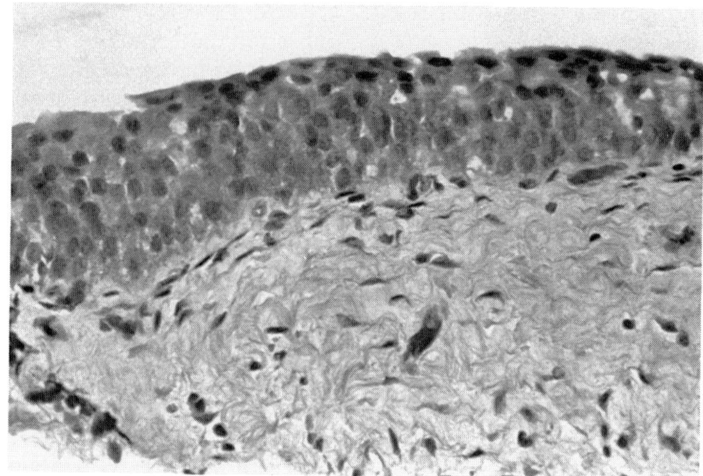

**Fig 1.** Normal bladder epithelium is composed of three to seven layers of umbrella (superficial cells) and intermediate cells resting on a basal cell layer.

deep muscle (detrusor) on pathologic specimen in order to accurately stage TCC.[41] Submucosal vascular spares apparently may allow for tumor metastasis even in the absence of underlying muscle invasion.

A similar anatomic arrangement of layers is present in the upper urinary tract with the exception of the markedly reduced deep muscle mass. This diminished barrier to tumor extension explains the ready access of tumor to the para-ureteral space.

## Abnormalities of the Urothelial Layer

Abnormalities of the urothelial layer can range from hyperplasia to carcinoma. Hyperplasia may be further subdivided into epithelial hyperplasia, which is characterized by an increase in the number of cells without nuclear or architectural abnormalities, inverted papilloma, von Brunn's nests, and cystitis cystica.

**Fig 2.** The submucosal layer contains muscularis mucosa (of various degrees of completeness) and multiple vascular spaces.

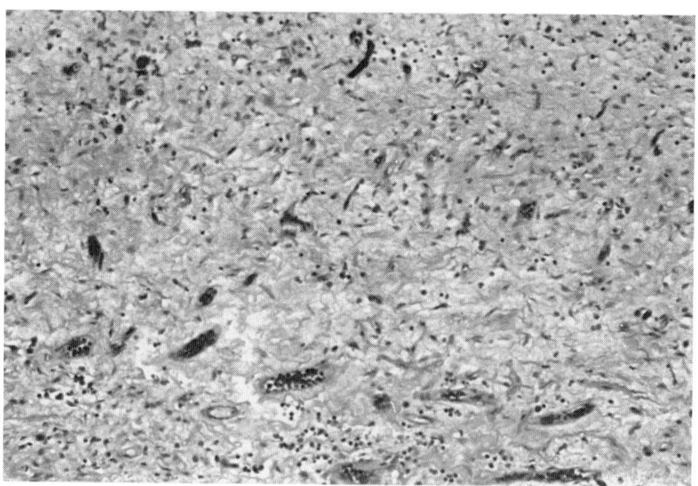

### Hyperplasia

*Inverted Papilloma.* Inverted papilloma is a rare benign proliferative lesion generally associated with chronic infection and/or bladder outlet obstruction. It occurs primarily in older men with prostatism and most often is located on the trigone and bladder neck area.[42] Inverted papilloma often contains areas of cystitis cystica or squamous metaplasia and is characterized by its benign cytologic appearance. Two basic types of inverted papilloma have been reported: trabecular and glandular. The trabecular type arises as a proliferation of the basal cells of the epithelium. The glandular type has been considered to be a form of cystitis glandularis and, as such, has been considered preneoplastic by some authors.[43] The treatment for inverted papilloma, therefore, is the same as that for low-grade TCC in that biopsy and fulguration or transurethral resection should be accomplished with subsequent periodic cystoscopic examinations.[42] Recurrence is rare, but malignant transformation has been reported.[44]

*Von Brunn's Nests.* Von Brunn's nests are clusters of benign transitional cells situated in the submucosal layer of the bladder. They are thought to result from an inward budlike proliferation of the basal cells of the urothelium.[45]

*Cystitis Cystica.* Cystitis cystica is a cystoscopic and histologic descriptive term for von Brunn's nests that have undergone central liquification.[43] It is characterized by submucosal nests of peripherally located transitional cells surrounding a central region of eosinophilic liquification.

**Urothelial Metaplasias.** Urothelial metaplasias are commonly subdivided to include cystitis glandularis, nephrogenic adenoma, and squamous metaplasia.

*Cystitis Glandularis.* Cystitis glandularis is similar histologically to cystitis cystica except that the transitional cell lining of the microcyst has undergone glandular metaplasia.[46] Cystitis glandularis may have a papillary appearance on cystoscopic examination. It is believed to be a precursor of urothelial adenocarcinoma.[47]

*Nephrogenic Adenoma.* Nephrogenic adenoma is a rare lesion that derives its name from its histologic similarity to primitive renal collecting tubules. It generally arises as a result of transformation of normal epithelium in response to trauma, infection, or ionizing radiation. Although typically little nuclear atypia or mitotic activity is present, this tumor has been known to recur in approximately 50% of patients.[48] Nephrogenic adenoma is more common in men and may produce dysuria and urinary frequency. Its papillary appearance on cystoscopic evaluation may lead to its confusion with papillary TCC. It is treated by biopsy and fulguration or transurethral resection.

A malignant counterpart of nephrogenic adenoma, mesonephric adenocarcinoma, has been reported.[48] This well-differentiated tumor resembles nephrogenic adenoma histologically and clinically except that infiltration of cells beyond the lamina propria is noted. It is frequently located on the trigone and is generally managed by radical excision. Tumor invasion into bladder muscle has been demonstrated.[48]

*Squamous Metaplasia.* Squamous metaplasia denotes the replacement of normal transitional cell epithelium by mature nonkeratinizing squamous epithelium. This lesion is common on the trigone of women. It has been called ''vaginalization'' of the bladder neck and appears to occur under hormonal influence.[49] Although this histologic change is present in nearly 50% of adult women, it occurs in less than 10% of men.[50] Squamous metaplasia in the absence of cellular atypia or marked keratinization would appear to be a benign condition in either sex.

**Dysplasia.** Dysplasia of the bladder may take the form of atypical hyperplasia, mild atypia, moderate atypia, or severe atypia. In addition, leukoplakia of the bladder may occur. Dysplastic urothelium exhibits histologic changes that are intermediate between normal urothelium and carcinoma in situ. It is generally felt that lesions on the severe end of this spectrum are neoplastic rather than dysplastic.[51] Morphologically, urothelial dysplasia is characterized by enlargement of the nuclei, which are basally situated, notched, and spherical with a loss of normal cellular polarity. Mitosis and increased numbers of cell layers may occur, but are not consistent findings.[51]

**Superficial Carcinomas.** Superficial carcinomas of the bladder urothelium include carcinoma in situ and cancers involving the epithelium and submucosal layers. Histologically, these cancers are either transitional cell, squamous, or adenocarcinomas.

*Carcinoma In Situ.* Histologically, carcinoma in situ is characterized by a poorly differentiated cancer involving only the urothelium. A loss of cellular cohesiveness, widening of the intracellular spaces, separation of cells from the basement membrane, and a loss of the superficial umbrella cell layer is characteristic. Carcinoma in situ may occur focally or diffusely within the urothelium. It is often associated with high-grade and high-stage transitional cell cancers. Although carcinoma in situ may occur in the absence of visible bladder tumor, its association with either a concurrent or prior bladder tumor significantly increases the risk of progression to muscle invasion of a non-muscle-invasive (superficial) TCC.[52,53] In patients having a concurrent tumor, the presence of carcinoma in situ is associated with an approximately 80% likelihood of cancer progression to muscle invasion. Likewise, in a patient with a prior history of bladder cancer, the presence of carcinoma in situ is associated with an approximately 40% risk of progression.

The cystoscopic appearance of carcinoma in situ is often misleading in that a normal-appearing epithelium is the most common finding. A reddened or velvety patch of erythematous mucosa should, however, suggest the possibility of carcinoma in situ. Carcinoma in situ, like papillary urothelial cancer, is more common in men than in women. Because carcinoma in situ frequently presents with irritative voiding symptoms, the patient is often misdiagnosed as suffering from prostatism, urinary tract infection, or neuropathic bladder dysfunction. Cytopathologic studies of urine or bladder exfoliative bladder specimens are positive in 85% to 90% of patients with carcinoma in situ.

The natural history of carcinoma in situ is unpredictable. Early in its evolution, carcinoma in situ may produce no symptoms, and, in fact, patients with focal asymptomatic carcinoma in situ have been reported to generally display a protracted clinical course with a low likelihood of development of invasive bladder cancer.[54,55] In contrast, patients with diffuse or symptomatic carcinoma in situ, especially in association with a history of bladder cancer, often display a poor prognosis despite definitive therapy.[56] Approximately 20% of patients, for example, who undergo cystectomy for diffuse carcinoma in situ are found to have microscopic evidence of muscle invasion.[57]

*Papillary Transitional Cell Carcinoma.* More than 99% of bladder tumors are carcinomas. Transitional cell carcinoma represents approximately 90% of these tumors. Transitional cell carcinoma is generally graded on a scale of 1 to 3 (some systems grade from 1 to 4). Grade I TCCs differ from normal epithelium by having an increased number of epithelial cell layers. With increasing grade, abnormalities of nuclear morphology, loss of cellular polarity, abnormalities of the normal cellular maturation from the basal to superficial layers, nuclear crowding, and increased nuclear to cytoplasmic ratio are seen. In addition, prominent nucleoli with clumping of the chromatin and an increased number of mitoses may be appreciated.[58]

Bladder cancer grading was first described by Broders in 1922.[59] Although there remains no uniformly accepted grading system for bladder cancer, there is a striking correlation between tumor grade and tumor stage in most systems that are employed.[60] In most grading systems, well-differentiated (grade 1) TCCs display a thin

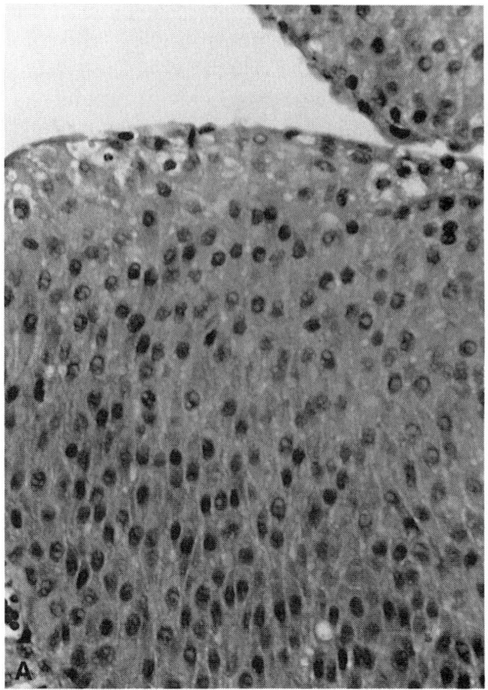

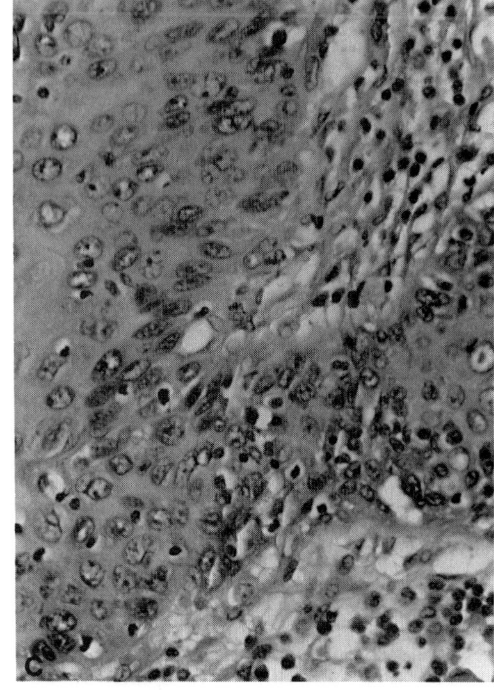

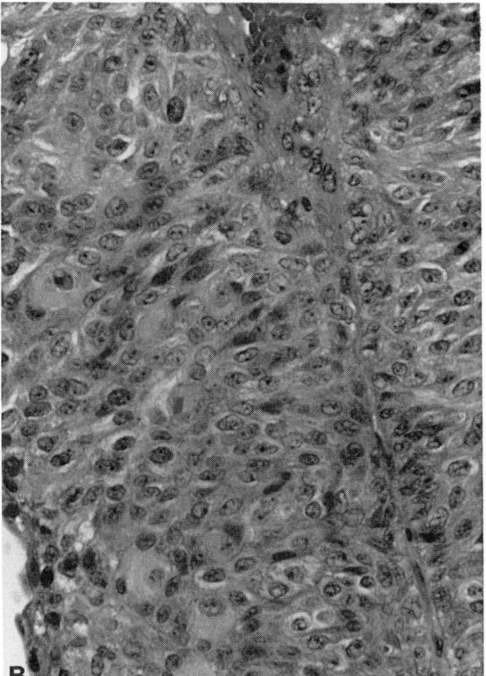

**Fig 3.** Grading of transitional cell carcinoma: **A,** grade I: thin fibrovascular stalk with an increased number of cell layers (>7); **B,** grade II: wide fibrovascular core, disturbance of basal to surface maturation, loss of cellular polarity, increased nuclear to cytoplasmic ratio, and frequent mitotic figures; **C,** grade III: lack of differentiation of cells from basement membrane to surface, marked nuclear pleomorphism, high nuclear to cytoplasmic ratio, and frequent mitotic figures.

fibrovascular stalk with an increase in the number of cell layers beyond the seven-cell thickness that typifies normal epithelium. Only slight cellular anaplasia and a mild disturbance of the basal to surface cellular maturation with rare mitotic figures are noted (Fig 3A).

Moderately differentiated carcinomas (grade 2) have a wide fibrovascular core, a greater disturbance of basal to surface maturation, and a loss of cellular polarity. The nuclear to cytoplasmic ratio is increased and nuclear pleomorphism and prominent nucleoli are seen. Mitotic figures are frequent (Fig 3B).

Poorly differentiated tumors (grade 3) are characterized by a lack of differentiation of cells as they progress from the basement membrane to the surface. Marked nuclear pleomorphism, a high nuclear to cytoplasmic ratio, and frequent mitotic figures are noted (Fig 3C).

***Nontransitional Cell Carcinomas (Squamous Cell Carcinoma, Adenocarcinoma).*** In the United States, squamous cell carcinomas account for approximately 3% to 7% of bladder cancers.[58,61] These tumors are commonly associated with a chronic inflammatory process involving the urothelium, including the presence of a chronic foreign body, (eg, an indwelling catheter), urinary tract calculi, or recurrent urinary tract infections. Generally, a greater proportion of patients with squamous cell carcinoma as compared to TCC present with advanced disease at the time of diagnosis. Stage for stage, however, the prognosis of patients with squamous cell carcinoma is comparable to that of patients with TCC.[62,63] In Egypt, more than 75% of bladder cancers are squamous cell in origin.[64] These so-called bilharzial cancers occur in patients 10 to 20 years younger than TCC patients and are generally exophytic, nodular, fungating lesions that are histologically well differentiated and appear to have a relatively lower incidence of lymph node and distant metastasis.[64]

Adenocarcinoma of the bladder is a rare lesion accounting for less than 2% of all bladder cancers.[61] These highly invasive tumors do not typically present as superficial lesions. Primary adenocarcinomas can occur anywhere within the bladder and are believed to occur in response to chronic inflammation.[65] Risk factors include bladder exstrophy, schistosomiasis, and perhaps coffee drinking.[61,65,66] Histologically, adenocarcinomas may be varied in appearance, including signet ring and colloid carcinomas. Most are mucin producing.[58] Adenocarcinomas are usually poorly differentiated and muscle-invasive.

Adenocarcinomas arising in the urachus represent the most common type of cancer arising in this structure. Generally, these tumors arise outside the bladder and invade through the urothelium with extension into the bladder. These tumors are typically mucin producing and advanced at the time of presentation. The prognosis of urachal adenocarcinomas is worse than for primary bladder adenocarcinoma.[67] Unexpectedly wide and deep infiltration of tumor is not uncommon on histologic examination of the surgical specimen. For this reason, partial cystectomy has been associated with local recurrence rates of 15% to 50%.[68] Therefore, the recommended treatment for all but the smallest, most well-differentiated tumors is radical cystectomy and bilateral pelvic lymphenectomy with en bloc excision of the urachus. Radiation therapy is not effective in treating this lesion.[69]

Table 2 summarizes this classification of urothelial histologic abnormalities, including hyperplastic, metaplastic, dysplastic, and neoplastic bladder lesions.

## NATURAL HISTORY

The natural history of superficial TCC includes recurrence and muscle invasion leading to potential metastasis and patient death. Transitional cell carcinomas involving only the epithelial and submucosal layers are a heterogeneous group of tumors that exhibit a broad spectrum of biologic potential. Although only 10% to 15% of patients with well-differentiated superficial

**TABLE 2. Classification of Urothelial Histologic Abnormalities**

1. Normal urothelium
2. Hyperplasia
   a. epithelial
   b. inverted papilloma
   c. von Brunn's nests
   d. cystitis cystica
3. Metaplasia
   a. cystitis glandularis
   b. nephrogenic adenoma
   c. squamous metaplasia
4. Dysplasia
   a. atypical hyperplasia
   b. atypia (mild, moderate, and severe)
5. Carcinoma
   a. in situ
   b. transitional cell
   c. squamous cell
   d. adenocarcinoma

tumors progress to muscle invasion, invasive progression rates as high as 45% to 50% have been reported for high-grade lesions involving the submucosal layer.[52,70,71]

## Recurrence

Approximately 70% of patients with superficial TCC will display one or more recurrence of tumor if treated by endoscopic resection alone.[52] Factors associated with increased risk of recurrence are shown in Table 3. It is believed that most recurrences are new tumors that arise in other areas of dysplastic epithelium. Some recurrences, however, undoubtedly result from inadequate treatment of preexisting tumors or from tumor cell implantation.[72] Grade seems to be an important indicator of recurrence. Seventy-five percent of patients with grade I tumors are likely to be disease-free at 12 months, compared with only 55% of patients with grade III tumors.[73,74] Tumor grade is also associated with signs of urothelial abnormalities at other sites in the bladder. For example, one series showed significant distant urothelial abnormalities in association with 15% of grade 1 tumors, 59% of grade 2, and 77% of grade 3.[75] The prevention of tumor recurrence is a major goal in the therapy of TCC.

## Progression to Muscle Invasion

Approximately 10% to 15% of patients presenting with superficial TCCs can be expected to progress to muscle invasion. Patients with high-grade tumors invading the lamina propria, however, may display progression rates as high as 45% to 50%.

| TABLE 3. Factors Influencing Time to Recurrence of Superficial TCCs |
|---|
| Number of visible tumors |
| Previous recurrence |
| Stage |
| Grade |
| Presence of dysplasia/hyperplasia in random biopsies |
| Size of largest tumor |
| DNA ploidy |

| TABLE 4. Risk Factors for Muscle Invasion |
|---|
| Stage |
| Grade |
| Carcinoma in situ |
| ABO (H) blood group |
| Chromosome analysis |
| DNA ploidy |

Factors associated with an increased risk of muscle invasion progression are shown in Table 4.[76] Lutzeyer et al reported death rates at 3 years for superficial TCC of 3% for patients with grade 1 stage cancers as compared to 43% for patients with grade 3 stage lesions.[77] Moreover, Anterstrom et al further subdivided patients with TCC by tumor stage and grade and has demonstrated an increased mortality rate with increasing stage and grade of superficial TCCs.[78] In fact, once a tumor has demonstrated its aggressiveness by invasion of the lamina propria, it has already expressed its ability to metastasize. A 20% incidence of lymphatic involvement by tumors involving only the lamina propria was reported by Jewett et al.[79] Undifferentiated tumors are also more likely to shed cells into lymphatics and blood vessels, thereby increasing the likelihood of metastases.[80]

**Carcinoma in Situ.** Carcinoma in situ of the bladder occupies a controversial area in the spectrum of bladder cancers. Patients with focal asymptomatic carcinoma in situ may have a relatively good prognosis whereas patients with diffuse carcinoma in situ, as stated previously, often display microscopic invasion at the time of cystectomy and are at high risk for the subsequent development of muscle-invasive cancers if cystectomy is not undertaken.

**Tumor Markers.** Markers felt to be associated with an increased risk of progression to muscle invasion in patients with superficial urothelial tumors are shown in Table 4. Cellular differentiation is an important predictor of progression as described earlier. In one study, for example, 19% of grade 1 superficial tumors progressed to muscle invasion as compared with 69% of grade 3 tumors.[81]

The presence or absence of blood group antigens on the surface epithelium has also been correlated with subsequent muscle invasion. Thus the presence of blood group antigens in a low-grade urothelial cancer is associated with a very low likelihood of progression (3% to 5%).[82] In contrast, the absence of blood group antigens is associated with a 65% chance of progression.[82] The presence of blood group antigens in urothelial cancers can be determined by red cell adherence or immunoperoxidase testing.[83] A schematic representation of the red cell adherence test is shown in Figure 4.

The Thomsen–Friedenreich antigen (T antigen) is another surface antigen that appears to be independent of the blood group antigens. It is masked in normal urothelium.[84] In one study, for example, patients with loss of blood antigen who had normal T antigen expression had few recurrences and only a 16% incidence of subsequent invasion.[85] On the other hand, patients with abnormal T-antigen expression (defined as T-antigen–positive or cryptic T-antigen–negative) display a nearly 65% incidence of recurrence with invasion.[86]

**Fig 4.** Schematic representation of the standard red cell adherence test.

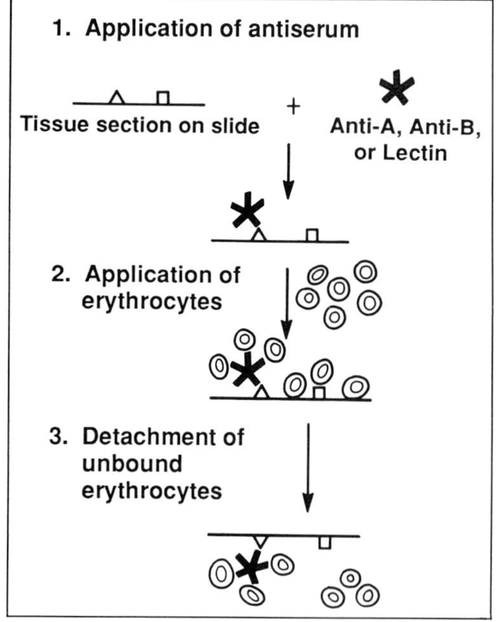


Tumor karyotype and marker chromosomes may also predict tumor aggressiveness. An increase in the modal chromosome number is associated with tumor dedifferentiation.[87] Of more importance may be the presence of a marker chromosome. In superficial cancers, the patients without marker chromosomes generally do well whereas those with markers do poorly.[88]

Monoclonal antibodies prepared against tumor-associated antigens from a variety of superficial bladders with a proven history of clinical aggressiveness may allow for identification of patients at low and high risk for progression.[89,90]

## DIAGNOSIS

### Signs and Symptoms

Hematuria is the most common presenting symptom of urothelial cancer, occurring in 85% of patients with bladder cancer.[91] There is no correlation between the size or stage of the tumor and the degree of hematuria seen. The next most common symptom is vesical irritability with urinary frequency, urgency, and dysuria. This latter symptom complex is frequently associated with diffuse carcinoma in situ.[56] Patients with hematuria and/or vesical irritability that cannot be explained on the basis of a documented urinary tract infection and do not resolve after treatment of this urinary tract infection must be investigated with excretory urography and cystoscopic examination. In addition, urinary cytologies including bladder wash cytologies are indicated. The mean duration of symptoms before diagnosis of tumor is between 3 and 8 months.[91,92]

Patients presenting with ureteral obstruction and flank pain are often found on histologic evaluation to have a muscle invasive bladder cancer. However, superficial urothelial cancers of the upper urinary tract may cause obstruction of the kidney without being associated with underlying muscle invasion (Fig 5). Upper tract cancers

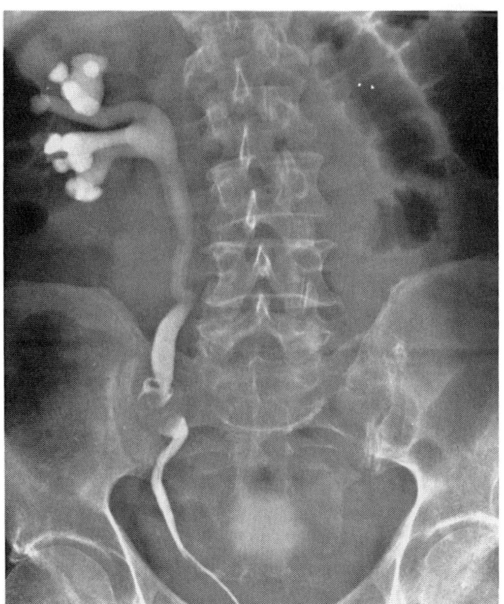

**Fig 5.** Retrograde pyelography revealing a large defect. Excretory urography (IVP) revealed significant obstruction of the right kidney. Histology revealed a grade II transitional cell cancer with no muscle invasion and no associated carcinoma in situ. Segmental ureterectomy was performed.

present with hematuria in 50% to 67% of patients. Other presenting signs and symptoms are flank pain and abdominal pain (20% to 40%), and, less commonly, an abdominal mass or hydronephrosis. Frequency, dysuria, and weight loss also may occur.[93]

## Excretory Urography

Excretory urography (by intravenous pyelography, or IVP) is an essential facet of the evaluation of patients with presumed urothelial carcinoma whether presenting with hematuria, vesical irritability, or other symptoms. It is important to completely identify the entire upper urinary tract on the excretory urogram. Although large bladder tumors may be visualized as filling defects within the bladder or an irregularity of the bladder contour on the cystogram phase of the urogram, the excretory urogram is not an adequate test of bladder carcinoma.

## Cystoscopy, Biopsy, and Transurethral Resection

**Cystoscopy.** Cystoscopy remains a mainstay in the diagnosis of TCC of the bladder. It is critical at the time of cystoscopic examination to identify any abnormalities involving the bladder and to map them carefully for future reference (Fig 6). Lesions should be identified as papillary, sessile, or nodular. The size of the lesion should be noted as this provides important prognostic information. Any slightly raised, velvety, or erythematous areas must be biopsied as they may portend carcinoma in situ. At the time of cystoscopy, bimanual examination of the bladder should be performed in patients with suspected carcinoma.

**Bladder Biopsy.** Biopsy of any and all abnormal areas of the bladder should be accomplished using either a cold cup biopsy forcep (with subsequent fulguration) or a transurethral resectoscope. Small lesions are more amenable to cold cup biopsy, so that coagulation artifact can be avoided. It is critical in any biopsy of a bladder lesion to ensure the presence of the underlying musculature within the biopsy specimen so that accurate staging of the bladder tumor can be possible. Although there are conflicting opinions about the proper technique for transurethral resection of large bladder tumors, the traditional teaching has been to resect the superficial portion of the tumor, sending it as a separate specimen, and then to resect the deep portion along with the underlying bladder muscle, sending it as a "deep specimen." This allows the pathologist additional facility in identifying evidence of underlying muscle invasion.

In the presence of a documented bladder tumor, selected random cold cup mucosal biopsies from areas adjacent to the tumor, as well as the opposite bladder wall, dome, trigone, and prostatic urethra, may be indicated. The rationale for obtaining random bladder biopsies is that they provide information of significant importance regarding the likelihood of tumor recurrence. These biopsies may be shown to reveal dysplasia in approximately 25% of patients

Bladder mapping: Outline and number all tumors, suspicious areas and selected mucosal biopsies. Report location, type of procedure, and shape for each number site.

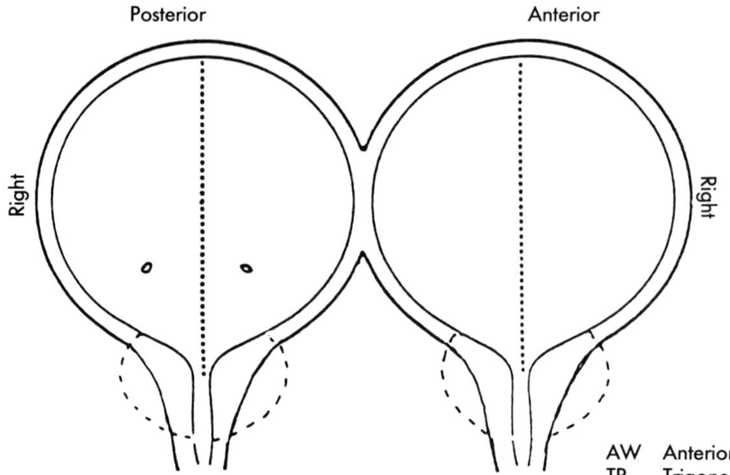

PW Posterior wall
RW Right wall
LW Left wall
RU Right ureteral orifice
LU Left ureteral orifice
U Urethra

AW Anterior wall
TR Trigone
D Dome
N Neck
PU Prostatic urethra
PS Prostatic substance

| | Tumor or Biopsy Site | | | | | | | |
|---|---|---|---|---|---|---|---|---|
| Number | | | | | | | | |
| Location | | | | | | | | |
| Procedure<br>Tumor biopsy | | | | | | | | |
| Adjacent to tumor biopsy | | | | | | | | |
| Suspicious area biopsy | | | | | | | | |
| Selected mucosal biopsy | | | | | | | | |
| Resection | | | | | | | | |
| Fulguration | | | | | | | | |
| Shape<br>Flat | | | | | | | | |
| Sessile | | | | | | | | |
| Papillary | | | | | | | | |
| Bullous Edema | | | | | | | | |

Size of largest tumor: ☐☐.☐ cm

Bladder status at follow-up: (Mark all appropriate)
☐ No visible tumor
☐ Suspicious area(s)
Tumor visible: ☐ Same site(s) ☐ Adjacent site(s) ☐ New site(s) ☐ None specified

**Fig 6.** A bladder map. Note tabulation of biopsy sites and a description of the lesion.

with carcinoma in situ and approximately 20% of patients with superficial bladder cancers.[94] However, some investigators believe that random bladder biopsies are unnecessary, and, in fact, may be hazardous because they denude the overlying urothelium and create potential areas for tumor cell implantation. These authors generally suggest that urinary cytology is a better indicator of the presence of concurrent carcinoma in situ than are selected random bladder biopsies.[95]

Because less than 15% of normal-appearing mucosa on cystoscopic examination will reveal significant histologic abnormalities on biopsy, staining of the bladder mucosa with various compounds (tetracycline, hematoporphyrins, acridine orange, or methylene blue) has been advocated as a means of detecting subclinical bladder cancer. These methods have not achieved general usage, however, because of the lack of sensitivity and specificity of this staining.[96,97]

When superficial tumors are seen to arise in or about the area of the ureteral orifice, one must suspect the possibility of seeding of tumor from the upper urinary tract. In this case, careful excretory urography and/or retrograde urography and ureteroscopy may be necessary to identify these upper tract lesions. If the tumor occurs at the site of the ureteral orifice, resection of the tumor can be accomplished with resection of a part of the underlying ureteral submucosal tunnel. This may give rise to ureteral reflex, but if the resection is performed using a cutting current, ureteral obstruction is less likely than when extensive cauterization is performed around the ureteral orifice. If upper tract evaluation is required in a patient with a tumor at or near a ureteral orifice, it is preferable to complete resection of the tumor prior to performing necessary upper tract studies in an effort to decrease the rate of implantation of tumor into the upper urinary tract. Placement of a ureteral catheter and/or guidewire prior to resection may, however, be helpful to allow for subsequent adequate upper tract drainage by ureteral catheterization and/or inspection of the upper urinary tract radiographically or ureteroscopically.

Because of the thin underlying muscular layer, tumors arising within a bladder diverticulum should generally be staged by cold cup biopsy and not by transurethral resection, which is more likely to lead to perforation. In addition, these tumors are typically best treated by partial or total cystectomy rather than transurethral resection.

Resection of tumors on the lateral bladder wall may be difficult because of stimulation of the obturator nerve. This stimulation results in contraction of the adductor muscles of the thigh. If this problem is noted, resection of the area should be performed with the patient under general anesthesia while employing intravenous muscle relaxation (pancuronium) to minimize the risk of inadvertent bladder perforation.

After resection of the bladder tumor, a urethral catheter should be left in place for some time. Although there is great controversy regarding this interval, the duration should be varied depending on the operator's impression as to the depth of resection. In general, a urethral catheter is left in place for approximately 1 to 2 days if superficial muscle has been resected and for 3 to 5 days if the resection has been deep or inadvertently carried through the entire bladder thickness. If continuous bladder irrigation is felt to be necessary because of bleeding after resection of the bladder tumor, care must be taken to ensure that overdistention of the bladder does not occur secondary to occlusion of the urethral catheter as this may result in perforation of the bladder.

### Evaluation of the Upper Urinary Tract

As mentioned previously, the mainstay for the evaluation of the upper urinary tract in patients with urothelial cancer is excretory urography. This should be accomplished in such a way that the upper urinary tract, including both ureters, can be carefully evaluated for any possible displacement of the collecting system and/or filling defects. If excretory urography does not evaluate the entire upper urinary tract, retrograde ureterography should be accomplished at the time of cystoscopic examination. Various techniques are available including cone tip (bulb tip) retrograde urography or the placement of a retrograde catheter into the renal pelvis. The latter technique allows for greater ease in the collection of urinary cytologic specimens.

In cases where retrograde urography does not supply information regarding a potential filling defect, or in cases of known urothelial cancer, ureteroscopy may be indicated. This can be accomplished using a flexible and/or rigid ureteroscope. Biopsy, either cytologic or histologic cold culp, should be obtained of any abnormal lesions seen during ureteroscopy.

Brush biopsies for cytologic evaluation of potential upper tract lesions should be accomplished under fluoroscopic control whenever possible. This minimizes the risk of perforation of the upper urinary tract that may occur during blind manipulation of the brush biopsy catheter.

## Urinary Cytology

Urinary cytology is a useful technique for identifying malignant cells that are exfoliated into the urine or that are obtained by washing with normal saline from the upper or lower urinary tract. Malignant transitional cells have enlarged nuclei with irregular, coarsely textured chromatin. Cytologic identification of these tumors is easier in patients with poorly differentiated cancers than well-differentiated tumors that are cytologically normal in appearance, more cohesive, and not readily shed into the urine (Fig 7). Thus, low-grade papillary tumors most often display a negative cytology, whereas 50% of grade 2 and the majority of grade 3 tumors are associated with a positive cytology.[98] On the other hand, urinary cytology, even in the face of high-grade tumors, may be falsely negative in 20% of cases. False-positive cytologic findings, which have been reported in 1% to 12% of patients, are usually due to severe atypia, inflammation, or changes induced in the urothelium by radiation therapy. To date, routine screening of urine for detection of urothelial cancer has not been shown to be cost-effective unless high-risk populations are studied.[99]

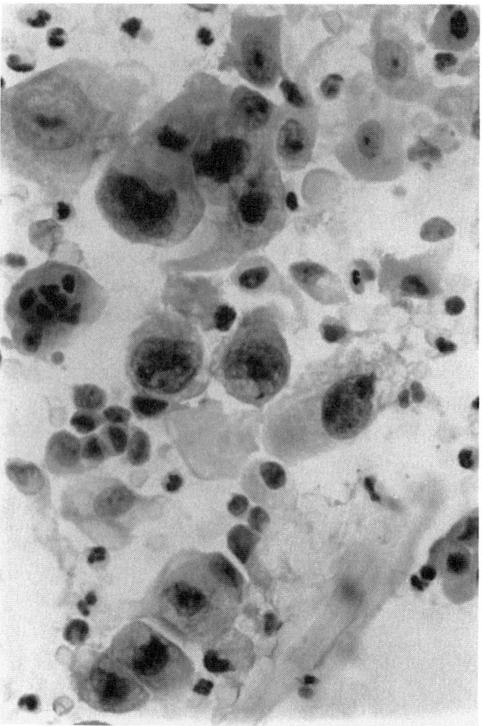

**Fig 7.** Urinary cytology. This microphotograph shows a high-grade transitional cell carcinoma (grade III) composed of single cells with hyperchromatic nuclei, irregular nuclear envelope, and increased nuclear to cytoplasmic ratio.

## Flow Cytometry

Flow cytometry is a technique that allows for the evaluation of large numbers of cells that are passed in single file through a light source after the cells have been stained with a fluorescent compound. Typically, urinary flow cytometry is directed at the identification of the DNA content of the urothelial cells. Most superficial low-grade tumors are diploid, thus leading to false-negative results. This problem is further complicated by the presence of inflammatory cells and other cellular debris within the urinary specimen that may make the identification of small populations of aneuploid tumor cells difficult.[100] In contrast, aneuploidy is common in high-grade lesions. Flow cytometry is capable of detecting carcinoma in situ with an accuracy of over 90%.

Theoretically, the advantage of flow cytometry is that quantitative data are generated. The major disadvantage of flow cytometry is its high cost and questionable reproducibility. The future of flow cytometry would seem to be directed to the use of multiparameter studies.[100] Simultaneous measurement of DNA ploidy and the expression of other antigens of differentiation, eg, cytokeratins, may allow for the identification of smaller numbers of aneuploid tumor cell populations within an exfoliated urinary specimen.

It has been reported that saline bladder washings are generally more accurate than voided urine for detection of bladder cancer because the mechanical action of the barbotage encourages tumor cell shedding and provides more adequately preserved cells for examination.[101,102] At present, however, voided urinary cytology continues to be the procedure of choice in most institutions because of the long experience with voided urinary cytology and because it is noninvasive and widely available.[103]

It is not unusual for a patient with a low-grade papillary tumor to have an occult (high-grade) carcinoma in situ elsewhere in the urinary tract. Therefore, urinary cytologic study after transurethral resection of a bladder tumor is important because a positive urinary cytology will suggest either incomplete resection of the tumor and/or the presence of residual carcinoma in situ.

## STAGING

An accurate staging of urothelial cancers is critical to the development of a carefully planned therapeutic approach to these tumors. The mainstay of staging is a thorough biopsy of the identified lesions, including resection of underlying bladder muscle. Computerized tomography (CT) scanning, ultrasound, and magnetic resonance imaging (MRI) may also be used to evaluate the local extent of bladder tumors, although all of these studies provide limited accuracy in determining the presence or absence of microscopic muscle invasion or minimal extravesical tumor spread.[104] Furthermore, postoperative changes induced by transurethral resection and/or other therapies, including radiation and chemotherapy, may make interpretation of these studies extremely difficult.

In general, if adequate histologic biopsies identify a superficial urothelial cancer, CT scanning will probably provide limited useful clinical information. The major usefulness of CT scanning would be to detect regional lymph nodes. It is important to recognize that enlarged lymph nodes do not always indicate the presence of metastases and that CT scans have failed to detect lymph node metastasis in 40% to 75% of node-positive patients in some studies.[105]

### Staging Systems

Two principal staging systems for bladder cancer remain in use in the United States. In recent years, the conversion to the International Union Against Cancer (UICC) and the American Joint Committee on Cancer Staging and End Results (AJC Staging Systems) has been rapid.[106] In the past, most urologists used the Jewett–Strong system as modified by Marshall.[107] Table 5 describes and compares these two staging systems.

**TABLE 5. Staging Systems of Bladder Cancer**

| Jewett–Strong–Marshall 1952 | Stage Description | AJC-UICC 1987 | |
|---|---|---|---|
| | | Clinical | Pathologic |
| No tumor-definitive specimen | | T0 | PO |
| 0 | Carcinoma in situ | Tis | Pis |
| | Papillary tumor–no invasion | Ta | Pa |
| A | Papillary tumor–lamina propria invasion | T1 | P1 |
| B1 | Superficial | T2 | P2 |
| B2 | Deep muscle invasion | T3a | P3 |
| C | Invasion of perivesical fat | T3b | |
| | Invasion of contiguous viscera | T4 | P4 |
| D1 | Involvement of pelvic nodes | | N1–3 |
| | Involvement of juxtaregional nodes | | N4 |
| D2 | Distant metastases | | M1 |

The Jewett–Strong–Marshall staging system classifies superficial tumors involving only the urothelium as stage 0 or carcinoma in situ. Tumors involving the lamina propria are classified as stage A. The AJC–UICC classification is subdivided into clinical and pathologic stages. (Clinical staging is referred to as the T stage and pathologic staging as the P stage.) Clinical carcinoma in situ is stage Tis, noninvasive papillary tumors involving only the urothelium as stage Ta, and tumor with lamina propria invasion as stage T1. The pathologic counterparts in this system are identical.

## MANAGEMENT OF SUPERFICIAL UPPER URINARY TRACT CANCERS (Tis, Ta, T1)

Urothelial lesions of the upper urinary tract may or may not occur in association with synchronous or metachronous urothelial carcinoma of the bladder. Upper urinary tract cancers are most frequently transitional cell carcinomas. Upper tract urothelial lesions occur in association with prior bladder cancer in only 2% to 5% of patients, whereas patients with an initial upper tract lesion develop tumors in the bladder in 50% to 75% of cases. These data imply that urothelial cancer is a field disease. Approximately 80% of renal pelvic transitional cell tumors are papillary and grade I or II.[108] High-grade lesions are therefore infrequent but are associated with rapid invasion and a poor prognosis. Because of the relatively thin ureteral muscle layer (as compared with bladder), tumor penetration results in a higher stage of disease more quickly.[109]

The diagnosis of upper urinary tract cancers relies on the evaluation of the upper urinary tract as previously discussed. Although microscopic or gross hematuria occurs in 50% to 67% of patients with upper urinary tract cancers, up to 15% of the patients are asymptomatic and the diagnosis is established serendipitously as a result of studies initiated for other reasons. Flank pain occurs in 30% to 40% of patients and is usually a dull ache, although acute renal colic and the passage of long, thin clots indicative of upper tract bleeding may occur. A palpable flank mass is present in less than 15% of patients and usually indicates an extensive lesion.

Excretory urography reveals an abnormal filling defect suspicious for intrinsic lesion in 50% to 75% of patients with upper urinary tract cancers. A large variety of other lesions can produce similar filling defects including nonopaque calculi, blood clots, sloughed renal papillae, fungus balls, fibroepithelial polyps, hemangiomas, and extrinsic compression by renal vessels. Ultrasonography or CT scanning can be used to reliably distinguish a radiolucent stone from other causes of a filling defect. Indications for upper urinary tract endoscopy have been discussed previously. Percutaneous nephrostomy has also been advocated by some authors. However, as with other antegrade studies, the risk of tumor spillage contraindicates this approach except in highly selected patients.[110]

### Treatment of Upper Tract Cancers

To date, there have been no controlled randomized series that have evaluated the optimum therapy for upper tract urothelial cancer. In particular, the treatment of cancers that do not invade the muscle or renal parenchyma can be approached in several different fashions, including ureteroscopic or nephroscopic biopsy and fulgeration, segmental ureterectomy or pyelectomy, simple nephrectomy, and radical nephroureterectomy. Patients with low-grade, low-stage lesions may be appropriately treated by local therapies including endoscopic biopsy and fulgeration and/or segmental resection of the lesion. If local therapy is employed, care must be taken to analyze the surrounding tissues and to assess the entire upper urinary tract carefully using all available modalities. Carcinoma in situ of the upper tract may occur in conjunction with a papillary urothelial cancer. If carcinoma in situ of the upper urinary tract is found in a patient with a low-grade, low-stage lesion, nephroureterectomy is generally preferable in a patient with an otherwise normal contralateral kidney.

In patients with high-grade lesions of the

upper urinary tract, simple nephrectomy and subtotal ureterectomy results in a substantial local recurrence in the renal bed (30% to 40%) and distal ureteral stump (30% to 60%).[111,112] These patients are therefore probably best treated by nephroureterectomy with removal of the associated bladder cuff. The role of formal retroperitoneal lymphadenectomy in this setting is undetermined. It would appear to be unnecessary in patients with low-stage, low-grade disease, and may be only of prognostic value in high-grade, high-stage lesions. With improvement in adjunctive therapy, eg, MVAC chemotherapy, the presence or absence of regional lymphatic metastases may direct the use of these therapies.

The standard surgical approaches to nephroureterectomy are a retroperitoneal flank incision plus a second low midline or Gibson incision, a single extended flank incision, or a single transperitoneal abdominal incision. The kidney, ureter, and bladder cuff should be delivered as a single unit whenever possible. The entire ureter, including the intramural portion, should be removed to prevent recurrence.[113] The retention of a ureteral stump has been associated with an overall 20% likelihood of recurrence in the stump (30% to 60% for high-grade cancers).[93]

Intravesical therapeutic agents will be discussed in detail later. These agents may play a role in the treatment of upper urinary tract urothelial cancers. Both BCG and thiotepa may be given safely by a percutaneous route to patients with upper urinary tract cancers. In addition, reflux of an intravesical agent into the ureter may be possible in some patients where vesicoureteral reflux has occurred.

### Prognosis of Upper Tract Cancers

The 5-year survival rate for all patients with transitional cell upper tract tumors approaches 50% to 60%.[114] High-grade and high-stage tumors are associated with a poorer prognosis. In one series, grade I and II tumors had a 63% 5-year survival compared with a 13% survival for grade III and IV lesions.[115] Squamous cell cancers are associated with a dismal prognosis with few 5-year survivals.[116]

## MANAGEMENT OF SUPERFICIAL BLADDER CANCER (STAGES Tis, Ta, AND T1)

Approximately 70% to 80% of bladder cancer patients have low-grade superficial tumors at the time of their initial presentation. The great majority of these patients can be treated adequately by simple transurethral resection or biopsy and fulgeration. The overall 5-year survival rate of patients with superficial cancers treated with transurethral resection alone approaches 70%.[118,119] Nonetheless, because of the high likelihood of recurrence of superficial bladder cancers (approximately 50% to 75%), many trials have been undertaken to define the efficacy of intravesical therapy, not only to destroy existing bladder cancer (definitive) but also to reduce the recurrence rate (suppressive therapy). Intravesical therapy will be discussed in greater detail later in this chapter.

It is important to recognize that this group of superficial cancers is a very heterogeneous group in terms of the likelihood that the patient will progress to muscle invasion, and, in fact, succumb to the bladder cancer. For example, the patient with a grade I Ta lesion, although prone to recurrence, has only approximately a 2% chance of progressing to muscle invasion. Similarly, patients with a grade II Ta lesion have only approximately a 6% chance of proceeding to muscle invasion. It is therefore possible to withhold intravesical therapy in this group of patients unless they present initially with four or more tumors or develop multiple rapid recurrences of their cancer. On the other hand, the unusual patient with a high-grade low-stage cancer (grade III, stage Ta) is very prone to progress to muscle invasion and should be treated with intravesical therapy at the time of initial presentation. Similarly, patients with invasion of the lamina propria are generally treated with intravesical chemotherapy at initial presentation.

The frequency of upper tract surveillance after diagnosis of superficial bladder cancer remains debatable. A recent review revealed the development of upper tract disease in 4.8% of cases with a mean time to upper tract disease of 5.4 years.[119] Excretory urography is probably warranted every 1 to 2 years after initial treatment. Patients with reflux are at higher risk of upper tract recurrence and may be evaluated more frequently using voiding cystourethrography.[120]

External beam irradiation therapy has not been proven effective in controlling superficial bladder cancer and does not prevent the recurrence of new lesions.[121] It has been reported that interstitial radiation therapy preceded by low-dose preoperative external beam radiation therapy may be more effective than transurethral resection in controlling small superficial bladder cancers.[122,123]

Patients with carcinoma in situ present an interesting and difficult problem. Patients with focal, asymptomatic carcinoma in situ are probably at only modest risk of progression to muscle invasion. These patients may be treated by local therapies including transurethral resection, laser therapy, or phototherapy using hematoporphyrin derivatives. However, most studies favor the use of intravesical therapy in patients with focal carcinoma in situ especially if cytologies are not cleared after tumor resection.

Patients with diffuse or symptomatic carcinoma in situ should be treated with intravesical therapy at the time of initial presentation. Careful reassessment using endoscopically controlled biopsies and urinary cytologies is critical in this group of patients.

It would appear that BCG immunotherapy is superior to other intravesical therapies in the treatment of carcinoma in situ. Failures of intravesical therapy are common in this group and one must always remember the extremely high tendency for these patients to proceed to muscle invasion. There is also a high reported incidence of ureteral and prostatic urethral recurrence during intravesical therapy for carcinoma in situ, so that these areas of the urothelium must be carefully evaluated, including sequential prostatic urethral biopsies.

Recent studies have shown that the presence of a recurrent stage T1 TCC occurring at the 3-month cystoscopy after a single 6-week course of BCG therapy is an extremely poor prognostic sign that is associated with a high incidence of progression to muscle invasion and a high mortality rate.[124] In this situation, early cystectomy may be beneficial. Other authors favor the use of a second 6-week course of BCG therapy.[125]

Recently Malkowicz et al analyzed the result of cystectomy for patients with high-grade superficial bladder cancer.[126] They reviewed 160 patients who underwent cystectomy and were found to have pathologic stage $P_2$ or less, including 11 patients with positive nodes. The survival rates at 95% confidence limits were 100% for stage $P_{0/a}$, 80% for stage $P_1$, and 76% for stage $P_2$. This study suggested that cystectomy is highly effective in curing patients with high-grade superficial disease, including those with lymph node metastases.

Most studies suggest that preoperative radiation therapy does not enhance survival of patients with superficial bladder cancer who are treated with cystectomy.

## Intravesical Therapy

The use of intravesical therapy employing either chemotherapeutic agents or immunotherapeutic agents has arisen in response to the extremely common problem of recurrence in patients with superficial bladder cancer and the definite (10% to 15%) risk of progression to muscle invasion. Intravesical agents have been used as definitive therapy for the treatment of tumor left in the bladder after transurethral resection as well as in an attempt to decrease the rate of subsequent recurrence in patients who have had complete resection of all cystoscopically visible tumor. The results of definitive therapy have generally shown 30% to 60% complete response rates for the various agents tested (Table 6).

**Triethylene Thiophosphoramide (Thiotepa).** The modern era of intravesical therapy began with the use of thiotepa in the 1960s.[127]

**TABLE 6. Agents for Intravesical Chemotherapy-Definitive Treatment**

| Agent | CR (%) | PR (%) | CR + PR (%) |
|---|---|---|---|
| Thiotepa | 30–41 | 35–53 | 72–85 |
| Mitomycin C | 47–49 | 30–35 | 79–82 |
| Adriamycin | | | 45–71 |
| BCG | 17–83 | 10–27 | 58–83 |

CR = Complete response; PR = Partial response.

Thiotepa is an alkylating agent that derives its activity from its ability to cause cross-linking of nucleic acids and proteins. Thiotepa has been used in varying dose schedules. Typically, doses of 30 mg in 30 mL of saline or 60 mg and 60 mL of saline (1 mg/mL) are instilled in the bladder and allowed to be retained in the bladder for 2 hours. Therapies are usually given weekly for 6 to 8 weeks followed by monthly therapies for 1 to 2 years.

The National Bladder Cancer Collaborative Group A (NBCCGA) demonstrated that thiotepa given in doses of 30 or 60 mg following complete endoscopic resection of all visible bladder tumor reduced the recurrence rate to 47% in treated patients as compared to 73% in patients treated by transurethral resection alone (follow-up 2 years).[128] Most of this benefit occurred in patients with low-grade tumors. Patients with high-grade tumors did not appear to derive a significant benefit.[128] Thiotepa has been used in the treatment of carcinoma in situ with limited success.[129] A randomized clinical trial comparing BCG with thiotepa in the treatment of superficial bladder cancer suggested that thiotepa was less effective than BCG therapy.[130]

The toxicity of thiotepa is primarily related to myelosuppression, which occurs in 15% to 20% of patients. It is believed that this myelosuppression occurs because the low molecular weight of thiotepa (198 d) allows for ready systemic absorption through the urothelium. A major advantage for thiotepa is that it is relatively inexpensive as compared to other intravesical chemotherapies.

**Mitomycin C.** Mitomycin C is an antitumor antibiotic that is poorly absorbed (<1%) through the urothelium because of its high molecular weight (334 d).[131] Hence myelosuppression is rare. Like other antitumor antibiotics, it exerts its primary mechanism of action in the inhibition of DNA synthesis.

The optimum dosing schedule is 40 mg/week for 8 weeks, followed by maintenance therapy every month. Complete tumor responses have approximated 40%.[132,133] Mitomycin, unlike thiotepa, is effective in high-grade tumors.[132]

The principal side effects of mitomycin C are chemical cystitis (10% to 15%) and rash (5% to 15%).[134] It is an expensive agent when used in doses necessary for intravesical therapy.

Mitomycin C is effective in preventing recurrences in patients with completely resected cancers.[135,136]

Mitomycin C has also been shown to be effective in patients who have failed prior thiotepa therapy.[132,137,138] A recent trial comparing mitomycin C with BCG intravesical therapy by the Southwest Oncology Group revealed an advantage for BCG over mitomycin C in the prevention of bladder cancer recurrence (unpublished data).

**Doxorubicin (Adriamycin).** Adriamycin is a tumor antibiotic that is minimally absorbed through the urothelium because of its high molecular weight (580 d). Although various treatment schedules have been used, available data suggest that a 50-mg dosage should be used for intravesical therapy.

Toxicity associated with adriamycin includes a relatively marked chemical cystitis in many patients that may progress to permanent bladder contraction in some patients. In addition, adriamycin is considerably more expensive than thiotepa or BCG. No significant differences in response rates in patients with low-grade and/or high-grade lesions have been reported.[139] A recent randomized clinical trial comparing adriamycin with BCG therapy conducted by the Southwest Oncology Group suggests a clear superiority of BCG in preventing tumor recurrence in patients with completely resected transitional cell carcinomas. An increased interval to recurrence was also noted in this trial.[140]

**BCG (Bacille Calmette-Guérin).** Intravesical BCG therapy was introduced by Morales in 1976 using the Pasteur strain of BCG given both intravesically and intradermally. BCG is an attenuated tuberculin bacillus that is known to be effective in treating superficial cancers left in situ as well as in reducing the recurrence rate in patients whose tumor has been completely resected. Several different strains of BCG have been used including Pasteur, Tice, Dutch, Connaught, and Moreau. The viability and density of the tuberculin bacilli per mL of vaccine may vary with the strain used and may vary from lot to lot within the same strain.[141] Various routes of administration of BCG have been employed including intravesical, intradermal, and oral. All routes have been reported to be successful, but the optimum route is still debatable.

The mechanism of action of BCG is unknown. Clinical data support the development of an immune response to BCG. Several authors have reported increased urinary interleukin-2 levels after BCG therapy.[142,143] Intravesical BCG has also been shown to induce a chronic granulomatous response in the bladder in many patients.[144–147] Although there may be an increased trend for favorable response to BCG in patients who have either developed granulomas within the urinary tract or converted their purified protein derivative (PPD) test, this correlation is not reliably predictive for the individual patient.[148,149]

The principal toxicity of intravesical BCG therapy is vesical irritability. Patients commonly complain of dysuria, urinary frequency, hematuria, fever, malaise, nausea, chills, and arthralgia. Granulomatous prostatitis is a common occurrence following BCG therapy and approximately 6% of these patients have severe enough symptoms to require treatment with isoniazid (INH).[148] Recently, a small number of deaths have been reported in patients treated with BCG therapy due to apparent disseminated BCG infection.[150,151] A correlation between these deaths and the absorption of BCG organism at the time of a traumatic catheterization has been reported. If systemic BCG infection is suspected, rapid treatment with triple-drug therapy including isoniazid, rifampicin, and cycloserine should be instituted.[150,152]

Several prospective randomized trials have evaluated BCG for prophylaxis of recurrent tumors. Lamm et al reported that BCG reduced the tumor recurrence rate to 17% as compared to 42% in control patients treated with transurethral resection alone.[147] Other trials are summarized in Table 7. High-risk patients display a delay in disease progression, prolonged bladder preservation, and improved survival when treated with BCG.[157] Patients who have failed prior intravesical thiotepa have also been successfully treated with BCG.[130,146,158] Responses to BCG treatment appear to be durable rather than simply delaying eventual tumor recurrence.[159]

Intravesical BCG has been extensively evaluated for the therapy of carcinoma in situ. A complete response rate can be expected to occur in approximately 70% of treated patients.[160–163] Complete responses are usually associated with the resolution of irritative voiding symptoms.

The dilemma of how much BCG therapy to provide still remains. Some evidence points to the usefulness of a second induction course of BCG, particularly in patients who have responded to the initial treatment.[164]

## Interferon

Interferons are proteins that have been categorized as belonging to the group of biologic response–modifying agents. Interferons are capable of inducing a broad spectrum of immunologic modulations including the inhibition of tumor cell proliferation. In bladder cancer, the most commonly studied type of interferon is the alpha interferon. Alpha interferons have demonstrated activity in the treatment of superficial bladder cancer and carcinoma in situ.[165,166] In one study, the overall complete response rate was 44%. Although the appropriate dosing schedule remains un-

**TABLE 7. BCG Trials**

**Trials of BCG for Prophylaxis**

| Author | Rx | Number | Recurrence Rate (%) | Time to Recurrence |
|---|---|---|---|---|
| Melekos[153] | BCG | (67) | 33* | 13.4 ± 6 |
| | Control | (33) | 58 | 9.9 ± 5 |

**Prospective Trials of Prophylactic BCG vs Other Agents**

| Author | Rx | Reccurence Rate (%) | Recurrence/100 pt/mo |
|---|---|---|---|
| Martinez-Pineiro[154] | BCG | 13.4* | 0.53* |
| | Thiotepa | 35.7 | 1.55 |
| | Adriamycin | 44.2 | 1.7 |
| DeBruyne[155] | BCG | 0.33 | |
| | Mitomycin C | 0.29 | |
| Mori[156] | BCG | 19* | |
| | Adriamycin | 54 | |

* Statistically significant difference.

known, one randomized, controlled trial suggested that complete responses were more frequent in high-dose ($100 \times 10^6$ IU) as compared to low-dose ($10 \times 10^6$ IU) therapy (45% and 6%, respectively).[167]

### Hematoporphyrin Derivative Phototherapy

Hematoporphyrin derivative (HpD) is a mixture of porphyrins that appear to be preferentially concentrated in neoplastic or dysplastic tissues. When tissues containing this derivative are irradiated with a light of appropriate wavelength, death of sensitized cells occurs. Recent clinical trials of HpD therapy with subsequent illumination of the bladder with a krypton ion laser have revealed limited success in patients with small superficial tumors or carcinoma in situ. HpD is associated with generalized cutaneous photosensitivity, which is its primary toxicity and limits its clinical usefulness. Bladder contraction occurs in approximately 15% of patients.[168]

### Laser Therapy

Laser beam energy can be selectively absorbed by vascular tissues including TCCs. The Nd:YAG (neodymium:yttrium-aluminum-garnet) laser may be used in the bladder for the treatment of superficial bladder cancer. This laser has a significant depth of penetration (4 to 15 mm) and is not absorbed by water. The major theoretical advantages of laser therapy are that it may be performed through a small scope using local anesthesia, and it is associated with minimal bleeding or obturator nerve stimulation.[169,170] The major disadvantage of laser therapy is that tissue is not obtained for histologic evaluation.

## SUMMARY

The past decade has seen an explosion of knowledge regarding the diagnosis, staging, and management of superficial urothelial cancers of the upper urinary tract and bladder. Perhaps the greatest message that has been learned is the fact that these superficial tumors have a heterogeneous behavior depending on their individual stage, grade, and other markers of tumor aggressiveness. Careful understanding of these prognostic factors is therefore extremely important in determining the management plan for these patients. Generally, low-grade, low-stage tumors respond well to resection and fulguration. Although likely to recur, these lesions are unlikely to progress to muscle invasion and therefore do not often require the use of ancillary therapy including intravesical therapy. On the other hand, high-grade and/or high-stage superficial lesions are extremely aggressive and can be expected to progress to muscle invasion and cause patient death in a significant number of cases. Aggressive therapy is therefore warranted. Intravesical therapy at the time of presentation, careful monitoring, and early bladder removal when failure is documented are warranted.

## REFERENCES

1. Boring CC, Squires TS, Tong T. Cancer statistics, 1992. *CA*. 1992;42:19.
2. Blot WJ, Fraumeni JF Jr. Geographic patterns of bladder cancer in the United States. *J Natl Cancer Inst*. 1978;61:1017.
3. Hoover R, Fraumeni JF Jr. Cancer mortality in U.S. counties with chemical industries. *Environ Res*. 1975;9:196.
4. Rehn L. Uëber blasentumoren bei fuchsinarbëitern. *Arch Kind Chir*. 1895;50:588.
5. Case RAM, Hosker ME, McDonald DB, et al. Tumors of the urinary bladder in workmen engaged in the manufacture and use of certain dyestuff intermediates in the British chemical industry. *Br J Ind Med*. 1954;11:75–104.
6. Morrison AS, Cole P. Epidemiology of bladder cancer. *Urol Clin North Am*. 1976;3:13.
7. Cole P, Hoover R, Friedell GH. Occupation and cancer of the lower urinary tract. *Cancer*. 1972;29:1250.
8. Cole P. A population-based study of bladder cancer. In: Doll R, Vodopija I, eds. *Host–Environment Interactions in the Etiology of Cancer in Man*. Lyon: IARC; 1973:83.
9. Case RAM, Hosker ME, McDonald DB, et al. Tumors of the urinary bladder in workmen engaged in the manufacture and use of certain dyestuff intermediates in the British chemical industry. Part I. The role of aniline, benzidine, alpha-naphthylamine and beta-naphthylamine. *Br J Ind Med*. 1954;11:75.
10. Morrison AS. Advances in the etiology of urothelial cancer. *Urol Clin North Am*. 1984; 11:557–566.
11. Oyasu Y, Hopp ML. The etiology of cancer of the bladder. *Surg Gynecol Obstet*. 1974; 138:97.
12. Wolf H. Studies on the role of tryptophan metabolites in the genesis of bladder cancer. *Acta Chir Scand*. (Suppl). 1973;433:154.
13. Renwick AG, Thakara A, Lawrie CA, et al. Microbial amino acid metabolites and bladder cancer: no evidence of promoting activity in man. *Hum Toxicol*. 1988;7:267–272.
14. Lilienfeld AM, Levin JL, Moore GE. The association of smoking with cancer of the urinary bladder in humans. *Arch Intern Med*. 1956;98:129.
15. Cole P. Coffee drinking and cancer of the lower urinary tract. *Lancet*. 1971;1:1335–1337.
16. Wynder EL, Goldsmith R. The epidemiology of bladder cancer—a second look. *Cancer*. 1977;40:1246.
17. Augustine A, Herbert JR, Kabat GC, et al. Bladder cancer in relation to cigarette smoking. *Cancer Res*. 1988;48:4405–4408.
18. Hoffman D, Masuda Y, Wynder EL. α-naphthylamine and β-naphthylamine in cigarette smoke. *Nature*. 1969;221:254.
19. Kerr WK, Barkin J, Levers PE, et al. The effect of cigarette smoking on bladder carcinogens in man. *Can Med Assoc J*. 1865;93:1.
20. Hultergren H, Lagengren C, Ljungqvist A. Carcinoma of the renal pelvis in papillary necrosis. *Acta Clin Scand*. 1965;130:314.
21. McCredia M, Stewart JH, Ford JM, et al. Phenacetin-containing analgesics and cancer of the bladder or renal pelvis in women. *Br J Urol*. 1983;55:220.
22. Fokkens W. Phenacetin abuse related to bladder cancer. *Environ Res*. 1979;20:192–193.
23. Tosi SE, Movin LJ. Bladder tumor associated with phenacetin abuse. *Urology*. 1977;9:59.
24. Buck H, Hauser PK, Rudiger W. Uber die Ausseheidung eines noch nicht beschriebenen penacetin metaboliten bein menschen und beiden ratte. *Arch Pathol Pharmacol*. 1966;253:25.
25. Rathert P, Melchor H, Lutzeyer W. Phenacetin: a carcinogen for the urinary tract? *J Urol*. 1975;113:653.
26. Kunter AF, Hartge P, Hoover RN, et al. Urinary tract infection and risk of bladder cancer. *Am J Epidemiol*. 1984;119:510–515.
27. El-Masri WS, Fellows G. Bladder cancer after spinal cord injury. *Paraplegia*. 1981;19:265.
28. Melzak J. The incidence of bladder cancer in paraplegia. *Paraplegia*. 1966;4:85.
29. Lucas SB. Squamous cell carcinoma of the bladder and schistosomiasis. *East Afr Med J*. 1982;59:345–352.
30. Garvin DD, Weber CH Jr, Polsky MS. Carcinoma in the defunctionalized bladder: report of a case and review of the literature. *J Urol*. 1977;117:669.
31. Fairchild WV, Spence CR, Solomon HD, et al. The incidence of bladder cancer after cyclophosphamide therapy. *J Urol*. 1979; 122:163.
32. Pearson RM, Soloway MS. Does cyclophosphamide induce bladder cancer? *Urology*. 1978;11:437.
33. Elias AD, Eder JP, Sheat T, Begg CG, Frei E, Antman KH. High dose ofosfamide

with mesno-uroprotection. *J Clin Oncol.* 1990;8:170–178.

34. Cutler SH, Young JL Jr, eds. Third National Cancer Survey: incidence data. *Natl Cancer Inst Monogr.* 1975;41:1–454.
35. Benson RC Jr, Tomera KM, Kelalis PP. Transitional cell carcinoma of the bladder in children and adolescents. *J Urol.* 1983;130:54–55.
36. Risch HA, Burch JD, Miller AB, et al. Dietary factors and the incidence of cancer in the urinary bladder. *Am J Epidemiol.* 1988;127:1179–1191.
37. Duncan RE, Bennett DW, Evans AT, et al. Radiation-induced bladder tumors. *J Urol.* 1977;118:43–45.
38. Fraumeni JF Jr, Thomas LB. Malignant bladder tumors in a man and his three sons. *JAMA.* 1967;201:507–509.
39. McCullough DL, Lamm DL, McLaughlin AP III, et al. Familial transitional cell carcinoma of the bladder. *J Urol.* 1975;113:629–635.
40. Kadlubar FF, Talaska G, Lang NP, et al. Assessment of exposure and susceptibility to aromatic amine carcinogens. *IARC Sci Publ.* 1988;166–174.
41. Ro JY, Ayala AG, El-Naggar A. Muscularis mucosa of urinary bladder: importance for staging and treatment. *Am J Surg Pathol.* 1987;11:668–673.
42. DeMeester LJ, Farrow GM, Utz DC. Inverted papillomas of the urinary bladder. *Cancer.* 1975;36:505–513.
43. Kunze E, Schauer A, Schmitt M. Histology and histogenesis of two different types of inverted urothelial papillomas. *Cancer.* 1983;51:348–358.
44. Lazarevic B, Garret R. Inverted papilloma and papillary transitional cell carcinoma of urinary bladder. *Cancer.* 1978;42:1904–1911.
45. Patch FS, Rhea LJ. The genesis and development of Brunn's nests and their relationship to cystitis cystica glandularis and primary adenocarcinoma of the bladder. *Can Med Assoc J.* 1935;33:597–606.
46. Mostofi FK. Potentialities of bladder epithelium. *J Urol.* 1854;71:705–714.
47. Edwards PD, Hurm RA, Jaeschke WH. Conversion of cystitis glandularis to adenocarcinoma. *J Urol.* 1972;108:568–750.
48. Schultz RE, Bloch MJ, Tomaszewski JE, et al. Mesonephric adenocarcinoma of the bladder. *J Urol.* 1984;132:263–265.
49. Tyler DE. Stratified squamous epithelium in the vesical trigone and urethra: findings correlated with menstrual cycle and age. *Am J Anat.* 1962;111:319–335.
50. Wiener DP, Koss LG, Sabley B, et al. The prevalence and significance of Brunn's nests, cystitis cystica and squamous metaplasia in normal bladders. *J Urol.* 1979;122:317–321.
51. Murphy WM, Soloway MS. Urothelial dysplasia. *J Urol.* 1982;127:849–854.
52. Althausen AF, Prout GR Jr, Daly JJ. Noninvasive papillary carcinoma of the bladder associated with carcinoma in situ. *J Urol.* 1976;116:575–580.
53. Weinstein RS, Miller AW III, Pauli BV. Carcinoma in situ: comment of the pathobiology of a paradox. *Urol Clin North Am.* 1980;7:523–531.
54. Weinstein RS, Alroy J, Farrow GM, et al. Blood group isoantigen deletion in carcinoma in situ of the urinary bladder. *Cancer.* 1979;43:661–668.
55. Riddle PR, Chisholm GD, Trott PA, et al. Flat carcinoma in situ of bladder. *Br J Urol.* 1976;47:829–833.
56. Utz DC, Hanash KA, Farrow GM. The plight of the patient with carcinoma in situ of the bladder. *J Urol.* 1970;103:160–164.
57. Farrow GM, Utz DC, Rife CC. Morphological and clinical observations of patients with early bladder cancer treated with total cystectomy. *Cancer Res.* 1976;36:2495–2501.
58. Koss LG. *Tumors of the Urinary Bladder, Fascicle 11—Atlas of Tumor Pathology.* Washington, DC: Armed Forces Institute of Pathology; 1975:1–120.
59. Broders AC. Epithelioma of the genito-urinary organs. *Ann Surg.* 1922;75:574–604.
60. Jewett HJ, Strong GH. Infiltrating carcinoma of the bladder: Radiation of depth of penetration of the bladder wall to incidence of local extension and metastases. *J Urol.* 1946;55:336–372.
61. Kantor AF, Hartge P, Hoover RN, et al. Epidemiological characteristics of squamous cell carcinoma and adenocarcinoma of the bladder. *Cancer Res.* 1988;48:3853–3855.
62. Richie JP, Waisman J, Skinner DG, et al. Squamous cell carcinoma of the bladder: treatment by radical cystectomy. *J Urol.* 1976;115:670–672.
63. Johnson DE, Shoenwald MB, Ayala AG, et al. Squamous cell carcinoma of the bladder. *J Urol.* 1976;115:542–544.
64. El-Bolkainy MN, Mokhtar NM, Ghoneim MA, et al. The impact of schistosomiasis on the pathology of bladder carcinoma. *Cancer.* 1981;48:2643–2648.
65. Bennett JK, Wheatley JK, Walton KN. 10-Year experience with adenocarcinoma of the bladder. *J Urol.* 1984;131:262–263.
66. Anderstrom C, Johansson SL, von Schultz L. Primary adenocarcinoma of the urinary bladder: a clinicopathologic and prognostic study. *Cancer.* 1983;52:1273–1280.
67. Mostofi FK, Thomson RV, Dean AL Jr. Mucous adenocarcinoma of the urinary bladder. *Cancer.* 1955;8:741–758.
68. Magri J. Partial cystectomy: review of 104 cases. *Br J Urol.* 1962;34:74–86.

69. Sheldon CA, Clayman RV, Gonzalez R, et al. Malignant urachal lesions. *J Urol.* 1984;131:1–8.

70. Heney NM, Ahmed S, Flanagan M, et al. Superficial bladder cancer: progression and recurrence. *J Urol.* 1983;130:1083–1086.

71. Green LF, Hanash KA, Farrow GM. Benign papilloma or papillary carcinoma of the bladder? *J Urol.* 1973;110:205–207.

72. Page BH, Levison VB, Curwen MP. The side of recurrence of non-infiltrating bladder tumors. *Br J Urol.* 1978;50:237–242.

73. Cutler SJ, Heney NM, Friedell GH. Longitudinal study of patients with bladder cancer: factors associated with disease recurrence and progression. In: Bonney W, Prout G, eds. AUA Monographs, vol I: *Bladder Cancer.* Baltimore: Williams & Wilkins; 1982:35.

74. Anderson CK. Current topics on the pathology of bladder cancer. *Proc Roy Soc Med.* 1973;66:283.

75. Heney NM, Daly J, Prout GR, et al. Biopsy of apparently normal urothelium in patients with bladder cancer. *J Urol.* 1978;120:559.

76. Soloway MS. Diagnosis and management of superficial bladder cancer. *Semin Surg Oncol.* 1989;5(4):247–254.

77. Lutzeyer W, Rubben H, Dahm H. Prognostic parameters in superficial bladder cancer: an analysis of 315 cases. *J Urol.* 1982;127:250–252.

78. Anterstrom C, Johansson S, Nilsson S. The significance of lamina propria invasion on the prognosis of patients with bladder tumors. *J Urol.* 1980;124:23–26.

79. Jewett HJ, King LR, Shelley WM. A study of 365 cases of infiltrating bladder cancer: relation of certain pathological characteristics to prognosis after extirpation. *J Urol.* 1964;92:668.

80. Kleinerman J, Liotta L. Release of tumor cells. In: Day S, ed. Progress in Cancer Research and Therapy. vol 5. New York: Raven Press; 1977:135.

81. Limas C, Lange PH, Fraley EE, et al. A, B, H antigens in transitional cell tumors of the urinary bladder: correlation with the clinical course. *Cancer.* 1979;14:2099.

82. Catalona WJ. Practical utility of specific red cell adherence test in bladder cancer. *Urology.* 1981;18:113.

83. Flanigan RC, King CT, Clark TD, Cash JB, Greenfield BJ, Sniecinski IJ, Primus FJ. Immunohistochemical demonstration of blood group antigens in neoplastic and normal human urothelium. *J Urol.* 1983;130:499–503.

84. Coon J, Weinstein RS, Summers J. Blood group precursor T antigen expression in human urinary bladder carcinoma. *Am J Clin Pathol.* 1982;77:692.

85. Weinstein RS, Coon JS, Pauli BU. Characterization of urinary bladder cancer cells. In: Smith PH, Prout GR, eds. *Bladder Cancer.* London: Butterworth; 1984:12.

86. Summers JL, Coon JS, Ward RM, et al. Prognosis in carcinoma of the urinary bladder based on tissue ABH and T antigen status and karyotype of the initial tumor. *Cancer Res.* 1983;43:934.

87. Falor WH, Ward RM. DNA banding patterns in carcinoma of the bladder. *JAMA.* 1973; 226:1322.

88. Summers JL, Falor WH, Ward R. A 10-year analysis of chromosomes in non-invasive papillary carcinoma of the bladder. *J Urol.* 1981;125:177.

89. Huland E, Huland H, Schneider AW. Quantitative immunocytology in the management of patients with superficial bladder carcinoma. I. A marker to identify patients who do not require prophylaxis. *J Urol.* 1990;144:637–639.

90. Flam TA, Chopin DK, Leleu C. Immunohistochemical markers defined by monoclonal antibodies and response to bacillus Calmette–Guérin endovesical immunotherapy for superficial bladder tumors. *Eur Urol.* 1990;17:338–342.

91. Varkarakis MJ, Gaeta J, Moore RH, et al. Superficial bladder tumor: aspects of clinical progression. *Urology.* 1974;4:414.

92. Marshall VF. Symposium on bladder tumors: current clinical problems regarding bladder tumors. *Cancer.* 1956;9:543.

93. Strong DW, Pearse HD. Recurrent urothelial tumors following surgery for transitional cell carcinoma of the upper urinary tract. *Cancer.* 1976;38:2178.

94. Vicente-Rodriguez J, Chechile G, Algaba F, et al. Value of random endoscopic biopsy in the diagnosis of bladder carcinoma in situ. *Eur Urol.* 1987;13:150–152.

95. Harving N, Wolf H, Melsen F. Positive urinary cytology after tumor resection: an indicator for concomitant carcinoma in situ. *J Urol.* 1988;140:495–497.

96. Fukui T, Yokokawa M, Mitani G, et al. In vivo staining test with methylene blue for bladder cancer. *J Urol.* 1983;130:252–255.

97. Benson RC, Farrow GM, Kinsey JH, et al. Detection and localization of in situ carcinoma of the bladder with hematoporphyrin derivative. *Mayo Clin Proc.* 1982;57:548–555.

98. Eposti PL, Zajicek J. Grading of transitional cell neoplasms of the urinary bladder from smears of bladder washings: a critical review of 326 tumors. *Acta Cytol.* 1972;16:529.

99. Gamarra MC, Zein T. Cytologic spectrum of bladder cancer. *Urology.* 1984;23:23–26.

100. Flanigan RC, Nuzzarello J, Shankey VT. Current perspectives in the clinical relevance of flow cytometry in bladder cancer. In: Rous SN, ed. *Urology Annual.* vol 4. New York: Appleton & Lange; 1990:87–99.

101. Friedell GH, Hawkins IR, Ahmed SW, Schmidt JD. The role of urinary tract cytology in the detection and clinical management of bladder cancer. In: Bonney WW, Prout GR, eds. *Bladder Cancer*. AUA Monographs. Baltimore: Williams & Wilkins; 1982:49.

102. Trott PA, Edwards L. Comparison of bladder washings and urine cytology in the diagnosis of bladder cancer. *J Urol*. 1973;110:664–666.

103. Badalament RA, Fair WR, Whitmore WF Jr, et al. The relative value of cytometry and cytology in the management of bladder cancer: the Memorial Sloan-Kettering Cancer Center experience. *Semin Urol*. 1988;6:22–30.

104. Koss JC, Arger PH, Coleman BG, et al. CT staging of bladder carcinoma. *Am J Roentgen*. 1981;137:359–362.

105. Lantz EJ, Hattery RR. Diagnostic imaging of urothelial cancer. *Urol Clin North Am*. 1984;11:576–583.

106. Hermanek P, Sobin LH, eds. UICC—International Union Against Cancer TNM Classification of Malignant Tumors. ed. 4. Heidelberg: Springer-Verlag; 1987:133–135.

107. Marshall VF. The relation of the preoperative estimate to the pathologic demonstration of the extent of vesical neoplasms. *J Urol*. 1952;68:714–723.

108. Broders AC. Epithelioma of the genito-urinary organs. *Ann Surg*. 1922;75:574.

109. Bennington JL, Beckwith JB. Tumors of the kidney, renal pelvis, and ureter. In: *Atlas of Tumor Pathology,* Fascicle 12. Washington, DC: Armed Forces Institute of Pathology; 1975.

110. Smith AY, Vitale PJ, Lowe BA. Treatment of superficial papillary transitional cell carcinoma of the ureter by vesicoureteral reflux of mitomycin C. *J Urol*. 1987;138:1231–1233.

111. Johansson S, Wahlqvist L. A prognostic study of urothelial renal pelvic tumors. *Cancer*. 1979;43:2525.

112. Cummings KB. Carcinoma of the bladder: predictors. *Cancer*. 1980;45:1849–1855.

113. Strong DW, Pearse HD, Tank ES Jr, et al. The ureteral stump after nephroureterectomy. *J Urol*. 1976;115:654.

114. Axtell LM, Lourie WI Jr. Cancers of the urinary organs. In: National Cancer Institute: Cancer Patient Survival: Report No. 5 (DHEW Publication No. NIH 77–992). Bethesda: U.S. Department of Health, Education and Welfare, National Cancer Institute, 1976;206–220.

115. McDonald JR, Priestley JT. Carcinoma of the renal pelvis: histopathologic study of seventy-five cases with special reference to prognosis. *J Urol*. 1944;51:245.

116. Wagle DG, Moore RH, Murphy GP. Squamous cell carcinoma of the renal pelvis. *J Urol*. 1974;111:453.

117. Nichols JA, Marshall VF. The treatment of bladder carcinoma by local excision and fulguration. *Cancer*. 1956;9:559–565.

118. Barnes RW, Bergman RT, Hadley HT, et al. Control of bladder tumors by endoscopic surgery. *J Urol*. 1967;97:864–868.

119. Smith H, Weaver D, Barjenbruch O. Routine excretory urography in follow-up of superficial transitional cell carcinoma of bladder. *Urology*. 1989;34:193–196.

120. DeTorres Mateos IA, Banus Gasso JM, Redorta JP, Robles JM. Vesicorenal reflex and upper tract transitional cell carcinoma after transurethral resection of recurrent superficial bladder carcinoma. *J Urol*. 1987;138:49.

121. Goffinet DR, Schneider JJ, Glatstein EJ, et al. Bladder cancer: results of radiation therapy in 384 patients. *Radiology*. 1975;117:149–152.

122. Van der Werf-Messing BHP. Carcinoma of the urinary bladder treated by interstitial radiotherapy. *Urol Clin North Am*. 1985;11:659–670.

123. Russell KJ, Koh WJ, Russell AH. Combined intracavitary and external beam irradiation for superficial transitional cell carcinoma of the bladder: an alternative to cystectomy for patients with recurrence after intravesical chemotherapy. *J Urol*. 1989;141:30–32.

124. Herr H. Progression of stage T1 bladder tumors after intravesical bacillus Calmette-Guérin. *J Urol*. 1991;145:40–44.

125. Catalona WJ, Hudson MA, Gillen DP, Andriole GL, Ratliff TL. Risks and benefits of repeated courses of intravesical bacillus Calmette-Guérin therapy for superficial bladder cancer. *J Urol*. 1987;137:220–224.

126. Malkowicz SB, Nichols P, Lieskovsky GN, et al. The role of radical cystectomy in the management of high grade superficial bladder cancer (PA, P1, PIS and P2). *J Urol*. 1990;144:641–645.

127. Jones HC, Swinney J. Thiotepa in the treatment of tumors of the bladder. *Lancet*. 1961;2:615–618.

128. Prout GR Jr, Koontz WW Jr, Coombs J, et al. Long-term fate of 90 patients with superficial bladder cancer randomly assigned to receive or not to receive thiotepa. *J Urol*. 1983;130:677–680.

129. Koontz WW, Prout GR Jr, Smith W, et al. The use of intravesical thiotepa in the management of non-invasive carcinoma of the bladder. *J Urol*. 1981;125:307–312.

130. Brosman SA. Experience with bacillus Calmette-Guérin in patients with superficial bladder carcinoma. *J Urol*. 1982;128:27–30.

131. van Helsdingen PJ, Rikken CH, Sleeboom HP, et al. Mitomycin C resorption following repeated intravesical instillations using different instillation trones. *Urol Int*. 1988;43:42–46.

132. Soloway MS. Learning to integrate systemic chemotherapy into a treatment plan for patients with advanced bladder cancer. *J Urol.* 1985;133:440–441.

133. Lamm DL. Intravesical therapy of superficial bladder cancer. In: AUA Update, series 2. Houston: American Urologic Association, 1983;2–7.

134. Flanigan RC, King CT, Clark TD, et al. Immunohistochemical demonstration of blood group antigens in neoplastic and normal human urothelium: a comparison with standard red cell adherence. *J Urol.* 1983;130:499.

135. Flanigan RC, Ellison MF, Butler KM, Gonnella LG, McRoberts JW. A trial of prophylactic thiotepa or mitomycin C intravesical therapy in patients with recurrent or multiple superficial bladder cancers. *J Urol.* 1986;136:35–37.

136. Huland H, Otto U, Droese J, et al. Long-term mitomycin C instillation after transurethral resection of superficial bladder carcinoma: influence on recurrence, progression, and survival. *J Urol.* 1984;132:27–29.

137. Issell BF, Prout GR Jr, Soloway MS, et al. Mitomycin C intravesical therapy in noninvasive bladder cancer after failure on thiotepa. *Cancer.* 1984;53:1025–1028.

138. Prout GR Jr, Griffin PP, Nocks BN, et al. Intravesical therapy of low stage bladder carcinoma with mitomycin C: comparison of results in untreated and previously treated patients. *J Urol.* 1982;127:1096–1098.

139. Lundbeck F, Mogensen P, Jeppersen N. Intravesical therapy of noninvasive bladder tumors with doxorubin and urokinase. *J Urol.* 1983;130:1087–1089.

140. Mori K, Lamm DL. A trial of BCG versus adriamycin in superficial bladder cancer: a Southwest Oncology Group study. *Urolosica Internationalis.* 1986;4:254–259.

141. Kelley DR, Ratliff TR, Catalona WJ, et al. Intravesical BCG therapy for superficial bladder cancer; effect of BCG viability on treatment results. *J Urol.* 1985;134:48.

142. DeJong WH, DeBoer EC, Van der Meijden AP. Presence of interleukin-2 in urine of superficial bladder cancer patients after intravesical treatment with bacillus Calmette-Guérin. *Cancer Immunol.* 1990;31:182–186.

143. Haaff EO, Catalona WJ, Ratliff TL. Detection of interleukin-2 in the urine of patients with superficial bladder tumors after treatment with intravesical BCG. *J Urol.* 1986;136:970–974.

144. Morales A. Long term results and complications of intravesical BCG therapy for cancer. *Proc Am Urol Assoc.* 1983:177.

145. Brosman SA. BCG in the management of superficial bladder cancer. *Urology.* 1984; 23(Suppl):82–87.

146. Shellhammer PF, Ladaga LE, Fillion MB. Bacillus Calmette-Guérin (BCG) for superficial transitional cell carcinoma (TCC) of the bladder. *J Urol.* 1986;135:261–264.

147. Lamm DL, Thor DE, Stogdill VD, et al. Bladder cancer immunotherapy of superficial bladder cancer. *J Urol.* 1980;124:38–42.

148. Lamm DL, Stogdill VD, Stogdill BJ. Complications of BCG immunotherapy in patients with bladder cancer. *Proc Am Urol Assoc.* 1984:140A.

149. Dresner SM, Haaff EO, Ratliff TL, et al. Bacillus Calmette-Guérin intravesical therapy for superficial bladder cancer. *Urology Grand Rounds.* 1984:1–7.

150. Sakamoto GD, Burden J, Fisher D. Systemic bacillus Calmette-Guérin infection after transurethral administration for superficial bladder cancer. *J Urol.* 1989;142:1073–1075.

151. Steg A, Leleu C, Debrue B. Systemic bacillus Calmette-Guérin infection in patients treated by intravesical BCG therapy for superficial bladder cancer. *Prog Clin Biol Res.* 1989;310:325–334.

152. Lamm DL. Editorial comment. *J Urol.* 1989;142:1074–1075.

153. Melekos MD. Intravesical bacillus Calmette-Guérin prophylactic treatment for superficial bladder tumors: results of a controlled prospective study. *Urol Int.* 1990;45:137–141.

154. Martinez-Pineiro JA, Jimenez Leon J, Martinez-Pineiro L Jr, Fitter L, et al. Bacillus Calmette-Guérin versus doxorubicin versus thiotepa: a randomized prospective study in 202 patients with superficial bladder cancer. *J Urol.* 1990;143:502–506.

155. DeBruyne FMJ, van der Meijden APM, Geboers AH, Franssen MPH, et al. *J Urol.* 1988;XX I. No. 3(Suppl):20–25.

156. Mori K, Lamm DL, Crawford ED. A trial of bacillus Calmette-Guérin versus adriamycin in superficial bladder cancer: a southwest oncology group study. *Urol Int.* 1986;41:254–259.

157. Herr HW, Laudone VP, Badalament RA, et al. Bacillus Calmette-Guérin therapy alters the progression of superficial bladder cancer. *J Clin Oncol.* 1988;6:1450–1455.

158. Netto NR Jr, Lemos GC. A comparison of treatment methods for the prophylaxis of recurrent superficial bladder tumors. *J Urol.* 1983; 129:33–34.

159. Sarosdy MF, Lamm DL. Long-term results of intravesical bacillus Calmette-Guérin therapy for superficial bladder cancer. *J Urol.* 1989; 142:719–722.

160. Morales A, Ersil A. Prophylaxis of recurrent bladder cancer with bacillus Calmette-Guérin. In: Johnson DE, Samuels ML, eds. *Cancer of the Genitourinary Tract.* New York: Raven Press; 1979:121–132.

161. Lamm DL, Thor DE, Stogdill VD, et al. Bladder cancer immunotherapy. *J Urol.* 1982; 128:931–935.

162. Herr HW, Pinsky CM, Whitmore WF Jr, et al. Effect of intravesical bacillus Calmette-Guérin (BCG) on carcinoma in situ of the bladder. *Cancer.* 1983;51:1323–1326.

163. DeKernion JB, Huang M, Lindner A, et al. Management of superficial bladder tumors and carcinoma in situ with intravesical bacille Calmette-Guérin (BCG). *J Urol.* 1985;133:598–601.

164. Bretton PR, Herr HW, Kimmel M. The response of patients with superficial bladder cancer to a second course of intravesical bacillus Calmette-Guérin. *J Urol.* 1990;143:710–713.

165. Williams RD, Pitts WC, Kempson RL. Alpha-interferon in superficial bladder cancer: a Northern California Oncology Group Study. *J Clin Oncol.* 1988;6:476–483.

166. Shortliffe L, Freiha F, Higgins M, et al. Intravesical alpha 2 interferon therapy for superficial bladder cancer (abstract 203). Presented at meeting of the European Association of Urologists; 1984; Copenhagen.

167. Chodak GW. Intravesical interferon treatment of superficial bladder cancer. *Urol Suppl.* 1989;34:84–86.

168. Nseyo UO, Dougherty TJ, Sullivan L. Photodynamic therapy in the management of resistant lower urinary tract carcinoma. *Cancer.* 1987;60:3113–3119.

169. McPhee MS, Arnfield MR, Tulip J, et al. Neodymium:YAG laser therapy for infiltrating bladder cancer. *J Urol.* 1988;140:44–46.

170. Hofstetter A, Frank F, Keditsch E, et al. Endoscopic neodymium-YAG laser application for destroying bladder tumors. *Eur Urol.* 1981;7:278–282.

# 30

# Invasive Bladder Cancer

*Kevin R. Loughlin and Jerome P. Richie*

## INTRODUCTION

Bladder cancer represents one of the greatest challenges to the practicing urologist. In 1993 there were 52,300 new cases of bladder cancer diagnosed in the U.S. Bladder cancer is almost three times more common in men (39,000) than in women (13,300).[1] The incidence of bladder cancer is higher in white Americans (17.5 per 100,000) than in black Americans (9.9 per 100,000).[2] Bladder cancer is generally a disease of older individuals, with the median age of diagnosis being between 67 to 70 years of age.[3]

## ETIOLOGY

The etiology of bladder cancer is most likely multifactorial. In 1895, Rehn first proposed a relationship between aniline dyes and bladder cancer.[4] Modern reports have identified 2-naphthylamine, 4-aminobiphenyl naphthol, and 2 amino-1-naphthol as urothelial carcinogens.[5] In addition, dietary nitrites and nitrates have been implicated as additional bladder carcinogens.[6]

Cigarette smoking has been reported as increasing the risk of bladder cancer fourfold.[7] Analgesic abuse with phenacetin has been reported to increase the risk of transitional cell cancer of the renal pelvis and bladder.[8] Artificial sweeteners such as saccharin and cyclamate have been shown to be bladder carcinogens in rodents.[9] However, epidemiologic studies in humans remain unconvincing for a link between increased risk of bladder cancer and use of artificial sweeteners.

Patients who have been treated with cyclophosphamide have an increased risk of subsequent bladder cancer.[10] The cumulative risk of bladder cancer after cyclophosphamide exposure has been reported to be 3.5% at 8 years and 10.7% at 12 years.[11] Patients with bladder cancer have also been reported as having increased urinary tryptophan metabolite levels.[12,13] Other studies have correlated high tryptophan metabolite levels with increased recurrence rates.[14] Pyridoxine administration, which normalized urinary tryptophan metabolite levels, was shown in some reports to reduce tumor recurrence.[15]

## CLINICAL PRESENTATION

Hematuria is the hallmark presenting symptom of bladder cancer. Hematuria is the presenting complaint in 75%–85% of patients with bladder cancer.[16,17] The amount or frequency of hematuria does not correlate with the potential extent or stage of bladder carcinoma. All patients over the age of 40 who present with hematuria deserve a complete evaluation, which will usually include a urine culture, urine cytology, intravenous pyelogram (IVP), and cystoscopy. The need for evaluation of patients less than 40 years of age remains controversial, particularly in young females, but the safest course is to completely evaluate all patients with hematuria.

## DIAGNOSTIC PROCEDURES

### Intravenous Pyelogram

The IVP is an integral part of the evaluation of hematuria and bladder cancer. It screens the upper tracts for urothelial carcinoma of the renal pelvis or ureters. In addition, it can detect ureteral obstruction, which may be a sign of extravesical disease. The IVP also gives an indication of the relative function of each kidney. Finally, if attention is paid to the cystogram phase of the IVP, some bladder tumors can be identified radiographically.[18]

### Urine Cytology

Urine cytology is a useful adjunct in the diagnosis of bladder cancer. However, a false-negative rate of 20% in urine cytology has been reported.[3,16] False-positive cytology results may occur in 1%–12% of specimens and are usually due to inflammation or postchemotherapy or radiation changes.[19]

### Cystoscopy

The cystoscopic examination is the most important diagnostic procedure. An experienced endoscopist will evaluate the size, number, and location of the bladder lesions. He will also note their pattern of growth, specifically whether the tumor(s) appear papillary or sessile. In addition, areas of erythema should be biopsied to rule out the possibility of carcinoma in situ. If bladder diverticuli are present, they should be inspected carefully for tumors. Cold cup biopsies should be performed on all suspicious lesions and these biopsies should be submitted separately to the pathologist for careful histologic review. Four to six random biopsies should be taken of apparent uninvolved mucosa to rule out atypia or carcinoma in situ. Large papillary or sessile tumors should be removed using the resectoscope. Because of the cautery effect, these specimens are the least useful to the pathologist for determining histologic grade or level of invasion. After completion of the use of cautery to remove the bulk of the tumor(s), the cold cup biopsy forceps should again be used to biopsy the base of the tumor to check for the depth of invasion.

## STAGING

Accurate staging is paramount to the optimal treatment of bladder cancer. There are two current staging systems that are commonly used in discussions of bladder cancer. The so-called American system was first described by Jewett and Strong[20] in 1946. This staging system was based on the premise that bladder cancer could be divided into three pathologic stages: invasion of the submucosa (stage A), invasion of the muscularis (stage B), and invasion of the perivesical tissue (stage C).[21] In 1952, Marshall[22] added stage 0 to denote tumors not invading the lamina propria. Stage D disease was subsequently added and subdivided to include stage D1 (metastatic disease confined to the pelvis) and stage D2 (metastatic disease beyond the pelvis).

In 1978, Denoix[23] introduced the TNM system of staging bladder cancer which has been adopted by the Union International Contre le Cancer (UICC). This classification is based on the extent of the primary tumor (T), regional nodes (N), or metastases (M). The TMN classification is gaining increasing acceptance as the most commonly used staging system. Figure 1 illustrates the two staging systems.

## LOCAL STAGING

Historically, exact correlation between clinical and pathologic staging of bladder cancer occurred in only 35% of cases.[24] However, with the development of more sophisticated radiologic modalities, local staging accuracy continues to improve. Although, as previously mentioned, an IVP should be part of the evaluation of hematuria, its accuracy in staging of bladder

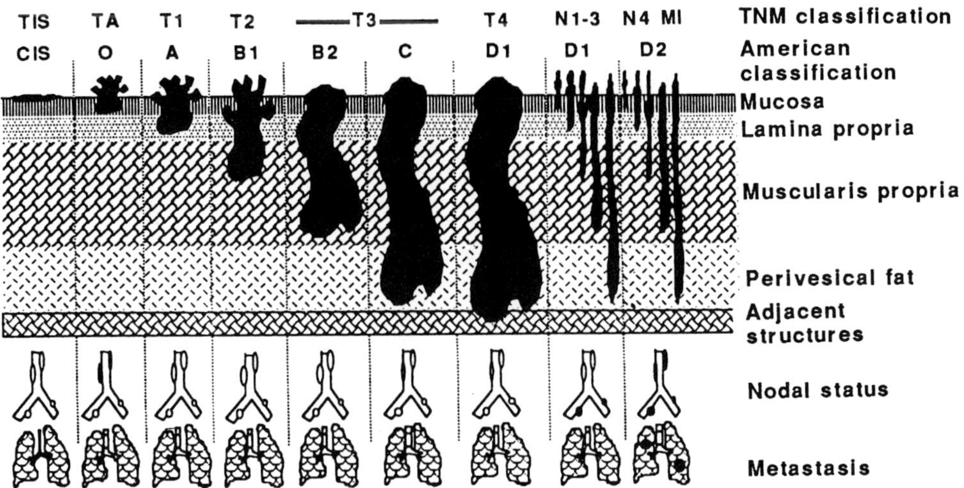


**Fig 1.** The Jewett–Marshall and the TNM (VICC) staging systems. [From See and Fuller, with permission.[24]]

cancer is limited. Hatch and Barry[25] found that 35 of 38 patients (92%) with bladder cancer who had ureteral obstruction by IVP had muscle-invasive tumors. However, Lang[26] found that only 7 of 88 patients with invasive bladder tumors had ureteral obstruction on urogram for a sensitivity of only 8%.

Ultrasound imaging has also been applied to the staging of bladder cancer. The technology has progressed from transabdominal to transrectal to transurethral ultrasound imaging. See and Fuller[24] reviewed combined series utilizing a transurethral technique and found a 90% sensitivity and 76% specificity for the ultrasonic diagnosis of muscle-invading tumors.

Transurethral resection has been considered the most straightforward staging technique. However, transurethral resection has its own set of limitations. Herr et al.[27] reviewed the staging accuracy of transurethral resection of bladder tumors subsequent to neoadjuvant chemotherapy and prior to cystectomy. They reported that 32% of the patients determined to have stage T0/T1,2 disease by transurethral resection of bladder tumors were found to have residual tumor of P2 or greater in the cystectomy specimen. Incomplete tumor resection and sampling error remain the greatest limitations of accurate staging via transurethral resection.

Computerized tomography (CT) has also been applied to the staging of bladder carcinoma. Voges et al.[28] found that CT overstaged 67% of patients with superficial disease and 20% of patients with invasive disease. In addition, Voges et al.[28] reported that CT understaged 30% of the patients with invasive disease. See and Fuller[24] reviewed five large series that utilized CT scans in identifying extravesical tumor spread in lesions that were T3b or greater. They found an overall sensitivity of 83% and specificity of 82%.

Magnetic resonance imaging (MRI) has recently emerged as another alternative for staging invasive bladder cancer. However, See and Fuller[24] again compared cumulative series using CT vs. MRI for staging of bladder cancer. The sensitivity of MRI vs. CT was 73% vs. 70% and the specificity was 84% vs. 81% in terms of staging the extent of the local lesion. However, from their literature review, See and Fuller[24] found that MRI may be more accurate in staging lymph node involvement than CT scan. In their review of the literature, See and Fuller[24] found 52% understaging and 6% overstaging of nodal status with CT scan and only 26% understaging and 0% overstaging of nodal involvement with

MRI. A recent report[29] using gadolinium-DTPA–enhanced MRI suggests that the accuracy of MRI staging of bladder cancer may continue to improve.

## TREATMENT OF LOCALLY INVASIVE BLADDER CANCER

### Cystectomy

In the modern era, radical cystectomy has emerged as the gold standard for the treatment of locally invasive bladder cancer. Improved surgical technique and postoperative care has lowered perioperative complication rates from 35% prior to 1970 to 10% in modern series.[30] Similarly, the operative mortality has decreased from 20% to 2%. Radical cystectomy is intended to be an extirpative procedure that will provide clear sugical margins and prevent local recurrence. Richie et al.[31] reported 5-year survival rates after cystectomy of 39.9% and 40.4% for patients with stage B1 and B2 disease, respectively. In a more recent series, Pagano and associates[32] reported 5-year survival rates of 68% and 67% for patients with P2 and P3a disease.

When metastatic disease spreads to the pelvic nodes, survival rates diminish significantly. Lerner et al.[33] reviewed 12 series in the literature from 1962 to 1992 and found 5-year survival rates of 4%–36%. Although it is still the topic of much debate, most urologists advocate adjuvant chemotherapy in the presence of nodal disease.

A radical cystectomy with construction of a urinary conduit is a major surgical undertaking. The technique of radical cystectomy described below is essentially that as developed and popularized by Skinner.[34] The patients are given a standard mechanical and antibiotic bowel prep as well as preoperative hydration. After satisfactory endotracheal anesthesia has been achieved, the patient is placed in the hyperextended supine position. A Foley catheter is placed to drain the bladder.

A midline or left paramedian incision is made from 2 in. above the umbilicus to the symphysis pubis. The peritoneal cavity is entered in the usual manner and then a careful exploratory laparotomy is performed. The presence of metastatic bladder cancer or significant nonurologic disease is assessed at this time.

The surgeon then mobilizes the ascending colon and the peritoneal attachments to the small bowel mesentery (Figure 2). The left colon and sigmoid are then mobilized off the sacral promontory and distal aorta up to the origin of the inferior mesenteric artery. At this point, a self-retaining retractor is placed and the right colon and small bowel are packed upward into the epigas-

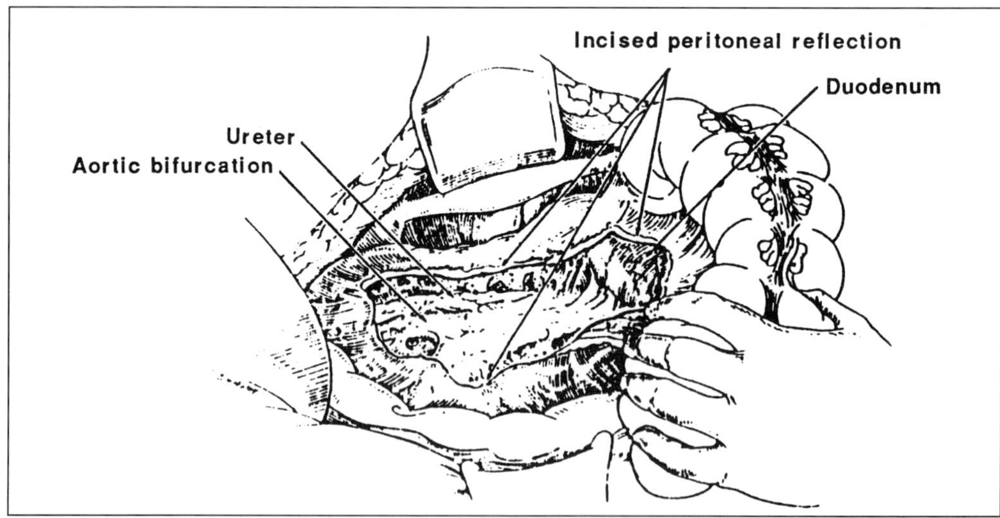


**Fig 2.** Mobilization of ascending colon and small bowel mesentery. [From Skinner DG, with permission.[34]]

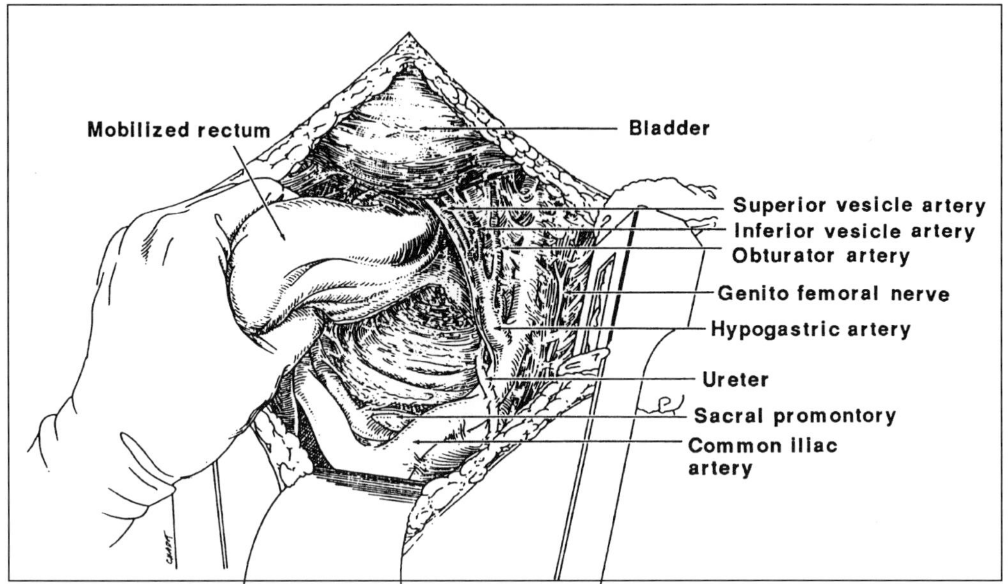


**Fig 3.** Identification of ureters crossing common iliac arteries. [From Skinner DG, with permission.[34]]

trium with lap pads. The next step is to identify and divide the ureters, usually beyond the point where they cross the common iliac arteries (Figure 3). Right angle hemoclips are placed on the proximal ureter to prevent urine leakage into the peritoneal cavity. A small portion of the proximal ureter is sent for frozen section to rule out occult carcinoma. The ureters are then packed out of the operative field in a cephalad direction.

The surgeon next focuses his attention on the pelvic node dissection. The limits of the dissection extend from 2 cm above the aortic bifurcation superiorly over the iliac vessels to the genitofemoral nerve laterally. All lymphatic tissue is dissected off the external iliac artery and vein. The circumflex iliac vein represents the distal limit of dissection along the artery and Cooper's ligament is the medial distal extent of the dissection. The lymph node of Cloquet or Rosenmuller is the distal limit of the dissection medial to the external iliac artery. The obturator fossa is then exposed and after the obturator nerve has been identified, all obturator nodal tissue is removed.

After the node dissection is completed, the surgeon's attention is turned to the identification and division of the bladder pedicles. The lateral pedicle arises off the hypogastric artery. The medial branches of the hypogastric artery that constitute the lateral pedicle of the bladder are ligated between large surgical clips sequentially down to the endopelvic fascia (Figure 4).

Once the two lateral pedicles have been divided, attention is focused on the posterior pedicle. The peritoneum lateral to the rectum is incised and the incision is extended anteriorly into the cul-de-sac to meet the incision from the opposite side (Figure 5). The plane between the posterior leaf of Denonvilliers' fascia and the anterior rectal wall is then developed. The rectum is mobilized away from the bladder, seminal vesicles, and prostate. At this point, the posterior pedicle is defined and divided between surgical clips.

In the female, the posterior pedicle and cardinal ligaments are clipped and divided beyond the cervix. After this maneuver, the posterior vaginal wall is opened and a sleeve of anterior vaginal wall left on the posterior wall of the bladder. Otherwise, the radical female cystectomy is similar to

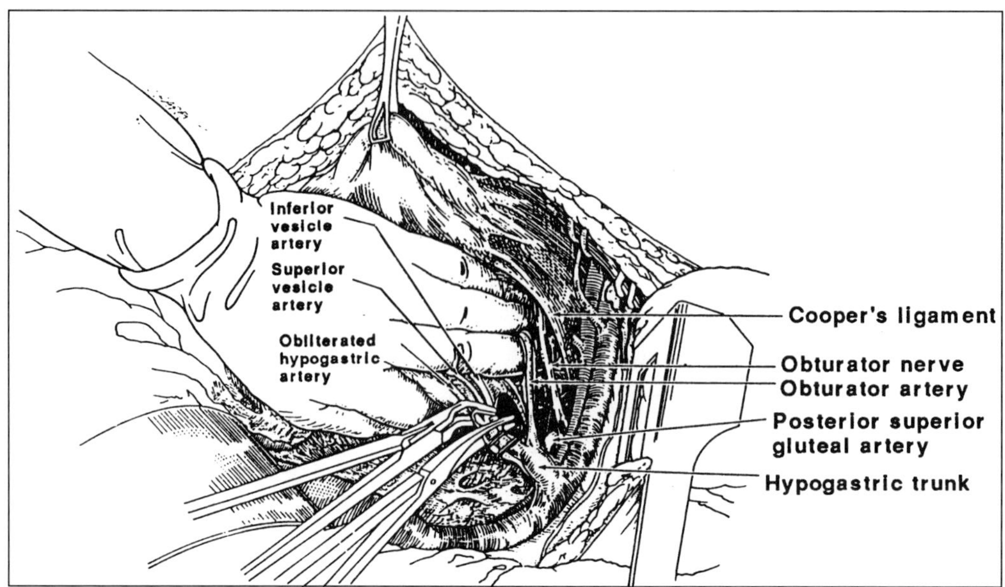


**Fig 4.** Division of lateral pedicle. [From Skinner DG, with permission.[34]]

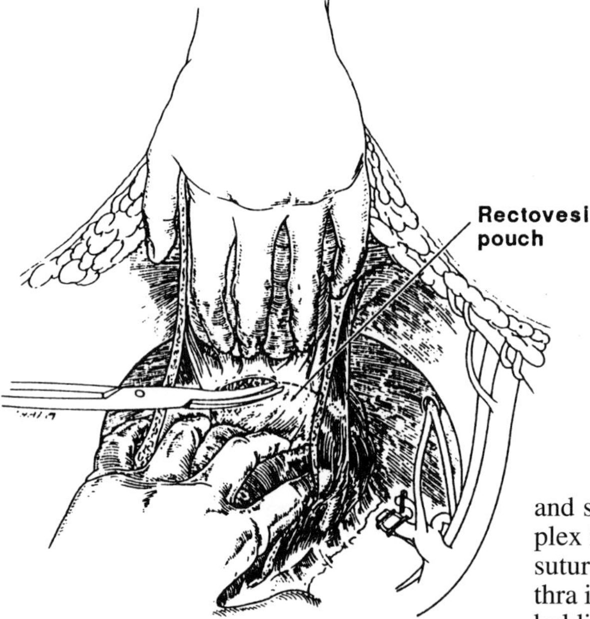


**Fig 5.** Division of peritoneal reflection to develop plane between bladder and rectum. [From Skinner DG, with permission.[34]]

the procedure performed in the male.

After the posterior and lateral pedicles have been divided, the surgeon's attention is turned to the anterior bladder wall. This portion of the procedure is very similar to that of a radical retropubic prostatectomy. The puboprostatic ligaments are stretched and sharply divided. The dorsal vein complex is identified and controlled with 0 silk sutures and divided. At this point the urethra is clearly seen and is the only structure holding the bladder in place. Many surgeons advocate instillation of 1% formalin into the bladder before dividing the urethra to prevent the possibility of tumor seeding if spillage occurs. After the bladder is removed, the deep pelvis is checked for hemostasis. At this point the construction of the urinary conduit commences and these techniques are discussed in other chapters.

### Partial Cystectomy

Fundamental to the application of partial cystectomy to the treatment of invasive bladder cancer is an understanding of the "field change" that can occur in the bladder urothelium. Because whatever etiologic factors that cause bladder cancer can theoretically effect all portions of the urothelium, the optimal candidates for a partial cystectomy are patients with a single invasive lesion without evidence of secondary lesions or carcinoma in situ elsewhere in the bladder. Ideally, partial cystectomy is best applied to lesions in the dome or posterior wall where good margins can be achieved. Sweeney et al.[35] stated the following relative contraindications to partial cystectomy: presence of multiple tumors, carcinoma in situ, cellular atypia, prostatic invasion, inability to achieve clear surgical margins, the need for ureteral reimplantation, prior therapy, inadequate bladder volume, and extravesical tumor extension.

Despite careful patient selection, partial cystectomy is still associated with increased recurrence rates. Sweeney et al.[35] reviewed the literature and reported recurrence rates of 38%–78% following partial cystectomy. In the same review, Sweeney et al.[35] found that 0%–17% of patients who had undergone partial cystectomy ultimately required radical cystectomy and urinary diversion. With these caveats in mind, patients who opt for partial cystectomy should be aware of the published recurrence rates and the potential need for subsequent total cystectomy. Obviously, all patients should be followed with regular cystoscopic examinations after partial cystectomy.

### Transurethral Resection

Herr[36] presented the following rationale for transurethral resection in the management of muscle-invading (T2,T3) bladder cancer. In carefully selected patients, survival rates free of disease after transurethral resection are comparable to those of more radical treatments. In addition, in approximately 10% of patients who undergo radical cystectomy, no residual tumor will be found in the surgical specimen. Finally, the patient benefits from the enhanced quality of life provided by having an intact bladder.

Herr[36] also advocates restaging the invasive bladder cancer with a second transurethral resection several weeks after the first resection to rule out more diffuse or extensive disease that would mitigate against conservative management. The same admonitions regarding patient selection for partial cystectomy apply to those selected for transurethral resection. In particular, patients with multiple tumors, carcinoma in situ, or prostatic invasion are not candidates for transurethral resection. In addition, radiographic staging–included pelvic CT scan should exclude local extension beyond the bladder wall.

Herr[37] reported on 45 patients with muscle-invasive disease who were managed with transurethral resection with intravesical therapy as necessary. These patients were followed from 3 to 7 years (median 5.1 years). Thirty patients were free of disease either without further therapy or with intravesical therapy for recurrent superficial bladder cancer. Of the 15 failures, 11 patients required cystectomy and 4 developed metastatic disease.

Selection of surgical treatment for invasive bladder cancer continues to evolve. A radical cystectomy remains the surgical treatment of choice for invasive bladder cancer, although partial cystectomy and transurethral resection are alternatives in carefully selected patients.

### Chemotherapy

Several chemotherapeutic agents have emerged as being effective against bladder cancer. Cisplatin, methotrexate, and vinblastine (CMV) as well as the addition of doxorubicin (M-VAC) have achieved complete responses in some patients with invasive bladder cancer. Chemotherapy has the potential to affect metastatic disease as well as the primary lesion. Meyers et al.[38] reported on the use of CMV for the treatment of metastatic bladder cancer. In the Meyers series,[38] of 17 patients who had not undergone cystectomy, 11 had a complete response of the bladder lesion. Further clinical studies with M-VAC following transurethral resection of the tumor have resulted in about a 50% clinical complete response and a 25%–30% pathologic complete response.[39–41]

These initial studies regarding the use of modern chemotherapy regimens are encouraging, but the exact role of chemotherapy in the treatment of bladder cancer remains to be defined. Studies by Shipley et al.[42] suggest that combined chemotherapy and radiation therapy may achieve cure as well as bladder preservation in some patients. Since cisplatin is considered a radiosensitizer,[43] it may potentiate the effect of radiotherapy and make combination therapy more attractive.

### Radiation Therapy

Radiation therapy has been used in the treatment of invasive bladder cancer both as a definitive primary treatment and as a preoperative adjunct to radical surgery. Radiation therapy is usually reserved in the U.S. for patients who are felt not to be good operative candidates. However, in Britain radiation therapy has been widely used as primary treatment for invasive bladder cancer.[44] Quilty et al.[44] report a 25% 5-year local control rate for stage T1–T3 tumors treated with 50–57.5 Gy over 4 weeks. In patients with T4 tumors, the 5-year local control rate was only 16%. Other series utilizing primary radiation alone for muscle invasive tumors report a 5-year survival rate of about 40%.[45–47]

In addition to definite radiation, preoperative radiation has also been used by some investigators prior to radical cystectomy. The rationale for such therapy has been pathologic downstaging and to decrease tumor seeding at the time of surgery. Parsons and Million[48] reviewed historical series comparing radiation followed by radical cystectomy. Although these series suggest a survival advantage in those patients receiving preoperative radiation, the argument for preoperative radiation appears less cogent in the era of modern chemotherapy, which not only potentially provides local control but also limits distant spread of disease as well. In a recent review of the subject, Wesson[49] concludes that radiation therapy can no longer be recommended as a curative single modality for bladder cancer. However, radiation therapy may continue to have a role in combination with chemotherapy as adjuvant preoperative therapy or as part of bladder preservation protocols.[42]

## SUMMARY

Invasive bladder cancer presents a formidable surgical and therapeutic challenge to the urologist. Continued efforts will need to be focused on a better understanding of factors contributing to the etiology and progression of bladder cancer. Surgery remains the cornerstone of therapy for invasive bladder cancer, but the role of adjuvant therapy requires continued investigation.

## REFERENCES


1. Boring CC, Squires TS, Tong T. *Cancer Stat.* 1993;43:7–26.
2. 1987 Annual Cancer Statistics Review. Including Cancer Trends: 1950–1985, NIH Publication No. 88-2789. Bethesda, Maryland, U.S. Dept. of Health and Human Services, National Cancer Institute.
3. Catalona WJ. Urothelial tumors of the urinary tract. In: Walsh PC, Retik AB, Stamey TA, Vaughan ED, eds. *Campbell's Urology.* Philadelphia: WB Saunders; 1992:1094–1158.
4. Rehn L. Veber blasentumoren bei fuchsinarbeitern. *Arch Kind Chir.* 1895;50:588.
5. Morrison AS, Cole P. Epidemiology of bladder cancer. *Urol Clin North Am.* 1976;3:13–29.
6. Chapman JW, Connolly JG, Rosenbaum L. Occupational bladder cancer: a case-control study. In: Connolly JG, ed. *Carcinoma of the Bladder.* New York: Raven Press; 1981:45.
7. Burch JD, Rohan TE, Howe GR. Risk of bladder cancer by source and type of tobacco exposure: a case-control study. *Int J Cancer.* 1989;44:622–628.
8. Piper JM, Tonascia J, Metanoski GM. Heavy phenacetin use and bladder cancer in women aged 20 to 49 years. *N Engl J Med.* 1985;313:292–295.
9. Sontgu JM. Experimental identification of genitourinary carcinogens. *Urol Clin North Am.* 1980;7:803–807.

10. Morrison AS. Advances in the etiology of urothelial cancer. *Urol Clin North Am.* 1984;11: 557–566.
11. Pedersen-Bjerguard J, Ersboll J, Hansen VL. Carcinoma of the bladder after treatment with cyclophosphamide for non-Hodgkins lymphoma. *N Engl J Med.* 1988;318:1028–1032.
12. Brown RR, Price JM, Friedell GH. Tryptophan metabolism in patients with bladder cancer: geographic differences. *J Natl Cancer Inst.* 1969; 43:295–299.
13. Wolf H. Studies on the role of tryptophan metabolites in the genesis of bladder cancer. *Acta Clin Scand.* 1973;(Suppl)433:154–158.
14. Tevlings FAG, Peters HA, Hop WCJ. A new aspect of urinary excretion of tryptophan metabolites in patients with cancer of the bladder. *Int J Cancer.* 1978;21:140–146.
15. Byar D, Blackhard C. Comparisons of placebo, pyridoxine, and topical thiotepa in preventing recurrence of stage 1 bladder cancer. *Urology.* 1977;10:556–561.
16. Olsson CA. Management of invasive carcinoma of the bladder. In: deKernian JB, Paulson DF, eds. *Genitourinary Cancer Management.* Philadelphia: Lea and Febiger; 1987.
17. Varkarakis MJ, Gaeta J, Moore GH. Superficial bladder tumor: aspects of clinical progression. *Urology.* 1974;4:414–420.
18. De Felippo N, Fortunato RP, Mellins HZ, Richie JP. Intravenous urography: important adjunct for diagnosis of bladder tumors. *Br J Urol.* 1984; 56(5):502–505.
19. Koshikawa T, Leyn H, Schenck V. Difficulties in evaluating urinary specimens after local mitomycin therapy of bladder cancer. *Diag Cytopathol.* 1989;5:117–121.
20. Jewett HJ, Strong GH. Infiltrating carcinoma of the bladder, relation of depth of penetration of the bladder wall to incidence of local extension and metastases. *J Urol.* 1946;55:366–372.
21. Richie JP. Radical cystectomy: innovations and results. In: Raghavan D, ed. *The Management of Bladder Cancer.* Edward Arnold Publishers, London: Edward Arnold; 1988.
22. Marshall VF. The relation of the pre-operative estimate of the pathologic demonstration of the extent of vesical neoplasms. *J Urol.* 1952;68: 714–718.
23. Denois PF. *TNM Classification of Malignant Tumors.* 3rd Ed. Geneva: International Union Against Cancer; 1978.
24. See WA, Fuller JR. Staging of advanced bladder cancer: current concepts and pitfalls. *Urol Clin North Am.* 1992;19(4):663–683.
25. Hatch TR, Barry JM. The value of excretory urography in staging bladder cancer. *J Urol.* 1986;135:49.
26. Lang EK. The roentgenographic assessment of bladder tumors: A comparison of the diagnostic accuracy of roentgenographic techniques. *Cancer.* 1969;23:717–722.
27. Herr HW, Whitmore WF Jr, Morse MJ. Neoadjuvant chemotherapy in invasive bladder cancer. The evolving role of surgery. *J Urol.* 1990;144: 1083–1088.
28. Voges GE, Tauschke E, Stockle M. Computerized tomography: an unreliable method for accurate staging of bladder tumors in patients who are candidates for radical cystectomy. *J Urol.* 1989;142:972–974.
29. Tachibana M, Baba S, Deguchi N, et al. Efficacy of gadolinium-diethletruiminepentacetic acid enhanced magnetic resonance imaging for differentiation between superficial and muscle-invasive tumor of the bladder: a comparative study with computerized tomography and transurethral ultrasonography. *J Urol.* 1991;145:1169–1173.
30. Skinner D, Lieskovsky G. Management of invasive and high grade bladder cancer. In: Skinner DG, Lieskovsky G, eds. *Diagnosis and Management of Genitourinary Cancer.* Philadelphia: WB Saunders; 1988:295–312.
31. Richie JP, Skinner DG, Kaufman JJ. Radical cystectomy for carcinoma of the bladder: 16 years of experience. *J Urol.* 1975;113:186–189.
32. Pagano E, Bassi P, Galetti TP. Results of contemporary radical cystectomy for invasive bladder cancer. A clinicopathological study with an emphasis on the inadequacy of the tumor, nodes, and metastases classification. *J Urol.* 1991; 145(1):45–50.
33. Lerner SP, Skinner E, Skinner DG. Radical cystectomy in regionally advanced bladder cancer. *Urol Clin North Am.* 1992;19(4):713–723.
34. Skinner DG. Radical cystectomy. In: Crawford ED, Borden TA, eds. *Genitourinary Cancer Surgery.* Philadelphia: Lea and Febiger; 1982:207–216.
35. Sweeney P, Kursh ED, Resnick MI. Partial cystectomy. *Urol Clin North Am.* 1992;19(4):701–711.
36. Herr HW. Transurethral resection in regionally advanced bladder cancer. *Urol Clin North Am.* 1992;19(4):695–700.
37. Herr HW. Conservative management of muscle-infiltrating bladder tumors: prospective experience. *J Urol.* 1987;138:1162–1163.
38. Meyers FJ, Palmer JM, Freiha FS. The fate of the bladder in patients with metastatic bladder cancer treated with cisplatin, methotrexate and vinblastine: a Northern California Oncology Group study. *J Urol.* 1985;134:1118–1121.
39. Herr HW. Neoadjuvant chemotherapy for invasive bladder cancer. *Semin Surg Oncol.* 1989;5: 266–271.
40. McCullough DL, Cooper RM, Yeaman CD. Neoadjuvant treatment of stage T2 bladder cancer with cis-platinum, cyclophosphamide and doxorubicin. *J Urol.* 1989;141:849–852.

41. Scher HI, Yagoda A, Herr HW. Neoadjuvant M-VAC (methotrexate, vinblastine, doxorubicin and cisplatin) effect on the primary bladder lesion. *J Urol.* 1988;139:470–474.
42. Shipley WV, Prout GR, Einstein AB. Treatment of invasive bladder cancer by cisplatin and radiation in patients unsuited for surgery. *JAMA.* 1987;258:931–935.
43. Walther PJ. Combined treatment approaches in regionally advanced bladder cancer. *Urol Clin North Am.* 1992;19(4):761–774.
44. Quilty PM, Duncan W, Chisholm GD, et al. Results of surgery following radical radiotherapy for invasive bladder cancer. *Br J Urol.* 1986;58:396–405.
45. Duncun W, Quilty PM. The results of a series of 963 patients with transitional cell carcinoma of the urinary bladder primarily treated by radical megavoltage X-ray therapy. *Radiother Oncol.* 1986;7:299–310.
46. Goftinet DR, Schneider MJ, Glatstein EJ, Ludwig H, Ray GR, Dunnick NR, Bagshaw MA: Bladder cancer: results of radiation therapy in 384 patients. *Radiology.* 1975;177:149–153.
47. Hope-Stone HF, Blandy JP, Oliver RTD. Radical radiotherapy and salvage cystectomy in the treatment of invasive carcinoma of the bladder. In: Oliver RTD, Hendry WF, Bloom HJG, eds. *Bladder Cancer: Principles of Combination Therapy.* London: Butterworths; 1981:127–138.
48. Parsons JT, Million RR. Planned preoperative irradiation in the management of clinical stage B2-C (T3) bladder carcinoma. *Int J Radiat Oncol Bul Phys.* 1987;14:797–802.
49. Wesson MF. Radiation therapy in regionally advanced bladder cancer. *Urol Clin North Am.* 1992;19(4):725–734.

# 31

# Urinary Tract Reconstruction with Intestinal Segments

*Michael O. Koch*

## INTRODUCTION

This chapter will review techniques for urinary tract reconstruction using intestinal segments. Continent urinary diversions, both cutaneous and with anastomosis to the urethra, are discussed in Chapter 6.

The successful use of intestinal segments for urinary tract reconstruction requires an understanding of basic intestinal anatomy and physiology. This is the initial focus of this chapter. Following this, surgical principles and techniques appropriate for intestinal segments as they are used in the urinary tract are reviewed. Emphasis is placed on basic anatomic and physiologic principles as these surgical techniques are described. Various uses for intestine in the urinary tract including conduits, ureteral replacement, and augmentation cystoplasty are presented. Finally, the long-term complications of the use of intestine in the urinary tract and their pathophysiology are discussed.

## INTESTINAL ANATOMY AND PHYSIOLOGY

All segments of intestine with the exception of the esophagus and duodenum have been used in urinary tract reconstruction. In this section the pertinent anatomy and physiology of each intestinal segment will be reviewed.

### Gastric Anatomy

The stomach, like most intestinal segments, is composed of an outer longitudinal muscle layer and an inner circular muscle layer. In addition, there is an inner oblique muscle layer just inside the circular layer. These fibers are particularly dense at the gastroesophageal junction and fan out anteriorly and posteriorly, paralleling the lesser curvature of the stomach. The muscular thickness of the stomach wall exceeds that of other intestinal segments.

The arterial supply of the stomach originates from the celiac trunk (Fig 1). The left gastric artery is usually the first branch off of the celiac trunk and courses to the left along the posterior surface of the lesser omentum until it reaches the gastroesophageal junction. When the left gastric artery reaches the stomach, it gives off small branches to the lower esophagus; then it courses inferomedially along the lesser curvature, giving off small gastric branches to both the anterior and posterior surfaces of the stomach. This anastomoses with the right gastric artery, which is a smaller vessel originating from the hepatic artery supplying the right side of the lesser gastric

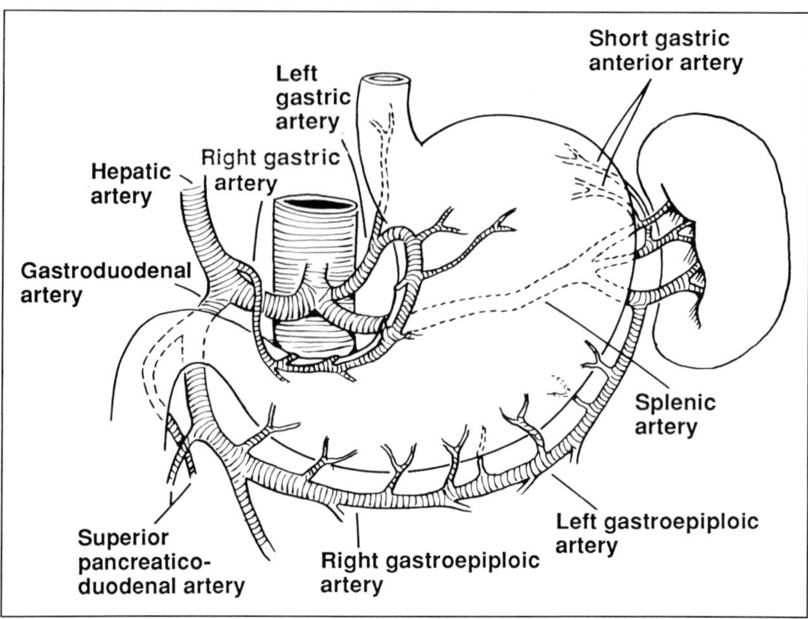


**Fig 1.** Normal gastric blood supply. Note the supply of the greater gastric curvature from the left and right gastroepiploic arteries.

curvature. The greater curvature of the stomach is supplied by the left and right gastroepiploic arteries. The left gastroepiploic artery originates from the splenic artery and courses from left to right along the greater curvature of the stomach through the greater omentum, giving off branches to the anterior and posterior surfaces of the stomach as it goes. The right gastroepiploic artery is a terminal branch of the gastroduodenal artery that courses posterior to the first portion of the duodenum. The right gastroepiploic artery is usually predominant and courses through the greater omentum giving off branches to the anterior and posterior gastric surfaces. The right and left gastroepiploic arteries anastomose along the greater gastric curvature and both vessels give off omental branches that loop down through the greater omentum. In addition to these major vessels, the fundal portion of the stomach receives additional blood supply via the short gastric vessels, which are branches off the splenic artery coursing through the gastrolienal ligament. Throughout the stomach there is abundant collateral circulation.

**Motility.** Physiologically the stomach has been described as having two distinct portions. The distal two thirds of the stomach will periodically undergo intense phasic contractions whereas the proximal one third does not. The proximal one third of the stomach functions in a reservoir fashion while the distal two thirds plays an active role in the grinding and emptying of food.

Two vagal reflexes are believed to modulate this differential gastric motility. *Receptive relaxation* refers to the reduction of intragastric pressure that occurs when the throat or esophagus is mechanically stimulated. When the stomach is filled with water, intragastric pressure rises very little. This is termed *gastric accommodation.* These reflexes are believed to be mediated via the release of vasoactive intestinal peptide (VIP) and are abolished by proximal vagotomy. As the fundus of the stomach is distended, antral peristalsis increases.

This is also vagally mediated. These unique motility patterns and reflexes become important to the urologist when the stomach is utilized for bladder augmentation.

**Digestive Function.** Water, hydrogen, chloride, sodium, potassium, pepsinogens, and intrinsic factor are normally secreted by the stomach. Gastric secretions vary among various portions of the stomach (Fig 2). Parietal cells located in the fundus and body of the stomach secrete hydrochloric acid and intrinsic factor. Pepsinogens are secreted as inactive precursors by chief cells located in the fundus and body of the stomach but also by other cells throughout the rest of the stomach. These pepsinogens are converted to active enzymes (pepsins) by the action of hydrochloric acid. Gastrin, produced by gastrin cells in the antrum and pylorus, is secreted both into the lumen and into the portal circulation.

Hydrochloric acid secretion by the parietal cell is the result of a unique hydrogen-potassium-ATPase pump. This energy-dependent pump, located on the apical membrane of the mucosal cell, exchanges one absorbed potassium for a secreted hydrogen ion. Chloride and potassium are both secreted into the lumen through a symport system. The substituted benzimidazoles (eg, omeprazole) are effective inhibitors of the potassium-hydrogen ion exchange port.

Fig 2. Site of acid- (shaded area) and gastrin-producing cells in the stomach.

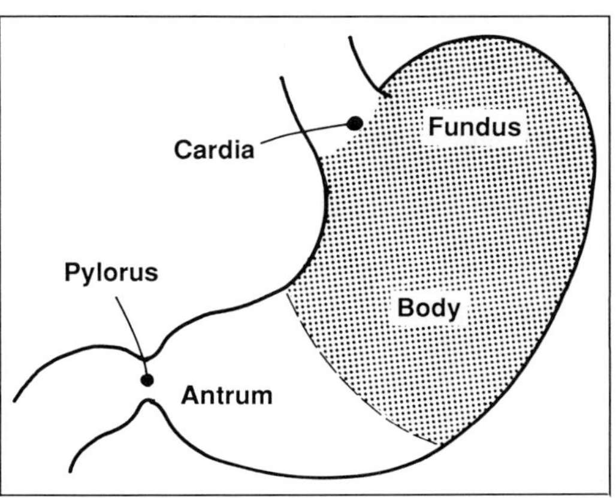


The rate at which the parietal cells in the fundus and body secrete acid is regulated by several substances including histamine, acetylcholine, and gastrin. Gastrin released from the gastrin cells in the antrum and pylorus stimulates gastric acid secretion from the parietal cells. As gastric pH decreases, gastrin release from the antrum is inhibited, resulting in decreased acid secretion from the fundus and body of the stomach. Interruption of this feedback loop may result in excessive gastrin production, such as following partial antrectomy and Bilroth II gastrojejunostomy, or possibly after gastrocystoplasty whereby the gastric mucosa is continuously bathed in relatively alkaline fluid.

## Small Intestine

**Anatomy.** Jejunum and ileum are both utilized in urinary tract reconstruction. Jejunum begins at the ligament of Treitz and comprises the first two fifths of the small intestine; ileum comprises the last three fifths, although there is no clear point of delineation between the two segments. The external muscular layer of the small intestine has two layers: an outer thinner layer of longitudinally oriented muscle and a thicker inner layer of circular muscle. These two layers are separated by the myenteric plexus.

All of the small intestinal blood supply is derived from the superior mesenteric artery (Fig 3). The superior mesenteric artery passes superior and anterior to the third portion of the duodenum. Located in the base of the mesentery of the small intestine, it courses inferiorly for a short distance before giving off branches to the pancreas and duodenum (inferior pancreaticoduodenal), ascending colon (ileocolic and right colic), and transverse colon (middle colic). As it courses through the root of the small bowel mesentery, it gives off a series of jejunal and ileal branches that supply the entire small intestine. These branches then divide into secondary arcades before entering the bowel wall. Once these vessels

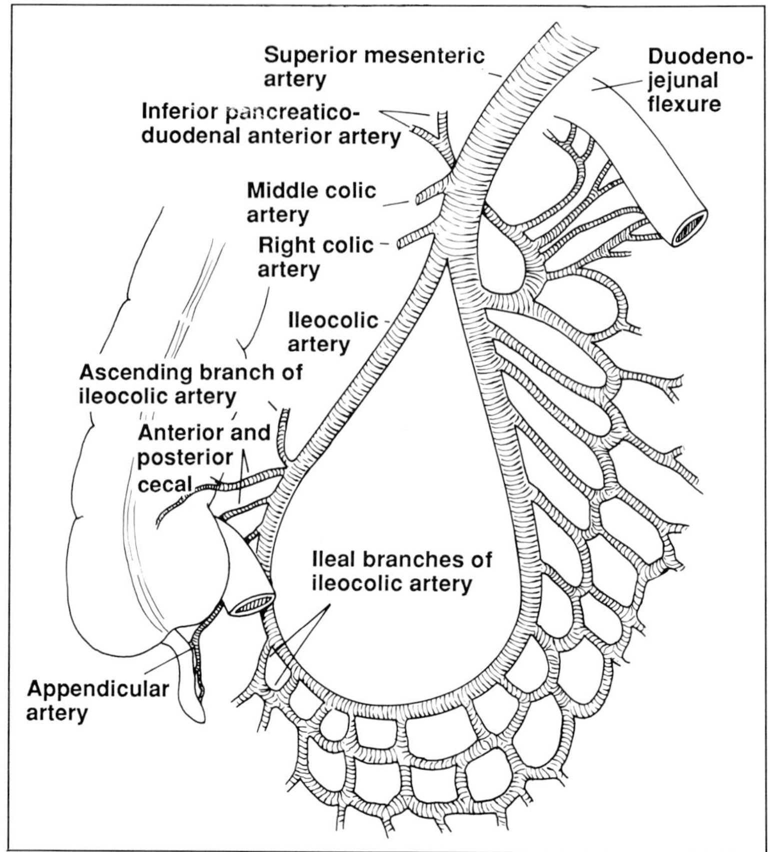


**Fig 3.** Normal small intestinal and cecal blood supply from the superior mesenteric artery.

enter the bowel, there is extensive collateralization throughout the submucosal layer that allows the mesentery to be stripped from significant lengths of bowel (up to 8 cm) without devascularizing the segment. This has important implications in urinary tract reconstruction and does not apply to other segments of bowel (eg, the colon).

**Motility.** Small intestinal contractions are phasic and tend to propagate in an oral-to-aboral direction. These phasic contractions are termed *migrating motility complexes* (MMC). The neurohumoral mechanisms that control the amplitude and frequency of MMCs are not known; however, the presence of intraluminal contents and distention of the lumen are stimulatory.

### Digestive Function

***Ileum.*** The ileum functions primarily to absorb any carbohydrates, fats, amino acids, or peptides that are not absorbed in the proximal small intestine. It also is the primary site of absorption of bile salts and vitamin $B_{12}$. It has the capability to absorb and secrete large amounts of salts and water. This capability is very pertinent to urinary tract reconstruction with intestine and will be reviewed in some depth.

The majority of electrolyte transport in ileum is thought to occur via transcellular processes. A significant paracellular pathway also exists in the ileum, particularly in comparison to the colon, which has relatively tight intraepithelial junctions. The intestinal brush border is composed of a

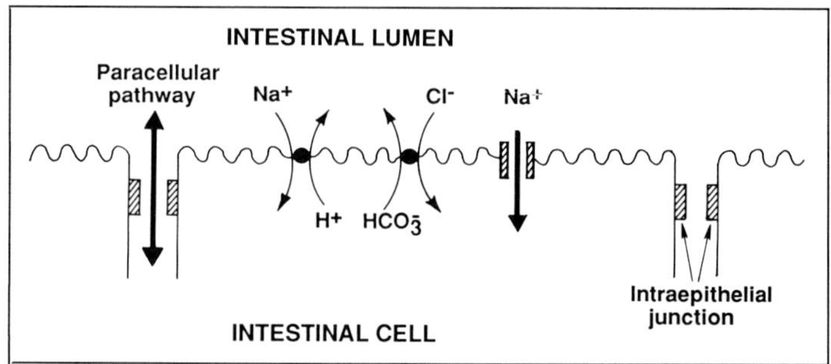


**Fig 4.** Basic mechanisms of electrolyte absorption in the ileum and colon.

number of ports that cotransport or countertransport electrolytes in an electroneutral fashion, and it also contains electrogenic conductance channels that allow movement of ions in an uncoupled fashion (Fig 4). These ports and channels are proteins embedded in the lipid bilayer that composes the cell membrane.

Sodium absorption in the small intestine has been well studied. An important mechanism of sodium entry is by $Na^+$-$H^+$ ion exchange. This countertransport system is linked, perhaps via an effect on intracellular pH, to a $Cl^-$-$HCO_3$ anion exchange system. The net effect of these two countertransport systems operating in tandem is neutral $Na^+Cl^-$ absorption. The absorption of other ions such as potassium and ammonium (which has particular pertinence to urinary tract reconstruction) is not as well understood. Multiple transport systems for potassium have been described in other epithelia including potassium conductance channels and an Na-$K^+$-$2Cl^-$ cotransport system. In certain epithelia such as kidney, ammonium ions have been shown to share these potassium transport pathways.

***Jejunum.*** Fluid and electrolyte transport in the jejunum differs markedly from that in the ileum. Jejunum functions primarily to reabsorb digested carbohydrates and bicarbonate that was secreted in the duodenal and pancreatic secretions. In contrast to the ileum and colon, while there is a sodium-hydrogen ion exchange port that accounts for the majority of sodium absorption, there is no chloride-bicarbonate exchange port (Fig 5). Hydrogen ion secreted in the jejunum in exchange for sodium is thought to titrate luminal bicarbonate to carbon dioxide and water, which are then absorbed passively. Also of importance are the relatively loose intraepithelial junctions in this segment of intestine. This results in large fluxes of solutes and water via paracellular pathways. This is of major importance when jejunal segments are used in the urinary tract. Finally, the jejunum is the major

**Fig 5.** Basic mechanisms of sodium and bicarbonate absorption in the jejunum.

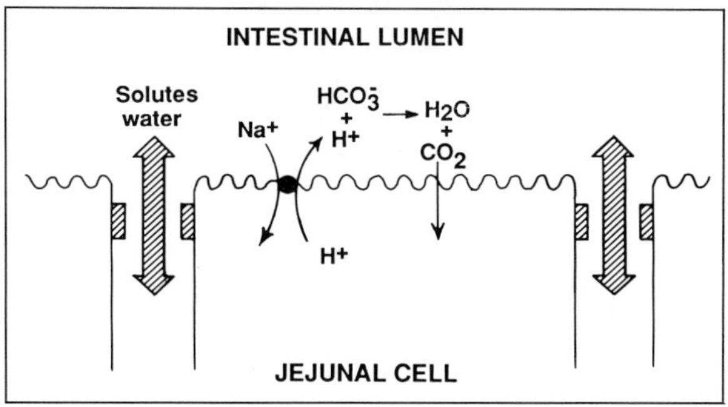

site for absorption of calcium, iron, folic acid, digested carbohydrates, fats, peptides, and amino acids.

## Colon

**Anatomy.** The colon, like the small intestine, has an outer longitudinal and inner circular muscle layer. In the bulk of the colon, the outer longitudinal muscle layer is separated into three distinct bands, the taeniae coli. The taeniae coli coalesce as they approach the rectosigmoid junction to form a complete outer longitudinal coat.

The blood supply to the right side of the colon is derived from the initial branches of the superior mesenteric artery, ie, the ileocolic artery and the right colic artery. The left side of the colon and a portion of the transverse colon are supplied by the inferior mesenteric artery arising from the aorta just below the duodenum (Fig 6). The inferior mesenteric artery gives off the left colic artery, which supplies the descending colon and frequently supplies branches to the sigmoid colon. The left colic artery anastomoses with the middle colic artery through the marginal artery. Distally the inferior mesenteric artery continues into the pelvis to give rise to the superior rectal artery and superior hemorrhoidal vessels. The lowest portion of the rectum is supplied by the inferior and middle hemorrhoidal vessels, which originate from the terminal branches of the hypogastric artery.

**Motility.** Colonic motility differs considerably from small intestinal motility and also varies along the length of the colon. All portions of the colon exhibit some element of forward peristalsis; however, the right colon is characterized by unique antiperistaltic contractions that drive the intestinal chyme back toward the ileocecal junction. These antiperistaltic contractions allow the right colon to serve as both a mixing and a storage organ. The transverse and descending colon are characterized more by slow tonic contractions that separate the feces into globular masses as it is dehydrated. The entire colon also exhibits a pattern of mass contraction. During a mass contraction, an entire section of the colon contracts while all other peristaltic

**Fig 6.** Normal blood supply and normal colonic vascular supply.

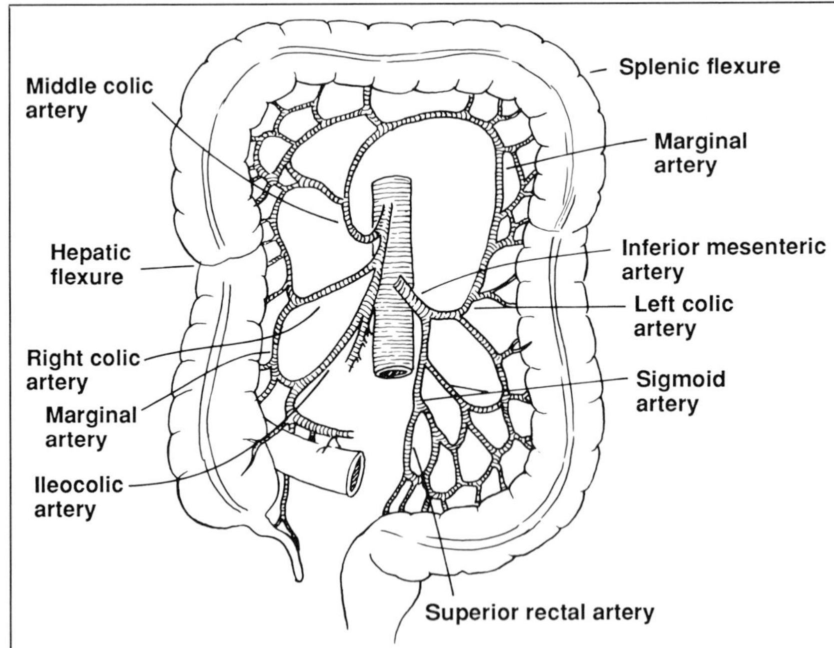

patterns cease. The pattern of mass contraction is unique to the colon and is the primary mechanism responsible for the aboral propulsion of colonic contents. The neurohumoral mechanisms that control colonic motility are poorly understood.

The ileocecal junction constitutes a unique area of small and large intestinal anatomy that has properties useful for urinary tract reconstruction. This area actually consists of the terminal segment of ileum that protrudes into the cecal lumen. While this area is usually referred to as an ileocecal valve, it actually functions as a sphincter. With distention of the terminal ileum, ileocecal valve pressures decrease, while increased pressures in the cecum result in increased ileocecal valve pressures. This zone of increased pressures is approximately 4 cm in length.

**Digestive Function.** The colon functions primarily to desiccate the feces and form it into globular masses. In health, it is not felt to be the site of any important solute absorption. Because of its relatively tight intraepithelial junctions compared to other intestinal segments, the colon is capable of reabsorbing salt and water against large electrochemical and osmotic gradients.

The basic transport processes are very similar to ileum, although variable in terms of the importance of each type of port or channel.

## PRINCIPLES OF UROLOGIC SURGERY WITH INTESTINAL SEGMENTS

### Preoperative Bowel Preparation

A preoperative mechanical and antibiotic bowel preparation is the standard of care for all patients undergoing a colorectal operation. The role of bowel preparation in operations on the ileum is less clear. Prior to the routine use of bowel preparation in colorectal operations, infectious complications occurred in 30% to 40% of patients. With preoperative mechanical and oral antibiotic bowel preparation, the incidence of these complications is reduced to less than 5% in most series.

The rationale for both mechanical and oral antibiotic bowel preparation was established in the original work of Nichols et al.[1] This study scientifically and quantitatively examined the effects of mechanical and antibiotic bowel preparations on both aerobic and anaerobic bacterial colony counts in different segments of the intestine. The small intestine contains relatively few bacteria of any kind (Fig 7). When the ileocecal valve is crossed, however, there is a significant increase in aerobic, and, in particular, anaerobic bacterial colony counts. Anaerobic bacteria are felt to play an important role in the development of anastomotic leaks and abscess formation after colorectal operations. A mechanical bowel preparation that includes the administration of cathartics and enemas does not appreciably reduce aerobic or anaerobic bacterial counts. In fact, in certain circumstances, mechanical bowel preparations may actually increase bacterial counts (vide infra). The primary purpose of a mechanical bowel preparation, then, is to reduce the likelihood of fecal spillage intraoperatively.

In contrast, an oral antibiotic bowel preparation has profound effects on bacterial colony counts. Neomycin has good activity against aerobic bacteria but only moderate activity against anaerobes. With the addition of erythromycin base that is poorly absorbed and has significant activity against anaerobes, there is a significant reduction in the colony counts in all areas of the intestine. The persistently elevated aerobic colony counts with the administration of neomycin and erythromycin in the study by Nichols et al were due to fungi, so that all bacterial counts with this regimen were less than 100 bacteria/mL. The implications of this study, then, are that surgical morbidity in these cases would be reduced by a combined mechanical and antibiotic bowel preparation.

Clinical studies have in fact confirmed these implications. In a prospective, randomized trial, Washington et al[2] compared mechanical preparation alone, with mechanical preparation combined with antibiotic preparation with neomycin or neomycin plus tetracycline. In the latter

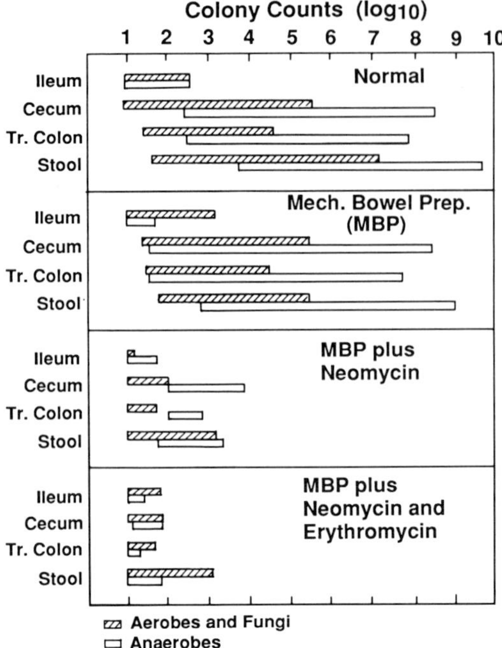


**Fig 7.** Bacterial colony counts in the small and large intestine. Note an absence of change in quantitative colony counts with mechanical bowel preparation alone. Neomycin results in significant reduction in aerobic and fungal colony counts. The addition of erythromycin provides a reduction in anaerobic bacterial colony counts.

regimen, tetracycline was employed for its anaerobic coverage. A mechanical preparation with combined neomycin and tetracycline given orally yielded clearly superior results with a tenfold reduction in the wound infection rate, a twofold reduction in septicemia, and a sevenfold reduction in fistula rate. Other large series find very similar results with the substitution of oral metronidazole for anaerobic coverage in these regimens.[3]

**Mechanical Bowel Preparation.** Various forms of mechanical bowel preparation have been utilized. Traditional methods employ both oral cathartics and enemas (Table 1). This may be physically exhausting as well as dehydrating to the patient. This method does result in a highly satisfactory mechanical preparation in the vast majority of patients, however. Due to the prolonged need for preoperative hospitalization and the adverse physiologic effects of the standard Nichols–Condon type of mechanical bowel preparation, alternative methods of bowel preparation were sought.

Whole-gut irrigation was a response to these needs. This refers to several methods of lavaging the intestinal tract over a relatively brief period of time with a variety of solutions either orally ingested or administered via nasogastric tube. The original form of whole-gut irrigation was by the administration of 9 to 12 L of lactated Ringer's solution or saline via a nasogastric tube over a 3-hour period.[4,5] The large volume of irrigation fluid required with this method resulted in significant nausea and vomiting in some patients and most patients had significant fluid retention. In one series employing whole-gut irrigation that pro-

**TABLE 1. Mechanical Bowel Preparations**

| | Day 1 | Day 2 | Day 3 | Day of Surgery |
|---|---|---|---|---|
| Nichols–Condon[1] | Low-residue diet; bisacodyl 1 PO at 6 PM | Low-residue diet; $MgSO_4$ 50%, 30 cm$^3$ PO at 10 AM, 2 PM, 6 PM; saline enemas until clear | Clear liquid diet; $MgSO_4$ 50%, 30 cm$^3$ PO at 10 AM, 2 PM; neomycin/erythromycin base, 1 g of each PO at 1, 2, and 11 PM | |
| Golytely[3] | Regular diet | Liquid evening meal | Golytely, 4–6 L until rectal effluent clear; neomycin 2 g, metronidazole 2 g orally at 7 and 11 PM | |

phylactically used both metoclopramide and furosemide to minimize nausea and fluid retention, 87% of patients tolerated the preparation with no complaints, with another 10% having only minor complaints of nausea and vomiting.[6] This resulted in a satisfactory bowel preparation in 90% of patients.

Because of the variable tolerance of whole-gut irrigation with saline or lactated Ringer's solution and because of the need for a nasogastric tube with this method, orally ingested solutions were developed. The first of these was a 10% mannitol solution. This solution is sweet to the taste and usually only 1 L is needed. Mannitol acts as an osmotic agent pulling fluid into the intestinal lumen resulting in a catharsis. This is a highly effective method of bowel preparation; however, it suffers from several problems.[7] An oral mannitol preparation is dehydrating as are other cathartic preparations. More importantly, an increased wound infection rate has been reported with mannitol that is thought to be due to bacterial metabolism of mannitol and bacterial overgrowth.[8] In addition, bacterial metabolism of the mannitol results in the production of high levels of colonic hydrogen gas. Several cases of intraoperative colonic explosions after mannitol bowel preparations have been reported.[8–10]

To overcome these difficulties, Davis et al[11] developed an isotonic whole-gut irrigation using polyethylene glycol in a balanced electrolyte solution (Golytely). Generally, 240 mL is ingested every 10 minutes until the rectal effluent is clear. Usually 2 to 3 L of solution must be ingested to reach this end point. A randomized trial comparing Golytely with 10% mannitol for bowel preparation found that Golytely is probably better in terms of the bowel preparation, results in minimal physiologic alterations, is better tolerated, results in lower colonic hydrogen gas levels, and, finally, is associated with lower wound infection rates.[12] The only disadvantage of Golytely is the large volume of fluid that must be ingested. Recent studies have confirmed the efficacy of Golytely bowel preparation in infants and children.[13,14] Studies that have prospectively compared 1-day Golytely preparation to the traditional 2-day mechanical bowel preparation using oral cathartics and enemas have found comparable patient tolerance and efficacy.[3]

**Parenteral Antibiotic Therapy.** The need for perioperative parenteral antibiotic coverage remains controversial. Studies that utilize parenteral antibiotics in addition to oral antibiotic regimens have generally shown minimal if any benefit.[3] Alternatively, series that have utilized parenteral antibiotics in combination with mechanical bowel preparations without oral antibiotic therapy have yielded very acceptable infectious complication rates.[6] As with oral antibiotic therapy, however, the antibiotic spectrum should include both aerobic and anaerobic bacteria. For example, one study of parenteral metronidazole alone resulted in wound infection and intra-abdominal abscess rates of 22% and 9%, respectively.[6] With the addition of ampicillin to this regimen, these rates were both reduced to 2%. Trials using second-generation cephalosporins as single agents in combination with mechanical bowel preparation have also demonstrated significant efficacy.[15]

Parenteral antibiotic therapy does have several potential advantages over oral therapy. Sterilization of the colonic contents with oral antibiotics can select out resistant organisms, promote the development of pseudomembranous enterocolitis, and result in the overgrowth of fungal organisms. Some studies have shown a superiority of parenteral antibiotic therapy in terms of wound infection rates.[15] Parenteral antibiotic therapy is associated with many of the same complications, however, and has the disadvantage of being significantly more expensive. One of these forms of antibiotic therapy should be used in all patients undergoing intestinal surgery; use of both oral and parenteral antibiotic therapy is not necessary.

## INTESTINAL ANASTOMOSES

### Fundamental Principles of Surgery

A multitude of techniques have been developed for fashioning a bowel-to-bowel anastomosis, with many of the techniques that are utilized today having their origins in the late 1800s. While there are advocates of single- or double-layer closures, running or continuous closures, and stapling techniques, all of these techniques are based on surgical principles that were established by our surgical predecessors. It is imperative that urologists understand these fundamental principles of intestinal surgery so that they can utilize intestine in a safe manner for urinary tract reconstructive procedures. With these principles in mind, the urologist can select those techniques of intestinal surgery that suit his or her own preferences and abilities.

These fundamentals of intestinal surgery are adequate exposure, containment of fecal spillage, good vascular supply, accurate tension-free anastomosis of the intestinal layers with a water-tight mucosal closure, and closure of all mesenteric defects. These issues will be discussed separately.

The intestinal segment should be mobilized sufficiently to afford exposure during the performance of the intestinal anastomosis. With the exception of the low sigmoid and rectal area, and the duodenum, all intestinal segments can usually be sufficiently mobilized to allow the performance of the anastomosis with the intestine at the level of the anterior abdominal wall. Sufficient mobilization is also critically important to prevent tension on the anastomosis. A sufficient amount of mesentery (0.5 to 1.0 cm) should also be dissected off the area of intestinal transection to facilitate the placement of the sutures along these edges. The majority of leaks from intestinal anastomoses are due either to a poor blood supply or to poor suture placement at the mesenteric edge of the anastomosis.

Since the contents of both small and large intestine contain significant amounts of bacteria, even after an effective mechanical and antibiotic bowel preparation, fecal spillage should be minimized. After adequate mobilization of the intestine, the area of the anastomosis should be walled off with laparotomy pads or surgical towels, and noncrushing linen-shod clamps should be placed across the proximal and distal intestine. It is the practice of many urologists to irrigate out intestinal segments with antibiotic solutions intraoperatively. This author's preference is to refrain from this technique as it probably does not significantly reduce bacterial colony counts and it most certainly increases the risk of fecal spillage. When fecal spillage does occur, however, copious irrigation with a solution containing antibiotics is most appropriate. It is clear that significant fecal spillage has an adverse effect on the healing of intestinal anastomoses. This is particularly important in an intestinal anastomosis that has a tenuous blood supply.

A good vascular supply is vitally important to the healing of any type of intestinal anastomosis. Certain areas of intestinal transection are recognized as high risk in terms of their blood supply. It is important when isolating a terminal ileal segment, for instance, not to transect the ileum within 6 to 8 in. of the ileal-cecal junction. This area of ileum is supplied through an arcade from the ileal-cecal artery that may be tenuous. Similarly, in irradiated patients, there are two separate areas of small intestine that are most likely to lie within the pelvis and therefore suffer significant radiation injury. These segments are the last 2 feet of the terminal ileum and an approximately 5-foot section of small bowel located 6 feet distal to the ligament of Treitz. Three tenuous areas of blood supply are recognized in the colon. The junction of the sigmoidal and superior hemorrhoidal arteries is considered a particularly tenuous area. It should be recalled that the middle and inferior hemorrhoidal vessels originate from the terminal branches of the hypogastric artery while the sigmoidal and superior hemorrhoidal vessels are the terminal branches of the inferior mesenteric artery. Both the inferior mesenteric artery and the hypogastric artery are commonly involved with atherosclerotic changes. The practice of many urologists of hypogastric artery ligation immediately prior to cystectomy further jeopardizes bowel anastomoses in this area. The midpoints between the middle colic and right colic arteries and the middle colic and left colic arteries are also considered relatively tenuous areas.

It is important for the urologist to consider not only the blood supply to the isolated intestinal segment that they plan to use for the urinary tract reconstruction but also the blood supply of the intestinal anastomosis. In most individuals the appropriate area for intestinal transection and mesenteric division can be selected by transillumination of the mesentery with the overhead lights or a surgical headlight. This allows visualization of the vascular arcades. When transillumination is not possible due to a thick mesentery, palpation of a strong pulsating vessel may suffice. It is important not to divide more mesentery than necessary for the surgical procedure. For instance, when fashioning the standard ileal conduit, the distal mesenteric incision must usually be fairly deep in order to gain sufficient length to create the ostomy while the proximal mesenteric incision can usually be very shallow as the length is not needed in this location. Certainly, the most important finding to suggest a well-vascularized anastomosis is fresh bleeding and pink viable tissue at the site of intestinal transection. Finally, when tying intestinal sutures, the goal is to approximate, not strangulate, the tissue. A sewn intestinal anastomosis improperly performed can cause delayed necrosis of the anastomotic tissue, resulting in an intestinal leak.

The concept of correct apposition of the intestinal layers has been known for some time. The importance of serosa-to-serosa apposition was first demonstrated by Lembert when he was still a surgical resident in 1825.[16] Techniques that depended on a mucosa-to-mucosa repair or that did not provide correct apposition of like intestinal layers were shown to be unsound. As the importance of the individual layers became recognized, the submucosa emerged as the most important layer in contributing strength to intestinal anastomoses. Halsted, practicing at Johns Hopkins Hospital in the late 1800s, popularized this concept and a number of surgeons developed suturing techniques based on its application. Both everting and inverting anastomotic techniques are acceptable.

Finally, all mesenteric defects should be closed to minimize the risk of internal herniation with all types of intestinal anastomoses.

## Surgical Techniques

In the following section a number of anastomotic techniques will be described. It is less important that the reader utilize these specific techniques rather than consider them as examples of anastomotic techniques based on the previously described surgical principles. Both sutured and stapled techniques will be briefly described.

**Standard Two-Layer Sutured Enteroenterostomy.** This technique applies for both small intestinal and large intestinal anastomoses. In addition, it may be used with gastric closures after the excision of a gastric segment. Prior to the division of the bowel, noncrushing clamps should be placed across the proximal and distal intestinal segments in order to prevent fecal spillage. Care should be taken not to place the linen-shod clamps across the mesentery lest they injure the vascular supply. It is best to place a 3.0 silk stay suture at the mesenteric and antimesenteric borders of the anastomosis to facilitate the alignment and orientation of the segments to be sewn together. A row of 3.0 silk sutures utilizing a noncutting intestinal needle are placed approximately 2 mm apart on the posterior surface (Fig 8). This suture should incorporate the serosa, muscle, and submucosa but should not extend full thickness into the intestinal lumen. The suture should be tied so that there is approximation but not strangulation of the tissue. Once the posterior wall of silk sutures is tied, a 3.0 absorbable suture is placed in a running fashion from the midpoint of the posterior wall up toward both the antimesenteric and mesenteric borders and then along the anterior surface of the anastomosis. This inner-running chromic suture should incorporate the mucosa and a small amount of

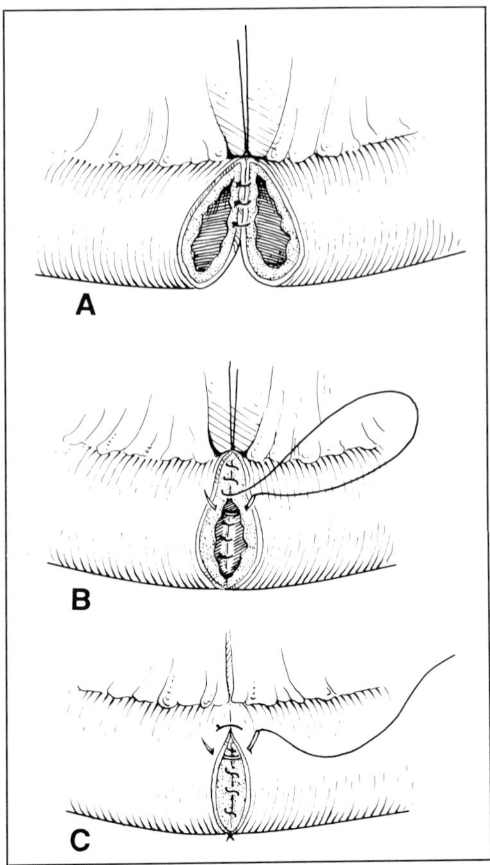


**Fig 8.** Two-layer, end-to-end, sewn intestinal anastomosis. **A,** the seromuscular layer on the back wall of the intestinal segments is sewn using interrupted 3.0 silk; **B,** the inner mucosal layer is closed on both the front and back walls using a running 3.0 chromic suture; **C,** the front wall is closed using interrupted 3.0 silk sutures.

the submucosa. Some surgical descriptions have this inner layer including all intestinal layers. As the junction of the posterior wall and anterior wall is encountered, one may convert to a Connell type of suture for the anterior closure. A simple running suture will suffice as long as the surgeon is careful not to compromise the intestinal lumen by purse-stringing the anastomosis. Once this inner layer of chromic closure is completed, an anterior wall of interrupted 3.0 silk sutures is placed in an identical fashion to the posterior layer. The patency of this anastomosis can be confirmed by palpation of the anastomosis between thumb and forefinger. In the situation where one is performing an end-to-end anastomosis between small and large intestine, it is frequently necessary to extend the incision on the small intestine along the antimesenteric border so that the length of the anastomotic suture lines at both ends of the intestine to be anastomosed are similar.

**Enteroenterostomy Using Single-Layer Sutured Anastomosis.** This technique is identical to the two-layer technique with the exception that the inner chromic layer is omitted and the silk layer incorporates a very small amount of mucosa. First, the 3.0 silk stay sutures are placed at the antimesenteric and mesenteric borders to align the ends of the severed intestine. The linen-shod clamps are again placed to minimize spillage. The 3.0 silk sutures are placed approximately 2 mm apart and are oriented so that they pass through the serosa, muscular layer, submucosa, and incorporate just a very slight amount of mucosa (Fig 9). As these are tied, a surgical assistant inverts the intestinal mucosa so that there is accurate apposition of the layers of the bowel wall. Some surgeons prefer to use a Gambee stitch when performing a single-layered closure. This facilitates the inversion of the intestinal mucosa and also assures accurate apposition of the intestinal layers (Fig 10).[17] Again, a patent anastomosis is confirmed by feeling the lumen between the thumb and forefinger. The mesenteric defect should be closed.

**Stapled Anastomoses.** A number of stapling techniques are available for fashioning intestinal anastomoses. There are three primary stapling devices that can be utilized. The first is a device available in several lengths that lays down four separate rows of staples and divides the intestinal segment between these two sets of rows of staples (GIA, linear stapler). The second device, also available in a variety of sizes, lays down two linear rows of staples (TA, thoracoabdominal stapler). It is utilized primarily for dividing an intestinal segment when it is only necessary to close off one end. The third device lays down two con-

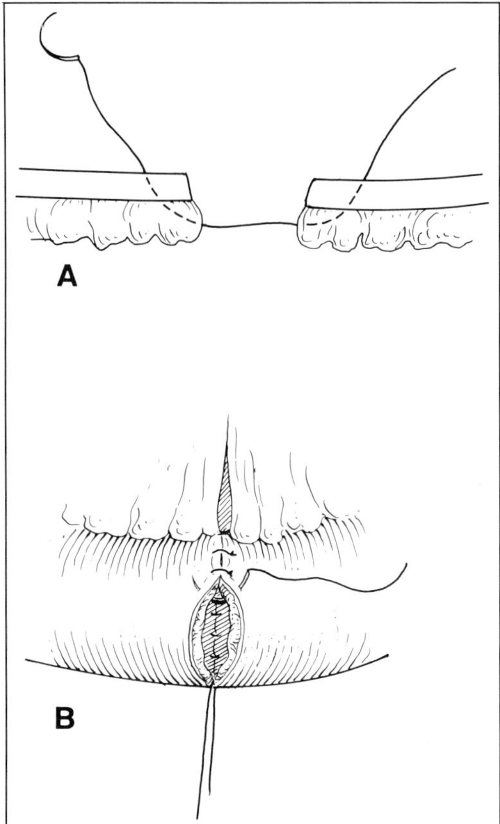


Fig 9. Single-layer intestinal anastomosis. **A**, the stitch should be triangulated so that it includes approximately 2 mm width of seromuscular layer and a small portion of the mucosa; **B**, after closing the back wall with interrupted 3.0 silk sutures, the front wall is closed in a similar fashion with interrupted 3.0 silk sutures.

centric circular rows of staples while removing the inner annulus (EEA, end-to-end anastomotic stapler). It is utilized primarily for low rectal resections and can be utilized for the performance of an end-to-side intestinal anastomosis. The theoretical benefits of a stapled anastomosis are that it provides a better blood supply to the healing margin, that it may be less time consuming to perform than a sutured anastomosis, and that a wider lumen is created. The theoretical disadvantage when stapled segments are utilized in the urinary tract is the formation of stones on staples that may be exposed to urine. While the majority of intestinal anastomoses are performed utilizing a metallic staple, absorbable staples are available. The majority of these, however, are bulky, which has limited their widespread acceptance.

A number of studies have compared the use of staplers to suturing techniques. In one large prospective trial comparing a two-layered hand-sewn closure with a stapled closure, complication rates were determined to be similar but the time required to complete the stapled anastomosis was 10 minutes less than the hand-sewn anastomosis.[18] Of note, however, when total operative time was compared between the two groups, no differences were detected. It is important to stress again, however, that the basic principles of intestinal surgery should be followed regardless of the method of anastomosis. These principles include good approximation of viable bowel, the absence of tension, adequate blood supply, adequate bowel preparation, a watertight anastomosis, avoidance of contamination, and satisfactory hemostasis. In contrast to hand-sutured techniques, stapling gives the surgeon less ability to modify his or her technique according to the peculiarities of the intestinal segment being utilized. For instance, the standard gastrointestinal anastomotic staplers have manufacturers' recommendations on the thickness limits of tissues. It behooves the surgeon to be aware of these recommendations so that stapling devices are not used in tissue that might be too thick or too thin (such as irradiated or edematous bowel) and that could lead to surgical failure.[19] Two specific stapling techniques are described below.

Fig 10. The Gambee stitch.

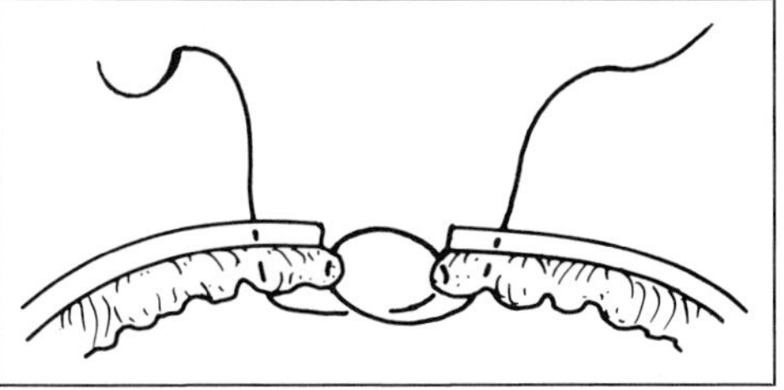

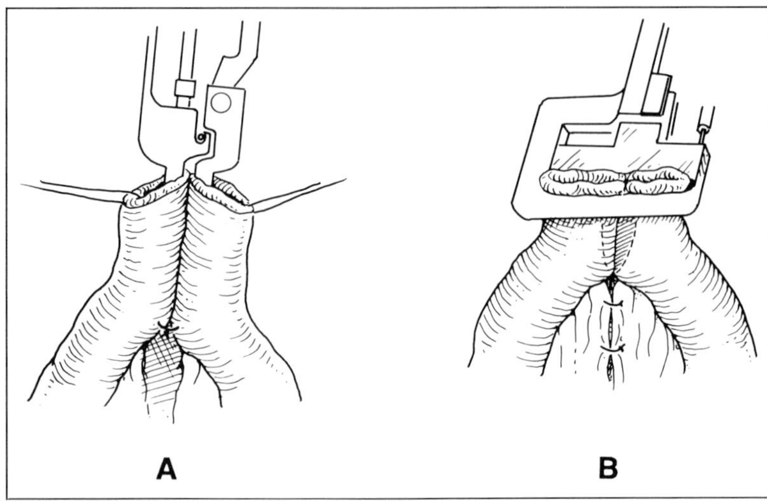


**Fig 11.** End-to-end staple intestinal anastomosis. **A,** antimesenteric borders of the intestine are approximated and held in place using interrupted silk suture. The approximated edges are then stapled and divided using a GIA stapling device; **B,** the opened end of the intestinal segments is then closed using the TA stapling device.

***End-to-End Ileoileal or Ileocolonic Staple Anastomosis.*** First, the antimesenteric borders of the intestinal segments should be aligned (Fig 11). It is convenient to place a holding suture at their juncture on the antimesenteric edge at the severed ends of the intestinal segments. In addition, several other stay sutures can be placed on the antimesenteric border several centimeters from the cut edges. The gastrointestinal anastomotic stapler is positioned with one arm down both intestinal lumens along the antimesenteric border. Care should be taken at this point to ensure that the stapling device is at the antimesenteric border and that none of the mesentery is going to be incorporated into the stapling line. The anastomotic stapler is then locked and fired. With the advancement of a knife, two separate stapled rows are placed and the anastomosis is divided between these rows. Although many surgeons place additional rows of interrupted silk sutures to reinforce the staple lines, this technique is probably unnecessary and results in narrowing of the intestinal lumen. Moreover, it negates the time-saving benefit of a stapled anastomosis. The transanastomotic stapling device is then used to close the ends of the intestinal segments and complete the anastomosis. It is critically important that the staple lines overlap and that the staple lines at this point include all of the intestinal layers. While originally there were concerns that the overlapping staple lines in this location might result in delayed necrosis and an intestinal leak, large series in humans have failed to confirm any adverse effect from this practice.

***Stapled Ileocolonic End-to-Side Anastomosis.*** The EEA circular stapling device may be used for this purpose. A convenient spot on the colon several centimeters from the transected colon is cleared of omentum and fat. Sizing devices for the ileum are available to select the proper diameter device. A 3.0 or 4.0 monofilament suture is used to place a purse string in the colon and the proximal end of an EEA stapling device is inserted through the opened colonic lumen with the post of the device placed out through an incision made in the center of the purse string (Fig 12). An additional purse string is then placed around the transected edge of the small intestinal

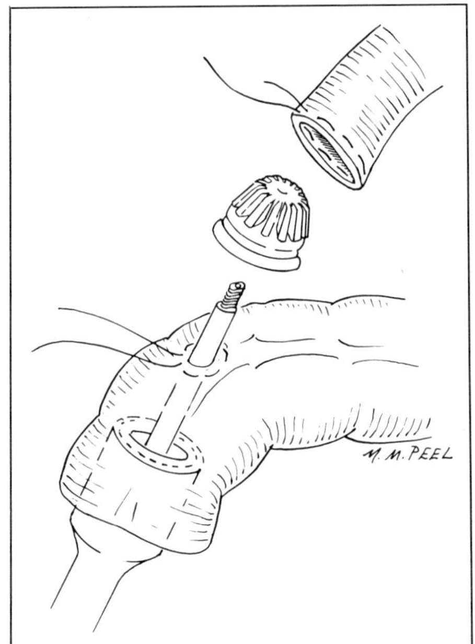


**Fig 12.** End-to-side ileocolonic anastomosis. A purse string suture is placed both in the colon and in the divided end of the ileal segment. The post of the EEA device is then placed out through an incision made in the center of the colonic purse string at which point the anvil is placed on the EEA. The anvil is then inserted into the small intestinal segment and both purse string sutures are tied. The EEA is then fired, providing a double layer of circular staples and excising a small doughnut of tissue. As the EEA is released and removed, a complete doughnut of tissue should be recovered.

lumen. The anvil of the stapling device is then attached to the post and the small intestinal segment is gently pulled over the top of this anvil, at which point this purse string suture is tied. The colonic purse string suture is then tied and the device is tightened and fired. This technique places a double circular row of staples and a doughnut of tissue is excised. The stapling device is then removed from where it was inserted in the colonic lumen. The end of the severed colon is then closed using a TA stapling device.

**Ureterointestinal Anastomosis.** A number of techniques for anastomosing the ureter to the intestine have been described. In general, colonic and gastric segments lend themselves more to tunneled nonrefluxing techniques while the thinner nature of the small intestine makes this more difficult.

***Nonrefluxing Techniques.*** The importance of a nonrefluxing ureterointestinal anastomosis is controversial in certain situations and clear cut in others. In the patient with a ureterosigmoidostomy, a refluxing ureteral anastomosis has significant morbidity due to the reflux of infected urine into the upper collecting system. The higher pressures seen with continent cutaneous urinary diversions or with orthotopic neobladders also make a nonrefluxing system preferable. With a conduit diversion, however, this issue is less clear. The sentinel work in this area by Richie and Skinner demonstrated that in dogs only 7% of nonrefluxing colon conduits demonstrated pyelonephritic scarring at 3 months while 83% of refluxing anastomoses demonstrated scarring.[20] Clinical series have failed to confirm any difference in the incidence of renal deterioration when refluxing and nonrefluxing systems are considered, however.[21] While nonrefluxing intestinal anastomoses in conduits may prevent the reflux of infected or contaminated urine into the upper collecting system, it also results in a higher incidence of ureterointestinal strictures that might account for the increased renal deterioration in some series. The purpose of constructing a nonrefluxing anastomosis is primarily to prevent bacterial colonization of the upper urinary tracts. Unfortunately, the creation of a successful antirefluxing anastomosis in a urinary conduit does not prevent bacterial colonization of the renal pelvis. Three quarters of patients with nonrefluxing enterocystoplasties and an additional patient with a nonrefluxing colon conduit had positive renal pelvic cultures on percutaneous renal pelvic aspiration in one series.[22] Consequently, the benefit of a nonrefluxing anastomosis in the adult diversion is questionable. In children or young adults in whom prolonged follow-up is likely, however, there may be a benefit.

Multiple techniques for the creation of a submucosal tunnel in the colon have been described. Colonic reimplantations may be fashioned extraluminally or transluminally. With either technique, an incision, typically in the tenia, is fashioned and the mucosa is dissected off of the seromuscular tissue. Several authors have described injection of saline submucosally to facilitate this dissection. Once the mucosa is dissected off of the seromuscular layers, the spatulated ureter is anastomosed in a full-thickness fashion to the mucosa (Fig 13). The ureter may be brought in through one of the ends[23] of the seromuscular incision or may be brought in laterally through a separate incision in the seromuscular layer.[24] In either situation, it is important to have a tunnel length that is approximately 4 to 5 times the ureteral diameter. The anastomosis itself should be fashioned with absorbable suture material. It is helpful to secure the ureter along its course in the tunnel as the tenia is closed to prevent separation and to maintain the tunnel length should tension occur. A transcolonic technique has also been described (Fig 14).[25] This type of technique may be particularly helpful during the performance of a ureteral reimplantation in a continent colonic reservoir. First, a small enterotomy is made and the ureter is brought into the intestinal lumen. From the luminal side, a submucosal tunnel is fashioned. The ureter is then placed through this submucosal tunnel, spatulated, and sutured to the mucosa.

Several techniques for the fashioning of a nonrefluxing anastomosis of the ureter to the small bowel have been reported. The technique of LeDuc et al establishes a nonrefluxing anastomosis by bringing the ureter intraluminally and then laying it in a trough that has been denuded of mucosa (Fig 15).[26] To accomplish this, however, an incision must be made that is approximately 4 to 5 cm along the antimesenteric border in order to gain adequate exposure. The spatulated ureter is laid in this mucosal trough and anastomosed to the inner lumen of the small bowel using interrupted absorbable sutures. It is then secured at its entrance point at the enterotomy and after the implantation of the second ureter the bowel wall is closed. The mucosa then reepithelializes over the top of this implanted ureter. Success rates of 85% and stricture rates of only 1.5% have been reported with this technique.[26] Another technique de-

**Fig 13.** Extraluminal ureterocolonic nonrefluxing anastomosis. **A,** the tinea is incised and lateral flaps are developed. A small incision through the mucosa is made into the intestinal lumen; **B,** the ureteral mucosal anastomosis is then fashioned using interrupted fine absorbable sutures; **C,** the tinea is then closed over the top of the implanted ureter; **D,** an alternative technique is to bring the ureters through the lateral tineal flaps. The anastomosis is then fashioned and the flaps are pulled back over as in **C.** This allows both ureters to be implanted through a single tineal incision.

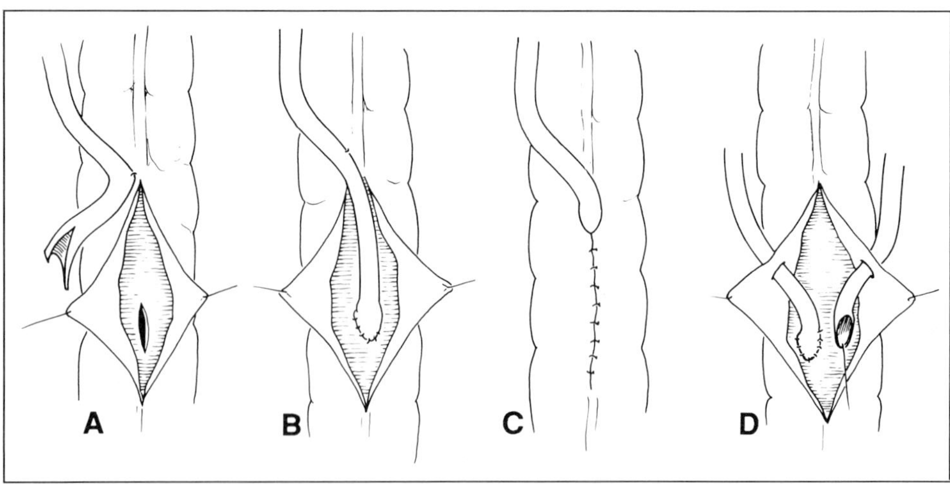

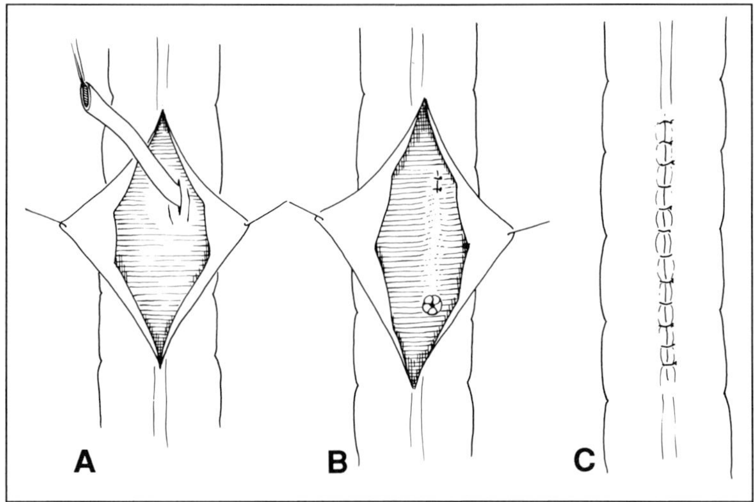


**Fig 14.** Transcolonic nonrefluxing ureteral reimplantation. **A,** the colon has been opened and the ureter has been brought into the colonic lumen through a posterior enterotomy; **B,** a submucosal tunnel is then made and the ureter is pulled down through this, at which point it is spatulated and anastomosed distally and the original enterotomy is closed using interrupted absorbable suture; **C,** the anterior enterotomy is then closed.

scribed involves the fashioning of a nipple valve from the spatulated ureter (Fig 16).[27] In this technique, an approximately 0.5-cm longitudinal incision is made in the ureter to spatulate it and the ureteral wall is turned back on itself, creating a nipple. The nipple should be approximately twice as long as it is wide. This is then sutured in this po-

**Fig 15.** Camey–LeDuc technique for nonrefluxing ureteroileal anastomosis. **A,** approximately 4–6 cm of antimesenteric ileal wall is opened and an approximately 4-cm incision in the posterior mucosa is made by sharp dissection; **B,** the ureter is then brought through a full-thickness enterotomy at the top of this mucosal incision, at which point it is secured using fine interrupted absorbable suture to the seromuscular layer. The ureter is then placed in this trough, which has been denuded of mucosa; **C,** the ureter is then secured in place along this mucosal trough using interrupted fine absorbable sutures; **D,** A cross-sectional appearance of the ureter once trough has been created.

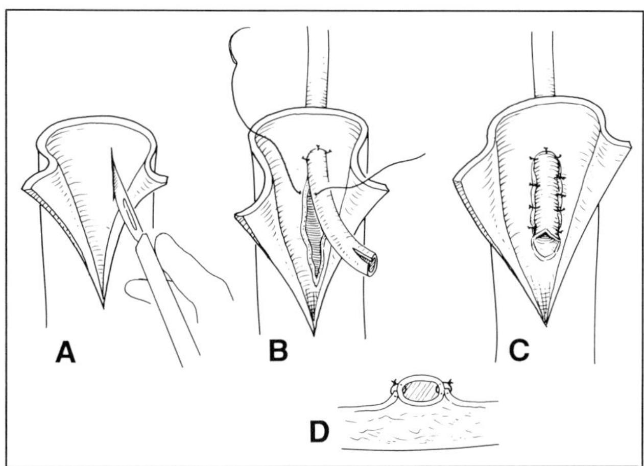

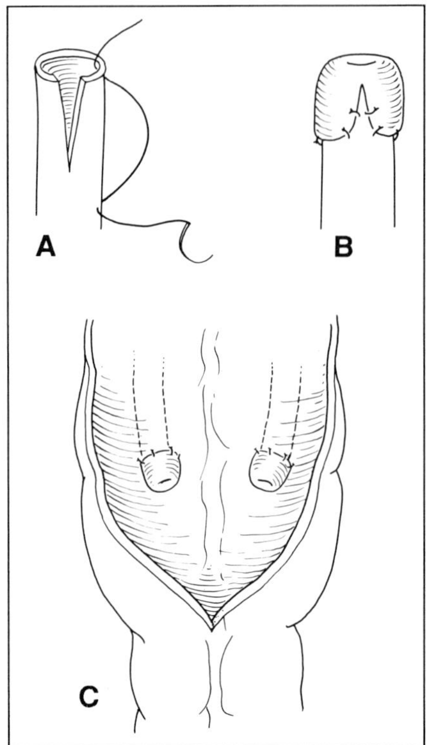


**Fig 16.** Ureteral nipple valve construction. **A,** the ureter is spatulated on one wall and then a suture is used to create the nipple effect; **B,** appearance of the ureter after the nipple valve has been created; **C,** appearance of the ureters once they have been implanted into the intestine in a nipple fashion.

sition with absorbable sutures and placed through the enterotomy where it is sutured to the intestine. In most series, the results in terms of preventing reflux with this technique are not as good as those with other techniques; however, there appears to be a relatively low incidence of stenosis.

An alternative technique for fashioning a nonrefluxing anastomosis is to create a nipple valve from the intestinal segment rather than the ureter. This can be accomplished by cleaning the ileal segment of mesentery. Because of vessels that run longitudinally within the submucosa of the small intestine, up to 8 cm of small intestine can be cleaned of its mesentery. The midpoint of this section of intestine that has been cleaned of mesentery is then grasped on the luminal side with a Babcock clamp and inverted on itself (Fig 17). The intestine must then be sutured in this position either intraluminally or at the seromuscular surface to prevent eversion of the nipple over time. It is also helpful to place a strip of polyglycolic acid mesh on the external surface of this inverted nipple valve to prevent eversion. A number of stapling techniques to prevent this eversion have also been described and are covered in the chapter on continent urinary diversions (Volume 2, Chapter 6). At this point, the ureters are implanted in a refluxing fashion proximal to the nipple.

***The Refluxing Anastomosis.*** A refluxing ureteral intestinal anastomosis will suffice in many circumstances. Two basic techniques have been described. The original Bricker anastomosis[28] involved excising a full-thickness segment of intestinal wall (Fig 18). The ureter is then spatulated and anastomosed in a full-thickness–to–full-thickness fashion to the intestinal wall. This anastomosis may be done in an interrupted or a continuous fashion. If this is accomplished in a continuous fashion, it is best to place the original stitches in the heel of the spatulated ureter and to run the anastomosis toward the toe. An alternative approach described by Wallace[29] involves first suturing the medial walls of the ureter together with absorbable sutures (Fig 19). A single enterotomy is then made and the lateral edges of the ureters are anastomosed to the intestinal segment. The advantage of this technique is a lower incidence of stricture compared to the Bricker anastomosis in which two separate anastomoses are fashioned.

***Complications.*** The complications of any form of ureterointestinal anastomosis are urinary leak, development of an anastomotic stricture, and, in the case of a nonrefluxing anastomosis, the persistence of reflux. The majority of ureterointestinal reimplantations have leakage rates of 2% to 3%. Refluxing anastomotic techniques have stricture rates of 4% to 20%, although this rate is considerably less with the Wallace technique. Nonrefluxing techniques

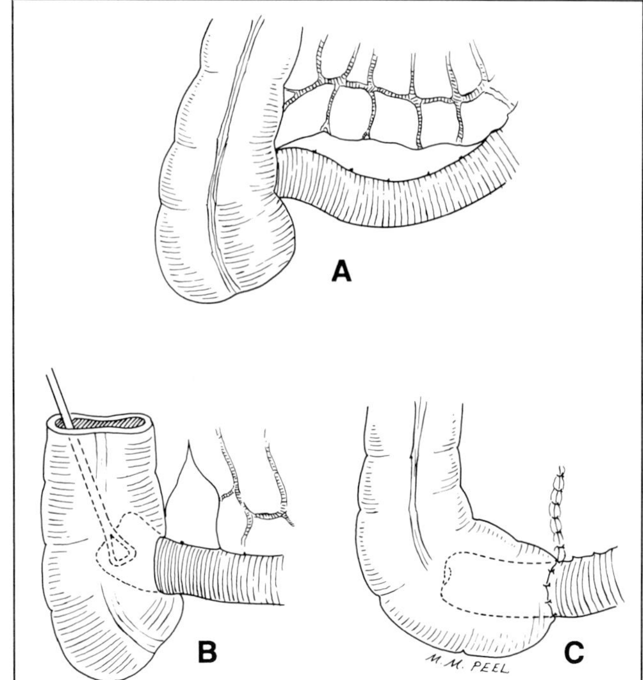


**Fig 17.** Ileocecal intussusception. **A,** approximately 6–8 cm of the terminal ileum is separated from its mesenteric blood supply; **B,** a Babcock clamp is used to grasp this ileal segment at the midportion of the ileum, which has been separated from its mesentery, and then to intussuscept the ileum into the cecum; **C,** the intussuscepted ileum is then secured in place using interrupted fine absorbable sutures from the ileal to cecal seromuscular layers.

**Fig 18.** Standard Bricker ureteroileal anastomosis. **A,** first the ureter is tacked with a fine absorbable suture to the butt end of the ileal conduit; **B,** a full-thickness incision is then made through the antimesenteric border of the ileal segment and the ureter is spatulated; **C,** the ureteral anastomosis is then fashioned using fine absorbable interrupted sutures. Generally the ureter is stented with a silastic stent.

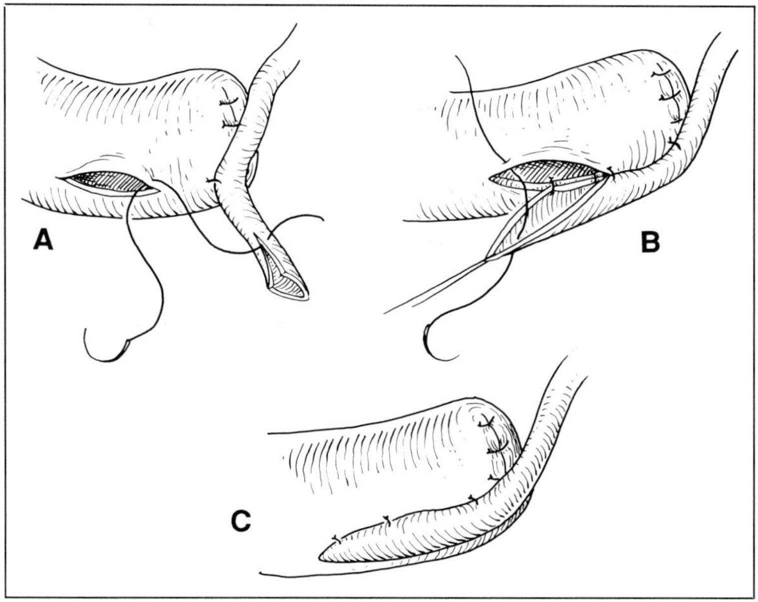

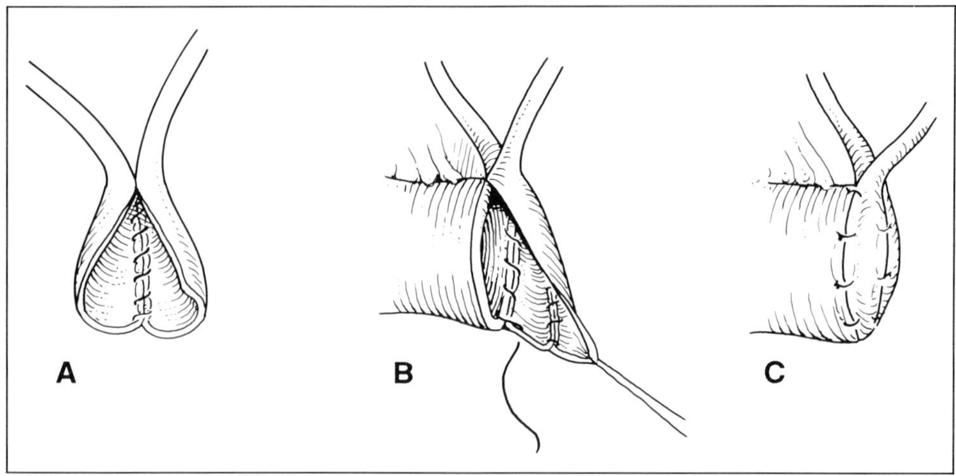


**Fig 19.** Wallace ureteroileal anastomosis. **A,** first the ureters are spatulated and the medial edges of the spatulated ureters are sewn together using interrupted absorbable sutures; **B,** the lateral and distal edges of the joined ureters are then anastomosed to the opened end of the ileal conduit; **C,** appearance once the anastomosis is complete.

have a higher incidence of ureteral stricture ranging from 14% to 25%. The literature suggests that the use of soft silastic stents through an anastomosis for a period of time postoperatively diminishes the incidence of both strictures and leaks.[30,31] In contrast, in older series using nonsilastic stents there is a significant incidence of anastomotic stricture. Currently available data suggest that a soft-stenting ureteral catheter should be used perioperatively.

## CONDUIT DIVERSIONS

### Ileal and Colon Conduits

The history of the development of the ileal conduit is quite interesting and instructional, particularly for those who consider themselves aficionados of the "newer forms of urinary diversion."[28,32] In 1949, Bricker reported on his attempts to use the ileocecal segment in order to create continent urinary diversions. At that time, the primary form of urinary diversion after removal of the bladder was bilateral ureterosigmoidostomy. Significant metabolic problems with urinary diversion into the intact sigmoid colon were just being recognized.[33] Bricker's primary interest in his original publication was in the development of a continent means of urinary diversion in patients in whom ureterosigmoidostomy was not possible. He employed two different surgical procedures using isolated ileocecal segments. The first involved implantation of the ureters into the ileal limb and using the appendix as a stoma through which a catheter continuously dwelled in the cecum and was intermittently drained. In the other procedure, the ureters were implanted in the cecum and the terminal ileum was brought out as a stoma. With both of these procedures, he was unable to successfully achieve complete continence. The first ileal conduit was reported by Bricker in 1950,[28] and in this specific incidence the tumor fortuitously involved both the sigmoid colon and the cecum, so that urinary diversion through an ileocecal segment was not possible. Consequently, the only available intestinal segment was an isolated segment of terminal ileum. The other often overlooked but equally important point at this time is that suitable ostomy appliances were just being developed. Prior to their development a cutaneous urostomy was not possible.

Bricker's initial results with the ileal conduit were most encouraging. This appeared to be a superior form of urinary diversion such that Bricker remarked in his publication in 1950 that "at the present time we are ready to drop the project of trying to develop a continent intra-abdominal pouch in favor of this method which provides for prompt elimination of the urine without stagnation into an extra-abdominal urinary reservoir which is convenient, sanitary, and under the control of the patient." He went on to remark that "we believe that the day of 'dunking' and 'tunneling' ureters is past." It appears that we have now come full circle.

**Surgical Techniques.** First, an approximately 6- to 8-in. length of terminal ileum is isolated. The small intestinal continuity should be reestablished according to the preference of the surgeon. The butt end of the ileal conduit should then be closed using absorbable sutures. If a stapling device was used to isolate this ileal segment, the staple lines should not be inverted with a reinforcing layer of sutures as this exposes the metallic sutures to the urinary stream. Stone formation on staples is uncommon as long as the normal everting staple line is not inverted by the placement of this additional layer of sutures. Typically, the ileal conduit comes to rest in the right lower quadrant with the butt end of the conduit at the sacral promontory. The left ureter should usually be tunneled underneath the sigmoid mesentery if the sigmoid colon is still present. After the left ureter is brought posterior to the sigmoid mesentery, bilateral ureteroenterostomies are performed. It is generally best to spatulate the ureter to minimize the formation of a cicatrix. Both running and interrupted suture techniques are reasonable with no data supporting one technique over the other. The placement of a tacking suture from the butt end of the ileal conduit to the sacral promontory will prevent the development of tension on the anastomoses at a later point. It is critically important that the conduit be oriented in an isoperistaltic fashion. The distal end of the ileal conduit is then brought out through a previously selected site on the anterior abdominal wall. This may be done in either the right or the left lower quadrants as well as the upper quadrants. Generally, the mobility of an ileal conduit is such that there is a great deal of flexibility in the selection of the site for the stoma. In fashioning the stoma, a circular segment of skin should be excised while the subcutaneous fat is bluntly separated. It is best to make a cruciate incision in the anterior rectus fascia. The distal end of the ileal conduit is then brought through the fascia and secured to the fascia either at the peritoneal surface or at the level of the anterior rectus fascia.

The development of the stoma is a critically important step in this process as many of the long-term problems that patients have with ileal conduits are the result of this step in the operation. Most enterostomal therapists prefer an everted rosebud type of stoma. This is accomplished utilizing an everting suture that goes from the skin to the seromuscular layer and then to the cut end of the ileal segment (Brooke's technique) (Fig 20). It is critically important to not place the seromuscular part of this stitch too proximal as it will cause inversion of the skin around the stoma making the use of a flat ostomy appliance very difficult. This eversion of the stoma should be accomplished using an interrupted suture technique. An alternative to the Brooke technique is to create a loop stoma as originally described by Turnbull (Fig 21).[34] There are several advantages to this technique. In the obese individual with a foreshortened mesentery, the use of a loop end ileostomy type of stoma usually yields increased conduit length. This frequently may be necessary to allow the conduit to reach the skin level. Once the bowel is brought to the skin level, it may be opened either transversely or longitudinally to create a rosebud stoma. Studies that have compared loop end stomas to end ileostomy stomas report a lower incidence of stomal stenosis with the former technique.[35]

**Results.** A number of publications have appeared on the long-term results of ureteroileal and ureterocolonic conduit diversions. There are both immediate and long-term complications. The immediate complications include wound infection (11% to 30%), acute pyelonephritis (1.5% to 22%), ureteral obstruction (1.8% to 18%), and operative mortality (3.3% to

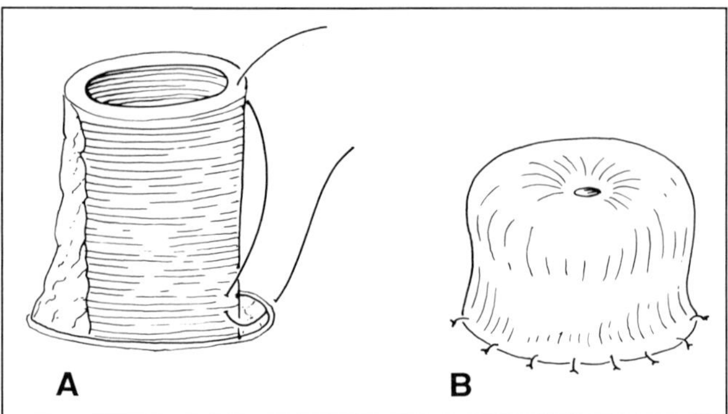


**Fig 20.** Standard Brooke technique for creation of bud stoma. **A,** an absorbable suture is used to go through the dermal layer to the seromuscular layer of the bowel and then out to the end of the divided intestinal segment; this everts the segment and creates a bud stoma (**B**). Care should be taken not to place the suture too proximally on the ileal conduit, as this will invert the skin edges and make the fitting of an appliance difficult.

14%).[36] In most series that review ureterointestinal conduits performed in conjunction with radical exenterative surgery, the creation of the urinary diversion is associated with a very significant part of the complications in these procedures.

The long-term complications of ileal con-

**Fig 21.** Turnbull technique for creation of a stoma. **A,** a Babcock clamp is used to grasp the ileal segment on its antimesenteric border. This provides additional length for the creation of a bud stoma; **B,** once the ileal segment is brought out through the stoma site, it can be opened longitudinally or transversely and a bud stoma can be created; **C,** note the presence of two lumens on such a stoma, one of which is blind-ending.

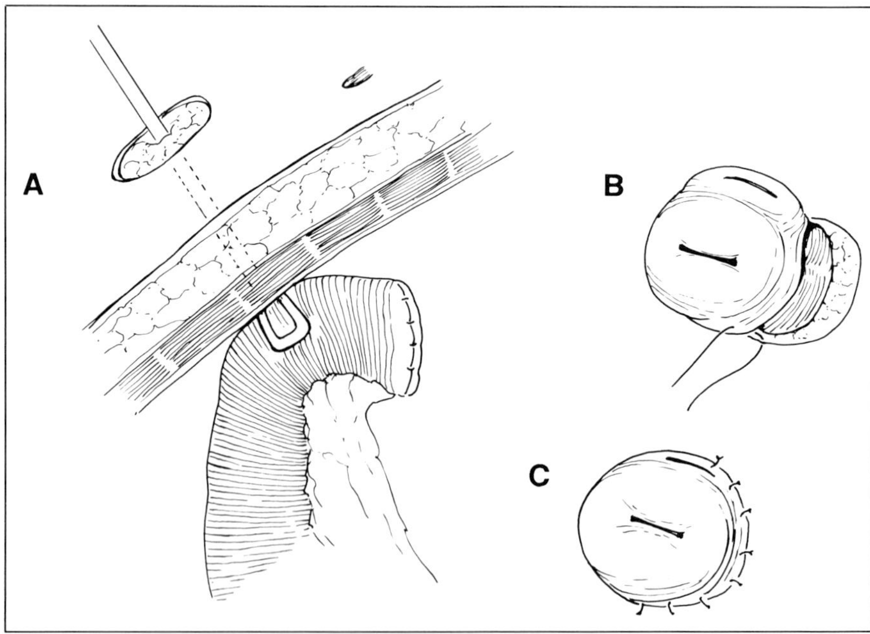

duits in adults are perhaps even more disappointing. It should be expected that up to 15% of patients will develop an intestinal obstruction, 6% to 10% will demonstrate radiographic findings consistent with chronic pyelonephritis, 6% to 8% will develop nonfunctioning kidneys, 17% of the renal units will develop hydronephrosis, 2% to 18% of patients will develop ureteral obstruction, 3% to 6% will develop stomal stenosis, and 3% to 5% will develop renal calculi. These results constitute a particular problem in children. Multiple series have reported the long-term outcome of children undergoing ileal conduit urinary diversion for both benign and malignant conditions and the long-term complication rates are extremely high (Table 2). Stomal stenosis represents the biggest problem and may actually be lessened by the currently available stomal appliances. However, of greatest concern is the fact that the long-term outcome in terms of preservation of renal function is not good. The series by Orr et al,[42] Dunn et al,[43] Shapiro et al,[44] and Koch et al[45] all have follow-ups in excess of 10 years. With this length of follow-up, renal deterioration occurs in 20% to 60% of patients with a significant percentage of patients in many series progressing to end-stage renal disease.

Studies that have compared their more recently diverted patients to their long-term diverted patients have shown a progressive decrease in renal function over time following ileal conduit urinary diversion. These changes may exert other untoward effects on these children in the long term. In the series by Malek et al,[46] 42 children were examined for metabolic abnormalities after chronic urinary diversion. Approximately 70% of patients demonstrated some hyperchloremia and/or mild to moderate acidosis. General height and growth rates in these children were also examined and typically children who had some element of azotemia or problems with stomal obstruction or calculi experienced decreased growth rates. A more recent study examining these children in depth with regard to their general health and growth found diminished linear growth rates measured by upper extremity morphometric parameters.[45]

Because of the problems with ileal conduits, nonrefluxing sigmoid conduits became popular in the 1970s. Unfortunately, the long-term results in terms of preservation of the upper urinary tract showed only modest improvement with sigmoid conduits. Technical difficulties with the ureteral intestinal nonrefluxing implantation may have accounted for some of these problems. In series such as the one from Althausen et al[47] and Husmann et al,[48] where the incidence of persistence reflux after urinary diversion is relatively low (less than 10%), the incidence of renal deterioration is similar to or slightly better than long-term follow-up with ileal conduits (Table 3). Therefore, while this remains controversial, it seems prudent to at least attempt to construct a nonrefluxing anastomosis in patients in whom a long life

**TABLE 2. Long-Term Follow-up of Ileal Conduits in Children (%)**

| Series | Stomal Stenosis | Ureteroileal Stricture | Renal Deterioration | Calculi | Intestinal Obstruction |
|---|---|---|---|---|---|
| Middleton et al[37] | 56 | 9 | 38 | 7 | 4 |
| Arnarson et al[38] | 35 | 12 | 11 | 8 | 15 |
| Schwartz et al[39] | 38 | 12 | 16 | 15 | 14 |
| Pitts et al[40] | 24 | 8 | 14 | 8 | — |
| Cass et al[41] | 19 | 6 | 37 | 2 | 1 |
| Orr et al[42] | 33 | 7 | 61 | 14 | — |
| Dunn et al[43] | 37 | 4 | 28 | 15 | — |
| Shapiro et al[44] | 34 | 20 | 19 | 8 | 13 |
| Koch et al[45] | 37 | 17 | 57 | 43 | — |

**TABLE 3. Long-Term Follow-up of Nonrefluxing Colon Conduits (%)**

| Series | Stomal Stenosis | Uretero-colonic Stricture | Reflux | Renal Deterioration | Calculi | Intestinal Obstruction |
|---|---|---|---|---|---|---|
| Althausen et al[47] | 3 | 9 | <10 | 9 | 4 | 6 |
| Husmann et al[48] | 8 | 14 | 8 | 26 | — | — |
| Elder et al[49] | 62 | 22 | 58 | 50 | 15 | — |
| Morales et al[50]* | — | 13 | — | 26 | 4 | 7 |
| Hill et al[51] | 34 | — | 48 | 36 | 2 | 2 |

* Includes some refluxing ureteral-intestinal anastomoses.

expectancy is anticipated. However, the advantage of a nonrefluxing anastomosis is certainly modest.

Mansson et al[52] conducted a study with long-term follow-up of ileal conduits, comparing them to both refluxing and nonrefluxing colon conduits as well as continent cecal reservoirs. In all populations studied, there was a gradual decrease in glomerular filtration rate over time that was relatively mild. They were unable to detect any advantages or disadvantages to any form of urinary diversion. Consequently, the changes that are seen may be due less to the specific surgical technique employed rather than to the fact that the urine was forced to drain through or into an intestinal segment.

Difficulties with the intestinal stoma are without question the most common complications to occur after urinary diversion through an intestinal conduit. These include bleeding and dermatitis at the stoma, the development of parastomal hernias or prolapse, and, most commonly, stomal obstruction and stenosis. Many of these complications can be reduced by proper construction of the stoma. Preoperative evaluation by either the surgeon or the enterostomal therapist is critical. As mentioned previously, the conduit should traverse the rectus sheath. Conduits that are located lateral to the rectus sheath are particularly prone to the development of parastomal hernias. The location for the stoma should be selected by examination of the patient in the recumbent, sitting, and standing positions. The stomal location should be a sufficient distance from any skin folds or previous scars. The conduit should not be angulated as it traverses the rectus sheath or subcutaneous tissues. It is also important not to place a stoma at or just above the belt line. This causes compression of the collection device or pressure directly over the stoma and will result in appliance leakage.

The most common problem with urinary stomas is the development of stomal stenosis, which is generally attributed to a parastomal dermatitis. This dermatitis is felt to result from exposure of the stoma and peristomal skin to a persistent alkaline urine.[53–55] The use of the currently available stoma appliances when properly fitted will minimize the incidence of these complications. A number of techniques have been reported for the acidification of the patient's urine. These include the administration of oral vitamin C, the use of an aspirin tablet placed in the ostomy bag, and rinsing of the ostomy appliance with a vinegar solution. These techniques may all be helpful.

Parastomal hernias generally occur when the conduit is not placed directly through the anterior rectus sheath. They usually occur at and around the site where the mesentery traverses the abdominal wall. While frequently asymptomatic, there is a tendency for them to generally enlarge over time and intestinal obstruction may occur. These hernias may be repaired by laparotomy through the patient's original incision with closure of the abdominal wall defect. If the rectus sheath was not traversed, the stoma site should be changed. It is this author's preference to approach most parastomal hernias through an infra- or suprastomal transverse incision. This affords excellent exposure of the hernia site, minimizes intraperitoneal dissection, and allows one to accomplish a secure repair. The use of reinforcing permanent mesh materials is rarely necessary; however, the use of polyglycolic acid mesh materials may be helpful in preventing early recurrence of the hernias.

## ILEAL URETERS

The first ileal interposition procedure for ureteral replacement was performed in the human by Schoemaker in 1909 and described in a report by Melnikoff in 1912.[56] Schoemaker had performed this procedure for a woman with tuberculous ureteral strictures. He accomplished this in two stages, first by the creation of a diverting ileal conduit followed 1½ years later by urinary undiversion accomplished by placing the conduit into the bladder.

Clark and Mahoney were the first investigators in this country to use ileum as a ureteral replacement in an experimental study in dogs.[57] More recent studies have been conducted to examine the effect of the ileal length and the need for a nonrefluxing anastomosis. It has been suggested that the use of a refluxing ileal ureter might predispose the upper urinary tract to the high intravesical pressures. Martinez et al[58] demonstrated that under normal and diuretic conditions renal pelvic pressures were no different than those of controls. However, during voiding, there was an increase in intrapelvic pressures on the side with the ileal ureter. Fortunately, this did not result in morphologic changes in the kidney. Hinman and Oppenheimer[59] suggested that the ileal ureter actually acts as a capacitance vessel that dampens any detrusor pressures and prevents transmission to the renal pelvis. They also demonstrated that when the pressure at the distal end of the ileal segment exceeds 15 cm $H_2O$, the ileal segment is no longer capable of directional fluid transport. Above this pressure, peristalsis will cease. In addition, antegrade peristalsis is more effective in a longer segment. Segments 18 to 20 cm in length effectively block the retrograde transmission of detrusor pressures until the detrusor pressure exceeds 15 cm $H_2O$. These findings emphasize the importance of only using ileal ureters in the situation where there is normal detrusor function and a compliant bladder. A number of investigators have advocated the use of tapered ileal segments to minimize fluid and electrolyte shifts. Experimental studies in dogs[60] have not demonstrated any benefit to tapering ileal segments with regard to fluid and electrolyte shifts.

Ureteral substitution with ileal segment is appropriate for most causes of extensive ureteral loss, transitional cell carcinoma of the ureter in solitary renal units, and severe metabolic stone disease. Ureteral replacement with ileum should be used as a last resort.

### Surgical Techniques

The surgical approach can be through a midline transperitoneal incision or through a sigmoid-shaped incision that starts from the tip of the eleventh or twelfth rib and courses anteriomedially down toward the midline (Fig 22). First, the proximal ureter above the abnormal area should be dis-

**Fig 22.** Positioning an incision for a patient for an extraperitoneal approach for the construction of an ileo-ureter.

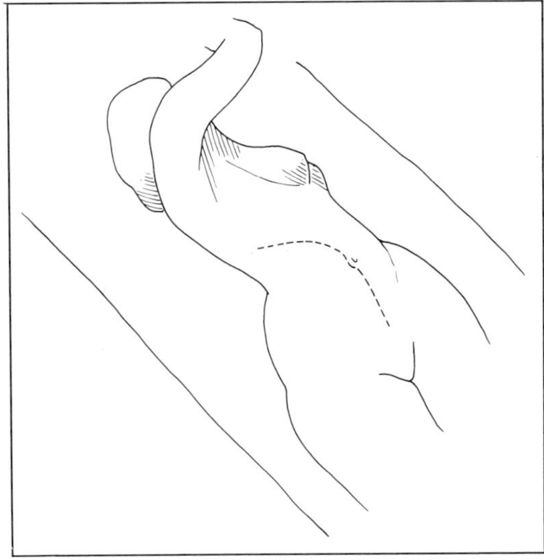

sected free and divided in an area where it appears to have a good blood supply. In cases where the ileal ureter is being performed because of severe stone disease, the anastomosis should be directly to the renal pelvis (Fig 23). The length of the ureteral deficit should then be estimated. An appropriate length of terminal ileum should be isolated on a healthy vascular pedicle. The enteroenterostomy is fashioned by standard techniques. Frequently, it is difficult to straighten out the ileal segment in order to allow it to reach both the renal pelvis and the bladder. Several steps may be helpful in this regard. Because of the longitudinal submucosal vessels in the ileum, it is possible to divide the mesentery along the distal and/or proximal end to the bowel in order to straighten out the ileal segment. This division should obviously be minimized. In addition, both the uretero- or pyeloileal anastomosis and the ileovesical anastomosis may be performed to the antimesenteric border of the intestine. This will frequently achieve a few extra centimeters in length. The performance of a vesicopsoas hitch if possible is also desirable. This allows the anastomosis between the bowel and the bladder to be performed in a fixed orientation so that kinking and obstruction of the ileal segment does not occur with bladder filling. For left ureteral substitutions, a small defect should be made in the sigmoid mesocolon and the ileal segment should be brought through this defect so that it lies in the retroperitoneal space. For right ureteral replacements, the cecum and ascending colon should be mobilized so that the ileal segment can be placed posterior to this segment of bowel. First, the proximal ureteroileal anastomosis is fashioned by spatulating the ureter or renal pelvis along its anterior surface. A single layer of full-thickness anastomosis is then fashioned using an absorbable suture of the surgeon's choice. The ileovesical anastomosis is then fashioned in an identical fashion. While a nonrefluxing ureteroileal or ileovesical reimplantation may intuitively seem desirable, the experimental studies and clinical studies do not confirm the necessity of this. The anastomosis should be stented and it is preferable to have a nephrostomy tube left indwelling postoperatively. It is critically important to close all of the mesenteric defects after this procedure. A horizontal position of the isolated ileal segment makes this particularly prone to the development of internal hernias.

**Fig 23.** Anastomosis of the ileo-ureter direct to the renal pelvis.

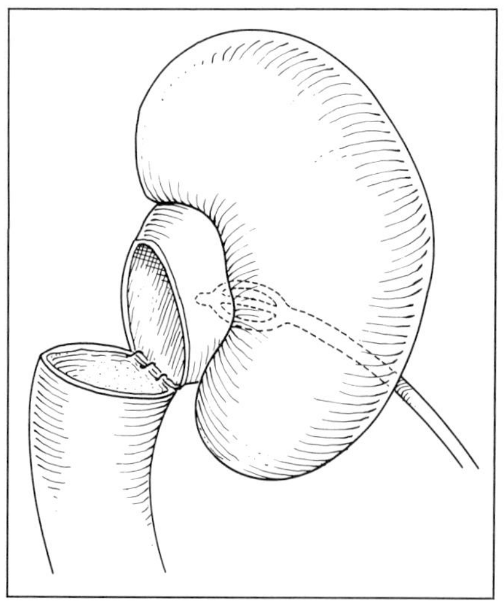

## Clinical Series

The group at the University of California at Los Angeles reported their first four cases and a review of the literature using isolated ileal segments for ureteral repair in 1956.[61] This same group published the largest series in the literature in 1979 when they reported on 92 cases in which the ureter was replaced by ileum.[62] Indications for the operation in this series included recurrent urinary calculi in 44 patients, ureteral stricture or fistula in 26 patients, ureteral carcinoma involving solitary kidneys in 2 patients, and a variety of congenital abnormalities in 11 patients. These patients were assessed in terms of perioperative renal function changes and the radiographic appearance of their upper urinary tracts. Of those patients with a preoperative serum creatinine less than 2 mg/dL, 88% had successful outcomes. Of their 11 patients with serum creatinines in excess of 2 mg/dL preoperatively, 45% developed acid–base abnormalities and subsequently required conversion to a cutaneous ileal diversion. Of note, 55 patients were evaluated by cystogram and 40 had vesicoileal reflux. In patients with vesicoileal reflux, the serum creatinine and the pyelographic appearance was unchanged or improved in 98%. In contrast, in the 15 patients who had no postoperative vesicoileal reflux, only 60% did well. The technical points that were emphasized in this report were that (1) the bladder must work properly and be capable of effective emptying, (2) intestinal segments should be anastomosed in an isoperistaltic fashion, (3) a nephrostomy tube should be placed intraoperatively to protect the anastomosis, and (4) the intestinal segment should be retroperitonealized. In addition, they recommended that this procedure not be performed in patients with preoperative serum creatinine levels greater than 2 mg/dL.

Several subsequent studies have confirmed the efficacy of the replacement of the ureter with ileal segments.[63–69] There have also been a number of series that have reported significant failure rates following ureteral replacement with ileum. Creevy[70] reported on 14 cases of ureteral replacement with ileum and found four failures. In these failures, he noted increasing dilatation of the ileal segment with the development of serum electrolyte changes and renal insufficiency. Tanagho[71] also reported on five patients in whom an ileal replacement of the ureter resulted in progressive dilatation of the ileal segment followed by renal deterioration and serum electrolyte and acid–base abnormalities. In a report on the use of the ileoureter for bilharzial stricture, Bazeed et al[72] reported deterioration in renal function in 34% of patients and pyelographic deterioration of renal function in 44%. Renal function was very poorly preserved in patients who had low creatinine clearances preoperatively.

Recollection of the experimental studies previously cited in this section allow one to draw some conclusions regarding the pitfalls of ureteral replacement with ileum. Ileal segments do not function well in the presence of high urinary pressures. In the series of ureteral substitutions with ileal segments reported by Boxer et al,[62] the ileal segments were used primarily for isolated ureteral defects in patients with no bladder pathology. In patients with congenital lesions of the ureter and associated bladder abnormalities, the results are uniformly poor. In the series reported by Tanagho in which all five patients had unsatisfactory results, all of these patients had some type of bladder pathology such as a neurologic lesion, congenital abnormalities, or scarring from previous surgery. Moreover, in the studies on the use of ileal ureter following bilharzial stricture disease, some degree of bladder abnormality was likely in most patients. The large series from Boxer et al demonstrates that in the properly selected patient with a normal detrusor and bladder outlet, ileal segments can function extremely well even in the presence of vesicoileal reflux. The patient with preexisting renal insufficiency is unquestionably at increased risk of developing electrolyte abnormalities including hyperchloremic metabolic acidosis. This acidosis can generally be controlled by alkali replacement in the form of bicarbonate or citrate salts. It is highly probable that reducing the mucosal surface area by tapering the ileal segment or using as short an ileal segment as possible will reduce these aberrations. Actual laboratory evidence for this concept is lacking, however. The concept of creating a nonrefluxing ileovesical anastomosis remains controversial. In the absence of high intravesical pressures, vesicoileal ureteral reflux has not been demonstrated to have any adverse effect. In the patient with high intravesical pressures, this condition should be addressed either pharmacologically with anticholinergic medication or with intestinal cystoplasty at the same time as the ureteral replacement with ileum.

## AUGMENTATION CYSTOPLASTY

Intestinal segments have been used to augment the capacity of the bladder since the late 19th century. The first ileal cystoplasty was performed in 1899 by Mikulicz.[73] Since that time, multiple surgical techniques with various intestinal segments have been utilized for the reconstruction of the bladder. Many early investigators demonstrated the efficacy of augmentation cystoplasty in patients who had low bladder capacities attributed to neurogenic causes, radiation cystitis, and tuberculosis.[74–78] Unfortunately, most of these studies preceded the widespread acceptance of clean intermittent catheterization. The majority of the failures reported in these early series were due to incomplete emptying and either radiographic deterioration of the upper urinary tract or progressive azotemia and electrolyte abnormalities. Many of these failures may have been due to poor emptying of the augmented bladder. The concept of clean intermittent catheterization gained widespread acceptance after the initial report of Lapides et al in 1972[79] and the follow-up report in 1975.[80] With the acceptance of clean intermittent catheterization, augmentation cystoplasty gained increasing popularity and it has found widespread use for the management of both children and adults with neurogenic bladder disease. There appears to be little difference in results depending on which intestinal segment is used; rather the selection of the intestinal segment depends more on the par-

**Fig 24.** Construction of a cup patch ileocystoplasty. **A,** first the ileum is opened on its antimesenteric border; **B,** the medial edges of the ileum, which has been folded into a U-shaped pattern, are then anastomosed; **C,** the ileum is then folded in a cephalad-to-caudad direction to create a cup effect; **D,** the cup patch is then anastomosed to the bivalved bladder.

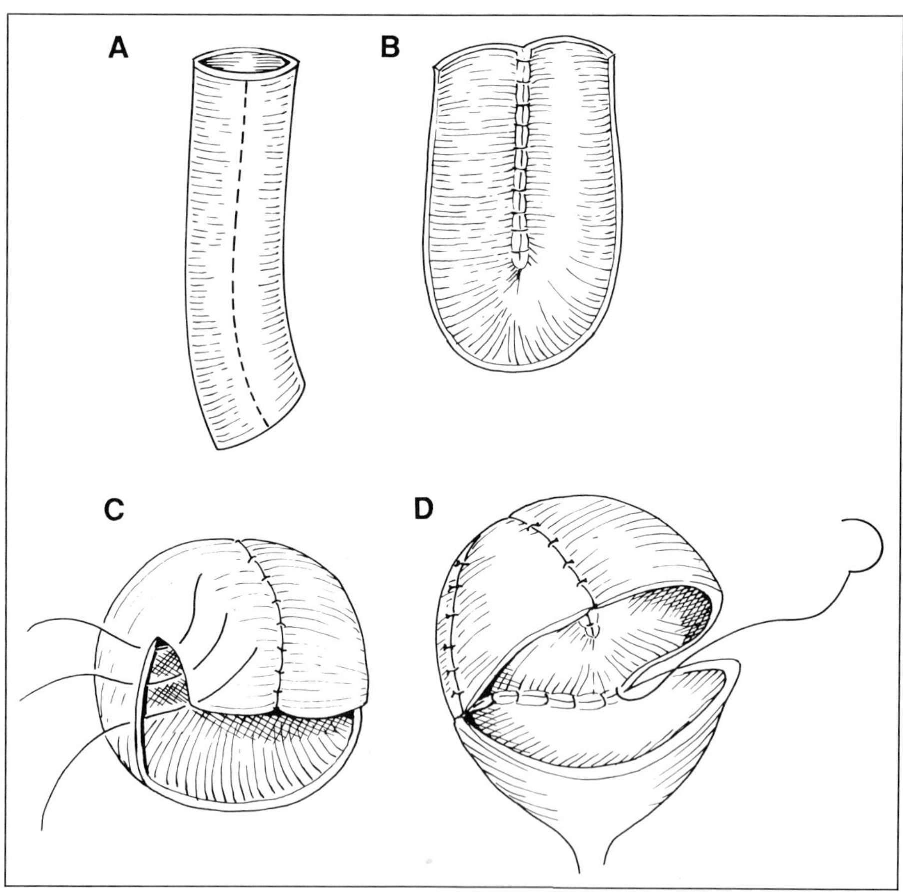

ticular anatomy of the case, including the pertinent intestinal anatomy and the amount of augmentation necessary.

## Surgical Techniques

**Ileal Cystoplasty.** The technique of ileocystoplasty, as popularized by Goodwin et al,[81] includes isolating a 20- to 25-cm segment of terminal ileum as one would do for an ileal conduit. The exact amount of ileum to be isolated depends somewhat on the preexisting bladder capacity. After completing the enteroenterostomy, the isolated ileal segment is opened along its antimesenteric border and the medial edges of the "U" are sewn together using an absorbable suture (Fig 24). We prefer a monofilament slowly absorbed suture such as polyglactin. Once the medial edges are sewn together, the intestine is again folded in a cephalad-to-caudad direction to complete the formation of a cup. It is very important to adequately dissect and open the bladder. Most authors prefer to open the bladder in a "clam shell" fashion. This means opening the bladder along a sagittal plane from the neck of the urethra up through the dome and then back down all the way to the bladder trigone. This leaves two lateral halves to the bladder with intact blood supply. This is necessary in order to prevent an hourglass deformity where the intestinal segment is sewn to the bladder (Fig 25). An hourglass deformity results from a constriction at the site of anastomosis of the intestinal segment to the bladder. This results in poor emptying and a compartmentalized bladder. While some authors recommend resection of all of the bladder above the trigone, this is probably unnecessary in most patients with the possible exception of patients with interstitial cystitis in which this procedure is being done for relief of pain. Once the bladder is adequately opened, the ileovesical anas-

**Fig 25.** Appearance of an hourglass deformity after augmentation cystoplasty. **A,** note the tapering and two-compartment effect due to a narrow anastomosis between the augmented bladder and the intact original bladder. This causes very poor emptying of the system; **B,** postdrainage film demonstrating large poorly emptying upper intestinal compartments.

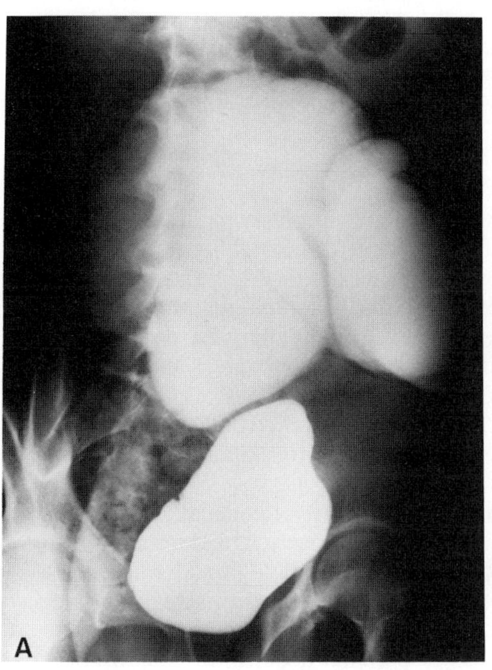


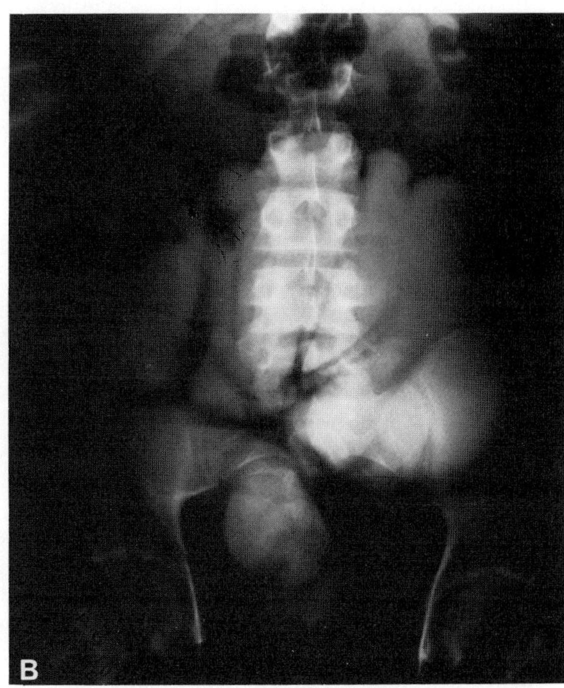

tomosis is again performed using an absorbable suture. It is generally preferable to place a suprapubic tube for postoperative drainage. It is best to bring this through the wall of the bladder, which is generally thickened in most patients in whom this procedure is being performed. This prevents a postoperative leak. The tube should not be placed through the suture line; however, in many cases it may be necessary to place it through the intestinal segment as the bladder itself will not reach the anterior abdominal wall. It is generally best to leave the bladder decompressed for 1 to 3 weeks.

In the patient with lower ureteral strictures or ureterovesical reflux, some form of ureteral reimplantation should be considered at the time of augmentation cystoplasty. The ileum does not generally lend itself to ureteral reimplantation, although techniques such as the one described by LeDuc et al[26] have been described. If the bladder wall is healthy, a tunneled reimplantation may be performed at this time. If the bladder is thickened or fibrotic, however, the ureter should be reimplanted into the intestinal segment. It is generally preferable to use a colonic segment or gastric segment if this is necessary as these intestinal segments have a thicker wall and lend themselves to the creation of a nonrefluxing ureterovesical anastomosis.

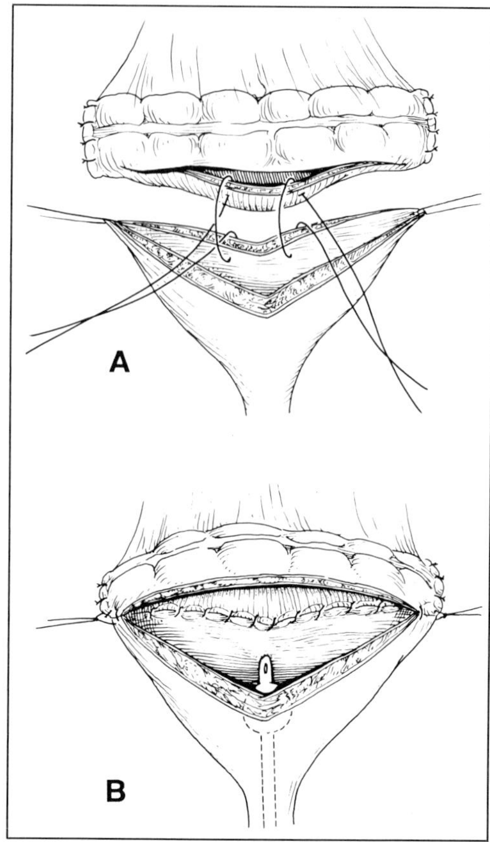


**Fig 26.** Sigmoid augmentation cystoplasty. **A,** a segment of a sigmoid colon has been isolated and opened on its antimesenteric border; **B,** it is then anastomosed to the bivalved bladder using interrupted absorbable sutures.

**Sigmoid Cystoplasty.** Sigmoid cystoplasty offers a number of advantages. First, the sigmoid segment is in close proximity to the bladder, and, particularly in patients with redundant sigmoid, involves relatively minimal dissection and an easy colovesical and colocolonic anastomosis. A simple patch technique is usually employed. With this technique, a 10- to 15-cm segment of sigmoid colon is isolated on a vascular pedicle (Fig 26). The colocolostomy is then fashioned according to one of the techniques previously described. After opening the bladder using a clam shell technique, the sigmoid colon segment is opened on its antimesenteric border. Generally with sigmoid segments, the segment is not folded and is simply used in a patch technique. A sigmoid cystoplasty frequently does not enhance the bladder capacity to the same degree as an ileocystoplasty or ileocecal cystoplasty as there is a more limited amount of bowel available to work with. In patients with particularly redundant sigmoid colons, however, there may be comparable results. A major advantage of the sigmoid colon cystoplasty is the thickness of the sigmoid colon wall, which lends itself to a tunneled ureteral reimplantation.

**Ileocecal Cystoplasty.** Ileocecal cystoplasty has gained popularity for bladder augmentation and for complete bladder replacement. The advantages of this segment are its mobility, its large capacity, and its usefulness in patients needing the creation of a nonrefluxing ureteral reimplantation and/or with deficient ureteral length. The ileocecal segment is supplied by the ileocecal artery. If a large capacity is necessary, the entire ascending colon can be utilized. In this case, it is best to divide the ileocecal segment between the right and middle colic arteries. A corresponding segment of terminal ileum is taken as well and then an ileal transverse or ascending anastomosis is performed. If there is insufficient length in the ileocecal mesentery to allow the intestinal segment to reach the bladder, the right colic artery can be divided leaving the entire segment based on the ileocecal artery and the marginal artery of Drummond. The right colic artery should be clamped with a noncrushing clamp prior to division in order to assess its importance in supplying the ascending colon. For the actual performance of the augmentation, two options are available. The ileocecal valve can be utilized to prevent vesicoureteral reflux with the cecal segment used for the bladder augmentation. Gil-Vernet was the first to popularize this procedure in 1956.[82] Generally, the creation of a nonrefluxing ureteral reimplantation involves intussusception and reinforcement of the ileocecal valve. This was generally accomplished by stripping the mesentery off of the terminal ileum for a 6- to 8-cm length. A number of techniques have since been described for preventing slippage of this intussusception. King et al[83] described a technique whereby the mucosal surface of the intussuscepted segment could be incised along with a corresponding area on the wall of the cecal segment and then sutured in such a position to prevent slippage (Fig 27). Al-

**Fig 27.** King technique for stabilization of an intussuscepted ileocecal segment. **A,** a 6- to 8-cm segment of terminal ileum is isolated from its mesenteric blood supply. An anterior cecal incision is then made; **B,** the ileum is then intussuscepted and an incision made into the seromuscular layer through the mucosa on both the intussuscepted ileal segment and the posterior cecal wall; **C,** the two areas that have been denuded of the mucosa are then anastomosed together.

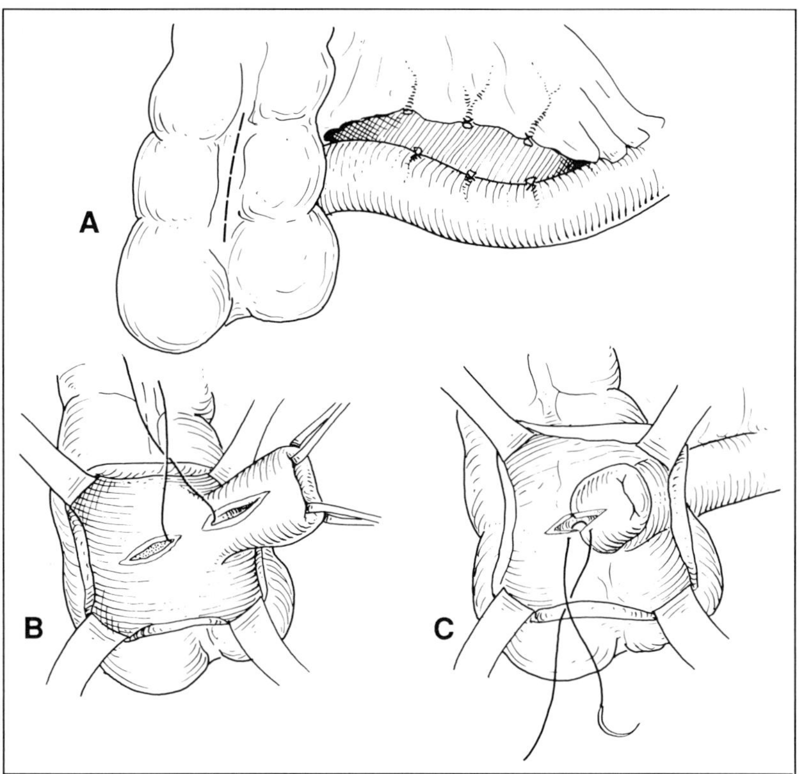

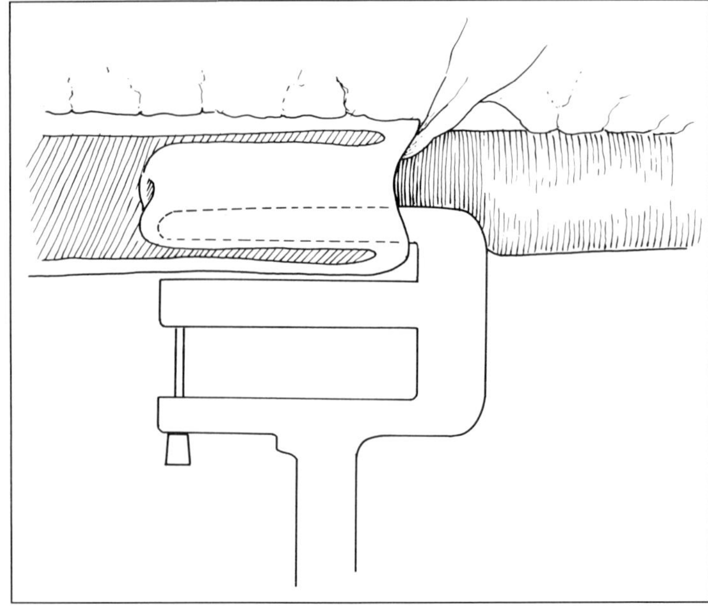

**Fig 28.** Alternative technique for stabilization of an intussuscepted ileal segment. The ileum is intussuscepted and a TA stapling device is placed from the outside of the ileal segment up into the nipple valve where the two edges are stapled together.

**Fig 29.** LeBag technique for creation of a urinary reservoir. **A,** an ileocecal segment is isolated on its mesenteric blood supply and then opened on its antimesenteric surface; **B,** the medial edges of the ileum and ascending colon are then anastomosed using a running absorbable suture. The anterior and superior edges are then also anastomosed as necessary to create the reservoir.

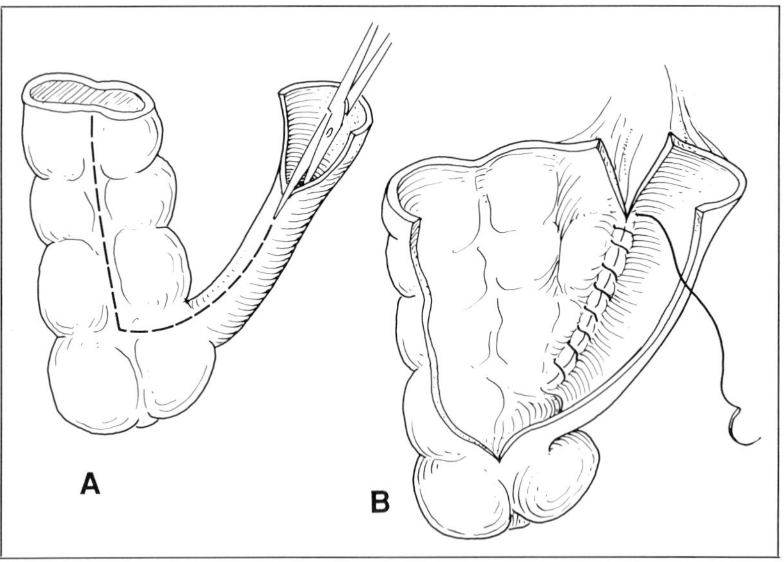

ternatively, the intussusception can be stapled in position from the outside of the intussusception (Fig 28). Many authors prefer to reinforce the intussuscepted segment by a 2- to 3-cm band of polyglycolic acid mesh that is sutured to the serosal surface of both cecum and ileum. The cecal segment is then opened and anastomosed to the bivalved bladder as previously described. The ureters are then implanted in the proximal ileal limb. A number of authors have described high-pressure tonic contractions within the cecal segment when it is utilized in this fashion. The intact cecum is capable of generating intraluminal pressures of 40 cm $H_2O$. This can result in both incontinence, and, over the long term, loss of the intussusception effect on terminal ileum, then ultimately renal damage.

An alternative procedure is to detubularize the ileocecal segment according to the technique of Light et al[84] or Thuroff et al.[85] With this procedure, the cecal segment is opened along its antimesenteric border along with the corresponding segment of ileum either in a U-shape configuration (Fig 29) or an S-shaped configuration (Fig 30). The medial edges of adjacent bowel are then sewn together and the bowel is rolled to form a spherical reservoir. This is then anastomosed to the bivalved bladder. The ureters can then be tunneled through the cecal wall to create a nonrefluxing anastomosis. The advantages of this procedure are the reliability of the ureteral reimplantation and the large spherical reservoir that it creates. Intraluminal pressures with these configurations are extremely acceptable and the ureteral implantation is highly successful.

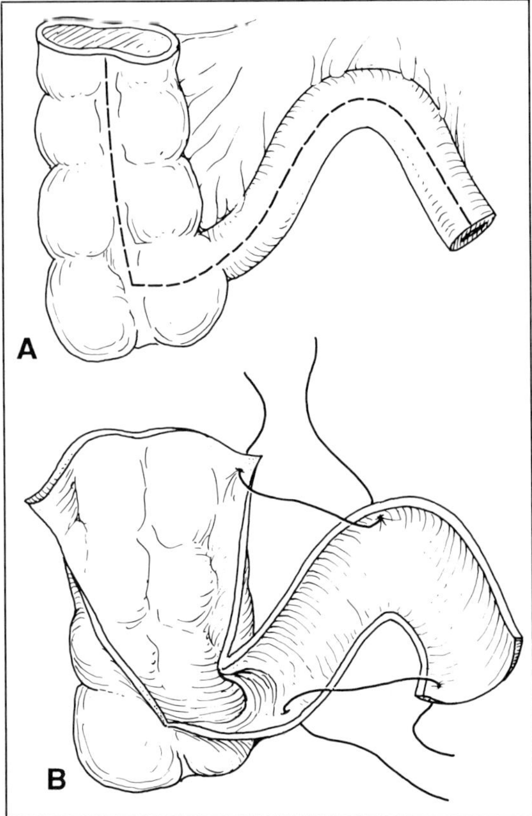


**Fig 30.** Mainz pouch technique for creation of a urinary reservoir. **A,** an ileocecal segment is isolated for the creation of the reservoir and opened on its antimesenteric surface. This is folded in an S-shaped fashion; **B,** the adjoining edges of the ileocecal segment and the folded ileal segment are then anastomosed to create the reservoir. The anterior surface is closed last.

***Results of Ileal or Colonic Augmentation Cystoplasty.*** A number of papers have confirmed the results of intestinal cystoplasty. Smith et al[78] reported on their results of augmentation cystoplasty in 74 patients, age 5 to 81 years. Their indications for cystoplasty were very diverse with the most common indication being interstitial cystitis followed by a neurogenic or defunctionalized bladder. In addition, they performed this procedure for patients with radiation, chemical, and tuberculous cystitis. These authors found no difference in whether or not the patient had the bladder removed prior to cystoplasty. Most patients voided normally. A number of complications were encountered including progressive uremia in two patients, small bowel obstructions, bladder calculi, and ureteral stricture. They considered the results good or excellent in only 57% of patients. Patients with radiation fibrosis and cystitis of the bladder seemed to do particularly poorly. It should be noted in this series that many of these patients had their procedures performed before the general acceptance of clean intermittent catheterization. Papers since this time have examined the use of intestinal cystoplasty combined with clean intermittent catheterization in both children and adults.[86,87] Results in these series have been more encouraging, with the vast majority of these patients having their procedures performed for neurovesical disease or for congenital bladder abnormalities. In review of 129 consecutive young patients with an average age of 13 years who underwent intestinocystoplasty at Indiana University, renal function was maintained or improved in 91% of patients and urinary continence was achieved in 82% of patients. The overall success rate of intestinocystoplasty in this series was 84%.

An additional complication that warrants mention are the reports of spontaneous bladder rupture after enterocystoplasty. There are 12 reported cases in the literature, all in children with augmented bladders who were also on clean intermittent catheterization programs. It has been reported with all forms of bladder augmentation with the exception of gastrocystoplasties. These patients generally present with classical symptoms of peritonitis occasionally heralded by bloody urine. The etiology of this problem is unclear. Unfortunately, cystograms were nondiagnostic or negative in approximately 50% of the reported cases in the literature. Conservative management generally fails and these patients require exploratory laparotomy with debridement of the necrotic-appearing bladder tissue and closure. Of the 12 cases reported in the literature, two patients died of sepsis secondary to the peritonitis.[88,89] While the initial cases in the literature were thought to be associated with noncompliance with intermittent catheterization, a number of these cases have occurred in patients who were completely compliant and who had low residual urines. There are no reported cases in the literature of patients who spontaneously void, strongly suggesting that the intermittent catheterization has a significant etiologic role.

**Gastrocystoplasty.** Recently, there has been significant interest in the use of gastric segments for bladder augmentation. These segments have a number of theoretical and, perhaps, practical advantages. Use of ileal or colonic segments for bladder reconstruction results in a hyperchloremic metabolic acidosis in many patients. This acidosis is usually mild and in the vast majority of patients may be clinically insignificant. In patients with significant renal impairment, however, clinical signs and symptoms of acidosis are more likely. In addition, over the long term, the effects of chronic metabolic acidosis are unknown. In contrast to ileal and colonic segments, which reabsorb urinary acids and secrete bicarbonate, the gastric segments acidify the urine. Initial studies in dogs showed that augmentation cystoplasty with a gastric segment does not result in any significant absorption of chloride or ammonium and therefore does not predispose to acidosis.[90,91] Clinical studies have confirmed this benefit. In an initial report from Adams et al at Indiana University, an isolated segment of stomach was used for bladder augmentation in ten patients.[92] The majority of these patients had neurogenic vesical disease or bladder exstrophy. The indications for the use of gastrocystoplasty included significant renal dysfunction and acidosis in six of these patients and/or insufficient large or small intestine secondary to a cloacal exstrophy in six others. With somewhat limited follow-up, these patients all demonstrated a mild correction in their serum total $CO_2$ values after bladder reconstruction compared to their preoperative values. An additional advantage of the stomach in these patients was the thick wall of the stomach, which allows a tunneled ureteral reimplantation.

***Surgical Technique.*** A gastric segment can be based on either the right or the left gastroepiploic artery (Fig 31). Generally, a segment of stomach is taken from the midportion of the greater curvature of the stomach. Care should be taken not to include the full width of the stomach. The size of the segment must be individualized but generally lengths of 7 to 10 cm along the greater curvature are taken. Once the decision has been made to use the right or left gastroepiploic arcade as a base for this,

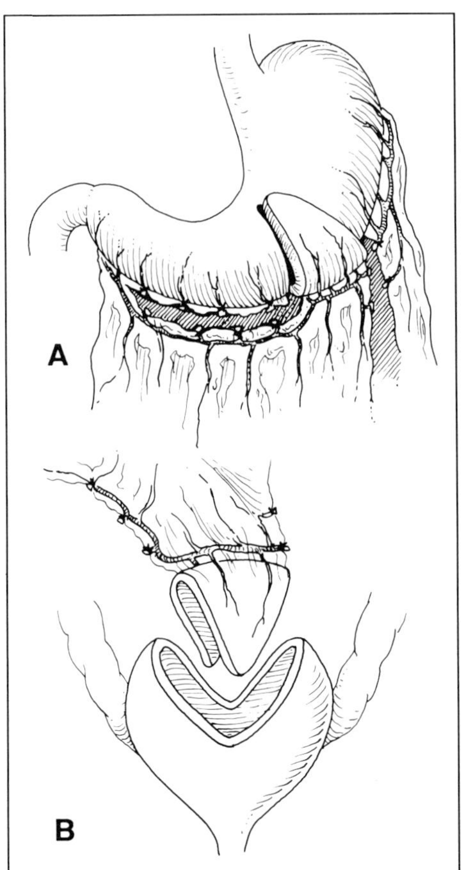


**Fig 31.** Gastrocystoplasty. **A,** gastrocystoplasty is based on the right gastroepiploic artery. The left gastroepiploic artery is divided. The perforating gastric vessels from the right gastroepiploic artery to the stomach are also divided, leaving it only attached at the segment of the stomach that is to be used for the cystoplasty; **B,** the segment is then rotated down on its intact blood supply and anastomosed to the bivalved bladder.

the short gastric perforating vessels that run from the gastroepiploic artery to the stomach are taken on the side on which the pedicle is to be placed. The gastroepiploic artery is then divided on the opposite side and the omentum is mobilized. The gastric closure is then performed using a two-layer technique (Fig 31). It is important to perform the mucosal closure using a locking absorbable suture to prevent postoperative gastric bleeding. The isolated gastric segment can then be tunneled down through the mesocolon and the wedge-shaped gastric segment fits nicely for bladder augmentation.

A number of long-term potential complications are possible with gastrocystoplasty. These patients are prone to salt and chloride loss and this predisposes them to metabolic hypochloremic, hypokalemic alkalosis during any acute gastrointestinal illnesses. The propensity for the augmented bladder or for the remaining stomach to form gastric ulcers has been a concern of several authors. Fasting serum gastrin levels in the report by Adams et al[92] were all normal or minimally elevated. Urine pH values remain low and many of these patients maintain a sterile urine in contrast to patients with ileal or colocystoplasties who are usually chronically colonized with bacteria.

## LONG-TERM METABOLIC COMPLICATIONS OF USING INTESTINE IN THE URINARY TRACT

### Ileal and Colon Diversions

A number of long-term complications of the use of intestinal segments in the urinary tract are being reported with increasing frequency. These complications include acid–base disturbances that result in bone mineral changes, vitamin and fatty acid deficiencies, and the induction of neoplasms in the intestinal segment.

The acidosis associated with urinary diversion was first described by Boyd in 1931.[93] Its frequency was not really appreciated until Ferris and Odel reported two series in the early 1950s.[94,95] These series of ureterosigmoidostomy patients demonstrated an alarmingly high incidence of both acidosis and hyperchloremia and reported a subset of patients who developed a syndrome that included severe watery diarrhea, dehydration, lethargy, and azotemia. Multiple theories were put forward in the ensuing decade to propose a pathophysiology for this. The syndrome was commonly reported in the setting of renal insufficiency or during episodes of acute pyelonephritis, which strongly suggests that renal compromise plays some role. More recently, studies by Koch and McDougal demonstrated that the majority of the acidosis following urinary diversion through intestinal segments is the result of the reabsorption of urinary ammonium by the intestinal segment and to a lesser degree by the secretion of bicarbonate by the intestinal segment into the urine.[96] These findings have been confirmed more recently in an intestinal perfusion model and appear to be the case for both ileum and colon.[97] While there are quantitative and qualitative differences between ileum and colon, they are relatively small and the primary mechanisms involved in the acidosis are quite similar. The mechanism by which urinary ammonium is absorbed is currently unknown. The conventional theory is that ammonium is absorbed as a nonionized species; however, recent laboratory studies suggest that this may not be the case. Until more precise information is available, the cellular mechanisms for ammonium absorption and the acidosis of urinary diversion will remain unclear.

Management of this acidosis consists of (1) establishing maximal urinary drainage, (2) administrating alkali supplementation as bicarbonate or citrate salts, (3) ensuring volume repletion, (4) administering potassium supplementation, and (5) restricting chloride. In calculating the alkali supplementation, it is helpful to realize that an adult consuming an average American diet containing meats generates 1 to 1.5 mEq of acid per kilogram of body weight per day, which must be excreted.

While the majority of the severe acidosis syndromes that have been reported have been seen following ureterosigmoidostomy, this syndrome can also occur following ileal conduit urinary diversion, colon conduits, intestinocystoplasty, and continent urinary diversions. Following an ileal conduit urinary diversion, hyperchloremic metabolic acidosis has been reported in between 1.7% to 29% of patients.[44,46,98–108] Clinically significant hyperchloremic metabolic acidosis is uncommon, however, following ileal conduit urinary diversion in the absence of renal insufficiency, stomal stenosis, or uretero-intestinal anastomotic strictures. While an early transient hyperchloremic metabolic acidosis is seen in as many as 70% of patients,[100] persistent long-term significant metabolic acidosis is seen in a minority of patients (less than 10%). Most of these patients are easily managed with oral alkali. The reported incidence of metabolic acidosis after colon conduit urinary diversion ranges from 0 to 11.5%.[47,109–113] While this incidence is somewhat less for colon conduits, differences in renal function between different series may account for this. Elder and associates[110] reviewed their long-term results with colon conduits in 41 children and reported an approximately 12% incidence of hyperchloremic metabolic acidosis. This incidence correlated well with the presence of stasis and renal insufficiency.[114]

Metabolic complications have also been reported following intestinocystoplasty. According to Mitchell and Piser,[87] even patients with normal renal function tend to develop hyperchloremia and patients with preexisting renal insufficiency are at risk for acidosis. Theoretically, patients should be more predisposed to the development of significant acidosis following intestinocystoplasty and continent urinary diversion than after conduit diversion. The reabsorption of ammonium and secretion of bicarbonate is a time-dependent process and the total rate of reabsorption is dependent on the surface area of bowel that is exposed. Whitmore and Gittes[115] reported a 15-year experience with cecal and ileocecal cystoplasty and noted that 19% of patients had a metabolic acidosis. All of these patients had some degree of preexisting renal dysfunction. The incidence of metabolic acidosis depends in large degree on the methodology used to detect it. Nurse and Mundy[116] described a prospective study of 48 patients with various types of cystoplasties looking for metabolic complications. All of their patients had abnormal blood gases with most exhibiting a metabolic acidosis with respiratory compensation. Thirty percent of their patients were also hyperchloremic. The incidence of metabolic acidosis was highest in patients with ileocecoplasty and least with ileocystoplasty, although it is difficult to correct this for the amount of bowel surface area and for renal function. Patients with significant preexisting renal function and particularly patients with preexisting acidosis thought to be of renal origin are at distinctly increased risk for the development of significant metabolic acidosis postoperatively. It is this subset of patients that may be better managed by augmentation cystoplasty using the stomach. Both experimentally and clinically, gastrocystoplasty tends to correct preexisting acidosis.[91,92] Over the last decade, there has been an increasing emphasis on construction of continent modes of urinary diversion. The continent ileal reservoir as described by Kock and associates[117] and popularized in this country by Skinner and coworkers has a reportedly low incidence of metabolic complications.[118] This is somewhat surprising because of the prolonged contact of the urine with the intestinal mucosa and because of the large surface area of the ileal mucosa involved. Skinner et al reported a low incidence of complications even in patients with preexisting renal insufficiency. In a prospective study of patients who underwent continent ileal reservoir urinary diversion, only 13% exhibited an acidosis and occasional hyperchloremia. This was normally during periods of renal deterioration associated with azotemia secondary to dehydration and/or urinary obstruction.[118] The study did not measure arterial blood gas values. Koch and associates[119] studied a group of patients with continent colonic urinary diversions under baseline conditions and under conditions of acid loading. Significant metabolic acidosis was not found in these patients either. The only detectable abnormalities were urinary acidification and concentrating defects. It is evident from these two studies that most patients have enough renal reserve to compensate for reabsorbed urinary acids through the intestinal segment. It is only under conditions of renal dysfunction that significant acid–base abnormalities develop.

A related syndrome to the hyperchloremic metabolic acidosis is ammoniogenic coma of urinary diversion. Studies in animals with chronic urinary diversion have provided evidence of chronic ammonium absorption and hepatic compensation.[96] Reabsorbed urinary ammonia or ammonium enters the portal circulation and is rapidly cleared by the liver via the ornithine cycle. In the ornithine cycle, reabsorbed ammonium is metabolized to urea. With hepatic dysfunction or with increased ammonia reabsorption due to urea-splitting organisms such as *Proteus* in the urinary tract, a syndrome of ammoniogenic coma may be encountered. This was first described by McDermott in 1957.[120]

## Jejunal Conduits

In contrast to the low incidence of metabolic abnormalities seen following ileal and colonic urinary diversion, jejunal conduits are associated with a high incidence of metabolic complications. This is usually referred to as the "jejunal conduit syndrome." This syndrome is characterized by hyperkalemia, hyponatremia, hypochloremia, and clinical signs of volume depletion.[121,122] Acidosis is usually present; however, alkalosis has been reported as well. This syndrome is thought to be due to sodium chloride wasting from secretion into the urine by the jejunal segment. Chronic salt loss results in volume depletion with contraction alkalosis or, under conditions of severe volume contraction, hypochloremic acidosis. More recent authors[123] have reported lower incidences of jejunal conduit syndrome (25%). If this procedure is performed only in patients with normal baseline renal function and very short segments of jejunum, this syndrome can be minimized. In these series, however, they prophylactically administered oral electrolyte therapy with sodium chloride to minimize the risk of salt wasting. Most authors advocate the use of jejunal segments only in situations where no other bowel segments are available.

## Miscellaneous

It should be recognized that any time an intestinal segment is utilized in the urinary tract, any substance that is excreted in the urine may be absorbed. This is evident in a variety of situations. For instance, in diabetics, glucose excreted into the urine is rapidly reabsorbed by ileal segments making the measurement of urinary glucose values inaccurate.[124] In addition, patients receiving chemotherapeutic drugs and Dilantin have been found to have impaired excretion and this has been attributed to reabsorption by the intestinal segment.[125,126]

**Bone Mineral Changes.** With an acute acid challenge, the normal renal physiologic response is to buffer the excreted acid with urinary phosphate and sulfate. Phosphate is derived primarily from bone. As an acidosis becomes chronic, however, such as the acidosis induced by ammonium reabsorption through a urinary diversion, acid is excreted primarily with ammonia.[127] Ammonia is generated in the distal tubular cell by the conversion of glutamine to α-ketoglutarate. Ammonia is then transported into the tubule lumen where it binds with urinary acid and is excreted as ammonium. In the setting of urinary diversion through intestinal segments, however, large amounts of urinary ammonium are reabsorbed. In an experimental model in which a dog ureter was replaced by ileum,[96] approximately 80% of ammonium excreted by the kidney was reabsorbed before it was eliminated through the bladder. This forces an increased amount of acid to be excreted with titratable acids, ie, phosphate and sulfate. Experimental studies in animals have suggested that there may be significant acid–base abnormalities in the absence of changes in serum electrolytes and that these may result in significant changes in bone mineral content.[128,129]

The first report of hyperchloremic metabolic acidosis associated with urinary diversion was in a child who had undergone ureterosigmoidostomy and who, in addition to having this chronic acidosis, developed active metabolic bone disease.[93] Since that initial report, it has become well recognized that osteomalacia may result from chronic acidosis associated with urinary diversion. While this has been most frequently reported with ureterosigmoidostomy, it has been reported with other forms of diversion as well.[130,131] Most recently, Koch and associates demonstrated that there are significant long-term metabolic effects of urinary diversion and in particular bone growth abnormalities in a population of myelomeningocele patients treated with urinary diversion when compared to a control group of patients treated with intermittent catheterization.[45] Bone changes were reflected in decreased upper extremity linear growth. Patients with urinary diversion had decreased lengths of all upper body linear growth measurements and a significantly greater percentage of patients with urinary diversions fell at or below the tenth percentile standards. These changes were seen in the absence of serum electrolyte, vitamin $D_3$, or parathormone abnormalities.

The real implications of studies such as this are unknown. It is likely that these changes in bone mineral content will only be seen with prolonged follow-up. Urinary diversions that incorporate large segments of bowel, particularly when coupled with renal dysfunction, should result in the most significant changes over the long term. Children and young adults with urinary diversion should be carefully followed and abnormalities in systemic electrolytes should be aggressively corrected.

**Vitamin and Fatty Acid Alterations.** Urinary diversions that utilize large segments of terminal ileum predispose patients to deficiencies of both vitamin $B_{12}$ and the lipid-soluble vitamins. In a population of patients who had undergone external beam radiation therapy followed by ileal conduit urinary diversion for carcinoma of the bladder, 25% of patients demonstrated vitamin $B_{12}$ deficiency.[132] This malabsorption of vitamin $B_{12}$ was confirmed by a Schilling test. Serum folate levels in the same group were normal and serum hemoglobin values correlated with abnormalities in vitamin $B_{12}$. More recent studies have examined vitamin $B_{12}$ deficiency in patients undergoing bladder replacement or augmentation with ileal segments. These patients had serum determinations of both vitamin $B_{12}$ and carotene, which is a precursor for fat-soluble vitamin

A and is used as a screening test for fat malabsorption.[133] In urinary diversion procedures that utilize a small segment of terminal ileum and incorporate the terminal ileum, ileocecal valve, and a portion of ascending colon, vitamin $B_{12}$ deficiency appears to be uncommon.[134] The incidence of vitamin $B_{12}$ deficiency following Kock pouch urinary diversion utilizing 80 cm of terminal ileum is reportedly low with only anecdotal cases reported. However, follow-up is probably too short to know the long-term consequences of utilizing such large segments of terminal ileum for urinary tract reconstruction. It should be recognized that the minimal daily requirement of vitamin $B_{12}$ is only 2.5 μg and that the total body stores of vitamin $B_{12}$ are 1 to 5 mg, with the liver being the predominant storage site. Vitamin $B_{12}$ is excreted exclusively in the bile and the vitamin is conserved by uptake in the terminal ileum where it is returned to the liver through the enterohepatic circulation. Because of the low minimum daily requirement, even in the absence of any vitamin $B_{12}$ absorption, it may take up to 3–6 years for vitamin $B_{12}$ deficiency to manifest. With partial absorption, this time interval will be even more prolonged.

In addition to vitamin $B_{12}$ absorption, the terminal ileum is responsible for the reabsorption of bile salts that are also returned to liver through the enterohepatic circulation. When the length of ileal resection exceeds 100 cm, considerable amounts of bile salts may be lost. Bile salts are necessary for the solubilization of fats by micelle formation in the jejunum.[135] In the absence of bile salts, free fatty acids pass into the colon. When unabsorbed bile salts and fatty acids enter the colon, both induce a secretory diarrhea. In addition, fat malabsorption leads to deficiencies of the fat-soluble vitamins A, D, E, and K. A secretory diarrhea may be induced by both resection of large amounts of terminal ileum and resection of the ileocecal valve which diminishes intestinal transit time and allows unabsorbed free fatty acids and bile salts to pass into the colon.

Initial treatment in these patients should be directed toward decreasing the bile salt load to the colon. Bile salt content in the bowel may be minimized by the administration of cholestyramine, which binds free bile salts and is highly effective in reducing bile salt–induced secretory diarrhea. Patients with significant steatorrhea should be placed on a low-fat diet. If these measures are unsuccessful, intestinal motility and transit time may be diminished by the administration of loperamide, codeine, or diphenoxylate. Patients with large volumes of secretory diarrhea are predisposed to volume depletion, acidosis, and hypokalemia.

Studies in the general surgical literature also suggest that patients who have had large amounts of ileum resected are predisposed to gallstone formation. In 1967, Hofmann and Borgstrom[135] suggested that chronic bile salt loss due to ileal resection could lead to decreased bile salt concentration in the bile and cholesterol precipitation. Several studies have demonstrated that there is an increased risk of gallstone formation when greater than 30% to 45% of ileum is resected. Interestingly, many of the stones in these patients were pigmented stones, not cholesterol.[136] Many of the currently performed urinary diversions such as the Koch pouch use large amounts of terminal ileum. The long-term incidence of gallstones in these patients is currently unknown; however, the amount of ileum utilized in these procedures is comparable to that reported in the general surgical series, which found increased gallstone formation following ileal resection. In a review of 90 children undergoing cholecystectomy at one hospital that has a large population of children with urinary diversions, none had undergone a previous urinary intestinal diversion.[137] This suggests that the clinical incidence of this phenomenon is fairly low.

**Carcinogenesis.** Until the early 1950s, ureeterosigmoidostomy was the primary means of urinary diversion. Initial problems with fluid and electrolyte balance in these patients were reported in 1950. However, these problems were fairly easily managed in most patients. In 1979, Leadbetter and associates[138] reported the first case of ureterosigmoidostomy associated with the development of an adenocarcinoma at the site of the ureteral reimplantation. Multiple case reports ensued. In a review of ureterosigmoidostomy in exstrophy patients in 1990, Husmann and Spence[139] reported on 94 patients who developed colonic tumors. In this population, the average age at diagnosis of tumor was 33 years and the average latency between the performance of the ureterosigmoidostomy and the development of tumor was 26 years. Two thirds of the tumors reported were malignant and one third were benign polyps. A very striking finding was that in 17% of the patients, the ureterosigmoidostomy had actually been taken down and the patients had some other form of urinary diversion at the time they presented with a urocolonic tumor. All of these lesions appeared at an anastomotic site where a ureteral stump had been left behind. In this particular subset of patients, colonic mucosa was in contact with the urine for only an average of 8 years. Perhaps most alarming, death from carcinoma occurred in 33% of patients. A significant number of the patients had metastases to regional lymph nodes at the time of presentation. These patients usually presented with urinary obstruction or bloody diarrhea. This single complication of ureterosigmoidostomy caused the procedure to be largely abandoned. Patients who currently have ureterosigmoidostomies must be followed with aggressive surveillance programs.

Perhaps equally concerning are the increasing number of reports of patients with malignancies developing in bladder augmentations and intestinal conduits. In a review article published in 1990, Filmer and Spencer[140] summarized the 14 patients reported to have developed malignancies in bowel used for bladder augmentation. In addition, there have been four cases of cancer in colon conduits and one cancer in an ileal conduit reported in the literature. In the bladder augmentation group, all types of intestinal segments had been used including ileum, cecum, and sigmoid colon. As in the ureterosigmoidostomy population of patients, the interval between bladder augmentation and diagnosis of tumor ranges between 5 and 29 years with a mean of 18 years. Perhaps most alarming is that of these 14 patients summarized, 9 had undergone ileocystoplasty and developed malignancies in the ileum. Adenocarcinoma of the ileum is extremely rare in the general population.

A number of mechanisms have been proposed for the pathogenesis of these malignancies. The original laboratory investigation of Crissey and associates[141] in 1980 demonstrated that when urine is diverted by vesicosigmoidostomy into the intact large bowel, neoplastic changes occurred in the colonic epithelium in a large percentage of animals. When proximal colostomy was performed simultaneously with a urinary diversion, however, no tumors developed. These investigators concluded that the mixing of the fecal and urinary streams was necessary for the induction of these tumors. Multiple etiologies have been subsequently proposed. Intestinal neoplasms in the intact intestine are thought to be induced by carcinogens in the diet. Urinary diversion through intestine may actually produce these carcinogens. Nitrate is normally excreted by the kidney into the urine and gram-negative bacteria are able to reduce nitrate to nitrite and furthermore catalyze the conversion of nitrite and urinary amines to *N*-nitrosamines. Nitrosamines are highly mutagenic and induce tumor in many animal species. High levels of nitrosamines are present in the rectal fluid of humans after ureterosigmoidostomy.[142,143] In addition, high levels of nitrosamines have been observed in the urine from ileal and colon conduits[144] and after augmentation cystoplasty.[145] Unfortunately, pharmacologic agents that are known to inhibit the formation of nitrosamines have not demonstrated any decrease in the frequency of tumor formation in animal models.[146,147]

An inflammatory response to chronic infection or surgery may also contribute to the development of neoplastic changes. Inflammatory cells secrete growth factors that may cause tumor induction. It has been theorized that increased cellular proliferation adjacent to a healing intestinal urinary anastomosis may induce increased susceptibility to neoplastic transformation.

The goblet cells of the colonic mucosa produce neutral and acid mucins. Chemical changes have been demonstrated in the type of mucin produced following urinary diversion through intestinal segments. In animals treated with colon carcinogens and in humans, there are foci of increased sialomucin production[148–151] in areas adjacent to induced carcinomas. There is also an increase in sialomucins in the sigmoid colon after ureterosigmoidostomy and in colon segments used as conduits, continent reservoirs, or augmentation cystoplasties.[152–154]

Another substance thought to be a marker for the development of intestinal tumors is ornithine decarboxylase. Ornithine decarboxylase activity has been reported to be elevated in colon adenomas and carcinomas compared to normal colonic mucosa.[155–157] Ornithine decarboxylase is thought to catalyze the conversion of ornithine to putrescine. The exact cellular function of putrescine is unclear; however, it is proposed to be an obligatory step in the development of carcinoma. When animals are given colonic carcinogens, a rise in colonic mucosal ornithine decarboxylase generally precedes the appearance of tumors.[158] In one animal study of ureterosigmoidostomy, ornithine decarboxylase levels at the site of the intestinal anastomosis were shown to be higher than in normal colon and these changes preceded the development of neoplasms.[159]

It is not currently known whether changes in sialomucin production and ornithine decarboxylase activity are actually pathogenic or whether they represent markers for the development of urocolonic neoplasms. Nevertheless, while the incidence of tumor induction following ileal and colon conduit diversion appears to be relatively low, the incidence after bladder augmentation or continent urinary diversion is currently unknown and will only become known when significant follow-up is available. It is highly probable that a significant risk will be associated with these forms of urinary diversion and that this may alter our approach to current forms of urinary diversion as it has with ureterosigmoidostomies in the past.

## ACKNOWLEDGMENTS

The author thanks Mary Margaret Peel and Ann Rees from the Medical Illustrations Department at the Nashville Veteran's Affairs Hospital for providing the medical illustrations for this chapter.

## REFERENCES

1. Nichols RL, Condon RE, Gorbach SC, Nyhus LM. Efficacy of preoperative antimicrobial preparation of the bowel. *Ann Surg*. 1972; 176(2):227–232.
2. Washington JA, Dearing WH, Judd ES, Elveback LR. Effect of preoperative antibiotic regimen on development of infection after intestinal surgery: prospective randomized, double-blind study. *Ann Surg*. 1974;180(4):567–572.
3. Wolff BG, Beart RW, Dozois RR, Pemberton JH, Zinsmeister AR, Ready RL, et al. A new bowel preparation for elective colon and rectal surgery: a prospective, randomized clinical trial. *Arch Surg*. 1988;123:895–900.
4. Hewitt J, Rigby J, Reeve J, Cox AG. Whole-gut irrigation in preparation for large bowel surgery. *Lancet*. 1973;2:337–340.
5. Crapp AR, Powis SJA, Tillotson P, Cooke WT, Alexander-Williams J. Preparation of the bowel by whole-gut irrigation. *Lancet*. 1975;2:1239–1240.
6. Gottrup F, Diederich P, Sorensen K, Nelson SV, Ornsholt J, Brandsborg O. Prophylaxis with whole gut irrigation and antimicrobials in colorectal surgery. *Am J Surg*. 1985;149:317–322.
7. Jagelman DG, Fazio VW, Lauery IC, Weakley FL. A prospective, randomized, double blind study of 10% mannitol mechanical bowel preparation combined with oral neomycin and short-term perioperative intravenous Flagyl as prophylaxis in elective colorectal resections. *Surgery*. 1985;98:861–865.
8. Keighley MR, Taylor EW, Hares MM, et al. Influence of oral mannitol bowel preparation on colonic microflora and the risk of explosion during endoscopic diathermy. *Br J Surg*. 1981;68:554–600.
9. Zanoni CE, Bergamini C, Bertoncini L, Garbini A. Whole-gut lavage for surgery: a case of intra-operative colonic explosion after administration of mannitol. *Dis Colon Rectum*. 1982;25:580–581.

10. van Coevora F, Taat CW, Boissevain AC, Jas B, et al. Preoperative whole gut irrigation with mannitol. *Neth J Surg.* 1982;34(5):225–228.
11. Davis GR, Santa Ana CA, Morawski SG, Fordtrau JS. Development of a lavage solution associated with minimal water and electrolyte absorption or secretion. *Gastroenterology.* 1980;78:991–995.
12. Beck DE, Fazio VW, Jagelman DG. Comparison of oral lavage methods for pre-operative colonic cleansing. *Dis Colon Rectum.* 1986;29(11):699–703.
13. Tuggle DW, Hoelzer DJ, Tunnell WP, Smith EI. The safety and cost-effectiveness of polyethylene glycol electrolyte solution bowel preparation in infants and children. *J Pediatr Surg.* 1987;22(6):513–515.
14. Vila JJ, Gutierez C, Garcia-Sala C, Ruiz S. Whole bowel irrigation: experience in pediatric patients. *J Pediatr Surg.* 1987;22(5):447–450.
15. Slama TG, Carey LC, Fass RJ. Comparative efficacy of prophylactic cephalothin and cefamandole for elective surgery. *Am J Surg.* 1979;137:593–596.
16. Hardy KJ. A view of the development of intestinal suture. Part II. Principles and techniques. *Aust NZ J Surg.* 1990;60:377–384.
17. Gambee LP. A single layer open intestinal anastomosis applicable to the small bowel as well as large intestine. *World J Surg Obstet Gynecol.* 1951;58:1.
18. Didolcar MS, Reed WP, Elias EG, Schnaper LA, Brow SD, Chaudhary SM. A prospective randomized study of sutured versus stapled bowel anastomoses in patients with cancer. *Cancer.* 1986;57:456–460.
19. Chassin JL, Rifkind KM, Turner JW. Errors and pitfalls in stapling gastrointestinal tract anastomoses. *Surg Clin North Am.* 1984; 64:441–449.
20. Richie JP, Skinner DG. Urinary diversion: the physiologic rationale for non-refluxing colonic conduits. *Br J Urol.* 1975;47:269–275.
21. Hill JT, Ransley PG. The colonic conduit: a better method of urinary diversion? *Br J Urol.* 1983;55:629–631.
22. Gonzalez R, Reinberg Y. Localization of bacteriuria in patients with enterocystoplasty and non-refluxing conduits. *J Urol.* 1987;138: 1104–1105.
23. Leadbetter WF, Clarke BG. Five years experience with ureteroenterostomy by the "combined" technique. *J Urol.* 1954;73:67–82.
24. Pagano F. Ureterocolonic anastomoses: description of a technique. *J Urol.* 1980;123:355–356.
25. Goodwin WE, Harris AP, Coffman JJ, Beal JM. Open transcolonic ureterointestinal anastomosis. *Surg Gynecol Obstet.* 1953;97:295–300.
26. LeDuc A, Camey M, Teillac P. An original anti-reflux ureteral ileal implantation technique: long-term follow-up. *J Urol.* 1987;137:1156–1158.
27. Turner-Warwick RT, Ashken MH. The functional results of partial, subtotal, and total cystoplasty with special reference to ureterocecocystoplasty, selective sphincterotomy, and cystocystoplasty. *Br J Urol.* 1967;39:3–12.
28. Bricker EM. Bladder substitution after pelvic evisceration. *Surg Clin North Am.* 1950; 30:1511–1521.
29. Wallace DM. Ureteroileostomy. *Br J Urol.* 1970;42:529–534.
30. Regan JB, Barrett DM. Stented versus non-stented ureteroileal anastomoses: is there a difference with regard to leak and stricture? *J Urol.* 1985;134:1101–1103.
31. Beddoe AM, Boyce JG, Remy JC, Fruchter RG, Nelson JH Jr. Stented versus non-stented transverse colon conduits: a comparative report. *Gynecol Oncol.* 1987;27:305–313.
32. Bricker EM, Eisman B. Bladder reconstruction from cecum and ascending colon following resection of pelvic viscera. *Ann Surg.* 1950; 132(1):77–84.
33. Ferris DO, Odell HM. Electrolyte pattern of the blood after bilateral ureterosigmoidostomy. *JAMA.* 1950;142:634–641.
34. Turnbull RB Jr, Hewitt CR. Loop-end myotomy ileostomy in the obese patient. *Urol Clin North Am.* 1978;5:423.
35. Emmott D, Noble MJ, Mebust WK. A comparison of end versus loop stomas for ileal conduit urinary diversion. *J Urol.* 1985;133:588.
36. Sullivan JW, Grabstald H, Whitmore WF Jr. Complications of ureteral ileal conduit with radical cystectomy: review of 336 cases. *J Urol.* 1980;124:797–801.
37. Middleton AW, Hendren WH. Ileal conduits in children at the Massachusetts General Hospital from 1955 to 1970. *J Urol.* 1976;115:591–595.
38. Arnarson O, Straffon RA. Clinical experience with the ileal conduit in children. *J Urol.* 1969;102:768–771.
39. Schwartz GR, Jeffs RD. Ileal conduit urinary diversion in children: computer analysis of follow-up from 2 to 16 years. *J Urol.* 1975;114:285–288.
40. Pitts WR, Muecke EC. A 20-year experience with ileal conduits: the fate of the kidneys. *J Urol.* 1979;122:154–157.
41. Cass AS, Luxenberg M, Gleich P, Johnson CF. A 22-year follow-up of ileal conduits in children with a neurogenic bladder. *J Urol.* 1984;132:529–531.
42. Orr JD, Shand JEG, Walters DAH, Kirkland IS. Ileal conduit urinary diversion in children. An assessment of the long-term results. *Br J Urol.* 1981;53:424–427.

43. Dunn M, Roberts JBM, Smith DJB, Slade N. The long-term results of ileal conduit diversion in children. *Br J Urol.* 1979;51:458–461.

44. Shapiro SR, Lebowitz R, Colodny AH. Fate of 90 children with ileal conduit urinary diversion of a decade later: analysis of complications, pyelography, renal function and bacteriology. *J Urol.* 1975;114:289–295.

45. Koch MO, McDougal WS, Hall MC, Hill DE, Braren HV, Donofrio MN. Long-term metabolic effects of urinary diversion: a comparison of myelomeningocele patients managed by clean intermittent catheterization and urinary diversion. *J Urol.* 1992;147:1343–1347.

46. Malek RS, Burke EC, Deweerd JH. Ileal conduit urinary diversion in children. *J Urol.* 1971;105:892–900.

47. Althausen AF, Hagen-Cook K, Hendren WH. Non-refluxing colon conduit: experience with 70 cases. *J Urol.* 1978;120:35–39.

48. Husmann DA, McLorie GA, Churchill BM. Non-refluxing colonic conduits: a long-term life table analysis. *J Urol.* 1989;142:1201–1203.

49. Elder DD, Moisey CU, Rees RWM. A long-term follow-up of the colonic conduit in children. *Br J Urol.* 1975;51:462–465.

50. Morales P, Golimbu M. Colonic urinary diversion: 10 years of experience. *J Urol.* 1975;113:302–307.

51. Hill JT, Ransley PG. The colonic conduit: a better method of urinary diversion? *Br J Urol.* 1983;55:629–631.

52. Mansson W, Ahlgren G, White T. Glomerular filtration rate up to ten years after urinary diversion of different types: a comparative study of ileocolonic conduit, refluxing and antirefluxing ureteral anastomoses, and continent cecal reservoir. *Scand J Urol Nephrol.* 1989;23:195–200.

53. Jeter KF, Lattimer JK. Common stomal problems following ileal conduit urinary diversion. *Urology.* 1974;3(4):399–403.

54. Esho J, Cass AS. The management of stomal encrustation in children. *J Urol.* 1972;108:797–799.

55. Jeter K, Bloom S. Management of stomal complications following ileal or colonic conduit diversions in children. *J Urol.* 1971;106:425–428.

56. Melnikoff AE. On the replacement of the ureter by an isolated segment of small intestine. *Rev Clin Urol.* 1912;1:601.

57. Clark BG, Mahoney DT. Effect upon the kidney of replacing the lower half of the ureter with terminal ileum: an experimental study. *J Urol.* 1960;84:268.

58. Martinez J, Kaplan N, Boyarsky S. Laboratory and clinical studies of ureteral replacement by ileum. *J Urol.* 1965;93:185.

59. Hinman F, Oppenheimer R. Functional characteristics of the ileal segment as a valve. *J Urol.* 1958;80:448.

60. Waters WB, Whitmore WF, Lage AL, et al. Segmental replacement of the ureter using tapered and non-tapered ileum. *Invest Urol.* 1981;18:258.

61. Moore ED, Woodward ER, Goodwin WE. Isolated loops for ureteral repair. *Surg Gynecol Obstet.* 1956;102:87.

62. Boxer RJ, Fritzsche P, Skinner GG, et al. Replacement of the ureter by small intestine: clinical application and results of the ileal ureter in 89 patients. *J Urol.* 1979;121:728.

63. Ghoneim MA, Shoukry I. The use of ileum for correction of advanced or complicated Bilharzial lesions of the urinary tract. *Int Urol Nephrol.* 1972;1:25.

64. Amin HA. Experience with the ileal ureter. *Br J Urol.* 1976;48:19.

65. Baum WC. The clinical use of terminal ileum as a substitute ureter. *J Urol.* 1954;72:16.

66. Kvarstein B, Mathisen W. Total replacement of the ureter with a segment of ileum. *Scand J Urol Nephrol.* 1980;14:47.

67. Dowd JB, Chen F. Ileal replacement of the ureter in the solitary kidney. *Surg Clin North Am.* 1971;51:739.

68. Dufour B, Blondel P, Bonaud P, Claude JM. Renoureteral bypass in obstructions and losses of substances of the initial ureter. *Eur Urol.* 1980;6:14.

69. Monnig JA, Dale G, Bicknell SL. The ileal ureter in recurrent urolithiasis. *J Urol.* 1976;116:699.

70. Creevy CD. Misadventures on replacement of ureters with ileum. *Surgery.* 1965;58:497.

71. Tanagho EA. A case against incorporation of bowel segments into the closed urinary system. *J Urol.* 1975;113:796.

72. Bazeed MA, El-Rakhawy M, Ashamalla A, et al. Ileal replacement of the Bilharzial ureter: Is it worthwhile? *J Urol.* 1983;130:245.

73. Mikulicz J. Zur operation der angeborenen Blasenspalte. *Zentralbl Chir.* 1899;26:641.

74. Couvelaire R. La petite vessie des tuberculeaux génitourinaires. Essai de classification, place et variantes des cystointestinoplasties. *J d'Urol.* 1950;56:381.

75. Cibert J. Bladder enlargement through ileocystoplasty. *J Urol.* 1953;70:600.

76. Hradec EA. Bladder substitution: indications and results in 114 operations. *J Urol.* 1965; 94:406.

77. Küss R, Bitker M, Camey M, Chatelain C, Lassau JP. Indications and early and late results of intestinocystoplasty: review of 185 cases. *J Urol.* 1970;103:53.

78. Smith RB, Van Cangh P, Skinner DG, Kaufman JJ, Goodwin WE. Augmentation entero-

cystoplasty: a critical review. *J Urol.* 1977;118(1):35–39.

79. Lapides J, Diokno AC, Silver SJ, Lowe BS. Clean intermittent catheterization in the treatment of urinary tract disease. *J Urol.* 1972;107:458.
80. Lapides J, Diokno AC, Gould FR, Lowe BS. Further observations on self catheterization. *J Urol.* 1975;116:169.
81. Goodwin WE, Turner RD, Winter CC. Results of ileocystoplasty. *J Urol.* 1958;80(6):461–466.
82. Gil-Vernet JM Jr. The ileocolic segment in urologic surgery. *J Urol.* 1965;94:418.
83. Kim KS, Susskind MR, King LR. Ileocecal ureterosigmoidoscopy: an alternative to conventional ureterosigmoidoscopy. *J Urol.* 1988;140:1494–1498.
84. Light JK, Engelmann MH. LeBag: total replacement of the bladder using an ileocolonic pouch. *J Urol.* 1986;136:27–31.
85. Thuroff JW, Alken P, Riedmiller H, Engelmann U, Jacobi GH, Hohenfellner R. The Mainz pouch (mixed augmentation ileum and cecum) for bladder augmentation and continent diversion. *J Urol.* 1986;136:17–26.
86. Mitchell ME, Kulb TB, Backes DJ. Intestinocystoplasty in combination with clean intermittent catheterization in the management of vesical dysfunction. *J Urol.* 1986;136:288–291.
87. Mitchell ME, Piser JA. Intestinocystoplasty and total bladder replacement in children and young adults. Follow-up in 129 cases. *J Urol.* 1987;138:579–584.
88. Sheiner JR, Kaplan GW. Spontaneous bladder rupture following enterocystoplasty. *J Urol.* 1988;140:1157–1158.
89. Elder JS, Snyder HM, Hulbert WC, Duckett JW. Perforation of the augmented bladder in patients undergoing clean intermittent catheterization. *J Urol.* 1988;140:1159–1162.
90. Piser JA, Mitchell ME, Kulb TB, Rink RC, Kennedy HA, McNulty A. Gastrocystoplasty and colocystoplasty in canines: the metabolic consequences of acute saline and acid loading. *J Urol.* 1987;138:1109–1113.
91. Kennedy HA, Adams MC, Mitchell ME, et al. Chronic renal failure and bladder augmentation: stomach versus sigmoid colon in the canine model. *J Urol.* 1988;140:1138.
92. Adams MC, Mitchell NE, Rink RC. Gastrocystoplasty: an alternative solution to the problem of urological reconstruction of the severely compromised patient. *J Urol.* 1988;140:1152.
93. Boyd JD. Chronic acidosis secondary to ureteral transplantation. *Am J Dis Child.* 1931;42:366–371.
94. Ferris DO, Odel HM. Electrolyte pattern of the blood after bilateral ureterosigmoidostomy. *JAMA.* 1950;142:634–641.
95. Odel HM, Ferris DO, Priestly JT. Further observations on the electrolyte pattern of the blood after bilateral ureterosigmoidostomy. *J Urol.* 1951;65:1013–1020.
96. Koch MO, McDougal WS. The pathophysiology of hyperchloremic metabolic acidosis after urinary diversion through intestinal segments. *Surgery.* 1985;98(3):561–570.
97. Koch MO, Gurevitch E, Hill DE, et al. Urinary solute transport by intestinal segments: a comparative study of ileum and colon. *J Urol.* 1990;143:1275–1279.
98. Arnarson O, Straffon RA. Clinical experience with ileal conduit in children. *J Urol.* 1969;102:768.
99. Bowles WT, Tall BA. Urinary diversion in children. *J Urol.* 1967;98:597.
100. Castro JE, Ram MD. Electrolyte imbalance following ileal urinary diversion. *Br J Urol.* 1970;42:29.
101. Cohen SM, Persky L. A ten year experience with ureteroileostomy. *Arch Surg.* 1967; 95:278.
102. Creevy CD. Renal complications after iliac diversion of urine in non-neoplastic disorders. *J Urol.* 1960;83:394.
103. Harbach LB, Hall RL, Cockett ATK, et al. Ileal loop cutaneous urinary diversion: a critical review. *J Urol.* 1971;105:511–515.
104. Remigailo RB, Lewis EL, Woodard JR, et al. Ileal conduit urinary diversion: a ten year review. *Urology.* 1976;7:343–348.
105. Retik AB, Perlmutter AD, Gross RP. Cutaneous ureteroileostomy in children. *N Engl J Med.* 1967;277:217.
106. Schmidt JD, Hawtrey CE, Flocks RH, et al. Complications, results, and problems of ileoconduit diversion. *J Urol.* 1973;109:210–216.
107. Smith ED. Follow-up studies of 150 ileoconduits in children. *J Pediatr Surg.* 1972;7:1.
108. Stevens PS, Eckstein HB. Ileoconduit urinary diversion in children. *Br J Urol.* 1977;49:370.
109. Beckly S, Wajsman Z, Pontes JE, et al. Transverse colon conduit: a method of urinary diversion after pelvic irradiation. *J Urol.* 1982;128:464–468.
110. Elder DD, Moisey CU, Rees RWN. A long-term follow-up of colon conduit operation in children. *Br J Urol.* 1979;51:462.
111. Husbann DA, McLorie GA, Churchill BN. Non-refluxing colon conduits. A long-term life table analysis. *J Urol.* 1989;142:1201.
112. Moralies P, Golimbu N. Colonic urinary diversion. Ten years of experience. *J Urol.* 1975;113:302.
113. Schmidt JD, Hawtrey CE, Buchsbaum HJ. Transverse colon conduit. A preferred method of urinary diversion for radiation treated pelvic malignancies. *J Urol.* 1975;113:308.

114. Hendren WH, Radopoulous D. Complications of ileal loop and colon conduit urinary diversion. *Urol Clin North Am.* 1983;10:451.

115. Whitmore WF, Gittes RF. Reconstruction of the urinary tract by cecal and ileocecal cystoplasty. A review of a 15 year experience. *J Urol.* 1983;129:494.

116. Nurse DE, Mundy AR. Metabolic complications of cystoplasty. *Br J Urol.* 1989;63:165.

117. Kock NG, Nilson AE, Norlan L, et al. Urinary diversion via continent ileum reservoir: clinical experience. *Scand J Urol Nephrol.* (Suppl) 1978;49:23.

118. Boyd SD, Lieskovsky G, Schiff WM, Kanellos AW, Skinner DG, Klimaszewski AD. *Urology.* 1989;33(2):85–88.

119. Koch MO, McDougal WS, Reddy PK, Lange PH. Metabolic alterations following continent urinary diversion through colonic segments. *J Urol.* 1991;145:270–273.

120. McDermott WV. Diversion of urine to the intestines as a factor in ammoniogenic coma. *N Engl J Med.* 1957;256:460–462.

121. Clark SS. Electrolyte disturbance associated with jejunal conduit. *J Urol.* 1974;112:42.

122. Golimbu M, Morales P. Electrolyte disturbances in jejunal urinary diversion. *Urology.* 1973;1:432.

123. Klein EA, Monte JE, Montigue D, et al. Jejunal conduit urinary diversion. *J Urol.* 1986; 135:244–246.

124. Sridhar KN, Samuell CT, Woodhouse CRJ. *Br Med J.* 1983;287:1327–1329.

125. Fossa SD, Heilo A, Bormer O. Unexpectantly high serum methotrexate levels in cystectomized bladder cancer patients with an ileal conduit treated with intermediate doses of the drug. *J Urol.* 1990;143:498–501.

126. Savariragen F, Dixey GN. Syncope following ureterosigmoidostomy. *J Urol.* 1969;101:844.

127. Lemann J, Litzow JR, Lennon EJ. The effects of chronic acid loads in normal man: Further evidence for the participation of bone mineral in the defense against chronic metabolic acidosis. *J Clin Invest.* 1966;45:1608.

128. McDougal WS, Koch MO, Shands C, Price RR. Bony demineralization following urinary intestinal diversion. *J Urol.* 1988;140:853.

129. Koch MO, McDougal WS. Bone demineralization following ureterosigmoid anastomosis: an experimental study in rats. *J Urol.* 1988;140:856.

130. Salahudeen AK, Eliott RW, Ellis HA. Osteomalacia due to ileal replacement of ureters: a report of two cases. *J Urol.* 1984;131:335.

131. Hossain M. The osteomalacia syndrome after colocystoplasty: a cure with sodium bicarbonate alone. *Br J Urol.* 1970;42:243.

132. Kinn AC, Lantz B. Vitamin $B_{12}$ deficiency after radiation for bladder carcinoma. *J Urol.* 1984;131:888–890.

133. Canning DA, Perman JA, Jeffs RD, Gearhart JP. Nutritional consequences of bowel segments in the lower urinary tract. *J Urol.* 1989;142:509–511.

134. Mansson W, Colleen S, Sundin T. Continent caecal reservoir in urinary diversion. *Br J Urol.* 1984;56:359–365.

135. Hofmann AF, Borgstrom B. Physical chemical state of lipids in intestinal content during their ingestion and absorption. *Gastroenterology.* 1962;21:43.

136. Pitt HA, Lewinski MA, Muller EL, et al. Ileal resection induced gallstones: altered bilirubin or cholesterol metabolism? *Surgery.* 1984; 96:154.

137. Frexes-Steed M, Neblett WW, Holcomb GW. Spectrum of biliary disease in childhood. *South Med J.* 1986;79(11):1342–1349.

138. Leadbetter GW, Zickerman P, Pierce E. Ureterosigmoidostomy and carcinoma of the colon. *J Urol.* 1979;121:732.

139. Husmann DA, Spence HM. Current status of tumor of the bowel following ureterosigmoidostomy: a review. *J Urol.* 1990;144:607–610.

140. Filmer RB, Spencer JR. Malignancies in bladder augmentations and intestinal conduits. *J Urol.* 1990;143:671–678.

141. Crissey MM, Gittes RF, Steel JD. Rat model of carcinogenesis in ureterosigmoidostomy. *Science.* 1980;207:1079.

142. Stewart M, Hill MG, Pugh RCB, et al. The role of N-nitrosamine in carcinogenesis at the ureterocolonic anastomosis. *Br J Urol.* 1981;53:115.

143. Cohen MS, Hilz ME, Davis CP, et al. Urinary carcinogen (nitrosamine) production in a rat animal model for ureterosigmoidostomy. *J Urol.* 1987;138:449.

144. Stewart M. Urinary diversion and bowel cancer. *Bowel Cancer Ann Roy Coll Surg Eng.* 1986;68:98.

145. Nurse DE, Mundy AR. Assessment of the malignant potential of cystoplasty. *Br J Urol.* 1989;64:489.

146. Shands C III, McDougal WS, Wright EP. Prevention of cancer at the urothelial enteric anastomotic site. *J Urol.* 1989;141:178.

147. Stribling MD, Cohen MS, Fagan JD, et al. The effect of ascorbic acid on urinary nitrosamines in tumor development in a rat model for ureterosigmoidostomy. *J Urol.* 1989;141:304A (abstr).

148. Flipe MI. Mucous secretion in rat colonic mucosa during carcinogenesis induced by dimethylhydrozine: a morphological and histochemical study. *Br J Cancer.* 1985;32:60.

149. McGarrity TJ, Via EA, Colony PC. Qualitative and quantitative changes in sialomucins during 1,2-dimethylhydrozine induced colon carcinogens in the rat. *JNCI.* 1987;79:1375.

150. Shamsuddin AK, Trump BF. Colon epithelium II: In vivo studies of colon carcinogenesis: Light microscopic histochemical and ultrastructural studies of histogenesis and azoxymethane induced colon carcinomas in Fischer 344 rats. *JNCI*. 1981;66:389.

151. Dawson PM, Habib NA, Rees HC, et al. The influence of sialomucin at the resection margin on local tumor recurrence and survival in patients with colorectal cancer: a multivaried analysis. *Br J Surg*. 1987;74:366.

152. Mansson W, Willen R. Mucosal morphology and histochemistry of the continent cecal reservoir for urine. *J Urol*. 1988;139:1199.

153. Marcheggiano A, Iannoni C, Pallone F, et al. Abnormal patterns of colonic mucin secretion after ureteral sigmoidostomy. *Human Pathol*. 1984;15:647.

154. Strachan JR, Rees HC, Williams G. Histochemical changes after ureterosigmoidostomies and colonic diversion. *Br J Urol*. 1985;57:700.

155. LaMuraglia GM, Lacaine F, Malt RA. High ornithine decarboxylase activity and polyamine levels in human colorectal neoplasia. *Ann Surg*. 1986;204:89.

156. Porter CW, Herrera-Ornelas L, Pera P, et al. Polyamine biosynthetic activity in normal and neoplastic human colorectal tissues. *Cancer*. 1987;60:1275.

157. Rozhin J, Wilson PS, Bull AW, et al. Ornithine decarboxylase activity in the rat and human colon. *Cancer Res*. 1984;44:3226.

158. Luk GD, Hamilton SR, O'Ceallaigh D, et al. A oxymethane (AOM) induces a generalized biphasic increased in intestinal ornithine decarboxylase (ODC) during colon carcinogenouses. *Gastroenterology*. 1982;82:1121.

159. Weber TR, Westfall HS, Steinhardt GF, et al. Malignancy associated with ureterosigmoidostomy: detection by mucosa ornithine decarboxylase. *J Pediatr Surg*. 1988;23:1091.

# 32

# Continent Diversion—Neobladders

*Stephen F. Bardot and James E. Montie*

## HISTORY

One of the early landmarks of childhood development is the attainment of fecal and urinary continence. Although this occurs early in human development, it is a late evolutionary step and one that separates man from beast. Since the middle of the 19th century, the quest for continent urinary diversion after removal of the bladder has also been an evolutionary process.

The first ureterosigmoidostomy was performed by Simon in 1851 for bladder extrophy.[1] Although there were rare successes reported with this procedure in the following years, patients usually succumbed to infectious complications.[2] The procedure became more successful after Coffey described a nonrefluxing, tunnelled ureterocolic anastomosis in 1911.[3] Reports from other authors followed, detailing improved mucosa-to-mucosa anastomotic techniques that helped avoid obstructive complications.[4,5]

Despite these modifications, patients undergoing ureterosigmoidostomy were troubled by pyelonephritis, hydronephrosis, incontinence, and metabolic acidosis. Publications began to describe the long-term complications.[6]

In 1950, two important papers helped shape the future of permanent urinary diversion. Bricker, unsuccessful in attempts to construct a continent urinary diversion, described the ileal conduit.[7] He emphasized meticulous care in constructing a two-layer mucosa-to-mucosa ureterointestinal anastomosis. Although, with the addition of a bowel anastomosis, the ileal conduit was technically more challenging than the ureterosigmoidostomy, it allowed for separation of the urinary and fecal streams. The Bricker procedure was associated with a low incidence of anastomotic obstruction and metabolic acidosis, problems which had so troubled those treated with ureterosigmoidostomy. The ileal conduit gradually became the preferred technique for permanent urinary diversion.

Also in 1950, Gilchrist described his technique of continent urinary diversion based on an isolated ileocecal segment.[8] The bowel was not detubularized and relied on the ileocecal valve, the oblique course of the efferent limb through the abdominal wall, and the antiperistaltic action of the ileum for continence. Later, Sullivan reported good long-term results with this technique, with a 90% continence rate.[9] However, others were not able to achieve success with this method.[10,11]

Innovative work by Camey and Kock continued to stimulate the search for a safe and reliable technique of continent diversion. In 1959, Camey began creating bladder substitutes based on anastomosing a loop of ileum to the urethral stump.[12] Kock, after achieving success in creating a continent ileostomy, turned his attention to creating a continent urinary diversion based on a detubularized pouch constructed from ileum with a cutaneous stoma.[13]

Numerous factors have led to the precipitous increase in efforts to create a continent diversion, including dissatisfaction with the need for an external appliance and numerous reports of long-term stomal complications and upper tract deterioration in the ileal conduit.[14–16] In addition, a decrease in the use of preoperative radiation therapy prior to cystectomy has led to the availability of healthier bowel tissue for use in construction of a continent diversion. Finally, the recognition of the safety and efficacy of intermittent catheterization has led to its rapid acceptance and adaptation in emptying a continent urinary reservoir.

## URETERAL REIMPLANTATION

A variety of techniques are available for constructing a continent urinary diversion; most attempt to create a nonrefluxing ureterointestinal anastomosis. The reconstructive urologist may use several methods to create a ureteral anastomosis. Although the individual techniques vary considerably, there are certain points common to all. A meticulous dissection of the ureter—with preservation of its vascular adventitia—is necessary to prevent ischemia and subsequent obstruction. A mucosa-to-mucosa anastomosis without tension is also important. Many surgeons rely on postoperative ureteral stenting to permit satisfactory healing and ensure adequate upper tract drainage.

The extracolonic technique described by Leadbetter and Goodwin's intracolonic implantation have been successfully used to create many continent diversions.[17,18] This procedure, based on a submucosal tunnel, is usually straightforward when the reservoir uses tissue from the large bowel, which has a thicker muscular wall. However, the technique is less applicable to small bowel because of the less substantial muscular layer and the mucosal adhesions of the valvulae conniventes. The tunnel techniques rely on a flap–valve mechanism to prevent reflux. Hydrostatic pressure in the reservoir causes coaptation of the intramural ureteral walls against the backing of the muscularis mucosa; this is the same physiologic principle as that present at the normal ureterovesical junction.

LeDuc described the technique of implanting the ureter in a nonrefluxing fashion into small bowel.[19] The technique is based on creating a 3 cm mucosal trough and securing the distal ureter into this sulcus. With time, the ileal mucosa grows over the ureter, forming a submucosal tunnel. LeDuc described the results of this technique in conjunction with the Camey continent diversion. He related that obstructive complications occurred in only 1.5% of the anastomoses; however, reflux was present in 19% of the patients. This high rate of reflux is undoubtedly related to the nondetubularized nature of the Camey diversion. LeDuc's technique has been used in detubularized reservoirs with tissue from both the large and small bowels with a much lower rate of reflux.[20,21] The simplicity of this technique and its applicability to both large and small bowel have led to an increase in its use in a variety of continent urinary diversions.

The second technique that may be used with both large- and small-intestine tissue is the split-cuff nipple. Turner-Warwick originally described the technique in 1967 in a cystoplasty study.[22] More recently, Stone described its use in 18 patients undergoing supravesical diversion.[23] With this technique, the ureter is spatulated and folded back upon itself (Fig 1). To prevent reflux, a 2:1 ratio of nipple length to ureteral diameter is necessary. This technique may also be used with dilated ureters, as long as the 2:1 ratio is maintained. Stone reported mild reflux in one patient and no cases of obstructive complications. However, the split-cuff technique should be used with caution in patients with a thick-walled ureter. Also, with a markedly dilated ureter, adequate ureteral length may not be available to be used during the split-cuff technique. Both the LeDuc anastomosis and a split-cuff nipple offer the ad-

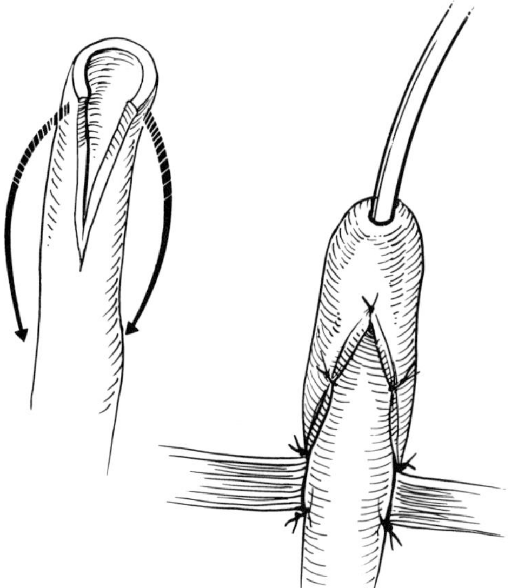

**Fig 1.** The split-cuff nipple technique. After spatulation, the ureter is folded back upon itself over an 8 F infant feeding tube. The nipple is then brought through an enterotomy and secured with serosal sutures.

vantage of sacrificing no bowel tissue to create the antireflux mechanism.

The afferent limb of a continent reservoir may also be based on the ileocecal valve or remodeled ileum. Gil-Vernet was the first to describe the use of the ileocecal valve to prevent reflux.[24] The ureters can be anastomosed to the ileal stump using either a Bricker or Wallace anastomosis. Dependence on the unreinforced ileocecal valve to prevent reflux is prone to failure, particularly in a nondetubularized reservoir under higher pressures. Rendleman studied the integrity of reservoirs created from the ileocecal valve and found a 75% incidence of reflux at pressures greater than 50 cm of water.[25] Gittes introduced a reinforcement procedure to improve the antireflux ability of the ileocecal valve.[26] Then, Hendren augmented the ileocecal valve by intussusception of a segment of ileum through the valve. The mesentery was stripped from the terminal 6–8 cm of ileum, this section of small bowel was intussuscepted through the ileocecal valve, and was fixed in place with serosal sutures. The procedure has been modified, as Hendren now stabilizes the nipple with staples.[27]

Kock, in 1973, described a continent fecal diversion based on an intussuscepted ileal valve[28]; Leisinger also used this technique to create a continent ileal bladder. Two ileal nipples were used, one to prevent reflux and one as the continent efferent limb.[29] Both Kock and Skinner have modified the intussuscepted ileal valve and used the technique in a large number of patients. While the efferent nipple valve has been a frequent source of complications and reoperations, the afferent nipple valve has proven to be very reliable. Reflux is prevented in 98% of patients and obstruction is uncommon.

Studer recently described an alternate method to prevent reflux.[30] An afferent limb consisting of 18–20 cm of ileum is used with a nontunnelled ureteroileal anastomosis (Fig 2). Reflux is minimized by the isoperistaltic action of this long segment of ileum.

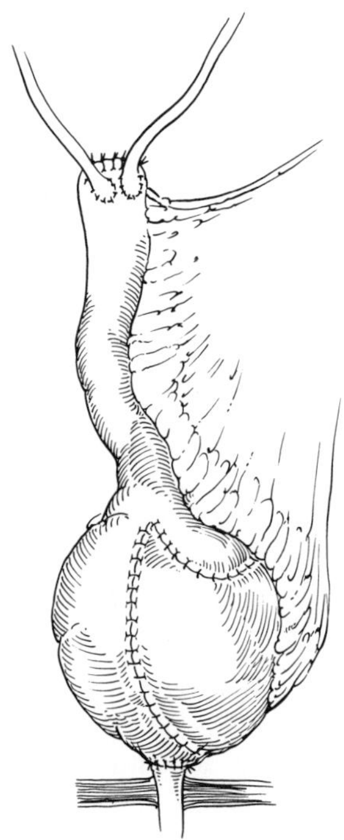

**Fig 2.** Afferent limb described by Studer; ureters are implanted in a direct, non-tunnelled fashion into an 18–20 cm limb of ileum.

Urine storage at pressures greater than 40 mm Hg has been associated with upper tract deterioration. Recently, the need for an antireflux anastomosis has been questioned when used in patients with a low-pressure, continent urinary reservoir, as nontunnelled anastomoses are predicted to have a lower rate of anastomotic obstruction. Lockhart used a direct anastomosis while creating 91 detubularized right colonic reservoirs.[31] Reflux occurred in 6 ureters (6.5%) and obstruction in 3. Long-term follow-up will be needed to determine if renal deterioration occurs.

## RESERVOIR CLASSIFICATION

The urologist is faced with a myriad of techniques of continent urinary diversion which have been described in the literature.[32] For clarity, it is helpful to categorize continent diversions into groups which have similar functional and anatomic characteristics. One classification that is readily apparent to both the urologist and to the patient is the method by which the continent reservoir is emptied. The neobladder is anastomosed to the intact urethra and relies on the external urinary sphincter for continence. Cutaneous reservoirs have an external stoma, through which the reservoir is emptied via intermittent catheterization. A third group of rectal reservoirs relies on the rectal sphincter for continence. Further subdivisions within these broad categories can be made on an anatomic basis. This classification system not only helps clarify the differences between the variety of techniques but also has clinical utility. Although excellent success has been achieved with a number of continent diversions, there is no single technique that represents the best choice for every patient. Continent diversions based entirely on small bowel have often been successful. However, they would be contraindicated in the patient with preexistent short-gut syndrome. Likewise, when considering a continent urinary diversion in patients with meningomyelocele sacrifice of the ileocecal valve and use of a long segment of large bowel may result in fecal incontinence. A broad classification system is also helpful when presenting alternatives to the patient. While most patients who choose a continent urinary diversion are primarily interested in avoiding an external appliance, there are some who would prefer to void through the urethra, even at the risk of possible nocturnal incontinence, as opposed to having an external stoma which needs to be emptied by intermittent catheterization. In the following sections, representative examples of each type of reservoir will be discussed.

### Neobladders

The ultimate goal of reconstructive surgery following cystectomy is to create a system that replicates the function of the normal bladder as closely as possible. This system would be continent, compliant, and allow a convenient drainage interval. At the same time, it would have a low rate of complications requiring reoperation and would not lead to metabolic or infectious complications. The neobladder has come the closest to achieving this goal. Unfortunately, use of this procedure is not recommended in all patients. It may be used only in the male patient with an intact urethra.

**Ileal Neobladders.** Tizzoni and Foggi first attempted to create a neobladder in 1888.[33] In a staged procedure in a dog, ureters were drained into a segment of bowel, which was anastomosed to the urethra. In 1951, Couvelaire described the first successful use of a neobladder in a human.[34] His approach was modified by Camey and LeDuc, who first described their procedure in 1979.[12] The Camey reservoir consists of a 35–40 cm U-shaped segment of ileum with the apex of the U anastomosed to the membranous urethra (Fig 3). The authors note that in 15% of patients this procedure is not possible, due to a short small-bowel mesentery which prevents anastomosis to the urethra. The ureters are anastomosed in a nonrefluxing fashion to the end of each of the ileal limbs. Lilien recently reviewed the results of this procedure in 84 patients.[35] Daytime continence was achieved in over 90% of the patients. However, nocturnal incontinence occurred in half the patients,

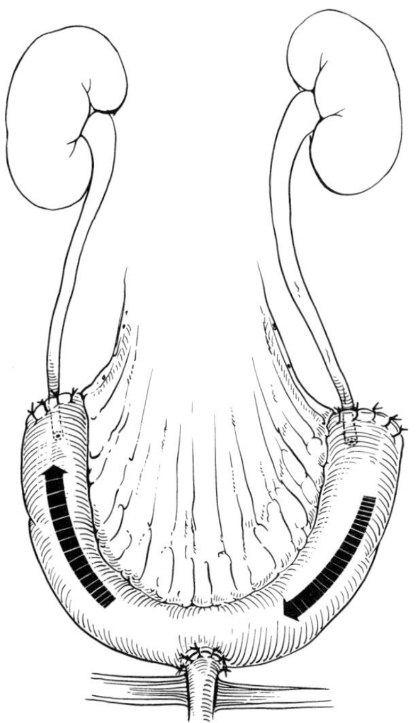

**Fig 3.** Camey U-shaped loop is anastomosed to urethra at apex of U. Peristaltic action of ileum is indicated by arrows.

and patients should be encouraged to void every 2–3 hours at night to avoid this problem. Reflux was present in 15% of the patients. Camey reported that 70% of patients had sterile urine. With long-term follow-up, renal impairment had developed in five patients. The higher pressures resulting from the use of nondetubularized bowel undoubtedly contribute to the development of reflux and incontinence. Roehrborn subsequently performed urodynamic studies on 14 patients with Camey ileobladders.[36] In this group, 11 patients were continent during the day; however, all patients had nocturnal enuresis. Urodynamic study revealed phasic contraction waves with maximum pressures of 30–65 cm of water. The waves occurred at a frequency of 1 per minute. The mean capacity of the Camey reservoir was 362 mL, and unlike detubularized reservoirs, the capacity did not increase with time. The pioneering work by Camey has not led to the widespread use of his technique in the urologic community, but it did show the feasibility and safety of creating a continent urethral reservoir.

Since the innovative work by Camey, other investigators have described ileal neobladders. Although a variety of techniques are used, all ileal neobladders use a reservoir created from detubularized ileum. Tscholl, in 1987, described seven successful cases of ileal bladder replacement based on the S-pouch that has been successfully used in anorectal reconstruction.[37] Fifty-five cm of ileum is formed into an S-shaped configuration with three 12-cm limbs. The most dependent portion is anastomosed to the urethral stump. A nipple valve is used to prevent reflux in the afferent limb. Although follow-up was short in Tscholl's series, daytime continence was good. However, two patients had stress incontinence. All patients were dry at night, although most patients had to void at least once a night to remain dry. Interestingly, one female patient was continent after anastomosis of the pouch to the urethral stump.

Ghoneim described a similar experience with the hemi-Kock reservoir.[38] The procedure was performed in 16 men following radical cystoprostatectomy. A 45-cm segment of ileum was used to construct the neobladder. The proximal third of the small bowel was used to create an intussuscepted nipple valve to prevent reflux, and the remaining two thirds was detubularized and folded into a U-shaped configuration for the reservoir. All patients were continent during the day. Four patients (25%) experienced nocturnal enuresis. Three patients became continent at night during therapy with desmopressin and/or imipramine. Four patients had reoperations for nipple valve malfunction. Urodynamics were performed in this study and revealed pressures lower than 40 cm water at a capacity of 300 $cm^3$.

Studer, after preliminary animal experiments, described a successful technique for creating an ileal neobladder.[30,39] After a nerve-sparing radical cystoprostatectomy in 22 patients, the pouch was created from a detubularized segment of 50–65 cm of ileum. Continence was good in 18 patients in whom the pouch was anastomosed directly to the urethra. However, in four patients, a short (2–5 cm), intact ileal segment was anastomosed to the urethra. This small segment of tubularized bowel resulted in incontinence and poor emptying in all four patients and required revision in two. Urodynamic studies revealed peristaltic waves in this short section with pressures up to 80 cm water.

Wenderoth and associates described using a different technique to create an ileal neobladder in a large series of patients. The reservoir was constructed from 60–80 cm of ileum, and the ileocecal valve and distal 15 cm of ileum were not used to create this reservoir, in an attempt to prevent diarrhea and vitamin B12 deficiency. After detubularization, a W-shaped plate is formed, anastomosed to the urethra, and closed, to create a spherical reservoir. The average maximum capacity of the reservoir is 750 mL, with an average maximum pressure of 26 cm water. Eighty-two percent of patients were continent both day and night. Age was noted to be a risk factor for incontinence in this study; while 89% of the patients under 70 years old were continent both day and night, 50% of patients over 70 were incontinent.[40]

**Ileocecal Neobladder.** The ileocolic segment is also frequently used to create a neobladder. Use of the larger diameter right colon allows the creation of a larger volume reservoir while sacrificing a shorter length of the gastrointestinal tract. Also, the ileocecal valve is available for antireflux or efferent limb use.

Gilchrist initially described use of the ileocecal segment in the creation of a neobladder.[41] The ileal end of the intact segment was anastomosed to the urethra, and although the ileocecal valve was plicated to facilitate continence, high-pressure contractions in the isolated segment caused problems. Light described the use of a detubularized ileocolic segment to create a neobladder in 1986.[42] Using this technique, a 20 cm or longer segment of cecum, with an equal length of ileum, is detubularized into two plates and reconfigured to form a bivalved reservoir. The proximal ileum is left intact, to be used for anastomosis to the urethral stump. In the four cases described, two had an artificial urinary sphincter placed at the time of surgery and the remaining two patients experienced some degree of incontinence following creation of the neobladder. Marshall, in a recent series, successfully used an ileocolonic segment to create a neobladder in 20 patients.[43] Fifteen cm of cecum and segment of ileum at least 30 cm in length are used to create the reservoir.[44] The bowel is placed in an inverted-N configuration and detubularized, and the most dependent portion of the cecum is selected for urethral anastomosis. After urethral anastomosis and ureteral implantation, the pouch is closed in a spherical configuration. Marshall related good results; 19 patients were able to void volitionally and none of the patients required the use of absorbent pads for incontinence either during the day or night. Two patients required reoperation for late complications, including one with rupture of the neobladder during chemotherapy.

**Sigmoid Neobladders.** Reddy has used the sigmoid colon to create a neobladder; in one series, a neobladder was constructed from tubularized sigmoid colon in ten patients and from an ileal-patched cecal reservoir in seven.[45,46] The sigmoid bladder was constructed from 35–45 cm of bowel anastomosed to the urethra with a configuration similar to that described by Camey. The patched cecal reservoir had median pressures of 25 cm of water, while median pressures in the reservoir created from intact sigmoid colon was 50 cm of water. All of the patients with patched reservoirs were dry during the day, while 30% of those with sigmoid reservoir experienced urinary leakage. Only one of the patients in this series was dry at night. In more recent work, the authors detubularized the sigmoid bowel in a series of 27 patients.[47] Although less bowel tissue was used, with detubularization, a larger capacity, lower pressure neobladder was created. In addition, continence was improved; 60% of the patients were dry at night. After one year of follow-up, complications had resulted in only one reoperation, which was performed to correct a ureteroenteric obstruction.

The function of the continent neobladder most closely mirrors that of the normal bladder. The neobladder, free of external appliance or stoma and emptied by volitional voiding, is also the most socially and psychologically acceptable alternative. Numerous authors, using a variety of techniques, have reported mixed results. However, certain basic points are evident. A meticulous dissection of the prostatic apex, as described by Walsh, is essential to success.[48,49] Second, use of tubularized bowel will result in a high rate of nocturnal enuresis. Finally, use of ileum in the neobladder, whether to construct the entire reservoir or simply a portion of the wall, seems to give the best results in terms of continence.

## Cutaneous Abdominal Stoma

Continent cutaneous diversions are those which are drained via an abdominal stoma. Cutaneous diversions generally do not cause the nocturnal enuresis which can occur in reservoirs that are anastomosed to the urethra. These diversions also have broader applicability, since they are not dependent on the presence of a functional urethra. Also, the urologist has more freedom in selecting a stoma site, since an external appliance is not necessary. Placement of the stoma in the base of the umbilicus has been advocated by several authors, and use of this site can facilitate catheterization in the patient with limited mobility. An umbilical stoma also decreases the length of efferent limb necessary in the obese patient. Due in part to some of these advantages, creation of a continent urinary diversion using an abdominal stoma is a common technique today.

**Cutaneous Stoma: Ileum.** After achieving success in constructing a continent ileostomy for patients with inflammatory bowel disease, Kock turned his attention to developing a continent urinary reservoir. After initial laboratory experiments, Kock reported the results in 12 patients of the continent reservoir he developed.[13,50] Kock's goal of creating a high-volume, low-pressure, nonrefluxing system was achieved, although seven patients required reoperation to achieve continence. The first report from the United States was Gerber's experience with seven patients.[51] In 1984, Skinner and colleagues described results in 51 patients.[52] This group has since published results—with the world's largest experience with this technique—in 489 patients.[53]

The Kock pouch is constructed with 70–80 cm of ileum. The terminal ends are intussuscepted to form the afferent and efferent nipple valves, while the central 40-cm segment is used to construct a spherical reservoir after detubularization (Fig 4). The Kock pouch has good functional characteristics, and is capable of storing 800–1000 $cm^3$ of urine at low pressure. The reservoir is emptied every 4–6 hours by intermittent catheterization. Malfunction of the efferent nipple valve has been the principal cause for reoperation in all series. A number of modifications to the Kock pouch

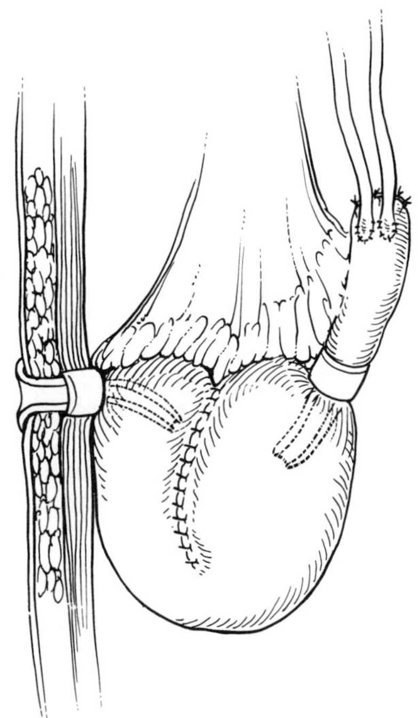

**Fig 4.** A schematic diagram of the completed Kock pouch.

have been described in the last decade, in attempts to improve the function of the efferent nipple.[54–56] Efforts have been aimed at decreasing the bulk of the mesentery of the small bowel included in the intussusception and improving the fixation of the valve. Some authors have stripped the mesentery of the bowel.[57] Kock, concerned about devascularization of the bowel, stripped the fat and peritoneum of the mesentery while preserving the blood supply.[54] A sleeve or collar of material is used to reinforce the nipple valve; materials that have been used include a fascial strip, collagen fleece, Marlex mesh, and polyglycolic acid mesh. Use of a stapling instrument has proven to be a very reliable form of nipple fixation. Three to four rows of staples are used, with at least one row used to fix the nipple to the reservoir wall. However, use of the stapling device can lead to additional problems. The stabilizing pin on the TA55 device can lead to formation of a pinhole fistula which bypasses the intussuscepted valve. Stone formation has been reported to occur in over 16% of patients with Kock pouch diversions, and these stones usually form on exposed staples, particularly at the tip of the nipple valve. In addition, a Marlex collar can erode into the pouch and stones can form on Marlex present in the reservoir. Stone formation can be decreased if no staples are placed in the tip of the nipple and if an absorbable material is used to form the collar instead of Marlex.[58]

Clinical experience in the largest number of patients and the longest follow-up has been reported with the use of the Kock pouch. Good results have been reported at the centers which perform a large number of this procedure. However, due to the complexity of the procedure, initial experience at most centers has resulted in a significant reoperation rate.[13,52,57]

**Cutaneous Stoma: Ileocecum.** Over the last 40 years, numerous authors have described using the ileocecal segment to create a continent urinary diversion. The ileocecal segment has been popular for several reasons, including the fairly constant vascular anatomy, the large cecal volume, and the presence of the ileocecal valve. After initial pioneering work by Gilchrist and associates, a variety of techniques have been developed to use this segment as a continent reservoir.[8,59] Both Zingg and Mansson attempted to augment the continence of the ileocecal valve by intussusception of ileum into the reservoir.[60,61] These early efforts utilized the intact cecum as the reservoir. However, Mansson has recently published details of an updated technique. The cecum is now detubularized to increase the compliance of the reservoir. Also, the efferent nipple is stabilized with staple fixation and an anchoring fascial collar in a manner similar to that advocated by Kock and Skinner.[62] The author describes a reliable technique of continent diversion; only one of 14 patients required reoperation for nipple malfunction.

The Mainz pouch, initially described by Thuroff and associates in 1985, has been shown to provide an adaptable and reliable continent diversion.[63] This pouch is based on a detubularized, 10 to 15-cm length of cecum, with a contiguous segment of ileum twice that length. When used to form a neobladder or for bladder augmentation, the entire section is detubularized and anastomosed to the urethral stump or remaining bladder wall. When a cutaneous stoma is needed, the proximal 6- to 8-cm of ileum is intussuscepted through the intact ileocecal valve. The intussusception is fixed with staples, not only to the ileocecal valve but also to the posterior wall of the reservoir, resulting in a very stable efferent limb. The most recent report details these results in a series of 51 patients with cutaneous stomas.[64] In the initial series, when suture fixation was used to stabilize intussusception, seven of eight patients required operative revision of the nipple valve. However, using the current technique, the efferent limb has proven to be very reliable. Forty-nine patients achieved continence in the most recent series.

In 1985, Rowland and associates described a continent reservoir based on the ileocecal segment, the Indiana pouch.[11] Initial attempts using the intact cecum resulted in an unacceptable level of incon-

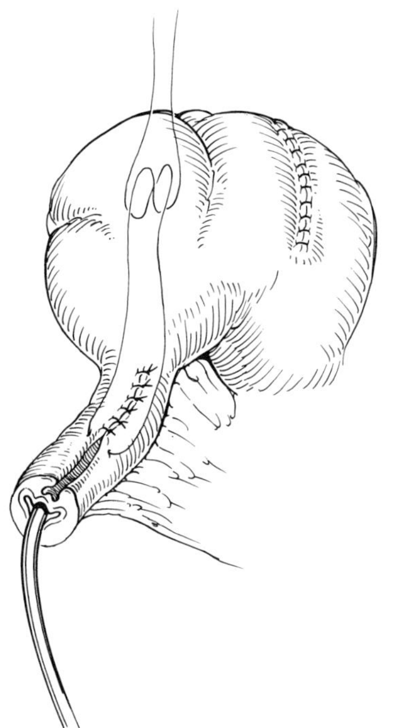

**Fig 5.** Indiana pouch; plication of the terminal ileum over a 12 F catheter to create the efferent limb. The GIA stapling device is now widely used to taper the ileal limb.

tinence. However, the procedure was successfully modified with the use of either an ileal patch or a Heineke-Mikulicz reconfiguration of the cecum to disrupt the circular muscle fibers of the colon. The efferent limb was created by plicating the ileum over a 12 F catheter (Fig 5). Results have been good, with a continence rate of over 90% and a low reoperation rate.[65] The simplicity of the technique, along with the excellent results, have led to broad acceptance in the urologic community. The procedure has undergone subsequent modifications by Rowland and at other centers.[66] Generally, the reservoir is now constructed entirely from the right hemi-colon, and the ileal patch is used only if there is an inadequate length of colon available. In the initial description, the ileum was plicated around the catheter with interrupted silk sutures. The gastrointestinal anastomosis (GIA) stapling device can also be used to effectively taper the ileum of the efferent limb.[21] Both the Goodwin and LeDuc techniques have been used with success to create the ureterocolic anastomosis.[31] Several centers have reported using the Indiana pouch or a reservoir with minor modifications, and results have been consistent, with continence achieved in over 90% of patients and a low reoperation rate of approximately 10%.[21,31,67]

## Rectosigmoid Reservoirs

A number of techniques rely on the anal sphincter for continence. This option has been employed in ureterosigmoidostomy, and in the creation of a rectal bladder. Although ureterosigmoidostomy is less commonly performed today, at some centers it is the procedure of choice in selected patients.[68,69] However, ascending urinary tract infections have plagued patients who have undergone ureterosigmoidostomy. In spite of the use of a nonrefluxing ureterointestinal anastomosis and suppressive antibiotics, acute pyelonephritis occurs in 20% to 57% of patients.[70] Following ureterosigmoidostomy, most patients will have some degree of metabolic acidosis and will require chronic bicarbonate replacement.

More recently, another complication has been noted in patients after ureterosigmoidostomy: the development of adenocarcinoma of the bowel arising from the site of ureterocolic implantation. There is a long latency period before the adenocarcinoma develops, particularly in younger patients. In patients over 40 years of age, Leadbetter reported a mean lag time of 8 years, with a range of 5–14 years.[71] In the younger patient with a longer life expectancy the risk is higher, although the latency period is longer. Husman described 94 patients who developed tumors after ureterosigmoidostomy for extrophy of the bladder.[72] Husman related a mean latency period of 26 years with a range of 3 to 53 years; the mean age of development of colon tumor was 33 years. Estimates of the relative risk for development of adenocarcinoma of the colon following ureterosigmoidostomy have varied widely, and range from about 350 times that of the normal population to as high as 7000 times in young adults.[69,73]

The etiology of the urocolonic tumors is uncertain, but several theories have been advanced. One theory advocates the production of nitrites and carcinogenic nitrosamines by enteric bacteria.[74] The second theory involves free radical production by phagocytes that induces DNA damage.[75] Although the etiology has not been elucidated, it is apparent that the risk of development of neoplasia is a direct function of the length of time following ureterosigmoidostomy.

In spite of these problems, in a motivated patient with a normal anal sphincter, and normal renal function, ureterosigmoidostomy may still be an attractive option. Suppressive antibiotics and bicarbonate replacement have helped reduce the risk of infectious and metabolic complications. Patients require regular urograms to access the upper tracts and regular endoscopy of the rectum to detect the development of adenocarcinoma after ureterosigmoidostomy.[76]

The anal sphincter has been used in a number of continent diversions besides ureterosigmoidostomy, with variable success. Creation of a rectal bladder has been used commonly in Egypt. The rectal bladder differs significantly from ureterosigmoidostomy in that the fecal and urinary streams are separated by the use of a terminal colostomy. In early work by Ghoneim, early postoperative mortality was 17%.[77] The mortality rate has decreased in subsequent reports. However, late complications, including recurrent pyelonephritis in 30% and nocturnal enuresis in 40% of patients, have been noted.[78] Despite these complications, Ghoneim related that this diversion was particularly useful in Egypt, where stomal appliances and proper stomal care are unavailable to many patients.

In 1962, Modelski described a procedure in which the rectosigmoid is divided, the ureters are implanted in a nonrefluxing fashion, and the terminal sigmoid is anastomosed end-to-side to the rectum.[79] Several subsequent studies by other authors have detailed the use of this procedure in a small number of patients.[80,81] The procedure is troubled by two factors which it has in common with ureterosigmoidostomy. One, urine may freely reflux throughout the colon leading to metabolic acidosis, and two, the diversion is not detubularized, resulting in nocturnal enuresis.

Kock and Ghoneim described an innovative technique which avoided the problems of the previous rectal bladder while using the anal sphincter for continence.[82] Reflux of urine into the proximal colon was prevented by an intussuscepted sigmoid valve. Also, an ileal patch was used to augment the rectum and lower the pressure in the system (Fig 6). Ureteral anastomosis was performed by three techniques in the 19 cases described: if the ureter was of normal caliber, a Goodwin technique was used, or the ureters were implanted directly into the intussuscepted sigmoid valve; if ureteral dilation was present, an intussuscepted ileal valve was incorporated into the patch to prevent reflux. In this study, all 19 patients were continent both day and

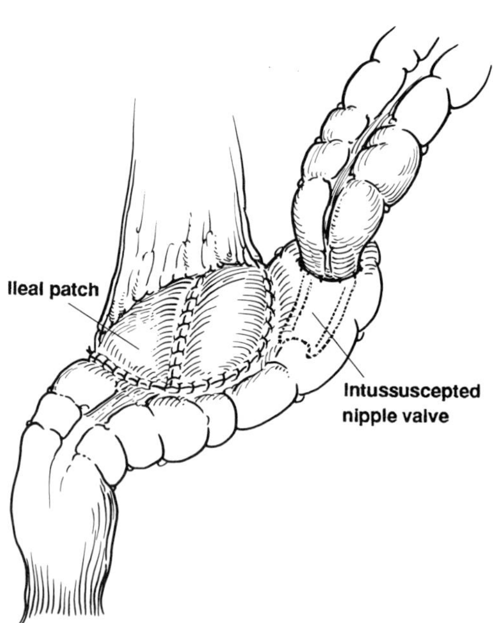


**Fig 6.** The augmented and valved rectosigmoid reservoir with ileal patch attached.

night. At 6 months postoperatively, the capacity of the reservoir was 700 mL. The mean peak pressure was 18 cm of water, while the highest pressure recorded was 30 cm of water. Although follow-up is short (3–14 months), the results are encouraging. Kock recommends yearly endoscopy of the rectum to screen for the development of adenocarcinoma.

## CONTINENCE MECHANISMS

In the preceding sections, the continence mechanism or efferent limb of the various reservoirs was described. Due to their adaptability and applicability in a number of reservoir systems, the Mitrofanoff principle and the Benchekroun "ink well" valve merit separate discussion. Benchekroun inverted a length of ileum into its own lumen and sutured the inner wall together over half the circumference. The valve functions much like an ink well. The entrance of urine and mucous into the space between the walls collapses the inner layer.[83] Results in 136 patients were described in 1989.[84] The valve needed operative revision in 17% of the cases and continence was achieved in over 88% of the patients. Particularly noteworthy is the wide applicability of the procedure: the "ink well" valve was used during the creation of ileal, ileocecal, and rectal reservoirs.

In 1980, Mitrofanoff described a novel continent urinary diversion. The distal end of the isolated appendix was implanted in a submucosal tunnel (in a nonrefluxing fashion) into the bladder, and the proximal end of the appendix was used as a stoma for catheterization. Mitrofanoff also described use of the distal ureter to create the efferent limb; a transureteroureterostomy was used to drain the kidney, and the distal ureter was used to create the stoma.[85] Duckett expanded the use of the Mitrofanoff principle to both bladder augmentation and formation of a continent cecal pouch.[86] Although results in a large series of patients have not been reported, the Mitrofanoff principle has proven to be reliable and flexible in its application.

## COMPLICATIONS OF CONTINENT URINARY DIVERSION

With extended follow-up, renal deterioration has been noted with ureterosigmoidostomy and the creation of an ileal conduit. Although continent urinary diversion results in an improved quality of life, this should not be achieved with the penalty of progressive renal impairment or metabolic complications. Chronic metabolic acidosis is common following ureterosigmoidostomy. Several factors influence the development of this abnormality, including the surface area of the bowel exposed to urine, the length of exposure, and the patient's underlying renal function. In patients with a ureterosigmoidostomy, the entire surface of the colonic mucosa is exposed to urine over a long period of time. This undoubtedly explains the metabolic acidosis observed in many of these patients. Although the amount of bowel used to construct different continent reservoirs varies, considerably less mucosa is exposed to urine after reservoir creation than following ureterosigmoidostomy. It appears that, in the patient with normal renal function, mild metabolic acidosis can occur following continent urinary diversion. However, this abnormality decreases with time. Thuroff noted that although most patients with a Mainz pouch required alkalinization postoperatively, after 1 year, none of the patients required this therapy.[64] Akerlund and associates followed 17 patients whose urine had been diverted with a Kock reservoir for over 5 years. The patients all had a normal base excess and arterial pH. A subtle defect in acid handling was noted in six patients when challenged by an acute acid load.[87] Kock evaluated 13 patients who had undergone either creation of an Indiana pouch or neobladder diversion. After a mean follow-up of 1 year, all patients were well compensated from an acid-base standpoint.[88] It appears that patients with normal renal function do not develop significant metabolic acidosis following continent urinary diversion. However, patients with impaired renal function will be at higher risk for this complication. Adams and Mitchell suggested the use of a segment of the stomach in constructing a continent urinary reservoir in this group of compromised patients.[89]

The distal ileum is the site for intestinal absorption of vitamin B12 and reabsorption of bile salts, and the nutritional consequences of resection of this segment to create the continent reservoir has been questioned. Canning assayed B12 and carotene levels in 26 patients following reconstructive surgery to screen for B12 deficiency or fat malabsorption; none of the patients demonstrated low levels of vitamin B12 or carotene.[90] Ackerlund found subnormal vitamin B12 levels in 35% of patients more than 5 years following Kock pouch urinary diversion, but none of these patients had signs of vitamin B12 deficiency.[87]

Renal deterioration has been reported to occur in 17% to 41% of patients following construction of an ileal conduit.[15,91] The influence of a nonrefluxing continent urinary diversion on renal function will have to be compared to this standard. However, few long-term studies are available. After a mean follow-up of 6.6 years, Ackerlund found a decrease in renal function in only one of 17 patients. However, after 5 to 11 years of follow-up, upper tract dilation was present in 29 patients.[87] Additional long-term studies are needed to determine the degree of upper tract preservation following the various continent diversions.

The pioneering work by Camey, Kock, Ghoneim, and others has led to the increasing use of continent urinary diversion today. Patient demand and surgical creativity will undoubtedly lead to further innovation. The relative merits of the various continent diversions await data from long-term follow-up in large series of patients. It is apparent that, with proper patient selection, and by creating a reservoir adhering to the principles set forth by Hinman,[92] continent urinary diversion represents a significant improvement in reconstructive surgery.

## REFERENCES


1. Simon MR. Ectropia vesicae (absence of the anterior walls of the bladder and pubic abdominal parietes); operation for directing the orifices of the ureters into the rectum; temporary success; subsequent death; autopsy. *Lancet*. 1852;2:568.
2. Tuffier T. De la deviation par le rectum du cours de l'urine: uretero-enterostomie, cysto-enterostomie. *Bull Soc Anat*. 1892;1:67.
3. Coffey RC. Physiologic implantation of the severed ureter or common bile duct into the intestine. *JAMA*. 1911;56:397.
4. Leadbetter WF. Consideration of problems incident to performance of ureteroenterostomy: report of a technique. *J Urol*. 1951;65:818.
5. Mathisen W. A new method for ureterointestinal anastomosis, a preliminary report. *Surg Gynecol Obst*. 1953;96:255.
6. Ferris DO, Odel HM. Electrolyte pattern of the blood after bilateral ureterosigmoidostomy. *JAMA*. 1950;142:634.
7. Bricker EM. Bladder substitution after pelvic evisceration. *Surg Clin North Am*. 1950; 30:1511.
8. Gilchrist RK, Merricks JW, Hamlin MH, Rieger IT. Construction of a substitute bladder and urethra. *Surg Gynecol Obst*. 1950;90:752.
9. Sullivan H, Gilchrist RK, Merricks JW. Ileocecal substitute bladder: long term followup. *J Urol*. 1973;109:43.
10. Bricker EM, Eiseman B. Bladder reconstruction from cecum and ascending colon following resection of pelvic viscera. *Ann Surg*. 1950; 132:77.
11. Rowland RG, Mitchell ME, Bihrle R. The cecoileal continent urinary reservoir. *World J Urol*. 1985;3:185.
12. Camey M, LeDuc A. L'entérocystoplastie avec cystoprostatectomie totale pour cancer de la vessie. *Ann Urol*. 1979;13:114.
13. Kock NG, Nilson AE, Nilsson LO, Norlén LJ, Philipson BM. Urinary diversion via a continent ileal reservoir: clinical results in 12 patients. *J Urol*. 1982;128:469.
14. Schwarz GR, Jeffs RD. Ileal conduit urinary diversion in children: computer analysis of follow-up from 2 to 16 years. *J Urol*. 1975; 114:285.
15. Pitts WR Jr, Muecke EC. A 20-year experience with ileal conduits: the fate of the kidneys. *J Urol*. 1979;122:154.
16. Smith ED. Follow-up studies on 150 ileal conduits in children. *J Pediatr Surg*. 1972;7:1.
17. Leadbetter WF, Clarke BG. Five years experience with ureteroenterostomy by the "combined" technique. *J Urol*. 1954;73:67.
18. Goodwin WE, Hauns AP, Kaufman JJ, Beal JM. Open, transcolonic ureterointestinal anastomosis: a new approach. *Surg Gynecol Obst*. 1953;97:295.

19. LeDuc A, Camey M, Teillac P. An original antireflux ureterointestinal implantation technique: long-term followup. *J Urol.* 1987;130:1156.

20. Hautmann RE, Egghart G, Frohneberg D, Miller K. The ileal neobladder. *J Urol.* 1988;139:39.

21. Bejany DE, Politano VA. Stapled and nonstapled tapered distal ileum for construction of a continent urinary reservoir. *J Urol.* 1988; 140:491.

22. Turner-Warwick RT, Ashken MH. The functional results of partial, subtotal and total cystoplasty, with special reference to ureterocaecocystoplasty, selective sphincterotomy and cystoplasty. *Br J Urol.* 1967;39:3.

23. Stone AR, MacDermott JP. The split-cuff ureteral nipple reimplantation technique: reliable reflux prevention from bowel segments. *J Urol.* 1989;142:707.

24. Gil-Vernet JM. Technique for construction of a functioning artificial bladder. *J Urol.* 1960; 83:39.

25. Rendleman DF, Anthony JE, Davis C Jr, Buenger RE, Brooks AJ, Beattie EJ Jr. Reflux pressure studies on the ileocecal valve of dogs and humans. *Surgery.* 1958;44:640.

26. Gittes RF. Bladder augmentation procedures. In: Libertino JA, Zinman L, eds. *Reconstructive Urologic Surgery: Pediatric and Adult.* Baltimore: Williams & Wilkins Co; 1977:210–220.

27. Hendren WH. Techniques for urinary undiversion. In: King LR, Stone AR, Webster GD, eds. *Bladder Reconstruction and Continent Urinary Diversion.* Chicago: Yearbook Medical Publishers; 1987:101–126.

28. Kock NG. Continent ileostomy. *Prog Surg.* 1973;12:180.

29. Leisinger HJ, Säuberli H, Schauwecker H, Mayor G. Continent ileal bladder: first clinical experience. *Eur Urol.* 1976;2:8.

30. Studer UE, Ackerman D, Casanova GA, Zingg EJ. Three years experience with an ileal low pressure bladder substitute. *Br J Urol.* 1989; 63:43.

31. Lockhart JL, Pow-Sang JM, Persky L, Kahn P, Helal M, Sanford E. A continent colonic reservoir: the Florida pouch. *J Urol.* 1990;144:864.

32. Goldwasser B, Hanani J. Continent urinary diversion. In: Paulson DF, Webster GD, eds. *Problems in Urology.* Philadelphia: JB Lippincott Company; 1987;1:375.

33. Tizzoni G, Foggi A. Die Wiederherstellung der harnblase experimentalle untersuchungen. *Zentralbl Chir.* 1888;15:1921.

34. Couvelaire R. Le réservoir iléal de substitution après la cystectomie totale chez l'homme. *J d'Urol Nephrol.* 1951;57:408.

35. Lilien OM, Camey M. 25-year experience with replacement of the human bladder (Camey procedure). *J Urol.* 1984;132:886.

36. Roehrborn CG, Tiegland CM, Sagalowski AI. Functional characteristics of the Camey ileal bladder. *J Urol.* 1987;138:739.

37. Tscholl R, Leisinger HJ, Hauri D. The ileal S-pouch for bladder replacement after cystectomy: preliminary report of 7 cases. *J Urol.* 1987;138:344.

38. Ghoneim MA, Kock NG, Lycke G, Shehab El-Din AB. An appliance free sphincter controlled bladder substitute: the urethral Kock pouch. *J Urol.* 1987;138:1150.

39. Studer UE, deKernion JB, Zimmern PE. A model for a bladder replacement plasty by an ileal reservoir: an experimental study in dogs. *Urol Res.* 1985;13:243.

40. Wenderoth UK, Bachor R, Egghardt G, Frohneberg D, Miller K, Hautmann RE. The ileal neobladder: experience and results of more than 100 consecutive cases. *J Urol.* 1990;143:492.

41. Gilchrist RK, Merricks JW. Construction of a substitute bladder and urethra. *Surg Clin North Am.* 1956;36:1131.

42. Light JK, Engelmann UH. LeBag: total replacement of the bladder using an ileocolonic pouch. *J Urol.* 1986;136:27.

43. Marshall FF, Mostwin JL, Radebaugh LC, Walsh PC, Brandler CB. Ileocolic neobladder post-cystectomy: continence and potency. *J Urol.* 1991;145:502.

44. Marshall FF. Creation of an ileocolic bladder after cystectomy. *J Urol.* 1988;139:1264.

45. Reddy PK, Lange PH, Fraley EE. Bladder replacement after cystoprostatectomy: efforts to achieve total continence. *J Urol.* 1987;138:495.

46. Reddy PK, Lange PH. Bladder replacement with sigmoid colon after radical cystoprostatectomy. *Urology.* 1987;29:368.

47. Reddy PK, Lange PH, Fraley EE. Total bladder replacement using detubularized sigmoid colon: technique and results. *J Urol.* 1991;145:51.

48. Walsh PC, Donker PJ. Impotence following radical prostatectomy: insight into etiology and prevention. *J Urol.* 1982;128:492.

49. Walsh PC, Lepor H, Eggleston JC. Radical prostatectomy with preservation of sexual function: anatomical and pathological considerations. *Prostate.* 1983;4:473.

50. Kock NG, Nilson AE, Norlén N, Sundin T, Trasti H. Changes in renal parenchyma and the upper urinary tracts following urinary diversion via a continent ileum reservoir. An experimental study in dogs. *Scan J Urol Nephrol.* 1978; 49(suppl):11.

51. Gerber A. The Kock continent ileal reservoir for supravesical urinary diversion. An early experience. *Am J Surg.* 1983;146:15.

52. Skinner DG, Boyd SD, Lieskovsky G. Clinical experience with the Kock continent ileal reservoir for urinary diversion. *J Urol.* 1984; 132:1101.

53. Skinner DG, Lieskovsky G, Boyd S. Continent urinary diversion. *J Urol.* 1989;141:1323.

54. Kock NG, Norlen L, Philipson BM, Åkerlund S. The continent ileal reservoir (Kock pouch) for urinary diversion. *World J Urol.* 1985;3:146.
55. Boyd SD, Skinner DG, Lieskovsky G. Ongoing experience with the Kock continent ileal reservoir for urinary diversion. *World J Urol.* 1985;3:155.
56. Skinner DG, Lieskovsky G, Boyd SD. Continuing experience with the continent ileal reservoir (Kock pouch) as an alternative to cutaneous urinary diversion: an update after 250 cases. *J Urol.* 1987;137:1140.
57. deKernion JB, DenBesten L, Kaufman JJ, Ehrlich R. The Kock pouch as a urinary reservoir. *Am J Surg.* 1985;150:83.
58. Ginsberg D, Huffman JL, Lieskovsky G, Boyd S, Skinner DG. Urinary tract stones: a complication of the Kock pouch continent urinary diversion. *J Urol.* 1991;145:956.
59. Ashken MH. An appliance-free ileocecal urinary diversion: preliminary communication. *Br J Urol.* 1974;46:631.
60. Zingg E, Tscholl R. Continent cecoileal conduit: preliminary report. *J Urol.* 1977;118:724.
61. Månsson W, Colleen S, Sundin T. Continent caecal reservoir in urinary diversion. *Br J Urol.* 1984;56:359.
62. Månsson W, Davidsson T, Colleen S. The detubularized right colonic segment as urinary reservoir: evolution of technique for continent diversion. *J Urol.* 1990;144:1359.
63. Thüroff JW, Alken P, Engleman U, Riedmiller H, Jacobi GH, Hohenfellner R. The Mainz pouch (mixed augmentation ileum'n zecum) for bladder augmentation and continent urinary diversion. *Eur Urol.* 1985;11:152.
64. Thüroff JW, Alken P, Riedmiller H, Jacobi GH, Hohenfellner R. 100 cases of Mainz pouch: continuing experience and evolution. *J Urol.* 1988;190:283.
65. Rowland RG, Mitchell ME, Bihrle B, Kahnoski RJ, Piser JE. Indiana continent urinary reservoir. *J Urol.* 1987;137:1136.
66. Ahlering TE, Weinberg AC, Razor B. A comparative study of the ileal conduit, Kock pouch and modified Indiana pouch. *J Urol.* 1989; 142:1193.
67. Ahlering TE, Weinberg AC, Razor B. Modified Indiana pouch. *J Urol.* 1991;145:1156.
68. Duckett JW, Gazak JM. Complications of ureterosigmoidostomy. *Urol Clin North Am.* 1983;10:473.
69. Spirnak JP, Caldamone AA. Ureterosigmoidostomy. *Urol Clin North Am.* 1986;13:285.
70. Golomb J, Klutke CG, Raz S. Complications of bladder substitution and continent urinary diversion. *Urology.* 1989;35:329.
71. Leadbetter GW, Zickerman P, Pierce E. Ureterosigmoidostomy and carcinoma of the colon. *J Urol.* 1979;121:732.
72. Husman DA, Spence HM. Current status of tumors of the bowel following ureterosigmoidostomy: a review. *J Urol.* 1990;144:607.
73. Eraklis AJ, Folkman MJ. Adenocarcinoma at the site of ureterosigmoidostomies for extrophy of the bladder. *J Pediatr Surg.* 1978;13:730.
74. Davis CP, Cohen MS, Anderson MD, Gruber MB, Warren MM. Urothelial hyperplasia and neoplasia. Detection of nitrosamines and interferon in chronic urinary tract infections in rats. *J Urol.* 1985;134:1002.
75. Dull BJ, Gittes RF, Goldman P. Nitrate production and phagocyte activation: differences among Sprague-Dawley, Wistar-Furth, and Lewis rats. *Carcinogenesis.* 1988;9:625.
76. Gleeson MJ, Griffith DP. Urinary diversion. *Br J Urol.* 1990;66:113.
77. Ghoneim MA. The rectosigmoid bladder for urinary diversion. *Br J Urol.* 1970;42:429.
78. Ghoneim MA, Shehab-El-Din AB, Ashamallah AK, Gaballah MA. Evolution of the rectal bladder as a method for urinary diversion. *J Urol.* 1981;126:737.
79. Modelski W. The transplantation of the ureters into the partially excluded rectum. *J Urol.* 1962;87:122.
80. Leiter E, Brendler H. Method of urinary diversion which preserves continence: description of a surgical technique and postoperative electrolyte study. *J Urol.* 1964;92:37.
81. Kamidono S, Yoshinori O, Hamami G, Hikosaka K, Kataoka N, Ishigami J. Urinary diversion: anastomosis of the ureters into a sigmoid pouch and end-to-side sigmoidorectostomy. *J Urol.* 1985;133:391.
82. Kock NG, Ghoneim MA, Lycke KG, Mahran MR. Urinary diversion to the augmented and valved rectum: preliminary results with a novel surgical procedure. *J Urol.* 1988;140:1375.
83. Benchekroun A. Continent caecal bladder. *Eur Urol.* 1977;3:248.
84. Benchekroun A, Essakalli N, Faik M, Marzouk M, Hachimi M, Abakka T. Continent urostomy with hydraulic ileal valve in 136 patients; 13 years experience. *J Urol.* 1989;142:46.
85. Mitrofanoff P. Cystostomie continente trans-appendiculaire dans le traitment des vessies neurologiques. *Chir Pediatr.* 1980;21:297.
86. Duckett JW, Snyder HM III. Continent urinary diversion: variations on the Mitrofanoff principle. *J Urol.* 1986;136:58.
87. Åkerlund S, Delin K, Kock NG, Lycke G, Philipson BM, Volkman R. Renal function and upper tract configuration following urinary diversion to a continent ileal reservoir (Kock pouch): a prospective 5- to 11-year followup after reservoir construction. *J Urol.* 1989;142:964.
88. Koch MO, McDougal WS, Reddy PK, Lange PH. Metabolic alterations following continent urinary diversion through colonic segments. *J Urol.* 1991;145:270.

89. Adams MC, Mitchell ME, Rink RC. Gastrocystoplasty: an alternative solution to the problem of urologic reconstruction in the severely compromised patient. *J Urol.* 1988;140:1152.

90. Canning DA, Perman JA, Jeffs RD, Gearhart JP. Nutritional consequences of bowel segments in the lower urinary tract. *J Urol.* 1989;142:509.

91. Schmidt JD, Hawtrey CE, Flocks RH, Culp DA. Complications, results and problem of ileal conduit diversion. *J Urol.* 1973;109:210.

92. Hinman F Jr. Selection of intestinal segments for bladder substitution: physical and physiological characteristics. *J Urol.* 1988;139:519.

# 33

# Testicular Tumor

*Richard S. Foster, John P. Donohue, Richard Bihrle, and Randall G. Rowland*

## INTRODUCTION

Testicular tumors are the most common type of solid tumors found in men between the ages of fifteen and forty.[1] Although once lethal when found to be metastatic, advances in medical and surgical therapy have rendered testicular tumors curable in most cases. The evolution of therapy for these tumors is due in large part to cooperation between medical and surgical oncologists. This chapter will trace the evolution of the therapy for this disease and describe current therapy on a stage-by-stage basis.

## EPIDEMIOLOGY

The incidence of testis cancer varies depending on the population studied, and is higher in white than in non-white populations. The yearly incidence varies between three and six cases per 100,000 men.[2] It is generally believed that the incidence has increased through the latter portion of the twentieth century, although increased awareness and improved diagnostic techniques may be factors in this apparent increase.

Ninety-seven percent to 98% of all testicular tumors are of germ-cell origin.[3] Seminoma is the most common histologic type, accounting for approximately 40% of cases in patients with normal testicular descent and for approximately 60% of cases in patients with a history of cryptorchidism. Other primary cell types include embryonal, teratocarcinoma, and teratoma. Choriocarcinoma is the least common histologic type, accounting for less than 5% of patients in most series.[4] Mixed tumors (tumors of more than one primary histologic type) account for approximately 25% of cases in most series.

Testicular tumors appear to be slightly more common on the right testis than on the left. The reason for this right-sided predisposition is not known.

Cryptorchidism, a history of trauma, and infertility have each been associated with testis cancer.[5] Cryptorchidism increases the risk of developing testis cancer approximately 35-fold; early orchiopexy is not thought to change this predisposition, although this has not been proven. Trauma is not a causative factor per se, but is generally acknowledged to be the impetus for examination of the testicle. Infertile men have a higher incidence of carcinoma in situ of the testis. Roughly 60% of patients diagnosed with testis cancer have been found to have abnormal semen analyses.[5]

## CLINICAL PRESENTATION

Localized testis cancer most commonly presents as scrotal enlargement with the accompanying symptoms of a sensation of fullness in the scrotum or, occasionally, discomfort. Another common presentation is an asymptomatic scrotal mass discovered by a sexual partner.

Metastatic testis cancer most commonly presents as back pain. An asymptomatic abdominal mass is another common presentation. Other presentations include supraclavicular or neck adenopathy and hemoptysis.

The differential diagnosis of a scrotal enlargement in young male patients includes epididymitis. If the patient is thought to have epididymitis, he should be treated with short-term antibiotic therapy and soon be re-examined to determine whether the enlargement is resolving. In the absence of improvement, radical orchiectomy should be considered—the original diagnosis of epididymitis may have been incorrect, and the patient may actually be suffering from a testicular tumor.

Physical examination of a scrotal enlargement should include palpation of the spermatic cord and cord structures and a careful examination of the testis. The groove between the epididymis and the testis proper should be identified with the index finger and thumb, followed by palpation of the testis. Small tumors, which may present as a subtle change in consistency, manifest as increased firmness in the testis.

Special mention should be made of the clinical situation in which a young male patient presents with an acute hydrocele. If transillumination confirms a hydrocele, consideration must be given to the possibility of the hydrocele being of reactive rather than idiopathic origin. Scrotal ultrasonography is useful when the testis proper cannot be easily palpated due to the presence of the hydrocele. An intratesticular mass on ultrasonography confirms the diagnosis of testicular tumor and mandates an inguinal exploration instead of the scrotal approach normally used for repair of hydrocele.

Finally, if a suspicious mass is noted in the scrotum, a useful adjunct is to determine serum levels of alpha-fetoprotein and beta-human chorionic gonadotropin (β-hCG). Since the levels of these proteins are elevated in approximately 80% of all patients with nonseminomatous tumors, elevation of one of these markers in the presence of a scrotal mass confirms the diagnosis of testis tumor. Lack of elevation of either of these markers, however, does not preclude the diagnosis of testis tumor in patients with a scrotal mass.

## PATHOLOGY

In the United States, the most common system of classification of testicular tumors is that of Dixon and Moore.[3] This classification is based on the fact that seminomatous and nonseminomatous tumors both originate from totipotential stem cells but take separate paths of differentiation. It is a functional classification, as the treatment of early-stage disease is different depending on whether the tumor is a seminoma or a nonseminoma. In the remainder of this chapter the American classification will be used.

### Seminoma

Approximately 40% of primary germ-cell tumors of the testis are seminomatous.[3] This tumor type characteristically presents in older patients as compared with nonseminomatous tumors. Approximately 10% of seminomas are associated with low-level elevations of serum β-hCG. Serum levels of alpha-fetoprotein are never abnormal in a typical pure seminoma, and elevation of alpha-fetoprotein eliminates the diagnosis of pure seminoma.

Three histologic varieties of seminomatous tumors have been described, including classical, anaplastic, and spermatocytic. In the past, anaplastic tumors were felt to confer a poor prognosis; however, this is no longer felt to be the case. The spermatocytic seminoma usually presents in older patients and rarely metastasizes.

### Nonseminoma

Nonseminomatous tumors present with serum elevations of alpha-fetoprotein and/or β-hCG in roughly 70% to 80% of cases. The subtypes of nonseminomas include embryonal carcinoma, yolk-sac carcinoma, choriocarcinoma, and teratoma. Embryonal carcinoma is the most common single histologic type, but combinations of the subtypes are frequent. It should be mentioned that the presence of immature teratoma in the primary testicular specimen confers the same prognosis as does that of mature teratoma.

### Nongerminal Tumors

Various types of nongerminal primary testicular tumors account for approximately 3% of all cases of testis cancer. The most common of these are Leydig-cell and Sertoli-cell tumors. The malignancy rate associated with these tumors is reported to be approximately 10%.[6] These tumors may be associated with increased production of various hormones, and a young patient with a nongerminal tumor may present with precocious sexual development.

## DISEASE STAGING

The accuracy of clinical staging in patients with testicular cancer is only about 60% to 80%.[7,8] (This will be discussed more fully under treatment of patients with clinical stage A disease.) The staging system used at Indiana University is presented in Table 1. However, it should be added that any evidence of visceral metastasis is considered to be indicative of stage C disease.

Disease staging in patients who have undergone radical inguinal orchiectomy for testis cancer includes a determination of serum alpha-fetoprotein, β-hCG, abdominal computed tomography (CT) scanning, and either chest CT scanning or whole-lung tomography. Serum markers are especially useful in patients with clinical stage A tumors who are considered for observation protocols. The half-life of alpha-fetoprotein is approximately 5 days and the half-life of β-hCG is approximately 1 day; determination of the serum values of these substances at several points in time after orchiectomy can indicate whether the levels are falling appropriately for the absence of residual tumor.

Other tests, including lymphangiography and magnetic resonance imaging (MRI) may also be used. Lymphangiography is not routinely used at Indiana University in patients with clinical stage A seminoma since the results of this test will not alter treatment. Although MRI may prove useful in the future, at this time routine use is not recommended.

## TREATMENT

### Initial Surgical Treatment

The inguinal approach should be used to examine any suspected testicular or paratesticular tumor; the rationale behind this approach is to avoid cross-contamination of the scrotum and hence the inguinal lymphatics. Testicular tumors are uncharacteristic in that surgical cure is possible even after metastasis has occurred. Therefore, it is logical to avoid contamination of more than one lymphatic drainage area. By making an inguinal incision, the chance of spilling tumor is low because the primary tumor is distant from the initial incision site.

The surgeon should approach the procedure in this situation with the intent of

**TABLE 1. Clinical Stages of Testis Tumors**

| Disease Stage | Clinical Presentation |
|---|---|
| A | Tumor limited to the testis alone |
| B | Tumor in both testis and retroperitoneal lymph nodes |
| | B-1 Microscopic metastases to retroperitoneal nodes (1–6 nodes) |
| | B-2 Tumor of retroperitoneal lymph nodes 2–6 cm in greatest dimension by CT or >6 microscopic nodes |
| | B-3 Tumor of retroperitoneal lymph nodes >6 cm in greatest dimension by CT |
| C | Tumor above the diaphragm or involving abdominal solid organs |

performing radical inguinal orchiectomy. The patient should be so informed prior to the procedure and should not be given the impression that the procedure will merely be exploratory. Because roughly 97% to 98% of all solid intratesticular lesions represent malignancy, there is no need for biopsy in a patient with a normal contralateral testicle and a clearly intratesticular lesion.

The procedure is begun with an inguinal incision which is carried down sharply until the aponeurosis of the external oblique is visualized. The aponeurosis is then incised, following the direction of its fibers, to expose the spermatic cord with its enveloping cremasteric fibers. These fibers are divided, after which both blunt and sharp dissection are used to elevate the cord from the inguinal floor. Next, the cord is separated into its vasal and vascular components, clamped, and divided. The stump should be controlled using ties and suture ligatures, and the vascular portion of the cord stump should be pushed through the internal ring into the retroperitoneum to facilitate removal at the time of retroperitoneal lymphadenectomy, should this be required. The cord is then grasped and traction is gently applied as the external spermatic fascia is divided at the inferior portion of the testicle. The gubernaculum is divided sharply, after which the specimen is removed. After irrigation of the wound, the aponeurosis of the external oblique is closed, as is Scarpa's fascia and the skin. If a patient elects placement of a testicular prosthesis, it is positioned in the most dependent portion of the hemiscrotum prior to closure. Antibiotic irrigation is then used.

Despite the availability of scrotal ultrasonography, sometimes the diagnosis of an intratesticular lesion is in doubt. In such cases, an inguinal exploration should be performed and the cord should be clamped with a non-crushing clamp prior to mobilization of the testis and lesion. After draping a separate field into which the testis is placed, the testis is carefully palpated. If the lesion is discovered to be intratesticular, then radical orchiectomy is performed. However, if palpation does not clearly define the nature of the lesion, the tunica vaginalis and tunica albuginea can be opened and biopsy performed. It should be stressed, however, that biopsy is highly unusual—the majority of procedures result in radical inguinal orchiectomy without the necessity for biopsy.

If a patient is found to already have undergone a scrotal orchiectomy, hemiscrotectomy must be considered because of the potential for tumor implantation in the scrotum that could lead to contamination of the inguinal lymphatic areas. Some researchers have advocated not only hemiscrotectomy but also immediate inguinal lymphadenectomy in this situation. It is now clear, however, that the majority of cases of scrotal orchiectomy for testicular tumor do not result in scrotal contamination and subsequent inguinal lymphatic contamination. Therefore, our current practice is to perform limited hemiscrotectomy alone.

## Seminoma

**Clinical Stage A.** Modern radiographic staging reveals clinical stage A seminoma in approximately 70% to 80% of patients. Abdominal radiotherapy has been the traditional treatment for these patients, at a typical dosage of 2500 cGy. Lymphangiography may be used as a diagnostic adjunct to plan radiotherapy.

The rationale for using radiotherapy to treat patients with low-stage seminoma is that this tumor type is extremely sensitive to radiation therapy in dosages that are associated with very low morbidity. Side effects of radiation therapy include mild nausea and diarrhea; however, abdominal radiotherapy is generally well tolerated in patients with this disease. Survival is expected in more than 95% of cases. Analysis of relapse patterns indicate that there is no benefit in extending the radiotherapy field to include areas above the diaphragm.

Several investigators have proposed the use of observation alone to treat patients with clinical stage A seminoma.[9] In this model, patients receive treatment only at relapse; the pathologic stage A patients thereby avoid radiotherapy. This approach must be compared critically to the extremely effective, low-morbidity approach of administering radiotherapy to the abdomens of all clinical stage A patients.

**Clinical Stage B.** Low-volume clinical stage B disease is managed very effectively with abdominal radiotherapy. Eighty percent to 90% of patients with low volume retroperitoneal disease will be cured with radiotherapy.[10] However, increasing amounts of retroperitoneal disease diminishes the cure rate achieved with radiotherapy. Because chemotherapy is extremely successful in this setting, high-volume retroperitoneal disease is best treated with platinum-based chemotherapy.

**Clinical Stage C.** Standard platinum-based chemotherapy is the treatment of choice for patients with stage C seminoma. Cure rates of 80% to 90% can be expected in patients with disseminated disease. There is currently controversy regarding the management of a patient with stage C seminoma who has a radiographic mass after standard chemotherapy for seminoma. Some clinicians advocate post-chemotherapy resection to determine if active cancer remains, while others have found the residual masses to consist universally of fibrosis/necrosis and therefore argue against post-chemotherapy dissection of pure seminomatous tumors.[11,12]

## Nonseminoma

**Clinical Stage A.** Roughly 70% of patients who present with clinical stage A nonseminoma are found to indeed have pathologically confirmed stage A disease. The traditional approach to treatment of patients with clinical stage A nonseminoma has been radical retroperitoneal lymphadenectomy. The rationale for this approach is to identify the 30% of patients with pathologic stage B disease and to eliminate areas of metastases. Because effective chemotherapy was not available, the dissection was extensive and involved the removal of all lymphatic tissue from the renal hilum to the bifurcation of the common iliac from ureter to ureter. This full bilateral dissection cured between 50% and 70% of patients with retroperitoneal disease. The principal morbidity associated with this procedure was loss of emission/ejaculation, which occurred because retroperitoneal sympathetic nerves were interrupted. Both the thoracoabdominal and transabdominal approaches were used. The technique of retroperitoneal lymph-node dissection (RPLND) has been well described.[13] Briefly, the split and roll technique is used to clear the great vessels of overlying lymphatic tissue. Lumbar arteries and veins are divided, freeing the great vessels from the posterior body wall. Lymphatic tissue is then harvested in four packages: the right paracaval, the interaortocaval, the left periaortic, and the presacral packages.

Two factors subsequently led investigators to question the need for full bilateral dissection in each patient: the development of effective platinum-based chemotherapy and the emergence of mapping studies which showed that the site of small-volume retroperitoneal disease could be predicted reliably.[14] It became clear that low-volume disease arising from a left-sided primary tumor occurred in only the left periaortic and interaortocaval zones; low-volume retroperitoneal disease arising from a right-sided primary tumor could be predictably found in the interaortocaval and precaval zones. Modified dissections were proposed in an effort to maintain the efficacy of RPLND yet limit the principal morbidity loss of emission and ejaculation. The templates used for a right- and left-modified RPLND are shown in Figure 1.

The right-sided modified dissection was found to preserve emission/ejaculation in roughly 60% to 70% of patients, while the left-sided modified dissection preserved emission/ejaculation capability in only approximately 30% to 40% of cases (Foster RS, et al. Unpublished data). These modified dissections clearly represented an advance in patient management, but a significant number of men still suffered loss of emission/ejaculation as a result of therapy for their testicular cancer.

The "surveillance" strategy arose out of an effort to limit the morbidity of treatment. Because 70% of men presenting with clinical stage A disease have pathologic confirmation of this stage, subjecting all such men to RPLND results in "unnecessary"

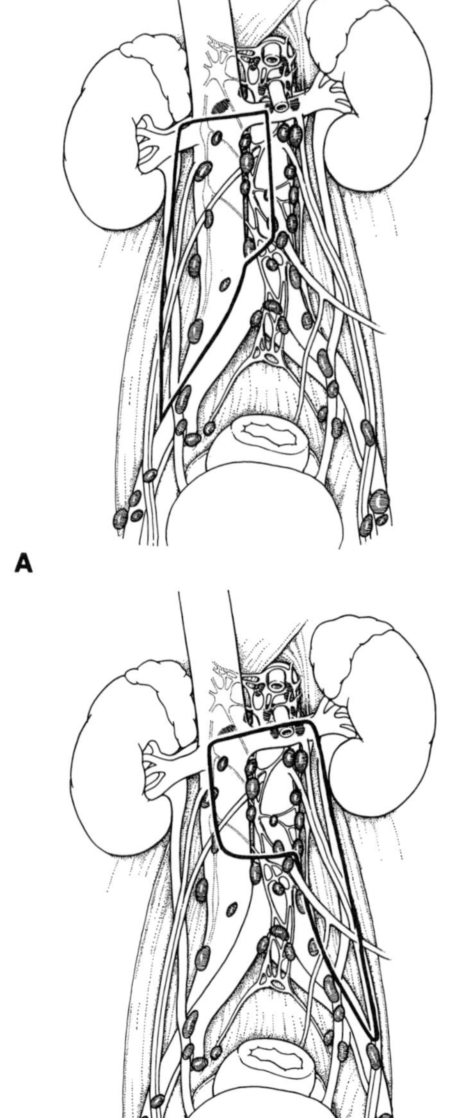


**Fig 1.** A, template for right-sided, nerve-sparing RPLND; B, template for left-sided, nerve-sparing RPLND.*

surgery. In addition, some of these men lose the ability for emission/ejaculation as a result of modified or full-bilateral dissection. Thus, surveillance of all men with clinical stage A disease by monitoring serial marker determinations and radiographic imaging has been proposed. Platinum-based chemotherapy is used to treat the 30% to 40% of patients who experience relapse.[15]

Surveillance is an effective method of management in most patients. Results of surveillance protocols from various institutions have shown cure rates of approximately 96%. It is clear, however, that not all patients are rescued with platinum-based chemotherapy and that, ultimately, the chance of cure with the surveillance strategy as now practiced in the U.S. is lower than with immediate RPLND. Attempting to define the cohort of patients destined to fail under the surveillance strategy is an area of active investigation. Various parameters of the histology of the primary tumor, such as vascular invasion or pure embryonal histology, tend to portend a higher risk of retroperitoneal disease.[15] Other predictors of metastasis are being sought.

The surveillance strategy has attempted to maintain the efficacy of treatment but minimize its morbidity. It clearly reduces morbidity in some patients, but has not proven to be as effective as immediate RPLND.

In 1990, Donohue and colleagues described a nerve-sparing method of RPLND. This method was developed in an attempt to maintain the high cure rate of immediate RPLND while decreasing its morbidity.[20] Retroperitoneal sympathetic efferent fibers can be reliably located during RPLND; in the nerve-sparing dissections, these fibers are prospectively dissected from retroperitoneal tissue and lymphadenectomy is carried out (based on the templates and mapping studies described in Figs 1 and 2). This technique preserves emission/ejaculation in greater than 99% of cases. Additionally, the efficacy of RPLND is maintained.[20]

The survival of patients with clinical stage A nonseminomatous testis cancer at Indiana University was 99.1% from 1965

* The illustrations used in this chapter are the property of the Medical Illustrations Department at the Indiana University School of Medicine. Permission to publish should be obtained through Craig Gosling at (317) 274–4423.

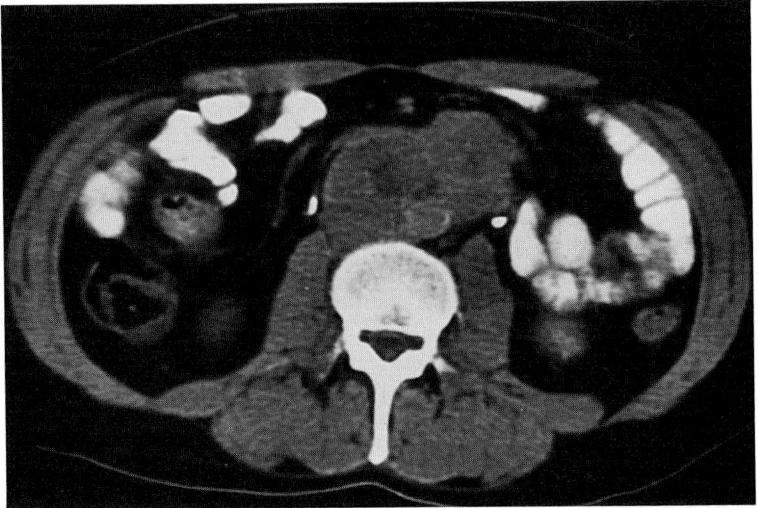

**Fig 2.** CT scan showing retroperitoneal residual tumor in patient with normal serum markers after chemotherapy.

**TABLE 2. Primary RPLND in Clinical Stage A NSGC Testis Cancer Results, 1965–1989**

| Disease Extent (Pathologic Stage) | Patients N | (%) | Relapse N | (%) | Survival % | Deaths N |
|---|---|---|---|---|---|---|
| Pathologic stage A | 324 | (70) | 35 | (11) | 99.1 | 2* |
| Pathologic stage B (No adjuvant chemotherapy) | 74 | (16) | 25 | (34) | 98.6 | 1† |
| Pathologic stage B (Adjuvant chemotherapy) | 66 | (14) | 3 | (4) | 98.5 | 1† |
| All cases | 464 | | 63 | (14) | 99.1 | 4 |

* One cancer death, one postoperative death.
† Two cancer deaths.

to 1989 (Table 2). Early in this series, patients were managed with full bilateral RPLND; later, patients were managed with a modified dissection or a nerve-sparing modified dissection.

Table 3 shows the results of various surveillance series from around the world. Overall survival rates range between 95% and 99%, and the relapse rate ranges between 25% and 35%.

A patient presenting with clinical stage A nonseminomatous testis cancer must be advised of his treatment options. Surveillance is appealing since it avoids unnecessary surgery in the group of patients (70% of all patients) who are pathologic stage A.

**TABLE 3. Morbidity and Mortality Associated with the Surveillance Strategy**

| Author | Patients | Relapse (%) | Survival (%) | Deaths |
|---|---|---|---|---|
| Freedman[15] | 259 | 32 | 98.8 | 3 |
| Raghavan[16] | 46 | 28 | 95.6 | 2 |
| Thompson[17] | 36 | 33 | 97.2 | 1 |
| Liedke[18] | 107 | 35 | 99.1 | 2 |
| Sogani[19] | 102 | 25 | 97.1 | 3 |

However, the patient must be informed that his ultimate chance of dying of testis cancer may be increased with this option. The benefits of RPLND must also be presented: 1) precision in disease staging and definition of subsequent treatment requirements; 2) therapeutic benefit if the nodes are positive; 3) ease of follow-up, since retroperitoneal relapse is extremely rare; and 4) alteration of the disease model in the event of relapse.

After RPLND, relapse occurs not in the retroperitoneum but in the lungs. Metastases to the lungs are easier to detect and treat than the relapse form on a surveillance protocol involving retroperitoneum plus lungs. Chemotherapy achieves cure with minimal pulmonary disease in almost all cases; the efficacy of chemotherapy in patients with both retroperitoneal and pulmonary disease is not as great.[21]

**Clinical Stage B.** The relapse rate after RPLND in patients with pathologic stage B disease is directly related to the volume of retroperitoneal disease. Approximately 25% of patients who have microscopic disease experience relapse. In patients with moderate disease, the relapse rate is approximately 40%, and in patients with high-volume retroperitoneal metastasis, the relapse rate is even higher. Because of the high relapse rate in patients with high-volume retroperitoneal disease, systemic chemotherapy is the appropriate initial therapy.

If no gross disease is noted in the retroperitoneum at RPLND, a modified nerve-sparing RPLND is performed. Mapping studies have shown that if microscopic disease is present it occurs within the confines of the templates previously described.[14] If gross disease is palpated, the traditional approach has been full bilateral RPLND with consequent loss of emission/ejaculation. However, nerve-sparing approaches are beginning to be used in patients with gross retroperitoneal disease. Defining exactly which patients with gross retroperitoneal disease can be managed with a nerve-sparing approach is an area of current investigation.

Because of the 25% to 50% recurrence rate in RPLND in pathologic stage B testis cancer, it was questioned whether postoperative adjuvant chemotherapy should be administered. A multicenter, randomized study showed no difference in survival between patients who received two courses of platinum-based chemotherapy post-RPLND and those who were given three or four courses of chemotherapy at relapse.[22] The current policy at Indiana University is to individualize the treatment of patients with pathologic stage B disease post-RPLND. The patient is given his options and allowed to decide whether adjuvant chemotherapy will be administered. Qualification to this policy must be made if the patient is felt to be unreliable or is not able to be closely followed; adjuvant chemotherapy is recommended for these patients. On the other hand, if a patient is reliable and has access to follow-up, it is entirely reasonable to avoid chemotherapy that may be unnecessary.

The results of RPLND in patients with clinical stage B nonseminomatous testis cancer at Indiana University are depicted in Table 4. The overall survival of 98% is extremely good; note that survival is similar

**TABLE 4. Primary RPLND in Clinical Stage B—Results, 1979–1989**

| Disease Extent | Patients N (%) | Relapse N (%) | Survival % | Deaths* N |
|---|---|---|---|---|
| Pathologic Stage A | 32 (23) | 2 (6) | 100 | 0 |
| Pathologic Stage B (No Adjuvant) | 49 (35) | 18 (37) | 96 | 2 |
| Pathologic Stage B (Plus Adjuvant) | 59 (42) | 0 (5) | 98.3 | 1 |
| All Cases | 140 | 20 (14) | 98 | 3 |

* Cause of deaths: cancer (1), postoperative complications (1), chemotherapy-related (1).

in both the patients who received adjuvant chemotherapy and in those who did not.

**Clinical Stage C.** Patients presenting with clinical stage C (and high-volume clinical stage B) disease are candidates for primary platinum-based chemotherapy. The initial study of 50 patients who were administered cisplatin, vinblastine, and bleomycin (PVB) chemotherapy was published in 1977.[23] This report detailed principles of combination chemotherapy as well as the method of using surgical resection of residual disease after chemotherapy. Thirty-eight of the patients obtained complete remissions with chemotherapy or a combination of chemotherapy and surgery. The report proved the efficacy of PVB chemotherapy, but associated morbidity was substantial.

Subsequent attempts to use platinum-based chemotherapy have focused on maintaining the efficacy of therapy but minimizing morbidity, and many excellent studies have been carried out, both at individual institutions and under the aegis of cooperative oncology groups. Discussion of these studies in detail is beyond the scope of this chapter. However, several conclusions regarding chemotherapy, as it exists at this point in time, may be described.

It is now clear that maintenance chemotherapy after standard platinum-based induction chemotherapy is not necessary. Also, etoposide (VP-16) has been substituted for vinblastine in initial platinum-based chemotherapy because it has demonstrated similar efficacy with lower morbidity.

Predictive factors of response to chemotherapy in patients with disseminated testis cancer have also been defined. "Poor risk" patients (patients generally considered to have a poor prognosis) are those with high volumes of metastatic disease, high elevations of tumor markers, extragonadal primary lesions, and visceral organ involvement. All other patients ("good risk" patients) are likely to respond to chemotherapy.

Good risk patients at Indiana University are now treated with three courses of platinum, VP-16, and bleomycin as opposed to the former standard therapy of four courses of platinum/vinblastine/bleomycin because a Southeastern Cancer Group study demonstrated lower morbidity and equivalent efficacy with three compared to four courses.[21] Standard therapy of poor risk patients currently involves four courses of platinum, VP-16, and bleomycin. However, treatment of this category of patients is an area of active investigation. Newer strategies may eventually involve the use of various platinum analogues, autologous bone marrow support, and various factors to stimulate marrow recovery.

## Post-Chemotherapy RPLND

The primary candidates for post-chemotherapy RPLND are patients treated with primary induction chemotherapy whose serum markers have normalized but who have persistent radiographic abnormalities (Fig 2). It is now clear that the pathologic identity of the residual tumor may be one of three types: fibrosis/necrosis, teratoma, and active carcinoma.

Resection of fibrosis/necrosis tissue is not therapeutic; indeed, it may be said, at least retrospectively, that surgery in this situation is unnecessary. However, prediction of which patients harbor only fibrosis/necrosis tissue post-chemotherapy is currently not possible. Needle biopsy or biopsy at laparotomy does not adequately determine the tumor histology, since these masses are typically heterogeneous. Prediction of the pathologic entity of fibrosis/necrosis may be made in only those patients who had a pathologically pure tumor type at orchiectomy (pure embryonal, for example, with no teratoma) and who have normalized serum markers along with a greater than 90% volumetric reduction in the radiographic tumor.[24] At Indiana University these patients are sometimes followed expectantly. It should be stressed, however, that this group of patients is a small and select cohort of the entire group of post-chemotherapy patients. Therefore, the patient with normal serum markers and persistent radiographic abnormality is usually subjected to post-chemotherapy RPLND.

The second pathologic entity found at post-chemotherapy RPLND is teratoma. Teratoma is a benign tumor, although it continues to enlarge if not resected; teratoma does not respond to any variety of chemotherapy. It is now known that the risk of recurrence of teratoma is lowest when the volume of teratoma resected at post-chemotherapy RPLND is low. Therefore, waiting and allowing a teratoma to grow is not wise. It is also clear that patients who have multiple recurrences of teratoma have an increased risk of developing sarcoma with each subsequent recurrence.[25] Therefore, teratoma should be resected when it is at the lowest possible volume.

Finding carcinoma in this situation is an indication for additional chemotherapy. Indeed, in this patient cohort, the survival is approximately 60% to 70% if post-chemotherapy RPLND is performed and two subsequent courses of chemotherapy are administered.[26]

Post-chemotherapy RPLND should also be used in patients whose serum markers do not normalize after primary platinum-based chemotherapy and who subsequently undergo salvage platinum-based chemotherapy with normalization of markers. The technical considerations of RPLND are not different in this group of patients. Rare patients, however, may benefit from post-chemotherapy RPLND when an elevation in serum markers persists after all chemotherapeutic alternatives have been exhausted. This highly select group of patients includes those who have been known to have had retroperitoneal localized disease only, with no history of other disseminated disease. It should be stressed, however, that operating on post-chemotherapy patients with concomitant elevation of serum markers is highly unusual.

The technique of post-chemotherapy RPLND has been described.[27] Briefly, a full bilateral RPLND is performed after division of lumbar arteries and veins. Sympathetic fibers are removed, although we have begun to use nerve-sparing techniques in the post-chemotherapy setting in a select group of patients and have had good results. Patients who initially present with disseminated disease may have disease in various sites after chemotherapy. The surgical approach is dictated by the site of disease: retroperitoneal disease can usually be resected via a transperitoneal approach; mediastinal and retrocrural disease is usually approached via a thoracoabdominal or thoracic approach (Figs 3, 4, 5); cervical and high mediastinal disease is approached via median sternotomy or neck dissection. It should be stressed that post-chemotherapy RPLND is, by-and-large, a vascular procedure. Mobilizing the great vessels is of prime importance with this technique. This mobilization may be extremely time-intensive and difficult, and the surgeon embarking on post-chemotherapy RPLND should be thoroughly familiar with techniques of vascular control.

If the diagnosis of nonseminomatous germ-cell cancer was made by means other than radical inguinal orchiectomy, the post-chemotherapy patient who has not had the primary tumor removed should undergo an inguinal orchiectomy. This should be carried out regardless of whether the patient has experienced an apparent complete response to chemotherapy. In 40% to 50% of these patients teratoma or carcinoma will be found in the testicle which is removed after chemotherapy.[28] This finding suggests that a blood-testis barrier exists to prevent passage of chemotherapeutic agents into the testis.

The morbidity of post-chemotherapy RPLND is greater than that associated with primary RPLND performed in patients with clinical stage A or stage B disease.[29] Various factors account for this increased morbidity, including the fact that pulmonary toxicity associated with bleomycin can make fluid management difficult in these patients. Great care must be exercised in monitoring pulmonary function in post-chemotherapy RPLND patients who have received prior therapy with bleomycin. Noncardiogenic pulmonary edema can be a devastating complication in this group of patients.

The adherence of tumor to the great vessels in the retroperitoneum cannot be reliably predicted following chemotherapy. In some post-chemotherapy patients, dissecting tumor from the great vessels is not

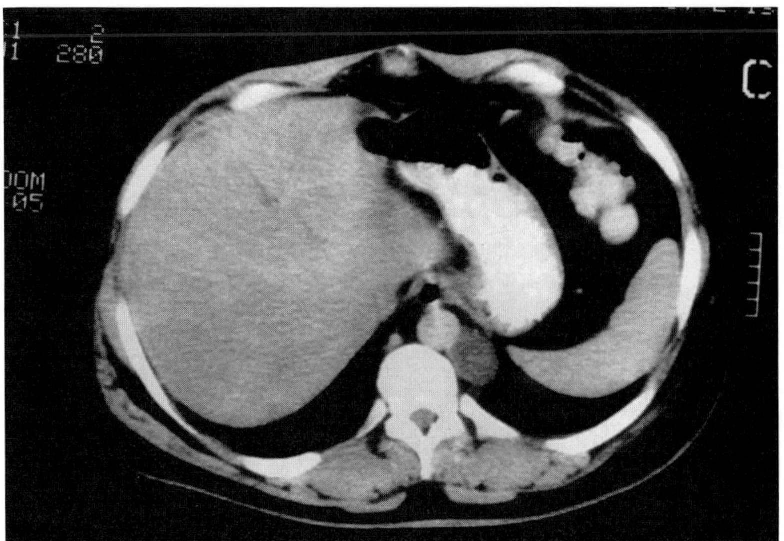

Fig 3. CT scan of post-chemotherapy patient showing persistent left retrocrural tumor.

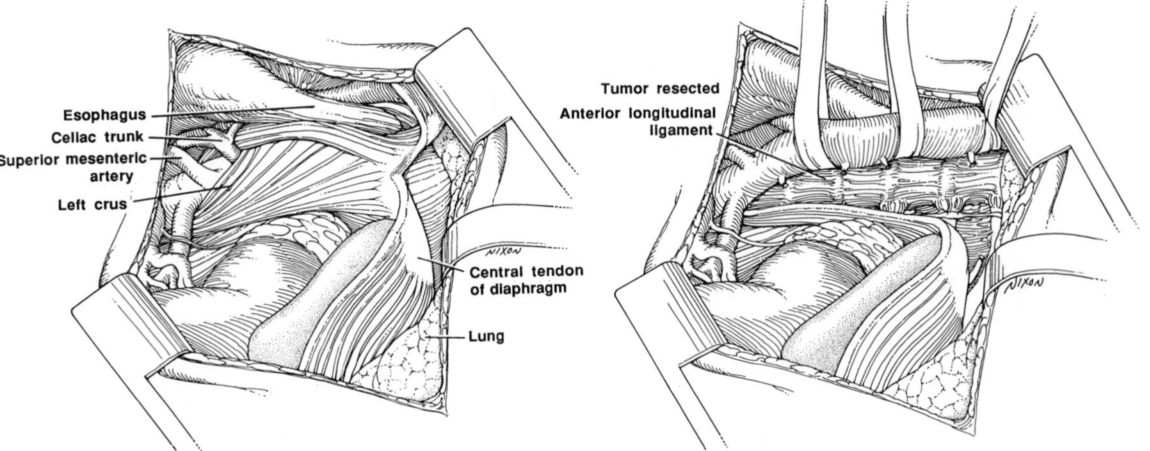


Fig 4. Left thoracoabdominal exposure for resection of left retrocrural disease.

Fig 5. Left thoracoabdominal exposure with incision through crus and aorta mobilized.

difficult; in others, the amount of reaction makes identification of planes extremely tenuous. Care should be taken to preserve the adventitia of the great vessels because our experience indicates that the adventitia is very important in maintaining the integrity of the vessels and in repairing intraoperative injury to the vessel.

Because these procedures are sometimes long, patients are routinely monitored overnight in the intensive care unit. Fluids are administered cautiously, and respiratory function is monitored accurately.

## FOLLOW-UP OF SURGICAL PATIENTS

Patients who have undergone primary RPLND for clinical stage A or stage B disease should be seen one month after surgery. The following are usually monitored on a monthly basis for the first year postoperatively: chest x-ray, serum alpha fetoprotein, and serum β-hCG. Since recurrence in the second postoperative year is less likely, these same tests are performed on a bimonthly basis. Retroperitoneal recurrence is rare; therefore CT scans of the abdomen are not routinely obtained. Recurrences after 2 years are extremely rare.

Post-chemotherapy RPLND patients should be followed in a similar fashion. The necessity for obtaining CT scans in these patients is dependent on the individual situation. If teratoma was present in the resected material, CT scans are usually obtained on a regular basis. Frequency of CT scanning is contingent on the amount of teratoma resected and should be individualized.

## REFERENCES

1. Patton JF, Hewitt CB, Mallis N. Diagnosis and treatment of tumors of the testis. *JAMA.* 1959;17:2149.
2. Clemmensen J. A doubling in mortality from testis carcinoma in Copenhagen 1943–1962. *Acta Path Microbiol Scand.* 1968;72:348.
3. Dixon FJ, Moore RA. Tumors of the male sex organs. In: *Atlas of Tumor Pathology,* section VIII, Fasciles 31b and 32. Washington, DC: Armed Forces Institute of Pathology; 1952.
4. Johnson DE. Epidemiology. In: Johnson DE, ed. *Testicular Tumors.* 2nd ed. Flushing, NY: Medical Examination Publishing Co Inc; 1976;37.
5. Lange PH, et al. Fertility issues in the therapy of nonseminomatous testicular tumors. *Urol Clin North Am.* 1987;14:731.
6. Silverberg S, Thompson J, Higashig G, Baskin A. Malignant interstitial cell tumor of the testis: case report and review. *J Urol.* 1966; 96:356–363.
7. Ellis JH, Bies JR, Kopecky KK, et al. Comparison of the NMR and CT imaging in the evaluation of metastatic retroperitoneal lymphadenopathy form testicular carcinoma. *J Comput Assist Tomogr.* 1984;8:709.
8. Richie JP, Farnick MB, Finberg H. Computerized tomography: how accurate for abdominal staging of testis tumors? *J Urol.* 1982;127:715.
9. Oliver R. Limitations to the use of surveillance as an option in the management of stage I seminoma. *Int J Androl.* 1987;10:263.
10. Gregory C, Peckham M. Results of radiotherapy for stage II testicular seminoma. *Radiother Oncol.* 1986;6:285.
11. Motzer R, Bosl G, Heelan R, et al. Residual mass: an indication for further therapy in patients with advanced seminoma following systemic chemotherapy. *J Clin Oncol.* 1987;5:1064.
12. Schultz S, Einhorn L, Conces D, Williams S, Loehrer P. Management of postchemotherapy residual mass in patients with advanced seminoma: Indiana University experience. *J Clin Oncol.* 1989;7:1497.
13. Donohue JP. Retroperitoneal lymphadenectomy: the anterior approach including bilateral and suprahilar dissection. *Urol Clin North Am.* 1977;4:509.
14. Donohue JP, Maynard B, Zachary M. The distribution of nodal metastases in the retroperitoneum from nonseminomatous testis cancer. *J Urol.* 1982;128:315.
15. Freedman L, Parkinson M, Jones W, et al. Histopathology in the prediction of relapse of patients with stage I testicular teratoma treated by orchiectomy alone. *Lancet.* 1987;2:294.
16. Raghavan D, Colls B, Leir J, et al. Surveillance for Stage I nonseminomatous germ cell tumours of the testis: the optimal protocol has not yet been developed. *Br J Urol.* 1988;61:522–526.
17. Thompson PI, Nixon J, Harvey VJ. Disease relapse in patients with stage I nonseminomatous germ cell tumours of the testis on active surveillance. *J Clin Oncol.* 1988;6:1597–1603.
18. Liedke S, Allhoff EP, Jones U. Wait and see in NSGCT clinical stage I: a critical assessment after eight years. *J Urol.* 1990;143(4):397A.
19. Sogani PC, Fair WR. Surveillance alone in the treatment of clinical stage I nonseminomatous germ cell tumour of the testis (NSGCT). *Sem Urol.* 1988;6:53–56.
20. Donohue JP, Foster RS, Rowland RG, Bihrle R, Jones J, Geier G. Nerve-sparing retroperitoneal lymphadenectomy with preservation of ejaculation. *J Urol.* 1990;144:287.
21. Einhorn L, Williams S, Loehrer P, et al. Evaluation of optimal duration of chemotherapy in favorable prognosis disseminated germ cell tumors; a Southeastern Cancer Study Group protocol. *J Clin Oncol.* 1989;7:387.
22. Williams SD, Stablein DM, Einhorn LH, et al. Immediate adjuvant chemotherapy versus observation with treatment at relapse in pathological stage II testicular cancer. *N Engl J Med.* 1987;317:1433–1438.
23. Einhorn LH, Donohue JP. Cis-diammine dichloroplatinum, vinblastine, and bleomycin

combination chemotherapy in disseminated testicular cancer. *Ann Intern Med.* 1977;87:293.

24. Donohue JP, Rowland RG, Kopecky KK, et al. Correlation of computerized tomographic changes and histologic findings in 80 patients having radical retroperitoneal lymph node dissection after chemotherapy for testis cancer. *J Urol.* 1987;137:1176.
25. Loehrer PJ, Williams SD, Clark SA, et al. Teratoma following chemotherapy for nonseminomatous germ cell tumor (NSGCT): a clinicopathologic correlation. *J Urol.* 1986;135:1183.
26. Nichols C, Gupta S, Loehrer P, Williams S, Birch R, Einhorn L. Outcome in patients with residual germ cell cancer after post chemotherapy surgery. *Proc Am Soc Clin Oncol.* 1987;6:100.
27. Donohue JP, Einhorn LH, Williams SD. Cytoreductive surgery for metastatic testis cancer: considerations of timing and extent. *J Urol.* 1980;123:876.
28. Griest A, Williams SD, Einhorn LH, Donohue JP, Rowland RG, Estes N. Pathologic findings at orchiectomy following chemotherapy for disseminated testicular cancer. *Proc Am Soc Clin Oncol.* 1983;2:139.
29. Bihrle R, Donohue JP, Foster RS. Complications of retroperitoneal lymph node dissection. *Urol Clin North Am.* 1985;15:2.

# 34

# Benign and Malignant Tumors of the Penis, Urethra, Epididymis, and Seminal Vesicles

*W. Scott McDougal*

## BENIGN AND MALIGNANT TUMORS OF THE PENIS

### Benign Soft Tissue Tumors of the Penis

Benign soft tissue tumors of the penis occur very infrequently and are half as common as their malignant counterparts. They are classified according to the tissue of origin as either angiomatous, neurogenous, myogenous, or fibrous.

**Angiomatous Tumors.** Tumors of angiomatous origin are the most common type of benign tumor. They include capillary or cavernous hemangiomas, sclerosing hemangioma, glomus tumor, and lymphangiomas. Their etiology is controversial. Some suggest that they represent true neoplasms, whereas others feel they are merely a herniation of the corpus spongiosum.[1] They are usually found on the glans and appear as a nontender mass that is superficial, easily compressible, and bluish in color. Local excision or laser ablation is curative.[2]

**Neurogenous Tumors.** The most common type of tumor in this group is the neurofibroma, which may be associated with von Recklinghausen's disease or may occur independently. Malignant degeneration does not occur in the solitary neurofibroma but may occur in the plexiform neurofibroma.[3]

Neurolemmomas also have been reported. These lesions present as nonpainful hard masses on the glans or shaft or the penis.[3] Excision is curative.

**Myogenous Tumors.** Leiomyomas present as a slow-growing, painless, well-circumscribed mass. The average age of patients with this tumor is 41 years.[2] Local excision is curative.

**Fibrous Tumors.** Dermatofibromas present as hard, nontender localized masses. Local excision is the preferred therapy.

### Premalignant Lesions of the Penis

**Erythroplasia of Queyrat, Carcinoma In Situ, Bowen's Disease.** Erythroplasia of Queyrat is a form of epithelial dysplasia described by Queyrat in 1911. It is apparent that carcinoma in situ and Bowen's disease are the same lesion originally described by Queyrat. The lesion presents in patients—-

usually uncircumcised—of all ages. It appears on the glans as a red, velvety, thickened plaque that occasionally is ulcerated. Complete excision is the preferred treatment, but cryotherapy, laser ablation, and topical application of thiocolciram cream (0.5% Colemid) and 5-fluorouracil also have been used successfully.[4]

A variant of this disorder, known as Bowenoid papulosis, presents as multiple elevated red-to-violescent, slightly scaly, and sometimes verrucous or velvety areas that are generally asymptomatic and located on the shaft or the glans penis. It resembles condylomata acuminata or seborrheic keratosis. Most patients have been circumcised, and the delay in seeking medical attention generally is 3–18 months. The lesion is an intraepithelial carcinoma of the penis. Human papilloma virus (HPV) has been demonstrated intranuclearly in some of these lesions and DNA fragments of the HPV virus have been found in other patients.[5] Simple excision, cryosurgery, the laser, and 5-fluorouracil all have been successfully employed. Recurrence is common despite local therapy.[6–8]

There does not appear to be a significant association between Bowen's disease of the glans penis (erythroplasia of Queyrat or carcinoma in situ) and other malignancies. It has been proposed that perhaps a common carcinogen may be responsible for the penile lesion as well as the visceral lesion in those rare patients in whom two malignancies coincidentally occur.[4,9] Bowen's disease located elsewhere in the body, however, is associated with visceral malignancies approximately 25% of the time.

**Leukoplakia.** Leukoplakia appears as a whitish, macular lesion often found adjacent to squamous cell carcinoma. It is associated with chronic irritation, infection, and, like squamous cell carcinoma, a lack of hygiene. It may progress to squamous cell cancer, although this tendency is poorly documented.[10] The lesion should be completely excised.

**Balanitis Xerotica Obliterans.** Balanitis xerotica obliterans, or lichen sclerosus et atrophicus, is a chronic inflammatory process characterized by urethral meatal involvement; it often presents as a whitish plaque that burns and is pruritic. It has been noted in 3.6% of circumcision specimens.[11] Histologically there is a loss of rete pegs with thinning of the epidermis. Grossly, the epidermis appears thin and scaly, and it is prone to ulceration, cracks, and fissures. Since it is a progressively sclerosing disease, meatal involvement may result in a meatal stricture. Simple dilatation is not likely to be successful, and wedge meatotomy may be required. If the lesion is located on the prepuce, circumcision is curative. Nonoperative treatment with sublesional injections of triamcinolone acetonide has been used with some success. The relationship of this lesion to malignancy is controversial because in only a few cases has the association between this disease and squamous cell carcinoma been noted.[12]

**Pseudoepitheliomatous Hyperplasia.** This lesion usually occurs in proximity to or overlying an inflammatory or ulcerative lesion. It is characterized by epithelial hyperplasia and microscopically identified by thickening of the epidermal layer and elongation of the rete pegs. A chronic inflammatory infiltrate is also present. Although slight, there is a tendency to carcinomatous change.

**Buschke–Lowenstein Tumor.** Buschke–Lowenstein tumor, also known as verrucous carcinoma, invasive penile condylomatosis, and giant condyloma acuminatum, was first described by Buschke in 1896 and was described in greater detail by Lowenstein in 1939. A variant of epidermoid carcinoma, it generally appears as a slow-growing, warty, fungating, ulcerating mass. The mean age at presentation is 36 years. In approximately two thirds of patients the course is indolent, whereas in the other third the lesion may be rapidly and relentlessly locally destructive.[13] The tumor has been found in the oral cavity, larynx, nasal fossa, vagina, vulva, scrotum, and perineum as well as on the penis.

Microscopically, it has an undulating, densely keratinized outer layer covering large fungating papillary frons and a sharply circumscribed deep margin composed of rows of bulbous, extremely well-oriented rete ridges. The rete ridges are composed of large, well-differentiated squamous epithelial cells.

The lesion generally occurs in uncircumcised men.[14] The rapidly progressive tumors often result in adjacent tissue destruction with urethral fistulization, erosion, and abscess formation. These lesions are locally aggressive but do not metastasize. In no case has this lesion been demonstrated to produce distant metastases, provided radiotherapy has not been previously employed. There are reports, however, of this tumor occurring on areas other than the penis and being irradiated with resultant malignant degeneration of the tumor. Radiation is not indicated because of this fact and because it is uniformly unsuccessful on penile lesions. Rarely, squamous cell carcinoma has been noted to coexist with this lesion.[2]

The treatment is wide surgical excision, and as long as the surgeon ensures that the margins are free of disease, eradication is the rule.

## Malignant Tumors of the Penis

**Epidermoid Carcinoma of the Penis.** Carcinoma of the penis in North America is an uncommon lesion, accounting for less than 0.5% of all male malignancies[15] and occurring with a frequency of 0.8 cases per 100,000 population.[16] The incidence of this tumor on the North American continent has declined steadily over the past several decades.[17] It is considerably more common in other parts of the world, accounting for 10%–18% of all male cancers in patients living in Burma, Indochina, mainland China, and India.[18] On this continent, the lesion occurs predominantly in whites. Combining the series of Beggs et al.,[19] Hardner et al.,[20] Johnson et al.,[21] and Narayana et al.,[17] 86% of the patients (479 of 557) were white; 13% (74 of 557) were black, and 1.0% (4 of 557) were Asian.

Mean age at the time of presentation is 58 years with a range of 15–95 years.[17,21–23] Most cases occur, however, between the ages of 40 and 70 years.[24] The youngest reported patient was 2 years old. However, he did not have a squamous cell carcinoma but rather an ''embryonal carcinoma of the corpus cavernosum.''[25] In other parts of the world where the disease is more common, the average age at time of presentation is younger. In India, for example, most patients present at about 45 years of age.[25]

***Etiology.*** Carcinoma of the penis invariably occurs in the uncircumcised male. Indeed, the world's literature contains reports of only nine cases of carcinoma of the penis in patients who were circumcised at birth.[26] The importance of the foreskin and the age at which it is removed is emphasized by the fact that cancer of the penis is exceedingly rare in Jews who practice circumcision at birth, more common in Muhammedans who circumcise between ages 3 and 10 years, and most common in Hindus who do not practice circumcision.[27] Thus, circumcision protects against the disease if done during infancy but is of little benefit if obtained in boyhood and of no benefit if obtained during adulthood. This fact is borne out by the finding that 5%–12% of patients with carcinoma of the penis have been circumcised usually in adulthood, rarely in boyhood, and almost never before age 5 years.[21,28,29] Phimosis is present in approximately half of patients and underscores the chronic irritation that most likely plays a primary role in the genesis of the disease.

Trauma and venereal disease also have been implicated in the pathogenesis. More recently, human papilloma virus has been implicated in the etiology of these lesions.[30] Viral infestation associated with poor hygiene may increase contact time. With poor hygiene and the presence of foreskin, carcinogens remain in contact with the glans and foreskin for long periods, thus inducing malignant changes in the epidermis.

On occasion, the tumor is preceded by or associated with a premalignant lesion. In 17% of the cases reported by Hanash et

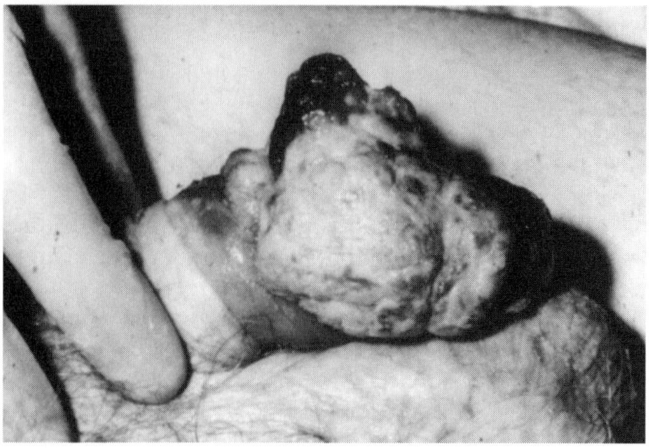

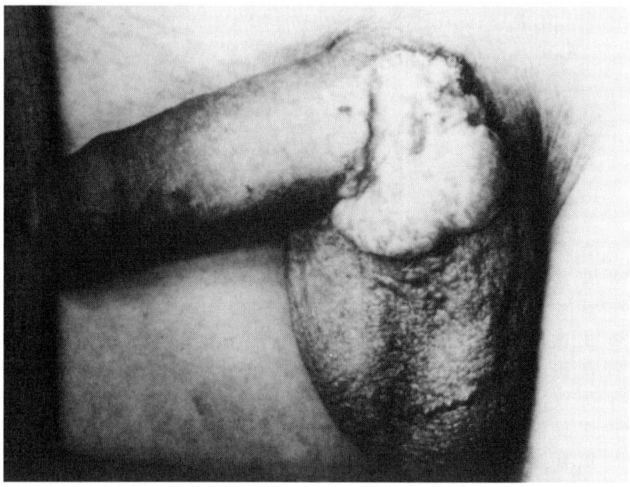

**Fig 1. A**: Gross appearance of squamous cell carcinoma of the penis, of glans, and **B**: of the base of the penis.

al.,[10] leukoplakia was associated with the tumor; in 4%, erythroplasia of Queyrat was associated; and in 2%, Paget's disease was found concomitantly. However, most patients give no history of a premalignant lesion from which the cancer arose.

***Natural History.*** Carcinoma of the penis begins as a small lesion that grows slowly and progresses in an orderly fashion. As the lesion grows, it may be either ulcerative and plaque-like, or frondular and exophytic (Fig 1). It occurs most commonly on the glans penis.[17] Metastases occur by lymphatic spread initially, but when the corpora cavernosa are invaded, bloodborne metastases can occur. Bloodborne metastases are generally a late manifestation of the disease. The lymphatic drainage of the foreskin and skin of the penis is to the superficial and deep inguinal nodes. Since there is crossover of lymphatics, location on one side of the penis is no guarantee that spread will be to the ipsilateral nodes. The glans, corpora, and urethra drain into the deep inguinal and external iliac nodes.

As the lesion grows, it invariably destroys the local tissues, which become infected and purulent. The regional lymph nodes enlarge early, probably secondary to infection and, later in the course, because of metastatic disease. The inguinal nodes are generally involved first, then the iliac and paraaortic nodes. It is important to note, however, that when the glans and corpora are involved, metastases may go directly to the iliac nodes without passing through the inguinal nodes. The tendency for regional lymphatic spread is not related to the size of the primary lesion, but does correlate with the patient's age, site of the primary lesion, and histologic differentiation of the tumor. Thus, young patients and those with lesions on the glans are more likely to metastasize, whereas patients with exceedingly well-differentiated tumors are less likely to have metastatic lymph node involvement.[27] As local invasion progresses and bloodborne spread occurs, distant metastases to, in decreasing order, the lungs, liver, and thyroid gland may be found. If uncontained, local growth and inguinal node spread result in local invasion of the scrotum, perineum, bone, and femoral blood vessels. A cause of death in many patients is exsanguination secondary to erosion into the femoral vessels.[15] Others usually die of inanition.[19]

Patients with carcinoma of the penis who receive no treatment die of their disease relatively soon after diagnosis. Of 16 patients who received no treatment, most were dead within 3 years of diagnosis and all succumbed by 5 years.[24] Rarely, long-term survivals have been recorded in patients who have lived with their disease. Furlong and Uhle[31] reported a patient who died 12 years after presenting with inguinal metastases.

***Signs and Symptoms.*** The most common presenting complaint is a growth or swelling on the penis that is noted by the patient. Other symptoms and signs in decreasing order of occurrence include ulceration, bleeding, pain, discharge, phimosis, voiding difficulties, hematuria, groin swelling, and pruritus.[17] It is important to point out that phimosis occurs in many patients and often obscures the lesion. Invariably there is a delay in seeking medical attention even when the lesion is not obscured by phimosis. Fewer than half of the patients seek medical attention less than 6 months from the time of discovery. Fifteen to twenty percent of patients delay for more than a year.[17]

Approximately half of the patients who present with cancer of the penis have palpably enlarged nodes, and only half of the nodes that are enlarged contain tumor. Conversely, approximately 20% of patients with palpably negative nodes at presentation harbor tumor.[19,20,22,32]

Rarely, patients with large, bulky tumors have hypercalcemia in the absence of bony metastases. The etiology of the hypercalcemia is unclear, but it has been noted to disappear when the tumor mass and soft tissue metastases are surgically removed.[33]

***Diagnosis and Staging.*** The diagnosis is made by biopsy. In patients with phimosis, the lesion may be unsuspected preoperatively. It is important to emphasize that histologic confirmation of the diagnosis must be obtained before any treatment is rendered since syphilis, local infection, and benign tumors can all simulate the malignant condition.

Squamous cell carcinoma is clearly the most common histologic type of cancer of the penis and is characterized by irregular nests of epidermal cells with disruption of the basement membrane and infiltration of the dermis to varying depths. Keratinous nests of ''epithelial pearls'' and intracellular bridges are often observed (Fig 2). Local invasion is common, but direct invasion of the urethra is rare.[34] The tumors may be graded histologically as very well, moderately, and poorly differentiated. Histologic differentiation is based on the degree of keratinization, the number of mitotic cells per high-power field, the presence of cellular atypia, and the presence of inflammatory cells. The potential for metastatic spread is greater with the less differentiated tumors.[35] Preputial cancers seem more benign with a lesser chance for metastases than lesions located on the glans.[27]

Once the histologic diagnosis is made, the patient is staged according to a modification of the classification proposed by Jackson.[36] Since the stage is critically important in determining the type of therapy

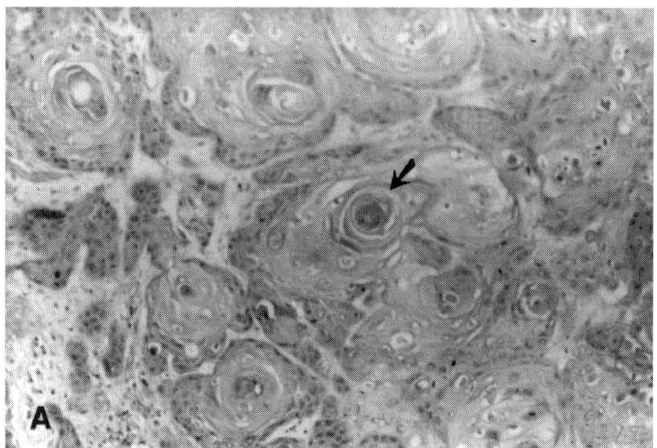


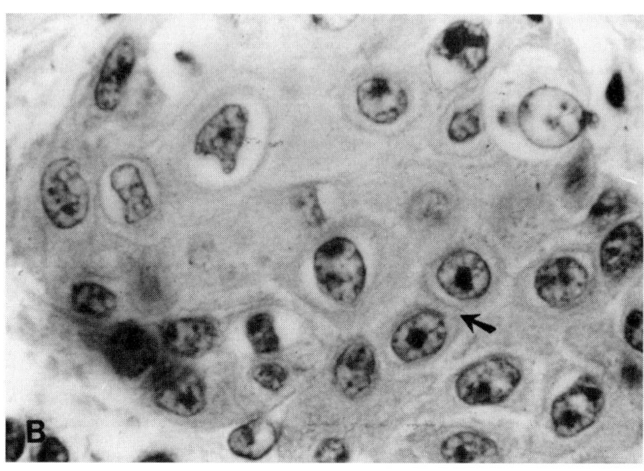


**Fig 2.** Histologic appearance of squamous cell carcinoma. Note in **A** the epithelial "pearl" *(arrow)* and in **B** the intracellular bridges *(arrow)*.

the patient should receive, we have found that a modification of the original Jackson classification is necessary (Table 1). Stage I comprises well-differentiated squamous cell tumors that do not invade deep to the dermis in patients with no evidence of regional lymphatic involvement. Stage II lesions are locally invasive without clinical evidence of regional lymph node involvement. This stage is subdivided into stage IIA, which includes invasive lesions that are well differentiated and do not involve the corpus spongiosum or the corpus cavernosum, and stage IIB, comprising all invasive tumors that are poorly differentiated irrespective of depth of invasion and all tumors that involve the corpus spongiosum or corpus cavernosum irrespective of the degree of differentiation. Stage III lesions are those in which there are palpably positive inguinal lymph nodes that are amenable to surgical removal. Stage IV disease includes those with any of the following: inoperable groin nodes, and/or distant metastases. To place the patient in the appropriate clinical stage, a chest roentgenogram, liver function studies, and an abdominal computerized axial tomogram for paraaortic and pelvis lymph node involvement are obtained. Lymphangiography has limited usefulness in this disease.

Because some nonpalpable groin nodes contain tumor, surgical staging by selected inguinal lymph node biopsy has been suggested as a method for increasing the accuracy of diagnosis. Cabanas[37] suggested that a sentinel node in the groin located on the anteromedial aspect of the superficial

**TABLE 1. Stages of Malignant Tumors of the Penis**

| | |
|---|---|
| Stage I | Superficial carcinoma, no subcutaneous tissue invasion, no invasion of corpora cavernosa, corpora spongiosum, or scrotum. No involvement of inguinal lymph nodes. Well differentiated. |
| Stage IIA | Locally invasive, no invasion of the corpora spongiosum or corpora cavernosa. No lymph node involvement. Well or moderately differentiated. |
| Stage IIB | All tumors invasive to corpora spongiosum and corpora cavernosa. All poorly differentiated tumors irrespective of depth of invasion. No lymph node involvement. |
| Stage III | Palpably positive regional lymph nodes that are surgically resectable. |
| Stage IV | Includes any of the following: inoperable lymph nodes, positive pelvic lymph nodes, distant metastases. |

epigastric vein just above and medial to the epigastric–saphenous junction was the first site of drainage of the lymphatics from the penis. Of 31 patients with a negative sentinel lymph node, 28 survived 5 years. Only six of these patients, however, had an inguinal lymphadenectomy that confirmed the absence of other positive nodes. Fifteen patients had positive sentinel lymph nodes; and in 12 of these, no other nodes were positive when an inguinal lymphadenectomy was performed. Seventy percent of this group survived 5 years. Unfortunately, Cabanas does not tell us the cause of death in the three patients with negative sentinel lymph node biopsies. If they died of cancer, the 10% false-negative rate with biopsy does not appear to justify its use when there is only a 20% false-negative rate with clinical palpation alone.

Several facts appear to discourage reliance on this technique as a reliable method of predicting inguinal node spread. First, micrometastases may bypass the superficial nodes and drain directly to the deep inguinal nodes or may bypass the groin altogether and drain directly into the iliac nodes. Second, in one report[38] the sentinel node was biopsied and found to be negative, yet a short 3 months later, both groins were so replaced with tumor that the nodes were unresectable. Also, Fegen and Persky[39] noted that one of two biopsies they performed was falsely negative. Third, others have used random open biopsies of the nodes or needle aspiration with variable success. It appears that inguinal node biopsy has little to offer in either the staging or the treatment of this disorder.

***Treatment of Primary Lesion.*** Once the diagnosis of squamous cell carcinoma is confirmed, the primary lesion may be treated by local excision, laser, cryotherapy, circumcision, radiation, partial penectomy, or total penectomy. The type of procedure performed depends on the stage and location of the primary lesion. Antibiotics should be administered following removal of the growth to promote wound healing since the area is invariably infected. The antibiotics will also reduce the size of groin nodes enlarged because of infection, thereby allowing for more accurate clinical staging.

For stage I tumors, which are confined to the foreskin, circumcision appears to provide the best chance for removal with the least deformity, provided a 2-cm margin can be obtained. If adequate margins cannot be obtained, recurrence is assured. Hardner et al.[20] reported on three patients treated with circumcision in whom adequate margins were not obtained, and in all three the tumor recurred. Skinner et al.[15] noted only one recurrence in six patients treated by circumcision and Williams[40] noted one recurrence in nine patients treated with circumcision. It is clear that circumcision applied primarily to preserve cosmetic appearance rather than performed only when adequate surgical margins can be obtained is doomed to failure.

Noninvasive lesions may be locally excised provided they meet the stage I criteria (Table 1). Invasive lesions of the glans and all stage II tumors require partial or total penectomy, depending on what is necessary to ensure a 2-cm margin free of tumor. Lesser procedures guarantee failure, eg, glandular lesions treated by local excision have a 40% recurrence rate.[10] A composite of several series in the literature reveals that patients who have a partial penectomy have a 2% (4 of 218) chance of local recurrence,[13,20,40,41] while those undergoing a total penectomy rarely if ever have local recurrence (0 of 17).[16,40]

Cryosurgery also has been used to eradicate the primary lesion. In the series by Madej and Meyza,[42] 15 patients with stage I and II disease were treated with cryotherapy with no evidence of recurrence. The advantage of this form of therapy is that the lesion can be removed with the greatest preservation of normal penile tissue. The method is cumbersome and, in our experience, may require more than one treatment.

The Nd:YAG laser has been used effectively to eradicate local disease, particularly in patients too debilitated to undergo a major surgical procedure. Generally several treatments are required. This therapy is not recommended for invasive lesions in the patient in whom cure is sought. It has been used quite effectively for invasive disease, for those in whom palliation is the goal.

Extirpative surgery is less morbid for invasive lesions and has a lesser chance of resulting in locally recurrent disease. If local recurrence does occur, resection apparently does not significantly lessen the patient's chance of survival.[43]

The use of radiation therapy to treat these lesions has met with variable success. Small localized lesions treated with irradiation are eradicated in 90% of the cases.[44] However, if all stages of primary lesions are considered, about 50% of patients treated with radiotherapy are refractory to treatment or experience a local recurrence.[20,45] In patients with tumors that involve the corpora (stage IIB), severe strictures of the urethra often develop following therapy. Although Williams[40] noted that irradiation of the primary lesion failed in 44% of the patients, when amputation was employed for the failures, survival was said to be unaffected. It is difficult, however, to confirm this from the data presented. The complications of radiation include a 4% (4 of 92) incidence of necrosis, an 11% (10 of 92) incidence of leg edema, a 15% (14 of 92) incidence of sepsis, and a 20% (18 of 92) incidence of urethral stenosis.[40]

***Treatment of Groin Nodes.*** Carcinoma of the penis is one of the few diseases in which removal of regional nodes involved with metastatic cancer can result in cure. Indeed, in patients with surgically proven positive inguinal nodes treated by lymphadenectomy, there is a 50% (68 of 137) 5-year survival rate (Table 2). Of patients with surgically proven positive inguinal nodes in whom only the primary lesion is removed, 95% are dead in 3 years.[24] Thus, it is clear that the patient with positive inguinal nodes will benefit greatly from a node dissection. What is not clear is whether patients with clinically negative regional nodes should undergo a prophylactic inguinal lymphadenectomy.

Baker et al.[46] reviewed 122 cases and noted that, according to 5-year survival sta-

**TABLE 2. Cancer-Free Survival According to the Method of Treatment for Various Stages of Penile Cancer[a]**

| Stage | Local Resection | Amputation | Amputation + Immediate Lymphadenectomy | Amputation + Delayed Lymphadenectomy |
|---|---|---|---|---|
| I | 69%(11/16)[40] | 89%(24/27)[16,41] | 80%(4/5)[16,17] | |
| I & IIA, B | 33%(2/6)[22] | 86%(185/214)[15,19,24,27,37] | 71%(20/28)[19,24,47] | |
| IIA, B | — | 68%(25/37)[16,17,41] | 66%(2/3)[17] | |
| III | 0%(0/1)[24] | 5%(1/21)[19,24,41] | 50%(68/136)[15-17,19,24,27,37,40,41] | 42%(15/36)[15,17,19,27,41] |
| IV | 0%(0/10)[24] | 0%(0/4)[19,41] | | |

[a]The data are expressed as percent survival (number surviving/total number of patients). Superscripts denote references from which patient data were obtained.

tistics, prophylactic lymphadenectomy could not be justified. Furthermore, they found no difference in survival between patients who had superficial and those who had superficial plus deep node dissections, and no difference between those whose node dissections were prophylactic and those whose nodes were dissected once clinical evidence of positive nodes became evident. They also noted that if two or more nodes were positive, the patient died within 5 years.

These conclusions appear tenuous to me for the following reasons. Two of their four patients with pathologically positive deep inguinal nodes that were removed survived 5 years. If the contention of Baker et al. that there is no difference in survival between patients undergoing superficial node dissections and those receiving superficial plus deep dissections is correct, then if the two patients who had deep nodes involved with tumor had not received a deep node dissection, tumor would have been left behind and, according to the investigators' conclusions, they would have had an equal chance of surviving when compared to the group as a whole. But since we know that positive nodes left behind and untreated result in the patient's demise within 3 years, their conclusion does not seem credible. The statement that waiting for nodes to appear and then removing them is just as successful as removing them before they become grossly enlarged does not seem consistent with their finding that patients who had two or more positive nodes are not cured irrespective of therapy. It would seem that the longer one waited for microscopic metastases to become evident, the more likely that the tumor would spread to involve more than two nodes.

Baker et al.'s conclusion that there is no place for prophylactic inguinal lymphadenectomy in view of the morbidity is a direct outgrowth of a similar conclusion made earlier by Beggs and Spratt, who reviewed many of the same patients.[19] Beggs and Spratt based their conclusion on the observation that two patients who initially were thought not to have inguinal metastases died of progressive inguinal disease. They suggested that since lymphadenectomy cures 50% of patients with positive nodes, they reasonably could expect only one of the patients to have lived if both had a lymphadenectomy. One patient out of their entire series constituted 1.2% of the population. Since the operative mortality was slightly higher than this, if all patients were treated surgically, one would anticipate a mortality of such a magnitude that somebody else would have died for the one patient who survived because of the lymphadenectomy. The authors concluded that to the population at large, prophylactic lymphadenectomy did not result in an increased survival because patients saved by lymphadenectomy would be offset by patients dying from operative mortality. This spurious argument is based on too few patients being inappropriately compared with the whole population and insufficient data.

Another argument used to support not performing a lymphadenectomy in patients without clinically palpable metastatic disease comes from the survival statistics of patients who were first thought to have negative nodes, so had only local therapy, but who eventually developed metastatic disease and then underwent a (delayed) lymphadenectomy. A composite of these reports reveals a 42% (15 of 36) 5-year survival rate in patients who underwent delayed lymphadenectomy (Table 2), which compares favorably with the 50% 5-year survival rate of patients whose nodes were positive for tumor at presentation and who then underwent a lymphadenectomy as part of the primary therapy. Unfortunately, it is not with patients who present initially with positive nodes that delayed lymphadenectomy should be compared, but rather with patients who first had lymphadenectomy with palpably negative nodes that pathologically were positive. There have not been enough data to make a valid comparison; however, from the few cases reported and from our own experience, it does appear now that the 5-year survival rate is much better than 42% and approaches 70% in patients with clinically negative nodes who underwent inguinal lymphadenectomy and whose nodes were found pathologically to be malignant.[48]

To compound the problem, on the average, 49% (36 of 74) of patients with palpable nodes do not have tumor present,[19–21] whereas 20% of patients without palpable nodes harbor tumor. However, this 20% figure includes both patients with stage I and stage II disease. When patients with stage II disease are evaluated for the presence of microscopic disease, between 38% and 66% of those who have clinically negative nodes at the time of initial presentation are found to have metastatic nodal disease in the groin.[17,41,47] As noted above, it has been suggested that the clinical error could be eliminated by the use of sentinel node biopsy. As previously pointed out, this technique seems less helpful than was originally thought and, in some hands, as accurate as clinical assessment alone.[48]

Table 2, a composite of data from the literature, shows survival statistics according to pathologic stage and treatment modality. An analysis of these data helps to elucidate the most appropriate form of therapy for each stage. Unfortunately, it is often not possible from the reports to differentiate between stages I and II and therefore where they could not be differentiated they were combined.

Patients with stage I and II disease who have a prophylactic lymphadenectomy or in whom amputation alone is performed have approximately an 83% 5-year survival rate with lymphadenectomy and a 68% 5-year survival rate with amputation alone. Clinical stage I and II patients undergoing amputation followed by delayed lymphadenectomy when nodes become apparent have a 52% 5-year survival rate. Although this survival rate is not much different from the 50% 5-year survival rate in patients thought initially to have positive nodes who undergo an immediate lymphadenectomy, the delayed lymphadenectomy group should not be compared with clinical stage III patients, but rather with clinical stage I and II patients who have microscopically positive nodes at the time of diagnosis. Following nodes until they become clinically positive allows the disease to become untreatable in a finite number of patients. Indeed, one of the most common causes of treatment failure is the development of inoperable nodes while the patient is being followed. This occurred in 22% (6 of 27) of those followed by Uehling.[49]

Other studies have also confirmed that survival is directly related to the number of positive groin nodes at the time of dissection. The chance that the nodes will be positive is directly related to the depth of invasion[50] and the differentiation of the tumor.[35]

Patients with clinical stage I and IIA disease have a very low incidence of undetected positive inguinal nodes, whereas patients with clinical stage IIB disease have much higher incidences of undetected positive nodes. Indeed, data from our series would suggest a greater than 66% chance of positive nodes in this group (Stage IIB) of patients who have clinically nonpalpable nodes. In view of the data, our treatment preference for inguinal nodes is as follows. In stage I and IIA disease, patients with lesions that are localized, superficial, and well differentiated do not require lymphadenectomy but are followed expectantly. Indeed, the majority of patients with clinical stage I tumors who receive local therapy alone and survive 5 years have no recurrence of their disease. For stage IIB disease where the incidence of undetected positive nodes is high, it seems prudent to perform an ilioinguinal lymphadenectomy. With modern surgical techniques, the morbidity of this type of lymphadenectomy is minimal. Stage III patients should have an ilioinguinal node dissection and stage IV patients should receive chemotherapy (see *Chemotherapy* below).

Since lymphatic drainage theoretically can bypass the inguinal region and proceed directly to the iliac nodes, an ilioinguinal node dissection should be performed rather than an inguinal dissection alone for patients who have pathologic evidence of positive inguinal lymph nodes. Also, in collected series in which inguinal and iliac nodes were looked at separately, 34% (33 of 97) of patients with positive inguinal nodes had positive iliac nodes.[28,34,41,49] Moreover, patients with stage III disease who have an inguinal dissection survive an average of 5 years, whereas those who undergo an ilioinguinal dissection survive an average of 9 years.[20] Others also have reported cures in patients in whom the iliac nodes were positive.[41] Both groins should be dissected since 60% (18 of 30) of patients with one groin positive have bilateral disease.[27]

***Radiation Therapy.*** Several decades ago, radiation therapy was thought to be as efficacious as surgery in the eradication of this disease.[36] Engelstad[51] noted that 76% (28 of 37) of his patients were cured with radiotherapy. More recent studies have failed to substantiate its superiority over surgery for either local disease eradication or nodal disease control. Treatment with radiotherapy results in 5-year survival rates of 46% for stage I, 44% for stage II, and 0% for stage III,[24,40] compared with surgical therapy which results in 80%–90% survival rates for stage I and IIA, 70% for stage IIB, and 50% for stage III. Others have had similar experiences. Beggs and Spratt[19] noted that only one of eight patients was cured with radiotherapy. If surgery is combined with radiotherapy and employed when radiation fails, 62% (16 of 26) of stage I and II patients survive 5 years and 25% of stage III patients survive 5 years.[24] Moreover, the small stage I lesion located on the foreskin or frenulum appears to be treated as well by radiotherapy as by surgery. Radiotherapy is of less benefit for treating the primary disease of stage II patients and of no benefit for treating nodal metastases.[52] The advantages of radiotherapy include preservation of the part with minimal destruction, but the complications are many including urethral stricture, sepsis, edema, and local necrosis. Some, however, maintain that failure of the patient to respond to radiotherapy in no way jeopardizes his or her chances for surgical cure.

***Chemotherapy.*** Bleomycin, cisplatin, and methotrexate have all been used with success as single agents and in combination for the treatment of cancer of the penis. Bleomycin in some series has been shown to have a 50%–70% response rate and methotrexate has demonstrated a 38% response rate.[53,54] These high response rates have not been confirmed by others. Cisplatin has a 33% response rate.[55] A recent report suggests a 25% partial response rate for 5-fluorouracil in combination with cisplatin.[56] This is a more realistic assessment of expected response in this disease. These drugs are used in stage IV disease and, although some patients respond, the effect on most is palliative only.

***Technique of Lymphadenectomy.*** Removal of the superficial and deep inguinal nodes in continuity with the iliac nodes, the classic ilioinguinal lymphadenectomy, is performed in the following manner (Fig 3). Preoperatively, the patient is hydrated, a mechanical bowel cleansing is performed, and the lower extremities are wrapped with pneumatic compression stockings. We prefer to perform the dissection in the groins simultaneously through an oblique/transverse incision 4 cm below and parallel to the inguinal ligament. If the nodes are attached to the dermis, an ellipse of overlying skin is removed. Skin flaps are developed deep to the superficial fascia and extend to the inguinal ligament cephalad, the junction of the adductor longus and sartorius caudad, the lateral border of the sartorius laterally, and the medial border of the adductor muscles medially.

Dissection begins at the inguinal ligament. Once the tissue is freed from the ligament, lateral and medial dissection exposes the femoral vessels. The main saphenous vein may be preserved by careful dissection, although its five branches at the fossa ovalis will need to be sacrificed. The tissue is dissected and left attached to a pedicle entering the empty space medial to the femoral vein.

Subsequently, through a lower midline extraperitoneal incision, the iliac nodes are dissected from the hypogastric artery cephalad to Cooper's ligament caudad, and from the obturator nerve posteriorly and the bladder medially to the psoas muscle and genitofemoral nerve anteriorly and laterally. The tissue specimen then may be removed en bloc by connecting through the empty space both inguinal and iliac nodes. The sartorius is transposed over the femoral vessels and sutured to the inguinal lig-

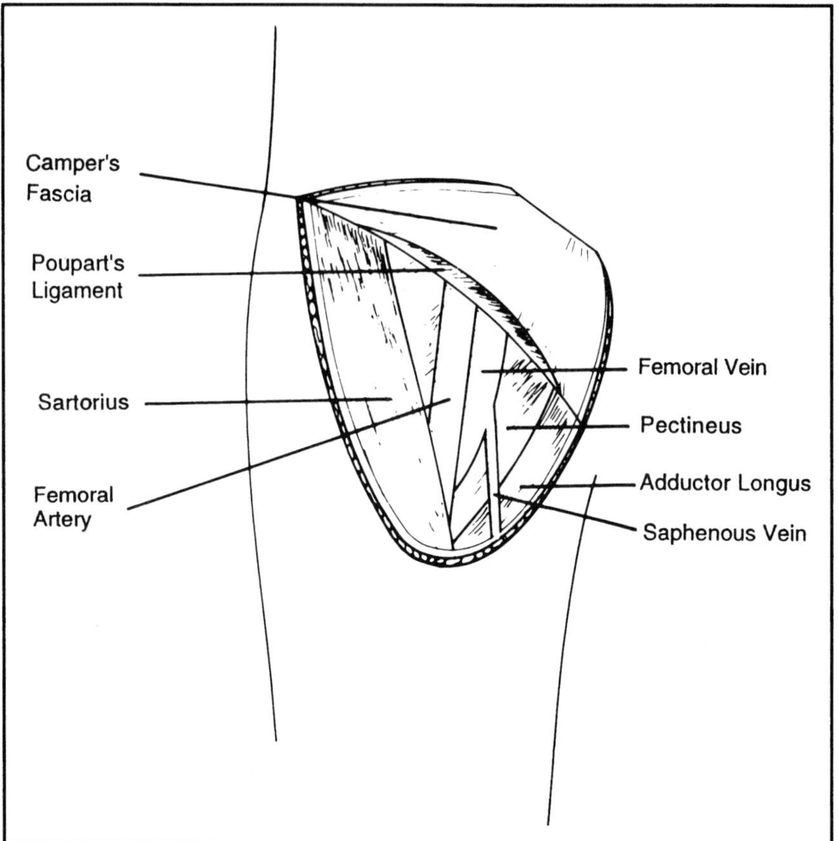


**Fig 3.** Limits of dissection for an inguinal node dissection. The femoral dissection extends from the lateral border of the sartorious to the medial half of the adductor longus and from the junction of the two muscles caudad to Pupart's ligament cephalad. All the tissue confined within these borders and extending from the femoral vessels dorsally to the superficial fascia ventrally is removed.

ament. The wounds are drained with suction catheters and dressings are applied.

We do not use prophylactic heparinization in either the preoperative or postoperative period. We have found it to be associated with a higher incidence of lymphocele formation. The patients ambulate on the fifth postoperative day and continue to wear elastic stockings for a minimum of 3 months postoperatively.

In the last 10 patients in whom this technique was employed, we have not observed flap necrosis requiring a split-thickness skin graft. In 3 of the 20 groins, 1 cm of skin along the incision line was lost, but it subsequently granulated and scarred without requiring grafting. Most patients experienced lymphedema, but none was incapacitated, and there were 8 instances of groin seromas that responded to sequential aspirations during the immediate postoperative period. Others have reported similarly good results.[56,57] Complications that have been observed following this dissection include infection, lymphedema, flap necrosis, seroma, hernia, femoral artery rupture, and pulmonary emboli.

**Adenocarcinoma.** Extremely rare, adenocarcinomas occur with a frequency of 1 per 250 cases of cancer of the penis.[27] They are treated similarly to anterior urethral adenocarcinomas that originate from Littre's and Cowper's glands. Adenocarcinomas of urethral origin are discussed below in the section on urethral tumors.

**Sarcomas.** Malignant soft tissue tumors, although rare, are more common than benign soft tissue tumors. Angiosarcomas[58] (including Kaposi's sarcoma) and fibrosarcomas[59] predominate, while leiomyosarcomas[60] and neurofibrosarcomas occur less commonly. These lesions tend to present as fixed, painful masses with infiltrating margins (Kaposi's sarcoma, however, presents as a nonpainful nodular lesion). They are usually located on the glans penis or prepuce and appear as a bluish, poorly circumscribed cutaneous and/or subcutaneous nodule.[2] These malignant soft tissue tumors have a tendency for rapid growth, and multiple local recurrences are frequent. Leiomyosarcomas are most prone to multiple local recurrence, whereas fibrosarcomas are more likely to be aggressive with a greater tendency to metastasize early.[2]

Treatment is total excision with as much surrounding healthy tissue as possible. These tumors spread both by the lymphatic and hematogenous routes.[61,62] In view of this and because so few cases are reported, the role of lymphadenectomy remains controversial.[2] Kaposi's sarcoma has been shown to respond to radiation. This may be very efficacious in patients whose immune status is compromised.

**Malignant Melanoma.** Malignant melanoma of the penis has been reported in less than 100 patients thus far.[63,64] The average age at diagnosis is 56 years with the youngest patient being 13 years of age. The lesion has been observed only once in the black population. The glans is the most common site, accounting for two thirds of the lesions. The prepuce is the next most common site. Penile melanoma metastasizes early, with 60% of patients having metastatic disease at the time of diagnosis and 43% having positive groin nodes.[63,64] Even with radical extirpative surgery, node dissection, and chemotherapy, survival is poor.[64,65]

**Metastatic Tumors to the Penis.** Metastatic lesions to the penis arise three quarters of the time from the genitourinary tract with the prostate predominating, followed by the bladder and kidney. Metastases from the testes, rectosigmoid colon, lung, and secondary lymphoma all have been reported. Patients generally present with an asymptomatic nodule, but about one third of the time priapism is the presenting complaint.[66,67]

## BENIGN AND MALIGNANT TUMORS OF THE URETHRA

### Benign Tumors of the Male Urethra

**Polyps.** Urethral polyps occur most often in males and are found predominantly in the posterior urethra. They occur in both children and adults who usually complain of urinary obstruction, hematuria, or hematospermia. In the very young, obstructive symptoms predominate and may be severe enough to cause urinary retention or hydroureteronephrosis.

The diagnosis is made by voiding cystourethrography or endoscopy and confirmed by pathologic examination. Urethral polyps are divided into three types based on their histologic appearance: fibrous polyps, villous polyps, and papillary hyperplasia.[68] Fibrous polyps, also referred to as congenital, solitary, or pedunculated polyps, have a fibrovascular stroma covered by transitional cell epithelium. They occur mainly in infants and children, with an age range reported between 2 and 46 years[69] and an average age at presentation of 9.7 years.[70] As in all polyps of the male urethra, they occur predominantly around the verumontanum. Of the 38 reported cases of fibrous polyps in two series only three were in the anterior urethra.[71,72] The origin of the polyp is unclear, but some have proposed a defect in the urethral wall as the cause. Transurethral resection is curative.

Villous polyps, often referred to as ectopic prostatic tissue, glandular polyps, adenomatous polyps, or papillary adenoma, have a fibrovascular connective tissue core that may be composed of prostate-like glandular cells covered with a papillary columnar epithelium. Although villous polyps are benign, recurrences have been reported.[73] They occur primarily in young adults in the posterior urethra and are located adjacent to the verumontanum. Various authors have suggested that they represent ectopic prostatic tissue.[74,75] In some countries, they appear to be a common cause of hematospermia and hematuria.[76] The lesions are treated by transurethral excisional biopsy and fulguration.

Papillary hyperplasia, sometimes referred to as polypoid urethritis, papillary pseudotumor, and proliferative papillary urethritis, is characterized by transitional cell epithelium, prostatic ductal epithelium, or acinar epithelium that covers an edematous inflamed fibrovascular stroma.[68] The lesions are thought to be a hyperplastic reaction to inflammation. The diagnosis is made by biopsy. These lesions are treated by transurethral fulguration and/or correction of the underlying inflammatory disorder.[77]

**Other Benign Lesions.** Other benign lesions of the male urethra include angiomas and leiomyomas. Patients with these lesions present with symptoms of obstruction, a palpable mass, and/or hematuria. Local excision results in cure.

**Condylomata Acuminata.** Condylomata acuminata are not uncommonly found in the urethra. Patients often complain of urethral discharge that may be bloody, dysuria, and warts on the external genitalia. Condylomata are caused by a human papovavirus that is sexually transmissible. They appear as papillary frond-like lesions and have a tendency to spread and to recur despite excision, fulguration, or chemical destruction. If they involve the bladder as well, they may cause severe irritative and obstructive symptoms and occasionally sepsis. Rarely, cystoprostatourethrectomy may be required for control. More commonly, urethral lesions can be treated successfully by excision and fulguration. The latter modality is limited by scar formation and can lead to a stricture if used extensively. Colchicine, thiotepa, sodium oxychlorosene, and 5-fluorouracil all have been successfully employed in their eradication.

### Benign Tumors of the Female Urethra

**Prolapsed Urethral Mucosa.** Urethral prolapse occurs in patients of all ages. Patients complain of spotting, dysuria, hematuria, obstructive symptoms, and, occasionally, a palpable mass at the meatus that may be painful. Prolapse of a portion of urethral mucosa, referred to as a urethral caruncle, occurs at the external meatus and is usually the result of chronic inflammation.

Whether caruncles are premalignant lesions remains controversial,[78] but they often occur in patients of the same age range as patients with urethral carcinoma.[79,80]

The treatment is local care and correction of chronic infection. The lesions should be excised if carcinoma is suspected or in patients in whom local symptoms cannot be controlled by conservative measures.

Prolapse of the entire circumference of the urethra occurs primarily in black girls younger than 5 years and in elderly patients. The patients present with symptoms of obstruction, a painful mass, and spotting. A discolored or necrotic-appearing mass protrudes from the urethral meatus and may have an appearance similar to malignant melanoma. The lesion is excised if necrotic.

Pedunculated fibrous polyps, similar histologically to those discussed in males, have been reported to protrude from the urethral meatus in women. Patients present with bleeding, obstructive symptoms, and a palpable mass. Treatment is by excision.

**Leiomyoma.** Patients with leiomyomas have symptoms of obstruction, recurrent urinary tract infections, dyspareunia, and a palpable mass. The average age of the patient at presentation in the 14 documented cases was 34 years.[81] Simple surgical excision, generally transvaginally, is the treatment of choice.[82] There has been one reported case of recurrence after local excision; this patient was adequately treated by a wider local excision.[83]

Other benign tumors in females include angiomas, fibrocystic masses, and masses composed of hyperplastic glandular tissue resembling male prostate tissue.[84] Local excision is curative.

## Cancer of the Urethra

Primary carcinoma of the urethra unassociated with bladder cancer is an exceedingly rare lesion. It is the only urothelial tumor that occurs more commonly in women than in men. The peak incidence is in the sixth decade, with most patients presenting between the ages of 50 and 70 years.[85] It has been reported, however, in a patient 18 years of age.[86] Survival depends on the location and stage of the tumor rather than the cell type. If the tumor is left untreated, death occurs generally within 1 year as a result of chronic infection, sepsis, inanition, or hemorrhage. Distant metastases are late occurrences.[87]

**Etiology.** Urethral carcinoma is frequently associated with chronic irritation, particularly in males. A history of infection, inflammation, and trauma with stricture disease is often obtained. Since the site of irritation is most frequently the bulbomembranous portion of the urethra, also the most frequent site of urethral cancer, the suggestion has been made that perhaps squamous cell carcinoma is a result of the irritative lesion.

Adenocarcinomas may arise from Cowper's glands in the membranous urethra, the most frequent location of this pathologic type of tumor in males, and from Littre's glands in the male and Skene's glands in the female, both of which are distributed throughout the urethra. Adenocarcinoma arising from Cowper's glands carries a dismal prognosis.

Transitional cell cancers may be induced by environmental toxins and oncologic viruses similar to transitional cell tumors of the bladder and upper urinary tract. This is emphasized by the fact that most urethral transitional cell carcinomas are associated with similar lesions of the bladder and upper urinary tract.

**Pathology.** Epithelial cancers are much more common in the urethra than are sarcomas. The histologic types of epithelial urethral cancer encountered most commonly include squamous cell carcinoma, transitional cell carcinoma, adenocarcinoma, and undifferentiated carcinoma. Very rarely malignant melanoma, clear cell adenocarcinoma, and cloacogenic carcinoma occur. Sarcomas that have been reported include fibrosarcoma, lymphosarcoma, myxosarcoma, and large cell, small cell, and spindle cell sarcomas.[79] Squamous cell carcinoma is the most common lesion in both males and females, accounting for 60%–75% of the cases. Transitional cell carcinoma occurs in 10%–15% of patients and is the second most common type in males. Adenocarcinoma, however, is the second most common type in females, occurring about 20% of the time. It is the third most common type in males, occurring 6% of the time. Undifferentiated tumors account for about 1%–6% of cases.[88–90]

There are about 60 reports of carcinoma arising in urethral diverticula in females.[91] The pathologic type is most commonly adenocarcinoma (46%) or transitional cell carcinoma (38%). Squamous cell carcinoma is the least common, occurring in only 12% of these patients.[92,93]

Urethral tumors arise from the mucosa, which is composed of different cell types depending on the region of the urethra. This accounts for the various histologic types, their incidence, and their location. In the male, the meatal urethra is lined by squamous epithelium, the penile and bulbomembranous urethra by stratified or pseudostratified columnar epithelium, and the prostatic urethra by transitional cell epithelium. In the female, the distal two thirds of the urethra is lined by squamous epithelium, while the proximal one third contains transitional cell epithelium. Since the most common type of tumor is the squamous cell carcinoma and since the epithelium from which it arises is in the bulbomembranous portion of the urethra in males and the distal two thirds of the urethra in females, it stands to reason that the most frequent location of urethral cancer in males is the bulbomembranous urethra (accounting for 50%–75% of the tumors), and in females the distal two thirds of the urethra. Lesions in females that arise in the proximal one third of the urethra are usually of transitional cell origin. Anterior urethral neoplasms in males are located in the meatus or fossa navicularis in most patients.

At the time of diagnosis, most primary urethral carcinomas have invaded locally; however, distal or anterior urethral lesions are usually less advanced locally than posterior or proximal urethral lesions. They are more likely to involve inguinal nodes, however. Distant metastases are rare, occurring in 10% of males[87] and 14% of females.[94] The lungs, liver, and bones are the common sites of metastatic spread.

Transitional cell cancer may occur primarily in the urethra or it may be associated with vesical tumors. Five to seven percent of patients with vesicle transitional cell carcinomas have synchronous or metachronous urethral involvement, while carcinoma in situ occurs in the urethra in 12% of these patients.[95,96] Since de novo transitional cell cancers make up only 10%–15% of all primary urethral cancers, their incidence is considerably less than that of the tumors associated with bladder cancer. Transitional cell tumors occur with decreasing frequency from bladder to meatus: 48% are located in the prostatic urethra, 6% in the anterior urethra, and 46% throughout the entire urethra.[95]

**Symptoms.** Both males and females may have symptoms of obstruction, a palpable mass, periurethral abscess, urethral discharge, urethral or vaginal bleeding, hematuria, urethral fistula, perineal pain, urinary retention, symptoms of urinary tract infection, pruritus, or tenesmus. Males may present with a "pepper pot" or "watering can" perineum, and females with dyspareunia, urethral prolapse, urethral polyps, a caruncle, or erosions. Unfortunately, even with these symptoms, patients often do not present for 5–18 months after their onset.[87,97]

**Diagnosis and Staging.** The diagnosis of urethral cancer is made by biopsy. Patients with multiple perineal fistulas (pepper pot or watering can perineum) should have deep biopsies of the area. Cancers that cause these conditions can be particularly difficult to diagnose and will elude the clinician unless he or she persistently and aggressively biopsies these patients.

Inguinal adenopathy is usually indicative of metastatic disease. Grabstald et al.[94] reported that 92% of their patients who had clinically positive nodes had pathologically positive nodes. Others, however, found a slightly lesser incidence of pathologically positive nodes in the presence of clinically palpable adenopathy. In the male, the penile urethra drains to the deep inguinal and external iliac nodes, whereas the bulbomembranous and prostatic urethra drain to the external iliac, obturator, internal iliac, and presacral nodes. In the female, the distal third of the urethra drains to the inguinal nodes and the proximal urethra to the pelvic nodes. Thus, lesions in the anterior urethra (penile urethra in the male and distal urethra in the female) require careful evaluation of the inguinal nodes, but more proximal lesions would not be expected to involve these nodes. Since survival depends on the stage and location rather than the specific histologic type, it is critical to stage the patients accurately. Table 3 illustrates the staging system advocated by Grabstald and associates.[94]

**TABLE 3. Stages of Malignant Tumors of the Urethra**

| | |
|---|---|
| Stage 0 | In situ cancer confined to the mucosa. |
| Stage A | The tumor is into but not beyond the lamina propria. |
| Stage B | The lesion invades but is not beyond the substance of the corpus spongiosum or prostate in the male or periurethral musculature in the female. |
| Stage C | There is direct extension into tissues beyond the corpus spongiosum or periurethral musculature. |
| Stage $D_1$ | Regional nodal metastases. |
| Stage $D_2$ | Distant metastases. |

**Treatment of Urethral Carcinoma in Males.** Failure of therapy generally stems from failure to control the disease locally. Conversely, local control of the disease often means cure. The treatment and survival depend on the location of the tumor. Anterior urethral cancers of squamous cell, adenocarcinoma, or undifferentiated type are treated by partial or total penectomy, depending on the extent of the primary lesion. Local recurrence is rare with penectomy.[87,98] If radiation is chosen as the primary therapy there is a local failure rate as high as 90%.[99]

Bilateral ilioinguinal node dissection should be performed if there are clinically palpable groin nodes. Unlike penile carcinoma, the overwhelming majority of clinically positive groin nodes are found to be pathologically positive.[94] Although patients with positive nodes have a poor prognosis, some have survived 5 years following node dissection.[87,98] The overall 5-year survival rate for anterior urethral carcinoma is 50%.

Transitional cell carcinoma that arises de novo and is noninvasive has been reported in the anterior urethra in three patients. Local transurethral resection of the tumor was successful in eradicating the disease in all three.[100]

Posterior urethral lesions generally present in a more advanced stage than do anterior urethral lesions and, therefore, the prognosis is considerably less favorable irrespective of treatment modality. The standard therapy for invasive squamous cell carcinoma, adenocarcinoma, undifferentiated carcinoma, and transitional cell carcinoma is total penectomy with en bloc prostatoseminal vesiculectomy, cystectomy, and pelvic lymph node dissection. Even with this type of radical surgery, 5-year survival rates of only 8% have been reported.[89] These discouraging results have prompted others to be more aggressive surgically since radiotherapy and chemotherapy are of little benefit. Three patients are alive and well with no evidence of disease 18–60 months after extended radical exenteration. The procedure involves removing the bladder, prostate, seminal vesicles, entire urethra, penis, scrotum, and perineal skin overlying the tumor en bloc with the symphysis pubis and medial 1 in. of the inferior pubic rami to include a portion of the attached striated muscles of the pelvic floor.[99]

We have proposed a slight modified approach that preserves the appearance of the phallus without compromising the extensive dissection required. We have found that this surgery is more readily accepted by patients as it preserves the male appearance. The pelvic lymph nodes, bladder, prostate, corpora cavernosa, corpus spongiosum, and fossa navicularis, including all of Buck's fascia and subcutaneous fat, are removed with this technique. Only the penile skin, glans penis, and one testis and spermatic cord are preserved. If neither testis can be preserved, the procedure can be modified (see below). If the tumor cannot be excised without a sufficient margin adjacent to the pubic rami and symphysis, they may be excised en bloc as well. The corporal bodies and fossa navicularis are removed with an inverting technique similar to that described by Whitmore and Mundt (personal communication) for urethrectomy (Fig 4A).

The perineal incision begins just anterior to the anus and includes a wide margin around the tumor, extends around the edge of the scrotum, and comes together in the midline on the ventral surface of the penis. A plane then is developed between the penile skin and Buck's fascia overlying the corporal bodies. The penis is inverted until both corpora cavernosa and the corpus spongiosum including the fossa navicularis are removed. The bulk of the glans penis is preserved. The scrotal tissue down to the tunica vaginalis is removed with the specimen. The testis and spermatic cord are transplanted into the penile skin tube (Fig 4B). The tunica albuginea is fixed to the cut edge of the glans penis to prevent later retraction of the testis. If both testes must be sacrificed because of tumor involvement, the penile skin tube may be filled with a rectus abdominis muscle flap rotated caudad and based on the inferior epigastric vessels. The reconstructed phallus is drained with a penrose drain for several days (Fig 4C).[101]

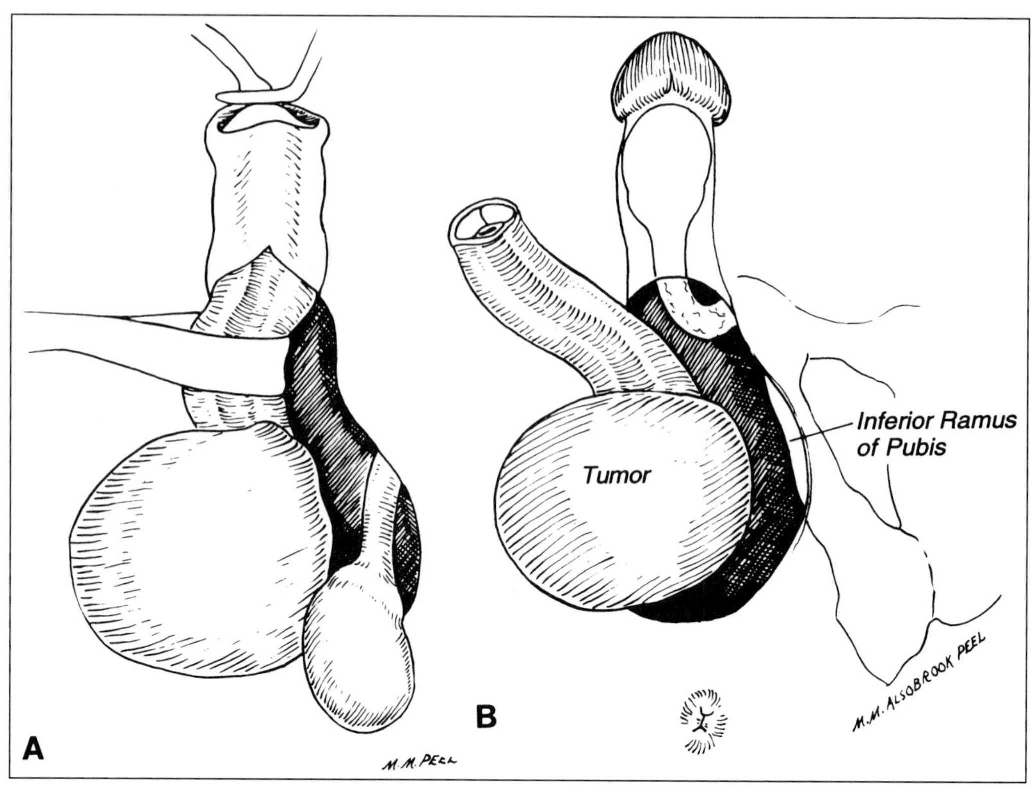


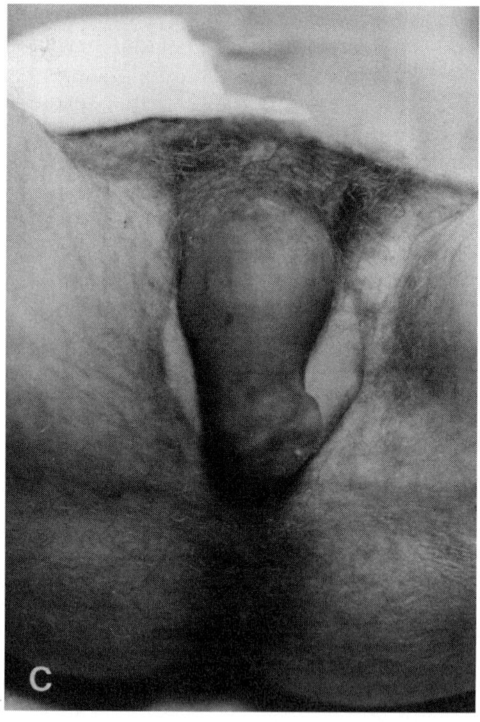


**Fig 4. A**. The technique of removing the corpora cavernosa and corpora spongiosum from the glans penis and skin of the penile shaft. A right angle clamp is placed at the meatus on the urethral catheter and the corpora are dissected from the overlying skin by progressively inverting the tissues. [From *J Urol.* (1989; 141:1201), with permission.] **B**. Upon completion of removing the corpora cavernosa and corpora spongiosum with its contained urethra from the penile skin tube a testicle is placed in the skin tube and sutured to the corpora spongiosum of the glans. [From *J Urol.* (1989; 141: 1201), with permission.] **C.** Gross appearance of the phallus following healing. Note that behind the phallus is a gracilis musculocutaneous flap that was used to close the perineal defect. [From *J Urol.* (1989; 141: 1201), with permission.]

The perineal defect is closed with a gracilis myocutaneous flap (Fig 4C) or an inferiorly based rectus muscle flap over which a split-thickness skin graft is placed. It is important to note that proper excision of the tumor will create a large soft tissue defect that cannot be primarily closed and will require a rotated flap. It is a mistake to believe that in this disease an excision that allows for primary closure would have an adequate soft tissue excision.

Transitional cell carcinoma arising in the posterior (prostatic) urethra accounts for 15% of the primary neoplasms of the male urethra. It is resistant to endocrine therapy, does not result in an elevation of acid phosphatase, and responds poorly to both radiation and surgery.[102] If superficial, it can be controlled by transurethral resection in 50% of cases. Superficial transitional cell carcinomas of the urethra associated with bladder neoplasms are also successfully treated by transurethral resection. In one series, 15% of patients had their urethral cancer eradicated by one transurethral resection and fulguration, whereas 50% had recurrent disease and required repeated fulgurations.[95]

Although well-differentiated superficial tumors may be treated successfully locally, once invasion occurs the prognosis is very poor. Therefore, these tumors must be followed very carefully. If there is a change in size or number with a worsening of the grade in the recurrent lesion or if invasion or a poorly differentiated neoplasm is noted in patients with either a primary or recurrent lesion, cystoprostatourethrectomy should be performed without delay. Particular attention should be paid to those patients who have multiple tumors at the bladder neck since they are more likely to develop subsequent invasive urethral involvement.[95]

**Treatment of Urethral Cancer in Females.** For the purposes of treatment, urethral cancers in females are divided according to whether they are confined to the distal third of the urethra, in the proximal two thirds of the urethra, or in a urethral diverticulum.

Tumors occurring in the distal third of the urethra generally are found earlier with less extensive disease. Twenty-five percent of these patients have positive inguinal nodes at the time of diagnosis.[103] For superficial localized lesions confined to the urethra, distal urethrectomy results in a 70% cure.[102] Radiotherapy also has been used very successfully in the treatment of these lesions irrespective of cell type.[104–106] Local application of interstitial radiation has given the best results.[94] Complications of radiotherapy occur about 42% of the time and include stricture; enterovaginal, vesicovaginal, and urethrovaginal fistulas; ulcers, vaginal stenosis; incontinence; radiation cystitis and enteritis; osteomyelitis pubis; and small bowel obstruction.[90,107]

Invasive lesions (stages B and C) should be treated with an anterior exenteration. If the groin nodes are clinically positive, an ilioinguinal node dissection also should be performed. Although there are too few reported cases to give meaningful 5-year survival rates, isolated case reports have been encouraging.[108,109] Radiotherapy, either locally or by external beam, appears less successful than surgery for these stages and is of little benefit as a primary modality.[110]

Lesions that involve more than the distal third or involve the proximal portion of the urethra are treated as though the entire urethra were involved. The prognosis is very poor with many authors reporting no survivors.[109] With radical surgery, however, others have reported 5-year survival rates between 10% and 21%.[111] Anterior exenteration with ilioinguinal node dissection if the groin nodes are palpable is the treatment of choice.

Locally invasive disease may require pubectomy as described above. As in males, failure to control the disease locally accounts for most failures. Indeed, 67% of patients dying of their disease following surgery die of complications of local recurrence.[112]

As in the male, adequate soft tissue removal will require rotation of a flap to cover the defect. We prefer the gracilis myocutaneous flap.

Tumors confined to diverticula may be treated by local excision with success provided they do not involve the peridiverticular soft tissues. Six of nine patients reported have been successfully treated by local excision.[93,113] The most common pathologic type is adenocarcinoma; however, once invasive, adenocarcinomas are more likely to metastasize than invasive squamous cell carcinoma. If the disease is beyond the confines of the diverticula, an exenterative procedure should be performed as described above.[114,115] Indeed, in one reported series 86% of urethral cancers in women invaded the periurethral tissue. More than half of the tumors were adenocarcinomas. Only 2 of 12 patients were free of disease with a relatively short follow-up.[116]

**Melanoma of the Urethra.** Melanoma of the urethra appears in males and females, with the majority occurring in patients between the ages of 60 and 80 years.[117] It presents as an enlarging, macular-pigmented lesion that may cause a mass, dysuria, hematuria, bloody discharge, melanuria, and obstructive symptoms.[63] There have been 36 cases reported in males. In males, the average age at presentation is 58 years,[118] and only 22% survive their disease.[63] The majority of lesions (60%) are located in the distal urethra, but they may occur throughout the entire urethra. There is generally a 2-year delay between onset of symptoms and treatment, which perhaps accounts for the relatively poor survival. The lesion has a similarly exceedingly poor prognosis in females. Only 3 of the 38 females with melanoma of the urethra described in the literature have survived.

The lesion appears radioresistant.[118] The treatment is pelvic exenteration with ilioinguinal node dissection.[119] Immunotherapy in the form of bacillus Calmette-Guérin and chemotherapy including dacarbazine, cyclophosphamide, and methyl-CCNU have been used with minimal success.[53]

## BENIGN AND MALIGNANT TUMORS OF THE EPIDIDYMIS

Benign and malignant tumors of the epididymis are exceedingly rare lesions that can be very difficult to diagnose accurately. Indeed, they are often misdiagnosed as inflammatory lesions. This is perhaps due to the rarity of these tumors combined with the very common occurrence of inflammatory lesions that often present on physical examination as an epididymal mass. Both benign and malignant tumors may appear as a painful, hard, paratesticular mass, or they may be asymptomatic and found incidentally. Similarly, epididymitis due to infection or chemical irritation, epididymal sperm granulomas, granulomatous epididymitis, polyarteritis nodosa,[120] and sarcoidosis[121,122] also may present as asymptomatic or painful scrotal masses. Perhaps the most useful diagnostic tool is ultrasound, which helps localize the mass to the epididymis and helps in the differential diagnosis, particularly in defining whether there is a discrete mass as opposed to diffuse inflammation and whether the mass is cystic or solid (Fig 5). The literature indicates that 25% of epididymal tumors are malignant,[123] but this figure is most likely an overestimate resulting from the propensity to report each malignant case encountered but not benign lesions. Analysis of reviews from one institution in which both benign and malignant lesions are reported reveals an incidence of malignancy of about 5%, a figure more in keeping with most urologists' clinical experience.[124]

### Benign Tumors of the Epididymis

**Adenomatoid.** The adenomatoid tumor, sometimes called an adenofibroma or mesothelioma, has a peak incidence between the third and fifth decades of life. This solid neoplasm is the most common benign tumor of the epididymis, accounting for 60% of all solid masses of extratesticular scrotal tissue. It occurs twice as often on the left as on the right side and most commonly occurs in the lower pole of the epididymis. In about 20% of patients, it is associated with a hydrocele.[124] It is of uncertain origin, but recent evidence indicates that it may be derived from coelomic epithelium.[125] The tumor also occurs in women and may be located in the uterus, fallopian tubes, and ovaries. Male patients present with a painless, hard epididymal mass. Ultrasonography generally reveals a solid mass 1–2 cm in diameter in the lower

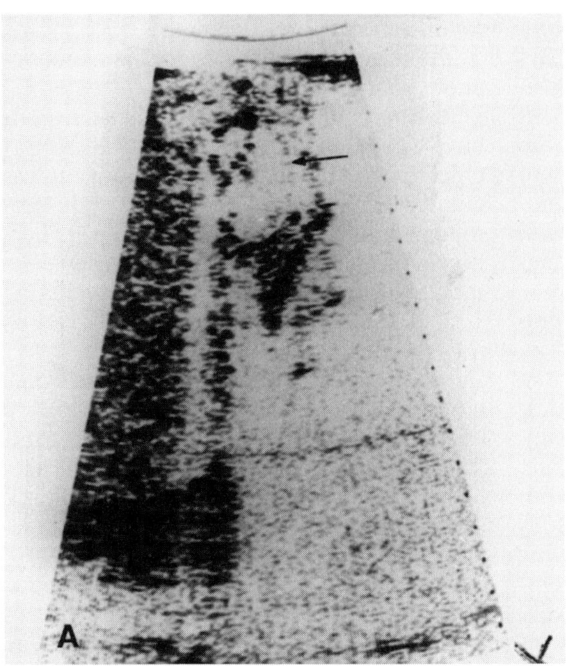


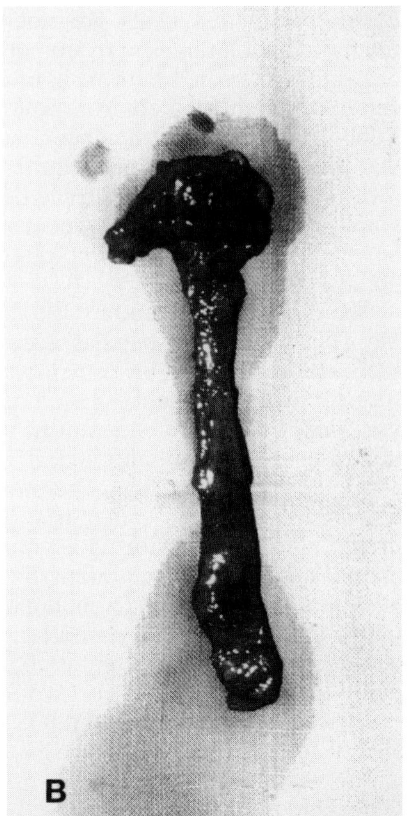


**Fig 5. A:** Ultrasonogram of an epididymal cyst *(arrow).* Note lack of internal echoes and posterior enhancement of the echoes. **B:** Gross specimen.

pole of the epididymis. Surgical excision is diagnostic and curative.

**Leiomyoma.** Leiomyomas are the second most common solid tumor of the epididymis, accounting for about 10% of all primary epididymal neoplasms.[123] Their peak incidence is in the fifth decade of life, and they are found bilaterally in about 15% of the cases. Half the patients have an associated hydrocele.[126] The lesions generally present as a painless mass. Ultrasound reveals a solid mass in the epididymis and a hydrocele about the testicle. Surgical excision is diagnostic and simultaneously therapeutic.

**Cystadenoma.** The cystadenoma has been referred to as an adenoma, a papillary adenoma, and a hamartoma and is associated 50% of the time with the Lindau–von Hippel disease.[127] Indeed, when the lesion is bilateral, other manifestations of this syndrome are invariably present. When the lesion is unilateral and no other manifestations of the Lindau–von Hippel disease are found, some authors suggest that the cystadenoma may be the single manifestation or forme fruste of the syndrome.[128] The tumor accounts for less than 10% of epididymal masses. Unlike adenomatoid tumors, which occur in the tail of the epididymis, cystadenomas are most commonly found in the head. They occur in patients from 16 to 57 years, range in size from 1 to 5 cm in diameter,[118] and are asymptomatic 75% of the time. One third are bilateral. In patients with Lindau–von Hippel disease, ultrasound suggests the diagnosis by revealing a solid and occasionally a cystic mass. For symptomatic lesions, simple excision is curative.

**Fibroma.** Fibromas are exceedingly rare lesions that may grow to considerable size. Ultrasound presumably would reveal a solid mass, and surgical excision is diagnostic and curative.

**Cysts.** Epididymal cysts are not uncommonly found on physical examination. Because they may feel hard, it is often difficult to differentiate them from solid masses solely by their feel. It has been suggested that exposure to diethylstilbestrol in utero results in an increased incidence of epididymal cysts.[129–131] More recent studies, however, cast serious doubt on this hypothesis.[132]

The diagnosis is made by ultrasonography (Fig 5). No treatment is necessary in most cases. It must be remembered that surgical exploration and excision of epididymal masses most often result in interruption of epididymal tubules and, in essence, a vasectomy on that side. Therefore, with ultrasonography the diagnosis is confirmed, and if the lesion is asymptomatic there is no need for exploration. Symptomatic cysts have been treated nonoperatively with success by needle aspiration and injection of a sclerosing solution.[133] It is likely that this treatment also would result in obstruction of epididymal tubules on the side of the lesion.

**Other Benign Tumors.** There have been isolated reports of lymphangioma, hemangioma, cystic embryoma, cholesteatoma, teratoma, lipoma, hamartoma, dermoid cyst, and adrenal cortical adenoma.[123,134]

## Malignant Tumors of the Epididymis

Malignant tumors of the epididymis occur much less commonly than the infrequently occurring benign tumors. They are likely to present as painful masses and therefore more likely to be confused with inflammatory conditions of the epididymis. Primary malignant tumors of the epididymis are of two pathologic types: sarcomas and carcinomas. Sarcomas occur about twice as frequently as carcinomas. The average age at the time of presentation of patients with these tumors is 41 years.[126]

**Sarcoma.** Leiomyosarcomas have been reported in 11 patients. The mitotic rate noted histologically is an important criterion of malignancy and the potential for metastasis.[135] Fibrosarcomas occur with about equal frequency whereas rhabdomyosarcomas are decidedly more rare. These tumors metastasize by the hematogenous route; therefore, lymphadenectomies performed in patients with these lesions have not been found helpful. Radical orchiectomy is the treatment of choice. It was curative in five of six patients with leiomyosarcomas.[135] Sarcomas as a group, however, generally run an exceedingly malignant course with survivals averaging 1–2 years.[126]

**Carcinoma.** Carcinomas of the epididymis have been reported but can be confirmed in only a few patients. They present as a painful mass between 20 and 40 years of age. Most patients die of their disease within 2 years of diagnosis despite radical orchiectomy.

**Other Malignant Tumors.** Primary histiocytic lymphoma has been reported in one patient. The site of origin was the epididymis, and the patient was cured by radical orchiectomy and radiation therapy.[136] A retinal anlage tumor, seminoma, and malignant teratoma also have been reported.[124,137]

**Metastatic Lesions to the Epididymis.** The gastrointestinal tract including the stomach, ileum, and pancreas is the most common site of origin of tumors metastatic to the epididymis closely followed in frequency by the kidney and prostate.[138–142] Metastatic lesions to the epididymis indicate a very poor prognosis. Indeed, patients with metastatic prostate cancer to the epididymis have a poorer prognosis than do patients with metastatic prostate cancer to other organs.[143]

# BENIGN AND MALIGNANT TUMORS OF THE SEMINAL VESICLES

Benign and malignant lesions of the seminal vesicles occur very infrequently. They present as masses in the retrovesical space and must be differentiated from the more common mass lesions that occur in contiguous structures, particularly the prostate, bladder, rectosigmoid colon, and pelvic peritoneal reflection. Intravenous pyelography may suggest the diagnosis by demonstrating a distorted bladder that is raised asymmetrically from its base. The studies most helpful in establishing a diagnosis are rectal ultrasonography, computerized axial tomography, and magnetic resonance imaging (MRI) with a surface rectal coil that locates the lesion and determines whether it is cystic or solid. The advantage of rectal ultrasound and MRI with a surface rectal coil is that they can be slightly more accurate in differentiating primary prostatic lesions from seminal vesicle masses when the latter are adjacent to the prostate. Angiography may be helpful in selected circumstances by demonstrating neovascularity and suggesting the diagnosis of malignancy. Pathologic diagnosis of solid lesions may be obtained by needle biopsy, which is best performed under the direction of either rectal ultrasound or computerized axial tomography.

### Benign Tumors of the Seminal Vesicles

**Benign Solid Tumors.** Solid benign lesions of the seminal vesicles are exceedingly rare, are usually asymptomatic, and are almost always found incidentally. Tumors that have been reported as single case reports include an angioma, lipoma, leiomyoma, cystadenoma, cystomyoma, and fibroma.[144,145] Local excision is curative.

**Cysts.** Patients with cysts of the seminal vesicles and ejaculatory ducts generally have hematospermia, painful ejaculation, irritative urinary tract symptoms, or outlet obstruction, but sometimes the lesion is asymptomatic and discovered incidentally. The cysts are classified into one of three types depending on their etiology: ejaculatory duct, Mullerian, or retention. Ejaculatory duct cysts are of Wolffian duct origin, are congenital, and generally occur unilaterally, although one case of bilateral involvement has been reported.[146] There have been a total of four cases reported. Successful treatment has consisted of aspiration, dilatation of the os,[147] transurethral incision of the floor overlying the cyst, and surgical excision (see Surgical Therapy, below).

Mullerian duct cysts are congenital and arise from remnants of the Mullerian duct that during embryogenesis failed to regress completely. They are midline in location and do not contain spermatozoa. Treatment is by aspiration or surgical excision (see Surgical Therapy, below).

Retention cysts are the most common of the cystic lesions. They arise from the seminal vesicles, are generally located lateral to the midline, and may contain spermatozoa. They occur in patients between ages 20 and 70 years old and contain from a few milliliters to 5 L of fluid.[148] If aspirated, they often recur and are best managed by surgical excision.

### Malignant Tumors of the Seminal Vesicles

There are three types of malignant tumors of the seminal vesicles: sarcomas, carcinomas, and metastatic implants.

**Sarcomas.** Sarcomas are the least common of the malignant tumors, and since it is often impossible to be certain that they actually arise from the seminal vesicle, they are best referred to as retrovesicle sarcomas. Pleomorphic cell sarcoma[144] and fibrosarcoma[145,149,150] have been reported. The tumors present with a soft, retrovesicle mass that may cause obstructive symptoms, perineal discomfort, constipation, or tenesmus. Treatment consists of radical excision, usually a radical cystoprostatovesiculectomy but a posterior exenteration may be required as well. The tumors are surrounded by a pseudocapsule and, if shelled out, local recurrence is assured.

**Carcinomas.** There have been about 40 cases of adenocarcinoma of the seminal vesicle reported in the literature. Such tumors occur between the ages of 24 and 90 years, with a mean age of 62 years and a peak incidence between 60 and 90 years. Because of the frequent extension of other contiguous tumors, particularly prostate, to the seminal vesicle, rigid pathologic criteria have been established that must be met to confirm a seminal vesicle origin. The neoplasm must be a papillary or anaplastic carcinoma localized primarily to the seminal vesicle with no other primary tumors present.[151] If the tumor is anaplastic, evidence of mucin production is necessary.[152] Of some help in differentiating these tumors from prostate cancer is that they do not stain for prostatic acid phosphatase (PAP) or prostate-specific antigen (PSA) as most prostate tumors do, and they may stain for carcinoembryonic antigen, which suggests either a seminal vesicle or gastrointestinal tract origin rather than prostate.[152]

Grossly, the tumors are usually surrounded by a fibrous capsule with frequent local extension to the opposite vesicle, prostate, and bladder. The rectum may be displaced, but invasion of its wall is a late occurrence.[153] Patients with carcinoma of the seminal vesicle often present late in their disease with symptoms of urinary outlet obstruction. Indeed, many are anuric.[153] Thirty percent have evidence of ureteral obstruction.[152] Some patients have a painless, soft mass, and very few have had hematospermia.[154]

An interesting presentation is that of the "phantom tumor." These patients may pass fragments of tumor and yet conventional studies of the urinary tract fail to detect the site. Occasionally, the tumor is visualized protruding from the ejaculatory duct and on subsequent urethroscopy no evidence of tumor is noted.[155]

On physical examination, a nontender, soft mass is palpated cephalad to the prostate. The diagnosis is suspected by intravenous pyelography, which reveals distortion of the floor of the bladder and, frequently, hydronephrosis; computerized axial tomography and rectal ultrasound, which reveal a solid retrovesical mass; and seminal vesiculography, which reveals an irregular border of the vesicle. Angiography reveals irregular neoplastic vessels with arteriovenous shunting.[156] Needle biopsy of the mass is diagnostic.

The prognosis is poor since often at the time of presentation metastases have occurred. In decreasing order of frequency of occurrence, the metastatic deposits occur in the lymph nodes, lungs, and liver. Occasionally, osteolytic bone metastases are noted.[155]

Treatment is by radical surgery, which should include the prostate and ejaculatory ducts since the latter may be involved with tumor, and often the bladder, since it is frequently involved by contiguous extension. Hormonal therapy (diethylstilbestrol) and hormonal ablation (orchiectomy) have been used in four patients with dramatic success.[152,155] Indeed, the long-term survivors of this disease have been for the most part treated with radical extirpative surgery coupled with hormonal manipulation. Radiation therapy does not appear helpful in this disease.

Secondary metastases are not uncommon, particularly from the prostate, and generally are an indication of a poor prognosis. Other organs that have been reported metastatic to the vesicle in decreasing order of occurrence include the bladder, testis, and rectum.[157]

## Surgical Therapy

Benign solid tumors and cysts of the seminal vesicles that require surgical excision may be approached by the perineal route, transsacrally (Kraeske's approach), transvesically, or retropubically. The perineal approach is more likely to result in impotence, and exposure may be somewhat limited, particularly if the tumor originates from the cephalad portion of the vesicle. On the other hand, small cysts that arise from the ejaculatory ducts may be conveniently approached by this route.

The Kraeske approach affords superb exposure with the flexibility for removing one or both seminal vesicles and surrounding tissue. It involves removing the coccyx, displacing the rectum laterally, and approaching the vesicles from their posterior surface (Fig 6). It is somewhat limited in that node dissections and exenterative surgical procedures cannot be performed.

The retropubic approach allows for removal of extensive tumors but is cumbersome for the small isolated lesion in which only the affected vesicle is to be removed. Approaching the lesion from the lateral aspect of the bladder may be awkward and,

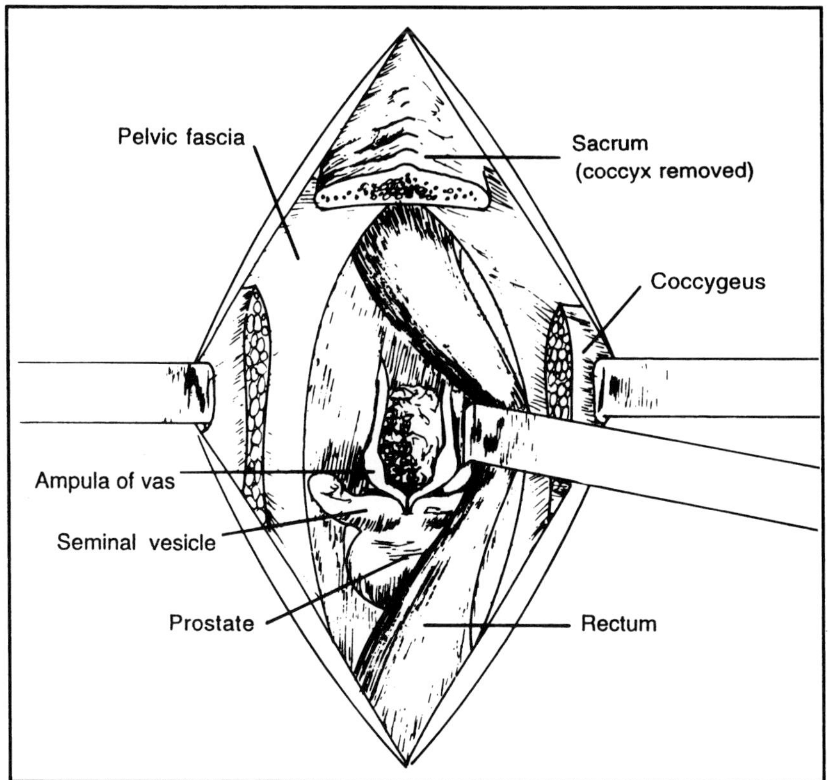


**Fig 6.** The Kraeske approach. A vertical incision is made over the proximal coccyx and extended over the sacrum. The coccyx is excised after detachment of the anal coccygeal raffe from its inferior aspect and the coccygeus from its lateral aspect. The pelvic fascia is incised, the rectum retracted to the side, the rectovesical fascia incised, and the posterior aspect of the seminal vesicles exposed.

therefore, to gain adequate exposure a transvesical approach may be necessary. The lateral neurovascular bundle containing nerves from the pelvic plexus that innervate the corpora and course adjacent to the prostate and lateral to the seminal vesicle should be identified and preserved if potency is to be maintained. For malignant lesions, the retropubic approach is preferred since these lesions often require en bloc removal of the vesicles, bladder, prostate, and, rarely, the rectum.

## REFERENCES

1. Senoh K, Miyazaki T, Kikuchi I, et al. Angiomatous lesions of glans penis. *Urology.* 1981; 17:194.
2. Dehner LP, Smith BH. Soft tissue tumors of the penis. A clinicopathologic study of 46 cases. *Cancer.* 1970;25:1431.
3. Elliott FG, Eid TC, Lakey WH. Genitourinary neurofibromas: clinical significance. *J Urol.* 1981;125:725.
4. Sonnex TS, Ralfs IG, DeLanza MP, et al. Treatment of erythroplasia of Queyrat with liquid nitrogen cryosurgery. *Br J Dermatol.* 1982;106: 581.
5. Gross G, Hagedorn M, Ikenberg H, et al. Bowenoid papulosis. Presence of human papillomavirus (HPV) structural antigens and of HPV 16–related DNA sequences. *Arch Dermatol.* 1985;121:858.
6. Kossow AS, Cotelingam JD, MacFarland F. Bowenoid papulosis of the penis. *J Urol.* 125: 124, 1981.
7. Peters MS, Perry HO. Bowenoid papules of the penis. *J Urol.* 1981;126:482.
8. Wade TR, Kopf AW, Ackerman AB. Bowenoid papulosis of the penis. *Cancer.* 1978;42:1890.

9. Bender ME, Katz HI, Posalaky Z. Carcinoma in situ of the genitalia. *JAMA.* 1980;243:145.
10. Hanash KA, Furlow WL, Utz DC, et al. Carcinoma of the penis: a clinicopathologic study. *J Urol.* 1970;104:291.
11. Herschorn S, Colapinto V. Balanitis xerotica obliterans involving anterior urethra. *Urology.* 1979;14:592.
12. Jamieson NV, Bullock KN, Barker THW. Adenosquamous carcinoma of the penis associated with balanitis xerotica obliterans. *Br J Urol.* 1986;58:730–731.
13. Ananthakrishnan N, Ravindran R, Veliath AJ, et al. Lowenstein–Bushke tumour of penis—a carcinomimic. *Br J Urol.* 1981;53:460.
14. Kraus FT, Perez-Mesa C. Verrucous carcinoma. Clinical and pathologic study of 105 cases involving oral cavity, larynx, and genitalia. *Cancer.* 1966;19:26.
15. Skinner DG, Leadbetter WF, Kelley SB. The surgical management of squamous cell carcinoma of the penis. *J Urol.* 1972;107:273.
16. Norman RW, Millard OH, Mack FG, et al. Carcinoma of the penis: an 11-year review. *Can J Surg.* 1983;26:426.
17. Narayana AS, Olney LE, Loening SA, et al. Carcinoma of the penis. Analysis of 219 cases. *Cancer.* 1982;49:2185.
18. Reddy CR, Raghavaiah NV, Mouli KC. Prevalence of carcinoma of the penis, with special reference to India. *Int Surg.* 1975;60:474.
19. Beggs JH, Spratt JS Jr. Epidermoid carcinoma of the penis. *J. Urol.* 1964;91;166.
20. Hardner GJ, Bhanalaph T, Murphy GP, et al. Carcinoma of the penis: analysis of therapy in 100 consecutive cases. *J Urol.* 1972;108:428.
21. Johnson DE, Fuerst DE, Ayala AG. Carcinoma of the penis. Experience with 153 cases. *Urology.* 1973;1:404.
22. Kossow JH, Hotchkiss RS, Morales PA. Carcinoma of the penis treated surgically: analysis of 100 cases. *Urology.* 1973;2:169.
23. Derrick FC Jr, Lych KM Jr, Kretkowski RC, et al. Epidermoid carcinoma of the penis: computer analysis of 87 cases. *J Urol.* 1973;110:303.
24. Staubitz WJ, Lent MH, Oberkircher OJ. Carcinoma of the penis. *Cancer.* 1955;8:371.
25. Kini MG. Cancer of the penis in a child aged two years. *Indian Med Gaz.* 1944;79:66.
26. Boczko S, Freed S. Penile carcinoma in circumsised males. *NY State J Med.* 1979;79:1903.
27. Ekstrom T, Edsmyr F. Cancer of the penis. A clinical study of 229 cases. *Acta Chir Scand.* 1958;115:25.
28. Gursel EO, Georgountzos C, Uson AC, et al. Penile cancer: clinicopathologic study of 64 cases. *Urology.* 1973;1:569.
29. Salaverria JC, Hope-Stone HF, Paris AM, et al. Conservative treatment of carcinoma of the penis. *Br J Urol.* 1979;51:32.
30. Thomas JA. Penile carcinoma and viruses. *J Urol.* 1982;128:307.
31. Furlong JH, Uhle AW. Cancer of penis. A report of 88 cases. *J Urol.* 1953;69:550.
32. Kuruvilla JT, Garlick FH, Mammen KE. Results of surgical treatment of carcinoma of the penis. *Aust NZ J Surg.* 1971;41:157.
33. Block NL, Rosen P, Whitmore WF. Hemipelvectomy for advanced penile cancer. *J Urol.* 1973;110:703.
34. Riveros M, Gorostiaga R. Cancer of the penis. *Arch Surg.* 1962;85:377.
35. Maiche AG, Pyrhonen S, Karkinen M. Histologic grading of squamous cell carcinoma of the penis: a new scoring system. *Br J Urol.* 1991; 67:522.
36. Jackson SM. The treatment of carcinoma of the penis. *Br J Surg.* 1966;53:33.
37. Cabanas RM. An approach for the treatment of penile carcinoma. *Cancer.* 1977;39:456.
38. Perinetti E, Crane DB, Catalona WJ. Unreliability of sentinel lymph node biopsy for staging penile carcinoma. *J Urol.* 1980;124:734.
39. Fegen P, Persky L. Squamous cell carcinoma of the penis. Its treatment with special reference to radical node dissection. *Arch Surg.* 1969;99:117.
40. Williams JL. Carcinoma of the penis. *Proc R Soc Med.* 1975;68:781.
41. DeKernion JB, Tynberg P, Persky L, et al. Carcinoma of the penis. *Cancer.* 1973;32:1256.
42. Madej G, Meyza J. Cryosurgery of penile carcinoma. Short report on preliminary results. *Oncology.* 1982;39:350.
43. Murrell DS, Williams JL. Radiotherapy in the treatment of carcinoma of the penis. *Br J Urol.* 1965;37:211.
44. Grabstald H, Kelley CD. Radiation therapy of penile cancer. *Urology.* 1980;15:575.
45. Green JP, Lowry RO, Valth JM. Carcinoma of the penis: radiotherapeutic approach for the primary lesion. *Radiol Clin Biol.* 1970;39:1.
46. Baker BH, Spratt JS, Perez-Mesa C, et al. Carcinoma of the penis. *J Urol.* 1976;116:458.
47. McDougal WS, Kirchner FK Jr, Edwards RH, et al. Treatment of carcinoma of the penis: case for primary lymphadenectomy. *J Urol.* 1986; 136:38.
48. Srinivas U, Josi A, Agarwal B, et al. Penile cancer: the sentinel lymph node controversy. *Urol Int.* 1991;47:108–109.
49. Uehling DT. Staging laparotomy for carcinoma of the penis. *J Urol.* 1973;110:213.
50. Horenblas S, VanTinteran H, Delemane JFM, et al. Squamous cell carcinoma of penis. III. Treatment of regional lymph nodes. *J Urol.* 1993;149:492.

51. Engelstad RB. Treatment of cancer of the penis at the Norwegian Radium Hospital. *AJR.* 1948; 60:801.
52. Krieg RM, Luk KH. Carcinoma of the penis. Review of cases treated by surgery and radiation therapy 1950–1977. *Urology.* 18:149, 1981.
53. Sklaroff RB, Yagoda A. Methotrexate in the treatment of penile carcinoma. *Cancer.* 1980; 45:214.
54. Sklaroff RB, Yagoda A. cis-Diaminedichloride platinum II (DDP) in the treatment of penile carcinoma. *Cancer.* 1979;44:1563.
55. Meyers FJ. Penile cancer chemotherapy. Recent results. *Cancer Res.* 1983;85:143.
56. Whitmore WF, Vagaiwala MR. A technique of ilioinguinal lymph node dissection for carcinoma of the penis. *Surg Gynecol Obstet.* 1984; 159:573.
57. Groshong LE. A technique for radical groin dissection. *Surg Gynecol Obstet.* 1973;136:986.
58. Wasmer JM, Block NL, Politano VA, et al. Penile angiosarcoma presenting in bladder. *Urology.* 1981;18:179.
59. Wilson LS, Lockhardt JL, Bergman H, et al. Fibrosarcoma of the penis: case report and review of the literature. *J Urol.* 1983;129:606.
60. McDonald MW, O'Connell JR, Manning JT, et al. Leiomyosarcoma of the penis. *J Urol.* 1983; 130:788.
61. Weinberger GI, Wajsman Z, Beckley S, et al. Primary sarcoma of penis. *Urology.* 1982;19: 193.
62. Zungri E, Algaba F, Santaularia JM. Epithelioid sarcoma of penis. *Eur Urol.* 1983;9:53.
63. Begun FP, Grossman HB, Diokno AC, et al. Malignant melanoma of the penis and male urethra. *J Urol.* 1984;132:123.
64. Stein BS, Kendall AR. Malignant melanoma of the genitourinary tract. *J Urol.* 1984;132:859.
65. Khezri AA, Dorinis A, Roberts JBM. Primary malignant melanoma of the penis. Two cases and a review of the literature. *Br J Urol.* 1979; 51:147.
66. Ordonez NG, Ayala AG, Bracken RB. Renal cell carcinoma metastatic to penis. *Urology.* 1982;19:417.
67. Trulock TS, Wheatley JK, Walton KN. Secondary tumors of penis. *Urology.* 1981;17:563.
68. Glancy RJ, Gaman AJ, Rippey JJ. Polyps and papillary lesions of the prostatic urethra. *Pathology.* 1983;15:153.
69. Zulian RAS, Brito RR, Borges HJ. Transurethral resection of pedunculated congenital polyps of the posterior urethra. *Br J Urol.* 1982; 54:45.
70. Downs RA. Congenital polyps of the prostatic urethra. A review of the literature and reports of 2 cases. *Br J Urol.* 1970;42:76.
71. Foster RS, Weigel JW, Mantz FA. Anterior urethral polyps. *J Urol.* 1980;124:145.
72. Falkowski WS, Cook WA. Anterior urethral polyps: an unusual cause of hematuria in a child. *J Urol.* 1981;125:744.
73. Mori K, Spiro LH, Hect H, et al. Recurrent intraurethral proliferation of ectopic prostatic tissue associated with hematuria. *J Urol.* 1975; 114:316.
74. Nesbit RM. The genesis of benign polyps in the prostatic urethra. *J Urol.* 1962;87:416.
75. Butterick JD, Schnitzer B, Abell MR. Ectopic prostatic tissue in urethra: a clinicopathological entity and a significant cause of hematuria. *J Urol.* 1971;105:97.
76. Baroudy AC, O'Connell JP. Papillary adenoma of the prostatic urethra. *J Urol.* 1984;132:120.
77. Schinella R, Thurm J, Feiner H. Papillary pseudotumor of the prostatic urethra: proliferative papillary urethritis. *J Urol.* 1974;111:38.
78. Monaco AP, Murphy GB, Bowling W. Primary cancer of the female urethra. *Cancer.* 1958;11: 1215.
79. Fagan GE, Hertig AT. Carcinoma of the female urethra. Review of the literature; report of 8 cases. *Obstet Gynecol.* 1955;6:1.
80. Allen R, Nelson RP. Primary urethral malignancy: review of 22 cases. *South Med J.* 1978; 71:547.
81. Unni Mooppan MM, Kim H, Wax SH. Leiomyoma of the female urethra. *J Urol.* 1979;121: 371.
82. Smith HW, Campbell EW Jr. Benign periurethral masses in women. *J Urol.* 1976;116:451.
83. Merrell RW, Brown HE. Recurrent urethral leiomyoma presenting as stress incontinence. *Urology.* 1981;17:588.
84. Marshall FC, Melicow MM. Neoplasms and caruncles of the female urethra. *Surg Gynecol Obstet.* 1960;110:723.
85. Bolduan JP, Farah RN. Primary urethral neoplasms: review of 30 cases. *J Urol.* 1981;125: 198.
86. Dean AL. Carcinoma of the male and female urethra: pathology and diagnosis. *J Urol.* 1956; 75:505.
87. Kaplan GW, Bulkley GJ, Grayhack JT. Carcinoma of the male urethra. *J Urol.* 1967;98:365.
88. Silverman ML, Eyre RC, Zinman LA, et al. Mixed mucinous and papillary adenocarcinoma involving male urethra, probably originating in periurethral glands. *Cancer.* 1981;47:1398.
89. Levine RL. Urethral cancer. *Cancer.* 1980;45: 1965.
90. Johnson DE, O'Connell JR. Primary carcinoma of female urethra. *Urology.* 1983;21:42.
91. Clayton M, Siami P, Guinan P. Urethral diverticular carcinoma. *Cancer.* 1992;70:665–670.
92. Cea PC, Ward JN, Lavengood RW, et al.

Mesonephric adenocarcinomas in urethral diverticula. *Urology.* 1977;10:58.

93. Evans KJ, McCarthy MP, Sands JP. Adenocarcinoma of a female urethral diverticulum: a case report and review of the literature. *J Urol.* 1981; 126:124.
94. Grabstald H, Hilaris B, Henschke U, et al. Cancer of the female urethra. *JAMA.* 1966;197:835.
95. Hamilton-Stewart PA, Anderson CK, Williams RE, et al. Urethral tumours. *Br J Urol.* 1978; 50:583.
96. Schellhammer PF, Whitmore WF. Urethral meatal carcinoma following cystourethrectomy for bladder carcinoma. *J Urol.* 1976;115:56.
97. Ray B, Canto AR, Whitmore WF. Experience with primary carcinoma of the male urethra. *J Urol.* 1977;117:591.
98. Bracken RB, Henry R, Ordonez N. Primary carcinoma of the male urethra. *South Med J.* 1980; 73:1003.
99. Bracken RB. Exenterative surgery for posterior urethral cancer. *Urology.* 1982;19:248.
100. Harty JI, Mojsejenko IK. Transitional cell carcinoma of the anterior urethra. *J Surg Oncol.* 1982;21:121.
101. McDougal WS, Koch MO. Phallic reconstruction during exenterative surgery for invasive urethral carcinoma. *J Urol.* 1989;141:1201.
102. Grabstald H. Tumors of the urethra in men and women. *Cancer.* 1973;32:1236.
103. Antoniades J. Radiation therapy in carcinoma of the female urethra. *Cancer.* 1969;24:70.
104. Turner AG, Hendry WF. Primary carcinoma of the female urethra. *Br J Urol.* 1980;52:549.
105. Staubitz WJ, Carden LM, Oberkircher OJ, et al. Management of urethral carcinoma in the female. *J Urol.* 1955;73:1045.
106. Prempree T, Wizenberg MJ, Scott RM. Radiation treatment of primary carcinoma of the female urethra. *Cancer.* 1978;52:1177.
107. Bracken RB, Johnson DE, Miller LS, et al. Primary carcinoma of the female urethra. *J Urol.* 1976;116:188.
108. Benson RC Jr, Runda JC, Buchler DA, et al. Primary carcinoma of the female urethra. *Gynecol Oncol.* 1982;14:313.
109. Blath RA, Boehm FH. Carcinoma of the female urethra. *Surg Gynecol Obstet.* 1973;136:574.
110. Rhamy RK, Boldus RA, Allison RC, et al. Therapeutic modalities in adenocarcinoma of the female urethra. *J Urol.* 1973;109:638.
111. Ziegerman JH, Gordon SF. Cancer of the female urethra—a curable disease. *Obstet Gynecol.* 1970;36:785.
112. Hopkins SC, Vider M, Nag SK, et al. Carcinoma of the female urethra: reassessment of modes of therapy. *J Urol.* 1983;129:958.
113. Marshall S, Hirsch K. Carcinoma within urethral diverticula. *Urology.* 1977;10:161.
114. Reheis JP, Goldstein IS, Mogil RA. Papillary adenocarcinoma arising in a urethral diverticulum accompanied by adenocarcinoma of the bladder: case report and review of the literature. *J Urol.* 1981;126:695.
115. Tesluk H. Primary adenocarcinoma of female urethra associated with diverticula. *Urology.* 1981;17:197.
116. Mayer R, Fowler JE, Jr, Clayton M. Localized urethral cancer in women. *Cancer.* 1987;60: 1548–1551.
117. Katz JI, Grabstald H. Primary malignant melanoma of the female urethra. *J Urol.* 1976;116: 454.
118. Weiss J, Elder D, Hamilton R. Melanoma of the male urethra: surgical approach and pathological analysis. *J Urol.* 1982;128:382.
119. Godec CJ, Cass AS, Hitchcock CR, et al. Melanoma of the female urethra. *J Urol.* 1981;126: 553.
120. McLean NR, Burnett RA. Polyarteritis nodosa of epididymis. *Urology.* 1983;21:70.
121. Amenta PS, Gonick P, Katz SM. Sarcoidosis of testes and epididymis. *Urology.* 1981;17:616.
122. Hefferman JC, Blenkinsopp WK. Epididymal sarcoidosis. *Br J Urol.* 1978;50:211.
123. Broth G, Bullock WK, Morrow J. Epididymal tumors. 1. Report of 15 new cases including review of literature. 2. Histochemical study of the so-called adenomatoid tumor. *J Urol.* 1968; 100:530.
124. Beccia DJ, Krane RJ, Olsson CA. Clinical management of nontesticular intrascrotal tumors. *J Urol.* 1976;116:476.
125. Soderstrom KO. Origin of adenomatoid tumor. A comparison between the structure of adenomatoid tumor and epididymal duct cells. *Cancer.* 1982;49:2349.
126. Longo VJ, McDonald JR, Thompson GJ. Primary neoplasms of the epididymis. Special reference to adenomatoid tumors. *JAMA.* 1951; 147:937.
127. Gruber MB, Healey GB, Toguri AG, et al. Papillary cystadenoma of epididymis: component of von Hippel–Lindau syndrome. *Urology.* 1980;16:305.
128. Price EB Jr. Papillary cystadenoma of the epididymis. A clinicopathologic analysis of 20 cases. *Arth Pathol.* 1971;91:456.
129. Whitehead ED, Leiter E. Genital abnormalities and abnormal semen analyses in male patients exposed to diethylstilbestrol in utero. *J Urol.* 1981;125:47.
130. Stillman RJ. In utero exposure to diethylstilbestrol: adverse effects on the reproductive tract and reproductive performance in male and female offspring. *Am J Obstet Gynecol.* 1982; 142:905.
131. Conley GR, Sant GR, Ucci AA, et al. Seminoma and epididymal cysts in a young man

with known diethylstilbestrol exposure in utero. *JAMA.* 1983;249:1325.

132. Leary FJ, Resseguie LJ, Kurland LT, et al. Males exposed in utero to diethylstilbestrol. *JAMA.* 1984;252:2984.
133. Macfarlane Jr. Sclerosant therapy for hydroceles and epididymal cysts. *Br J Urol.* 1983;55: 81.
134. Gray CP, Biorn CL, Drinker HR. Tumors of the epididymis. *J Urol.* 1961;86:620.
135. Farrell MA, Donnelly BJ. Malignant smooth muscle tumors of the epididymis. *J Urol.* 1980; 124:151.
136. Schned AR, Variakojis D, Straus FH, et al. Primary histiocytic lymphoma of the epididymis. *Cancer.* 1979;43:1156.
137. Salm R. Papillary carcinoma of the epididymis. *J Pathol.* 1969;97:253.
138. Addonizio JC, Thelmo W. Epididymal metastasis from prostatic carcinoma. *Urology.* 1981; 18:490.
139. Cia EMM, Billis A, Moriyama H, et al. Metastasis in epididymides from papillary adenocarcinoma of prostate. *Urology.* 1981;18:607.
140. Faysal MH, Strefling A, Kosek JC. Epididymal neoplasms: a case report and review. *J Urol.* 1983;129:843.
141. Wachtel TL, Mehan DJ. Metastatic tumors of the epididymis. *J Urol.* 1970;103:624.
142. Brotherus JV. Metastatic tumors of the epididymis and the spermatic cord. *J Urol.* 1960;83: 171.
143. Johansson JE, Lannes P. Metastases to the spermatic cord, epididymis, and testicles from carcinoma of the prostate. Five cases. *Scand J Urol Nephrol.* 1983;17:249.
144. Lazarus JA. Primary malignant tumors of the retrovesical region with special reference to malignant tumors of the seminal vesicles: report of a case of retrovesical sarcoma. *J Urol.* 1946; 55:190.
145. Buck AC, Shaw RE. Primary tumours of the retrovesical region with special reference to mesenchymal tumours of the seminal vesicles. *Br J Urol.* 1972;44:47.
146. Elder JS, Mostwin JL. Cyst of the ejaculatory duct/urogenital sinus. *J Urol.* 1984;132:768.
147. Lund AJ, Cummings MM. Cyst of the accessory genital tract: a case report with a review of the literature. *J Urol.* 1946;56:383.
148. Lawson LJ, MacDougall JA. Multilocular cyst of the seminal vesicle. *Br J Urol.* 1965;37:440.
149. Williamson RCN, Slade N, Feneley RCL. Seminal vesicle tumours. *J R Soc Med.* 1978;71: 286.
150. Tripathi VNP, Dick VS. Primary sarcoma of the urogenital system in adults. *J Urol.* 1969;101: 898.
151. Dalgaard JB, Giertsen JC. Primary carcinoma of the seminal vesicle. *Acta Pathol Microbiol Scand.* 1956;39:255.
152. Benson RC Jr, Clark WR, Farrow GM. Carcinoma of the seminal vesicle. *J Urol.* 1984;132: 483.
153. Smith BA Jr, Webb EA, Price WE: Carcinoma of the seminal vesicle. *J Urol.* 1967;97:743.
154. Ewell GH. Seminal vesicle carcinoma. *J Urol.* 1963;89:908.
155. Rodriguez-Kees OS. Clinical improvement following estrogenic therapy in a case of primary adenocarcinoma of the seminal vesicle. *J Urol.* 1964;91:665.
156. Goldstein AG, Wilson ES. Carcinoma of the seminal vesicle: with particular reference to the angiographic appearances. *Br J Urol.* 1973;45: 211.
157. Dawson EK, Mekie DE. Primary carcinoma of the seminal vesicles. *J R Coll Surg Edinb.* 1965; 10:235.

# 35

# Prostate Cancer Detection and Screening

*Gerald L. Andriole*

## INTRODUCTION AND RATIONALE FOR SCREENING

Prostate cancer poses a significant public health problem in the U.S. Prostate cancer is now the most common cancer affecting men in this country and is estimated to be the second leading cause of cancer death.[1] In 1993, it is predicted that more than 160,000 new cases of prostate cancer will be diagnosed. This represents almost 30% of all new cancers diagnosed, excluding basal and squamous cell cancers of the skin. It is anticipated that more than 35,000 men are expected to die of prostate cancer. The incidence and the mortality rate of prostate cancer have been rising over the past few years and are anticipated to continue to rise as the American population ages and individual life expectancy increases.

Traditionally, prostate cancer was detected on the basis of an abnormal digital rectal exam and/or patient symptoms such as hematuria, bladder outlet obstruction, or irritative lower urinary tract complaints. When these symptoms and findings have been used as indications to perform prostate biopsy, only about two thirds of the newly diagnosed cases of prostate cancer were clinically localized to the prostate at the time of detection. Moreover, when patients judged to have clinically localized prostate cancer found in this manner underwent surgical staging with pelvic lymphadenectomy and radial retropubic prostatectomy, fewer than half were found to have pathologically organ-confined disease. Therefore, overall, only about one third of newly diagnosed cases of prostate cancer were detected before the disease had left the prostate. Since it has become apparent that pathologically organ-confined prostate cancer is the only stage of this disease that can be reliably cured by either radical prostatectomy or radiation therapy, the only practical means of decreasing the mortality from prostate cancer is to strive to detect pathologically organ-confined tumors more commonly. Recent innovations using serologic testing with prostate specific antigen and prostatic biopsy techniques that employ transrectal ultrasound guidance have made the detection of pathologically organ-confined prostate cancer feasible.

In addition to having a valid rationale for screening, successful screening programs should fulfill three additional criteria that have been enumerated by the World Health Organization.[2] These are that the disease should be common and have serious consequences for the population; that detection of the disease at a preclinical, early stage is possible; and that treatment of the disease at this early stage is curative. It is becoming increasingly apparent that prostate specific antigen (PSA)–based screening for prostate cancer fulfills each of these criteria.

## CONSIDERATIONS AGAINST IMPLEMENTING PROSTATE CANCER SCREENING

There are two main arguments that are frequently cited as reasons to urge caution before implementing widespread prostate cancer screening. These are that screening programs may detect prostate cancer that is not pathologically organ-confined and therefore not potentially curable and that the cancers that are pathologically organ-confined at the time of detection may be slow-growing, biologically insignificant tumors for which treatment is unnecessary. These concerns are often referred to as lead time bias and length-time bias, respectively. In the former circumstance, earlier detection of cancers for which therapy is not effective may give the *appearance* of improved survival from the time of detection, but in fact there may be no change in the overall length of the individual's life. In the latter circumstance, since slowly growing, potentially latent tumors have a longer preclinical course than biologically significant tumors, they may be more likely to be detected by screening. This may be especially true if repetitive examinations are performed over several years of the individual's life. Since slowly growing tumors are *least* likely to cause symptoms or to be fatal, detection of these tumors may actually result in increased morbidity and mortality over that expected from their natural history. In this regard, prostate cancer may be especially prone to screening-induced length-time bias. While approximately 30% of men over 50 years of age have autopsy evidence of prostate cancer, fewer than 5% are expected to die from it. Therefore, it is clear that if every cancer were detected and treated, a significant proportion of patients would undergo unnecessary treatment as a consequence of aggressive screening.

There are other theoretical issues that suggest caution before implementing widespread screening for prostate cancer. These include the morbidity of screening; the unnecessary anxiety induced by screening, especially if a high proportion of men are found to have an abnormal or falsely positive initial screen; the false sense of security if the initial screen is falsely negative but prostate cancer is truly present; the economic cost of screening; and the morbidity and mortality of treatment for tumors detected by screening.[3] Regrettably, in 1993, the actual risk and clinical impact of these potential adverse occurrences cannot be quantitated with very much certainty.

## CHOICE OF PROSTATE CANCER SCREENING MODALITY

The optimal means of screening for prostate cancer has been the subject of great interest to the urologic community for the past several years. Digital rectal examination, transrectal ultrasonography, and serum PSA testing have been evaluated individually and in combination as a means of achieving early detection of prostate cancer. While no uniformly agreed on approach has been established, most authorities currently feel that the digital rectal exam and serum PSA testing should be performed initially with ultrasound and ultrasound-guided biopsy of patients found to have abnormal PSA and/or digital rectal exam as a secondary procedure. Serial evaluation with serum PSA and/or digital rectal examination may be performed on a 6- to 12-month basis.

### Digital Rectal Examination

Screening performed by digital rectal examination alone has historically been associated with very low detection rates. These range between 1 and 2.5%.[4] Many of the tumors detected by digital rectal exam–based screening have been found to be clinically advanced and therefore, are not curable at the time of diagnosis. This has been found to be true even if repeated digital rectal examination screening is performed on an annual basis.[5] Because of these findings, ie, the relative low detection rate of digital rectal exam for potentially curable (pathologically localized) prostate cancer, its rather low specificity (high false-positive rate, even when performed by urologists), and the marked patient dissatisfaction caused by this examination, repeated digital rectal examination alone is not an appropriate means of screening for prostate cancer.

### Transrectal Ultrasound

Transrectal ultrasound–based screening has more recently been evaluated and has, in general, been associated with higher cancer detection rates than digital rectal examination–based screening. In the best studies, detection rates approaching 5% have been achieved.[4] These relatively high cancer detection rates, however, typically occur at the expense of biopsying a high proportion of men undergoing screening. This has been reported to approach about 30% of the population. This statistic belies the somewhat subjective nonspecific nature of transrectal ultrasonographic interpretation. Because of this, the fact that a considerable proportion of tumors are ultrasonographically isoechoic with respect to the normal tissues of the prostate, and the expense and patient dissatisfaction associated with this procedure, transrectal ultrasonography alone has also been judged to be an inappropriate initial diagnostic tool for widespread prostate cancer screening.

On the other hand, it is important to note that transrectal ultrasonography is an essential secondary part of screening for prostate cancer. This occurs because ultrasound-guided biopsies of the prostate are unsurpassed for their ability to thoroughly evaluate the prostate with minimal morbidity and almost no mortality. Three specific types of ultrasound-guided biopsies of the prostate may be performed on the individual patient. These include *random* ultrasound-guided biopsies that are systematically spread throughout both lobes of the prostate, *directed* biopsies that are obtained from sites within the prostate that are sonographically abnormal and consistent with prostate cancer, and *geographic* biopsies of the prostate that are taken in the region of the prostate that corresponds with a palpable prostatic abnormality. Performing these types of prostatic biopsy on individual patients undergoing screening often results in taking six or more cores. Additionally, under some circumstances, eg, if a second set of ultrasound-guided biopsies is necessary, biopsies of the central and transition zones of the prostate (that typically are not sampled during the initial evaluation) may be readily obtained if ultrasound guidance is employed. These could be especially helpful in detecting prostate cancer in men with suspicious screening findings but whose initial biopsies of the peripheral zone are not positive for prostate cancer.

### Prostate-Specific Antigen (PSA)

Prostate-specific antigen (PSA) was identified by Wang et al.[6] PSA is a single polypeptide chain of 240 amino acids with an estimated molecular weight of approximately 34,000. This protein is functionally and immunologically distinct from prostatic acid phosphatase. The exact physiologic role of PSA is not certain, but it appears to have protease activity for some seminal vesical proteins and is thought to have a role in the liquefaction of the seminal coagulants. In contrast to prostatic acid phosphatase, PSA is found only within the prostate, within the epithelial cells of the prostatic acini and ducts. The mechanism by which PSA enters the serum in patients with normal prostates, with benign prostatic hyperplasia (BPH), or with prostate cancer is not known. On a cell-per-cell basis, it is estimated that BPH cells produce more PSA than prostate cancer cells but that more of the PSA produced by cancer cells enters the circulation because of the disorganized nature of the neoplastic glands.

As a screening tool, serum PSA has many advantages over either the digital rectal examination or transrectal ultrasonography (Table 1). These include the facts that PSA is relatively inexpensive, and is an objective and quantitative test that is often, from the patient's point of view, preferable to either of the other primary screening modalities. Additionally, serum PSA testing does not require a specially skilled examiner. Because of this, less professional time may be required in PSA-based screening programs than those based on sonography or digital rectal examination.

**TABLE 1. Rationale for PSA-Based Screening Rather than Digital Rectal Examination or Transrectal Ultrasonography**

- Objective
- Quantitative
- Enhanced patient tolerance
- Independent of examiner's skill
- Relatively inexpensive
- More specific and accurate

PSA, prostate-specific antigen.

These features, coupled with the known clinical superiority of PSA over digital rectal exam and ultrasonography in detecting prostate cancer among patients undergoing urologic evaluation for symptomatic diseases,[7] have made serum PSA the primary screening tool of choice for patients with prostate cancer.

## INITIAL RESULTS OF A SERUM PSA-BASED SCREENING PROGRAM

For approximately 2 years, beginning in the summer of 1989, slightly more than 10,000 men over the age of 50 were enrolled in a PSA-based screening program at Washington University in St. Louis. Men over the age of 50, without a history of prostate surgery or prostate cancer, volunteered to be evaluated with a serum PSA level. During this study, men whose PSA levels were less than 4 ng/mL are asked to return every 6 months for a repeat PSA level. Men whose serum PSA levels exceed 4 ng/mL returned for a repeat level within a few weeks. If the repeat level is also elevated above 4 ng/mL, these men undergo digital rectal examination and transrectal ultrasonography. Suspicious abnormalities on either the digital rectal examination or the transrectal ultrasound are then biopsied with transrectal ultrasound guidance.[8]

The initial results of this study have been published.[8] About one third of the volunteers were between the ages of 50 and 60, one half between 60 and 70, and the remainder over 70 years of age. Overall, approximately 12% of volunteers were found to have an initial serum PSA level above 4 ng/mL. The probability of an elevated serum PSA level correlates with advancing age, but for a given PSA level the probability of cancer is similar for men of all ages, confirming that serum PSA levels are a much more powerful predictor of the presence of prostate cancer than patient age.

About one third of men with an elevated serum PSA have been found to have prostate cancer on the basis of the initial evaluation. This translates to an overall 3% cancer detection rate on the initial evaluation. This detection rate was achieved by biopsying about 9% of the population. Some of the men with elevated serum PSA levels did not undergo biopsy because both the digital rectal exam and the ultrasound were judged to be normal. The probability of prostate cancer varied directly with the degree of PSA elevation. If the initial PSA level was between 4 and 10, about 25% of the men had prostate cancer whereas nearly 60% of men whose PSA was above 10 had prostate cancer (Table 2). Overall, the digital rectal exam was normal in 40% of men who were found to have prostate cancer.

**TABLE 2. Detection of Prostate Cancer on Initial Evaluation in a PSA-Based Screening Program**

| | |
|---|---|
| Among all volunteers | ~3.0% |
| Among biopsied volunteers | 34% |
| If PSA < 4 ng/mL | 30% |
| PSA 4–10 ng/mL | 21% |
| PSA > 10 ng/mL | 57% |

PSA, prostate-specific antigen.

For a short time, men with initial PSA values between 2.9 and 4 were also evaluated with digital rectal examination and ultrasonography. Only 7% of the men in this group were found to have prostate cancer. Because of this low detection rate, men with initial PSA values in this range are no longer referred for rectal examination or ultrasound biopsy of the prostate.

### Stage of Cancers Detected on Initial Evaluation

Nearly all of the cancers (more than 95%) detected on initial evaluation were clinically localized to the prostate gland. Clinical staging included digital rectal examination findings, serum enzymatic prostatic acid phosphatase testing, radionuclide bone scan, and, in some cases, pelvic imaging with either CT or MRI. Pathologic staging from bilateral pelvic lymph node dissection and radical retropubic prostatectomy has shown that men with a PSA level between 4 and 10 ng/mL have pathologically organ-confined disease about 70% of the time. On the other hand, only slightly more than 40% of men with cancer and a PSA level >10 ng/mL have been found to have pathologically organ-confined disease. Overall, about 65% of the cancers detected on initial evaluation were pathologically organ-confined if the PSA was >4 ng/mL. All of the men with cancer and a PSA between 2.8 and 4 ng/mL who underwent a radical prostatectomy were found to have pathologically organ-confined disease (Table 3).

**TABLE 3. Pathologic Organ-Confined Prostate Cancer in PSA-Based Screening**

| PSA (ng/mL) | % Pathologic Organ-Confined |
|---|---|
| 2.8–4.0 | 100 |
| 4.0–10 ng/mL | 67 |
| >10 ng/mL | 44 |

PSA, prostate-specific antigen.

### Clinical Significance of Tumors Detected by Screening

While there is no unequivocal means of determining the true biological significance of an individual prostate cancer, the Gleason tumor score and the tumor volume seem to represent two of the most important predictors of the overall disease significance. In this regard, it is reassuring that more than 90% of the cancers detected through initial PSA screening were present bilaterally throughout the prostate, indicating a relatively high tumor volume, and/or were moderately or poorly differentiated, ie, the Gleason score was ≥5. Additional evidence that the large majority of tumors detected by PSA-based screening are apt to be clinically significant may be derived from consideration of the fact that the 3% detection rate represents only 1 of 10 cancers *expected* to be present in this population based on the reported 30% autopsy prevalence of prostate cancer. It seems most likely that only the larger cancers among each 10 that are present are actually being detected with the ultrasound sampling techniques being employed. A third reason to believe that the large majority of tumors detected in this manner are clinically significant may be derived from detailed analysis of final tumor grade and stage in men who were initially found to have the most minute amount of cancer at the time of detection. When men with impalpable, well-differentiated prostate cancer that involved less than half of one biopsy core underwent radical prostatectomy, nearly every such patient was found to have significantly higher grade and/or higher stage cancer when the entire prostate was available for inspection. Detailed analysis of 24 such men suggests that when the final pathologic stage and grade are known, only two or three such patients could be considered to have focal or incidental prostate cancer. Taken together, these arguments suggest that the large majority of cancers detected by this form of PSA-based screening are apt to be biologically and clinically important.

## RESULTS OF SERIAL SCREENING

Serial evaluation of volunteers with repeat serum PSA levels is an integral part of screening for prostate cancer with PSA testing. Men whose initial PSA level is less than 4 ng/mL but whose subsequent level rises above 4 ng/mL are found to have prostate cancer about one third of the time. Most significantly, more than three quarters of the cancers detected along this group of patients are pathologically organ-confined. In an analogous manner, patients whose initial serum PSA is greater than 4 but whose initial biopsy is negative for cancer are found to have prostate cancer between 25% and 30% of the time if a second, third, or fourth prostatic biopsy is

**TABLE 4. Proportion of Prostate Cancers That Are Pathologically Organ-Confined by Method of Detection**

| | |
|---|---|
| Clinical abnormality | 40–45% |
| Initial PSA screening | 60–65% |
| Serial PSA screening | 70–75% |

PSA, prostate-specific antigen.

performed. When cancer is detected on a subsequent biopsy, it was pathologically organ-confined almost 75% of the time. Taken together, these results suggest that serial PSA screening may be associated with the highest probability of detecting pathologically organ-confined prostate cancer (Table 4).

## POTENTIAL ROLE OF MEASUREMENTS IN SERIAL PSA SCREENING

The ideal method of follow-up for patients with persistent serum PSA elevation and an initially negative prostatic biopsy has not been fully established. In the PSA-based screening program, repeat biopsies of the prostate have been recommended every 6 months for patients who have had persistently elevated PSA values. Serial reevaluation of men in this fashion will theoretically diagnose 100% of the clinically detectable cases of prostate cancer occurring among this group of men. This approach, however, exacts a fairly significant cost to the patient in terms of discomfort, morbidity, and expense. Identification of other tools that may guide the selection of only certain men in this category for repeated biopsy would be beneficial. PSA rate of change (PSA velocity) and/or PSA density (serum PSA level ÷ prostate volume) have been investigated for their use in this setting.

### PSA Rate of Change

PSA velocity may be a useful means of determining if an individual has prostate cancer.[9] This long-term retrospective study suggested that men ultimately found to have prostate cancer generally had serum PSA levels rising at a greater rate than men with BPH or normal prostates. Patients with cancer typically had a PSA rate of change exceeding 0.75 ng/mL per year. Unhappily, over the relatively short duration of the current PSA screening trial, PSA velocity has not been useful. In this trial, men who have ultimately been found to have prostate cancer on the basis of *serial* reevaluation of the prostate have had almost an identical rate of PSA change when compared to those individuals who have not been found to have prostate cancer in spite of undergoing multiple biopsies of the prostate. The lack of usefulness of PSA rate of change over the short-term duration of this trial could be due to the 10%–20% biological variation of serum PSA values. Much longer follow-up may be necessary to precisely clarify the role of PSA rate of change in the serial evaluation of men in early detection and screening programs.

### PSA Density

PSA density could improve the clinician's ability to distinguish patients with elevated PSA who have BPH from those who have prostate cancer.[10] The rationale for using PSA density is that by considering the size of the prostate, elevations of serum PSA secondary to BPH may be factored out of the total serum PSA level. In the PSA screening program, an initial PSA density >0.15 has been associated with a 50% rate of positive serial biopsy while men with a PSA density <0.1 have infrequently (less than 10% of the time) had prostate cancer, even if repeated biopsies were taken. These results seem to suggest that PSA density could be a potentially useful means of predicting which patients with elevated serum PSA and an initially negative biopsy of the prostate should undergo repeated serial biopsy of the prostate gland.

## IMPACT OF PSA-BASED SCREENING ON STAGE OF PROSTATE CANCER AT DETECTION

An important aspect of successful screening is the ability to detect cancer at a time when intervention alters the disease's natural course. For prostate cancer, this may be translated as requiring that prostate cancer be detected when it is pathologically organ-confined. When compared to a contemporary group of symptomatic men who have been diagnosed with prostate cancer, men in the serum PSA-based screening program are much more likely to have pathologically organ-confined prostate cancer. Patients whose prostate cancer is detected because of urologic symptoms in the current series have been found to have pathologically organ-confined disease about 40% of the time. If prostate cancer is detected in a screening program because of an initially elevated PSA level, about 65% of such tumors are pathologically organ-confined. However, when prostate cancer is detected on the basis of serial PSA evaluation, including those who are undergoing repeated biopsy of the prostate, the tumor is found to be pathologically organ-confined nearly 75% of the time. Therefore, repeated measurement of serum PSA levels and repeated evaluation of the prostate nearly doubles the proportion of patients with pathologically organ-confined prostate cancer at the time of detection.

The importance of detecting prostate cancer when it is pathologically organ-confined may be appreciated by examining the long-term (more than 5 years) outcome of patients with clinically localized prostate cancer who have undergone radical prostatectomy. At 5 years, fewer than 5% of men whose tumors were pathologically organ-confined have had any evidence of treatment failure including a detectable postradical prostatectomy PSA level. While nearly 40% of men who had non-pathologically organ-confined prostate cancer and a radical prostatectomy have some evidence of disease persistence,[11] it is important to determine through longer follow-up that men whose PSAs remain undetectable at 5 years will continue to have undetectable PSA values for the long term.

## THE ADDITION OF DIGITAL RECTAL EXAMINATION SCREENING TO PSA-BASED SCREENING

Over the past year, a second PSA-based screening program has been undertaken employing both an initial serum PSA level and a digital rectal exam. If either test is abnormal, patients undergo ultrasound-guided biopsies of the prostate. Experience with patients screened in this manner has shown that approximately 10%–15% have an elevated serum PSA and that almost 15% have a suspicious digital rectal exam. Since many men with an elevated serum PSA also have suspicious digital rectal exams, overall about 20% of patients are referred for ultrasound-guided biopsy of the prostate. For men who have both an elevated PSA and a suspicious digital rectal examination, biopsy shows prostate cancer about 50% of the time. If the serum PSA is elevated above 4 ng/mL but the digital rectal exam is not suspicious for prostate cancer, only 20% of men have prostate cancer. If the rectal examination is suspicious but the serum PSA is within the normal range, prostate cancer is present only 10% of the time. Overall, about 25% of cancers detected in the screening program would have been missed if PSA-based screening alone were performed. Conversely, if digital rectal exam–based screening alone were performed, about one third of the cancers would not be detected. This comparative study demonstrates that the digital rectal exam and serum PSA may be viewed as complementary diagnostic tests for prostate cancer but that, overall, serum PSA seems to detect more cancers than digital rectal examination.

The combination of an initial serum PSA and a digital rectal exam results in a higher overall cancer detection rate compared with using either modality alone. Combined modality screening resuls in a 4%–5% detection rate (Table 5). This has been

**TABLE 5. Comparison of Prostate Cancer Screening Modalities**

| | Initial Test | |
|---|---|---|
| Factor | PSA Alone | PSA and DRE |
| Detection rate on initial evaluation | ~3% | ~4.5% |
| Biopsy rate | ~9% | ~20% |
| No. patients undergoing biopsy per case CaP | ~3 | ~5 |

PSA, prostate-specific antigen; DRE, digital rectal examination.

achieved at the expense of biopsying about 20% of the population. This means that to find a single case of prostate cancer, nearly five men must undergo a biopsy of the prostate. This compares unfavorably to screening with PSA alone where only about three patients are required to undergo biopsy to find one case of prostate cancer. It is also important to consider that the addition of the digital rectal exam to PSA-based screening results in more biopsies per case of pathologically organ-confined prostate cancer than PSA screening alone. This occurs because cancers that are palpable are apt to have spread beyond the prostate, whereas impalpable cancers that produce minimal serum PSA elevations are usually pathologically organ-confined.

## ECONOMIC COSTS OF SCREENING

The economic cost of screening has been estimated to exceed several billion dollars annually. Certain considerations may lower this estimate and place it in a more appropriate prospective. First, the cost to diagnose a case of prostate cancer using PSA-based screening is about $2000. This is less than 20% of the cost to diagnose a case of breast cancer in mammography-based screening programs. Second, since effective screening for prostate cancer detects pathologically localized disease in a higher proportion than the traditional indications, the cost of treating prostate cancer may be lower if screening is employed. This occurs because the global cost of radical prostatectomy is approximately $2000. Conversely, if a man is found to have prostate cancer, he incurs the same initial diagnostic costs as those evaluated in the screening program who often undergo several treatments that may include one or more transurethral resections of the prostate to control local disease, with each procedure costing approximately $1000. Palliative radiation therapy to either the primary tumor or to symptomatic metastases may also be adminstered at a cost that approaches $2 per centiGray. Additionally, hormonal therapy may be necessary for some patients with advanced prostate cancer. This could cost up to $7000 per year if combined androgen deprivation with a luteinizing hormone–releasing hormone analog and flutamide is preferred. These considerations suggest that the total cost of screening for prostate cancer must be balanced against some potential savings that may occur because of detection and treatment of organ-confined disease.

## RESULTS OF OTHER SCREENING STUDIES

Brawer et al.[12] measured serum PSA values in 1249 men over 50 years of age and performed digital rectal exam and ultrasound-guided biopsy in those whose PSA levels exceeded 4 ng/mL. Their results mirror the Washington University experience in that cancer was detected in about 2.5% of patients and was clinically localized in 95% of them. Labrie et al.[13] screened about 1000 randomly selected men using digital rectal examination, ultrasound, and PSA. In evaluating these patients, various serum PSA value cutoffs were tested to determine the ideal level to optimize prostate cancer detection. When 3 ng/mL was employed as the upper limit of normal, the accuracy of PSA testing approached 88%. This accuracy and associated specificity of almost 90% exceeds that reported in most other series. Using a PSA of 3 ng/mL as the upper limit of normal resulted in 19% of the population as having an "elevated" PSA (vs. 12% if 4 ng/mL was considered the upper limit of normal). Five additional cancers were detected in men with PSA values between 3 and 4 ng/mL. The American Cancer Society[14] trial employing PSA, digital rectal examination, and ultrasonography as the primary screening tools yields a higher cancer detection rate, but at the expense of many TRUS evaluations in men with PSA values below 4 ng/mL (approximately 18 to find one cancer).

## CURRENT GUIDELINES

Although no screening trial has demonstrated a reduction in prostate cancer mortality, the evidence is accumulating that early detection and treatment with radical prostatectomy will alter the natural course

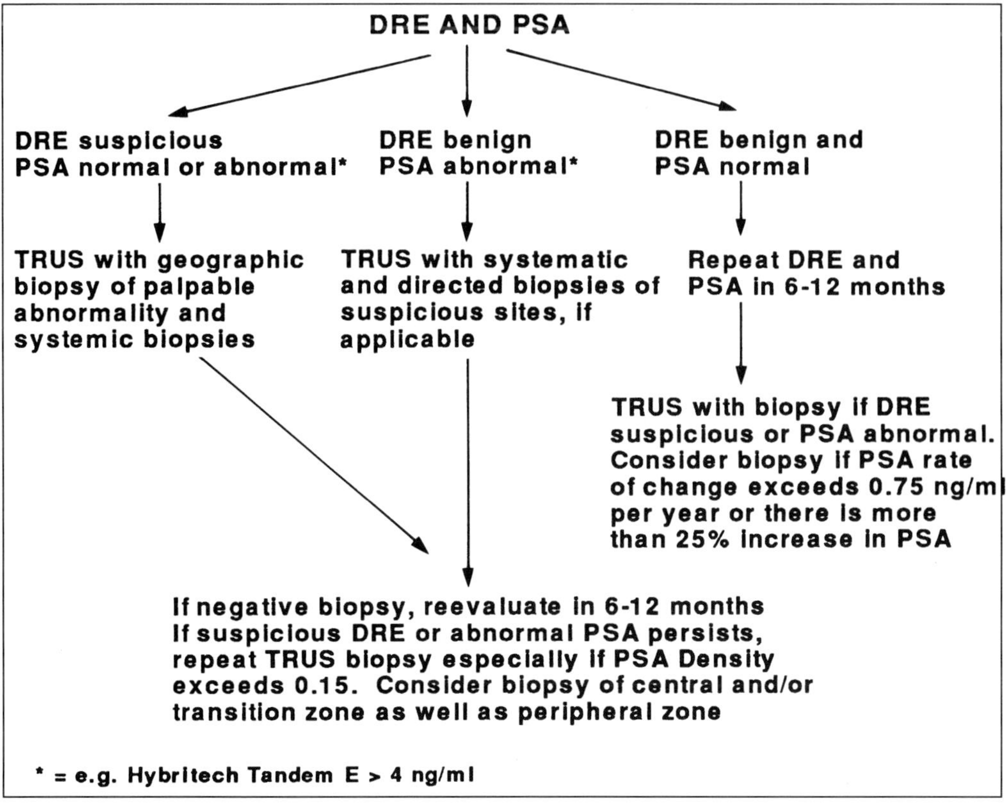


Fig 1.

of this disease and that at least some patients destined to die of prostate cancer will benefit. However, this issue has never been adequately studied. Therefore, the overall efficacy of prostate cancer screening at the moment remains unproven. A randomized prospective trial to address this issue is underway at several sites throughout the U.S. and is sponsored by the National Cancer Institute.[15]

Currently it seems most appropriate to limit screening for prostate cancer to men whose life expectancy exceeds 10 years, since expectant management of prostate cancer, especially if it is well-differentiated, has been associated with excellent survivals within a decade of diagnosis.[16] It has been recommended that screening begin at the age of 50 for most men, except those with a family history of prostate cancer, in whom screening should begin at the age of 40. Although this is no uniformly agreed on screening protocol, one logical diagnostic algorithm is proposed (Fig 1).

## REFERENCES


1. Boring CC, Squires TS, Tong GT. Cancer statistics 1993. *CA.* 1993;43(1):7–26.
2. Wilson J, Jungner G. Principles and practice of screening for disease. *Public Health Papers 34.* Geneva: World Health Organization; 1968.
3. Prorok PC, Connor RJ, Baker SG. Statistical considerations in cancer screening programs. *Urol Clin North Am.* 1990;17(4):699–708.
4. Optenberg SA, Thompson IA. Economics of screening for carcinoma of the prostate. *Urol Clin North Am.* 1990;17(4):719–737.
5. Gerber GS, Thompson IM, Thisted R, Chodak GW. Disease-specific survival following routine prostate cancer screening by digital rectal examination. *JAMA.* 1193;269:61.
6. Wang MC, Valenzuela LA, Murphy GP, Chu TM. Purification of a human prostate specific antigen. *Invest Urol.* 1979;17:159.
7. Cooner WH, Moseley BR, Rutherford CL, et al.

Clinical application of transrectal ultrasonography for prostate specific antigen: the search for prostate cancer. *J Urol.* 1988;139:758–764.

8. Catalona WJ, Smith DS, Ratliff TL, et al. Measurement of prostate specific antigen in serum as a screening test for prostate cancer. *N Engl J Med.* 1991;324:1156–1161.
9. Carter HB, Pierson JD, Medder, EJ, et al. Longitudinal evaluation of prostatic specific antigen levels in men with and without prostate disease. *JAMA.* 1992;267:2215.
10. Benson MC, Whang IS, Pantuk A, et al. Prostate specific antigen density: a means of distinguishing benign prostate hypertrophy in prostate cancer. *J Urol.* 1992;147:815–816.
11. Brendler CB, Walsh PC. The role of radical prostatectomy in the treatment of prostate cancer. *CA.* 1992;42:212–222.
12. Brawer MK, Chetner MP, Beatie J, et al. Screening for prostatic carcinoma with prostate specific antigen. *J Urol.* 1992;147:841.
13. Labrie F, Dupont A, Suburu R, et al. Serum prostate specific antigen as pre-screening test for prostate cancer. *J Urol.* 1992;147:846.
14. Babaian RJ, Mettlin C, Kane R, et al. The relationship of prostate specific antigen to digital rectal examination and transrectal ultrasonography: findings of the American Cancer Society National Prostate Cancer Detection Project. *Cancer.* 1992;69:1195–1200.
15. Kramer BS, Gohagan J, Prorok PC, Smart C. A National Center Institute sponsored screening trial for prostatic, lung, colorectal, and ovarian cancers. *Cancer.* 1993;71:589–593.
16. Johansson JE, Adami HO, Andersson SW, et al. High 10 year survival rate in patients with early untreated prostatic cancer. *JAMA.* 1992;267:2191.

# 36

# Localized Carcinoma of the Prostate

*Joseph A. Smith, Jr.*

In the United States and many European countries, carcinoma of the prostate is the second most common cancer and the third leading cause of cancer death in men. In the United States alone, it is estimated by the American Cancer Society that there will be over 100,000 new cases of prostatic cancer in 1991 and nearly 30,000 deaths.[1]

## SYMPTOMS OF PROSTATE CANCER

Knowledge of the symptoms that may be associated with carcinoma of the prostate may help the clinician to establish the diagnosis and institute appropriate therapy. Unfortunately, most localized prostatic cancers that are amenable to potentially curative therapy produce no symptoms. Locally advanced carcinoma of the prostate may cause symptoms of bladder outlet obstruction that mimic those seen in patients with benign prostatic hyperplasia (BPH). As the cancer enlarges, the flow of urine is restricted and the patient may complain of hesitancy, dribbling, urinary frequency, nocturia, and a feeling of incomplete emptying. These symptoms may develop and progress more rapidly in patients with carcinoma of the prostate than in those with BPH, but distinction between the two is not possible based solely on symptoms and patient history. Hematuria, either gross or microscopic, may be seen occasionally in patients with prostatic cancer, but this is neither a sensitive nor a specific finding. Urinary tract infections may occur, especially if there is poor bladder emptying. Independent of the effects of various treatments, there is generally no association between localized carcinoma of the prostate and sexual potency.

## DETECTION OF PROSTATE CANCER

### Digital Rectal Examination

Historically, digital palpation of the prostate has been the method used for early detection of prostate cancer.[2] Areas of induration, nodularity, or irregularity in the prostate are considered suspicious for the presence of carcinoma. Nevertheless, digital rectal examination has been recognized as a relatively insensitive and nonspecific method for detection of prostate cancer. Moreover, a significant number of patients with palpable abnormalities of the prostate have extracapsular disease at the time of detection.[3]

Most screening and early-detection studies using digital rectal examination have shown a detection rate of around 1% to 2% of the population examined.[4] However, the incidence of disease detection is directly

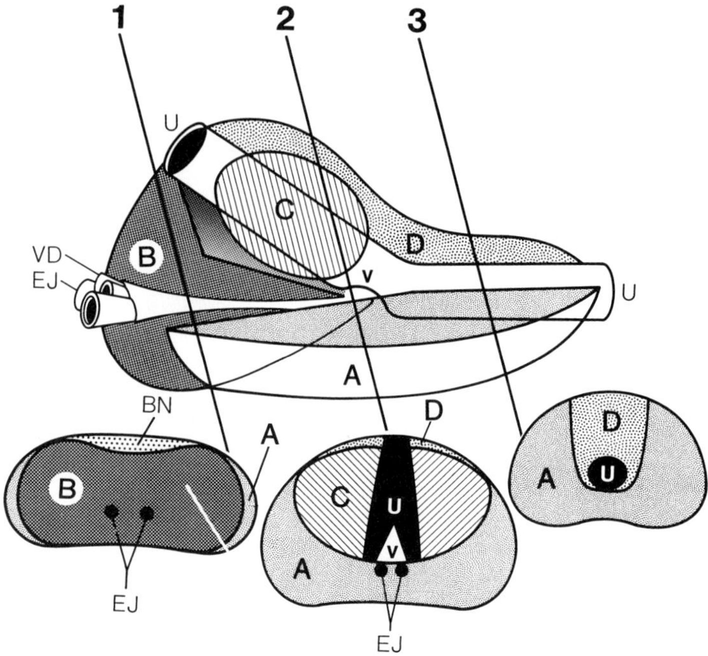


**Fig 1.** Zonal anatomy of the prostate in sagittal view. A = peripheral zone; B = central zone; C = transition zone; D = anterior fibromuscular stroma; U = urethra; V = verumontanum; VD = vas deferens, EJ = ejaculatory ducts; BN = bladder neck.

related to the frequency with which biopsy is performed. In most historic series, biopsy has been performed in a relatively small number of patients. However, the morbidity and expense of biopsy have decreased in recent years, and prostate biopsy is now performed more readily.

## Transrectal Ultrasonography

Although digital rectal examination has been the primary method for detection of prostate cancer, its limitations are well recognized. Only a minority of prostate cancers are palpable. In addition, only a relatively small portion of the gland is accessible for evaluation by digital palpation. Transrectal ultrasonography has emerged as the best imaging modality currently available for the prostate.[5] Transrectal ultrasonography has been available in some form for more than 25 years. Improvements in equipment, including the use of real-time imaging and high-frequency transducers, have helped define prostate anatomy as well as the echo characteristics of prostate cancer.

In 1968, McNeal reported for the first time the existence of histologic heterogeneity in the glandular tissue of the prostate.[6] This histologic variation causes differences in the reflection of sound waves, allowing identification of these various tissue zones by ultrasonography (Fig 1). The tissue immediately surrounding the ejaculatory duct, referred to as the central zone, is histologically different from the remaining gland and is the site of origin of only a small number (around 5% to 10%) of prostate cancers.

The peripheral zone of the prostate is composed of small, round, regular acini with smooth walls. The epithelium consists of simple, columnar pale cells and basal small nuclei. The peripheral zone makes up nearly 70% of a normal prostate gland and is the origin of some 70% to 80% of prostate adenocarcinomas.[7]

The transition zone surrounds the urethra from the upper end of the verumontanum proximally to the bladder neck. The histology and architecture of the transition zone closely resemble that of the peripheral zone, but the glandular tissue lies anterior and closely follows the course of the sphincter toward the bladder neck. The transition zone constitutes less than 5% of the normal prostate and is the site of origin of BPH. Some 10% to 20% of prostate cancers arise in the transition zone. Because of their central location, transition-zone tumors are often nonpalpable.

The ultrasonic characteristics of carcinoma of the prostate have changed with the development of higher frequency transducers. Early investigators using B-mode and initial gray-scale imaging techniques reported that prostatic carcinoma appeared as hypoechoic areas. Large prostate cancers can replace all of the normally isoechoic peripheral zone, thereby obliterating any ultrasound reference for contrast with normal tissues. With the development of 5- and 7-MHz transducers, it became evident that most peripheral-zone tumors were hypoechoic.[8] Although it is now commonly accepted that peripheral-zone cancers are hypoechoic in the substantial majority of patients scanned with contemporary 7-MHz transducers, tumors located in other zones of the prostate show more variation. The echo pattern of anteriorly located tumors is difficult to define; this difficulty is reflected by the decreased sensitivity and specificity of transrectal ultrasonography in detecting transition-zone tumors. The normally hypoechoic texture of the transition zone, enlargement by BPH, calcifications, and scarring from previous transurethral instrumentation or infections all contribute to the difficulty in interpreting the results of transrectal ultrasonography of the transition zone (Fig 2). In such cases, other sonographic characteristics assume increased importance, including overall prostate shape, symmetry, and the anterior-posterior dimension of the gland. Capsular boundary echoes also are important. Distortion or absence of normal internal echoes are significant features in the evaluation of the anterior prostate.

Undoubtedly, transrectal ultrasonography is capable of imaging some prostate cancers that are not palpable. In addition, most palpable tumors are visible by ultrasonography (Fig 3). This knowledge has naturally led to the evaluation of transrectal ultrasonography for early detection of prostate cancer. Watanabe and coworkers used ultrasound for screening of prostate cancer in 1396 men.[9] Cancer was identified in only 0.6%. However, these studies were performed using a chair-mounted scanner and

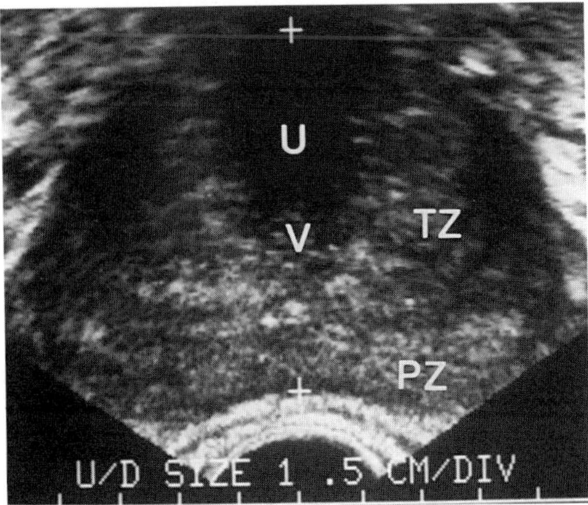


**Fig 2.** Transrectal ultrasound scan of the prostate in a man with benign hyperplasia. The enlarged transition zone compresses the peripheral zone. U = urethra; V = verumontanum; TZ = transition zone; PZ = peripheral zone.

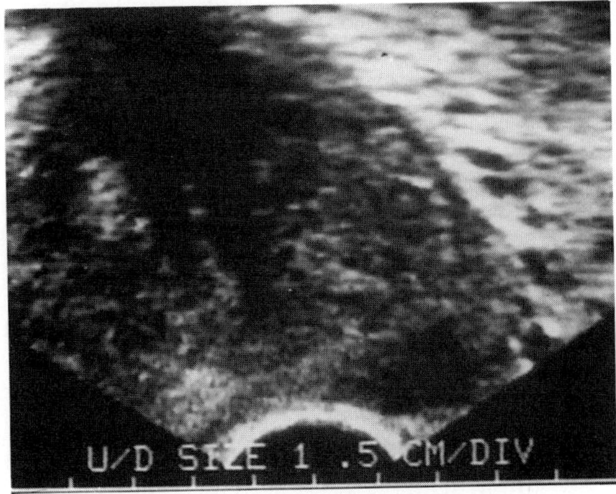


**Fig 3.** Transverse image of the prostate showing a hypoechoic area in the peripheral zone corresponding to a palpable, well-differentiated adenocarcinoma.

a 3.5-MHz transducer. Lee and coworkers evaluated 784 self-referred men using transrectal ultrasonography and digital rectal examination. Ultrasound detected cancer in 2.6% of patients as compared with 1.3% of those evaluated by digital palpation.[10] Cooner et al performed ultrasonography in 1867 men.[11] Biopsy was performed in 835 patients (46%), and 263 cancers were detected, yielding a detection rate of 14.6%.

These data suggest that evaluation of men using transrectal ultrasonography detects prostate cancer more often than does digital palpation. In fact, there is almost a doubling of the detection rate, from around 2% to almost 4%. However, two primary issues remain unanswered. The rate of detection of prostate cancer clearly is related to the frequency and number of biopsies, independent of findings on ultrasound or rectal examination. The morbidity and expense of prostate biopsy have decreased with the introduction of automatic biopsy guns, and most contemporary series of ultrasonography have made ready use of biopsy in the presence of any index of suspicion for cancer. In reported series of digital rectal examination for screening or early detection of prostate cancer, only a small percentage (around 5%) of patients undergo biopsy, whereas in recent ultrasound series, as many as 40% to 50% of patients are biopsied. The impact of this increased frequency of biopsy on the higher detection rates seen with ultrasound studies can be neither ignored nor calculated.

Transrectal ultrasonography used alone is a relatively imprecise method for early detection of prostate cancer. In the series of Lee and associates, only 5% of patients with an abnormal ultrasound examination but a normal level of prostate-specific antigen (PSA) and digital rectal examination had carcinoma confirmed by biopsy.[12] Furthermore, no patient with normal marker levels, normal rectal examination, and an ultrasound lesion less than 1 cm in size was found to have cancer. Thus, although ultrasonography clearly is capable of imaging some nonpalpable tumors, the procedure currently does not seem indicated for early detection of prostate cancer, if both PSA levels and rectal examination are normal.

### Prostate-Specific Antigen (PSA)

PSA is a serine protease enzyme whose function is thought to be lysis of the seminal coagulum. PSA is not cancer-specific, and is present in benign as well as malignant prostatic epithelia.[13] This enzyme has been identified in cells of bladder cystitis cystica and in periurethral glands, but has not been seen in tissues other than cloacal in origin.

The establishment of a normal range for the level of PSA is problematic because of the high prevalence of pathologic lesions of the prostate other than carcinoma. BPH and prostatitis can cause elevations in PSA levels, decreasing the specificity of PSA as a screening tool.[14] For PSA to be detected in the serum, marker-secreting tissue must be present in the patient and the molecule must obtain access to the systemic circulation. Although PSA is present in high concentrations in benign prostatic epithelium, the molecule enters the serum more readily from prostatic carcinoma cells. Despite a lack of specificity for cancer cells, PSA is useful for early detection of carcinoma of the prostate. Catalona et al found that 22% of patients with PSA levels between 4 ng/mL and 10 ng/mL (hybritech) were proven to have prostate cancer on biopsy. If the level of PSA was greater than 10 ng/mL, 67% of men had biopsies positive for prostate cancer. Overall, these researchers found evaluation of PSA to be a better method for detecting prostate cancer than digital rectal examination.[15]

### Prostate Biopsy

Biopsy of the prostate can be performed by the transurethral, perineal, or transrectal routes. Transurethral biopsy of the prostate usually samples only the transition zone and is neither an efficient nor effective method for detection of most prostate cancers. Transperineal biopsy has been used frequently and avoids transgression of the rectal wall. Increasingly, though, prostate biopsy is being performed by the transrectal route, using an automatic, spring-loaded gun (Fig 4). This has decreased not only the discomfort and expense of the procedure but also the morbidity. If pre-biopsy antibiotics are given, the incidence of sepsis related to the transrectal biopsy is min-

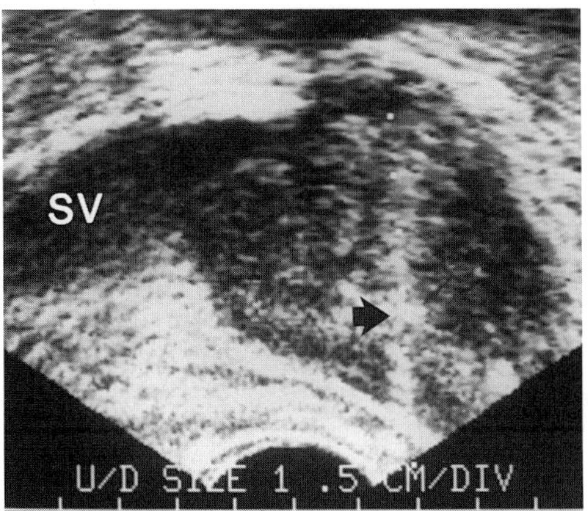


**Fig 4.** Sagittal view of the prostate showing the hyperechoic path of a transrectal needle biopsy. Precise localization of the needle can be accomplished with ultrasound (arrow). SV = seminal vesicle.

imal. When used with ultrasonography, transrectal biopsy can allow precise sampling of various anatomic areas of the prostate.

Fine-needle aspiration of the prostate is a low-morbidity procedure. In the hands of an experienced cytopathologist, the false-positive rate for aspiration biopsy of the prostate should be extremely low. In such hands, false-negative rates with transrectal aspiration biopsy are no higher than those associated with core biopsy. Currently, however, most centers in this country obtain core biopsies of the prostate, and the popularity of fine-needle aspiration has diminished as a result of the low morbidity associated with spring-loaded biopsy guns.

## STAGING

Staging of prostatic cancer involves determination of the size and local extent of the tumor as well as detection of distant foci either in lymphatic, bone, or soft tissue. Selection of therapy for patients with prostatic cancer is directly dependent upon the stage of the tumor.[16] Various staging classifications for prostatic cancer have been described, but the one proposed by Whitmore and modified by Jewett has endured as one that sufficiently categorizes patients for treatment purposes. Another commonly used staging system is that proposed by the Union Internationale Contre Le Cancer (UICC), sometimes called the TNM system. There have been recent efforts to consolidate these two systems and to define tumors which are detected because of ultrasonographic or PSA abnormalities in patients with palpably normal prostates. A brief description of the stages follows.

### Stage A (UICC Stage T0)

Stage A adenocarcinoma of the prostate is defined as a tumor detected by histologic examination of a prostatectomy specimen when the procedure was performed for presumed BPH. Thus, although often considered a clinical stage, it is by definition a pathologic diagnosis. Increasingly, nonpalpable tumors are being detected by ultrasonography and PSA abnormalities and there is no current staging classification that specifically categorizes these tumors. Because of differences in prognosis and, therefore, in treatment implications, stage A prostatic cancer is further subdivided into stage $A_1$ and stage $A_2$.

**Stage $A_1$ (UICC Stage T0a).** Various criteria are used to define stage $A_1$ carcinoma of the prostate. In general, the foci of microscopic carcinoma are quantified either numerically or as a percentage of the total prostatic tissue. Most commonly, less than 5% cancerous involvement of the total prostatic tissue resected is considered to indicate stage $A_1$ disease. High-grade tumors often are excluded from this category, regardless of the total number of foci or percent involvement.

**Stage $A_2$ (UICC Stage T0b).** Greater than 5% total cancerous involvement of the prostatic specimen or more than 5 microscopic foci of carcinoma is considered to denote stage $A_2$ disease. Also, all high-grade carcinomas should be considered stage $A_2$.

### Stage B

Stage B carcinoma of the prostate is defined as a palpable nodule or area of induration that apparently is confined within the capsule of the prostate.

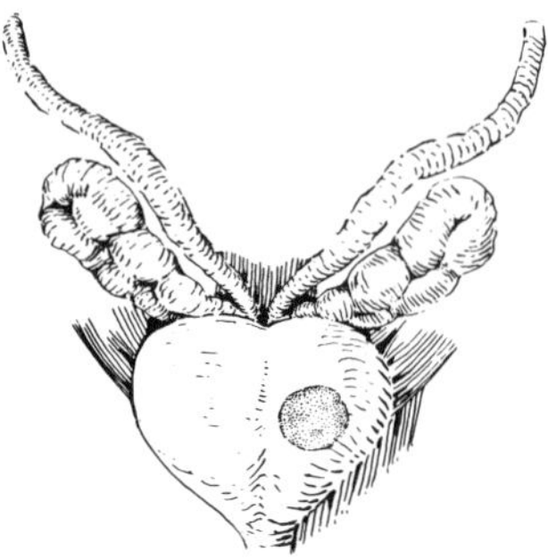

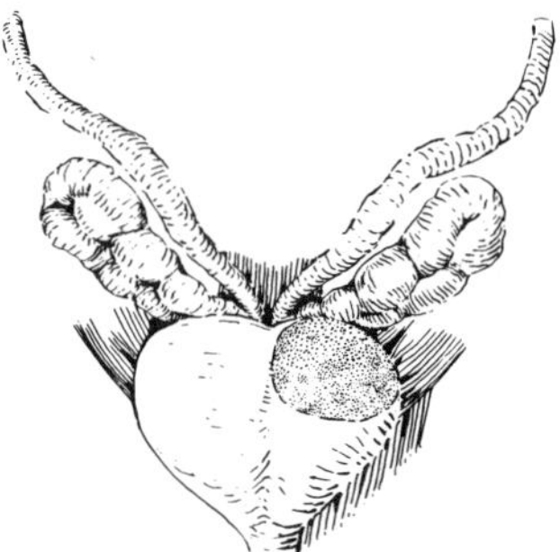

**Fig 5.** Schematic drawing of stage $B_1$ prostate cancer. On the left is a classic nodule surrounded by normal-feeling prostate. The lesion on the right is located near the base of the prostate, but is <2 cm in size and confined to one lobe.

**Stage $B_1$ (UICC Stage T1a or T1b).** The classic stage $B_1$ adenocarcinoma of the prostate is described by Jewett as a nodule of less than 1½ cm in size that is surrounded by palpably normal prostatic tissue. Currently, most urologists broaden this category somewhat to include small nodules located at the periphery of the prostate if they seem to be palpably confined within the capsule and are less than 2 cm in size (Fig 5).

**Stage $B_2$ (UICC Stage T1c or T2).** A palpable nodule that exceeds 2 cm in size but that still seems to be confined within the capsule of the prostate is considered stage $B_2$ adenocarcinoma (Fig 6).

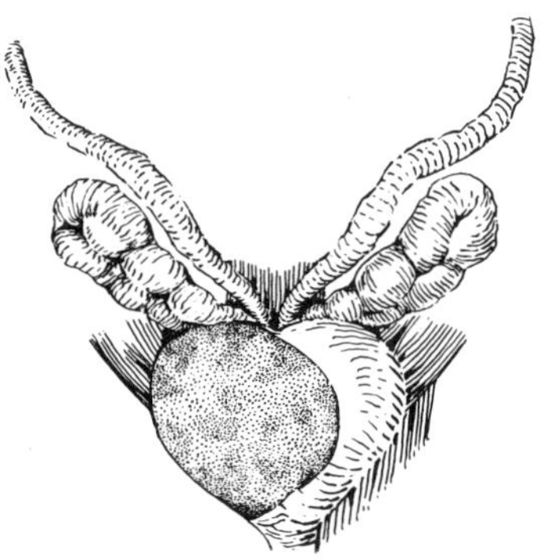

**Fig 6.** Schematic drawing of stage $B_2$ adenocarcinoma of the prostate. The nodule is >2 cm in size and involves both lobes of the prostate, but there is no palpable evidence of extracapsular extension.

## Stage C

Stage C prostatic cancers are those that have not metastasized to distant areas or lymph nodes but that have extended locally beyond the confines of the prostatic capsule. Most commonly, stage C tumors extend laterally or through the apex into the muscles of the pelvic floor, or superiorly into the seminal vesicles and bladder base.

**Stage $C_1$ (UICC Stage T3).** Stage $C_1$ includes tumors with minimal amounts of palpable extracapsular extension.

**Stage $C_2$ (UICC Stage T4).** Stage $C_2$ tumors are large (> 5 cm), and may cause symptomatic bladder outlet or ureteral obstruction.

## Stage D

Stage D tumors are those that have metastasized beyond the periprostatic region.

**Stage $D_1$ (UICC Stage T0 to T4, N+).** Stage $D_1$ tumors are those that have spread to involve the pelvic lymph nodes but are not detected in any other distant site. By the Whitmore–Jewett system, the extent of the primary tumor is irrelevant in defining stage if the nodes are positive. In the UICC system, the size and extent of the primary tumor is defined under the T category.

**Stage $D_2$ (UICC Stage T0 to T4, N+, M+).** This category includes prostatic tumors that have metastasized beyond the pelvic lymph nodes. Stage $D_2$ usually identifies patients with bone metastases, but it also includes those with soft-tissue metastases and lymph-node involvement outside of the pelvis.

## STAGING LOCAL EXTENT

### Digital Palpation

Not all prostatic cancers are palpable. Increasingly, localized tumors are being detected by other methods. However, most clinically significant tumors are evident as an area of induration or nodularity within the prostate. Overstaging in prostatic cancer is relatively infrequent, although periprostatic bleeding shortly after a biopsy may obscure tissue planes. On the other hand, understaging is an important issue: in historical series the incidence of understaging of stage B tumors has been significant. With the use of whole-mount histologic sections of the prostate, over ½ of palpable stage $B_2$ tumors are found to have histologic evidence of capsular invasion. Seminal-vesicle involvement has been noted in as many as 15% to 20% of patients with clinical stage $B_1$ tumors and up to half of those with the clinical diagnosis of stage $B_2$ lesions. Thus, the accuracy of digital palpation of the prostate alone as a means of staging local extent of prostate cancer has been questioned. Nevertheless, careful digital examination of the prostate remains the most important staging maneuver in apparently localized carcinoma of the prostate.

### Ultrasound

Transrectal ultrasonography provides information about tumor volume and location that may be helpful in staging known carcinoma of the prostate. Initially, the overall shape and symmetry of the prostate should be considered. Undoubtedly, tumor volume is an important feature. McNeal and associates have shown that lesions greater than 3 $cm^3$ usually exhibit capsular penetration or seminal-vesicle invasion, whereas tumors less than 1 $cm^3$ in volume often are confined within the capsule.[7] The capsular or boundary echoes of the prostate can be ascertained using either a transaxial or sagittal view. Bulging, thickening, irregularity, interruption, and asymmetrical contour have all been associated with capsular invasion.[8]

Changes in the seminal vesicles associated with early tumor involvement are not well understood. Certainly, abnormal internal echoes, anterior displacement, or disparity in size and shape may increase the level of suspicion. Symmetry is best evaluated on a transaxial scan. Most often, normal seminal vesicles are symmetric and vary little in size, even after ejaculation.[17] A normal fat plane exists between the seminal vesicle and the base of the prostate; this is best evaluated using a sagittal image. The entrance of the seminal vesicles into the ejaculatory ducts forms a beak; failure to demonstrate this normal finding has been described as an early sign of seminal-vesicle invasion (Fig 7).[8]

Rifkin and associates reported the results of a study performed by the Radiologic Diagnostic Oncology Group (RDOG).[18] They compared transrectal ultrasonography to magnetic resonance imaging in staging patients with apparent stage B carcinoma of the prostate prior to radical prostatectomy. Both methods were found to be imprecise; transrectal ultrasonography had a sensitivity of only 56% and a specificity of 64%, while magnetic reso-

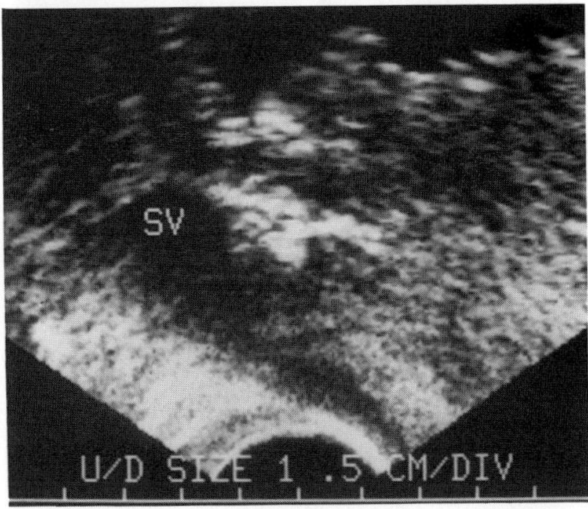


**Fig 7.** Sagittal image of the prostate in a patient with a palpable prostate cancer. The hypoechoic peripheral-zone lesion obliterates the normal plane with the seminal vesicle (SV).

nance imaging was slightly better, with a sensitivity of 61% and a specificity of 72%. In the opinion of these investigators, neither modality was proven to be clinically beneficial in staging carcinoma of the prostate.

## Lymph-Node Staging

The first echelon of metastasis beyond the prostate is usually the pelvic lymph nodes. When definitive local therapy is being contemplated for an otherwise localized prostate cancer, detection of pelvic lymph-node metastasis becomes critical. A number of potential methods for evaluation of the pelvic lymph nodes have been described. Noninvasive staging techniques such as computed tomography (CT) scanning or lymphangiography may be useful in higher stage or grade tumors, which may have gross nodal metastasis (Fig 8). False-positive studies can be eliminated by confirmatory fine-needle aspiration or biopsy of suspicious nodes. The primary limitation of both CT scanning and lymphangiography when used to stage lymph nodes in patients with prostate cancer is an inordinately high false-negative rate. Only around ¼ of patients with histologically proven lymph-node metastases have preoperative identification of lymph-node metastasis by lymphangiography or CT scanning.[19]

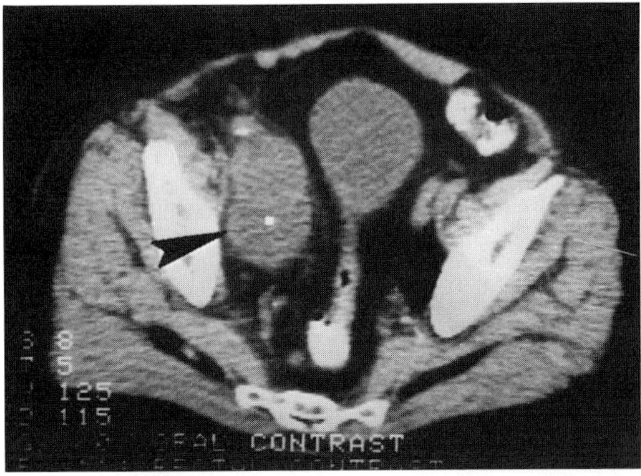


**Fig 8.** CT scan showing a large pelvic lymph-node mass (arrow) in a patient with high-grade carcinoma and palpable seminal-vesicle invasion. Although CT scan may identify gross nodal disease in a patient such as this, CT scans are less helpful in patients with clinically localized disease, since nodal metastases usually are microscopic only.

**Pelvic Lymph-Node Dissection.** Because of the inaccuracies of staging of pelvic lymph nodes, lymph-node dissection has been used for staging purposes in patients with apparently localized prostate cancer. The incidence of pelvic lymph-node metastases identified after surgical lymphadenectomy is dependent upon the stage and grade of the primary tumor.[20] Pelvic nodal metastasis is rare in true stage $A_1$ tumors. On the other hand, up to 25% of patients with stage $A_2$ carcinoma can be expected to have metastatic pelvic lymph nodes detected by a node dissection. The incidence of pelvic-node metastasis is around 12% in patients with stage $B_1$ tumors, but may be as high as 30% in patients with stage $B_2$ lesions. Finally, more than half of patients with palpable extracapsular tumor extension can be expected to have pelvic node metastasis.

Improvements in laparoscopic equipment and technique have led recently to the use of laparoscopic pelvic lymph-node dissection. Only very limited and preliminary data are available. In general, this has been a lengthy procedure and it has not yet been demonstrated definitively that all of the nodes of interest are removed satisfactorily by laparoscopy. Undoubtedly, with further refinement in instrumentation and technique, results will improve.

The most commonly defined surgical boundaries for lymph-node dissection are located in a triangle subtended by the inferior border of the external iliac vein, the obturator nerve, and the endopelvic fascia. The lymph nodes lie superior to the obturator vessels and the obturator nerve. Involvement of the external iliac lymph nodes or nodes superior to the bifurcation of the common iliac artery is unusual without simultaneous metastatic disease within the anatomic boundaries described above. Therefore, if a lymphadenectomy is performed for staging purposes, removal of the lymphatic tissue surrounding the external iliac artery and extending over the psoas muscle to the genitofemoral nerve is unnecessary.

## DEFINITIVE LOCAL THERAPY FOR PROSTATE CANCER

There are, perhaps, fewer areas in medicine that generate more disagreement than the appropriate management of localized prostatic cancer. To a great extent, the confusion surrounding this subject is due to the variable natural history of the disease and its occurrence in a patient population that generally is of an advanced age and in which many competing causes of death exist. Very few randomized studies have been conducted to compare the various treatments for localized prostatic cancer. Comparisons between retrospective series often are invalid because of variability in patient selection and staging. Therefore, there are no definitive data that allow the clinician to make dogmatic recommendations regarding selection of therapy. Although patient wishes clearly should be paramount in selecting therapy and even in deciding the indication for treatment, it is incumbent upon the clinician to make well-informed recommendations that encompass the specifics of the individual patient's situation.

Survival statistics alone do not allow firm conclusions regarding the most efficacious treatment for localized prostate cancer. The natural history of untreated disease is an important consideration.[21] Several studies suggest a low rate of disease progression and an even lower rate of death from carcinoma of the prostate in patients with stage $A_1$ tumors.[22] Cantrell and associates originally published data showing only a 2% progression rate for patients with stage $A_1$ carcinoma.[23] In a follow-up to this study, it was reported that 16% of patients at risk for 8 years or longer experienced disease progression.[24] However, almost half of the patients were excluded from analysis because they died from other causes within 8 years or had not been followed for a full 8 years. Lowe et al retrospectively analyzed stage $A_1$ patients and found that 9% experienced disease progression during a median follow-up of 9 years, using extent of tumor alone as a criterion for stage $A_1$ disease.[25] However, death from prostatic cancer occurred in only 1% of these patients.

Stage $A_2$ prostate cancer represents a much more lethal disease as compared to stage $A_1$ cancer. This is evidenced by the increased volume of residual tumor that remains in these patients after radical prostatectomy and the nearly 25% incidence of pelvic lymph-node metastasis.[26]

The natural history of stage B cancer of the prostate is not well documented. Whitmore followed a selected group of men who had clinical stage B prostate cancer and who did not receive treatment.[27] The expected 15-year survival rates were 45% for patients with stage $B_1$ tumors and 38% for those with stage $B_2$ lesions. An overall prostate cancer mortality rate of 24% was observed.

### Radical Prostatectomy

Radical prostatectomy implies surgical removal of the entire prostate gland and prostatic capsule, as well as of the seminal vesicles. Generally, patients with tumor that apparently is confined within the capsule of the prostate are candidates for radical prostatectomy. Increasingly, radical prostatectomy is being performed in patients with higher stage disease and even in those with positive pelvic lymph nodes, based on the belief that early adjuvant hormonal therapy improves long-term survival.

Radical prostatectomy was first popularized by Young in 1905, who used the perineal route.[28] In 1948, radical retropubic prostatectomy was described by Millen.[29] The surgical specimen is similar with both approaches, and neither has been shown to have any therapeutic advantage over the other. The choice depends to some extent on the preference and experience of the individual surgeon, although radical retropubic prostatectomy has been used more frequently in recent years. Staging pelvic lymph-node dissection can be performed simultaneously and through the same incision.

**Radical Perineal Prostatectomy.** The radical perineal approach for prostatectomy has been used less frequently in recent years because, when associated with pelvic lymph-node dissection, the procedure requires two incisions. Further refinements in laparoscopic lymph-node dissection may

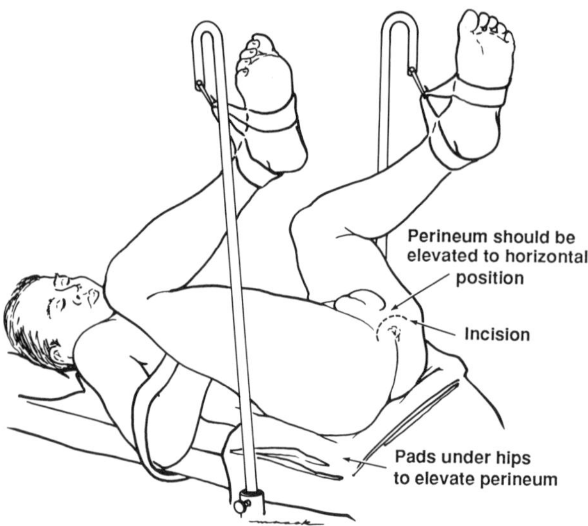


**Fig 9.** Patient position for radical perineal prostatectomy. The perineum should be elevated to a position horizontal with the table.

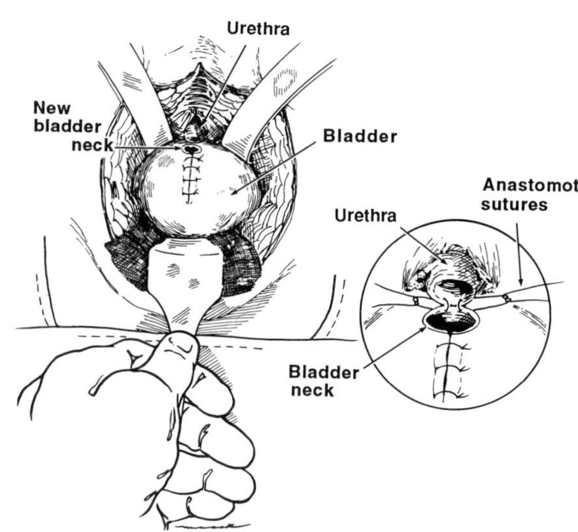


**Fig 11.** Vesicourethral anastomosis after radical perineal prostatectomy. Excellent exposure with precise suture placement can be achieved.

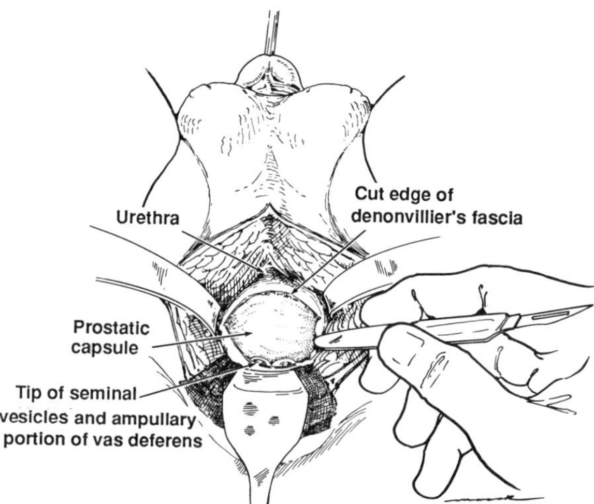


**Fig 10.** Schematic drawing of prostatic exposure during radical perineal prostatectomy. Incision in Denonvillier's fascia exposes the posterior capsule of the prostate and the rectum is retracted inferiorly.

increase the appeal of radical perineal prostatectomy.

Patients are placed in an exaggerated lithotomy position and an inverted ''U'' incision is made, with the apex of the incision several cm anterior to the anal verge (Fig 9). Rectal laceration during dissection of the prostatic apex is a major concern (Fig 10). The primary advantage of radical perineal prostatectomy is that, if lymph-node staging is not necessary or is performed by less invasive techniques, an abdominal incision is avoided. No increased incidence of deep venous thrombosis has been identified despite the exaggerated lithotomy positioning. Blood loss is usually less than after radical retropubic prostatectomy, and excellent exposure for the vesicourethral anastomosis is obtained (Fig 11).

**Radical Retropubic Prostatectomy.** Radical retropubic prostatectomy is performed through an incision extending from the pubic symphysis to the umbilicus. Pelvic lymphadenectomy is first completed and then the bladder is mobilized from the pubic symphysis. The prostate can be removed in a retrograde manner after dividing the puboprostatic ligaments and the urethra or by first dividing the bladder neck (Fig 12). Walsh has described a technique for preservation of sexual potency during radical retropubic prostatectomy.[30] The nerves which apparently are responsible for erec-

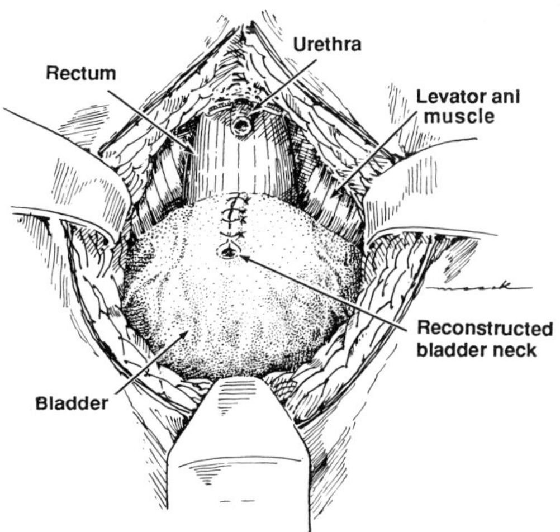


**Fig 12.** Pelvis after radical retropubic prostatectomy and reconstruction of the bladder neck. A posterior-based racket-handle closure of the bladder has been achieved and a tension-free anastomosis to the urethra can be obtained under direct vision.

tile function lie posterolateral to the urethra, and can be dissected free from the prostate, avoiding damage to the nerves during ligation of the pedicle.[31]

### Complications of Radical Prostatectomy

*Urinary Incontinence.* Perhaps the most feared complication of radical prostatectomy is urinary incontinence.[32] Incontinence is reported to occur in from zero to more than 50% of patients who have undergone radical prostatectomy. However, most contemporary series have shown an incidence of significant postoperative incontinence of less than 5%.[32] Return of urinary control after radical prostatectomy is a gradual process. The substantial majority of patients regain relatively good control within 2 to 3 months of surgery, although the ultimate potential for recovery may not be realized until up to 1 year postoperatively. Moderate amounts of stress incontinence may be treated satisfactorily by sympathomimetic drugs or bladder antispasmodics. If more marked incontinence occurs and is persistent, insertion of an inflatable artificial urinary sphincter can be successful.

*Impotence.* Previously, the incidence of erectile impotence after radical prostatectomy exceeded 90%. In 1982, Walsh and Donker described the pelvic anatomy of the parasympathetic nervous system and identified the nerves that appear to be responsible for potency.[31] A technique was developed in which the neurovascular bundle containing these nerves could be preserved.[30] In a recent update of his series, Walsh reported that potency was preserved overall in 72% of patients with clinical stage A or B prostate cancer.[33] Catalona has reported that potency was preserved in 71% of his patients with clinical stage $A_1$ tumors and 67% of those with clinical stage $B_1$ disease.[34] Preservation of potency was seen in 64% of those with clinical stage $B_2$ tumors. However, in patients with stage $B_2$ lesions, only 24% had preservation of potency with complete tumor excision, raising questions about whether preservation of the neurovascular bundle should be attempted in patients with higher stage tumors.

**Adjuvant Therapy after Radical Prostatectomy.** In nearly 50% of patients with stage $B_2$ adenocarcinoma of the prostate, radical prostatectomy results in incomplete tumor excision.[35] This is evidenced not only by positive surgical margins but also by residual detectable levels of PSA. After complete excision of the prostate, PSA levels should be undetectable. The use of postoperative radiation therapy appears to be associated with a lower local recurrence rate.[36,37] However, the effect of postoperative radiation therapy in preventing systemic recurrences is less certain.[38,39] Most studies have identified decreased local recurrence when radiation is used, but have reported no apparent survival benefit. The addition of postoperative radiation therapy may adversely affect potency, and the effects on urinary incontinence or the incidence of urethral stricture are uncertain.[40] Ongoing randomized studies are attempting to address these issues.

Adjuvant hormonal therapy may also be used after radical prostatectomy. Zincke retrospectively reviewed patients with stage $D_1$ disease treated by radical prostatectomy and orchiectomy. This investigator reported 5- and 10-year progression-free survival rates superior to those achieved with alternative treatment, including rates observed with delayed endocrine therapy.[41] However, there are no well-designed, randomized studies confirming the therapeutic benefit of either radical prostatectomy or early hormonal therapy in patients with prostate cancer which extends locally outside the capsule or which has metastasized to the pelvic lymph nodes.

## Radiation Therapy

Orthovoltage irradiation initially found limited acceptance as a treatment for prostatic cancer, primarily because of the damage to skin and subcutaneous tissue that occurred when potentially lethal doses were delivered to prostatic cancer cells. Cobalt-60 units and, more recently, linear accelerators allow delivery of potentially lethal doses of radiation with less fibrosis and radiation damage to the skin. There is no consensus regarding the optimal technique for delivery of external irradiation for prostate cancer. Most often, 4- to 6-mmeV linear accelerators are used as an energy source for treatment of prostate cancer; the energy beam from a linear accelerator can be precisely focused, reducing treatment morbidity resulting from damage to normal structures.

The portal size and total dose is of critical importance in determining treatment outcome and subsequent complications. The maximum dose of radiation that can be delivered to the tumor without producing permanent damage to normal tissue is desirable. Dose fractionation decreases side effects and may improve therapeutic efficacy.[42] Portals that encompass the entire prostate and periprostatic region should be used, but the actual field size varies depending upon patient size. There is no evidence that irradiation of the pelvic lymph nodes improves survival in patients with either low-stage tumors or proven pelvic lymph-node metastasis.[43]

### Complications of External Irradiation

*Radiation Cystitis.* Acute radiation cystitis, manifested by urinary frequency, urgency, and nocturia, occurs in approximately 40% of patients. Hematuria, either microscopic or gross, may also be seen. Symptoms of acute radiation cystitis may occasionally be severe and are cause for treatment interruption in up to 5% to 10% of patients. In the majority of patients, symptoms resolve in 3 months, but chronic symptomatic radiation cystitis occurs in around 10% of patients receiving curative doses of external irradiation.[44]

*Gastrointestinal Complications.* Radiation enteritis, resulting in diarrhea, anorexia, and nausea, occurs primarily in patients receiving radiation to large pelvic fields. About 40% of patients in whom significant amounts of small bowel are included in the radiation field develop symptomatic acute radiation enteritis.[45] Symptoms resolve in most patients within 3 months, but around 10% have persistent chronic symptoms, primarily diarrhea, related to radiation enteritis and proctitis.

**Impotence.** Slightly more than half of patients with normal sexual function before treatment retain their sexual potency after definitive doses of external irradiation for prostate cancer. However, with longer term follow-up and late fibrosis of pelvic nerves and vessels, this figure increases.

**Results.** There have been a number of reports on the incidence of positive biopsies after external irradiation. Some authors have considered that post-irradiation biopsies lack prognostic significance, whereas others have concluded that irradiation alone is rarely capable of sterilizing prostate cancer.[46,47] It is becoming increasingly evident that patients with positive biopsies have a worse prognosis than those whose biopsies are normal 18 months after therapy.[48] In addition, positive biopsies are seen in a significant number of patients undergoing biopsy 18 months after treatment.[49]

Despite the concerns regarding positive biopsies, long-term survival statistics after radiation treatment for prostate cancer appear to be comparable to most alternative treatments. Bagshaw and colleagues have reported the largest and most extensively studied series of patients treated with radiation therapy for localized prostate cancer.[50] The mean follow-up is 8 years. Fifteen-year survival in patients with stage $B_1$ tumors was 52%. However, the only randomized, prospective study comparing external irradiation and radical prostatectomy, that conducted by the Uro-Oncology Research Group, showed a statistically significant improvement in the time to first evidence of disease failure for patients undergoing radical prostatectomy when compared to patients who received external irradiation.[51]

**Interstitial Irradiation.** Compared to external radiation sources, interstitial implantation of radioactive substances into the prostate has the potential advantage of delivering a higher dose of ionizing radiation to the prostate while limiting the effect on adjacent organs. Also, the long half-life of some isotopes theoretically may be advantageous in treating tumors with long doubling times. Primarily, three different isotopes have been used to treat prostatic cancer. Each has distinct energy specifications and effects upon prostatic cancer.

***Iodine 125.*** The use of interstitial implantation of iodine 125 for the treatment of prostatic cancer was initiated and popularized at Memorial Sloan-Kettering Cancer Center in the early 1970s.[52] The rationale for the use of iodine 125 was based on the long half-life of the isotope coupled with its relatively low energy. Thus, high doses of radiation are delivered to the prostate over a prolonged period, while the adjacent structures receive more limited amounts.

Iodine 125 emits pure gamma radiation with a half-life of around 60 days. Thus, the useful life of the isotope or the period for which effective doses of radiation may be emitted is 1 year. The relatively low energy of iodine 125, along with its long half-life, increases the safety and ease with which health care personnel can handle the isotope. The half-value layer in tissue is only 1.7 cm. This layer limits the amount of radiation delivered to the rectum and bladder when the seeds are implanted in the prostate.

The geometry of the implant is important, and a relatively uniform distribution of the seeds within the prostate and tumor should be attempted. Postoperative computerized dosimetric analysis should be performed to determine the isodose curves (Fig 13). The 160-Gy curves should encompass the entire prostate and tumor volume. The rectum and bladder usually fall well outside the 160-Gy curve and often receive less than 40 Gy of brachytherapy.[53]

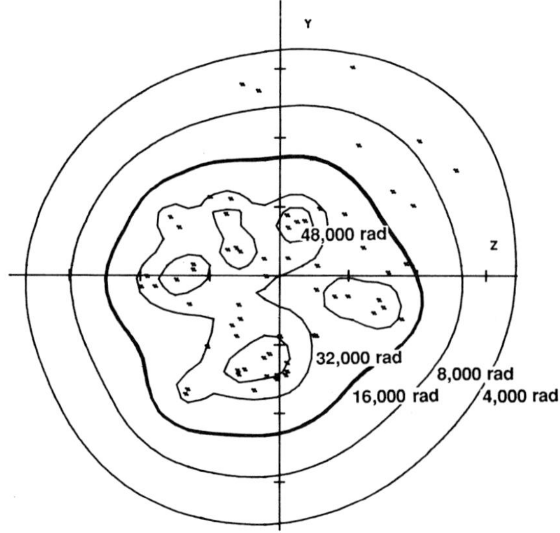


**Fig 13.** Computerized dosimetry isodose curves after iodine 125 implantation of the prostate. The 160-Gy line encompasses the entire prostate volume while the rectal wall receives less than 40 Gy. Isolated areas of higher dose intensity are present within the prostate.

Previously, iodine 125 seeds were usually implanted after retropubic exposure of the prostate. Follow-up studies have shown an increased incidence of local failure after iodine 125 seed implantation via the retropubic approach.[54,55] More recently, ultrasound-directed placement of seeds has been performed. Whether this will improve the local control rates because of better geometric placement of seeds remains to be determined.

***Interstitial Gold 198.*** Interstitial implantation of gold 198 in the prostate with external beam irradiation was developed by Carlton and colleagues in 1972 as a treatment for localized prostate cancer.[56] Gold

198 has properties that present advantages and disadvantages. Both beta- and gamma-irradiation are emitted, and the half-value layer in tissue is 4.5 cm. In addition, the isotope has a relatively short half-life of less than 3 days. The relatively high energy requires protection for personnel involved with its use. However, geometric placement of seeds is not critical because of the high energy.

Gold 198 seeds are used primarily to deliver a boost of irradiation to the prostate, and supplemental external irradiation is used after the radiation energy from the seeds is exhausted. Supplemental external irradiation is delivered at least 3 weeks after the implant.

***Iridium 192.*** Iridium 192 emits gamma energy. The half-life of this isotope is 75 days and its half-value layer in tissue is 6 cm. The technique for implantation involves after-loading of needles placed intraoperatively. The iridium-192 needles are left in place for approximately 40 to 50 hours and are then removed. Thirty to 35 Gy are delivered to the prostate and periprostatic tissue over this period. About 2 weeks later, supplemental external irradiation is delivered to 8 × 8 cm portals. The reported experience with iridium-192 implantation in the prostate is insufficient to allow any conclusions regarding its efficacy or role in the treatment of prostate cancer.[57]

### Laser Treatment

Application of Nd:YAG laser energy has gained popularity in Scandinavia and other parts of Europe as a treatment for carcinoma of the prostate.[58] Energy is applied transurethrally and through a cystotomy to allow better access to the posterior prostate. Clinical follow-up is limited, but a low incidence of posttreatment positive biopsies has been observed.

## REFERENCES


1. Cancer Statistics 1991. *CA.* 1991;36:16–17.
2. Guinan P, Bush I, Ray V, et al. The accuracy of the rectal examination in the diagnosis of prostate carcinoma. *N Engl J Med.* 1980;303:499.
3. Chodak GW, Keller P, Schoenberg HW. Assessment of screening for prostate cancer using the digital rectal examination. *J Urol.* 1989; 141:1134–1138.
4. Chodak GW, Schoenberg HW. Early detection of prostate cancer by routine screening. *JAMA.* 1984;252:3261–3264.
5. Hernandez AD, Smith JA Jr. Transrectal ultrasonography for the early detection and staging of prostate cancer. *Urol Clin North Am.* 1990;17:745–757.
6. McNeal JE. Regional morphology and pathology of the prostate. *Am J Clin Pathol.* 1968;49:347–357.
7. McNeal JE, Kindrachuk RA, Frieha FS, et al. Patterns of progression in prostate cancer. *Lancet.* 1986;1:60–63.
8. Lee F, Torp-Pedersen ST, Siders DB, et al. Transrectal ultrasound in the diagnosis and staging of prostatic carcinoma. *Radiology.* 1989; 170:609–615.
9. Watanabe H, Igari D, Takahashi Y, et al. Transrectal ultrasonography of the prostate. *J Urol.* 1975;114:734–739.
10. Lee F, Gray JM, McLeary RD, et al. Transrectal ultrasound in the diagnosis of prostate cancer: location, echogenicity, histopathology and staging. *Prostate.* 1985;7:117–129.
11. Cooner WH, Mosley BR, Rutherford CL, et al. Clinical application of transrectal ultrasonography and PSA in the search for prostatic cancer. *J Urol.* 1988;139:758–761.
12. Lee F, Torp-Peterson ST, Littrup PH, et al. Hypoechoic lesions of the prostate: clinical relevance of tumor size, DRE and PSA. *Radiology.* 1989;170:29–32.
13. Stamey TA, Yang N, Hay AF, et al. Prostate specific antigen as a serum marker for advanced adenocarcinoma of the prostate. *N Engl J Med.* 1987;317:909.
14. Brawer MK. Laboratory studies for the detection of carcinoma of the prostate. *Urol Clin North Am.* 1990;17:745–757.
15. Catalona WJ, Smith DS, Ratliff TL, et al. Management of prostate specific antigen in serum as a screening test for prostate cancer. *N Engl J Med.* 1991;324:1156–1161.
16. Smith JA Jr. Staging of prostate cancer. In: Smith JA Jr, Middleton RG. *Clinical Management of Prostatic Cancer.* Chicago: Year Book Medical Publishers; 1987;23–53.
17. Hernandez AD, Urry RI, Smith JA Jr. Ultra-

sonographic characteristics of the seminal vesicles after ejaculation. *J Urol.* 1990;144:1–3.

18. Rifkin MD, Serhouni EA, Gatsonis CA, et al. Comparison of early magnetic resonance imaging and ultrasonography in staging early prostate cancer. *N Engl J Med.* 1990;323:621–626.
19. Correa RJ Jr, Kidd CR, Burnett L, et al. Percutaneous pelvic lymph node aspiration in carcinoma of the prostate. *J Urol.* 1981;126:190–191.
20. Smith JA Jr, Seaman JP, Gleidman JB, et al. Pelvic lymph node metastasis from prostatic cancer: influence of tumor grade and stage in 452 consecutive patients. *J Urol.* 1983;130:290–292.
21. Johansson JE, Andersson SO, Krusemo UB, et al. Natural history of localized prostatic cancer. *Lancet.* 1989;1:799–803.
22. Parfitt HE Jr, Smith JA Jr, Gliedman JB, et al. Accuracy of staging in $A_1$ carcinoma of the prostate. *Cancer.* 1983;51:2346–2350.
23. Cantrell BB, DeKlerk DP, Eggleston JC, et al. Pathologic factors that influence prognosis in stage A prostatic cancer: the influence of extent versus grade. *J Urol.* 1981;125:516–520.
24. Epstein JI, Walsh PC, Eggleston JC. Prognosis of untreated stage $A_1$ prostate carcinoma: a study of 94 cases with extended follow-up. *J Urol.* 1986;135:242A.
25. Lowe BA, Listrom MB. Incidental carcinoma of the prostate: an analysis of the predictors of progression. *J Urol.* 1988;140:1340–1344.
26. Parfitt HE Jr, Smith JA Jr, Seaman JP, et al. Surgical treatment of stage $A_2$ prostatic carcinoma: significance of tumor grade and extent. *J Urol.* 1983;129:763–765.
27. Whitmore WF Jr: The natural history of low stage prostatic cancer. *Urol Clin North Am.* 1990;17:689–697.
28. Young HH. The early diagnosis and radical cure of carcinoma of the prostate: being a study of 40 cases and presentation of a radical operation which was carried out in 4 cases. *Bull Johns Hopkins Hosp.* 1905;16:315–321.
29. Millen T. *Retropubic Urinary Surgery.* Baltimore: Williams & Wilkins Co; 1947:86–94.
30. Walsh PC, Mastwin JL. Radical prostatectomy and cystoprostatectomy with preservation of potency: results utilizing a new nerve sparing technique. *Br J Urol.* 1984;56:694–697.
31. Walsh PC, Donker PJ. Impotence following radical prostatectomy: insight into etiology and prevention. *J Urol.* 1982;128:492–497.
32. Smith JA Jr, Middleton RG. Radical prostatectomy for stage $B_2$ prostatic cancer. *J Urol.* 1982;127:702–703.
33. Walsh PC, Epstein JI, Lowe FC. Potency following radical prostatectomy with wide unilateral excision of the neurovascular bundle. *J Urol.* 1987;138:823–827.
34. Catalona WJ. Patient selection for, results of, and impact on tumor resection of potency sparing radical prostatectomy. *Urol Clin North Am.* 1990;17:745–757.
35. Montie JE: Positive margins after radical prostatectomy. *Urol Clin North Am.* 1990;17:803–812.
36. Jacobson GM, Smith JA Jr, Stewart JR. Postoperative radiation therapy for pathologic stage C prostate cancer. *Int J Radiat Oncol Biol Phys.* 1987;13:1021.
37. Lange PH, Moon TD, Narayan P. Radiation therapy as adjuvant treatment after radical prostatectomy: patient tolerance and preliminary results. *J Urol.* 1986;136:45.
38. Paulson DF, Stone AR, Walther PJ, et al. Radical prostatectomy: anatomical predictors of success or failure. *J Urol.* 1986;136:1041.
39. Anscher MS, Prosnitz LR. Postoperative radiotherapy for patients with carcinoma of the prostate undergoing radical prostatectomy with positive surgical margins, seminal vesicle involvement and/or penetration through the capsule. *J Urol.* 1987;138:1407.
40. Gibbons RP, Cole BS, Richardson EG, et al. Adjuvant radiotherapy following radical prostatectomy: results and complications. *J Urol.* 1986;135:65.
41. Zincke H. Extended experience with surgical treatment of stage $D_1$ adenocarcinoma of the prostate. *Urology.* 1989;33:27.
42. Hanks GE, Leibel SA, Krall JM, et al. Patterns of care studies: dose response observation for local control of adenocarcinoma of the prostate. *Int J Radiol Oncol Biol Phys.* 1985;11:153–157.
43. Smith JA Jr, Middleton RG. Impact of external irradiation on disease-free survival and local symptoms in patients with pelvic lymph node metastases from prostatic cancer. *J Urol.* 1984;131:705–708.
44. Ray GR, Cassady R, Bagshaw MA. Definitive radiation therapy of carcinoma of the prostate: a report on 15 years of experience. *Radiology.* 1973;106:407–418.
45. Perez CA, Bauer W, Garza R, et al. Radiation therapy in the treatment of localized carcinoma of the prostate. *Cancer.* 1974;34:1059–1068.
46. Cox JD, Stoffel TJ. The significance of needle biopsy after irradiation for stage C adenocarcinoma of the prostate. *Cancer.* 1977;40:156.
47. Freiha F, Bagshaw MA. Carcinoma of the prostate: results of post-irradiation biopsy. *Prostate.* 1984;5:19.
48. Scardino PT, Frankel JM, Wheeler TM, et al. The prognostic significance of post-irradiation biopsy results in patients with prostatic cancer. *J Urol.* 1986;135:510.
49. Kabalin JN, Hodge KK, McNeal JE, et al. Identification of residual cancer in the prostate following radiation therapy: role of transrectal ultrasound guided biopsy and prostate specific antigen. *J Urol.* 1989;142:326.

50. Bagshaw MA, Cox RS, Ramback JE. Radiation therapy for localized prostate cancer. *Urol Clin North Am.* 1990;17:787–802.

51. Paulsen DS, Sin GH, Hinslow W, the Uro-Oncology Group. Radical surgery versus radiotherapy for stage $A_2$ and B adenocarcinoma of the prostate. *J Urol.* 1982;128:502–505.

52. Whitmore WR Jr, Hilaris B, Grabstald H. Retropubic implantation of Iodine 125 in the treatment of prostate cancer. *J Urol.* 1972;109:918–920.

53. Whitmore WF Jr. Interstitial radiation therapy for carcinoma of the prostate. *Prostate.* 1980; 1:157–168.

54. Grossman HB, Batata M, Hilaris B, et al. I-125 implantation for carcinoma of the prostate: further follow-up of first 100 cases. *Urology.* 1982;20:591–598.

55. Herr HW. Preservation of sexual potency in prostatic cancer patients after pelvic lymphadenectomy and retropubic I-125 implantation. *J Urol.* 1979;121:621–623.

56. Scardino PT, Guerriero WG, Carlton CE Jr. Surgical staging and combined therapy with radioactive gold groin implantation and external irradiation. In: Johnson DE, Boileau MA, eds. *Genitourinary Tumors: Fundamental Principles and Surgical Techniques.* New York: Grune & Stratton; 1982:75–90.

57. Tansey LA, Shanberg AM, Syed AM, et al. Treatment of prostatic carcinoma by pelvic lymphadenectomy, and temporary iridium 192 implant and external irradiation. *Urology.* 1983; 21:594–598.

58. Beisland HO, Sander S. First clinical experiences on Neodymium:YAG laser irradiation of localized prostate cancer. *Scand J Urol Nephrol.* 1986;20:113–117.

# 37

# Advanced Carcinoma of the Prostate

*Michael J. Schutz and E. David Crawford*

In 1991, prostate cancer was diagnosed in approximately 122,000 men, and was the most common cancer in men. This neoplasm is the second leading cause of cancer deaths; and more than 32,500 men died of the disease in the United States in 1991.[1] Over 25% of patients present with distant metastatic disease (stage D2), and are not candidates for surgical extirpation.[2] This chapter will review current diagnostic and treatment modalities for stage D2 carcinoma of the prostate.

## PRESENTATION

Patients with stage D2 carcinoma of the prostate commonly present with back pain, anemia, and prostatism. Alternatively, the disease may progress to stage D2 in a man with known prostate cancer. Other presenting signs and symptoms include pathologic fracture, renal failure, urinary retention, bone pain, paraplegia, and enlarged supraclavicular or inguinal lymph nodes.[3] In addition, the authors have noted an increase in the number of men with advanced disease who are asymptomatic.

## DIAGNOSIS

The diagnosis of prostate cancer is made through histologic identification of the malignancy. Tissue for examination can be obtained in a number of ways. In the past, it was obtained by performing open perineal prostate biopsy on suspicious lesions. However, this procedure is rarely used today because of the associated morbidity. Currently, transrectal or transperineal core needle biopsy is used to detect prostate cancer. These procedures initially made use of Vim-Silverman needles, which obviated the need for open biopsy. Subsequent refinements to the core-needle biopsy technique include the development of the Tru-Cut biopsy needle and spring-loaded mechanisms for delivering the needle into the prostate. As a result of these improvements, prostate biopsies may now be performed on an outpatient basis, without anesthesia.

Other diagnostic methods include ultrasonography and fine-needle aspiration cytology. The use of prostate ultrasound to facilitate accurate biopsy of prostate nodules has recently been evaluated by Weaver et al.[4] These researchers performed biopsies, assisted by either transrectal ultrasonographic or digital guidance, on 51 men. Forty-one percent of the nodules were found to be positive with transrectal ultrasound guidance, as opposed to 18% of digitally guided biopsies.[4]

Fine-needle aspiration cytology is performed transrectally, and may have sensitivity and specificity equivalent to that of core-needle biopsy. However, the pathologist must be experienced to adequately evaluate the biopsy, as there is much less tissue obtained with this method when compared to core-needle biopsy, and because the glandular architecture is obliterated with aspiration.[5,6]

## STAGING

Once the diagnosis of prostate cancer is made, either through transperineal or transrectal needle biopsy, transurethral or open prostatectomy, or biopsy of a site of metastases, the patient must be evaluated to determine the extent of disease. Physical examination may reveal adenopathy; rectal examination will reveal the extent of the primary lesion. Tests used to determine the disease stage in patients with prostate carcinoma include serum markers and radiologic studies such as bone scan, chest x-ray, excretory urography, computed tomography (CT) scan, and magnetic resonance imaging (MRI) scan.

### Serum Markers

Serum markers used to evaluate patients with prostate cancer include acid and alkaline phosphatase and prostate specific antigen (PSA).

Monitoring acid phosphatase levels has been used in the management of patients with carcinoma of the prostate for more than 50 years. The early tests, using enzymatic techniques, found that 70% of men with metastatic prostate cancer had elevated levels of acid phosphatase. Now immunoassays to measure the prostatic fraction of acid phosphatase (PAP) are available; these tests are more sensitive for advanced disease. Approximately 90% of men with metastatic prostate cancer have elevated PAP levels. However, 15% of men without prostate cancer also demonstrate elevated acid phosphatase levels (Table 1).[7]

In the past, the serum level of alkaline phosphatase was also used as a marker for prostate cancer. While the level is frequently elevated in patients with prostate cancer, elevated alkaline phosphatase is a nonspecific finding that infrequently provides more information than other serum markers.[7] Elevated liver function indices may indicate hepatic metastases, but isolated hepatic metastases are rarely seen in patients with prostate cancer.

Recently, serum PSA levels have been used to diagnose prostate cancer. PSA is a protein produced in prostatic epithelial cells, but serum prostate-specific antigen elevation is not specific to patients with prostate cancer[8]; those with benign prostatic hyperplasia, prostatitis, and prostatic infarction may demonstrate elevated serum PSA levels.[7] Serum PSA levels generally increase with the severity of disease, but levels vary between patients. Thus, there is no specific range of PSA levels that directly correlates to each stage of disease.[9] At this time, the best use for PSA is as a marker to monitor the patient's response to treatment.

Recently, attempts have been made to use PSA to stratify patients with prostate cancer at risk for bony metastases at diagnosis. PSA values of <20 ng/mL by the Hybritech assay have been associated with a 0.3% incidence of osseous metastases in a series of over 300 patients.[10] Further studies are needed to confirm this finding and may eliminate the need for bone scan in these patients.

### Radiologic Studies

The chest radiograph is an inexpensive, easy test which not only gives information about possible prostate cancer metastases but also about the patient's cardiovascular health. Six percent of patients with prostate cancer demonstrate intrathoracic metastases at presentation. This figure rises to 25% of patients with stage D disease. The signs and symptoms of intrathoracic metastases can manifest as pleural effusion, reticular opacities, mediastinal adenopathy, and lung nodules.[11]

Excretory urography still plays an important role in the evaluation of patients with prostate cancer. It is a relatively inexpensive test that reveals a great deal of information. The scout film will reveal osseous metastases to the pelvis, lumbar spine, and femoral heads (Fig 1). Irregularities of the bladder base, hydroneph-

**TABLE 1. Disorders Associated with an Elevation of Serum Acid Phosphatase***

| Organ Site | Condition |
|---|---|
| Prostate | Carcinoma |
| | Infarction |
| | Rectal examination/prostatic massage |
| | Endoscopic manipulation |
| | Urinary retention |
| Reticuloendothelial system | Acute and chronic lymphocytic leukemia |
| | Acute and chronic myelogenous leukemia |
| | Hairy cell leukemia |
| | Gaucher's disease |
| | Niemann-Pick disease |
| | Eosinophilic granuloma |
| | Reticulum cell sarcoma |
| | Hodgkin's disease |
| | Multiple myeloma |
| | Malignant lymphoma |
| | Thrombocytopenia |
| | Polycythemia vera |
| Carcinomas with hepatic/skeletal metastases | Breast |
| | Stomach |
| | Colon |
| | Kidney |
| | Adrenal cortical |
| | Melanoma |
| | Lung |
| Liver | Viral hepatitis |
| | Cirrhosis |
| | Biliary tract obstruction |
| | Chlorpromazine hepatitis |
| Kidney | Chronic glomerulonephritis |
| | Gouty nephropathy |
| Skeletal system (primary) | Paget's disease |
| | Osteogenesis imperfecta |
| | Osteogenic sarcoma |
| | Osteopetrosis |
| | Osteoporosis |
| Skeletal system (secondary) | Primary hyperparathyroidism |

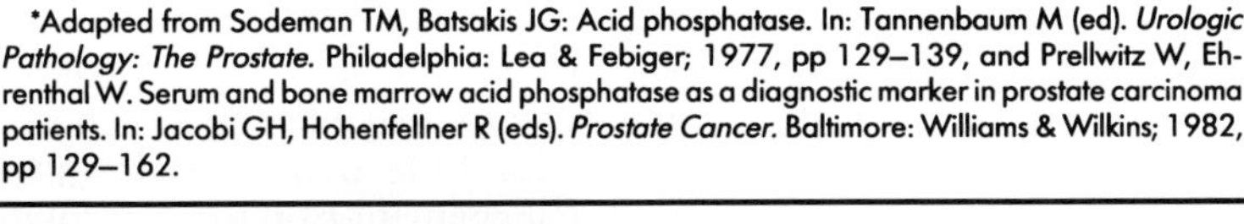
*Adapted from Sodeman TM, Batsakis JG: Acid phosphatase. In: Tannenbaum M (ed). *Urologic Pathology: The Prostate.* Philadelphia: Lea & Febiger; 1977, pp 129–139, and Prellwitz W, Ehrenthal W. Serum and bone marrow acid phosphatase as a diagnostic marker in prostate carcinoma patients. In: Jacobi GH, Hohenfellner R (eds). *Prostate Cancer.* Baltimore: Williams & Wilkins; 1982, pp 129–162.

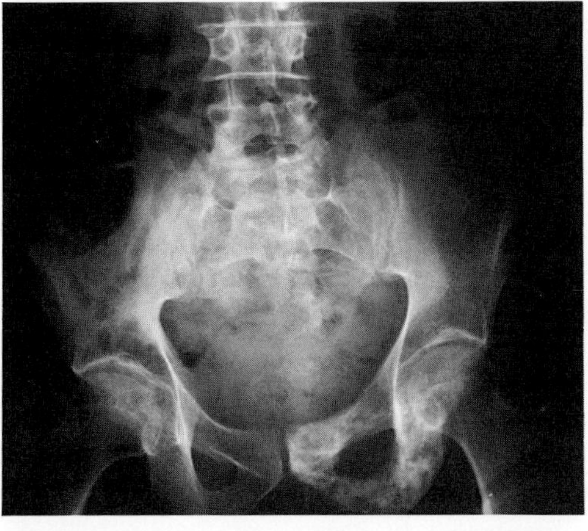

**Fig 1.** Plain pelvic x-ray showing replacement of left superior and inferior pubic rami with osteoblastic metastases from prostate cancer.

rosis, deviation of the ureter by lymph node enlargement, or nonfunction of one or both kidneys can also be detected by excretory urography.

Radionuclide bone scan is one of the most important tests in the evaluation of patients with prostate cancer. Seventy percent to 80% of patients with prostate cancer will develop bone metastases. The most

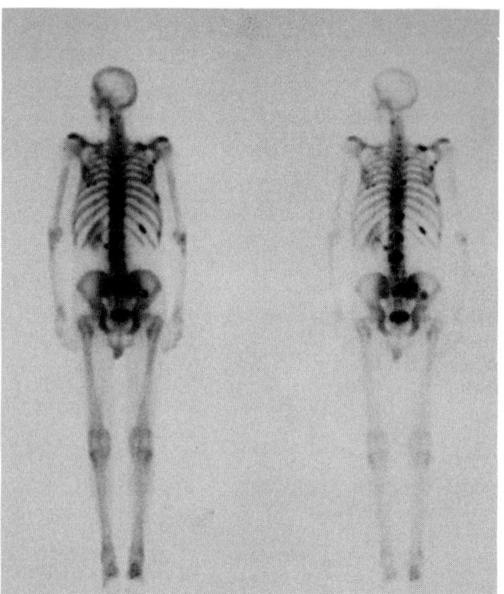

**Fig 2.** Bone scan with areas of uptake of radionuclide noted in the cervical, thoracic, lumbar, and sacral spine, left 7th rib, right 6th and 11th ribs, right scapula and clavicle, right ilium and sacroiliac joint.

common sites for these metastases include the pelvis, spine, ribs, and skull. Skeletal x-rays were initially used to evaluate patients for osseous metastases, and were able to reveal a classic osteoblastic lesion. However, skeletal x-rays are not very sensitive in finding early bone lesions, because 30% to 50% of the bone mineral must be lost before the lesion is detected on x-ray.[12,13]

Bone scans were first introduced in the 1950s, but widespread use did not occur until the 1970s, when technetium-99m ($^{99}$Tc) polyphosphate was introduced. This radionuclide is available in a kit form which has a shelf life of 6 weeks; when activated, it has a short half-life—6 hours. Ten to 20 MCi are injected intravenously (IV) and either a gamma camera or a rectilinear scanner can be used to collect counts approximately 2 to 4 hours after injection. Two mechanisms have been proposed for the uptake of radionuclide by bone. One theory suggests that $^{99}$Tc is absorbed to the hydroxyapatite crystal of the bone and the other is that $^{99}$Tc is incorporated into immature collagen in new bone formation. Any process that increases blood flow to the bone and bone turnover will appear with increased radionuclide uptake or a "hot spot."[12]

Metastatic lesions will appear on the bone scan as patchy, asymmetric areas of radionuclide uptake (Fig 2). Extensive bony deposits can appear as a "super scan." Super scans occur when the isotope is almost completely taken up by the skeleton. These scans may look almost normal, with the increased activity spread throughout the skeleton, except there is no renal excretion. False-negative rates of up to 8% have been reported and may be due to super scans or to lesions that do not provoke an osteoblastic response.[11] False-positive results can occur in patients with old fractures, arthritis, osteomyelitis, primary skeletal neoplasms, metabolic skeletal disorders, or Paget's disease.[12] Plain radiographs can be helpful in assessing individual areas, as single lesions noted on bone scan can be malignant in up to 50% of cases. CT or MRI scans may also be helpful in determining the disease etiology if plain radiographs are inconclusive. MRI has a 98% accuracy in differentiating benign from malignant causes of collapsed vertebrae.[14]

CT scan has been used in the evaluation of patients with metastatic prostate cancer. Autopsy studies have shown 35% incidence of hepatic metastases, 17% incidence of adrenal metastases, and 10% incidence of renal or retroperitoneal metastases; most were clinically silent.[15] Routine use of CT scan to image the abdomen and pelvis provides little additional information in the management of the patient with metastatic prostate cancer. However, pelvic and abdominal CT scan may be useful in patients with minimally elevated PAP, elevated PSA, and negative bone scan to assess for the presence of pelvic or retroperitoneal adenopathy prior to surgery or radiation therapy. CT scan should not be used routinely, because microscopic metastases are not identified by this method, and lymph nodes are not always enlarged as a result of metastatic disease. However, fine-needle aspiration of enlarged lymph nodes as an adjunct to CT scan may help to improve

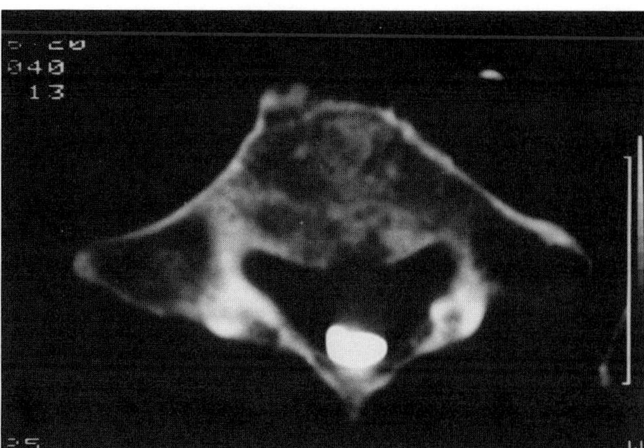

**Fig 3.** CT scan of lumbar spine showing extensive replacement of body of vertebrae with prostate cancer.

disease staging. Patients who present with neurologic symptoms, ie, paraplegia or muscle weakness, may benefit from CT myelography if MRI is not available (Fig 3). Because it is difficult to image the entire spine with either CT or MRI, neither method is optimal for evaluating spinal involvement or revealing clinically undetected lesions at other levels.[16]

MRI has drawbacks similar to those of CT in staging prostate cancer, and the best use of MRI is to evaluate metastatic disease to the spine (Fig 4). It is less invasive and more sensitive in detecting paraspinal masses than myelography. However, poor-quality images may result from patient motion and other spinal metastases may easily be overlooked. Myelography can be used as an adjunct examination in any cases in which the results of MRI are suspect.[16]

## THERAPY

In patients with advanced disease, palliation is a reasonable objective. Manipulation of androgens has been the mainstay of therapy for metastatic prostate cancer for the past 50 years.

In 1941, Huggins and Hodges showed that prostate cancer is androgen-dependent and that androgen deprivation leads to a decrease in acid phosphatase levels and significant tumor response in a majority of patients.[17] Extensive data have been accumulated over a number of years concerning the use of androgen deprivation in the treatment of patients with metastatic prostate cancer. Between 60% and 80% of men respond to hormonal therapy,[18] and a median survival of 24 months is observed in patients treated with androgen-deprivation therapy.[19–21] Therapeutic modalities used to treat patients with prostatic cancer include hormonal therapy, radiotherapy, cytotoxic chemotherapy, and immunotherapy. Each will be discussed below.

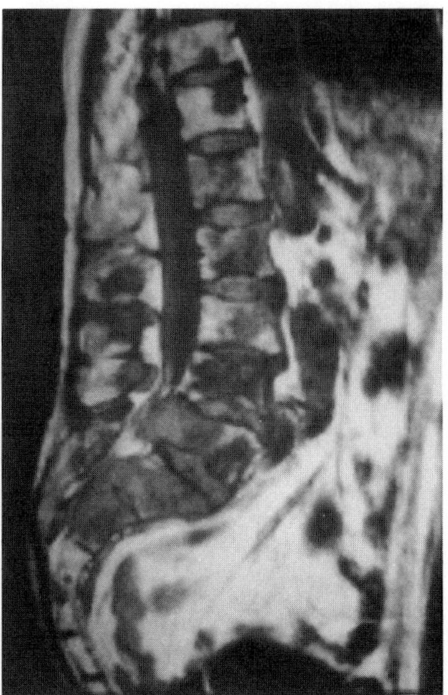

**Fig 4.** MRI of lower spine with metastatic deposit from L5 extending into the spinal canal.

### Assessment of Response to Therapy in Prostate Cancer

Assessing the efficacy of systemic therapy for prostate cancer is difficult and generally includes evaluation of disease sites as well as any changes in survival that occur in response to treatment.

Bone is the predominant site of metastases, and often diffuse osteoblastic lesions occur that are difficult to assess prospectively in a reliable and reproducible manner.[22] Lesions that appear on bone scan are often difficult to quantitate and follow. Physical examination of the prostate is also difficult to quantitate; furthermore, even if this type of examination could be quantitated for response, the response of the prostate may not be representative of the response of the metastatic lesions.

Response to therapy is somewhat easier to assess in patients with bidimensionally measurable disease. However, the measurable site is usually not the dominant site of metastases, and it may not provide a true indication of response to therapy. Serum markers also provide some information about the effectiveness of treatment, but may be inaccurate as the tumor progresses and becomes more poorly differentiated.

The National Prostate Cancer Project (NPCP) attempted to quantitate responses to treatment and has published a list of criteria for response (Appendix).[21] The criteria stratify responses according to the ability to evaluate disease—measurable vs evaluable—in an attempt to better define responses in patients with heterogeneous metastatic deposits. Currently, most investigators use these or similar criteria to assess response to therapy.

The stable-disease category given in the NPCP criteria poses a problem, because patients in this category are usually considered to be responders. However, prostate cancer usually progresses slowly. Thus, a treatment may be instituted, the patient reevaluated, and no evaluable change in disease found, yet it cannot be proved whether the lack of progression is related to the therapy or to the natural history of the cancer. If a patient in the stable-disease category is counted as a responder but does not show improved survival as a result of therapy, should this indicate the efficacy of treatment? This is why survival is also used to determine the efficacy of treatment in patients with prostate cancer.

### Prognostic Factors

Many factors influence patient survival and the time to disease progression in patients with metastatic prostate cancer (Table 2). Histologic grade, DNA ploidy, hemoglobin level, pretreatment testosterone levels, performance status, extent of bony metastases, changes in pre- and posttreatment acid phosphatase and prostate-specific antigen levels, and nuclear androgen-receptor content have been shown to influence survival or response in patients with stage D2 prostatic cancer.

Gleason et al reviewed the Veterans Administration Cooperative Urologic Research Group (VACURG) data, and found that patients with a Gleason pattern score of 8 to 10 had a higher death rate than those with lower Gleason scores.[23] Other researchers have reported that aneuploidy is associated with a clinically aggressive course and relative hormonal insensitivity.[24] These investigators showed that 14% of aneuploid tumors exhibited hormone responsiveness as compared with 93% of diploid or tetraploid tumors.

Schmidt and coworkers found that low hemoglobin levels are an adverse prognostic sign for survival in patients with prostatic cancer.[21] In addition, serum testosterone levels <300 ng/dL impaired performance status (ECOG performance status of 2 to 4), or more than six sites of metastases as revealed by bone scan have been associated with decreased time to progression and survival.[25] Patients with elevated acid phosphatase levels that failed to normalize or to approach 50% of pretreatment levels also were found to have a poor prognosis.[6] PSA changes after the initiation of hormonal therapy are predictive of response in patients with stage D2 prostate cancer. Miller et al found that a decrease of PSA to normal levels (<4.0 ng/mL by Tandem R assay) correlates with a 36-month mean survival, while mean survival in patients with persistently elevated PSA values (>4.0 ng/mL) was 16 months.[26]

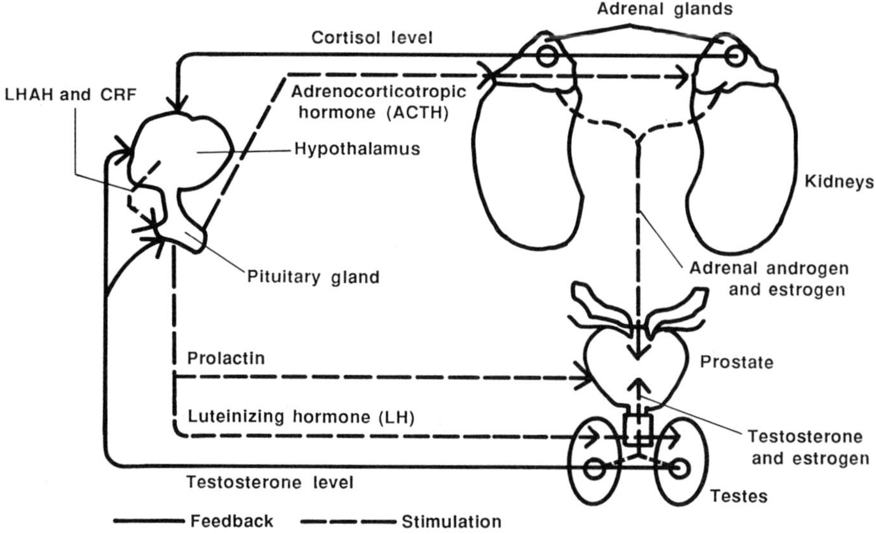


**Fig 5.** Hypothalamic-pituitary-testicular axis. [From Crawford ED and Davis MA; unpublished data (1991).]

| **TABLE 2. Prognostic Factors in Metastatic Prostate Cancer** |
|---|
| • Histologic grade<br>• DNA ploidy<br>• Hemoglobin level<br>• Pretreatment testosterone levels<br>• Performance status<br>• Extent of bony metastases<br>• Changes in pre- & posttreatment acid phosphatase levels<br>• Changes in pre- & posttreatment PSA levels<br>• Nuclear androgen receptor content |

Trachtenberg and Walsh measured the number of androgen receptors in the cytosol and nucleus as well as total androgen receptors in 23 previously untreated patients with stage D prostate cancer.[27] No correlation was found between androgen-receptor content and histologic tumor grade. However, a significant correlation was observed between nuclear androgen-receptor content and the duration of response and survival. Patients with receptor values <110 fmol/mg DNA were found to have a mean duration of response of 7 months; all experienced relapse within 1 year and mean survival was 15 months. In contrast, patients with receptor values >110 fmol/mg DNA had a mean duration of response of 17 months and mean survival of 25 months. While not clinically useful at present, these results indicate future avenues of investigation to determine which patients will respond to hormonal therapy. Those who will not respond to hormonal therapy will require other forms of therapy.

## Androgen Production and Effect

**Hypothalamic-Pituitary-Testicular Axis.** The hypothalamic-pituitary-testicular axis is responsible for testosterone production in the adult male (Fig 5). Reduced levels of serum testosterone (T) stimulate the arcuate nucleus of the hypothalamus to release luteinizing-hormone–releasing hormone (LHRH). LHRH is transported to the pituitary gland, where it stimulates the release of luteinizing hormone (LH). Next, LH is transported to the Leydig cells of the testes, where it initiates the synthesis and release of T. T then produces feedback inhibition of the production and release of LHRH in the hypothalamus.[28] Approximately 90% of circulating T is produced by the testes. The remainder of the circulating T is produced by the adrenal gland. Almost half (44%) of the circulating T is bound to sex-steroid–binding globulin,

54% is bound to albumin and other proteins, while 2% remains unbound and active.[29]

The role of adrenal androgens in prostate cancer is not clear. The testes account for 90% of androgen production. The adrenals are responsible for the remaining androgen production in the form of androstenedione and dehydroepiandrosterone (DHEA). After medical or surgical castration, circulating levels of androgens persist and dihydrotestosterone (DHT) remains detectable in the prostate tissue.[30] These androgens are thought to be responsible for further stimulation of the cancer cells after castration.[31]

**Effect of Testosterone in the Prostate.** Unbound testosterone passively diffuses through the prostate cell membrane into the cytoplasm. T is then converted into dihydrotestosterone (DHT) by the enzyme 5α-reductase.

DHT diffuses into the nucleus and binds to its receptor. DHT-receptor complex then attaches to acceptor sites on DNA and initiates the transcription of mRNA, which leads to protein synthesis and cell growth.[32,33]

## Methods of Hormonal Therapy

Androgen deprivation can be accomplished in four ways:

1) Orchiectomy and removal of the major source of T.
2) Interruption of the hypothalamic-pituitary-testicular axis.
3) Inhibition of cellular binding of T.
4) Direct inhibition of androgen synthesis.

### Methods of Androgen Deprivation

***Orchiectomy.*** Orchiectomy continues to represent the gold standard of hormonal ablation to which all other forms of hormonal therapy are compared. Removal of the testes results in a 90% reduction in circulating T in 3 hours. After orchiectomy, T levels are reduced to 10 to 50 ng/100 mL.[34] Orchiectomy offers the following advantages over other forms of androgen deprivation: 1) patient compliance, 2) reduced cost as compared with long-term medical castration, and 3) the reduction in T is almost immediate and is prolonged. Adverse effects include psychological trauma, hot flashes, and impotence. Infection and bleeding are infrequently seen.

Subcapsular or subepididymal orchiectomy may be performed, with removal of all androgen-producing tissue. Subepididymal orchiectomy is easily performed with local or regional anaesthesia using a transcrotal incision. After the testis is delivered through the wound, the attachments between the epididymis and testis are divided with electrocautery. Any bleeding points are controlled with cautery or ligatures. The visceral tunica vaginalis is approximated over the exposed edge of the epididymis. This procedure is usually performed on an outpatient basis. The continued sensation of the tunica albuginea or epididymis in the scrotum helps reduce the psychological trauma of orchiectomy.

***Interruption of the Hypothalamic-Pituitary-Testicular Axis.*** Two main classes of compounds are currently in use to disrupt this axis: estrogens and related compounds and LHRH agonists.

ESTROGENS. Estrogens have been known to reduce acid phosphatase levels and, by inference, prostate cancer, since Huggins and Hodges injected estrogen into men with metastatic prostate cancer and measured the responses.[17] Estrogens affect the progression of prostatic cancer by a number of mechanisms:

1) Binding to T receptors in the hypothalamus and inhibiting the release of LHRH.
2) Increasing levels of sex-steroid–binding globulin and decreasing the level of free T.
3) Interfering with 5α-reductase and reducing the levels of DHT.
4) Interfering with the binding of DHT to the androgen receptor.[35]

Estrogens also promote release of prolactin, which enhances the transport of T into prostate cells. Animal studies also suggest that estrogens may stimulate prostatic growth. With the doses used clinically, direct excitatory effects on the prostate are not seen.[36]

The most commonly used estrogen is diethylstilbestrol (DES). DES is available as an oral preparation that is simple to use, and eliminates the need for surgery. Other estrogens are available, including Premarin, ethinyl estradiol and chlorotrianisene (TACE) in oral form; polyestradiol phosphate (Estradurin) for intramuscular depot administration every 3 to 4 weeks; and DES diphosphate (Stilphostrol) for IV use.[30,37] DES in a dose of 3 mg per day will produce castrate levels of testosterone in 7 to 21 days.[18]

Estramustine phosphate is formed when nitrogen mustard is linked to phosphorylated estradiol; reports have shown that 50% of patients with hormone-refractory prostate cancer will respond to this drug.[36] However, no advantage has been shown with this compound vs other estrogens in the survival of untreated patients or in patients with progression of disease despite hormone therapy.[36]

Many side effects are associated with estrogen therapy, including nausea, vomiting, fluid retention, gynecomastia, loss of libido, azoospermia, and impotence. Gynecomastia can be prevented by utilizing pretreatment breast radiation with 800 to 1500 rads.[38] The most serious side effect associated with the use of estrogens is the increased incidence of cardiovascular complications, including myocardial infarction, cerebrovascular accident, deep venous thrombosis, congestive heart failure, and peripheral vascular disease. Cardiovascular complications were observed in 25% of patients with prostate cancer who were treated with estrogen during the first year of therapy, as opposed to no patients treated with orchiectomy.[39] This complication was first described in the VACURG study in patients receiving high-dose (5 mg/d) estrogen therapy.[40] Lower doses (1 mg/d) were not associated with increased side effects; however, incomplete androgen suppression occurred in some patients.[41] A dose of 3 mg DES has been shown to be associated with approximately the same cardiovascular risks as a 1 mg dose of DES; however, the higher dose more reliably reduces the T level to the anorchic state.[38] Because of the increased cardiovascular risks and the availability of other nonsurgical forms of testosterone suppression, the use of estrogens is less common today than in the past.

LHRH Agonists. LHRH is a decapeptide which was first identified and synthesized in the early 1970s.[42] Since then, analogues have been produced with greater than 100 times the potency of the naturally occurring compound by substituting amino acids at the 6, 9, and 10 positions of the natural molecule.[30]

The arcuate nucleus of the hypothalamus is the major source of LHRH, and it releases LHRH every 60 to 90 minutes in a pulsatile manner. These pulses stimulate the pituitary gland to release LH.[28] Administration of LHRH agonists such as leuprolide, goserelin, nafarelin, or buserelin initially produces a surge of LH release and subsequent T production. This "flare" period lasts approximately 1 week. After the fourth week of treatment, castrate levels of T are achieved and remain as long as the therapy is continued.[20]

The advantages of therapy with LHRH agonists as compared with DES are that LHRH agonists do not produce peripheral edema, gynecomastia, and cardiovascular side effects. The major side effects associated with LHRH agonists are the flare period, hot flashes, and impotence.[20] These agents also require parenteral administration. The flare associated with LHRH agonists is usually not significant; however, patients with impending spinal cord compression or ureteral obstruction may progress with the flare to paraplegia or complete ureteral obstruction. In these cases, another form of androgen deprivation, either orchiectomy or combination therapy with an antiandrogen, is indicated.[37,43–45]

According to the results of several randomized, multicenter comparative trials, the safety and efficacy of LHRH agonists is comparable to that of orchiectomy and may be greater than that of estrogen therapy. In 1984, a multicenter, prospective, randomized trial compared the effects of leuprolide and DES in 199 patients with untreated stage D2 carcinoma of the prostate.[20] Serum testosterone reductions were delayed in the leuprolide-treated group, but anorchic levels were achieved by week 4.

Reductions in acid phosphatase levels were also delayed in the leuprolide group, but by week 12, there was no difference in PAP levels between the study groups. Objective response rates were 85% for the DES group as compared with 86% in the leuprolide group. Median times to disease progression were similar in both groups, and after 1 year, 87% of patients who received leuprolide were alive vs 78% of those who received DES. DES-treated patients had significantly higher incidences of peripheral edema, nausea, vomiting, and gynecomastia. In addition, there was a trend toward more serious complications such as venous thrombosis, pulmonary embolism and phlebitis in DES-treated patients, but the trend was not statistically significant. Patients receiving leuprolide had a significantly greater incidence of hot flashes.

Goserelin was compared to orchiectomy in a multicenter, randomized study of 292 patients.[46] Response rates were equivalent: 89% of patients in the goserelin group responded as compared with 94% of those in the orchiectomy group. No significant difference was noted in time to disease progression or survival rates. Buserelin and orchiectomy were compared in 59 patients with stage D2 prostate cancer. After 8 weeks of therapy, no difference was found in the serum T levels between the treatment groups. Response rates were similar; 94% of patients treated with orchiectomy responded vs 93% of those who received buserelin. Relapse rates and death rates were also equivalent.[19]

LHRH agonists are peptides and break down when administered orally. In the past, nasal sprays and daily injections have been used, but this frequent administration may result in reduced compliance. In addition, nasal agents may be poorly absorbed, limiting their usefulness.[43,44] New formulations have been developed which require monthly injections, and new dosage forms are being tested to reduce the frequency of injection to every 3 months. A biodegradable, biocompatible matrix of lactide-glycolide copolymer containing 10.8 mg of goserelin can be given by injection once every 3 months, and has been shown to produce responses comparable to the 1-month depot of 3.6 mg of goserelin in patients with advanced prostate cancer.[47]

***Inhibition of Cellular Binding of T.*** Antiandrogens are another weapon in the armamentarium of drugs for hormonal therapy of adenocarcinoma of the prostate. There are two types of antiandrogens: steroidal and nonsteroidal. Both classes of antiandrogens have demonstrable activity against prostate cancer.

Steroid antiandrogens are represented by three compounds: cyproterone acetate (CPA), medroxyprogesterone acetate, and megesterol acetate (Megace). These progestational agents have both central and peripheral actions.

CPA is a synthetic 21-carbon hydroxyprogesterone derivative with many modes of action. At doses of 200 mg per day, CPA causes a decrease in LH release, thereby reducing T production. This effect diminishes after several months, leaving only peripheral effects. When given in combination, DES (0.1 mg per day) plus CPA induces castrate levels of T. This synergistic activity continues throughout treatment, and no late rise of T is noted.[48]

The predominant action of CPA is the competitive inhibition of DHT binding to androgen receptors. Such inhibition results in marked reduction of DHT/nuclear androgen-receptor complexes, and androgen-dependent DNA and RNA synthesis is inhibited. Protein synthesis is reduced, and cells become senescent and die.[22] The response rates to CPA therapy are similar to those reported with orchiectomy or estrogen therapy in patients with prostate cancer.[22] The side effects associated with steroidal antiandrogens include gynecomastia, fluid retention, impotence, and a 10% incidence of cardiovascular complications.[44] The salt and water retention associated with CPA was less than that observed with DES; therefore, the risk of congestive heart failure is less for patients treated with CPA.[22]

The mechanism of action of Megace is similar to that of CPA. The rise in plasma T reported in patients undergoing long-term megesterol therapy at doses of 120 mg per day is also blocked with low-dose (0.1 mg/

day) DES. Response rates are equivalent to those of orchiectomy or estrogen therapy, and side effects are lower as compared with DES.[49]

Nonsteroidal antiandrogens such as flutamide, nilutamide, and ICI 176,334 (Casodex), have no steroidal activity and therefore no central activity. These compounds have potent antiandrogen effects, but no other hormonal activity. It is thought that these agents act by inhibiting DHT binding by androgen binding sites in the prostate cell.[50,51] In humans, serum T and LH levels rise with antiandrogen therapy and plasma T levels are not decreased. Some investigators have reported a rise in plasma testosterone following flutamide therapy.[35] This effect was not seen with Casodex.[50]

Flutamide is a synthetic nonsteroidal antiandrogen approved for use in the United States. During the first passage through the liver, it is metabolized to the active metabolite, 2-hydroxyflutamide.[52] The current recommended dosage is 250 mg three times per day. Side effects associated with flutamide include diarrhea, flushing, and occasional reversible hepatotoxicity. Gynecomastia has also been reported, and is related to the increased LH and T levels associated with flutamide monotherapy. Increased levels of T lead to increased aromatization to estradiol, which produces gynecomastia.

Response rates in patients treated with flutamide alone are comparable to those of orchiectomy in clinical trials, and range between 66% and 85%.[53–55] These compounds offer the advantage of maintenance of potency during monotherapy.[55] In Sogani's series, 86% of men who were potent prior to therapy remained potent throughout the study period.[35] The maintenance or even increase in serum T with treatment is thought to be the mechanism for continued potency with flutamide monotherapy. At present, the only approved use for flutamide in the United States is in combination with LHRH agonist therapy.

Nilutamide is another antiandrogen which, unlike flutamide, does not require conversion to the active metabolite in the liver. It is an effective antiandrogen, and has activity similar to that of flutamide. Nilutamide has been associated with alcohol intolerance, difficulty with visual adaptation to the dark, and several cases of interstitial pneumonitis which resolved on withdrawal of the drug.[44]

Casodex is another nonsteroidal antiandrogen currently undergoing clinical trials. The half-life of Casodex is 6 days. This long half-life allows for daily dosing. In contrast, flutamide has a short half-life, and must be given three times per day.[50] Thus, patient compliance is less of a concern in those patients treated with Casodex. Even if the patient misses a dose of Casodex, serum concentrations remain until the next dose and sufficient antiandrogen activity is available to antagonize the effects of the patient's androgens.[56] Preliminary results from the clinical trials indicate that Casodex produces response rates similar to those of standard hormonal therapy.[57] Survival data is not available, however, as the studies have not yet sufficiently matured. The most common side effects associated with Casodex therapy are breast swelling and tenderness (reported to occur in 50% of patients) and hot flashes (reported to occur in 20% of patients). Impotence was reported in fewer than 5% of patients.[57] Phase III trials are in progress to compare Casodex to orchiectomy and LHRH agonists.

***Inhibitors of Steroid Synthesis.*** Aminoglutethimide, ketoconazole, and spironolactone inhibit multiple enzymes in steroid synthetic pathways and block the production of T by blocking the cytochrome P-450 system.[58]

Aminoglutethimide is a potent inhibitor of adrenal steroidogenesis. It blocks several enzymes of the cytochrome P-450 pathway, including the conversion of cholesterol to pregnenolone, and the hydroxylation of desoxycortisol, cortisol, and corticosterone.[35] When used therapeutically, corticosteroids must be given concomitantly to prevent hypoadrenalism and to interrupt the stimulation of adrenocorticotropic hormone.[18] Nausea occurs in many patients during therapy with aminoglutethimide.

Aminoglutethimide has been used primarily in patients with disease progression despite previous hormonal therapy. Crawford et al treated 129 patients with prostate cancer whose disease progressed despite hormonal therapy, and Drago et al reported the results of treatment of 43 patients with aminoglutethimide.[59,60] Response rates of 40% were noted in these patients. However, some authors felt these responses were due to the effects of the glucocorticoid replacement alone.[61]

Ketoconazole is an imidazole derivative which becomes active after oral administration. Ketoconazole inhibits the 17–20 desmolase and 17-hydroxylase enzymes of the steroid synthesis pathway.[43,58] Patients administered ketoconazole (400 mg every 8 hours) were found to achieve castrate levels of T in 4 to 8 hours.[58] A reduction of 75% of adrenal androgen production was also noted.[35] Ketoconazole has also been used to block the flare associated with LHRH agonists. Side effects associated with ketoconazole include hypoadrenalism, nausea, and rare instances of hepatotoxicity.[58]

Marked subjective responses in patients who had previously undergone hormonal therapy have been reported.[62] This effect may be mediated by other cytochrome P-450–dependent intracellular systems. A significant cytostatic effect of ketoconazole was noted in vitro using androgen-independent prostate cancer-cell lines which were exposed to clinical therapeutic concentrations. Newer analogues of ketoconazole, with more specific and longer durations of action, are being investigated.[58,63]

***Total Androgen Suppression.*** The adrenal androgens, DHEA and androstenedione, are converted peripherally to T and DHT. Harper et al reported that adrenal androgens contribute between 16% and 20% of the total DHT in the prostate.[64] Up to 50% of intraprostatic DHT remains after orchiectomy, estrogen, or LHRH therapy.[30] Thus, even though 90% of circulating T is removed, a significant level of DHT remains in prostatic tissue.

The possible role of adrenal androgens in metastatic prostate cancer was first investigated by Huggins and Scott in 1945 when they performed bilateral adrenalectomy on four patients. Unfortunately, all four patients died of adrenal insufficiency.[65] Miller and Hinman published their results of "medical adrenalectomy" in 1954.[66] Patients who had failed previous hormonal therapy were given 50 mg cortisone daily in four divided doses. These doses were titrated to effect. Most of the salutory effects were noted at the initial dose. A few patients received 100 mg cortisone per day, and one patient received 200 mg cortisone per day for a prolonged period. The results of oral cortisone administration were compared with results from 26 patients from four institutions who had undergone bilateral surgical adrenal removal. The authors reported "clinical remission" in 8 of 10 patients receiving cortisone. Of the 22 patients who were evaluated after undergoing bilateral adrenalectomy, 20 were judged to have achieved clinical remission. The other four surgical patients died of postoperative complications. The length of remission in patients treated with cortisone was short, ranging from 17 to 180 days (average 82 days), and was comparable to those who received bilateral adrenalectomy.[66] It should be noted that this investigation was performed in an era without bone scans, and the ability of the investigators to objectively evaluate treatment response was limited.

Approximately 30% of patients with advanced prostate cancer who develop disease progression after initial ablation of gonadal androgen respond to surgical or medical adrenalectomy.[35]

The first hypophysectomy for metastatic prostate cancer was performed in 1948. Hypophysectomy has been shown to produce objective remissions in patients previously considered to be nonresponders. However, these responses have been of short duration.[67]

Two theories exist to explain the clinical relapse that most patients experience after conventional androgen deprivation with orchiectomy or estrogen therapy. One theory proposes that prostate cancer cells are heterogeneous in their growth requirements for androgens. According to this theory, relapse occurs when the population of androgen-insensitive cells grow to a critical size after hormone therapy. This suggests that further androgen blockade, specifically adrenal androgen blockade, would have little effect on response or survival. The other theory suggests that cancer cells are capable of adapting to survive in androgen-poor environments.

Coffey and Issacs studied Dunning R-3327 rats with prostatic adenocarcinomas, and reported a heterogeneous cell composition within the tumor.[68] Approximately 80% of cells were found to be androgen sensitive while the remaining 20% were androgen insensitive. These researchers proposed that the relapse of prostate cancer that follows castration occurs as a result of continued growth of the androgen-insensitive cell lines. Mechanisms by which this may occur include genetic instability or multifocal tumor origin. The idea of genetic instability assumes that the cancer began as a single cell, and that as growth continued, the progeny cells became unstable and developed into a wide variety of cell types with different DNA. Thus, certain tumor-cell properties become altered, including hormonal responsiveness. A multifocal origin of cancer cells may also account for different growth-factor requirements. Multifocal tumors have been noted in radical prostatectomy specimens examined by whole-mount techniques, and may have different grades and biologic potentials. This heterogeneity in the primary prostatic tumor can lead to many cell lines with differing responses to therapy.

On the other hand, environmental pressures may produce adaptations in tumor cells such that the cells remain differentiated and require androgens for full growth while androgens are present. When androgens are removed from the tumor cell's environment, the cells undergo adaptations that enable them to continue to grow. Preincubation of androgen-sensitive, Shionogi mouse mammary cancer cells for 15 days in the absence of androgens causes the development of a cell line that is resistant to the effects of androgens (Fig 6).[69] However, androgen sensitivity is maintained by incubation of these cells with flutamide, which implies that the administration of antiandrogens might preclude or delay the development of androgen resistance and improve the response to androgen withdrawal.

This theory forms the basis for total androgen suppression: lowering serum T to castrate levels and blocking the adrenal androgens with antiandrogens may reduce the adaptation of hormone-resistant clones. As previously mentioned, a significant amount of DHT from the adrenal glands is found in prostate cancer cells after orchiectomy or estrogen treatment. However, the lowest amount of androgen capable of stimulating human prostate tumor growth is not known. Thus, the goal of total androgen suppression is the removal of all gonadal and adrenal androgens from the prostate tumor cell to further retard growth.

Labrie has been one of the most strident advocates of complete androgen blockade, and has utilized medical or surgical castration combined with a nonsteroidal an-

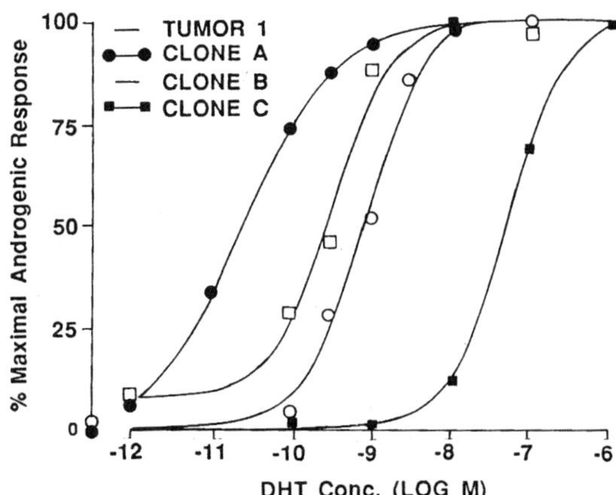


**Fig 6.** Effect of increasing concentrations of DHT on the maximal androgenic response (DNA content) in the three clones obtained from a Shionogi mouse mammary tumor. To facilitate visualization of differences in androgen sensitivity, all data are expressed as a percentage of the maximal response to DHT. [From Labrie F, Veilleux R, A wide range of sensitivities to androgens developed in cloned Shionogi mouse mammary tumor cells, *Prostate* (1986;8:296), with permission from Wiley-Liss, A Division of John Wiley & Sons, Inc.]

tiandrogen to achieve complete androgen suppression.[70] In 1987, Labrie and colleagues reported encouraging results from an uncontrolled study of patients with metastatic disease. Patients with stage D2 carcinoma of the prostate (N = 154) were treated with the combination of leuprolide and flutamide for an average of 22 months. Using five previously published studies as controls, Labrie et al reported complete response rates (according to NPCP criteria) of 29.2%. This result is 6.3 times greater than the response rate (4.6%) achieved in the control studies. Only 4.5% of the patients receiving combined therapy did not respond, as compared with 18% of patients who received monotherapy. In addition, duration of response was longer in patients who received combination therapy.[70]

In 1985, the National Cancer Institute sponsored a large intergroup study of patients with stage D2 adenocarcinoma of the prostate that compared leuprolide monotherapy to combined leuprolide and flutamide therapy (Fig 7). The study was double-blinded and randomized. After 3 years, patients in the combination treatment arm showed a statistically significant increase in time to disease progression and survival. These advantages were most pronounced among patients with minimal disease and good performance status.[71] Flutamide was shown to exert the greatest effects during the first 3 months of study. A reasonable explanation for this unexpected finding may be that the improvement observed in patients in the two treatment arms was due to the early prevention of disease progression by flutamide. The best responses were seen in patients with minimal disease and good performance status, with median survival in this group not yet reached after 60 months.

Denis et al evaluated the safety and efficacy of orchiectomy as compared with that of Zoladex and flutamide in 327 patients with metastatic prostate cancer.[72] The mean period of follow-up was 2.5 years. These investigators found that time to disease progression was greater in patients in the combination therapy group, but reported no difference in survival rates between the groups. Iversen et al studied 262 patients with untreated advanced carcinoma of the prostate who also received either orchiectomy or Zoladex and flutamide.[73] The median period of follow-up in this study was 39 months. In contrast to Denis et al, these researchers found no differences in time to disease progression or survival between the two treatment groups.

Beland et al compared the effects of orchiectomy plus nilutamide with those of orchiectomy alone in 208 patients.[74] No statistically significant difference in time to progression or survival was observed between the two groups. However, median survival in nilutamide-treated patients was 5.4 months longer (24.3 versus 18.9 months); statistical significance may develop as the follow-up period lengthens. The study design allowed the administration of nilutamide to patients in the orchiectomy monotherapy group after evidence of disease progression developed. This may interfere with obtaining statistically significant differences in results.

Additional multicenter, randomized trials are now in progress to further clarify this issue.

## Radiotherapy

Radiation therapy has been used to treat prostate cancer for many years, and patients with metastatic prostate cancer can benefit from this type of therapy in a number of ways. Local radiation therapy to areas of painful metastases (usually bony sites) often results in palliation of the pain.

Hemibody radiation therapy may be used in patients who have previously received treatment with hormonal therapy and who have numerous sites of painful bony metastases, as radiotherapy to each individual site of metastasis would necessitate several weeks of treatment. Hemibody radiation was initially described in the 1970s. The maximum dose of total-body radiation may not exceed 300 cGy because of the risk of lethal bone marrow damage. Hemibody radiation protects the unirradiated bone marrow and allows repopulation of the treated areas. Radiation therapy at doses of 600 to 800 cGy will result in a cell kill of one to three logs. This amount of cell kill results in pain relief that lasts an average of 5 to

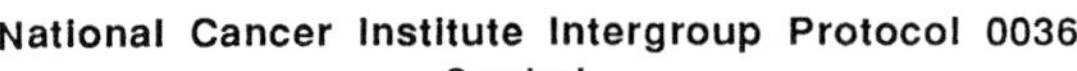


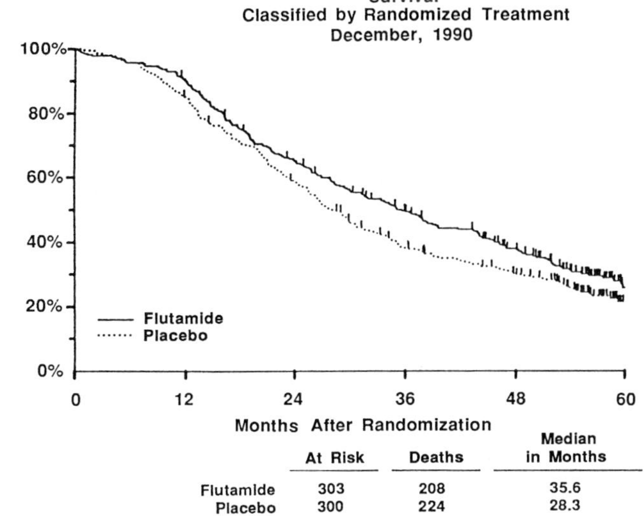


| | At Risk | Deaths | Median in Months |
|---|---|---|---|
| Flutamide | 303 | 208 | 35.6 |
| Placebo | 300 | 224 | 28.3 |

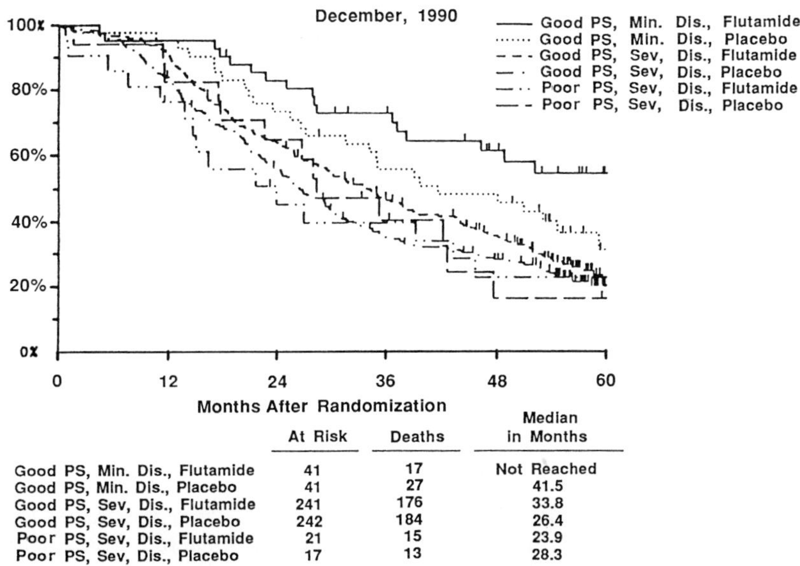


| | At Risk | Deaths | Median in Months |
|---|---|---|---|
| Good PS, Min. Dis., Flutamide | 41 | 17 | Not Reached |
| Good PS, Min. Dis., Placebo | 41 | 27 | 41.5 |
| Good PS, Sev, Dis., Flutamide | 241 | 176 | 33.8 |
| Good PS, Sev, Dis., Placebo | 242 | 184 | 26.4 |
| Poor PS, Sev, Dis., Flutamide | 21 | 15 | 23.9 |
| Poor PS, Sev, Dis., Placebo | 17 | 13 | 28.3 |

**Fig 7.** A, survival of patients from intergroup study 0036: leuprolide and placebo vs leuprolide and flutamide; B, survival of patients from intergroup study 0036 stratified by performance status, amount of disease, and randomized treatment.

6 months. The treatment can be given to the other half of the body 4 to 6 weeks after the initial treatment if the blood counts have returned to baseline levels.

Side effects include acute radiation syndrome, which is similar to a stress reaction caused by a lack of adrenal reserve. It usually appears in 1 to 2 hours and resolves in 8 to 10 hours, and most commonly occurs after radiation of the upper half of the body. Other toxicities include bone marrow suppression and radiation pneumonitis.[75]

## Cytotoxic Chemotherapy

Hormonal manipulation is the first line of therapy for patients with prostate cancer; once hormonal therapy has failed, median survival is 6 months.[76] There are few alternatives for patients who do not respond to hormonal therapy, and any responses achieved after the tumor has become refractory to hormones are usually of short duration.[59,62,76] Cytotoxic chemotherapy is usually reserved for use in hormone-refractory patients because of the low morbidity associated with hormonal therapy and the toxic side effects of cytotoxic chemotherapy. In addition, the results of cytotoxic chemotherapy when treating patients with metastatic prostate cancer have been disappointing.

In the mid-1970s, the NPCP began to evaluate chemotherapeutic agents alone and in combination in multicenter, randomized trials. Unfortunately, objective responses were observed in fewer than 10% of patients, and median survival was identical between experimental and control groups.[77] These results were later confirmed by Eisenberger and coworkers, who recently reviewed the results of uncontrolled, single-agent and multiagent trials of cytotoxic chemotherapy, and found the objective response rate to be 7.5%.[78] Stable disease was reported in 8% of patients (Fig 8). However, the total objective response rate is probably lower because not all responses were judged according to NPCP criteria. Even when responses were noted, there was no significant impact on survival.

Chemotherapy has also been attempted in concert with hormonal therapy. A Southwestern Oncology Group (SWOG) trial of endocrine therapy combined with either initial chemotherapy or chemotherapy at the time of disease progression was recently completed.[79] Patients initially treated with combination therapy had a slightly higher initial response rate, but the time to disease progression and survival were the same for both groups. Chemotherapy has been attempted following androgen stimulation of the tumor, to enhance the response.[80] Responses were found to be similar in both groups and survival was unaffected.

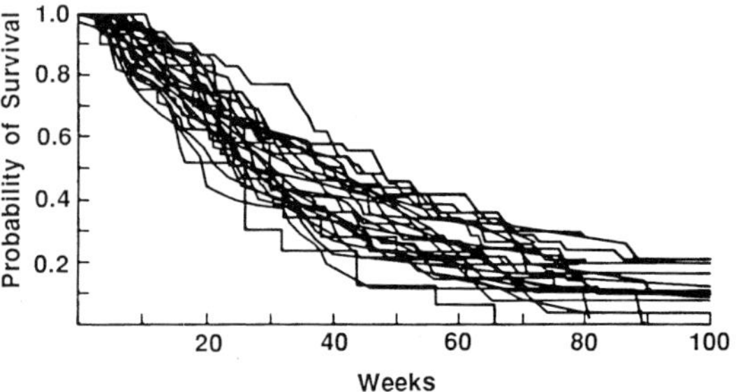


**Fig 8.** Survival curves from all studies with 20 or more patients with hormone-refractory prostate cancer who received cytotoxic chemotherapy. [From Eisenberger MA, Bezerdjian L, Kalash S, A critical assessment of the role of chemotherapy for endocrine resistant prostatic carcinoma, *Urol Clin North Am* (1987;14(4):703), with permission.]

There are many reasons for this dismal experience. Most patients who receive chemotherapy have already received extensive treatment and have extensive disease. Performance status is also usually impaired in patients with progressive metastatic disease. Extensive pretreatment, extensive disease, and diminished performance status have all been shown to be adverse prognostic factors for outcome in other, more chemosensitive tumors, and there is no reason to expect any different effect of these factors on outcome in prostate cancer.[22]

## Immunotherapy

Immunotherapy has been used in patients with prostate cancer since 1962, when Johnston administered Coley's toxin to a patient who had symptomatic relief until the tumor recurred.[81] Subsequent investigators have used bacillus Calmette-Guerin (BCG), administered both systemically and intralesionally, with poor results.[81]

Biologic response modifiers have been investigated for use in metastatic prostate cancer. The response of prostate cancer to interferons has been mixed. α- and β-interferon have been studied in vitro on prostate cancer cell lines PC-3 and DU-145, and produced reductions in cell growth.[82,83] Steroid receptor content was also reduced after interferon therapy, and this reduction may allow the use of interferon to regulate cell proliferation and hormone sensitivity.[83] In a 1991 study, γ-interferon and tumor necrosis factor were combined in the treatment of Dunning rat prostate cancers. Significant antiproliferative effects were noted, and survival was increased in the combination treatment group.[84]

The clinical experience with interferon has not been as encouraging. β-interferon was used in patients who had failed to respond to previous hormonal therapy. No regression of tumor was noted but three of 16 patients treated had stable disease. Side effects of chills and fever were noted in 10 of the 16 patients.[85]

The use of combination immunotherapy and chemotherapy has been studied in the laboratory. Hybrid monoclonal antibodies which recognize specific prostatic antigens were bound to the cellular toxin ricin. This conjugated antibody toxin, when used in combination with vinblastine or bleomycin chemotherapy, resulted in increased cell death.[86]

Investigations into other forms and combinations of immunotherapy, such as the use of tumor-infiltrating lymphocytes, monoclonal antibodies, and various growth factors, are in progress. The clinical utility of these agents is still being defined, but possible uses include directed therapy against metastatic deposits and an imaging modality to detect microscopic metastases.

## REFERENCES


1. Boring CC, Squires TT, Tong T. Cancer statistics, 1991. *CA.* 1991;41:19–37.
2. Jones WG. Is there a place for chemotherapy on advanced prostatic cancer. *Am J Clin Oncol.* 1988;11(suppl 2):S98–S100.
3. McCullough DL. Diagnosis and staging of prostatic cancer. In: Skinner DG, Lieskovsky G, eds. *Diagnosis and Management of Genitourinary Cancer.* Philadelphia: WB Saunders; 1988;405–416.
4. Weaver RP, Noble MJ, Wergel JW. Correlation of ultrasound guided and digitally directed transrectal biopsies of palpable prostatic abnormalities. *J Urol.* 1991;145:516–518.
5. Narayan P, Jajodia P, Stein R. Core biopsy instrument in the diagnosis of prostate cancer: superior accuracy to fine needle aspiration. *J Urol.* 1991;145:795–797.
6. Kozlowski JM, Grayhack JT. Carcinoma of the prostate. In: Gillenwater JY, Grahack JT, et al, eds. *Adult and Pediatric Urology.* Chicago: Year Book Medical Publishers; 1987:1126–1219.
7. Lightner DJ, Lange PH. Tumor markers in the management of urologic neoplasm. *AUA Update Series.* 1987;6:lesson 36.
8. Wang MC, Papsidero LD, Kuriyama M, Valenzuela LA, Murphy GP. Prostate antigen: a new potential marker for prostatic cancer. *Prostate.* 1981;2:89–96.
9. Partin AW, Carter HB, Chan DW, et al. Prostate specific antigen in the staging of localized prostate cancer: influence of tumor differentiation, tumor volume and benign hyperplasia. *J Urol.* 1990;143:747–752.
10. Chybowski FM, Larson Keller JJ, Bergstralh EJ, Oesterling JE. Predicting radionuclide bone scan findings in patients with newly diagnosed, untreated prostate cancer: prostate specific antigen is superior to all other clinical parameters. *J Urol.* 1991;145:313–318.
11. McCarthy P, Pollack HM. Imaging of patients with stage D prostatic carcinoma. *Urol Clin North Am.* 1991;18:35–54.
12. Spirnak JP, Resnick MI. Clinical staging of prostatic cancer: new modalities. *Urol Clin North Am.* 1984;11:221–235.
13. Whitmore WF. Natural history and staging of prostate cancer. *Urol Clin North Am.* 1984; 11:205–220.
14. Wajsman Z, Klimberg IW. Staging evaluation and follow up of patients with advanced prostatic carcinoma. *Semin Urol.* 1988;4:249–261.
15. Saitoh H, Hida M, Shimbo T, Nakamura K, Yamagata J, Satoh T. Metastatic patterns of prostate cancer: correlation between the sites and number of organs involved. *Cancer.* 1984; 54:3078–3084.
16. Flynn DF, Shipley WU. Management of spinal cord compression secondary to metastatic prostatic carcinoma. *Urol Clin North Am.* 1991; 18:145–152.
17. Huggins C, Hodges CV. Studies on prostatic cancer. 1. The effect of castration, of estrogen and of androgen injection on serum phosphatases in metastatic carcinoma of the prostate. *Cancer Res.* 1941;1:293–297.
18. Crawford ED, Nabors W. Hormone therapy of advanced prostate cancer: where we stand today. *Oncology.* 1991;5:21–37.

19. Koutsilieris M, Faure N, Tolis G, Laroche B, Robert G, Ackman CFD. Objective response and disease outcome in 59 patients with stage D2 prostatic cancer treated with either buserelin or orchiectomy. *Urology*. 1986;27:221–228.

20. The Leuprolide Study Group. Leuprolide versus diethylstilbestrol for metastatic prostate cancer. *N Engl J Med*. 1984;311:1281–1286.

21. Schmidt JD, Johnson DE, Scott WW, et al. Chemotherapy of advanced prostatic cancer. *Urology*. 1976;7:602–610.

22. Eisenberger MA, Abrams JS. Chemotherapy for prostatic carcinoma. *Semin Urol*. 1988;4:303–310.

23. Gleason DF, Mellinger GT, The Veterans Administration Cooperative Urological Research Group. Prediction of prognosis for prostatic adenocarcinoma by combined histologic grading and clinical staging. *J Urol*. 1974;111:58–64.

24. Tavares AS, Costa J, Costa Maia J. Correlation between ploidy and prognosis in prostatic carcinoma. *J Urol*. 1973;109:676–679.

25. Soloway MS. The importance of pretreatment testosterone and other prognostic variables in the response to androgen deprivation therapy. In: Frohmuller HGW, Wirth MP, eds. *Uro-Oncology: Current Status and Future Trends*. New York: Wiley-Liss; 1990;141–148.

26. Miller JI, Ahmann FR, Drach GW, Bottaccini MR. PSA levels predict duration of remission and survival post hormone therapy of metastatic prostate cancer. *J Urol*. 1991;145:384A. Abstract.

27. Trachtenberg J, Walsh PC. Correlation of prostatic nuclear androgen receptor content with duration of response and survival following hormonal therapy in advanced prostatic cancer. *J Urol*. 1982;127:466–471.

28. Vigersky RA. Pituitary-testicular axis. In: Lipshultz LI, Howards SS, eds. *Infertility in the Male*. New York: Churchill Livingstone; 1983;19–41.

29. McClure RD. Endocrine investigation and therapy. *Urol Clin North Am*. 1987;14:417–488.

30. Nabors W, Crawford ED. Metastatic prostate cancer hormonal treatment. *World J Urol*. 1990;8:34–39.

31. McConnell JD. Physiologic basis of endocrine therapy for prostatic cancer. *Urol Clin North Am*. 1991;18:1–13.

32. Quarmby VE, Kemppainen JA, Sar M, Lubahn DB, French FS. Expression of recombinant androgen receptor in cultured mammalian cells. *Mol Endocrinol*. 1990;4:1399–1407.

33. Evans RM. The steroid and thyroid hormone receptor superfamily. *Science*. 1988;240:889–895.

34. Maatman TJ, Gupta MK, Montie JE. Effectiveness of castration versus intravenous estrogen therapy in producing rapid endocrine control of metastatic cancer of the prostate. *J Urol*. 1985;133:620–621.

35. Sogani PC, Fair WR. Treatment of advanced prostatic cancer. *Urol Clin North Am*. 1987;14:353–372.

36. Foote JE, Crawford ED. Combined hormonal therapy in the management of adenocarcinoma of the prostate. *Probl Urol*. 1990;4:473–488.

37. Grayhack JT, Keeler TC, Kozlowski JM. Carcinoma of the prostate: hormonal therapy. *Cancer*. 1987;60:589–601.

38. Resnick MI. Hormonal therapy in prostatic carcinoma. *Urology*. 1984;24(suppl 5):18.

39. Henriksson P, Johansson S. Prediction of cardiovascular complications in patients with prostatic cancer treated with estrogen. *Am J Epidemiol*. 1987;125:970–978.

40. Byar CP. The Veterans Administration Cooperative Urological Research Group's studies of cancer of the prostate. *Cancer*. 1973;32:1126–1130.

41. Prout GR, Kliman B, Daly JJ, MacLaughlin RA, Griffin PP, Young HH. Endocrine changes after diethylstilbestrol therapy. Effects on prostatic neoplasm and pituitary gonadal axis. *Urology*. 1976;7:148–155.

42. Schally AV, Nair RMG, Redding TW, Arimura A. Isolation of the luteinizing hormone and follicle stimulating hormone-releasing hormone from the porcine hypothalamus. *J Biol Chem*. 1971;246:7230–7236.

43. Brendler CB. The current role of hormonal therapy in the clinical treatment of prostatic cancer. *Semin Urol*. 1988;4:269–278.

44. Trachtenberg J. Hormonal management of stage D carcinoma of the prostate. *Urol Clin North Am*. 1987;14:685–692.

45. Labrie F, Dupont A, Belanger A, et al. New approach in the treatment of prostate cancer: complete instead of partial withdrawal of androgen. *Prostate*. 1983;4:579–594.

46. Peeling WB. Phase I studies to compare goserelin (zoladex) with orchiectomy and with diethylstilbestrol in the treatment of prostatic carcinoma. *Urology*. 1989;33(suppl):45–52.

47. Dijkman GA, Fernandez del Moral P, Plusman JWMH, et al. A new longer acting LHRH analog depot: preliminary results of a Dutch open phase II clinical study on a 10.8 mg Zoladex 3 monthly depot. *Eur Urol*. 1990;18(suppl 3):22–25.

48. Goldenberg SL, Bruchovsky N. Use of cyproterone acetate in prostate cancer. *Urol Clin North Am*. 1991;18:111–122.

49. Geller J. Megesterol acetate plus low dose estrogen in advanced prostatic carcinoma. *Urol Clin North Am*. 1991;18:83–91.

50. Furr BJA. Casodex: preclinical studies. *Eur Urol*. 1990;18(suppl 3):2–9.

51. Suffrin G, Coffey DS. Flutamide: mechanism of action of a new nonsteroidal antiandrogen. *Invest Urol*. 1976;13:429.

52. Schulz M, Schmoldt A, Donn F, Becker H. The pharmacokinetics of flutamide and its major metabolites after a single oral dose and during

chronic treatment. *Eur J Clin Pharmacol.* 1988;34:633 636.

53. Irwin RJ, Prout GR. A new antiprostatic agent for treatment of prostatic carcinoma. *Surg Forum.* 1973;24:536.

54. Pavone-Macaluso M, Serretta V, et al. Is there a role for pure antiandrogen in the treatment of advanced prostatic carcinoma? In: Frohmuller HGW, Wirth MP, eds. *Uro-Oncology: Current Status and Future Trends.* New York: Wiley-Liss; 1990:149–157.

55. Prout GR, Irwin RJ, Kliman B, Daly JJ, MacLaughlin RA, Griffin PP. Prostatic cancer and SCH-13521. Histological alterations and pituitary gonadal axis. *J Urol.* 1975;113:834–840.

56. Cockshot ID, Cooper KD, Sweetmore DS, Blacklock NJ, Denis L. The pharmacokinetics of casodex in prostate cancer patients after single and during multiple dosing. *Eur Urol.* 1990; 18(suppl 3):10–17.

57. Newling DWW. The response of advanced prostatic cancer to a new non-steroidal anti-androgen: results of a multicenter open phase II study of casodex. *Eur Urol.* 1990;18(suppl 3): 18–21.

58. Trachtenberg J. Hormonal management of stage D carcinoma of the prostate. *AUA Update Series.* 1990;9:lesson 30.

59. Crawford ED, Ahmann FR, Davis MA, Levasseur YJ. Aminoglutethimide in metastatic adenocarcinoma of the prostate. *Prog Clin Biol Res.* 1987;243A:283–288.

60. Drago JR, Santen RJ, Lipton A, et al. Clinical effect of aminoglutethimide medical adrenalectomy in the treatment of 43 patients with advanced prostatic carcinoma. *Cancer.* 1984; 53:1447.

61. Plowman PN, Perry LA, Chard T. Androgen suppression by hydrocortisone without aminoglutethimide in orchiectomized men with prostate cancer. *Br J Urol.* 1987;59:255–257.

62. Gerber GS, Chodak GW. Prostate specific antigen for assessing response to ketoconazole and prednisone in patients with hormone refractory metastatic prostate cancer. *J Urol.* 1990; 144:1177–1179.

63. Trachtenberg J, Pont A. Ketoconazole therapy for advanced prostate cancer. *Lancet.* 1984; 2:433.

64. Harper ME, Pike A, Peeling WB, Griffiths K. Steroids of adrenal origin metabolized by human prostatic tissue both in vivo and in vitro. *J Endocrinol.* 1974;60:117–125.

65. Huggins C, Scott WW. Bilateral adrenalectomy in prostatic cancer: clinical features and urinary excretion of 17-ketosteroids and estrogen. *Ann Surg.* 1945;122:1031.

66. Miller GM, Hinman F Jr. Cortisone treatment in advanced carcinoma of the prostate. *J Urol.* 1954;72:485.

67. Brendler H. Adrenalectomy and hypophysectomy for prostate cancer. *Urology.* 1973;2:99.

68. Coffey DS, Issacs JT. Prostate tumor biology and cell kinetics theory. *Urology.* 1981;27(suppl 3):40–53.

69. Luthy I, Labrie F. Development of androgen resistance in mouse mammary tumor cells can be prevented by the antiandrogen flutamide. *Prostate.* 1987;10:89.

70. Labrie F, Dupont A, Giguere M, et al. Combination therapy with flutamide and castration (orchiectomy or LHRH agonist): the minimal endocrine therapy in both untreated and previously treated patients. *J Steroid Biochem.* 1987;27:525–532.

71. Crawford ED, Eisenberger MA, McLeod DG, et al. A controlled trial of leuprolide with and without flutamide in prostatic carcinoma. *N Engl J Med.* 1987;321:419–424.

72. Denis L, Smith PH, Carniero De Moura JL, et al. Orchiectomy versus Zoladex plus flutamide in patients with metastatic prostate cancer. *Eur Urol.* 1990;18(suppl 3):34–40.

73. Iversen P, Danish Prostatic Cancer Group. Zoladex plus flutamide vs. orchidectomy for advanced prostatic cancer. *Eur Urol.* 1990; 18(suppl 3):41–44.

74. Beland G, Elhilali M, Fradet Y, et al. Total androgen ablation: Canadian experience. *Urol Clin North Am.* 1991:18:75–82.

75. Kuban DA, Schellhammer PF, El-Mahdi AM. Hemibody irradiation in advanced prostatic cancer. *Urol Clin North Am.* 1991;18:131–137.

76. Lyss AP. Systemic treatment for prostate cancer. *Am J Med.* 1987;83:1120–1127.

77. Eisenberger MA, Bezerdjian L, Kalush S. A critical assessment of the role of chemotherapy for endocrine resistant prostate cancer. *Urol Clin North Am.* 1987;14:695–706.

78. Eisenberger MA, Bezerdjian L, Kalush S, et al. A critical assessment of the role of chemotherapy for endocrine resistant prostatic carcinoma. *AUA Update Series.* 1988;7:lesson 28.

79. Osborne CK, Blumenstein B, Crawford ED, et al. Combined versus sequential chemo-endocrine therapy in advanced prostate cancer: final results of a randomized Southwest Oncology Group study. *J Clin Oncol.* 1990;8:1675–1682.

80. Manni A, Bartholomew M, Caplan R, et al. Androgen priming and chemotherapy in advanced prostate cancer: evaluation of determinants of clinical outcome. *J Clin Oncol.* 1988;6:1456–1466.

81. Donovan JF, Lubaroff DM, Williams RD. Immunotherapy of prostate cancer. *Prob Urol.* 1990;4:489–505.

82. Okutani T, Nishi N, Kagawa Y, et al. Role of cyclic AMP and polypeptide growth regulators in growth inhibition by interferon in PC-3 cells. *Prostate.* 1991;18:73–80.

83. Sica G, Fabbroni L, Castagnetta L, Cacciatore M, Pavone-Macaluso M. Antiproliferative effect of interferons on human prostate carcinoma cell lines. *Urol Res.* 1989;17:111–115.

84. van Moorselaar RJA, Hendriks BT, van Stratum P, van der Meide PW, Debruyne FMJ, Schalken JA. Synergistic antitumor effects of rat gamma interferon and human tumor necrosis factor alpha against androgen-dependent and -independent rat prostatic tumors. *Cancer Res*. 1991;51:2329–2334.

85. Bulbul MA, Huben RP, Murphy GP. Interferon beta treatment of metastatic prostate cancer. *J Surg Oncol*. 1986;33:231–233.

86. Webb KS, Liberman SN, Ware JL, Walther PJ. In vitro synergism between hybrid immunotoxins and chemotherapeutic drugs: relevance to immunotherapy of prostate carcinoma. *Immunol Immunother*. 1986;21:100–106.

# 38

# Chemotherapy for Genitourinary Malignancies

*Lori M. Minasian, Robert J. Motzer, Howard I. Scher, and George J. Bosl*

## INTRODUCTION

Genitourinary tumors are of particular interest to the medical oncologist because of their diversity in biologic potential and sensitivity to treatment. This varies from germ cell tumors, which are curable with systemic chemotherapy, to renal cell tumors, which are uniformly refractory to chemotherapy. This chapter summarizes the experience with chemotherapy for the four genitourinary tumors (germ cell tumors, transitional cell carcinoma of the bladder, prostate carcinoma, and renal cell carcinoma) and reviews the basic principles of clinical trial methodology.

## PRINCIPLES OF CHEMOTHERAPY

The efficacy of a chemotherapy agent is based on two factors: (1) the enhanced growth fraction of malignant cells (the percentage of cells that are actively in the cell cycle and capable of injury by cell cycle–specific cytotoxic agents) and (2) the lack of intrinsic or acquired resistance of the malignant cells to the cytotoxic agent. Single agents that show antitumor activity are often combined into drug regimens with the intent of improving efficacy and achieving long-term remissions. For a combination regimen to be optimal in general, (1) each agent must have independent activity against the tumor, (2) each agent should have a different mechanism of action, (3) the toxicities of the agents should not overlap permitting use of maximal doses, and (4) whenever possible there should be in vitro evidence of synergism between the agents.[1]

Combination chemotherapy is given in several settings. Induction chemotherapy is given as the primary treatment for a patient with advanced disease. Maintenance chemotherapy is given over a prolonged time interval after a patient has achieved a complete response to induction. Salvage chemotherapy is given when a patient has failed induction. Adjuvant chemotherapy refers to use of chemotherapy after the primary tumor has been surgically resected, but the patient has a high risk for recurrence despite the absence of clinically detectable disease. Neoadjuvant chemotherapy is given as initial therapy to reduce tumor bulk to determine sensitivity in vivo and possibly enhance the efficacy of subsequent primary therapy such as surgery or radiation.

## CLINICAL TRIAL METHODOLOGY

Clinical trials are the primary means of investigating the efficacy of chemotherapy. Three phases of clinical trials are used to evaluate chemotherapeutic agents.[1] A phase I trial is designed to identify a safe and tolerable dose of a new agent. Three to four patients are treated at one dose level and if no toxicity is observed the dose is increased in successively smaller increments. In this manner, a maximum tolerated dose is established. Generally, patients with any tumor type may participate. A phase II trial is designed to identify the activity of a drug in a defined patient population with a particular tumor type. Here a specific dose and schedule is used based on an earlier phase I trial. The intent is to determine efficacy and thereby decide if further testing is worthwhile. A phase III trial is designed to determine (1) the effects of treatment relative to the natural history of the disease, (2) whether a new treatment is more effective than standard therapy, or (3) whether a new treatment is as effective as standard therapy but associated with less toxicity.

A phase II trial requires a clearly defined end point to accurately evaluate efficacy. For solid tumors, the patients must have disease that can be measured either by physical exam or radiographically so that the response of the tumor to the agent can be followed. The clinical response is then determined to be a complete response, partial response, stable disease, or progression as defined in Table 1. The most important indicator for the success of chemotherapy is the proportion of patients who achieve a complete response.

## GERM CELL TUMORS

The successful treatment of metastatic germ cell tumors (GCTs) is a major achievement in medical oncology. As a result, GCTs represent a model for a curable cancer. Early on, chemotherapy agents including dactinomycin, chlorambucil, and methotrexate[2] each showed antitumor activity. Following the example of combining antibiotics in the treatment of tuberculosis, these agents were combined and served as the prototype for the use of combination chemotherapy in other malignancies.[2] With the advent of cisplatin-based chemotherapy, 70% to 80% of patients with metastatic disease were cured with chemotherapy and adjunctive surgery.[3,4] More recently, investigations have been directed at tailoring treatment to favorable and unfavorable prognostic groups and the development of effective salvage therapy.

### Single-Agent Trials

As shown in Table 2, many chemotherapeutic agents have shown antitumor activity[2,5–21] in GCTs. In the 1960s and early 1970s, chemotherapy with dactinomycin,[2] methotrexate,[2] chlorambucil,[2] vinblastine,[10] and bleomycin[5] alone or in combination achieved major responses, but complete responses were infrequent and rarely durable. The most important discovery of the early trials was cisplatin, the most effective agent in the treatment of GCT. For the first time long-term remissions were possible. More recently, etoposide (VP-16) was found to be an effective single agent in the treatment of patients after failure with cisplatin-based therapy.[17,22,23] In vivo synergism between etoposide and cisplatin was shown in animal models[24] and became the basis for further combination trials. The other two drugs

| TABLE 1. Standard Response Criteria |
|---|
| Complete Response (CR): Complete disappearance of all clinical evidence of tumor on physical examination, x-ray, and biochemical evaluation for 1 month. |
| Partial Response (PR): Greater than 50% decrease on physical examination or radiography of the summed products of the perpendicular diameters of all measured lesions. No simultaneous increase in size of any lesion or appearance of any new lesions may occur. |
| Stable Disease (STAB): Less than 25% decrease or increase in tumor size or biochemical abnormalities for a minimum of 3 months. |
| Progression (PROG): Less than 25% decrease in tumor size for less than 3 months or greater than 25% increase in the sum of all measurable lesions, appearance of new lesions, or mixed response. |

**TABLE 2. Single Agents Used in Chemotherapy for GCT**

| Agent | Patients (No.) | PR/CR (No.) | Response (%) |
|---|---|---|---|
| | **Pre-cisplatin** | | |
| Actinomycin D[2] | 32 | 7 | 22 |
| Bleomycin[5] (± vinblastine) | 42 | 20/4 | 57 |
| Cyclophosphamide[6,7] | 10 | 1/1 | 20 |
| Adriamycin[8] | 20 | 3/0 | 15 |
| 6-Mercaptopurine[2] | 8 | 1 | 12 |
| Mithramycin[9] | 44 | 9/11 | 45 |
| Vinblastine[10] | 32 | 12/4 | 50 |
| | **Platinum Agents** | | |
| Cisplatin[11] | 11 | 7/2 | 81 |
| Carboplatin[12,13]* | 42 | 2/1 | 7 |
| Iproplatin[14]* | 23 | 0 | 0 |
| DACCP[15]* | 9 | 0/0 | 0 |
| | **Nonplatinum Agents** | | |
| Cis-retinoic acid[16]* | 15 | 0/0 | 0 |
| Etoposide[17]* | 85 | 26/3 | 34 |
| Ifosfamide[18,19]* | 117 | 22/2 | 17 |
| Mitoguazone[20]* | 14 | 0 | 0 |
| Vindesine[21]* | 19 | 3/0 | 16 |

PR = Partial response; CR = Complete response. DAACP = 1,2-Diaminocyclohexane-(4-carboxyphthalato)platinum(II).
*Agents investigated in patients who were cisplatin-refractory.

that showed efficacy in patients refractory to cisplatin were ifosfamide[18] and carboplatin,[12] both of which have since been included in combination therapy.

## Cisplatin, Vinblastine, and Bleomycin Chemotherapy Regimens

Antitumor activity shown for cisplatin, vinblastine, bleomycin, alone (PVB) or in combination with cyclophosphamide and dactinomycin (VAB) prompted their further investigation in combination chemotherapy. From the early 1970s to the mid-1980s, successive trials were conducted at Memorial Sloan-Kettering Cancer Center (MSKCC) (the VAB series,[3,25–29] summarized in Table 3) with parallel studies conducted at Indiana University (the PVB series). The culmination of the VAB studies was the VAB-6 regimen in which 78% of patients achieved a complete response and only 12% of the patients relapsed.[3]

The VAB trials showed that (1) high-dose cisplatin (≥100 mg/m$^2$) is the most effective agent (70% to 80% of patients can be expected to achieve a durable complete response to cisplatin-based chemotherapyapy[3]), (2) serum tumor markers, α-fetoprotein (AFP), and human chorionic gonadotropin (HCG) are critical for proper patient management,[30] (3) surgical excision of apparent residual disease after chemotherapy is often necessary,[3] and (4) maintenance chemotherapy was not required for a durable response. Most of the regimens used in the 1960s and early 1970s included long-term maintenance chemotherapy for up to 21 months. A randomized study of 113 patients showed no advantage to maintenance chemotherapy.[38] No increased relapse rate or decreased initial response rate was seen, and subsequently patients no longer received maintenance chemotherapy. In addition, the VAB studies lead to the identification of prognostic

**TABLE 3. Combination Chemotherapy Trials in GCT at MSKCC**

| Setting | Therapy | Patients (No.) | CR (%) | Durable CR (%) |
|---|---|---|---|---|
| Induction | VAB-1[25] | 47 | 15 | 71 |
| | VAB-2[26] | 50 | 50 | 44 |
| | VAB-3[27] | 74 | 61 | 69 |
| | VAB-4[28] | 41 | 80 | 91 |
| | VAB-5[29] | 38 | 47 | 89 |
| | VAB-6[3] | 161 | 78 | 88 |
| Induction | | | | |
| Good Risk | EP/VAB-6[30] | 164 | 95 | 84 |
| | EP/EC[31] | 192 | 90 | 94 |
| Induction | | | | |
| Poor Risk | VAB-6[3]* | 29 | 43 | 29 |
| | VAB-6/EP[32] | 39 | 51 | 33 |
| | EBC[33] | 32 | 57 | 44 |
| Salvage | | | | |
| | EP[34] | 45 | 18 | 9 |
| | VIP[35] | 42 | 25 | 15 |
| | AuBMT[36] | 16 | 50 | 18 |

CR = Complete response; EP = Etoposide + cisplatin; EC = Etoposide + carboplatin; EBC = Etoposide + bleomycin + carboplatin; VIP = Etoposide + ifosfamide + cisplatin; AuBMT = High-dose carboplatin + etoposide + cyclophosphamide with autologous bone marrow transplant.

*Twenty-nine patients from the original VAB-6 article[21] updated for presentation.

features in GCTs and subsequent clinical trials have been directed to GCTs with stratification by favorable and unfavorable predicted outcomes.

**Serum Markers.** The role of the serum markers, AFP and HCG, is unique in medical oncology. In GCT, these markers are important in diagnosis, as prognostic indicators, in monitoring responses to treatment, and in the detection of early relapse. Over 70% of patients presenting with disseminated nonseminomatous GCT will have one or the other elevated.[37] Radioimmunoassays have made it possible to detect these markers at ng/mL concentrations.[39,40] The kinetics of both markers have been studied and the biologic half-lives are well described; 5 to 7 days for AFP and 18 to 48 hours for HCG.[41] Additionally, the serum lactate dehydrogenase (LDH) level is often elevated in patients with disseminated GCT, and serves as another important tumor marker, although not as specific as AFP or HCG. When the serum markers LDH and HCG are elevated at diagnosis, patients have a less favorable prognosis.[42]

A recent analysis showed that the rate of serum tumor decline during chemotherapy is predictive of tumor response and patient survival.[43] All patients with nonseminomatous germ cell tumor who received high-dose cisplatin from 1979 to 1988 at MSKCC were followed with sequential serum tumor markers. Patients whose AFP half-life was longer than 7 days or whose HCG half-life was longer than 3 days had significantly inferior survival and achieved a complete response less frequently.[43] Hence, the rate of serum tumor marker decline can be used to identify early treatment failure during induction chemotherapy and allow consideration for a change in therapy.

## Prognostic Factors

One of the major goals in the investigation of GCT has been the identification of prognostic factors with treatment tailored to a patient's prognosis. Many studies of pretreatment clinical characteristics have identified extent of disease and elevated serum tumor markers as significant predictors of response and survival. In a multivariate analysis of prognostic factors of all patients with disseminated testicular nonseminomatous GCT treated at MSKCC from 1975 to 1981, a mathematical model was identified that correctly predicted 94% of all complete responses and 83% of all outcomes.[42] The variables that achieved statistical significance were the logarithm of the serum LDH, the logarithm of the serum HCG, and the total number of metastases. In using this model, if the calculated probability of achieving a complete response yielded a value ≥0.5, the patient was henceforth considered "good risk." If the predicted probability was <0.5, the patient was considered "poor risk." Once patients were stratified according to predicted prognosis, the goal of clinical trials was tailored to each subgroup. The goal of therapy in good-risk patients is to reduce toxicity without compromising efficacy. The goal of therapy in poor-risk patients is either to find new effective drugs or to intensify current drug regimens that could lead to more durable complete responses.

Histology becomes a prognostic factor if the tumor is a pure seminoma. Patients with advanced seminoma do well regardless of primary site and have been considered "good risk." In a retrospective series of patients with advanced seminoma,[44] 88% achieved a complete response, of which 85% were durable.

Primary extragonadal tumors occur in 1% to 2% of germ cell tumors.[38] Several analyses done at MSKCC have shown an inferior complete response proportion and more frequent relapses in patients with extragonadal nonseminomatous primaries.[3,46–48] Hence, all patients with nonseminomatous extragonadal primaries are considered "poor risk." This observation has been supported by some[49–51] and disputed by others.[52,53]

**Good-Risk Trials.** For those patients who have favorable prognostic features, clinical trials have been directed at maintaining efficacy and reducing treatment-related morbidity. In the early 1980s, cisplatin and etoposide was shown to be a highly effective salvage regimen.[34] This prompted a randomized prospective phase III trial that compared VAB-6 to the two-drug regimen of cisplatin and etoposide as initial therapy for good-risk patients (summarized in Table 3). The therapeutic results were identical (complete responses in 92% of patients) with a significant reduction in toxicity in patients treated with the two-drug regimen.[30]

The second good-risk trial at MSKCC was a comparison of etoposide with cisplatin versus etoposide with carboplatin (an analog of cisplatin with less nephrotoxicity and neurotoxicity). This trial showed that both regimens produced the same proportion of complete responses. However, the relapse proportion in patients treated with carboplatin was higher than that in patients treated with cisplatin.[31] Therefore, the standard chemotherapy regimen at MSKCC for disseminated disease in patients with favorable prognostic features remains four cycles of cisplatin and etoposide.

The Indiana University group conducted a randomized prospective phase III clinical trial to compare PVB to PEB (cisplatin, etoposide, and bleomycin) as initial therapy. There was a statistically significant reduction in neuromuscular toxicity in the etoposide arm.[4] A recent study compared three cycles to four cycles of PEB in patients with a favorable prognosis by the Indiana University criteria and found that three cycles were as effective as four.[52] A standard regimen for patients with favorable prognostic factors by the Indiana University criteria is three cycles of cisplatin, etoposide, and bleomycin.

**Poor-Risk Trials.** Twenty percent to 30% of patients with advanced GCT will either relapse or never achieve a complete response. The goal in this group is early identification with the investigation of more intensive therapy. The results of the major poor-risk trials[32,33] conducted at MSKCC are shown in Table 3. About 33% of patients considered poor risk achieved a durable complete response to cisplatin-based therapy. The proportion of patients achieving a durable complete response had not significantly improved with VAB-6 alternating with etoposide and cisplatin or carboplatin, bleomycin, etoposide as compared to VAB-6 alone. In an ongoing trial at MSKCC, poor-risk patients are treated with conventional cisplatin-based chemotherapy. If their markers are not declining appropriately by the expected half-life, then therapy is changed to high-dose etoposide and carboplatin chemotherapy and autologous bone marrow transplantation. Completion of this trial is needed to determine if this approach will result in an improved survival.

## Salvage Chemotherapy

The first effective salvage regimen for patients who failed to achieve a durable complete response to cisplatin, vinblastine, and bleomycin-based chemotherapy was cisplatin and etoposide. In those patients who had (1) never received cisplatin or (2) previously had a complete response to cisplatin chemotherapy, 47% achieved a complete response.[34] In those who had never responded to cisplatin therapy no complete responses were seen. More recently, the combination of cisplatin, etoposide, and ifosfamide (VIP) has been found to be an effective salvage regimen.[35,55,56] Durable complete responses were achieved and the inclusion of ifosfamide added efficacy to etoposide and cisplatin.[35] Again, in an analysis of patients treated with first-line salvage therapy, the importance of prior response to cisplatin was shown as an important prognostic factor in cisplatin-based salvage therapy. In those patients who had previously achieved a complete response to cisplatin-based chemotherapy, an overall survival of 38% was seen as opposed to 12% in those who never attained a complete response.[57]

For those patients who fail salvage chemotherapy with VIP, chemotherapy with high-dose carboplatin and etoposide followed by autologous bone marrow transplant can achieve a durable complete response and is the treatment of choice.[36,58] The substantial morbidity in some series[58] may be reduced by the use of hematopoietic growth factors and by transplanting patients with poor prognostic features who have not been heavily pretreated.[36]

## Adjuvant Chemotherapy

Single-arm studies have shown that almost all patients with stage II disease are cured after retroperitoneal lymph node dissection with adjuvant chemotherapy.[59,60] An alternative approach to adjuvant chemotherapy is careful observation with treatment reserved for relapse. In a recent prospective randomized trial,[61] patients with pathologic stage II were randomized to either observation alone or two cycles of adjuvant cisplatin-based chemotherapy. In the observation group 48% of patients with any positive lymph nodes relapsed as opposed to the adjuvant group in which only 2% relapsed.[61] However, there was no difference in long-term survival compared to the adjuvant group. A retrospective analysis of patients with pathologic stage IIA ($\leq$ five nodes involved, all nodes $<$2 cm in diameter) was conducted at the Dana Farber Cancer Center.[62] Of the 39 patients observed following retroperitoneal lymph node dissection, only three (8%) relapsed. All three were rendered disease-free after cisplatin-based chemotherapy.[62]

Therefore, two options exist for GCT patients with pathologic stage II disease. First, they may be treated with two cycles of adjuvant chemotherapy. Second, they may be closely observed with chemotherapy reserved for the 50% who will relapse. Observation should be considered in patients with stage IIA as they have a low likelihood of relapse.

## Adjunctive Surgery

Surgical resection of metastatic sites plays a critical role in the management of patients with nonseminomatous GCT. After completion of chemotherapy, patients are restaged with tumor markers and radiologic studies. Those patients with residual radiographic abnormalities and normal markers undergo surgical resection of residual disease. In a series of 133 patients with nonseminomatous GCT who had adjunctive surgery,[63] the histologic findings at exploration included fibrotic or necrotic tissue (38%), mature teratoma (30%), and malignant tumor (32%). If viable tumor is found, complete resection of the metastatic disease and an additional two cycles of chemotherapy resulted in long-term survival for 65% of patients.[64,65] Patients who required surgery for residual disease after chemotherapy were at higher risk for relapse than patients who achieved a complete response to chemotherapy alone.[64]

A recent analysis[66] of patients undergoing retroperitoneal lymph node dissection at MSKCC from 1979 to 1988 was conducted to determine prognostic factors for finding residual disease at surgery. The 185 patients with prechemotherapy masses >3 cm were treated with either cisplatin- or carboplatin-based chemotherapy. A multivariate analysis identified the prechemotherapy LDH and AFP as well as the size and amount of tumor shrinkage as the best predictive factors for necrotic debris at surgery.[66] No criteria could predict a negative pathology with sufficient accuracy to avoid surgical resection of residual disease. Therefore, a retroperitoneal lymph node dissection should be considered in all patients after chemotherapy if the pretreatment nodal disease was >3 cm in diameter or if there are residual radiographic abnormalities.

### Conclusions

In summary, 70% to 80% of patients presenting with metastatic GCT can be rendered disease-free with cisplatin-based chemotherapy. Serum tumor markers are important tools in both prognosis and management. Patients should be stratified by prognostic group in order to receive optimal therapy. Serum markers should be followed closely and can be used early on to predict treatment failure. In those who relapse, chemotherapy with etoposide and ifosfamide and high-dose carboplatin with autologous bone marrow transplant are effective salvage therapies, although both regimens achieve a durable complete response in only a minority of patients. And finally, surgery for residual disease after chemotherapy is necessary to determine the histology of the residual matter and can lead to long-term cure.

## TRANSITIONAL CELL CARCINOMA OF THE BLADDER

Within the past 10 years, cisplatin-based combination regimens have been developed that can result in complete or partial responses in 45% to 70% of patients treated[67] with metastatic urothelial tumors. However, few patients with metastatic transitional cell carcinoma (TCC) have long-term remissions and most of these patients will not survive 5 years after diagnosis. Current clinical trials are in the process of defining the most effective chemotherapy regimen in metastatic disease and determining whether chemotherapy given before or after surgical resection can prolong overall survival.

### Single-Agent Trials

Many single agents have been investigated in patients with advanced TCC. Selected agents are shown in Table 4.[68] The most active single agents for TCC of the urinary tract are cisplatin and methotrex-

**TABLE 4. Single-Agent Trials for Urothelial Tract Tumors**

| Agent | Patients (No.) | Response* (%) |
|---|---|---|
| Methotrexate | | |
| "Low dose" | 236 | 29 |
| "High dose" | 57 | 28 |
| Adriamycin | 274 | 17 |
| Vinblastine | 38 | 16 |
| Cyclophosphamide | 98 | 31 |
| Mitomycin C | 42 | 12 |
| Fluorouracil | 141 | 16 |
| Cisplatin | | |
| Single institution | 206 | 34 |
| Randomized trials | 316 | 17 |
| Neoadjuvant | 184 | 41 |
| Overall | 640 | 28 |
| Carboplatin | 186 | 11 |
| CHIP | 39 | 18 |
| Gallium nitrate | 31 | 29 |

* Complete and partial response.
Adapted from Seidman,[68] with permission.

**TABLE 5. MVAC Regimen**

| | Day (doses in mg/m²) | | | |
|---|---|---|---|---|
| **Agent** | **1** | **2** | **15** | **22** |
| Methotrexate | 30 | | 30* | 30* |
| Vinblastine | | 3 | 3* | 3* |
| Adriamycin | | 30† | | |
| Cisplatin | | 70‡ | | |

*These doses are withheld if WBC <2500/mm³, or platelets <100,000/mm³, or mucositis is present.
† Adriamycin dose is reduced to 15 mg/m² in patients who have had >20 Gy prior pelvic irradiation.
‡ Stop protocol when creatinine clearance <40 mL/min.

ate.[69] In patients with cisplatin-refractory disease, gallium nitrate has activity.[70] While single agents can produce tumor regression, complete responses are achieved only with combination regimens.

## Combination Regimens

The effective combination regimens used in patients with metastatic disease are based on cisplatin and methotrexate.[67,71] The most efficacious regimen is the four-drug combination MVAC (methotrexate, vinblastine, adriamycin, and cisplatin, with doses and schedule shown in Table 5).[72] In 124 patients with advanced urothelial tract carcinoma, significant tumor regression (complete and partial responses) was achieved in 72% of patients treated with MVAC.[72] Of particular importance, 36% of patients achieved a complete response and of those patients, 55% had a greater than 3-year survival. Figure 1 shows the survival distributions of patients at MSKCC with a median 74-month follow-up. The median survival of patients with advanced nodal disease was 32.9 months with 32% of patients alive at 6 years.[68] The median survival of patients with metastatic disease was 12 months with 17% alive at 6 years.[68] Those patients who had a major response to chemotherapy had a significantly higher likelihood of prolonged survival. Responses were seen in all sites of metastases with intra-abdominal nodes the most sensitive and liver disease the least sensitive.

While nodal disease alone may predict

Fig 1. Survival of patients treated with MVAC. □, advanced nodal (22 patients, 7 censored); ○, metastatic (110 patients, 15 censored); tick mark, last follow-up. (From Seidman,[68] with permission.)

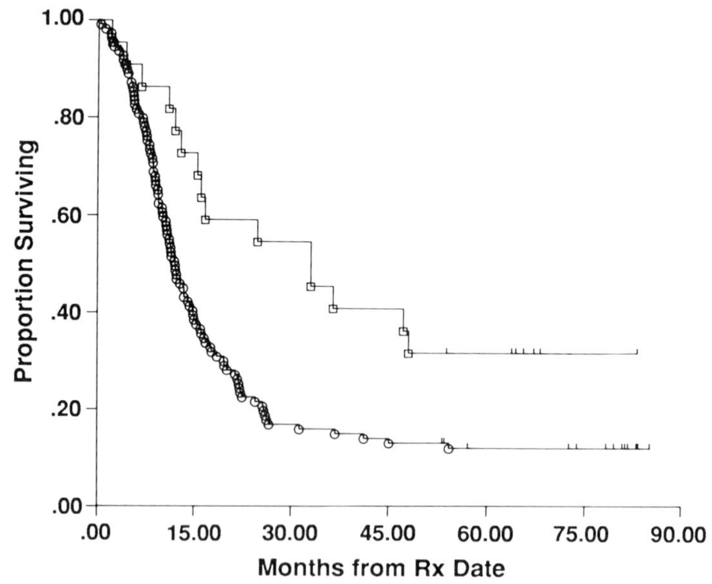

improved response to MVAC chemotherapy, it was not shown to be an independent prognostic factor for survival.[73] The only variables that were statistically significant predictors for improved survival with MVAC chemotherapy were a normal serum alkaline phosphatase and a high Karnofsky performance status[73] at the time of diagnosis. Additionally, metastatic disease to the liver was a poor prognostic factor.

The reported toxicities of the MVAC regimen include mucositis and myelosuppression with associated neutropenic sepsis. The myelosuppression has resulted in 25% of patients developing nadir sepsis.[72] This toxicity can result in significant morbidity and require frequent dose attenuation. Hematopoietic growth factors, specifically granulocyte colony stimulating factor (GCSF), administered with MVAC chemotherapy resulted in significant reduction of both mucositis and myelosuppression.[74] Thus, the toxicities that can prevent full administration of chemotherapy can be ameliorated with GCSF.

Two randomized prospective clinical trials have been conducted to compare MVAC to other agents. One trial compared MVAC to single-agent cisplatin. Although more toxic, the combination was superior to single-agent cisplatin in both overall response proportion (9% for cisplatin and 33% for MVAC) and survival.[75] This response proportion for MVAC was less than that reported in single-arm studies. A possible explanation for this discrepancy in response proportion is the multi-institutional design of the trial and the frequent dose attenuation performed in this trial. The second trial randomized 110 patients to either MVAC or CISCA (cisplatin, cyclophosphamide, adriamycin). The combined overall response proportion was significantly higher for MVAC (65%) than for CISCA (46%).[76] With an 18-month median follow-up, the 2-year survival for the MVAC group was 32% as compared to 8% for the CISCA group.[76]

In summary, MVAC chemotherapy is an effective regimen that results in a major response in 70% of treated patients with advanced TCC. The toxicities that prevent delivering full dose and schedule can be ameliorated with GCSF. However, only a small proportion of patients will achieve a durable complete response. Future trials will be designed to investigate new regimens with the intent to increase efficacy.

### Salvage Chemotherapy

Several agents either alone or in combination have demonstrated activity in patients who have failed cisplatin-based combination therapy (MVAC). With single-agent gallium nitrate, a 17% response proportion was achieved.[70] With the combination of 5-fluorouracil (5FU) and interferon-$\alpha$, a response proportion of 30% (9 of 30 patients previously treated had a partial response) was achieved.[77] In addition, dose intensification of MVAC therapy showed activity in patients who had previously failed either MVAC or CISCA regimens given at conventional doses.[78]

### Adjuvant Chemotherapy

No consensus exists on the benefit of adjuvant chemotherapy following a cystectomy for patients with TCC and poor prognostic features. The primary end point of adjuvant chemotherapy clinical trials is disease-free survival. Several early trials have not shown a survival benefit.[79–83] These trials were limited by the inclusion of small numbers of patients, the lack of uniform pathologic criteria for high risk of recurrent disease, and the suboptimal chemotherapy doses and schedules.[68]

Two recent studies have suggested a survival advantage in some patients receiving adjuvant chemotherapy. In the MD Anderson trial,[84] patients were determined to be high-risk for relapse after cystectomy if there was nodal metastasis, invasion of adjacent organs, extravesicular tumor invasion, or histologic evidence of vascular invasion. If none of the above criteria was met, the patient was considered low risk. Three groups were analyzed: (1) 71 high-risk patients who received adjuvant CISCA, (2) 61 high-risk patients who either refused adjuvant chemotherapy or were excluded due to other medical illnesses, and (3) 260 low-risk patients. There was a survival advantage in the high-risk group for those receiving chemotherapy.[84] However, this trial was not a randomized or a prospective study, the two high-risk groups were not truly comparable, and the survival benefit was seen in subset analysis only. In the second trial,[85] 498 patients who underwent radical cystectomy and lymph node dissection were considered for the trial. Of the 229 patients with pathologic stage P3, P4, N+, or M0, 160 were eligible based on pathology, lack of positive lymph nodes above the aortic bifurcation, and informed consent. Only 91 were randomized to observation or chemotherapy. While a survival advantage for those receiving chemotherapy was shown, the number of patients in each arm was small and different chemotherapy agents, doses, and schedules were used.

To define the role of adjuvant chemotherapy in patients with locally advanced TCC, randomized prospective trials are warranted with larger numbers of patients, specific pathologic criteria for deciding patient enrollment, and conformity of chemotherapy regimen.

## Neoadjuvant Chemotherapy

The intent of neoadjuvant is to downstage the primary tumor and either make an unresectable lesion amenable to surgery or allow for organ preservation (partial as opposed to complete cystectomy).[86] Patients who respond to therapy are then treated to maximal response, and those who do not respond go directly to primary therapy.

Factors such as patient selection, different chemotherapy doses and schedules, and different institutional policies have made the interpretation of clinical trials of neoadjuvant therapy difficult. The original pathology is critical in patient selection as the response to chemotherapy is based on depth of tumor invasion on urologic assessment.[87–89] In a trial of neoadjuvant MVAC, the proportion of complete responses for those patients with $T_2$ (tumor invades superficial muscle) disease was 43% as compared to 8% for those with $T_4$ disease (tumor locally invades adjacent tissue).[87] In addition to patient selection, the chemotherapy given in neoadjuvant trials has varied significantly. The results of several trials of neoadjuvant chemotherapy followed by definitive surgery are shown in Table 6. MVAC has been the regimen used in almost half the trials conducted. The overall proportion of patients with a pathologic complete response at surgery was 28%.[68] Different institutional policies make intergroup studies difficult to assess. A patient at MSKCC with "muscle-invasive disease" undergoes a repeat cystoscopy and biopsy. If no disease is documented, the patient may be observed and cystoscopy repeated in 6 weeks.[90] If muscle invasion is again documented, the patient is considered for neoadjuvant chemotherapy.[68] Uniform pathologic criteria for entry and chemotherapy regimens are required for definitive assessment of whether neoadjuvant therapy is beneficial.

Neoadjuvant chemotherapy can result in tumor downstaging that may allow for bladder preservation.[90] Patients still require primary therapy as clinical staging to detect the extent of disease is often inaccurate. Close monitoring by cystoscopy is required as there is a risk for the appearance of a

**TABLE 6. Results of Selected Neoadjuvant Trials Showing Complete Pathologic Responses in the Bladder Using Combination Chemotherapy**

| Agent(s) | Trials (No.) | Patients (No.) | CR (%) |
|---|---|---|---|
| CDDP/5FU | 1 | 16 | 43 |
| CDDP/MTX | 4 | 110 | 25 |
| CMV | 5 | 107 | 30 |
| CAP | 4 | 83 | 22 |
| MVAC | 11 | 228 | 28 |

CR = Complete response; CDDP/5FU = Cisplatin + 5-fluorouracil; CDDP/MTX = Cisplatin + methotrexate; CMV = Methotrexate + vinblastine + adriamycin + cisplatin; CAP = Cyclophosphamide + doxorubicin + cisplatin; MVAC = Methotrexate + vinblastine + adriamycin + cisplatin.

Adapted from Seidman,[68] with permission.

new primary lesion.[88,89] Response to neoadjuvant chemotherapy has prognostic significance.[91] In a summary series of 125 patients treated with cisplatin-based chemotherapy followed by radical surgery, 91% of patients with an overall response as compared to 37% of nonresponders had a disease-free survival of at least 25 months.[92]

### Conclusions

In summary, transitional cell carcinoma is sensitive to chemotherapy. With MVAC chemotherapy, 70% of patients can achieve a significant response. The toxicities that preclude giving full dose and schedule of MVAC can be ameliorated with hematopoietic growth factors. To date, few patients will have long-term survival despite achieving a complete response. Thus, further clinical trials aimed at identifying new agents and intensifying current regimens in order to improve efficacy are needed.

## PROSTATE CARCINOMA

The first-line treatment for metastatic prostate cancer is androgen ablation. In hormone-refractory patients, chemotherapy has been of marginal benefit. While many agents have been investigated, efficacy has been difficult to show. Conventional response criteria for phase II trials requires bidimensionally measurable disease. The most prevalent metastatic site for prostate cancer is bone, usually manifested as osteoblastic lesions that are not measurable in two dimensions. Hence, efficacy is difficult to quantitate and survival has become the end point of some clinical trials. To date, no randomized clinical trial has shown a survival benefit for chemotherapy.[93]

### Single-Agent Trials

Numerous single-agent phase II trials have been conducted. The results of MSKCC trials[94–102] in patients with bidimensionally measurable disease are shown in Table 7. No complete responses were seen and only a few patients have achieved a partial response with any of the agents tested. In addition, the median survival for all treated patients with hormone-refractory disease was found to be 6.3 months in a review of single-agent chemotherapy trials at MSKCC.[103] The disappointing results of the agents studied in phase II trials at MSKCC and elsewhere emphasize the need for continued investigation of new agents and alternative approaches to therapy.

**TABLE 7. Single-Agent Trials in Bidimensionally Measurable Prostate Cancer at MSKCC**

| Agent | Patients (No.) | PR (%) | 95% CI |
|---|---|---|---|
| Cisplatin[94] | 22 | 12 | 4–34 |
| Neocarcinostatin[95] | 20 | 0 | 0 |
| Amsacrine[96] | 18 | 0 | 0 |
| Adriamycin[97] | 39 | 5 | 0–12 |
| Mitoguazone[98] (MGBG) | 25 | 24 | 11–44 |
| VP-16[99] | 20 | 5 | 0–24 |
| Gallium nitrate[100] | 20 | 10 | 2–32 |
| DFMO/MGBG[101] | 14 | 0 | 0–23 |
| Trimetrexate[102] | 31 | 17 | 3–30 |

PR = Partial response; CI = Confidence interval; VP-16 = Etoposide; DFMO = Difluoromethylornithine.

Adriamycin (doxorubicin) was investigated in several trials that suggested antitumor activity.[104,105] However, the criteria for evaluating response differed by study and often included patients without bidimensionally measurable disease. In most of the patients treated, ancillary factors such as response to pain, changes in performance status, and hemoglobin concentration were subjectively graded to assess response.[104,105] A phase II clinical trial of adriamycin in 41 hormone-refractory patients with bidimensionally measurable disease showed an overall response of 5% with only two patients achieving a partial response.[97] This trial suggested that adriamycin has minimal benefit in the treatment of patients with hormone-refractory prostate cancer.

Suramin has been investigated as an antineoplastic agent because of its ability to inhibit the binding of growth factors to their receptors[106] and the production of adrenal steroids.[107] Suramin has shown in vitro and in vivo antitumor activity against prostate cancer cells.[108–110] In early trials,[111,112] a partial response of 40% was reported in patients with measurable disease. In a summary of several trials, 21 of 73 patients with measurable disease (19% with 95% confidence limits from 18% to 39%) showed a greater than 50% reduction in tumor size[113] and 46 of 97 patients with an elevated serum prostate-specific antigen (PSA) (47% with 95% confidence limits from 37% to 57%) showed a greater than 50% reduction in PSA.[113] Therefore, suramin may be an active agent in patients with prostatic cancer and warrants further study. Efficacy may be dependent on drug exposure period and schedule.[114]

## Combination Therapy

Given the modest activity of individual agents, it is not surprising that randomized trials of combination chemotherapy have failed to show any benefit over single agents. Combination regimens with chemotherapy and hormonal therapy have also been investigated. One study[115] prospectively randomized patients with metastatic disease who had not previously been treated to one of three treatment arms: (1) orchiectomy or diethylstilbestrol (DES), (2) DES plus cyclophosphamide, or (3) cyclophosphamide plus estramustine. No difference in overall response was seen. The median survival was 92, 91, and 94 weeks, respectively.[115] This study suggests that the addition of chemotherapy to hormonal therapy is no better than hormonal therapy alone in patients with hormone-naive prostate cancer.

More recently the combination of estramustine and vinblastine has been investigated. Estramustine, a nitrogen mustard with an estrogen moiety attached, acts as an antimitotic agent. It binds to microtubule-associated proteins to inhibit assembly and disrupt microtubule organization.[116] Vinblastine binds to tubulin and destroys the spindle required for mitosis. Synergism between these two agents has been shown in prostate cancer cell lines.[117] A recent clinical trial[117] showed activity of this combination. Twenty-five patients with hormone-refractory disease and elevated PSA received estramustine and vinblastine. Of the five patients with measurable disease, 2 had a partial response[117] and 13 had a greater than 50% reduction in PSA.[117] Similar results (3 of 7 patients with measurable disease had a partial response, and 11 of 22 had a greater than 50% reduction in PSA) were seen in another study with a slightly different dose schedule of estramustine and vinblastine.[118] Further study of this combination is warranted in an expanded series of patients.

## Prognostic Factors

Alternative approaches to standard response criteria in determining efficacy are needed. One approach is to identify posttreatment prognostic factors that correlate with survival and can be substituted for response as an end point of agent efficacy. The Veteran's Administration Cooperative Urologic Research Group prospectively investigated selected criteria for prognostic significance.[119] Eighty-eight patients with hormone-refractory disease were treated with a five-drug regimen (melphalan, methotrexate, 5-fluorouracil, vincristine, and prednisone). Of the several factors examined only normalization of serum acid phosphatase and serum alkaline phosphatase were predictive of prolonged survival. A reduction in the serum levels that did not fully normalize was not predictive. This and other retrospective analyses have revealed a broad range of different prognostic factors from the pretreatment serum acid phosphatase,[119–121] hemoglobin,[121] subjective degree of pain,[120,121] pretreatment serum alkaline phosphatase,[119,121] and performance status.[122] However, no uniform criteria have been accepted or reproducibly shown to correlate with survival. Most of these analyses were conducted prior to the frequent use of the PSA.

The PSA is elevated in more than 90% of patients with hormone-refractory prostate cancer. Its most established use is in the monitoring of patients after primary therapy for localized disease.[123] More recently, it has been investigated as a means of following response to androgen therapy.[124,125] Two retrospective analyses have shown that changes in serum PSA after hormonal therapy correlated with survival. One analysis[125] showed a prolonged remission and survival benefit in those patients who normalized their PSA (<4 ng/mL) after either orchiectomy, DES, or Lupron. In another analysis[124] 60% of patients with the lowest value of serum PSA (<2.3 ng/mL) were alive at 24 months after therapy as compared to 35% of patients with a nadir value >10 ng/mL.

Changes in serum PSA levels have been shown to correlate with regression of measurable disease in patients treated with androgen ablation[126] and in survival in hormone-refractory patients treated with chemotherapy.[127] Of the 114 patients at MSKCC treated on seven different chemotherapy clinical trials, all were followed with serial PSA levels during therapy. A reduction in serum PSA level of greater than 50% correlated with prolonged survival. The median survival of patients with 50% reduction in PSA was 20 months as compared to 8 months for those with less than a 50% reduction.[127] Hence, changes in PSA may be a more rapid means of assessing the antitumor activity of new agents.

### Small Cell Carcinoma

A minority of patients with prostate cancer have a histologic subtype of small cell carcinoma that expresses neuroendocrine features. The clinical presentation of patients with small cell carcinoma of the prostate is typically visceral metastases with relatively few bone metastases, which differs from the usual presentation of adenocarcinoma.[128] The identification of these patients is important as this tumor is more responsive to chemotherapy.[128] In a recent clinical trial[129] 21 patients with this variant were treated with either etoposide and cisplatin or etoposide, adriamycin, and cyclophosphamide. The overall response proportion was 62% with two patients achieving a complete response, one of whom was alive without disease at 25 months.[129] Hence, chemotherapy may have significant impact on patients with this subtype. Confirmatory trials are underway and investigation is being directed at better understanding the tumor biology.

### Conclusions

In summary, few agents have activity in hormone-refractory prostate cancer. Although initial results with suramin and estramustine and vinblastine are promising, further investigation is warranted. The degree and duration of decline in PSA may aid in monitoring response to chemotherapy. The subtype of small cell carcinoma of the prostate is an important entity because of its sensitivity to chemotherapy. At this time, patients with metastatic prostate cancer who have failed hormonal therapy should be offered investigational therapy.

## RENAL CELL CARCINOMA

Renal cell carcinoma is a chemotherapy-resistant tumor. Early clinical trials of chemotherapy and hormonal therapy used subjective or poorly defined objective criteria for response. When strict criteria (as shown in Table 1) are used or stable disease is excluded, the response proportions are significantly less than originally reported.

### Single-Agent Trials

Table 8 shows the phase II single-agent trials[130–144] conducted at MSKCC since 1977. None of the agents tested shows activity greater than 5%. In a recent review[145] 2120 patients from 39 phase II trials of single agents (objective response proportions ranged from 0% to 19%) were combined for an overall response proportion of 8.7%.

One agent that has been extensively studied is vinblastine. In a review[146] of 135 patients treated with vinblastine an overall response proportion of 25% was noted. This proportion includes patients with stable disease. If only patients with complete and partial responses are considered, the proportion of responses decreases to 19%.[146] Most regimens consist of once-a-week dosing. An alternative schedule of

**TABLE 8. Single-Agent Trials in Renal Cell Carcinoma at MSKCC 1977–1984**

| Agent | Patients (No.) | Response* (%) |
|---|---|---|
| AMSA[130] | 21 | 0 |
| Bisantrene[131] | 26 | 0 |
| Cisplatin[132] | 9 | 0 |
| 10-Deazaaminopterin[133] | 17 | 0 |
| Demethoxydaunorubicin[137] | 19 | 0 |
| Didemnin[135] | 23 | 5% |
| Elliptinium[136] | 8 | 0 |
| 4-Epi-adriamycin[137] | 19 | 0 |
| Gallium nitrate[138] | 8 | 0 |
| Mitoguazone[139] | 31 | 0 |
| *N*-methylformamide[140] | 16 | 0 |
| PALA[141] | 15 | 0 |
| Trimetrexate[142] | 14 | 0 |
| Vinblastine[143] | 9 | 0 |
| Vindesine[144] | 17 | 0 |

* Complete and partial response.
AMSA = 4′-(9-acridinylamino)-methanesulfon-*m*-anisdide; PALA = N-phosphoacetyl-L-aspartate.

vinblastine as a 5-day infusion given every 3 weeks was shown to have greater toxicity without improved efficacy.[147,148]

A 5-fluorouracil-related metabolite, 5-fluoro-2-deoxyuridine (FUDR), has been tested in renal cell carcinoma. Because its plasma half-life is approximately 10 minutes, FUDR has been given as a continuous infusion. With this regimen, the gastrointestinal toxicity, particularly diarrhea, nausea, and vomiting, can be severe and dose limiting. This toxicity can be ameliorated and possibly the delivery of the agent made more effective by giving circadian patterning continuous infusion (adjusting the delivery of the drug such that more than half the daily dose is given between 3 PM and 9 PM).[149] An early trial[149] randomized 30 patients to receive either a fixed rate or a variable (circadian patterning) rate of continuous infusion FUDR. Each patient received the same overall daily dose. Significantly more moderate to severe diarrhea ($p < 0.05$) was seen with the fixed rate infusion. The overall response proportion seen was 23%.[149] This response proportion has not been replicated in a recent trial that reported a response proportion of 14%[150] for circadian rhythm FUDR. A randomized prospective clinical trial is indicated to determine whether FUDR administered by circadian rhythm is more effective than a continuous dose schedule.

## Combination Therapy

Combination regimens have not demonstrated greater efficacy than single agents[146] alone in the treatment of metastatic renal cell carcinoma. A trial of carmustine in combination with vinblastine was reported to have a response proportion of 24%. Subsequent phase II clinical trials of this combination with standard response criteria have shown no better than 6%.[151,152] When vinblastine was added to other agents, an overall response proportion (only complete and partial responses) of 6% was seen.[146] When noneffective agents were added to vinblastine, dose reductions due to cumulative toxicity were often required and response proportions were less than with vinblastine alone.[146] Because of lack of effective combination chemotherapy regimens, cytotoxic agents have been combined with hormones and cytokines in order to enhance a therapeutic effect.

Trials of hormonal therapy were prompted by the observation that cultured renal cell carcinoma cells were inhibited by androgens.[153] Early trials that demonstrated responses to progesterones[154] and androgens[153] employed subjective response criteria. When strict criteria are used, these initial studies have an overall response proportion of 1.8%.[146] Using standard criteria for response, phase II studies of tamoxifen alone[155] and tamoxifen with medroxyprogesterone acetate[156] showed no complete or partial responses at all. One trial with medroxyprogesterone and combination chemotherapy had shown some activity[157] (four out of eight patients had at least a partial response), but the numbers of patients were small and subjective criteria for response were used. However, subsequent studies with chemotherapy and hormonal therapy have failed to demonstrate antitumor activity.[153,158]

Chemotherapy and cytokines have been tested in patients with advanced renal cell carcinoma. Single-agent trials of alpha interferon in patients with metastatic renal cell carcinoma have shown an overall response of 10% to 20%.[159–161] In vitro studies[162,163] have suggested synergism between alpha interferon and vinblastine. In clinical trials[160,164–167] greater toxicity was seen without improved efficacy. Furthermore, the sequential delivery of vinblastine followed by interferon showed no benefit over concomitant administration.[164]

## Drug Resistance

One possible explanation for the highly resistant nature of renal cell carcinoma is the multidrug resistance (*MDR1*) gene.[168,169] *MDR1* is expressed as a P-glycoprotein within the plasma membrane of cells and acts to efflux drugs out of the cell.[170,171] Cancer cells that exhibit *MDR1* expression display cross-resistance to many different chemotherapeutic agents. In cell lines selected for drug resistance, expression of the *MDR1* gene correlates with the level of drug resistance.[172,173] *MDR1* expression has been found on normal kidney cells as well as renal cell carcinoma cells,[168] and may account for the high de novo incidence of *MDR1* expression in renal cell carcinoma.

Resistance to chemotherapy may be reversed by blocking *MDR1* expression. In cell cultures, resistance to vinblastine can be overcome with a wide variety of agents including verapamil,[174] quinidine,[174,175] steroids,[176] and tamoxifen.[176] These agents can bind to the P-glycoprotein and inhibit the efflux of vinblastine.[177] Clinical trials are currently ongoing to study whether the addition of *MDR1* blocking agents in combination with cytotoxic agents will improve objective responses.

## Observation Only

Spontaneous remissions are well recognized in patients with renal cell carcinoma. A retrospective review[178] found a 0.8% proportion of spontaneous remissions. In an attempt to establish the frequency of such occurrences, 73 patients with metastatic disease were prospectively observed.[179] Most of them progressed after 1 to 3 months. Notably, three complete responses and two partial responses (lasting 10, 52, 120, 4, and 42 months, respectively) were seen without any therapeutic intervention.[179] In this small population, a 7% incidence of unexplained response was seen. In addition, four patients had stable disease for greater than 12 months. The inclusion of patients with stable disease in phase II trials can inflate response proportions. Therefore, a small percentage of patients may be followed with response or stable disease to observation and be spared the morbidity of therapy. Patients in phase II trials should be restricted to those with symptomatic disease or in whom clear evidence of progression is documented.

## Conclusions

Renal cell carcinoma is highly resistant to chemotherapy. Early clinical trials that showed responses often incorporated either subjective or poorly defined objective criteria. The only extensively studied cytotoxic agent is vinblastine, and its response proportions have been modest at best. Combination therapy is not more effective than single-agent therapy. One mechanism for this resistance is the *MDR1* and its P-glycoprotein expression as an efflux pump. Current trials with vinblastine and *MDR1* blocking agents are ongoing. Patients with metastatic renal cell carcinoma should be offered investigational therapy.

## ACKNOWLEDGMENTS

Supported in part by the American Cancer Society grant for Immunology, the Mortimer J Lacher Research Fund, the Sheila Waldman Fund, and the Barbara Lubin Goldsmith Foundation.

## REFERENCES


1. DeVita VT. Principles of chemotherapy. In: DeVita VT, ed. *Cancer: Principles and Practice of Oncology*. Philadelphia: JB Lippincott; 1989:276–287.
2. Li MC, Whitmore WF, Golbey R, et al. Effects of combination drug therapy on metastatic cancer of the testis. *JAMA*. 1960;174:145.
3. Bosl GJ, Gluckman R, Geller N, et al. VAB-6: an effective chemotherapy regimen for patients with germ cell tumor. *J Clin Oncol*. 1986;4:1493–1499.
4. Williams SD, Birch R, Einhorn LH, et al. Treatment of disseminated germ cell tumors with cisplatinum, bleomycin and either vinblastine or etoposide. *N Engl J Med*. 1987;316:1435–1440.
5. Blum RH, Carter SK, Agre K. A clinical review of bleomycin: a new antineoplastic agent. *Cancer*. 1973;31:903–914.
6. Mullins GM, Colvin M: Intensive cyclophosphamide (NSC-26271) therapy for solid tumors. *Cancer Chemother Rep*. 1975;59:411–419.
7. Buckner CD, Clift RA, Fefer A, et al. High-dose cyclophosphamide (NSC-26271) for the treatment of metastatic testicular neoplasms. *Cancer Chemother Rep*. 1974;58:709–714.
8. Monfardini S, Bajetta E, Musumeci R, Bonadonna G. Clinical use of adriamycin in advanced testicular cancer. *J Urol*. 1972; 108:293–296.
9. Kennedy BJ. Mithramycin therapy in testicular neoplasms. *Cancer*. 1970;26:755–766.
10. Samuels ML, Lanzotti VJ, Holoye PY, et al. Vinblastine in the management of testicular cancer. *Cancer*. 1970;25:1009–1017.
11. Higby DJ, Wallace HJ, Albert DJ, et al. Diaminodi-chloroplatinum: a phase I study showing responses in testicular and other tumors. *Cancer*. 1974;33:1219–1251.
12. Motzer RJ, Tauer K, Bosl GJ, et al. A phase II trial of carboplatin in patients with advanced germ cell tumors refractory to cisplatin. *Cancer Treatm Rep*. 1987;71:197–198.
13. Trump DL, Elson P, Brodovsky H, et al. Carboplatin in advanced, refractory germ cell neoplasms: a phase II Eastern Cooperative Oncology Group study. *Cancer Treatm Rep*. 1987;71:989–990.
14. Drasga RE, Williams SD, Einhorn LH, et al. Phase II evaluation of iproplatin in refractory germ cell tumors: a Southeastern Cancer Study group trial. *Cancer Treatm Rep*. 1987;7:863–864.
15. Chun H, Bosl GJ, Golbey RB. Phase II trial of 1,2-diaminocyclohexane-(4-carboxyphthalato) platinum (II) in patients with refractory germ cell tumors. *Cancer Treatm Rep*. 1985;69:459–460.
16. Gold E, Bosl GJ, Whitmore WF, et al. Phase II trial of 13 cis-retinoic acid in the treatment of patients (PTS) with advanced germ cell tumors. *Proc Am Assoc Cancer Res*. 1983;24:150 (Abstract C-552).
17. Vogelzang NJ, Raghaven D, Kennedy BJ. VP-16-213 (etoposide): the mandrake root from Issyk-Kul. *Am J Med*. 1982;72:136–144.
18. Wheeler BM, Loehrer PJ, Williams SD, et al. Ifosfamide in refractory male germ cell tumors. *J Clin Oncol*. 1986;4:28–34.
19. Scheulen ME, Niederle N, Bremer K, et al. Efficacy of ifosfamide in refractory malignant diseases and uroprotection by mesna: results of a phase II study with 151 patients. *Cancer Treatm Rep*. 1983;10 (Suppl A):93–101.
20. Chun H, Bosl GJ. Phase II trial of mitoguazone in patients with refractory germ cell tumors. *Cancer Treatm Rep*. 1985;69:461–462.
21. Bosl GJ. Treatment of germ cell tumors at Memorial Sloan-Kettering Cancer Center: 1960 to present. In: Garnick MB, ed. *Genitourinary Cancer*. New York: Churchill Livingstone, 1985:45–61.
22. Fitzharris EM, Kaye SB, Saverymuttu S, et al. VP-16-213 as a single agent in advanced testicular tumors. *Eur J Cancer*. 1980;16:1193–1197.
23. Cavalli F, Klept O, Revard J, et al. A phase II study of oral VP-16-213 in patients with nonseminomatous testicular cancer (abstr). *Proc Am Assoc Cancer Res Am Soc Clin Oncol*. 1980;21:137.
24. Schabel M Jr, Trader MW, Laster WR, et al. cis-Dichorodiammineplatinum (II): combination chemotherapy and cross resistance studies with tumors of mice. *Cancer Treatm Rep*. 1979;63:1593–1597.
25. Wittes RE, Yagoda A, Silvay O, et al. Chemotherapy of germ cell tumors of the testis: induction of remissions with vinblastine, actinomycin D, and bleomycin. *Cancer*. 1976; 37:637–645.

26. Cheng E, Cvitkovic E, Wittes R, et al. Germ cell tumors: VAB II in metastatic testicular cancer. *Cancer.* 1978;42:2162–2168.
27. Reynolds TG, Vugrin D, Cvitkovic E, et al. VAB-3 combination chemotherapy of metastatic testicular cancer. *Cancer.* 1981;48:888–898.
28. Vugrin D, Cvitkovic E, Whitmore W, et al. VAB-4 combination chemotherapy in the treatment of metastatic testis tumors. *Cancer.* 1981;47:833–839.
29. Vugrin D, Whitmore W, Golbey R: VAB-5 combination chemotherapy in prognostically poor risk patients with germ cell tumors. *Cancer.* 1983;51:1072–1075.
30. Bosl GJ, Geller N, Bajorin D, et al. A randomized trial of etoposide + cisplatin versus vinblastine, + bleomycin + cisplatin + cyclophosphamide + dactinomycin in patients with good-prognosis germ cell tumors. *J Clin Oncol.* 1988;6:1231–1238.
31. Bajorin DF, Sarosdy MF, Bosl GJ, et al. A randomized trial of etoposide + carboplatin (EC) versus etoposide + cisplatin (EP) in patients (PTS) with metastatic germ cell tumor (GCT). *Proc Am Soc Clin Oncol.* 1991;10:535.
32. Bosl GJ, Geller NL, Vogelzang NJ, et al. Alternating cycles of etoposide + cisplatin and VAB-6 in the treatment of poor risk germ cell tumors. *J Clin Oncol.* 1986;10:1493–1499.
33. Motzer RJ, Cooper K, Geller N, et al. Carboplatin, etoposide, bleomycin for patients with poor-risk germ cell tumors. *Cancer.* 1990;65:2465–2470.
34. Bosl GJ, Yagoda A, Golbey RB, et al. Role of etoposide-based chemotherapy in the treatment of patients with refractory or relapsing germ cell tumors. *Am J Med.* 1985;78:423–427.
35. Motzer RJ, Cooper K, Geller NL, et al. The role of ifosfamide plus cisplatin-based chemotherapy as salvage therapy for patients with refractory germ cell tumors. *Cancer.* 1990;66:2476–2481.
36. Motzer RJ, Gulati SC, Crown JP, et al. High-dose chemotherapy and autologous bone marrow rescue for patients with refractory germ cell tumors: early intervention is better tolerated. *Cancer.* 1992;69:550–556.
37. Bosl GJ, Geller NL, Cirrincione C, et al. Serum tumor markers in patients with metastatic germ cell tumors of the testis. *Am J Med.* 1983;75:29–35.
38. Einhorn LH, Williams SD, Troner M, et al. The role of maintenance therapy in disseminated testicular cancer. *N Engl J Med.* 1981;305:727–731.
39. Vaitudaitis JL, Braunstein G, Ross G. A radioimmunoassay which specifically measures HCG in the presence of human luteinizing hormone. *Am J Obstet Gynecol.* 1972;113:751–758.
40. Waldman TA, McIntire KR. The use of radioimmunoassays for alpha-fetoprotein in the diagnosis of malignancy. *Cancer.* 1974;34:1510–1515.
41. Lange PH, Vogelzang NJ, Goldman A, et al. Marker half-life analysis as a prognostic tool in testis cancer. *J Urol.* 1981;128:708–711.
42. Bosl GJ, Geller NL, Cirrincione C, et al. Multivariate analysis of prognostic variables in patients with metastatic testicular cancer. *Cancer Res.* 1983;43:3403–3407.
43. Toner G, Geller NL, Tan C, et al. Serum tumor marker half life during chemotherapy allows early prediction of complete response and survival in nonseminomatous germ cell tumors. *Cancer Res.* 1990;50:5904–5910.
44. Motzer RJ, Bosl GJ, Geller NL, et al. Advanced seminoma: the role of chemotherapy and adjunctive surgery. *Ann Intern Med.* 1988;108:513–518.
45. Collins DH, Pugh RCB. Classification and frequency of testicular tumors. *Br J Urol.* 1964;36 (Suppl):1–11.
46. Israel A, Bosl GJ, Golbey RB, et al. The results of chemotherapy for extragonadal germ-cell tumors in the cisplatin era: the Memorial Sloan-Kettering Cancer Center experience (1975–1982). *J Clin Oncol.* 1985;3:1073–1078.
47. Martini N, Golbey R, Hajdu S, et al. Primary mediastinal germ cell tumors. *Cancer.* 1974;33:736–769.
48. Reynolds TG, Yagoda A, Vugrin D. Chemotherapy of mediastinal germ cell tumors. *Semin Oncol.* 1979;6:113–115.
49. Feun LG, Samson MK, Stephans RL. Vinblastine, bleomycin, cis-diaminedichloroplatinum in disseminated seminoma. *Cancer Clin Trials.* 1980;3:307–313.
50. Garnick MB, Canellos GP, Richie JP. Treatment and surgical staging of testicular and primary extragonadal germ cell tumors. *JAMA.* 1981;250:1733–1741.
51. Logothetis CJ, Samuels M, Selig JJ, et al. Improved survival with cyclic chemotherapy for nonseminomatous germ cell tumors of the testis. *J Clin Oncol.* 1985;3:316–325.
52. Birch R, Williams S, Cone A, et al. Prognostic factors for favorable outcome in disseminated germ cell tumors. *J Clin Oncol.* 1986;4:400–407.
53. Hainsworth JD, Einhorn LH, Williams SD. Advanced extragonadal germ cell tumors: successful treatment with combination chemotherapy. *Ann Intern Med.* 1982;93:7–11.
54. Einhorn L, Williams SD, Loehrer PJ, et al. A comparison of four versus three courses of cisplatin, VP-16, and bleomycin in favorable prognosis disseminated germ cell tumors. *J Clin Oncol.* 1989;7:387–391.
55. Harstrick A, Schmoll HJ, Wilke H, et al. Cisplatin, etoposide, and ifosfamide salvage ther-

apy for refractory germ cell carcinoma. *J Clin Oncol.* 1991;9:1549–1555.

56. Loehrer PJ, Lauer R, Einhorn LH, et al. Salvage therapy in recurrent germ cell cancer: ifosfamide and cisplatin plus either vinblastine or etoposide. *Ann Intern Med.* 1988;109:540–546.
57. Motzer RJ, Geller NL, Tan CCY, et al. Salvage chemotherapy for patients with germ cell tumors: the Memorial Sloan-Kettering Cancer Center experience (1979–1989). *Cancer.* 1991;67:1305–1310.
58. Nichols C, Tricot G, Williams S, et al. Dose-intensive chemotherapy in refractory germ cell cancer—a phase I/II trial of high-dose carboplatin and etoposide with autologous bone marrow transplantation. *J Clin Oncol.* 1989;7:932–939.
59. Motzer RJ, Bosl GJ. The role of adjuvant chemotherapy in patients with stage II nonseminomatous germ cell tumors. *Urol Clin North Am.* (in press).
60. Weissbach L, Hartlapp JH. Adjuvant chemotherapy of metastatic stage II nonseminomatous testis tumor. *J Urol.* 1991;146:1295–1298.
61. Williams SD, Stablein DM, Einhorn LH, et al. Immediate adjuvant chemotherapy versus observation with treatment at relapse in pathologic stage II testicular cancer. *N Engl J Med.* 1987;317:1433–1438.
62. Richie JP, Kantoff PW. Is adjuvant chemotherapy necessary for patients with stage BI testicular cancer? *J Clin Oncol.* 1991;9:1393–1396.
63. Brenner J, Vugrin D, Whitmore W. Cytoreductive surgery for advanced nonseminomatous germ cell tumors of the testis. *Urology.* 1982;19:571–575.
64. Geller NL, Bosl GJ, Chan EYW. Prognostic factors after complete response in patients with metastatic germ cell tumors. *Cancer.* 1989; 63:440–445.
65. Hendry WF, Goldstraw P, Peckham MJ. The role of surgery in the combined management of metastases from malignant teratomas of the testis. *Br J Urol.* 1987;59:358–362.
66. Toner GC, Panicek DM, Bosl GJ, et al. Adjunctive surgery after chemotherapy for nonseminomatous germ cell tumors: recommendations for patient selection. *J Clin Oncol.* 1990;8:1683–1694.
67. Yagoda A. Chemotherapy of urothelial tract tumors. *Cancer.* 1987;60:574–585.
68. Seidman AD, Scher HI. The evolving role of chemotherapy for muscle infiltrating bladder cancer. *Semin Oncol.* 1991;18:585–595.
69. Yagoda A. Chemotherapy of metastatic bladder cancer. *Cancer.* 1980;45:1879–1888.
70. Seidman AD, Scher HI, Heinemann MH, et al. Continuous infusion gallium nitrate for patients with advanced refractory urothelial tract tumors. *Cancer.* 1991;68:2561–2565.
71. Stoter G, Splinter TAW, Child JA, et al. Combination chemotherapy with cisplatin and methotrexate in advanced transitional cell cancer of the bladder. *J Urol.* 1987;137:663–666.
72. Sternberg CN, Yagoda A, Scher HI, et al. Methotrexate, vinblastine, doxorubicin, and cisplatin for advanced transitional cell carcinoma of the urothelium. *Cancer.* 1989;64: 2448–2458.
73. Geller NL, Sternberg CN, Penenberg P, et al. Prognostic factors for survival of patients with advanced urothelial tumors treated with methotrexate, vinblastine, doxorubicin, and cisplatin chemotherapy. *Cancer.* 1991;67:1525–1531.
74. Gabrilove JL, Jakubowski A, Scher HI, et al. Effects of granulocyte colony-stimulating factor on neutropenia and morbidity due to chemotherapy for transitional-cell carcinoma of the urothelium. *N Engl J Med.* 1988;318:1414–1422.
75. Loehrer PJ, Elson P, Kuebler JP, et al. Advanced bladder cancer: a prospective intergroup trial comparing single agent cisplatin (CDDP) versus MVAC combination therapy (INT 0078). *Proc Am Soc Clin Oncol.* 1990; 9(abstract):132.
76. Logothetis CJ, Dexeus FH, Finn L, et al. A prospective randomized trial comparing MVAC and CISCA chemotherapy for patients with metastatic urothelial tumors. *J Clin Oncol.* 1990;8:1050–1055.
77. Logothetis CJ, Hossan E, Sella A, et al. Fluorouracil and recombinant interferon alfa-2a in the treatment of metastatic chemotherapy-refractory urothelial tumors. *JNCI.* 1991;83:285–288.
78. Logothetis CJ, Dexeus FH, Sella A, et al. Escalated therapy for refractory urothelial tumors: methotrexate-vinblastine-doxorubicin-cisplatin plus unglycosylated recombinant human granulocyte-macrophage colony-stimulating factor. *JNCI.* 1990;82:667–672.
79. Merrin C, Beckley S. Adjuvant chemotherapy for bladder cancer with doxorubicin hydrochloride and cyclophosphamide: preliminary report. *J Urol.* 1978;119:62–63.
80. Richards B, Akdas A, Corberr P, et al. Adjuvant chemotherapy following radical radiotherapy in $T_3$ bladder carcinoma. *Recent Results Cancer Res.* 1978;68:334–337.
81. Einstein AB, Coombs J, Pearse H, et al: Cisplatin (CP) adjuvant therapy following pre-operative radiotherapy plus radical cystectomy (RT = RCy) for invasive bladder carcinoma: a randomized trial of the National Bladder Cancer Group (NBCG). *Am Urol Assoc.* 1985;133:222 (abstract #433).
82. Skinner DG, Daniels JR, Lieskovsky G. Current status of adjuvant chemotherapy after radical cystectomy for deeply invasive bladder cancer. Urology. 1984;24:46–52.

83. Socquet Y. Surgery and adjuvant chemotherapy with high-dose methotrexate and folinic acid rescue for infiltrating tumors of the bladder. *Cancer Treatm Rep.* 1978;65:187–189.

84. Logothetis CJ, Johnson DE, Chong C, et al. Adjuvant cyclophosphamide, doxorubicin, and cisplatin chemotherapy for bladder cancer: an update. *J Clin Oncol.* 1988;6:1590–1596.

85. Skinner DG, Daniels JR, Russell CA, et al. The role of adjuvant chemotherapy following cystectomy for invasive bladder cancer: a prospective comparative trial. *J Urol.* 1991; 145:459–467.

86. Scher HI: Chemotherapy for invasive bladder cancer: neoadjuvant versus adjuvant. *Semin Oncol.* 1990;17:555–565.

87. Scher HI, Herr HW, Sternberg C, et al. M-VAC (methotrexate, vinblastine, adriamycin, and cisplatin) and bladder preservation. In: Splinter T, Scher H, eds. *Neoadjuvant Chemotherapy of Invasive Bladder Cancer.* New York: Alan R. Liss; 1990:179–186.

88. Scher HI, Yagoda A, Herr HW, et al. Neoadjuvant MVAC (methotrexate, vinblastine, doxorubicin, cisplatin) effect on primary bladder lesions. *J Urol.* 1988;139:470–474.

89. Shipley WU, Kaufman DS, Heney NM. Radiation therapy in bladder cancer: can its integration with chemotherapy and transurethral surgery make cystectomy unnecessary? *Oncology.* 1990;4:25–32.

90. Herr HW. Conservative management of muscle-infiltrating bladder cancer: prospective experience. *J Urol.* 1987;138:1162–1163.

91. Logothetis CJ, Samuels ML, Selig DE, et al. Combined intravenous and intra-arterial cyclophosphamide, doxorubicin, and cisplatin (CISCA) in the management of select patients with invasive urothelial tumors. *Cancer Treatm Rep.* 1985;69:33–36.

92. Scher HI, Yagoda A, Herr HW, et al. Neoadjuvant MVAC (methotrexate, vinblastine, doxorubicin, cisplatin) for extravesicular urinary tract tumors. *J Urol.* 1988;139:475–477.

93. Eisenberger MA, Simon R, O'Dwyer PJ, et al. A reevaluation of nonhormonal cytotoxic chemotherapy in the treatment of prostatic carcinoma. *J Clin Oncol.* 1985;3:827–841.

94. Yagoda A, Watson RC, Natale RB, et al. A critical analysis of response criteria in patients with prostatic cancer with cis-diamminedichloride platinum II. *Cancer.* 1979;44:1553–1562.

95. Natale RB, Yagoda A, Watson RC, et al. Phase II trial of neocarzinostatin in patients with bladder and prostatic cancer: toxicity of a five-day IV bolus schedule. *Cancer.* 1980;45:2836–2842.

96. Natale RB, Yagoda A, Watson RC. Phase II trial of AMSA (4[9-acrinylamino methanesulfon-m-anisidide]) in prostatic cancer. *Cancer Treatm Rep.* 1982;66:208–212.

97. Scher HI, Yagoda A, Watson RC, et al. Phase II trial of doxorubicin in bidimensionally measurable prostate carcinoma. *J Urol.* 1984; 131:1099–1102.

98. Scher HI, Yagoda A, Ahmed T, et al. Methygyoxal-bis(guanylhydrazone) in hormone-resistant adenocarcinoma of the prostate. *J Clin Oncol.* 1985;3:224–228.

99. Scher HI, Sternberg C, Heston WD, et al. Etoposide in prostatic cancer: experimental studies and phase II trial in patients with bidimensionally measurable disease. *Cancer Chemother Pharmacol.* 1986;18:24–26.

100. Scher HI, Curley T, Geller N, et al. Gallium nitrate in prostatic cancer: evaluation of antitumor activity and effects on bone turnover. *Cancer Treatm Rep.* 1987;71:887–893.

101. Scher HI, Smart-Curly T, Heston WDW, et al. Phase I-II trial of alpha-difluoromethylornithine (DFMO) [MDL 71,782] and mitoguazone (MGBG) in hormone refractory prostatic cancer (PC). *Proc Am Assoc Cancer Res.* 1988;29:204 (abstr).

102. Scher HI, Curly T, Geller N, et al. Trimetrexate in prostatic cancer: preliminary observations on the use of prostate-specific antigen and acid phosphatase as a marker in measurable hormone-refractory disease. *J Clin Oncol.* 1990;8:1830–1838.

103. Petrylak DP, Scher HI, Li Z, et al. Prognostic factors for survival of patients treated with single-agent chemotherapy for bidimensionally measurable hormone refractory metastatic prostatic carcinoma. *Proc Am Assoc Cancer Res.* 1990;31:225.

104. Eagan RT, Hahn RG, Myers RP. Adriamycin (NSC-123127) versus 5-fluorouracil (NSC-19893) and cyclophosphamide (NSC-26271) in the treatment of metastatic prostate cancer. *Cancer Treatm Rep.* 1976;60:115–117.

105. Torti FM, Aston D, Lum BL, et al. Weekly doxorubicin in endocrine-refractory carcinoma of the prostate. *J Clin Oncol.* 1983;1:477–482.

106. Scher HI, Curley T, Yeh S, et al. Therapeutic alternatives for hormone-refractory prostatic cancer. *Semin Urol.* 1992;10:55–64.

107. Ashby H, DiMattina M, Linehan M, et al. The inhibition of human adrenal steroidogenic enzyme activities by suramin. *J Clin Endocrinol Metab.* 1989;68:505–598.

108. Berns EMJJ, Schurmans ALG, Bolt J, et al. Antiproliferative effects of suramin on androgen responsive tumor cells. *Eur J Cancer.* 1990;26:470–474.

109. Kim JH, Sherwood ER, Krengel SS, et al. Cytostatic and cytotoxic effects of suramin on human prostate cancer cell lines, PC3 and DU145. *J Urol.* 1990;143:213–216.

110. LaRocca RV, Danesi R, Cooper MR, et al. Effect of suramin on human prostate cancer cells in vitro. *J Urol.* 1991;145:393–398.

111. Ahman FR, Schwartz J, Dorr R, et al. Suramin in hormone resistant metastatic prostate cancer: significant anticancer activity but unanticipated toxicity. *Proc Am Soc Clin Oncol.* 1991; 10:178.

112. Meyers CE, LaRocca R, Stein C, et al. Treatment of hormonally refractory prostate cancer with suramin. *Proc Am Soc Clin Oncol.* 1990; 9:133.

113. Scher HI. Prostatic cancer: where do we go from here? *Current Op Oncol.* 1991;3:568–574.

114. Scher HI, Jodrell DI, Iversen JM, et al. Use of adaptive control with feedback to individualized suramin doses. *Cancer Res.* 1992;52:64–70.

115. Murphy GP, Beckley S, Brady MF, et al. Treatment of newly diagnosed metastatic prostate cancer patients with chemotherapy agents in combination with hormones versus hormones alone. *Cancer.* 1983;51:1264–1272.

116. Stearns ME, Wang M, Tew K, et al. Estramustine binds a MAP-1 like protein to inhibit microtubule assembly in vitro and disrupt microtubule organization in DU 145 cells. *J Cell Biol.* 1988;107:2647–2656.

117. Seidman AD, Scher HI, Petrylak D, et al. Estramustine and vinblastine: use of prostatic specific antigen as a clinical end point for hormone-refractory prostatic cancer. *J Urol.* 1992; 147:931–934.

118. Amato RJ, Logothetis CJ, Dexeus FH, et al. Preliminary results of a phase II trial of estramustine (EMCYT) and vinblastine (VLB) for patients with progressive hormone-refractory prostate carcinoma (HRPC). *Proc Am Assoc Cancer Res.* 1991;32:86 (abstr 1111).

119. Paulson DF, Berry WR, Cox EB, et al. Treatment of metastatic endocrine-unresponsive carcinoma of the prostate gland with mutagenic chemotherapy: indicators of response to therapy. *JNCI.* 1979;63:615–622.

120. Berry WR, Laszlo J, Cox E, et al. Prognostic factors in metastatic and hormonally unresponsive carcinoma of the prostate. *Cancer.* 1979;44:763–775.

121. Emrich LJ, Priore RL, Murphy GL, et al. Prognostic factors in patients with advanced stage prostate cancer. *Cancer Res.* 1985;45:5173–5179.

122. Mulders PFA, Dijkman GA, Fernandez de Moral P, et al. Analysis of prognostic factors in disseminated prostatic cancer: an update. *Cancer.* 1990;65:2758–2761.

123. Brawer MK, Lange PH. PSA in the screening, staging and follow-up of early-stage prostate cancer. A review of recent developments. *World J Urol.* 1989;7:7.

124. Cooper EH, Armitage TG, Robinson MRG, et al. Prostate specific antigen and the prediction of prognosis in metastatic prostatic cancer. *Cancer.* 1990;(Suppl 5) 66:1025–1028.

125. Miller JI, Ahmann FR, Drach GW, et al. The clinical usefulness of serum prostate specific antigen after hormonal therapy of metastatic prostate cancer. *J Urol.* 1992;147:956–961.

126. Ahman FR, Marx P, Ahman M. Predicting response to therapy in metastatic prostate cancer with serum prostate specific (PSA) levels. *Proc Am Soc Clin Oncol.* 1990;9:134 (abstr 521).

127. Kelly WK, Scher HI, Mazumdar, et al. Prostate specific antigen (PSA) as a measure of disease outcome in metastatic hormone refractory prostate cancer (PC). *Proc Am Soc Clin Oncol.* 1992;11:199 (abstr 609).

128. Oesterling JE, Hauzer CG, Farrow GM. Small cell anaplastic carcinoma of the prostate: a clinical, pathological, and immunohistological study of 27 patients. *J Urol.* 1992;147:804–807.

129. Amato RJ, Logothetis CJ, Hallinan R, et al. Chemotherapy for small cell carcinoma of prostatic origin. *J Urol.* 1992;147:935–937.

130. Schneider RJ, Woodcock TM, Yagoda A. Phase II trial of 4′-(9-acridinylamino) methanesulfon-m-anisidide (AMSA) in patients with metastatic hypernephroma. *Cancer Treatm Rep.* 1980;64:183–185.

131. Scher HI, Ahmed T, Yagoda A, et al. Experimental studies and phase II trial of bisantrene in advanced urothelial malignancies. *Cancer Invest.* 1985;3:123–127.

132. Yagoda A. Phase II trials with cis-dichlorodiammineplatinum(II) in the treatment of urothelial cancer. *Cancer Treatm Rep.* 1979;63:1565–1572.

133. Scher HI, Yagoda A, Ahmed T, et al. Phase II trial of 10-deazaaminopterin for advanced hypernephroma. *Anticancer Res.* 1984;4:409–410.

134. Scher HI, Yagoda A, Golbey RB, et al. Phase II trial of 4-demethoxydaunorubicin (DMDR) for advanced hypernephroma. *Cancer Chemother Pharmacol.* 1985;14:79–80.

135. Motzer R, Scher H, Bajorin D, et al. Phase II trial of didemnin B in patients with advanced renal cell carcinoma. *Invest New Drug.* 1990;8:391–392.

136. Sternberg CN, Yagoda A, Casper E. Phase II trial elliptinium in advanced renal cell carcinoma and carcinoma of the breast. *Anticancer Res.* 1985;5:415–418.

137. Benedetto P, Ahmed T, Yagoda A, et al. Phase II trial of 4′epi-adriamycin in advanced hypernephroma. *Am J Clin Oncol.* 1983;6:211–214.

138. Schwartz S, Yagoda A. Watson RC. Phase I-II trial of gallium nitrate for advanced hypernephroma. *Anticancer Res.* 1984;4:317–318.

139. Zeffren J, Yagoda A, Watson RC, et al. Phase II trial of methylglyoxal bis-guanyhydrazone in advanced renal cell cancer. *Cancer Treatm Rep.* 1981;65:525–527.

140. Sternberg C, Yagoda A, Scher HI. Phase II trial of n-methyl-formamide in renal cancer. *Cancer Treatm Rep.* 1986;70:681–682.

141. Natale RB, Yagoda A, Kelsen DP, et al. Phase II trial of PALA in hypernephroma and urinary bladder cancer. *Cancer Treatm Rep.* 1982; 66:2091–2092.

142. Yagoda A, Scher HI, Bosl GJ. Phase II trial of trimetrexate in patients with advanced renal cell carcinoma. *Eur J Cancer.* 1989;25:753–754.

143. Zeffren J, Yagoda A, Kelsen D, et al. Phase I-II trial of a 5 day continuous infusion of vinblastine sulfate. *Anticancer Res.* 1984;4:411–414.

144. Wong PP, Yagoda A, Currie VE, et al. Phase II study of desacetyl vinblastine amide sulfate (vindesine) in the therapy of advanced renal carcinoma. *Cancer Treatm Rep.* 1977;61: 1727–1729.

145. Yagoda A. Chemotherapy of renal cell carcinoma: 1983–1989. *Semin Urol.* 1989;7:199–206.

146. Hrushesky WJ, Murphy GP. Current status of therapy for advanced renal cell carcinoma. *J Surg Oncol.* 1977;9:277–288.

147. Crivellari D, Tumolo S, Frustaci S, et al. Phase II study of five-day continuous infusion of vinblastine in patients with metastatic renal-cell carcinoma. *Am J Clin Oncol.* 1987;10:231–233.

148. Kluebler JP, Hogan TF, Trump DL, Bryan GT. Phase II study of continuous 5-day vinblastine infusion in renal adenocarcinoma. *Cancer Treatm Rep.* 1984;68:925–926.

149. Von Roemeling R, Hrushesky WJ. Circadian patterning of continuous floxutidine infusion reduces toxicity and allows higher dose intensity in patients with widespread cancer. *J Clin Oncol.* 1989;7:1710–1719.

150. Damascelli B, Marchiano A, Spreafico C, et al. Circadian continuous chemotherapy of renal cell carcinoma with an implantable infusion pump. *Cancer.* 1990;66:237–241.

151. Hahn RG, Begg CB, Davis T. Phase II study of vinblastine-CCNU, triazinate, and dactinomycin in advanced renal cell carcinoma. *Cancer Treatm Rep.* 1981;65:711–713.

152. Sommer HH, Fossa SD, Lien HH. Combination chemotherapy of advanced renal cell carcinoma with CCNU and vinblastine. *Cancer Chemother Pharmacol.* 1985;14:227–278.

153. Harris DT. Hormonal therapy and chemotherapy for renal cell carcinoma. *Semin Oncol.* 1983;10:422–430.

154. Bloom HJG. Medroxyprogesterone acetate (provera) in the treatment of metastatic renal cancer. *Br J Cancer.* 1971;25:250–265.

155. Glick JH, Wein A, Torri S, et al. Phase II study of tamoxifen in patients with advanced renal cell carcinoma. *Cancer Treatm Rep.* 1980; 64:343–344.

156. Fuks JZ, Aisner J, Van Echo DA, et al. Phase II study of medroxyprogesterone acetate with tamoxifen in advanced renal cell cancer. *Cancer Treatm Rep.* 1982;66:1773–1774.

157. Katakkar SB, Franks CR. Chemo-hormonal therapy for metastatic renal cell carcinoma with adriamycin, hydroxyurea, vinblastine and medroxyprogesterone acetate. *Cancer Treatm Rep.* 1978;62:1379–1380.

158. Bell DR, Aroney RS, Fisher RJ, et al. High-dose methotrexate with leucovorin rescue, vinblastine, and bleomycin with or without tamoxifen in metastatic renal cell carcinoma. *Cancer Treatm Rep.* 1984;68:587–590.

159. Krown SE. Interferon treatment of renal cell carcinoma: current status and future prospects. *Cancer.* 1987;59:647–651.

160. Minasian LM, Motzer RJ, Krown SE, et al. Interferon-α 2a (IFN-α) in 160 patients (pts) with advanced renal cancer (RCC). *Proc Am Soc Clin Oncol.* 1992;11:203 (abstr 625).

161. Muss HB. Interferon therapy for renal cell carcinoma. *Semin Oncol.* 1987;(Suppl 2) 13:36–42.

162. Aapro MS, Alberts DS, Salmon SE. Interactions of human leukocyte interferon and vinca alkaloids and other chemotherapeutic agents against human tumors in clonogenic assays. *Cancer Chemother Pharmacol.* 1983;10:161–166.

163. Sidky YA, Borden EC, Schmid SM, et al. In vitro and in vivo antitumor effects of treatment with vinblastine (VBL) is enhanced by combination with interferons (IFN). *Proc Am Assoc Cancer Res.* 1987;28:380 (abstr).

164. Dexeus F, Logothetis C, Chong C, et al. Phase II study in metastatic renal cell carcinoma (RCC) comparing combination chemotherapy (CT) versus interferon (IFN) alternating with combination chemotherapy. *Proc Am Soc Clin Oncol.* 1988;7:131 (abstr).

165. Fossa SD, De Garis ST, Heier MS, et al. Recombinant interferon alfa-2a with or without vinblastine in metastatic renal cell carcinoma. *Cancer.* 1986;57:1700–1704.

166. Neidhart JA, Anderson SA, Harris JE, et al. Vinblastine fails to improve response of renal cancer to interferon alpha-nl: high response in patients with pulmonary metastases. *J Clin Oncol.* 1991;9:832–837.

167. Schornagel J, Verwey J, ten Bokkel Huinink W, et al. Phase II study of recombinant interferon alpha-2 (IFN) and vinblastine (VLB) in advanced renal carcinoma (RCC). *Proc Am Soc Clin Oncol.* 1987;6:106 (abstr).

168. Fojo AT, Shen DW, Mickley LA, et al. Intrinsic drug resistance in human kidney cancer is associated with expression of a human multidrug-resistance gene. *J Clin Oncol.* 1987; 5:1922–1927.

169. Rothenberg M, Ling V. Multidrug resistance: molecular and clinical relevance. *JNCI.* 1989;81:907–910.

170. Fojo A, Akiyama SI, Gottesman MM, et al. Reduced drug accumulation in multiply drug-resistant human KB carcinoma cell lines. *Cancer Res.* 1985;45:3002–3007.

171. Kartner N, Riordan JR, Ling V. Cell surface P-glycoprotein associated with multi-drug resistance in mammalian cell lines. *Science.* 1983;221:1285–1288.

172. Shen DW, Fojo A, Chin JE, et al. Human multidrug-resistant cell lines: Increased MDR1 expression can precede gene amplification. *Science.* 1986;232:643–645.

173. Shen DW, Fojo A, Roninson IB, et al. Multidrug-resistance in DNA mediated transformants is linked to transfer of the human MDR1 gene. *Mol Cell Biol.* 1986;6:4039–4045.

174. Tsuruo T, Iida H, Kitatani Y, et al. Potentiation of vincristine and adriamycin effects in human hematopoietic tumor cell lines by calcium antagonists and calmodulin inhibitors. *Cancer Res.* 1983;43:2267–2272.

175. Tsuruo T, Iida H, Kitatani Y, et al: Effects of quinidine and related compounds on cytotoxicity and cellular accumulation of vincristine and adriamycin in drug-resistant tumor cells. *Cancer Res.* 1984;44:4303–4307.

176. Chabhner BA, Fojo A. P-glycoprotein and its allies—the elusive foes. *JNCI.* 1989;81:910–913.

177. Cornwell MM, Pastan I, Gottesman MM. Certain calcium channel blockers bind specifically to multidrug-resistant KB carcinoma membrane vesicles and inhibit binding to P-glycoprotein. *J Biol Chem.* 1987;262:2166–2170.

178. Montie JE, Stewart BH, Straffon RA, et al. The role of adjunctive surgery in renal cell carcinoma. *J Urol.* 1977;117:272–274.

179. Oliver RTD, Nethersell ABW, Bottomley JM. Unexplained spontaneous regression and alpha-interferon as treatment for metastatic renal carcinoma. *Br J Urol.* 1989;63:128–131.

# 39

# Radiation Therapy in Urologic Disease

*William T. Sause and Jennifer Fischbach*

## INTRODUCTION

Ionizing radiation has been used to eradicate malignant tumors for approximately 90 years. The first reported use of radium in the treatment of a patient with cervical carcinoma was credited to Margaret Cleaves, an American physician, in 1903. An American surgeon, Dr. Nicholas Sinn, was the first to publish therapeutic results with external beam irradiation in the treatment of a spleen in a patient with leukemia. It remained for the Europeans, however, to apply and optimize this new tool in the treatment of malignant diseases.[1]

The development of radium applications for carcinoma of the cervix began at the Institute of Radium in Paris in 1919 under Regaude, Lacassagne, and their associates. The clinic organization was consistent with what is now called a modern tumor clinic. The surgeon, urologist, dentist, and radiotherapist saw the patients in consultation. At that time, all patients with cancer of the cervix were treated with radiation. Their technique, which remains essentially unchanged since the late 1920s, has been successfully utilized in the treatment of thousands of carcinomas of the cervix.[2] Table 1 reflects the survival figures for those patients with invasive carcinoma of the cervix treated from the early 1900s to the 1980s.[1,3]

The French were also the first to define the application of external beam radiation therapy in the treatment of carcinoma of the larynx. In Coutard's classic article published in 1930, he describes his experience from 1920 to 1926 in the treatment of hypopharyngeal carcinomas. This was the first large series in which external beam radiation therapy alone was utilized as a potentially curative modality in head and neck cancer. Coutard observed a cure rate of approximately 30% in those patients heretofore treated with an aggressive surgical approach (Table 2).[4,5] These early successes with tumors in the head and neck area, larynx, hypopharynx and oral cavity, and gynecologic sites were probably due to their favorable anatomic locations, suitable for x-ray equipment available at that time, rather than any inherent radiosensitivity. The radiobiological properties of low-energy x-ray machines resulted in the development of unusual treatment schedules designed to avoid moist desquamation of the skin. The inadequacy of equipment and incorrect clinical observations resulted in the elucidation of erroneous radiobiologic principles that have impacted modern radiation therapy. Two classic premises that have been responsible for perpetuating erroneous utilization of irradiation are that cells having a greater reproductive capacity and greater doubling time are preferentially killed with irradiation and that tumors are inherently radiosensitive or radioresistant.[6]

**TABLE 1. Cure Rates of Patients with Cervix Cancer (%)**

| Study | Stage I | Stage II |
|---|---|---|
| Institute of Radium | | |
| 1919 | 57 | 36 |
| 1933 | 81 | 51 |
| Patterns of Care USA | | |
| 1983 | 90 | 75 |

When one corrects for the size and anatomic location of the tumor, there is little clinical evidence supporting a concept that the common epithelial neoplasms respond differently from one another in regard to their inherent radiosensitivity. The availability of modern equipment has resulted in a better understanding of principles of clinical radiobiology.

Treatment in the latter part of this century has been optimized with the use of modern megavoltage irradiation equipment. The major advantage of this equipment is skin sparing. This allows radiation to be delivered at depth without creating intolerable skin reactions. Modern equipment is also isocentrically mounted so that treatment can be delivered with optimal sparing of critical structures.

The field of irradiation has made great strides in this century and the remainder of this chapter will deal with current concepts regarding radiobiology, physical application of irradiation, and specific tumors of the genitourinary system.

Clinical evidence of the effects of ionizing radiations on a variety of malignant tumors and normal tissues accumulated rapidly in the early 1900s. Development of more rational approaches to tumor therapy and efforts to improve the therapeutic ratio require an understanding of the physical basis of ionizing radiations and their interaction with biological material.

**TABLE 2. Cure Rates of Hypopharynx Cancer (%)**

| Study | Cure Rate |
|---|---|
| Coutard[5]—tonsil | |
| France 1926 | 46 |
| Million[4] T2 tonsil | |
| USA 1984 | 78 |

## PHYSICAL BASIS OF RADIATION ONCOLOGY

Ionizing radiations are part of the continuous spectrum of electromagnetic (EM) radiation that includes visible light, infrared, radio and electrical waves, as well as ultraviolet light. All types of EM radiation consist of photons, discrete packets or quanta of energy that travel at the speed of light and have wave properties. The x-ray and γ-ray photons carry more energy than visible light or heat, and differ only in their origin, not in physical or biological properties. X-rays result from energy losses from electrons stopped in an absorbing material whereas γ-rays are emitted from the nucleus of a natural or artificial material during the decay process.

Another type of radiation used experimentally or for radiotherapy is particulate radiation, which includes electrons, protons, α particles (He nuclei), neutrons, negative π-mesons, and heavy charged particles (Table 3). The charged particles may be *directly ionizing,* ie, produce chemical and biological changes by direct interaction with the atomic nucleus. X-rays and γ-rays are absorbed in biological matter and result in displacement of a bound orbital electron, giving up energy to produce fast-moving,

**TABLE 3. Types of Ionizing Radiation**

| Radiation | Charge |
|---|---|
| **Electromagnetic** | |
| x Rays | None |
| γ Rays | None |
| **Particles** | |
| Electrons | Negative |
| Protons | Positive |
| Neutrons | None |
| α Particle (He nuclei) | Positive |
| Negative π mesons | Negative |
| Heavy charged ions (C, Ne, Ar) | Positive |

charged particles that interact with tissue to produce chemical and biological changes (*indirectly ionizing*). Neutrons are uncharged and cause ionization due to secondary particles created during their absorption in matter.

X-ray photons interact with matter, ionize atoms, and lose energy by one of three processes: the photoelectric effect, the Compton effect, and pair production. The relative importance of these processes depends on the energy of the photons and the composition of the absorbing material. At lower energies (10 to 100 keV), energy loss is primarily by the photoelectric effect in which all of the photon energy is given up to an inner shell electron, which is released from orbit and accelerated causing secondary ionization. From 100 keV to 3 MeV, energies more commonly used in radiotherapy, photons lose energy by Compton scattering where only a fraction of the photon energy is lost to an outer shell, "free" electron resulting in forward scattering of reduced energy photons and accelerated electrons. At energies greater than 1.02 MeV, pair production occurs where the x-ray photons interact with the nucleus, producing an electron and a positron. This is of major importance only with x-rays greater than 20 MeV. All three processes produce secondary electrons that move through tissue and give up energy by interactions with other atoms and molecules, resulting in further ionizations and excitations.

Charged particles, such as electrons, protons, or α particles, interact directly with the nucleus and give up energy by ionization throughout the entire length of their track as they travel through the biological material. The rate of energy loss is dependent on the velocity and charge of the particle, increasing at lower speed and higher charge.

The efficiency of biological damage varies among the different types of ionizing radiation even though they all eventually result in the production of energetic electrons. The difference in efficiency results from the average density of energy deposition along the path of the particle, or loss of energy per unit distance, referred to as the linear energy transfer (LET) of the radiation. In this concept, energy loss or depositions by charged particles in biological material is inversely related to their velocity. As the particle slows down, it loses energy more rapidly, reaching a maximum rate of energy loss in the region known as the Bragg peak just before it comes to rest. LET varies along the length of the track. Heavier charged particles such as photons and α particles travel in straight lines with little deflection and have a pronounced Bragg peak. Electrons, having less mass, give up energy more uniformly along their track with no evidence of a Bragg peak.

The importance of the concept of LET is that the biological effect of radiation dose depends on its LET or pattern of energy deposition. Irradiation of tissue with x-rays or γ-rays results in a random distribution of electron tracks with a range of LET values producing a similar LET spectrum at all depths. In contrast, for a monoenergetic beam of heavier charged particles, the Bragg peak occurs at a similar region in tissue for all particles (Fig 1). This aspect of heavy-particle irradiation has potential therapeutic applications.

Because of the various methods of photon, neutron, and charged particle absorption, different patterns of penetration occur through an absorbing medium. Charged particles have a finite range. Cobalt 60 and higher energy photons deliver a maximum dose at a particular depth below the surface dependent on energy due to forward scattering of electrons and secondary photons. This property is advantageous in clinical use and is responsible for sparing of superficial overlying tissues. This occurs to a minor degree with electrons and neutrons and is essentially absent for heavier charged particles.

Better methods of radiation measurement were developed along with better sources of ionizing radiation, with the description of the roentgen in 1928, the rad in 1954, and, more recently, the gray (the international unit of radiation dose). The unit of radiation exposure (the roentgen) was based on a measurement of ionization produced in a given volume of air at standard temperature and pressure. The unit of

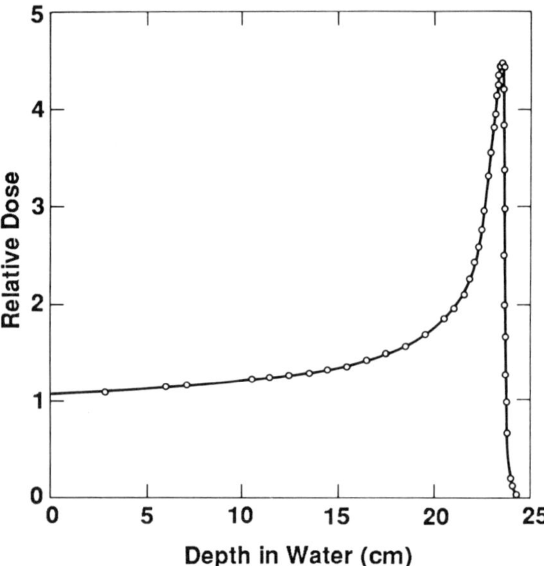


**Fig 1.** Depth-dose curve for 187-MeV protons from the Uppsala synchrocyclotron. [From *Br J Radiol* (1961;34:143–151), with permission.]

absorbed dose or energy absorbed per unit mass, the rad, is that dose resulting in an energy deposition of 100 erg/g. The new SI unit is the gray (Gy), 1 J/kg, which is equivalent to 100 rads.

## RADIOBIOLOGY

The total amount of energy absorbed is not as important for the biological effects of ionizing radiation as the specific ionization in critical target molecules. These effects may be due to direct energy absorption with ionization and excitation occurring within these target molecules, or may be indirectly caused by the formation of reactive radicals, such as the hydroxyl radical, within other molecules primarily in cellular water, and their interaction with critical target molecules. The end result may be altered cellular and tissue function expressed hours, days, or years later.

### Determination of Critical Target Molecules

Initially, the biological effects of radiation were measured by animal death, destruction of seed germination, plant growth retardation, or observation of skin erythema.[7] Beginning in the 1950s, in vivo and in vitro assay methods of tumor and normal tissue were developed.[8] Such methods led to determination of critical target structures at the cellular level for ionizing radiation.

Radiation causes cellular and tissue damage through damage to any molecule, but it is generally believed that damage to DNA itself and chromosomal DNA is most crucial in cell killing.[9] Such damage may include single- or double-strand breaks, change in or loss of bases, or crosslink formation between DNA strands or other molecules. The exact nature of DNA damage responsible for cell killing remains unclear; DNA repair processes exist and expression of DNA damage is very complex. Thus DNA repair capacity can influence cellular radiosensitivity.

Damage to cellular macromolecules results in a wide range of effects, such as chromosome aberrations, inhibition of continued reproductive ability, and delayed progression of cells through the cell cycle or mitotic delay. Assays for clonogenic or proliferative capacity include in vitro plating assays of irradiated single-cell suspensions, in vivo–in vitro assays for sensitivity of tumor cells grown after being irradiated in vivo, and assays of estimation of cell

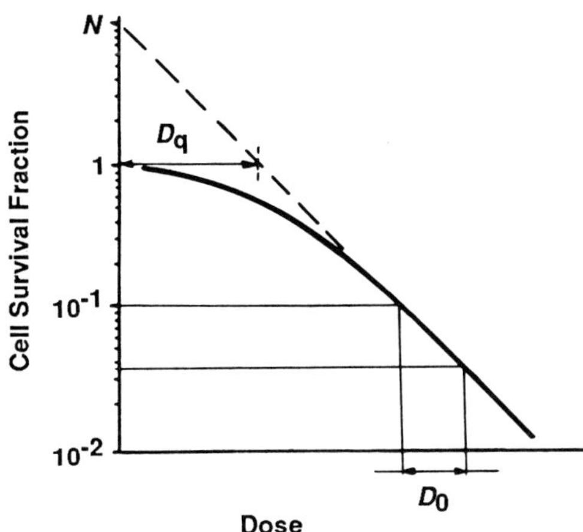


**Fig 2.** Parameters of a typical cell survival curve. [From Nias AHW, *An Introduction to Radiobiology* (Chichester: John Wiley & Sons; 1990), with permission.]

survival by in vivo transplantation of irradiated and control cells.

Such techniques have been used to obtain survival curves for many normal and malignant cell populations (Fig 2). These curves are obtained from culture of irradiated and normal cells and counting the number of colonies developed. For x-rays and γ-rays, survival curves for most mammalian cells have evidence of a shoulder at low doses, while at higher doses the curve becomes steeper with survival decreasing exponentially with dose. No consistent differences are apparent between normal and malignant cells. In most instances, response differences of cells and tissues must be explained on a basis other than the inherent basic radiosensitivity of the cells. The slope ($D$) of the exponential region of the survival curve is similar for most mammalian cells, but the shape and size of the shoulder varies considerably between different cell lines, reflecting the ability of the cells to accumulate and repair radiation damage.[10]

## Influential Factors of Biological Effects

Various factors can influence the response of cells to radiation treatment. The biological effect of radiation depends on the effective LET, characterized by a parameter known as relative biological effectiveness (RBE), which is defined as the ratio of the dose of a standard type of radiation to a test radiation giving the same biological effect. The relationship between RBE and LET is complex. RBE increases with LET to a maximum of about 100 keV/mm, and then decreases with higher LET because of an "overkill phenomenon." The RBE of high-LET radiation compared with low-LET radiation increases as the dose per fraction decreases, since the dose–response curve for low-LET radiation has a broader shoulder than for high-LET radiation (Fig 3).

**Presence of Oxygen.** Biological effects of radiation are also influenced by the presence of oxygen. Cells irradiated with low-LET radiation in the presence of oxygen are approximately three times more sensitive than those irradiated in its absence[7] (Fig 4). Oxygen acts as a radiation sensitizer and is characterized by the oxygen enhancement ratio (OER) defined as the ratio of doses required to give the same biological effect in the absence or the presence of oxygen. The OER is reduced for high-LET radiation. Most normal tissues contain few hypoxic cells, but most tumors contain a significant fraction (10% to 20%) of hypoxic cells that are resistant to radiation.[11,12]

**Cell Cycle and Cell Age.** Position in the cell cycle and cell age also influences radiosensitivity; cells in S phase are often more resistant than those in G2/m phases with some variation between cell types (Fig 5). This variation in response as a function of cell age can have important clinical implications, since cells in the most sensitive phases of the cycle will be selectively killed, leading to partial synchronization of surviving cells and more or less sensitivity to subsequent exposures. Cellular repair capacity also influences cell survival and is responsible for the clinical observation that a larger total radiation dose is tolerated when fractionated.[13,14] Such repair, termed "sublethal damage repair," is one of the

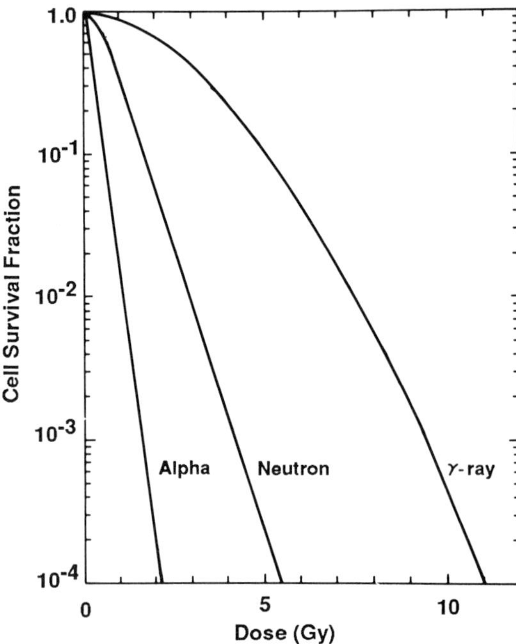


**Fig 3.** Typical mammalian cell survival curves for radiations varying in their linear energy transfer. [From Hill RP, Tannock IF, *The Basic Science of Oncology* (Oxford: Pergamon Press; 1987), with permission.]

most important modifying responses following radiation injury and occurs at both the DNA and chromosome level. A second type of repair, called "potentially lethal damage repair," occurs when environmental conditions are varied after radiation exposure.

**Tissue Tolerance.** Radiation treatment of tumors within the body requires that the radiation must pass through normal tissues. Radiation injury in normal tissues and in tumors differs because of the ability of normal tissue to respond to injury with physiologic mechanisms of adaptation, including shortening of cell cycle and recruitment of cells into the cell cycle from the tissue itself or adjacent tissue.[13] Tumors lack such control mechanisms but may show increased proliferation at certain stages following radiation injury. A typical radiation treatment field also encompasses a margin of normal tissue around known tumor extent. Since radiation damages both normal and tumor tissue, radiation dose is limited by normal tissue tolerance and risk of complications. The balance between the prob-

**Fig 4.** Data for survival curves of mammalian cells exposed to x-rays under aerobic and hypoxic conditions (1 rad = 0.01 Gy). OER, oxygen enhancement ratio. [From Holleb AI, Fink DJ, Murphy GP, *American Cancer Society Textbook of Clinical Oncology* (Atlanta: The American Cancer Society; 1991), with permission.]

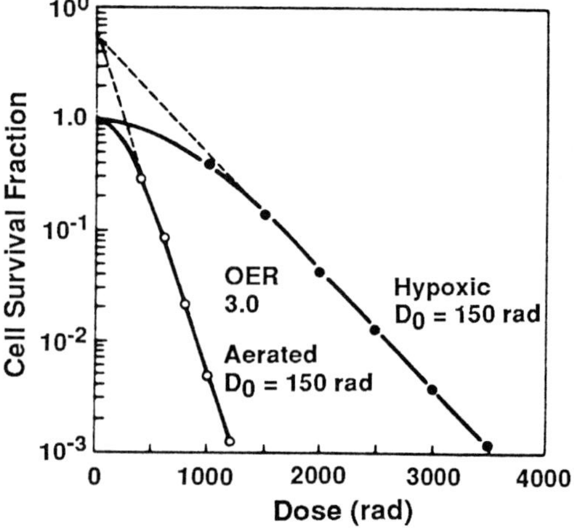

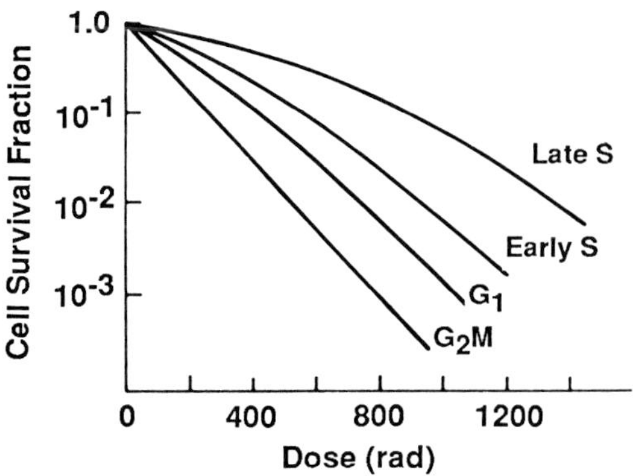


**Fig 5.** Variation in pattern of radiosensitivity according to cell cycle age (1 rad = 0.01 Gy). [From Holleb AI, Fink DJ, Murphy GP, *American Cancer Society Textbook of Clinical Oncology* (Atlanta: The American Cancer Society; 1991), with permission.]

ability of tumor control and the risk of normal tissue complications is a measure of the therapeutic ratio. As stated by Kramer in 1976, "Improvements in the therapeutic ratio can come from either a reduction in normal tissue injury or an increase in the effectiveness of tumor treatment."[15] Increasing tumor dose relative to normal tissue implies improvements in the physical aspects of radiation therapy such as high-energy x-ray equipment, more sophisticated treatment planning, or use of high-LET radiation. Increasing the tumor response requires an understanding of cellular and tissue response to irradiation.

The response of normal tissues to irradiation in single doses is qualitatively the same as to fractionated doses. Fractionation of radiation therapy, giving 20–30 individual dose fractions of 1.8–2.5 Gy over 4–6 weeks, developed from early clinical observations showing greater tumor control at acceptable levels of normal tissue damage. The underlying biological effects occurring during fractionation and influencing the shape of isoeffect curves were later identified from experimental studies of cells in culture and animal models. These are the "four R's" of radiation therapy likely to influence response to fractionated treatment: repair of radiation damage, repopulation of damaged tissue by proliferation of surviving cells, redistribution of proliferating cells through the cell cycle, and reoxygenation of hypoxic cells. Repair and repopulation occur in tumors and normal tissue, and allow cells and tissue to tolerate a larger total dose when fractionated.[13,14] The shoulder on the survival curve is indicative of the ability to accumulate and repair radiation damage. Repopulation decreases early normal tissue damage and response of tumors to a greater extent than it decreases late normal tissue damage, which occurs in late-responding, slowly proliferating tissues. Reoxygenation occurs primarily in tumors and is theoretically responsible for the improved therapeutic ratio resulting from increased sensitivity of tumor during fractionation. The mechanism of reoxygenation is poorly understood and different mechanisms may be involved in different tumors. While repair and repopulation increase the total dose required to achieve a given level of biological damage during fractionated treatment, redistribution and reoxygenation would reduce the required total dose for such an isoeffect.[14] These relationships have been expressed by a number of mathematical equations such as the nominal standard dose (NSD) equation, designed to predict isoeffective treatments.[16] Factors influencing tissue or tumor survival in a fractionated course of radiation are complex and any mathematical consideration of time–dose–fractionation relationship is limited in applicability. Differences in isoeffect relationships for early and late damage implies that reducing fraction size will reduce late tissue damage to a greater extent than rapidly proliferating tissue or tumors.

## Modifiers of Radiation Response

Modifiers of radiation response have included various approaches to improve the therapeutic ratio including changes in LET and dose rate, hypoxic cell sensitizers, radioprotectors, cytotoxic drugs and nucleic acid analogs, heat, and the host immune response. Attempts have been made to reduce resistance of hypoxic tumor cells by increasing oxygen delivery. Clinical trials with hyperbaric oxygen have shown limited success and have not demonstrated substantial benefit. An alternative approach has been the development of drugs known as hypoxic cell radiosensitizers, which mimic the radiosensitizing properties of oxygen.[17] Some hypoxic cell radiosensitizers have undergone clinical trials and more are in progress. Only a few trials have shown any significant improvement in tumor control with substantial neurotoxicity demonstrated. Current trials are focusing on agents with less toxicity or more effective sensitization, such as SR 2508 and Ro 03-8799. Alternatively, radioprotective drugs have the potential to improve therapeutic gain by protecting normal tissues relative to tumors. Again, success in the clinical situation has been variable and toxicity in humans dose limiting.

High-LET radiations are also being studied in an effort to improve the therapeutic ratio through improved depth–dose distributions for deep-seated tumors compared to x-rays or γ-rays and specific radiobiological properties such as a reduced OER, reduced capacity for repair following high-LET radiation, and decreased variation in cell cycle–dependent radiosensitivity.[18] Altered fractionation schedules have been used to exploit differences in repair capacity between early- and late-responding tissues. Hyperfractionation refers to a treatment course giving the same or increased total dose in multiple smaller fractions without prolonging the overall treatment time. Accelerated fractionation delivers the same total dose as conventional irradiation but with a shortening of overall treatment time.[19]

The clinical application of these principles of radiation physics and radiobiology is a complex process involving evaluation of tumor extent, knowledge of the natural history and pathologic characteristics of the disease, definition of therapeutic aims, selection of appropriate treatment modalities, determination of radiation dose and treatment volume, and clinical evaluation of the patient during treatment.

## CARCINOMA OF THE PROSTATE

Treatment for carcinoma of the prostate with irradiation has been performed for over 80 years. Early investigators placed radium sources through urethral catheters for the treatment of carcinoma of the prostate.[20] Combined brachytherapy and external beam radiation therapy was performed on many patients in several institutions such as the University of Iowa.[21] Interstitial irradiation in the treatment of prostate cancer has continued through the 1990s.[22] With the advent of megavoltage irradiation in the 1950s and 1960s, treatment for carcinoma of the prostate with high-energy external beam irradiation has also become popular.[23,24]

Modern radiotherapy can be delivered with a variety of techniques. The technical aspects of the radiation delivery are critical, but to the practicing physician the most important questions relate to the efficacy of therapy and the attendant complications associated with treatment. In this section, issues regarding complications and therapeutic efficacy of treatment will be addressed. Discussion regarding the volume of tissue to be treated and the preferred method of radiation delivery to the prostate will be included.

### Results of Therapy

Table 4 reflects the survival of those patients treated for stages A, B, and C carcinoma of the prostate. Five-year survival

**TABLE 4. Radiation Therapy Results for Stages A, B, C**

| Study | Survival % | | |
|---|---|---|---|
| | 5 Yr. | 10 Yr. | 15 Yr. |
| **Stages A and B** | | | |
| Bagshaw[25] | 80 | 58 | 35 |
| Perez[26] | 76 | 56 | |
| Zagars[27] | 93 | 70 | |
| **Stage C** | | | |
| Bagshaw[25] | 64 | 35 | 18 |
| Hanks[24] | 58 | 38 | |
| Zagars[28] | 72 | 47 | 27 |

for stage A and B carcinoma range from 70% to 90% and 10-year survivals are in the range of 50% of 60%.[25–27] For stage C carcinoma, the 5-year survivals are in the range of 60% to 70% and the 10-year survivals in the range of 30% to 40%.[24,25,28] The Radiation Therapy Oncology Group (RTOG) has analyzed the results of those patients with early stage, minimal tumor volume disease. Clinical stages T1B, T2 patients with prostate cancer who were included from RTOG protocol 77–06 were analyzed. Those patients who would otherwise be amenable to surgical resection and who had negative surgical lymph node staging were included. The 10-year actuarial survival for this group of patients is exceptionally good[29] (Fig 6). These results with irradiation compare favorably with those patients treated with surgical resection. All of the data included above represent an uncontrolled retrospective clinical analysis.

The only reported prospective randomized trial involving irradiation and surgery in carcinoma of the prostate was conducted by Paulsen.[30] In that study, 97 patients with stage A2 or B disease were randomized to irradiation or prostatectomy. In this analysis, those patients receiving radical prostatectomy exhibited a disease-free survival of 76% while those patients undergoing external beam irradiation exhibited a disease-free survival of 57%. The results of irradiation in this trial are inferior to similar groups of patients reported in single institutions[31] (Fig 7). This small prospective trial awaits confirmation as some technical aspects of the trial have been questioned.

## Dose-Response

The dose of external beam radiation necessary to control a patient with carcinoma of the prostate has been addressed by several investigators. The USA Patterns of Care Study (PCS) was able to evaluate local dose relative to the size of the tumor and amount of radiation delivered. Table 5 depicts the PCS data. Stage B tumors required doses of greater than 6000 cGy whereas stage C tumors required doses as high as 7000 cGy to control disease with a high probability.[32] Perez et al were also able to show a dose–response curve of local failure in the dose of external beam irradiation. Those patients with stage C carcinoma required greater than 6500 cGy to control the tumor 75% of the time.[33]

Attempts to increase the dose of radiation that can be delivered to the tumor volume have been attempted with a variety of techniques. Currently, interstitial irradiation

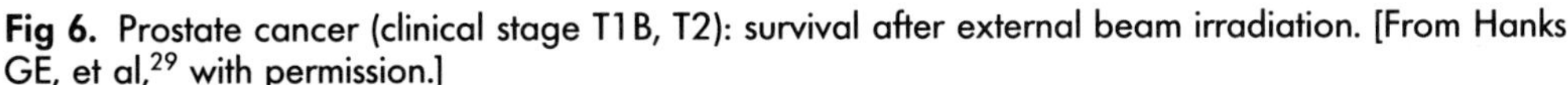
**Fig 6.** Prostate cancer (clinical stage T1B, T2): survival after external beam irradiation. [From Hanks GE, et al,[29] with permission.]

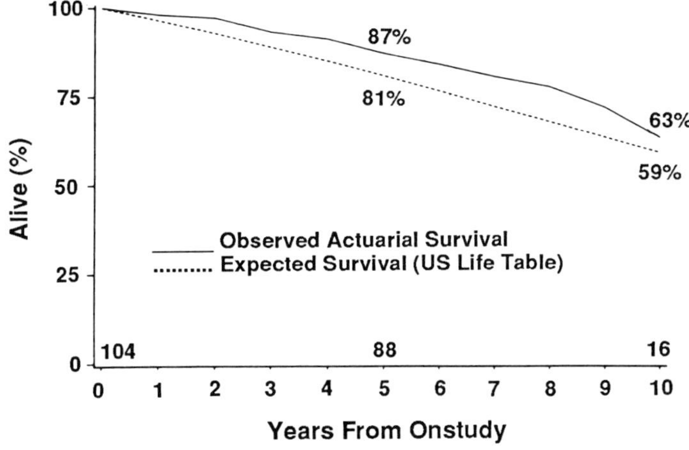

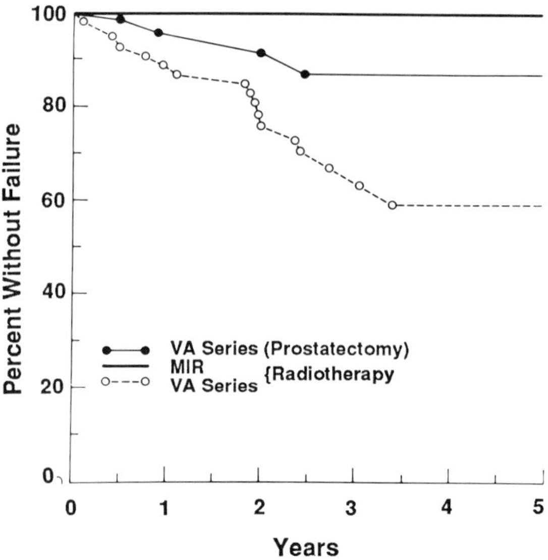


**Fig 7.** Mallinckrodt Institute of Radiology (MIR), Washington University School of Medicine, data superimposed over VA Uro-Oncology Group data. [From *Int J Radiat Oncol Biol Phys* (1987; 13(5):661), with permission.]

has achieved renewed interest as a mechanism of increasing the irradiation to the prostate. However, those patients who are good candidates for interstitial irradiation have relatively small-volume disease. Puthwala and his colleagues have reported a biopsy-proven local control rate of 89% in patients with relatively small tumors of the prostate, stages A and B, treated with iridium 192 implants.[22] I-125 implants have been used for a number of years. There appear to be comparable local control rates with I-125 and external beam irradiation for those patients with small-volume disease. In patients with A2 or B glands, local failure is probably equal to either I-125 or external beam irradiation. Patients with stage C disease are not good candidates for interstitial treatment either with I-125 or iridium 192. The control rate with external beam treatment appears better[34,35] (Table 6).

## Radiation Technique

Modern advances in the use of computer-guided three-dimensional radiation therapy treatment planning may allow a higher amount of external beam irradiation to the prostate gland while sparing normal tissue. This technique, also called conformal therapy, has been preliminarily reported by Hanks et al.[36] One is able to deliver a substantially higher dose of external beam irradiation with a minimum of complications.

The presence of positive lymph nodes in patients with adenocarcinoma of the prostate varies with the grade of the tumor and the size of the primary lesion. As the tumor

**TABLE 5. Infield Clinical Recurrence of Prostate Cancer (%)**

| Dose | Stage B | Stage C |
|---|---|---|
| <6000 cGy | 25 | 25 |
| 6500–6999 cGy | 13 | 23 |
| ≥7000 cGy | 14 | 17 |

**TABLE 6. Local Failure of Type of Irradiation (%)**

| Stage | I-125 | External Beam |
|---|---|---|
| A2, B1 | 10 | 6 |
| C | 33 | 21 |

**TABLE 7. Incidence of Nodes at Lymphadenectomy (%)**

| Stage | Well Differentiated | Poorly Differentiated |
|---|---|---|
| B1 | 4 | 33 |
| C | 50 | 93 |

size increases, the likelihood of nodal metastases also increases. As the grade of the tumor increases, the incidence of nodal metastases also increases[32] (Table 7). Radiation therapy utilized in other disease sites, such as gynecologic and head and neck malignancies, has been shown to cure a small but measurable group of patients with known nodal metastases.

Theoretically, irradiation applied to the pelvis or to the pelvis and periaortic lymph nodes may result in tumor sterilization in some patients with positive nodes and improve the cure rate. McGowan reported an uncontrolled trial that suggests that those patients treated with more generous fields have a better outcome than those treated with small fields.[38] He suggests that this is due to nodal tumor eradication. Bagshaw also suggested that those patients with B2 tumors who have their regional lymph nodes irradiated have improved survival.[39] Other investigators, including Zagars, Neglia, and Sause,[28,40,41] report no improved survival in patients if positive lymph nodes are irradiated. Stanford University also conducted a prospective randomized trial in patients with stage B disease.[25] Preliminary data suggest that those patients with treated pelvic lymph nodes do not exhibit a higher survival. Two large studies conducted by the RTOG suggest no improvement in survival if the patients were electively treated to the pelvis or pelvis plus periaortic lymph nodes[42,43] (Figs 8 and 9). The value of irradiation in the patients with positive lymph nodes remains to be defined. Certainly, if there is improvement in survival, it is relatively modest and a large prospective trial with long follow-up would be needed to demonstrate such an improvement.

Documented local failures following definitive irradiation have received a great deal of attention in the past few years. An initial report of 46 patients by Cox and Stoffel suggested that those patients with positive biopsies had a clinical course similar to those without a positive biopsy.[44]

**Fig 8.** Survival of patients treated on RTOG protocol 77-06 by treatment arm (prostate field versus prostate and pelvic field). [From Asbell SO, et al,[43] with permission.]

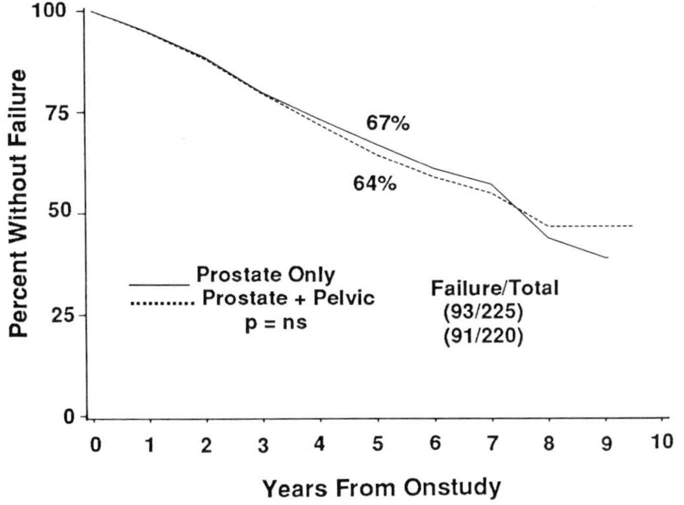

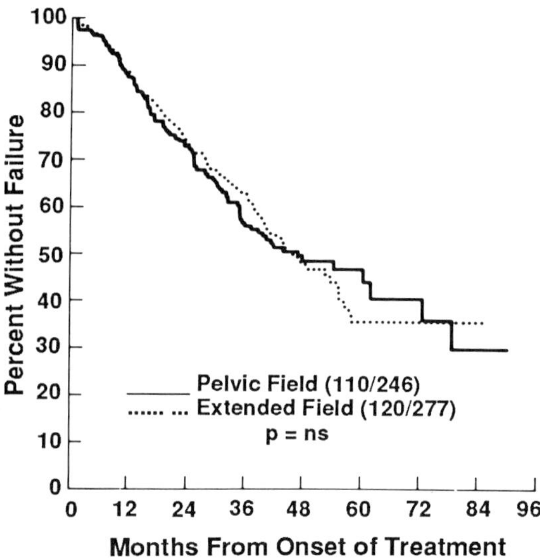


**Fig 9.** Survival of patients treated on RTOG protocol 75-06. Patients were randomized to receive pelvic irradiation followed by a boost to the prostate or pelvic and para-aortic irradiation followed by a boost to the prostate. [From Pilepich MV, et al,[42] with permission.]

Since that time, several investigators have reported information to the contrary. Scardino and Wheeler in a large study suggested that the incidence of positive biopsies was directly related to the size of the tumor at the initiation of treatment and that the survival was detrimentally affected by the presence of a positive biopsy[45] (Table 8). Stamey et al and Kabalin et al reported a very high incidence of positive biopsies following serum PSA evaluation and ultrasonically directed biopsy of tissue.[46,47] The significance of these positive biopsies remains unclear and will await further follow-up and evaluation. Serum prostate specific antigen (PSA) levels can be measured following definitive irradiation. Levels can continue to decline up to 1 year following treatment.[48] Stamey et al report that more than 80% of patients will exhibit a decrease in PSA level.[46] Those patients who exhibit progressively rising PSA levels at 3-month intervals represent a high-risk group for clinical recurrence.

**TABLE 8. Postirradiation Positive Biopsies**

| Stage | % |
|---|---|
| A2 | 35 |
| B1N | 11 |
| B1 | 21 |
| B2 | 33 |
| C | 55 |

External beam irradiation represents one of the most useful palliative tools available in those patients with metastatic carcinoma of the prostate.[49] Relatively modest doses of irradiation in the range of 2000 to 3000 cGy delivered over 2 to 3 weeks can result in marked symptomatic relief in over 80% of those patients with osseous metastases. The use of radiation should not be overlooked in clinical situations in which pain relief is indicated.

## Complications

The risks of complications with irradiation are related to the volume of normal tissue treated and the radiation dose. Treatment of prostate cancer demands a high dose of radiation therapy delivered to both the prostate and adjacent normal tissues. The majority of complications will occur in the rectum, bladder, and associated structures. Tables 9 and 10 list the incidence of complications as well as the relationship to the volume treated.[50] As noted, the incidence of severe genitourinary complications is 7.7% with most of those being grade III. The incidence of gas-

**TABLE 9. Incidence of Urinary Sequelae by Grade: Studies 7506 and 7706**

| | Grade | | | Total |
|---|---|---|---|---|
| Toxicity | 3<br>No. (%) | 4<br>No. (%) | 5<br>No. (%) | No. (%) |
| Cystitis | 23 (2.3) | 4 (0.4) | 0 | 27 (2.6) |
| Hematuria | 30 (2.9) | 2 (0.2) | 0 | 32 (3.1) |
| Urethral stricture | 45 (4.4) | 2 (0.2) | 0 | 47 (4.6) |
| Bladder contracture | 5 (0.5) | 2 (0.2) | 0 | 7 (0.7) |
| Total | 74 (7.3) | 5 (0.5) | 0 | 79 (7.7) |

trointestinal complications is approximately 3%. The relationship of total dose to complications is noted in Table 11.[50] These data are taken from large RTOG trials involving approximately 600 patients. Sexual impotence has been observed in approximately 35% to 40% of formerly potent patients treated with external beam irradiation. This is somewhat higher than the rate of approximately 15% to 20% reported with interstitial irradiation.[29,51] Patient characteristics such as age and degree of sexual activity may influence the comparison between interstitial and external beam irradiation. It has been reported that men who are more vigorously sexually active have a greater likelihood of maintaining their sexual potency.

Irradiation plays a major role nationally in the management of prostate cancer. The optimal delivery technique of irradiation and selection of cases to which irradiation should be applied remains to be defined.

## CARCINOMA OF THE BLADDER

Carcinoma of the bladder represents a therapeutic challenge. Fifteen thousand to twenty thousand cases of invasive bladder cancer will develop in the USA annually and at least half of those patients with invasive tumors will develop systemic disease irrespective of local therapy.[52] Cystectomy represents the most effective means of obtaining local control, but it incurs the morbidity of bladder removal and has no impact in control of systemic disease. Radiation therapy may play a role in augmenting local treatment in highly invasive tumors or allowing bladder preservation in some patients. Augmentation of traditional irradiation with interstitial im-

**TABLE 10. Incidence of Intestinal Sequelae by Grade: Studies 7506 and 7706**

| | Grade | | | Total |
|---|---|---|---|---|
| Toxicity | 3<br>No. (%) | 4<br>No. (%) | 5<br>No. (%) | No. (%) |
| Diarrhea | 3 (0.3) | 1 (0.1) | 0 | 4 (0.4) |
| Proctitis | 12 (1.2) | 4 (0.4) | 0 | 16 (1.6) |
| Rectal/anal stricture | 2 (0.2) | 2 (0.2) | 0 | 4 (0.4) |
| Rectal bleeding or ulcer | 12 (1.2) | 4 (0.4) | 1 (0.1) | 17 (1.7) |
| Obstruction/perforation | 0 | 5 (0.5) | 1 (0.1) | 6 (0.6) |
| Total | 21 (2.1) | 11 (1.1) | 2 (0.2) | 34 (3.3) |

**TABLE 11. Pretreatment- and Treatment-Related Factors Predicting for Late Morbidity**

| Factors | Level of Significance for Urinary Morbidity (Grades 3, 4, 5) | Level of Significance for Intestinal Morbidity (Grades 3, 4, 5) |
|---|---|---|
| Laparotomy | NS | NS |
| Stage | NS | NS |
| Positive LN[a] | NS | NS |
| Diastolic BP ≥90 | NS | NS |
| Previous TUR | NS | NS |
| >70-Gy dose to prostate | .03 | NS |
| 4 fields vs. AP/PA | NS | NS |
| Energy of accelerator | NS | NS |

[a] Data from 7506 only as these patients were ineligible for 7706.

plants, chemotherapy, or radiosensitizers may expand the role of traditional radiotherapy. By and large, radiation therapy has been used to treat those patients with at least T2 lesions. There has been some utilization of irradiation for those lesions of earlier stage but in general these patients are handled adequately with transurethral resection. External beam irradiation for early lesions requires doses of irradiation of 6500 to 7000 cGy. Most reported series for early lesions are small and control rates are approximately 50%.[53–55] The morbidity incurred from external beam irradiation for little therapeutic benefit over surgical resection has limited its usefulness in these early lesions.[56] Interstitial implants of early lesions have gained some popularity in Europe. The Rotterdam Institute reports on the largest series of selected cases. Selection criteria are strict for those patients undergoing interstitial therapy. Selection is limited to superficial tumor of less than 5 cm in size. In general, interstitial therapy is proceeded by external beam treatment that varies with the T stage of the tumor. Table 12 reflects the survival and bladder-free relapse rate of selected tumors from Rotterdam.[57–59]

## Results of Therapy

Radiotherapy is most commonly utilized worldwide in muscle invasive, locally advanced bladder cancer. Multiple investigators have reported series of patients treated primarily with radiotherapy. Survival ranges from approximately 40% to less than 10% as the stage and grade of the tumor increases. A great deal of effort and analysis has been done to predict which patients will exhibit a good result from irradiation. Such factors as age, hematocrit, stage, papillary histology, grade, size, location, completeness of transurethral resection of the bladder (TURB), and ureteral status have all been analyzed. Little consensus has been achieved among investigators regarding which factors are of prime importance. The major predictors for high survival following cystectomy, ie, tumor grade and stage, are also predictive of a good result with radiotherapy. Table 13 reflects representative survival data from external beam irradiation.[60–63]

**TABLE 12. Survival and Bladder-free Relapse Rate at Rotterdam Radiotherapy Institute**

| Stage | No. Pts. | 5-Yr Bladder-Free Relapse (%) |
|---|---|---|
| T1 | 196 | 82 |
| | | 10-Yr survival |
| T2 | 328 | 69 |
| T3 | 63 | 59 |

**TABLE 13. Survival for External Beam Irradiation (%)**

| Study | T2 | T3A | T3B | T4 |
|---|---|---|---|---|
| Miller[62] | 24 | 21 | 18 | 9 |
| Goffinet[61] | 42 | 35 | 20 | 8 |
| Fish and Fayos[63] | 43 | 26 | 13 | 11 |
| Bloom[60] | | 29 | | |

Overall, the results of external beam irradiation for bladder cancer are suboptimal. Local recurrence in a deeply invasive bladder tumor occurs approximately two thirds of the time. Although some patients can exhibit a useful response to treatment, our ability to predict which patients will benefit is difficult and unreliable. Cystectomy undoubtedly offers the optimal means of local control in deeply invasive tumors. Randomized trials conducted by Miller and Bloom et al attest to the improvement of cystectomy and irradiation over irradiation alone for local control.[60,62]

## Combined Modality Therapy

In the past several years, several institutions have reported excellent response rates to cytotoxic chemotherapy. Complete response rates with a variety of chemotherapy regimens have been reported in the range of 30% to 50%.[64–67] Most combinations include cisplatin and the most enthusiastically reported combination includes methotrexate, vincristine, adriamycin, and cisplatin (M-VAC).[68] The enthusiasm for cytotoxic chemotherapy has resulted in several protocols utilizing concurrent or sequential chemotherapy/radiotherapy treatment in advanced bladder cancer. The National Bladder Cancer Group reported a 4-year survival of 20% in 48 T3 and T4 lesions and 60% in 22 T2 lesions with concurrent cisplatin and full-dose irradiation.[69] There is little doubt that the combination of chemotherapy and radiation therapy has increased the complete response to therapy[70] (Table 14).

Although the complete response to local therapy is improved, it remains unclear as to whether we can maintain these complete responses and preserve the bladder. In an attempt to answer these questions and preselect patients for bladder preservation, a national protocol has been promulgated through the Radiation Therapy Oncology Group. Patients are treated with combination chemotherapy and radiation therapy up to 4000 cGy (Fig 10). If at 4000 cGy less than a complete response is achieved, cystectomy is performed. This allows cystectomy prior to full-dose radiation therapy and the attendant complications of such therapy. The protocol is ongoing and results are pending final analysis. This is an attempt to attain local control comparable to that of cystectomy while preserving the bladder in some patients.

## Preoperative Irradiation

The use of preoperative irradiation in bladder cancer is being utilized with less frequency. Although downstaging frequently occurs with preoperative treatment, it has been difficult to prove a survival benefit to its utilization. A recent Southwest Oncology Group (SWOG) study utilizing 2000 cGy in 1 week suggested no benefit to preoperative treatment although some low-stage tumors were included in the trial.[71] Prior to the SWOG trial five previous prospective trials produced inconclusive and contradictory data.[72–76] When one

**TABLE 14. Invasive Bladder Cancer: Complete Response by Treatment**

| Treatment | Complete Response (%) | No. Studies |
|---|---|---|
| Chemotherapy alone | 10–50 | 10 |
| Radiotherapy alone | 40–60 | 4 |
| Concurrent chemotherapy and radiotherapy | 60–85 | 7 |

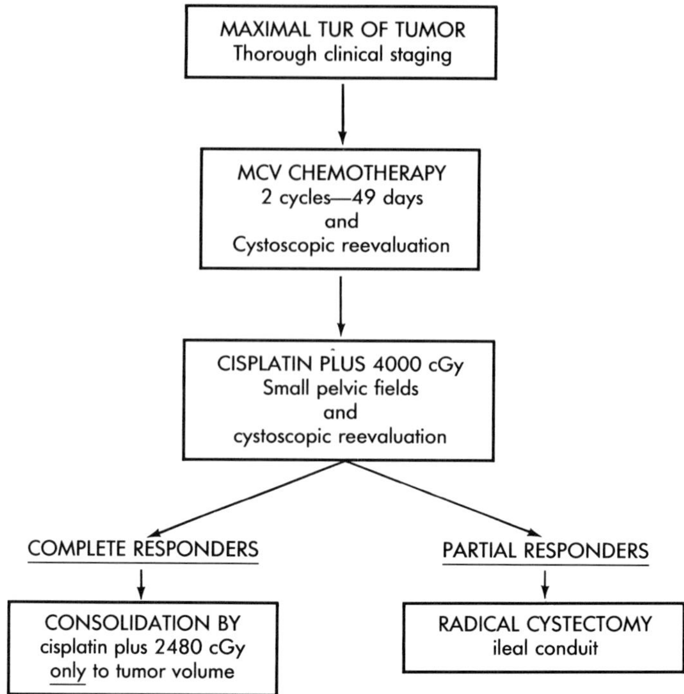


**Fig 10.** Treatment schema for invasive bladder cancer used by both the Massachusetts General Hospital and the Radiation Therapy Oncology Group. TUR, transurethral resection; MCV, methotrexate 30 mg/$m^2$, cisplatin 70 mg/$m^2$, vinblastine 3 mg/$m^2$.

analyzes the serial results of several institutions, there appears to be an improvement with the addition of high-dose preoperative irradiation. Whether this difference can be explained on the basis of better patient selection and improved surgery remains unclear.[77]

## Complications

A worrisome feature of primary irradiation for bladder cancer is the occurrence of chronic bladder injury. The late effects of irradiation are usually manifested at 2 to 4 years following therapy.[78] Bladder thickening and contracture with diminished bladder capacity represent the hallmark of radiation injury. Duncan and Quilty report the largest series of patients treated with primary irradiation.[79] Their patients received 275 cGy per fraction for 20 fractions, and such a schedule would predict for a higher complication rate than most modern schemes. They report an 11% incidence of severe complications. Miller reports a severe incidence of bladder injury of 13% in patients receiving 6000 to 6600 cGy.[62]

Irradiation represents a viable alternative to cystectomy in patients with deeply invasive bladder tumors.[80] The emergence of protocols incorporating chemotherapy and irradiation may allow comparable cure rates to cystectomy with bladder preservation in selected patients. It remains for ongoing clinical trials to define the optimal role of radiation therapy in the management of patients with bladder cancer.

## CANCER OF THE TESTES

### Seminoma

Radiotherapeutic management of testicular seminoma generally has been successful with most series demonstrating cure rates greater than 90%.[81–84] Initial management includes obtaining serum markers of α-fetoprotein and β-HCG (human chorionic gonadotropin) followed by radical inguinal orchiectomy. Pathologic diagnosis and stage of disease define further management. The majority of patients with seminoma present with early stage disease and postorchiectomy external beam irradiation to the retroperitoneal lymph nodes offers high cure rates with minimal morbidity. Traditionally, radiation therapy has been used to treat all but stage IV seminoma.

### Stage I

Management of stage I seminoma includes adjuvant irradiation of the first echelon of draining lymph nodes beyond those nodes involved after noninvasive staging with CT scanning and lymphangiography. Despite these excellent results, there is some controversy about the optimal management of early stage seminoma. Standard treatment for patients with stage I seminoma is postoperative irradiation of the periaortic and ipsilateral pelvic lymph nodes. Results are presented in Table 15.[82,85–88] Availability of sophisticated, noninvasive staging procedures, effective irradiation and systemic chemotherapy for salvage after relapse, and the low risk of retroperitoneal disease in well-staged patients have led some investigators to propose observation after orchiectomy without adjuvant irradiation.[89–91] At present, standard therapy remains adjuvant irradiation following orchiectomy to periaortic and pelvic lymph nodes.

In the past it was recommended that irradiation treatment volumes include the inguinal regions or scrotum if previous inguinal surgery or a transscrotal approach for orchiectomy was performed, based on an assumed risk of scrotal and/or inguinal relapse. Scrotal and/or inguinal relapse is extremely unusual and recent studies do not confirm an increased risk of relapse in such patients.[92,93] As treatment-related morbidity is significant, modification of treatment volumes to include those sites is not recommended. Prophylactic mediastinal irradiation for stage I seminomas is also not recommended in view of the rarity of subsequent mediastinal relapse.[94,95]

### Stage II

Optimal management of stage II seminoma has become increasingly controversial. Survival and cure rate with postorchiectomy radiation therapy for patients with minimal disease (stage IIA) is above 90% and similar for those obtained in stage I seminoma treated in a similar manner.[90–92,96] For patients with bulky retroperitoneal metastases (stage IIB) survival with irradiation alone is in the range of 60%.[90,96,97] Results for all stage II treated with postorchiectomy irradiation are presented in Table 16. This is prior to the

**TABLE 15. Results of Irradiation in Stage I Seminoma**

| Study | No. Patients | 5-Yr Survival (%) |
|---|---|---|
| Maier and Sulak[85] | 284 | 97 |
| Hamilton[82] | 232 | 98 |
| Earle[86] | 71 | 100 |
| Zagars[87] | 161 | 95 |
| Hanks[88] | 229 | 98 |

**TABLE 16. Results of Irradiation in Stage II Seminoma**

| Study | No. Patients | 5-Yr Survival (%) |
|---|---|---|
| Maier and Sulak[85] | 34 | 76 |
| Peckham[94] | 63 | 79 |
| Zagars[96] | 48 | 88 |
| Thomas[92] | 86 | 74 |

emergence of successful multiagent chemotherapy. Study of patterns of failure following irradiation for stage IIB seminoma suggests that approximately one third of patients will develop metastatic disease outside the treated irradiation volume.[90,96,97] Patients with stage IIA and IIB disease have a low incidence of distant metastases whether or not they are given prophylactic mediastinal irradiation. The necessity of prophylactic mediastinal irradiation for these patients remains controversial and data from several series suggest that supradiaphragmatic relapse is rare in the absence of mediastinal irradiation.[83] The limited value of extended field irradiation may be offset by the rare patient who suffers a relapse and is subsequently unable to tolerate effective aggressive combination chemotherapy, and many radiation oncologists no longer recommend its use.[98]

Optimal management for patients with stage IIC bulky retroperitoneal disease (5 to 10 cm in transverse diameter) is extremely controversial and several different approaches have been recommended. These include infradiaphragmatic irradiation only followed by chemotherapy containing cisplatin for relapse; infradiaphragmatic and subdiaphragmatic irradiation and chemotherapy for subsequent relapse; or initial combination chemotherapy followed by observation, consolidation irradiation, or surgical resection of residual disease. Selection of a treatment approach may be influenced by size and location of the retroperitoneal disease. If the treatment volume would necessitate inclusion of a kidney or a significant portion of the liver, then initial combination chemotherapy may obviate the potential morbidity of radiation therapy in such situations. Although an unusual presentation, patients with masses greater than 10 cm (stage IID) should be treated with cisplatin-containing combination chemotherapy since results with radiation therapy alone are disappointing.[99,100]

### Stages III and IV

Advanced seminoma is a rare disease and current standard therapy would be cisplatin-containing chemotherapy regimens. Although radiation therapy may cure one third of patients with stage III and IV disease, and was standard treatment prior to the availability of modern chemotherapy, the majority of patients require salvage therapy and extended field irradiation may interfere with administration of effective doses of chemotherapy. In general, a policy of observation after appropriate chemotherapy and a radiographic complete remission is recommended. Surgical removal or routine irradiation of radiographic disease does not appear to be indicated since the majority of these residual masses represent fibrosis only.[101,102]

### Results of Therapy

Results of radiation therapy alone for management of patients with early stage testicular seminoma are excellent with overall survival rates of approximately 85%. The use of cisplatin and combination chemotherapy regimens for more advanced disease has improved survival to over 95%. Outcome of treatment is dependent on stage and extent of disease at presentation. Radiation therapy has been the treatment of choice in patients with stage I and stage II disease less than 5 cm in diameter. Optimal management of patients with more bulky disease remains controversial but the various approaches that have been used have comparable results.[103]

### Complications

Complications and long-term sequelae of standard infradiaphragmatic irradiation for early stage seminoma is related to dose, with essentially no major complications seen below 2500 cGy to approximately 2% between 2500 cGy and 3500 cGy, and rising to 6% over 4000 cGy.[82,84,104] Doses above 2500 cGy do not appear necessary for cure. Many patients with testicular seminoma have some impaired spermatogenesis at the time of initial presentation and irradiation may further impair fertility. Careful shielding of the remaining testes may reduce the dose from 1% to 2% of the prescribed dose.[105]

### Nonseminomatous Germ Cell Tumors

Management of nonseminomatous germ cell tumors with histologic confirmation after radical inguinal orchiectomy has changed with the development of effective cisplatin-based chemotherapy and the radical retroperitoneal lymphadenectomy. Survival of patients with disseminated nonseminomatous germ cell tumors is approximately 70% to 80% at the present time.[106,107] Radiation therapy has essentially no role in the initial management of disseminated nonseminomatous tumors except for palliation and management of metastases where surgical resection would be difficult. This relatively minor role for radiation therapy is based on the availability of highly effective combination chemotherapy and salvage therapy and excellent results with surgical resection of residual disease, not on any inherent radioresistance of nonseminomatous germ cell tumors. In the Royal Marsden Hospital experience, irradiation was effective in preventing retroperitoneal recurrence in stage I and stage II tumors with minimal disease but less effective in patients with bulky retroperitoneal metastases.[108]

In general, radiation therapy is reserved for patients with radiographic evidence of residual masses following chemotherapy that are not amenable to surgical resection, although there are some advocates for its use in stage I and II disease.[108,109] Postorchiectomy surveillance has been recommended as an acceptable alternative to retroperitoneal lymphadenectomy for patients with stage I and stage II disease.[110,111] Both approaches appear to have similar cure rates. In general, the high risk of dissemination has diminished the role of local therapies for nonseminomatous tumors.

## RENAL CELL CARCINOMA

Standard treatment in patients with localized renal cell carcinoma has been surgical with a radical nephrectomy. A benefit to survival from any adjuvant therapy has been difficult to demonstrate. Radiation therapy has been used preoperatively and postoperatively as a definitive treatment for medically inoperable patients and for palliation of symptoms related to metastatic disease. The role of preoperative and postoperative irradiation has not been well defined. The studies have been few and the results have been inconclusive. An increased resectability rate and improved local control have been reported with little impact on overall survival. The reports of any benefit with postoperative irradiation have come from only one nonrandomized trial[112] while two randomized studies[113–115] demonstrated no benefit from postoperative irradiation and had high complication rates (Table 17). Any demonstrated benefit may have been compromised by the irradiation technique or dose. Dose-limiting structures in the upper abdomen limit the ability to deliver high doses of radiation and reported complications have been significant.[113–115]

Results of studies of preoperative irradiation showed increased resectability and improved survival at 2 years for stage II and stage III patients with renal cell carcinoma.[116] Juusela et al showed no survival advantage for patients receiving preoper-

**TABLE 17. Postoperative Adjuvant Irradiation in Renal Cell Carcinoma**

| Study | No. Patients | Treatment | 5-Yr Survival (%) | Local Recurrence (%) |
|---|---|---|---|---|
| Rafla[112] | 96 | Nephrectomy | 37 | 25 |
| | 94 | RT + nephrectomy | 57 | 7 |
| Finney[113] | 48 | Nephrectomy | 47 | 7 |
| | 52 | RT + nephrectomy | 36 | 7 |
| Kjaer[114] | 33 | Nephrectomy | 62 | 3 |
| | 32 | RT + nephrectomy | 38 | 0 |

**TABLE 18. Preoperative Irradiation for Renal Cell Carcinoma**

| Study | Stage | Treatment | 5-Yr Survival Rate (%) |
|---|---|---|---|
| van der Werf-Messing[116] | I | Nephrectomy | 88 |
| | | RT + nephrectomy | 85 |
| | II | Nephrectomy | 64 |
| | | RT + nephrectomy | 62 |
| | III | Nephrectomy | 29 |
| | | RT + nephrectomy | 27 |
| Rubin[118] | | Nephrectomy | 52 |
| | | RT + nephrectomy | 68 |
| Juusela[117] | | Nephrectomy | 63 |
| | | RT + nephrectomy | 47 |

ative radiation.[117] Rubin and others showed improved survival at 2 years for those receiving preoperative radiation.[118] These are summarized in Table 18. To date, the efficacy of preoperative or postoperative irradiation with radical nephrectomy has not been well defined and should be the subject of future studies.

For patients with metastases from renal cell carcinoma, palliative nephrectomy may alleviate symptoms of pain, hemorrhage, hypercalcemia, or hypertension but is not recommended with the goal of inducing spontaneous regression of metastases.[119]

The role of radiation therapy for hematogenous metastases of renal cell carcinoma to bone, lung, and brain is nearly always palliative. Patients with metastatic renal cell carcinoma and presenting with a solitary metastasis may have a 30% to 40% chance of surviving 5 years.[120] Although the majority will develop multiple metastases, a course of palliative irradiation designed to ensure a long disease-free survival should be delivered.[121] External beam irradiation for other symptomatic metastases can produce subjective improvement in symptoms in the majority of patients.[122,123]

## CANCER OF THE URETER

Management of renal pelvis or ureteral carcinoma has also been primarily surgical with little data on the role of adjuvant irradiation. A retrospective review by Brookland and Richter demonstrated a lower incidence of local recurrence and increased 5-year survival in patients with locally advanced or high-grade transitional cell carcinoma of the renal pelvis and ureter.[124] A significant number of patients in this poor-risk group with poor prognostic factors developed distant metastases. Reports from Brady et al[125] and Babaian et al[126] suggest that postoperative irradiation may benefit poor-risk patients following nephroureterectomy. Patients with locally advanced disease or documented regional lymph node metastases may be candidates for postoperative irradiation.[127] In addition, there are ongoing studies combining local irradiation with adjuvant cisplatin-based chemotherapy regimens.[128] Results supporting use of combination chemotherapy and radiation therapy in the primary management of renal pelvis and ureteral carcinoma are not available. Promising results from combined modality therapy in other urothelial sites offer support for its use in these sites but will require multi-institutional studies in a protocol setting.

### Complications

Acute side effects and long-term sequelae from irradiation of the upper abdomen and pelvis are similar to those expected for other tumor sites in these areas. These include nausea, vomiting, diarrhea, and abdominal cramping. Long-term sequelae include radiation injury of the small bowel but the extremely high complication rates reported by Finney[113] and Kjaer et al[114] in postoperative irradiation for renal cell carcinoma should not be considered typical.

## CARCINOMA OF THE PENIS

General management of penile carcinoma includes treatment of the primary tumor and regional lymphatics. A surgical approach, utilizing partial or total penectomy with or without inguinal and pelvic lymph node dissection, has been the most commonly accepted treatment. Radiation therapy with external irradiation or brachytherapy techniques has also been used effectively in the management of the primary lesion and metastases to regional lymph nodes. A major advantage of radiotherapeutic management of the primary tumor in carcinoma of the penis is functional organ preservation. A favorable anatomic location rather than any particular radiosensitivity allowed for the use of irradiation as a treatment modality early in the history of radiation therapy. As early as 1924, Barringer and Dean treated such patients with partial amputation of the penis and radiation therapy to the regional lymph nodes.[129] Many variations in techniques including interstitial implants, molds and contact therapy, orthovoltage and megavoltage equipment, and dose were used. These early series were associated with wide variation in tumor dose and a high incidence of normal tissue injury. Modern series show significant increases in local control and corresponding decreases in treatment-related sequelae.

A high percentage of patients with carcinoma of the penis present with palpable lymphadenopathy but the incidence of inflammatory inguinal lymphadenopathy varies from 13% to 82%.[129,130] The incidence of metastases to the clinically uninvolved nodes is approximately 20%.[131,132] Appropriate management of clinically uninvolved lymph nodes remains unresolved with some authors advocating immediate lymphadenectomy[133] and others management by observation with a therapeutic lymphadenectomy if nodal involvement becomes apparent.[134]

Elective regional node irradiation remains controversial. Several series suggest a benefit for irradiation in the clinically uninvolved groin[131,135] but routine prophylactic regional lymph node irradiation has not been recommended. Irradiation of clinically involved regional lymph nodes in patients with carcinoma of the penis can be effective for local control and can be curative. Staubitz et al reported on 13 patients with documented regional lymph node involvement treated with radiation therapy, with 5 of 13 patients surviving 5 years.[136]

### Results of Therapy

A large proportion of patients with penile carcinoma have been treated surgically with local control rates of 25% to 80%, dependent on primary tumor stage and regional lymph node involvement. Results of radiation therapy from several authors have been similar and are summarized in Table 19. Five-year survival rates ranging from 44% to 100% are reported in several small series treated with a variety of irradiation techniques including molds, interstitial implants, and external beam treatment. Doses of 6000 to 7000 cGy are required depending

**TABLE 19. Results of Radiation Therapy for Penile Carcinoma**

| Study | Tumor Control | | Complications |
|---|---|---|---|
| | Stage I–II | Stage III–IV | |
| Jackson[137] | 20/45 (44%) | | 2/45 (4%) |
| Haile and Delclos[142] | 18/18 (100%) | 2/2 (100%) | |
| Kelley[143] | 10/10 (100%) | | |
| Sagerman[155] | 9/12 (75%) | 1/3 (33%) | |
| Salaverria[134] | 12/13 (92%) | | |

on the volume treated. Tumor control is closely associated with stage.[136]

### Complications

Treatment-related complications are similar to those for irradiation of male urethral carcinoma and include acute reversible moist desquamation of the penile skin and edema of the subcutaneous tissues. Late telangiectasia is common and usually asymptomatic. Ulceration and necrosis are rare with modern techniques.

## CARCINOMA OF THE MALE URETHRA

Carcinoma of the male urethra is uncommon and treatment approaches have included surgical management such as transurethral resection or penectomy. For tumors of the distal urethra, results of surgical resection or radiation therapy are similar.[138] Lesions of the prostatic urethra are treated with radiotherapeutic techniques similar to those used for carcinoma of the prostate. However, results of radiation therapy in male urethral carcinoma are difficult to evaluate since most patients are treated surgically[139] and radiation therapy series have few patients for evaluation. As with surgery, radiation therapy results are dependent on location with anterior lesions having a more favorable prognosis than posterior sites.

Unlike penile carcinoma, clinically involved nodes at the time of diagnosis usually represent metastases rather than inflammatory changes. Management of regional lymph nodes has been by bilateral lymphadenectomy and radiation therapy has been used infrequently in these patients.[140,141]

Irradiation techniques for management of penile carcinoma and male urethral carcinoma are similar and treatment-related sequelae are also similar. Acute reactions from irradiation of the penis as well as the male urethra include moist desquamation of the skin and edema of the subcutaneous tissues. Routine circumcision prior to initiation of radiation therapy is recommended and will help minimize such treatment-related morbidity. Ulceration and skin necrosis are rare. The frequency of urethral strictures ranges from 0 to 40% in reported series.[135,142–145]

Radiation therapy has been useful in the treatment of carcinoma of the penis in terms of both the primary tumor and regional lymph node disease. Its major advantage has been organ and functional preservation. However, the role of radiation therapy in male urethral carcinoma is less well defined because of the rarity of the disease.

## CANCER OF THE FEMALE URETHRA

Therapeutic approaches to the management of carcinoma of the female urethra vary with the extent of local and regional disease and individual physician preferences.

Small tumors at the meatus or in situ involvement of the distal half of the urethra may be treated with local excision, fulguration, or laser coagulation.[146,147] For larger than stage I (disease limited to distal one half of urethra) interstitial irradiation[148] or a combination of interstitial and external beam irradiation[149] offers an alternative to surgical resection. Interstitial implants have used radium needles, or, more recently, afterloading $^{192}$Ir implants. Doses of 60 to 70 Gy are administered to the target volume over 6 to 7 days. For patients treated with a combination of external beam and interstitial irradiation, the external beam portal includes inguinal and pelvic lymph nodes as well as the perineum. Doses of 45 to 50 Gy to the pelvic and inguinal nodes and an interstitial implant raising the tumor dose to 70 to 80 Gy are delivered. Elective inguinal node irradiation is recommended for invasive lesions; with palpable inguinal adenopathy, ipsilateral node dissection and/or irradiation is indicated. Tumors involving the entire urethra (stages II, III, and IV) are usually associated with extensive periurethral, vaginal, and/or vulvar or bladder involvement and a high probability of regional lymph node metastases. The best results have been obtained with a combination of preoperative irradiation and radical surgery with urinary diversion.[150] Local recurrence after surgical excision may be treated with irradiation and further surgical resection.

Cure rates of 70% to 90% have been obtained with radiation therapy alone for small tumors of the distal urethra.[147,151–153] Results are less satisfactory for more extensive tumors involving the entire urethra. Bracken et al treated 81 patients with 5-year survival rates of 25% stage III and 20% stage IV.[146] Weghaupt et al reported a 5-year survival rate of 50% for patients with tumors of the proximal urethra treated with irradiation or a combination of irradiation and surgery.[154]

Complications from irradiation or a combination of modalities can be significant.[146,151] These include urethral strictures, incontinence, cysts, vaginal stenosis, fistula formation, and bowel obstruction. Reported complication rates vary from 20% to 40%.[150–153]

## SUMMARY

Radiation therapy has evolved substantially during the past 50 years. Undoubtedly, improvement in delivery systems and an improved understanding of biology will refine the utilization of this modality. Radiation therapy will continue to play a major role in the management of many genitourinary tumors. This chapter was designed to provide the practicing urologist with an overview of the basic science of therapeutic radiology and outline the major indications for its application in clinical practice.

## REFERENCES

1. Cantril ST. *Radiation Therapy in the Management of Cancer of the Uterine Cervix*. Springfield, IL: Charles C Thomas; 1950:44–50.
2. O'Brien FW. The radium treatment of cancer of the cervix, a historical review. *Am J Roentgenol Radium Ther Nucl Med*. 1947;57(3):281.
3. Hanks GE, Herring DF, Kramer S. Patterns of Care outcome studies: results of the national practice in cancer of the cervix. *Cancer*. 1983;51:959.
4. Million RR, Cassisi NJ. Oropharynx. In: Million RR, Cassisi NJ, eds. *Management of Head and Neck Cancer: A Multi-disciplinary Approach*. Philadelphia: JB Lippincott; 1984:299–314.
5. Coutard H. Roentgen therapy of epitheliomas of the tonsillar region, hypopharynx and larynx from 1920 to 1926. *Roent Ther Epithel*. 1932;28(3):313.
6. Fletcher GH. Cancer of the uterine cervix, Janeway lecture, 1970. *Am J Roentgenol Radium Ther Nucl Med*. 1971;3(2):225.
7. Read J: Mode of action of x-ray doses given with different oxygen concentrations. *Br J Radiol*. 1952;25:336.
8. Puck TT, Marcus PI. Action of x-rays on mammalian cells. *J Exp Med*. 1956;103:653.
9. Elkind MM, Whitemore GF. *The Radiobiology of Cultured Mammalian Cells*. New York: Gordon and Breach; 1967.
10. Deacon S, Peckham MS, Steel CG. The radioresponsiveness of human tumors and the initial slope of the cell survival curve. *Radiother Oncol*. 1984;2:317.
11. Bush RS, Jenkin RDT, Allt WEC. Definitive evidence of hypoxic cells influencing cure in cancer therapy. *Br J Cancer*. 1978;37(S3):302.
12. Thomlinson RH, Gray LH. The histological structure of some human lung cancers and the possible implications for radiotherapy. *Br J Cancer*. 1955;9:539.
13. Ang KK, Landuyt W, Rijnders A, et al. Differences in repopulation kinetics in mouse skin during split course multiple fractions per day or daily fractionated irradiation. *Int J Radiat Oncol Biol Phys*. 1985;10:95.
14. Fowler JF, Stern BE. Dose-time relationships in radiotherapy and the validity of cell survival curve models. *Br J Radiol*. 1963;36:163.
15. Kramer S: Research plan for radiation oncology committee on radiation oncology studies. *J Cancer*. 1976;37(2):2031.
16. Orton CG, Ellis F. A simplification in the use of the NSD concept in practical radiotherapy. *Br J Radiol*. 1973;46:529.
17. Dische S. Chemical sensitizers for hypoxic cells: a decade of experience in clinical radiotherapy. *Radiother Oncol*. 1985;3:97.
18. Duncan W. A clinical evaluation of fast neutron therapy. In: Steel GG, Adams GE, Peckham MS, eds. *The Biological Basis of Radiotherapy*. Amsterdam: Elsevier; 1983:277–286.
19. Withers HR. Biologic basis for altered fractionation schemes. *Cancer*. 1985;55:2086.
20. Paschkis R, Tittinger W. Radiumbehandlung eines prostatasarkoms. *Weiner klische Wochenschrift* Nr. 48, 1910.
21. Flocks RH. Interstitial irradiation therapy with a solution of Au 198 as part of combination therapy for prostatic carcinoma. *J Nucl Med*. 1964;5:691.
22. Syed AMN, Puthwala AA, Tansey LA, et al. Management of prostate carcinoma: Combination of pelvic lymphadenectomy, temporary Ir-192 implantation and external irradiation. *Radiology*. 1983;149:829.

23. Bagshaw MA. Potential for radiotherapy alone in prostate cancer. *Cancer*. 1985;55:2079.
24. Hanks GE. External-beam radiation therapy for clinically localized prostate cancer: Patterns of Care studies in the United States. *NCI Monogr*. 1988;7:75.
25. Bagshaw MA, Cox RS, Ray GR. Status of radiation therapy of prostate cancer at Stanford University. *NCI Monogr*. 1988;7:45.
26. Perez CA, Pilepich MV, Garcia D, et al: Definitive radiation therapy in carcinoma of the prostate localized to the pelvis: experience at the Mallinckrodt Institute of Radiology. *NCI Monogr*. 1988;7:85.
27. Zagars GK, von Eschenbach AC, Johnson DE, Oswald MJ. The role of radiation therapy in stages A2 and B adenocarcinoma of the prostate. *Int J Radiat Oncol Biol Phys*. 1988; 14:701.
28. Zagars GK, von Eschenbach AC, Johnson DE, Oswald MJ. Stage C adenocarcinoma of the prostate: an analysis of 551 patients treated with external beam radiation. *Cancer*. 1987; 60:1489.
29. Hanks GE, Asbell S, Krall JM, et al. Outcome for lymph node dissection negative T-1b, T-2 (A-2,B) prostate cancer treated with external beam radiation therapy in RTOG 77-06. *Int J Radiat Oncol Biol Phys*. 1991;21:1099.
30. Paulson DF. Randomized-series of treatment with surgery versus radiation for prostate adenocarcinoma. *NCI Monogr*. 1988;7:127.
31. Perez CA, Garcia D, Simpson JR, et al. Factors influencing outcome of definitive radiotherapy for localized carcinoma of the prostate. *Radiother Oncol*. 1989;16:1.
32. Hanks GE, Leibel SA, Krall JM, Kramer S. Patterns of Care studies: dose–response of observations for local control of adenocarcinoma of the prostate. *Int J Radiat Oncol Biol Phys*. 1985;11:153.
33. Perez CA, Pilepich MV, Zivnuska F. Tumor control in definitive irradiation of localized carcinoma of the prostate. *Int J Radiat Oncol Biol Phys*. 1986;12:523.
34. Kuban DA, El-Mahdi AM, Schellhammer PF. 192-Ir interstitial implantation for prostate cancer. What have we learned 10 years later? *Cancer*. 1989;63:2415.
35. Robey EDL, Schellhammer PF. Local failure after definitive therapy for prostatic cancer. *J Urol*. 1987;137:613.
36. Hanks GE, Martz JH, Diamond JJ. The effect of dose on local control of prostate cancer. *Int J Radiat Oncol Biol Phys*. 1988;15:1299.
37. Middleton RG. Value of and indications for pelvic lymph node dissection in the staging of prostate cancer. *NCI Monogr*. 1988;7:41.
38. McGowan DG. The value of extended field radiation therapy in carcinoma of the prostate. *Int J Radiat Oncol Biol Phys*. 1981;7:1333.
39. Bagshaw MA. Radiotherapeutic treatment of prostate carcinoma with pelvic node involvement. *Urol Clin North Am*. 1984;11:297.
40. Neglia WJ, Hussey DH, Johnson DE. Megavoltage radiation therapy for carcinoma of the prostate. *Int J Radiat Oncol Biol Phys*. 1977;2:873.
41. Sause WT. The role of radiation therapy in the management of advanced prostate cancer. *Semin Urol*. 1988;6(4):279.
42. Pilepich MV, Krall JM, Johnson RJ, et al. Extended field (periaortic) irradiation in carcinoma of the prostate: Analysis of RTOG 75-06. *Int J Radiat Oncol Biol Phys*. 1986;12:345.
43. Asbell SO, Krall JM, Pilepich MV, et al. Elective pelvic irradiation in stage A2, B carcinoma of the prostate: analysis of RTOG 77-06. *Int J Radiat Oncol Biol Phys*. 1988;15:1307.
44. Cox JD, Stoffel TJ. The significance of needle biopsy after irradiation for stage C adenocarcinoma of the prostate. *Cancer*. 1977;40:156.
45. Scardino PT, Wheeler TM. Local control of prostate cancer with radiotherapy: frequency and prognostic significance of positive results of postirradiation prostate biopsy. *NCI Monogr*. 1988;7:95.
46. Stamey TA, Kabalin JN, Ferrari M. Prostate specific antigen in the diagnosis and treatment of adenocarcinoma of the prostate. III. Radiation treated patients. *J Urol*. 1989;141:1084.
47. Kabalin JN, Hodge KK, McNeal JE, et al. Identification of residual cancer in the prostate following radiation therapy: role of transrectal ultrasound guided biopsy and prostate specific antigen. *J Urol*. 1989;142:326.
48. Russell KJ, Duantov C, Hafermann MD, et al. Prostate specific antigen in the management of patients with localized adenocarcinoma of the prostate treated with primary radiation therapy. *J Urol*. 1991;146:1046.
49. Sause WT, Richards RS, Plenk HP. Prostate carcinoma: five-year follow-up in surgically staged patients with extended field radiation. *J Urol*. 1986;135:517.
50. Lawton CA, Minhee Won MA, Pilepich MV, et al. Long-term treatment sequelae following external beam irradiation for adenocarcinoma of the prostate: analysis of RTOG studies 7506 and 7706. *Int J Radiat Oncol Biol Phys*. 1991;21:935.
51. Sogani PC, DeCosse JJ Jr, Montie J, et al. Carcinoma of the prostate: treatment with pelvic lymphadenectomy and 125-I implants. *Clin Bull*. 1979;9:24.
52. Silverberg E, Lubera JA. Cancer statistics, 1989. *CA*. 1989;39:3.
53. Sawczuk IS, Olsson CA, deVere White R. The limited usefulness of external beam radiotherapy in the control of superficial bladder cancer. *J Urol*. 1988;61:330.

54. Whitmore WF, Prout GR Jr. Discouraging results of high dose external beam radiation therapy in low stage (O and A) bladder cancer. *J Urol.* 1982;127:902.

55. Quilty PM, Duncan W. Treatment of superficial (T1) tumors of the bladder by radical radiotherapy. *Br J Urol.* 1986;58:174.

56. Goodman GB, Hislop TG, Elwood JM, et al. Conservation of bladder function in patients with invasive bladder cancer treated by definitive irradiation and selective cystectomy. *Int J Radiat Oncol Biol Phys.* 1981;7:569.

57. Van der Werf-Messing B, Menon RS, Hop WCJ. Carcinoma of the urinary bladder category T3 NX M0 treated by the combination of radium implant and external irradiation: second report. *Int J Radiat Oncol Biol Phys.* 1983;9:177.

58. Van der Werf-Messing B, Star WM, Menon RS. T3 NX M0 carcinoma of the urinary bladder treated by the combination of radium implant and external irradiation. A preliminary report. *Int J Radiat Oncol Biol Phys.* 1980;6:1723.

59. Van der Werf-Messing B, Menon RS, Hop WCJ. Cancer of the urinary bladder category T2, T3, (NX M0) treated by interstitial radium implants: second report. *Int J Radiat Oncol Biol Phys.* 1983;9:481.

60. Bloom HJG, Hendry WF, Wallace DM, et al. Treatment of T3 bladder cancer: controlled trial of preoperative radiotherapy and radical cystectomy versus radical radiotherapy: second report and review. *Br J Urol.* 1982;54:136.

61. Goffinet DR, Schneider MJ, Galstein EJ, et al. Bladder cancer: results of radiation therapy in 384 patients. *Radiology.* 1975;117:149.

62. Miller LS. Bladder cancer: superiority of preoperative irradiation and cystectomy in clinical stages B2 and C. *Cancer.* 1977;39:973.

63. Fish JC, Fayos JW. Carcinoma of the urinary bladder. *Radiology.* 1976;118:179.

64. Meyers FJ, Palmer JM, Freiha FS, et al. The fate of the bladder in patients with metastatic bladder cancer treated with cisplatin, methotrexate, and vinblastine: a Northern California Oncology Group study. *J Urol.* 1985; 134:1118.

65. Logothetis CJ, Samuels ML, Odgen S, et al. Cyclophosphamide, adriamycin, and cisplatin chemotherapy for patients with locally advanced urothelial tumors with or without nodal metastases. *J Urol.* 1985;134:460.

66. Scher H, Herr H, Sternberg C, et al. Neoadjuvant chemotherapy for invasive bladder cancer: experience with the M-VAC regimen. *Br J Urol.* 1989;64:250.

67. Kaufman DS, Prout GR Jr, Shipley WU, et al. Upfront MCV chemotherapy plus cisplatin and radiotherapy: its efficacy in successful bladder preservation in 50 patients with invasive cancer. *Proc Am Soc Clin Oncol.* 1989;8:129.

68. Sternberg CN, Yagoda A, Scher HI, et al. Patterns of response, survival and relapse in advanced urothelial cancer following M-VAC therapy. *Proc Am Soc Clin Oncol.* 1989;8:129.

69. Soloway MS, Einstein AB, Corder MP. A comparison of cisplatin and the combination of cisplatin and cyclophosphamide in advanced urothelial cancer: a National Bladder Cancer Group study. *Cancer.* 1983;52:767.

70. Shipley WU, Kaufman DS, Heney NM. Can chemo-radiotherapy plus transurethral tumor resection make cystectomy unnecessary for invasive bladder cancer? *Oncology.* 1990; 4(7):25.

71. Crawford ED, Das S, Smith JA Jr. Preoperative radiation therapy in the treatment of bladder cancer. *Urol Clin North Am.* 1987;14:781.

72. Slack NH, Bross IDJ, Prout GR Jr. Five-year follow-up results of a collaborative study of therapies for carcinoma of the bladder. *J Surg Oncol.* 1977;9:393.

73. Awaad HK, El-Baki HA, El-Bolkainy N, et al. Preoperative irradiation of T3 carcinoma in bilharzial bladder: A comparison between hyperfractionation and conventional fractionation. *Int J Radiat Oncol Biol Phys.* 1979;5:787.

74. Ghoneim, MA, Ashamallah AK, Awaad HK, et al. Randomized trial of cystectomy with or without preoperative radiotherapy for carcinoma of the bilharzial bladder. *J Urol.* 1985;134:266.

75. Anderstrom C, Johansson S, Nillsen S, et al. A prospective randomized study of preoperative irradiation with cystectomy or cystectomy alone for invasive bladder carcinoma. *Eur Urol.* 1983;9:142.

76. Blackard CE, Byar DP, and Veterans Administration Cooperative Urological Research Group. Results of a clinical trial of surgery and radiation in stages II and III carcinoma of the bladder. *J Urol.* 1972;108:875.

77. Parsons JT, Million RR. Planned preoperative irradiation in the management of clinical stage B2-C (T3) bladder carcinoma. *Int J Radiat Oncol Biol Phys.* 1988;14:797.

78. Rubin P, Casarett GW. *Clinical Radiation Pathology.* Philadelphia: WB Saunders; 1968: 334–374.

79. Duncan W, Quilty PM. The results of a series of 963 patients with transitional cell carcinoma of the urinary bladder primarily treated by radical megavoltage x-ray therapy. *Radiother Oncol.* 1986;7:299.

80. Russell KJ. Radiation therapy of urinary bladder cancer. In: Crawford ED, Das S, eds. *Current Genitourinary Cancer Surgery.* Philadelphia: Lea & Febiger; 1990:534–551.

81. Caldwell WL, Kademian MT, Friar Z, Davis TE. The management of testicular seminomas. *Cancer.* 1980;7(S)45:1768.

82. Hamilton C, Horwich A, Easton D, et al. Radiotherapy for stage I seminoma testis: results

of treatment and complications. *Radiother Oncol.* 1986;6:115.

83. Thomas GM. Controversies in the management of testicular seminoma. *Cancer.* 1985;55:2296.
84. Fossa SD, Aass N, Kaahluus O. Radiotherapy for testicular seminoma stage I: treatment results and long-term post-irradiation morbidity in 365 patients. *Int J Radiat Oncol Biol Phys.* 1989;16:383.
85. Maier JG, Sulak MH. Radiation therapy in malignant testes tumors seminoma. *Cancer.* 1973;32:1212.
86. Earle JD, Bagshaw MA, Kaplan HS. Supervoltage radiation therapy of testicular tumors. *Am J Roentgenol.* 1973;117:653.
87. Zagars GK, Babaian RJ. Stage I testicular seminoma: rationale for post-orchiectomy radiation therapy. *Int J Radiat Oncol Biol Phys.* 1987;13:155.
88. Hanks GE, Herring DF, Kramer S. Patterns of Care outcome studies: results of the national practice in seminoma of the testis. *Int J Radiat Oncol Biol Phys.* 1981;7:1413.
89. Peckham MJ, Hamilton CR, Horwich A, Hendry WF. Surveillance after orchiectomy for stage I seminoma of the testes. *Br J Urol.* 1987;59:343.
90. Oliver RTD. Limitations to the use of surveillance: An option in the management of stage I seminoma. *J Androl.* 1987;10:263.
91. Horwich A, Peckham MJ. Surveillance after orchiectomy for clinical stage I germ cell tumors of the testis: EORTC Genitourinary Group Monograph 5. *Progr Controv Oncol Urol.* 1988;2:471.
92. Thomas GM, Sturgeon JF, Alison R, et al. A study of postorchiectomy surveillance in stage I testicular seminoma. *J Urol.* 1989;142:313.
93. Kennedy CL, Hendry WF, Peckham MJ. The significance of scrotal interference in stage I testicular cancer managed by orchiectomy and surveillance. *Br J Urol.* 1986;58:705.
94. Peckham MJ. Testicular tumors: investigation and staging. In: Peckham MJ, ed. *The Management of Testicular Tumors.* London: Edwin Arnold; 1981:89–101.
95. Thomas GM, Rider WD, Dembo AJ, et al. Seminoma of the testis: results of treatment and patterns of failure after radiation therapy. *Int J Radiat Oncol Biol Phys.* 1982;8:165.
96. Zagars GK, Babaian RJ. The role of radiation therapy in stage II testicular seminoma. *Int J Radiat Oncol Biol Phys.* 1987;13:163.
97. Dosoretz DE, Shipley WU, Blitzer PH, et al. Megavoltage irradiation for pure testicular seminoma: results and patterns of failure. *Cancer.* 1981;48:2184.
98. Sause WT. Testicular seminoma: analysis of radiation therapy for stage II disease. *J Urol.* 1983;130:702.
99. Mason BR, Kearsley JH. Radiotherapy for stage II testicular seminoma: the prognostic influence of tumor bulk. *Clin Oncol.* 1988; 6:1856.
100. Zagars GK, Babaian J. The role of radiation in stage II testicular seminoma. *Int J Radiat Oncol Biol Phys.* 1987;13:163.
101. Peckham MJ, Horwich A, Hendry WF. Advanced seminoma: treatment with cisplatin based combination chemotherapy or carboplatin (JM8). *Br J Cancer.* 1985;52:7.
102. Stomper PC, Jochelson MS, Friedman EL, et al. CT evaluation of advanced seminoma treated with chemotherapy. *Am J Roentgenol.* 1986;146:746.
103. Thomas GM. Consensus statement on the investigation and management of testicular seminomas. EORTC Genito-Urinary Group Monograph 7. In: Newling DW, Jones WG, eds. *Prostate Cancer and Testicular Cancer.* New York: Wiley-Liss; 1990.
104. Coia LR, Hanks GE. Complications from large field intermediate dose infradiaphragmatic radiation: an analysis of the Patterns of Care outcome studies for Hodgkin's disease and seminoma. *Int J Radiat Oncol Biol Phys.* 1988;15:29.
105. Fraas BA, Kinsella TJ, Harrington FS, et al. Peripheral dose to the testes: The design and clinical use of a practical and effective gonodal shield. *Int J Radiat Oncol Biol Phys.* 1985;11:609.
106. Hainsworth JD, Greco FA. Testicular germ cell neoplasm. *Am J Med.* 1983;75:817.
107. Loehrer PJ, Williams SD, Einhorn LH. Testicular cancer: the quest continues. *JNCI.* 1988;80:1373.
108. Tyrell CJ, Peckham MJ. The response of lymph node metastases of testicular teratoma to radiation therapy. *Br J Urol.* 1976;48:363.
109. Rorth M, von der Maase H, Nielsen ES, et al. Orchidectomy alone versus orchidectomy plus radiotherapy in stage I nonseminomatous testicular cancer: a randomized study by the Danish Testicular Carcinoma Study Group. *Int J Androl.* 1987;10(1):255.
110. Hoskin P, Dilly S, Eastors P, et al. Prognostic factors in stage I non-seminomatous germ cell testicular tumors managed by orchiectomy and surveillance: implications for adjuvant therapy. *J Clin Oncol.* 1986;4:1031.
111. Sogani PC, Whitmore WF, Herr HW, et al. Orchiectomy alone in the treatment of clinical stage I non-seminomatous germ cell tumor of the testis. *J Clin Oncol.* 1984;2:267.
112. Rafla S. Renal cell carcinoma. Natural history and results of treatment. *Cancer.* 1970;25:26.
113. Finney R. An evaluation of postoperative radiotherapy in hypernephroma treatment: a clinical trial. *Cancer.* 1973;32:1332.

114. Kjaer M, Fredericksen PL, Engelholm SA. Postoperative radiotherapy in stage II and III renal adenocarcinoma. A randomized trial by the Copenhagen Renal Cancer Study Group. *Int J Radiat Oncol Biol Phys*. 1987;13:665.

115. Finney R. Radiotherapy in the treatment of hypernephroma. A clinical trial. *Br J Urol*. 1973;45:258.

116. van der Werf-Messing B. Carcinoma of the kidney. *Cancer*. 1973;32:1056.

117. Juusela H, Melmio K. Alfthan O, et al. Preoperative irradiation in the treatment of renal adenocarcinoma. *Scand J Urol Nephrol*. 1977;11:277.

118. Rubin P, Keller BO, Cox C, et al. Preoperative irradiation in renal carcinoma: evaluation of radiation treatment plans. *Cancer*. 1975; 123:114.

119. deKernian JB, Ramming KP, Smith RB. The natural history of metastatic renal cell carcinoma: a computer analysis. *J Urol*. 1978; 120:148.

120. Kjaer M. The treatment and prognosis of patients with renal adenocarcinoma with solitary metastasis: 10 year survival results. *Int J Radiat Oncol Biol Phys*. 1987;13:619.

121. Onufrey V, Mohiuddin M. Radiation therapy in the treatment of metastatic renal cell carcinoma. *Int J Radiat Oncol Biol Phys*. 1985;11:2007.

122. Fossa SD, Kjolbseth I, Lungd G. Radiotherapy of metastasis from renal cancer. *Eur Urol*. 1982;8:340.

123. Halpern EC, Harisiadis L. The role of radiation therapy in the management of metastatic renal cell carcinoma. *Cancer*. 1983;51:614.

124. Brookland RK, Richter MP. The postoperative irradiation of transitional cell carcinoma of the renal pelvis and ureter. *J Urol*. 1985;133:952.

125. Brady LW, Gislasan GJ, Faust DS, et al. Radiation therapy: a valuable adjunct in the management of carcinoma of the ureter. *JAMA*. 1968;206:2871.

126. Babaian RJ, Johnson DE, Chan RC. Combination nephroureterectomy and postoperative radiotherapy for infiltrative ureteral carcinoma. *Int J Radiat Oncol Biol Phys*. 1980;6:1229.

127. Brady LW, Manning DM. The role of radiation therapy in primary carcinoma of the ureter. In: Bergman H, ed. *The Ureter*. 2nd ed. New York: Springer-Verlag; 1981:417.

128. Sternberg CN, Yagoda A, Scher HI, et al. Preliminary results of M-VAC for transitional cell carcinoma of the urothelium. *J Urol*. 1985;133:403.

129. Barringer BS, Dean AL Jr. Epithelioma of the penis. *J Urol*. 1924;11:497.

130. Srinivias V, Morse MJ, Herr HW, et al. Penile cancer: relation of extent of nodal metastases to survival. *J Urol*. 1987;137:880.

131. Persky L, deKernion JB. Carcinoma of penis. *Cancer*. 1986;36:258.

132. deKernion JB, Tynberg P, Persky L, et al. Carcinoma of penis. *Cancer*. 1973;32:1256.

133. Fraley EE, Zhang G, Sazama R, Lange PH. Cancer of penis. Prognosis and treatment plans. *Cancer*. 1985;55:1618.

134. Salaverria JC, Hope-Stone HF, Paris AMI, et al. Conservative treatment of carcinoma of the penis. *Br J Urol*. 1979;51:32.

135. Ekstrom T, Edsmyr F. Cancer of the penis: a clinical study of 29 cases. *Acta Chir Scand*. 1958;115:25.

136. Staubitz WJ, Lent MH, Oberkirchir OJ. Carcinoma of the penis. *Cancer*. 1955;8:371.

137. Jackson SM. The treatment of carcinoma of the penis. *Br J Surg*. 1966;53:33.

138. Ray B, Canto AR, Whitmore WF. Experience with primary carcinoma of the male urethra. *J Urol*. 1977;117:591.

139. Bracken RB, Henry R, Ordanez N. Primary carcinoma of the male urethra. *South Med J*. 1980;73:1003.

140. Kaplan GW, Bulkley GJ, Grayhack JT. Carcinoma of the male urethra. *J Urol*. 1967; 98:365.

141. Pointau RCS, Poole-Wilson DS. Primary carcinoma of the urethra. *Br J Urol*. 1968;40:682.

142. Haile K, Delclos L. The place of radiation therapy in the treatment of carcinoma of the distal and of the penis. *Cancer*. 1980;45:1980.

143. Kelley CD, Arthur K, Rogoff E, et al. Radiation therapy of penile cancer. *Urology*. 1974; 4:571.

144. Mandler JI, Pool TL. Primary carcinoma of the male urethra. *J Urol*. 1966;96:67.

145. Newaisby GA, Deeley TJ. Radiotherapy in the treatment of carcinoma of the penis. *Br J Radiol*. 1968;41:519.

146. Bracken RB, Johnson DE, Miller LS, et al. Primary carcinoma of the female urethra. *J Urol*. 1976;116:188.

147. Antioniades J. Radiation therapy in carcinoma of the female urethra. *Cancer*. 1969;24:70.

148. Pierquin B, Chassange D, Cox JD. Toward consistent local control of certain malignant tumors: endoradiotherapy with iridium 192. *Radiology*. 1971;99:661.

149. Hopkins SC, Vider M, Nag SK, et al. Carcinoma of the female urethra: reassessment of the nodes of therapy. *J Urol*. 1983;129:958.

150. Johnson DE, O'Connell JR. Primary carcinoma of the female urethra. *Urology*. 1983;21:42.

151. Taggart CG, Castro JR, Rutledge FN. Carcinoma of the female urethra. *Am J Roentgenol*. 1972;114:145.

152. Prempree T, Amoremaru R, Patanaphau J. Radiation therapy in primary carcinoma of the female urethra. *Cancer*. 1984;54:729.

153. Prempree T, Wizenberg MJ, Scott RM. Radiation treatment of primary carcinoma of the female urethra. *Cancer*. 1978;42:1177.

154. Weghaupt K, Gerstner GJ, Kucera H. Radiation therapy for primary carcinoma of the female urethra: a survey over 25 years. *Gynecol Oncol*. 1984;17:58.

155. Sagerman RH, Yu WS, Chung CT, Puranik A. External beam irradiation of carcinoma of penis. *Radiology*. 1984;152:183.

# 40

# Urologic Laser Surgery

*Ralph C. Benson, Jr., Joseph A. Smith, Jr., and Barry S. Stein*

## LASER PHYSICS

The word *laser* is an acronym that stands for light amplification by the stimulated emission of radiation. Laser is light energy that is part of the electromagnetic wave spectrum (Fig 1). Most commercially available lasers today are within either the visible or the infrared light spectra.[1]

### Principles of Stimulated Emission

The same principles of physics apply to all of the available laser wavelengths. In a normal population of atoms, the majority will be in the resting state, $E_0$ (Fig 2). A small percentage of atoms will be at the next higher energy level, $E_1$, and a decreasing percentage is present at ever-increasing energy levels to $E_n$. It is possible, by the addition of optical, chemical, or electrical energy from a pump (external) source, to raise the atoms in the resting state to higher energy levels. This occurrence is known as the spontaneous absorption of energy (Fig 3). When this occurs, more atoms are in the excited or high-energy state than in the resting state, which is an unstable situation known as a population inversion (Fig 4). Such unstable atoms tend to give off their extra packet of optical energy and return back to the resting state, which is known as spontaneous emission (Fig 5). Regardless of what type of energy source was used to create the population inversion, when the atoms release their extra photon of energy, it is of a wavelength determined by the atoms involved. For example, with a neodymium: yttrium-aluminum-garnet (Nd:YAG) laser, the neodymium atoms are raised to higher energy levels with the use of a krypton lamp. When the process of spontaneous emission occurs, the extra photons of energy that are given off are those of neodymium energy. As these extra photons of neodymium energy strike other excited neodymium atoms, they force the excited neodymium atoms to give off their extra energy and return to the resting state. This process is known as stimulated emission (Fig 6). Both photons of neodymium energy are emitted exactly in phase. Thus, one incoming photon has been amplified to two outgoing photons.[2]

As this process is repeated, more photons are recruited into the beam, and the process of light amplification by stimulated emission is produced. All this activity takes place within a laser cavity (Fig 7). The laser cavity is a cylinder that is closed at both ends by mirrors. The mirror in the back is a fully reflecting mirror, whereas the mirror in the front has a small aperture in the middle, through which the laser beam can be released. Any atoms traveling parallel to the laser cavity may be reflected back and forth between the mirrors at the ends. In addition, an energy pump of some sort, such as the krypton lamp used in the neodymium laser, is needed in order to create

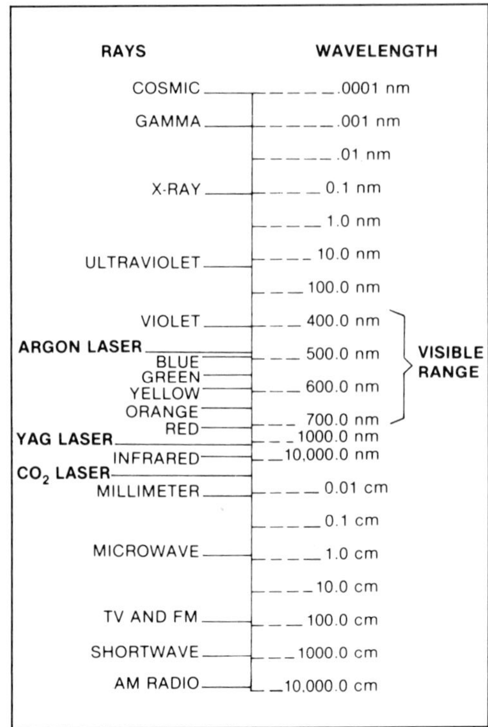


**Fig 1.** Electromagnetic wave spectrum, showing location of medical laser wavelengths.

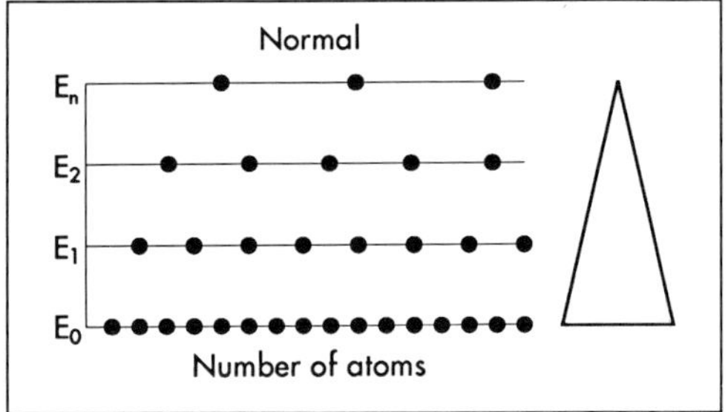


**Fig 2.** Energy state of normal population of atoms. [From Stein B S and Kendall AR, Lasers in urology: I. Laser physics and safety, *Urology* (1984; 23:405), with permission.]

the population inversion. As the atoms are raised to higher energy levels, they begin to bounce around within the laser cavity. Most of the energy escapes tangentially into the interstices surrounding the cavity and must be removed by a heat sink (Fig 8). A small percentage of the beam, however, is trapped between the mirrors and continually bounces back and forth, running parallel to the cavity. These photons of energy that are trapped between the mirrors continue to recruit more and more of the excited atoms by the process of stimulated emission, and thus continue to amplify their beam.[2]

By using a foot petal, the surgeon has three options as to how the beam can be released from the cavity (Fig 9)[3]: (1) In the continuous wave (CW) mode, the beam continues to be emitted at a steady rate for as long as the foot pedal is depressed. The level of energy emitted is determined by

**Fig 3.** Absorption of energy. A photon (P) of light gives off energy to an atom in the resting state ($E_0$). The $E_0$ atom absorbs this energy and is now at a higher energy level ($E_1$). [From Stein BS, Kendall AR, Lasers in urology: I. Laser physics and safety, *Urology* (1984; 23:405), with permission.]

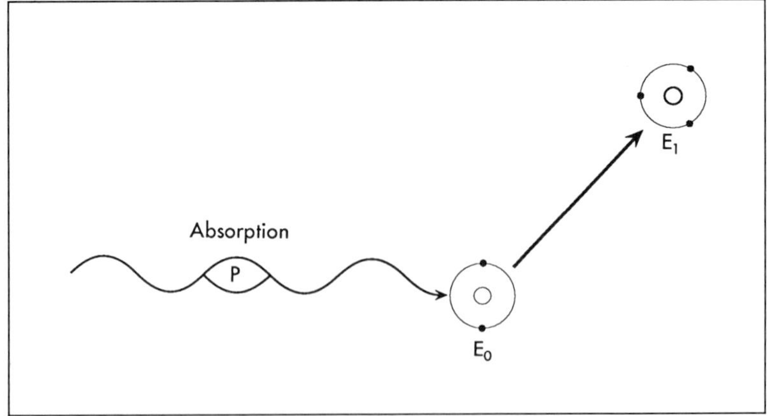

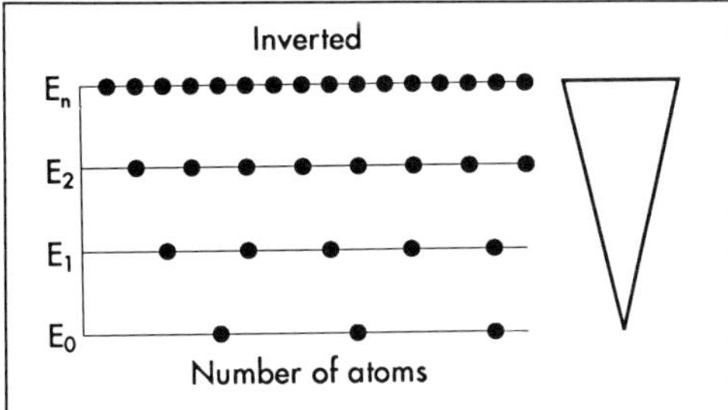


**Fig 4.** Energy state of inverted population of atoms, with most atoms at higher energy levels. [From Stein BS, Kendall AR, Lasers in urology: I. Laser physics and safety, *Urology* (1984; 23:405), with permission.]

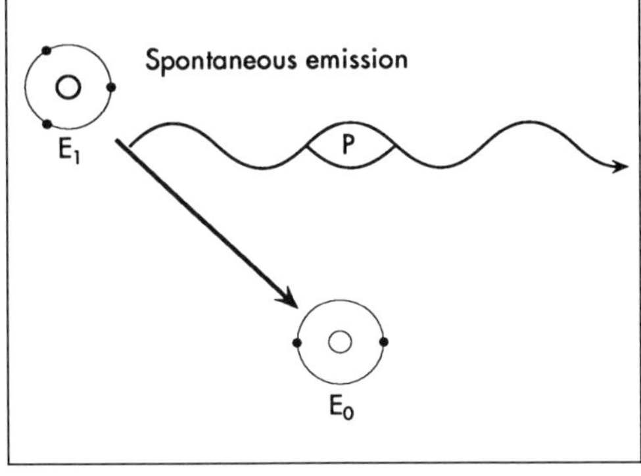


**Fig 5.** Spontaneous emission of energy. Higher energy level ($E_1$) atom spontaneously discharges photon of energy (P) and drops down to the ground state ($E_0$). [From Stein BS, Kendall AR, Lasers in urology: I. Laser physics and safety, *Urology* (1984; 23:405), with permission.]

the power setting on the machine. (2) In the pulse mode, the pulse is released for a limited period of time, as determined by the machine setting. There is then a fixed interval between pulses. In the interval between pulses, it is possible for the power in the laser cavity to climb higher than it does in the CW mode. Thus, higher peak powers are possible when using a pulsed setting. (3) In the Q switched mode, a shutterlike device similar to the one in a camera allows for the escape of energy in exceedingly narrow pulses. In this situation, the power achieved within the laser cavity between pulses is extremely high.[2] This is the type of laser used frequently in ophthalmologic procedures, and the powers in these lasers tend to be measured in milliwatts. High power and short pulse durations are the hallmark of ophthalmologic lasers, but in general these lasers are not useful for urologic applications.

## Unique Properties of the Laser

Three properties make the laser unique. First, the light is monochromatic (Fig 10). As opposed to light from a tungsten lamp,

**Fig 6.** Stimulated emission of radiant energy. When an atom at higher energy state ($E_1$) is struck by a photon of light of the same wavelength, it gives off a second photon of energy identical to the first and drops down to the $E_0$ level. [From Stein BS, Kendall AR, Lasers in urology: I. Laser physics and safety, *Urology* (1984; 23:405), with permission.]

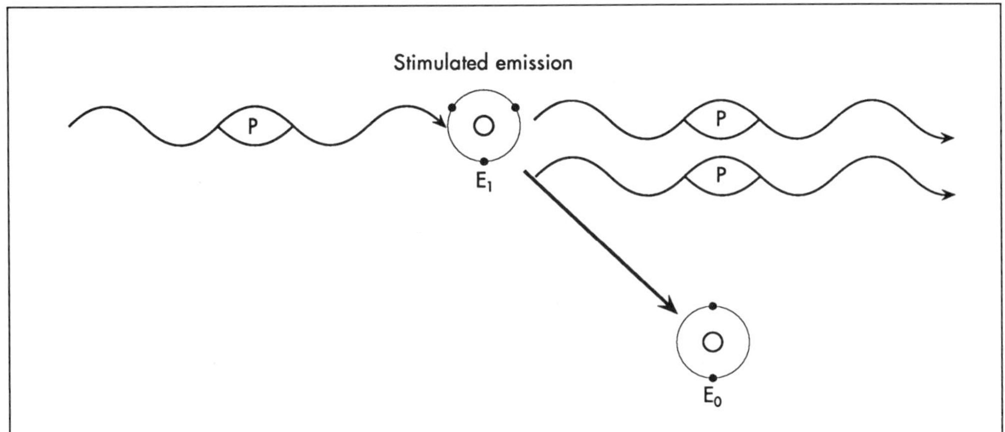

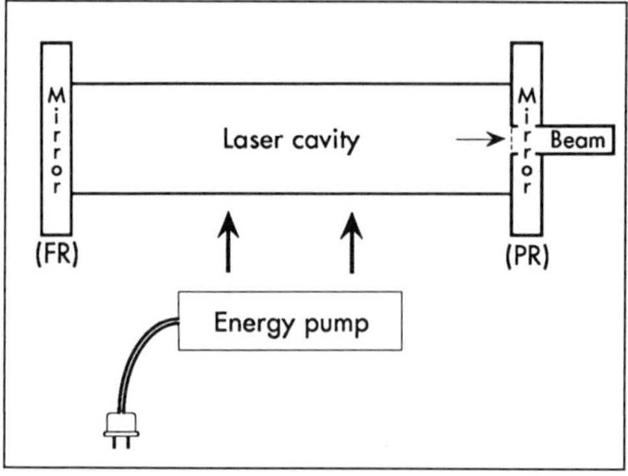


Fig 7. Diagram of typical laser. FR = fully reflecting; PR = partially reflecting; → = aperture. [From Stein BS, Kendall AR, Lasers in urology: I. Laser physics and safety, *Urology* (1984; 23:405), with permission.]

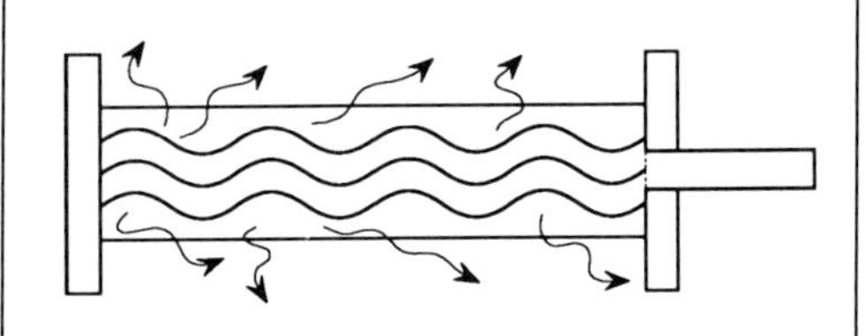

Fig 8. Amplified beam travels parallel to laser cavity reflected by mirrors. Arrows are excited photons not traveling parallel to cavity, which are lost to surrounding laser cavity. [From Stein BS, Kendall AR, Lasers in urology: I. Laser physics and safety, *Urology* (1984; 23:405), with permission.]

which emits over the entire visible spectrum, the laser emits light over a very narrow, well-defined wavelength. Second, the light is coherent (Fig 11). Normal light is incoherent, which means that the peaks and valleys of the sine wave curves do not necessarily coincide perfectly. Because of the properties of stimulated emission, laser light is perfectly in phase; ie, each peak and valley of the sine wave curves align exactly. Finally, the laser beam is nondivergent (Fig 12). Standard tungsten light emits diffusely, whereas the quartz fiber laser beams define as 8° divergence. With a $CO_2$ laser, it is possible to achieve less than 1° of divergence.[2]

## Biophysical Principles

Three major types of medical lasers are available commercially today, all named for the medium in the laser cavity. The carbon dioxide laser has a wavelength in the far infrared region of the spectrum at 10 600 nm (Table 1). Ninety-seven percent of its energy is absorbed at the point of contact, with a penetration of only 0.1 mm.

Fig 9. Types of laser delivery. [From Fuller TA, Fundamentals of lasers in surgery and medicine, in Dixon JA, (ed.), *Surgical Applications of Lasers* (Chicago, Ill: Year Book Medical Publishers; 1983), with permission.]

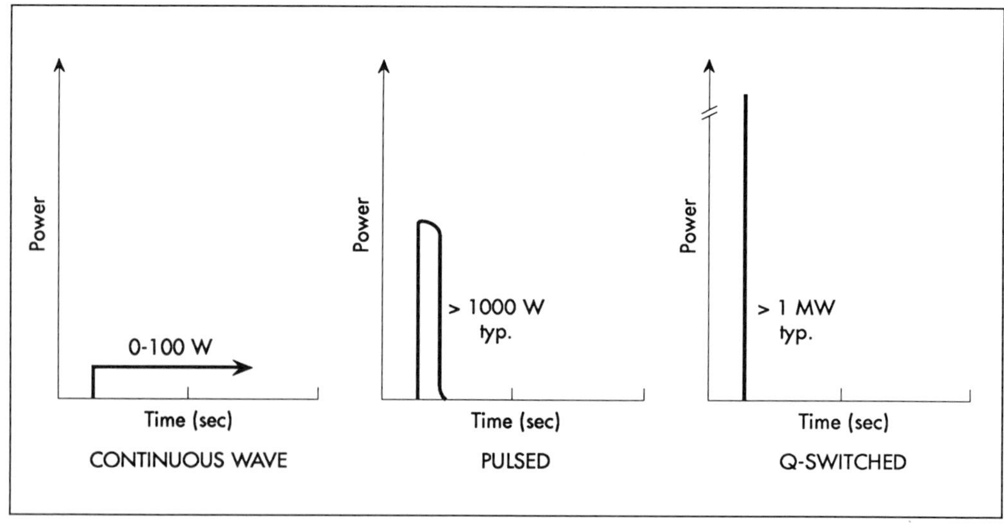

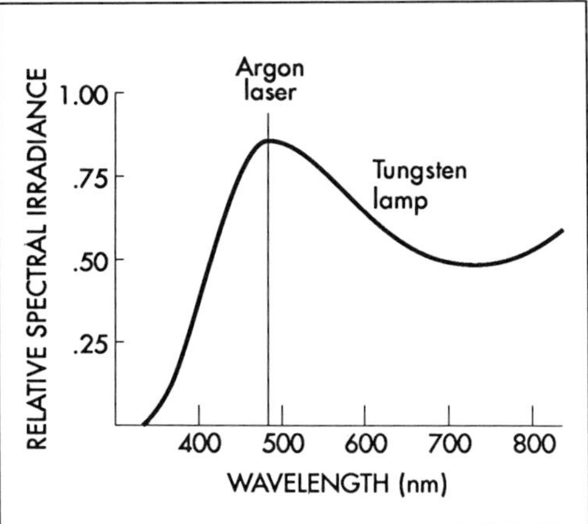


**Fig 10.** Monochromaticity of lasers (example is argon) compared with tungsten lamp. [From Stein BS, Kendall AR, Lasers in urology: I. Laser physics and safety, *Urology* (1984; 23:405), with permission.]

To date, this laser cannot be transmitted via fiber optics, and the beam must be directed by a series of mirrors.

The argon laser emits light with a wavelength in the blue-green portion of the electromagnetic spectrum. Approximately 55% of the power is reflected back from the tissue, and the remainder is absorbed. The argon laser is absorbed by hemoglobin or melanin selectively, and does not penetrate more than 1.0 mm. It is possible to use fiber optics for the transmission of the argon laser.

The Nd:YAG laser is within the near-infrared region of the spectrum at 1060 nm. Fifty percent of its energy is reflected back from the tissue, while the other 50% is absorbed. It is not absorbed preferentially by any pigment. Its penetration is 4 mm into tissue, and the energy can easily be transmitted through thin quartz fibers.[4]

In order to select the laser properly for a given application, it is necessary to consider the overlap of the optical wavelength of the laser with the hemoglobin and water optical absorption curves (Fig 13). The argon laser operates in the area of the optical spectrum in which the hemoglobin absorption curve is at its maximum, so this laser is highly absorbed by the pigment hemoglobin in preference to absorption by surrounding tissues. The potassium, titanyl-phosphate (KTP) laser is a modified Nd:YAG laser that emits light at 532 nm, and thus is similar in properties to the argon laser. The hemoglobin optical curve decreases by 600 nm, which is just above the argon wavelength. The $CO_2$ laser, in the far-infrared region of the spectrum, lies at the point at which the optical absorption of the water curve is at its maximum. The water curve begins to increase past 1000 nm, peaks at approximately 2000 nm, and remains at this level throughout the infrared spectrum. This is precisely the area in which the $CO_2$ laser is operative. Thus, a $CO_2$ laser will not penetrate water or any tissue containing water. The Nd:YAG laser, operating in the near-infrared region, lies at the point at which both the hemoglobin and water curves are at their lowest. Thus, an Nd:YAG laser will penetrate both

**Fig 11. Left:** Noncoherent light with random orientation. **Right:** Coherent laser with light in phase. [From Stein BS, Kendall AR, Laser physics and safety, *Urology* (1984; 23:405), with permission.]

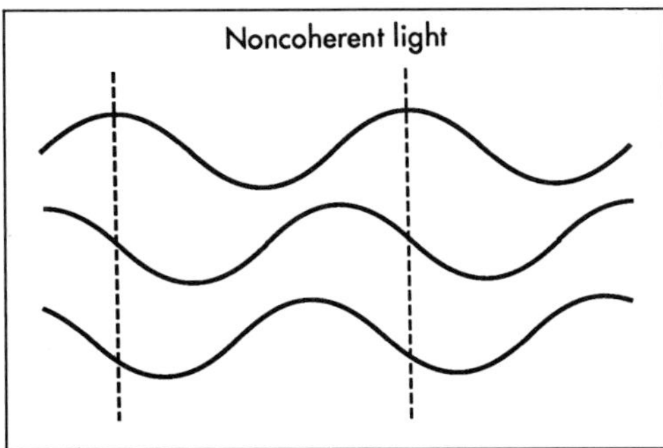


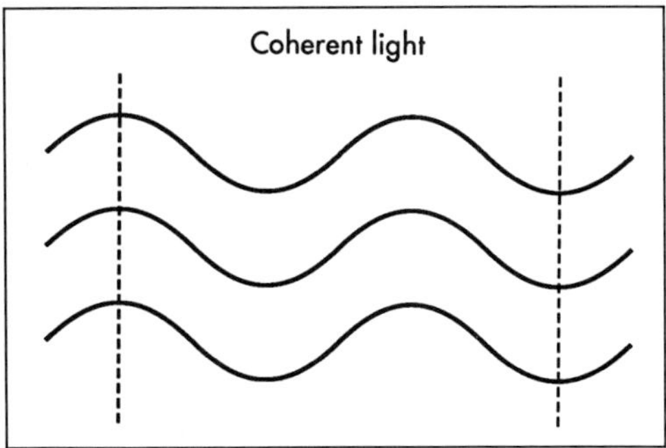

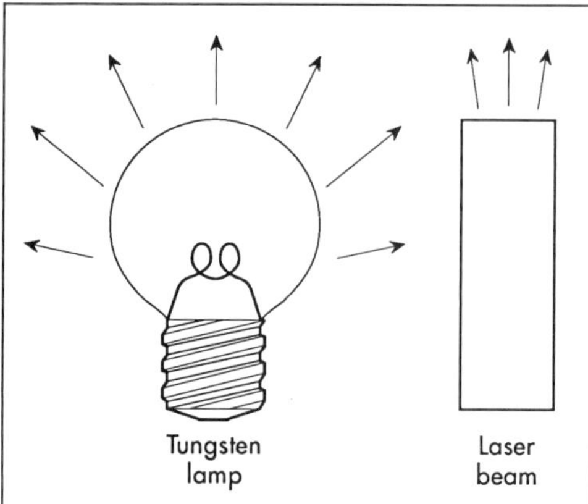


**Fig 12.** Nondivergent laser beam compared with widely divergent tungsten lamp. [From Stein BS, Kendall AR, Lasers in urology: I. Laser physics and safety, *Urology* (1984; 23:405), with permission.]

hemoglobin and water without a significant decrease in its energy.[2]

All three of these lasers work fundamentally by thermal action. When tissue is heated by any of these lasers up to 60°C, there is no permanent or visible damage to the tissue (Fig 14). By 65°C, denaturation of protein occurs. The tissue will visibly turn white or grey and will disintegrate approximately 4 to 7 days later. This is the temperature range in which the Nd:YAG laser works. Once tissue has been heated to 90 to 100°C, there is tissue drying, some shrinkage, and permanent damage due to dehydration. Over 100°C, carbonization or blackening of tissue occurs. As the temperature rise continues, there is evolution of smoke and gas with tissue vaporization. This is the temperature range in which the $CO_2$ and argon laser work.[5]

The only laser system that does not work by thermal activity is the argon-pumped dye laser combined with hematoporphyrin derivative (Fig 15). In this laser system, hematoporphyrin derivative is administered intravenously 48 hours prior to therapy. The hematoporphyrin derivative in certain organ systems of the body, including the bladder, is concentrated within the tumor cells in preference to the normal cells. When exposed to red light, the hematoporphyrin derivative is excited and cleaves oxygen to form singlet oxygen within the mitochondria, leading to cell death. This is a nonthermal effect.[6]

## Tissue Interaction

The typical commercial laser has a front panel that allows for setting of wattage, pulse duration, and accumulation of total joules delivered. Unfortunately, there is a great discrepancy between the numbers that may be set on the dials and the actual amount of energy that is delivered to the tissue. A number of local tissue properties such as color, presence of hemoglobin, and degree of local circulation (which may act as a heat sink), as well as the power density and lens system, all may modify the actual delivery of the laser energy.

In order to understand the principles of tissue interaction, one must understand the nomenclature of physics as it applies to lasers. Power is measured in watts, and the pulse or radiation time is measured in seconds. When the amount of power in watts is multiplied by the time in seconds, watts-seconds or joules are measured, which is the amount of energy being delivered (Table 2).

**TABLE 1. Medical Lasers**

| Type | Wavelength (nm) | Depth Penetration (mm) | Special Properties | Delivery |
|---|---|---|---|---|
| $CO_2$ | 10,600 | 0.1 | Absorbed by water | Mirrors |
| Argon | 455–515 | 1.0 | Absorbed by hemoglobin | Fiber |
| KTP | 532 | 1–2 | | Fiber |
| Nd:YAG | 1060 | 4.0 | Not affected by water or hemoglobin | Fiber |

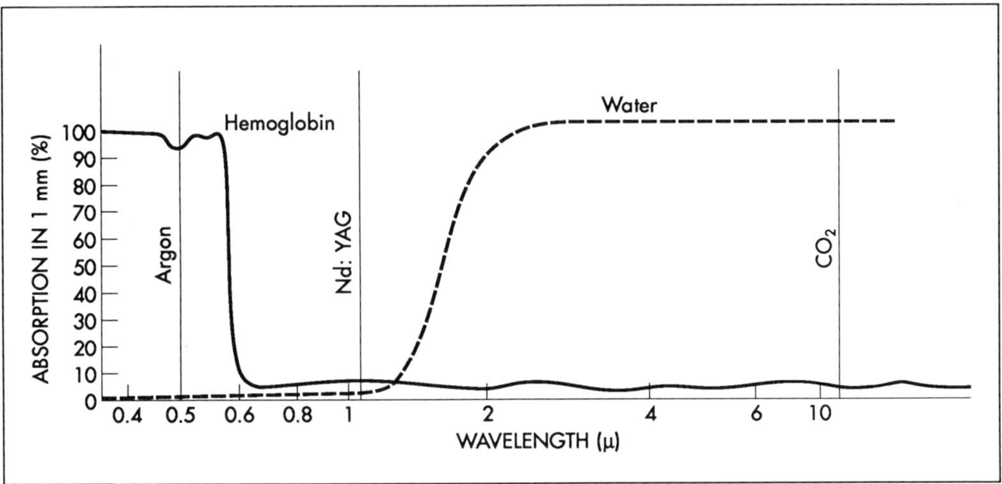


**Fig 13.** Absorption of hemoglobin and water as a function of three common medical lasers. [From Stein BS, Kendall AR, Lasers in urology: I. Laser physics and safety, *Urology* (1984; 23:405), with permission.]

One must then take into consideration the area over which that energy is delivered. The amount of watts divided by the area over which it is delivered

$$\frac{W}{CM^2}$$

is known as the power density or power intensity of the laser beam. When the time factor is considered

$$\frac{W \cdot S}{CM^2}$$

the energy density or irradiation dose is determined. Thus, the power density is defined as the concentration of energy of the laser beam and is expressed in watts divided by centimeters squared of the spot size. The formula

$$\frac{W \cdot 100}{(r)^2}$$

calculates the power density.

It is important to recognize that the denominator of this formula includes the radius of the spot size squared. Thus, as the radius of the spot size doubles, the amount of energy delivered falls not by a factor of 2, but by a factor of 4. The spot size is defined as the beam diameter at the focal point for the given lens system. As the tissue surface moves closer or farther away from a focused laser beam, the beam increases in size in both directions (Fig 16), making it extremely critical to know the exact location of the focal point.[7] In addition, all of these calculations are based on a static, round spot produced by a head-on laser beam. As the beam is angulated, as would be common in the treatment of a bladder tumor, an ellipse rather than a circle is formed, and the actual amount of energy delivered varies in ways that are impossible to measure (Fig 17). In addition, when "painting" with the fiber as one would do to treat a bladder tumor, the formula for power density becomes

$$\frac{W \cdot 100}{(r)}$$

Instead of measuring the laser energy delivered by the machine, it would be more useful to measure the laser energy as received by the tissue. This is known as radiant exposure, and is the amount of energy per unit area of tissue surface exposed.

Unfortunately, this measurement can only be produced at the bench in a laboratory and cannot be measured accurately in the human subject undergoing a laser

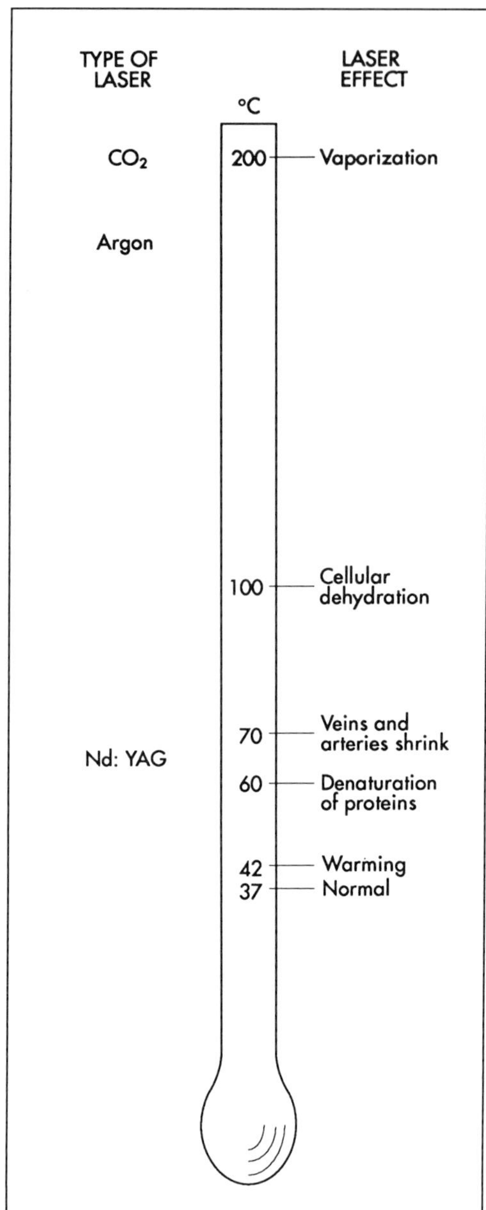


**Fig 14.** Thermal effects of lasers. [From Stein BS, Kendall AR, Lasers in urology: I. Laser physics and safety, *Urology* (1984; 23:405), with permission.]

treatment. Thus, the amount of laser energy described in articles in terms of joules and number of pulses delivered does not necessarily reflect the amount of laser energy received by the tissue.

## Depth of Penetration

Another important principle in understanding tissue interaction is that of depth of penetration. It has already been discussed that the $CO_2$ laser penetrates to 0.1 mm, the argon laser 1.0 mm, and the Nd:YAG laser approximately 4.0 mm. These are principles of physics, however, and they do not necessarily apply directly to the use of lasers in human tissue. One commonly misunderstood point relates to depth of penetration. The depth of penetration has come to be understood as the depth to which the laser produces the desired effect on tissue. However, this is not the correct interpretation of this term.

The depth of penetration or extinction length is that tissue thickness at which 90% of the laser beam has been absorbed. This does not imply, however, that the laser is still active enough at 90% of its absorption to effect a significant temperature rise and thus create tissue effects. It must be understood, therefore, that the depth of penetration is based on the calculation of the laser energy penetration, not laser effect. Fig 18 shows that as the Nd:YAG laser beam penetrates, diffusion takes place laterally, and the amount of temperature rise decreases proportionally with penetration. Thus, there will be an area at which penetration by the definition of physics is still occurring, but significant temperature rise is not. This is dependent on the coefficient of absorption, which, in turn, is dependent on the wavelength of the laser, the chemical composition of the tissue, and the color of the tissue. In general, the shorter the laser wavelength (ie, the closer to the ultraviolet region), the greater the depth of penetration.

In Fig 19, a liver model is used to demonstrate the effect of one pulse of the $CO_2$ laser. In this case, the theoretical 0.1 mm penetration has been achieved as measured with an in-line reticular micrometer. Eight pulses would be expected to penetrate approximately 0.8 mm. However, as is evident in Fig 20, this is not the case. The penetration is between 4.0 and 5.0 mm, although it is broader at the surface than

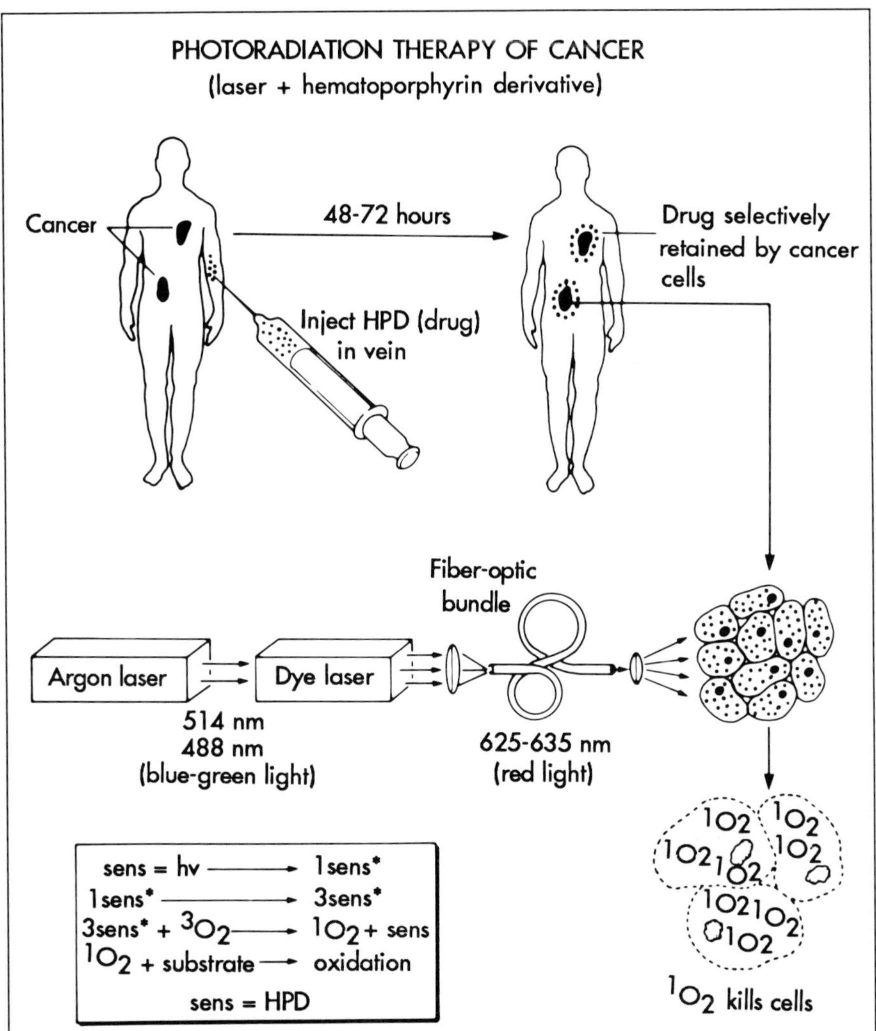


**Fig 15.** Argon-pumped dye laser in concert with hematoporphyrin derivative. [From Berns MW, Wilson M, Rentzepis P, et al, Cell biology of hematoporphyrin derivative (HPD), *Lasers Surg Med* (1983; 2:261), with permission.]

**TABLE 2. Physics of Laser Energy**

| Term | Abbreviation | Definition | Formula |
|---|---|---|---|
| Watts | W | Power setting | |
| Seconds | S | Time setting | |
| Watt-seconds or joules | W-S<br>J | Energy | W · S |
| Power density | PD | Amount of power delivered over a given area | $\frac{W}{cm^2}$ or $\frac{W \cdot 100}{ii(r)^2}$ |
| Energy density | ED | Amount of energy delivered over a given area | $\frac{W \cdot S}{cm^2}$ or $\frac{J}{cm^2}$ |

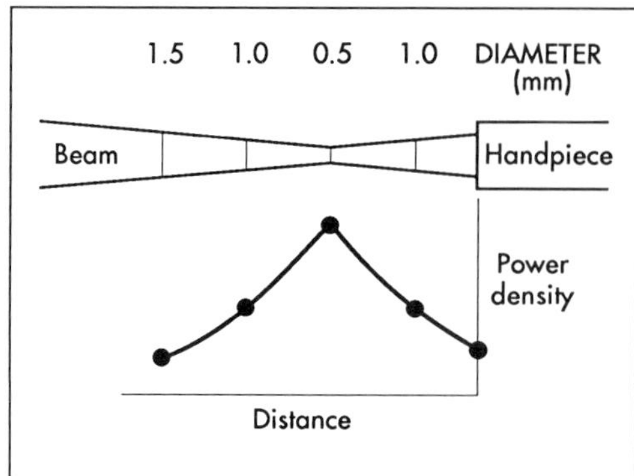


**Fig 16.** Focusing handpiece. [From Stein BS, Treatment of lesions of the external genitalia, in Smith JA, (ed), *Lasers in Urologic Surgery* (Chicago; Year Book Medical Publishers; 1985), with permission.]

as it descends. It is possible with the use of high-power $CO_2$ or repeat pulses to exceed the theoretical penetration at any given time. In Fig 21, the depth of penetration in liver with the argon laser is approximately 1.0 mm. It is evident here that although some vaporization has taken place, there is also a zone of coagulation of protein that adds to the depth of laser injury. The last example demonstrates the effect of the Nd:YAG laser on the liver (Fig 22). Here the effect is largely coagulation of protein, although when the laser is used in open applications, some tissue vaporization is produced. However, the degree of penetration is not significantly greater than it is with the argon laser.[8]

Because of these discrepancies in expected dose penetration, we performed studies that examined the degree of penetration possible with the various lasers. Fig 23 shows the effect of 60 J as delivered by the argon laser with 3 W for 20 seconds. It is possible to exceed 1 mm of penetration and have tissue effects well into the superficial muscle of the bladder in this dog model. It has become evident by such tissue studies that time is a more effective indicator of laser penetration than is watt setting. One hundred joules of laser energy can be delivered in a number of ways, including 100 W for 1 second, 50 W for 2 seconds, and 25 W for 4 seconds. We believe that 25 W for 4 seconds produces a far more effective penetration of laser effect than 100 W for 1 second. The increase of time is more significant than the increase in power.

We performed studies both endoscopically and openly on dog bladder and kidney using the Nd:YAG and $CO_2$ lasers.[9] Fig 24 is an example of the greatest depth of penetration that could be obtained endoscopically in the dog bladder using 50 W for 4 seconds with room-temperature solutions. These depths of penetration are less than 3.0 mm. Fig 25 demonstrates the results of treating the dog bladder as we would human tissue, until the visible surface color changes occur. In this case, the depth of penetration is not substantially below the submucosal tissue. Similar results were achieved with the use of the Nd:YAG

**Fig 17. Left:** Circular spot results from straight-on application of laser. **Right:** Elliptical spot results from angulation of beam.

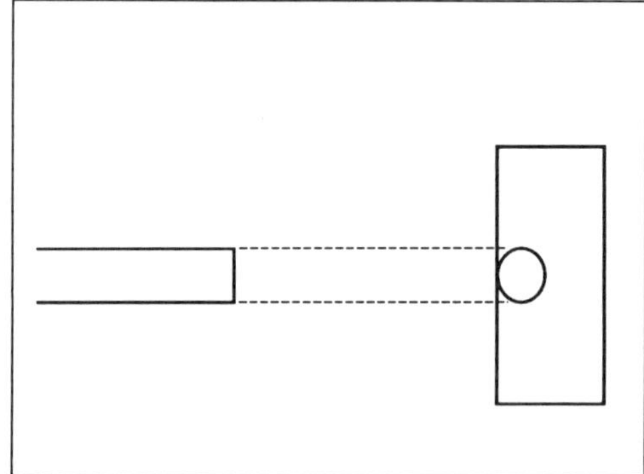

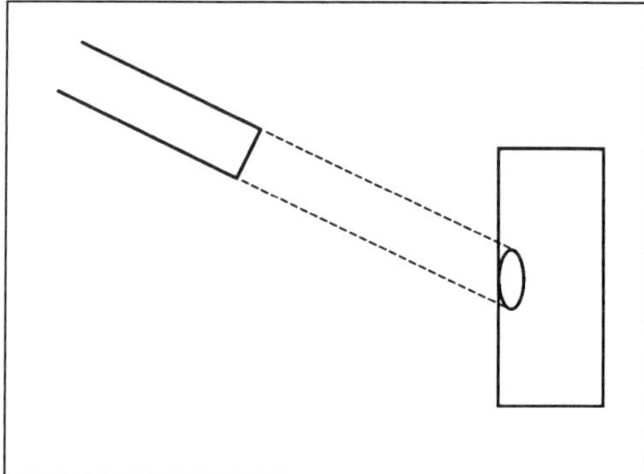

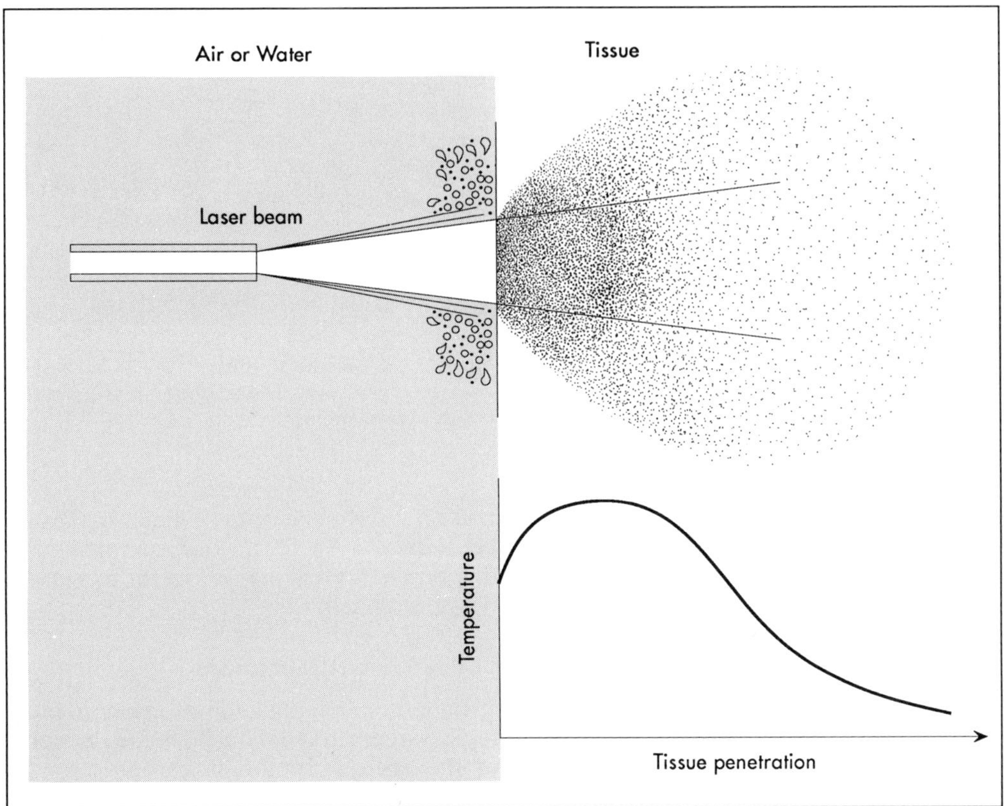


**Fig 18.** Depth of penetration of Nd:YAG laser. Note decrease in temperature rise with penetration. [From Stein BS, Kendall AR, Lasers in urology: I. Laser physics and safety, *Urology* (1984; 23:405), with permission.]

laser in the kidney. By contrast, the results with the $CO_2$ laser were linear; the higher the power used, the greater the vaporization that resulted. Five watts of laser power were just enough to make an evident change in the tissue (Fig 26), where 30 W of laser power were enough to vaporize a substantial area (Fig 27).

**Fig 19.** $CO_2$ laser effect on 5 W at ½-second pulse on animal liver. Depth of penetration is approximately 0.1 mm.

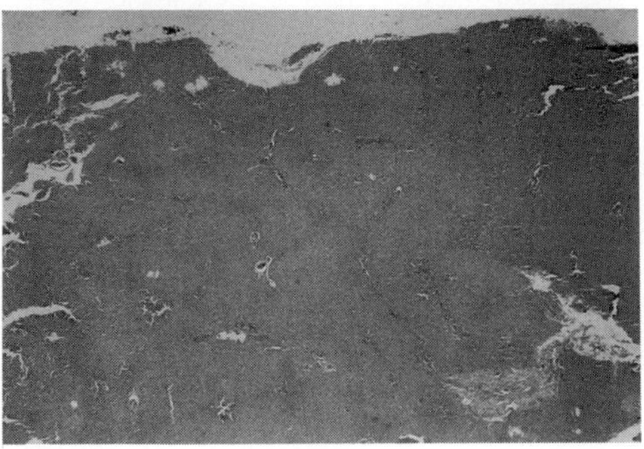

Fig 28 reveals that the greatest depth of penetration found with the Nd:YAG laser was less than 3.0 mm, and was achieved with 4 seconds at 50 W. We also noted that when using irrigation solutions of different temperatures, the solutions at room temperature provided the maximum amount of penetration. We feel that some cooling effect of the surface is provided by room-temperature solutions, which allow for greater penetration by decreasing the amount of vaporization at the surface. This has been called the "blooming effect" by Staehler and associates.[5] The $CO_2$ laser curves show this linear relationship (Fig 29). It is of interest to note that Fig 30

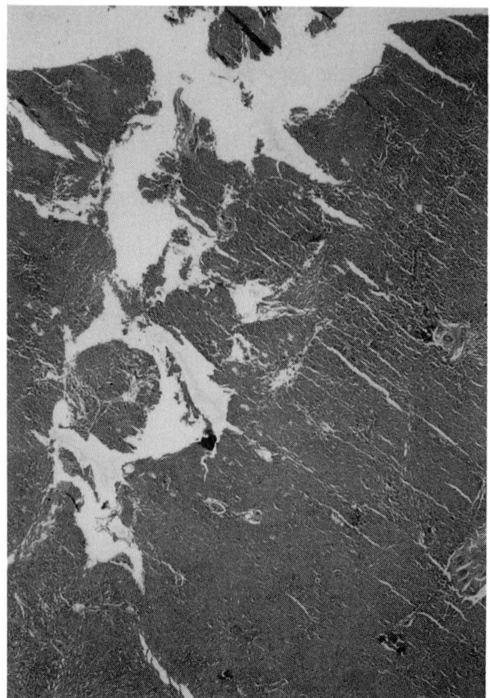

**Fig 20.** $CO_2$ laser effect of 8 pulses at 5 W for ½ second each on animal liver. Maximal depth of penetration is approximately 5 mm.

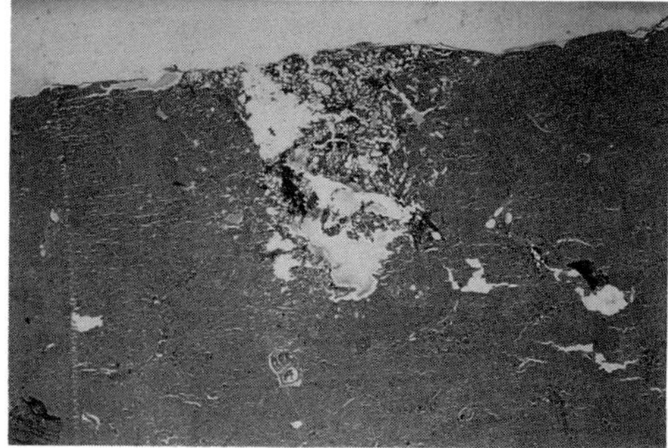

**Fig 22.** Nd:YAG laser effect of 40 W for 2 seconds on animal liver. Maximal depth of penetration is approximately 1.5 mm.

shows both the luminal and serosal surface of a bladder that was treated with the Nd:YAG laser prior to cystectomy. Substantial laser injury is demonstrated to, but not completely through, the deep muscle of the bladder in a U-shaped manner. This was achieved by multiple treatments over the same area. The recommendation of multiple treatments with several seconds in between to allow for the tissue temperature to return to normal may allow for increased depth of penetration.[10]

## Endoscopic Applications

Endoscopic application of lasers in urologic surgery requires a fiber for delivery of the energy. Prototype carbon dioxide laser cystoscopes have been developed,[11] but they have not proven to be clinically useful. Moreover, fibers for conduction of $CO_2$ energy have not been perfected. Although the blue-green color of an argon laser is selectively absorbed by hemoglobin, light at this wavelength has not shown any particular advantages in urologic surgery. Frequency doubling crystals applied to Nd:YAG lasers produce light with a

**Fig 21.** Argon laser effect of 3 W for 10 seconds on animal liver. Maximal depth of penetration is approximately 1 mm.

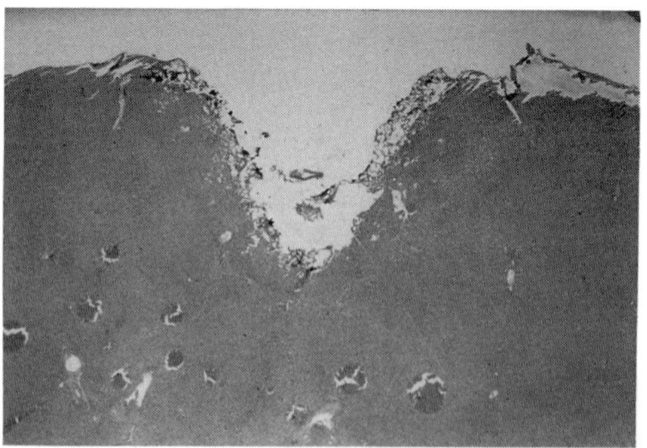

**Fig 23.** Argon laser effect on 3 W for 20 seconds on dog bladder. Penetration extends well into superficial muscle.

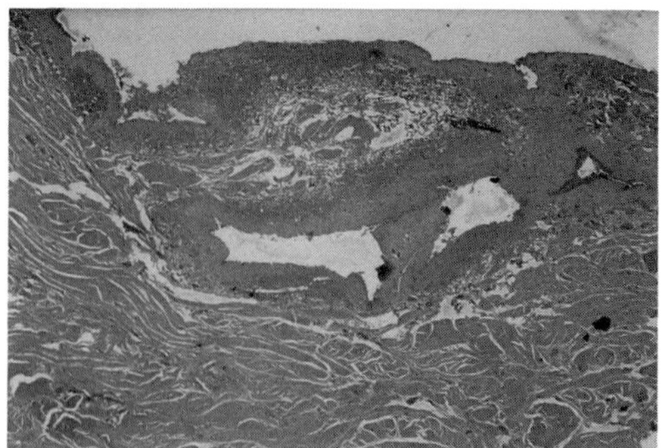

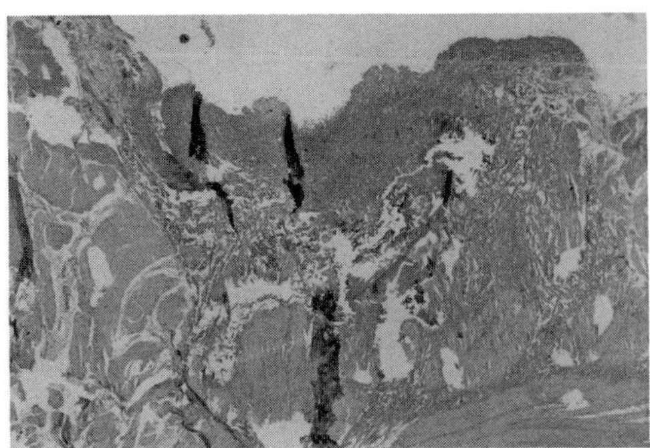

**Fig 24.** Nd:YAG laser effect of 50 W for 4 seconds endoscopically on dog bladder. Depth of penetration is 2.76 mm.

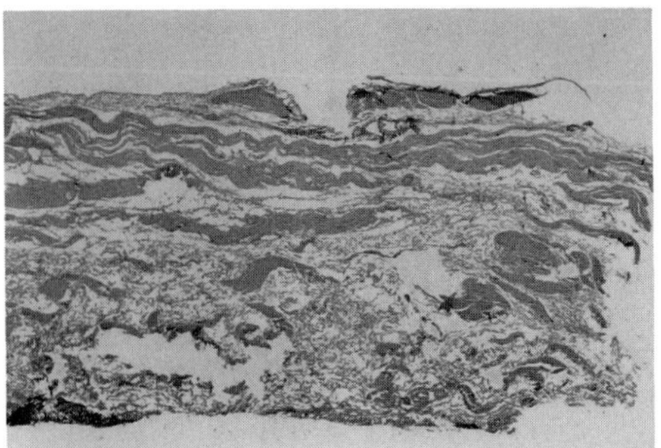

**Fig 26.** $CO_2$ laser effect of 5 W for ½ second on dog bladder. [From Stein BS, Laser dosimetry with the Nd:YAG and $CO_2$ lasers in the bladder and kidney, *Laser Surg Med* (1986; 6:353–363), with permission.]

wavelength of 532 nm. The tissue effects are similar to those of an argon laser, and clinical experience in urology is extremely limited. Therefore, for the most part, endoscopic applications of laser energy in urology to date have involved the 1060 nm wavelength of a Nd:YAG laser.

The small flexible fiber for delivery of Nd:YAG laser energy can be inserted through the working channel of a standard cystoscope (Fig 31). Modified Albarran inserts have been developed by most major instrument companies and provide a water tight entry port as well as a stabilized tip (Fig 32). When flexible instruments are used, a 400-μm laser fiber should be employed in order to permit full deflection of the instrument tip.

**Fig 25.** Nd:YAG laser effect of 40 W used on dog bladder until grey-white mucosal color change was seen. Depth of penetration is only to submucosal area. [From Stein BS, Laser dosimetry with the Nd:YAG and $CO_2$ lasers in the bladder and kidney. *Laser Surg Med* (1986; 6:353–363), with permission.]

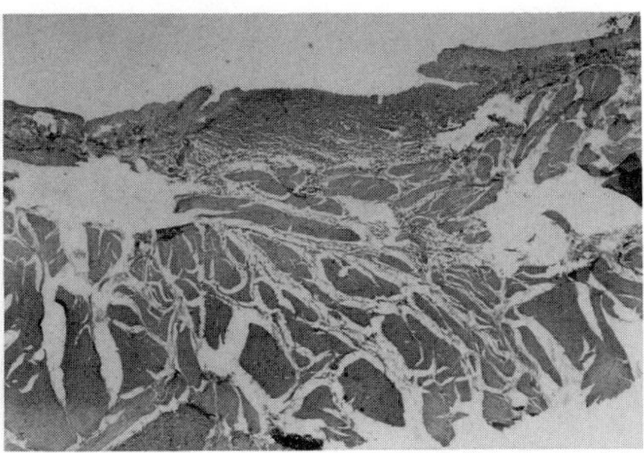

## URETHRA

### Urethral Condyloma Acuminata

Although intraurethral extension of condyloma acuminata is relatively uncommon, treatment by standard methods has been disappointing. Intraurethral 5-flourouracil cream has not been particularly effective in treating gross lesions, and electrocautery resection generally is unsatisfactory. The irregular thermal injury that results from electrocautery is prone to cause stricture formation.

**Fig 27.** $CO_2$ laser effect of 30 watts for ½ second on dog bladder. [From Stein BS, Laser dosimetry with the Nd:YAG and $CO_2$ lasers in the bladder and kidney, *Laser Surg Med* (1986; 6:353–363), with permission.]

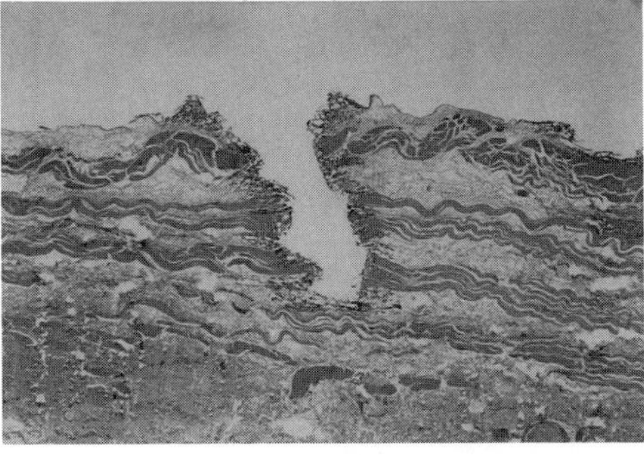

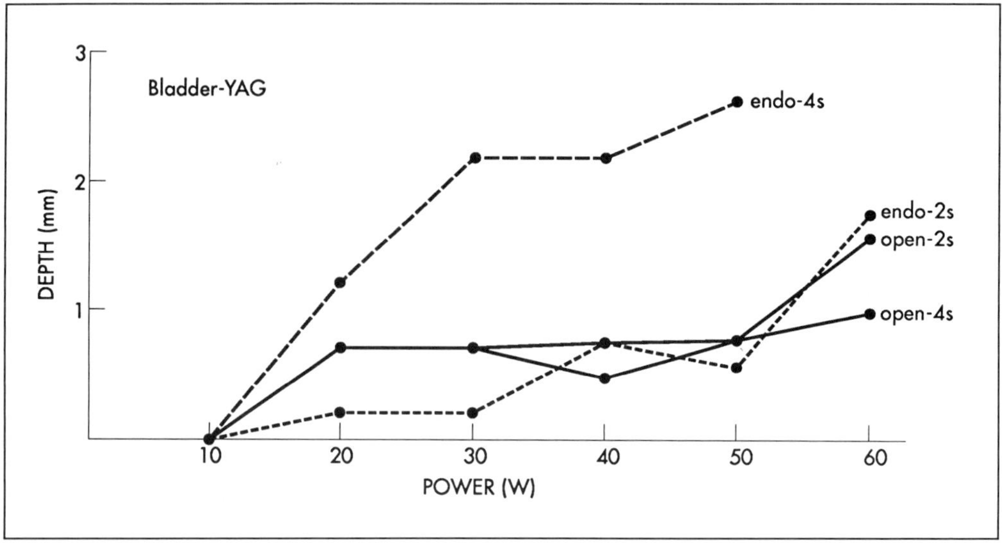


**Fig 28.** Curves of depth of penetration of Nd:YAG laser endoscopically used on dog bladder with varying irrigation fluid temperature. [From Stein BS, Laser dosimetry with the Nd:YAG and $CO_2$ lasers in the bladder and kidney, *Laser Surg Med* (1986; 6:353–363), with permission.]

A number of investigators have reported excellent results using Nd:YAG laser treatment of condylomata extending along the entirety of the urethra.[12] Most often, condylomata are located at the urethral meatus or in the fossa navicularis. There is some difficulty in visualizing these lesions endoscopically because of their location, and pediatric cystoscopes are helpful. Along more proximal portions of the urethra, visualization is easy, and the fiber should be directed to within 1 mm or 2 mm of the surface of the lesion. A power output of 35 W is chosen, and the condyloma is treated until it undergoes a white discoloration indicative of adequate thermal ne-

**Fig 29.** Curves of depth of penetration of $CO_2$ openly on dog bladder with varying tissue temperatures. [From Stein BS, Laser dosimetry with the Nd:YAG and $CO_2$ lasers in the bladder and kidney, *Laser Surg Med* (1986; 6:353–363), with permission.]

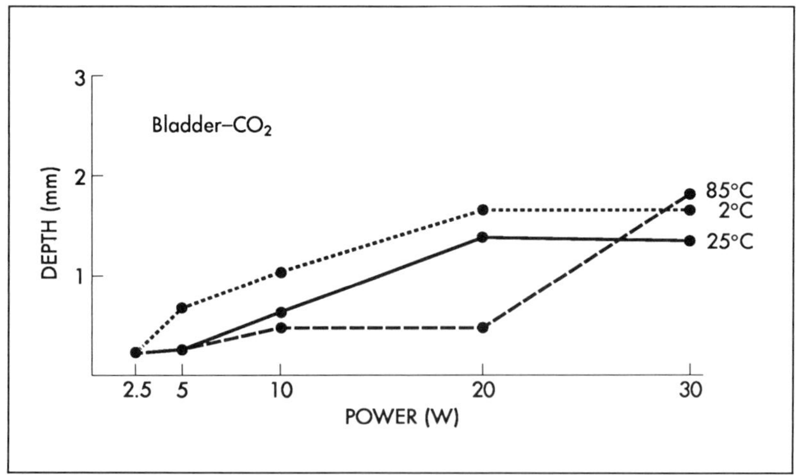

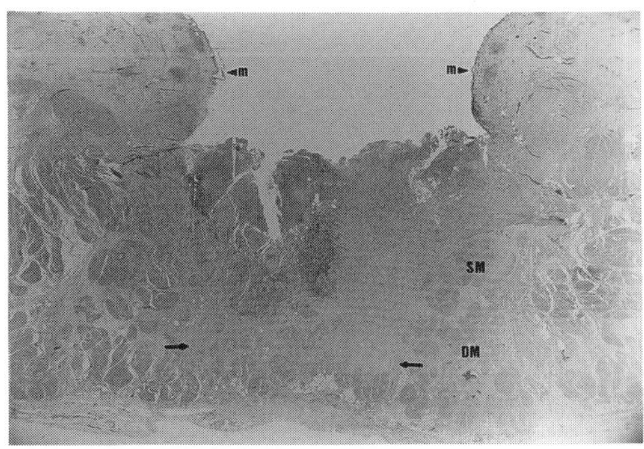


**Fig 30.** Histologic section of bladder, showing invasive bladder cancer treated with Nd:YAG laser before cystectomy.

crosis (Fig 33). Stricture formation after treatment has not been observed in proximal portions of the urethra, although fossa navicularis strictures have been seen after extensive laser treatment. Depending upon the number of lesions treated and their location, intraurethral 5-flourouracil cream is used postoperatively to help prevent recurrence.

## Urethral Stricture

Evidence that the thermal injury which results from Nd:YAG laser irradiation may heal with less collagen deposition and more elastic fibers than a comparable electrical injury has formed the theoretical basis for laser treatment of benign urethral strictures.[13] Two basic techniques have been used in various series. Most commonly, a circumferential application of laser energy to the entire strictured area is performed. A power output of 45 W is used. Since minimal tissue vaporization occurs during endoscopic Nd:YAG laser treatment, dilation of the urethra is performed after treatment, to afford immediate symptomatic relief. The laser coagulated tissue sloughs secondarily, and a postoperative Foley catheter is not required. Although the initial reported results were good, over half of the patients had a recurrence of their stricture

**Fig 31.** Fiber for conduction of laser energy. The fiber tip is flexible, allowing projection of energy onto the tissue surface. When flexible cystoscopes are used, a 400 μm fiber is necessary to allow full deflection of the instrument tip.

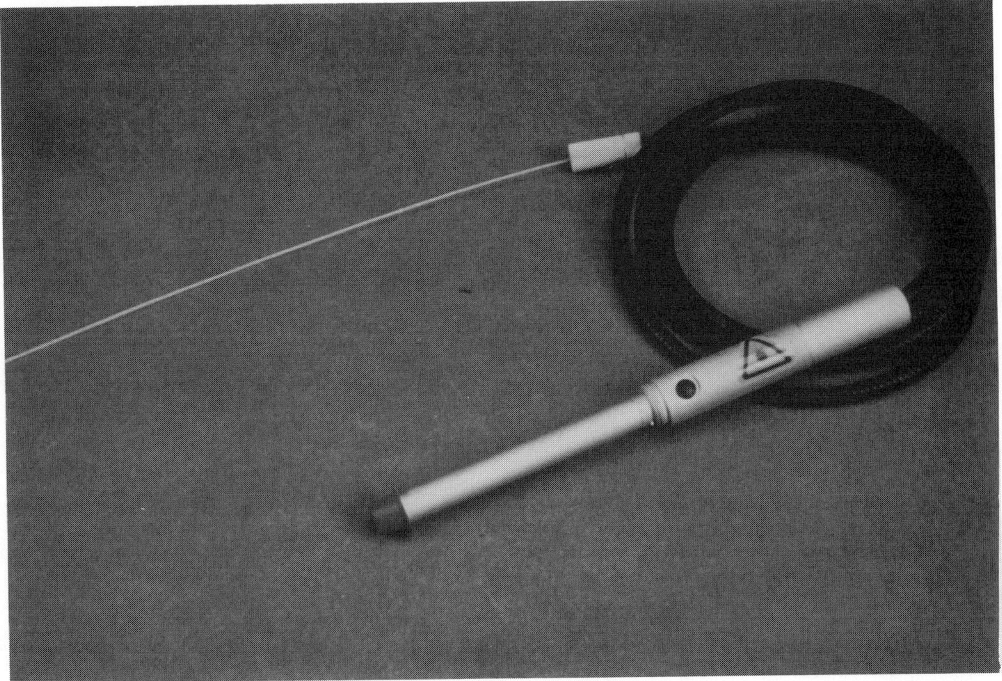

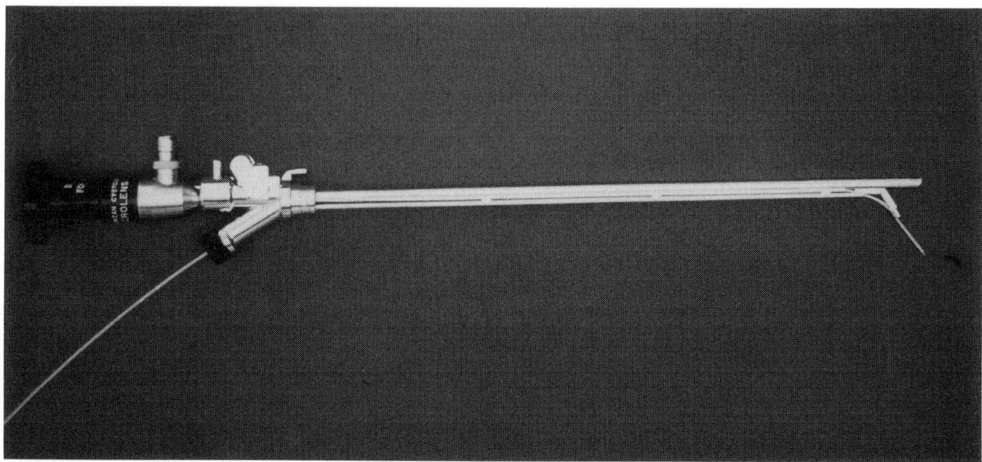

**Fig 32.** Cystoscope with modified Albaran insert for laser treatment. A watertight entry port is provided along with a stabilized tip for deflection of the laser fiber.

within 6 months, especially in complicated strictures.[14,15] Therefore, it was concluded that this technique offered no substantial advantages over alternative methods of treatment, including simple dilation or direct vision urethrotomy.

An alternative approach to urethral strictures is to perform a laser urethrotomy using either a bare fiber or, preferably, contact tips. The tips are constructed of sapphire or a similar material and greatly increase the power density (Fig 34). They are designed for contact between the fiber tip and the tissue. The chisel shaped tip provides the best combination of cutting action and hemostasis. Nevertheless, the treatment is relatively slow compared to a urethrotomy, and the cutting action is less effective. Results have been no better than those obtained by direct vision cold knife urethrotomy.[15,17] However, Shanberg et al. and Tansey feel that they have obtained

**Fig 33. Left:** Condyloma acuminata along pendulous urethra. **Right:** After Nd:YAG laser treatment, the lesions have a typical appearance. Slough occurs 3 to 4 days later. Postoperative stricture formation has not been observed except in the fossa navicularis or at the urethral meatus.

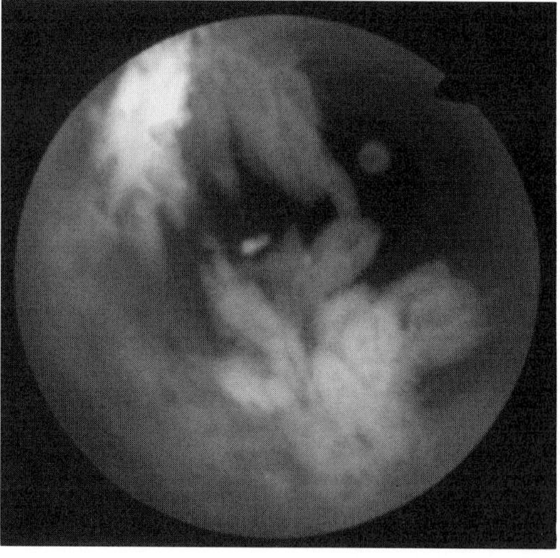

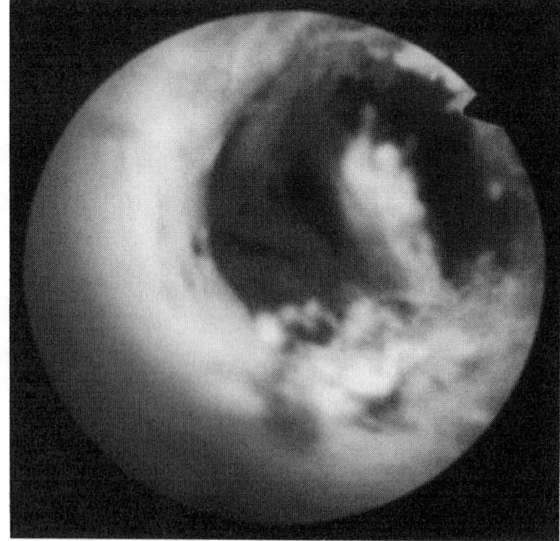

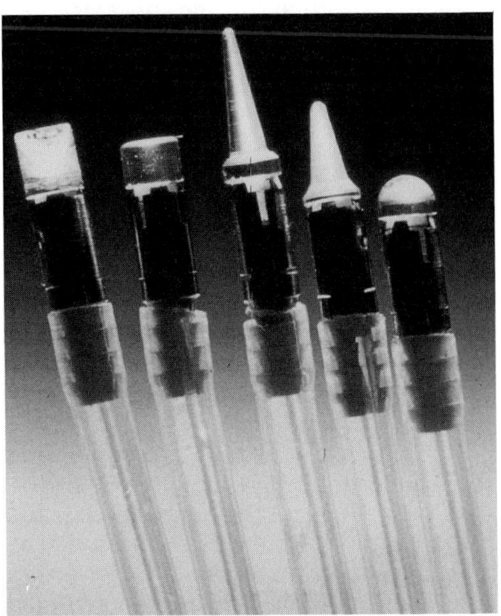

**Fig 34.** Sapphire tips for a Nd:YAG laser fiber. These tips are designed for contact between the fiber and tissue. The energy density and, thereby, cutting effect of the laser is enhanced.

good results in patients failing alternative treatment.[16]

Presently, it seems fair to state that treatment with Nd:YAG laser has not demonstrated any advantages over standard therapy for benign urethral strictures.

The argon and KTP lasers, both in the blue-green range, have recently been tried in the treatment of stricture disease. Since these lasers have both vaporization and coagulation properties, they have theoretical advantages over the Nd:YAG laser in the treatment of strictures. Most recently, Adkins has investigated the use of the argon laser for urethral and vesical neck strictures. A total of 17 patients was studied. A 300-μm fiber was used as it provided a higher power density than the larger fibers. The maximum power (14 W) was used, and a single urethrotomy made at the 12 o'clock position. The majority of patients had failed other treatments. A total of 88% of the group had "good" or "acceptable" results, with an average of 8 months follow-up.[18]

Shanberg and associates have studied the use of the 532-nm KTP laser for urethral strictures. A total of 20 patients was evaluated, all of whom had previously failed by more conventional treatments. A 400-μm fiber was used with power settings of 9 W. Grooves were placed in 4 to 5 quadrants, and the laser used to vaporize tissue between the grooves. Success rates of 68% were reported, with follow-up between 6 and 14 months.[19]

## Prostate

Considering that no clinically useful technique for laser removal of benign prostatic tissue has been developed, the idea of a laser prostatectomy has received a great deal of attention. This has been influenced by the hope that lasers could offer a means for complete vaporization of obstructing prostatic tissue with excellent hemostasis. The reality is that lasers which produce relatively good hemostasis, such as a Nd:YAG laser, exert their primary tissue effects through coagulation. Therefore, they have proven to be unsuitable for removal of large volumes of obstructive tissue.

Shanberg and Tansey reported a technique of laser prostatotomy.[20] The results have been relatively good in patients with small prostates, but there is no evidence that this technique is superior to an electrocautery incision through the bladder neck and prostate.

Kandel and associates described a method of Nd:YAG laser prostatectomy in dogs whereby relatively high power outputs were used and the fiber placed in direct contact with the tissue.[21] Postoperative urethrograms showed apparent good vaporization of the prostatic fossa. Despite this, it seems unlikely that this treatment will be as effective as transurethral electrocautery resection of the prostate for bulk tissue removal.

Sander and Beisland investigated the use of a Nd:YAG laser for carcinoma of the prostate.[22] A thorough transurethral electrocautery resection of the prostate was performed preliminarily. Subsequently, a cystoscope was inserted through a suprapubic cystotomy incision. This allowed direct access to the posterior capsule of the prostate. Laser energy was then applied to the prostatic fossa. No treatment complications were observed. Patient follow-up was short, so no conclusions can be drawn regarding treatment efficacy. However, it seems unlikely that the 3 mm to 4 mm of tissue penetration which can be achieved with a Nd:YAG laser will result in thorough coagulation of the prostatic capsule. Furthermore, access to the entire prostatic fossa is quite limited, and uniform distribution of the laser energy is extremely difficult to achieve.

## BLADDER

### Benign Diseases

A number of benign lesions of the bladder have been treated with Nd:YAG laser energy, with varying results. Large bladder hemangiomas have been treated successfully without bleeding. In certain patients, the need for segmental cystectomy or total cystectomy may be avoided.[23] Somewhat less successful has been the treatment of bleeding from radiation cystitis or cytoxan induced cystitis. Although the laser is capable of ablating focal areas of inflamed mucosa and thereby improving bleeding, the diffuse nature of these diseases does not lend itself well to the focal treatment afforded by a Nd:YAG laser.

The success of laser treatment of interstitial cystitis has been difficult to determine. The ambiguous definition of the disease and the potential influence of other treatments, such as bladder dilation, which may occur during cystoscopy, compound the difficulty in interpreting results. Nevertheless, subjective improvement in bladder symptoms has been observed in the majority of patients treated, and there have been reports suggesting that functional bladder capacity is increased. A power output of 30 to 35 W is used and any area suggestive of a Hunner's ulcer is thoroughly ablated. Areas of obvious inflammation are treated, as well as the bladder trigone. Considering the thin wall of the female bladder and the fact that the areas of inflammation may occur on the intraperitoneal portion of the bladder, care should be taken to avoid excessive energy in a given area, in order to decrease the chance of bowel injury due to forward scatter of the laser beam.

### Superficial Bladder Cancer

The most widespread endoscopic use of lasers in urology has been in the treatment of superficial bladder cancer. The use of lasers has been predicated by theoretical therapeutic advantages over standard therapy as well as demonstrated practical improvements and decreased patient morbidity.

It has been theorized that the noncontact thermal destruction of tumor cells that occurs with Nd:YAG laser energy leads to a lower overall recurrence of tumors than after electrocautery resection. Experimental results and clinical observation suggest that at least some recurrences of bladder cancer are because of implantation of viable tumor cells which may be dislodged at the time of electrocautery resection. See and Chapman demonstrated in an experimental model that the implantation of tumor cells onto a laser created injury is equal to that of a comparable electrocautery injury of the bladder.[24] However, they also found that there were significantly fewer viable cells available for implantation after laser treatment compared to electrocautery resection. Therefore, there does seem to be some experimental basis for the clinical theory of a decreased recurrence rate.

Examination of various clinical series yields conflicting results. Hofstetter and Frank claim a recurrence rate of only 8% after laser treatment.[13] Malloy et al found an 18% recurrence at one year in their laser treatment patients, but this increased with further follow-up.[25] We have treated 137 patients with superficial transitional cell carcinoma of the bladder with a Nd:YAG laser. All patients had a history of recurrent bladder cancer treated by electrocautery resection. At one year, 37% of patients had developed a tumor recurrence in an area of the bladder remote from the site of the previous tumor. Four percent of patients had persistent tumor at the site of laser treatment.

In collaboration with other European investigators, Hofsetter has attempted a randomized prospective trial comparing lasers and electrocautery.[26] Although the claim is that there is a statistically significant decrease in the recurrence rate in patients treated with laser, the series is small and confused by the addition of mitomycin-C in some patients.

Overall, the effect of a Nd:YAG laser on the recurrence rate of superficial bladder cancer remains unknown. It seems unlikely that any difference in recurrence rates will be as striking as claimed by some authors. However, the question must remain open until adequate randomized studies have been performed.

Another potential property of laser energy that has been exploited in the treatment of bladder cancer is the ability to seal lymphatic vessels. In animal models, a Nd:YAG laser appeared to be capable of blocking the lymphatic uptake of a vital dye injected into the bladder.[27] However, further studies using a more sensitive radioisotope for detection of lymphatic uptake have not been able to confirm this. Moreover, the potential therapeutic benefit of sealing lymphatic vessels around the periphery of a tumor has not been demonstrated.

A pertinent issue that has arisen is the ability to stage adequately tumors treated with laser energy. During treatment, the tumor undergoes a coagulation necrosis and material is not retrieved routinely for histologic examination. After laser therapy, the coagulated material does maintain some of its architectural integrity, and some histologic detail can be discerned if the coagulated material is removed and fixed properly. However, detail is rarely sufficient for optimal staging.

In the experience at the University of Utah only 3 of 121 patients treated with the Nd:YAG laser for superficial disease had muscle invasive recurrences at 9, 17, and 46 months. All of the recurrences were in new areas not previously treated with the laser. We believe that significant understaging is not a clinical problem if appropriate patient selection criteria are maintained. In these patients, the most important criteria appear to be history of low-grade and stage lesions, tumors less than 2 cm in size, and gross appearance of a papillary lesion. Cytology and biopsy may provide confirmatory evidence of the low grade of the tumor.[28]

Preliminary electrocautery resection can be used to debulk a tumor prior to laser therapy and in order to retrieve a specimen for histologic examination. However, this may negate any potential therapeutic advantages of laser treatment, and it also eliminates some of the practical advantages. Probably the best method for staging is to take preliminary cold-cup biopsies from the base of the tumor. This will establish the diagnosis of transitional cell carcinoma, allow an assignment of tumor grade, and give some information regarding infiltration of the tumor. However, it remains a less than optimal way for staging of bladder tumors. Therefore, when there is a real suspicion of invasion, such as with higher grade tumors or those with a more sessile appearance, intitial treatment should be by electrocautery resection rather than laser energy.

Laser treatment may be performed in any area suitably equipped for cystoscopy in which adequate electrical power supply and water for cooling of the laser are available. Standard rigid cystoscopes with a modified laser insert or flexible cystoscopes may be used. The operating surgeon and other personnel in the immediate operating area should wear appropriate eye protection. Alternatively, a lens cap with an appropriate filter may be used once the fiber is inserted through the cystoscope.

The tip of the fiber is positioned 1 mm or 2 mm away from the surface of the tumor. Tumors greater than 2 cm are extremely difficult to treat with laser energy alone. The primary limiting factor is the depth of the exophytic portion of the tumor, since 3 mm to 5 mm of penetration can be anticipated. As the superficial areas of the tumor are treated, the debris can be dislodged with the tip of the fiber or cystoscope to expose the deeper portions of the tumor. Debris that sticks to the tip of the fiber should be removed with a saline soaked sponge.

A power output of 35 W to 40 W is chosen. Treatment is continued in a given area until a white color indicative of adequate thermal necrosis is observed (Fig 35). Treatment is best performed as a dynamic process rather than a series of adjacent static impulses. To accomplish this, it often is better to operate the laser with a continuous output rather than on a defined pulse duration. The beam should not be held in contact with a given area for more than 3 or 4 seconds. Visible changes in the tumor determine treatment adequacy.

Bleeding is usually negligible or nonexistent during treatment, and significant delayed bleeding has not been observed. The tumor sloughs within a week after treatment, although complete re-epithelization of the bladder may not occur for several months. A pale white scar is seen at the site of laser therapy after healing is complete (Fig 36).

On many patients, treatment can be performed without an anesthetic. The decision to proceed under local anesthesia depends partly upon the number and size of tumors, their location within the bladder, and the patient's anticipated pain tolerance. The laser energy itself is perceptible as a burning sensation, but usually the amount of discomfort is slight and can be easily tolerated.

**Fig 35.** Typical appearance of a superficial bladder tumor after Nd:YAG laser therapy. The characteristic white discoloration is indicative of adequate thermal necrosis.

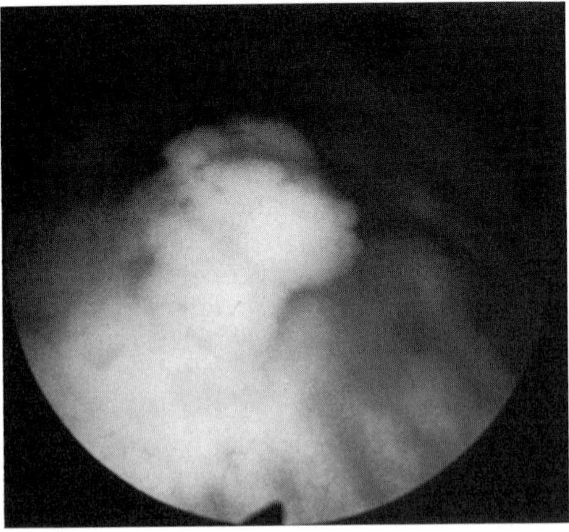

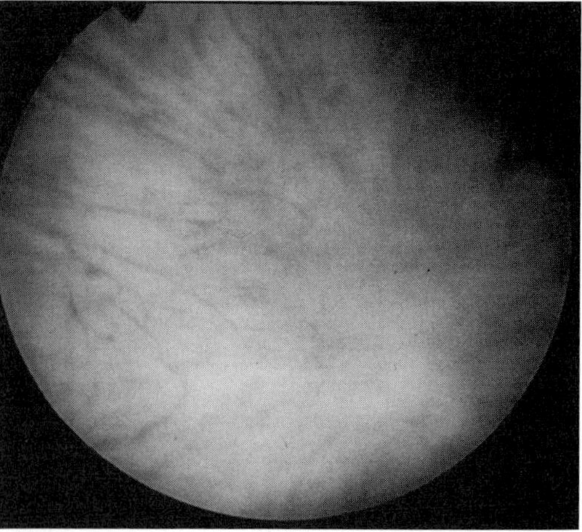

**Fig 36.** Scar of bladder wall 6 weeks after laser treatment of a superficial bladder cancer.

Even though a transmural injury may be created, the bladder maintains its structural and architectural integrity. Therefore, a Foley catheter is not necessary postoperatively.

The factors discussed in the preceding paragraphs combine to make laser treatment of superficial bladder cancer an easy, outpatient procedure. Patients may return immediately to their pretreatment activity. Bladder spasms are usually minimal, and the use of flexible instruments can further decrease the discomfort of the cystoscopy.

The potential complication of greatest concern is thermal damage to adjacent organs, in particular, the small bowel. Some 20% to 30% of the laser energy is transmitted as forward scatter. The bowel wall appears to be more susceptible to laser injury than the bladder wall. Moreover, small areas of perforation of the bladder may remain subclinical. Although bowel perforation is an uncommon complication, there are scattered reports throughout the world literature. Most often, clinical signs of peritonitis are evident within 24 hours of surgery, although they have been seen as long as 1 week later.

Several considerations may help decrease the low (less than 1%) incidence of bowel perforation. Energy densities should not be excessive and treatment should be terminated in a given area when the characteristic visible changes are observed. The female bladder is often thinner and perhaps more susceptible to perforation. Special caution is appropriate when treating lesions on the intraperitoneal portion of the bladder, especially if there has been previous pelvic surgery, irradiation, or inflammatory disease that may result in adhesions between the bladder dome and the peritoneal contents.

Tumors overlying the ureteral orifice or extending just inside the intramural ureter may be treated with laser energy. There are no reports of stenosis of the ureteral orifice or ureteral obstruction after laser treatment. The thin wall of bladder diverticula raises concern for treatment of any tumors within bladder diverticula. However, successful Nd:YAG laser treatment of small tumors within bladder diverticula has been accomplished. A coagulation necrosis without perforation of the diverticulum is observed and a shriveling effect is often seen.

## Invasive Bladder Cancer

The ability of a Nd:YAG laser to produce a transmural coagulation of the bladder wall without perforation forms the basis for laser treatment of invasive bladder cancer. In a controlled setting, a Nd:YAG laser can penetrate 3 mm to 5 mm in tissue with reasonable reproducibility.

Several factors influence the tissue effects of a laser. Some of these are under precise control, whereas others are not. The power output and the pulse duration are predetermined by turning the appropriate controls on the instrument panel. However, the denominator in the equation that determines energy density is the spot size of the laser beam, ie, the area of tissue being treated. There is a 5° to 8° angle of divergence from flexible laser fibers. Therefore, the spot size is influenced by the distance between the fiber tip and the bladder wall, angulation at the point of impact, irregularities in the bladder wall, and fiber damage. Each of these factors is difficult to control in a clinical endoscopic setting. Thus, the energy density and depth of penetration of a Nd:YAG laser in a clinical setting are imprecisely controlled (Fig 37).

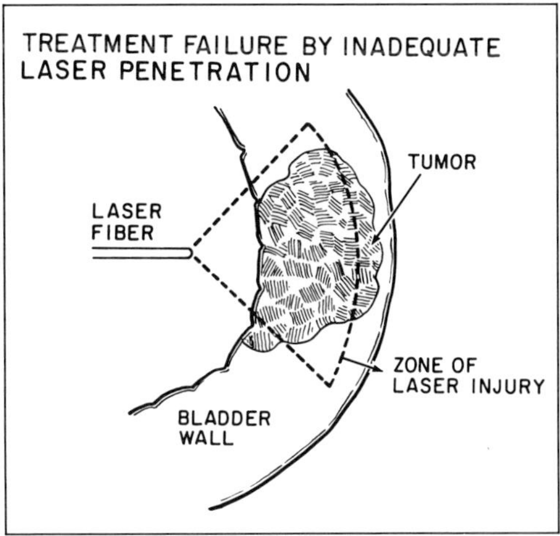


**Fig 37.** Reproducible, transmural thermal injury in the bladder is difficult to achieve in a clinical endoscopic setting, raising the possibility of undertreatment of invasive bladder cancer.

Another factor that limits the use of a Nd:YAG laser in treatment of invasive bladder cancer is the recognition that up to one third of invasive bladder cancers are clinically understaged (Fig 38). Although a Nd:YAG laser can theoretically eradicate a tumor of up to stage T3A (stage B2), lesions that extend into the perivesical fat probably are not amenable to primary treatment by endoscopic laser application.

The technique that has been used for en-

**Fig 38.** Up to one third of invasive bladder cancer is understaged clinically.

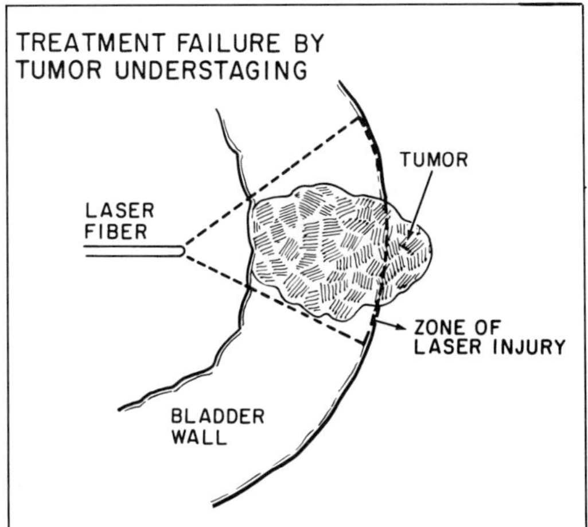

doscopic application in the treatment of invasive bladder cancer involves a preliminary electrocautery resection. This is performed to establish the diagnosis as well as to debulk the tumor. It is best to wait several days between resection and treatment in order to allow all of the overlying blood clots to close, but treatment can be initiated at the time of resection if bleeding is minimal. Visible changes in the tumor crater are unreliable predictors of penetration depth. Therefore, a systematic application of energy over the entire tumor crater, as well as the surrounding more normal appearing mucosa, should be performed. Since transmural penetration is the goal, power outputs of 40 W to 50 W are used, and treatment is maintained in a given area for 3 or 4 seconds. Healing is usually relatively delayed and re-epithelialization may not be complete for 3 or 4 months. Sometimes, a dystrophic calcification is seen overlying the area of laser treatment. Most often, though, a pale white scar is evident if all of the tumor has been eliminated. A concern has been that re-epithelialization could occur while viable tumor persists in deeper layers of the bladder. Although this clearly is possible, it has not been observed or, at least, recognized.

The results from the University of Utah confirm both the capabilities and limitations of laser treatment of invasive bladder cancer.[29] In patients with clinical stage T2 tumors, repeat resection or biopsies from the tumor base have been negative after 3 months in 80% of the patients. None of these patients have developed tumor at the site of laser treatment with longer follow-up. As stage increases, the results become much less impressive. Fewer than half of the patients with deep-muscle invasion have had their tumor eliminated by laser therapy. In patients with bulky tumors, treatment has been performed with palliative intent. There are no objective measures by which to judge the success of therapy. However, it appears that laser treatment is only modestly successful in this setting. McPhee and associates from Edmonton, Canada, have published results very similar to the Utah study. No local recurrences were noted in the T2 group of patients (total of 12). As the stage increases, the percentage of recurrences likewise increases, reaching 100% recurrences in the six patients with stage T4 lesions.[30]

Hofstetter and colleagues have used a combined endoscopic approach with an open incision. This allows packing of the bowel away from the bladder wall and, if desired, external application of energy to the bladder wall. A pelvic lymph node dissection is also performed at the time of treatment, but this adds no real therapeutic benefit to the procedure. Although this seems reasonable in selected patients, the location of most invasive bladder tumors on the trigone limits access to them from an open approach such as this.

Overall, the results of laser treatment of invasive bladder cancer do not seem to justify it as a reasonable alternative to cystectomy in patients who are candidates for a radical surgery. On the other hand, in a patient who is a poor surgical candidate, laser therapy may offer a reasonable alternative treatment with low morbidity.

## OPEN APPLICATIONS WITH THE LASER

### Condyloma Acuminata

A major advance represented by the laser is the treatment of genital lesions and particularly condyloma acuminata. Prior to this time, the treatment of podophyllum-resistent condyloma generally required electrofulguration. For extensive lesions or those located on the glans this was potentially a disfiguring procedure. In addition, lesions of the urethral meatus or intraurethral lesions were most difficult to treat. All three laser modalities have been used to treat these lesions; however, the carbon dioxide ($CO_2$) and Nd:YAG lasers are most frequently used today.

### Diagnosis

It is extremely important for the urologist today to understand the needs of the gynecologist in evaluating male partners of women found to have vaginal or cervical condyloma or cervical dysplasia. Although there is some debate as to the percentage of male partners who are subsequently found to have genital condyloma, the etiologic relationship is inarguable. Failure of the urologist to properly screen the male consorts of women with cervical condyloma or dysplasia will lead to the gynecologist assuming this role. Two recent studies have underscored the importance of examining the male not only grossly, but microscopically as well. Our current technique, similar to that reported by Rosemberg,[31] is to incubate the genitalia with 3% acetic acid impregnated gauze and examine the patient under magnification. In our hands, this is performed by soaking 4 × 4 gauze in 3% acetic acid and wrapping the penis and scrotum in the gauze for 3 to 5 minutes. Following this, the excess acetic acid is wiped off, as it may prove caustic. The patient is then examined with 6 × 6 magnifying surgical loupes. According to previous series, between 36% and 89% of men will be found to have white plaques after acetic acid incubation, proven by biopsy to be flat condyloma.[31,32] Between 14% and 16% of men will also be found to have papillary exophytic lesions. Carpinello and associates have labeled this procedure magnified penile surface scanning (MPSS).[32] A recent follow-up study by Rosemberg on 199 patients has maintained the importance of a thorough examination, including acetic acid incubation.[33] In addition, urine for cytology may be useful to screen for patients who may have intraurethral condyloma. In our experience, urethroscopy has not been worthwhile unless a meatal condyloma or voiding symptoms are present. In addition, the perineum and perianal region should be closely examined to rule out condyloma acuminata in those areas, since lingual condyloma are becoming an increasing problem. When in doubt as to the diagnosis of a lesion, it is possible to infiltrate the lesion with 1% lidocaine and use a 2-mm skin punch to perform biopsy.

## Selection Criteria

At this point in time, we are faced with the specter of cervical carcinoma in the woman as being the potential consequence of incompletely treated condyloma acuminata in the male. In addition, carcinoma of the penis or rectum in the male has, on occasion, been associated with larger condylomata. Because of the recurrence rates after topical treatment with podophyllin or electrofulguration. We treat all but the smallest of condyloma with the laser as primary treatment. Small lesions less than 5 mm in diameter or 3 mm in height, or those located on the glans, are treated with the $CO_2$ laser. This is more controlled since there is less tissue penetration. Larger lesions, particularly those on the penile shaft, the perianal areas, or the lingual areas are better treated with the Nd:YAG laser, which is more penetrating.

## Technique

The genitals are first wrapped in acetic acid–impregnated gauze, as described previously. After incubation and examination with optical loupes, determination is made as to the degree of involvement of the penis with condyloma. At this time, a decision can be made as to direct injection of lesions with 1% lidocaine, or the use of a penile block (as for circumcision) for extensive areas. Perianal lesions, as well as those on the tongue, require general anesthesia.

The $CO_2$ laser vaporizes in a U-shaped crater. Because of this, intervening ridges may be missed.[34] For this reason, we have used three passes: one vertical, one horizontal, and one oblique, to completely irradicate the area of condyloma. A wet sponge is ued to wipe off carbonized surface tissue and to protect adjacent areas. The treatment of small lesions is begun with 2 W, using a focused laser beam. After the entire condyloma is vaporized, the beam is defocused by enlarging the spot, and the base is treated to irradicate any viral particles in the base of the lesion. Larger condyloma may be treated with the $CO_2$ laser, starting initially at 5 W to 10 W of power and decreasing to 2 W to 5 W as the base of the lesion is encountered. Topical bacitracin ointment is applied as a dressing.

When using the Nd:YAG laser, the anesthetic needs are the same. It is not ne-

**TABLE 3. $CO_2$ Laser for Condyloma Acuminata**

| Author | # Patients | Cure Rates |
|---|---|---|
| Amagi, et al[35] | 43 | Not stated |
| Rosemberg[36] | 61 | 88% |
| Lundquist-Lindstedt[37] | 150 | 95% |
| Stein[38] | 100 | Study in progress |

cessary to make three passes, since the laser effect is one of wide necrosis rather than a narrow crater of vaporization. We have been using the contact laser scalpel at settings of 20 W to 22 W. Following treatments with the laser scalpel, the bare fiber can be used in the defocused beam to treat the base of the lesion as described above.

## Results

The $CO_2$ laser has been the most widely used in the treatment of condyloma of the genitalia. Table 3 reviews four of the larger series in the urologic literature.[35,36,37,38] Cure rates after a single treatment ranged from 88% to 95%. Extensive lesions are better treated in multiple sittings at least 4 weeks apart. To date, we have treated over 200 patients with the $CO_2$ laser in an outpatient office setting, without complications. In his most recent review, Rosemberg reports a 75% to 82% cure rate of flat and raised lesions respectively. This compares to his recurrence rates of 40% using only an eye cautery.[33]

Only two studies have been reported on the use of the Nd:YAG laser for condyloma. Hofstetter and Frank treated 30 patients with only two recurrences.[39] We have reported on the treatment of 38 patients with the Nd:YAG laser, only one of whom had a recurrence in the laser treated area, although several had recurrences elsewhere.[38]

## Premalignant and Malignant Penile Lesions

The use of the laser for premalignant and superficially invasive penile cancer may preclude penile amputation. Obviously, careful patient selection is required, with adequate biopsies to ensure that the depth of invasion is less than 2 mm to 3 mm. Although in the literature both the $CO_2$ and Nd:YAG lasers have been used for this indication, we believe the Nd:YAG laser is preferable because of its greater depth of penetration without tissue disruption.

The largest series reported to date includes 19 patients with penile dysplasia, carcinoma in situ, or early invasive disease treated with the $CO_2$ laser.[40] The duration of follow-up was short, but no recurrences have been reported.

Numata and associates from Japan report on three patients treated with the Nd:YAG laser for penile carcinoma.[41] In their series, high power settings were used, up to 80 W, with the use of a topical black cream to increase local absorption. Extensive damage to the glans and penile skin was noted, including a complete sloughing of the glans in one case. Use of high power settings and topical creams is to be condemned. Hofstetter and Frank reported on 17 patients treated with the Nd:YAG laser at 40 W of power.[39] Of the 11 patients followed for more than 10 months, only 1 had a local recurrence and all patients had excellent cosmetic results. Hofstetter and Frank did have several deaths from metastatic disease, which emphasizes the importance of proceeding to treat the lymph node drainage as usual, whether the primary lesion was treated with laser or amputation.

We have treated four patients with penile carcinoma with the Nd:YAG laser at 40 W. It is important to treat in this setting with the penis immersed in water, to increase the penetration of the laser without increasing the surface temperature. These patients have had excellent local results.

## RENAL PARENCHYMAL SURGERY

### Carbon Dioxide Laser

Any discussion of the use of the $CO_2$ laser for renal surgery must be prefaced by the statement that it is impossible to use this instrument on renal parenchyma without first clamping the renal pedicle. Although the $CO_2$ laser is an effective cutting device, the relatively high-pressure arteries and larger-caliber renal vessels certainly exceed the coagulative abilities of this laser, so that complete hemostasis within the renal parenchyma cannot be accomplished. In addition, once the renal-collecting system is entered, extreme care must be taken to evacuate all urine because of the high absorption of $CO_2$ energy by water.

Mulvaney and Beck[42] first reported an attempt at wedge resection of the canine kidney with a 50 W $CO_2$ laser; they found the incision to be slow and hemostasis unsatisfactory. Hughes and Scott[43] also examined the use of the $CO_2$ laser for partial nephrectomy in seven dogs, in the hope that the procedure could be performed faster and with less renal ischemia time and blood loss than with conventional surgery. After transection of the parenchyma, the cut surface of the kidney was coagulated with the unfocused laser beam. The average time of ischemia was 15 minutes and renal damage was limited to a 1-mm to 2-mm area of coagulation necrosis. No closure of the collecting system was performed other than laser coagulation, and subsequent x-ray evaluation indicated that urinary extravasation was not a problem. The authors were generally impressed by the ease with which the $CO_2$ laser could be used to perform partial nephrectomy in the dog. These observations were later confirmed in cats by Meiraz et al;[44] the authors make the important point that although the $CO_2$ laser can seal vessels only up to a diameter of 0.5 mm, when blood flow is stopped temporarily while the tissue is divided, empty vessels up to 2 mm can be sealed. In 1982, Barzilay et al,[45] reported on a careful comparative study on the use of the $CO_2$ laser in partial nephrectomies in dogs. They compared the $CO_2$ laser with the scalpel and the electric knife in the performance of partial nephrectomy in 20 dogs. Although sutures were needed in addition to the unfocused $CO_2$ laser beam for control of bleeding in the partial nephrectomies performed with the laser, the authors concluded that the $CO_2$ laser "shortens the time of operation by facilitating hemostasis, diminished blood loss, and does not interfere with the final kidney function."

On the basis of the results of these animal studies, a number of investigators have used a $CO_2$ laser to perform partial nephrectomy and nephrolithotomy in humans. Pariente and d'Ovidio[46] did $CO_2$ laser nephrectomies for renal calculi and reported that "the incision of the renal parenchyma was always bloodless though we never practiced the clamping of the renal pedicle." This is a rather surprising observation, and is contrary to the experience of most laser users. Barzilay et al[47] performed three partial nephrectomies (two patients with calculi, one with a calculus and xanthogranulomatous pyelonephritis) and one anatrophic nephrolithotomy using the $CO_2$ laser, and were satisfied that the operation resulted in a minimum of blood loss and parenchymal damage. In using the $CO_2$ laser for partial nephrectomy, Hall[48] reported that hemostasis was adequate, but that the incision was slow and prolonged renal ischemia times.

Rosemberg and Lutz[49] and Rosemberg[50] reported on the successful performance of three anatrophic nephrolithotomies (staghorn calculus) and three partial nephrectomies (one congenital arteriovenous fistula, one segmental chronic atrophic pyelonephritis and calculus, and one bilateral renal mass). The surgical procedures were performed during regional hypothermia, but no mention of occlusion of the renal vessels was made. Incision of the renal parenchyma with the $CO_2$ laser beam was slow in the first three cases, taking approximately 15 minutes. The average power was 28 W, with an optical spot size of 2 mm corresponding to a power density of 700 $W/cm^2$. Because of the slowness, the power densities were increased in the second three cases to 1000 to 1250 W/cm$^2$; this increase lowered the parenchymal incision time to 6 minutes. Total operation time ranged between 110 and 120 minutes and the average estimated loss of blood was 160 mL per case.

The cumulative experience with the $CO_2$ laser in renal surgery is somewhat contradictory, but theoretical considerations and practical experience seem to indicate that the instrument has little to offer over conventional surgery. With this laser, making the incision is slow, large vessels bleed readily (although small vessels are well controlled), and the articulated arm of the instrument makes its use somewhat awkward.

## Nd:YAG Laser

Unlike the $CO_2$ laser, the Nd:YAG laser has received relatively little use in renal surgery. Application of Nd:YAG energy causes protein denaturation, which results in deep thermal coagulation but no effective tissue vaporization. Therefore, one would expect that even with a focused-beam incision in the renal parenchyma healing would be very slow and there might be extensive thermal damage to adjacent tissue. The Nd:YAG laser is effective in coagulating vessels up to 3 mm or 4 mm in diameter. Therefore, for hemostasis, it may be preferable to use the Nd:YAG laser to coagulate a specific vessel on the cut surface of the kidney rather than to use cautery or a suture ligature. High-power densities are required for this procedure and use of a 60 W to 80 W for 1 to 3 seconds may be necessary. These energies may cause excessive tissue heating and resultant tissue explosion. Heating can be avoided by irrigation of the cut surface of the kidney with saline. In addition, when cold knife incisions are made in the renal parenchyma, the brisk bleeding that occurs if the renal pedicle is not clamped may make effective application of the Nd:YAG laser to the bleeding site difficult. When the renal pedicle is clamped, the surface of the renal parenchyma can be coagulated; however, retraction of vessels may necessitate high powers to control bleeding, with resultant excessive tissue damage.

In 6 dogs, Benderev and Schaeffer[51] performed partial nephrectomy using 100 W of focused Nd:YAG power to determine its hemostatic capabilities, safety, and effect on renal function and histologic pattern. These studies were carried out with the renal pedicle clamped and with renal cooling. The renal-collecting system was not closed. Hemostasis was reported to be excellent, but urinomas occurred in 2 dogs and the zone of necrosis produced by the laser energy penetrated as far as 7 mm. Because of this unacceptable amount of tissue necrosis, Melzer et al[52] combined the use of the Cooper Cavitron ultrasonic surgical aspirator for parenchymal dissection with the Nd:YAG laser for vessel coagulation. Twenty partial nephrectomies were performed in 10 dogs with the combination of these two instruments after the renal vessels had been isolated and temporarily occluded. Blood loss and total operating time were less than those in a control series of partial nephrectomies performed with a scalpel. The authors concluded that the combination of the Cavitron ultrasonic surgical aspirator and the Nd:YAG laser appears to offer advantages over either method used alone or over standard techniques for partial nephrectomy. Since their original report, this combination of technologies has been used to perform three successful partial nephrectomies in humans.

Hofstetter and Frank[53] have advocated Nd:YAG treatment of the renal parenchyma adjacent to an area where a small malignant renal lesion has been "shelled out" or removed by wedge resection. This practice seems warranted, especially when an adequate free-tissue margin is questioned. Malloy[54] has used a similar technique while doing partial nephrectomies for renal cell carcinoma in patients with a solitary kidney or in patients with bilateral renal cell carcinoma. In this use of the Nd:YAG laser in combination with blunt dissection, the laser allows sealing of the lymphatics and small vessels around the tumor before excision and limits the blood loss while the tumor is being surgically elevated and removed.

Landau and associates recently studied the sapphire contact tips for use in partial nephrectomy. Both the laser scalpels and endoscopic types of tips were evaluated. Neither probe was found to represent an advantage in regard to blood loss, ischemia time, or total time until hemostasis.[55]

## Endoscopy of the Ureter and Renal Collecting System

With the realization that Nd:YAG laser photocoagulation appears to result in less scarring in the urinary tract than electrocoagulation, combined with the recent availability of instruments that allow transurethral access to the ureter and renal-collecting systems, has come the possibility of Nd:YAG laser treatment of transitional cell carcinoma of the ureter and renal pelvis. Clinicians have noted for several years that Nd:YAG treatment of transitional cell tumors overlying the ureteral orifices did not result in stenosis of the orifice—an observation which led naturally to progression of laser therapy in a retrograde fashion up the urinary tract.

In 1983, Rothenberger et al reported on the treatment of 4 patients with low-grade transitional cell carcinoma of the distal ureter with the Nd:YAG laser via the ureteroscope.[56] All patients were found to have no evidence of recurrent disease 18 months post-treatment. This initial experience has been expanded upon with 12 patients with a total of 16 biopsy-proved noninvasive tumors having been treated with 40 W of power and 1- to 3-second pulses. Follow-up has averaged 23 months with no local recurrences having been noted.[57,58] Benson has had a similar, though smaller experience, with 5 patients with noninvasive ureteral tumors and 2 patients with tumors of the renal pelvis or upper pole infundibulum who were treated with Nd:YAG laser surgery (20 W of power on continuous mode). With a mean follow-up of 12 months, no instances of ureteral stenosis or local tumor recurrence have been noted.[59]

Recently, consideration has been given to the percutaneous approach of selected upper tract lesions that are not accessible transurethrally. Patient selection is of utmost importance, and at present it seems reasonable to consider only patients with low-grade noninvasive lesions in solitary kidneys or those with bilateral synchronous tumors as candidates for this approach. Korth has treated 5 patients for transitional cell carcinoma with good local control but with the eventual development of distal metastatic disease in 2 of the 5 patients.[60]

Benson has treated 5 patients who fit the above criteria, with evidence of local recurrence having been noted in 1 of the 5 at 12 months (mean follow-up 24 months).[59] No patients in the United States or Europe have thus far been reported to have experienced tumor seeding in the percutaneous tract.

The possible advantages for the percutaneous treatment of tumors in the renal collecting system of selected patients are obvious: (1) possible avoidance of renal dialysis; (2) sparing of renal parenchyma; (3) patient preference for percutaneous versus open renal surgery and resultant diminished morbidity and cost. However, the disadvantages are also obvious: (1) the long-term treatment outcomes are unknown; (2) tumor seeding of the percutaneous tract is possible; (3) the technique requires expertise in both percutaneous and laser techniques. Until the long-term outcome of percutaneous laser treatment of the upper tract transitional cell carcinoma is known, a plea must be made for strict adherence to patient selection criteria and rigorous follow-up examinations.

Although the entire ureter and a significant amount of the renal-collecting system are accessible for endoscopic treatment with the Nd:YAG laser, specifications for safe laser application have not been established. Studies on the dog with doses of 35 W for 2 seconds resulted in perforation and urinary extravasation.[61] Although experience is limited, this has not been the case in humans who have been treated. No doubt the reason for this discrepancy is that in practice it is impossible to deliver laser energy in a perpendicular manner to the ureter with existing endoscopic instrumentation. Tumors are treated tangentially, with resultant lower and safer power densities being achieved. With the ongoing improvement in flexible and rigid endoscopic instrumentation for evaluation of the ureter and renal-collecting system, use of the Nd:YAG laser for the treatment of noninvasive transitional cell carcinoma of the upper tracts is likely to increase.

## Calculi

Tanahashi et al first reported the satisfactory disintegration of known urinary calculi transplanted into the canine bladder using 50 W to 70 W of Nd:YAG power.[62] However, Pensel et al were less successful in destroying bladder calculi with the laser.[63]

It became apparent a few years ago that it may be possible to fragment ureteral calculi via a ureteroscope using either Q-switched Nd:YAG laser or tunable pulsed-dye laser energy passed down a fiber.[64,65] A fiber small enough to pass through the working ports of standard ureteroscopes for use with the Q-switched Nd:YAG laser has only recently become available (200 U), and therefore clinical results using this laser system are not as yet available, although the technology appears promising.

Watson et al were the first to use a flash lamp–pumped tunable dye laser to fragment stones in vitro,[66] and this same group demonstrated that ureteral stone fragmentation could be successfully achieved in animals without thermal tissue injury.[67] This experience naturally progressed to the use of similar technology for the fragmentation of ureteral calculi in man.[68] The laser system in common use is a flash lamp–pumped pulsed dye laser emitting at a wavelength of 504 nm (Cumarin green dye) for 1-microsecond duration at a frequency of 5 to 10 Hz and laser energies of 40 to 62 mJ/pulse transmitted via a 250-μm diameter silicone-coated quartz fiber. The fiber can be passed through a 4-F ureteral catheter or a specially designed stone basket, both of which are easily accepted by a 9.5-F rigid or a 9-F flexible ureteroscope. It is mandatory that the fiber be in direct contact with the calculus for adequate fragmentation (Fig 39). It is postulated that the absorption of laser pulse by the stone causes a plasma to form at the surface of the calculus. This plasma is a rapidly expanding cavity of ions and electrons that collapses rapidly after the laser pulse, producing a mechanical shock wave. Since saline irrigating solution around the stone conforms this shock wave, the stone itself is subject to high pressures, and stone fragmentation

**Fig 39. Left:** Photograph of stone impacted in a ureteral orifice. **Right:** Action photograph of pulsed dye laser fiber (bottom of photo) in contact with stone demonstrating fragmentation.

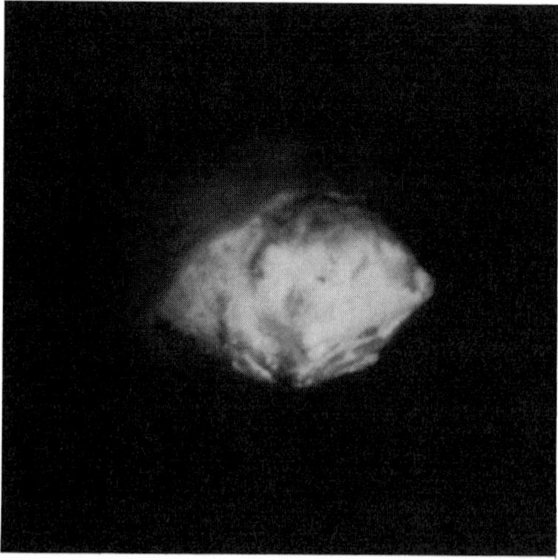

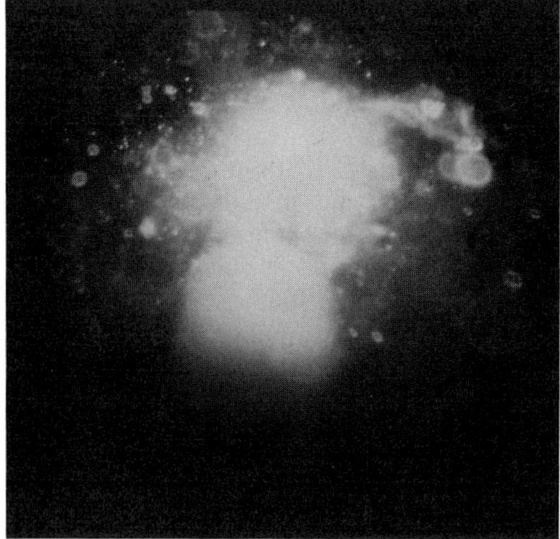

occurs. Dretler has reported on laser photofragmentation of ureteral calculi in 73 patients with ureteral calculi ranging in size from 5 mm × 5 mm to 10 mm × 30 mm and 2 patients with Steinstrasse.[69] In 70 cases, the patients were partially or entirely freed of stones. There were three equipment failures necessitating another form of lithotripsy, and two stones (one of brushite and one of cystine) that did not respond to laser energy (and required ultrasonic lithotripsy). One of the major disadvantages of this technique lies in the fact that the patient must pass stone fragments. However, this shortcoming may be balanced by the distinct advantage that the laser energy can be delivered through a flexible fiber, which makes the majority of the urinary tract easily accessible.

In his most recent review, Dretler presented results on a total of 157 patients treated with the laser lithotripter for renal or ureteral calculi. In 106 (68%) cases, the laser was sufficient to complete fragment the stone. In 34 cases, extracorporeal shock wave lithotripsy (ESWL) was needed to complete adequate fragmentation. In only 10 cases (6%) was the laser totally unsuccessful at stone fragmentation.[70]

Bagley and associates have reported their results using a new laser, the pulsolith (Technomed). This laser uses an identical technology to the Candela unit. Bagley treated 56 patients with 70 ureteral and renal calculi with a 100% fragmentation rate.[71]

It should also be mentioned that it is possible to generate extracorporeal shock waves using laser light, which can be focused down to a very small point.[72] The high-intensity light in a water media strips electrons off the hydrogen and oxygen atoms of the water molecule, forming a plasma (ionized gas) bubble that expands to produce the shock wave in much the same way a shock wave is produced by the electrohydraulic method. The theoretical advantages of this technique includes better focusing and lack of need for coordinating the shock wave with the electrocardiogram (ECG). This would make it possible to increase the frequency of the shock waves beyond the pulse rate, allowing the option of either shortening the length of treatment or reducing the strength of the individual shocks. Perhaps in the next few years, when laser technology has advanced further, it will be possible to use laser light to create a clinical useful extracorporeal lithotripter.

## Hematoporphyrin Derivative (HpD) Photodynamic Therapy

Lasers may be used endoscopically in urology for the production of reactions that are not related to the hyperthermic effect of the laser, but rather to the spectral output of the light the laser produces. Absorption of light by one molecule leading to the chemical alteration of another molecule is termed a photosensitized reaction. The light-absorbing molecule is termed the photosensitizer and the other molecule is termed the substrate of the reaction. Photosensitizers, light, and oxygen have been known for years to be toxic to cells.[73] On the basis of this principle, a new approach to the treatment of various malignant lesions has emerged. It has been variously termed "phototherapy," "photoradiation therapy," "photodynamic therapy," and "photochemotherapy."

Although no photosensitizing drug is currently taken up or retained selectively only by malignant tissue, several potentially useful photosensitizers are available for which such a tumor-specific characteristic has been claimed. These include berberine sulfate, flourescin, eosin, tetracycline, acridine orange, sulfonated aluminum phthalocyanine, and several porphyrins.[73–80] Certainly the porphyrins have been the drugs most completely investigated and they appear, at present, to be the most useful.

Hematoporphyrin is a product extracted by alcohol and sulfuric acid from hemoglobin, and was first discovered in the second half of the 19th century. Early investigators noted that hematoporphyrin tended to localize in malignant tissues as could be noted from the fact that tumor cells would fluoresce a salmon-red color when exposed to ultraviolet light. However, observed tumor fluorescence was frequently inconsistent, often with unreliable results. It was then ascertained that the hematoporphyrin product which was commercially available contained a mixture of porphyrins with varying localizing properties that in some cases exceeded those of pure hematoporphyrin. This prompted Lipson to report on a method of preparing an acetic and sulfuric acid derivative of naturally occurring hematoporphyrin called hematoporphyrin derivative (HpD) that showed greater affinity for malignant tissue than hematoporphyrin.[76] It was subsequently found that HpD was not only a tumor localization agent but also an active photosensitizing agent in that cytotoxicity would occur in cells that had taken up HpD if they were exposed to wavelengths of light that corresponded to the absorption spectrum of HpD.

These early observations prompted exploration of the use of HpD first as a tumor localization agent for transitional cell carcinoma of the bladder. Subsequent flourescence bladder-mapping studies established that HpD does, indeed, localize preferentially in malignant and severly dysplastic transitional cells.[81] This fact, plus the knowledge that activation of intracellular HpD with light of appropriate wavelength results in cytotoxicity, prompted trials of HpD photodynamic therapy in patients with focal or diffuse resistant cancer (Tis) of the bladder. Production of the desired photochemical cytotoxic effect requires that the spectral output of the delivered light be matched closely with the absorption levels of HpD and that the total energy density irradiating the cells be sufficient [energy density in joules per square centimeter ($J/cm^2$) is the product of the power intensity in watts per square centimeter and the irradiation time in seconds]. Red light (630 nm) has been most often used in the clinical setting because it penetrates tissue for approximately 1 cm. A suitable optical fiber is inserted through an open channel of the endoscope and light of sufficient power is delivered into the bladder. The major problem is the focusing of light of high-power density into the proximal end of this fiber. Focusing enough power from external light sources, such as incandescent lamps and mercury arcs, into this filter is not technically possible. Most clinical studies use lasers for this purpose because of their high-power density, beam of small diameter, and high coupling efficiency to optical fibers which allow light to be conveniently delivered to many areas.

An argon ion laser pumped-dye laser system is the instrument most often used in the clinical setting. These instruments are all similar and use a 5-W to 20-W argon ion laser to pump a dye laser operating with a dye (rhodamine B or DCM) to produce light near 630 nm. The distal end of the fiber can be varied to accommodate the particular therapeutic situation: an optically flat end to produce an expanding cone of light; a rounded tip to further expand the spot; a cylindrical tip to diffuse the light within a narrow beam; or a ''light-bulb'' tip for use in large, hollow organs such as the bladder.

The timing of light delivery after HpD administration has varied from 48 to 72 hours after administration. The proper light dose for maximal effect in the bladder is unknown, but doses should approximate 100 to 200 $J/cm^2$ for focal-tumor therapy and 15 to 20 $J/cm^2$ for whole-bladder therapy.

In 1976, Kelly and Snell[82] reported on the first treatment of a human bladder carcinoma by transmission of white light (mercury vapor lamp) transurethrally through a quartz rod after intravenous administration of HpD. The patient had multicentric noninvasive tumors, but only a small area was illuminated. Two days after treatment, there was histologic evidence of tumor necrosis in the treated area and unaltered tumor in the untreated areas. In 1983, Benson et al and two groups in Japan published results of HpD phototherapy using an argon ion pumped-dye laser as a source of red light.

Tsuchiya and associates[83] treated 6 patients with Ta and T1 disease and 2 patients with T2 tumors. Patients were given HpD intravenously at a dose of 2.5 mg/kg of body weight, and light (630 nm) was delivered 48 to 72 hours thereafter. The dose rate for Ta and T1 lesions was 120 to 360 $J/cm^2$ and for T2 lesions was 240 to 360

J/cm$^2$. Follow-up ranged from 6 to 18 months. All patients with Ta and T1 disease remained tumor free. One T2 tumor persisted and one tumor recurred at 6 months.

Hisazumi and coworkers[84] administered HpD, 2 to 3.2 mg/kg of body weight, to 9 patients with Ta and T1 lesions. Forty-eight to 72 hours later, red light was administered in a dose of 100 to 250 J/cm$^2$. These authors claimed complete tumor remission in 5 of 6 patients with tumors 1 cm or smaller in diameter, but had less success with tumors greater than 1 cm in diameter.

Benson et al have directed treatment attempts primarily at patients with recurrent resistant Tis in whom all conservative treatment measures, including electrofulguration and various intravesical chemotherapeutic agents, have failed.[85,86] Fifteen patients with focal resistant Tis were treated and followed up for at least 6 months. All treated patients had biopsy and cytologic evidence of disappearance of the lesion in the treated area at the 3-month follow-up cystoscopic examination. Eight patients had one or more recurrent lesions, either in the treated area or at a remote site, in follow-up that ranged from 6 to 38 months. One patient underwent cystectomy and urinary diversion because of progression to T1 disease after multiple recurrences. Metastatic disease did not develop in any patient.

Reviewing the published recurrence rates for focal treatment of transitional cell carcinoma of the bladder with HpD phototherapy clearly shows that they are not significantly different from those with conventional electrofulguration. For this reason, several groups have investigated ways to deliver light of appropriate dosage to the entire bladder in hopes of reducing recurrences. Jocham and coworkers and Baghdassarian et al introduced the possibility of the use of a lipid-diffusing medium, but no results of clinical trials in humans have been published.[87,88] Hisazumi and colleagues[84] devised a laser light–scattering optic coupled with a driving instrument that irradiates the entire bladder in sequential segmental strips. Two patients had been treated with an argon ion pumped-dye laser as a light source, a dose of approximately 10 J/cm$^2$ being delivered to the entire bladder. Early results in 2 patients appeared encouraging, because urinary cytologic findings returned to normal after treatment. This group has recently reported on the use of this technique in 24 patients with multifocal carcinoma in situ and/or dysplasia of the bladder mucosa associated with or without multicentric concurrent superficial tumor. Total bladder treatment was performed using their optical diffusion device 48 hours after intravenous injection of 4 mg/kg of HpD.[89] In 6 of the 24 patients treated with whole bladder photodynamic therapy (PDT) using 10, 20, or 30 J/cm$^2$ of light energy, there was no recurrence with the mean tumor-free time of 7.5 months, and there was no significant relationship between the recurrence rate and total light energy used. These authors stress that if papillary lesions are present with Tis, the papillary lesions should be focally treated with 100 J/cm$^2$ prior to whole-bladder therapy.

A simpler, less cumbersome approach to whole-bladder treatment has evolved in the United States. This approach utilizes a fiber with a modified tip, in the form of a light bulb, which has been perfected to deliver fairly uniform light to the entire bladder. Benson has reported one or more whole-bladder treatments in 22 patients who were followed for a minimum of 3 months.[84,89-92] In the 16 patients with Tis alone, 14 of 16 had a complete response and 2 had a partial response. The partial responders had disappearance of their disease in the majority of the bladder, but persisted in having biopsy positive carcinoma at the bladder neck. Recurrences have been noted in 6 of the 14 complete responses to date. Four patients had both Tis and Ta lesions, and all experienced disappearance of their Tis, but 2 of 4 had persistence of the Ta disease. Two patients had Tis plus T2 disease and both had persistence of the invasive component of their tumor. Similar response rates in patients with resistant Tis treated with this technique have more recently been reported by other authors.[93,94]

Adverse effects of treatment have been minimal. Cutaneous photosensitivity (sunburn) is a risk, and patients must remain out of direct and indirect sunlight for 4 to 6 weeks. Irritative bladder symptoms and reduced bladder capacity have been noted in patients who have had whole-bladder treatments, but those adverse effects have not lasted more than 2 months.

Relatively few patients with transitional cell carcinoma of the bladder have been treated with HpD phototherapy, and it clearly must continue to be considered an experimental technique. Several practical problems, such as optimal drug dosage, light wavelength, timing of light delivery, and light dose for the various stages of carcinoma to be treated, are yet to be resolved. Once these unanswered questions are successfully addressed, HpD and light may offer the urologist the possibility of an additional means to diagnose and treat transitional cell carcinoma of the bladder.

## Tissue Welding

One of the more promising future uses of laser technology in urology may be tissue welding. The Nd:YAG laser, the $CO_2$ laser, and the argon laser have all been successfully used in the animal laboratory for the welding of small blood vessels (arteries and veins), peripheral nerves, skin, and the vas deferens. Although reports are encouraging, few comparative studies have been performed; therefore, these techniques await refinement and judicious scrutiny before they can be considered superior to current microvascular techniques. Theoretically, laser welding may be superior to microsurgery because anastomosis might be less time consuming, require less surgical dexterity, and result in a stronger tissue bond. Although no vascular welding studies directly pertaining to urology have been performed, a number of reports indicate that laser welding of vessels is feasible.

Jain and Gorish[95] and Jain[96] were the first to report on microvascular repair of arteries and veins with the Nd:YAG laser, and they compared its efficacy with that of bipolar coagulation and microsuture technique. When rat vessels ranging in size from 0.3 mm to 1.1 mm were treated, no vessels between 0.7 mm to 1.1 mm in diameter became occluded after laser repair. In addition, for vessels as small as 0.3 mm in diameter, laser welding was the only technique that significantly preserved vessel patency. If the vessel edges tended to gape, a small piece of vein or muscle was placed over the area to be welded and was fused to the vessel wall. Tensile strength measurements of the laser-repaired veins and arteries showed that there was no disruption with intraluminal pressures as high as 300 mm Hg. Frazier et al have substantiated the usefulness of the $CO_2$ laser–assisted microvascular anastomoses.[99] Stein and Cooley, however, raise some concern about the thickness of the muscle wall of the vas deferens after laser welding. In their study on laser welding in rats, the muscle-wall thickness was significantly reduced in laser-welded vas deferens as compared to microsutured anastamosis.[97] Of interest is the work by Poppas et al on protein solder. They agree that the strength of the laser weld may be weaker than standard anastamoses. They have used a protein solder to give additional strength to their laser welds.[98] Further investigations in this area are clearly warranted. Using low-power $CO_2$ laser radiation (70 mW), and a 150-μm spot size, successful end-to-end anastomoses of the femoral arteries (mean diameter 1.6 mm) were performed in miniature swine. Laser-assisted anastomoses took less time to perform, and all were functional and free of stenosis at the 3-month postoperative examination.[100]

Of particular interest to the urologist is the possibility of using the laser to assist in vasovasostomy. Lynne et al[101] used a specially constructed optical bench and a continuous-wave, RF-excited $CO_2$ laser delivering from 100 to 200 mW of energy with a beam spot size of 0.2 mm to 0.5 mm to weld the edges of rata vasa held in approximation with three sutures. The wall of the healed vasa was thin in the region of anastomosis, but no sperm granulomas and very little inflammatory response were noted in the surrounding scar tissue. Rosemberg et al[102] using 1.8 W of power from a continuous-wave $CO_2$ laser with a spot size of 2 mm and a pulse duration of 0.2 seconds performed similar experiments in dogs. They concluded that speed of performance, patent vas lumen, and lack of sperm granuloma formation supported the $CO_2$ laser's ability to simplify the technique of vasovasostomy (Fig 40).

This same group has performed vasovasostomy using the $CO_2$ laser coupled with an operating microscope on 14 patients who had vasectomy performed from 1 to 13 years prior to reversal. The average power density was 45 W/cm$^2$. Sperm counts of $>$ 20 million per cm$^3$ were obtained in 86% of patients with a pregnancy rate of 43% if the vasectomy was performed $<$ 10 years prior to reversal. With $>$ 10 year intervals, 43% of patients had counts $>$ 20 million per cm$^3$ with a 0% pregnancy rate.[103] Although results such as these are encouraging, extended experience will be needed to determine if laser welding will result in improved clinical results for vasovasostomy.

Additional uses for the tissue welding in urology may exist. It is possible to use low-power $CO_2$ laser energy to weld the bladder of a rat with resultant adequate tensile strength to avoid urinary extravasation. In addition, preliminary experience with the use of similar techniques to perform ureteroureterostomies have been reported.[104,105] Although treatment parameters have varied, it appears that a power density of approximately 40 to 50 W/cm$^2$ should be used. As is true with any $CO_2$ laser–assisted tissue welding, adequate tissue approximation and a meticulously dry field are absolutely necessary.

## Newer Technology and Laser Wavelengths

Conventional noncontact open Nd:YAG laser surgery is time consuming, requires relatively high powers of laser energy with resultant excessive tissue damage, cannot be performed with sterile delivery systems, and is associated with excessive production of smoke. In addition, a major problem is damage to the fiber tip or handpiece if it comes into contact with blood or tissue. Many of these problems may have been solved by the recent development of contact fiber tips and contact ''scalpels'' for the use with the Nd:YAG laser. The contact tips made from a synthetic sapphire crystal, which has optical properties, geometric design, thermal conductivity, and high melting temperature (2030°C to 2050°C), have proved more effective than the current conventional noncontact method of delivering laser energy through a quartz fiber.[106] Advantages include greater precision, sterility, avoidance of tip melting, and a requirement of lower Nd:YAG laser energy with reduced tissue damage. Because these tips focus laser energy, lower power settings can be used to deliver higher power densities to a more limited area (less forward scatter). The result is more vaporization potential with minimal surrounding coagulative tissue destruction. It would appear that the best endoscopic use of these contact tips might be for the treatment of small genital skin lesions or perhaps for transurethral incision of urethral strictures. Unfortunately, no comparative studies have been performed, and therefore it is difficult to claim that these tips offer any advantage to noncontact Nd:YAG therapy.

A Nd:YAG laser can emit not only at 1.06-μm, but also at 1.32-μm wavelengths. This longer wavelength, which is still not appreciably absorbed by water, appears to have the possibility of deeper tissue penetration than the Nd:YAG laser emitting at 1.06-μm.[107] It was the original hope that the 1.32-μm wavelength would carry with it the coagulative properties of a 1.06-μm YAG plus more of the vaporization potential of the longer wavelength $CO_2$ laser. In actuality, this laser appears to offer little benefit over the conventional YAG laser and has not found use in urology at the present time.

The potassium-titanyl-phosphate (KTP) laser is a frequency-doubled Nd:YAG laser producing all of its output at 535 nm, which is in the green portion of a visible spectrum. The output is a train of light pulses at a frequency of 25 000 Hz and a pulse duration of about 200 ns. The Nd:YAG laser rod is continuously pumped with a krypton arc lamp and Q-switched. The original Nd:YAG wavelength of 1064 nm is frequency-doubled with a KTP crystal to produce the 532-nm output. The green light

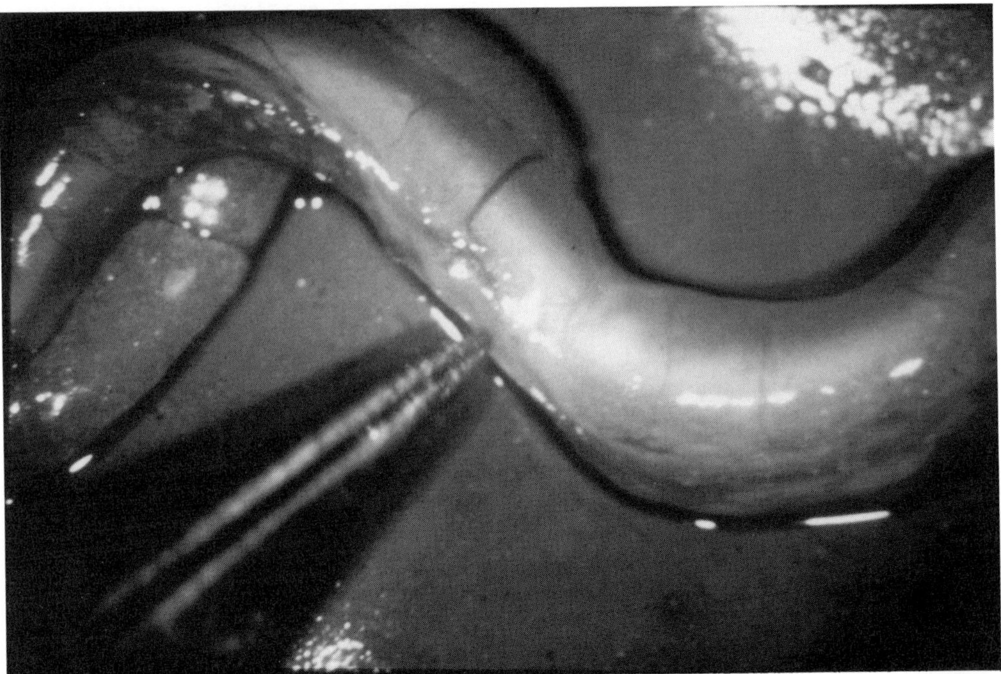

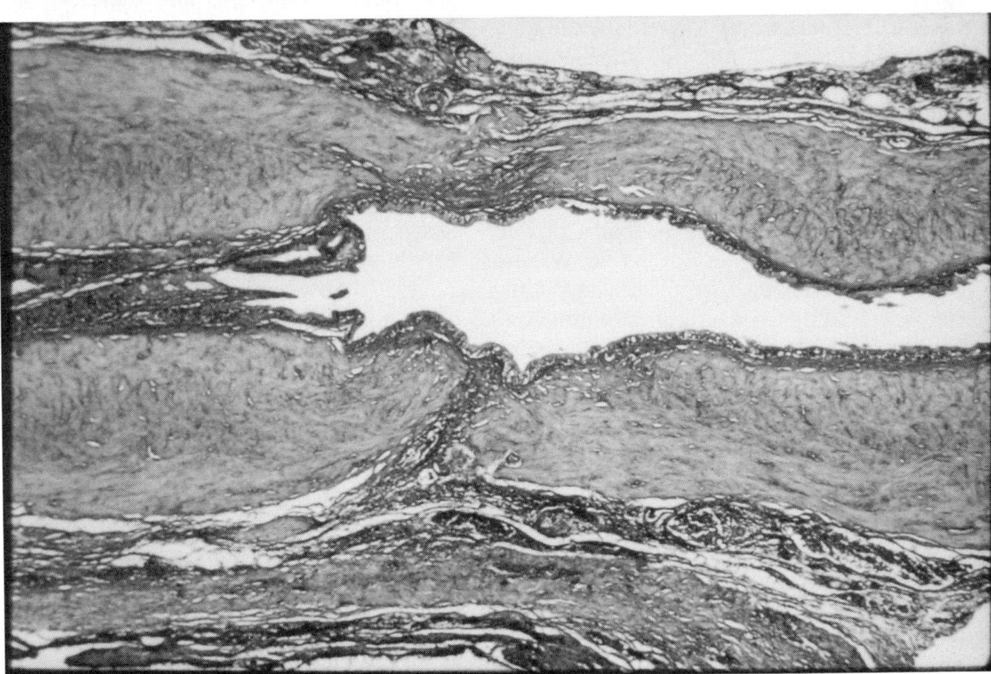

**Fig 40. Top:** Laser-assisted rat vas deferens anastomosis 3 months postoperative. Forceps pointing at narrowed area of anastomosis. (Magnification × 10.) **Bottom:** Photomicrograph of longitudinal section through area of laser-assisted rat vas deferens anastomosis. Area shows minimal narrowing and fibrosis. (Trichione stain. × 25.)

is directed through a series of fiber optics from the source to the end output and can be passed through a 600- or a 400-μm quartz fiber. This wavelength of light is 90% absorbed by melanin and hemaglobin (similar to argon), and minimally absorbed by water. The currently available medical KTP laser delivers a maximum of approximately 15 W of power. By varying power output and spot size (power density), one can theoretically, with this laser, achieve either cutting, coagulation, or vaporization. This laser has had fairly extensive use in gynecology (endometriosis), dermatology (hemangiomas and tatoos), and ear, nose, and throat (ENT) (primarily ablative applications). The use of the KTP laser in urology has been minimal. Shanberg and associates have reported 10 patients with urethral strictures that were treated using this laser modality with apparent good results.[108] Theoretically, because of the minimal amount of forward scatter produced by this laser, it could be an improvement over other available laser technologies for the treatment of stricture disease. The KTP laser might also be used either to photocoagulate or vaporize bladder tumors. Because of its minimal penetration (maximum 2 mm), this laser could provide a very reasonable margin of safety when treating noninvasive disease and could obviate the possible complications of bowel perforation. Other obvious miscellaneous uses for this laser in urology would include hemangiomas of the bladder, carcinoma in situ of the bladder, and hemangiomas of the penile skin because of their red color and subsequent high absorbency of this laser wavelength.

## REFERENCES


1. Smith JA, Dixon JA. Tissue effects of lasers in the genitourinary system. In: Smith JA, ed. *Lasers in Urologic Surgery*. Chicago, Ill: Year Book Medical Publishers; 1985.
2. Stein BS, Kendall AR. Lasters in urology. I: Laser physics and safety. *Urology,* 1984; 23:405.
3. Fuller TA. Fundamentals of lasers in surgery and medicine. In: Dixon JA, ed. *Surgical Applications of Lasers*. Chicago, Ill: Year Book Medical Publishers, 1983.
4. Hofstetter A, Frank F. *The Neodymium:YAG Laser in Urology*. Basel, Switzerland: F Hoffman LaRoche and Co Ltd; 1980.
5. Staehler G, Halldorsson T, Langerholc J, Bilgram R. Dosimetry for neodymium:YAG laser applications in urology. *Laser Surg Med.* 1980; 1:191.
6. Berns MW, Wilson M, Rentzepis P, et al. Cell biology of hematoporphyrin derivate (HPD). *Laser Surg Med.* 1983;2:261.
7. Stein BS, Kendall AR. Lasers in urology. II: Laser therapy. *Urology*. 1984;23:411.
8. Stein BS. Unpublished work.
9. Stein BS. Laser dosimetery studies with the Nd:YAG and $CO_2$ lasers: bladder and kidney. *Laser Surg Med.* 1986;6:353–363.
10. Stein BS. Laser physics and tissue interaction. *Urol Clin North Am.* 1986;3:365.
11. Willscher MK. Endoscopic delivery of $CO_2$ laser energy. In: Smith JA, ed. *Lasers in Urologic Surgery*. Chicago, Ill: Year Book Medical Publishers; 1985; chap 11.
12. Stein BS, Kendall AR. Lasers in urology. II: Laser Therapy. *Urology*. 1984;23:411.
13. Hofstetter A, Frank F. Laser uses in urology. In: Dixon JA, ed. *Surgical Application of Lasers*. Chicago, Ill: Year Book Medical Publishers; 1983; chap 8.
14. Smith JA Jr, Dixon JA. Nd:YAG laser treatment of benign urethral strictures. *J Urol.* 1984;131:1080–1082.
15. Bloiso G, Warner R, Cohen M. Treatment of urethral diseases with neodymium:YAG laser. *Urology*. 1988;32:106–110.
16. Shanberg AM, Chalfin SA, Tansey LA. Nd: YAG laser: new treatment for urethral stricture disease. *Urology*. 1984;24:15.
17. Smith JA. Treatment of benign urethral strictures using a sapphire tipped neodymium:YAG laser. *J Urol.* 1989;142:1221–1222.
18. Adkins WC. Argon laser treatment of urethral stricture and vesical neck contracture. *Laser Surg Med.* 1988;8:600–603.
19. Shanberg A, Baghdassarian R, Tansey L, Sawyer D. KTP 532 laser in treatment of urethral strictures. *Urology*. 1988;32:517–520.
20. Shanberg AM, Tansey LA. The use of Nd: YAG laser in prostatotomy. *J Urol.* 1985; 133:196A.
21. Kandel LB, Harrison LH, McCullough DL, et al. Transurethral laser prostatectomy. *J Urol.* 1986;135:110A.
22. Sander S, Beisland H. Laser in the treatment of localized prostatic cancer. *J Urol.* 1984; 132:280–281.
23. Smith JA Jr, Dixon JA. Laser treatment of massive bladder hemangioma. *Urology*. 1984; 24:134.
24. See WA, Chapman WH. Tumor cell implantation following neodymium:YAG bladder in-

jury: a comparison to electrocautery injury. *J Urol.* 1987;137:1266–1269.

25. Malloy TR, Wein AO, Shanberg AM. Superficial transitional cell carcinoma of the bladder treated with a Nd:YAG laser. *J Urol.* 1984;131:251.
26. Hofstetter A. Laser treatment of bladder cancer. Presented at University of Pennsylvania Laser Update: November, 1986; Philadelphia, Pa.
27. Zimmerman I, Stern J, Frank F, et al. Interception of lymphatic drainage by Nd:YAG laser in rat urinary cancer. *Laser Surg Med.* 1984;4:169.
28. Smith JA, Middleton RG. Adequacy of tumor staging after laser treatment of superficial transitional cell carcinoma of the bladder. *J Endourol.* 1988;2:403–406.
29. Smith JA Jr. Laser treatment of invasive bladder cancer. *J Urol.* 1986;135:55–57.
30. McPhee MS, Arnfield MR, Tulip J, Lakey WH. Neodymium:YAG laser therapy for infiltrating bladder cancer. *J Urol.* 1988;140:44–46.
31. Rosemberg SK. Subclinical papilloma viral infection of male genitalia. *Urology.* 1985; 26:554.
32. Carpiniello V, Sedlacek TV, Cunnane M, et al. Magnified penile surface scanning in diagnosis of penile condyloma. *Urology.* 1986; 28:190.
33. Rosemberg SK. Sexually transmitted papillomaviral infections. III: Management of male partner. *Urology.* 1988;31:375–378.
34. Rosemberg SK, Fuller T, Jacobs H. Continuous wave carbon dioxide laser treatment of giant condylomata acuminata of the distal urethra and perineum: technique. *J Urol.* 1980;126:827.
35. Amagi T, Onoe Y, Okada K, et al. Laser application for urological diseases. Presented at the Fourth Congress of the International Society for Laser Surgery and Medicine. 1981; Tokyo.
36. Rosemberg SK. The use of the $CO_2$ laser in urology. *Laser Surg Med.* 1983;3:114.
37. Lundquist SG, Lindstedt EM. Laser treatment of condylomata acuminata. *Laser Surg Med.* 1983;3:152.
38. Stein BS. Laser treatment of condylomata acuminata. *J Urol.* 1986;136:593.
39. Hofstetter A, Frank F. *The Neodymium-YAG Laser in Urology.* Basle, Switzerland, Roche; 1980.
40. Bandieramonte G, Lepera P, Marchesini R, Andreola S, Pizzocaro G. Laser microsurgery for superficial lesions of the penis. *J Urol.* 1987;138:315–319.
41. Numata I, Tanahashi Y, Harada K, et al. Laser therapy for carcinoma of the penis. Presented at the Fourth Congress of the International Society for Laser Surgery and Medicine; 1981; Tokyo.
42. Mulvaney WP, Beck CW. The laser beam in urology. *J Urol.* 1968;99:112.
43. Hughes BF, Scott WW. Preliminary report on the use of the $CO_2$ laser surgical unit in animals. *Invest Urol.* 1972;9:353.
44. Meiraz D, Peled I, Gassner S, et al. The use of the $CO_2$ laser for partial nephrectomy: an experimental study. *Invest Urol.* 1977;15:262.
45. Barzilay B, Lojovetzky G, Perlberg S, et al. Comparative experimental study on the use of the carbon dioxide laser beam in partial nephrectomy. *Laser Surg Med.* 1982;2:73.
46. Pariente R, d'Ovidio M; cited by Willscher MK. Endoscopic delivery of $CO_2$ laser surgery. In: Smith JA, ed. *Lasers in Urologic Surgery.* Chicago, Ill: Year Book Medical Publishers; 1985;138–150.
47. Barzilay B, Lijovetzky G, Shapiro A, et al. The clinical use of $CO_2$ laser beam in the surgery of kidney parenchyma. *Laser Surg Med.* 1982;2:81.
48. Hall RR. Report to the standing committee on urological instruments: lasers in urology. *Br J Urol.* 1982;54:421.
49. Rosemberg SK, Lutz SJ. Some clinical applications of carbon dioxide laser in urologic surgery. *Urology,* 1984;23:240.
50. Rosemberg SK. Clinical experience with carbon dioxide laser in renal surgery. *Urology.* 1985;25:115.
51. Benderev TV, Schaeffer AJ. Efficacy and safety of the Nd:YAG laser in canine partial nephrectomy. *J Urol.* 1985;133:1108.
52. Melzer RB, Wood TW, Landau ST, et al. Combination of CUSA and neodymium:YAG laser for canine partial nephrectomy. *J Urol.* 1985; 134:620.
53. Hofstetter A, Frank F. Laser use in urology. In: Dixon JA, ed. *Surgical Application of Lasers.* Chicago, Ill: Year Book Medical Publishers; 1983;146–162.
54. Malloy TR. Laser treatment of ureter and upper collecting system. In: Smith JA, ed. *Lasers in Urologic Surgery.* Chicago, Ill: Year Book Medical Publishers; 1985;82–83.
55. Landau ST, Wood TW, Smith JA. Evaluation of sapphire tip Nd:YAG laser fibers in partial nephrectomy. *Laser Surg Med.* 1987;7:426–428.
56. Rothenberger K, Pensel J, Hofstetter A, et al. Transurethral laser coagulation for treatment of urinary bladder tumors. *Laser Surg Med.* 1983;2:255.
57. Hofstetter A. Laser application for destroying ureter tumors. *Laser Surg Med.* 1983;2:255A.
58. Bowering R, Hofstetter A, Keiditsche E, et al. Treatment of ureteral tumors by endoscopic neodymium:YAG laser irradiation. *J Urol.* 1985;133(4)(pt 2):236A.
59. Benson RC. Mayo Clinic, Jacksonville, Fla. Personal communication.

60. Korth K. Frieburg, West Germany. Personal communication.

61. Smith JA, Lee RG, Dixon JA. Tissue effects of neodymium:YAG laser photoradiation of canine ureters. *J Surg Oncol.* 1984;27:168.

62. Tanahashi Y, Numata Kambe K, Harada K, et al; cited in Hall RR. Report to the standing committee on urological instruments: lasers in urology. *Br J Urol.* 1982;54:421.

63. Pensel J, Frank F, Rothenberger KH, et al; cited in Hall RR. Report to the standing committee on urological instruments: lasers in urology. *Br J Urol.* 1982;54:421.

64. Watson GM. Laser fragmentation of urinary calculi. In: Smith JA, ed. *Lasers in Urologic Surgery*. Chicago, Ill: Year Book Medical Publishers, 1985;125–138.

65. Hofmann R, Hartung R, Braun J, et al. Laser-induced shock wave lithotripsy. *J Urol.* 1987;13:279A.

66. Watson GM, Dretler SP, Parrish JA. The pulsed dye laser fragmentation of urinary calculi. *J Urol.* 1987;137:386–389.

67. Watson GM, Murray S, Dretler SP, et al. Laser fragmentation of ureteral calculi. *J Urol.* 1986;135:210A.

68. Dretler SP, Watson G, Parrish J, et al. Laser fragment of ureteral calculi: initial experience. *J Urol.* 1987;137:386.

69. Dretler SP. Laser photofragmentation of ureteral calculi: analysis of 75 cases. *J Endourol* 1987;1(1):9–14.

70. Dretler SP. Techniques of laser lithotripsy. *J Endourol.* 1988;2:123–128.

71. Bagley DH, Grasso M, Shalaby M, El-Akkad MA. Ureteral laser lithotripsy using the pulsolith. *J Endourol.* 1989;3:91–98.

72. Chapman W, Mayo M, Brooks R, et al. An outline of the physics of the Dormia lithotripter and some possible alternatives. In: de Vere White R, Palma JM eds. *New Techniques in Urology*. Mount Lisco, Wy: Futima Publishing Co; 1987; Chap 6:63–73.

73. Blum HF. *Phodynamic Action and Diseases Caused by Light.* New York: Reinhold;1941.

74. Auler H, Banzer G. Untersuchungen über die rolle der prophyrine bei geschwulsterkranken menschen und tieren. *Z Krebsforsch.* 1942; 53:65.

75. Figge FHJ, Weiland GS, Manganiello LOJ. Cancer detection and therapy: affinity of neoplastic embryonic and traumatized tissues for porphyrins and metalloporphyrins. *Proc Soc Exp Biol Med.* 1948;68:640.

76. Lipson RL. *The Photodynamic and Fluorescent Properties of a Particular Hematoporphyrin Derivative and Its Use in Tumor Detection.* Rochester, Minn: Mayo Graduate School of Medicine; 1959. Thesis.

77. Mellors RC, Glassman A, Papanicolau GN. A microgluorometric scanning method for the detection of cancer cells in smears of exfoliated cells. *Cancer.* 1952;5:458.

78. Moore GE. *Diagnosis and Localization of Brain Tumors: A Clinical and Experimental Study Employing Fluorescent and Radioactive Tracer Methods.* Springfield, Ill: Chas C Thomas;1953.

79. Policard A. Etude sur les aspects offerts par des tumeurs experimentales examinees a la luminere de Wood. *Compi Rend Soc Biol.* 1924;91:1423.

80. Tomson SH, Emmett EA, Fox SH. Photodestruction of mouse epithelial tumors after oral acridine orange and argon laser. *Cancer Res.* 1974;34:3124.

81. Benson RC Jr, Farrow GM, Kinsey JH, et al. Detection and localization of in situ carcinoma of the bladder with hematoporphyrin derivative. *Mayo Clin Proc.* 1982;57:548.

82. Kelly JF, Snell ME. Hematoporphyrin derivative: A possible aid in the diagnosis and therapy of carcinoma of the bladder. *J Urol.* 1976;115:150–151.

83. Tsuchiya A, Obara N, Miwa M, et al. Hematoporphyrin derivative and laser photoradiation in the diagnosis and treatment of bladder cancer. *J Urol.* 1983;130:79–82.

84. Hisazumi H, Misaki T, Miyoshi N. Photoradiation therapy of bladder tumors. *J Urol.* 1983;130:685.

85. Benson RC Jr. Photochemotherapy of bladder cancer. In: Spitzy KH, Karrer K, eds. Proceedings of the 13th International Congress on Chemotherapy: August 28–September 2, 1983; Vienna, Austria.

86. Benson RC Jr, Kinsey JH, Cortese DA, et al. Treatment of transitional cell carcinoma of the bladder with hematoporphyrin derivative phototherapy. *J Urol.* 1983;130:1090.

87. Jocham D, Staehler G, Chausz C, et al. Integral dye-laser irradiation of photosensitized bladder tumors with the aid of a light-scattering medium. In: Doran DR, Gomer CJ, eds. Porphyrin localization and treatment of tumors. New York, NY: Alan P. Liss; 1984;249–256.

88. Baghdassarian R, Wright MW, Vaughn SA, et al. The use of lipid emulsion as an intravesical medium to disperse light in the potential treatment of bladder tumors. *J Urol.* 1985;133:126.

89. Misaki T, Hisazumi H, Hirata A, et al. Photodynamic therapy for superficial bladder tumors. First International Conference on the Clinical Applications of Photosensitization for Diagnosis and Treatment; April 30–May 2, 1986; Tokyo, Japan.

90. Benson RC Jr. Endoscopic management of bladder cancer with hematoporphyrin derivative phototherapy. In: Symposium in Advances in the Management of Urothelial Cancer. *Urol Clin North Am.* 1984;11(4)(Nov):637–642.

91. Benson RC Jr. Treatment of diffuse transitional

cell carcinoma in situ by whole bladder hematoporphyrin derivative photodynamic therapy. *J Urol.* 1985;134:675–678.

92. Benson RC Jr. Photodynamic therapy in bladder cancer. Clayton Foundation Conference on Photodynamic Therapy; February 15–19, 1987; Los Angeles, Calif.
93. Shumaker BPS, Hetzel FW, Mattielo J. The practical clinical use of laser photodynamic therapy in the treatment of bladder carcinoma in situ. The First International Conference on the Clinical Applications of Photosensitization for Diagnosis and Treatment; April 30–May 2, 1986; Tokyo, Japan.
94. Nseyo UO, Dougherty TJ, Boyle DE, et al. Whole bladder photodynamic therapy for transitional cell carcinoma of the bladder. *Urology.* 1985;26:274–280.
95. Jain KK, Gorish W. Microvascular repair with neodymium-YAG laser. *Acta Neurochirurgia (Wein).* 1979;28(suppl)260.
96. Jain KK. Sutureless microvascular anastomosis using a neodymium-YAG laser. *J Microsurg.* 1980;1:436.
97. Stein BS, Cooley BC. Carbon dioxide laser-assisted microscopic vasovasostomy. *J Endourol.* 1988;2:299–307.
98. Poppas DP, Schlossberg SM, Richmond IL, Gilbert DA, Devine CJ. Laser welding in urethral surgery: improved results with a protein solder. *J Urol.* 1988;139:415–417.
99. Frazier OH, Painviw GA, Morris JR, et al. Laser-assisted microvascular anastomoses: angiographic and anatomopagthologic studies on growing microvascular anastomoses: preliminary report. *Surgery.* 1985;(May):585–590.
100. Gomes OM, Macruz R. Armelin E, et al. Vascular anastomosis by argon laser beam. *Tex Heart Inst J.* 1983;10:145.
101. Lynne CM, Carter M, Morris J, et al. Laser-assisted vas anastomosis: a preliminary report. *Laser Surg Med.* 1983;3:261.
102. Rosemberg SK, Elson L, Nathan LE Jr. Carbon dioxide laser microsurgical vasovasostomy. *Urology.* 1985;25(1):53.
103. Rosemberg S. Further clinical experience with $CO_2$ laser in microsurgical vasovasostomy. *Sterility & Fertility.* 1988;32:225–227.
104. Seidmon J. Ureteral welding with the $CO_2$ laser. *J Urol.* 1986(April);135:172A.
105. Merguerian PA, Rabinowitz R. The $CO_2$ laser in the sutureless welding anastomosis of dismembered rabbit ureters. *J Urol.* 1986 (April);135:171A.
106. Daikuzono N, Joffe SN. Artificial sapphire probe for contact photocoagulation and tissue vaporization with the Nd:YAG laser. *Med Instrum.* 1985;19:173.
107. Stokes L, Auth D, Tanaka O, et al. Biomedical utiligy of 1.34 μm Nd:YAG laser radiation.
108. Shanberg A, Tansey L, Baghdassarian R. Use of the KTP 532 in the treatment of urethral stricture disease. *J Urol.* 1987(April); 137:166A.

# 41

# Laparoscopic Urologic Surgery

*Louis R. Kavoussi and Kevin R. Loughlin*

## INTRODUCTION

Laparoscopic surgery has been an integral part of gynecologic practice for several decades. However, it is only relatively recently that it has begun to be applied to the other surgical specialties including urology. This type of surgical approach has several advantages over traditional open surgery due to its minimally invasive nature, resulting in less postoperative discomfort, less disfigurement, and quicker convalescence.

Unfortunately, most urologic surgeons have not had formal instruction in laparoscopic surgery during their training and may not be familiar with instrumentation and operative techniques. It is extremely important to understand and master the basic principles of laparoscopic surgery in order to avoid serious complications. This chapter will attempt to serve as an introduction to laparoscopic urologic surgery. Basic techniques in the performance of laparoscopy will be reviewed and current applications of laparoscopic surgery in urology will be presented.

## PATIENT SELECTION

Patient selection is crucial to assure a successful outcome of any urologic laparoscopic procedure and one needs to recognize instances in which this procedure is contraindicated. All patients should be evaluated by the anesthetic team preoperatively and be deemed adequate candidates for a general endotracheal anesthesia.

Patients who have had multiple prior abdominal surgeries or peritonitis should be approached with great caution since they have a high likelihood of having multiple adhesions to the abdominal wall making trocar placement dangerous. Likewise, for similar reasons, patients with dilated bowel secondary to functional or mechanical obstruction should not undergo laparoscopic surgery. Laparoscopic surgery should also be avoided in patients with severe cardiopulmonary disease since the pneumoperitoneum may further embarrass ventilation and cause compression of the vena cava, which may markedly decrease venous return to the heart.[1] Moreover, uncorrected coagulopathy or hypovolemic shock are considered absolute contraindications to laparoscopic surgery.

There are certain relative contraindications to laparoscopic surgery including the existence of large abdominal masses or aneurysms. Patients who are markedly obese also fall into this category, since the higher pressure required to achieve an adequate pneumoperitoneum could cause problems with venous return and ventilation. Likewise, patients with mild chronic obstructive pulmonary disease (COPD) and pulmonary hypertension should be considered relative risks for laparoscopic surgery.

## PATIENT PREPARATION

All patients should be fully informed of the nature and risks of operative laparoscopy including the possibility of requiring an emergent laparotomy. This latter risk is not uncommon, especially when one is first beginning to perform this type of surgery.

Bowel preparation varies with surgeon preference and operative procedure. For relatively minor pelvic procedures such as the laparoscopic lymph node dissection or varix ligation, two Fleet enemas the night prior to the planned surgery are sufficient. This helps decompress the bowel, particularly the sigmoid colon and rectum, to facilitate pelvic dissection. For patients undergoing more advanced laparoscopic procedures (ie, nephrectomy, nephroureterectomy, retroperitoneal node dissection, ureteral surgery), a full bowel preparation should be implemented. This decompresses the bowel to increase the working space within the intra-abdominal cavity and allows for conservative management in the event of a bowel injury. At our institution, Brigham and Women's Hospital, the full bowel preparation consists of a clear liquid diet and 4 L of GoLytely the day before surgery. One gram each of neomycin and erythromycin is also administered in three divided doses on the day before surgery. All patients should be typed and screened for blood in the event of unexpected hemorrhage. For more advanced procedures, a cross-match should be completed. Preoperatively patients are given one parenteral dose of a broad-spectrum antibiotic (cephalozin 1 g). All patients should be evaluated by the anesthetic team preoperatively and be deemed adequate candidates for a general endotracheal anesthesia.

Patients are initially placed in the supine position on the operating table. Lower extremity sequential compression stockings should be utilized to decrease the risk of venous thrombosis. An indwelling Foley catheter is placed to drain the bladder. Likewise a nasogastric tube is positioned to keep the stomach decompressed. The table is initially placed in 10° Trendelenburg position to shift the bowel from the pelvis prior to Veress needle placement. The patient should undergo a full abdominal preparation in the event that an emergency laparotomy is required. Also, in this regard a full laparotomy set should be available in the operating room. Figure 1 indicates physician positioning for urologic laparoscopic pelvic procedures.

Laparoscopic procedures should be done under a general endotracheal anesthetic. This allows for controlled ventilation, ensures adequate oxygenation, and minimizes the risk of hypercarbia.

## ESTABLISHING THE PNEUMOPERITONEUM

The first step in performing laparoscopy is achieving the pneumoperitoneum. The surgeon's hand dominance dictates where he or she should stand relative to the patient. A right-handed physician should stand on the patient's left side, and a left-handed physician on the patient's right side. The patient's abdomen should be palpated to rule out any underlying masses (ie, aortic aneurysm, tumor) before passing the insufflation needle or trocars.

The most common needle used for insufflation is the Veress needle (Fig 2). The Veress needle is constructed of an outer sheath with a sharp beveled edge and a retractable inner blunt tip. When pressure

**Fig 1.** The physician location for urologic laparoscopic pelvic procedures. The surgeon stands on the opposite side of the pelvis from which the pathology is being approached. His assistant stands across the table, and, if a cameraman is present, he is positioned above the surgeon.

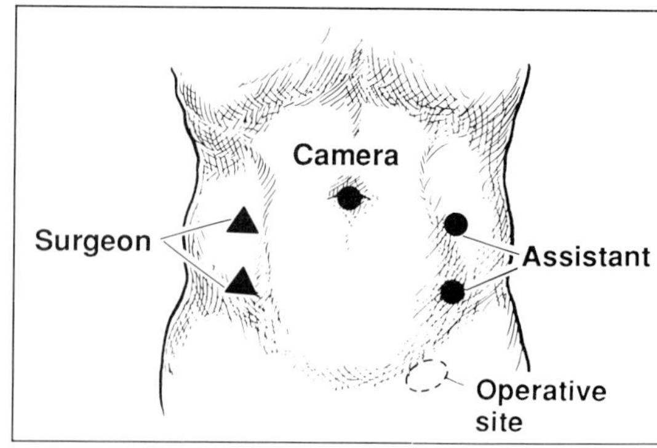

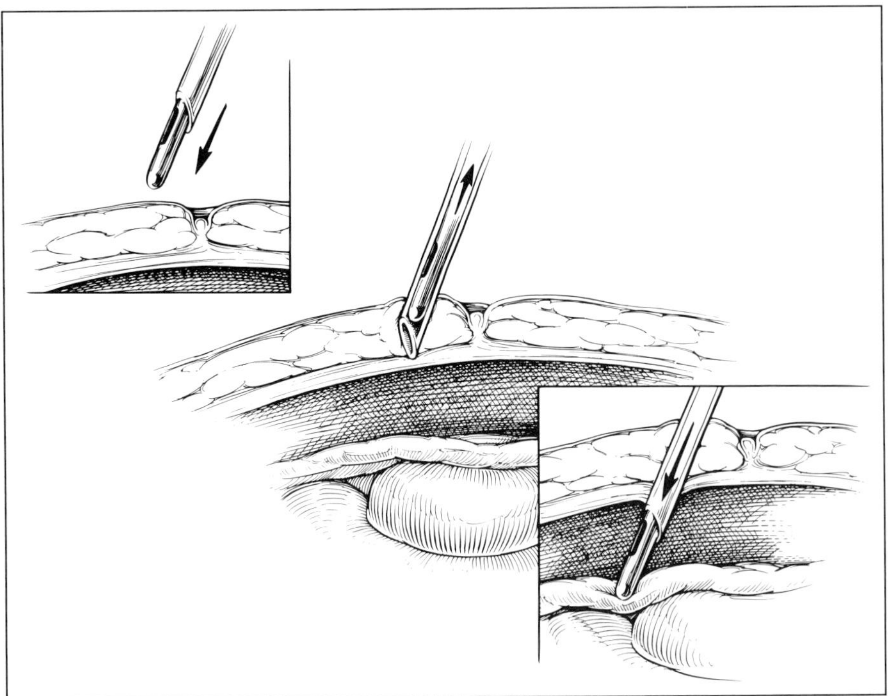

**Fig 2.** The Veress needle for insufflation is shown. The inner core is spring-loaded and retracts when it meets resistance to expose the outer beveled needle.

is applied to the tip of the needle, the blunt core retracts exposing the sharp outer tip that pierces through the abdominal fascia. Once the needle penetrates the peritoneal cavity, the blunt core snaps forward to protect underlying structures from injury. The Veress needle is of a small bore (usually 14 gauge) and comes in standard lengths of 12 and 15 cm. Both disposable and reusable Veress needles are available. The reusable needles tend to dull with use.

The Veress needle should be tested for patency and proper function prior to use. It is usually inserted through the base of the umbilicus since this is where the peritoneum is most adherent to the abdominal fascia. The lower edge of umbilicus is tented upward when passing the needle. Since the aortic bifurcation usually directly underlies the umbilicus, the needle should be angled slightly toward the pelvis. Usually two clicks can be heard as the blunt core of the needle springs forward when passing through the abdominal wall fascia and peritoneum.

When scars are present in the area of the umbilicus, an alternate location of the needle placement is necessary to avoid injury to the underlying viscera. The needle may be placed in the mammary lines above the level of the umbilicus, the cul-de-sac, or the superumbilical midline.

Once the needle is passed through the abdominal wall, one must ensure that it is in the proper location prior to insufflation. The needle should move freely in the peritoneal cavity. Saline (5 $cm^3$) injected through the needle should flow easily and not aspirate. Incorrect needle placement may be identified by aspirating fluid, bowel content, gas, urine, or blood. A drop of saline placed at the opening of the Veress needle should flow easily into the peritoneal cavity while lifting the abdominal wall. Once one is relatively certain the needle is in the proper position, insufflation may commence.

Currently two gases are commonly utilized for laparoscopic insufflation: carbon dioxide and nitrous oxide. Carbon dioxide is the more frequently used since it dissolves rapidly in the bloodstream, decreasing the risk of pulmonary embolization. Furthermore, unlike nitrous oxide, carbon dioxide does not support combustion, so that electric cautery and laser can be used safely in its presence.

The main drawbacks of carbon dioxide are that it is a peritoneal irritant which, if significantly absorbed, can cause life-threatening metabolic disorders.[2] Due to these shortcomings, some laparoscopists have used nitrous oxide as the insufflant. It is not a peritoneal irritant and does not result in metabolic abnormalities. Unfortunately, nitrous oxide is somewhat less soluble in blood than carbon dioxide and theoretically there is a higher risk of gas embolism. Moreover, there is a small but real risk of explosion with the use of nitrous oxide in the presence of electric cautery. This gas may be well suited for short procedures performed under a local anesthetic.

The insufflant gas is transmitted from the source (gas tank) to the intraabdominal cavity by an insufflator. The insufflator is an electronic valve that gates the flow of pressurized gas from the tank into the patient's abdomen (Fig 3). All modern insufflators simultaneously measure intra-abdominal pressure and can be set such that gas flow into the peritoneal cavity shuts off if the measured pressure is increased above a preset value.

The initial gas flow setting should be 1 L/min, and at this rate the intra-abdominal pressure should measure less than 10 mm Hg. Higher pressures indicate improper needle placement and the needle should be repositioned accordingly. When 500 $cm^3$ of gas has been insufflated, a gradual increase in tympany can be observed over the four abdominal quadrants and at this point the flow rate can be increased to 10 L/min. The amount of gas necessary to achieve adequate pneumoperitoneum varies with patient body habitus, but averages anywhere from 4 to 8 L in the adult male. Insufflation is complete when the preset intra-abdominal pressure has been reached and no further gas enters the peritoneal cavity.

The intra-abdominal pressure should be maintained at less than 15 mm Hg during the procedure. At prolonged higher pressures the patient is at increased risk of gas absorption and hypercarbia.[1,2] Impaired ventilation may occur due to increased pressure on the diaphragm. This may necessitate increasing ventilatory pressure and put the patient at risk for developing pneumothorax. Moreover, the increased pressure decreases venous return secondary to caval compression.[1]

For pediatric applications, the pressure should be maintained at less than 10 mm Hg. Higher pressures are problematic, and, especially in infants, can lead to difficulties with ventilation, impaired venous return, and hypercarbia.

In preparing for initial trocar placement the intra-abdominal pressure may be tran-

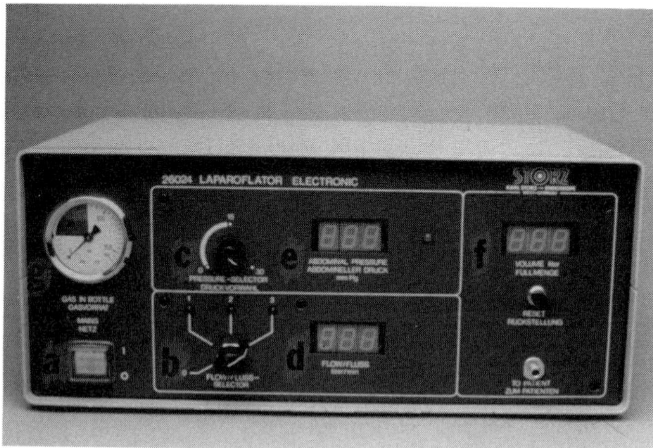


**Fig 3.** All insufflators have certain basic controls: A, power switch; B, flow control; C, pressure setting above which insufflator will stop flow of gas; D, monitor of flow rate; E, monitor of intra-abdominal pressure from tank; F, monitor of amount of gas utilized; G, gauge of line pressure from tank.

siently elevated to 25 mm Hg to allow the peritoneum to adhere closely to the posterior fascia. Care must be taken to lower the pressure once the initial camera trocar is in position.

## TROCAR PLACEMENT

Trocars are the surgeon's access into the peritoneal cavity and are designed to serve several important functions (Fig 4A). First, they are means to maintain the pneumoperitoneum once the Veress needle is removed. Trocars also allow passage of the laparoscope and surgical instruments into the intra-abdominal cavity. Finally, the trocars are the avenue by which dissected tissue can be removed from the operative site.

The basic trocar is a hollow tube with a valve mechanism built into the handle and a sharpened removable inner obturator. The internal valve in conjunction with a series of gaskets prevents gas from leaking out of the peritoneal cavity. Most trocars contain an external one-way valve with a Luer-lock fitting. This can be connected to the insufflator tubing to maintain gas flow for pneumoperitoneum during the procedure.

Disposable and nondisposable trocars are available from a variety of manufacturers. The nondisposable trocars are made of metal and thus are heavier than their plastic disposable counterparts. The metal reusable trocars are also radiopaque and are a disadvantage if one needs to perform intraoperative radiography. The tips of the nondisposable units tend to dull with use and need to be sharpened periodically. Data exist demonstrating that increased force is necessary to introduce these trocars through the fascia compared to disposable trocars.[3]

An important feature of the disposable trocars is a plastic safety shield over the obturator (Fig 4B). This shield retracts as pressure is applied exposing the sharp tip. Once the obturator has pierced the fascia, the outer safety shield snaps back forward and locks into position to protect underlying structures from injury by the obturator tip.

There are several techniques for trocar placement. The most common method of trocar insertion commences once adequate pneumoperitoneum has been achieved. The patient is placed in steep Trendelenburg position and an incision is made in the umbilical area just sufficient to admit the trocar. The incision should be taken through the subcutaneous layer and then a straight clamp can be used to spread away underlying superficial abdominal wall vessels. At this point some surgeons will make a small incision in the abdominal wall fascia to decrease the force necessary to push the trocar through the abdominal wall. The surgeon should hold the trocar in the dominant hand and stand on the patient's opposite side (ie, a right-handed surgeon should be on the patient's left, and a left-handed surgeon should be on the patient's right). Towel clips may be applied on either side of the incision to elevate the abdominal wall to facilitate trocar placement. The index finger should be extended along the side of the shaft to prevent the trocar from advancing too deeply once the peritoneal cavity is entered. Alternatively, the nondominant hand may be utilized as a brake. The trocar is placed in the incision and is pushed into the peritoneum utilizing a rotation motion while applying constant pressure forward. Once the peritoneal cavity is entered and the obturator removed, carbon dioxide should be heard escaping from the trocar when the valve is opened. The insufflator is then connected via tubing to the Luer-lock fitting on the trocar. Once the initial trocar is in position, the laparoscope is introduced and the abdominal cavity inspected to rule out any injury that may have occurred during Veress needle or trocar placement.

Some surgeons will place the initial trocar without first creating a pneumoperitoneum.[4] The skin incision is made and the abdominal wall lifted with the nondominant hand while forward pressure is exerted on the trocar. This potentially decreases risks involved in creating the pneumoperitoneum.

An alternative method for placing the initial trocar is via an open technique.[5] This is useful in patients who have had prior abdominal surgery and some surgeons pref-

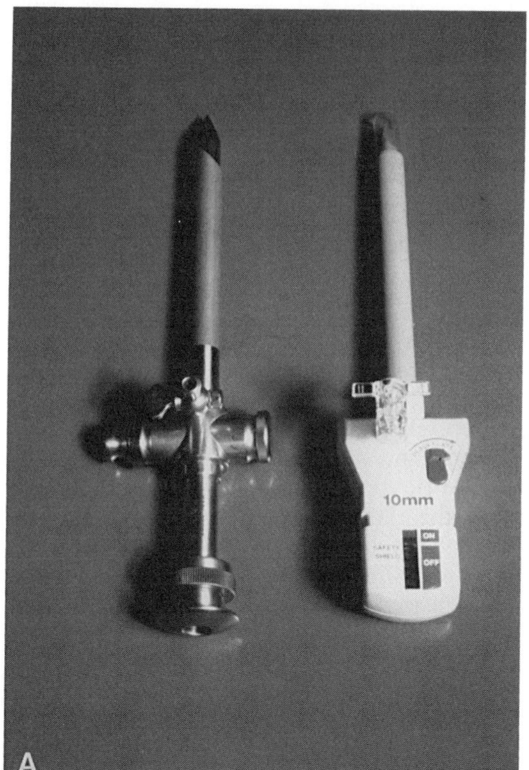


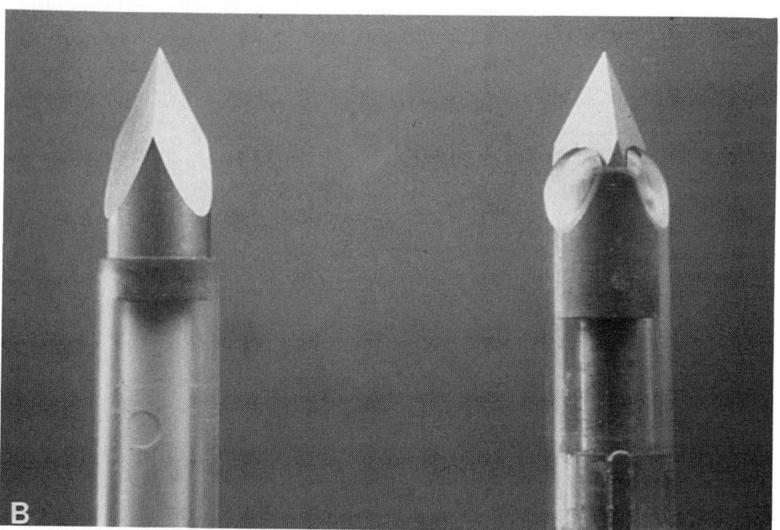

**Fig 4. A,** disposable (right) and nondisposable (left) trocars. As the plastic protector sheath meets resistance it retracts, exposing the sharpened inner tip **(B).**

erentially use this approach in all patients undergoing laparoscopy. A specially designed Hassan cannula that has a blunt obturator and adjustable outer sleeve is utilized (Fig 5). Placement involves first making a 2- to 3-cm skin incision down to the level of the fascia. A zero silk suture is placed on either side of the fascia, which is then incised. The peritoneum is then grasped and incised just wide enough to allow the trocar to enter. A finger is placed in the peritoneal cavity to be sure there is

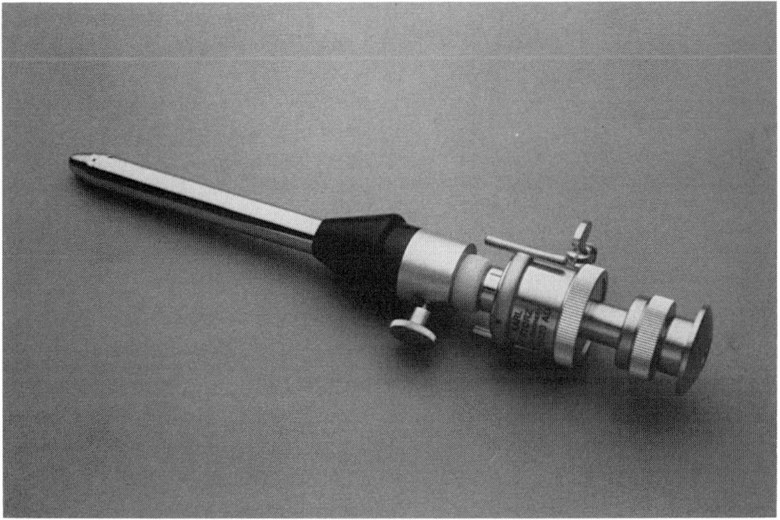

**Fig 5.** The Hassan cannula is a specially designed laparascope.

no underlying adherent bowel. The Hassan trocar is placed in the opening of the peritoneum and the sleeve on the trocar is cinched down while the fascial stitches are pulled up. The stitches are then wrapped around holders built onto the trocar or sleeve to fix the cannula in place and seal the peritoneal cavity.

Once the laparoscope is in position, additional trocar sites may be placed under direct vision. Again, in patients who have had prior surgery, scars should be avoided since there is a high likelihood of injury to underlying viscera. Location of accessory trocars varies with the surgical procedure being performed. For diagnostic laparoscopy, the umbilical camera trocar may be sufficient. Alternatively, an additional trocar site may be necessary to pass instruments, retract bowel, or take biopsies.

When choosing sites for accessory trocars, care must be taken not to place these too close together or between the camera port and the operative site. In general, when working in the pelvis a diamond or fan configuration for trocars will allow maximal access for dissection (Fig 6). Similarly, when working on the upper ureter or kidney

**Fig 6.** The diamond and fan trocar configurations for pelvic urologic procedures. The squares represent 10-mm ports, the circles represent 5-mm ports.

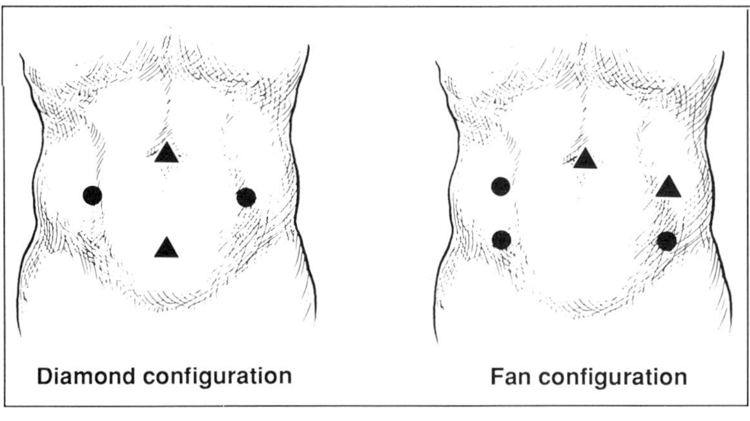

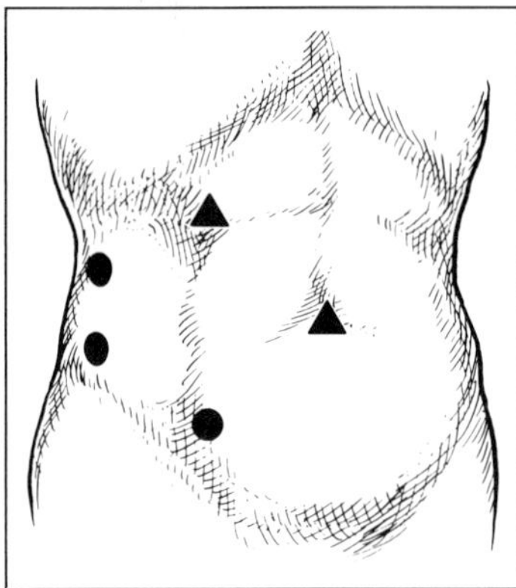

**Fig 7.** Trocar configuration utilized while approaching the flank or retroperitoneum. Triangles represent 12-mm ports, circles represent 5-mm ports.

a diamond configuration in the flank area is advisable (Fig 7).

Once a trocar site is chosen, the light from the endoscope should be shown underneath the planned puncture site to identify overlying superficial abdominal wall vessels. The peritoneal surface should also be inspected to avoid inadvertently injuring an epigastric vessel. An incision is made along Langer's lines to optimize the postoperative cosmetic result. Secondary trocars are passed as was the initial trocar. To avoid injury to underlying structures, care must be taken to continuously observe the position of the tip while the trocar is being placed.

If a trocar is accidentally pulled from the abdominal cavity, the obturator should be replaced and the trocar guided through the original puncture site under endoscopic control. A variety of methods have been developed to prevent trocars from inadvertently coming out of the intraperitoneal cavity during dissection. Special sleeves or self-retaining trocars are available that screw into the abdominal wall to minimize problems with trocar slippage. Newer trocars are available with balloons or malecot tips that prevent inadvertent removal from the abdominal cavity. We preferentially use a 2–0 Vicryl suture to secure the trocar to the abdominal wall.[6]

Occasionally gas will leak around the trocar site leading to problems maintaining a pneumoperitoneum. A purse string stitch placed about the trocar may be helpful to obtain a seal. Alternatively, bone wax or petroleum jelly gauze can be wrapped around the insertion site to prevent loss of pneumoperitoneum.

## CONCLUSION OF LAPAROSCOPIC PROCEDURES

Several steps must be followed when concluding any diagnostic or therapeutic laparoscopic procedure. The abdomen must be thoroughly inspected to ensure that no inadvertent vascular or bowel injury has been caused during the operation. Surgical areas should be inspected for adequate hemostasis. It is helpful to lower the intra-abdominal pressure to below 7 mm Hg and observe the operative site for bleeding that may have been tamponaded by the pneumoperitoneum.

All trocar sites including the initial camera port should be inspected prior to closure. Trocars should be removed under direct vision since a trocar may tamponade an abdominal wall blood vessel. If a hematoma or bleeding is noted around a port site, one should suspect an injury to an underlying abdominal wall vessel.

Prior to removing the final trocar, $CO_2$ should be removed from the peritoneal cavity since it is an irritant and may cause postoperative abdominal or shoulder pain (due to diaphragmatic irritation). The final trocar should be slipped over the laparoscope and the laparoscope backed out slowly through the port site. In this way no bowel is pulled into the incision and inspection of the tract for bleeding can be performed.

The anterior fascia of the larger trocar sites (ie, greater than or equal to 10 mm) should be closed under direct vision. Port sites should be irrigated as with any surgical procedure and checked for adequate hemostasis. The skin may then be reapproximated with tape strips or subcuticular suture.

## POSTOPERATIVE CARE

The nasogastric tube and Foley catheter can be removed in the recovery room once the patient is deemed stable. Two doses of broad-spectrum antibiotic are given postoperatively. Oral intake can usually resume the evening of surgery for most pelvic laparoscopic procedures. For more involved retroperitoneal operations, feeding can begin once signs of bowel activity return.

Postoperative pain is usually minimal. If a patient requires significant narcotic analgesia in the postoperative period, one should suspect an underlying pathologic process. Patients are allowed to resume usual activities as tolerated.

## COMPLICATIONS

Complications can occur during one of four phases of laparoscopy: needle or trocar placement, insufflation, dissection, and closure. Moreover, as with any surgical procedure, anesthetic complications can occur. Patient positioning is crucial, and all patients should be adequately secured to the operation table. Appropriate padding should be utilized to avoid neuromuscular injury.

### Needle and Trocar Injuries

While passing the Veress needle or trocar, it is possible to injure underlying structures and several precautions need to be taken to avoid these injuries.[7] As stated above, a Foley catheter and oral gastric tube are placed to decrease the possible risk of injuring a visceral structure during needle or trocar placement.

Prior to placing any needles, the abdomen should be inspected and palpated. Placement of needles or trocars in the area of a mass should be avoided. Additionally, any scars noted on the abdominal wall from prior surgery should be avoided since underlying bowel or omentum may be adherent. After the Veress needle is placed, tests as outlined above should be performed to assure that it is in proper position.

When placing trocars, a finger should be placed alongside the sheath to serve as a brake to prevent advancing too deeply and causing injury to the underlying structures. Using disposable trocars with a safety shield as the initial trocar for blind placement may be helpful in decreasing injury to underlying structures.

Despite these precautions, injuries may occur to underlying structures. A viscus may be perforated by either a Veress needle or a trocar[7,8] (Fig 8). A Veress needle injury to the bowel is usually small enough to heal with conservative management. However, if a trocar is passed through a bowel the safest course of action is to perform an open repair.

Bladder injuries may present with intra-

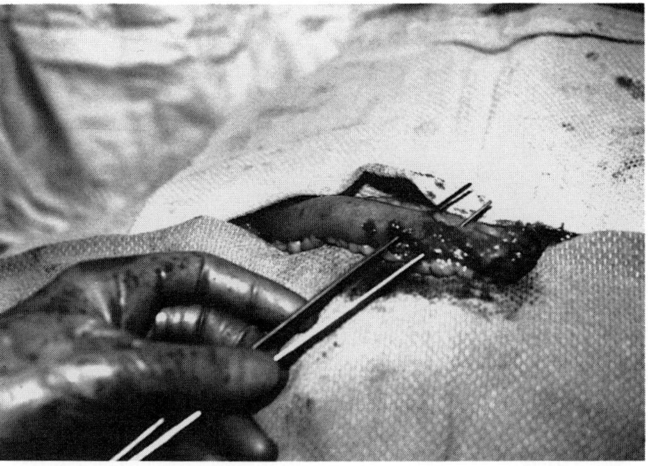

**Fig 8.** Photograph of a through-and-through bowel injury due to a trocar. In this instance, resection of the bowel with reanastomosis was necessary.

operative hematuria or pneumaturia noted in the Foley drainage system.[9] If suspected, methylene blue can be instilled into the bladder and any leakage into the peritoneal cavity can be identified laparoscopically.

A Veress needle injury to the bladder usually heals spontaneously. If a trocar is passed through the bladder, attempts at laparoscopic repair may be undertaken. Endoscopic clips can be applied to reapproximate the edges of small bladder injuries; otherwise laparoscopic suturing or open repair is required.[10]

Unfortunately, many times bowel and bladder injuries are not noted until the postoperative period. With bowel injuries, a patient may have persistent pain, fever, and peritoneal signs. In this circumstance the patient should undergo immediate exploration and repair. Bladder injuries can also be missed intraoperatively. If hematuria develops postoperatively a cystogram should be obtained. When extravasation is noted, conservative management consisting of antibiotics and catheter drainage may be attempted; however, in some instances patients require secondary laparoscopic or open repair.

Vascular injuries are the second most common complication reported in the gynecologic literature.[11] If upon placement of the Veress needle, blood is aspirated, the safest course of action is to leave the needle in place and perform a laparotomy. The needle will lead the surgeon directly to the area of injury. If the needle passes in and out of a vessel one may not note intraperitoneal bleeding but may notice a retroperitoneal hematoma. A trocar passed through a major vascular structure represents a true laparoscopic emergency and immediate laparotomy should be performed.

Not uncommonly, anterior abdominal wall vessels are injured by trocar placement. If bleeding is minor, fulguration can be attempted laparoscopically. If the bleeding is moderate or severe, a transcutaneous stitch may be passed using either a Keith needle or a Stamey needle[12] (Fig 9). This stitch can be tied over a bolster placed on the abdominal wall and removed 2 weeks

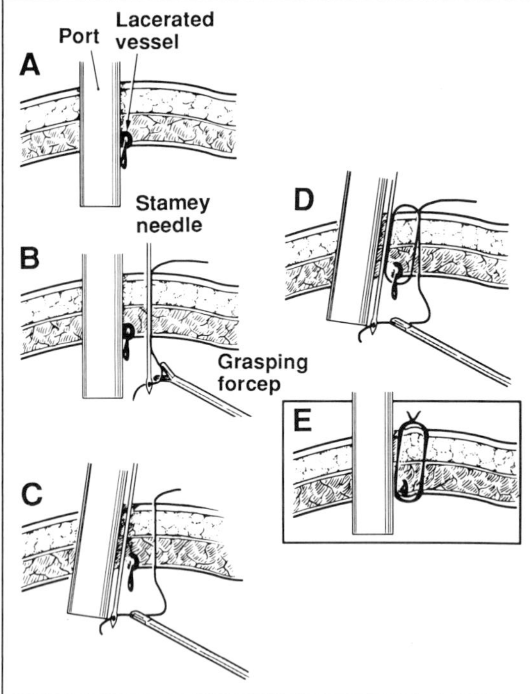


**Fig 9.** Percutaneous suturing technique when treating bleeding from an abdominal wall vessel.

postoperatively. In some instances a cut-down may need to be performed to control bleeding.

### Insufflation Injuries

Complications due to insufflation may result in technical difficulties while performing the procedure as well as injury to the patient. Incorrect Veress needle positioning can result in subcutaneous emphysema, preperitoneal insufflation, or insufflation of a viscus. If the Veress needle is placed in the subcutaneous or preperitoneal position, insufflation will result in an increase in the distance between the peritoneal cavity and the anterior abdominal wall. This will make subsequent trocar placement difficult. Gas insufflated into subcutaneous tissue will usually absorb but may result in postoperative pain and ecchymosis. With severe subcutaneous emphysema, hypercarbia may occur.[13] Usually this can be compensated by adequate ventilation; however, acidosis with associated metabolic abnormalities may occur. If a needle is inadvertently placed in a viscus, marked bowel distension may result. In this case the laparoscopic procedure should be aborted and either an open laparotomy performed or the patient rescheduled for a laparoscopy at a future date.

During prolonged procedures in which high insufflation pressures are utilized, cardiopulmonary problems may occur including difficulty with ventilation, decreased venous return, pneumothorax, pneumopericardium, hypotension, and cardiovascular collapse.[14,15] In patients with large hiatal hernias it is possible that pressures can push abdominal contents into the chest cavity and also impede ventilation and cardiac output.

Increased absorption of carbon dioxide can result in a gas pulmonary embolism.[2,13–18] Gas embolism during laparoscopy is a life-threatening situation and must be recognized quickly to avoid patient demise. Acute cardiovascular collapse may be the first sign of a gas embolism.[14,15] Just prior to this event, the anesthesiologist may notice a mill-wheel murmur and the end-tidal $CO_2$ may rapidly decrease due to the gas lock in the pulmonary artery.[1,17] If a gas embolism occurs, one should immediately desufflate the abdomen and begin cardiopulmonary resuscitative measures. It is helpful to place the patient in the left lateral decubitus position to prevent gas from entering the pulmonary artery. A central line may be placed to aspirate gas. Sternotomy with cardiopulmonary bypass and open evacuation of the gas has also been reported.[18]

In order to prevent the aforementioned insufflation injuries, it is extremely important to try to confirm that the Veress needle is in proper location prior to initiating insufflation. As previously stated, pressures less than 15 mm Hg in adults and 10 mm Hg in children should be utilized during laparoscopy.

### Dissection Injuries

Dissection injuries are similar to those seen during needle and trocar placement. Injuries may occur to the bowel, vascular structures, ureter, or bladder. Again, depending on the type and extent of injury, either laparoscopic repair or open surgical revision may be necessary. If a vascular injury occurs, one may need to perform an emergent open laparotomy. Quick entry into the abdominal cavity can be accomplished by torquing the laparoscope up against the anterior abdominal wall and cutting down on top of the laparoscope with a skin knife.

Ureteral injuries may occur during laparoscopic dissection.[19,20] If these are minor in nature and discovered at the time of the surgery, conservative management with stenting may be effective. However, if complete transection occurs, one may need to perform open laparotomy and repair. In some instances ureteral injuries are not detected until the postoperative period. Again, if the patient is stable, conservative management with either percutaneous drainage or stenting may be attempted. If patients have marked peritoneal signs, open laparotomy is preferable.

Electrocauteral injuries may also occur during dissection.[21] If there is any breakage of the insulation along the shaft of electrocautery instruments, inadvertent injury may occur to structures in contact with the instrument. Moreover, the insulation usually does not run to the tip of most electrocautery instruments; thus the entire tip of the instrument must be in view prior to the application of current. It is important to realize that electrocautery instruments cause an increase in temperature at the site of the fulguration and thermal injury to structures in close proximity is possible. The extent of a thermal injury is usually more severe than initially apparent. Thus, if thermal injury occurs, open surgical repair with wide debridement should be strongly considered.

### Closure Injuries

Care must be taken when terminating laparoscopic procedures to avoid several complications.[22] The abdomen must be inspected to rule out any injury that may have occurred during dissection. Incisional hernias can occur through larger (ie, greater than 10 mm) trocar sites. Port sites should be palpated with a finger prior to closure to ensure that no bowel is protruding. When closing the fascia, only the anterior layer should be reapproximated. Attempts at taking deep bites may result in passing a suture through a loop of bowel, resulting in bowel injury. Some laparoscopists will close these larger ports under direct vision of the laparoscope to assure that the suture is not inadvertently passed into the bowel.

Prior to removing all ports, each site should be inspected to exclude the possibility of any bleeding that may have been tamponaded by the trocar. Moreover, it is important to inspect the trocar site that has been used for the laparoscope. Prior to removing the last port, it is important to remove all carbon dioxide from the abdomen.

Trocar sites should be irrigated thoroughly and inspected for adequate hemostasis to prevent postoperative problems with wound infections. The skin of larger trocar sites may be sutured closed, whereas smaller ones can be reapproximated with tape strips.

## CURRENT INDICATIONS FOR LAPAROSCOPY IN UROLOGY

Laparoscopic surgery has been applied to several areas in urology. The initial application was in pediatric urology to evaluate patients with nonpalpable testes.[23–25] This technique has proven valuable in helping to localize cryptorchid testes in select patients as well as aiding the surgeon in planning the incision for orchiopexy. Other pediatric applications include evaluating intersex conditions and performing the first stage of a Fowler–Stephen orchiopexy by clipping the spermatic vessels laparoscopically.[26,27] More recently, Jordan and associates reported on performing a complete laparoscopic orchiopexy[28] and Atala and associates devised a laparoscopic model to correct reflux.[29]

The latest applications of operative laparoscopic surgery in urology have been as a diagnostic tool in evaluating the pelvic node status in patients with prostate, bladder, or penile carcinoma.[30,31] With surgical experience, this appears to be a very safe and effective technique, giving equivalent information to what is obtained with open node dissection with much less morbidity and quicker convalescence. Furthermore, diagnostic lymphadenectomy has been expanded and cases have been reported of retroperitoneal node dissections in patients with low-stage testicular carcinoma.[32]

Laparoscopic varicocele ligation is another current common application of operative laparoscopy.[33–35] Symptomatic varicoceles and those associated with infertility have been successfully ablated with this technique. Again, early data demonstrate equivalent results as that obtained with open varix ligation.

Laparoscopic nephrectomy has been reported by Clayman and associates.[35] This was performed primarily for benign renal disease. Patients as young as 6 months of age have successfully undergone the procedure and more recently it has been applied to patients with renal malignancies.[36]

Other applications in which laparoscopic surgery has been performed include ureterolysis, ureteroureterostomy, radical prostatectomy, ureterolithotomy, unroofing of symptomatic renal cysts, unroofing of pelvic lymphoceles, bladder diverticulectomy, bladder suspension, partial cystectomy, partial nephrectomy, ureteral reimplantation, and ileal conduits.[37–44] More than likely, by the time of publication of this chapter, further applications will have been reported.

## CONCLUSIONS

From the available experience in urology, the advantages of laparoscopic surgery include a decrease in postoperative pain, quicker convalescence, and a better cosmetic result when compared with the traditional open surgical procedures. Unfortunately, several drawbacks remain that somewhat limit the widespread utilization of laparoscopic urologic surgery. First, there is a great learning curve, and it is still unclear how much experience the surgeon requires to perform any given laparoscopic procedure safely. Second, there is a lack of purpose-built instrumentation to perform many urologic procedures. Visualization devices (ie, camera, video monitors) allow the surgeon only a limited, two-dimensional view of the operative field. Tactile information normally obtained through palpation is now blunted and transmitted to the surgeon via instruments.

Long-term complications of laparoscopic urologic surgery are yet to be defined. From the gynecologic literature, risks appear to be minimal; however, the newer urologic procedures are much more involved than the diagnostic and minor surgical procedures that have been performed for several decades. Further data are required before the true complication rate is assessed. Finally, and most importantly, the efficacy of laparoscopic procedures is unknown when compared to that of open traditional surgery. These aforementioned concerns may well be addressed in the near future to allow the application of laparoscopic surgery to treat a wider variety of disease entities, including malignancy. As technology advances and surgeons become more comfortable with basic laparoscopic techniques, this form of minimally invasive therapy will likely become a major part of standard urologic practice.

## REFERENCES


1. Monk TG, Weldon BC. Anesthetic considerations for laparoscopic surgery. *J Endourol.* 1992;6:89.
2. Sosa RE, Weingram J, Poppas D, Lyons J. Physiological considerations in laparoscopic surgery in urology. *J Endourol.* 1992;6:85.
3. Corson SL, Batzer FR, Grocial B, Maislin G. Measurement of force necessary for laparoscopic trocar entry. *J Reprod Med.* 1989;34:282.
4. Jarrett JC II. Laparoscopy: direct trocar insertion without pneumoperitoneum. *Obstet Gynecol.* 1990;75:725.
5. Hassan HM. A modified instrument and method for laparoscopy. *Am J Obstet Gynecol.* 1971;110:886.
6. Kavoussi LR, Clayman RV. Trocar fixation during laparoscopy. *J Endourol.* 1992;6:71.
7. Feldblum PJ. Laparoscopic sterilizations requiring laparotomy. *Am J Obstet Gynecol.* 1982;142:712.
8. Thompson BH, Wheeless CR. Gastrointestinal complications of laparoscopy sterilization. *Obstet Gynecol.* 1973;41:669.
9. Loffer FD, Port D. Indications, contraindications and complications of laparoscopy. *Obstet Gynecol Surv.* 1975;30:407.
10. Kavoussi LR, Loughlin KR, Chandhoke PJ, Clayman RV, Chodak G, Rukstalis D, et al. Complications of laparoscopic pelvic lymph node dissection. *J Urol.* 1992;147:451A.
11. Hulka JF. *Textbook of Laparoscopy.* New York: Grune and Stratton; 1985:119–130.
12. Green LS, Loughlin KR, Kavoussi LR. Management of epigastric vessel injury during laparoscopy. *J Endourol.* 1992;6:99.
13. Kent RB. Subcutaneous emphysema and hypercarbia following laparoscopic cholecystectomy. *Arch Surg.* 1991;126:1154.
14. Ostman PL, Pantie-Fisher FH, Faure EA, Glosten B. Circulatory collapse during laparoscopy. *J Clin Anesthesiol.* 1990;2:129.
15. Brantley JC, Riley PM. Cardiovascular collapse during laparoscopy. A report of two cases. *Am J Obstet Gynecol.* 1988;159:735.
16. Yacoub OF, Cardona I, Coverler LA, Dodson MG: Carbon dioxide embolism during laparoscopy. *Anesthesiology.* 1982;57:533.
17. Shulman B, Aronson HB. Capnography in the early diagnosis of carbon dioxide during laparoscopy. *Can Anaesth Soc J.* 1984;31:455.

18. Diakun TA. Carbon dioxide embolism: successful resuscitation with cardiopulmonary bypass. *Anesthesiology*. 1974;74:1151.
19. Grainger DA, Soderstrom RM, Schiff SF, Glickman MG, Decheney AH, Diamond MP. Ureteral injuries at laparoscopy: insights into diagnosis, management and prevention. *Obstet Gynecol.* 1990;75:839.
20. Gomel V, Christopher J. Intraoperative management of ureteral injury by operative laparoscopy. *Fertil Steril.* 1991;55:416.
21. Schwimmer WB. Electrosurgical burn injuries laparoscopy sterilization. Treatment and prevention. *Obstet Gynecol.* 1974;44:526.
22. Thomas AG, McLymont F, Moshipur J: Incarcerated hernia after laparoscopic sterilization: a case report. *J Reprod Med.* 1990;35:639.
23. Castilho LN. Laparoscopy for the nonpalpable testis: how to interpret the endoscopic findings. *J Urol.* 1990;144:1215.
24. Cortesi N, Ferrari P, Zambarda E, Manenti A, Baldina A, Pignatti-Morano F. Diagnosis of bilateral abdominal cryptorchidism by laparoscopy. *Endoscopy*. 1976;8:33.
25. Das S. Laparoscopic evaluation of nonpalpable testes. *Urology*. 1991;37:460.
26. Bloom DA. Two step orchiopexy with pelviscopic clip ligation of the spermatic vessels. *J Urol.* 1991;145:1030.
27. Gans SL, Berci G. Peritoneoscopy in infants and children. *J Pediatr Surg.* 1973;8:399.
28. Jordan GH, Robey EL, Winslow BH. Laparoendoscopic surgical management of the abdominal/transinguinal undescended testicle. *J Endourol.* 1992;6:157.
29. Atala A, Kavoussi LR, Goldstein DS, Retik AB, Peters CA. Laparoscopic correction of vesicoureteral reflux in an animal model. *J Endourol.* 1992;6:S168.
30. Schuessler WW, Vancaillie TG, Reich H, Griffith DP. Transperitoneal endosurgical localized prostate carcinoma. *J Urol.* 1991;145:988.
31. Winfield HN, Donovan JF, See WA, Loening SA, Williams RD. Urological laparoscopic surgery. *J Urol.* 1991;146:941.
32. Hulbert JC, Fraley EE. Laparoscopic retroperitoneal lymphadenectomy: new approach to pathologic staging of clinical stage I germ cell tumors of the testis. *J Endourol.* 1992;6:123.
33. Matsuda T, Horii Y, Higashi S, Oishi K, Takeuchi H, Yoshida O. Laparoscopic varicocelectomy: a simple technique for clip ligation of the spermatic vessels. *J Urol.* 1992;147:636.
34. Aaberg RA, Vancaillie TG, Schuessler WW. Laparoscopic varicocele ligation: a new technique. *Fertil Steril.* 1991;56:776.
35. Clayman RV, Kavoussi LR, Soper NJ, Dierks SM, Meretyk S, Darcy MD, et al. Laparoscopic nephrectomy. *N Engl J Med.* 1991;324:1370.
36. Clayman RV, Kavoussi LR, Albala DM, Chandhoke P, Soper NJ, and Figenshau RS. Laparoscopic nephrectomy: initial clinical series. *J Urol.* 1992;147:432A.
37. Nezhat C, Nezhat F, Green B, Gonzalez G. Laparoscopic ureteroureterostomy. *J Endourol.* 1992;6:143.
38. Albala DM, Schuessler WW, Vancaille TG. Laparoscopic bladder neck suspension. *J Endourol.* 1992;2:137.
39. Lee CK, Smith AD. Percutaneous transperitoneal approach to the pelvic kidney for endourologic removal of calculus: three cases with two successes. *J Endourol.* 1992;6:133.
40. Castilho Nogueira L, Ferreira U, Netto Rodrigues N. Laparoscopic pediatric orchiectomy. *J Endourol.* 1992;2:153.
41. Kozminski M, Parjamian KO. Case report of laparoscopic ileal loop conduit. *J Endourol.* 1992;6:147.
42. Kavoussi LR, Clayman RV, Brunt LM, Soper NJ: Laparoscopic ureterolysis. *J Urol.* 1992;147:425.
43. Bardot SF, Montie JE, Jackson CL, Seiler JC: Laparoscopic surgical technique for internal drainage of pelvic lymphocele. *J Urol.* 1992;147:908.
44. Figenshau RS, Albala DM, Clayman RV, Kavoussi LR, Chandhoke PS, Stone AM. Laparoscopic nephroureterectomy: initial laboratory experience. *Min Invas Ther.* 1991;1:93.

# 42

# Male Infertility

*Mark Sigman and Larry I. Lipshultz*

## INTRODUCTION

During the 1970s, the two-career family became a popular model of the American family. As a result, childbearing was often delayed, with couples attempting to conceive in their 30s instead of their 20s. Unfortunately, many couples found themselves unable to conceive and faced the possibility of childless marriages. This, combined with the rapid technological advances in the diagnosis and treatment of various forms of infertility, resulted in infertility evolving from a condition causing embarrassment and rarely discussed to one that has become highly publicized in the media. As a result, many couples' values have changed from the pursuit of individual careers in the 1970s to the pursuit of parenthood in the 1980s.

Approximately 15% of couples trying to conceive for the first time will be unable to do so within 1 year. Twenty percent of these cases are due solely to a male factor; in an additional 30% the male factor is contributory. Thus, in approximately 50% of infertile marriages a male factor is at least partially responsible. In the past, it has been recommended that a couple not pursue an infertility evaluation until after 1 year of unprotected intercourse. With the advancing age of many couples attempting conception, we feel that any couple questioning their fertility status should undergo at least a basic initial evaluation at the time of presentation. This evaluation should be performed simultaneously on both the male and the female.

The evaluation of the infertile male should proceed as with the evaluation of any other medical problem. A thorough history and physical examination with particular attention to the genitalia should be performed. This should be followed by appropriate laboratory tests, which will result in placing the patient in a diagnostic category. Appropriate therapy should then be instituted. Of equal importance, the urologist should counsel the couple as to when to pursue adoption or therapeutic donor insemination. Unduly prolonged, futile treatments not only result in a large financial burden but can result in a high psychological cost to the couple.

The ability to accurately diagnose and treat the infertile male rests upon a sound knowledge of normal reproductive endocrinology and physiology.

## ENDOCRINOLOGY OF MALE REPRODUCTION

The Gonadotropin-releasing hormone (GnRH) is a decapeptide produced in hypothalamic neurosecretory cells. GnRH is released in a pulsatile pattern every 70 to 90 minutes into the portal circulation, where it reaches the pituitary gland.[2–4] This pulsatile secretion of GnRH results in the release of the two glycopeptide gonadotropins, follicle-stimulating hormone (FSH), and leuteinizing hormone (LH) from the anterior pituitary. The episodic nature of GnRH secretion is necessary for stimulation of gonadotropin secretion. Following secretion, FSH and LH travel in the peripheral circulation to the gonad, where they bind to specific cell surface receptors. LH binds to specific receptors on the Leydig's cells present in the interstitial tissue of the testis, resulting in an increase in intracellular cyclic adenosine monophosphate (cAMP). This leads to an increase in testosterone synthesis.[5,6] Testosterone is required for the initiation of spermatogenesis; however, in the absence of FSH, spermiogenesis (the maturation of spermatids into mature sperm) does not go to completion. FSH binds to the surface of Sertoli cells stimulating intracellular cAMP production where, by poorly understood mechanisms, spermatogenesis is stimulated to completion.[7] Testosterone in the peripheral circulation results in feedback inhibition of LH secretion at the hypothalamic-pituitary level.

Inhibin, a protein composed of two polypeptide chains, is produced by the Sertoli cells.[8] This hormone feeds back to the hypothalamic-pituitary axis resulting in inhibition of FSH secretion. Inhibin binds to specific membrane receptors on pituitary gonadotrops.[9] This is followed by an increase in cyclic guanosine monophosphate (cGMP), which most likely acts as the second messenger in inhibition of FSH secretion by inhibin.[10] In the presence of normal spermatogenesis, hormone levels are kept in balance (Table 1). In the absence of adequate Leydig's-cell and Sertoli-cell function (primary testicular failure), gonadotropin levels rise. Similarly, in the presence of hypothalamic or pituitary dysfunction resulting in inadequate levels of gonadotropins, stimulation of the gonads does not occur, resulting in low peripheral levels of testosterone as well as an absence of spermatogenesis. These patients will have small testes.

The pulsatile secretion of GnRH results in an episodic secretion of LH and FSH. This results in a considerable variation in the serum concentrations of these hormones. Goldzieher et al determined that a single random blood sample would be within 20% of the true mean value 30% to 50% of the time for LH and FSH and 70% of the time for testosterone.[11] It had thus been recommended that for proper hormonal determination three blood samples taken at 15-minute intervals and subsequently pooled should be used for hormonal analysis. However, from a practical clinical point of view, it is uncommon for a single hormonal measurement to incorrectly determine a patient's hormonal status. That is, while a patient's absolute hormonal level may not be precise using one blood sample, it will still be in the normal range if the patient is normal and will usually be in the abnormal range if the patient's true levels are abnormal. Thus, one hormonal determination is usually adequate. If the values are abnormal or do not fit the clinical situation, three blood samples may be obtained.[12] Gonadotropin and testosterone levels remain low throughout early childhood. Beginning from approximately 6 to 8 years of age, LH and FSH levels increase. This is followed by an increase in testosterone levels beginning at 10 to 12 years of age.[13] Gonadotropin and androgen levels remain relatively constant during the reproductive years. However, later in life gonadotropin levels rise while testosterone levels decrease.[14] These changes are due primarily to decreased

**TABLE 1. Hormone Levels in Normal and Pathologic States**

| Condition | FSH | LH | T |
|---|---|---|---|
| Normal function | Normal | Normal | Normal |
| Primary testicular failure | Increased | Increased | Decreased |
| Hypothalamic or pituitary disease | Decreased | Decreased | Decreased |

numbers of Leydig's cells and degeneration of seminiferous tubules. However, there may be additional thalamic or pituitary changes as well.

## Spermatogenesis

The parenchyma of the testis consists of a highly complex system of seminiferous tubules surrounded by connective tissue containing lymphatics, blood vessels, and Leydig's cells. The seminiferous tubules form loops that connect to a single duct, the tubulus rectus. This tube connects with the rete testis, which empties into the epididymal duct through several ductuli efferentes.

Seminiferous tubules consist of a basement membrane composed of collagen fibers, mucopolysaccharides, contractile myoid cells, and fibroblasts. The precise role of these peritubular cells remains unclear.[15] Sertoli's cells and germ cells in various stages of spermatogenesis are found within the seminiferous tubule. The Sertoli cells line the seminiferous tubules. These cells form complicated cytoplasmic extensions that surround the germ cells. The Sertoli cells form the basis of the "blood testis barrier," which is due to Sertoli:Sertoli tight junctional complexes dividing the germinal epithelium into basal and adluminal compartments. The composition of the fluid from these two compartments is quite different.[16] The Sertoli cells nurture the developing germ cells. In addition, they are complex secretory cells, secreting different compounds into the basal and adluminal compartments.

Spermatogonia form the stem cells of the testis. Type A spermatogonia divide, either replenishing their supplies or differentiating into type B spermatogonia.[17] Differentiation and mitotic division of type B spermatogonia produce preleptotene spermatocytes. The preleptotene spermatocytes and both types of spermatogonia are found within the basal compartment of the seminiferous tubule. As the preleptotene spermatocytes replicate their DNA in preparation of meiosis, they pass from the basal compartment across the blood-testis barrier into the adluminal compartment (Fig 1).[18] The leptotene primary spermatocytes then pass through the zygotene and pachytene stages, during which they contain a tetraploid number of chromosomes. After passing through the first meiotic division, the pachytene spermatocytes become secondary spermatocytes containing a diploid number of chromosomes. The secondary spermatocytes undergo the second meiotic division, producing round spermatids containing a haploid number of chromosomes (Fig 2).

During division and differentiation of spermatocytes into mature sperm, the cells retain cytoplasmic bridges, the function of which remains unclear. In addition, the spermatids are connected to Sertoli cells via ectoplasmic specializations.[19] During spermiogenesis the acrosome is formed, the nucleus elongates, and the flagella is developed. If a portion of a seminiferous tubule is examined, one finds that germ cells are not randomly distributed but form a number of well-defined patterns. These patterns or stages represent the various cells of the seminiferous tubules in different stages of development.

Clermont has defined six stages of spermatogenesis in the human.[17] In the rat, a transverse section through a seminiferous tubule will reveal that all portions of the wall are in the same stage of spermatogenesis. In contrast, the human seminiferous tubule contains sections of differing stages of spermatogenesis.

It has been determined that spermatogenesis takes approximately 74 days in man. The mature spermatozoa measures approximately 60 μm wide. The sperm head contains the nucleus, consisting of highly condensed chromatin, and an apical acrosome, which is a membrane-bound organelle. The acrosome contains the enzymes required for sperm penetration of the zona pellucida of the egg. The head is attached to the flagella by a midpiece containing helically arranged mitochondria. Mitochondria surround a set of outer dense fibers as well as a precisely organized arrangement of microtubules in the characteristic 9+2 pattern. The mitochondria supply the energy for flagellar motion. The

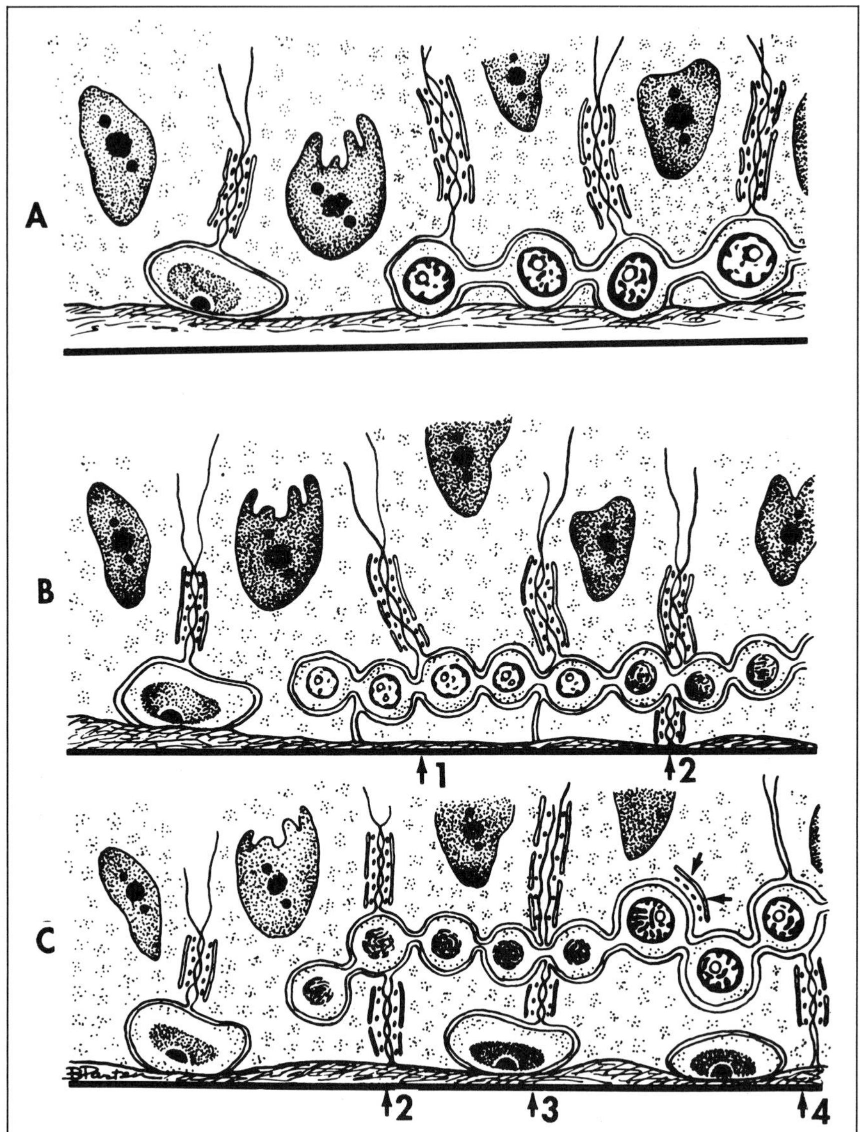


**Fig 1.** A demonstration of the passage of spermatocytes across the blood-testis barrier. **A:** A cohort of spermatogonia are below the Sertoli tight junctional complexes. **B–C:** As the spermatogonia divide and mature, they pass through these tight junctional complexes. [Reprinted with permission from Huckins C, Adult spermatogenesis: characteristics, kinetics, and control, in Lipshultz LI, Howards SS (eds), *Fertility in the Male* (New York, NY: Churchill Livingstone; 1983; copyright Lipshultz LI).]

axonemal structure, together with the fibrous sheath, continue through the principal piece of the flagella. The outer dense fibers terminate as the axoneme continues into the endpiece.

Following release into the seminiferous tubule, mature sperm travel from the caput to the cauda epididymis in approximately 14 to 18 days. The sperm then enter the vas deferens traveling to the ampullary portion of the vas in approximately 4 days. Sperm entering the caput of the normal

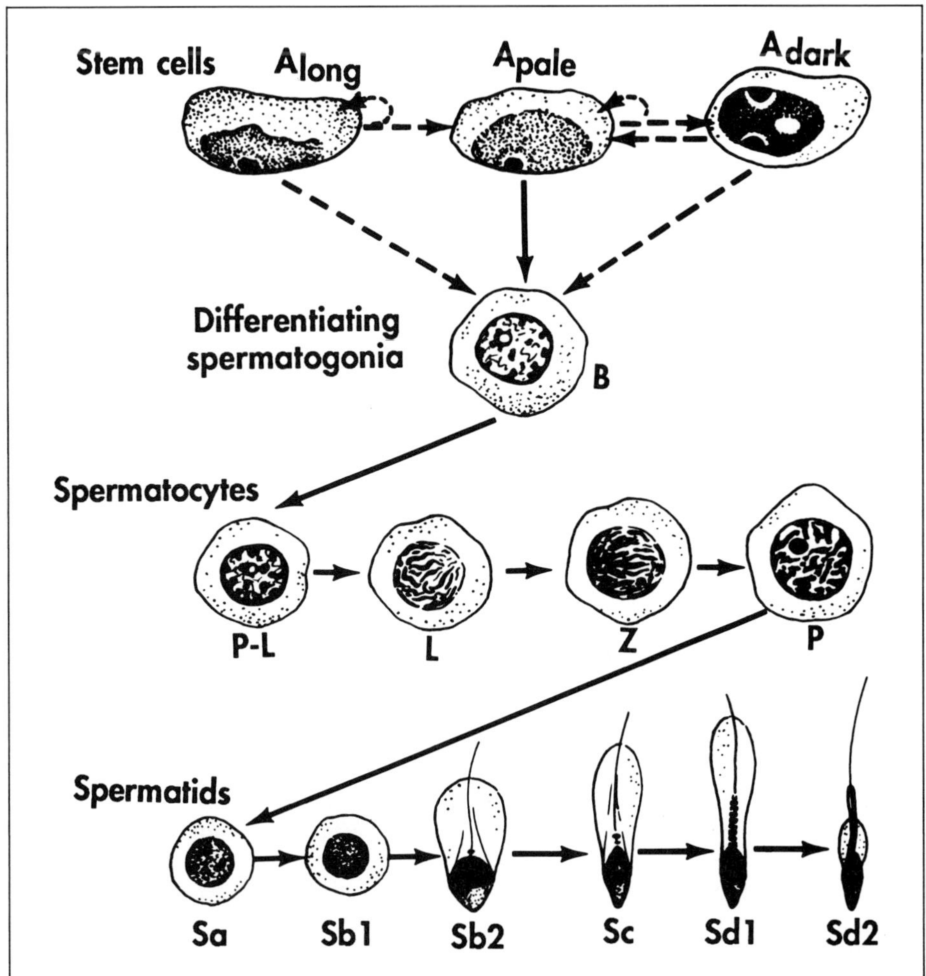


**Fig 2.** The various types of germ cells as they mature from stem cells through mature spermatozoa. [Reprinted with permission from Huckins C, Adult spermatogenesis: characteristics, kinetics, and control, in Lipshultz LI, Howards SS (eds), *Fertility in the Male* (New York, NY: Churchill Livingstone; 1983; copyright Lipshultz LI).]

epididymis are nonmotile and attain motility after maturing and passing through the length of the epididymis.

**Seminal Fluid and Accessory Glands.** The seminal fluid is composed of secretions from the testis, epididymis, bulbourethral glands (Cowper's glands), Littre's glands (periuretheral glands), prostate, and seminal vesicles. During ejaculation, fluid is released from the glands in a specific sequence. Prior to the expulsion of the major portion of the ejaculate, there is a small amount of secretion from the bulbourethral glands. The initial portion of the ejaculate derives primarily from prostatic secretions. This is followed by the midportion of the ejaculate, containing the highest concentration of sperm along with secretions from the testis, epididymis, and vas deferens. Seminal-vesicle secretions account for the last fraction of the ejaculate. Out of the total ejaculate, Cowper's-glands secretions account for 0.1 to 0.2 mL, prostatic secretions account for 0.5 mL, whereas seminal-vesicle secretions account for 1.5 to

2.0 mL. Following ejaculation, semen forms a coagulum that liquifies over a 5- to 20-minute period. Proteins secreted by the seminal vesicles are responsible for coagulation, whereas prostatic secretions account for subsequent liquefaction.[20,21]

The seminal vesicles are paired structures. Vasography has determined normal dimensions of 4.0 to 5.0 cm in length by an average width of 2.0 cm. Transrectal ultrasonography has demonstrated that the combined width of the seminal vesicle and ampulla normally exceeds 2.5 cm, and the anterioposterior thickness normally is between 0.7 and 1.5 cm.[21] Fructose is a major component of seminal vesicle secretions. Fructose will be absent from semen in patients with bilateral absence of the seminal vesicles. Additional compounds secreted by the seminal vesicles include prostaglandins, various proteins, ascorbic acid, and substrates for the clotting process.

The prostate gland is responsible for secretion of seminal acid phosphatase, alkaline phosphatase, citric acid, amylase, β-glucuronidase, albumin, calcium, zinc, and magnesium. In addition, the prostate is responsible for secretion of spermine and spermidine, which are basic polyamines. It is believed that spermine is involved in sperm energy metabolism as well as acrosomal protein activation.[23,24] The role that zinc plays in fertility is unclear. However, it appears that zinc may be involved with antibacterial factors in the prostate.

The epididymis is responsible for the majority of carnitine found in the seminal plasma. It may be involved in fatty-acid transport in the mitochondria.[25] The bulbourethral glands are paired structures found in the urogenital diaphragm as outgrowths of the membranous urethra. Their small-volume secretions may function as a lubricant for the urethra during ejaculation.[26]

**Capacitation and the Acrosome Reaction.** Freshly ejaculated sperm or sperm aspirated from the epididymis will not fertilize mature eggs unless they have undergone a period of maturation, termed capacitation. Once capacitated, sperm have the ability to bind to, penetrate, and fuse with oocytes. During capacitation, many membrane events occur such as an increase in the permeability to small molecules, a decrease in the negative surface charge, changes in antigens, ATPase activation, modified lectin binding, and increase in membrane fluidity.[27] Capacitation normally occurs inside the female reproductive tract over a 4- to 6-hour period, as determined by animal experiments. Semen processing in in vitro fertilization may allow for capacitation to occur in as short as a 1- to 3-hour period when sperm are exposed to appropriate media.

The acrosome reaction involves a fusion between the plasma membrane and the outer acrosomal membrane. This results in the formation of a series of vesicles and the extrusion of the acrosomal contents. The acrosome reaction may be induced by the zona pellucida as well as by ionophores. Only capacitated sperm are able to acrosome-react.[28] An increase in intracellular calcium is the primary signal for inducing the acrosome reaction.[29] During the acrosome reaction, hyaluronidase, acrosin (a protease) as well as other enzymes, are released. These enzymes allow sperm to penetrate the cumulum oophorus cells surrounding the ovum as well as the zona pellucida (a glycoprotein layer surrounding the oocyte). Once a sperm has penetrated the zona pellucida and entered the perivitelline space, the zona pellucida undergoes a reaction that prevents penetration by additional spermatozoa resulting in a block to polyspermy.

## Ejaculation

Ejaculation consists of three phases: seminal emission (passage of sperm from the vas deferens and ejaculatory ducts into the posterior urethra), bladder-neck closure, and antegrade ejaculation (the passage of semen from the urethra out the urethral meatus). Afferent sensory stimuli from the genitalia are relayed to the cerebral cortex via the pudendal nerve. Efferent nerve fibers travel through the anterolateral columns of the spinal cord emerging through T11-L3 sympathetic ganglia. This results in contraction of the vas deferens stimulating expulsion of semen from the cauda epididymis to the ampulla of the vas. Subsequent smooth-muscle contraction in the ampulla, prostate, and seminal vesicles, along with partial closure of the bladder neck, produces deposition of semen in the posterior urethra. Additional parasympathetic sacral nerve stimuli as well as stimulation from pelvic nerves causes clonic contraction of the striated smooth muscle of the pelvis and urethra, resulting in rhythmic projectile ejaculation through the urethra.

## EVALUATION OF THE INFERTILE MALE

### History

At the basis of any type of evaluation for male infertility should be the standard techniques for evaluating medical problems in general: the performance of a complete history and physical examination. A thorough history should detail the duration of the couple's infertility as well as any prior pregnancies and any previous treatments. In addition, difficulty in achieving prior pregnancies should be noted. Details of the couple's sexual history should be explored. Any history of erectile dysfunction should be addressed. The couple's frequency of intercourse during the periovulatory period needs to be discussed. Not uncommonly, it is found that the couple is having intercourse either too frequently or too infrequently. In addition, the couple should understand the menstrual cycle—specifically that the fertile period is in the middle of the menstrual cycle, not at the end. Since sperm survive in normal cervical mucus and in the cervical crypts for approximately 2 days, intercourse every 48 hours is most effective around the ovulatory peak. This will assure that viable spermatozoa are present during the 12- to 24-hour period during which the oocyte will be within the fallopian tube and capable of being fertilized. The use of lubricants for intercourse should be addressed. In vitro testing has determined that commonly used lubricants such as K-Y Jelly, Lubifax, Surgilube, Keri Lotion, and saliva result in a deterioration of motility.[30–33] Several natural lubricants, such as vegetable oil, safflower oil, peanut oil, raw egg white, and petrolatum jelly have not impaired in vitro sperm motility. Couples should be cautioned to only use a vaginal lubricant if necessary and then a minimal amount of one that does not affect sperm motility.

Details of the patient's childhood medical history should be elucidated. Cryptorchidism, whether unilateral or bilateral, has been associated with infertility. Approximately 30% of men with unilateral cryptorchidism and 50% with bilateral cryptorchidism will have sperm densities below 12 to 20 million per mL.[34] Defects in spermatogenesis are present regardless of the time of orchiopexy.[35] Testicular trauma, or a history of torsion of the testis, should be noted since both may result in atrophic testicles and predispose the patient to the development of antisperm antibodies. Delayed or incomplete progression through puberty may suggest an endocrinopathy. A history of inguinal herniorrhaphy may suggest the possibility of vasal ligation. Bladder surgery, such as Y-V plasties of the bladder neck, were often done in combination with ureteral reimplantation. This results in an incompetent bladder neck, causing retrograde ejaculation. Systemic illnesses, such as diabetes mellitus or multiple sclerosis, may predispose a patient to the development of ejaculatory dysfunction or erectile abnormalities.

Approximately 60% of testicular cancer patients have oligospermia at the time of presentation.[36–38] Following chemotherapy, radiotherapy, or retroperitoneal node dissection, these patients' fertility status may be further impaired. A radiated or chemotherapeutically treated testicle may take 4 to 5 years to resume spermatogenesis.[38–40] Additionally, chemotherapy or radiotherapy for other malignant diseases may also result in an impairment of spermatogenesis. A classical retroperitoneal node dissection as performed for testicular carcinoma results in a disruption of the sympathetic nerves causing anejaculation or retrograde ejaculation. Recently, modifications using nerve-sparing techniques have resulted in the majority of patients retaining ejaculatory competence.[41] Mumps obtained prepubertally does not affect the testis. After the age of 11 or 12, 30% of patients affected with the mumps virus develop unilateral mumps orchitis whereas 10% of the patients develop it bilaterally.[42] Severe atrophy of the testis often results. Any recent high fever should be noted since this may result in a temporary impairment of spermatogenesis that may not be apparent until 1 to 3 months after the event, depending upon the stage of spermatogenesis that was affected. Thus, if a patient presents with an abnormal semen analysis and a significant medical illness in the 3 months prior to his visit, follow-up semen analyses over a 3- to 6-month period should be obtained before a conclusion can be reached as to his baseline level of spermatogenesis. Exposure to pesticides as well as other potentially gonadotoxic agents should be identified. Medications, such as cimetidine, nitrofurantoin, and sulphasalazine as well as cocaine, marijuana, nicotine, and caffeine, have been implicated as impairing spermatogenesis.[43–48] The cessation of ingestion of these substances will usually result in a return to normal spermatogenesis. Recently, with the widespread use of anabolic steroids in sports, athletes have presented with infertility. The androgenic component of the steroids may result in a state of hypogonadotropic hypogonadism. Cessation of these agents will usually, but not always, result in a return of normal hormonal function.[49]

The testes normally are 1°F to 2½°F cooler than body temperature. It has been demonstrated that experimental hyperthermia will result in an impairment of semen quality and spermatogenesis.[50] Consequently, the use of hot tubs or saunas should be discontinued in patients with suboptimal semen analyses. While smoking has been linked to abnormalities in the semen analyses, not all studies agree upon this point. A family history of intersex disorders may suggest androgen-receptor abnormalities. Cystic fibrosis may be associated with epididymal or vasal abnormalities, and a history of this disease or trait should be noted. Finally, a review of systems should be obtained with particular attention directed toward any genital urinary symptoms. In addition, a history of frequent respiratory infections suggests the possibility of immotile cilia syndrome or Kartagener's syndrome if associated with situs inversus. These patients will present with immotile sperm. Similarly, patients with Young's syndrome will present with a history of frequent respiratory infections and azoospermia due to epididymal inspissation resulting in azoospermia. Impaired visual fields, severe headaches, or galactorrhea raises the possibility of a central nervous system tumor whereas anosmia suggests Kallmann's syndrome with hypogonadotropic hypogonadism.

### Physical Examination

Following a detailed history, a general physical examination should be performed with specific attention to the genitalia. As mentioned previously, situs inversus raises the possibility of Kartagener's syndrome and immotile cilia. The location of the urethral meatus should be noted since hypospadias may not allow for cervical deposition of semen. Severe penile chordee may interfere with intercourse. The evaluation of the scrotal contents should be performed with the patient standing in a warm room, allowing for relaxation of the cremasteric muscle. The testes should be palpated and their dimensions measured to the nearest millimeter with calipers, or their volume should be determined with an orchidometer. In normospermic men, the length of the testis is greater than 4.0 cm with a volume greater than 20 mL.[51,52] A unilateral or bilateral decrease in testicular size may be associated with impaired spermatogenesis.[53] The epididymis should also be carefully palpated to assure its presence as well as the completeness of its length. Induration and cystic abnormalities should be noted as these may represent areas of potential obstruction. The presence of the vas deferens should be determined. The spermatic cords should be examined for the presence of a varicocele. Asymmetry in the spermatic cords accentuated by Valsalva's maneuver should be noted. In patients with strong creamateric reflexes in whom the testes ride high in the scrotum, slight traction on the testes will assist in the examination of the spermatic cords. The varicocele should be graded according to its size. Grade I or small varicoceles are only palpable with Valsalva's maneuver. Grade II or moderate varicoceles are palpable with the patient in the standing position. Grade III or large varicoceles are visible through the scrotal skin. Lipomas of the spermatic cord will cause thickening and asymmetry of the cords. However, the asymmetry will persist in the supine position whereas a varicocele will decrease in size. Bilateral thickening of the spermatic cords that decreases in the supine position suggests bilateral varicoceles. Some investigators use other diagnostic methods to identify subclinical varicoceles—varicoceles not palpable on physical examination. While venography has been the gold standard for diagnosis, it is an invasive examination and not without risks.[54] In addition, the position of the catheter, the pressure of injection, and the judgment of the examiner may affect the outcome. Scrotal ultrasound directly demonstrates dilated veins in the scrotum.[55] A varicocele is diagnosed when there are more than three veins, at least one of which has a diameter larger than 3 mm. With a Doppler stethoscope a venous rushing may be heard in varicocele patients.[56–60] Contact scrotal thermography relies on a higher temperature in the scrotum or testicle of the varicocele patient for the diagnosis of varicoceles.[61,62] Recently, color duplex scrotal ultrasonography has been applied to the diagnosis of clinical and subclinical varicoceles. While the results are comparable to traditional real-time ultrasound examination of the scrotum, differentiation of veins from arteries has improved the ease of this technique.

The use of these techniques has resulted in subclinical varicoceles being identified in up to 91% of patients with idiopathic infertility,[56,59,63] and bilateral varicoceles demonstrated in up to 58% of patients.[56,59] This is a marked difference from the 10% incidence of bilateral varicoceles found on clinical examination. There are no controlled studies documenting an improved pregnancy rate following the diagnosis and treatment of subclinical varicoceles. In view of this we do not advocate pursuing the diagnosis of nonpalpable varicoceles.

Finally, the patient's pattern of androgenization should be noted as decreased body hair, gynecomastia, and eunuchoid proportions suggest the diagnosis of delayed maturation due to an endocrinopathy.

### Laboratory Evaluation

Following a thorough history and physical examination of the infertile male, appropriate laboratory testing should be performed. The cornerstone of the laboratory evaluation consists of the semen analysis. It is important to differentiate between an average semen analysis and the minimal seminal parameters required for fertility. Studies of fertile populations have demonstrated mean sperm densities between 70 and 80 million per $cm^3$.[64] It is important to realize that while this represents a mean of the fertile population, it is not the minimal sperm density required for initiating a pregnancy. It has become clear by means of in vitro fertilization that while human ova are fertilized by one sperm, 50,000 to 500,000 sperm may be required for this penetration.[65] In addition, clinical studies have suggested that only 1 out of every 5000 sperm in the vagina reach the cervical mucus and 1 out of every 14 million in the vagina reach the ova duct.[66] Studies of infertile populations have demonstrated that as semen quality decreases, the chances of initiating pregnancy also decrease. Thus, it is found that many patients are subfertile, but not sterile. Limits of adequacy have been established (Table 2).[67,68] Finally, data from in vitro fertilization of human ova have demonstrated that the standard semen parameters do not

**TABLE 2. Minimum Semen Parameters Associated With Normal Fertility**

| | |
|---|---|
| Volume | 1.5–5.0 mL |
| Density | $\geq 20 \times 10^6$ sperm/mL |
| Motility | $\geq$ 60% |
| Forward progression | > 2.0 |
| Morphology | $\geq$ 60% normal forms |

adequately measure the fertility potential of individual sperm since equal numbers of motile sperm from oligospermic patients result in lower fertilization rates than equal numbers of motile sperm from normospermic patients.[65]

**Collection of Semen.** Semen specimens should be collected into a clean, wide-mouthed container. The specimen should be collected after 2 to 3 days of abstinence and should arrive at the laboratory within 2 hours of collection. Masturbation is the preferred method of collection; however, special condoms designed for semen collection may be used, allowing the couple to have intercourse. These condoms are specifically designed not to contain spermatotoxic ingredients. Coitus interruptus should be discouraged since part of the specimen may be lost with this technique. Once the specimen is collected, it should be kept at body temperature by placing it in the patient's pocket during transport to the laboratory. The bottle should be labeled with the patient's name, the date, and the time of collection as well as the abstinence period. We suggest the evaluation of 2 to 3 specimens to determine a baseline since semen parameters may vary significantly from one specimen to another. In those occasional cases in which parameters differ markedly in the initial set of specimens, several more specimens obtained over a 2- to 3-month period should be obtained.

**Physical Characteristics of Semen.** Fresh semen forms a thick coagulum that liquefies over a 5- to 25-minute period. Following liquefaction, the volume of the ejaculate should be measured to the nearest millimeter and semen viscosity should be determined. Liquefied semen should be capable of being poured drop by drop. Hyperviscous semen will form thick strands when attempts are made to pour it. Liquefied semen is a slightly translucent, whitish liquid. Any abnormal color, such as a pink tinge, should be noted as this may suggest hematospermia.

**Sperm Concentration.** The semen specimen should be well mixed prior to performing a sperm count. A normal specimen should contain at least 20 million sperm per mL. There are several devices commonly used to perform sperm density determination. A Neubauer standard blood cell counting chamber may be used. A specimen is diluted 1:20 in a test tube with distilled water to immobilize the spermatozoa. A drop of this specimen is examined microscopically on the counting chamber. Spermatozoa are counted within 5 blocks containing 16 squares each. All spermatozoa within this area and touching the lower and right-hand sides of each block are included. This number, multiplied by $10^6$, represents the count per milliliter. Two sets of 5 blocks should be counted and an average taken. For specimens with low sperm densities, a 1:10 dilution should be used and an appropriate modification of the calculation performed. Recently, the Makler chamber has become popular for performing semen analyses (Sefi Medical Industries, Israel). This device has the advantage of allowing the examination of undiluted semen. The number of sperm in 10 blocks is counted and represents the number of sperm, in millions, per milliliter. The percent motility may also be determined from the same slide. Using the above techniques, variations of 10% to 20% in counts of the same specimen may be obtained.[69] Viscous specimens may be drawn into a 5 mL syringe and forcibly ejected through an 18- to 19-gauge needle several times. The specimen will no longer be viscous and may be counted more accurately.[17] If no sperm are seen, the specimen should be centrifuged at ≥600 g for 10 minutes and the pellet examined for the presence of sperm.

**Sperm Motility and Forward Progression.** The fresh specimen should be examined by placing a drop of semen on a clean slide and covering it with a cover slip. This examination may be done under 400 × power. The percentage of sperm that are moving in 10 random fields should be determined. In oligospermic specimens the actual number of moving sperm may be counted whereas in higher-density specimens this parameter must be estimated. It has been found that estimates performed by skilled technicians are quite consistent. Notation should be made of the quality of forward movement of the sperm. This is measured on an arbitrary scale of forward progression. Forward-progression rating consists of 0 (no sperm movement), 1 (sperm moving in place), 2 (sperm moving with slow, meandering, forward direction), 3 (sperm moving in a relatively straight line with moderate speed), 4 (sperm moving in a straight line with high speed).[71] While occasional clumps of agglutinated sperm may be seen, frequent sperm agglutination should be noted as this may indicate the presence of antisperm antibodies. The presence of other cell types should also be determined. Both immature germ cells and white blood cells will appear as round cells in the unstained wet mount semen specimen. The number of these cells per high-powered field should be determined. While there appears to be considerable overlap in the concentration of white blood cells in the fertile and infertile populations, excessive white cells suggest the presence of an infection or an inflammation. The concentration of immature germ cells may vary with the number of sperm. However, there is considerable patient-to-patient variation, and the significance of this finding remains unclear.[72] In a normal specimen, 60% or more of the sperm should be motile and the forward progression of the majority of the moving sperm should be 2.5 or greater. The motility determination should be performed within 2 hours of semen collection. Prolonged periods of abstinence may result in specimens demonstrating poor motility. It should be remembered that nonmotile sperm are not necessarily nonviable sperm since vital stains have demonstrated that these sperm may be alive.[73,74]

**Sperm Morphology.** The morphology of the sperm cells should be examined since this may be a sensitive indicator of fertility and spermatogenesis.[74,76] Sperm morphology may be rapidly assessed in a wet mount specimen with phase-contrast microscopy. However, more detailed morphology requires the use of a stained specimen. The Papanicolaou stain has routinely been used, but a more rapid technique employing a hematoxin stain that gives adequate, although not quite as fine, cellular detail has emerged. Recently, prestained slides (Blustan; Irving Scientific, Calif) allow for a very rapid and reasonably accurate evaluation of sperm morphology. One hundred cells should be examined and classified as normal (oval head), amorphous (irregular head), tapered, double-headed, and immature. Immature spermatozoa have retained cytoplasm surrounding the midpiece. In addition, tail defects should be noted. Normal specimens contain up to 40% abnormal forms. The morphological classification in an individual patient remains remarkably consistent from specimen to specimen.[75] Testicular stress such as radiation, varicocele, or testicular infection may result in increased numbers of immature forms identified in the semen.

**Other Seminal Characteristics.** While the pH of semen may be determined and usually varies between 7.6 and 7.8, this is usually of no clinical value. The pH of seminal vesicle fluid is usually above 7 whereas prostatic fluid is usually less than 7. Thus, patients with absence or dysfunction of the seminal vesicles may produce a semen specimen with a low pH. However, this condition is more readily diagnosed by seminal volume and transrectal ultrasonography. Similarly, the seminal vesicles produce fructose, which may be easily measured in the semen. Absence or dysfunction of the seminal vesicles may be accompanied by an absence of fructose in the semen. While this compound was commonly measured in the past, transrectal ultrasonography has supplanted this procedure in most centers.

**Computer-Assisted Semen Analysis.** Since a properly performed semen analysis is a subjective and time-consuming procedure requiring a trained observer, computers have been used in an attempt to improve upon the speed and objectivity of the analysis. Commercial systems include Cellsoft (Cryo Resources), Hamilton-Thorn motility analyzer (Hamilton-Thorn Research),

TS 1500 Sperm Motion Analysis System (TS Scientific), and Celltrack (Motion Analysis Corporation). These systems digitize an image from a microscope and record it on a video camera and monitor. The digitized image is then analyzed by a computer using proprietary algorithms. Unfortunately, these systems have not provided the simple, rapid, and accurate analyses hoped for. Vantman et al found that cell counts were overestimated by 30% when there were 11 to 60 cells per high-powered field.[77] Most significantly, azoospermic samples were read as containing $3.6 \times 10^6$ sperm per high-powered field. In addition, motility was underestimated due to the inclusion of noncell particles and cell-to-cell collisions. Other investigators have found similar problems with the use of other systems.[78] One advantage of the computerized systems is that parameters may be determined that cannot be measured manually. These measurements include curvilinear velocity, linear velocity, linearity lateral head displacement, flagellar bead frequency, and circular movement analysis. Presently, it is unclear which, if any, of these measurable parameters will be clinically useful in separating the fertile from infertile population beyond what can be determined with manual semen analysis. Recent systems can also determine sperm morphology. However, there is inadequate data to assess their accuracy. While computerized semen analysis systems are useful in the research setting, they have not proven themselves of use in a routine clinical arena.

**White Blood Cell Staining of Semen.** As mentioned previously, leukocytes present as round cells when examined under wet mount microscopy. Pyospermia has been associated with infection and infertility.[79–81] Traditional staining techniques, such as the Papanicolaou stain, require a highly trained observer to differentiate leukocytes from immature germ cells. Recently, immunohistochemical techniques employing monoclonal antibodies against white blood cell surface antigens have been used for this purpose. Leukocytes are easily differentiated due to their red-brown staining pattern.[82] The semen also may be stained by the peroxidase technique, which will identify granulocytes but may miss samples that primarily contain macrophages. In this procedure, peroxidase-positive white blood cells stain a dark brown color.[83] Greater than 1 million white blood cells per milliliter has been considered pathologic. However, recent data has brought this number into question.[72]

**Genital Tract Cultures.** Epidemiologic studies have demonstrated a correlation between the incidence of genital tract infection and infertility.[84] Unfortunately, the data directly linking the presence of specific organisms to male infertility remains confusing.[85] Cultures of human semen have often shown the presence of a variety of organisms including aerobic and anaerobic organisms as well as mycoplasma.[86–93] In a patient with clinical evidence of a genital urinary infection such as prostatitis, urethritis, or cystitis, appropriate treatment should be rendered. However, in patients with no clinical evidence of an infection and no evidence of pyospermia, routine genital tract bacterial culturing is not indicated.

Mycoplasma have been cultured from the genital tracts of infertile couples.[94] Initial uncontrolled studies reported increased pregnancy rates following treatment of infected infertile couples.[95,96] These data have not been borne out by controlled studies, and the data examining the relationship between seminal parameters and the presence of mycoplasma are conflicting. Chlamydia are obligate intracellular bacteria that are agents in the most prevalent sexually transmitted disease in the United States. This organism is a common cause of nongonococcal urethritis and epididymitis. Chlamydia has been cultured from the urine, expressed prostatic secretions, and semen.[92,97] Presently, mycoplasma and chlamydia cultures should be performed in patients with clinical evidence of an inflammatory or infectious process. Further studies are required to document the utility of cultures in patients without evidence of disease. If cultures are to be performed, swabs from the urethra should be sent for chlamydia and mycoplasma, and semen may be sent for bacterial cultures. In patients with evidence of cystitis, urine cultures should also be obtained.

**Cervical Mucus Interactions.** Following intercourse, sperm must travel through the cervical mucus. The quality of this interaction is measured by the postcoital test. The examination is performed in the preovulatory phase of the menstrual cycle, just prior to ovulation. Typically, the couple will have intercourse in the morning, and several hours later a specimen of cervical mucus is examined under a microscope. While there is no consensus as to the grading system, a normal test is often defined as one in which more than 10 to 20 sperm are seen per high-powered field, the majority of which have progressive motility. Indications include hyperviscous semen, a normal semen analysis in a couple with unexplained infertility, abnormal anatomy of the penis, and decreased volume of semen with good sperm density. While a normal postcoital test suggests that there is not a cervical factor involved in the couple's infertility, there are many reasons for an abnormal postcoital test. Antisperm antibodies in the semen or cervical mucus, inappropriate timing of the postcoital test, anatomic abnormalities, inappropriately performed intercourse, and an abnormal semen specimen may all result in an abnormal postcoital test. In vitro cervical mucus tests have been developed in an attempt to standardize the cervical mucus–sperm interaction. By placing cervical mucus under a cover slip or in a capillary tube adjacent to a drop of sperm, these tests evaluate the ability of sperm to penetrate the mucus. Recently, bovine cervical mucus has been used in in vitro testing to completely remove the female factor from the evaluation. Studies have demonstrated that the migration of sperm into human and bovine cervical mucus appears to be similar.[98–101] The results of cervical mucus penetration tests generally correlate with the quality of the semen specimen, particularly with the motility parameters. Of note, however, there are patients with normal semen parameters but poor cervical mucus interaction tests.[102,103] Presently, the role of cervical mucus penetration tests in the evaluation of the infertile male remains unclear. While the postcoital test is the simplest and most physiologic, it suffers from poor reproducibility due to the many factors affecting its outcome. The in vitro cervical mucus tests eliminate some of the difficulties of the postcoital test but still are affected by the quality of the female cervical mucus. As more data on bovine cervical mucus interaction tests accumulate, it may be found that the test allows for the use of mucus of consistent quality, completely eliminating the effect of the female on the results. Presently, the postcoital test should be used as the initial screening test. If this is abnormal, one may give consideration to performing an in vitro cervical mucus interaction test. The couple's individual circumstances, as well as the availability of different tests at different institutions, will determine which in vitro test will be chosen.

**Endocrine Evaluation.** Primary hormonal abnormalities are unusual causes of male infertility, accounting for less than 3% of cases. In addition, they are rare in patients with sperm concentrations greater than 5 million sperm per milliliter.[104] There is controversy as to what should constitute a minimum endocrine evaluation. Some investigators suggest that measurement of serum FSH is sufficient to screen infertile men with otherwise unremarkable history and physical examinations. In most cases, the addition of testosterone, LH, and prolactin determinations will not add significant clinical information. If a significant abnormality in the FSH level is found, the additional hormone determinations may be obtained. Other investigators feel that a complete hormonal evaluation should be performed in most patients. If this approach is taken, it must be realized that this additional information will rarely add clinically useful information. Prolactin should be measured in any patient with symptoms of a central nervous system tumor such as impaired visual fields or severe headaches. Hypogonadotropism (coupled with low androgen levels) is commonly found in hyperprolactinemic patients with pituitary tumors. More commonly, mild elevations of prolactin are found with no identifiable tumor identified (idiopathic hyperprolactenemia). These patients will have normal gonadotropins and testosterone levels. While it has been suggested that prolactin may have a direct testicular effect, definitive evidence is lacking.[105] Until large controlled studies are performed, the treatment of isolated mild hyperprolactenemia should be considered an empiric therapy for male infertility. Recently, the GnRH stimulation test has been used to investigate the infertile male. An exaggerated elevation in gonadotropins in response to the GnRH stimulation is believed to result from abnormal testicular hormone production and spermatogenesis. Studies by Hudson and colleagues have found that varicocele patients with exaggerated gonadotropin responses demonstrate significant improvements in semen parameters following a varicocele repair. Patients without exaggerated gonadotropin responses respond poorly to varicocele repair.[106–110] Others have found normal gonadotropin responses to GnRH in varicocele patients.[111] Presently the use of this test in the varicocele patient remains a research tool.

**Antisperm Antibodies.** It has been known for many years that the presence of antisperm antibodies may adversly affect fertility. Rumke, et al found that pregnancy rates dropped significantly with agglutinating titers above 1:64.[112] Unfortunately, there is, as yet, very little consensus as to which antibody assays are the most appropriate and at what levels these tests are considered positive. As a result, many different assays are used to determine the presence of antisperm antibodies. Until recently, the presence of antibodies was most commonly determined from a serum sample. These tests required the antibodies to either cause agglutination of sperm, or immobilization. Recent experience with Immunobead assay has demonstrated that antisperm antibodies present in the serum may not be bound to the sperm. It is generally believed that if antibodies are not present on the spermatozoal surface, they are clinically insignificant.[113,114] Thus, current assays have shifted the focus from the indirect detection of antisperm antibodies in serum to direct assays measuring sperm-bound antibodies. In the mixed agglutination reaction, red blood cells coated with human antibodies are mixed with semen to be tested. The addition of antihuman antiserum will cause cross-linking and agglutination of the red blood cells and sperm. Recently, a modification of this assay, called the Sperm Mar test (Ortho Diagnostic Systems, Beerse, Belgium), has been developed. This test employs IgG-coated polystyrine microspheres and anti-IgG antiserum to create the mixed agglutination reaction. Enzyme-linked immunosorbent assays have also been applied to the detection of antisperm antibodies. The Immunobead assay has become commonly used for the determination of antisperm antibodies. Micron-sized polyacrylamide beads, to which rabbit antihuman antibodies are linked, are added to spermatozoa to be tested. These beads will bind to the portion of the sperm containing the antisperm antibodies. This binding may be visualized under a phase-contrast microscope. The test has the advantage that the class of antibody can be determined as well as the site of binding. The assay is scored by counting the percentage of sperm that have beads bound to them. The level of binding considered clinically significant varies from 20% to 50% of sperm demonstrating immunobead binding.[115,116] The Immunobead assay may also be performed as an indirect assay by mixing antibody negative donor sperm with patient serum. Antisperm antibodies present in the serum will then bind to the sperm and the assay may then be performed as previously described. As noted above, indirect assays are not ideal since the false-positive rate may be high. A recent modification of the Immunobead, SpermCheck (Bio-Rad Laboratories, Hercules, Calif) uses monodispersed Latex microspheres of uniform size instead of the variable-sized polyacrylamide beads used in the standard Immunobead assay. This allows for microscopic examination under bright field conditions instead of phase microscopy resulting in a somewhat simplified assay. Preliminary results suggest that this assay gives nearly identical results to the standard Immunobead assay. Both this assay and the standard Immunobead assay require sperm to be washed prior to performing the assay. This is in contrast to the Sperm Mar assay, which may be performed directly on unwashed semen. However, the Immunobead and Sperm Mar do not give identical results; more studies are needed to determine which more accurately detects the presence of clinically significant antibodies.[117]

The pattern of bead binding may be important. Bronson et al found that fertility was not impaired in those patients who only demonstrated binding to the tip of the tail region. Other patterns of binding (head, midpiece, or total tail) all appear to have detrimental affects upon fertility.[116] Antisperm antibodies in the female will also impair fertility. Assays in the woman must be indirect assays and will suffer from the same difficulties as indirect assays in the male. There is no consensus as to whether it is most important to test cervical mucus, which can be technically difficult to work with, or serum. Some authors feel that if a woman is going to be tested with the indirect assay, her husband's sperm should be used as the donor sperm in the indirect assay.[118]

Due to the blood-testis barrier, the immune system in the normal male is not exposed to the germinal elements. Any process that disrupts this barrier may result in the development of antisperm antibodies (Table 3). Following vasectomy, approximately 60% of men will demonstrate antisperm antibodies in their serum.[119,120] The incidence of antisperm antibodies is higher in the presence of a sperm granuloma at the vasectomy site. This presumably sensitizes the immune system to sperm antigens.[121] Similarly, patients with acquired ductal obstruction were found to have antisperm antibodies in the serum.[122] Less than 1% of infertile men are found to have congenital absence of the vas deferens. These patients produce sperm that are unable to exit from the genital system. Amelar et al found that 62% of these patients demonstrated antisperm antibodies in the serum.[123] Patients' who have had torsion or significant trauma of the testis may also have disruption of the blood-testis barrier, resulting in the development of antisperm antibodies.

**TABLE 3. Predisposing Factors for the Development of Antisperm Antibodies in the Male**

Ductal obstruction
Vasectomy
Epididymal or testicular infection
Torsion of the testicle (?)*
Cryptorchidism (?)
Varicocele (?)

*(?) Indicates controversy as to the role of the condition in the production of antibodies.

Patients with impaired sperm motility or sperm agglutination, as well as any of the above-mentioned risk factors, should have an antisperm antibody assay. If possible, a direct assay testing the patients sperm should be performed. We do not recommend the preoperative testing of vasectomy patients about to undergo vasovasostomy since the results of this assay will not affect the decision to proceed with surgery. Couples with unexplained infertility, as well as those with abnormal postcoital tests, should be tested for antisperm antibodies.

**Sperm Penetration Assay.** The zona pellucida is a glycoprotein layer surrounding the ova of most species, and prevents cross-species fertilization. By removing the zona pellucida, Yanagimachi et al demonstrated that human sperm could fuse with hamster oocytes.[124] In the sperm penetration assay (SPA), human sperm that have been capacitated in vitro are incubated with zona-free hamster oocytes allowing interspecies sperm penetration to occur. For successful penetration, sperm must be able to undergo capacitation, the acrosome reaction, fusion with the oolema, and incorporation into the ooplasm. The test is scored by measuring the percentage of ova that have been penetrated or determining how many sperm have penetrated each ova. In centers that score the test by the percentage of ova penetrated, the lower limit of normal is commonly between 10% and 30% of ova penetrated. While the assay has been used in many centers, there is no standardization as to how the test should be performed and much disagreement as to how it should be interpreted. While there is generally some correlation between the results of the SPA and the standard semen parameters, some institutions have found no correlation with semen parameters.[125] The gold standard for validation of the sperm penetration assay is in vitro fertilization (IVF) of human oocytes. Conflicting results have been found when correlating the SPA with IVF.[126,127] By altering laboratory conditions, Smith et al found that they could obtain fertilization of most oocytes. They determined that a more sensitive indicator was the number of penetrations per egg. Using this index, they found that couples with a normal SPA had a 95% chance of fertilizing human ova in vitro whereas couples with a negative SPA had a 50% chance of fertilizing human ova in vitro.[128] This data make it apparent that the physician should be familiar with the laboratory that is performing the sperm penetration assay in order to be able to determine what conclusions can be drawn from the results. Investigators have evaluated the ability of the SPA to predict natural in vivo pregnancy following intercourse. While an early study showed no relation between pregnancy and the results of the SPA, this has not been confirmed by other investigators.[129] Corson et al found that conception was twice as likely in those couples with an SPA of greater than 11% of ova penetrated then for those with an SPA of less than 11%.[130]

In summary, it is clear that the ideal SPA has not been developed. However, changes in the assay continue to be incorporated and may, in time, produce more accurate and predictive assays. Proper interpretation depends upon knowledge of the laboratory that is performing the assay and an understanding of the assay's limitations.

**Evaluation of the Seminal Vesicles.** Fructose is produced in the seminal vesicles. Patients with ejaculatory-duct obstruction or seminal-vesicle dysfunction will demonstrate small seminal volumes and semen that does not coagulate. Traditionally, seminal-vesicle function has been based on the measurement of seminal fructose. Recently, transrectal ultrasonography (TRUS) has gained popularity in evaluation of both the prostate and seminal vesicles. In a study of infertile patients with low ejaculate volumes or nonpalpable vas deferens, seminal-vesicle abnormalities were identified in 75% of patients. Two thirds of patients with bilateral absence of the seminal vesicles demonstrated some fructose in the semen.[131]

**Testis Biopsy.** Testicular biopsies are primarily performed to differentiate between azoospermia due to abnormal spermatogenesis and ductal obstruction. This includes azoospermic patients with normal-size testes and FSH values less than 2 to 3 times normal. Patients with bilaterally atrophic testes and markedly elevated FSH values will almost universally demonstrate an absence of spermatogenic cells. These patients do not require testicular biopsies. Other relative indications include patients with severe oligospermia, normal-sized testes, and normal FSH values. A normal biopsy in these patients suggests the possibility of a partial ductal obstruction. In most patients with oligospermia, a testicular biopsy will not change clinical management and is not indicated. In patients with symmetric testes, unilateral biopsies should be performed in most instances. In patients with asymmetric testes, bilateral biopsies may be indicated. While some surgeons prefer to perform this procedure in the operating room, we have found that it can easily be performed in an office setting under local anesthesia without IV sedation (Fig 3). The skin of the scrotum over the testis is infiltrated with a 1:1 mixture of 1% Xylocaine and 0.5% Marcaine. A 2- to 3-cm incision is made over the testicle and carried down to the tunica vaginalis. The tunica vaginalis is then sharply incised and an eyelid retractor is placed in the incision exposing the tunica albuginea of the testis. At this point, additional local anesthesia should be dripped into the wound. The tu-

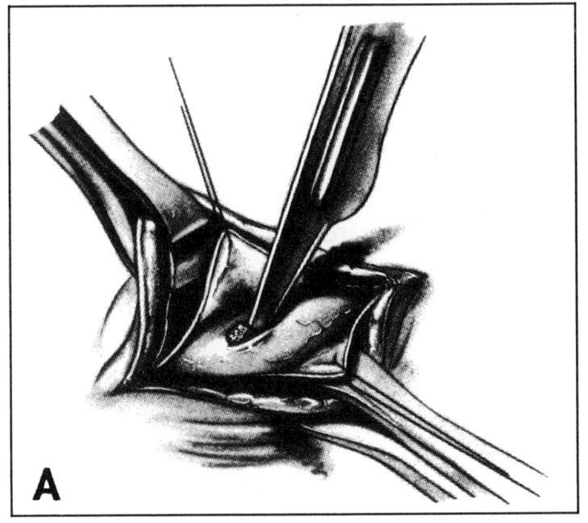


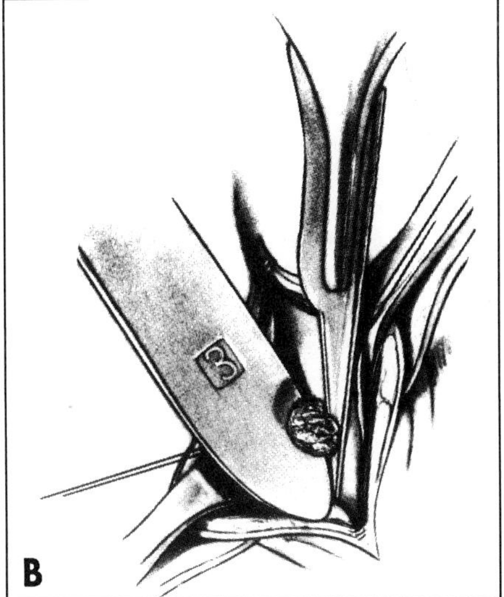


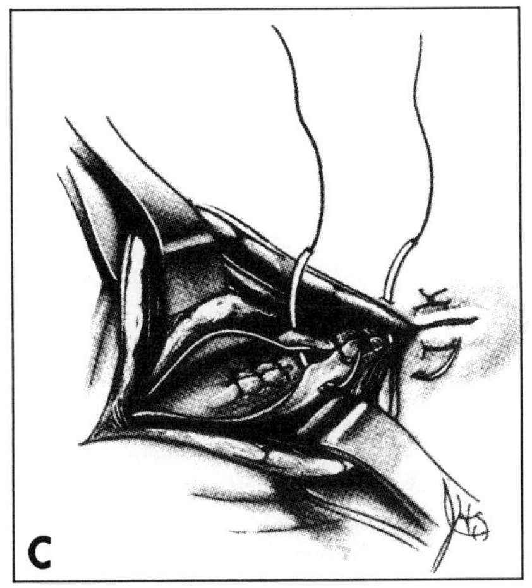


**Fig 3.** The testis biopsy. After the tunica vaginalis is exposed it is incised with a scapel blade (**A**). Seminiferous tubules are then excised (**B**). All layers are then closed with interrupted chromic sutures (**C**). [From Lipshultz LI, Howards SS, Surgical treatment of male infertility, in Lipshultz LI, Howards SS (eds) *Fertility in the Male.* (New York, NY: Churchill Livingstone; 1983; copyright Lipshultz LI).]

nica of the testis is then incised with an 11 blade. Slight pressure on the testis results in extrusion of seminiferous tubules through the tunical incision. These tubules are then sharply excised with curved iris scissors. The specimen should be lightly grasped with fine-toothed forceps. A testicular touch prep should then be performed by touching and gently rolling the specimen over a clear slide. The slide should quickly be sprayed with cytological fixative and allowed to dry. The specimen should then be promptly placed in Bouin's solution. Formalin should not be used as this results in marked distortion of the testicular histology. The incision in the tunica albuginea is closed with a figure-8 4–0 chromic suture. The tunica vaginalis, dartos muscles, and skin are closed in separate layers of chromic suture. A small telfa dressing and dry gauze should be applied to the scrotum with a scrotal support.

Light microscopic examination of the testicular biopsy usually reveals one of several histologic patterns. In the normal testis, germ cells in all stages of spermatogenesis should be present, although not necessarily all in the same tubule. The basement membrane should be thin and Leydig's cells should be present.

This pattern may be found in azoospermic patients with ductal obstruction.

Hypospermatogenesis refers to a reduction in all germinal elements in the seminiferous tubule. In this pattern, all stages of spermatogenesis are present, in reduced numbers, however. These patients will demonstrate oligospermia. This pattern is often found in conjunction with maturation arrest.

In maturation arrest, spermatogenesis precedes normally up to a certain point. In complete maturation arrest, no germinal elements are found beyond a specific stage. In early maturation arrest, no spermatids or mature sperm are found, while in late maturation arrest, all cells through the spermatid stage are present with no mature sperm being identified. A testicular touch prep will identify late stages of spermatogenic arrest since in permanent sections it may difficult to differentiate the two. On the touch prep, no mature spermatozoa will be found with complete maturation arrest. In partial maturation arrest, normal numbers of spermatogenic elements are found up to the stage of arrest. Beyond that stage, fewer numbers of germ cells will be present. Thus, patients with partial maturation arrest will demonstrate oligospermia.

End-stage testes typically demonstrate tubular and peritubular sclerosis. Sclerotic seminiferous tubules are found with no germ cells lining them. In addition, Leydig's cells will be absent from the sclerotic interstitium. The patient with this condition will present with bilaterally atrophic testes and elevated levels of gonadotropins. In Klinefelter's syndrome, tubular sclerosis may be found in association with hyperplastic nodules of Leydig's cells.

Sertoli-cell–only syndrome represents a condition in which seminiferous tubules contain only Sertoli's cells. The interstitium and basement membrane are usually minimally altered. Leydig's-cell function is normal in these patients. Serum FSH levels are typically markedly elevated due to the absence of spermatogenesis. Most cases of Sertoli-cell–only syndrome are idiopathic with no identifiable cause. Occasionally patients will have histories of exposure to chemotherapy, radiotherapy, or gonadotoxins. As can be seen from Table 4, a specific histologic pattern is generally not pathognomonic of one single disease process. Multiple etiologies may result in similar testicular biopsy. Similarly, a single etiology may yield biopsies showing several patterns of spermatogenic abnormalities. This has resulted in much difficulty in classifying testicular biopsies.

The purpose of the testicular touch prep is to identify the presence of mature sperm. This technique will differentiate ductal obstruction from complete late maturation arrest. Other investigators have used percutaneous fine-needle aspiration cytology to determine the presence of spermatogenesis.[132] The results are interpreted in a manner similar to the testicular touch prep. Fine-needle aspiration may also be combined with flow cytometry. The ploidy patterns obtained correspond with the state of spermatogenesis.[133]

**Vasography.** Vasography is indicated in azoospermic patients who have demonstrated spermatogenesis on testicular biopsies. In addition, it is used to identify

**TABLE 4. Disease States Associated With Various Histologic Testicular Biopsy Patterns**

| Pattern | Disease |
|---|---|
| Normal | Ductal obstruction<br>Congenital absence of vas<br>Ejaculatory duct obstruction |
| Hypospermatogenesis | Varicocele<br>Idiopathic<br>Heat (fever, hot tub)<br>Cryptorchidism |
| Maturation arrest | Varicocele<br>Idiopathic<br>Heat (fever, hot tub)<br>Hypogonadotropic hypogonadism |
| Sertoli only | Idiopathic<br>Cryptorchidism<br>Radiation<br>Chemotherapy |
| Tubular/Peritubular sclerosis | Infection<br>Trauma<br>Cryptorchidism<br>Radiation<br>Chemotherapy<br>Hypogonadotropic hypogonadism |

areas of partial obstruction in those rare cases in which this diagnosis is suspected. It may also be used to confirm the diagnosis of ejaculatory-duct obstruction, whether complete or partial. This procedure is generally performed in the operating room with the intention of correcting any obstruction found during the operative setting. Through a scrotal incision, the vas deferens is isolated and hemitransected. Using optical magnification, the distal end of the vas deferens is catheterized with a 25-gauge plastic angiocath. A 3 $cm^3$ syringe with saline is then used to irrigate the vas deferens. If the irrigant flows easily, ductal patency is indicated. Methyline blue may be combined with the saline. The bladder may then be catheterized with a red rubber catheter. Blue dye obtained from the bladder confirms ductal patency. If an obstruction is found, sterile renografin solution may be injected into the vas deferens to identify the site of obstruction. Retrograde vasography to visualize the proximal vas deferens and epididymis is contraindicated, as this may cause a blowout of the epididymis and subsequent epididymal obstruction. Any fluid from the proximal segment of the vas may be examined microscopically to determine the presence of spermatozoa. If sperm are found in this fluid, this rules out a proximal vas or epididymal obstruction. In azoospermic patients, a unilaterally patent vas will rule out ductal obstruction as the cause for azoospermia. Thus, bilateral vasograms are not required in these patients. If no distal obstruction is identified, the epididymis should be examined. The vasotomy site should be closed with several full-thickness 9–0 nylon sutures.

### Interpretation of the Semen Analysis

Following the history, physical examination, and laboratory evaluation of the infertile male, the patient will be placed into an etiologic category. The semen analysis will exclude some etiologies while raising the possibility of others. Absent ejaculation may be due to drug therapy, retroperitoneal or bladder neck surgery, vascular or neurologic abnormalities, as well as rare cases of psychological disturbances. In all cases of absent ejaculation and in cases of azoospermia with seminal volumes less than 1 mL, a postejaculate urine specimen should be obtained to rule out the possibility of a retrograde ejaculation. If significant numbers of sperm ($>10$ to 15 sperm per high-powered field) are identified, retrograde ejaculation is diagnosed. In patients with absent ejaculation in whom retrograde ejaculation is ruled out and a clear etiology for anejaculation (such as a history of a retroperitoneal node dissection) is not identified, transrectal ultrasonography should be performed to evaluate the seminal vesicles and ejaculatory ducts. Azoospermia may be due to chromosomal abnormalities, varicoceles, ductal obstruction, and idiopathic etiologies. Occasionally patients demonstrate nonmotile spermatozoa. This brings up the possibility of Kartagener's syndrome and immotile-cilia syndrome. In classic immotile cilia syndrome, cilia of the respiratory tract and flagella of the sperm demonstrate a microtubular defect in which there are no dynine arms. Patients will often have a history of chronic respiratory tract infections. Approximately 50% of these patients will have situs inversus in which case the syndrome is known as Kartagener's syndrome.[134]

Oligospermia may be due to the presence of a varicocele, cryptorchidism, or systemic infections, or result from drug therapy. In addition, oligospermia in many patients is idiopathic. Lastly, occasional cases of partial ductal obstruction are identified as previously mentioned. In those patients with normal semen analyses, attention should be directed toward the female to rule out an undiagnosed female factor. In addition, immunologic infertility should be addressed as well as the couple's coital habits. Using the results of the semen analyses and the remainder of the evaluation, the patient is then placed into an etiologic category and treatment instituted (Table 5).

## ETIOLOGY AND TREATMENT

The etiology of male infertility may be divided into pretesticular, testicular, and posttesticular dysfunctions.[135]

**TABLE 5. Classification of Infertile Men Following Evaluation**

| Diagnosis | % |
|---|---|
| Varicocele | 37.4 |
| Endocrine | 0.9 |
| Sexual dysfunction | 2.8 |
| Obstruction | 6.1 |
| Cryptorchid | 6.1 |
| Agglutinatin | 3.1 |
| Viscosity | 1.9 |
| Necrospermia | 0.5 |
| Volume | 4.7 |
| Testicular failure | 9.4 |
| Ejaculatory failure | 1.2 |
| High density | 0.5 |
| Idiopathic | 25.4 |

Reproduced with permission from Greenburgh SH et al, Experience with 425 subfertile male patients, *J Urol* (1978; 119(4):507–510). (Copyright by Williams & Wilkins, 1978.)

**TABLE 6. Pretesticular Causes of Male Infertility**

Hypogonadotropic hypogonadism
- Pituitary disease
  - Tumors
  - Infection
  - Iatrogenic (surgery, radiation)
  - Infarction
- Gonadotropin deficiency
  - FSH and LH deficiency (Kallmann's syndrome)
  - Isolated LH deficiency (fertile eunuch)
  - Isolated FSH deficiency
  - Congenital syndromes

Androgen excess
- Endogenous
  - Congential adrenal hyperplasia
  - Androgen-producing tumor
- Exogenous
  - Anabolic steroids
  - Other medical treatments

Estrogen Excess
- Endogenous
  - Cirrhosis of liver
  - Obesity (?)
  - Estrogen producing tumor

Hyperprolactinemia
- Idiopathic
- Pituitary tumor

Hyperthyroidism-hypothyroidism

Glucocorticoid excess

## Pretesticular Causes of Male Infertility

Pretesticular causes of male infertility refer to testicular dysfunction secondary to hormonal abnormalities (Table 6).

**Hypogonadotropic Hypogonadism.** Hypogonadotropic hypogonadism has a number of etiologies. Pituitary disease, resulting in a disruption of the hypothalamic pituitary gonadal axis, may result from tumors, infarction, surgery, radiation, or infectious etiologies.[136] The adult male with pituitary dysfunction may present with infertility or impotence. In addition, visual field abnormalities and severe headaches may also be presenting symptoms. The physical examination may demonstrate small, soft testes. Typically male secondary sexual characteristics will be present unless adrenal insufficiency exists. Hormonal evaluation will reveal low serum testosterone levels with low or normal serum gonadotropins. Thus, it is important to realize that a low serum testosterone associated with a normal LH is an abnormal finding and should be evaluated. The remainder of the pituitary hormones and their secondary endocrine functions should also be evaluated.

*Gonadotropin Deficiency.* Isolated FSH and LH deficiency is known as Kallmann's syndrome. This occurs in a familial and sporadic form. Gonadotropin deficiency leading to secondary testicular failure is the result of a genetic failure of GnRH secretion by the hypothalamus. It is associated with anosmia, which may be complete or partial. Other congenital anomalies include congenital deafness, harelip, cleft pallet, cranial facial asymmetry, renal abnormalities, cryptorchidism, and color blindness.[137] The hypogonadotropic syndrome may also exist without anosmia. Similarly, in families with Kallmann's syndrome, anosmia may be transmitted without hypogonadotropism. Patients may present in childhood with micropenis or cryptorchidism. However, most frequently, delayed development of puberty results in the patient presenting for medical evaluation. Physical examination may demonstrate the arms and legs to be longer than the trunk. In addition, the testes are prepubertal, usually being less than 2 cm in diameter. Treatment of the teenager consists of androgen replacement therapy with either testosterone or human chorionic gonadotropin (hCG). To initiate spermatogenesis, hCG must be given (2000 IU intramuscularly three times a week). Human chorionic gonadotropin alone will adequately virilize the male; however, in only about 20% of patients will spermatogenesis proceed to completion. In most patients, after approximately 6 months, FSH activity in the form of human menopausal gonadotropin (HMG) must be given. HMG (Pergonal, Serano) contains 75 IU of FSH and 75 IU of LH per vial. This will usually result in the completion of spermatogenesis. The dosage is ½ vial given intramuscularly three times per week.[138] Therapy must be continued for months before sperm may appear in the ejaculate. Following therapy, testicular volume will increase, although it still may remain below normal. Semen analyses typically reveal oligospermia with counts below 10 million sperm per milliliter. However, motility parameters are usually above 60%.[139] Many of these patients will be able to conceive despite low sperm densities. This is in contrast to idiopathic oligospermic patients who often are infertile with identical sperm densities. Recently, GnRH has been used in these patients.[140–142] This may be given as intermittent subcutaneous injections or via an infusion pump with pulses at 90-minute intervals.[143]

Isolated LH Deficiency. Individuals with isolated LH deficiency (fertile eunuchs) present with a variably eunuchoid habitis and low plasma testosterone and LH levels. FSH levels are typically normal. These patients may have large testes, and small-volume ejaculates that may contain a few spermatozoa.[144] Leydig's cells function normally, and these patients will respond to hCG injections with a rise in serum testosterone. It appears that the Leydig's cells secrete sufficient testosterone to support spermatogenesis. However, production is inadequate to supply sufficient peripheral levels of testosterone to promote virilization. Therapy in these patients consists of hCG injections.

Isolated FSH Deficiency. Isolated FSH deficiency is a rare disorder that is found in normally virilized patients who demonstrate normal levels of LH and testosterone. Testicular size in these patients is normal. However, sperm counts range from azoospermic to oligospermic.[144] Treatment consists of administration of hMG.[146] With the recent availability of pure FSH (Metrodin, Serano) these patients may be treated more specifically.

**Androgen Excess.** Both estrogens and androgens feed back to the pituitary, resulting in a decrease in gonadotropin production. Thus, androgen excess, whether endogenously produced from a metabolic abnormality or an androgen-producing tumor, or obtained exogenously, may result in a hypogonadal state. The most common cause for endogenous androgen excess is congenital adrenal hyperplasia. Of the five enzyme defects that may cause this syndrome, a congenital deficiency of 21-hydroxylase is the most common.

These patients develop precocious puberty and short stature. The penis may prematurely enlarge, however, the testes remain in a prepubertal state due to a lack of gonadotropin stimulation. Laboratory evaluation of these patients may reveal elevated urinary 17-ketosteroid and pregnanetriol levels. In addition, basal serum 17-hydroxy progesterone levels are often 50 to 200 × elevated.[147] Not all investigators have found fertility abnormalities in patients with congenital adrenal hyperplasia. It appears that in some cases in which untreated patients are fertile, the adrenal androgens are sufficient to stimulate the complete maturation of germ cells.[148] Treatment consists of glucocorticoid therapy, which results in a reduction in ACTH levels followed by a reduction in peripheral testosterone leading to a resumption of gonadotropin secretion. Occasionally patients will develop bilateral testicular adrenal rest tumors that resolve with hormonal therapy.[149–151]

Some patients demonstrate a partial 21-hydroxylase deficiency that does not develop until adulthood. These cryptic cases will not be clinically apparent because the mild androgen elevation is not evident in males. While anecdotal reports have suggested that some cases of male infertility may be due to cryptic 21-hydroxylase deficiency, studies of infertile populations have not revealed a significant incidence of this abnormality.[152]

Adrenal or testicular tumors may also result in excess endogenous androgen production. In the prepubertal patient, the testis will fail to mature. In the postpubertal patient, excess androgens will result in a hypogonadotropic state leading to tubular sclerosis and a loss of germ cells, which, if severe, may be nonreversible. The recent use of anabolic steroids by athletes has resulted in induced states of hypogonadotropic hypogonadism. While this is most commonly a temporary phenomenon that will reverse upon cessation of steroids, we have seen patients in whom pituitary suppression was permanent.

**Estrogen Excess.** Estrogens act on the pituitary, suppressing gonadotropin secretion, which results in secondary testicular failure. Estrogen-secreting tumors may develop in the adrenal cortex or in the testes as Sertoli-cell tumors or interstitial cell tumors. In addition, liver dysfunction may result in excess estrogens. While some investigators have found increased estrogen levels in morbidly obese patients, this has not been a universal finding.[153,154] Patients with estrogen excess may present with bilateral gynecomastia, impotence, and atrophic testes. Laboratory studies will reveal low levels of FSH, LH, and testosterone, and elevated levels of serum estrogens. In addition, elevated urinary excretion of 17-ketosteroids will be found.

**Hyperprolactinemia.** As mentioned previously, hyperprolactinemia may be associated with impotence and infertility. Other symptoms of hyperprolactinemia consist of gynecomastia and galactorrhea, which are uncommon in men. The evaluation should include a CT scan or MRI of the head. Treatment of macroadenomas consists of bromocryptine, surgery, or radiation therapy. Treatment of microadenomas is with bromocryptine alone. In idiopathic hyperprolactinemia, the medication may be withdrawn yearly to determine whether hyperprolactinemia returns.[155–159]

**Thyroid Abnormalities.** Both hyperthyroidism and hypothyroidism may be associated with infertility. These patients will have symptoms of thyroid dysfunction, and their initial presentation is generally not infertility.[160,161] Hyperthyroidism has effects at the pituitary and testicular level. Testicular biopsies may reveal maturation arrest.

**Glucocorticoid Excess.** Excess cortisol may be due to medical therapy or to endogenous production as in Cushing's syndrome. Infertility is due to a suppression of LH secretion at the pituitary due to the elevated levels of cortisol. This results in depressed levels of testosterone and testicular dysfunction.[162] Testicular biopsies demonstrate hypospermatogenesis or maturation arrest.[163,164] Treatment involves correction of the glucocorticoid excess.

## Testicular Causes of Male Infertility

**Chromosomal Abnormalities.** Chromosomal abnormalities have been found in approximately 6% of infertile men. The incidence increases as the count decreases with up to 21% of azoospermic men demonstrating karyotype abnormalities.[165] Most of the cases are found to have Klinefelter's or XYY syndrome (Table 7).

| TABLE 7. Testicular Causes of Male Infertility |
|---|
| Chromosomal abnormalities |
| Klinefelter's syndrome |
| XYY syndrome |
| Miscellaneous |
| Noonan's syndrome |
| Vanishing testis syndrome |
| Cryptorchidism |
| Orchitis |
| Mumps |
| Leprosy |
| Myotonic dystrophy |
| Gonadotoxins |
| Systemic illness |
| Sertoli-cell-only syndrome |
| Androgen abnormalities |
| Varicocele |
| Idiopathic |

***Klinefelter's Syndrome.*** Klinefelter's syndrome is the result of an extra X chromosome. Karyotypes will reveal either 47, XXY or 46, XY/47, XXY. It occurs in approximately 1 out of every 600 male births.[166,167] Prepubertal patients may be indistinguishable from normal pubertal boys. Once these patients enter puberty, they may not complete it. However, some patients develop complete virilization and present in adulthood with infertility, gynecomastia, and small, firm testes. Semen analysis will reveal azoospermia. Testicular biopsies demonstrate seminiferous tubular sclerosis. Occasionally, a few Sertoli cells or spermatozoa may be identified. Leydig's cells may appear prominent due to the absence of seminiferous tubules. Hormonal studies reveal elevated FSH levels while LH may be elevated or normal. Total testosterone levels may be normal due to an increase in testosterone binding globulin. However, free testosterone levels are commonly decreased. In most patients with the mosaic form of Klinefelter's, less severe abnormalities are found, and fertility in these patients has been reported.[168] There is no treatment for infertility in Klinefelter's-syndrome patients. While some authors recommend karyotype analysis in azoospermic patients with primary testicular failure, others feel this is not necessary since there is no treatment and the procedure may cause undue psychological stress to the patient.

***XYY Syndrome.*** The XYY karyotype occurs in 0.1% of male births.[169] Clinically, these patients are tall and demonstrate a range of fertility abnormalities. Testicular biopsies reveal patterns ranging from maturation arrest to germinal aplasia.[170–172] Hormonal evaluation usually reveals normal gonadotropins and testosterone levels.[173,174] Severe germinal aplasia may be associated with elevated levels of FSH. There is no treatment for infertile patients with this syndrome.

***Miscellaneous Chromosomal Abnormalities.*** While most patients with chromosomal abnormalities will have one of the above two syndromes, other abnormalities have been identified. In addition, testicular biopsies of infertile patients with normal somatic karyotypes have revealed meiotic abnormalities.[175–178] Down's syndrome may also be associated with testicular abnormalities.[179] Finally, abnormalities in mitotic and meiotic chromosomes have been reported in husbands of wives who had recurrent abortions.[180,181]

**Noonan's Syndrome.** The karyotype of patients with Noonan's syndrome is 46 XY. These patients have a phenotypic appearance of Turner's syndrome (XO) with short stature, hypertelorism, webbed neck, low-set ears, cubitus valgus, ptosis, and cardiovascular abnormalities.[182] In addition they may have cryptorchidism and associated testicular atrophy. Gonadotropin levels may be elevated as well. There is no treatment for these infertile patients.

**Vanishing Testis Syndrome.** This disorder occurs in XY males with nonpalpable absent testes. It is thought that while testicular tissue was present in utero, it was lost due to some event such as vascular injury, infection, or testicular torsion following gonadal differentiation. These patients will thus present with a male phenotype; however, they will not progress through puberty, due to a lack of androgen. Serum gonadotropins will be elevated while serum testosterone levels are low.[182] While virilization can be induced with testosterone, there is no treatment for infertility in these patients.

**Cryptorchidism.** Infertility in patients with cryptorchidism is common. Approximately 30% of men with unilateral cryptorchidism and 50% with bilateral cryptorchidism will have sperm densities below 12 to 20 million per milliliter.[184,185] Since infertility may occur in patients with unilateral cryptorchid testes, this data suggests that there is dysgenesis in both testes.[186,187] *The higher the cryptorchid testis, the more severe the testicular histology.* Thus, intra-abdominal testes may demonstrate an absence of germ cells in 90% of cases while only 20% to 40% of inguinal or prescrotal testes demonstrate absence of germ cells.[188] The mechanism of cryptorchidism remains unclear, with both mechanical and hormonal etiologies suggested. Therapy is aimed at correction of the cryptorchid testis at an early age. The evidence that testicular histologic changes occur within the first year of life have led to recommendations that the cryptorchid testis should be treated by 12 months of age. Fertility rates of patients with unilaterally cryptorchid testes that remain untreated were lower than fertility rates in patients with surgically corrected unilateral cryptorchidism.[185]

**Orchitis.** Postpubertal mumps results in orchitis in approximately 30% of patients.[188] In 10% to 30% of cases, there will be bilateral testicular involvement.[189,190] Testicular atrophy may result as early as a few months to several years after the infection. The atrophy is permanent and there is no treatment for cases which result in bilateral testicular atrophy. With the advent of mumps vaccine, this entity has become less common. Similarly, testicular and epididymal involvement may occur with syphilis. This results in diffuse interstitial inflammation with endarteritis and gumma formation. With increased awareness of sexually transmitted diseases, this entity has become rare. Other uncommon causes of orchitis include leprosy and untreated cases of gonorrhea.

**Myotonic Dystrophy.** This disease consists of myotonia, which is a condition of delayed muscle relaxation after contraction. In addition, patients demonstrate premature frontal baldness, posterior subcapsular cataracts, and cardiac conduction defects. Importantly, up to 80% of patients may develop testicular atrophy.[191] Testicular damage usually occurs in adulthood. Leydig's cells typically are uninvolved with biopsies demonstrating severe tubular sclerosis. Serum FSH will be elevated with severe tubular atrophy.[192] The disease is transmitted as an autosomal dominant trait with variable penetrance. Infertility is rarely the presenting symptom of this disease.[193] There is no therapy for the testicular dysfunction in these patients.

**Gonadotoxins.** Since the germinal epithelium consists of continually dividing cells, it is susceptible to injury by many agents that interfere with cell division. Drugs that interfere with androgen production or action may also affect fertility.

***Chemotherapy.*** Most chemotherapeutic agents adversely affect spermatogenesis.[194] Spermatogonia and spermatocytes up to the preleptotene stage are the most actively dividing and therefore the most susceptible to damage. Spermatids and mature spermatozoa are more resistant.[195] As long as the spermatogonial stem cells are not eradicated or permanently injured, they will slowly divide, eventually repopulating the seminiferous tubules, resulting in a resumption of spermatogenesis. The results in a particular patient vary with the type and combination of drugs used in therapy, the dose administered, and the age of the patient at the time treatment. Byrne, et al followed a large group of patients who survived childhood cancers. These investigators found that those patients treated with aklylating agents demonstrated fertility rates of 60% less than untreated controls.[196] With the increased use of multidrug regimens, it is difficult to ascribe testicular damage to one specific agent. Treatment of Hodgkin's disease with MOPP and MVPP and COPP regimens result in permanent sterility of 80% to 100% of patients.[197–204] Patients with non-Hodgkin's lymphoma and leukemia are treated with less toxic regimens and subsequently have a better prognosis for a resumption of spermatogenesis.[201,205] As mentioned previously, approximately 25% of testicular cancer patients had preexisting defects in spermatogenesis in the contralateral testis.[206] Newer chemotheric regimens including PVB, PVP-16, or POMB/ACE have allowed a resumption, of sperm production in 50% to 60% of patients.[207–212] It is important to realize that sperm production may not resume for up to 1 year after chemotherapy and maximal production may take several years.

***Drug Therapy.*** Many pharmacological agents have been found to affect fertility. Able, et al found that in animal experiments, cocaine ingestion was associated with the production of morphologically abnormal spermatozoa.[213] Heavy use of marijuana has been associated with decreased serum testosterone levels, gynecomastia, and a decrease in sperm concentration.[214,215] Alcohol has direct effects upon both the liver and the testes. Chronic alcoholics often demonstrate testicular atrophy. In a recent study, Marshburn looked at semen parameters as a function of the level of ethanol consumption in a group of infertile men. These investigators found no effect of the level of alcohol consumption on semen parameters. However, this study looked only at infertile populations and therefore the effect of ethanol may have been obscured by additional causes of infertility in these patients.[216] In the same study, coffee-drinking was correlated with increases in sperm density and decreases in normal morphologic forms. While cigarette use has been associated with a decrease in fertility in women, there is controversy as to whether there are significant effects in males.

Prenatal use of diethylstilbestrol (DES) has been associated with an increased incidence of epididymal cysts, testicular atrophy, and cryptorchidism.[217] Nitrofurantoin can cause a depression in spermatogenesis and maturation arrest at the primary spermatocyte stage.[218] This effect occurs only with high doses.[219] Finally, many other drugs, such as cimetidine, sulfur drugs, amebicide soil fumigants, lead, and arsenic have been associated with a depression of spermatogenesis.[220–224] It is important to determine which medications a patient has been taking at the time of his evaluation and to determine if these drugs have any adverse affects on spermatogenesis.

***Radiation Therapy.*** Ionizing radiation results in a dose-dependent effect on the testis.[225] Damage can occur with as little as 200 cGy to the testicles. Spermatogonia and spermatocytes are most sensitive with spermatids being more resistant. Recovery of spermatogenesis ranges from less than 1 year to over 5 years, depending on the dosage.

**Systemic Illness.** Patients with renal failure may demonstrate decreased libido, impotence, defects in spermatogenesis, and gynecomastia.[226,227] Hormonal studies reveal decreased plasma testosterone, increased gonadotropins, and a decrease in sperm production. This persists despite hemodialysis.[228,229] The cause of the testicular defect in these patients is unclear. Renal transplantation results in an improvement in testicular function and the return of sperm production.[230] As noted previously, febrile illnesses may temporarily suppress spermatogenesis. This effect may not be evident for several months.[231] Not surprisingly, cirrhosis of the liver is also associated with infertility. These patients may demonstrate impotence, gynecomastia, and testicular atrophy. Lastly, sickle-cell disease patients may demonstrate decreased testicular size and occasionally oligospermia.

**Sertoli-Cell–Only Syndrome.** Sertoli-cell–only patients present with bilaterally small testes on an otherwise normal physical examination. Semen specimens demonstrate azoospermia, and testicular biopsies reveal a complete absence of germ cells with seminiferous tubules lined by Sertoli cells. The interstitium is normal. Significantly, since the testes are not sclerotic, they are of reasonably normal consistency as compared with the firm testes found in Klinefelter's syndrome. Serum testosterone and LH are normal whereas FSH is usually elevated. The etiology of this syndrome is unknown. While seminiferous tubules containing only Sertoli cells may be found in other pathologic conditions such as following gonadotoxins or episodes of orchitis, the testes will demonstrate a mixed pattern of spermatogenic defects in these cases as well as significant amounts of sclerosis.

**Androgen Abnormalities.** Various defects in androgen action result in androgen-resistant syndromes. These patients are 46, XY males whose phenotypes range from pseudohermaphroditism to a normal male phenotype with infertility. Because the data regarding the incidence is unclear and there is no treatment for this condition, patients are generally not investigated for androgen resistance in the absence of other suggestive evidence.

**Varicocele.** The varicocele is the most common surgically correctable cause of male infertility, being found in approximately 30% of infertile males.[232–239] This incidence is significantly higher than the incidence of varicoceles in healthy asymptomatic men. A study of 1592 asymptomatic men identified varicoceles in 151 (9.5%). Of the 94 subjects in whom semen analyses were performed, 25% demonstrated a reduction in sperm count while 56% demonstrated decreased sperm motility. This incidence has been confirmed by other investigators.[240] Thus, it is clear that all varicoceles are not associated with semen abnormalities. Anatomically, a varicocele is an abnormal dilatation of the spermatic veins of the pampiniform plexus. Approximately 90% of varicoceles are left-sided. This may be related to different venous drainage patterns of the left and right testicular vein. Unilateral right-sided varicoceles are rare, and suggest the possibility of situs inversus or venous thrombosis.[241] Bilateral varicoceles constitute approximately 10% of the cases. There is controversy as to the pathophysiologic mechanisms responsible for abnormal spermatogenesis in varicocele patients. Zorgniotti and MacLeod reported that the intrascrotal temperatures of oligospermic patients with varicoceles were 0.6°C higher than those of a control group of patients without varicoceles.[242] In addition, recent studies examining the change in temperature from the supine to the standing position reported a 0.78°C-increase in temperature in the testis with a varicocele as compared with a decrease of 0.5°C in testes without varicoceles.[243] Other investigators have found no differences in testicular temperature between patients with and without varicoceles.[244,245] Other postulated mechanisms include reflux of renal and adrenal metabolites from the renal vein, decreased blood flow, and hypoxia.[246–248]

The semen analyses of patients with varicoceles was described by MacLeod in 1965. He found that 65% of patients demonstrated sperm densities of less than 20 million sperm per milliliter. Poor motility was more frequent, being found in 90% of patients. MacLeod also described a sperm morphologic pattern known as the "stress pattern." This consists of more than 15% tapered forms as well as increases in amorphous cells and increased numbers of immature germ cells. While this stress pattern is commonly found in varicocele patients, it is not pathognomonic of varicoceles being present in patients with viral illnesses and those that had ingested antispermatogenic compounds. Testicular biopsies in patients with varicoceles demonstrate hypospermatogenesis and/or maturation arrest and premature sloughing of spermatids into tubular lumen. This is believed to account for the seminal abnormalities.[249] The diagnosis of a varicocele rests on a thorough physical examination as previously mentioned. We feel that the data presently are insufficient to warrant investigations for subclinical varicoceles.

Recently, attention has been directed at the adolescent varicocele. Varicoceles are rare in the prepubertal age group while they are increasingly diagnosed as the child progresses through puberty.[250–252] By age 13, varicoceles are present in approximately 15% of males. Steeno, et al found that 34% of children with a grade II varicocele and 81% of children with a grade III varicocele demonstrated changes in testicular volume and consistency in the ipsilateral testis.[251] Hormonal studies of the varicocele patient are generally normal, although some patients may demonstrate elevations of FSH.[253] Cass and Belman treated 20 adolescents with grade II or III varicoceles and ipsilateral loss of testicular volume. Following varicocele repair, 16 of these patients demonstrated a significant increase in testicular volume.[254] Presently, attention is being directed at determining which adolescents with varicoceles will subsequently develop testicular atrophy. Presently, adolescents with grade II or III varicoceles and testicular atrophy should undergo varicocele correction.

Treatment of varicoceles consists of occlusion of the reflexing spermatic veins.

Both surgical ligation and radiographic occlusion have been used in this patient population. Although some investigators have suggested that medical therapy may be used in the treatment of varicoceles, there are no well-designed studies suggesting that medical therapy has any role in the initial treatment of the varicocele patient.[255] Following varicocele repair, Dubin and Amelar found motility improved in 70% of patients, sperm densities improved in 51% of patients, and morphology improved in 44% of patients.[256] Unfortunately, only 50% of couples will conceive.[237,239,256–263]

Radiographic occlusion has also been used to treat varicoceles. The success rate of this procedure varies with the skill of the radiologist. In those centers experienced in venographic occlusion, success rates in occluding the varicocele are up to 90%.[264] However, these high rates are not found by all investigators, with reported occlusion rates varying from 50% to 100%.[265] The recurrence rates after radiographic occlusion average 5%, whereas recurrence rates after surgery average approximately 10%. Thus, in the best of hands, success with radiographic occlusion equals that of surgical ligation. However, in many centers not experienced in this radiographic technique, this procedure is less effective than surgery. Additionally, Murray, et al studied the anatomy of recurrent varicoceles following surgical and radiographic occlusion.[266] These investigators found that recurrences following surgical correction tended to occur distally in the venous system whereas recurrences following radiographic occlusion occurred more proximally. Radiographic occlusion was more successful in treating recurrences following surgical ligation than treating recurrences following radiographic occlusion as the initial therapy. We therefore feel that in most instances, surgical therapy is the preferred initial treatment of varicoceles.

***Surgical Technique.*** The surgical correction of varicoceles involves the ligation of the refluxing testicular veins. There are three surgical approaches: a high-retroperitoneal approach, an inguinal approach, and a scrotal approach. In the high-retroperitoneal approach, a transverse abdominal incision is made 1 cm medial to the anterior/superior iliac spine. The external oblique fascia is incised in the direction of its fibers, and the internal oblique and transverse abdominis musculature are split in the direction of their fibers. The retroperitoneum is then entered by opening the transversalis fascia and reflecting the peritoneum medially. The spermatic vein is identified running in a vertical direction adjacent to the lateral reflection of the peritoneum. The veins are individually isolated and doubly ligated. It is not necessary to excise a portion of the vein. One or two branches of the spermatic vein are usually identified at this level. The abdominal musculature is reapproximated with 4.0 chromic sutures. The external oblique is approximated with a running 2.0 Polyglactin suture and the skin closed with a subcutaneous 4.0 Polyglactin suture (Fig 4).

For the inguinal approach to the varicocele, an oblique inguinal incision is made 2 cm above the pubic symphysis beginning medially at the lateral border of the insertion of the scrotal skin to the perineum and extending laterally. The external oblique fascia is then incised in the direction of its fibers over the spermatic cord. It is not necessary to open the external inguinal ring. The spermatic cord is then identified lying in the inguinal canal. Using the index finger and thumb, it is bluntly elevated from the inguinal canal and a Penrose drain placed under it. The spermatic fascia is then bluntly entered. The dilated spermatic veins are then easily visible. These are individually doubly ligated with 2.0 silk suture. Again, it is not necessary to remove a portion of the vein. We routinely use optical loops and/or a Doppler ultrasound to specifically identify and to avoid the testicular artery. At this level, there are usually between two and four veins requiring ligation. The spermatic cord is then placed back in the inguinal canal and the external oblique fascia closed with a running 2.0 Polyglactin suture. The wound is then closed in an identical manner to the high retroperitoneal approach (Fig 5).

The scrotal approach to varicocele repair

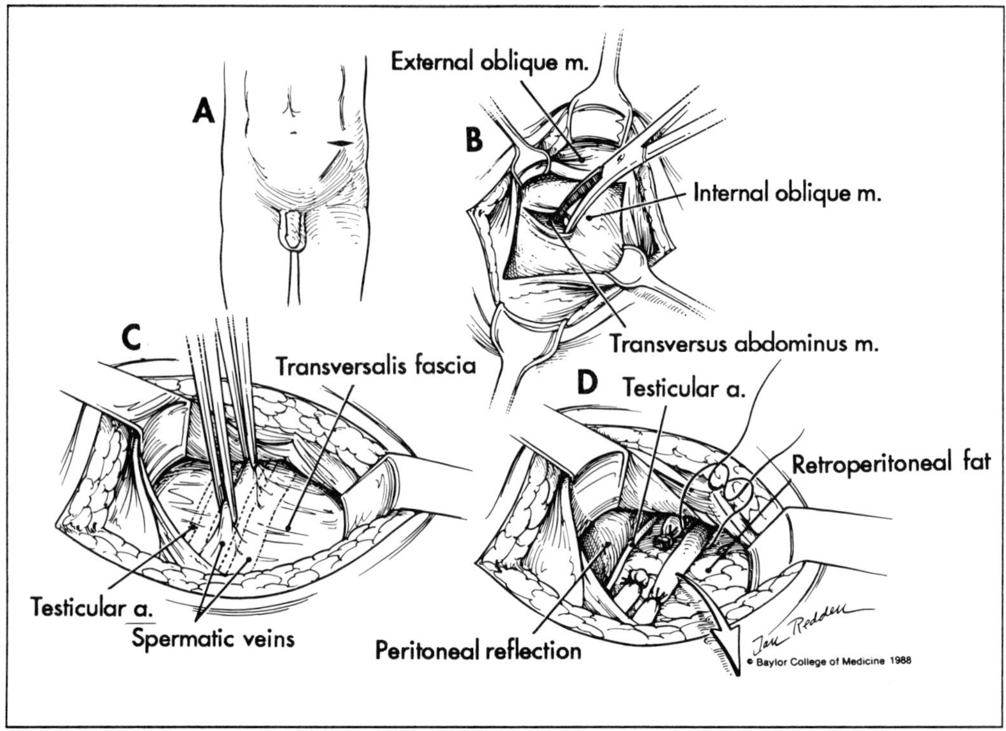


**Fig 4. A–D:** Technique for high retroperitoneal varicocele ligation. [Reproduced with permission from Sigman M, Lipshultz LI, Internal spermotic vein ligation, in Fowler JA (ed), *Mastery of Surgery: Urology* (Boston, Mass: Little, Brown & Co; 1990).]

involves using the operating microscope to individually ligate veins in the spermatic cord at the level of the scrotum. In most hands, this approach will be considerably more time consuming than the prior approaches and will yield similar success rates.

Postoperative complications are unusual. The most common complication in the Dubin and Amelar series was a hydrocele occurring in 3% of patients.[255] Other, less common, complications included wound infections, inguinal hematomas, epididymitis, atelectasis, and a bladder hernia injury. Following surgical correction, the average time to pregnancy was approximately 5 months.

While all three approaches give similar success rates, we find the inguinal approach easier and prefer this as the initial approach. In patients who have had hernia repairs or prior varicocele repairs with recurrence, a second surgical procedure may be employed. However, a different incision should be used to avoid traversing scar tissue and inadvertently injuring the contents of the spermatic cord. In these cases, a high-retroperitoneal approach or an inguinal approach, with the incision made over the pubic tubercle, may be employed. Radiographic occlusion may also be used in these patients. In the approach to the varicocele patient, it must be remembered that all varicoceles do not require correction. Indications include an infertile couple in which the male demonstrates a clinically detectable varicocele and an abnormal semen analysis. In addition, it is important to verify the wife's fertility status.

**Idiopathic Infertility.** Idiopathic male infertility refers to those patients with abnormal semen analyses and normal physical examinations, for which no etiology for the spermatogenic defect can be identified. While it has generally been considered that

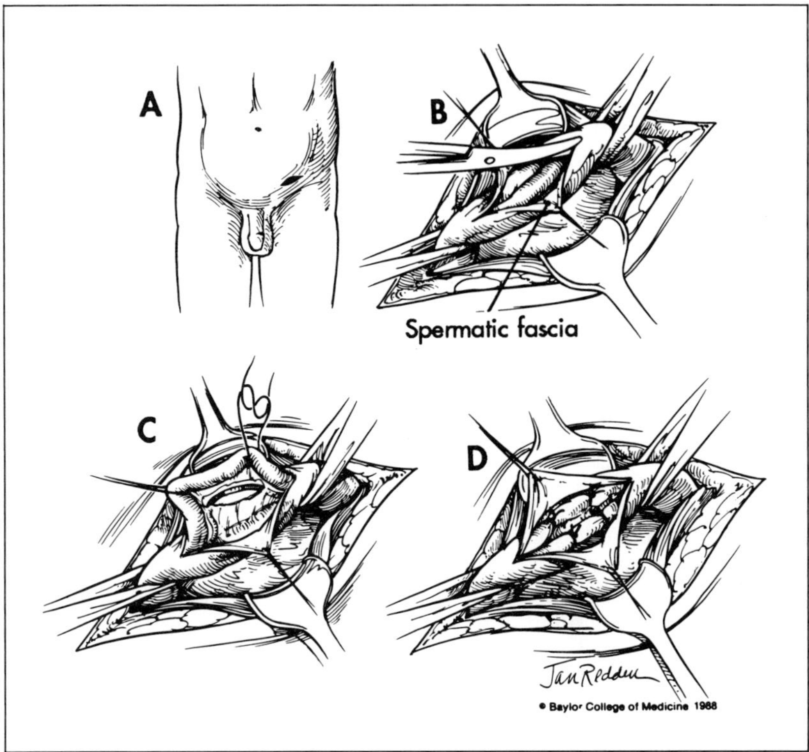


**Fig 5. A–D:** Technique for inguinal varicocele ligation. [Reproduced with permission from Sigman M, Lipshultz LI, Internal spermotic vein ligation, in Fowler JA (ed), *Mastery of Surgery: Urology* (Boston, Mass: Little, Brown & Co; 1990).]

these patients should have normal levels of gonadotropins and testosterone, we also include in this group patients with mild elevations of FSH but normal LH and testosterone levels. While some include patients with normal semen parameters but an abnormal sperm penetration test, this classification is not universally accepted.

Semen parameters in this group are variable. Greenburg, et al found that 43% of these patients demonstrated abnormalities of all sperm parameters, 39% had motility/viability abnormalities with normal sperm densities, 10% had isolated oligospermia, and 8% had isolated morphologic abnormalities.[267] Thus, while many physicians refer to this group of patients as having idiopathic oligospermia, it is clear that isolated oligospermia are not the most common abnormality. While patients with these seminal abnormalities are grouped into one classification, there are likely many different causes for these abnormalities. Therefore, one can expect that until individual etiologies are identified for these abnormalities, highly successful therapies will not be developed.

There are two approaches to the treatment of couples in which the male demonstrates idiopathic infertility. Pharmacologic therapy attempts to improve semen quality. Assisted reproductive techniques utilize the suboptimal semen specimen, but attempt to increase the chances of conception by manipulation of sperm and/or ova. Most commonly, initial therapy is directed at improving the quality of the semen. If this fails, the couple then may proceed with assisted reproductive techniques. However, in some instances, both therapies are initiated simultaneously. This section deals with the pharmacologic treatment of idiopathic male infertility.

***Antiestrogens.*** Antiestrogens act by blocking estrogen receptors in the hypothalamus.

A decrease in feedback inhibition of GnRH secretion by estrogens results. This causes an increase in gonadotropin secretion from the pituitary, which will result in increased testosterone production and, hopefully, improved spermatogenesis.

Clomiphene citrate has both antiestrogenic and estrogenic activity. It has been used in the treatment of male infertility for many years. While many dosages have been used, it appears that dosages greater than 100 to 200 mL per day yield no consistent change in sperm concentration, and in some cases result in suppression of spermatogenesis.[268] Lower dosages have resulted in improvement in sperm density in 4% to 89% and improved motility in 0% to 70% of patients. Although pregnancy rates have ranged from 0% to 90%, the majority of studies report rates of 30% or less.[269–280] Of the few controlled studies that have been performed, conflicting results have been obtained. Paulson,[281] Ronnberg,[279] Wang,[282] and Micic,[283] demonstrated favorable responses to Clomid therapy. However, in a recent study comparing clomiphene citrate (25 mg per day) to placebo for 12 months, a pregnancy rate of 44% was obtained in the placebo group compared with 9% in the clomiphene citrate group. All sperm counts in both placebo and treatment groups increased with time, emphasizing the importance of having a placebo arm. In addition, many of the studies, while demonstrating some improvement in sperm count, demonstrated no improvement in sperm motility. In conclusion, it appears that treatment with 25 to 50 mg of clomiphene citrate for a 6-month period may be beneficial in some patients. Unfortunately, no study has been able to identify which patients will respond to this treatment.

Tamoxifen, an oral antiestrogen, has also been used in the treatment of male infertility. Unlike clomiphene, it has no estrogenic activity. Most investigators have used regimens of 10 to 20 mg per day. Although some degree of improvement in sperm concentration has been reported (0% to 100%) there is usually no change in motility. Pregnancy rates range from 11% to 40%.[284–289] This indicates responses similar to that found with clomiphene studies. Similarly, it appears that a minority of patients may respond to tamoxifen; however, we are still unable to preselect this group of patients.

***Testolactone.*** Testolactone inhibits the peripheral conversion of androgens to estrogens. Since the majority of circulating estrogens in the male derive from peripheral conversion of androgens, and estrogens most likely have an adverse affect upon spermatogenesis, it is felt that a reduction in circulating estrogens may have a beneficial effect upon spermatogenesis. Uncontrolled studies suggested an improvement in sperm density following therapy with testolactone. However, a well-designed, double-blind placebo crossover study by Clark and Sherins[290] found that treated semen quality did not change during either treatment arm and no pregnancies occurred during the study. Thus, it appears that testolactone treatment no longer has a role in the treatment of idiopathic male infertility.

***Human Chorionic Gonadotropin.*** Human chorionic gonadotropin (hCG) is often given empirically to patients with idiopathic male infertility on the assumption that stimulation of testosterone synthesis may correct an intratesticular deficiency of this hormone. Dosages have ranged from 2500 to 5000 IU intramuscularly, 1 to 3 times per week, for 12 to 15 weeks. Improvement in sperm counts ranged from 17% to 35% and improvement in motility ranged from 22% to 94% of patients. Pregnancy rates ranged from 6% to 47%. It is difficult to draw conclusions from these uncontrolled studies, as the designs and treatment regimens differ significantly. It appears that motility increases more frequently than sperm density.[291–295] Human chorionic gonadotropin has also been used in patients with sperm densities of less than 10 million sperm per milliliter following varicocele ligation. In an uncontrolled study, it appeared that sperm density and pregnancy rates were improved as compared with no postoperative hormonal therapy. However, there have been no controlled studies to date that have confirmed this effect.[254] Some investigators have added human menopausal gonadotropin (hMG) to hCG in the hope that added FSH stimulation would result in improved spermatogenesis. Increased sperm counts have been demonstrated in approximately 50% of patients. However, conception rates have ranged from 0% to 17%.[296–299] These data indicate no benefit from the addition of hMG to hCG in the therapy for idiopathic male infertility.

***Gonadotropin-Releasing Hormone.*** Gonadotropin-releasing hormone (GnRH) is a more physiologic means of increasing gonadotropin levels. While some studies have demonstrated improved semen parameters, others have demonstrated no significant change and pregnancy rates have been inconsistent.[300–302] With the paucity of data on this therapy and the considerable expense involved, one must conclude that this therapy has yet to be proven useful in the treatment of idiopathic infertility.

***Testosterone Rebound.*** Early studies demonstrated that following testosterone administration to normal males for 12 or more weeks, most patients developed azoospermia. Following cessation of therapy, sperm densities usually returned to baseline levels.[303] Investigators found that in some oligospermic males sperm counts following cessation of therapy were higher than baseline levels. However, in 4% of patients, sperm counts did not return even to pretreatment levels.[303] Overall, the results have been disappointing, with improvement in sperm motility found in 0% to 25% of patients and pregnancy rates 3% to 9%.[304–306]

***Steroids.*** While steroids have a role in the treatment of immunologically mediated infertility, some investigators have used them in the treatment of idiopathic male infertility. However, results have been disappointing and we do not think there is a role for the use of steroids in this patient population.

***Kallikrein.*** Kallikreins are enzymes that stimulate the release of kinins from precursor molecules (kininogens). Although kallikrein is not available in the United States, European studies have noted that oral administration of the agent results in 67% of patients demonstrating an increase in sperm motility and pregnancy rates of 17% to 38%. There appear to be no predictive factors in determining a positive response to kallikrein.

***Pentoxifylline.*** Phosphodiesterase effects the breakdown of cyclic AMP, which is an important second messenger for polypeptide hormone action. Pentoxifylline, an inhibitor of phosphodiesterase, causes an increase in intracellular cyclic AMP concentration. Studies have demonstrated no consistent improvement in semen parameters. Of significance, pentoxifylline has been used for in vitro semen processing, resulting in increased fertilization rates when used with in vitro fertilization.[307,308]

***Prostaglandin Inhibitors.*** Prostaglandins have been found in large amounts in human semen. Several investigators have looked at the effect of nonsteroidal anti-inflammatory agents on prostaglandin concentrations as well as semen parameters. Both prostaglandin PGE and PGF are decreased after treatment with nonsteroidal anti-inflammatory agents. Barkay, et al examined 100 oligospermic patients treated with various doses of indomethacin and ketoprofen as compared with the placebo. They found that treatment increased sperm count and motility.[309] Of note, it has been found that these agents may increase gonadotropin levels while decreasing testosterone levels. At present, this data remains preliminary.[309–312]

***Miscellaneous Therapies.*** A number of other agents have been used empirically, with little or no effect. Among these are arginine, bromocriptine, thyroxin, and oxytocin.

### Posttesticular Causes of Infertility

Obstructions of the genital ducts constitute the majority of posttesticular causes of male infertility. Obstruction may occur at any level from the efferent ductuals to the ejaculatory duct. These obstructions may be congenital or acquired. Also included in this category are those patients with ejaculatory dysfunction in whom there is no anatomical obstruction but in whom the ejaculatory process functions abnormally (Table 8).

**Congenital Ductal Obstruction.** Congenital obstruction of the genital ducts is an uncommon cause of male infertility. Congenital absence of the vas deferens accounts for 11% to 50% of these cases.[313–315] Epididymal anatomy in these patients varies. Some may demonstrate full epididymides with a remnant of the convoluted portion of the vas, whereas others have only the caput portion of the epididymis formed. Often, the seminal vesicles are absent or atrophic. In addition, unilateral renal agenesis may also be present in some patients. Semen analyses will reveal a low volume azoospermic ejaculate that never coagulates. Early attempts at therapy were directed at the use of alloplastic spermatoceles. Unfortunately, these have not been successful as the devices often become occluded. In addition, nonmotile sperm were often obtained. Turner found pregnancy rates between 0% to 4% when reviewing published literature.[316]

Temple-Smith, et al first demonstrated the ability of sperm aspirated from the epididymis of a patient with secondarily obstructed azoospermia to fertilize human ova in vitro and result in conception.[317] Following this report, Silber applied this technique to patients with congenital absence of the vas.[318] In an initial report, 10 out of 32 couples (32%) conceived following epididymal sperm aspiration and in vitro fertilization. Other investigators have not found such promising results. While these data are preliminary, they offer promise for a treatment of this previously untreatable condition.[319]

**TABLE 8. Posttesticular Causes of Male Infertility**

| |
|---|
| Ductal obstruction |
| Congenital |
| Congenital absence of the vas |
| Ejaculatory duct obstruction |
| Young's syndrome |
| Acquired |
| Infection |
| Ligation of vas |
| Ejaculatory dysfunction |
| Miscellaneous |

Inflammatory conditions of the epididymis may also result in ductal obstruction and azoospermia. Both gonococcal and tuberculous epididymitis have been found as etiologic factors. The incidence of epididymal obstruction following epididymitis is not known since bilateral obstructions would need to occur before the patient would present with infertility. While these inflammatory causes have been common in the past, they are uncommon causes of obstruction at the present time.

Young's syndrome is a combination of obstructive azoospermia and chronic sinopulmonary infections. Azoospermia is due to obstruction of the epididymis by inspissated secretions. Spermatogenesis is normal in these patients. These patients differ from those with cystic fibrosis in that pancreatic function is normal, as is the sweat test. Fertility has been reported in some patients prior to the development of azoospermia. Poor results have been obtained following surgical vasoepididymostomies.[320,321]

With the advent of transrectal ultrasonography, the accuracy of diagnosis of obstruction of the ejaculatory ducts and seminal vesicles has improved. Obstruction may be congenital or secondary to infections. Treatment consists of incising the ejaculatory ducts cystoscopically. Following treatment, seminal volume and semen parameters markedly improve.

Vasectomy is the most common cause of ductal obstruction today. Most patients requesting vasectomy reversal have divorced and remarried. Evaluation of patients with ductal obstruction generally reveal normal testes associated with azoospermia. In most patients, testicular function is not grossly affected, following vasal occlusion. Gonadotropin and testosterone levels remained normal in most of these patients.[322,323] Treatment of ductal obstruction consists of surgery.

***Vasovasostomy.*** There have been many techniques described to perform vasovasostomies; however, they may be classified into three basic types. Macroscopic techniques use no optical magnification to perform the vasal anastomosis. These techniques do not guarantee a precise mucosal-to-mucosal anastomosis and have therefore frequently employed the use of intraluminal stents. While the results have varied between studies, both patency and pregnancy rates have generally been lower with macroscopic techniques as compared with techniques that employ optical magnification.[324]

Optical-loupe magnification allows for finer suture material to be used for the anastomosis. Patency rates have varied between 84% to 92% with pregnancy rates ranging between 54% and 70%.[324] Microscopic vasovasostomy is the preferred technique, allowing a precise mucosal-to-mucosal anastomosis. In addition, for an anastomosis involving the convoluted portion of the vas and vasoepididymostomies, the microscope is essential.

SURGICAL TECHNIQUE. Vasovasostomy may be performed under local, epidural, spinal, or general anesthesia. If local anesthesia is used, a block of the spermatic cord should be performed using 0.5% bupinicaine. The addition of IV sedation is recommended as it helps the patient remain still throughout the procedure. Following anesthesia, a vertical hemiscrotal incision is made. While some authors only expose the vas deferens and do not bring the testis through the wound, we find it advantageous to bring the testis, epididymis, and vas through the scrotal incision. The tunica vaginalis does not need to be entered if a vasoepididymostomy is not going to be performed. The site of the prior vasectomy is identified and a region of the vas proximal to this site is isolated. Care should be taken to avoid devascularizing a large segment of vas. Traction is then applied to the vas and it is sharply divided using a number 11 scalpel blade. Fluid from the testicular side of the vas should be examined microscopically. It is preferable to have a laboratory microscope in the operating room so that time is not wasted while the specimen travels to the pathology laboratory. The fluid may be collected using a 3-cm$^3$ syringe and a number 22 angiocath. The presence of sperm in this fluid indicates the absence of epididymal obstruction and is associated with improved patency rates. In cases in which no sperm are identified, consideration should be given to performing a vasoepididymostomy or exploring the vas deferens more proximally.

A portion of the vas deferens distal to the prior vasectomy site is then isolated in a similar manner and transected. Jeweler's forceps are then used to gently dilate this lumen. Frequently, the lumen is significantly smaller than the lumen of the vas proximal to the vasectomy site. The vas is then catheterized with a 22-gauge angiocath and irrigated with a syringe filled with saline. If the vas irrigates easily, distal patency is indicated. If there is any question as to whether the distal vas is patent, methylene blue may be added to the saline and the irrigation repeated. Methylene blue obtained from a catheter placed in the bladder confirms distal patency. If obstruction is found, a radiologic vasogram may be performed. If a decision is made to perform a vasovasostomy, the two ends of the vas deferens are placed in a vas clamp. Techniques of microsurgical anastomoses vary from a modified two-layer anastomosis and a complete two-layer anastomosis, to a modified three-layer anastomosis. In a recent study, the vasovasostomy study group compared the patency and pregnancy rates following modified two-layer and complete two-layer anastomoses. They found no difference in pregnancy or patency rates between these two procedures.[320] We prefer to use the complete two-layer anastomosis technique when there is a marked difference in size between the lumens of the two ends of the vas deferens. If no marked size difference exists, either technique may be used.

In the two-layer anastomosis, the two layers consist of a mucosa:mucosa anastomosis with a second layer of muscularis and adventitia. With the two ends of the vas deferens brought in proximity with a vas clamp (alternately 5–0 nylon sutures placed periadventitially may be used to loosely approximate the vas deferens), a back wall layer using 9–0 monofilament nylon suture is placed through the adventitia and muscularis of the vas. These sutures are tied with the knots on the outside. The mucosal anastomosis is then performed using 10–0 double armed nylon sutures. We have found the use of bicurved needles quite useful for this technique. Five to eight interrupted 10–0 nylon sutures are usually required to approximate the inner mucosal edges. It is usually advantageous to place the last three sutures without tying them until all mucosal sutures have been placed. Following the mucosal anastomosis, the front wall of the vas is approximated with additional 9–0 nylon sutures (Fig 6).

For the modified two-layer technique, 4–8 interrupted full-thickness 9–0 sutures are placed in the vas and tied. This is followed by placing partial thickness sutures (incorporating the muscularis and adventitia) between the full-thickness sutures (Fig 7). Hemostasis should be meticulously maintained with the use of bipolar electrocautery. The testis is then placed back into the scrotum. The dartos muscle and skin are then closed in separate layers.

Several factors have been found to affect the prognosis of vasovasostomies. The longer the time since vasectomy, the poorer the prognosis. Patency and pregnancy rates of 97% and 76% were obtained in those patients with an obstructed interval of less than 3 years. Rates of 88% and 53% were found for obstructive intervals of 3 to 8 years, 79% and 44% for intervals of 9 to 14 years, and 71% and 30% for intervals of 15 years or longer.[325] Similar results have been found by other investigators.[321] The presence of a sperm granuloma at the vasectomy site has been found to be a positive prognostic factor. It is felt that a sperm granuloma reflects sperm leakage from the vas deferens resulting in a lower intraluminal pressure in the vas, thereby preventing a blowout of the epididymis.[321] However, Belker, et al found no significance to the presence of a sperm granuloma.[326]

In those cases in which no sperm were found in the vas fluid, the color of the fluid had prognostic significance. In those cases in which the vas fluid was clear and watery, sperm was present in the semen postoperatively in all patients. In those cases in which the fluid was cloudy, 50% of patients demonstrated sperm in the ejaculate, whereas in those cases in which the fluid was creamy only 20% of patients demonstrated sperm in the semen postoperatively.[327] Finally, the experience of the surgeon plays an important role in success rates. Those surgeons who perform these techniques frequently will obtain more consistent results than those who perform it on an intermittent basis.

***Vasoepididymostomy.*** Initial attempts at vasal epididymal anastomoses involved macrosurgical techniques that relied on the creation of a fistula between the epididymis and the vas deferens. A portion of the epididymis was incised opening many tubules. The vas deferens was then anastomosed to the tunica of the epididymis. Patency and pregnancy rates following this technique averaged 43% and 17%.[328] Present techniques involve microsurgical specific tubule anastomoses. The vas deferens may be anastomosed in an end-to-end fashion with the epididymis or in an end-to-side fashion. Recent reports have demonstrated patency rates averaging 75% and pregnancy rates between 25% and 45%.[329–331]

SURGICAL TECHNIQUE. The vasoepididymostomy should be performed on the most distal portion of the epididymis in which sperm can be obtained. For the end-to-side anastomosis, a 1-cm incision is made in the tunica of the epididymis. Multiple epididymal loops will be identified. Using careful, sharp dissection, one loop should be freed from the surrounding connective tissue. The wall of the tubule is then incised using a Beaver blade. Fluid extruding from the tubule should be examined microscopically. If sperm are present, the anastomosis may then proceed. If no sperm are identified, a portion of the epididymis more proximally should be explored. A 10–0 nylon double-armed suture is then passed through the wall of the ep-

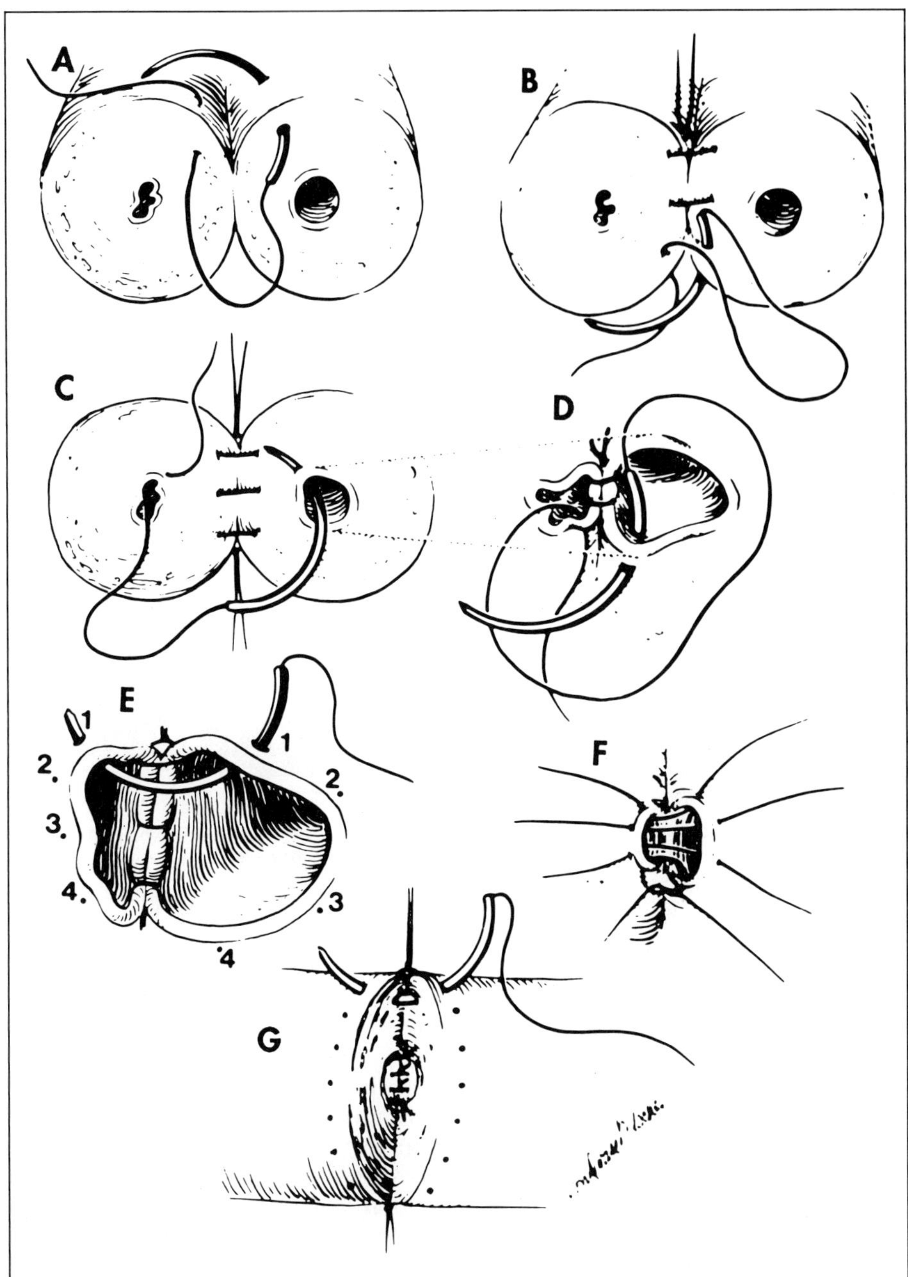


**Fig 6.** Technique of two-layer vasovasostomy. The back wall of the vas deferens is anastomosed with interrupted sutures **(A–B)**. The mucosal anastomosis is then performed with interrupted 10–0 sutures **(C–F)**. The front wall of the vas deferens is then approximated with interrupted 9–0 sutures **(G)**. [Reproduced with permission from Belker AM, Microsurgical two-layer vasovasostomy, *Urology* (1980; 16:376)

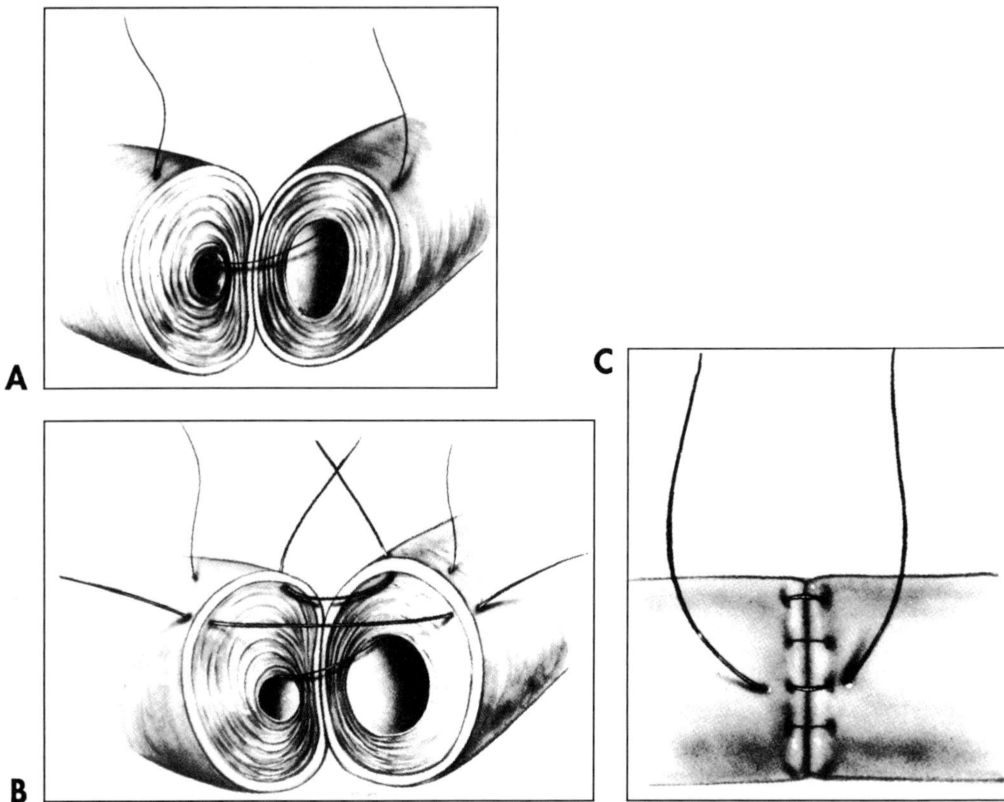


**Fig 7.** Technique of modified two-layer vasovasostomy. Four to six full-thickness sutures are placed through the vas deferens (**A**). These are followed by interrupted partial-thickness sutures, completing the anastomosis (**B–C**). [From Lipshultz LI, Howards SS, Surgical treatment of male infertility, in Lipshultz LI, Howards SS (eds), *Fertility in the Male.* (New York, NY: Churchill Livingstone; 1983; copyright Lipshultz LI).]

ididymis to aid in future identification. The distal vas deferens is then brought into proximity with the epididymal tunic. Using 9–0 nylon sutures, the anastomosis is begun, suturing the back wall muscular and adventitial layers of the vas to the epididymal tunic. The mucosa of the vas is then sutured to the edges of the epididymal tubule using the previously placed 10–0 nylon suture. A total of 4 to 6 sutures are used to complete the mucosal anastomosis. Additional 9–0 sutures are used to complete the anastomosis between the muscularis and adventitia of the vas and the tunica of the epididymis (Fig 8). To aid in the identification of the edges of the epididymal tubule, a drop of diluted methylene blue may be placed onto the epididymal tubule followed by saline irrigation. The outside edges of the epididymis will stain blue whereas the inner mucosa remains whitish-pink.

To perform an end-to-end vasoepididymostomy, the distal epididymis is freed from its mesentery connection to the testis. The epididymis is then transected at a distal portion and the extruding fluid examined for the presence of sperm. While many tubules will be transected, only one tubule will continue to produce fluid. If no sperm are found, the epididymis is transected at sequentially higher levels until sperm are identified. The distal cut end of the vas is then brought into proximity of the epididymis and the anastomosis performed. The mucosa of the vas is sutured directly to the epididymal tubule using 10–0 nylon sutures. The muscularis and adventitia of the

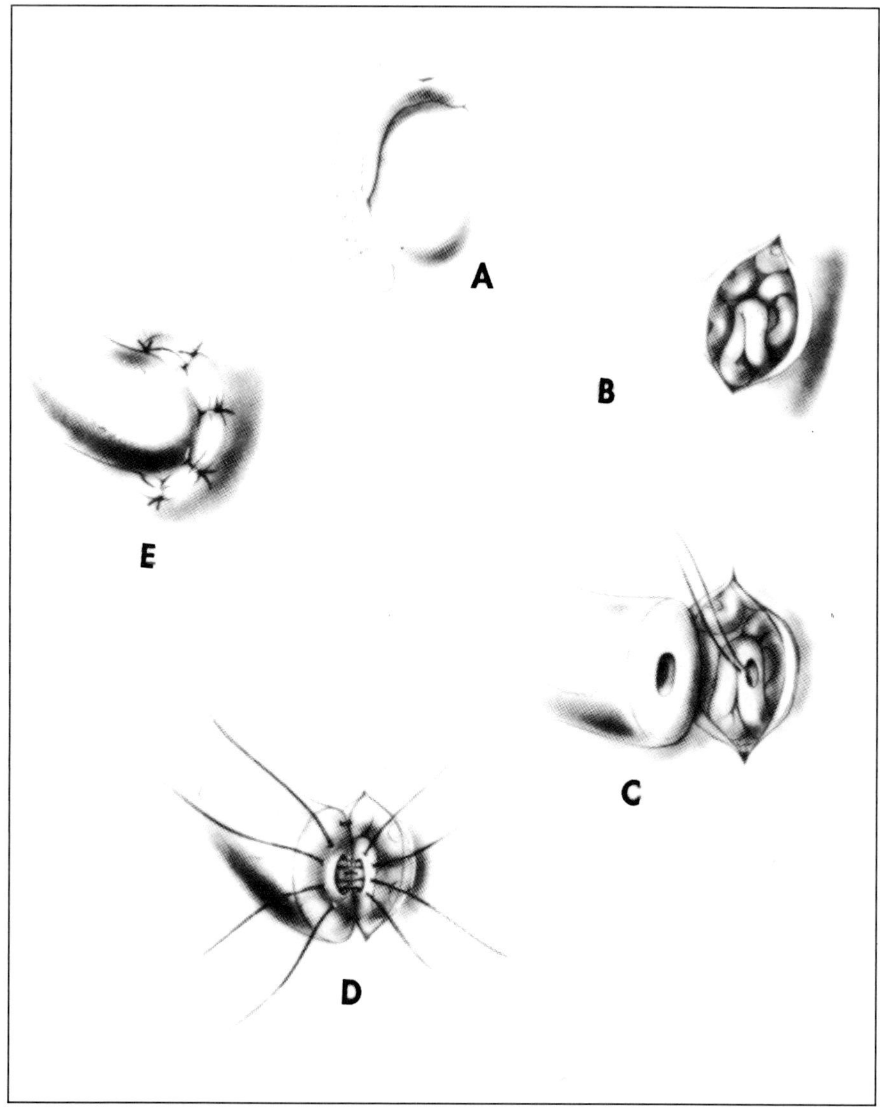


**Fig 8. A–E:** Technique of specific tubule end-to-side vasoepididymostomy. [Reproduced with permission from Thomas AJ, Vasoepididymostomy, *Urol Clin North Am* (1987; 14:527).]

vas are approximated to the epididymal tunic with interrupted 9–0 sutures (Fig 9). The testicle is then placed back into the scrotum and the wound closed as previously described.[332]

Pregnancy rates are higher the more distal the vasoepididymal anastomosis is performed. Silber reported pregnancy rates of 56% when the anastomosis was to the corpus epididymis as compared with a 31% pregnancy rate with anastomoses performed in the region of the caput epididymis.[329] Following vasoepididymostomies, sperm may not appear in the ejaculate for up to a year or more.[333] In addition, the quality of sperm may improve over time, possibly due to a recovery of epididymal function. Repeat vasovasostomies or vasoepididymostomies may be indicated in cases in which the initial

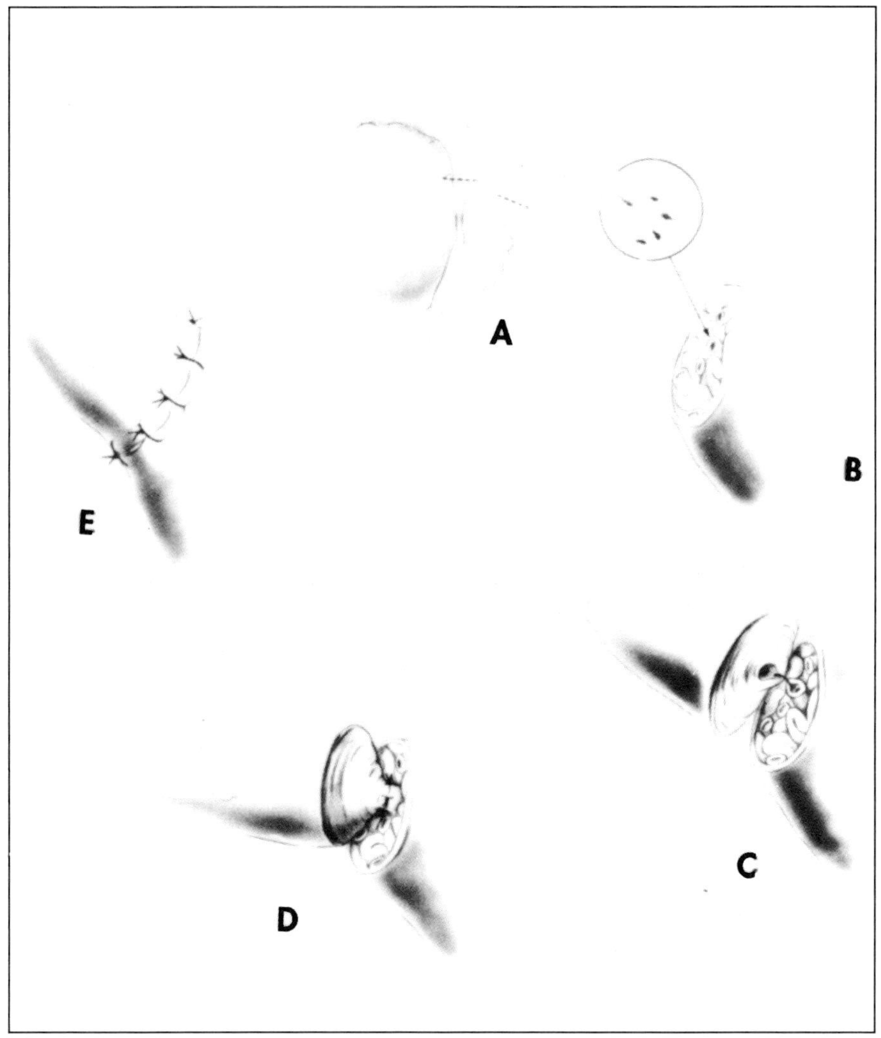


**Fig 9. A–E:** Technique of specific tubule end-to-end vasoepididymostomy. [Reproduced with permission from Thomas AJ, Vasoepididymostomy, *Urol Clin North Am* (1987; 14:527).]

procedure failed. Belker et al studied 219 repeat vasectomy reversals. They reported a 76% patency rate and a 31% pregnancy rate in this group of patients. These rates were significantly lower than the rates obtained after a first time vasectomy reversal.[334] Some investigators have advocated using lasers to assist in the performance of vasovasostomy citing increased surgical ease and shortened operative times.[335,336] Long-term follow-up is needed to determine whether this technique will result in pregnancy rates equal to those of traditional surgical approaches.

**Ejaculatory Dysfunction.** Ejaculatory dysfunction may be classified as retrograde ejaculation and lack of emission (ejaculatory failure). Retrograde ejaculation is diagnosed by examining a postejaculatory urine specimen. If significant numbers of sperm (>10–15 sperm per high-powered field) are identified, retrograde ejaculation is diagnosed. In most patients in whom retrograde ejaculation is not associated with a physical abnormality of the bladder neck (such as postsurgical changes), medical therapy may be attempted. This therapy may also be tried in patients with lack of emission. Therapy is directed at attempting to increase the tone of the internal sphincter and vas deferens. Pseudoephedrine hydrochloride (60 mg 4 times a day), ephedrine sulfate (25 to 50 mg 4 times a day), phenylpropanolamine hydrochloride (75 mg bid) and imipramine hydrochloride (25 mg bid) have been successfully used in some patients. Therapy should be continued for 2 weeks. In most patients with retrograde ejaculation with bladder neck scarring or in whom pharmacologic therapy has failed, sperm may be recovered from the bladder and used for insemination. Initial attempts may be directed at urinary alkinization. Sodium bicarbonate, in a dosage of 650 mg 4 times a day for 48 hours prior to collection, may be used. Water intake should be adjusted so that urine is in the isotonic range. Postejaculatory urine samples are then obtained, centrifuged, and sperm resuspended in sperm-washing media prior to insemination. If adequate sperm viability is not obtained by this method, more invasive methods may be used. Prior to ejaculation the bladder is emptied, then 30 to 60 $cm^3$ of a medium such as Hams F-10 media is instilled into the bladder. Following ejaculation, the patient may void this out, allowing for recovery of increased numbers of viable sperm.

***Electroejaculation.*** Recently, transrectal electrical stimulation has been used to induce ejaculation in cases of ejaculatory failure. While originally used in men with spinal-cord injuries, it is now being used in patients following retroperitoneal lymph node dissections, multiple sclerosis, transverse myelitis, other pelvic or retroperitoneal surgery, and diabetes mellitus. The rectal probe containing electrodes allows for the delivery of pulsed current to the periprostatic plexis. This will induce erections in most patients. Ejaculation is achievable in approximately 75% of patients.[337–339] In those patients with incomplete cord lesions or those patients post-retroperitoneal node dissections, general anesthesia will be required.[340] The semen obtained is washed and then used for intrauterine insemination. Semen quality varies from patient to patient. Those who have urinary tract infections or indwelling catheters demonstrate poorer semen parameters. Some investigators have found that vibratory stimulation of some spinal-cord-injured patients will induce ejaculation.[341] This technique may also be combined with electroejaculation. Further experience with these techniques will allow for a better estimation of expected conception rates.

## Assisted Reproduction Techniques

For those patients with idiopathic male infertility in whom no specific etiology can be found, or for those patients in whom an abnormal semen analysis persists after specific therapy, assisted reproductive techniques (ART) are indicated. These are techniques to improve conception rates by improving the ability of sperm to reach and fertilize ova and result in subsequent live births. There is a wide range of techniques employed in this group of patients. Some involve manipulation of sperm alone. Others involve manipulation of both sperm and eggs. Some techniques involve in vivo fertilization while others involve in vitro fertilization.

**Semen Processing.** All of the assisted reproductive techniques involve some form of semen manipulation. Semen processing involves removal of seminal plasma, while some procedures also select motile sperm and remove leukocytes and nonmotile sperm. This is accomplished through a variety of techniques ranging from simple sperm washing to more sophisticated swim-ups, sedimentation, and percol gradient centrifugations. By removing nonmotile sperm, the percentage of motile sperm in the processed specimen may be increased. While most investigators believe that it is important to remove nonmotile sperm and to allow in vitro sperm capacitation for in vitro fertilization technologies, there is no consensus as to whether this is required for intrauterine insemination. Recently, attempts have been made to increase the fertilizing capacity of sperm through the in vitro addition of various compounds, such as pentoxifylline. While the use of assisted techniques allows for conception with fewer numbers of sperm than would be required for natural conception, most investigators feel that following semen processing, 500,000 to 1 million motile sperm are needed to offer a significant chance of pregnancy.

**Intrauterine Insemination.** Intrauterine insemination is commonly employed in the treatment of both male and female factor infertility. The cervical mucus normally acts as both a barrier and a reservoir to sperm penetration. Only a small fraction of the sperm that present to the cervical mucus traverse it to reach the uterus. Intrauterine insemination bypasses the cervical mucus allowing for a higher concentration of motile sperm to reach the uterus and hopefully ascend the female reproductive tract. Indications include any abnormality preventing the deposition of semen in the region of the cervix (severe hypospadias, retrograde ejaculation), cervical mucus abnormalities, unexplained infertility, as well as male-factor infertility. There is considerable controversy as to the exact role of this technique in the treatment of male-factor infertility. In a review of 17 published series, Belker and Cook found the pregnancy rates ranged from 0% to 66%.[342] While the original studies employed deposition of raw semen into the uterus, this is no longer employed. Seminal prostaglandins may induce severe uterine cramping, and bacterial contamination of the semen may result in pelvic infection. Ovarian hyperstimulation has recently been used to induce the development of more than one mature egg per cycle. Preliminary controlled studies combining IUI and hyperstimulation have demonstrated pregnancy rates of 7% to 19% per cycle as compared with 0% to 2.2% pregnancy rates in nonstimulated cycles.[343–346]

**In Vitro Fertilization–Embryo Transfer.** In vitro fertilization–embryo transfer (IVF-ET) was originally used to treat female-factor infertility secondary to fallopian-tube obstruction. Many centers are now treating male-factor couples with this technique. This procedure requires several phases. In the first, hormonal stimulation is used to induce hyperovulation in the woman. Just prior to ovulation, oocytes are harvested from the ovary either laparoscopically or with the use of ultrasound-guided needle aspiration. A semen specimen is then collected and processed (commonly using the swim-up technique). Following oocyte retrieval and semen processing, the prepared sperm and oocytes are combined and incubated to allow fertilization to take place. Two to three days after ovum harvest, the developing embryos are injected into the uterus. While in the majority of non–male-factor couples, fertilization and embryos are achieved, in only 20% to 30% of these cases does a biochemical pregnancy result. This indicates that there is significant room for improvement in the techniques and methodologies of embryo transfer. Unlike non–male-factor couples, male-factor couples also demonstrate a defect in the ability of sperm to fertilize human ova in vitro. Fertilization rate is defined as the percentage of ova fertilized in vitro divided by the total number of oocytes inseminated. Experience has demonstrated that even if the motile sperm concentration is adjusted upward in male-factor patients, the sperm still do not function as well as sperm from non–male-factor patients. This results in persistant lower fertilization rates. Pregnancy rates also vary between male-factor and non–male-factor couples. An average of 16% of non–male-factor couples conceive per cycle as compared with 12% of male-factor couples. This difference arises from the increased rate of failure of fertilization in the male-factor couples. Once a couple has fertilized, many centers find that male-factor couples have better chance of implanting and proceeding to a subsequent pregnancy than non–male-factor couples. It is important to realize that a pregnancy rate is not the same as live birth. The 1989 IVF regestry reports a 9% live birth rate per egg-retrieval cycle for male-factor infertility couples. This is less than the live birth rate of 11% in non–male-factor couples.[347] The difference between live birth rates and pregnancy rates is due to the approximately 30% of abortions which occur after IVF. These are divided between subclinical and clinical abortions.

**Gamete Intrafallopian Transfer.** Gamete intrafallopian transfer (GIFT) is a technique in which ova are retrieved in a manner similar to IVF. However, sperm are mixed together with the ova and injected directly into the fallopian tube prior to fertilization. Since ova are normally fertilized by sperm in the fallopian tubes, this method has the theoretical advantage of allowing fertilization to occur in a more physiologic manner. In addition, no embryo culturing is involved. A disadvantage is that when couples undergo this procedure, the ability of the husband's sperm to fertilize the wife's oocytes is not determined. This is precisely the step that male-factor couples have difficulty with. The results of this procedure in male-factor couples has revealed pregnancy rates similar or higher than those found in IVF.

**Tubal-Transfer Techniques.** Tubal-transfer techniques combine the benefits of GIFT with the advantages of in vitro fertilization. Known by different names, [pronuclear stage tubal transfer (PROUST), zygote intrafallopian transfer (ZIFT), tubal embryo transfer (TET), tubal embryo stage transfer (TEST)] the techniques involve the in vitro fertilization of human eggs followed by placement of the embryo back into the fallopian tube. Several studies have demonstrated increased pregnancy rates using these techniques.[348]

**Micromanipulation.** While implantation rates have improved with the tubal-transfer techniques, fertilization rates remain a problem with male-factor patients. Various micromanipulation procedures have been used in attempts to increase fertilization rates in these patients. Since the zona pellucida around the ovum acts as a barrier to fertilization, attempts have been made to alter this structure. Zona drilling and partial zona dissection involve opening up a portion of the zona pellucida allowing sperm to fertilize the ova without having to traverse this structure. Malter and Cohen demonstrated a 68% fertilization rate in 18 couples undergoing IVF with micromanipulated oocytes as compared with a 47% fertilization rate in nonmicromanipulated controls.[349] Other techniques involve the microinjection of individual or few sperm into the perivitelline space (the space between the zona pellucida and the oocyte plasma membrane), or into the ooplasm directly. Further experience with these techniques is required to better determine which patients may benefit from this therapy.

With the plethora of therapies available to the infertile couple, it is imperative that the physician be familiar with these techniques. Specific therapy should be instituted in those cases in which a treatable abnormality is found. In those cases in which no identifiable or treatable condition is found, or in which the patient has not responded to specific therapy, the physician must help counsel the couple as to which therapeutic path to follow. The couple will need to decide between empiric medical therapy, therapeutic insemination with husband's semen, and in vitro technologies. In those cases in which no reasonable chance of conception can be expected, prolonged and unrewarding therapies should not be instituted and the couple should be encouraged to investigate therapeutic donor insemination and adoption. It is only with a thorough understanding of these options, that the physician can help the infertile couple arrive at a resolution to this frustrating condition.

## REFERENCES


1. Mosher WD. Reproductive impairments in the United States 1965–1982. *Demography*. 1985; 22:415.
2. Schally AV, Mair RMG, Arimura A, and Redding TW. Isolation of the luteinizing hormone and follicle-stimulating hormone releasing hormone porcine hypothalami. *J Biol Chem*. 1971; 246:7230.
3. Knobil E, Plant TM, Wildt L, Belchetz PE, Marshall G. Control of the Rhesus monkey menstrual cycle: permissive role of hypotha-

lamic gonadotropin-releasing hormone. *Science.* 1980; 207:1371.

4. Carmel PW, Arani S, Ferin M. Pituitary stalk portal blood collection in Rhesus monkeys: evidence for pulsatile release of gonadotropin-releasing hormones (GnRH). *Endocrinology.* 1976; 99:243.
5. Steinberger E, Steinberger A, Ficher M. Study of serpmatogenesis and steroid metabolism in cultures of mammalian testes. *Recent Prog Horm Res.* 1970; 26:547.
6. Hall PF, Irby DC, deKretser DM. Conversion of cholesterol to androgens by rat testes: comparison of intrastitial cells and seminiferous tubules. *Endocrinology.* 1969; 84:488.
7. Steinberger A, Elkington JSH, Sanborn BN, et al. Culture and FSH responses of Sertoli cells isolated from sexually mature rat testis. In: French FS, Hansson V, Ritzen EN, Mayfeh SH, eds. *Hormonal Regulation of the Spermato-genesis.* New York, NY: Plenum Press; 1975: 399.
8. Burger HG, McLachlan RI, Robertson DM, Bremner WJ, deKretser DM. Inhibin the regulation of testicular function historical and clinical aspects. *Ann NY Acad Sci.* 1989; 564:1.
9. Sairam MR, Ranganathan MR, Lamothe P. Purification and characterization of a follitropin suppressing principle from bull ejaculate. *Biol Reprod.* 1978: 18. Abstract #58.
10. Franchimont P, Croze F, Henderson K, Hazee-Hagelstein MT, Lecomte-Yerna MJ. Regulation of inhibin by granulosa cells in vitro. In: Sairam MR, Atkinson LE, eds. *Gonadal Protein and Peptides and Their Biological Significance.* World Scientific Publication; 1983: 127–139.
11. Goldzieher JW, Dozier TS, Smith KD, Steinberger E. Improving the diagnostic reliability of rapidly fluctuating plasma hormone levels by optimized multiple sampling techniques. *J Clin Endocrinol Metab.* 1976; 43:824.
12. Bain J, Langevin R, D'Costa M, SAnders RM, Hucker S. *Fert Steril.* 1988; 49:123.
13. Rifkind AB, Kulin HE, Ross GT. Follicle stimulating hormone (FSH) and leutinizing hormone (LH) in the urine of prepubertal children. *J Clin Invest.* 1967; 46:1925.
14. Albert A. Human urinary gonadotropins. *Rec Prog Horm Res.* 1956; 12:266.
15. Skinner MK, Fritz IB. Testicular peritubular cells secrete a protein under androgen control that modulates Sertoli cell functions. *Proc Natl Acad Sci USA.* 1985; 82:114.
16. Koskimies AI, Kormano M, Alfthan O. Proteins of the seminiferous tubule fluid in man—evidence for a blood testis barrier. *J Reprod Fertil.* 1973; 32:79.
17. Clermont Y. Renewal of spermatogonia in man. *Am J Anat.* 1966; 118:509.
18. Dym M, Cavicchia JC. Further observations on the blood testis barrier in monkeys. *Biol Reprod.* 1977; 17:390.
19. Phillips DM. Mammalian sperm structure. In: Hamilton DW, Greep RO, eds. *Handbook of Physiology, Section 7, Volume V, Male Reproductive System.* Baltimore, MD: Williams & Wilkins; 1975:405.
20. Amelar RD, Hotchkiss RS. The split ejaculate, its use in the management of male infertility. *Fertil Steril.* 1965; 16:46.
21. Eliasson R, Lindhomer C. Distribution and properties of the spermatozoa in different fractions of split ejaculates. *Fertil Steril.* 1972; 23:252.
22. Carter SSC, Shinohara K, Lipshultz LI. Transrectal ultrasonography in disorders of the seminal vessicles and ejaculatory ducts. *Urol Clin North Am.* 1989; 16:773.
23. Shah GV, Sheth AR, Mugatwala PP, Rao SS. Effect of spermine on adenyl cyclase activity of human spermatozoa. *Experientia.* 1975; 31:631.
24. Parrish KF, Polakoski KL. Effective of polyemines on the activity of acrosin and the activity of proacrosin. *Biol Reprod.* 1977; 17:417.
25. Wetterauer U, Heite HJ. Carnitine in seminal plasma. Its significance in diagnostic andrology. *Arch Androl.* 1980; 4:137.
26. Blank W. The role of the accessory glands in male infertility. *Semin Reprod Endocrinol.* 1988; 6:339.
27. Howards SS. The epididymis, sperm maturation, and capacitation. In: Lipshultz L, Howards SS, eds. *Infertility in the Male.* New York, NY: Churchill Livingstone; 1983; 131.
28. Byrd W, Wolf DP. Acrosomal status in fresh and capacitated human ejaculated sperm. *Biol Reprod.* 1986; 34:859.
29. Singh JP, Babcock BF, Lardy HA. Increased calcium ion influx is a component of capacitation of spermatozoa. *Biochem J.* 1978; 172:549.
30. Boyers SP, Corrales MB, Huszar G, DeCherney AH. The effects of lubrin on sperm motility in vitro. *Fertil Steril.* 1987; 47:882.
31. Goldenberg RL, White R. The effect of vaginal lubricants on sperm motility in vitro. *Fertil Steril.* 1975; 26:872.
32. Tagatz GE, Okagaki T, Sciarra JJ. The effect of vaginal lubricants on sperm motility and viability in vitro. *Am J Obstet Gynecol.* 1972; 113:88.
33. Tulandi T, Plouffe L Jr, McInnes RA. Effect of saliva on sperm motility and activity. *Fertil Steril.* 1982; 38:721.
34. Kogan SJ. Cryptorchidism. In: Kelalis PP, King LR, Belman AB, eds. *Clinical Pediatric Urology.* Philadelphia, Pa: WB Saunders; 1985:876.
35. Lipshultz LI, Caminos-Torres R, Greenspan

CS, Snyder PJ. Testicular function after orchiopexy for unilaterally undescended testes. *N Engl J Med.* 1976; 295:15.

36. Nijman JM, Koops H, Kremer J, et al. Gonadal function after surgery and chemotherapy in men with stage II and III non-seminimonous testicular tumors. *J Clin Oncol.* 1987; 5:651.
37. Carrol PR, Whitmore WF, Herr HW, et al. Endocrine and rxocrin profiles of men with testicular tumors before orchiectomy. *J Urol.* 1987; 137:420.
38. Rustin GJS, Pektasides D, Bagshawe KD, et al. Fertility and chemotherapy for male and female germ cell tumors. *Int J Androl.* 1987; 10:389.
39. McLeod J, Hotchkiss RS, Litterson BW. Recovery of male fertility after sterilization by nuclear radiology *JAMA.* 1964; 187:637.
40. Orecklin JR, Koffman JT, Thompson RW. Fertility in patients treated for malignant testicular tumors. *J Urol.* 1973; 109:293.
41. Jewett MAS. Nerve sparing technique for retroperitoneal lymphatinectomy in testis cancer. *Urol Clin North Am.* 1990; 17:449.
42. Werner CA. Mumps orchitis and testicular atrophy. *Ann Intern Med.* 1950; 32:1066.
43. Berul CI, Harclerode JE. Effects of cocaine hydrocloride on the male reproductive system. *Life Sci.* 1989; 45:91.
44. Kolodny RC, Masters WH, Kolodny RM, Toro G. Depression of plasma testostrone levels after chronic intensive marajuana use. *N Eng J Med.* 1974; 290:872.
45. Marshburn PB, Sloan CS, Hammond MG. Semen quality and association with coffee drinking, cigarette smoking and ethenol consumption. *Fertil Steril.* 1989; 52:162.
46. Abel EL, Moore C, Waselewsky D, Zajac C, Russell LD. Affects of cocaine hydrochloride on reproductive function and sexual behavior of male rats and on the behavior of their offspring. *J Androl.* 1989; 10:17.
47. VanThiel DH, Gavalet JS, Lester R, et al. Alcohol induced testicular atrophy. *Gastroenterology.* 1975; 69:326.
48. Ylikahri R, Huttunen M. Harkonen M, et al. Low plasma testosterone values during hangover. *J Steroid Biochem.* 1974; 5:655.
49. Holma PK. Effects of anibolic steroid (Metandienone) on spermatogenesis. *Contraception.* 1977; 15:151.
50. McLeod J, Hotchkiss RS. The effect of hyperpyrexia upon spermatozoa counts in men. *Endocrinology.* 1941; 28:760.
51. Carny SW, Tuttle W. The spermatogenic potential of the undescended testis before and after treatment. *J Urol.* 1960; 83:697.
52. Lubs HA Jr. Testicular size in Klinefelter's syndrome in men over 50. *N Engl J Med.* 1962; 267:326.
53. Lipshultz LI, Corriere JN Jr. Progressive testicular atrophy in the varicocele patient. *J Urol.* 1977; 117:175.
54. Seyferth W, Jecht E, Zeitler E. Percutaneous sclerotherapy of varicocele. *Radiology.* 1981; 139:335.
55. McClure RD, Hriacac H. Scrotal ultrasound in the infertile man: detection of subclinical unilateral and bilateral varicoceles. *J Urol.* 1986; 135:711.
56. Perrin P, Rollet J, Durand L. The Doppler stethoscope in the diagnosis of subclinical varicocele. *Br J Urol.* 1980; 52:390.
57. World Health Organization. Comparison among different methods for the diagnosis of varicocele. *Fertil Steril.* 1985; 43:575.
58. Natto NR Jr, Lemos GC, Barbosa EN. The value of thermography and of the Doppler ultrasound in varicocele diagnosis. *Int J Fertil.* 1984; 29:176.
59. Gonzalez R, Reddy P, Kaye KW, Marayan P. Comparison of Doppler examination and retrograde spermatic venography in the diagnosis of varicocele. *Fertil Steril.* 1983; 40:96.
60. Ponchietti R. Crarselli GF, Noci I, et al. Teletheromography and eco-Doppler. Evaluation of subclinical varicocele in infertile men. *Acta Eur Fertil.* 1983; 14:283.
61. Yamaguchi M, Sakatoku J, Takihara H. The application of intrascrotal deep temperature measurement for the noninvasive diagnosis of varicoceles. *Fertil Steril.* 1989; 52:295.
62. Lewis RW, harrison RN. Contact scrotal thermography: II. Use in the infertile male. *Fertil Steril.* 1980; 34:259.
63. Naryan P, Amplatz K, Gonzalez R. Varicocele in male subfertility. *Fertil Steril.* 1981; 36:92.
64. Greenberg SH. Varicocele and male fertility. *Fertil Steril.* 1977; 28:699.
65. Wolf DP, Byrd W, Dandekar P, Quigley MN. Sperm concentration in the fertilization of human eggs in vitro. *Biol Reprod.* 1984; 31:837.
66. Settladge DSF, Motoshima M, Treadway DR. Sperm transport from the external cervical os to the fallopian tubes in women: a time and quantitation study. *Fertil Steril.* 1973; 24:655.
67. McCleod J. Semen quality in 1,000 men of known fertility and 800 cases of infertile marriages. *Fertil Steril.* 1951; 2:115.
68. Sherins RJ, Howards SS. Male infertility. In: Harrison JH, Gittes RF, Perlmutter AD, et al. eds. *Campbell's Urology* Philadelphia, Pa: WB Saunders; 1978; 3:715.
69. Freund M, Carol B. Factors affecting haemocytometer counts of sperm concentration in human semen. *J Reprod Fertil.* 1964; 8:149.
70. Amelar RD. Coagulation liquification and viscosity of human semen. *J Urol.* 1962; 87:187.
71. Amelar RD, Dubin L, Schoenfeld C. Semen analysis. *Urology.* 1973; 2:605.

72. Wolf H, Politch JA, Martinez A, Haimovici F, Hale JA, Anderson DJ. Leukocytospermia is associated with poor semen quality. *Fertil Steril.* 1990; 53:528.

73. Phillips HJ: Evaluation of culture dynamics. Dye exclusion tests for cell viability. In: Krus PK, Patterson MK, eds. *Tissue Culture Methods and Applications.* new York, NY: Academic Press; 1973:406–408.

74. Talbot P, Chacon RS. A triple stain technique for evaluating normal acrosome reactions of human sperm. *J of Exp Zool.* 1981; 215:201.

75. McCleod J. Human seminal cytology as a sensitive indicator of the germinal epithelium. *Int J Fertil.* 1964; 9:1281.

76. Kruger TF, Acosta AA, Simmons KF, Swanson JR, Matta JF, Oehniger S. Predictive value of abnormal sperm morphology in in vitro fertilization. *Fertil Steril.* 1988; 49:112.

77. Vantman D, Koukoulis G, Dennison L, Zimmerman M, Sherins RJ. Computer assisted semen analysis. Evaluation of method and assessment of the influence of sperm concentration on linear velocity determination. *Fertil Steril.* 1988; 49:510.

78. Pedigo NG, Vernon MW, Curry TE Jr. Characterization of the computerized semen analysis system. *Fertil Steril.* 1989; 52:659.

79. Caldamone AA, Emilson LBV, Al-Juburi A, Cockett ATK. Prostatitis: prostatic secretory dysfunction affecting fertility. *Fertil Steril.* 1980; 34:602.

80. Berger RE, Karp LE, Williamson RA, Koehler J, Moore DE, Holmes KK. The relationship of pyospermia and seminal fluid bacteriology to sperm function as reflected in the Sperm Penetration Assay. *Fertil Steril.* 1982; 37:557.

81. Maruyama DK, Hale RW, Rogers BJ. Effects of white blood cells on the in vitro penetration of zona free hamster eggs by human spermatozoa. *J Androl.* 1985; 6:127.

82. Wolff H, Anderson DJ. Immunohistologic characterization and quantitation of leukocyte subpopulations in human semen. *Fertil Steril.* 1988; 49:497.

83. Endtz AW. A rapid staining method for differentiating granulocytes from germinal cells in Papanicolauo stained semen. *Acta Cytol.* 1974; 18:2.

84. World Health Organization. Infections, pregnancy and infertility. Perspectives on prevention. *Fertil Steril.* 1987; 47:964.

85. Hammill H, Sogor L. Infectious causes for male infertility: a revised look. *Semin Reprod Endocrinol.* 1988; 6:359.

86. Rehewy MSE, Hafez ESE, Thomas A, Brown WJ. Aerobic and anaerobic bacterial flora in semen from fertile and infertile groups of men. *Arch Androl.* 1979; 2:263.

87. Swensen CE, Toth A, Toth C, et al. Asymptomatic bacteriospermia in infertile men. *Andrologia.* 1980; 12:7.

88. Lewis RH, Harrison RM, Domonique GJ. Culture of seminal fluid in a fertility clinic. *Fertil Steril.* 1981; 35:191.

89. Busolo F, Zanchetta R, Lanzone E, Cusianato R. Microbial flora in semen of asymptomatic infertile men. *Andrologia.* 1982; 16:269.

90. Upadhya M, Hibbard BM, Walker SM. The effect of ureaplasma urealyticum on semen characteristics. *Fertil Steril.* 1984; 41:304.

91. Richmond SJ, Hilton AL, Clark SKR. Chlamydial infection: role of chlamydia subgroup A in non-gonococcal and post-gonococcal urethritis. *Br J Veneral Dis.* 1972; 48:437.

92. Enroth P, Ljungh-Wadstrom A, Moberg PJ, Norol CE. Studies on bacterial flora in semen for males in infertile relations. *Int J Androl.* 1978; 1:105.

93. Naessens A, Foulon W, Debrucker P, et al. Recovery of microorganisms in semen and relationship to semen evaluation. *Fertil Steril.* 1986; 45:101.

94. Friberg J: Mycoplasmas and infertility. *Curr Ther Res.* 1979; 26:760.

95. Friberg J, Gnarpe H. Mycoplasma and human reproductive failure: III. Pregnancies in "infertile" couples treated with Doxycycline for T-mycoplasma. *Am J Obstet Gynecol.* 1973; 116:23.

96. Kundsin RB. Mycoplasma infections of the female genital tract. In: Taylor ML, Green TH, eds. *Progress in Gynecology.* New York, NY: Grune & Stratton; 1976. Vol 6 p 291–306.

97. Ulstein M, Capell P, Holmes KK, et al. Nonsymptomatic genital tract infection in male infertility. In: Hafez ESE, eds. *Human Semen and Fertility Regulation in Men.* St. Louis Mo: BC Decker/CV Mosby; 1976:355.

98. Alexander MJ. Evaluation of male infertility with an in vitro cervical mucus penetration test. *Fertil Steril.* 1981; 36:201.

99. Gaddum-Rosse P, Blandau RJ, Lee WI. Sperm migration into cervical mucus in vitro: II. Human spermatozoa in bovine mucus. *Fertil Steril.* 1980; 33:644.

100. Mangione CM, Medley ME, Menge AD. Studies on the use of estrous bovine cervical mucus in the human sperm cervical mucus penetration technique. *Int J Fertil.* 1981; 26:20.

101. Moghissi KS, Siegel S, Meinhold D, Agronow SJ. In vitro sperm cervical mucus penetration: Studies in human and bovine cervical mucus. *Fertil Steril.* 1982; 37:823.

102. Keel BA, Kelly RW, Webster BW, Zumback KL, Roberts BK. Application of a bovine cervical mucus penetration test. *Arch Androl.* 1987; 19:33.

103. Takemoto FS, Rogers BJ, Wiltbank MC, Soderdahl DW, Vaughn WK, Hale RW. Comparison of the penetration ability of human

spermatozoa into bovine cervical mucus and zona free hamster eggs. *J Androl.* 1985; 6:162.

104. McClure RD. Endocrine investigations and therapy. *Uro Clin of North Am.* 1987; 14:471.

105. Padron RS, Mas J, deAcosta OM. Testicular response to human chorionic gonadotropin in men with non-tumoral hyperprolcatenemia. *Int J Androl.* 1984; 7:495.

106. Hudson RW, McKay DE. The Gonadotropin response of men with varicoceles to gonadotropin releasing hormone. *Fertil Steril.* 1980; 33:427.

107. Hudson RW, Perez-Marrero RA, Crawford VA, McKay DE. Hormonal parameters in incidental varicoceles and those causing infertility. *Fertil Steril.* 1986; 45:692.

108. Hudson RW, Perez-Marrero RA, Crawford VA, McKay DE. Hormonal parameters of men with varicoceles before and after varicocelectomy. *Fertil Steril.* 1985; 43:905.

109. Hudson RW, Crawford VA, McKay DE. The gonadotropin response of men with varicoceles to a 4 hour infusion of gonadotropin releasing hormone. *Fertil Steril.* 1981; 36:633.

110. Hudson RW. The endocrinology of varicoceles. *Fertil Steril.* 1988; 49:199.

111. Schiff I, Wilson E, Newton R, Shane J, Cates R, Ryan KJ, Maftolin F. Serum leutinizing hormone, follicle-stimulating hormone, and testosterone responses to gonadotropin-releasing factor in males with varicoceles. *Fertil Steril.* 1976; 27:1059.

112. Rumke P, Van Amstel N, Messa EM, Rezemar PD. Prognosis of fertility in men with sperm aglutinins in the serum. *Fertil Steril.* 1973; 24:305.

113. Sigman M, Basshum B, Lipshultz LI, Lamb DJ, Beck J, Lott N. Predictive value of the indirect immunobead assay in the male. Presented at the 45th annual meeting of the American Fertility Society. November 13–16, 1989; San Francisco, Calif.

114. Hellstrom WJ, Overstreet JW, Samuels SJ, Lewis EL. The relationship of circulating antisperm antibodies to sperm surface antibodies in infertile men. *J Urol.* 1980; 140:1039.

115. Clarke GN, Elliot PM, Smaila C. Detection of sperm antibodies in semen using the immunobead test: a survey of 813 consecutive patients. *Am J Reprod Immunol Microbiol.* 1985; 7:118.

116. Ayvaliotis B, Bronson R, Rosenfeld D, Cooper G. Conception rates in couples where autoimmunity to sperm is detected. *Fertil Steril.* 1985; 43:739.

117. Hellstrom JG, Samuels SJ, Waits AB, Overstreet JW. A comparison of the usefulness of the Sperm Mar and Immunobead tests for the detection of antisperm antibodies. *Fertil Steril.* 1989; 52:1027.

118. Bronson RA, Cooper GW, Rosenfeld DL. Correlation between regional specificity of antisperm antibodies to the spermatozoan surface and compliment-mediated sperm immobilization. *Am J Reprod Immunol.* 1982; 2:222.

119. Fuchs EF, Alexander NJ. Immunologic considerations before and after vasovasostomy. *Fertil Steril.* 1983; 40:497.

120. Ansbacher R. Sperm-aglutinating and sperm-immobilizing antibodies in vasectomized men. *Fertil Steril.* 1971; 22:629.

121. Silber SS. Microscopic vasectomy reversal. *Fertil Steril.* 1977; 28:1191.

122. Phadke AN, Padukone K. Presence and significance of autoantibodies against spermatozoa in the blood of men with obstructed vas deferens. *J Reprod Fertil.* 1974; 7:163.

123. Amelar RD, Dubin L, Schoenfeld CY. Circulating sperm-aglutinating antibodies in azoospermic men with congenital bilateral absence of the vasa deferentia. *Fertil Steril.* 1975; 26:228.

124. Yanagimachi R, Yanagimachi H, Rogers BJ. The use of zona-free animal ova as a test system for the assessment of the fertilizing capacity of human spermatozoa. *Biol Reprod.* 1976; 15:471.

125. Aitken JR, Best FSM, Richardson DW, Djahahanbakheh O, Templeton A, Lees MM. An analysis of semen quality and sperm function in cases of oligozoospermia. *Fertil Steril.* 1982; 38:705.

126. Swanson RJ, Mayer JF, Jones KH, Lanzendorf SE, McDowell J. Hamster ova/human sperm penetration: Correlation with count motility and morphology for in vitro fertilization. *Arch Androl.* 1983; 10:69.

127. Auzmanas M, Tureck RW, Blasco L, Kipf GS, Ribas J, Mastroianni L. The zono-free hamster egg penetration assay as a prognostic indicator in a human in vitro fertilization program. *Fertil Steril.* 1985; 43:433.

128. Smith RG, Johnson A, Lamb DJ, Lipshultz LI. Functional tests of spermatozoa. Sperm Penetration Assay. *Urol Clin North Am.* 1987; 14:451.

129. Aitken JR. Diagnostic value of the zona-free hamster oocyte penetration test and sperm movement characteristics in oligospermia. *Int J Androl.* 1985; 8:348.

130. Corson SL, Batzer FR, Marmar J, Maislin G. The human sperm-hamster egg penetration assay: prognostic value. *Fertil Steril.* 1988; 49:328.

131. Shinohara K, Lipshultz LI, Scardino PT. Transrectal ultrasonography of the seminal vesicles in the azoospermic patient. Presented to the south central section meeting of the American Urological Association, November, 1985; Guadalajara, Mexico.

132. Cohen MS, Frye S, Warner RS, Leiter E. Testicular needle biopsy in diagnosis of infertility.

ticular needle biopsy in diagnosis of infertility. *Urology*. 1984; 24:439.

133. Chan SL, Lipshultz LI, Schwartzendruber D. Deoxyribonucleic acid (DNA) flow cytometry: a new modality for quantitative analysis of testicular biopsies. *Fertil Steril*. 1984; 41:45.

134. Eliasson R, Mossberg B, Camner P, Afzelius BA. The immotile cilia syndrome: a congenital ciliary abnormality as an etiologic factor in chronic airway infections and male sterility. *N Eng J Med*. 1977; 297:1.

135. Wong Ting-Wa, Straus FH, Jones TM, Warner ME. Pathological aspects of the infertile testis. *Urol Clin of North Am*. 1978; 5:503.

136. Griffin JE, Wilson JD. Disorders of the testis in male reproductive tract. In Wilson JD, Foster DW, eds. *TExtbook of Endorcinology*. 7th ed. Philadelphia, Pa: WB Saunders Co; 1986.

137. Danish RK, Lee PA, Mazur T, et al. Micropenis: II. Hypogonadotropic hypogonadism. *Johns Hopkins Med J*. 1980; 146:177.

138. Finkel DM, Phillips JL, Snyder PJ. Stimulation of spermatogenesis by gonadotropins in men with hypogonadotropic hypogonadism. *N Engl J Med*. 1985; 313:651.

139. Paulsen CA, Espeland DH, Michals EL. Effects of HCG, HMG, HLH and HGH administration on testicular function. In: Rosenberg E, Paulsen CA, eds. *The Human Testis*. New York, NY: Plenum Press; 1970: 547.

140. Yashimoto Y, Moridera K, Imura H. Restoration of normal pituitary gonadotropin reserve by administration of lutenizing hormone-releasing hormone in patients with hypogonadotropic hypogonadism. *N Engl J Med*. 1975; 292:242.

141. Roth JC, Kelch RP, Kaplin SL, Grumbach MM. FSH and LH response to lutenizing hormone-releasing hormone factor in pre-pubertal children, adult males and patients with hypogonadotropic and hypergonadotropic hypogonadism. *J Clin Endocrinol Metab*. 1972; 35:926.

142. Mortimer CH, McNeilly AS, Fisher RA, Murray MAE, Besser GM. Gonadotropin-releasing hormone therapy in hypogonadal males with hypothalamic or pituitary dysfunction. *Br Med J*. 1974; 4:617.

143. Shargil AA. Treatment of idiopathic hypogonadotropic hypogonadism in men with lutenizing hormone-releasing hormone: a comparison of treatment with daily injections and with the pulsatile infusion pump. *Fertil Steril*. 1987; 47:492.

144. Faiman C, Hoffman DL, Ryan RJ, Albert A. The "fertile eunich" syndrome: demonstration of isolated lutenizing hormone difficiency by radioimmunoassay technique. *Mayo Clin Proc*. 1968; 43:661.

145. Maroulis GB, Parlow AF, Marshall JR. Isolated follicle-stimulating hormone deficiency in man. *Fertil Steril*. 1977; 28:818.

146. Al-Ansari AA, Khalil TH, Kelani Y, et al. Isolated follicle-stimulating hormone deficiency in men: successful long term gonadotropin therapy. *Fertil Steril*. 1984; 42:618.

147. Strott CA, Yoshimi T, Lipsett MB. Plasma progesterone and 17-hydroxy progestrone in normal men and children with congenital adrenal hyperplasia. *J Clin Invest*. 1969; 48:938.

148. Bonaccorsi AC, Adler I, Figueiredo JG. Male infertility due to congenital adrenal hyperplasia: testicular biopsy findings, hormonal evaluation, and therapeutic results in 3 patients. *Fertil Steril*. 1987; 47:664.

149. Kirkland RT, Keenan BS, Holcombe JH, Kirkland JL, Clayton GW. Treatment of congenital adrenal hyperplasia in men. *N Engl J Med*. 1979; 300:988. Letter.

150. Radfer N, Bartter FC, Easley R, Kolins J, Javapour N, Sherins RJ. Evidence for endogenous LH suppression in a man with bilateral testicular tumors and congenital adrenal hyperplasia. *J Clin Endocrinol Metab*. 1977; 45:1194.

151. Cutfield RG, Bateman JM, Odell WD. Infertility caused by bilateral testicular masses secondary to congenital adrenal hyperplasia (21-hydroxylase deficiency). *Fertil Steril*. 1983; 40:809.

152. Ojeifo JO, Winters SJ, Troen P. Basal and adrenocorticotropic hormone-stimulated serum 17 alpha-hydroxyprogesterone in men with idiopathic infertility. *Fertil Steril*. 1984; 42:97.

153. Schneider G, Kirschner MA, Berkowitz R, Ertel NH. Increased estrogen production in obese men. *J Clin Endocrinol Metab*. 1979; 48:633.

154. Hargreave TB, Elton RA, Sweeting VM, Basraliam K. Estradiol and male fertility. *Fertil Steril*. 1988; 49:871.

155. Masla A, Segal H, Polishuk MD, Ben-David M. Hyperprolactinemic male infertility. *Fertil Steril*. 1976; 27:1425.

156. Jordan RM, Kohler PO. Recent advances in diagnosis and treatment of pituitary tumors. *Adv. Intern Med*. 1987; 32:299.

157. Dollar JR, Blackwell RE. Diagnosis in management of prolactinomas. *Cancer Metastasis Rev*. 1986; 5:125.

158. Wang C, Lamb KSL, Mar JTC, Chan T, Liu TMY, Yeung RTT. *Clin Endocrinol*. 1987; 27:363.

159. Carter JN, Tyson JE, Tolis G, Vliet SV, Faiman C, Friesen HG. Prolactin-secreting tumors and hypogonadism in 22 men. *N Eng J Med*. 1978; 299:847.

160. Clyde HR, Walsh PC, English RW. Elevated plasma testosterone and gonadotropin levels in infertile males with hyperthyroidism. *Fertil Steril*. 1976; 27:662.

161. Kidd GS, Glass AR, Vigersky RA. The hypothalamic-pituitary testicular access in thy-

rotoxicosis. *J Clin Endrocrinol Metab.* 1979; 48:798.

162. Wong TW, Staus FH, Warner NE. Testicular biopsy in the study of male infertility. *Arch Pathol.* 1974; 98:1.

163. Gabrilove JL, Nicols GL, Sohval AR. The testis in Cushing's syndrome. *J Urol.* 1974; 112:95.

164. Mancini RE, Lavieri JC, Muller F, et al. Effect of prednisolone upon normal and pathologic human spermatogenesis. *Fertil Steril.* 1966; 17:500.

165. Kjessler B. *Fracteurs genetiques dans la subfertil male humaine. Fecondite et sterilite du male: acquisitions recentes.* Paris: Masson et Cie; 1972.

166. Paulsen CA, Gordon DL, Carpenter RW, et al. Klinefelter's syndrome and its variance: a hormonal and chromosomal study. *Rec Prog Horm Res.* 1968; 24:321.

167. MacLean N, Harnden DJ, Bond J, Court-Brown WM, Mantle, DJ. Sex-chromosome abnormalities in new born babies. *Lancet.* 1964; 1:286.

168. Foss GL, Lewis FJW. A study of 4 cases with Klinefelter's syndrome, showing motile spermatozoa in their ejaculates. *J Reprod Fertil.* 1971; 25:41.

169. Balodimos MC, Lisco H, Berwin I. Merrill W, Dingman JF. XYY karyotype in a case of familial hypogonadism. *J Clin Endocrinol.* 1966; 26:443.

170. Baghdassarian A, Bayard F, Borganakar S, Arnold EA, Solez K, Migeon CJ. Testicular function in XYY men. *Johns Hopkins Med J.* 1975; 136:15.

171. Skakkebaek NE, Zeuthen E, Neilsen J, Yde H. Abnormal spermatogenesis in XYY males: a report on 4 cases ascertained through a population study. *Fertil Steril.* 1973; 24:390.

172. Santen RJ, de Kretser DM, Paulson CA, Vorhees J. Gonadotropins and testosterone in XYY syndrome. *Lancet.* 1970; 2:371.

173. Ismail AAA, Harkness RA, Kirkham KE, Loraine JA, Whatmore PB, Brittain RP. Effective ofabnormal sex-chromosome compliments on urinary testosterone levels. *Lancet.* 1968; 1:220.

174. Lundberg PO, Helstrom J. Hormone levels in men with extra Y chromosomes. *Lancet.* 1970; 2:1133.

175. Koulischez L, Schoysman R. Chromosomes and human infertility. *Clin Genet.* 1974; 5:116.

176. Hulten M, Eliasson R, Tillinger KG. Low chiasma count and other meiotic irregularities in 2 infertile 46, XY men with spermatogenic arrest. *Hereditas.* 1970; 65:285.

177. Pearson PL, Ellis JD, Evans HJ. A gross reduction in chiasma formation during meiotic prophase and a defective DNA repair mechanism associated with a case of human male infertility. *Cytogenetics.* 1970; 9:460.

178. Skakkebaek NE, Bryant JI, Phillips J. Studies on meiotic and chromosomes in infertile men and controls with normal kariotypes. *J Reprod Fert.* 1973; 35:23.

179. Campbell WA, Lowther J, McKenzie I, Price WH. Serum gonadotropins in Down's syndrome. *J Med Genetics.* 1982; 19:98.

180. Blumberg BD, Shulkin JD, Rotter JI, Mohandas T, Kaback MM. Minor chromosomal variants and major chromosomal anomalies in couples with recurrent abortion. *Am J Hum Genetics.* 1982; 34:948.

181. Fortuny A, Carrio A, Soler A, Cararach J, Fuster J, Salami C. Detection of balanced chromosome rearrangements in 445 couples with repeated abortion and cytogenetic prenatal testing in carriers. *Fertil Steril.* 1988; 49:774.

182. Collins E, Turner G. The Noonan syndrome: a review of the clinical and genetic features of 27 cases. *J Pediatr.* 1973; 83:941.

183. Aynsley-Green A, Zachmann M, Illig R, et al. Congenital bilateral anorchia in childhood: a clinical, endocrine and therapeutic evaluation of 21 cases. *Clin Endocrinol.* 1976; 5:381.

184. Lipshultz LI, Caminos-Torres R, Greenspan C, Snyder, PJ. Testicular function after unilateral orchiopexy. *N Engl J Med.* 1976; 295:15.

185. Lipshultz LI. Cryptorchidism in the subfertile male. *Fertil Steril.* 1976; 27:69.

186. Charny CW. The spermatogenic potential of the undescended testis before and after treatment. *J Urol.* 1960; 83:697.

187. Sohval AR. Histopathology of cryptorchidism. *Am J Med.* 1954; 16:346.

188. Hadziselimovic F. *Cryptorchidism: Management and Implications.* New York, NY: Springer-Verlag New York; 1983.

189. Beard CM, Benson RC, Kelalis PP, Elveback LR, Kurland LT. The incidence of mumps orchitis in Rochester, Minnesota, 1935–1974. *Mayo Clin Proc.* 1977; 52:3.

190. Werner CA. Mumps orchitis and testicular atrophy. *Ann Intern Med.* 1950; 32:1066.

191. Drucker WD, Blanc WA, Rowland MM, et al. The testis in myotonic muscular dystrophy: a clinical and pathologic study with a comparison with Klinefelter's syndrome. *J Clin Endocrinol Metab.* 1963; 23:59.

192. Mahler C, Parizel G. Hypothalamic-pituitary function in myotonic dystrophy. *J Urol.* 1982; 226:233.

193. Fetterweit W, Mechanick JI. Myotonic dystrophy presenting as male infertility: A case report. *Int J Fertil.* 1987; 32:142.

194. Parvinen M, Lahdetie J, Parvinen LM. Toxic and mutogenic influences on spermatogenesis. *Arch Toxicol.* 1984 (suppl); 7:128.

195. Meistrich ML. Stage specific sensitivity of

spermatogonia to different chemotherapeutic drugs. *Bio Med Pharmacother.* 1984; 38:137.

196. Byrne J, Mulvihill JJ, Myers MH, Connelly R, et al. Affects of treatment on fertility in long-term survivors of childhood or adolescent cancer. *N Eng J Med.* 1987; 317:1315.
197. Kruser ED, Xiros N, Hetzel WD, et al. Reproductive and endocrine gonadal capacity in patients treated with COPP chemoterhapy for Hodgkins disease. *J Cancer Res Clin Oncol.* 1987; 113:260.
198. Redman JR, Bajorunas DR, Goldstein MC, et al. Semen cryoperservation and artificial inseminatin for Hodgkins disease. *J Clin Oncol.* 1987; 5:233.
199. daCunha MF, Meistrich ML, Fuller LN, et al. Recovery of spermatogenesis after treatment for Hodgkins disease: Limiting dose of MOPP chemotherapy. *J Clin Oncol.* 1984; 2:571.
200. Whitehead E, Shalet SM, Blackledge G, et al. The affects of Hodgkins disease and combination chemotherapy on gonadal function in the adult male. *Cancer.* 1982; 49:418.
201. Sherins RJ, DeVita VT. Effect of drug treatment for lymphoma on male reproductive capacity. *Ann Intern Med.* 1973; 79:216.
202. Waxman J, Terry YA, Wrigley PFN, et al. Gonadal function in Hodgkins disease: Long term follow-up of chemotherapy. *Br Med J.* 1982; 285:1612.
203. Roeser HP, Stocks AE, Smith AJ. Testicular damage due to cytotoxic drugs and recovery after cessation of therapy. *Aust MZ J Med.* 1978; 8:250.
204. Santoro A, Vivian S, Zucali R, et al. Comparative results and toxicity of MOPP vs ABVD combined with radiotherapy (RT) in PS II B, III (A,B) Hodgkins disease (HD) *Proc Am Soc Clin Oncol.* 1983; 2 (abstr):223.
205. Evenson DP, Arlin Z, Welt S, et al. Male reproductive capacity may recover following drug treatment with the L-10 protocol for acute lymphocytic leukemia. *Cancer.* 1984; 53:30.
206. Berthelsen JG, Skakkebaek NE. Gonadal function in men with testis cancer. *Fertil Steril.* 1983; 39:655.
207. Fossa SD, Ous S, Abyholm T, et al. Post treatment fertility in patients with testicular cancer: II. Influence of Cisplatin-based combination chemotherapy and retroperitoneal surgery on hormone and sperm production. *Br J Urol.* 1985; 57:210.
208. Drasga RE, Einhorn LH, William SD, et al. Fertility after chemotherapy for testicular cancer. *J Clin Oncol.* 1983; 1:179.
209. Hendry WF, Stedronska J, Jones CR, et al. Semen analysis in testicular cancer and Hodgkins disease: pre and post treatment findings and implications for cryopreservation. *Br J Urol.* 1983; 55:769.
210. Mijman JM, Koops H, Kremer J, et al. Gonadal function after surgery and chemotherapy in men with stage II and III nonseminomatous testicular tumors. *J Clin Oncol.* 1987; 5:651.
211. Rustin GJS, Pektasides D, Bagshawe KD, et al. Fertility and chemotherapy for male and female germ cell tumors. *Int J Androl.* 1987; 10:389.
212. Kreuser ED, Horsch U, Hetzel WD, et al. Chronic gonadotoxicity in patients with testicular cancer after chemotherapy. *Eur J Cancer Clin Oncol.* 1986; 22:289.
213. Abel EL, Moore C, Waselewsky D, Zajac C, Russell LD. Effects of cocaine hydrochloride on reproductive function and sexual behavior of male rats and on the behavior of their offspring. *J Androl.* 1989; 10:17.
214. Hembree WC, Zeidenberg P, Nahas G. Marijuana effects on human gonadal function. In Nahas G, Poton WDM, Idanpaan-Heittila J, eds. *Marijuana: Chemistry, Biochemistry and Cellular Effects.* New York: Springer-Verlag; 1976: 521.
215. Harmon J, Aliapoulios MA. Gynecomastia in marijuana uses. *N Eng J Med.* 1972; 287:936.
216. Marshburn PB, Sloan CS, Hammond MG. Semen quality and association with coffee drinking, cigarette smoking and ethanol consumption. *Fertil Steril.* 1989; 52:162.
217. Cosgrove, MD, Benton B, Henderson BE. Male genital urinary abnormalities and maternal diethylstilbestrol. *J Urol.* 1977; 117:220.
218. Nelson WD, Steinburger E. The effect of furadoxyl upon the testis of the rat. *Anat Rec.* 1952; 112:367.
219. Nelson WO, Bunge RB. The effect of therapeutic dosages of nitrofurantoin upon spermatogenesis in man. *J Urol.* 1957; 77:275.
220. Van Thiel DH, Gavaler JS, Smith WJ, et al. Hypothalamic-pituitary-gonadal dysfunction in men using cimetidine. *N Engl J Med.* 1979; 300:1012.
221. Toth A. Reversible toxic affect of salicylazosulfapyridene on semen quality. *Fertil Steril.* 1979; 31:538.
222. Lancranjan I, Popescu HI, Gavanescu O, et al. Reproductive ability of workmen occupationally exposed to lead. *Arch Environ Health.* 1975; 30:396.
223. White IG. The toxicity of heavy metals to mammalion spermatozoa. *Aust J Exp Biol Med Sci.* 1955; 33:359.
224. Lipshultz LI, Ross CE, Whorton D, et al. Dibromochloropropane and its effect on testicular function in man. *J Urol.* 1980; 124:464.
225. Rowley MJ, Leach DR, Warner GA, et al. Effect of greater doses of ionizing radiation on the human testis. *Radiat Res.* 1974; 59:665.
226. Elstein M, Smith EKM, Curtis JR. Reproductive potential of patients treated by maintenance hemodialysis. *Br Med J.* 1969; 2:734.
227. Swerdloff RS, Kantor G, Korenman SG: Go-

nadotropin disassociation in uremic gynecomastia: high plasma LH, low FSH and normal estradiol. *Clin Res.* 1970; 18:172.

228. Lin VS, Fang VS. Gonadal dysfunction in uremic men. A study of the hypothalamic-pituitary-testicular axis before and after renal transplantation. *Am J Med.* 1975; 58:655.
229. Chopp TR, Mendez N. Sexual function and hormonal abnormalities in uremic men on chronic dialysis and after renal transplantation. *Fertil Steril.* 1978; 29:661.
230. Handelsman DJ. Hypothalamic-pituitary gonadal dysfunction in renal failure, dialysis and renal transplantation. *Endocrinol Rev.* 1985; 6:151.
231. MacLeod J, Hotchkiss RS. The effect of hyperpyrexia upon spermatozoa counts in men. *Endocrinology.* 1941; 28:780.
232. Dubin L, Amelar RD. Etiologic factors in 1,294 consecutive cases of male infertility. *Fertil Steril.* 1971; 22:469.
233. Hendry F, Sommerville IF, Hall RR, et al. Investigation and treatment of the subfertile male. *Br J Urol.* 1973; 45:684.
234. Stewart BH. Varicocele in infertility: incidence and results of surgical therapy. *J Urol.* 1974; 112:222.
235. Johnson W. 120 infertile men. *Br J Urol.* 1975; 47:230.
236. Ridriguez-Rigau LJ, Smith KD, Steinburger E. Relationship of varicocele to sperm output and fertility of male partners in infertile couples. *J Urol.* 1978; 120:691.
237. Cockett ATK, Urry RL, Dougherty KA. The varicocele and semen characteristics. *J Urol.* 1979; 121:435.
238. Aafjes JH, van der Vijver JCM. Fertility of men with and without a varicocele. *Fertil Steril.* 1985; 43:901.
239. Marks JL, Mchahon R, Lipshultz LI. Predictive parameters of successful varicocele repair. *J Urol* 1986; 136:609.
240. Macleod J. Further observations on the role of varicocele in human male infertility. *Fertil Steril.* 1969; 20:545.
241. Grillo-Lopez AJ. Primary right varicocele. *J Urol.* 1971; 105:540.
242. Zorgniotti A, MacLeod J. Studies in temperature, human sperm quality and varicocels. *Fertil Steril.* 1973; 24:854.
243. Yamaguchi M, Sakatoku J, Takihara H. The application of intrascrotal deep body temperature measurement for the non-invasive diagnosis of varicoceles. *Fertil Steril.* 1989; 52:295.
244. Stephenson JD, O'Shaughnessy EJ. Hypospermia and its relationship to varicocele and intrascrotal temperature. *Fertil Steril.* 1968; 19:110.
245. Tessler AN, Krahn HP. Varicocele and testicular temperature. *Fertil Steril.* 1966; 17:201.
246. Comhaire F, Vermeulen A. Varicocele sterility: Cortisol and catecholamines. *Fertil Steril.* 1974; 25:88.
247. Saypol DC. Varicocele. *J Androl.* 1981; 2:61.
248. Chakraborty J, Sinha Hikim AP, Jhunjhunwala JS: Stagnation of blood in the microcirculatory vessels in the testes of men with varicocele. *J Androl.* 1985; 6:117.
249. Etriby A, Girgis SM, Hefnawy H, Ibrahim AA. Testicular changes in subfertile males with varicocele. *Fertil Steril.* 1967; 18:666.
250. Oster J: Varicocele in children and adolesents. *Scand J Urol Nephrol.* 1971; 5:27.
251. Steeno O, Knops J, DeClerck L, et al. Prevention of fertility disorders by detection and treatment of varicocele at school and college age. *Androl.* 1976; 8:47.
252. Berger OG. Varicocele in adolesents. *Clin Pediatr.* 1980; 19:810.
253. Swerdloff RS, Walsh PC. Pituitary and gonadal hormones in patients with varicocele. *Fertil Steril.* 1975; 26:1006.
254. Cass EJ, Belman AB. Reversal of testicular growth value by varicocele ligation. *J Urol.* 1987; 137:475.
255. Rodrigues-Metto N Jr, Fakioni EP, Lemos GC. Varicocele: clinical or surgical treatment. *Int J Fertil.* 1984; 29:164.
256. Dubin L, Amelar RD. 986 cases of varicocelectomy: A 12 year study. *Urology.* 1977; 10:446.
257. Tulloch WS. Varicocele in subfertility: results of treatment. *Br Med J.* 1955; 2:356.
258. Scott LS, Young D. Varicocele: a study of its effects on human spermatogenesis and of the results produced by spermatic vein ligation. *Fertil Steril.* 1962; 13:325.
259. Hanely HG, Harrison RG. The nature and surgical treatment of varicocele. *Br J Surg.* 1962; 50:64.
260. Charny CW, Baum S. Varicocele and infertility. *JAMA.* 1968; 204:1165.
261. Gunter D. The Palomo operation for varicocele and its affects on fertility. *Br J Urol.* 1975; 47:230.
262. Brown JS. Varicocelectomy in the subfertile male: a 10 year experience in 295 cases. *Fertil Steril.* 1976; 27:1046.
263. Glezerman M, Rakowszczyk M, Lunenfeld B, et al. Varicocele in oligospermic patients: pathophysiology and results after ligation and division of the internal spermatic vein. *J Urol.* 1976; 115:562.
264. Morag B, Rubinstein ZG, Goldwasser B, et al. percutaneous venography and occlusion in the management of spermatic varicoceles. *AJR.* 1984; 143:635.
265. Pryor JL, Howards SS. Varicocele. *Urol Clin North Am.* 1987; 14:499.
266. Murray RR Jr, Mitchell SE, Cadir S, et al.

Comparison of recurrent varicocele anatomy following surgery and percutaneous balloon occlusion *J Urol.* 1986; 135:286.

267. Greenburg SH, Lipshultz LI, Wein AJ. Experience with 425 subfertile male patients. *J Urol.* 1978; 119:507.

268. Heller CG, Rowley MJ, Heller CV. Clomiphene cirate: a correlation of its affect on sperm concentration and morphology, total gonadotropins, LH, estrogen and testosterone excretion and testicular cytology in normal men. *J Clin Endocrinol Metab.* 1969; 29:638.

269. Jungck EC, Roy S, Greenblatt RB, et al. Effect of clomiphene citrate on spermatogenesis in the human. *Fertil Steril.* 1964; 15:40.

270. Mellinger RC, Thompson RT. The effect of clomiphene citrate in male infertility. *Fertil Steril.* 1966; 17:94.

271. Mroueh A, Lytton B, Case N. Effect of clomiphene citrate on oligospermia. *Am J Obstet Gynecol.* 1967; 98:1033.

272. Palti Z. Clomiphene citrate in defective spermatogenesis. *Fertil Steril.* 1970; 21:838.

273. Foss GL, Tindal VR, Birkett JP. The treatment of subfertile men with clomiphene citrate. *J Reprod Fertil.* 1973; 32:167.

274. Check JH, Rakoff AE. Improved fertility in oligospermic males treated with clomiphene citrate. *Fertil Steril.* 1977; 28:746.

275. Paulson DJ, Wachsman J, Hammond CB, et al. Hypofertility and clomiphene citrate therapy. *Fertil Steril.* 1975; 26:982.

276. Paulson DF, Hammond CB, deVere-White R, et al. Clomiphene citrate: pharmacologic treatment of hypofertile male. *Urology.* 1977; 9:419.

277. Epstein JA. Clomiphene citrate in oligospermic infertile males. *Fertil Steril.* 1977; 28:741.

278. Charny CW. Clomiphene citrate therapy in male infertility: a negative report. *Fertil Steril.* 1979; 32:551.

279. Ross LA, Dandel GL, Prinz LM, et al. Clomiphene treatment of the idiopathic hypofertile male: high dose, alternate day therapy. *Fertil Steril.* 1980; 32:618.

280. Ronnberg L. The effect of clomiphene treatment on different sperm parameters in men with idiopathic oligozoospermia. *Andrologia.* 1980; 12:261.

281. Paulson DF. Cortisone acetate versus clomiphene citrate in pregerminal idiopathic infertility. *J Urol.* 1979; 121:432.

282. Wang C, Chan C-W, Wong K-K, Yeung K-K. Comparison of the effectiveness of placebo, colmiphene citrate, mesterolone, pentoxifylline, and testosterone rebound therapy for the treatment of idiopathic oligospermia. *Fert Steril.* 1983; 40:358.

283. Micic S, Dotlie R. Evaluation of sperm parameters in clinical trial with clomiphene citrate of oligospermic men. *J Urol.* 1985; 133:221.

284. Vermeulen A, Comhaire F. Hormonal effects of an antiestrogen, tamoxifen, in normal and oligospermic men. *Fertil Steril.* 1978; 29:320.

285. Willis KJ, London DR, Bevis MA, et al. Hormonal effect of tamoxifen in oligospermic men. *J Endocrinol.* 1977; 73:171.

286. Buvat J, Ardaenes A, Lemarie A, et al. Increased sperm count in 25 cases of idiopathic normogonadotropic oligospermia following treatment with tamoxifen. *Fertil Steril.* 1983; 39:700.

287. Danner C, Frick F, Maier F. Results of treatment with tamoxifen in oligozoospermic men. *Andrologia.* 1983; 15:584.

288. Dony JMJ, Smals AGH, Rolland R, et al. Effect of lower vs. higher doses of tomaxifen on pituitary-gonadal function and sperm indexes in oligozoospermic men. *Andrologia.* 1975; 17:369.

289. Brigante C, Motta G, Fusi F, et al. Treatment of idiopathic oligozoospermia with tomaxifen. *Acta Eur Fertil.* 1985; 16:361.

290. Clark RV, Sherins RJ. Treatment of men with idiopathic oligospermic infertility using the aromatase inhibitor, testalactone. Results of a double-blinded, randomized, placebo-controlled trial with crossover. *J Androl.* 1989; 10:240.

291. Misurale F, Cagnazzo G, Storace A. Asthenospermia and it's treatment with hCG. *Fertil Steril.* 1969; 20:650.

292. Homonnai ZT, Peled M, Paz GF. Changes in semen quality and fertility in response to endocrine treatment of subfertile men. *Gynecol Obstet Invest.* 1978; 9:244.

293. Cheval MJ, Mehan OJ. Chorionic gonadotropins in the treatment of the subfertile male. *Fertil Steril.* 1979; 31:666.

294. Margalioth EJ, Laufer N, Persistz E, et al. Treatment of oligoasthenospermia with human chorionic gonadotropin: Hormonal profiles and results. *Fertil Steril.* 1983; 39:841.

295. Pusch HH, Purstner P, Haas J. Treatment of asthenozoospermia with hCG. *Andrologia.* 1986; 18:201.

296. Troen P, Yanaihara T, Mankin H, et al. Assessment of gonadotropin therapy in infertile males. In: Rosenberg E, Paulson CA, eds. *The Human Testis.* New York, NY: Plenum Press; 1970.

297. Schirren C, Toyosi JO. Assessment of gonadotropin therapy in male infertility. In: Rosenberg E, Paulson CA, eds. *The Human Testis.* New York, NY: Plenum Press; 1970.

298. Sherins RJ. Clinical aspects of treatment of male infertility with gonadotropins: testicular response of some men given hCG with and without Pergonal. In: Mancini RE, Martini L, eds. *Male Fertility and Sterility.* London, Eng:

Academic Press; 1974. *Proceedings of the Serono Symposia* Vol 5, New York, Academic Press; 1974; pp 545–565.

299. Schill WB, Jungst D, Unterburger P, et al. Combined hMG/hCG treatment in subfertile men with idiopathic normogonadotropic oligozoospermia. *Int J Androl.* 1982; 5:467.
300. Zarate A, Valdes-Vallina F, Gonzales A, et al. Therapeutic effect of synthetic LH-RH in male infertility due to idiopathic azoospermia and oligospermia. *Fertil Steril.* 1973; 24:485.
301. Aparicio NJ, Schwarzstein L, Turner EA, et al. Treatment of idiopathic normogonadotropic oligoasthenospermia with synthetic lutinizing hormone releasing hormone. *Fertil Steril.* 1976; 27:549.
302. Fauser BCJM, Rowland R, Doney JMJ, et al. Long term, pulsatile, low dose, subcutaneous lutinizing hormone-releasing hormone administration in men with idiopathic oligozoospermia: failure of therapeutic and hormonal response. *Andrologia.* 1985; 17:143.
303. Charny CW, Gordon JA. Testosterone rebound therapy: a neglected modality. *Fertil Steril.* 1978; 29:64.
304. Charny CW. The use of androgen for human spermatogenesis. *Fertil Steril.* 1959; 10:557.
305. Rowley MJ, Heller CG. The testosterone rebound phenomenon in the treatment of male infertility. *Fertil Steril.* 1972; 23:498.
306. Lamensdorf H, Compere D, Begley G. Testosterone rebound therapy in the treatment of male infertility. *Fertil Steril.* 1975; 26:469.
307. Marrams P, Baraghini GF, Carani C, et al. Further studies on the affects of pentoxifylline on sperm count and sperm motility in patients with idiopathic oligoasthenozoospermia. *Andrologia.* 1985; 17:612.
308. Yovich JM, Edirisinghe WR, Cummins JN, Yovich JL. Preliminary results using pentoxifylline as a pronuclear stage tubal transfer (PROST) programmed for severe male factor infertility. *Fertil Steril.* 1988; 50:179.
309. Barkay J, Harpaz-Kerpel S, Ben-Ezra S, et al. The prostaglandin inhibitor effect of anti-inflammatory drugs in the therapy of male infertility. *Fertil Steril.* 1984; 42:406.
310. Conte D, Nordio M, Romanelli F, et al. Role of seminal prostaglandins in male fertility: II. Effects of prostaglandin synthesis inhibition on spermatogenesis in man. *J Endocrinol Invest.* 1985; 8:289.
311. Padron RS, Nodarse M. Effect of indomethacin on seman of infertile men. *Int J Androl.* 1979; 2:110.
312. Bendvold E, Gottlieb C, Svanborg K, et al. The effect of naproxen on the concentration of prostaglandins in human seminal fluid. *Fertil Steril.* 1985; 43:922.
313. El-Itreby AA, Girgis SM. Congenital absence of vas deferens in male sterility. *Int J Fertil.* 1961; 6:409.
314. Ameral RD, Hotchkiss RS. Congenital aplasia of the epididymides and vas deferentia: effects on semen. *Fertil Steril.* 1963; 14:44.
315. Charny CW, Gillenwater JY. Congenital absence of the vas deferens. *J Urol.* 1965; 93:399.
316. Turner TT. On the development and use of alloplastic sermatoceles. *Fertil Steril.* 1988; 49:387.
317. Temple-Smith PD, Southwick GJ, Yates CA, Trounson AO, De Kretser DN. Human pregnancy by in vitro fertilization (IFV) using sperm aspirated from the epididymis. *J In Vitro Fert Embryo Transfer.* 1985; 2:119.
318. Silber SJ, Balmaceda J, Borrero C, Ord T, Asch R. Pregnancy with sperm aspiration from the proximal head of the epididymis: a new treatment for congenital absence of the vas deferens. *Fertil Steril.* 1988; 50:525.
319. Silber SJ, Ord T, Balmacada J, Patrizio P, Asch RH. Congenital absence of the vas deferens: studies on the fertilizing capacity of human epididymal sperm. Presented at the 45th annual meeting of the American Fertility Society, November 13–16, 1989; San Francisco, Calif.
320. Hendry WF. The long term results of surgery for obstructive azoospermia. *Br J Urol.* 1981; 53:664.
321. Handlesman DJ, Conway AJ, Boylan LM, Turtle JR. Young's syndrome: obstructive azoospermia and chronic sinopulmonary infection. *N Engl J Med.* 1984; 310:3.
322. Johnsonbaugh RE, O'Connell K, Engel SB, et al. Plasma testosterone luteinizing hormone, and follicle-stimulating hormone after vasectomy. *Fertil Steril.* 1975; 26:329.
323. Rosemberg E, Marks SG, Howard PL, James LD. Serum levels of follicle stimulating and lutinizing hormones before and after vasecomty in men. *J Urol.* 1974; 111:626.
324. Yarbro ES, Howards SS. Vasovasostomy. *Urol Clin North Am.* 1987; 14:515.
325. Belker AM, Fuchs E, Konnak JW, et al. Results of 1247 first vasectomy reversals by the vasovasostomy study group. Presented at the 85th annual meeting of the American Urological Association, May 13–17, 1990; New Orleans, La.
326. Silber SJ. Microscopic vasectomy reversal. *Fertil Steril.* 1977; 28:11.
327. Belker AM. Microsurgical vasectomy reversal. *Infect in Urol.* 1989; 2:129.
328. Thomas AJ, Jr. Vasoepididymostomy. *Urol Clin North Am.* 1987; 14:527.
329. Silber SJ. Role of epididymis in sperm maturation. *Fertil Steril.* 1989; 33:147.
330. Fogdestan I, Fall M, Nilsson S. Microsurgical epididymovasostomy in the treatment of occlusive azoospermia. *Fertil Steril.* 1986; 46:925.

331. McLoughlin MG. Vasoepididymostomy: the role of the microscope. *Can J Surg.* 1982; 5:41.

332. Silber SJ. Microscopic vasoepididymostomy, specific anastomosis to the epididymal tubule. *Fertil Steril.* 1978; 30:565.

333. Schoysman R, Bedford JM. The role of human epididymis in sperm maturation and sperm storage as reflected in the consequences of epididymovasostomy. *Fertil Steril.* 1986; 46:293.

334. Belker AM, Fuchs EF, Konnak JW, et al. Results of 219 repeat vasectomy reversals by the vasovasostomy study group. Presented at the 85th annual meeting of the American Urological Association; May 13–17, 1990; New Orleans, La.

335. Shanberg A, Tansey L, Barhdassarian R, et al. Laser-assisted vasectomy reversal: Experience in 32 patients. *J Urol.* 1990; 143:528.

336. Lynne CM, Carter M, Morris J, et al. Laser-assisted vas anastomosis: a preliminary report. *Lasers Surg Med.* 1983; 3:261.

337. Brindley GS. Electroejaculation: its technique, neurologic implications, and uses. *J Neurol Neurosurg Psychiat.* 1981; 44:9.

338. Ohl DA, Bennett CJ, McCabe M, et al. Predictors of success in electroejaculation of spinal cord injured men. *J Urol.* 1989; 142:1483.

339. Shaban SF, Seager SW, Lipshultz LI: Electroejaculation. *Med Instrum:* 1988; 22:77.

340. Bennett CJ, Seager SWJ, McGuire EJ. Electroejaculation for recovery of sperm after retroperitoneal lymph node dissection: case report. *J Urol.* 1987; 137:513.

341. Brindley GS. Reflex ejaculation under vibratory stimulation in paraplegic men. *Paraplegia.* 1981; 19:299.

342. Belker AM, Cook CL. Sperm processing and intrauterine insemination for oligospermia. *Urol Clin North Am.* 1987; 14:597.

343. Cruz RI, Kemmann E, Brandeis VT, et al. A prospective study of intrauterine insemination of processed sperm from men with oligoasthenospermia in supraovulated women. *Fertil Steril.* 1986; 46:673.

344. Kemmann E, Bohrer M, et al. Active ovulation management increases the monthly probability of pregnancy occurrence in ovulatory women who receive intrauterine insemination. *Fertil Steril.* 1987; 48:916.

345. Melis GB, Poaletti AN, et al. Pharmacologic induction of multiple follicular development improves the success rate of artificial insemination with husband's semen in couples with male related or unexplained infertility. *Fertil Steril.* 1987; 47:441.

346. Nulsen JC, Metzger DA, Kuslis S, Luciano AA. Intrauterine insemination combined with human premenopausal gonadotropin (hMG) supraovulation in the treatment of infertility associated with antisperm antibodies in the male. Presented at the 45h annual meeting of the American Fertility Society, November 11–16; 1989; San Francisco, Calif.

347. Medical Research International and the Society for Assisted Reproductive Technology, The American Fertility Society. In vitro fertilization–embryo transfer in the United States: 1989 results from the IVF-ET registry. *Fertil Steril.* 1990; 53:13. 1991; 55:14.

348. Yovich JL, Yovich JM, Rohini W. The relative chance of pregnancy following tubal or uterine transfer procedures. *Fertil Steril.* 1988; 49:858.

349. Malter HE, Cohen J. Patrial zona dissection of the human oocyte: a nontramatic method using micromanipulation to assist zona pellucida penetration. *Fertil Steril.* 1989; 51:139.

# 43

# Biostatistical Concepts

*M. J. Egger*

## INTRODUCTION

The arrival of McLuhan's "global village" brings with it an immediacy and intensity of information about medical treatments and procedures which would have been unimaginable even 50 years ago. Computerized medical information databases facilitate retrieval of information from the current literature so quickly that, for example, abstracts on the use of ceftazidime in the treatment of spinal cord injured patients with urinary tract infections[1] can be printed out in one's office during a consultation. Computer-aided medical decision-making programs permit amplification of diagnostic skill by assigning an array of probabilities of having various diseases to a patient with a particular constellation of symptoms. These programs also provide suggestions for additional assessments or tests which would narrow the diagnostic possibilities or differentially refine the likelihood of a specific diagnosis. Another example of modern information capabilities is the Human Genome Project. It is likely that the entire human genome will be exhaustively mapped in the foreseeable future, base pair by base pair, and will be available for the use of those who can assimilate the details. Skills in the assimilation of a large and continuing volume of medical information include the informed utilization of statistics.

Although as an academic discipline, statistics is considerably younger than many medical specialties, statistical thinking permeates medicine. As embodied in games of chance, statistical thinking can be traced back to prehistory.[2] The same odds ratio applied to strategy in a game of chance is applicable to evaluation of the prognosis and choice of treatment protocol for a patient with a palpable lump in the prostate.

The potential for statistical summarization has advanced along with computers. The present discussion of statistics will be by no means exhaustive, but will focus on the conceptual framework underlying statistics as commonly used in medical research.

## PROBABILITY

One concept of a probability is the relative frequency of an event in an experiment repeated a large number of times under constant conditions. This concept can be made quite rigorous mathematically, and it forms the basis of frequentist statistics.[3] Archetypal **frequentist** probabilities include the probabilities of the events of "heads" on a coin toss, double-sixes on a toss of dice, or a straight-flush in poker. It is also reasonably simple to understand intuitively the probability that a live birth is male, the probability that a healthy child will creep before age 8 months, or the probability that repeated, unprotected coitus be-

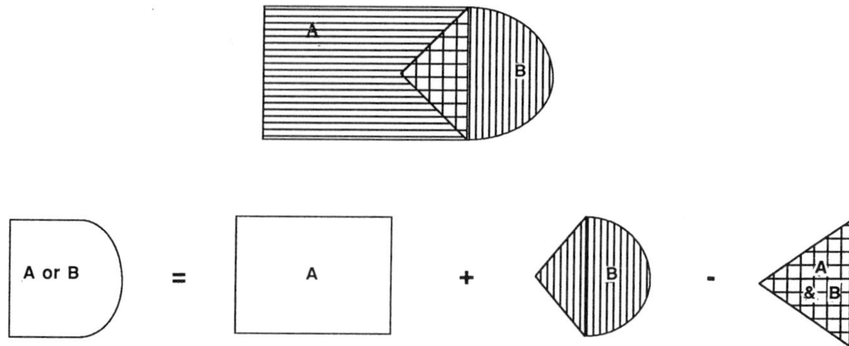


**Fig 1.** Calculating the probability of either or both of two events.

tween healthy heterosexuals who are 18 years old will result in pregnancy. It is trickier to hold the conditions constant—but is still intuitively reasonable—to speak about the probability of extracapsular extension in a patient with apparent stage $T_a$[7] prostate cancer, the probability that a urinary tract infection will respond to norfloxacin, or the probability of new urinary stone formation after a course of allopurinol plus thiazide. Much of statistics, as used in the medical literature, takes the frequentist approach to probability.

It might be argued that the relative frequency of an event is philosophically distinct from one's degree of belief in it. One way that **subjectivist** probability can be developed is in terms of one's willingness to take a bet based on the odds of occurrence of an event or its opposite. The odds, in this context, are the probability that the event will occur divided by the probability that it will not.

Substantial contributions to medical statistics, for example, computer-aided medical decision-making, have been made from a subjectivist or Bayesian framework.[4] A very readable introduction to the philosophical frameworks of frequentist vs subjectivist statistical inference is presented by Oakes.[5]

## Basic Properties of Probabilities

However the conceptual framework for probability is formalized, consistently developed probabilities have some properties in common. Probabilities of events take values between 0 (impossible, such as a woman having prostate cancer) and 1 (certain to occur, such as the ultimate death of any individual man). The probability that at least one of two events will occur is formally calculated by summing the individual probabilities and subtracting the probability of events occurring together. For example, the probability of having either nausea, dizziness, or both when taking norfloxacin is equal to the probability of nausea plus the probability of dizziness, minus the probability of both. The subtraction adjusts for the fact that the probability of both has been counted twice in the sum (Fig 1).

Finally, if two events are **independent,** ie, the occurrence of one does not help predict the occurrence of the other, the probability that they occur simultaneously is equal to the individual probabilities multiplied. This property is directly relevant to an understanding of the results of statistical tests: for example, the probability that two independent studies both made a Type I error (or erroneously concluded that an inefficacious treatment was effective) using a statistical test performed at the conventional 0.05 significance level, is $0.05 \times 0.05 = 0.0025$.

## Probability Distributions

A statistical model of a medical research problem can often be characterized in terms of a mathematically tractable **probability**

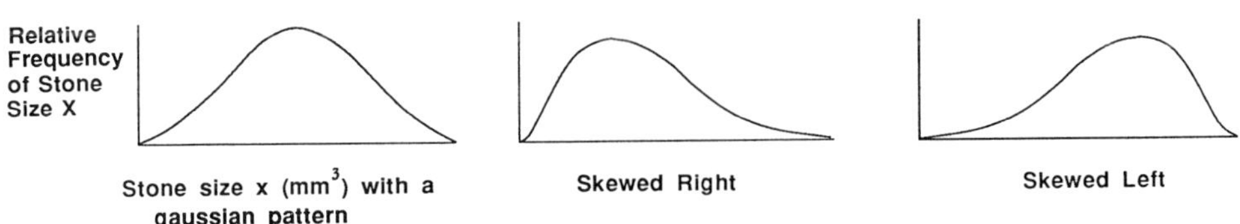


**Fig 2.** General shape of normal and skewed distributions.

**distribution,** or a formula for the assignment of probabilities to events. The binomial distribution and the normal, or Gaussian, distribution, are two of the many probability distributions which are commonly used to model research data. Yes-or-no determination of response to treatment for *n* independent subjects often leads to a binomial model of the number of responders, whereas a response measured along a continuum of values, such as size of urinary stones, might be modeled by a normal distribution if the size tends to cluster around a central value, with relative frequencies of stone sizes occurring in the notorious bell-shaped pattern of Figure 2.

Although probability distributions take a variety of shapes, the **central limit theorem** implies that the average of independent measurements of a variable, under fairly general conditions (eg, on a random sample of *n* patients) will tend to be approximately normal when *n* is large. One somewhat simple result of this theorem is that a great many statistical tests utilized in the medical literature can be referred to tables of the standard normal distribution in order to assess statistical significance of their results.

## SCREENING TEST PARAMETERS

Screening of asymptomatic individuals is performed in a variety of contexts: tuberculin tests, mammography, and serum cholesterol levels provide three examples. Screening may also be performed on symptomatic individuals whose exact diagnosis or extent of disease is still in question. Morrison[6] defines *lead time* as the time gained by screening, or the time from detection of disease in a particular individual to the time that diagnosis would have occurred without screening. If the effects of screening are measured by increased survival after diagnosis, this measure may be biased: patients may not live any longer, even though the doctor is aware of the disease earlier.

In addition, in the first years of a screening program, many existing (prevalent) cases of disease will be identified which would otherwise have been diagnosed later. In the second year, fewer of these will remain unidentified, and so screening programs will turn up a greater percentage of new (incident) cases. Early publicity may cause the population to use the screening program more enthusiastically, as was the case with mammography a number of years ago, when women of national prominence reported their breast cancers to the press. Such events can cause a surge and drop in the reported disease rate, independent of the actual value of the screening program. Evaluation of screening programs is discussed by Morrison.[6]

### Sensitivity, Specificity and Predictive Value

Rifkin et al compared the accuracy of magnetic resonance imaging (MRI) and ultrasonography (US) in staging early prostate cancer in patients thought to have a surgically resectable tumor.[7] Whether a patient had periprostatic extension of the cancer was assessed by pathology after radical prostatectomy. MRI and endorectal US were scheduled prior to surgery. Accuracy could thus be characterized by the **sensitivity** of an imaging technique, or its probability of detecting actual advanced disease, and the technique's **specificity,** or probability of accurately reporting localized disease. Thus, a screening test is **sensitive** among the truly positive patients, and **specific** in its accuracy among those who

| | | "Truth" by "Gold Standard" | | |
|---|---|---|---|---|
| | | + | − | Total |
| Conclusion of screening test | + | a | b | a + b |
| | − | c | d | c + d |
| | Total | a + c | b + d | n |

- Sensitivity = true-positive rate — a/(a + c)
- Specificity = 1 − false-positive rate — d/(b + d)
- Predictive value of a positive test — a/(a + b)
- Predictive value of a negative test — d/(c + d)
- Accuracy — (a + d)/n
- Frequency of a positive event in the study population — (a + c)/n
- Frequency of a negative event in the study population — (b + d)/n

**Fig 3.** Parameters of screening tests.

do not have the condition of interest. Figure 3 displays the estimators of parameters which are frequently reported in staging and diagnostic studies of screening tests.

In the Rifkin study, the sensitivity of US was reported to be 66% as compared to 77% for MRI. The specificity of US was a low 46% as compared to 57% for MRI. When the predictive value of a positive image was considered, positive pathology (ie, advanced disease) occurred in only 71% of patients, with a positive MRI, and in only 63% of patients with a positive US. The predictive value of a negative test was considerably lower: 49% for both MRI and US.

The equality of these parameters could be tested statistically for MRI as compared with US. Since both imaging techniques were performed on each patient, a reasonable test of, for example, sensitivity, might be McNemar's chi-squared test for paired proportions.[3] If patients had been randomized to receive one of the two techniques, a defensible argument could be made that the samples would be independent, and the usual Pearson's chi-squared test might be applied.[3]

## Dependency of Predictive Probability on Outcome Frequency in the Population

Bayes' theorem can be used to demonstrate that predictive values depend on the frequency of ''truly'' positive or negative events in the study population.[3] Thus, the predictive value of US or MRI in identifying patients with periprostatic extension of cancer might change in a population different from the one examined by Rifkin et al. If a physician has an index of suspicion that a particular patient has periprostatic extension of cancer, and a screening test is performed, the physician may wish to formally revise this prior probability by incorporating knowledge about the sensitivity and specificity of the screening procedure. The resulting **posterior probability** might be considered to be a kind of predictive value, adjusted for the prior probability instead of the population frequency of ''positives'' or ''negatives.'' Dawson-Saunders provides additional details and introduces extensions of this method.[8]

## Measurement of Screening Test Accuracy Using ROC Curves

''Accuracy'' is sometimes defined for a screening test, such as the one in Figure 3, to be the percentage of patients who were accurately staged or diagnosed. The concept of accuracy can be generalized through receiver-operating characteristic (ROC) curve methods, to distinguish the intrinsic accuracy of the staging modality as separate from the tendency of an individual clinician to give a conservative or liberal interpretation of the results.

**TABLE 1. Receiver-Operating Characteristic (ROC) Curves**

| | | "Truth" by "Gold Standard" + | − | Total |
|---|---|---|---|---|
| **Observer's degree of certainty, or confidence score** | 1. Certainly − | a1 | b1 | a1 + b1 |
| | 2. Probably − | a2 | b2 | a2 + b2 |
| | 3. Possibly + | a3 | b3 | a3 + b3 |
| | 4. Probably + | a4 | b4 | a4 + b4 |
| | 5. Certainly + | a5 | b5 | a5 + b5 |
| | Total | a1 + a2 + a3 + a4 + a5 | b1 + b2 + b3 + b4 + b5 | n |

**Dichotomized Tables for All Possible Cutpoints**

**"Truth"**

| | | + | − | | + | − | | + | − | | + | − |
|---|---|---|---|---|---|---|---|---|---|---|---|---|
| **Observer's dichotomized degree of certainty** | 1 | | | 1–2 | | | 1–3 | | | 1–4 | | |
| | 2–5 | | | 3–5 | | | 4–5 | | | 5 | | |

Classical ROC curve methods calculate the 2 × 2 table of Figure 3 for all possible dichotomizations of Table 1 and Figure 4, ie, for all of the possible cutpoints dividing the observer's confidence scores into "positives" and "negatives." The true-positive rate (sensitivity) is plotted versus the false-positive rate (1-specificity) for each 2 × 2 dichotomization of the table, and a smooth "binormal" curve is fitted, in the classical analysis. Examples are displayed in Figure 4.

The best possible imaging technique would have an ROC curve with very high true-positive rates for each possible value of the false-positive rate. The optimal curve would be located high and to the left in Figure 4. Then, one measure of accuracy of an imaging technique is the area under the ROC curve, which will be a value between 0 and 1. The area under the ROC curve can be shown to estimate the probability that a clinician's confidence score would be higher for a random positive pa-

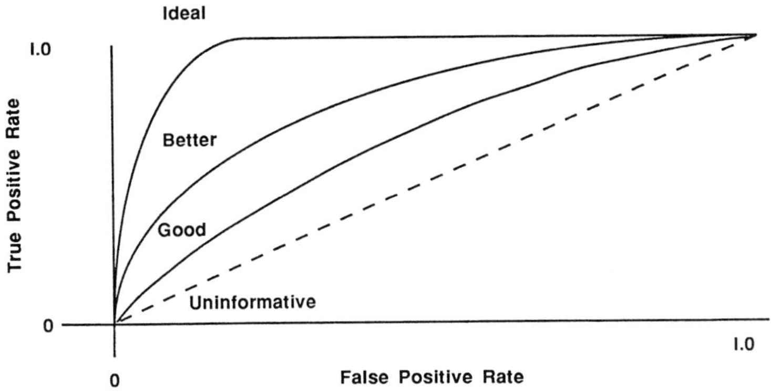


**Fig 4.** General shape of ROC curve plot.

tient than for a random negative patient. The area under the ROC curve thus combines and generalizes the concepts of sensitivity and specificity. The area under the ROC curves in the Rifkin study was 0.67 ± 0.05 for MRI and 0.62 ± 0.04 for US; these were not statistically significantly different.

ROC curves control for observer conservatism in the sense that two observers who differ only in their degree of conservatism will generate points on the same ROC curve. If one observer actually knows how to read the images more accurately than another observer, their readings will generate two different ROC curves, one higher than the other.

Kraemer[9] has discussed the extension of ROC curves to quality (Q) ROC curves to circumvent weaknesses of the classic model and to focus choice of, for example, an optimal imaging technique on the costs of false positives and negatives.

A brief, readable introduction to ROC curves is given by Dawson-Saunders,[8] and a more complete applied discussion is provided by Metz.[10] Other standard works in this area include those of Swets and Pickett,[11] Hanley and McNeil,[12] and McNeil and Hanley.[13]

## PHILOSOPHY OF STATISTICAL TESTING

Statistics play two major roles in medical research: to estimate unknown parameters and to test medical hypotheses which can be described in terms of a statistical model. Substantial portions of statistical theory are concerned with optimal properties of estimators and tests as well as development of procedures with optimal performance.

Statistical testing in the Neyman-Pearson tradition, as it is applied in the medical literature, can be capsulized as follows. A "null" hypothesis ($H_0$) about treatment effect (or noneffect) is proposed, and data are amassed against it. If the data are compelling, the null hypothesis is then rejected in favor of its opposite, or "alternative" hypothesis ($H_1$). If the amassed data are not impressive enough to reject the null

1. Interpret the medical research hypothesis in terms of statistical hypotheses:

   $H_0$: $\pi \leq 0.10$ (ie, response rate $\leq$ 10%)
   $H_1$: $\pi \geq 0.10$ (ie, response rate $>$ 10%)

2. Set a significance level $\alpha$ (eg, $\alpha = 0.05$)

3. Calculate test statistic $z$ and its tail probability. For this example,

$$Z = \frac{(p - \pi_0)}{\sqrt{\dfrac{\pi_0(1 - \pi_0)}{n}}} = 2.36, \text{ in this example, where:}$$

   $p$ = the observed response rate expressed as a proportion
   $n$ = the number of patients under study
   $\pi_0$ = the (null) hypothesized response rate

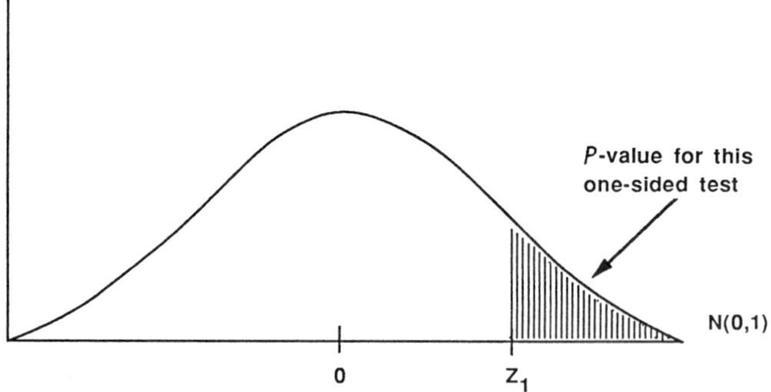


From a table of the standard normal distribution, the $P$-value is $P = .0091$.

4. Reject $H_0$ for $P < \alpha$
   Fail to reject $H_0$ for $P > \alpha$
   If $P = \alpha$, report borderline significance
   Here, reject $H_0$ since $P = .0091 < \alpha = 0.05$ and conclude that the response rate exceeds 10%

**Fig 5.** Outline of a one-sided statistical test. (For detailed formulae, see Rosner[3].)

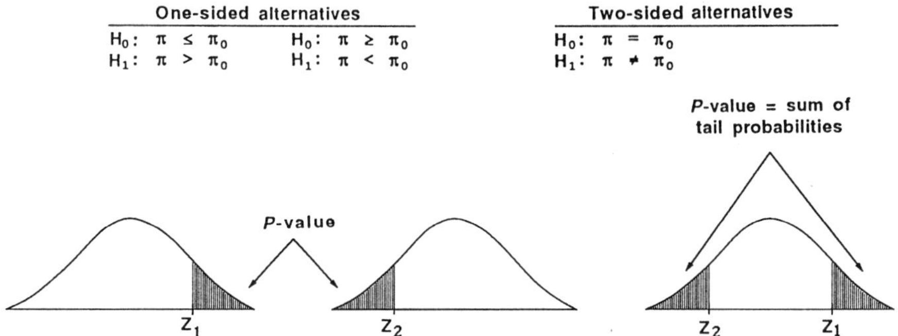


**Fig 6.** *P*-values for one-sided and two-sided tests.

hypothesis, one "fails to reject" it. This is similar to the familiar "proof by contradiction" of logic or geometry: one sets out to prove B by assuming not B, and proving that the assumption leads to a logical contradiction. In frequentist statistics, unlike pure logic, one cannot be absolutely certain that a contradiction has occurred. There is always at least a small chance that the amassed data are purely coincidental, however striking. For example, the probability that 50/50 patients respond to a treatment of no more than 10% efficacy (corresponding to the null hypothesis $H_0$: $\pi \leq 0.10$ versus an alternative hypothesis $H_1$: $\pi \geq 0.10$) is $10^{-50}$, not zero.

## Significance Levels and *P*-Values

In practice, the researcher determines a threshold probability, or **significance level,** below which he or she is willing to conclude that the data contradict the null hypothesis (ie, that the null hypothesis should be rejected), recognizing that one will have erroneously interpreted a coincidence as evidence of treatment efficacy a small percentage of the time.

Common significance levels are $\alpha = 0.05$, or $\alpha = 0.01$, and $10^{-50}$ is far below them, so in this example, one would conclude that the treatment has more than 10% efficacy. (In fact, one can reject a null hypothesis of less than 20%, 40%, 60% or even 90% response for such impressive data.)

If the data were less impressive, for example, if only 20 of the 50 patients responded, one would compute a slight variant, the *achieved significance level* or *P-value* to compare to the conventional significance level, say $\alpha = 0.05$. The calculation depends on the specific statistical model which seems to characterize the experiment. Computational details of various statistical tests are the subject of elementary statistics texts.[3] They have in common the calculation of a *test statistic,* here,

$$z = \frac{.20 - .10}{\sqrt{\frac{.10(.90)}{50}}} = 2.36$$

and its tail probability or *P*-value, here 0.0091. Since the *P*-value of 0.0091 is less than the significance level $\alpha = 0.05$, one would still reject the null hypothesis of no more than 10% efficacy, even though the data are somewhat less striking than the previous scenario. Figures 5 and 6 illustrate an outline of the logic of many common statistical test procedures.

## Risks of Erroneous Conclusions

Since the data cannot completely prove or disprove the null hypothesis, two types of erroneous conclusions are possible. Figure 7 illustrates that one of these is rejecting $H_0$ when it was really true, for instance, by concluding that an ineffective treatment is effective. This is termed a Type I error. Failing to reject $H_0$ when it was actually false, for example, by concluding that an effective treatment has no effect, is called a Type II error. The associated probabilities of such errors are denoted $\alpha$, the previously

| | 'TRUTH' H0 False | H0 True |
|---|---|---|
| Reject $H_0$ | Correct | Type I Error |
| Fail to Reject $H_0$ | Type II Error | Correct |

| Associated Probabilities | |
|---|---|
| $1 - \beta$ | $\alpha$ |
| $\beta$ | $1 - \alpha$ |

**Fig 7.** Types and probabilities of errors in statistical tests.

discussed significance level, and β, respectively. 1-β is termed the "power" or probability of correctly rejecting $H_0$. In practice it is calculated with respect to a specific, clinically important scenario, such as the event that the response rate is really 50%.

Statistical theory has been developed to allow the researcher to specify the maximum tolerable chance of Type I error in a study in advance and then to drive up the sample size $n$ to a value for which satisfactory power is available to detect clinically meaningful effects.

It is noteworthy that the typical significance levels, $\alpha = 0.05$ and $\alpha = 0.01$, are merely conventions. Typical requirements for power are $1 - \beta = 0.80$, 0.90, or 0.95 for scenarios of treatment effects which would be clinically meaningful.

The important distinction between clinical significance and statistical significance cannot be overstressed. For *any* pair of percentages of patients responding to two treatments, and a specified α, there is some $n$ for which this difference in response rates will achieve statistical significance, ie, will make the $P$-value less than α. This is a mathematical fact, unrelated to the clinical interpretation of the difference between treatments.

Similarly, for most treatment effects observed in practice, there is some $n$ small enough to fail to reject $H_0$.

For example, if 11.1% of the population will respond to drug A and 11.2% will respond to drug B, a very large $n$ will permit this clinically indistinguishable "difference" to be statistically significant. Conversely, a very small sample size would fail to detect statistically the difference between a response rate of 10% and a response rate of 90%.

Thus, effective incorporation of statistical hypothesis testing into medical research studies involves a calibration problem, which is solved by judicious choice of sample size at the time of study design. A number of outcomes which would be clinically meaningful are specified and the significance level and number of patients are then set so that statistically significant results will be clinically relevant (*also see* Sample Size Calculations, *below*).

## CONFIDENCE INTERVALS

Whether the null hypothesis is rejected or not, an additional dimension is added by confidence intervals, which display a range of plausible values for unknown parameters. For example, if an early study of the effects of a treatment on 14 patients concludes that an observed response rate of 40% is significantly greater than the historical 10% response rate, it is informative to add that a 95% confidence interval for the response rate is:

$$40\% \pm 1.96\sqrt{\frac{40\%(60\%)}{14}} = 40\% \pm 25.7\% = (14.3\%, 65.7\%).$$

That is, based on this sample, plausible values of the response rate are no less than 14.3% and no more than 65.7%. In fact, if this early study were repeated 100 times, one would expect the true response rate of this treatment to be outside the 95% confidence interval in only about five experiments.

Formulae for confidence intervals for means, for example, a mean laboratory value like prostate specific antigen (PSA), for median survival times of cancer patients, and other parameters are in standard texts.[3,8] Bayesian "credibility intervals" are an analog of the frequentist confidence interval.[14] In the Bayesian framework, a 95% credibility interval has 95% probability of containing the true response rate or other parameters, based on the posterior distribution of the true response rate, taking its prior distribution and the observed data into account.

## SAMPLE SIZE CALCULATIONS

### Calibration of Statistical and Clinical Significance

Sample size calculations are routinely performed first, as part of study design, and again, as a post-hoc check to verify that a study which failed to reject the null hypothesis had adequate power to detect clinically meaningful differences, if any existed.

Rosner's text[3] provides an excellent cross section of the necessary calculations, with additional tables available in Machin and Campbell[15] and elsewhere. Donner[16] reviewed key techniques, and Cohen[17,18] includes a variety of sample size tables for analysis of variance and regression, with effect sizes categorized as "small," "medium," or "large," according to the dictates of the author's experience in the behavioral sciences. Cohen notes that use of such conventions is less preferable than identification of effect sizes which are scientifically meaningful in one's own research area.

Blumenson[19] described the rate of decline in power when the size of a clinically meaningful difference is misspecified in the study design. Other papers discuss sample-size calculations for particular applications, such as the Mantel-Haenszel chi-square, logistic regression,[20] the logrank test,[21] and tests of interactions.[22]

Personal computer programs that aid calculations of sample size are regularly published. Some current examples include the Dupont POWER.FOR programs,[23] the Cohen calculations,[17,18] the Metz TESTPWR and ROCPWRPC,[24] and the well-known Rothman and Boyce case-control and cohort study programs for the scientific calculator.[25]

Sample size calculations are available not only to provide adequate power to detect clinically meaningful differences with statistical tests, but also to provide confidence intervals of a specified width.[26] Phase I, II, and III studies of drugs and treatment modalities have very different objectives, and correspondingly varied methods of demonstrating adequacy of sample size. Whitehead,[27] Buyse et al,[28] and Meinert[29] discuss some of the particular goals and the necessary sample size calculations at each phase.

Sample size calculations generally involve specification of an acceptable significance level, acceptable power, the size of the smallest effect which is still clinically meaningful, and either the response rate in untreated patients (or the reference group of patients) or the standard deviation of a continuous response such as PSA. In addition, the estimated sample size is often adjusted to allow for anticipated drop-out rates or protocol violations. Finally, an inflation factor may be added if the proposed statistical tests will be nonparametric or will include a continuity correction.[3] If any of these items is misspecified, statistically significant results will not be fully calibrated with results of clinical relevance.

Thus, it is also judicious to reevaluate the results of a nonsignificant study a second time, to determine whether unanticipated variability, increased drop-out, or other factors decreased the power to detect clinically meaningful treatment effects. A study achieving statistical significance had adequate power by definition; in this case, it is worth reviewing whether the admittedly statistically significant results were really of clinical merit.

Occasionally, sample size calculations are refined during the course of an ongoing study, but this is generally the case only when no informative pilot work exists, or a new or auxiliary hypothesis is being examined. There are cautions in the literature regarding fluctuations in repeated estimates of standard deviations based on accumu-

**TABLE 2. The Kaplan-Meier Survival Curve**

**Death/censoring**
**Times[1] (mo): 2 3 4 5+ 7 8+ 12 13+ 14+ 15+ 16 17 17+ 24+ 24+**

| Unique Death Times | No. Still at Risk | No. Dying | Probability of Dying | Probability of Surviving | Kaplan-Meier Cumulative Probability of Surviving |
|---|---|---|---|---|---|
| 2 | 15 | 1 | 1/15 | 14/15 | 14/15 = 0.93 |
| 3 | 14 | 1 | 1/14 | 13/14 | 13/14 × 0.93 = 0.87 |
| 4 | 13 | 1 | 1/13 | 12/13 | 12/13 × 0.87 = 0.80 |
| 7 | 11 | 1 | 1/11 | 10/11 | 10/11 × 0.80 = 0.73 |
| 12 | 9 | 1 | 1/9 | 8/9 | 8/9 × 0.73 = 0.65 |
| 16 | 5 | 1 | 1/5 | 4/5 | 4/5 × 0.65 = 0.52 |
| 17 | 4 | 2 | 2/4 | 2/4 | 2/4 × 0.52 = 0.26 |

[1] The time of each death or censored event is given, eg, the first death was at 2 months, the second and third at month 3 and 4 respectively, and the first censored event, denoted by +, was at 5 months' follow-up. Censored events might be due to the end of the study, drop-out, death from another cause, etc.

lating data, and their effects on sample size calculations.

## SURVIVAL-TYPE ANALYSES

Dawson-Saunders[8] provides a very readable introduction to the analysis of person-time data. A current example is the survival times of patients with metastatic renal carcinoma who have been treated with autolymphocyte therapy.[30] Statistical analysis of such data is complicated by the very factor which defines a successful treatment: patients may survive longer than the duration of the study. Since not everyone dies, this makes the use of an average time until death unsuitable to illustrate the effects of treatment. The event of interest (ie, death) is said to be **censored** in those patients for whom it was not actually observed. Censoring can also occur if patients die of other causes, move, or are otherwise lost to follow-up. For example, if one wishes to calculate a 2-year survival rate, ambiguities exist with respect to patients who were lost to follow-up or died of other causes before 24 months. These ambiguities may be finessed by the use of Kaplan-Meier and actuarial survival curves, the logrank test, Cox regression (to model the simultaneous effects of treatment and prognostic factors), and related techniques.[31]

### The Kaplan-Meier Survival Curve and Actuarial Probabilities

Table 2 displays hypothetical follow-up times and death times for 15 patients with metastatic renal carcinoma. In the example, 8 patients die in a 2-year period, 2 survive at least 2 years, and 5 are lost to follow-up before they died or were under observation for at least 2 years. The Kaplan-Meier survival curve estimates the probability of surviving past various times since entry. It is calculated by multiplying successive calculations of the cumulative probability of surviving from study entry past time $t$ by the probability of surviving each small interval of time. Thus, partial information provided by drop-outs is incorporated by multiplication into later estimates, where only a few people are still at risk. The results are plotted in Figure 8.

In Figure 8, the median survival time can be read from the curve as 17 months. The **actuarial probability** of surviving 12 months is similarly obtained as 0.65. This is in contrast to a simple proportion of those surviving 12 months, which might be estimated as 5/13 = 0.62, since two people were lost to follow-up before they had been observed for 12 months. The actuarial probability of surviving 24 months is

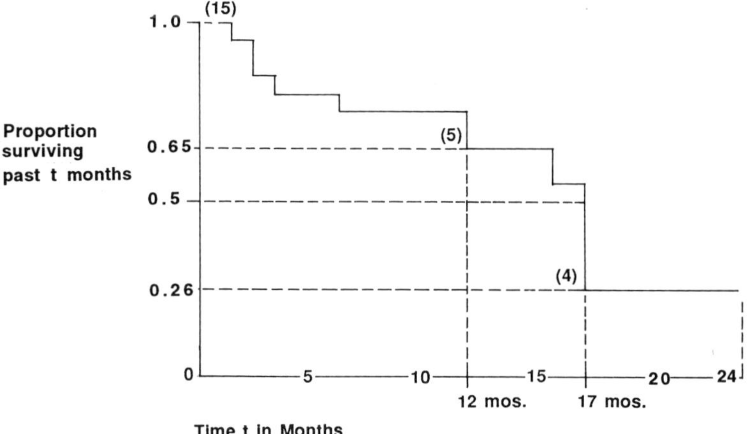


**Fig 8.** Kaplan-Meier Survival Curve. In parentheses are the numbers of patients still at risk at selected times.

0.26, in contrast to a naive proportion of 2/10 = 0.20.

It is not proper to extrapolate beyond the study's observation period, but it is noted that since all humans die, all survival curves eventually drop down to 0, unless the last event in the study is censored. Survival curves for two differentially effective treatments will thus be less distinguishable if the follow-up period is extended indefinitely.

Error bars for the Kaplan-Meier curve can be calculated using Greenwood's formula,[31] as was done by Graverson et al[32] in a report of 15-year follow-up on the effects of radical prostatectomy vs those of expectant primary treatment in patients with stage I and II prostate cancer. Such error bars become wider over the course of the study, as the number of patients still at risk decreases. For this reason, if error bars are not reported, the number of patients still at risk is often provided at selected time points as a visual aid regarding interpretation of apparent differences between two survival curves.

Statistical comparison of survival curves for two or more treatments is typically performed by the logrank test, a generalized Wilcoxon test, or their extensions.[8,31] The power of these tests depends on the number of events, for example, deaths.

Some studies report total survival, and others report cause-specific survival, censoring all deaths not due to the cause of interest. The latter may be influenced by the competing risks of other diseases. When time to local recurrence is the "survival time" variable, it is advisable to examine whether censoring other related events, like distant failures, may mask the real advantages or disadvantages of treatment.[33]

## REGRESSION MODELS

It is often useful to model a medical outcome by obtaining the sum of the hypothesized effects of demographic, prognostic, treatment, and concomitant factors measured in a particular study. Then, the magnitude of each effect is estimated, adjusting for the other factors in the model, and the effect size and statistical significance of each factor are calculated from the available data. For example:

- Prostate specific antigen level = effects of tumor stage + tumor size + age of patient + random variability.
- Expected logarithmic odds of response to treatment = effects of type of treatment + sex of patient + degree of spinal cord injury.
- Population conditional relative risk of death = effects of baseline conditional relative risk × type of treatment × tumor stage when treated.

Ordinary regression and analysis of variance techniques, logistic regression, and Cox proportional hazards regression are examples of statistical techniques that evaluate models of the simultaneous effects of several factors on clinical outcome. A nonsignificant effect is one that does not contribute substantially to explanation of the outcome. The validity of the results depends on whether all of the substantively important variables have been included in the model and whether the sample size was chosen with adequate statistical power so that statistically significant effects are calibrated with effects of medical importance. Additional discussion is provided by Rosner,[3] Dawson-Saunders,[8] and Anderson et al.[34]

The validity of the results may also depend on whether explanatory variables were themselves subject to misclassification or were measured with random variability, or so-called "errors in measurements." For example, sex is unlikely to be misclassified. Clinical stage of a tumor might vary slightly if the same patient is examined by different examiners or on different days. Laboratory values are measured with some variability, even within one laboratory, and the weekly frequency of eating saturated fat 3 years prior to diagnosis of cancer would be expected to be estimated with considerable variability.

## CLINICAL TRIALS

The current literature regarding procedural and statistical aspects of controlled clinical trials of new treatments and therapeutic modalities is continually growing. The details of coordination of a successful, controlled clinical trial, particularly a cooperative or network study, are extensive. Timely cooperation of all investigators within this substantial undertaking is critical, whether it be stimulated by the funding mechanism, the leadership of the principal investigator, or by the collegiality and collaborative interests of the investigative group. Adequate resources include a statistical and coordinating center, clinical coordinators at each site, and sufficient funding of each to ensure the smooth flow of accurate data gathered in compliance with a well-specified, prospectively written protocol. Several excellent references include the works of Meinert[29] and Buyse et al.[28]

Randomization of patients to treatment arms is a key issue, because the great majority of statistical analytic techniques are based on the concept of independent observations and random samples. An intuitive definition of independence has been given in the section on probability, but there is also a specific mathematical definition. When patients are enrolled into a study at clinical presentation, they cannot be said to be a random sample of the general population. Randomization into two treatment groups at least ensures that of this series of clinic patients, approximately half of those with any given prognostic characteristic will fall into one treatment group and about half will fall into the other. This limits the potential for serious imbalances between treatment groups, which can exist in nonrandomized studies.

Both randomized and nonrandomized studies can be subject to other types of biases, such as lack of generalizability, for example, if only stage $T_a$ and $T_c$ prostate cancer patients are enrolled in one experimental protocol and all stage $T_b$ patients are reserved for a competing study.[7] Sackett[35] details a variety of biases which may occur in clinical studies.

Double blinding of treatment arms is frequently useful to assure equal consideration of each treatment, particularly when one treatment is placebo.[29] For example, a patient receiving a well-advertised new treatment might inadvertently be scrutinized more closely for any inkling of improvement than a patient receiving placebo, who might be scrutinized more closely for signs of disease progression. A great many other statistical aspects of clinical trials are discussed in the literature, including stopping rules, interim analyses, subgroup analyses, concurrent versus historical controls, longitudinal analysis, multiple testing problems, and others, but they are beyond the scope of the present chapter.

[The assistance of Nancy Viscofsky, BS, in formatting figures and tables is gratefully acknowledged.]

## REFERENCES


1. Montgomerie JZ, Gilmore DS, Canawati HN, Morrow JW. Ceftazidime in treatment of urinary tract infection in patients with spinal cord injury; comparison with moxalactam. *Urology.* 1990; 35:93–95.
2. David F. *Games, Gods & Gambling. A History of Probability and Statistical Ideas.* Glasgow: Bell and Bain Ltd; 1962.
3. Rosner B. *Fundamentals of Biostatistics.* 3rd ed. Boston: PWS-Kent Publishing Company; 1990.
4. Weinstein MC, Fineberg HV, et al. *Clinical Decision Analysis.* Philadelphia: WB Saunders Company; 1980.
5. Oakes M. *Statistical Inference: A Commentary for the Social and Behavioral Sciences.* New York: John Wiley and Sons; 1986.
6. Morrison A. *Screening in Chronic Disease.* New York: Oxford University Press; 1985.
7. Rifkin M, Zerhouni EA, Gatsonis CA, et al. Comparison of magnetic resonance imaging and ultrasonography in staging early prostate cancer. *N Engl J Med.* 1990;323:621–626.
8. Dawson-Saunders B, Trapp RG. *Basic and Clinical Biostatistics,* Norwalk, Connecticut: Appleton & Lange; 1990.
9. Kraemer HC. Assessment of 2 × 2 associations: generalization of signal-detection methodology. *Am Statist.* 1988;42:37–49.
10. Metz CE. Some practical issues of experimental design and data analysis in radiological ROC studies. *Invest Radiol.* 1989;24:234–245.
11. Swets JA, Pickett RM. *Evaluation of Diagnostic Systems: Methods from Signal Detection Theory.* New York: Academic Press; 1982.
12. Hanley JA, McNeil BJ. The meaning and use of the area under a receiver operating characteristic (ROC) curve. *Diagn Radiol.* 1982; 143:29–36.
13. McNeil BJ, Hanley JA. A method of comparing the areas under receiver operating characteristic curves derived from the same cases. *Radiology.* 1983;148:839–843.
14. Rice J. *Mathematical Statistics and Data Analysis.* Pacific Grove: Wadsworth and Brooks/Cole Advanced Books & Software; 1988.
15. Machin D, Campbell MJ. *Statistical Tables for the Design of Clinical Trials.* Boston: Blackwell Scientific Publications; 1987.
16. Donner A. Approaches to sample size estimation in the design of clinical trials—a review. *Stat Med.* 1984;3:199–214.
17. Cohen J. *Statistical Power Analysis for the Behavioral Sciences.* 2nd ed. Hillsdale, NJ: Lawrence Erlbaum Associates, Inc; 1988.
18. Borenstein M, Cohen J. *Statistical Power Analysis: A Computer Program.* Hillsdale, NJ: Lawrence Erlbaum Associates, Inc; 1988.
19. Blumenson LE. Loss of power from an optimistic alternative hypothesis. *Stat Med.* 1988; 7:457–466.
20. Hsieh FY. Sample size tables for logistic regression. *Stat Med.* 1989;8:795–802.
21. Lakatos E. Sample size based on the log-rank statistic in complex clinical trials. *Biometrics.* 1988;44:229–241.
22. Lachenbruch PA. A note on sample size computation for testing interactions. *Stat Med.* 1988;7:467–469.
23. Dupont WD, Plummer WD. POWER.FOR: A computer program for power and sample size calculations, *Am Statist.* 1991;45:158.
24. Metz CE, Wang P, Kronman HB. A new approach for testing the significance of differences between ROC curves measured from correlated data. In: Deconinck F, ed. *Information Processing in Medical Imaging: Proceedings of the 8th Conference, Brussels, 29 August–2 September 1983.* Boston: Martinus Nijhoff Publishers; 1984:432–445.
25. Rothman KJ, Boice JD Jr. *Epidemiologic Analysis with a Programmable Calculator.* Boston: Epidemiology Resource Inc; 1982.
26. Bristol DR. Sample sizes for constructing confidence intervals and testing hypotheses. *Stat Med.* 1989;8:803–811.
27. Whitehead J. Sample sizes for phase II and phase III clinical trials: an integrated approach. *Stat Med.* 1986;5:459–464.
28. Buyse ME, Staquet MJ, Sylvester RJ. *Cancer Clinical Trials: Methods and Practice.* New York: Oxford University Press; 1984.
29. Meinert CL. *Clinical Trials: Design, Conduct, and Analysis.* New York: Oxford University Press; 1986.
30. Krane RJ, Carpinito GA, Ross SD, Lavin PT, Osband ME. Treatment of metastatic renal cell carcinoma with autolymphocyte therapy. *Urology.* 1990;35:417–422.
31. Lee ET. *Statistical Methods for Survival Data Analysis.* Belmont, CA: Lifetime Learning Publications; 1980.
32. Graverson PH, Nielsen KT, Gasser TC, Corle DK, Madsen PO. Radical prostatectomy versus expectant primary treatment in stage I and II prostatic cancer. *Urology.* 1990;36:493–498.
33. Gelman R, Gelber R, Henderson IC, Coleman CN, Harris JR. Improved methodology for analyzing local and distant recurrence, *J Clin Oncol.* 1990;8:548–555.
34. Anderson S, Auquier A, Hauck WW, Oakes D, Vandaele W, Weisberg HI. *Statistical Methods for Comparative Studies,* New York: John Wiley and Sons; 1980.
35. Sackett DL. Bias in analytic research. *J Chron Dis.* 1979;32:51–63.

# 44

# Urinary Tract Infections in Children

*Anthony A. Caldamone*

## INTRODUCTION

Urinary tract infections in children are common, second in occurrence only to infections of the respiratory tract. Infections may be associated with significant morbidity and result in permanent renal scarring especially in the very young child. Additionally, the incidence of a congenital anatomic abnormality in a child presenting with a urinary tract infection (UTI) warrants careful evaluation of such episodes.

The significance of pediatric urinary tract infections, therefore, cannot be overemphasized. While it is impractical and economically unrealistic to screen for urinary tract infections in all children, infection does warrant evaluation to disclose underlying abnormalities that may risk further infection and renal damage. Renal scarring is a significant cause of hypertension and is responsible for approximately 10% of all pediatric hypertension, and approximately 50% of severe pediatric hypertension. While hypertension is more commonly seen in children with bilateral renal scarring, children with a single renal scar are also at risk. Renal scarring can be expected to occur in 12% to 20% of all children with a symptomatic UTI.[1,2] These data emphasize the importance of an aggressive approach to the treatment and evaluation of all children with urinary tract infection.

## INCIDENCE AND PREVALENCE

The incidence of UTIs in the pediatric population is both age and sex dependent. It is essential that documentation of a significant bacterial colony count be done because, as has been shown by Heale, of those children presenting with a single symptom attributable to a possible UTI, only 14.4% had a positive culture.[3] Of those presenting with flank pain and dysuria, 33% had positive cultures while 31.5% were positive in those with recent onset incontinence. The prevalence of UTI in patients with symptoms suggestive of infection varies with age. A prevalence of 4% to 20% has been found by various authors in infants with nonspecific symptoms such as fever, jaundice, or failure to thrive.[4–6]

### Neonates and Infants

The incidence of urinary tract infection in neonates is gestational age dependent. Adelman et al found the incidence of bacteriuria in the preterm infant to be 2.4% to 3.4% and 0.7% to 1.1% in the full-term population as determined by suprapubic aspiration. In contrast to older children, the male infant has a higher incidence than the female infant, with a ratio ranging between 2.8 and 5.4 : 1.[7] The reason for this differential is not clear; however, Thrupp and

Edelman have each shown that this difference is even more dramatic in the premature and low-birth-weight neonate.[8,9]

Whether this finding has some relationship to circumcision practices will be discussed later. In addition, male neonates are more susceptible to sepsis from a UTI than are the neonatal females.[10] This male predominance occurs primarily in the first 3 months of life. According to Ginsburg and McCracken, up to 3 months of age, 75% of UTIs occurred in males, while by the ages of 3 to 8 months, males accounted for only 11% of cases.[11] The recurrence rate in infants has been reported by Bergstrom as 25%.[7]

It is thought that the hematogenous source of bacteria is more common than the ascending route in the neonate;[12] however, 85% to 90% of infecting bacteria are *Escherichia coli.*[11] This may be explained if the neonatal kidney is immature in its ability to prevent bacteria from being filtered from the blood into the urine, a function the mature kidney is capable of.[13]

Regarding the issue of asymptomatic bacteriuria in healthy neonates, Stamey found an incidence of 1.5% and 0.13% in males and females, respectively.[12] Similarly, Abbott demonstrated that 1.4% and 0.4% of consecutive neonatal males and females, respectively, had bacteriuria, with one third demonstrating symptoms.[14]

### Boys

Bacteriuria, both symptomatic and asymptomatic, in boys other than neonates is very low. Routine screening bacteriuria in this group has a prevalence of 0.2%.[15] Kunin et al found only 2 of 7,731 boys screened to have asymptomatic bacteriuria.[16] Winberg et al carried out a prospective study of 600 children with symptomatic UTI and demonstrated a cumulative incidence of UTI from 0 to 11 years of age of 1.1% for males, compared to 30% for females.[17] The incidence of the apparent first UTI decreases with age more rapidly in boys than girls. Three fourths of all boys who develop a UTI do so in the first year of life compared to only one third of girls.

### Girls

The incidence of bacteriuria in school-aged girls is 12% as demonstrated by Kunin in a classic study.[16] Based on extrapolation it was estimated that 5% of all school-aged girls would have bacteriuria sometime during their school years, with blacks having a somewhat lower risk than whites. In addition, Kunin noted a decreasing prevalence with age, 0.7% in 5- to 9-year-old girls and 0.5% in 10 to 14 year olds. This decreasing trend with age up to the sexually active years has been documented by other authors as well.[18–20] Thus, the incidence of apparent first UTI decreases with age. This was found to be true for males as well as females. Kunin's data also found a recurrence rate in this population of 80% for white girls and 60% for black girls.

## CLINICAL PRESENTATION

The presenting signs and symptoms of a UTI in a child vary significantly with the age at presentation, the severity of the infection, and the site of the infection (Table 1). A high index of suspicion is required to avoid delays in diagnosis and treatment in the pediatric age range as both symptoms and signs are often nonspecific and subtle, particularly in the younger child. Smellie et al reported that of 200 children subsequently proven to have a UTI, in only 9% of infants and 50% of older children had a UTI been the referring diagnosis.[20] Early diagnosis and prompt treatment are essential to prevent renal damage.

### Neonates

The neonatal group presents with the most obscure and least localizing manifestations of UTI. The most common signs include failure to thrive or weight loss, vomiting, diarrhea, or jaundice.[4,7,20,21] In the neonate, fever is a variable sign. Neurologic symptoms such as lethargy, fussiness, or seizures are also seen.

With the inability of the neonate to contain infection, both bacteriuria and sepsis are more common. Bacteremia occurs in approximately 25% of neonates with UTI.[11] Therefore, the urinary tract should

**TABLE 1. Presenting Symptoms of UTI in 200 Children**

| | Age Range (Percentage) | | | |
|---|---|---|---|---|
| Symptom | 0–1 Mo | 1–24 Mos | 2–5 Y | 5–12 Y |
| Failure to thrive/feeding problem | 53 | 36 | 7 | 0 |
| Jaundice | 44 | 0 | 0 | 0 |
| Irritability | 0 | 13 | 7 | 0 |
| Malodorous/cloudy urine | 0 | 9 | 13 | 0 |
| Diarrhea | 18 | 16 | 0 | 0 |
| Vomiting | 24 | 29 | 16 | 3 |
| Fever | 11 | 38 | 57 | 50 |
| Convulsions | 2 | 7 | 9 | 5 |
| Hematuria | 0 | 7 | 16 | 8 |
| Frequency/dysuria | 0 | 4 | 34 | 41 |
| Enuresis | 0 | 0 | 27 | 29 |
| Abdominal pain | 0 | 0 | 23 | 0 |
| Loin pain | 0 | 0 | 0 | 0 |
| Male/Female ratio | 3:1 | | 1:10 | 1:10 |

From Smellie JM et al, Clinical and radiological features of urinary tract infection in children, *Br Med J* (1964; 2:1222); modified from Bickerton MW, Duckett JW Jr, Urinary tract infections in pediatric patients, *AUA Update Series* (1985; 4:4).

be considered a source of sepsis or bacteremia in neonates, and a culture of the urine is mandatory in any neonate presenting with a nonspecific illness.

### Infants

The signs of UTI in the neonate remain nonspecific, although fever is more consistently found and sepsis less commonly seen.[17,20,40] Gastrointestinal symptoms and failure to thrive are commonly seen in this age group as well. In 1962, Neumann and Pryles reported an autopsy series in which only 17% of fatal cases of acute pyelonephritis in infants were diagnosed before death.[22] It is mandatory, therefore, that any infant who presents with unexplained fever have a urine culture.

### Toddlers

It is in the toddler age group that traditional urinary tract symptoms and signs may first become recognizable. Failure to toilet train at an appropriate age may be a sign of underlying chronic infection or a structural abnormality. Likewise, incontinence in a previously trained child may also herald a UTI. Parents should be questioned about the quality of the urinary stream, dribbling, or malodorous urine. Parental observations of the voiding pattern relative to frequency of voiding or damp diapers, dribbling, or prolonged voiding time were correlated by Randolph et al with the presence of bacteriuria.[23]

### Older Children

As the child becomes older, the presenting symptoms of a UTI become more typical of those seen in the adult population. Fever, frequency, dysuria, and enuresis are the most common complaints in this age group. As previously mentioned, dysuria is a common complaint and not in any way pathognomonic of a UTI, as it may be seen with vaginitis and irritative urethritis.

## PATHOGENESIS

### Route of Infection

Except in the neonate, the route of bacterial infection of the urinary tract is thought to be ascending, arising from colonization of the urethra.[7] Evidence indicates that girls with recurrent UTIs tend to have colonization of the introitus and perineum with organisms potentially pathogenic to the urinary tract.[24] This information is similar to that reported by Stamey in adult females.[12] Tuttle et al demonstrated a lower level of vaginal immunoglobulin A in girls with recurrent UTIs compared to controls with no bacteriuria.[25] It is theorized, therefore, that vaginal antibody levels may be the determining factor in introital colonization. Bacterial introital colonization may be an age-related phenomenon as well, in that Bollgren and Winberg reported that periurethral bacterial flora decreases over the first few years of life in both sexes.[26]

There is a variety of evidence indicating that the hematogenous spread is responsible for most urinary tract infections in the neonate. It has been shown that in neonates there is a high incidence of bacteremia associated with UTI, with symptoms at times preceding detectable bacteriuria.[7,11,27] Autopsy data by Porter and Giles demonstrated renal cortical infection in the absence of renal pelvic bacteriuria.[28] More recent data, however, implicates the ascending route, at least in male infants and neonates. It is interesting to note, however, that in a review of 100 infants with UTI by Ginsburg and McCracken, 95% of affected males were uncircumcised. One may infer, therefore, that bacterial colonization of the preputial sac may explain the previously curious male predominance of UTIs in the early infancy period.[26,29] This preputial colonization, while common in the young infant, decreases significantly after 5 years of age. It has also been shown that such colonization with gastrointestinal bacteria is a potential source of ascending infection.[17] It is possible that the source of preputial colonization in boys and perianal colonization in girls is maternal. Patrick has shown that 24% of infants were bacteriuric when delivered by mothers who were bacteriuric, compared to none in infants of nonbacteriuric mothers.[30] Three percent of these bacteriuric infants developed pyelonephritis, compared to 0.2% of controls. Wiswell has reported an increased incidence of UTI in the uncircumcised infant.[31,32] Of 5,261 infants reviewed, the incidence of UTI in uncircumcised males was 4.12% compared to 0.21% of circumcised males (0.4% in females). In a larger review of 422,328 infants, 1825 (0.43%) were hospitalized with a UTI in the first year of life, representing an overall incidence of 0.57% in the females, 0.11% in the circumcised males, and 1.12% in the uncircumcised males. This demonstrates a 10-fold higher incidence of UTI in the uncircumcised male. Over this 10-year period of study, there was a significant decrease in the circumcision rate from 85.4% to 73.9%, which was associated with a concomitant increase in the incidence of UTI in males. Although these data are striking, however, more information is required regarding the sequelae of these episodes of infection and the incidence of underlying uropathology.

## Host Factors

There are essentially four barriers to the development of urinary tract infection: the natural resistance of the perineum, bladder defense mechanisms, a competent antirefluxing ureterovesical junction preventing vesicoureteral reflux, and the anatomic structure of the renal papillae to prevent intrarenal reflux. We will examine aberrations of those host factors particularly significant in the child, such as underlying uropathology, heredity, and constipation.

The incidence of underlying uropathology in the child presenting with a urinary tract infection approaches 50% in certain study populations, with vesicoureteral reflux occurring in 35% overall.[33] Obstruction may be either mechanical or functional in nature. In various reported studies, mechanical obstruction occurs in 3% to 21% of children presenting with a UTI.[4,17,34] The more common obstructive lesions in children include ureteropelvic junction obstruction, ureterovesical junction obstruction, ectopic ureterocele (most often with duplication), and posterior urethral valves. Infection coupled with obstruction may cause a previously well-balanced ob-

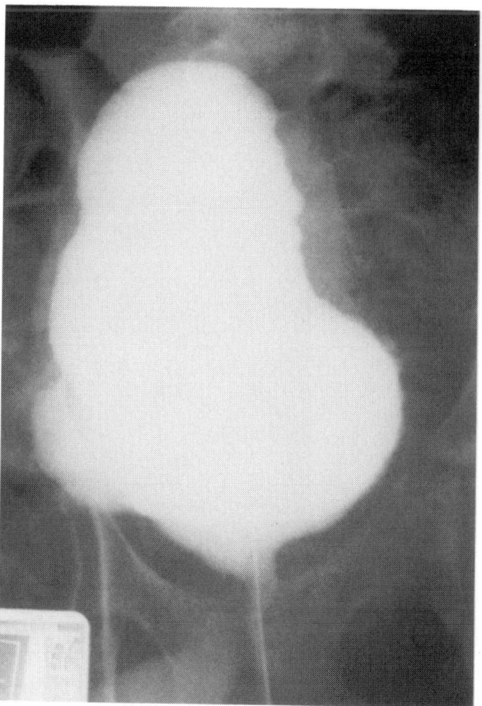

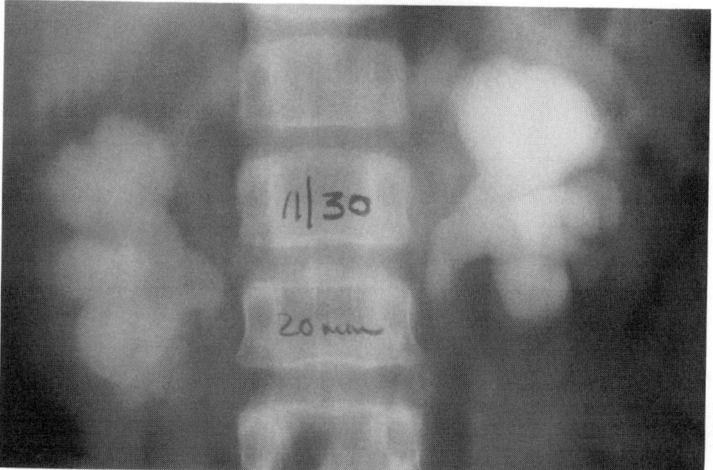

**Fig 1. A:** Cystogram in a boy with Hinman-Allen syndrome demonstrating a severely trabeculated bladder. **B:** Excretory urogram demonstrating hydronephrosis bilaterally.

struction to result in accelerated renal damage.[35]

The role of urethral stenosis in the female and its relationship to urinary tract infections deserves a word. It has been shown that females with recurrent UTIs have the same, or greater, calibrated urethral diameter as those without UTIs.[36] Additionally, urethral dilatation has not been shown to be effective in reducing bacteriuric episodes.[37]

Abnormal voiding dynamics in children

has also been found to be common in those with recurrent UTI. In a review of girls with UTIs, Lapides and Diokno found that 61% had detrusor instability and that 30% were abnormally infrequent voiders.[38] Children with dysfunctional voiding or Hinman-Allen syndrome, in which their detrusor contracts against a closed urethral sphincter, are particularly prone to recurrent UTIs.[39–43] These children may manifest uninhibited contractions, high intravesical filling and voiding pressures, poor bladder emptying, bladder trabeculation, vesicoureteral reflux, and hydronephrosis (Fig 1). Constipation and encopresis are commonly found in this group as well. Treatment aimed at correction of dysfunctional voiding pattern has been shown to reduce the incidence of recurrent UTIs.[44–46]

### Constipation

Constipation has been shown to increase the incidence of lower urinary tract infections. O'Regan et al identified a group of children with uninhibited bladder contractions and constipation leading to enuresis and encopresis.[47] Constipation may affect the lower urinary tract by direct mechanical compressions of the bladder (Fig 2), increased bacterial contamination of the perineum, and/or decreased voiding frequency.[48] Prospective studies found that a successful bowel regimen resulted in a significant decrease in recurrent UTI and enuresis.[49,50]

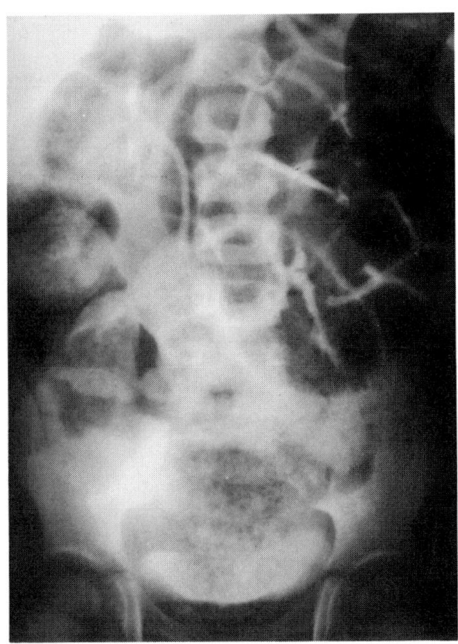

**Fig 2.** Excretory urogram in a 5-year-old female with recurrent UTIs and severe constipation.

### Hereditary Factors

Race is a factor in both the incidence of bacteriuria recurrence and, to a degree, the risk of vesicoureteral reflux. Kunin et al reported the prevalence rate of bacteriuria in white girls was 1.2% compared to 0.5% in black girls.[16] Additionally, the recurrence rate of bacteriuria is 80% in white girls versus 60% in black girls. Askari and Belman found a higher percentage of white girls requiring hospitalization for UTI.[51] Additionally, the incidence of vesicoureteral reflux is significantly lower in black girls compared to their white counterparts.

Bacteriuria tends to be more common in daughters of mothers who have bacteriuria and recurrent urinary tract infections as well as in female siblings of a proband with bacteriuria.[52] Similarly, vesicoureteral reflux has been shown by several studies to be more common in siblings of index refluxers.[53,54] This raises the controversial issue of screening for reflux in siblings. Some authors recommend nuclear cystography for such siblings, with results indicating that in 8% to 45% of siblings reflux will be demonstrated compared with 1% in the general population.

## LOCALIZATION OF INFECTION

The distinction between upper and lower tract infection in the child is important from a prognostic standpoint. Upper tract infections are responsible for renal scarring, especially in the young population, and are also more likely to be associated with a structural abnormality. Various criteria involving both direct and indirect methodology have been proposed to distinguish between upper and lower tract infections.

In the pediatric population, the distinction between upper and lower UTI is more often made on clinical findings. The presence of fever, flank or upper abdominal pain, and/or tenderness will most often indicate pyelonephritis and is rarely seen with cystitis. However, there is significant overlap between these two groups, and therefore one cannot rely on symptoms alone, especially in the younger child.

Direct methods of localization include bladder washout and ureteral catheterization techniques. The bladder washout test is performed by catheterization of the bladder and instillation of an antimicrobial into the bladder (to sterilize the lower tract), followed by saline washout.[55] Subsequent sequential urine samples are obtained representing upper tract source. This technique has been used in children with some success, although because in the pediatric patient general anesthesia may be required, its usefulness is limited. When dealing with children, one must be aware that vesicoureteral reflux can result in false-positive results with either of these direct methods.

Of the indirect methods available, erythrocyte sedimentation rate (ESR), C-reactive protein, and urinary lactic dehydrogenase (LDH-IV and V) correlate best with clinical findings and bladder washout studies. Significant overlap exists, however, in all of these parameters with upper and lower tract infections and, therefore, individually they are not absolutely reliable in the individual pediatric patient.[56]

Urinary concentrating ability has been shown to be impaired in the presence of renal inflammation; however, again, significant overlap has been demonstrated between upper and lower infection.[57–59]

Elevated serum levels of anti-Tamm-Horsfall (anti-TH) protein antibodies levels correlate well with acute pyelonephritis and vesicoureteral reflux, in contrast to acute cystitis.[60,61] In addition, very low levels are found in children with significant renal parenchymal scarring. However, since a rapid and reproducible assay for anti-TH antibody is not universally available, its clinical usefulness is limited at present.

In contradistinction to adults, urinary antibody–coated bacteria levels do not correlate as well with the presence of upper tract infection in children.[62–64] Both false-positive and false-negative results have been reported. False-negative results have been reported by Pulkkanen to be particularly high in the less-than-6-month-old child.[63]

In summary, both direct and indirect methodology for localization of a UTI have limited applicability in the pediatric age range—direct methods due to their need for catheterization and/or anesthesia, and indirect methods because of their poor reliability in children. In clinical practice, one relies on signs and symptoms to distinguish upper from lower tract infections. While there is significance in the distinction from a prognostic standpoint, either necessitates virtually identical radiographic evaluations (except in certain circumstances, specifically older age groups, which will be discussed later in this chapter).

## Pyelonephritis

Acute pyelonephritis in children other than neonates (among whom hematogenous spread is more common) occurs almost exclusively in the presence of obstruction or nonmechanical stasis syndromes and vesicoureteral reflux (Fig 3). The age of the patient is an important factor in the potential for renal scarring from pyelonephritis. Renal scarring occurs almost exclusively in children under 5 years with the infant under 1 year being most susceptible. Older children and adolescents are at low risk for renal damage from acute pyelonephritis. Reports indicate renal scarring in up to 41% of neonates with pyelonephritis.[65] Bailey reported that 39% of infants presenting with UTI and vesicoureteral reflux in the first year of life already had renal scarring at initial evaluation.[66] Winter reported that the mean age at first detection of renal scarring was 5.7 years (Fig 4), with approximately 75% presenting before six years of age.[67] Renal scarring occurs in 12% to 20% of all children with upper tract infections, with vesicoureteral reflux reported in at least 85% of children with renal scars.[2,68,69] The risk of renal scarring has been shown to vary with the grade of reflux.[70–73] The interna-

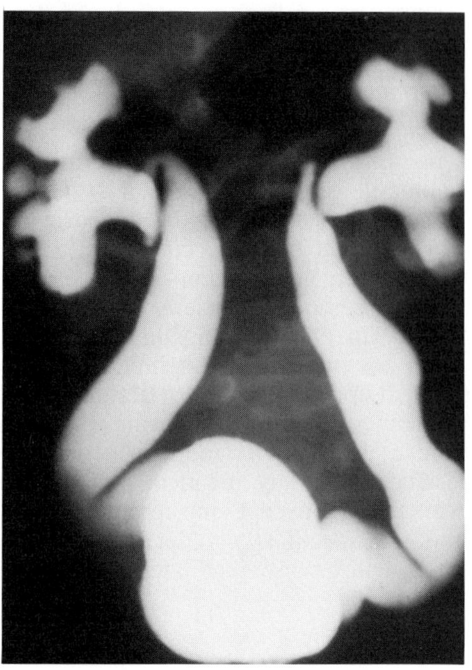

**Fig 3.** Voiding cystourethrogram (VCUG) in a 1-year-old boy with bilateral grade 5 reflux.

tional system for reflux is indicated in Fig 5.

Vesicoureteral reflux is the most common finding in association with urinary tract infection in children and its role in the etiology of pyelonephritis and renal scarring has been well established in both the laboratory and clinical arena.[15,17] In the absence of obstruction, pyelonephritis and renal scarring occur as a consequence of vesicoureteral reflux and intrarenal reflux in children (Fig 6). Intrarenal reflux is demonstrable on voiding cystourethrogram in up to 25% of children with moderate to severe grades of reflux.[68,72,74] As intrarenal reflux is more commonly seen in infants and young children, this group is at higher risk for the sequela of renal scarring.[2,75] Lower hydrostatic pressure is required to demonstrate intrarenal reflux in the infant group. Intrarenal reflux tends to occur more commonly in compound calyces with widely patent collecting ducts, which are more often found in the polar regions of the kidney.[35]

The ability of sterile reflux to induce renal scarring remains debatable. However, experimental evidence indicates that sterile-reflux-induced renal scarring occurs only in the presence of abnormal voiding dynamics with elevated bladder-filling and bladder-voiding pressures. Hodson was able to produce scarring in the presence of sterile reflux in a pig model with bladder outlet obstruction and high intravesical

**Fig 4.** Distribution of age at first detection of renal scarring. Average age = 5.7 years. [Reprinted with permission from Winter AL et al, acquired renal scars in children, *J Urol* (1983; 129:1190).]

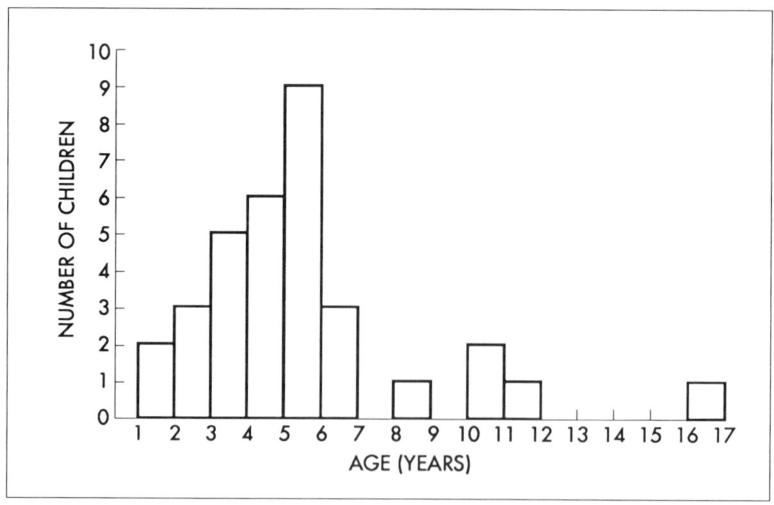

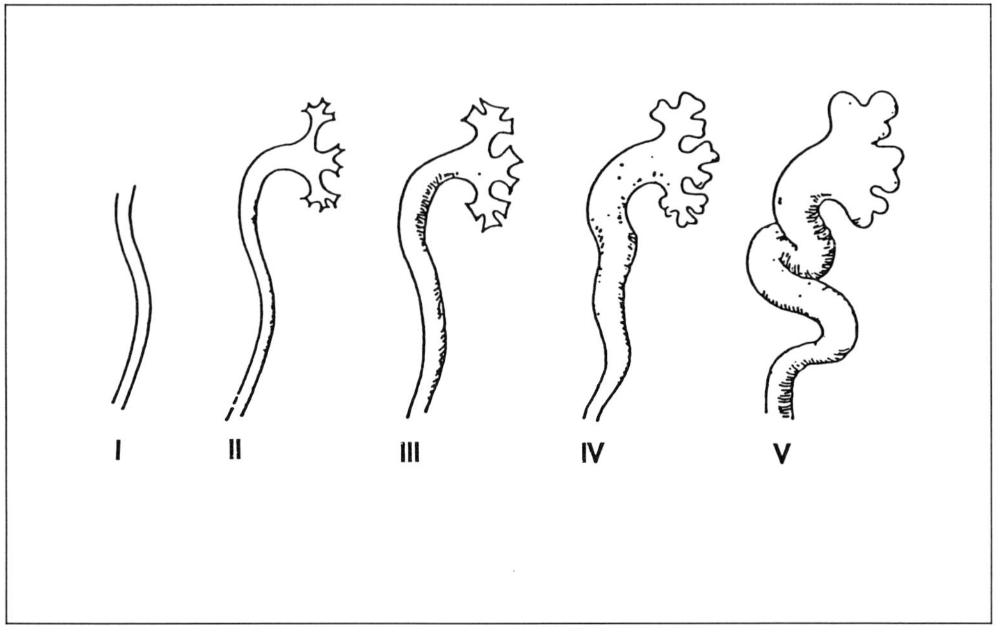


**Fig 5.** International classification of reflux. [From Duckett JW, Bellinger MF, A plea for standardized grading of vesicoureteral reflux, *Eur Urol* (1982; 8:125).]

**Fig 6.** Voiding cystourethrogram demonstrating left upper pole and lower pole intrarenal reflux.

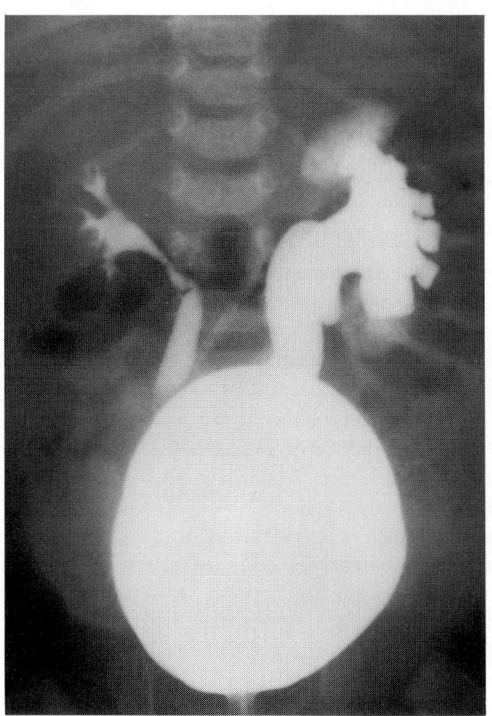

pressures. This would indicate that the child with vesicoureteral reflux and neuropathic bladder or bladder outlet obstruction (ie, posterior urethral valve, Hinman-Allen syndrome) is particularly at risk for renal scarring in the absence of symptomatic UTIs. The corollary of this argument is also clinically well founded. That is, in the absence of urinary tract infections, it is unusual for a child to develop new or progressive scars in face of normal bladder dynamics.[2,75] Long-term clinical reports are available to support this contention. Lenaghan et al found no new renal damage, loss of renal function, or loss of concentrating ability in 40 children followed with sterile reflux, whereas progressive renal damage occurred in approximately half of those refluxers with at least a single documented UTI.[71] Similar findings have been reported by Edwards et al.[70]

While the association of vesicoureteral reflux, urinary tract infection, and renal scarring is well established, recent studies have documented the development of infection-induced renal scarring in the absence of vesicoureteral reflux. Winter et al reported that in 43% of children with renal scarring subsequent to documented episodes of clinical pyelonephritis no evidence of vesicoureteral reflux was found.[75] Similarly, Winberg et al found that 30% of children with renal scarring had minimal or no vesicoureteral reflux.[76] It is likely that at least some of these cases may be explained by the vesicoureteral reflux being transient or intermittent in nature. Certain patients with a marginally competent antireflux mechanism may reflux only under certain conditions, such as in the presence of cystitis, which is known to be capable of shortening the intravesical ureteral tunnel due to mucosal edema. Therefore, patients who demonstrate recurrent upper tract infections in the absence of demonstrable reflux should be protected with prophylactic antibiotics similar to known reflux. One faces a clinical dilemma in this particular group, however, in that there is no clear end point to their prophylaxis except for the attainment of a lower renal-scarring risk for the age group.

Progressive renal scarring occurs almost exclusively as the result of repeated episodes of pyelonephritis rather than chronic indolent bacterial pyelonephritis.[2,77] Immunologic factors, however, may produce a progression of scarring in certain individuals, accounting for those older patients found to have advanced renal scarring in the absence of clinically evident infection.

## Acute Lobar Nephronia

An inflammatory process limited to one lobe of the kidney is termed focal bacterial nephritis, focal pyelonephritis, or acute lobar nephronia. This represents a compartmentalized inflammatory mass with poorly defined margins and calyceal distortion on excretory urogram.[78] CT scan demonstrates an area of decreased contrast enhancement. Radionuclide imaging with gallium may show that area to have increased uptake. The distinction from a solid tumor mass or an intrarenal abscess may be difficult, and one must rely on the clinical presentation of pyelonephritic signs or the response to antibiotic therapy to establish the diagnosis. Most cases demonstrate resolution on subsequent imaging in 4 to 6 weeks, although some may progress to abscess formation.

## Xanthogranulomatous Pyelonephritis

Xanthogranulomatous pyelonephritis (XGP) is an atypical severe chronic infection of the renal parenchyma, often mimicking other renal inflammatory processes or neoplasia, and characterized by phagocytosis of liberated lipids by macrophages, giving its characteristic appearance of foamy histiocytes. Its occurrence in children is uncommon, with less than 35 cases reported in the literature.[79,80] The disease in children differs from that in adults in that it may present in either a diffuse or focal form. The diffuse form is similar to its adult counterpart in that it presents as a systemic illness with a grossly enlarged nonfunctioning renal unit often with an underlying structural anomaly such as UPJ obstruction or ureterocele (Fig 7) and commonly associated with renal calculi.[79] The focal form is more unique to children and presents as an asymptomatic mass lesion with variable degrees of calyceal distortion often indistinguishable from Wilms' tumor. It is thought to represent an altered immune response to infection.

## Cystitis

Acute cystitis is a common childhood infection representing the majority of symptomatic urinary tract infections in the pediatric population. The recurrence rate, as previously noted, is high with approximately 80% of females developing a second infection, 10% doing so immediately following therapy for the first episode.[13] Outside of the newborn and infant age range, symptoms consist of frequency, urgency, incontinence, and squatting in response to urgency. The absence of fever, abdominal or flank pain, and nausea and vomiting make upper tract infection unlikely. Govan and Palmer demonstrated that only 6% of children with a UTI in the absence of reflux had systemic complaints

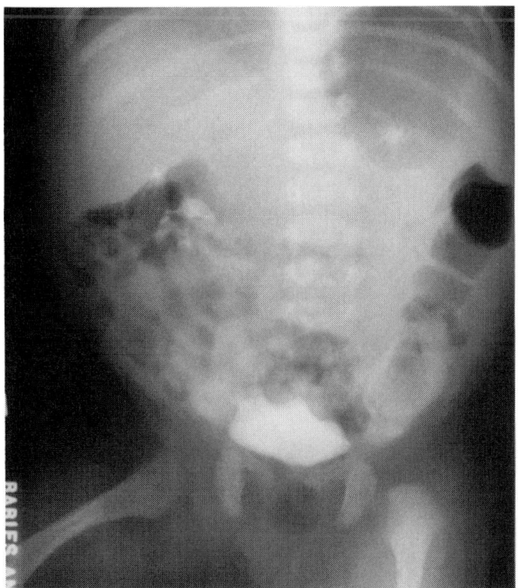

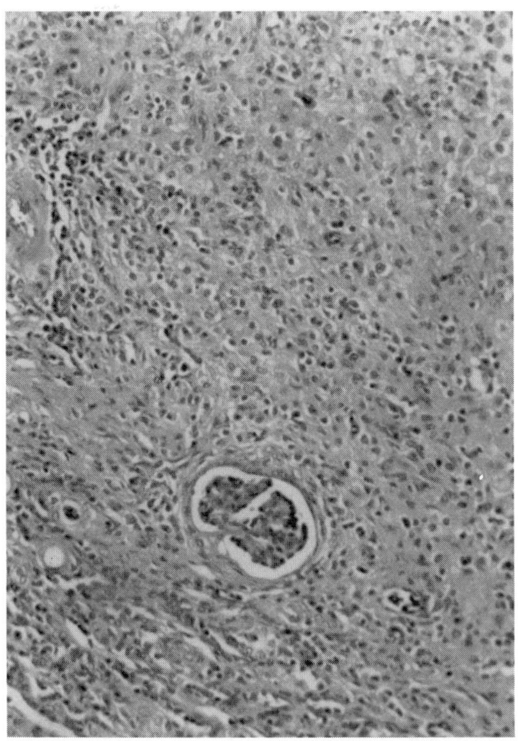

**Fig 7. A:** Excretory urogram in a 1-year-old girl with a ureterocele to a nonfunctioning right upper pole system. **B:** Histopathology of excised upper pole, demonstrating xanthogranulomatous pyelonephritis with classic foamy histocytes.

while in 80% of those with reflux, fever, and abdominal pain were present.[81]

Eosinophilic cystitis is an entity that has been seen in children presenting with chronic dysuria, hematuria, urgency, and frequency.[61,82,83] Although the etiology is poorly understood, a history of allergies is often present. Hellstrum has postulated an immune complex reaction that incites eosinophilic infiltration.[84] Filling defects in the bladder may be present on excretory urogram, and cystoscopy demonstrates inflammatory polypoid mucosal changes due to intense eosinophilic infiltration of the mucosa and muscularis with varying degrees of granulation and ulceration.[85] Peripheral eosinophilia may be present and is more commonly seen in the presence of a bladder mass. Biopsy is necessary to confirm the diagnosis and, in some cases, to exclude malignancy. Steroids, anti-inflammatory agents, and antibiotics have all been used with varying degrees of therapeutic success.

Viral cystitis presents as severe urgency, frequency, and gross hematuria with a negative routine bacterial urine culture. Mass lesions in the bladder may be seen on urography, and generally resolve along with the symptoms within 4 weeks.[13] The most common organisms are adenovirus 11 and 21. If the diagnosis can be made clinically, no further evaluation is required as viral cystitis does not generally portend a structural abnormality of the urinary tract.

## Asymptomatic Bacteriuria

The prevalence of asymptomatic bacteriuria in school-aged females is 0.5% to 1.6%.[16] In the absence of vesicoureteral reflux, the risk of upper tract damage is negligible.[86] Only those children with renal scars on presentation and vesicoureteral reflux will go on to develop new or progressive scarring. Therefore the presentation of asymptomatic bacteriuria warrants evaluation of the upper and lower urinary tracts. Lindberg et al reported that 21% of such girls had reflux and that 10% had demonstrable loss of renal parenchyma.[87] This study also found that approximately one third of patients with asymptomatic bacteriuria had a history consistent with previous unevaluated urinary tract infections. In those with anatomically normal urinary tracts and normal voiding dynamics, long-term treatment probably should be withheld as antibiotic therapy is likely to lead to reinfection with less sensitive and possibly symptom-producing organisms and no long-term sequelae in this specific patient population has been demonstrated.

## Epididymitis

Epididymitis is an unusual infection in the non–sexually active pediatric age group. In a report by Barber and Raper, of 136 cases of acute epididymitis there were no patients less than 14 years of age.[88] Reports vary considerably regarding the incidence of epididymitis in boys.[89–91] The most likely explanation is variability—the age range used for patient selection and whether or not the population at the upper end of the spectrum was sexually active. In the prepubertal age group, it should be considered an unusual cause of acute scrotal swelling, whereas its incidence increases in the adolescent population. Epididymitis may result from a structural abnormality of the lower urinary tract, although the incidence of underlying anatomic abnormalities also varies considerably. Once again, the incidence of underlying abnormalities will vary with the age group under consideration, with the prepubertal patient having a higher risk.[92–96] If one excludes epididymitis in the sexually active adolescent, the probability of an underlying structural abnormality likely justifies radiographic evaluation as with other urinary tract infections in children (Fig 8). Jarvi et al, in a review of 114 patients 17 years old and younger, found that structural abnormalities were either urological or anorectal and were all known prior to the episode of epididymitis.[97] There were no patients with underlying pathology that had not previously been apparent.

Epididymitis in infancy has also been evaluated by Jarvi et al.[98] Interestingly, they found no structural lesions in 9 infants with surgically proven epididymitis.

**Fig 8.** Age distribution of patients with epididymitis and distribution of those with underlying urogenital anomalies. [Reprinted with permission from Siegel A, Snyder H, Duckett JW, Epididymitis in infants and boys, *J Urol* (1987;138:1100–1103).]

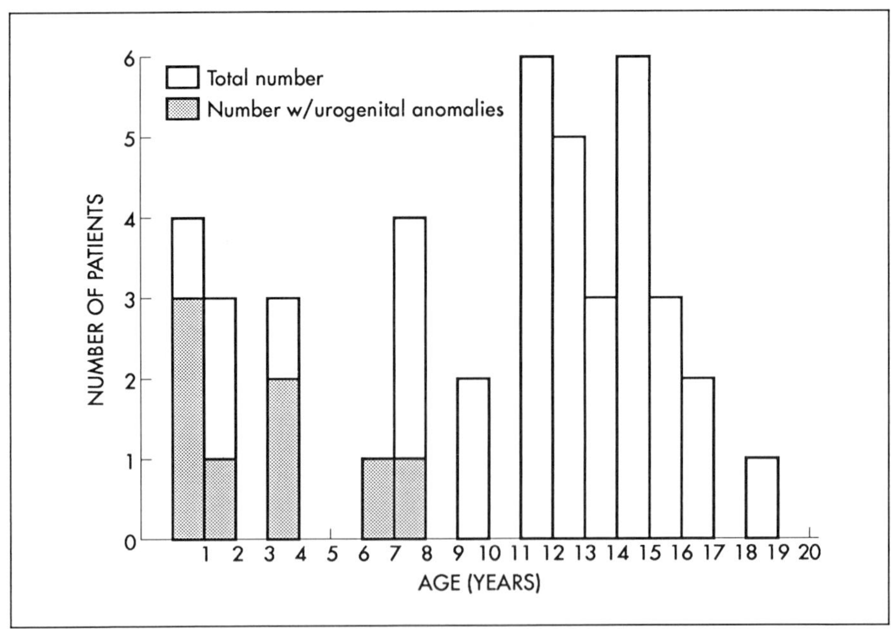

The most common presenting symptoms are those of scrotal swelling, pain, and erythema with voiding symptoms presenting rather infrequently. Pyuria on urinalysis, as well as a positive urine culture, are found infrequently as well. Treatment is based on the fact that in the sexually active patient bacterial epididymitis is most commonly due to *Chlamydia trachomatis* and *Neisseria gonorrhea* whereas in the prepubertal group it is most likely due to Gram-negative coliforms. The prognosis is optimistic in that the incidence of testicular atrophy in the pediatric age group is low.

## DIAGNOSIS AND SPECIMEN COLLECTION

The key to the diagnosis of a urinary tract infection is a positive urine culture of sufficient colony count, depending on the collection technique used. Reliance on symptoms suggestive of a UTI alone or the presence of pyuria and/or bacteria on urinalysis will result in many false-positive presumptions of UTI. Pyuria may occur in the absence of a bacterial UTI, as seen with gastroenteritis or dehydration. Symptoms of dysuria, frequency, and incontinence are nonspecific and not pathognomic of a UTI. These symptoms are indicative of lower genitourinary irritation and may be due to vaginitis, vulvitis, or nonspecific urethral irritation. Dickinson reported that of children presenting with lower tract symptoms, only 58% had bacteriuria.[99] Similar statistics have been reported by Heale: 14% of children with urinary complaints were culture positive, 33% culture positive of those with flank pain, and 31% positive with recent onset of incontinence.[3] Therefore, considering the implications of UTI in children and the necessity for urinary tract evaluation, a proven culture from a properly collected specimen is mandatory documentation.

The use of quantitative urine culture is based on the statistical probability of a colony count correlating with the presence of a UTI (Table 2). The traditional criterion for diagnosis of a UTI is a colony count of $10^5$ organisms per mL of a voided urine specimen. The probability of infection based on colony count, however, varies with the method of collection. This is particularly important in the pediatric patient.

In the neonate and infant the application of a collection bag to the perineum is often used. Its accuracy is limited by a high rate of contamination from both vaginal and fecal flora. Lincoln and Winberg found that 34% of uncircumcised male neonates had greater than $10^5$ bacteria/mL in a bagged specimen after routine cleansing of the genitalia.[29] Following more extensive cleansing of the preputial sac, only 8% grew greater than $10^5$ organisms/mL. Similar results were reported for neonatal girls. The risk of contamination is also related to the length of time the collection bag is on the perineum, with reliability of positive cultures falling significantly after 30 min-

**TABLE 2. Quantitative Colony Count and Probability of Infection**

| Method | Colony Count | Probability of Infection |
|---|---|---|
| Suprapubic aspiration | Any # Gram-negative or $>10^3$ Gram-positive | >99% |
| Catheterization | $>10^5$ | 95% |
| | $10^4$–$10^5$ | Likely |
| | $10^3$–$10^4$ | Suspicious |
| | $<10^3$ | Unlikely |
| Clean voided female | 3 specimens $>10^5$ | 95% |
| | 2 specimens $>10^5$ | 90% |
| | 1 specimen $>10^5$ | 80% |
| | $10^4$–$10^5$ | Suspicious |
| | $<10^4$ | Unlikely |
| Male (circumcised) | $>10^4$ | Likely |

utes.[100] Equally important is immediate plating or refrigeration of the specimen after the infant voids. Consequently, while a negative bagged specimen is reliable, a positive culture should be confirmed by catheterization or suprapubic aspiration prior to treatment. Edelmann et al found that of 53 positive cultures from bag specimens, only 75% were confirmed by suprapubic aspiration.[8]

Suprapubic aspiration is the most reliable method for obtaining an uncontaminated specimen and the one most applicable to neonates and young infants. It is particularly suitable for the young child as the bladder is still an abdominal organ at this age. Its complications are few if one adheres to the prerequisite of a palpable bladder prior to aspiration. Transient hematuria may occur in up to 3.2% of neonates,[101,102] although pelvic hematomas requiring transfusions as well as abdominal wall abscesses following puncture of the intestine have been reported.[103,104] The accuracy in obtaining a urine specimen by suprapubic aspiration is 90%; however, repeated attempts should be discouraged unless the bladder is palpable. Virtually any colony count of Gram-negative organisms or greater than $10^3$ Gram-positive organisms per mL is considered significant if obtained by bladder aspiration.

Bladder catheterization is a reliable method of obtaining an uncontaminated urine specimen except in the neonatal boy with an unretractable foreskin. Although the risk of contamination is higher than that with suprapubic aspiration, a palpable bladder is not a prerequisite. Therefore, in the ill infant without a palpable bladder or in the older child, a catheterization is ideal in obtaining a specimen urgently prior to instituting therapy. The risk of urethral trauma in the male is minimal if a well-lubricated 5F or 8F feeding tube is used. The procedure should be virtually atraumatic in the female.

Clean-voided specimens require a cooperative, toilet-trained child. Specimens are less likely to be contaminated in the circumcised male and are more reliable in older children; however, contamination with perineal flora should always be considered in girls. In a study of 120 patients in which clean-voided specimens were compared to suprapubic aspirates, only 42% of culture-positive clean-voided specimens in children less than 18 months old were confirmed by suprapubic aspiration, whereas the correlation increased to 71% in children 3 to 12 years of age.[105]

## RADIOGRAPHIC EVALUATION

There has been much debate as to the indications for evaluation in children with UTIs. The most common teaching has advocated evaluation for males after the first UTI and females after the third UTI.[106] Others recommend imaging in all children less than 3 years of age. There is sound evidence that the first documented urinary tract infection in most children should be evaluated radiographically. This is based on several factors. First, up to 80% of children with a urinary tract infection can be expected to have a second UTI. Second, those children with anatomic abnormalities are at high risk for developing renal damage with each subsequent infection. Early identification and treatment of those children at risk for upper tract damage has been shown to obviate or ameliorate renal parenchymal scarring and preserve renal function. Third, the incidence of an anatomic abnormality, most commonly vesicoureteral reflux, in a child with a single UTI is at least 30% and as high as 50% in children less than 3 years old.[20,106] Table 3 identifies the incidence of reflux from various studies evaluating children with their first UTI. Bourchier et al detected radiographic abnormalities in 47% of 100 infants with culture proven UTIs, 40% of boys and 63% of girls.[107] Vesicoureteral reflux or reflux neuropathy accounted for 77% of abnormalities and obstructive lesions 15% (Fig 9). Six of 10 preterm infants had positive radiographic findings, 5 of 6 were refluxers. Finally, in children where the incidence of undiagnosed febrile illnesses is so common, the chance of previously undocumented UTIs often makes one suspicious of the label "first infection." Winberg et al reported that 4.5% of girls presenting with their "first" UTI already had renal scarring as

**TABLE 3. First UTI and the Frequency of Reflux**

| Study (Reference) | Age Group | % with Reflux |
|---|---|---|
| Winberg (*) | Neonates | 100 |
| | <12 mo | |
| | Males | 30 |
| | Females | 57 |
| | 2–16 Y | |
| | Males | 18 |
| | Females | 32 |
| Maherzi (†) | Neonates | 35 |
| Ginsberg (‡) | <8 months | 21 |
| Rolleston (§) | <12 months | 42 |
| Kunin (‖) | School girls | 19 |
| Oxford-Cardiff (¶) | School girls | 34 |

From Hymes LC, Woodward JR, Urinary tract infection, in Libertino AB, et al (eds), *International Perspectives in Urology: Pediatric Urology* (Baltimore, Md: Williams & Wilkins; 1987:1–11).

* Winberg et al, Epidemiology of symptomatic urinary tract infection in children, *Acta Pediatr Scand* (1974; 252 (suppl):1).

† Maherzi M et al, Urinary tract infection in high-risk infants, *Pediatrics* (1978; 62:521).

‡ Ginsberg CM, McCracken GH, Urinary tract infections in young infants, *Pediatrics* (1982; 69:409).

§ Rolleston GL et al, Relationship of infantile vesicoureteral reflux to kidney damage, *Br Med J* (1970; 1:460).

‖ Kunin CM, The natural history of recurrent bacteriuria in school girls, *N Engl J Med* (1970; 282:1143).

¶ Oxford-Cardiff Bacteriuria Study Group, Sequelae of covert bacteriuria in school girls: a four year follow-up study, *Lancet* (1978; 1:889).

did 17% of those evaluated after a second UTI.[108] This supports the contention that in the majority of children with their first UTI, radiographic imaging is required. In addition, waiting for recurrence only increases the risk of upper tract damage.

One exception to this dictum may be the black female with an afebrile UTI. Kunin has noted that the prevalence and recurrence rate of UTI in black girls is significantly reduced compared to their counterparts.[109] Additionally, Askari and Belman reported that the incidence of vesicoureteral reflux in this group is significantly lower.[51] Consequently, it is reasonable to recommend ultrasound imaging alone for black girls with a clinically lower tract UTI, reserving voiding cystourethrogram for infants and those with a febrile UTI or recurrences.

The mechanics of the evaluation have undergone significant changes over recent years.[110] It is clear, however, that both upper and lower tract screening is required. Traditionally, this included voiding cystourethrogram and excretory urogram. In most centers, however, ultrasonography has replaced excretory urography for screening of the upper tracts. Additionally, one has the option of renal isotope scanning to image the renal parenchyma. Lower tract imaging can be accomplished by conventional contrast voiding cystourethrogram or by nuclear cystogram. Each of these options has features applicable to certain clinical settings.

## Lower Urinary Tract Evaluation

The purpose of lower tract evaluation is to gain information regarding bladder size, contour, wall thickness, presence of vesicoureteral reflux, and patency of the urethra (in males). A preliminary plain abdominal and pelvic view is helpful to examine the integrity of the spine and the amount of stool in the colon. A dynamic voiding study is mandatory, as vesicoureteral reflux may be only present on voiding and therefore missed on a static cystogram in approximately 20% of children. An expression cystogram under anesthesia can produce both false-positive and false-negative results in addition to adding needless risk. The advantages of radiographic contrast voiding cystourethrogram (VCUG) are a clear anatomic delineation of the bladder and urethra and the ability to grade the degree of vesicoureteral reflux by a standardized grading system (Fig 10), which provides the best single datum regarding spontaneous resolution rate.[111] The disadvantage in comparison to nuclear cystography is an up-to-50-times-increased radiation exposure.

The nuclear voiding cystogram is more sensitive in detecting vesicoureteral reflux in that it continuously monitors the upper tract, and requires a smaller radiation dosage.[65,112] Quantitation of the volume of reflux, bladder volume, volume at which reflux occurs, and bladder capacity is possible with nuclear cystography. Nasrallah

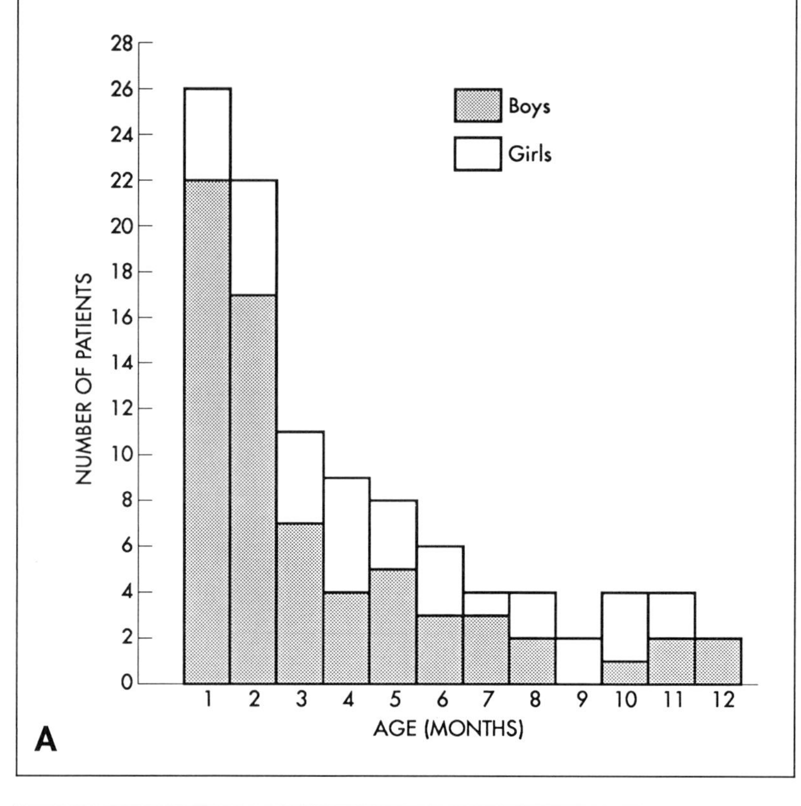


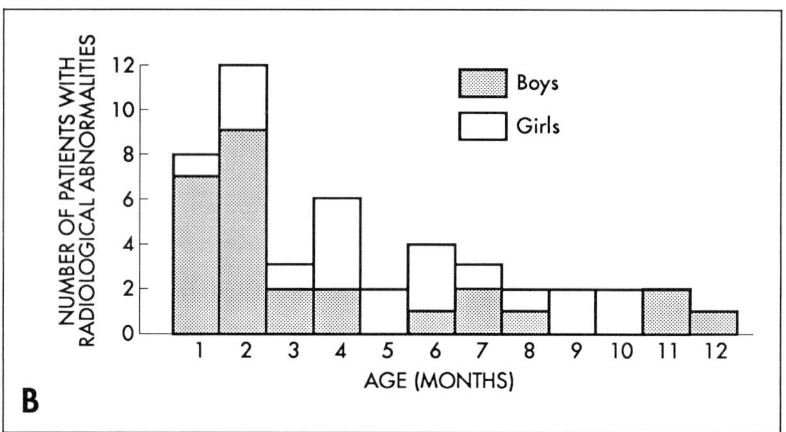


**Fig 9. A:** Age and sex distribution in 100 infants with urinary tract infections. **B:** Radiological abnormalities in 100 infants with urinary tract infections. [Reprinted with permission from Bouchier D, et al, Radiological abnormalities in infants with urinary tract infections, *Arch Dis Child* (1984; 59:620).]

et al have demonstrated a correlation between the bladder volume at which reflux occurs and the spontaneous resolution rate.[112] Its disadvantages are poor anatomic detail and an absence of urethral visualization, which is a factor in boys (Fig 11). Another practical disadvantage of using the isotope cystogram as the initial lower tract

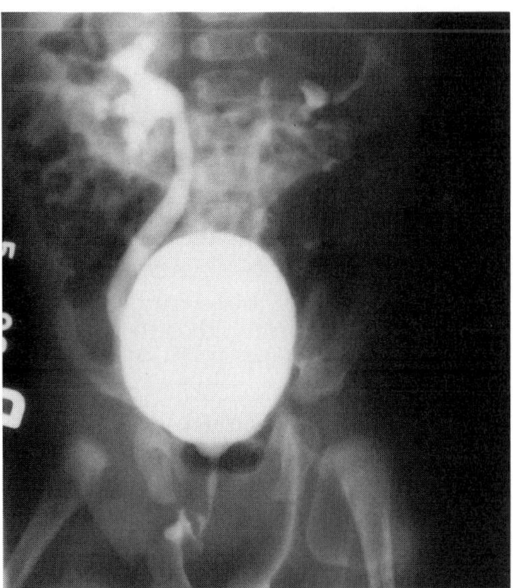

**Fig 10.** Voiding cystourethrogram in a 3-month-old female with bilateral reflux: grade 3 right and grade 2 left.

screening study is that it obviates a plain abdominal and pelvic film, thereby potentially causing clinically unsuspected spinal anomalies or constipation to be overlooked.

**Fig 11.** Nuclear voiding cystogram demonstrating bilateral reflux.

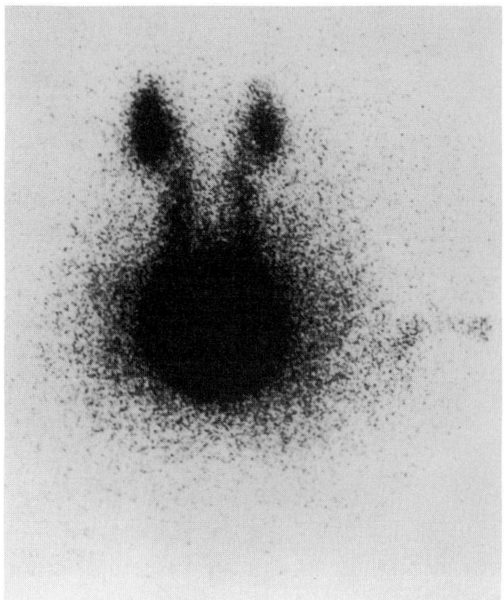

As urethral abnormalities in girls are very uncommon, this latter limitation is of little consequence in the female. The only anatomic abnormality that is potentially overlooked in not visualizing the female urethra is a refluxing ectopic ureter. In boys, however, urethral visualization is mandatory on the initial lower tract study. Therefore, it is reasonable to recommend a standard contrast VCUG as the initial lower tract study in boys and the isotope cystogram as the screening study in girls. Follow-up studies to monitor vesicoureteral reflux is best accomplished by isotope cystography in both sexes.

The routine use of cystoscopy in evaluating the pediatric UTI should be avoided. It provides little information to the workup of the child with a normal VCUG, as the chance of detecting an otherwise unsuspected abnormality is minimal.[113]

## Upper Urinary Tract Evaluation

Excretory urography has been the traditional study used for upper tract imaging in children with UTIs. It provides information regarding function, configuration, and renal scarring with reasonable anatomic detail in most children. In most centers, however, renal ultrasound has replaced the excretory urogram as the initial upper tract screening modality as it is ideally suited to the pediatric patient. Kangarloo et al have shown that ultrasound is as sensitive as the excretory urogram in detecting most renal abnormalities with the exception of the nondilated duplicated system or focal renal scarring.[114] Other reports have corroborated their findings.[48,115] Johnson et al found a 30% or greater increase in renal volume in 15 of 18 children with pyelonephritis.[115] Ultrasonography has a particular advantage in the young infant when compared to excretory urography, as poor renal concentrating ability and excessive bowel gas can often result in limited delineation of the kidneys with the latter study. Ultrasound is more useful in defining the anatomy of a nonfunctioning kidney as well. The major disadvantage of ultrasound is that it provides no measure of function.

Radioisotope renography is an additional means of visualizing the upper tracts. With newer computerized techniques, images can be produced that are capable of providing information about individual renal function, hydronephrosis, subtle degrees of renal scarring, and, with the aid of diuretics, the presence or absence of obstruction.[65]

## Tailoring the Radiographic Evaluation

To a certain degree, the protocol one chooses to electively evaluate the children with a UTI depends on the child's age, sex, and clinical presentation. Many reports in the literature condemn routine upper and lower tract imaging in all children with UTIs. Some authors advocate excretory urography only, avoiding the VCUG if the upper tracts are normal.[12,116] The rationale for this approach is that a normal urogram is unlikely to be associated with significant vesicoureteral reflux, and low grades of reflux are unlikely to produce renal damage. This approach, however, does not take into account that radiographically evident renal scarring may be delayed for 6 months to 2 years following an episode of pyelonephritis.[77] Furthermore, with significant vesicoureteral reflux, renal function based on an excretory urogram without a catheter in the bladder may be overestimated or underestimated (Fig 12). It is probably safe to take the opposite tack, however (that is, if the VCUG is normal, then the excretory urogram can be omitted).[117]

All children with a febrile UTI, and all infants, require both upper and lower imaging. This is best accomplished with an initial VCUG. If the VCUG is normal, then ultrasound should be used to screen the upper tracts for hydronephrosis. If reflux is present then a more functional image is required, leading one to use excretory urography or radioisotope renography—the latter being more sensitive in delineating renal scarring. If moderate to severe degrees of reflux are present, the excretory urogram should be performed with a catheter in the bladder for reasons mentioned. In the older

**Fig 12.** An excretory urogram in a 6-year-old boy with reflux, with (**A**) and without (**B**) a catheter draining the bladder.

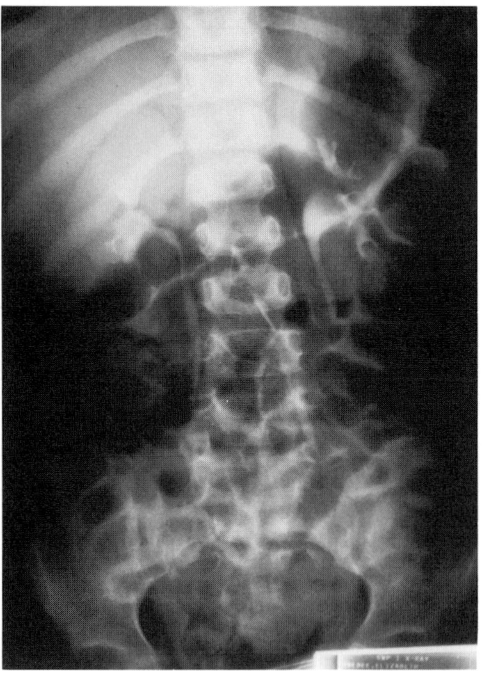

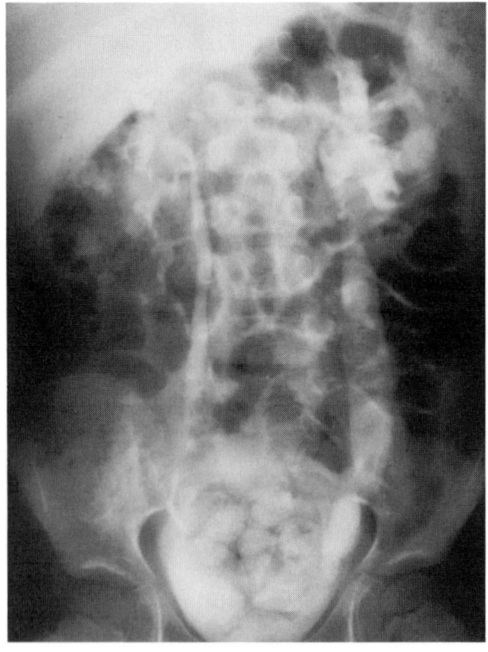

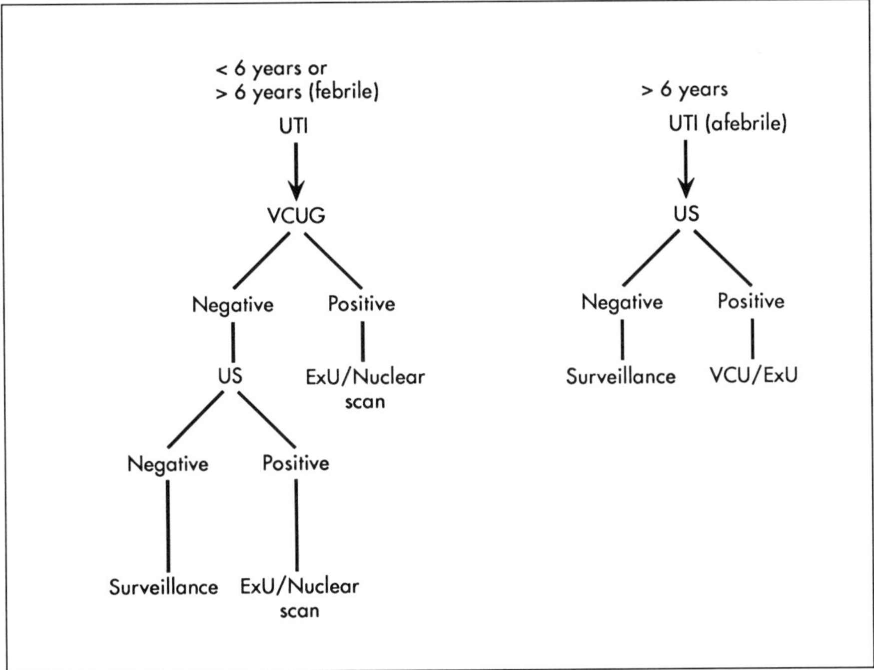


**Fig 13.** Algorithms for UTI evaluation.

girl (> 6 years) with an afebrile UTI screening with ultrasound alone probably suffices, avoiding the VCUG if the ultrasound is normal (Fig 13).

### Timing of Radiographic Evaluation

The timing of the radiographic imaging in relation to the UTI bears some consideration. Upper tract imaging can be done at any time, and is advisable that it be performed as soon as possible after treatment is instituted in the very ill child, looking for obstruction as the etiology. It had been advised that the VCUG be delayed 4 to 6 weeks following the acute episode to avoid discovering low grades of transient reflux resulting from edema of the bladder mucosa. While it is true that this type of reflux may not have the same risk of upper tract damage as reflux that occurs without bladder inflammation, it is desirable to identify this situation, as present recommendations are for prophylactic antibiotics as well. This transient, or occult, type of reflux may also explain the clinical situation of the child who presents with repeated febrile infections and no demonstrable reflux on VCUG. Consequently, the VCUG can be performed at any time after a negative urine culture is obtained. It is advisable to maintain the child on prophylactic antibiotic therapy following a febrile UTI until radiographic screening is completed.

## PRINCIPLES OF TREATMENT

The management of a child with a suspected UTI begins with obtaining a properly collected urine specimen as previously emphasized. Following this, antibiotic therapy is dictated on the clinical situation and degree of illness. Children who present with a febrile infection, and who are ill enough to require hospitalization, or those presenting with infection and an abdominal mass, should have obstruction screened for early in the therapeutic course. Ultrasound is best suited to this task in children, followed by functional evaluation with excretory urography or nuclear renography, should obstruction be suspected. A voiding cystourethrogram should be performed anytime after a negative culture is obtained.

Delay in the initiation of therapy in pyelonephritis has been shown experimentally by Miller and Philips to result in progressively more severe renal scarring.[67] Clinically Winberg et al demonstrated a four-times-higher incidence of renal scarring in girls in whom the first UTI was inadequately treated.[76] Unfortunately, due to the nonspecificity of symptoms in the infant age group, it is not uncommon for treatment to be delayed.

## Afebrile UTI

The child with a lower tract infection and normal radiographic studies is treated more or less based on symptomatology. (That is an exaggeration; albeit, the chances of renal damage in such a setting are minimal.) Follow-up cultures should be obtained 1 to 2 weeks following treatment and again 1 to 2 months later. In the younger child (< 5 years of age), it is best to obtain routine cultures every 3 months for 1 year as surveillance. In the older child, however, cultures need be done only when symptoms recur, as the risk of renal scarring is minimal. Available evidence indicates that not only is asymptomatic bacteriuria harmless in the older child, but that treatment of this group tends to select out more resistant and virulent organisms.[52,118]

Short-course therapy has gained popularity in adults and has some applicability in the pediatric group as well, with certain restrictions. The reports of short-course therapy in the pediatric population have been somewhat mixed.[119–121] Overall, short-course therapy, with a single dose or a 3-day course of antibiotics, has been shown to be as effective in eradication of bacteria as the traditional 7- to 10-day course; however, recurrence tends to occur more rapidly. It is appropriate, therefore, to consider short-course therapy in females older than 6 years with lower tract infections and previously documented normal urinary tract anatomy.

The choice of antibiotic therapy for the lower tract infection is based largely on user preference (Table 4). The traditional urinary antiseptics—such as nitrofurantoin, sulfanomides, and naladixic acid—should be emphasized as these tend to affect gastrointestinal flora to a minimal degree and, therefore, are less likely to encourage the proliferation of more resistant organisms. This latter scenario is seen commonly with synthetic penicillins, such as ampicillin and amoxicillin.

## Acute Febrile UTI

The child with a febrile UTI should be suspected of having pyelonephritis, and, therefore, receive prompt treatment with either oral or parenteral antibiotics—depending on the age of the child and associated symptoms such as nausea, vomiting, and dehydration—immediately after appropriate cultures have been obtained. It is in this setting that renal scarring is likely and, therefore, prompt treatment is necessary. As mentioned previously, once antibiotic therapy is started, an ultrasound should be obtained to rule out obstruction as an etiology. Once effective treatment is assured and antibiotic therapy is tailored based on sensitivities, it is prudent to maintain low-dose prophylaxis pending the voiding cystourethrogram.

## Prophylaxis

Low-dose prophylactic antibiotics are indicated in children with low to moderate grades of vesicoureteral reflux and those with normal anatomy and more than 4 to 5 recurrent UTIs per year. Whether the greater-than-6-years-old child with vesicoureteral reflux should be maintained on prophylaxis is controversial. It has been argued that since the risk of renal scarring from pyelonephritis is minimal beyond that age, prophylaxis is unwarranted. It may be appropriate to discontinue prophylaxis beyond age 6 in those children who have not previously demonstrated a tendency toward breakthrough infections.

Trimethoprim-sulfmethoxazole and nitrofurantoin have been shown to be effective and safe when used as continuous long-term prophylaxis.[122] Sulfamethoxazole alone is as safe but less effective, and synthetic penicillin (ampicillin and amoxicillin) are not effective as they tend to promote

**TABLE 4. Antibiotics Used for Pediatric Urinary Tract Infections**

| Agent | Therapeutic Dose | Suppressive Dose | Advantages | Disadvantages |
|---|---|---|---|---|
| Trimethoprim; Sulfa | 4 mg/kg Trimethoprim 20 mg/kg Sulfa po BID (suspension has 8 mg Trimethoprim + 40 mg Sulfa per cm³) | 2 mg/kg Trimethoprim + 10 mg/kg Sulfa po once daily | Effective against *E coli;* often effective against enterococci, *Proteus, Klelbsiella;* occasionally effective against *Pseudomonas* | Kernictreis in newborns with elevated bilirubin; contraindicated 2 mo; dose adjustments if creatinine clearance 30 mL/kg |
| Nitrofurantoin | 1–2 mg/kg po QID (suspension has 3 mg per cm³) | 1 mg/kg po once daily | Resistant strains rare; good for suppressive therapy | Not effective against Pseudo; nausea and unpleasant taste; not effective if creatinine clearance 40 cm³/min Contraindicated 1 mo |
| Ampicillin | 25 mg/kg po QID (suspension has 25 & 50 mg per cm³) | Not recommended 25 mg/kg po once daily is used | Good urinary levels; useful in renal failure; minimal toxicity | Many resistant strains—*Klebsiella, Pseudomonas* and *Enterobacter* usually resistant; hypersensitivity and diarrhea; suspension needs to be reconstituted every 14 days |
| Amoxicillin | 12 mg/kg po TID (suspension has 25 & 50 mg per cm³) | Not recommended 12 mg/kg po once daily is used | Same as Ampicillin; less diarrhea than Ampicillin | Same as Ampicillin |
| Penicillin G | 125–500 mg po QID (suspension has 25–50 mg per cm³) | 250 mg po BID | Good urine levels; effective against *E coli, Proteus* and some *Klebsiella;* minimal toxicity | Hypersensitivity; suspension needs to be reconstituted every 14 days |
| Gentamycin & Tobramycin | 1–2/kg q8 hr IM or IV | Not recommended | Effective against most *Proteus, E coli, Klebsiella* | Renal and eight nerve toxicity |

Modified from Bickerton MW, Duckett JW Jr, Urinary tract infections in pediatric patients, *AUA Update Series* (1985; 4:4).

the emergence of resistant bowel flora.[13] Generally one third to one quarter of the normal therapeutic dose given once daily is used for prophylaxis. Prophylaxis in the neonate and young infant requires special attention, as nitrofurantoin and sulfa antibiotics should be avoided, especially in those with immature liver function. Penicillin G or a synthetic penicillin is an excellent choice in this group as it has minimal toxicity and achieves good urinary levels.

In children with normal voiding dynamics without vesicoureteral reflux, breakthrough infections are uncommon.[123] Prophylaxis is effective in limiting recurrence rates. The duration of prophylaxis in the child without reflux, however, is empiric. Most choose 3 to 6 months without breakthrough infections as the period of prophylaxis. If recurrence develops after prophylaxis is discontinued, a therapeutic treatment course of 3 to 7 days is used followed by reinstitution of prophylaxis for 6 to 12 months. Approximately one third to one half of patients can be expected to recur after prophylaxis is discontinued.[45] Recurrence rates tend to decrease with increasing age.

## REFERENCES


1. Lindblad BS, Ekengrenk K. The long-term prognosis of nonobstructive urinary infection in infancy and childhood, after the advent of sulfonamides. *Acta Pediatr Scand* 1969; 58:25.
2. Smellie JM, Edwards D, Hunter N, et al. I.C.S.: Vesicoureteral reflux and renal scarring. *Kidney Int (suppl)* 1975; 8:65.
3. Heale WF, Weldon AP, Hewstone AS. Reflux nephropathy presentation or urinary infection in children. *Med J Aust* 1973; 1:1138.
4. Drew JH, Acton CM. Radiological findings in newborn infants with urinary infection. *Arch Dis Child.* 1976; 51:628.
5. Roberts KB, Charney E, Sweren RJ, et al. Urinary tract infections in infants with unexplained fever: a collaborative study. *J Pediatr.* 1983; 103:864–867.
6. Siegel SR, Sokoloff B, Siegel B. Asymptomatic and symptomatic urinary tract infection in infancy. *AJDC.* 1973; 125:45–47.
7. Bergstrom T, Larson H, Lincoln K, and Winberg J. Studies of urinary tract infections in infancy and childhood: XII. Eighty consecutive patients with neonatal infections. *Fetal Neonatal Med.* 1972; 80:858.
8. Edelmann CM Jr, Ogwo JE, Fine BP, et al. The prevalence of bacteriuria in full-term and preterm newborn infants. *J Pediatr.* 1973; 82:125.
9. Thrupp LD, Hodgman JE, Karelitz M, et al. Transurethral reflux during cleansing procedure for clean-voided urine specimen in low birth weight infants. *J Pediatr.* 1973; 82:1057.
10. Buetow KC, Klein SW, Lane RB. Septicemia in premature infants. *AJDC.* 1965; 110:29.
11. Ginsburg CM, McCracken GH. Urinary tract infections in young infants. *Pediatrics.* 1982; 69:409.
12. Stamey TA. Urinary tract infection in infancy and childhood. In: Stamey TA, ed. *Pathogenesis and Treatment of Urinary Tract Infections.* Baltimore, Md: Williams & Wilkins; 1980, 290.
13. Belman AB. Genitourinary infections: nonspecific infections. In: Kelalis PP, King LR, Belman AB, eds. *Clinical Pediatric Urology.* Philadelphia, Pa: W.B. Saunders Co; 1985; 1:235–255.
14. Abbot GD. Neonatal bacteriuria: a prospective study in 1,460 infants. *Br Med J.* 1972; 1:267–269.
15. Newcastle Asymptomatic Bacteriuria Research Group. Asymptomatic bacteriuria in school children in Newcastle-upon-Tyne. *Arch Dis Child.* 1975; 50:90.
16. Kunin CM, Deutscher R, Paquin A Jr. Urinary tract infection in school children: an epidemiologic, clinical and laboratory study. *Medicine.* 1964; 43:91.
17. Winberg J, Anderson JJ, Bergstrom T, et al. Epidemiology of symptomatic urinary tract infection in children. *Acta Pediatr Scand.* 1974; (suppl), 252:1.
18. Deluca FG, Fisher JH, Swenson O. Review of current urinary tract infections in infancy and early childhood. *N Engl J Med.* 1963; 268:75.
19. Meadow SR, White RHR, Johnston NM. Prevalence of symptomless urinary tract disease in Birmingham school children: I. Pyuria and bacteriuria. *Br Med J.* 1969; 3:81.
20. Smellie JM, Hodson CJ, Edwards D, et al. Clinical and radiological features of urinary tract infection in children. *Br Med J.* 1964; 2:1222.
21. Littlewood JM. 66 infants with urinary tract infection in the first month of life. *Arch Dis Child.* 1972; 47:218.
22. Neumann CG, Pryles CV. Pyelonephritis in infants and children: autopsy experience of the Boston City Hospital, 1933–1960. AJDC. 1962; 104:215–229.
23. Randolph MF, Morris KE, Gould EB. The first urinary tract infection in the female infant: prevelance, recurrence, and prognosis. A 10-year study in private practice. *J Pediatr.* 1975; 86:342–348.
24. Bollgren I, Winberg J. The periurethral aerobic flora in girls highly suceptible to urinary infections. *Acta Pediatr J Scand.* 1976; 65:74.
25. Tuttle JB Jr, Sarvas H, Koistinen J. The role of vaginal immunoglobulin A in girls with recurrent urinary tract infections. *J Urol.* 1978; 120:742.
26. Bollgren I, Winberg J. The periurethral aerobic bacterial flora in healthy boys and girls. *Acta Pediatr. Scand.* 1976; 65:74.
27. Craig WS. Urinary disorders occurring in the neonatal period. *Arch Dis Child.* 1935; 10:337.
28. Porter KA, Giles H. A pathologic study of five

cases of pyelonephritis in the newborn. *Arch Dis Child.* 1956; 31:303.

29. Lincoln K, Winberg J. Studies of urinary tract infections in infancy and childhood: II. Quantitative examination of bacteriuria in unselected neonates with special reference to the occurrence of asymptomatic infections. *Acta Pediatr Scand.* 1964; 53:307–316.
30. Patrick MJ. Influence of maternal renal infection on the fetus and infant. *Arch Dis Child.* 1967; 42:208.
31. Wiswell TE, Roscelli JD. Corroborative evidence for decreased incidence of urinary tract infections in circumcised male infants. *Pediatrics.* 1986; 78:96.
32. Wiswell TE, Smith FR, Bass JW. Decreased incidence of urinary tract infections in circumcised male infants. *Pediatrics.* 1985; 75:901.
33. Monahan M, Resnick JS. Urinary tract infections in girls: age of onset and urinary tract abnormalities. *Pediatrics.* 1978; 62:237.
34. Burbridge KA, Retik AB, Colodny AH, et al. Urinary tract infection in boys. *J Urol.* 1984; 132:641.
35. Ransley PG, Risdon RA. Reflux nephropathy: the effects of antibiotic treatment on the development of pyelonephritis scar. In: Losse H, Asscher AW, Lison AE, eds. *Urinary Tract Infection, IV, Pyelonephritis.* New York, NY: Thieme Stratton Inc; 1980, 32.
36. Immergut MA, Wahman GE The urethral caliber of female children with recurrent urinary tract infections. *J Urol.* 1968; 99:189.
37. Kaplan GW, Sammons TA, King LR. A blind comparison of dilatation, urethrotomy and medication alone in the treatment of urinary tract infection in girls. *J Urol.* 1973; 109:917–919.
38. Lapides J, Diokno AC. Persistence of the infant bladder as a cause for urinary infection in girls. *J Urol.* 1970; 103:243.
39. Allen TD. The non-neurogenic bladder. *J Urol.* 1977; 117:232.
40. Allen TD, Bright TC II. Urodynamic patterns in children with dysfunctional voiding problems. *J Urol* 1978; 119:247.
41. Hinman F. Urinary tract damage in children who wet. Pediatrics. 1974; 54:142.
42. Tanagho EA, Miller ER, Lyon RP, et al. Spastic striated external sphincter and urinary tract infection in girls. *Br J Urol.* 1971; 43:69.
43. VanGool J, Tanagho EA. External sphincter activity and recurrent urinary tract infections in girls. *Urology.* 1977; 10:348.
44. Koff SA, Murtagh DS. The uninhibited bladder in children: effect of treatment on recurrence of urinary infection and on vesicoureteral reflux resolution. *J Urol* 1983; 130:1138.
45. Spencer JR, Schaeffer AJ. Pediatric urinary tract infections. *Urol Clin North Am.* 1986; 13:661.
46. VanGool JD, Kuitjen RH, Donckerwolcke R, et al. Bladder sphincter dysfunction, urinary infection and vesicoureteral reflux with special reference to cognitive bladder training. *Contrib Nephrol.* 1984; 39:190.
47. O'Regan S, Yasbeck S, Schick E. Constipation, bladder instability, urinary tract infection syndrome. *Clin Nephrol.* 1985; 23:152.
48. Alon U, Pery M, Davidai G, et al. Ultrasonography in the radiological evaluation of children with urinary tract infection. *Pediatrics.* 1986; 78:58.
49. Fritz GK, Armbrust J. Enuresis and encopresis. *Psychiatr Clin North Am.* 1982; 5:283.
50. Neumann PZ, deDomenico IJ, Nogrady MD. Constipation and urinary tract infection. *Pediatrics.* 1973; 52:241.
51. Askari A, Belman AB. Vesicoureteral reflux in black girls. *J Urol.* 1982; 127:747.
52. Gillenwater JY, Harrison RB, Kunin CM. Natural history of bacteriuria in school girls. *N Engl J Med.* 1979; 301:396.
53. Jerkins GR, Noe HN. Familial vesicoureteral reflux: prospective study. *J Urol.* 1982; 128:774.
54. Van der Abbeale AD, Treves ST, Lebowitz RL, et al. Vesicoureteral reflux in asymptomatic siblings of patients with known reflux. Radionuclide cystography. *Pediatrics.* 1987; 79:147.
55. Fairly KF, Bond AG, Brown RB, et al. Single test to determine the site of infection of the urinary tract. *Lovett.* 1967; 2(1):427.
56. Hellerstein S, Duggan E, Welchert E, et al. Serum C-reactive protein and the site of urinary tract infection. *J Pediatr* 1982; 100:21.
57. Uehling DT. Effects of vesicoureteral reflux on concentrating ability. *J Urol.* 1971; 106:947.
58. Walker D, Richard G, Dobson D, et al. Maximum urine concentration. *Urology* 1973; 1:343.
59. Winberg J. Renal concentrating capacity during acute nonobstructive urinary tract infection in infancy and early childhood. *Acta Pediatr Scand.* 1958; 47:635.
60. Fasth A, Hanson LA, Jodal U, et al. Autoantibodies to Tamm-Horsfall protein associated with urinary tract infections in girls. *J Pediatr.* 1979; 95:54.
61. Hanson LA, Fasth A, Jodal U. Autoantibodies and Tamm-Horsfall protein, a tool for disguising level of urinary tract infection. *Lancet.* 1976; 1:226.
62. Hellerstein S, Kennedy E, Nussbaum L, et al. Localization of the site of urinary tract infections by means of antibody-coated bacteria in urinary sediment. *J Pediatr.* 1978; 92:188.
63. Pulkkanen J. Antibody-coated bacteria in the urine of infants and children with their first two urinary tract infections. *Acta Pediatr Scand.* 1978; 67:275.

64. Wientzen RL, McCracken GH, Petrucka ML, et al. Localization and therapy of urinary tract infections of childhood. *Pediatrics.* 1979; 63:467.
65. Majd M. Nuclear medicine. In Kelalis PP, Kings LR, Belman AB, eds. *Clinical Pediatric Urology.* Philadelphia, Pa: WB Saunders; 1985; 140–180.
66. Bailey RR. An overview of reflux nephropathy. In: Hodson J, Kincaid-Smith P, eds. *Reflux Nephropathy.* New York, NY: Masson Publishing USA; 1979;
67. Miller T, Philips S. Pyelonephritis: the relationship between infection, renal scarring and antimicrobial therapy. 1981; 19:654.
68. Cremin BJ. Observations on vesicoureteral reflux and intrarenal reflux: a review and survey of material. *Clin Radiol.* 1979; 30:607.
69. Shah KJ, Robins DG, White RHR. Renal scarring and vesicoureteral reflux. *Arch Dis Child.* 1978; 53:210.
70. Edwards DJ, Normand ICS, Prescod N, et al. Disappearance of vesicoureteral reflux during long-term prophylaxis of urinary tract infections in children. *Br Med J.* 1977; 1:285.
71. Lenaghan D, Whitaker JG, Jensen R, et al. The natural history of reflux and long-term effects of reflux on the kidney. *J Urol.* 1976; 115:729.
72. Rolleston GL, Shannon FT, Utley WLF. Relationship of infantile vesicoureteral reflux to kidney damage. *Br Med J.* 1970; 1:460.
73. Warshaw BL, Hymes LC, Woodard JR. Long-term outcome of patients with obstructive uropathy. *Pediatr Clin North Am.* 1982; 29:815.
74. Bourne H, Condon VR, Hoyt TS, et al. Intrarenal reflux and renal damage. *J Urol.* 1976; 115:304.
75. Winter AL, Hardy BE, Alton DJ, et al. Acquired renal scars in children. *J Urol.* 1983; 129:1190.
76. Winberg J, Bollgren I, Kallemius G, et al. Clinical pyelonephritis and focal renal scarring. *Ped Clin North Am.* 1982; 29:801.
77. Filly R, Friedland GW, Govan DE, et al. Development of progression of clubbing and scarring in children with recurrent urinary tract infections. *Radiology.* 1974; 113:145.
78. Siegel JJ, Glasier CM. Acute focal bacterial nephritis in children: significance of ureteral reflux. *AJR.* 1981; 137:257.
79. Bagley FH, Stewart AM, Jones PF. Diffuse xanthogranulomatous pyelonephritis in children: an unrecognized variant. *J Urol.* 1977; 118:434.
80. Yazaki T, Ishikawa S, Ogawa Y, et al. Xanthogrannulomatous pyelonephritis in childhood: Case report and review of English and Japanese literature. *J Urol.* 1982; 127:80.
81. Govan DE, Palmer JM. Urinary tract infection in children: the influence of successful antireflux operations in morbidity from infection. *Pediatrics.* 1969; 44:677.
82. Frensicci FJ. Eosinophilic cystitis: observations on etiology. *J Urol.* 1972; 107:595–596.
83. Middleton ALW. Eosinophilic cystitis in children: self-limited process. *J Urol.* 1984; 132:117–119.
84. Hellstrum HR. Eosinophilic cystitis—a study of 16 cases. *Am J Clin Pathol.* 1979; 72:777–784.
85. Brown E. Eosinophilic granuloma of the bladder. *J Urol.* 1980; 83:665–668.
86. Oxford-Cardiff Bacteriuria Study Group. Sequelae of covert bacteriuria in school girls: a four year follow-up study. *Lancet.* 1978; 1:889.
87. Lindberg U, Claessen I, Hanson L, et al. Asymptomatic bacteriuria in school girls. *J Pediatr.* 1978; 92:124.
88. Barber I, Raper FP. Torsion of the testis. *Br J Urol.* 36:35–41, 1964.
89. Caldamone AA, Valvo JR, Altebarmakian VK, Rabinowitz R. Acute scrotal swelling in children. *J Pediatr Surg.* 1984; 19:581–584.
90. Gislason T, Noronha RFX, Gregory JG. Acute epididymitis in boys: a 5-year retrospective study. *J Urol.* 1980; 124:533–534.
91. Likitnukul S, McCracken GH Jr, Nelson JD, Voheler TP. Epididymitis in children and adolescents. *AJDC.* 1987; 141:41–44.
92. Amar AD, Chabra K. Epididymitis in prepubertal boys. *JAMA.* 1969; 207:2397–2400.
93. Doolittle KH, Smith JP, Sylor ML. Epididymitis in the prepubertal boy. *J Urol.* 1966; 96:364–366.
94. Kaplan GW, King LR. Acute scrotal swelling in children. *J Urol.* 1970; 104:219–223.
95. Reisman DD. Epididymitis owing to ectopic ejaculatory duct: a case report. *J Urol.* 1977; 117:540–541.
96. Siegel A, Snyder H, Duckett JW. Epididymitis in infants and boys: underlying urogenital anomalies and efficacy of imaging modalities. *J Urol.* 1987; 138:1100–1103.
97. Jarvi K, Churchill BM, McLorie G. Diagnostic yield in childhood epididymitis. Presented at AUA, 83rd Annual Meeting; June 3–7, 1988; Boston, Mass. Abstract #3.
98. Jarvi K, Churchill BM, McLorie G, Alibadi H. Infantile epididymitis. Presented at AUA, 83rd Annual Meeting; June 3–7, 1988; Boston, Mass. Abstract #299.
99. Dickinson JA. Incidence and outcome of symptomatic urinary tract infection in children. *Br Med J.* 1979; 1:1330.
100. Randolph MF, Majors F. Office screening for bacteriuria in early infancy: collection of a suitable urine specimen. *J Pediatr.* 1970; 76:934.
101. Nelson JD, Peters PC. Suprapubic aspiration of urine in premature and term infants. *Pediatrics.* 1965; 36:132.

102. Saccharow L, Pryles CV. Further experience with the use of percutaneous aspiration of the urinary bladder: bacteriologic studies in 654 infants and children. *Pediatrics.* 1969; 43:1018.

103. Morrell RE, Duritz G, O'Horf C. Suprapubic aspiration associated with hematuria. *Pediatrics.* 1982; 69:455.

104. Polnay L, Fraser AM, Lewis JM. Complications of suprapubic bladder aspiration. *Arch Dis Child.* 1975; 50:80.

105. Aronson AS, Gustafson B, Svenningsen NW. Combined suprapubic aspiration and clean-voided urine examination in infants and children. *Acta Pediatr Scand.* 1973; 62:396–400.

106. Margileth AM, Pedriera FA, Hirschmann GH, et al. Urinary tract infections: office diagnosis and management. *Pediatr Clin North Am.* 1976; 23:721.

107. Bouchier D, Abbott GD, Maling TMJ. Radiological abnormalities in infants with urinary tract infections. *Arch Dis Child.* 1984; 59:620.

108. Winberg J, Bergstrom T, Jacobson B. Morbidity, age and sex distribution, recurrences and renal scarring in symptomatic urinary tract infection in childhood. *Kidney Int.* 1975; 8:S101.

109. Kunin CM. The natural history of recurrent bacteriuria in school girls. *N Engl J Med.* 1970; 282:1143.

110. Morrison SC, Caldamone AA. Imaging. In: Ashcraft KW, ed. *Pediatric Urology.* Philadelphia, Pa: WB Saunders Co; 1990; 1–34.

111. International Reflux Study Committee. Medical versus surgical treatment of primary vesicoureteral reflux. Prospective international study in children. *J Urol.* 1981; 125:277.

112. Nasrallah PF, Conway JJ, King LR, et al. Quantitative nuclear cystogram. Aid in determining spontaneous resolution of vesicoureteral reflux. *Urology.* 1978; 12:654.

113. Johnson DK, Kroovand RL, Perlmutter AD. The changing role of cystoscopy in the pediatric patient. *J Urol.* 1980; 123:232.

114. Kangarloo H, Gold RH, Fine RN, et al. Urinary tract infection in infants and children evaluated by ultrasound. *Radiology.* 1985; 154:367.

115. Johnson CE, DeBaz BP, Shurin PA, et al. Renal ultrasound evaluation of urinary tract infections in children. *Pediatrics.* 1986; 78:871.

116. Cavanagh PM, Sherwood T. Too many cystograms in the investigations of urinary tract infections in children? *Br J Urol.* 1983; 55:217.

117. Redman JF, Seibert JJ. The role of excretory urography in the evaluation of girls with urinary tract infection. *J Urol.* 1984; 132:953.

118. Cardiff-Oxford Bacteriuria Study Group. Long-term effects of bacteriuria on the urinary tract in school girls. *Radiology.* 1979; 132:343–350.

119. McCracken GH Jr, Ginsburg CM, Namasonthi V, et al. Evaluation of short term antibiotic therapy in children with uncomplicated urinary tract infections. *Pediatrics.* 1981; 67:796.

120. Pitt WR, Dyer SA, McNee JL. Single dose trimethoprim treatment of symptomatic urinary tract infections. *Arch Dis Child.* 1975; 50:80.

121. Shapiro ED, Wald EF. Single dose Amoxicillin treatment of urinary tract infection. *J Pediatr.* 1981; 99:989.

122. Smellie JM, Gruneberg RN. The treatment of childhood urinary tract infection with special reference to the use of trimethoprim and talampicillin for prophylaxis. In: Losse H, Asscher AW, Lison AE, eds. *Urinary Tract Infection, IV, Pyelonephritis.* New York, NY: Thieme Stratton Inc; 1980, 175.

123. Smellie JM, Katz G, Gruneberg RN. Controlled trial of prophylactic treatment in childhood urinary tract infections. *Lancet.* 1978; 2:175–178.

# 45

# Incontinence in Children

*Randy M. Rockney and Anthony A. Caldamone*

## INTRODUCTION

Incontinence problems are among the high-incidence, low-morbidity problems of children that are brought to the attention of physicians. Because incontinence involves excretory functions, it is often accompanied by a good deal of shame on the part of both parents and children. These problems are embarrassing and unpleasant for families to deal with. Symptomatic relief is very gratifying for child, family, and physician.

## URINARY INCONTINENCE

### The Development of Urinary Control

The achievement of urinary continence involves three factors that seem to occur sequentially: enlargement of bladder capacity, voluntary control of the periurethral striated muscle sphincter, and voluntary control of the spinal micturition reflex.[1]

In infancy, voiding occurs as a result of a spinal cord reflex arc, responding to bladder distension and resulting in detrusor contraction, coordinated with striated sphincter relaxation. Over the next 2 years, voiding continues in a reflex fashion, although not as frequently. This may represent some degree of early modulation of bladder contraction, but more likely it is due to an increase in bladder capacity relative to urine volume production.[2] Over the 2nd year of life some sensation of bladder fullness is thought to develop. Voluntary control of the striated muscle sphincter usually occurs by 3 years of age and allows one to initiate and terminate urination consciously. The ability to inhibit the spinal micturition reflex centrally is the final phase in the attainment of urinary continence. Children who are unable to inhibit a detrusor contraction when they are expected to be socially continent may elicit increased striated sphincter activity to prevent incontinence. Persistence of this pattern is thought to result in dysfunctional voiding or the Hinman-Allen syndrome.

The achievement of bowel and bladder control follows a reproducible sequence: nighttime bowel control, daytime bowel control, daytime urinary control, and nighttime urinary control.[3]

Most urinary incontinence that occurs in children can be defined as some form of enuresis. Anatomic or pathophysiologic etiologies for urinary incontinence are less common, and will be discussed after a discussion of enuresis.

### Enuresis

**Definitions and Epidemiology.** Enuresis is the involuntary voiding of urine beyond the age at which control of voiding is normally attained, usually expected by age 4 to 6 years or "school age." Primary enuresis is defined as wetting that occurs in children who never had control; whereas secondary enuresis is the situation in which the child had a consistent period of dryness (3 to 6 months) preceding the onset of the wetting, 20% to 25% of cases. Fifteen percent to 20% of enuretics have diurnal enuresis. Sixty percent of them stop wetting during the day before nighttime wetting stops.[4–6]

Enuresis occurs in 10% to 20% of 5 year olds with the prevalence in boys exceeding that in girls at all ages, in a ratio of about 3 to 2. Forsythe and Redmond's long-term follow-up of 1129 children with nocturnal enuresis not treated by the electric alarm showed that the annual spontaneous cure rate between 5 and 9 years was 14%, such that approximately 5% of 10 year olds wet the bed.[7] Between 10 and 19 years the annual spontaneous cure rate is 16%. Thirty-three patients (3%) still wet after 20 years in that series. Other series, including studies of military recruits, have shown that the prevalence of enuresis at ages 18 to 20 years is about 1%. The natural history of enuresis that persists into the adult years is unknown. It would be reasonable to postulate that the annual spontaneous resolution rate of 14% to 16% continues into adulthood because it is such a consistent rate at earlier ages. This question has not been studied systematically, however, and leaves unresolved the issue of whether there is something unique about adult enuretics. We are aware of anecdotal reports of adult enuretics including a 23-year-old woman who wet the bed at night until after she delivered her first baby; and two men in their 40s, uncles of a patient seen in our enuresis clinic, who were frequent wetters into their teen years and still wet on those nights after "they had been out drinking."

**Etiology.** Enuresis represents a symptom and not a specific disease entity. It follows, therefore, that there is no single explanation that fits all cases, and it is possible that more than one etiology may be operational in any individual case. Several theories have been proposed to explain enuresis: developmental delay, psychological factors/stress, genetic factors, sleep disorder, and structural and functional urinary tract abnormalities. While training and learning patterns are thought to play a major role in the achievement of daytime control, night control emerges more spontaneously, influenced only by negative factors.

**Urodynamic Findings.** The most consistent and reproducible finding in enuretic children who have been evaluated urodynamically is a reduction in functional bladder capacity.[8–10] Under anesthesia and with the use of intravenous anticholinergics, a normal bladder capacity is obtained in enuretics. Koff has demonstrated that the capacity of the bladder enlarges by about 1 ounce per year, and, therefore, an estimate of bladder capacity in ounces is the age of the child plus 2.[2]

Uninhibited bladder contractions, what might be thought of as an infantile voiding pattern, are found more commonly in enuretics as well.[11–13] Uninhibited contractions have also been documented during sleep urodynamics, usually occurring during lighter stages of sleep. They occur more frequently and are of greater amplitude in enuretic children.[14] The relationships between these contractions and wetting episodes is unclear, however.

It has been found by some investigators that adult enuretics have a higher percentage of abnormal urodynamic findings than that of the pediatric population.[15,16] As would be expected to follow, the incidence of daytime symptoms of frequency, urgency, and urgency incontinence appears to be higher as well.

### Etiologies of Enuresis

***Developmental Delay.*** The most commonly accepted theory of nocturnal enuresis is a developmental delay or maturational arrest in the attainment of central control of bladder function. Urodynamic findings of a reduced functional bladder capacity along with an increase in diurnal and nocturnal uninhibited bladder contractions tend to support this theory. These findings may reflect the persistence of an infantile bladder pattern and have been demonstrated in up to 85% of enuretics.[13] The observation that many enuretics also have significant daytime symptoms, which are seen more consistently in younger enuretics, also lends credence to this theory.[17] Similarly, the natural history of resolution of daytime symptoms followed by nighttime symptoms recapitulates the normal developmental process.

Nocturnal enuresis is often seen in association with other patterns of developmental delay such as delayed bowel sphincter control. There is a greater incidence of bedwetting in children who are also delayed in walking and talking.[18] These observations again support the theory that enuresis represents a maturational lag that may be seen in association with other developmental delay patterns.

***Psychological Factors/Stress.*** Generally, enuretics do not suffer from significant psychological disorders, although emotional disturbances have been found to be slightly higher in this population.[19] In many instances, cause and effect are not completely clear. The successful treatment of enuresis generally results in a positive psychologic effect, thereby dispelling the notion that enuresis represents a symptom of a psychologic disturbance.[20] Stress and/or anxiety at critical developmental periods may have an effect on the attainment of dryness, similar to their potential effects on other developmental milestones.[21]

That enuresis is more common in lower socioeconomic classes, stressful family circumstances such as broken homes, and following separation of child from mother all support the influence of negative reinforcement on the development of urinary control.[22–24] It is the contention of some that primary enuresis differs from secondary only in the timing of the stress, it often being more obvious in the latter.[25,26]

In the past, enuresis was often viewed as a symptom of underlying emotional stress. More recent studies, however, have indicated that enuretics are little different emotionally and behaviorally from nonenuretic children.[27] Nevertheless, children with enuresis may suffer from lowered self-esteem as a secondary effect of the chronic stress that derives from enuresis. It is likely that the effect of self-esteem becomes more pronounced the longer the symptom persists nd the more it frustrates the patient and his or her family. Moffatt et al studied 121 children aged 8 to 14 years who were randomly assigned to receive conditioning therapy or a 3-month waiting period for treatment of enuresis.[28] Those children in the treatment group showed significant improvements on the Piers-Harris Self-Concept scale when compared to controls. In addition, the changes were greatest for those who had the largest decreases in wetting frequency. Anyone who has worked with enuretic children and teenagers can attest to the positive feelings of both the patient and the family when significant improvement has occurred. When a child or adolescent experiences such an improvement under our management, we emphasize the value of looking on the experience as a paradigm for overcoming other difficult and seemingly hopeless problems in later life.

***Genetic Factors.*** There are oftentimes other family members with enuresis. Bakwin demonstrated that, compared to a 15% incidence of enuresis in children from nonenuretic families, 44% and 77% of children were enuretic when one or both parents, respectively, were enuretic.[29,30] Conversely, approximately a third of fathers and a fifth of mothers of enuretic children were themselves enuretic as children. Apparently a positive family history does not influence the spontaneous resolution rate. The parental attitude, however, is often considerably less anxious in those cases in which other family members were also enuretic.

***Sleep Disorder.*** Parents will often describe their enuretic child as an extremely sound sleeper. This may be more apparent than real in that they are unlikely to attempt to awaken their nonenuretic siblings. Controlled sleep lab studies indicate, however, that enuretics do not spend more time in stage 4 non-REM (deep) sleep than controls and that certain enuretics wet during lighter stages of sleep or during transition periods between stages of sleep.[31,32] More recently, studies indicate a random pattern of wetting irrespective of the stage of sleep and wetting is more often a function of the time spent in each stage.[33,34] Presently, therefore, it is concluded that enuretics and nonenuretics do not differ appreciably in their sleep pattern.

### *Anatomic and Pathophysiologic Etiologies of Urinary Incontinence*

ANATOMIC URINARY TRACT DISEASE. It is not unusual for a parent of an enuretic child to indicate that they are in your office "just to make sure everything is okay." It is important to them that an underlying anatomical abnormality is not overlooked. It was not many years ago that an extensive radiographic and cystoscopic evaluation of enuretics was undertaken for just that purpose. Well-documented studies indicate, however, that the incidence of underlying anatomical pathology does not warrant radiographic nor cystoscopic evaluation in most instances.[35,36] In the absence of significant daytime symptoms, a history of urinary tract infections, an abnormal voiding pattern, or a family history of an anatomical problem that tends to be genetic, anatomical evaluation is probably not warranted.[37] Similarly, the incidence of underlying pathology in adolescent enuretics is very low.[38] Treatment of various minor "disorders" such as meatal stenosis has been ineffective in resolving enuresis.[39]

In viewing children with urinary incontinence, one must be cognizant of various underlying structural abnormalities that may result in this symptom. There are certain "red flags" in the history or physical examination that might indicate the need for a more extensive evaluation for the possibility of an anatomical abnormality (Tables 1 & 2).

Anatomical causes of urinary incontinence can be divided into three categories:

| TABLE 1. "Red Flags" in the Patient History |
|---|
| Past history of uropathology |
| Daytime incontinence—significant |
| Family history of uropathology |
| Dribbling |
| Continuous wetting |
| UTIs |

| TABLE 2. "Red Flags" in the Physical Examination/Urinalysis |
|---|
| Neurologic abnormality |
| Spinal anomaly (sacral dimple) |
| Palpable bladder post void |
| Decreased urinary concentrating ability |
| Proteinuria/hematuria/pyuria |

1. extravesical urinary drainage;
2. bladder dysfunction resulting from obstruction or neurologic impairment;
3. reduced sphincter tone, which may be neurologic or anatomic.

Extravesical urinary drainage occurs when one or both ureters are ectopic in relationship to the bladder. This anomaly presents more commonly in females than males due to the fact that the ectopic ureter is more likely to drain distal to the urinary sphincter system. The most common symptom, therefore, would be continuous urinary leakage in spite of a normal voiding pattern. This also may be observed by examining the perineum of a little girl and actually seeing a dimple with urinary drainage or continuous leakage from a site other than the urethral meatus (Fig 1). The embryologic basis for this is related to the site of the ureteral bud on the wolffian duct. If the ureteral bud originates from a site more proximal than is normal on the wolffian duct, a longer segment of common excretory duct would be created. This longer segment must be absorbed into the trigone and bladder neck, and, if it is abnormally long, cannot be completely absorbed, therefore, leaving the ureter outside the bladder in location.

Understanding this embryologic arrangement, therefore, one can envision the fact that systems in which there is a complete duplication have a higher incidence of ectopia. The ectopia more commonly involves the upper pole segment since that is the segment that is generally more proximal on the wolffian duct, that is, further away from the common urogenital sinus. Often the upper pole is either small or dysplastic and with very poor function, and, therefore, poorly visualized radiographically, or large and hydronephrotic, pre-

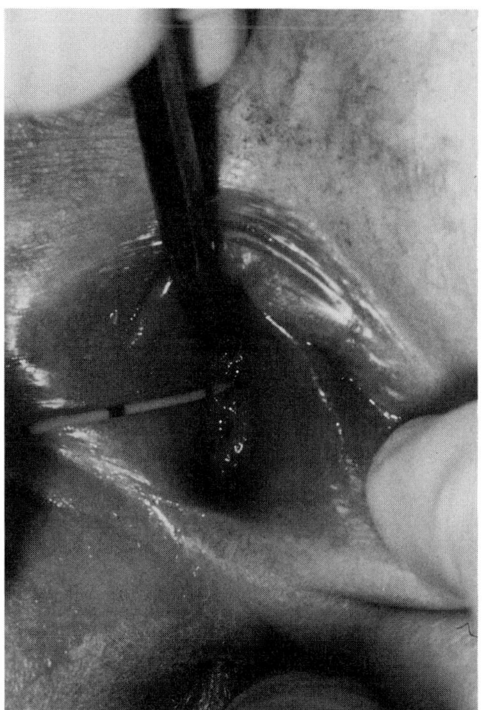

**Fig 1.** The perineum of a 4-year-old girl with continuous wetting. Upper sound is in urethral meatus. Gray catheter is in an ectopic ureteral orifice.

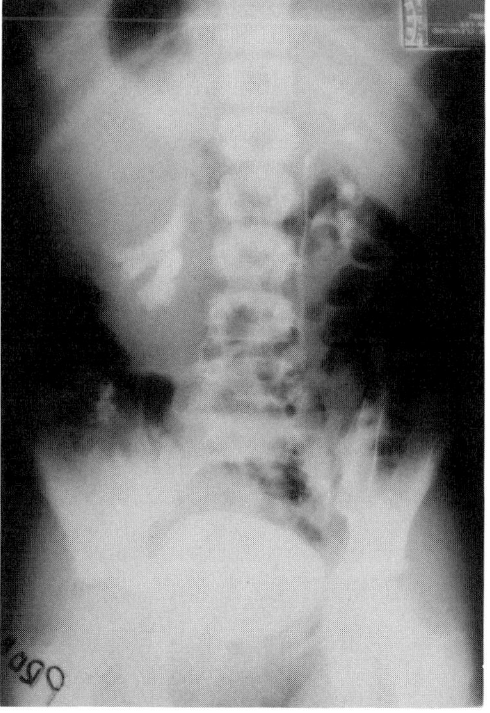

**Fig 2.** Intravenous pyelogram of a 6-year-old girl with continuous wetting and recurrent UTIs. Right system is duplicated with hydronephrotic upper pole; its ureter ended in the urethra.

senting as a mass effect in the upper pole region of the affected kidney (Fig 2). Under the circumstances of ureteral ectopia, the ureter with its affected upper pole segment is excised if it is demonstrated to have no function or be minimally functioning. If, on the other hand, there is a significant amount of function present, then the system can be preserved by either performing an ipsilateral ureteroureterostomy or a reimplantation of the affected ureter into the bladder.

Bladder dysfunction resulting from outlet obstruction or neurologic disease is generally in the form of hypertonicity. This is caused by trabeculation of the detrusor muscle, which leaves the bladder hyperactive. The opposite may occur, however, in that the outlet obstruction over longer periods of time may result in an atonic type of bladder that would empty quite poorly and result possibly in overflow incontinence. In children, however, the former situation (that of a hypertonic bladder) is more commonly seen. Examples of this situation include boys with posterior urethral valves, girls with outlet obstruction from a prolapsed ureterocele or a cecoureterocele, boys with an anterior urethral diverticulum, or, rarely, boys with obstruction from a large Cowper's duct cyst.

Neurologic impairment of the bladder and/or sphincter mechanism may also result in hypertonicity of the bladder and present with urinary incontinence. This is commonly seen in lower motor neuron types of lesions. In the pediatric population it is most commonly found in the myelomeningocele patient where a mixed pattern of hypertonicity and low urethral resistance is seen. A reduction in bladder capacity is also seen with certain anatomical conditions such as bilateral single ectopic ureters and in children who have exstrophy of the bladder that has been closed.

Reduced outlet resistance will also result

in incontinence that may be on an anatomical or structural or neurological basis. The structural causes for this again have a varied presentation including children with exstrophy and epispadias, and those children with poor formation of the trigone and bladder neck and sphincter mechanism on the basis of bilateral single ectopic ureters.

DYSFUNCTIONAL VOIDING. If one follows the previously described developmental sequence of the attainment of urinary incontinence to its extreme, then a dysfunctional pattern of voiding develops. This has been previously described by Hinman and Allen and often is referred to as the Hinman-Allen syndrome or nonneurogenic neurogenic bladder. This is a developmental abnormality in which a child attempts to be dry by tightening the external sphincter muscles instead of centrally inhibiting a detrusor contraction. This mechanism is used because they are unable to centrally inhibit a detrusor contraction on a maturational delay basis. In other words, a child feels that he or she should be dry but cannot prevent the detrusor from contracting and therefore tightens the external sphincter muscles in order to accomplish this. The result of this continence pattern, therefore, is a development of a functional outlet obstruction due to a spastic sphincter or a sphincter that is unable to relax when the detrusor does contract. The detrusor, therefore, must contract against a closed sphincter. That is the basis for the outlet obstruction. This outlet obstruction pattern, therefore, will mimic any type of anatomical outlet obstruction in its resulting effects on the bladder and potentially the upper tracts. The epitome of this situation, if you will, will result in hydronephrosis either on an obstructional basis or from vesicoureteral reflux (Fig 3).

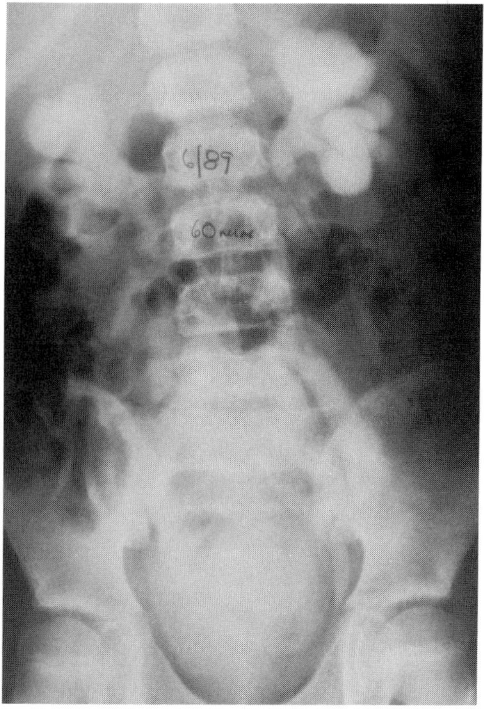


**Fig 3.** Intravenous pyelogram in a dysfunctional voider presenting at 11 years of age with day and night wetting and encopresis. This 60-minute film demonstrates bilateral hydroureteronephrosis with a thickened bladder.

The treatment of this developmental abnormality depends on the severity of the problem and the age at which it is diagnosed. The use of a timed voiding schedule along with anticholinergics is helpful. The next step would be reconditioning of the voiding pattern in a biofeedback type of mechanism. This does involve a very cooperative child and fairly long sessions of therapy. It has, however, proven successful. The next echelon of treatment would involve intermittent catheterization. This has a dual effect of affording complete bladder drainage at regular intervals along with teaching a child to relax his or her external sphincter, which is necessary for self-catheterization.[40] In years past, these children would be categorized as having idiopathic hydronephrosis and often went on to urinary tract diversion.

An additional facet of this syndrome is that of varying degrees of constipation and encopresis. This results from the same mechanism in terms of inability to relax the external sphincter with defecation, therefore resulting in fecal retention.

### Assessment

***Evaluation.*** As part of a large-population-based study involving parents of 1753 children aged 5 to 13 years, Foxman et al[41] found that only 38% of enuretics had seen a physician about their condition. This finding is troubling in that in more than half the cases the parents worried about the symptom and perceived that it distressed the child. It is our experience that the distress for the child or teenager and the parental anxiety increase with persistence of the symptom. Parents who worried more about their child's enuresis were more likely to seek medical care for the child.

Is medical evaluation and treatment of benefit to enuretics in view of the mostly self-limiting nature of enuresis and the annual spontaneous cure rate? Several studies indicated that there is strong evidence for the benefit of treatment with regard to both behavior and resolution of the symptom. Furthermore, studies have shown there is no risk of symptom substitution[42] after successful treatment and no risk of adverse effects of treatment for those who fail to respond.[43]

What is a reasonable approach to the assessment of urinary incontinence? The assessment of urinary incontinence begins with an extensive history, focusing on the symptom itself with particular attention to any red flags that might suggest the necessity of a more in-depth evaluation involving radiographic or urodynamic studies. It should be emphasized at the outset, however, that while many aspects of the past medical history are obtainable only from the parent of the patient, because of the symptom's sensitive nature the patient must be given the opportunity to discuss it alone with the physician.

We ask that a baseline (2-week) record of the wetting frequency be maintained prior to the first clinic visit for urinary incontinence. This alone, or the act of scheduling an appointment for an evaluation, has been curative in a number of patients, especially the older ones. We call this "the placebo effect." The baseline record helps us to assess any progress or improvement as the evaluation and treatment proceed.

***History.*** At the initial appointment everything relating to the symptom of urinary incontinence is discussed. Does the patient have primary or secondary incontinence? Does the wetting occur during the day, during the night, or anytime? What is the wetting frequency? Has the symptom improved over time or remained unchanged? Is there a history of a previous urinary tract infection or other symptoms like urinary hesitancy that are referable to the urinary tract? Does the child or teenager sleep in his own bed or have his own room? While not essential to diagnostic decisions, this question may be very important when therapeutic options are discussed. Does the child or teenager take responsibility for changing and washing the soiled bedclothes, or does the parent do it? These mundane functions may entail a significant amount of time, energy, and expense, especially for single-parent families with more than one enuretic.

A thorough past medical history and review of symptoms is essential as derangement of other organ systems may have some bearing on the symptom. Is there neurologic impairment? There is no patient more challenging than the incontinent child or teenager who demonstrates neurologic dysfunction on the basis of a past event and who also has a strong family history of enuresis. Such impairment should be obvious from the history and physical examination. In a study of enuretic adolescents Murphy et al demonstrated "there is no evidence for a subtle neurological factor in chronic enuresis."[44]

Incontinence, polyuria, and polydipsia should make one suspicious of diabetes mellitus or diabetes insipidus. It would be very unusual, however, for enuresis to be the only presenting symptom of either condition. What we have noticed is that known diabetics who are also enuretic experience an increased wetting frequency, as expected, when their diabetes is poorly controlled.

Upper airway obstruction, too, may be related to the symptom of enuresis. Weider and Hauri reviewed 35 children between the ages of 3½ and 11 years who had symptoms of upper airway obstruction and enuresis.[45] Surgical removal of the upper airway obstruction led to a significant decrease or complete cure of nocturnal enuresis in 26 patients. The beneficial response to surgery is attributed to altered sleep or arousal states.

It is crucial to inquire about the presence of constipation or encopresis. Of the first 125 patients presenting to our enuresis clinic, 18% were also encopretic. The dilated rectum with impacted feces can distort the posterior bladder wall, thus reducing functional bladder capacity. O'Regan et al have noted the association between bladder instability, recurrent urinary tract infections, vesicoureteral reflux, and constipation.[46] One must inquire about these symptoms referable to the gastrointestinal tract because neither the family nor the patient may mention them spontaneously. Aggressive management of the constipation or encopresis may cure the wetting problem and is essential in the management of those enuretics, mostly girls, who also have recurrent urinary tract infections with or without vesicoureteral reflux.

The physician must be alert to the possibility of any previous or ongoing inappropriate sexual contact. While certainly less important as an etiology than was once believed, the onset of enuresis or encopresis in a child should make the physician question the possibility of sexual abuse. In the adolescent or young adult attention to issues of sexuality is essential. We successfully managed a mentally retarded adolescent male who wet his bed while awake following masturbation.[47]

Discussion of the symptom with the patient and his or her family should also focus on the family history of enuresis. Our experience has shown that it is not unusual for the 17-year-old enuretic to learn for the first time that one of his parents was enuretic until a similar age when we discuss the family history of enuresis. A strong family history of the symptom can be reassuring to the parents and the patient as it helps them to understand the symptom and makes other etiologies for the enuresis less likely.

The parents' or caretakers' attitudes toward the symptom is also important. We routinely administer the Parents Statements on Enuresis Scale, a simple one page yes-no questionnaire, to both parents or caretakers as a means to assess their tolerance for the symptom of enuresis.[48] The authors who studied the value of this scale concluded: "The attitudinal variables measured were not found to be relevant to rate of therapeutic response, but intolerant mothers were more likely to withdraw their children prematurely from treatment." As many as 30% of patients entering treatment for enuresis may subsequently be withdrawn from treatment prematurely. Recognition of the problem may help to prevent this.

And finally, the patient and his or her family should be questioned about any previous evaluations and attempts at therapy. Almost all families have tried nighttime fluid restrictions and night lifting, usually without benefit. Many children may have been treated with conditioning therapies like the enuresis alarm at an earlier age. This is important information because the therapy may not have been directed by a physician or has been undertaken at a younger age when the child's motivation to eliminate the symptom was inadequate for the success of conditioning therapy. In like manner, previous attempts at pharmacotherapy may have involved doses that were too small or trials on medications that were too brief or not well monitored.

***Physical Examination.*** A thorough physical examination of the patient with urinary incontinence is essential to uncover findings that may have a bearing on diagnostic or therapeutic decision making. It can also be reassuring to the patient and the parents.

A mental status examination is important to determine the level of intellectual functioning and the motivation to work toward a cure, and to detect any evidence of psychopathology. It is important, too, to assess the patient's interactions with his or her parents or caretakers. The patient's psychosocial milieu is an important determinant of the likelihood of follow-through with diagnostic procedures and compliance with therapy.

Particular note of the quality of the voice, and other symptoms that might suggest the possibility of upper airway obstruction, is important. The abdomen should be examined for the presence of masses such as a distended bladder or, more often, a nontender sausage-shaped mass in the left lower quadrant that results from fecal impaction of the descending colon and rectum. An anal and rectal examination is necessary to assess perianal sensation, sphincter tone, and the degree of fecal impaction in the rectum. The genitalia should be examined to assess the size and position of the urethral meatus and to observe for any evidence of infection. An examination of the back might reveal the presence of a sacral dimple or another clue of the presence of a vertebral or spinal cord anomaly. A thorough neurologic examination helps to reassure everyone that there is no subtle neurologic dysfunction to account for the symptom.

Finally, voiding should be witnessed. In the adolescent or young adult this is understandably a sensitive procedure and should, if at all possible, be done by someone of the same sex as the patient. Observation should be made of the force and directionality of the urinary stream. In females, the seating position on the toilet should be noted as vaginal reflux with subsequent postvoid wetting may occur if the females sits too far forward on the toilet seat.

***Diagnostic Evaluations.*** Urinalysis should be performed on all patients. A urine specific gravity greater than 1.020 will rule out a concentrating defect and diabetes insipidus. The absence of glucosuria is helpful to rule out diabetes mellitus. Urine culture, too, should be performed. Bacteriuria is known to increase wetting frequency and is especially common in girls.

We screen all new patients with diurnal incontinence with uroflowmetry. This procedure is useful as a nonintrusive measurement of the hydrodynamic properties of the urinary stream. Normal parameters are available for boys between 2 and 12 years old and adults.[49] Any unusual patterns or peak flow rates that are more than two standard deviations from the mean prompt a repeat measurement at follow-up. A second abnormal study often indicates the need for a uroradiographic and urodynamic assessment.

There is controversy about the indications for uroradiographic evaluation of the enuretic patient. Redman and Seibert examined 138 enuretic children radiographically with an intravenous pyelogram (IVP) and voiding cystourethrogram (VCUG) to see if they met any of the following criteria: symptoms of hesitancy or straining to void, a diminished urinary stream size noted on multiple occasions, frequent dysuria, diurnal enuresis, reinitiation of wetting after a relatively long period of dryness (>6 months), infected urine on urine culture or a history of urinary tract infection, children ⩾ 6 years old who were deemed candidates for pharmacologic control, and all children ⩾ 8 years old presenting with enuresis "because of concern that the older child with enuresis was exceptional and would likely have a significant abnormality."[50] Of these patients, 21 were found to have a significant abnormality. The abnormalities were found in children with either a history of urinary tract infection, infected urine at the time of examination, or obstructive signs or symptoms.

Several authors have proposed other criteria for radiographic evaluation of the enuretic patient including failure to respond to an adequate therapeutic trial, diurnal enuresis, high anxiety level of the parents, and age greater than 12 years. The validity of these criteria is unproven.

No one would argue against the need for uroradiographic studies in the child with a history of a urinary tract infection or symptoms of abnormal or dysfunctional voiding. Of late, too, there has been a trend toward using ultrasonography and voiding cystourethrography as the initial radiographic assessments, reserving IVP for those patients who demonstrate an abnormality on either of the first two evaluations.[51] The noninvasive ultrasound study may be a reasonable first step for those enuretics with "soft" indications for uroradiographic assessment like failure to respond to an adequate therapeutic trial, high anxiety level of the parents, or age greater than 12 years. The yield for such indications is unknown.

We also find it useful to obtain a plain film of the abdomen in children who present with evidence of fecal retention or encopresis. This film can help to confirm the diagnosis of fecal retention and serves as a useful teaching tool for the patient and the family when planning therapy.

**Treatment.** The management of enuresis should be individualized based on the child's concerns, motivation, and intelligence. As there is no one theory to explain the etiology of enuresis, no one therapy is universally successful. Once the child and family circumstances are evaluated, one can propose an individualized treatment plan. Presently accepted treatment falls into two large categories: behavior modification and pharmacotherapy.

That is not to say that all enuretics require treatment. Many parents, once reassured that an underlying structural problem is very unlikely, do not request treatment or are not willing to accept either the risks or inconveniences associated with treatment. Hague et al reported that while parents expect their children to be dry at an earlier age than do physicians, parents are more likely to shun interventional therapy for bedwetting.[52]

The age at which enuresis is treated, again, should be individualized. Certainly if daytime symptoms are a significant component one may elect to treat at a relatively younger age. On the other hand, it is usually not necessary to consider treatment for the pure nighttime enuretic before 6 to 7 years of age. A reasonable guide is that treatment should be initiated when the child is significantly bothered by the symptom to become motivated enough to pursue a treatment plan. One should not be guided solely by the level of concern or motivation of the parents. As a rule, those families with a strong history of enuresis are likely to delay treatment as they are more comfortable with the spontaneous cure rate.

The efficiency of various treatment modalities is difficult to assess due to the spontaneous cure rate. Approximately 15% of enuretics per year resolve their symptoms spontaneously.[35] In addition, there is a significant placebo response that has been documented.[53]

Two measures that are often used by parents are waking a child during the night to void (night lifting) and decreasing fluid intake after supper. Whereas these measures may be effective in achieving a dry bed or decreasing the volume of voided urine, overall they have not been shown to have any therapeutic benefit in curing enuresis.[8]

One of the most important aspects of dealing with a bedwetter is that the child and parents be counseled on the etiology and natural history of enuresis. Enuretics must be reassured that they are not being lazy or misbehaving and that this symptom rarely indicates a serious disease. They should be informed of the "high incidence" of bedwetting in their age group and be reassured by knowledge of the spontaneous cure rate.

***Behavior Modification.*** Behavior modification has demonstrated some success in selected cases. It calls for significant cooperation and, therefore, motivation on the part of the patient. These techniques include timed voidings, positive reinforcement, bladder retention training, and conditioning therapy. Behavior modification techniques may be used alone or in combination with other therapy, most commonly pharmacotherapy.

MANAGEMENT OF DAYTIME ENURESIS. In the absence of an underlying anatomical abnormality, the majority of daytime incontinence occurs in children with uninhibited bladder contractions or children who have a reduced signal to bladder filling and may in addition have an inability to centrally suppress a detrusor reflex. Often these children will have no warning of a full bladder and will squat or use some other mechanism to tighten their perineal musculature to prevent wetting. Their ability to centrally inhibit bladder contraction—the normal mechanism by which we are continent—is somewhat delayed; therefore they use alternate means.

The situation can be managed by instituting a more frequent voiding schedule prior to wetting episodes caused by uninhibited contractions or due to a full bladder. A timed voiding schedule coupled with a motivational overplay is the most effective means. It is generally futile to have the parents constantly remind a child to go to the bathroom. This will often create a confrontational situation. If, on the other hand, the child is provided with a reminder, such as a wristwatch with an alarm, and some motivation to comply with it, such as a calendar chart with a predetermined reward, then the chances of success are increased significantly. This also takes the pressure off the parents to remind the child to void, and places complete responsibility with the child. If the child is not motivated enough to subscribe to this type of plan, then it is unlikely any other mechanism will help.

If, in spite of this schedule, the child still wets in between episodes of timed voiding, anticholinergic therapy may be indicated if the child is at an age where social continence is necessary.

Positive Reinforcement Therapy. Any reinforcement therapy requires a cooperative, motivated patient and a concerned physician who is able to develop a good rapport with the patient. Responsibility reinforcement allows the child to assume control of his or her program with positive reinforcement or response shaping based on behavior modification therapy. The child maintains a progress record (''star chart'') with a sequential reward system established for longer and longer dry intervals. In this way, the child assumes both the responsibility for wetting and the credit for dryness.The cure rate with motivational therapy is thought to be about 25% with an 80% improvement rate.[54] While improvement appears to be slower than with other treatment modalities, the relapse rate is lower than 5%.[55]

Bladder Retention Training. The finding of a reduced functional bladder capacity in many enuretics has prompted attempts to increase bladder capacity in treating enuretics. Various regimens have been proposed. Most of these involve forcing fluids (with or without diuretics), interrupting the urinary stream, lengthening the interval between daytime voidings, and recording the volumes of daytime voids.[56] With a goal of progressively larger voidings and progressively longer intervals between voids a positive reinforcement system is established. While the effectiveness of this approach has been reported as positive in terms of increasing voided volumes, it has not been met with success in curing nighttime enuresis. While it does follow that functional bladder capacity improves with the spontaneous cure of enuresis, therapies such as bladder conditioning or anticholinergic medications have not been successful in pure nocturnal enuresis.[57–59]

Conditioning Therapy. Success with the use of an alarm system triggered by wetting was first reported by Mowrer and Mowrer in 1938.[60] This system consists of a battery-operated alarm with either a pad or electrodes. When the pad or electrodes become wet, the alarm is triggered, which awakes the child and, in doing so, interrupts urination. The child is then instructed to arise and go to the bathroom to complete voiding. The theory underlying this technique is that the triggered alarm results in inhibition of micturition, which, when it happens repeatedly following the initiation of normal reflex voiding, results in inhibition of those factors responsible for triggering reflex voiding.[58]

The alarm system reportedly affords the best cure rates of bedwetters. Overall success rate approaches 70% with relapses expected in 30% of responders. A repeat course of treatment has been shown to be effective in many relapsers.

The most common causes of failure are noncompliance or lack of motivation and/or understanding by the patient or parents. It is not uncommon that the parents will report that the child sleeps through the alarm. If this occurs the parents should be instructed to awaken the child during the voiding episode. It is imperative that there be no delay between the alarm and arousing the child. It is helpful, therefore, to have a parent sleeping close by, at least during the induction phase of the treatment course. Suffice it to say, however, the patient and family must be well motivated and well selected before embarking on this treatment modality. This protocol requires close physician supervision and counseling for optimal results.

The length of treatment is rather long,

as a mean period of 16 to 17 weeks is required for a response.[61,62] The drop-out rate, therefore, is significant. Neither the age of the patient nor the amount or frequency of bedwetting appears to affect the success rate significantly.[58]

"Buzzer ulcers" have been reported in the past with the alarm and pad systems when body parts wet from urine come into prolonged contact with electrical current in the pad. With modern devices which are activated on smaller urine volumes, however, this complication is very unlikely. Most alarms in current usage utilize a single electrode clipped to the undergarment or a small pad that is sewn into the pajama bottoms. The proximity of the sensor to the urethral meatus appears to improve the success rate due to earlier triggering of the alarm. In the future, alarms which contain a tape cassette with a personalized message will be available.[63]

At present, the cost of most alarm systems averages $50 and may be beyond the means of many families. The cost of the alarm is rarely covered by third-party payors.

***Pharmacotherapy.*** Drug therapy for enuresis can be divided into agents that decrease urinary output, anticholinergics to increase bladder capacity or reduce uninhibited contractions, and tricyclic antidepressants.

AGENTS DECREASING URINARY OUTPUT. As previously mentioned, attempts at decreasing urinary output by limiting fluid intake or producing relative nocturnal dehydration by the use of daytime diuretics have not been met with success. It is likely that parental attempts at limiting fluid intake become a focus of contention with the child.

There is some evidence that the normal diurnal variation in antidiuretic hormone (ADH) levels may be altered in some enuretic patients.[64,65] Norgaard et al demonstrated absence of the normal nocturnal antidiuretic hormone level increase in enuretics studied.[65] This results in increased output at night that exceeds functional bladder capacity resulting in bedwetting. The authors suggest screening for diurnal diuresis in all enuretics to identify those with low nocturnal ADH levels.

Desmopressin acetate (DDAVP), a synthetic analog of the natural antidiuretic hormone, arginine vasopressin, was recently approved by the US Food and Drug Administration for treatment of primary nocturnal enuresis. DDAVP Nasal Spray, marketed by Rorer Pharmaceuticals, can be used for this indication. It is given intranasally at bedtime, plasma concentrations peak about 45 minutes after administration, and it has a duration of action of 8 to 10 hours, ranging from 6 to 24 hours.[66] Twelve placebo-controlled trials of Desmopressin in nocturnal enuresis, including three multicenter trials and involving a total of 516 patients, have been reported.[67] Improvement was measured in terms of percent fewer wet nights while taking Desmopressin. Improvement ranged from 10% to 65%. While not spectacular, these results must be viewed in light of the fact that most of the study participants had been tried unsuccessfully on numerous other forms of therapy for their enuresis. Success rates have been reported in up to 75% of patients in other studies.[68,69] In comparison to the alarm system, Wille found conditioning therapy to result in a higher long-term success rate whereas DDAVP had a more rapid response rate.[70] A double-blind trial in 28 children found that an alarm used in conjunction with DDAVP proved more effective than an alarm and placebo.[71] One study comparing DDAVP with imipramine showed similar efficacy of the two drugs.[72]

Adverse effects reported have included transient headache, epistaxis, nostril pain, conjunctivitis, nasal congestion, rhinitis, chills, dizziness, nausea, and abdominal pain.[66] Water intoxication, convulsion, and coma occurred in a 13-year-old enuretic child with cystic fibrosis after four doses of Desmopressin.[73] One 6 year old who took the drug for 8 days developed hyponatremia and had a grand mal seizure.[74] It has been our experience that the presence of nasal congestion makes it less likely for a child to have success with the use of Desmopressin. We have also noted anecdotally that older enuretics, specifically teenagers, have responded dramatically to DDAVP whereas younger children have not. It is possible that those with persistent primary enuresis may be the ones who have as an underlying reason for their enuresis the lack of the normal diurnal variation in the output of vasopressin.

The initial recommended dose of the nasal spray for children is 20 μg. at bedtime. Each nasal instillation delivers 10 μg. It is estimated that approximately 10% of the dose is absorbed from the nasal mucosa. After 3 days, if there is no response to 20 μg, the dose may be increased to 40 μg. It should be noted, however, that some patients may respond to as little as 10 μg daily, and there is one patient in our practice, a 19-year-old male, who insists that he requires 10 μg every other day—that any more is unnecessary and any less allows for breakthrough bedwetting. In 1990 the DDAVP Nasal Spray pump cost the pharmacist $88.60 for 50 doses of 10 μg. This means that, for the average patient, using DDAVP would cost approximately $100 to $200 per month, depending on the dose used.[66]

There is some indication that DDAVP is a useful pharmacotherapeutic adjunct in the treatment of nocturnal enuresis. It should be emphasized, however, that long-term experience with this medication is not yet available. The manufacturer recommends periodic serum electrolyte determinations.

ANTICHOLINERGIC AGENTS. Anticholinergic agents have not been successful in treating pure nocturnal enuresis, despite their ability to increase functional bladder capacity. They do have a role in patients with demonstrable uninhibited contractions or other urodynamic abnormalities. These patients may be suspected if there is a history of daytime incontinence, urgency, or frequency. Kass et al demonstrated a 90% response rate in those patients with documented uninhibited bladder contractions, compared to only 11% in those with normal cystometrograms.[37]

TRICYCLIC ANTIDEPRESSANTS. Imipramine (Tofranil) has been the most common frequently used medication for the treatment of nocturnal enuresis. It belongs to a class of tricyclic antidepressants that also includes desipramine (Pertofrance), amitriptyline (Elavil), and nortriptyline (Aventyl), all of which have some antienuretic effect. Imipramine was first reported to be successful in treating enuresis by MacLean in 1960.[75]

The overall success of imipramine varies from series to series depending on the age range of the patient population and patient compliance; however, a positive response can be expected in at least 50% of patients with a relapse rate of 60%.[39,76–78]

The effectiveness of imipramine does correlate with plasma levels.[76] The dosage range is 0.9 to 1.5 mg/kg/dose, which usually computes to 25 mg for children 5 to 8 years and 50 mg to 75 mg for older children. The achievement of therapeutic plasma levels at these dosages, however, is not optimal, which may explain the erratic response rate.[79]

The timing of administration is generally at bedtime, although some children who consistently wet shortly after bedtime may benefit from an earlier administration.[80] Once a response has been achieved, an arbitrary decision is made to discontinue treatment after a 3- to 6-month course. A tapering dosage schedule may reduce the relapse rate.[81]

The mechanism of action of imipramine on enuresis remains unclear. Imipramine has direct effects on the bladder, albeit a rather weak anticholinergic activity, along with an $\alpha$-adrenergic effect and a $\beta$-receptor enhancement. In addition, imipramine affects sleep patterns by decreasing REM sleep time. Which of these pharmacologic actions is responsible for its antienuretic effect, however, has not been determined.

***Hypnotherapy.*** Hypnosis and self-hypnosis has been reported to be successful in isolated series.[82,83] The data reported by Olness with self-hypnosis was quite remarkable with 31 of 40 cured and 6 improved. Of the 31 cures, 28 occurred within the first month of therapy. Lack of popularity of this modality, however, prevents more objective evaluation of these results.

*Diet.* Food allergies contributing to reduced bladder capacity and increased bladder instability have been reported to be an etiology of enuresis.[84,85] Attempts to correlate serum IgE levels with enuresis, however, have not been successful.[86,87] Serial elimination diets (dairy products, chocolate) may be attempted though success would be unusual. The elimination of caffeinated products, however, should be considered to avoid excessive urine output from the diuretic effect of caffeine.

## BOWEL INCONTINENCE

### The Development of Bowel Continence

A young infant has no difficulty passing stools, because she makes no attempt to exercise control over this function. By contrast, a 5-year-old child is able to perceive the urge to defecate, suppress the impulse to pass stool immediately, disengage from play, find a bathroom, ensure privacy, unfasten her clothes, climb upon the toilet, initiate the passage of stool, recognize when she is finished, dismount from the toilet, clean herself, refasten her clothes, unbolt the door, and emerge successfully to resume play. As can be appreciated, the successful completion of this complex series of events is the result of developmental skills that take years to master.[88]

The joy of changing a newborn's diaper when, if the child is breast-fed, the stools do not have an unpleasant odor, becomes a distasteful task for the parents of a 1 year old on solid foods.The child's sensitivity to the parents' facial expressions during the diaper change may actually contribute to the development of bowel continence. Later, the child's parents begin acquainting the child with the potty chair and suggest she pass her excreta into it. The child begins to be aware of the fecal urge, and connects it with the potty chair and the parents' request. Soon, she discovers her ability to exercise control over her pelvic floor muscles. In time, she will let her parents know about her urge to defecate—usually after the fact—but nevertheless an important step toward autonomy. Progress is only likely on good days when the emotional climate of the family is pleasant and calm, and not likely on days when either parent or child is distracted or uncomfortable. With time, the child's ability to perceive the urge to defecate and her skill at temporarily withholding stool improve. A delicate balance develops and exists between withholding and letting go of stool. Eventually, the child will be able to incorporate the expectation that she will pass stool into the toilet as one of her demands on herself. Toileting evolves from an act done to gain parental approval to something done for her own comfort. In this process, the parents' role is more that of a facilitator than a trainer.[88]

Any previous or ongoing impediment to the attainment of the skills necessary to achieve bowel continence can sabotage this process. This is especially likely when one considers how fraught with emotional peril the toilet-training process can be. The child may be perceived as resistant to the toilet-training process. The birth of a new sibling or the negativism of many toddlers may confound the process. Individual children may have idiosyncratic fears of the potty chair or the toilet, making the attainment of bowel continence difficult. The parents may be too coercive or too permissive in their toilet training. The child may have a tendency toward colonic inertia or constipation. A child may be developmentally unprepared to master the complex steps necessary to attain bowel continence. Any condition that leads to painful defecation such as passage of hard or large stools or an anal fissure may predispose the child to withhold stools (Table 3). As children grow older other contributing factors may potentiate the development of bowel incontinence.

### Encopresis

When bowel continence is not adequately established or when, after the establishment of bowel continence, the child becomes incontinent of stool, the condition termed encopresis exists. The term was coined in 1926 by Weissenberg to describe the fecal equivalent of enuresis. The def-

**TABLE 3. Critical Stages in the Potentiation of Encopresis***

| |
|---|
| Stage I potentiators (infancy and toddler years) |
| Simple constipation |
| Early colonic inertia |
| Congenital anorectal problems |
| Parental over-reaction |
| Coercive medical interventions |
| Stage II potentiators (training and autonomy: 3–5 y) |
| Psychosocial stresses during training period |
| Coercive or extremely permissive training |
| Idiosyncratic toilet fears |
| Painful or difficult defecation |
| Stage III potentiators (extramural function: early school years) |
| Avoidance of school bathrooms |
| Prolonged or acute gastroenteritis |
| Attention deficits with task impersistence |
| (?) Food intolerance, including lactase deficiency |
| Psychosocial stresses |

Reprinted with permission of the author and publisher from Levine MD, Encopresis, in Levine M et al (eds), *Developmental-Behavioral Pediatrics* (Philadelphia, Pa: WB Saunders; 1983).

* Children who ultimately develop encopresis are likely to have accumulated multiple risk factors on this list.

inition of encopresis, according to Levine, is "any child more than 4 years old who regularly passes formed, semi-formed, or liquid stools into the underwear or pajamas without an apparent or organic cause."[89] Encopresis is a common problem and one that is viewed with disgust and shame; so much so, that a lot of the child's and family's energy is spent trying to cover up the symptom. According to Levine, "In appreciating the tragedy of encopresis, one must conceptualize a human condition in which a child is ridiculed, shamed, or blamed (by himself and others) for something he did not cause and over which he has had little, if any, actual control."[89]

**Epidemiology.** Encopresis is present in 1½ to 2% of second-grade children.[3] This prevalence study comes from a homogeneous population in Europe and probably underestimates the prevalence of encopresis in low-income heterogeneous populations like those encountered in the United States. The male-to-female predominance of the condition is 5 or 6 to 1. In females with encopresis, one should look hard for the diagnosis of recurrent urinary tract infections.

**Pathophysiology.** The pathophysiology of encopresis invariably involves some degree of fecal retention. The proclivity toward fecal retention may be subtle and clinically elusive. In most instances, the child will have a dilated, stool-filled rectum, and will experience bowel incontinence due to one of two causes: (1) phenomenon whereby liquid stool percolates through the interstices of the hardened fecal mass in the rectum or (2) a process akin to glaciation whereby large amounts of stool, close to the anus, by having attained a critical mass or through normal activity, pass into the child's pants without the child's awareness (Fig 4). In most instances, there is no single, easily identifiable cause of the fecal incontinence. Rather, the etiology is multifactorial. Most children who develop encopresis will have accumulated multiple potentiating factors in the development of the problem (Table 3). Recognition of the potentiating factors can help the parents and child to understand the circumstances that may have brought on the condition and may be important in management.

***History.*** In taking a history from the family and the child who has a problem

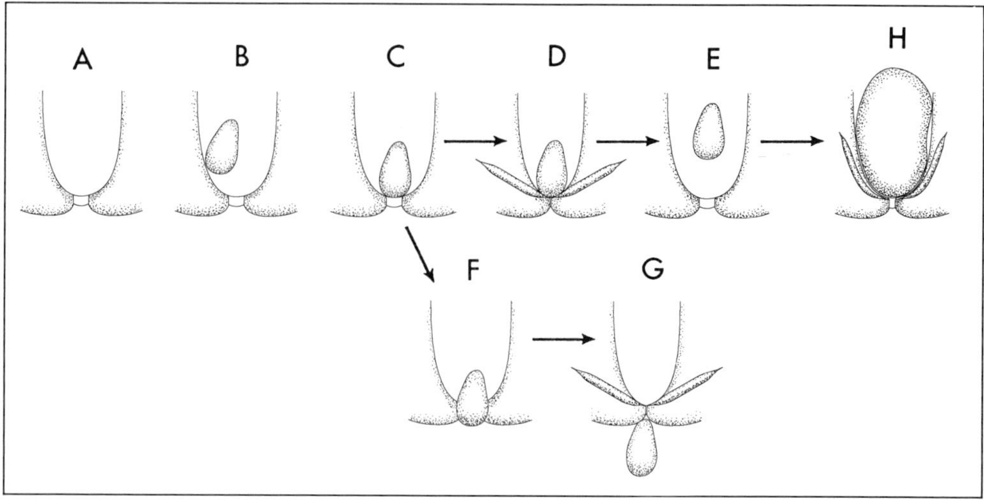


**Fig 4.** Diagrammatic representation of the sequence of events during defecation, fecal continence, and chronic fecal retention. **A, B, C, F, G:** Normal defecation. **A, B, C, D, E, H:** Pathway of fecal retention. [Reprinted from Fleisher DR, Diagnosis and treatment of disorders of defecation in children, *Pediatr Ann* (1976; 5:701), with permission of the author and the publisher (SLACK Incorporated, Thorofare, NJ).

with fecal soiling, the physician must be sensitive to the shame and perhaps anger experienced by all parties. The physician should also be aware that this may be the first time that this issue has been discussed publicly. Simple discussion of the problem can be therapeutic, especially if the physician asks questions that indicate how common the problem is and also show that the physician is aware of the circumstances leading to the problem and may have a practical solution to offer.

There are a number of historical features that are very common in children with fecal incontinence. Most children who soil do so between 3 PM and 7 PM. Fecal soiling is less likely at school or at night. If a child soils at either of those times, it is a poor prognostic sign. Children with this problem exercise an inordinate amount of energy to suppress the fecal urge. This is especially true during school when fecal incontinence would be devastating to the child's peer relationships. At the conclusion of the school day, however, there is a generalized release of inhibition and an increase in activity, both of which contribute to an increased likelihood for the soiling to occur. Most children with fecal soiling pass large stools. The caliber of the stool is merely a reflection of the size of the rectum, which is, in most cases, massively dilated with stool. In fact, many parents will state that they keep a stick or a toilet plunger readily available in the bathroom because when the child does pass stool into the toilet it is sometimes such a large amount that a parent must break it up in order to successfully flush it down the toilet. Another common historical feature is the tendency for children with fecal soiling to hide their soiled underpants. This is often what disturbs parents the most. At times, the parent may feel that the problem is getting better because there have been no soiled underclothes to wash. Unfortunately, however, the supply of underpants reaches critically low levels or the family dog discovers a cache of soiled underwear, to the parents' chagrin. Positive responses to any of these historical features are helpful in that both parent and child are made to recognize that the physician has encountered this problem on numerous occasions in the past.

Most children who have fecal soiling are not aware of the urge to defecate when the rectum is dilated with stool. The normal mechanism by which rectal fullness is appreciated is subverted. When these children pass stool, it is usually without control. It is important to ask the child in the parents' presence whether or not he or she is aware of the urge to defecate. When a child is incontinent of stool, he or she becomes aware of the stool's passage and may go through motions to try to withhold the stool, usually after the fact. At times, these motions are witnessed by the parent who may misinterpret them to mean that the child is willfully defecating into his or her pants. This misconception must be clarified to the parents. It is also apparent that the child who habitually soils his pants becomes inured to the fecal odor that is often attendant on his person. It is known that one can become habituated to an omnipresent odor.

***Physical Examination.*** Physical examination often reveals confirmatory evidence of the underlying pathophysiology. Many children with fecal soiling on the basis of chronic fecal retention will have a palpable, nontender or slightly tender, sausage-shaped mass in the left lower quadrant of the abdomen, which represents the stool-filled, dilated descending colon. In addition, the rectum is often full of stool and the anus may actually be patulous. This latter physical finding has been widely misinterpreted in the past to suggest that children with this condition have been sexually abused. The anal dilatation in most of these cases, however, is due to stretching of the anus that occurs as a result of the massive fecal retention in the rectum. Overinterpretation of this physical sign can lead to wrongful accusation of sexual abuse. Attention, too, should be paid to the height, weight, and the neurological examination to rule out other, more rare conditions that can cause problems with fecal incontinence due to fecal retention such as hypothyroidism or a neurologic deficit.

A flat plate of the abdomen is helpful in children with fecal soiling, both to confirm the diagnosis and to serve as a teaching tool for child and parent. Both parents and children can readily appreciate the stool that is visible on a flat plate of the abdomen. In most children with fecal soiling secondary to fecal retention, there is an abundant amount of stool apparent on a flat plate of the abdomen.

**Treatment.** Treatment begins during the evaluation process by an open discussion of the common historical points. Parents and child are made to feel reassured that they are not the only family suffering with this condition. It is useful to explain the pathophysiology of the condition using diagrams and the x-ray to help engage both the parents and the child in the therapeutic tasks necessary to remedy this problem.

The first stage in treating encopresis involves cleaning out the excess stool. There have been a number of regimens advocated for this process, including chronic mineral oil administration up to 1 ounce per year of age twice per day,[90] or daily enemas for 1 month followed by enemas every other day for another month.[46] The regimen advocated by Levine involves a 2-week cleanout program that involves sequential enemas, laxatives, and suppositories (Table 4). This approach is readily accepted by both parents and child, and produces good results with a minimum of disruption or inconvenience. At the completion of the

**TABLE 4. Encopresis Cleanout Regimen**

| | | | |
|---|---|---|---|
| Day 1 | Fleets enema (adult size) | Day 8 | Dulcolax suppository |
| Day 2 | Dulcolax suppository | Day 9 | Dulcolax tablet |
| Day 3 | Dulcolax tablet | Day 10 | Fleets |
| Day 4 | Fleet enema | Day 11 | Dulcolax suppository |
| Day 5 | Dulcolax suppository | Day 12 | Dulcolax tablet |
| Day 6 | Dulcolax tablet | Day 13 | Dulcolax tablet |
| Day 7 | Fleets enema | Return to clinic | |

Reprinted with permission of the author and publisher from Levine MD, Encopresis, in Levine M et al (eds), *Developmental-Behavioral Pediatrics* (Philadelphia, Pa: WB Saunders; 1983).

2-week cleanout period, most parents and children express satisfaction with the results. In most instances, the symptom is alleviated significantly. Parents also note that the child's color or appetite may have improved and that the child's clothes fit better. The child, too, may perceive many of these benefits. Paradoxically, it is this point in the treatment that is most fraught with risk for relapse. This occurs because of the high rate of symptom relief and the family's perception that the problem is completely alleviated. It is important to emphasize that, while there has been a good response and the colon has been cleaned out, the rectum remains stretched and dilated and probably does not function adequately. It is important to emphasize this because without attention to the next phase of treatment most children with this problem will gradually reaccumulate excess stool over a 6- to 12-month period and will have a relapse of their symptom. A recent approach to the cleanout in difficult to treat encopretics has involved the use of the balanced electrolyte solution, Go-Lytely.[91]

To assist the child in maintaining bowel continence, it is important to help the child develop good bowel habits. The goal of therapy is for the child to have no problems with fecal soiling and to experience regular, soft bowel movements. The child should have a bowel movement at least every other day. To help the child achieve this goal, a mild laxative like Senokot is recommended on an intermittent basis for approximately 1 month. A stool softener, most often mineral oil, is also recommended in order to help the child have regular bowel movements and to prevent reaccumulation of feces. The dose of mineral oil to be employed depends on the child. To begin, a dose of 2 tablespoons twice a day is recommended with the understanding that the mother will titrate that dose to help the child achieve regular, soft bowel movements but not to experience passage of soiled mineral oil, which would discourage the child. The child is encouraged to sit on the toilet twice a day for 5 to 10 minutes each time, ideally at a time when the child would ordinarily have a bowel movement. If the child is young or small, it is important to instruct the parent to make sure that the child's feet are flat on a hard surface while the child is stooling.

**Prognosis.** With this approach, approximately 80% of children with fecal soiling can achieve cure or significant improvement.[92] This leaves a substantial percentage who do not respond. Factors associated with lack of response or relapse include the following: poor compliance with either the cleanout or the maintenance regimen; in-school or nocturnal soiling; severe incontinence or constipation; a high loading of behavioral, developmental, or academic problems; or a lack of concern about the symptom (for example, children who do not hide their underwear). In many cases, repeating the above approach can be beneficial. Some children and their families, however, will not be helped by this approach, and cure will have to await readiness to comply with the cleanout and maintenance programs, or a resolution of social stresses that make resolution of the symptom unlikely.

## REFERENCES


1. Koff SA. Enuresis. In: Walsh PC, Gittes RF, Perlmutter AD, Stamey TA, eds. *Campbell's Urology*. Philadelphia, Pa.: WB Saunders Co; 1986; chap 54.
2. Koff SA. Estimating bladder capacity in children. *Urology*. 1983; 21:248.
3. Bellman M. Studies on encopresis. *Acta Pediatr Scand.* 1966; 170 (suppl):51.
4. Burke EC, Stickler GB. Enuresis: Is it being overtreated? *Mayor Clin Proc.* 1980; 55:118–119.
5. Smith LR. Nocturnal enuresis. Ped Rev 1980. 2(6):183–186.
6. Shaffer D. Enuresis. In: Rutter M, Hersov L, eds. *Child and Adolescent Psychiatry; Modern Approaches*. Boston, Mass: Blackwell Scientific Publishers; 1985:465–481.
7. Forsythe WI, Redmond A. Enuresis and spontaneous cure rate. Study of 1129 enuretics. *Arch Dis Child.* 1974; 49:259–263.
8. Starfield B. Functional bladder capacity in enuretic and non-enuretic children. *J Pediatr.* 1967;5:777.
9. Troup CW, Hodgson NB. Nocturnal functional bladder capacity in enuretic children. *J Urol.* 1971, 129:132.

10. Johnstone JMS. Cystometry and evaluation of anticholinergic drugs in enuretic children. *J Pediatr Surg*. 1972; 7:18.
11. Koff SA, Lapides J, and Paizza DH. The uninhibited bladder in children: a cause of urinary tract infection, obstruction and reflux. In: Hodson J, Kincaid-Smith P, eds. *Reflux Nephropathy*. New York, NY: Masson Publishing; 1979.
12. Pompeius R. Cystometry in pediatric enuresis. Scand. J. Urol., 1971; 5:222.
13. Mahony DT, Laferie RO, Blais DJ. Studies on enuresis. DX Evidence of a mild form of compensated detrusor hyperreflexia in enuretic children. *J Urol*. 1981; 126:520.
14. Grossman HB, Koff SA, Diokno AC. Cystometry in children. *J Urol*. 1977; 117:646.
15. Torrens MJ, Collins CD. The urodynamic assessment of adult enuresis. *Br J Urol*. 1975; 47:433.
16. Hindmarsh JR, Byrne PO. Adult enuresis—a symptomatic and urodynamic assessment. *Br J Urol*. 1980; 52:88.
17. Koff SA, Murtagh DS. The uninhibited bladder in children: effect of treatment on recurrence of urinary infection and on vesicoureteral reflux resolution. *J Urol*. 1983; 130:1138.
18. Stein ZM, Susser MW. Social factors in the development of sphincter control. *Dev Med Child Neurol*. 1967; 9:692.
19. Werry JS. Enuresis—a psychosomatic entity? *Can Med Assoc J*. 97:319, 1967.
20. Bindelglas PM, Dee G. Enuresis treatment with imipramine hydrochloride. a 10 year follow-up study. *Am J Psychiatry*. 1978; 135:12.
21. MacKeith RC. A frequent factor in the origins of primary nocturnal enuresis: anxiety in the third year of life. *Dev Med Child Neurol*. 1968; 10:465.
22. Essen J, Peckham C. Nocturnal enuresis in childhood. *Dev Med Child Neurol*. 1976; 18:577.
23. Miller FJW, Court SDM, Walton NG, Knox EG. Growing-up in Newcastle upon Tyne. London, Eng. Oxford University Press; 1960.
24. McKendry JBJ, William HAL, Broughton C. Enuresis—a study of untreated patients. 1968; 10:815.
25. Apley J, MacKeith R. *The Child and His Symptoms*. 2nd ed. Philadelphia, Pa: FA Davis Co; 1968.
26. MacKeith RC. Is maturation delay a frequent factor in the origins of primary nocturnal enuresis? *Dev Med Child Neurol*. 1972; 14:217.
27. Couchells SM, Johnson SB, Carter R, Walker D. Behavioral and environmental characteristics of treated and untreated enuretic children and nonenuretic controls. *J Pediatr*. 1981; 99:812–816.
28. Moffatt MEK, Kato C, Pless IB. Improvements in self-concept after treatment on nocturnal enuresis: Randomized controlled trial. *J Pediatr*. 1987; 110:647–652.
29. Bakwin H. Enuresis in twins. AJDC. 1971; 121:222.
30. Bakwin H. The genetics of enuresis. In: Kolvin I, MacKeith RC, and Meadow SR, eds. *Bladder Control and Enuresis*. London, Eng: W. Heinemann Medical Books; 1973:73–77.
31. Ritvo ER, Ornitz EM, Gottlieb F, Maron AF, Ditman KS, Blinn KA. Arousal and non-arousal enuretic events. *Am J Psychiatry*. 1969; 126:115.
32. Broughton RJ. Sleep disorders: disorders or arousal? *Science*. 1968; 159:1070.
33. Kales A, Kales JD, Jacobson A, Humphrey FJ, Soldatos CR. Effect of imipramine on enuretic frequency and sleep stages. *Pediatrics*. 1977; 60:431.
34. Mikkelsen EF, Rapoport JL, Nee L, et al. Childhood enuresis: I. Sleep patterns and psychopathology. *Arch Gen Psychiatry*. 1980; 37:1138.
35. Forsythe WI and Redmond A. Enuresis and spontaneous cure rate. Study of 1129 enuresis. *Arch Dis Child*. 1974; 49:259.
36. McKendry JBJ, Stewart DA. Enuresis. *Pediatr Clin North Am*. 1974; 21:1019.
37. Kass EJ, Diokno AC, Montealegre A. Enuresis: principle of management and result of treatment. *J Urol*. 1979; 121:794.
38. Murphy S, Chapman W. Adolescent enuresis: a urologic study. *Pediatrics*. 1970; 45:426.
39. Kunin SA, Limbert DJ, Platzker ACG, McKinley J. The efficacy of imipramine in the management of enuresis. *J Urol*. 1970; 104:612.
40. Snyder HM, Caldamone AA, Wein AJ, Duckett JW. The Hinman syndrome: alternatives for treatment. Presented at the American Urological Association 77th Annual Meeting; May 16–20, 1982; Kansas City. Abstract #1.
41. Foxman B, Valdez R, Brook R. Childhood enuresis: prevalence, perceived impact, and prescribed treatments. *Pediatrics*. 1986; 77(4):482–487.
42. Baker B. Symptom treatment and symptom substitution in enuresis. *J Abnorm Psychol*. 1969; 74:42–49.
43. Sacks S, DeLeon G, Blackman S. Psychological changes associated with conditioning functional enuresis. *J Clin Psychol*. 1974; 30:271–276.
44. Murphy S, Nickols J, Hammar S. Neurological evaluation of adolescent enuretics. *Pediatrics*. 1970; 45(2):269–275.
45. Weider D, Hauri P. Nocturnal enuresis in children with upper airway obstruction. International Journal of Pediatric Otorhinolaryngology 1985; 9:173–182.
46. O'Regan S, Schick E, Hamburger B, Yazbeck S: Constipation associated with vesicoureteral reflux. *Urology*. 1986; 28(5):394–396.

47. Rockney R, Fritz G, Caldamone A. Enuresis following masturbation in a mentally retarded adolescent: a case report. Journal of Adolescent Health Care 1989. In press.
48. Morgan R, Young G. Parental attitudes and the conditioning treatment of childhood enuresis. Behav. Res. and Therapy 1975; 13:197–199.
49. DiScipio W, Smey P, Kogan S, Donner K, Levitt S. Impromptu micturitional flow parameters in normal boys. *J Urol.* 1986; 136:1049–1051.
50. Redman J, Seibert J. The uroradiographic evaluation of the enuretic child. *J Urol.* 1979; 122:799–801.
51. Alon U, Pery M, Davidai G, Berant M: Ultrasonography in the radiographic evaluation of children with urinary tract infection. *Pediatrics.* 1986; 78(1):58–64.
52. Haque M, Ellerstein NS, Gundy JH, et al. Parental perceptions in enuresis, a collaborative study. *AJDC.* 1981; 135:809.
53. Mishra PC, Agarwal VK, Rahman H. Therapeutic trial of amytriptyline in the treatment of nocturnal enuresis—a controlled study. *Indian Pediatr.* 1980; 17:279.
54. Schmitt BD. Nocturnal enuresis: an update on treatment. *Pediatr Clin North Am.* 1982; 29:21.
55. Marshall S, Marshall HH, Lyon RP. Enuresis: an analysis of various therapeutic approaches. *Pediatrics.* 1973; 52:813.
56. Kimmel HD, Kimmel EC. An instrumental conditioning method for the treatment of enuresis. *J Behav Ther Exp Psychiatry.* 1970; 1:121.
57. Harris LS, Purohit AP. Bladder training and enuresis: a controlled trial. *Behav Res Ther.* 1977; 15:485.
58. Doleys DM. Behavioral treatments for nocturnal enuresis in children: a review of the recent literature. *Psychol Bull.* 1977; 1:30.
59. Lovering JS, Tallet SE, McKendry JBJ. Oxybutinin-Efficacy in the treatment of primary enuresis. *Pediatrics.* 1988; 82:104–106.
60. Mowrer OH, Mowrer WM. Enuresis—a method for its study and treatment. *Am J Orthopsychiatry.* 1938; 8:436.
61. Young GC, Morgan RTT. Conditioning techniques and enuresis. Med J. *Aust.* 1973; 2:329.
62. Forsythe WI, Redmond A. Enuresis and the electric alarm. Study of 200 cases. *Br Med J.* 1970; 1–211.
63. Schmitt BD. New enuresis alarms: safe, successful, and child-operable. *Contemp Pediatr.* 1986.
64. Puri VN. Urinary levels of antidiuretic hormone in nocturnal enuresis. *Indian Pediatr.,* 1980; 17:675.
65. Norgaard JP, Pederson EB, Djurhuus JC. Diurnal antidiuretic hormone levels in enuretics. *J Urol.* 1985; 134:1029–1031.
66. Anonymous. Desmopressin for nocturnal enuresis. *Med Lett Drugs and Ther.* 1990; 32:38.
67. Klauber GT. Clinical efficacy and safety of desmopressin in the treatment of nocturnal enuresis. *J Pediatr.* 1989; 1145:719.
68. Lenoir G. Les traittments del'enuresie. Paris Entretiens De Bichat, Expansion Scientifique Francaise, 1986:151–158.
69. Miller K, Goldberg S, Atkin B. Nocturnal enuresis: experience with longterm use of intranasally administered desmopressin. *J Pediatr.* 1989; 114S:723–726.
70. Wille S. Comparison of desmopressin and enuresis alarm for nocturnal enuresis. *Arch Dis Child.* 1986; 61:30–33.
71. Sukhai RN, Mol J, Harris AS. Combined therapy of enuresis alarm and desmopressin in the treatment of nocturnal enuresis. *Eur. J. Pediatr.* 1989; 148:465.
72. Holt J, Borresen B. Enuresis nocturna in school children in Bod. A therapeutic trial with a vasopressin analog: desmopressin and imipramine. *Tidsskr Nor Laegeforen.* 1986; 106:651.
73. Simmonds EJ, Mahony MJ, Little JM. Convulsion and coma after intranasal desmopressin in cystic fibrosis. *Br Med J.* 1988; 297:1614.
74. Bamford MFM, Cruickshank G. Dangers of intranasal desmopressin for nocturnal enuresis. *J Coll Gen Pract.* 1989; 39:345. Letter.
75. MacLean REG. Imipramine hydrocholoride (Tofranil) and enuresis. *Am J Psychiatry.* 1960; 117:551.
76. Rapoport JL, Mikkelsen EJ, Zavodil A, et al. Childhood enuresis: II. *Arch Gen Psychiatry.* 1980; 37:1146.
77. Hagglund TB, Parkkulaninen KV. Enuretic children treated with imipramine (Tofranil), *Ann Paediatr Fenn.* 1965; 11:53.
78. Blackwell B Currah J. The psychopharmacology of nocturnal enuresis. In: Kolvin I, MacKeith RC, Meadow SR, eds. *Bladder Control and Enuresis.* London, Eng: W. Heinemann Medical Books; 1973:231–257.
79. Jorgensen OS, Lober M, Christiansen JW, et al. Plasma concentration and clinical effect in imipramine treatment of childhood enuresis. *Clin Pharmacokinet.* 1980; 5:386.
80. Alderton HR. Imipramine in childhood enuresis: further studies on the relationship of time of administration to effect. *Can Med Assoc J.* 1970; 102:1179.
81. Martin GI. Imipramine pamoate in the treatment of childhood enuresis. A double-blind study. *JDC.* 1971; 122:42.
82. Collison DR. Hypnotherapy in the management of nocturnal enuresis. *Med J Aust.* 1970; 1:52.
83. Olness K. The use of self-hypnosis in the treatment of childhood nocturnal enuresis. *Clin Pediatr.* 1975; 14:273.
84. Esperanca M, Gerrard JW. Nocturnal enuresis. Comparison of the effect of imipramine and dietary restriction on bladder capacity. *Can Med Assoc J.* 1969; 101:721.

85. Zaleski A, Shokeir MK, Gerrard JW. Enuresis: familial incidence and relationship to allergic disorders. *Can Med Assoc J*. 1972; 106:30.

86. Kaplan G. Allergic origin of enuresis seen possible but unlikely. Pediatr. News. 1973; 7:12.

87. Siegel S, Rawitt L, Sokoloff B, et al. Relationship of allergy, enuresis and urinary infection in children 4 to 7 years of age. *Pediatrics*. 1976; 57:526.

88. Fleisher DR. Diagnosis and treatment of disorders of defecation in children. *Pediatr Ann*. 1976; 5:701.

89. Levine MD. Encopresis. In: Edited by Levine M, Carey W, Crocker A, Gross R, eds. *Developmental-Behavior Pediatrics*. Philadelphia, Pa: WB Saunders Company; 1983.

90. Davidson M, Kugler MD, Baver CH. Diagnosis and management in children with severe and protracted constipation and obstipation. *J Pediatr*. 1963; 62:261.

91. Ingebo KB, Hyman MB. Polyethylene Glycol-Electrolyte Solution for intestinal clearance in children with refractory encopresis. *AJDC*. 1988; 142:340.

92. Levine MD, Bakow H. Children with encopresis: a study of treatment outcome. *Pediatrics*. 1976; 58:845.

# 46

# Pediatric Genitourinary Emergencies

*Robert A. Mevorach, William C. Hulbert, Jr., and Ronald Rabinowitz*

## INTRODUCTION

Two classes of pediatric genitourinary emergencies can be identified. The first type can pose an immediate threat to the life of an infant or child, eg, severe posterior urethral valves with sepsis, or can risk permanent damage to the affected organ if not managed expediently, eg, as with testis torsion. The second type of diagnosis necessitates urgent evaluation because of either short- or long-term genitourinary or systemic consequences, eg, imperforate anus. Unfortunately, the outward signs of these problems are often common to both classifications and may also overlap with nonurgent or normal findings. A discussion of these nonspecific but important signs will be the focus of the first section, and then a discussion of specific diagnoses will complete the chapter.

## IMPORTANT SIGNS

### Abdominal Masses

A majority of abdominal masses in neonates and children arise from the genitourinary tract or retroperitoneal structures.[1] At least 50% of these masses in neonates take origin from the kidney.[2] Increasingly, these cystic masses or hydronephrosis may be identified on prenatal ultrasound screening examinations and subsequently confirmed on postnatal studies (Fig 1). If postnatal imaging fails to confirm fetal findings, especially if sonograms were initially obtained late in gestation, it is imperative to reexamine the child to assure that moderate hydronephrosis has not been masked by perinatal oliguria.[3] If a cystic mass or hydronephrosis is detected, expedient diagnosis is established through history, physical examination, and additional studies as indicated. The presence of bilateral hydronephrosis, or unilateral hydronephrosis with contralateral renal nonfunction, requires a more urgent evaluation than does unilateral hydronephrosis, particularly if the renal parenchyma is thinned. Unilateral hydronephrosis, no matter what the degree of abnormality, is not an emergency if the contralateral renal unit is functioning normally. Rarely, simple renal cysts may be detected during the course of evaluation. They usually require no further management.

Solid abdominal masses in neonates should be diagnosed prior to discharging the infant from the hospital. In children, solid abdominal masses are considered cancers until proven otherwise. Excretory urography and CT scanning accurately delineate the origin and character of solid

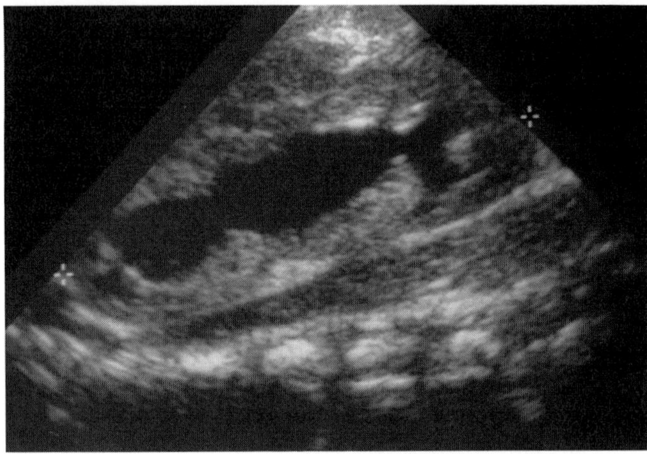

**Fig 1.** Longitudinal renal sonogram on day 1 of life, showing central hydronephrosis that involves the pelvis and calyces. This kidney was not palpable and the abnormality was discovered on prenatal ultrasound exams.

abdominal masses and have eliminated the "diagnostic celiotomy" except in disorders requiring biopsy prior to nonsurgical therapy.[4] Thorough history, physical examination, and imaging studies lead to the appropriate timing of both surgical and medical treatment of children with solid masses of the abdomen. Renal ectopia and fusion may present as abdominal masses, but once defined require additional care only if complicated by other anomalies (ie, tumor, obstruction, reflux).

## Hematuria

Microhematuria in the neonate and child must be investigated, and gross hematuria (visible to the naked eye) is a urologic emergency. The two most common reasons for hematuria are urinary tract infection and medical renal disease. Clues to the diagnosis are easily obtainable by an accurate history and microscopic and strip reagent urinalysis, and can allow further directed evaluation. In addition, patient and family anxiety can be addressed in a straightforward manner with this approach. Obvious bacterial infection can be treated and further evaluated with radiographs as appropriate; more urgent evaluation of the entire genitourinary system can proceed in the absence of signs of infection by ultrasonography or intravenous urography. Normal findings can be reassuring and can lead to pediatric nephrologic consultation to evaluate for medical renal disease. Small urothelial lesions or transitional cell tumors can be missed by this approach but are exceedingly rare. Cystoscopy, while certainly not routine for the majority of cases, may occasionally be used in older children with persistent findings and clinical indications. One common presentation of hematuria in young males should be mentioned because of the specific clinical picture that it paints, and because it should not prompt radiographic or cystoscopic evaluation. This is *idiopathic urethrorrhagia,* typified by postvoid dripping of gross blood from the meatus for a few moments and findings of brown or red blood spots, usually the size of a small coin and scattered on the inside front of the underwear. Dysuria may or may not be present. This condition resolves spontaneously and the etiology is unclear.

Worrisome urologic causes of hematuria include renal vascular insults, obstructive lesions of the collecting system, tumors, and trauma, and these will be addressed specifically.

## Febrile Urinary Tract Infection

Infection should be documented by culture whenever possible; it is a sign that there may be an underlying structural problem. For that reason, documented infection plays a key role in initiating a radiographic evaluation that will lead to proper diagnosis. Up to 60% of such neonates and 30% of older children will be found to have such a structural problem. Usually identification of the infection will allow prompt therapy pending definitive culture results, and if the clinical response is appropriate, further evaluation can be elective while the child is maintained on urinary prophylaxis. Immediate radiographic imaging is usually not recommended unless the child is an infant or the clinical course indicates a complicated urinary tract infection (ie, possible obstruction). Renal scarring and associated decreased renal function may be minimized by prompt intervention for children with urinary infection.

### Urinary Retention

Urinary retention is a much more common presenting symptom in the adult, but in the child it requires prompt intervention for simple relief and an urgent screen to rule out worrisome problems. Acute infection can lead to more or less voluntary holding of urine because of anticipated dysuria, and this can be significant; diagnosis is made by urinalysis and resolution during treatment. Neonates with this sign may have urethral obstruction. By 24 hours postnatally nearly 100% of infants have urinated.[5] If delay occurs, prerenal, postrenal, and renal causes must be excluded. While neonates are oliguric for the first few days of life, anuria is abnormal. Older children could have an obstructing tumor, urethral stricture with an acute-on-chronic presentation, neurologic problem, functional voiding disorder, or intra-abdominal inflammatory process, such as appendicitis.[6]

## SPECIFIC DIAGNOSES

### Life-Threatening Problems

**Posterior Urethral Valves.** There is a wide spectrum of severity in valve obstruction and therefore a similar variation in the clinical presentation. An abnormal urinary stream or pattern can be seen in some neonates, but the presence of a "good" stream or diapers that are sufficiently wet are not reliable signs for dismissing the possibility of bladder outlet obstruction in the male. Other signs can include sepsis, urinary ascites, pneumothorax, pneumomediastinum, or respiratory distress. Pulmonary hypoplasia may be an occult indication of bladder outlet obstruction, secondary to oligohydramnios. An abdominal mass may be present in up to 50% of patients. This percentage is decreasing as prenatal ultrasound is being used more frequently, and the diagnosis can now be suspected *in utero* and confirmed shortly after delivery. This outlet obstruction is suggested by the ultrasound finding of bilateral hydronephrosis, bladder distention, and dilatation of the posterior urethra (Fig 2A and B). Voiding cystourethrography is used to visualize the obstruction, identify reflux, and allow placement of a urethral feeding tube (Fig 2C). Emergent management of urethral valves hinges on establishing free urinary drainage; a 5 or 8 French feeding tube is best. It is important that the catheter not be coiled within the dilated posterior urethra, where it will drain intermittently and inadequately. As the obstruction is being relieved, the infant is cultured and treated with antibiotics, and monitored for compromise of renal function with serum urea nitrogen and creatinine levels. Acidosis and electrolyte imbalances must be corrected prior to consideration of surgical intervention to minimize anesthetic risks and to avoid mortality and additional renal morbidity, problems that have decreased over the past 20 years because of improved medical management. Early diagnosis provides the opportunity for prompt intervention to avert significant mortality from uremia or sepsis.[7]

Transurethral ablation of the valve leaflets is performed under direct vision with a cystoscope designed for the infant urethra. A vesicostomy may be utilized when the urethral caliber is too small to accommodate instruments for safe and complete valve ablation. Numerous techniques of "blind" valve rupture have been described in the literature, and valve disruption may also be performed via a prior vesicostomy.

The long-term prognosis for these children includes renal failure in up to 32% of patients.[8] Poor renal function outcome is more likely to be seen in those infants whose ultrasound images delineate loss of

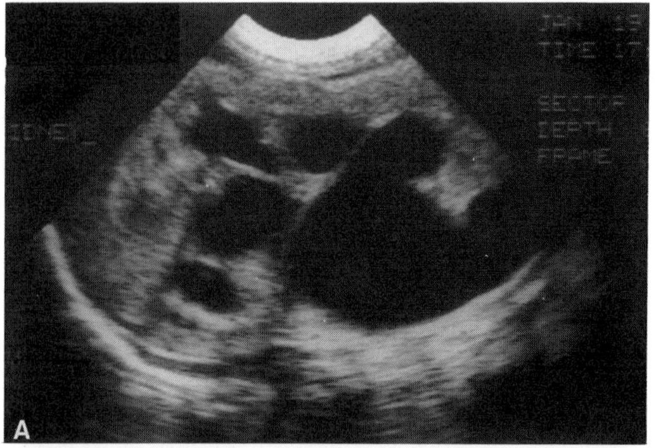

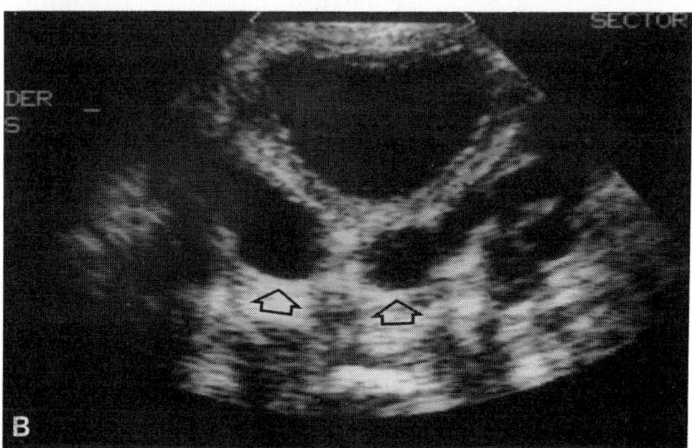


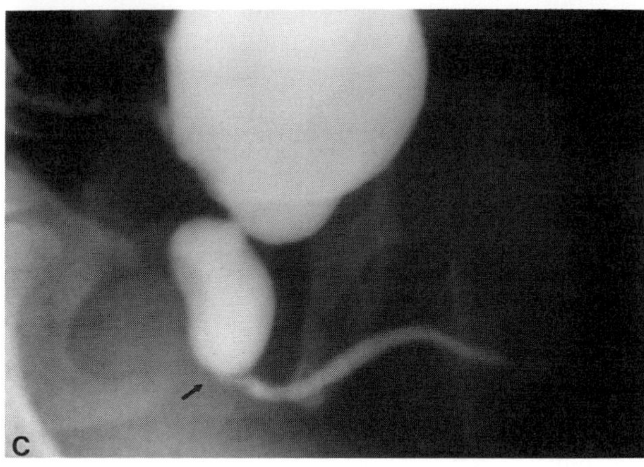

**Fig 2. A,** Longitudinal sonogram of the kidney with dilated pelvis, upper ureter, and calyces; **B,** transverse sonogram. The bladder is thick-walled with dilated ureters posteriorly (arrows); **C,** lateral view of a voiding cystourethrogram. The bladder neck is hypertrophied, the prostatic urethra is dilated, and there is an abrupt transition to the normal anterior urethra at the point of valve obstruction (arrow).

normal corticomedullary definition.[9] In addition, a nadir serum creatinine level greater than 0.7 mg/dL following adequate drainage of the bladder portends a poorer prognosis.[10] Management of the infant with persistent dilatation of the upper urinary tract and associated azotemia despite adequate valve ablation may include ureterostomy or pyelostomy, although controversy still exists regarding the benefit and necessity of this type of intervention.[11,12] Finally, the full valve bladder syndrome with detrusor dysfunction, decreased bladder compliance, and persistent upper tract dilatation may pose a long-term management dilemma in terms of both continence and renal function.

### Solid Abdominal Masses

***Wilms' Tumor.*** Wilms' tumor, or nephroblastoma, is the most common solid abdominal mass in childhood. Ultrasound imaging shows a solid mass distorting the normal architecture in the involved kidney. Cystic variants may be confused with a benign process at times. Misdiagnosis occurs in 1.4% of cases, usually due to confusion with neuroblastoma.[13] Excretory urography demonstrates nonvisualization of the involved kidney in 10% of children.[14] Computed tomography is beneficial in questionable cases and is useful while investigating the lungs and central nervous system for metastases (Fig 3). Bone scan may be warranted in clear cell sarcoma. Staging is performed at the time of urgent surgery. Current treatment protocols are designed to spare renal tissue and use combination chemotherapy and radiotherapy to achieve cures.[15]

***Neuroblastoma.*** Neuroblastoma is the single most common tumor of infancy and childhood. Abdominal presentation occurs in 60% of cases and only one of three is extra-adrenal. Masses frequently cross the abdominal midline, displacing the kidney and other organs on ultrasound imaging. While a homogeneous appearance is the rule, larger lesions may exhibit areas of necrosis. Urinary vanillylmandelic acid (VMA) and homovanillic acid (HVA) are uniformly elevated. CT and magnetic resonance scans are useful in assessing the extent and resectability of tumors. CT may detect intraspinal extension in 15% of masses (less in adrenal origin lesions); this knowledge is essential prior to surgery.[16]

Metastatic disease occurs in 90% of patients. Bone marrow aspiration or lymph node biopsy is used for diagnosis prior to initiation of chemotherapy or radiation treatment. This cancer bears a poor prognosis, with 2-year survival approximating 20%.[17]

***Congenital Mesoblastic Nephroma.*** Congenital mesoblastic nephroma (CMN) presents as an abdominal mass and is the most common solid tumor of the kidney in the neonate and young infant. Hypertension is also present in many cases. Ultrasound imaging demonstrates a homogeneous renal mass. Resection constitutes adequate therapy in management of these tumors. A less favorable prognosis is expected when the tumor displays histologic features of nuclear atypia, hypercellularity, and increased cell size.[18] Consideration should be

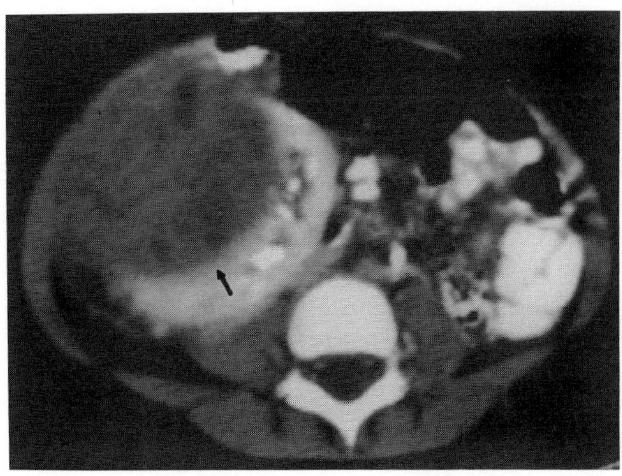

**Fig 3.** CT scan of right Wilms' tumor that displaces functioning renal tissue (arrow).

given to chemotherapy and radiation treatment for atypical CMN or in the older child.[19,20]

***Multilocular Cystic Nephroma.*** Multilocular cystic nephroma classically presents as an abdominal mass, with renal colic and hematuria[21] (Fig 4). While the origin of these lesions may be in question, their possible histologic and embryologic relation to Wilms' tumor has led to a recommendation for routine nephrectomy.[22] There are also histologic similarities to congenital mesoblastic nephroma.[23]

***Renal Cell Carcinoma.*** Renal cell carcinoma may occur in children, but it accounts for less than 8% of kidney tumors. The incidence in girls and boys is equivalent. Abdominal mass, palpable on exam, is a common presentation. Tumor calcification is demonstrated in 20% of lesions on ultrasound scanning or x-ray studies.[24] Urgent nephrectomy is appropriate care.

***Pheochromocytoma.*** Pheochromocytoma presents as a mass lesion in 6% of cases and occurs in infants as early as 1 month old.[25] These tumors arise from chromaffin tissue within the adrenal medulla and sympathetic ganglia. Classic presentation includes sustained hypertension, headache, and sweating as a result of elevated catecholamines produced by the tumor(s). Diagnosis is confirmed by determination of serum and urine catecholamines and VMA. In addition, ultrasound, excretory urography, and CT scanning detect abdominal masses, particularly in the suprarenal region, which is the primary site in 69% of tumors. Extra-adrenal tumors occur in 20% of cases and are multiple in the same percentage.[26] When a diagnosis is established, MIBG (methyliodobenzylguanidine) scanning is helpful in screening for multiple or suspected lesions.[26] α-Adrenergic blockade with restoration of intravascular volume prior to surgical excision is the appropriate therapy. Periodic follow-up is essential to detect hypertension, which may be the first evidence of recurrent disease.

***Adrenal Adenomas and Carcinoma.*** Adrenocortical tumors are rare in children, and approximately two thirds are associated with virilization. Cushing's syndrome, due to sustained hypersecretion of glucocorticoids, is often seen in the remainder. Treatment consists of complete surgical removal of the identified lesion. It is sometimes difficult to accurately assess the malignant potential of the lesion by pathologic evaluation; larger tumors carry a worse prognosis, in general.[27]

***Rhabdomyosarcoma.*** Rhabdomyosarcoma, the most common soft tissue sarcoma of childhood, may present as a suprapubic mass. This may be secondary to a bladder or uterine lesion, or due to a distended bladder secondary to outflow ob-

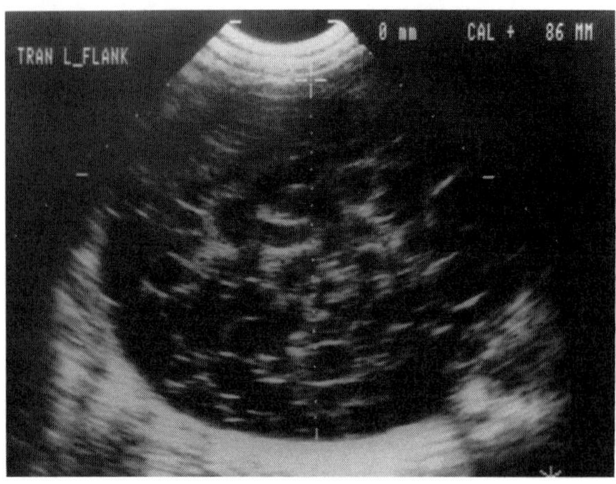


**Fig 4.** Left renal sonogram of multilocular cystic nephroma—a distinct appearance with multiple discrete cysts.

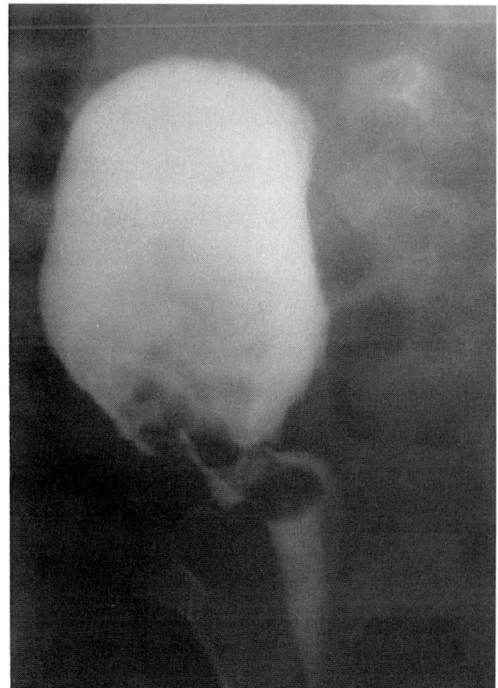

**Fig 5.** Rhabdomyosarcoma of bladder. Multiple filling defects on contrast voiding cystourethrogram (VCUG).

struction from a prostate tumor.[28] Catheterization with a feeding tube relieves urinary obstruction and allows renal function to normalize. Hematuria, stranguria, and constipation define the classical presenting symptoms (Fig 5). Palpable masses or visible lesions (as in vaginal rhabdomyosarcoma) are further evaluated by ultrasound and CT scans to define, if possible, the organ of origin. Abdominal and chest CT scans, bone marrow aspiration, and bone scan are utilized to evaluate for metastatic disease. Initial surgical intervention is for biopsy, transurethrally if feasible, as the mainstay of therapy is multiagent chemotherapy (vincristine, actinomycin D, and cyclophosphamide) and radiation therapy.[29] Partial responses are followed with extirpative surgery when feasible to maximize survival. The best survival rates have been obtained with exenterative surgery, but improvements in chemotherapy regimens have made bladder-conserving approaches possible, as above.

### Trauma

***Kidney.*** Injuries to the kidney in infants and children suffering from blunt trauma are associated with an underlying anomaly in up to 25% of cases.[30] Lack of perinephric fat, larger relative renal size, and nonrigid rib cage make injury from blunt trauma more likely than in the adult. Renal arterial or venous disruptions may be present with minimal or no hematuria, and should be suspected in major deceleration injuries. Computed tomography will demonstrate the degree of parenchymal disruption, nonfunction, and associated injuries. Emergent repair represents the only possible course for salvage of the involved kidney in vascular injuries. Injuries extending to the collecting system may be managed expectantly in selected cases. Emergent repair may decrease complications but may also end in preventable nephrectomy. Penetrating injuries require exploration more often, and arteriography is often helpful in man-

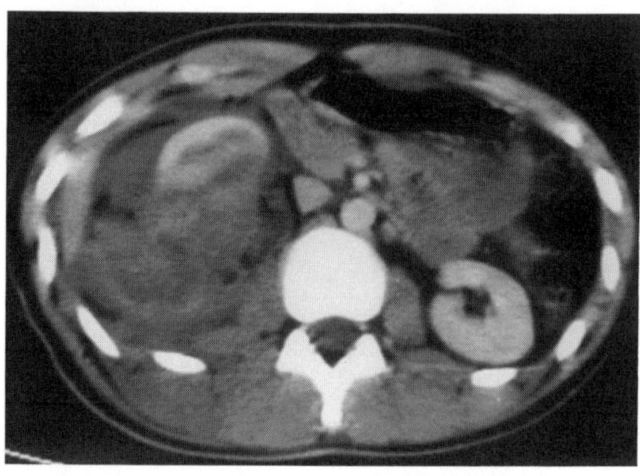

Fig 6. CT scan of a patient with a right flank stab wound with a large hematoma, anterior renal displacement, and laceration of the kidney.

agement, in addition to the previously described tests (Fig 6).

***Ureter.*** Ureteral injuries are rare, but must be suspected especially in blunt trauma associated with hyperextension or lateral flexion of the trunk. Extravasation or obstruction on excretory urography is suggestive of injury, and it is especially important to suspect a disruption at the ureteropelvic junction in such a situation. Prior to exploration a retrograde pyelogram (in the absence of other injuries) may identify a forniceal disruption and render exploration unnecessary.

***Bladder.*** The relatively intra-abdominal location of the pediatric bladder causes it to be more vulnerable to trauma. Most bladder disruptions are extraperitoneal and 70% are associated with pelvic fractures.[30] Most extraperitoneal and a few intraperitoneal ruptures may be managed with prolonged bladder drainage. Exploration for repair of typical intraperitoneal rupture and extraperitoneal injury with associated bony fragments is the appropriate therapy.

***Urethra.*** Acute disruptions of the urethra occur most commonly in males at the membranoprostatic junction. Suprapubic drainage is appropriate when gross blood is seen at the urethral meatus and when a retrograde urethrogram demonstrates extravasation. Urethral catheter placement is avoided in suspected injuries to protect the patient from increasing the extent of disruption. Reanastomosis of the disruption in the acute phase of injury is advocated by some, and there may be fewer late strictures using this approach. The need to enter the pelvic hematoma, possibly increasing the chance for infection, and the worry about iatrogenic injury to periurethral nerve bundles by this approach have led many surgeons to adopt suprapubic drainage with secondary repair as their preferred treatment.

***Penis.*** Blunt trauma to the penis usually results in minor injury with contusion and hematoma, but without corporal disruption. These injuries are managed with reassurance. A urethrogram is not warranted, and may precipitate retention. Major penile trauma is associated with disruption of the corpora cavernosum and/or spongiosum. These injuries necessitate a urethrogram followed by surgical repair to limit subsequent scarring and complications. Lacerations and skin avulsion are managed by debridement and primary repair. Avulsions that result in complete degloving or isolated distal skin islands are managed by debridement of the distal skin and split-thickness skin grafting. Removal of distal skin islands prevents complications of chronic lymphedema.

***Zipper Injuries.*** Zipper injuries of the penis occur when the glans, or, more commonly, the foreskin is caught by the zipper mechanism. Cutting the median bar of the zipper slide allows separation and release of the trapped skin. This results in a minimal abrasion to the area and can be performed with little or no sedation.[31–33]

**Adrenal Hemorrhage.** Adrenal hemorrhage may be massive and is a true urologic emergency. Birth trauma appears to be the most significant etiologic factor, but asphyxia, septicemia, and bleeding disorders may be contributory.[34] The right adrenal gland is more commonly affected, possibly related to direct transmission of vena caval pressure increases via the short central vein.[35] In theory, the relatively large and hypervascular neonatal adrenal is more at risk for injury than its more protected infant and childhood counterpart.[36] Hemodynamic instability from massive hemorrhage and adrenal rupture is initially managed with transfusion awaiting tamponade of bleeding. Surgery is reserved for those who fail to stabilize during nonoperative therapy or who experience repeated episodes of hemodynamic shock. Bilateral lesions may induce adrenal insufficiency.

In less emergent cases, diagnosis is supported by a palpable abdominal mass with localization to the suprarenal area on ultrasound imaging. Excretory urography may demonstrate displacement of the kidney by a nonenhancing mass, but nonvisualization of the ipsilateral kidney is often noted (possibly secondary to renal vein thrombosis). HVA and VMA levels in the urine are obtained to assess the possibility of hemorrhage into a neuroblastoma. With normal urine levels of VMA and HVA, adrenal hemorrhage may be from neuroblastoma in situ which is of questionable pathologic significance.[37] In cases where neuroblastoma is felt to be unlikely, serial radiographic imaging with resolution of the mass will confirm the diagnosis. Older children should be carefully evaluated because bleeding into or hemorrhage from an adrenal malignancy may occur.[38]

**Renal Vein Thrombosis.** Renal vein thrombosis classically presents in the neonate with gross hematuria, an abdominal mass, and dehydration or sepsis. Nephrotic syndrome, maternal diabetes, and shock are also associated factors. Renal vein thrombosis is diagnosed in one of five children with gross hematuria in the first month of life, and 50% of cases occur by 2 months of age. Thrombosis begins within small vessels in the kidney, propagating to the main renal vein and occasionally to the vena cava. Ultrasound examination will demonstrate an enlarged kidney that lacks evidence of hydronephrosis (Fig 7A); a clot within the renal vein may be demonstrated. Excretory urography or renal scintigraphy will show evidence of diminished renal function and perfusion (Fig 7B). Definitive diagnosis is achieved by venocavography or magnetic resonance imaging. Platelet count, fibrinogen level, and hematocrit are consistently decreased.

Treatment via supportive fluids, maintenance of electrolyte balance, and institution of systemic anticoagulation with heparin (only after documentation of normal fibrin-split products to exclude disseminated intravascular coagulation) may be helpful.[39] Urokinase instituted early in the course of care has likewise proven effective.[40,41] Bilateral severe disease should cause one to consider acute surgical excision of thrombus.[42] Some children suffer progressive azotemia, and this may occur in severe bilateral lesions. Long-term follow-up to detect hypertension and manage renal insufficiency is essential. Improved treatment will probably involve direct infusion or systemic application of thrombolytic agents, once the safety and efficacy of standardized doses are more well established.

**Renal Cortical Necrosis.** Renal cortical necrosis occurs as a result of renal ischemia. This may occur particularly in the neonate as a result of placental abruption, shock, dehydration, and hypoxemia.[43] Clinically the infants may display pallor or cyanosis and flaccidity. Effects are commonly bilateral, and pathologically there are areas of hemorrhagic necrosis isolated to the cortex reminiscent of the histology of renal vein thrombosis, from which it must be distinguished. Inferior venocavography serves to exclude renal vein thrombosis, and CT findings of nonenhancing renal cortex, enhancement of renal medulla, and

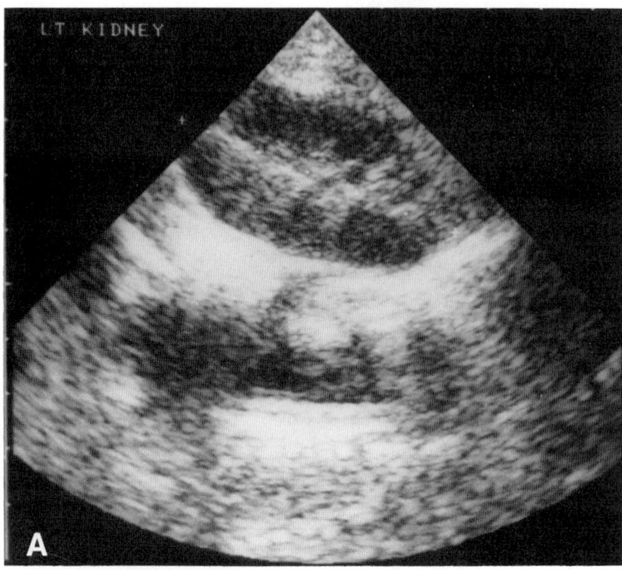


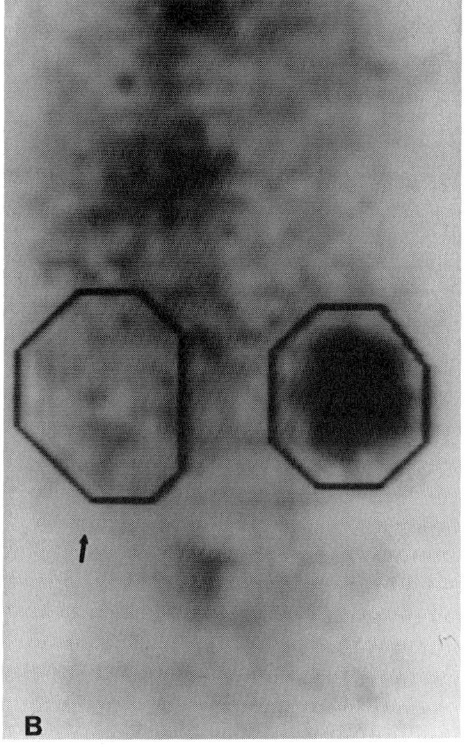


**Fig 7. A,** Longitudinal sonogram of left renal vein thrombosis in a newborn. There is enlargement of the kidney (55 mm compared to 39 mm on the normal contralateral side) and loss of cortico-medullary differentiation; **B,** Tc 99 DTPA renal scan of the same patient, demonstrating poor uptake in the effected left kidney (arrow). [From Kalalis PP, King LR, Belman AB, eds, *Clinical Pediatric Urology,* 3rd ed (Philadelphia: WB Saunders; 1992;2:1317, 1319), with permission.]

absent renal function may preclude biopsy for diagnosis.[44] Treatment is supportive but the outcome is usually fatal.

**Renal Artery Thrombosis.** Renal artery thrombosis is rare and its increasing incidence is probably due to umbilical artery catheterization.[45] Clinical signs include hypertension, hematuria, and congestive heart failure. Azotemia and proteinuria are present.[46] Nonvisualization of the involved kidney on excretory urography is a confirmatory finding. Survivors have been treated with unilateral nephrectomy, but intra-arterial thrombolytic therapy may be considered if rapid diagnosis is made.

**Child Abuse.** The National Center for Child Abuse and Neglect has defined sexual abuse as any contact or interaction between a child and an elder where the child is used for sexual stimulation of that individual or another.

Vaginal examination may suggest a possibility of abuse, but it is vital that measurements be extremely accurate because of the variability of normal hymenal diameter and introital appearance.[47,48] Laboratory examination of cervicovaginal secretions includes inspecting for spermatozoa, prostate specific antigen, acid phosphatase, and seminal vesical proteins.

Pregnancy and sexually transmitted diseases after rape can be devastating dilemmas for the traumatized child and adolescent. Pregnancy can be prevented by high-dose estrogens administered postcoitally in the majority of cases. Sexually transmitted diseases can be conveyed via the birth canal, but maternal history and exam in conjunction with knowledge of infection incubation periods should allow identification of abuse-related diseases. Definitive diagnosis is a prerequisite to filing charges of abuse.[49]

Appropriate training is available to increase awareness and understanding of the many manifestations of child abuse.[50]

**Perforation of Augmentation Cystoplasty.** Intestinal augmentation of the bladder in myelodysplastic children is now common practice. Due to the neurologic lesion present in these patients, most empty their augmented bladder by intermittent catheterization.[51] Perforation of an augmentation cystoplasty results in peritonitis, abdominal pain, and sepsis. Clinical symptoms may vary in degree, but a high index of suspicion must be maintained to prevent fatal outcome. Ventriculoperitoneal shunts must be tapped in cases of sepsis to exclude infection. The exact etiology of perforation has not been settled but infection, nondistensibility, adhesions, and sustained elevation of intravesical pressure may be culprits.[52] Catheter trauma, however, seems to have the most pervasive influence on perforation.[53]

Abdominal x-rays and ultrasound may detect intraperitoneal fluid, and this should cause the physician to suspect perforation. A cystogram may be normal, and proves to be diagnostic in only 20% of cases.[53]

Treatment requires emergent celiotomy under the coverage of broad-spectrum antibiotics, the selection of which can be guided by urine Gram stain. Repair of leaks at the time of surgery is facilitated by distention of the bladder with an indwelling catheter. Bladder drainage is maintained until full recovery, and the integrity of the repair should be verified by cystography prior to catheter removal.

### Risk to the Organ System or Systemic Problems

**Phimosis.** Only 4% of neonates are found to have fully retractable foreskin. Intervention for the nonphysiologic stenosed prepuce (phimosis) is warranted for treatment of balanitis or intractable preputial infection. Dorsal slit is performed in the presence of severe infection that is unresponsive to local measures and systemic antibiotics, with subsequent circumcision performed after resolution of inflammation. Rarely, the phimotic ring is so narrow that the flow of urine is impeded, and this would also constitute a need for treatment of the scar or a complete circumcision.

**Paraphimosis.** Preputial retraction proximal to the glans for a prolonged period of time causes edema within the foreskin and progressive constriction about the penis, restricting replacement of the prepuce. With time the glans may become engorged, and necrosis has been reported. Forcible reduction of the prepuce is accomplished by squeezing the swollen foreskin circumferentially to reduce distal edema. At this point, facing the patient and with forefingers on preputial edges and thumbs on the glans, the foreskin is replaced. *Rarely* the constricting band of tissue requires an incision to release the skin for reduction.

**Circumcision.** Whether prudent care or unnecessary surgery, circumcision can be a source of emergent complications. Infection, bleeding, and significant surgical trauma may result from this operation. Bleeding is usually nominal and relieved by local pressure. Massive bleeding may require surgical revision and transfusion.[54] Surgical trauma occurs primarily with the misuse of cautery and may prove disastrous.[55]

Urethral abnormalities and chordee should preclude neonatal circumcision until parents are counseled regarding the possible need for future surgical repair. Children with incontinence and/or neurologic deficits (ie, myelomeningocele) should be left uncircumcised as glanular erosion may become a problem if foreskin protection is eliminated.

**Acute Scrotum.** Acute scrotal pain or swelling in children is spermatic cord torsion until proven otherwise. Early exploration has been advocated in the literature even though 50% of interventions prove nontherapeutic.[56] In any event, suspected neonatal and childhood torsion demand emergency evaluation in order to maximize testicular salvage (Fig 8A–C).

The majority of cases of neonatal torsion present at birth and should be considered a prenatal event. Bilateral lesions have been reported and warrant emergent surgery.[57] Physical findings include swelling, scrotal discoloration, and testicular enlargement. Color Doppler imaging (CDI) may be used to detect subtle intratesticular blood flow, and direct exploration in equivocal cases, or those with delayed presentation, is advocated by many.[58] While controversy exists regarding the approach to surgical exploration (inguinal versus scrotal), the literature supports each option.[59] Contralateral orchidopexy, or at least reflection of the tunica vaginalis, has been suggested, but this remains controversial in the neonatal group, since most cases involve extravaginal torsion, and contralateral orchidopexy is designed to prevent intravaginal torsion. The need for contralateral orchidopexy has been well established in cases of torsion outside the neonatal group, since the incidence of asynchronous torsion can be up to 50%.[60,61] In the older child differential diagnoses include epididymo-orchitis, appendix torsion, and spermatic cord torsion. Epididymitis is exceedingly rare in the prepubertal male, and is characterized by gradual onset of discomfort, and leukocytes on urinalysis.[62] The presence of an active cremasteric reflex provides supportive evidence for absence of torsion and should stimulate reevaluation of those felt to have spermatic cord torsion.[63] Diagnostic imaging with scintigraphy is quite accurate, but nonspecificity of the "rim sign" has been reported.[64,65] CDI accurately depicts testicular ischemia and is 100% accurate in diagnosis of testicular torsion.[66] In addition, interobserver variability is decreased with CDI and the study is extremely expedient and reproducible.[67] CDI can also diagnose both epididymitis and torsion of the testicular appendage with little delay in therapy.[58]

Epididymoorchitis is managed with antibiotic therapy and scrotal rest. In the prepubertal male, genitourinary anomalies (ie, ureteral ectopia) should be sought in all cases of epididymitis that are associated with documented urinary tract infection.[68] Torsion of the appendix testis is managed with observation and analgesics, although surgical removal of the appendage may occasionally decrease the recovery period in some patients, but at the expense of the risk from anesthesia.

**Urolithiasis.** Two to three percent of all urinary calculi occur in children.[69] Neonatal renal calcification poses no immediate threat to the premature infant as long as there is no evidence for obstruction. A diagnosis suspected by abdominal x-rays is confirmed by ultrasound documentation of calcification about the renal papillae in one or both kidneys. Lasix and glucocorticoid therapy for bronchopulmonary dysplasia, relative hypophosphatemia, and low birth weight are risk factors for stone formation.[70–72] Parathormone levels are invariably normal, and infection is rarely found in these neonates. Observation is presently considered reasonable therapy although thiazide diuretics, used singly or in con-

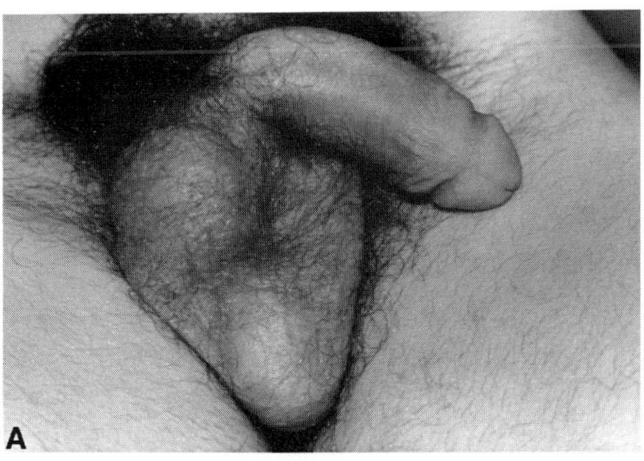

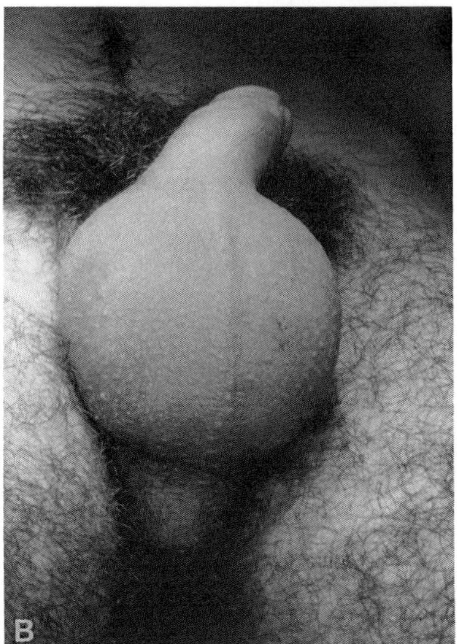

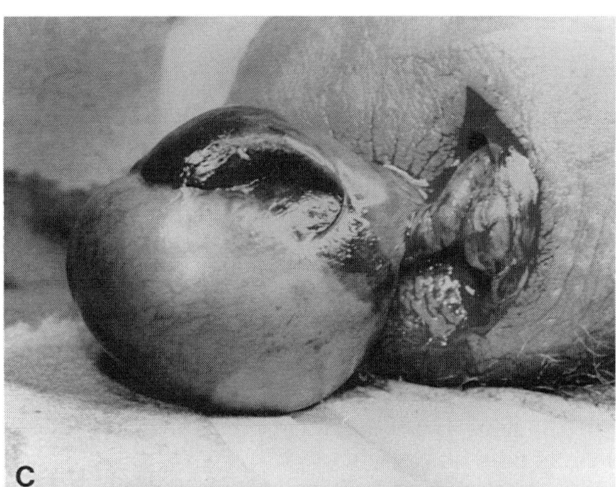

**Fig 8.** **A,** Early right testis torsion. There is no inflammation, the testis is elevated in the scrotum, and it is a bit swollen; **B,** 48-hour left testis torsion. The entire scrotum is erythematous and swollen; **C,** same patient as in **B.** The twisted spermatic cord is seen cephalad to the infarcted testis.

junction with phosphate supplements, have been shown to dissolve calcifications.[73]

Urolithiasis in children may cause hematuria both gross and microscopic. Bladder stones are the most common form of childhood calculus disease and is seen in endemic regions.[74] In Western society, one third of calculi are idiopathic and the remainder due to metabolic disorders.[75] Current therapy includes extracorporeal shock wave lithotripsy, endoscopic antegrade and retrograde stone manipulation, and open stone surgery. The latter treatment remains particularly helpful in removal of renal calculi associated with ureteropelvic junction obstruction at the time of repair and staghorn stones in association with infundibular stenosis.

**Ambiguous Genitalia.** Newborns with ambiguous genitalia pose a potential medical and a definite personal emergency. With thorough and compassionate evaluation these infants are spared medical complications and assigned a gender of rearing in an expedient fashion. Assignment of neutral names should be discouraged, and premature reporting of chromosomal sex should be avoided, as both actions may hinder parental adjustment to plans that sometimes pit genetic sex against the sex of rearing.

A history of prior neonatal deaths, family history of sterility or amenorrhea, maternal medication use during pregnancy, and gestational course all may suggest diagnoses. If bilateral inguinal or scrotal gonads are palpated, diagnosis in the neonate is that of a chromosomal male until otherwise proven. In contrast, bilateral impalpable gonads should suggest a female until further evaluation to detect a uterus, vaginal development, and absent testes is performed.[76] Phallic appearance is a highly misleading finding (Fig 9).

Laboratory evaluation includes 17-ketosteroid levels, buccal smear for Barr body (present in 20% of females), and peripheral leukocyte karyotyping. Ultrasound confirms the presence of uterus and internal Müllerian structures. A genitogram may accurately delineate urogenital sinus anatomy. Exploratory gonadal biopsy along with assays of tissue hormone receptors and tissue enzyme levels (ie, 5α-reductase activity) aids in appropriate gender assignment.

Congenital adrenal hyperplasia accounts for 90% of female pseudohermaphrodites and certain cases of male pseudohermaphrodites. With appropriate steroid replacement and genital reconstruction as warranted, these children may be reared in concert with their genetic sex. Enzymatic defects in the biosynthetic pathway of cortisol lead to accumulation of metabolically active precursors and deficiency of steroids that maintain normal fluid and electrolyte homeostasis. Deficiency of 21-hydroxylase and 3β-hydroxysteroid dehydrogenase leads to lack of mineralocorticoid activity and a relative salt-wasting condition. In 20% of these neonates, failure to diagnose and replace steroid deficiency will lead to vascular collapse within 2 weeks of birth. 11-Hydroxylase deficiency leads to increased levels of deoxycorticosterone, resulting in salt retention and hypertension. This hypertension may contribute to a patent ductus anteriosus, bronchopulmonary dysplasia, renal cortical necrosis, or necrotizing enterocolitis in the newborn. Treatment is by steroid replacement.

Evaluation of the upper urinary tract in patients with ambiguous genitalia may be reserved for those with additional anomalies of the urogenital and nongenitourinary systems.

## Need for Urgent Evaluation

**Bladder Exstrophy.** Classical bladder exstrophy consists of pubic diastasis, a midline abdominal wall defect, and exposed posterior bladder wall. The incidence is approximately 1 in 30,000 live births. Closure is performed within 72 hours of birth. Spina bifida, imperforate anus, vaginal malformations, and ventricular septal defects occur in nearly 10% of patients.

Long-term outcome with regard to renal function, continence, and potency is improved by early intervention.[77,78] Initial management of the exposed bladder is to

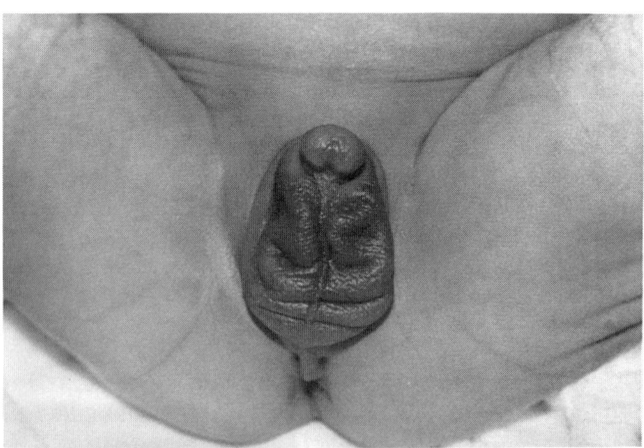

**Fig 9.** XX infant, 3 days old, with severely masculinized external genitalia due to congenital adrenal hyperplasia.

maintain a moist coverage to prevent trauma.

**Imperforate Anus.** Genitourinary abnormalities occur in up to 50% of cases of imperforate anus. The presence of a perineal fistula, anal stenosis, or anal fistula indicates a low defect; absence of an anal dimple or the finding of a "flat bottom" suggests a high anomaly that is associated with an increased incidence of urinary tract abnormalities.

Emergent urologic evaluation is warranted if urosepsis occurs or if evaluation demonstrates meconium, squamous cells, or gas in the urinary tract. These findings suggest an enterovesical (or urethral) fistula.[79] Care must be taken to follow these patients carefully, as they may develop hyperchloremic acidosis, and if infection intercedes they should be treated promptly.[80]

Renal agenesis, dysplasia, ureteropelvic junction obstruction, and horseshoe kidney have been associated frequently with supralevator lesions and less often with low malformations.[81] Genital tract anomalies, uterine and vaginal deformities, and hydrocolpos have been noted.[82]

Due to the significant incidence of genitourinary abnormalities in relation to imperforate anus, it benefits the patient to have the urologist involved in management and reconstructive plans.[83–85] Correction of imperforate anus may intimately involve the lower urinary tract, and the urologist should be available at surgery for consultation and assistance.[86]

**Myelomeningocele and Occult Spina Bifida.** Evaluation of patients with myelomeningocoele should be performed prior to closure of the spinal canal. Innervation of the genitalia, anal sphincter, and lower extremities should be documented. Emergent neurosurgical intervention to prevent infection or injury may preclude postvoid residual measurement and bladder outlet assessment. After recovery from the spinal closure, inadequate bladder emptying is managed with intermittent catheter drainage or vesicostomy as needed. Even if the preoperative ultrasound displayed no hydronephrosis, spinal shock after closure causes hydronephrosis in 3% of children, if only on a temporary basis.[87] If upper tract assessment is normal and there is little to no outlet resistance, Credé may be carefully substituted for the catheterizations. Renal function is monitored periodically and surgical intervention for reflux and incontinence is addressed later in childhood, as long as there is no functional deterioration. The presence of bladder emptying pressures greater than 40 cm $H_2O$ should prompt concern for eventual upper tract deterioration[88] and has led some to recommend active intervention to relieve these pressures even if the upper tracts are still normal.[89]

Occult spina bifida can be an insidious problem, marked only by urinary or bowel difficulties and cutaneous stigmata in the lumbar or sacral areas that are clues to the underlying neurologic disorder (Fig 10A, B). It is important to maintain a high level of awareness of the possibility of this diagnosis when faced with voiding complaints in an otherwise healthy individual. A negative neurologic exam, in addition to the standard office evaluation for such complaints, should be enough to rule out this possibility.

**Multicystic Dysplastic Kidney.** Multicystic dysplastic kidney (MCDK) is the most common cystic mass of the abdomen in neonates and the second most frequently encountered mass in infants.[90] The diagnosis is usually established by a characteristic appearance on ultrasound imaging, supported by renal scintigraphy documenting "nonfunction" of the mass[91] (Fig 11). Fewer than 13% of MCDKs are detected by palpation of an abdominal mass. The contralateral kidney should be examined for evidence of ureteropelvic junction obstruction, megaureter, or renal ectopia and fusion, or reflux, which may occur in 30% of cases.[92]

At the present time there are two equally divided schools of thought on the appropriate treatment of MCDK. Lesions may be observed for regression, reserving excision for those masses found to persist or enlarge on subsequent ultrasound studies. Based on case reports of hypertension, cyst

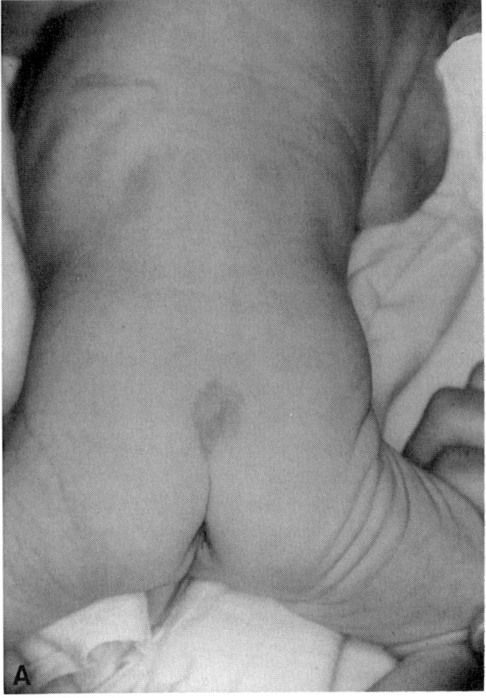


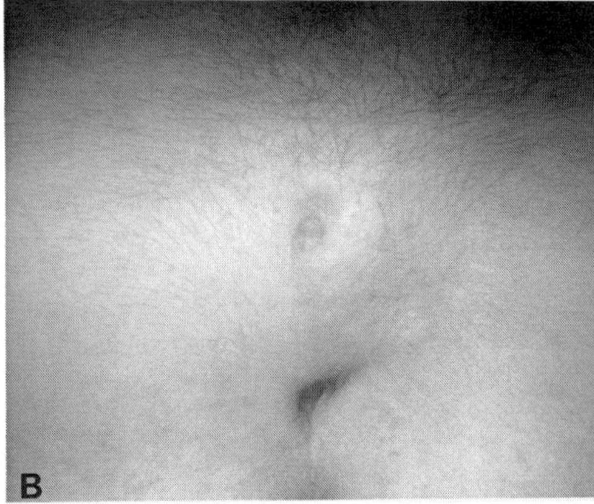


**Fig 10. A,** Neonate with lumbosacral hemangioma and congenital sacral cerebrospinal fluid fistula; **B,** 1-year-old female with a sacral dimple and cutaneous signs of spina bifida. [Fig 10A courtesy of William Chadduck, MD.]

infection, and documentation of nodular renal blastema in pathology specimens, recommendation has also been made for the routine resection of the MCDK in early infancy.[93,94]

**Ureteropelvic Junction Obstruction.** Ureteropelvic junction (UPJ) obstruction is the most common cause of hydronephrosis in neonates and infants.[95] In the absence of ascites or sepsis, the indication for emergent surgical repair is currently controversial. This debate is largely based on the questionable accuracy of currently utilized techniques (ie, renal scintigraphy, pressure flow studies) in the diagnosis of ''obstruc-

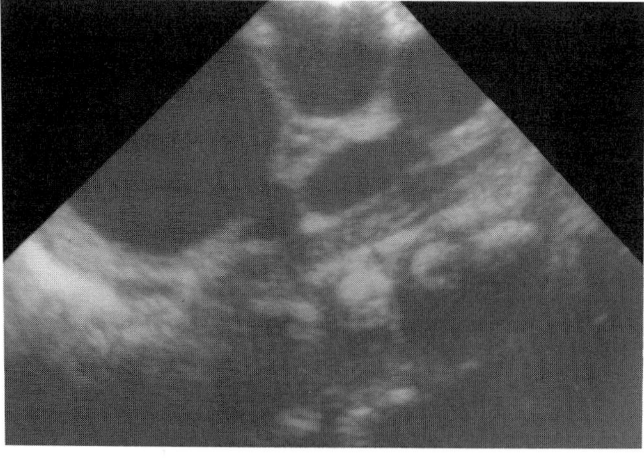

**Fig 11.** Sonogram of a multicystic dysplastic kidney. There are multiple noncommunicating cysts with some parenchyma seen.

tion in the neonate.'' The use of prophylactic antibiotics while the child is under evaluation or observation should be considered because the most common complication of UPJ obstruction in childhood is infection.[96] Vesicoureteral reflux with secondary UPJ obstruction should be assessed by conventional voiding cystourethrography. Excretory urography may contribute additional diagnostic information regarding a possible crossing vessel as a component of the obstruction, and also regarding ureteral integrity. Retrograde study of the ureter at the time of repair is sometimes advocated.[97]

The timing of surgical repair of physiologically significant obstruction is based on a desire to preserve renal function and prevent the risk of injury from prolonged drainage impairment or intercurrent infection. While an observation approach may avoid unnecessary operation on questionable lesions, a delay of surgery may have a negative impact on long-term results.[98] Postobstructive diuresis may occur in the perioperative period in the neonate.[99] Losses from this complication may be excessive, and lack of nephrostomy tube drainage may hinder diagnosis.

**Ectopic Ureterocele.** Ectopic ureterocele is the most common cause of bladder outlet obstruction in girls and is second to posterior urethral valves as a cause of obstruction in boys. Diagnosis is suggested by a history of poor or intermittent urinary stream. A family history of ureteral duplication in patients with obvious symptoms should suggest this diagnosis as well. The child may have previously experienced an episode of urinary tract infection or sepsis. Any neonatal girl with bladder distention, anuria, or ascites should be evaluated for the presence of an ectopic ureterocele.[7]

Ultrasound examination classically demonstrates hydronephrosis, accompanied by bladder distention with an intravesical lesion characterized by an echogenic rim protruding toward the bladder neck. Older children may form stones within a ureterocele, appearing as acoustic shadowing foci on ultrasonography.

The septic child requires supportive therapy with correction of acid–base and electrolyte imbalances and institution of broad-spectrum antibiotic coverage. While an ectopic ureterocele may obstruct the bladder outlet, it more commonly causes unilateral hydronephrosis with ureteral blockage. When conservative therapy fails to stabilize signs of systemic infection, emergent treatment of the ureterocele is warranted. Nephrostomy drainage via percutaneous access may provide ample relief of obstruction to allow patient recovery and elective definitive therapy. Endoscopic unroofing of an obstructive ureterocele has proven safe and efficacious. In addition, endoscopic incision potentially negates the need for further surgical procedures.[100,101] In order to avert further complications from the prolapsing walls of the ureterocele following incision, quite often a complete repair may be warranted. This surgery entails resection or drainage of the upper pole moiety of a duplex system, and marsupialization or excision of distal ureteral segment as a single or staged procedure.[102,103]

**Ectopic Ureter.** Ureters that enter the bladder caudal to their normal position on the trigone or end in other structures of mesonephric duct origin are considered to be ectopic.[104] Ectopia occurs more commonly in girls and in these neonates is likely to subtend the upper pole of a duplicated collecting system. In males the vast majority of ectopic ureters drain single collecting systems.[105] The child with an ectopic ureter draining a duplicated system will also have contralateral duplication 10% of the time, 80% without ectopia and 20% with ectopic insertion.[106] Rarely the ectopic ureter with its associated obstruction will originate in the lower pole moiety of a duplication while the upper pole ureter demonstrates reflux in violation of both statistics and the Meyer–Weigert law.[107,108]

Bladder neck ectopia may present as an abdominal mass or be mistaken for a massive retroperitoneal abscess.[108,109] Ureters that are ectopic outside of the urinary tract, and especially those with a more caudal insertion, are less likely to present as abdominal masses, as they commonly drain dysplastic kidneys or poorly functioning upper pole systems. Acute intervention is reserved for resistant infections or recurrent complications. Surgical procedures to establish renal drainage, when adequate parenchyma is present, or resect systems with little salvagable function (<10% perfused parenchyma) are pursued on an elective basis.

**Megaureter.** Primary megaureter represents an additional abnormality that may be diagnosed by palpation of an abdominal mass or on an ultrasound image as hydroureteronephrosis. In the diagostic evaluation, renal scintigraphy, voiding cystourethrography, and excretory urography are often complimentary and necessary to establish a "primary" etiology. Classification of megaureters as refluxing, obstructive, and nonrefluxing/nonobstructive may require an antegrade pyelogram and at times pressure-perfusion measurements.[110]

Acute intervention is most likely to be warranted in cases of obstructed megaureter, usually in the setting of urinary tract infection. Initial management with antibiotic therapy is supplemented with percutaneous nephrostomy drainage in recalcitrant cases. In order to optimize renal function and minimize any risk of complications, surgical repair in the neonate has been recommended to establish drainage, or, in cases of refluxing ureters, to prevent possible nephropathy. The need for aggressive neonatal intervention is not universally accepted.[111]

**Hydrocolpos (Hydrometrocolpos).** Hydrocolpos, cystic dilatation of the vagina, and hydrometrocolpos, distention of both vagina and uterus, occur secondary to vaginal obstruction in the neonate due to congenital anomalies. Simple hydrocolpos occurs as a result of an imperforate hymenal membrane, persistent vaginal septum, or primary vaginal atresia. Complex vaginal obstructions are associated with a urogenital sinus anomaly or cloacal malformation.[112]

Ultrasound examination delineates a midline cystic mass and is able to demonstrate a separate bladder in only 50% of complex cases.[113] In the neonate, most patients diagnosed with hydrocolpos have the simple variant. After the diagnosis is certain and a urogenital sinus or persistent cloaca has been ruled out, treatment is accomplished by incision of the obstructing membrane to allow drainage of secretions and preclude infection. Drainage decreases the potential for extrinsic compression of the distal urinary tract with subsequent obstruction and the risk of secondary infection or urosepsis. Patients with a transverse vaginal septum or partial vaginal agenesis may require a vaginal pull-through procedure with separate drainage of the uterus to achieve a successful outcome.

If no mass presents at birth, these conditions usually become clinically apparent as primary amenorrhea or abdominal mass at puberty (hematocolpos). Treatment considerations at that juncture are identical to those of the neonatal patients. Differential diagnosis must also include Mayer–Rokitansky–Kuster–Hauser syndrome and cervical dysgenesis. Ultrasound imaging assists in establishing a diagnosis.[114]

**Megalourethra.** Megalourethra is a rare malformation of the penile urethra. Physical examination detects a bulging urethra, penile deformity, and may also detect signs of the prune belly syndrome. Pathogenesis consists of an arrest of spongiosal development but the cavernosal bodies may also be malformed.[115] Other associated anomalies include hydronephrosis, vesicoureteral reflux, and renal dysplasia, and therefore full urinary tract investigation is mandated. Anuria may occur but is more likely to be associated with renal dysplasia than obstruction. Early diagnosis is essential to preclude inadvertent circumcision that may complicate subsequent urethroplasty.[116]

**Prune Belly Syndrome.** Prune belly syndrome requires prompt urologic evaluation; the immediate morbidity and mortality results from respiratory distress, cardiac anomalies, and uremia.[117,118] The classic triad includes hypoplastic abdominal musculature, urinary tract abnormalities, and undescended testes (Fig 12).

Patients may be classified into three general categories. The first is characterized

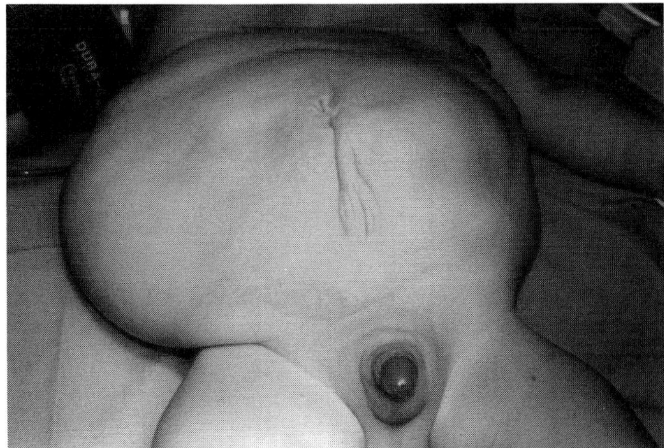

**Fig 12.** Six-month-old male with prune belly syndrome. Note the floppy abdomen, flared rib cage, and lack of fullness in the scrotum.

by urethral obstruction, oligohydramnios, and Potter's faces. Death usually results from pulmonary hypoplasia. The second group has mild impairment of renal function and may succumb in time to renal failure. The third group displays structural abnormalities of the urinary tract but has normal renal function. In these last patients, life expectancy is potentially normal if surgical and medical intervention is conducted judiciously to prevent pyelonephritis or nephropathy.[119]

Patients with this syndrome have a 50% incidence of patent urachus. Voiding cystourethrogram is usually diagnostic, but a fistulogram may be needed for definitive diagnosis. Relief of any urethral obstruction leads to spontaneous closure in most instances. If patency persists beyond 2 months, or if stones have formed (in the older child), formal excision may become necessary.

**Urethral Prolapse.** Urethral prolapse occurs predominantly in young black girls and may present as vaginal bleeding.[120] Pelvic inspection reveals protrusion of the urethral mucosa that is commonly friable and discolored. Treatment occasionally consists of excising the exuberant mucosa under anesthesia, but most patients respond easily to local therapy with sitz baths. Consideration of sexual abuse is always warranted, but this abnormality should not be confused with traumatic injuries.[121] It is important on inspection to differentiate this entity from prolapsed ureterocele and sarcoma botryoides.

## SUMMARY

This chapter has presented a grouping of clinical problems that are usually perceived as emergencies. Some need to be treated emergently or urgently, whereas others can undergo urgent evaluation prior to formulation of a management plan. Each of these entities is discussed in more detail elsewhere in this book.

## REFERENCES


1. Kasper TE, Osborne RW Jr, Semerdjian HS, Miller HC. Urologic abdominal masses in infants and children. *J Urol.* 1976;116:629–633.
2. Griscom NT. The roentgenology of neonatal abdominal masses. *Am J Roentgenol.* 1965; 93(2):447–462.
3. Zerin JW, Lebowitz RL. Pediatric uroradiology. AUA Update Series. Vol 8. Lesson 28. 1989.
4. Willi UV. Pediatric genitourinary imaging. *Curr Opin Radiol.* 1990;2:909–917.
5. Clark DA. Times of first void and first stool in 500 newborns. *Pediatrics.* 1977;60(4):457–459.
6. Dever DP, Hulbert WC, Emmens RW, Rabinowitz R. Appendiceal abscess masquerading as acute urinary retention in children. *Urology.* 1985;25(3):289–292.
7. Gonzalez R, Sheldon CA. Septic obstruction and uremia in the newborn. *Urol Clin North Am.* 1982;9(2):297–303.

8. Parkhouse HF, Barratt TM, Dillon MJ, et al. Long term outcome of boys with posterior urethral valves. *Br J Urol.* 1988;62:59.
9. Hulbert WC, Rosenberg HK, Cartwright PC, Duckett JW, Snyder HM. The predictive value of ultrasonography in evaluation of infants with posterior urethral valves. *J Urol.* 1992; 148:122–124.
10. Warshaw BL, et al. Prognostic features in infants with obstructive uropathy due to posterior urethral valves. *J Urol.* 1985;133:240.
11. Warshaw BL, Ettenger RB, Pennis AJ, et al. Progression to end-stage renal disease in children with obstructive uropathy. *J Pediatrics* 1992;100:183.
12. Scott JES. Management of congenital posterior urethral valves. *Br J Urol.* 1985;57:71.
13. D'Angio GJ, Breslow N, Beckwith JB, et al. Treatment of Wilms' tumor. Results of the Third National Wilms' tumor study. *Cancer.* 1989;64:349–360.
14. Mesrobian HJ, Kelalis PP. Wilms' tumor. AUA Update Series. Vol 19. Lesson 10. 1991:146–151.
15. Green DM, Finklestein JZ, Breslow NE, Beckwith JB. Remaining problems in the treatment of patients with Wilms' tumor. *Pediatr Clin North Am.* 1991;38(2):475–488.
16. Armstrong EA, Harwood-Nash DCF, Fitz CR, et al. CT of neuroblastomas and ganglioneuromas in children. *Am J Roentgenol.* 1981; 139:571–576.
17. Daneman A. Adrenal neoplasms in children. *Semin Roentgenol.* 1988;23(3):205–215.
18. Joshi W, Kasznica J, Walters TR. Atypical mesoblastic nephroma: Pathologic characterization of potentially aggressive variant of conventional mesoblastic nephroma. *Arch Pathol Lab Med.* 1986;110:100–106.
19. Beckwith JB, Weeks DA. Congenital mesoblastic nephroma: when should we worry? *Arch Pathol Lab Med.* 1986;110:98–99.
20. Chan HSL, Chen M, Mancer K, Payton D, Weitzman SS, Kotecha P, et al. Congenital mesoblastic nephroma: A clinicoradiologic study of 17 cases representing the pathologic spectrum of the disease. *J Pediatrics.* 1987;111:64–70.
21. Thijssen AM, Carpenter B, Jiminez C, Schillinger J. Multilocular cyst (multilocular cystic nephroma) of the kidney: a report of 2 cases with an unusual mode of presentation. *J Urol.* 1989;142:346–348.
22. Fowler M. Differentiated nephroblastoma: solid, cystic or mixed. *J Pathol.* 1971;105:215.
23. Aoyagi T, Kakudo K, Satoh S, et al. Multilocular cystic nephroma in an adult: immunohistochemical study. *J Urol.* 1987;138:397.
24. Booth CM. Renal parenchymal carcinoma in children. *Br J Surg.* 1986;73:313–317.
25. Stackpole RH, Melicow MM, Uson AC. Pheochromocytoma in children. *J Pediatrics.* 1963;63(2):315–330.
26. Whalen RK, Althausen AF, Daniels GH. Extra-adrenal pheochromocytoma. *J Urol.* 1992; 147:1–10.
27. Zimmerman D. Adrenal cortex. In: Kelalis P, King L, Belman B, eds. *Clinical Pediatric Urology.* 2nd ed. Philadelphia: WB Saunders; 1985:1235–1251.
28. Houghton PJ, Shapiro DN, Houghton JA. Rhabdomyosarcoma: from the laboratory to the clinic. *Pediatr Clin North Am.* 1991;38(2):349–364.
29. Loughlin KR, Retik AB, Weinstein HJ, Colodny AH, Shamberger RC, Delorey M, et al. Genitourinary rhabdomyosarcoma in children. *Cancer.* 1989;63:1600–1606.
30. Livne DM, Gonzalez ET. Genitourinary trauma in children. *Urol Clin North Am.* 1985;12:53–65.
31. Flowendrew R, Fishman IJ, Churchill BM. Management of penile zipper injury. *J Urol.* 1977;117:671.
32. Saraf P, Rabinowitz R. Zipper injury to the foreskin. *Am J Dis Child.* 1982;136:557–558.
33. Nolan JF, Stillwell J, Sands J Jr. Acute management of the zipper-entrapped penis. *J Emerg Med.* 1990;8:305–307.
34. Snelling CE, Erb IH. Hemorrhage and subsequent calcification of the suprarenal. *J Pediatrics.* 1935;6:22.
35. Goldhizer MA, Gordon MB. Syndrome of adrenal hemorrhage in the newborn. *Endocrinology.* 1932;16:165.
36. Smith JA, Middleton R. Neonatal adrenal hemorrhage. *J Urol.* 1979;122:674–677.
37. Guin GH, Gilbert EF, Jones B. Incidental neuroblastoma in infants. *Am J Pathol.* 1969; 51:126.
38. Khuri FJ, Alton DJ, Hardy BE, Cook GT, Churchill BM. Adrenal hemorrhage in neonates: report of 5 cases and review of the literature. *J Urol.* 1980;124:684–687.
39. Rasoulpour M, McLean RH. Renal venous thrombosis in neonates. *Am J Dis Child.* 1980;134:276–279.
40. Vogelzang RL, Moel DI, Cohn MD, Donaldson JS, Langman CB, Nemcek AA Jr. Acute renal vein thrombosis: successful treatment with intraarterial urokinase. *Radiology.* 1988;169:681–682.
41. Bromberg WD, Firlit CF. Fibrinolytic therapy for renal vein thrombosis in the child. *J Urol.* 1990;143:86–88.
42. Gonzalez R, Schwartz S, Sheldon CA, Fraley EE. Bilateral renal vein thrombosis in infancy and childhood. *Urol Clin North Am.* 1982;9(2):279–283.
43. Goergen TG, Lindstrom RR, Tan H, et al. CT appearance of acute cortical necrosis. *Am J Roentgenol.* 1981;137:176–177.

44. Jordan J, Low R, Jeffrey RB Jr. CT findings in acute renal cortical necrosis. *J Comput Assist Tomogr.* 1990;14(1):155–156.
45. Plummer LB, Mendosa SA, Kaplan GW. Hypertension in infancy: The case for aggressive management. *J Urol.* 1975;113:555.
46. Woodard JR, Patterson JH, Brinsfield D. Renal artery thrombosis in newborn infants. *Am J Dis Child.* 1967;114:191–194.
47. McCann J, Voris J, Simon M. Genital injuries resulting from sexual abuse: a longitudinal study. *Pediatrics.* 1992;89(2):307–317.
48. Gardner JJ. Descriptive study of genital variation in healthy, nonabused premenarchal girls. *J Pediatrics.* 1991;120(2):251–260.
49. Paradise JE. The medical evaluation of the sexually abused child. *Pediatr Clin North Am.* 1990;37(4):839–862.
50. Alexander RC. Education of the physician in child abuse. *Pediatr Clin North Am.* 1990;37(4):971–988.
51. Elder JS, Snyder HM, Hulbert WC, Duckett JW. Perforation of the augmented bladder in patients undergoing clean intermittent catheterization. *J Urol.* 1988;140(2):1159.
52. Sheiner JR, Kaplan GW. Spontaneous bladder rupture following enterocystoplasty. *J Urol.* 1988;140:1157.
53. Mevorach RA, Hulbert WC, Merguerian PA, Rabinowitz R. Perforation and intravesical erosion of a ventriculoperitoneal shunt in a child with an augmentation cystoplasty. *J Urol.* 1992;147(2):433, 444.
54. Wiswell TE, Geschke DW. Risks from circumcision during the first month of life compared to those for uncircumcised boys. *Pediatrics.* 1989;83(6):1011–1015.
55. Gearhart JP, Rock JA. Total ablation of the penis after circumcision with electrocautery: A method of management and long-term followup. *J Urol.* 1989;142:799–801.
56. Cass AS, Cass BP, Veeraraghavan K. Immediate exploration of the unilateral acute scrotum in young male subjects. *J Urol.* 1980;124:829–832.
57. LaQuaglia MP, Bauer SB, Eraklis A, Feins N, Mandell J. Bilateral neonatal torsion. *J Urol.* 1987;138:1051–1054.
58. Lerner RM, Mevorach RA, Hulbert WC, Rabinowitz R. Color Doppler US in the evaluation of acute scrotal disease. *Radiology.* 1990; 176:355–358.
59. Das S, Singer A. Controversies of perinatal torsion of the spermatic cord: A review, survey and recommendations. *J Urol.* 1990;143:231–233.
60. Brandt MT, Sheldon CA, Wacksman J, Matthews P. Prenatal testicular torsion: Principles of management. *J Urol.* 1992;147:670–672.
61. Hulbert WC. Management of torsion of the testicle recognized at birth. In: Gonzales ET Jr, Roth D, eds. *Common Problems in Pediatric Urology.* St. Louis: Mosby; 1991:325–332.
62. Doolittle KH, Smith JP, Saylor ML. Epididymitis in the prepubertal boy. *J Urol.* 1966;96:364–366.
63. Rabinowitz R. The importance of the cremasteric reflex in acute scrotal swelling in children. *J Urol.* 1984;132:89–90.
64. Valvo JR, Caldamone AA, O'Mara R, Rabinowitz R. Nuclear imaging in the pediatric acute scrotum. *Am J Dis Child.* 1982;136:831–835.
65. Vieras F, Kuhn CR. Nonspecificity of the "rim sign" in the scintigraphic diagnosis of missed testicular torsion. *Radiology.* 1983;146:519–522.
66. Middleton WD, Melson GL. Testicular ischemia: color Doppler sonographic findings in five patients. *Am J Roentgenol.* 1989;152:1237–1239.
67. Mevorach RA, Lerner RM, Greenspan BS, Russ GA, Heckler BL, Orosz JF, et al. Color Doppler ultrasound compared to a radionuclide scanning of spermatic cord torsion in a canine model. *J Urol.* 1991;145:428–433.
68. Siegel A, Snyder HM, Duckett JW. Epididymitis in infants and boys. Underlying urogenital anomalies and efficacy of imaging modalities. *J Urol.* 1987;138:1100–1103.
69. Vanlensieck W, Bastian HP. Clinical features and treatment of urinary calculi in childhood. *Eur Urol.* 1976;2:129–134.
70. Chevalier RL. Prenatal renal development and physiology. AUA Update Series. Vol 8. Lesson 8. 1989.
71. Karlen J, Aperia A, Zetterstrom R. Renal excretion of calcium and phosphate in preterm and term infants. *J Pediatrics.* 1985; 106(5):814–819.
72. Jacinto JS, Modaniou HD, Crade M, Strauss AA, Bosu SK. Renal calcification incidence in very low birth weight infants. *Pediatrics.* 1988;81:31–35.
73. El-Dahr S, Chevalier RL, Gomez RA. Hypercalciuria in the premature infant: Influence of diuretic therapy and phosphate depletion. *Am J Dis Child.* 1988;142:256–257.
74. Lyrdal F, Hofvander Y. Urinary bladder stones. *Trop Doctor.* 1988;18:102–104.
75. Diamond DA, Menon M. Pediatric urolithiasis. AUA Update Series. Vol 10. Lesson 40. 1991.
76. Snyder HM. Management of ambiguous genitalia in the neonate. In: King LR, ed. *Urologic Surgery in Neonates and Young Infants.* Philadelphia: WB Saunders; 1988.
77. Turner WR, Ransley PG, Williams DI. Patterns of renal damage in the management of vesical exstrophy. *J Urol.* 1980;124:412.
78. Connor JP, Hensle TW, Lattimer JK, Burbige K. Long-term followup of 207 patients with

bladder exstrophy: an evolution in treatment. *J Urol.* 1989;142:793–796.

79. Brock W, Pena A. Urologic implications of imperforate anus. AUA Update Series. Vol 10. Lesson 26. 1991.
80. Caldamone AA, Emmens RW, Rabinowitz R. Hyperchloremic acidosis and imperforate anus. *J Urol.* 1979;122:817–818.
81. Belman AB, King LR. Urinary tract abnormalities associated with imperforate anus. *J Urol.* 1972;108:823–824.
82. Fleming SE, Hall R, Gysler M, McLorie GA. Imperforate anus in females: Frequency of genital tract involvement, incidence of associated anomalies and functional outcome. *J Pediatr Surg.* 1986;21(2):146–150.
83. McLorie GA, Sheldon CA, Fleisher M, Churchill BM. The genitourinary system in patients with imperforate anus. *J Pediatr Surg.* 1987; 22(12):1100–1104.
84. Wiener ES, Kiesewetter WB. Urologic abnormalities associated with imperforate anus. *J Pediatr Surg.* 1973;8(2):151–157.
85. Parrot TS. Urologic implications of anorectal malformations. *Urol Clin North Am.* 1985; 12(1):13–21.
86. Persky L, Tucker A, Izant RJ Jr. Urological complications of correction of imperforate anus. *J Urol.* 1974;111:415–418.
87. Chiaramonte RM, Horowitz EM, Kaplan GA, et al. Implications of hydronephrosis in newborns with myelodysplasia. *JAMA.* 1987; 258:1630.
88. McGuire EJ, Woodside JR, Borden TA, et al. Prognostic value of urodynamic testing in myelodysplastic patients. *J Urol.* 1981;126:205.
89. Bauer S. Personal communication.
90. Gordon AC, Thomas DFM, Arthur RJ, et al. Multicystic dysplastic kidney: Is nephrectomy still appropriate? *J Urol.* 1988;140:1231.
91. Stuck KJ, Koff SA, Silver TM. Ultrasonic features of multicystic dysplastic kidney: expanded diagnostic criteria. *Ultrasound.* 1982; 143:217–221.
92. Peters CA, Mandell J. The multicystic dysplastic kidney. AUA Update Series. Vol 8. Lesson 7. 1989.
93. Susskind MR, Kim KS, King LR. Hypertension and multicystic kidney. *Urology.* 1989; 34:362.
94. Snyder HM, Duckett JW, Elder JS. Nodular renal blastema in a multicystic kidney. *Soc Pediatr Urol Newslett.*, April 18, 1986.
95. Brown T, Mandell J, Lebowitz RL. Neonatal hydronephrosis in the era of sonography. *Am J Roentgenol.* 1987;148:959–963.
96. Wolpert JJ, Woodard JR, Parrott TS. Pyeloplasty in the young infant. *J Urol.* 1989; 142:573–575.
97. Allen TD, Husmann DA. Ureteropelvic junction obstruction associated with ureteral hypoplasia. *J Urol.* 1989;142:353–355.
98. Roth DR, Gonzalez ET Jr. Management of ureteropelvis junction obstruction in infants. *J Urol.* 1983;129:108.
99. Boone TB, Allen TD. Unilateral post-obstructive diuresis in the neonates. *J Urol.* 1992; 147:430–432.
100. Tank ES. Experience with endoscopic incision and open unroofing of ureteroceles. *J Urol.* 1986;136:241–242.
101. Monfort G, Morrisson-Lacombe G, Coquet M. Endoscopic treatment of ureteroceles revisited. *J Urol.* 1985;133:1031–1033.
102. Decter RM, Roth DR, Gonzales T. Individualized treatment of ureteroceles. *J Urol.* 1989;142:535–537.
103. Scherz HC, Kaplan GW, Packer MG, Brock WA. Ectopic ureteroceles: surgical management with preservation of continence—review of 60 cases. *J Urol.* 1989;142:538–543.
104. Tessler AN, Mahmood P. Blind-ending duplication of ureter. *Urology.* 1973;1:46.
105. Shapiro E. The ectopic ureter. AUA Update Series. Vol 9. Lesson 31. 1990.
106. Malek RS, Kelalis PP, Strickler GB, et al. Observations on ureteral ectopy in children. *J Urol.* 1972;107:308–313.
107. Stephens FD. *Congenital Malformations of the Urinary Tract.* New York: Praeger; 1983:286.
108. Ahmed S, Pope R. Uncrossed complete ureteral duplication with upper system reflux. *J Urol.* 1986;135:128–129.
109. Uson AC, Womack CE, Berdon WE. Giant ectopic ureter presenting as abdominal mass in a newborn infant. *J Pediatrics.* 1972;90:473.
110. Stephens FD. The ABC of megaureters. In: Bergsma D, Duckett JW, eds. *Birth Defects* (original article series, vol 13). New York: Alan R. Liss; 1977.
111. Elder JS. Megaureter in children. AUA Update Series. Vol 7. Lesson 24. 1988.
112. Williams DI, Bloomberg S. Urogenital sinus in the female child. *J Pediatr Surg.* 1976; 11:51–56.
113. Nussbaum Blask AR, Sanders RC, Gearhart JP. Obstructed uterovaginal anomalies: demonstration with sonography. *Radiology.* 1991;179(1):84–85.
114. Nussbaum Blask AR, Sanders RC, Rock JA. Obstructed uterovaginal anomalies: demonstration with sonography. *Radiology.* 1991; 179(1):79–83.
115. Lockhart JL, Reeve HR, Krueger RP, et al. Megalourethra. *Urology.* 1978;12:51.
116. Appel RA, Kaplan GW, Brock WA, Streit D. Megalourethra. *J Urol.* 1986;135:747–751.
117. Geary DF, MacLusky IB, Churchill BM, McLorie G. A broader spectrum of abnormal-

ities in the prune belly syndrome. *J Urol.* 1986;135:324–326.

118. Manivel JC, Pettinato G, Reinberg Y, et al. Prune belly syndrome: clinicopathologic study of 29 cases. *Pediatr Pathol.* 1989;9:691.

119. Reinberg Y, Manivel JC, Pettinato G, Gonzalez R. Development of renal failure in children with the prune belly syndrome. *J Urol.* 1991; 145:1017 1019.

120. Abrams M, Lewis KH. Prolapse of the urethra in young girls. *J Urol.* 1954;72:222–225.

121. Johnson CF. Prolapse of urethra: confusion of clinical and anatomic characteristics with sexual abuse. *Pediatrics.* 1991;87(5):722–725.

# 47

# Anomalies of the Kidney

*Gianantonio Manzoni and Emilio Merlini*

## EMBRYOLOGY OF THE KIDNEY

Renal organogenesis begins by the third week of embryonal life with the development of the pronephros in the cervical region of the embryo. The pronephros arises from the mesodermic cells that form the nephrogenic ridge and is composed of seven tubules that fuse together forming the pronephric duct. This anlage is not apparent after the fifth week, but the pronephric duct persists and caudally it is in continuity with the mesonephric duct.

The mesonephros appears around the fourth week and is located immediately caudal to the last pronephric tubule; the duct grows distally and during its growth induces the differentiation of the mesodermic cells of the nephrogenic cord into mesonephric nephrons, which distally are in continuity with the mesonephric duct.

In humans, the mesonephros regresses by the eleventh week, when the metanephros begins to function; the mesonephric duct opens into the cloaca by the fifth week and at the same time the ureteric bud originates as a small diverticulum from the posterior surface of the distal part of the mesonephric duct, close to the urogenital sinus (anterior portion of the cloaca). The ureteric bud reaches the caudal portion of the mesonephric cord, whose cells cluster and surround the growing end of the bud, forming the metanephric blastema. By the sixth week the ureteral bud and the metanephros migrate cranially and nephrogenic differentiation of the blastema begins. The ureteral bud is essential to induce the metanephric blastema to differentiate into the definitive renal tissue.

Potter divided the development of the kidney into four phases.[1] In the first period (5th–14th week) the cranial end of the bud dilates forming an ampulla and undergoes dichotomous branching: the metanephric blastema proliferates and remains apposed to each new ampulla. Since branching is faster cranially and caudally, a reniform shape of the future kidney is established. The initial branches (three to five) dilate and form the renal pelvis and the major calyces; the next divisions (five to seven) form the collecting ducts and nephrogenic differentiation is started by the sixth division ampullae.

In the second and third phase (15th–36th week) the dichotomous branching continues and the ampullae grow peripherally inducing further generations of nephrons. After the 36th week (fourth phase) no more nephrons are induced, but the collecting tubules elongate, the proximal tubules convolute, and the loops of Henle penetrate deeper into the renal medulla, thereby contributing to the functional maturation of the kidney.

## RENAL AGENESIS

Renal agenesis is the complete absence of renal tissue and can occur bilaterally or unilaterally.

## Bilateral Renal Agenesis

Bilateral renal agenesis is rare; its incidence is 1 in 4800 births[2] and is more common in males (75%) with a familial occurrence reported.[3] Bilateral renal agenesis can be due either to a failure of the ureteral bud to develop and reach the metanephric blastema or to an absence of the nephrogenic ridge. Ashley and Mostofi showed that most anephric patients had at least a rudimentary ureter, while the structures of Wolffian origin were unaffected, thus demonstrating that the teratogenic accident occurs after the outpouching of the ureteral bud.[4] In a few cases gonads also were absent, indicating a failure of the nephrogenic ridge.

The kidneys and renal vessels are generally absent, and rarely some vestigial metanephric tissue can be found. The ureters are absent or rudimentary and the bladder is hypoplastic or absent while the adrenals are present and ovoid in shape.

Approximately 40% of the affected infants are stillborn, and those born alive don't generally survive beyond 2 days because of respiratory insufficiency. Newborns present with a typical appearance (Potter syndrome): the child has a low birth weight and looks prematurely senile, the space between the eyes is increased, and a prominent fold at the inner canthus is present; the nose is blunted; the ears are large, flabby, and low set; and a depression between lip and chin is evident. The hands are large and claw-like, while the legs are frequently bowed and clubbed. The deformations are caused by the intrauterine compression secondary to the oligohydramnios.[5] Lungs are hypoplastic, with a reduced number of bronchioles and immature alveolar tissue secondary to intrauterine compression and deficiency of amniotic fluid.[6] In approximately 50% of the patients malformations of the gastrointestinal or cardiovascular systems have been recorded. The malformation can be detected by prenatal ultrasound: absence of renal tissue, oligohydramnios, and nonvisualization of the bladder are diagnostic. After birth the diagnosis can be confirmed by ultrasonography or radionuclide studies (DMSA), while urography or arteriography are not necessary.

## Unilateral Renal Agenesis

Unilateral renal agenesis is relatively common (1/1000 live births) and is more frequently found in the male and on the left side. The condition is probably due to an early insult to the mesonephric duct and this can also explain the high incidence of coexisting genital malformations.[4] Recent evidence would suggest that some cases of apparent unilateral renal agenesis can result from the shrinkage and final disappearance of a multicystic kidney.[7] Associated genital malformations are more common in the female (40–50%) and can be secondary either to the absence of the ipsilateral Mullerian duct or to a fusion defect of the two Mullerian ducts.

The uterus can be unicornuate, septate, or didelphus, and the vagina can be normal, septate, completely duplicated with one obstructed system, or totally absent (Meyer–Rokitansky syndrome). A lower incidence of genital malformations (10–15%) is recorded in the male, where the Wolffian duct structures are defective. Absence of the vas, seminal vesicles, and ejaculatory ducts is a frequent finding; in either sex gonads are normal. Other system anomalies involve the cardiovascular, musculoskeletal, and gastrointestinal systems.[8] Despite early reports, there is no solid evidence of a greater susceptibility of the solitary kidney to infections; but an increased incidence of focal and segmental glomerular sclerosis induced by chronic hyperfiltration was recently reported in patients with a solitary kidney.[9]

Unilateral agenesis is symptomless and is generally found incidentally, although it should be looked for with hydrometrocolpos or hematocolpos in the female or absence of the vas or testis in the male. Ultrasonography and urography are generally sufficient to diagnose renal agenesis; radionuclides (DMSA) can be useful to distinguish this condition from a nonfunctioning kidney. At cystoscopy the usual findings are absence of the ureteric orifice and hypoplasia of ipsilateral hemitrigone. With modern imaging techniques cystoscopy is no longer necessary to confirm the diagnosis of a solitary kidney.

## SUPERNUMERARY KIDNEY

Supernumerary kidney is one of the rarest renal malformations; it is an accessory organ caudally or less commonly, cranially located to the normal ipsilateral kidney. The accessory kidney has its own capsule and blood supply and it can be drained by a separate ureter or by one of the two branches of a bifid ureter.[10] In many cases the supernumerary kidney is hydronephrotic and can cause urinary tract infections. Intravenous urography and radionuclide imaging are generally diagnostic. Some supernumerary kidneys have been correctly diagnosed only at operation.

## RENAL HYPOPLASIA

The term *hypoplasia* describes a small kidney resulting from a reduced number of otherwise normal nephrons. Such a miniature or ''dwarf'' kidney is rarely encountered because the vast majority of small kidneys, previously described as ''hypoplastic,'' are in fact either dysplastic or pyelonephritic. Small dysplastic kidneys are called ''hypodysplastic kidneys'' and are clinically and radiologically indistinguishable from pure hypoplastic organs. Only histology can reveal the structural features of dysplasia: primitive ducts, ductules, and glomeruli; areas of hyaline cartilage, and cortical cysts. Hypoplasia can be unilateral, bilateral, or segmental (Ask–Upmark kidney) and is thought to be caused by an inadequate branching of the ureteral bud with few reniculi. Hypoplastic kidneys present a reduced number of normal calices and their ureters' orifices can be either orthotopically or ectopically placed.[11]

The rare patients described with bilateral hypoplasia have usually presented with dehydration due to the inability of the reduced renal mass to maintain corporal homeostasis or with signs of renal tubular insufficiency.[12] A rare form of bilateral hypoplasia is oligomeganephronia, characterized by small kidneys with a reduced number of giant nephrons; its clinical presentation is renal insufficiency in the neonatal period which remains stable through childhood until adolescence, when renal failure supervenes.[13] Unilateral hypoplasia is usually asymptomatic. Segmental hypoplasia has been mainly described in severely hypertensive children and is characterized by a small kidney with one or more deep grooves on its lateral profile. Hypoplastic areas with thyroid-like tubules, sharply delimited from the adjoining normal parenchyma, are allocated under the grooves.[14] Its pathogenesis is unknown, but it could represent a segmental pyelonephritis secondary to vesicoureteric reflux.[15] When the lesion is unilateral and hypertension severe, nephrectomy is the treatment of choice.

## CYSTIC LESIONS OF THE KIDNEY

Cysts develop somewhat commonly in the kidney, can be congenital or acquired, solitary or multiple, and may involve one or both kidneys. The Committee on Terminology, Nomenclature, and Classification of the American Academy of Pediatrics (Section on Urology) has proposed a simple classification into two main groups: genetic and nongenetic renal cysts.[11] The first group comprises polycystic kidneys, both autosomal recessive and autosomal dominant variants; juvenile nephronophthisis—medullary cystic disease complex; the cysts associated with multiple malformations syndromes; and congenital nephrosis. The nongenetic group includes multicystic kidneys, multilocular cysts, simple renal cysts, medullary sponge kidneys, and acquired cystic diseases.

### Autosomal Recessive (Infantile) Polycystic Renal Disease

Recessive polycystic renal disease (RPK) is the most common renal cystic disease in children, occurring in about 1 in 10,000 live births, and includes a spectrum of phenotypically different manifestations, ranging from massive renal involvement in newborns to congenital hepatic fibrosis (CHF) in older children.[16] RPK is inherited as an autosomal recessive disease. The risk of its occurrence in siblings of affected children is 25%. The disease is characterized by the coexistence of renal and hepatic abnormalities; renal involvement is prominent in neonates and infants, whereas in children over 6 years of age kidneys are less affected and portal hypertension due to CHF is the predominating symptom. A continuum of clinical pictures exists among these two extremes and children suffering from both renal insufficiency and CHF have been reported.

RPK can be detected prenatally, but the most common presentation is that of a newborn with massively enlarged kidneys and pulmonary hypoplasia. In this setting respiratory insufficiency is the rule and is the leading cause of death in these newborns. Oliguria and Potter's face can also be present. Those who survive the perinatal period are affected by renal failure and severe arterial hypertension with congestive heart failure; in surviving patients the kidneys become progressively smaller because of a reduction in size of the cysts and interstitial fibrosis. Infants presenting before age 6 months show a less severe renal enlargement, but they still progress to renal insufficiency and systemic hypertension and develop hepatosplenomegaly. Older children fare better from the renal standpoint with only a mild renal insufficiency, but they are generally affected by severe CHF with portal hypertension and esophageal varices. Gross and microscopic findings vary with the age of children at presentation: in newborns both kidneys are massively enlarged (up to tenfold), but still remain reniform in shape; their outer surface is smooth and shows innumerable small cysts. The cut surface shows radially arranged dilated channels extending from the pelvis to the cortex, which appear microscopically as dilated collecting tubules and ducts. In older children the kidneys are smaller, ducts are less dilated, the cysts tend to be more rounded, and interstitial fibrosis is more intense; conversely, the liver is more severely affected, showing excessive periportal and interlobular fibrosis.

In RPK sonography reveals diffusely hyperechogenic enlarged kidneys with normal calices and pelvis. Intravenous urography may show, in delayed films, a dense nephrogram or, more commonly, the typical "sunray" picture due to the pooling of the contrast medium in the radially arranged dilated collecting ducts (Fig 1).

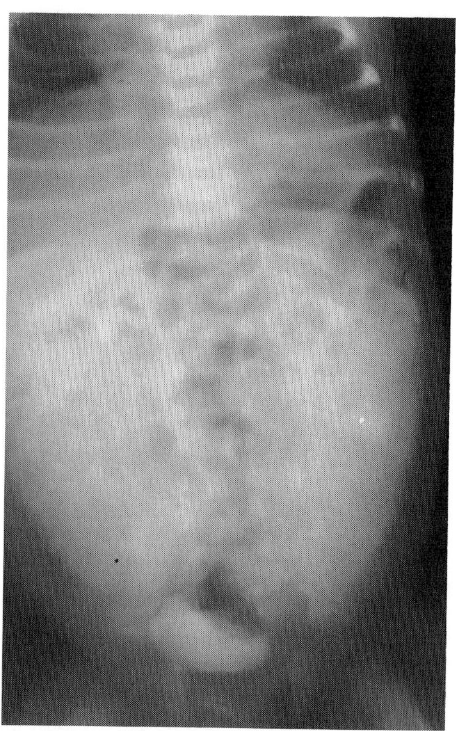

**Fig 1.** Excretory urogram of an infant with recessive (infantile) polycystic disease. Kidneys are enlarged and showing some streaky spotty parenchymal opacification.

There is no specific treatment for RPK and only supportive measures can be provided. At birth respiratory intensive care is needed and later on chronic renal dialysis and renal transplantation may be necessary, provided that the liver is not massively affected. Portal hypertension and esophageal varices may eventually require specific treatment.

### Autosomal Dominant (Adult) Polycystic Renal Disease

Dominant polycystic renal disease (DPK) is a cystic degeneration of both kidneys that normally becomes symptomatic in adulthood with less than 10% of cases presenting in the first decade of life. DPK is the third most common cause of ESRD in adults, with an incidence of 1 in 1250 live births. As a rule, it is bilateral, but in children the kidneys can be asymmetrically or asynchronously affected. Cysts can be found in the liver in 50% of cases and less commonly in the pancreas or ovaries; 30% to 40% of patients are also affected by berry aneurysms of the cerebral arteries that can cause subarachnoidal hemorrhage.

DPK is a dominantly inherited disease, with a penetrance of 100% by the eighth decade. Nevertheless, about one third of patients lack a positive family history. Reeders et al showed that the DPK locum is probably located on the short arm of chromosome 16.[17]

Macroscopically the kidneys are large, but retain their reniform shape and the cut surface reveals hundreds of fluid-filled cysts of different diameter; microscopically, cystic degeneration can involve the nephron or the collecting duct. Kanwar and Carrone described thickening and lamination of tubular basal membrane as an early lesion in DPK, suggesting that cyst formation may be ascribed to a decreased tubular compliance.[18]

Cysts begin to develop at variable ages and ultrasound has recently allowed early recognition of cysts in asymptomatic children from affected families. In one prospective study the average age at the discovery of the first cysts was 9.6 years,[19] but cysts have been exceptionally found at prenatal ultrasounds and about 30 cases of infants under 6 months have been reported in the literature.[20] Neonatal presentation often has a poor outcome while in older children the presenting symptoms are variable and usually mild. Infants are generally recognized because of a flank mass, while at a later age children present with microscopic hematuria, proteinuria, or hypertension. A urinary concentrating defect is always present and can be considered an early marker in children genetically at risk. In some patients the disease can become symptomatic in the fifth decade with flank and abdominal pain being the most common presenting symptoms. Urinary tract infection (UTI), macroscopic hematuria, and hypertension are other common complaints. Other patients remain asymptomatic and present with renal insufficiency in the sixth decade. Both groups slowly progress toward end-stage renal disease (ESRD).

Ultrasound is the most useful diagnostic tool in DPK since it is more sensitive than intravenous urography in detecting the early stages of the disease in asymptomatic individuals.[19] CT scan is invaluable in the differential diagnosis of DPK complications, such as cysts or parenchymal infections, calculi, and hemorrhage. Both ultrasound and CT scan have largely replaced intravenous urography in the diagnosis and follow-up of DPK patients.

Treatment aims to slow the progression of the disease toward renal failure, to prevent and treat complications, and to substitute function when renal failure supervenes. Conservative treatment implies dietary restrictions and pharmacologic treatment of hypertension. Renal infections are difficult to treat because few antibiotics reach therapeutically useful concentrations in the cyst fluid. Prolonged treatments and often dialysis are required.

ESRD patients require chronic hemodialysis and renal transplantation from cadaver donors most often, because of the familial nature of the disease; renal transplantation in DPK patients has achieved the same success rate as in non-DPK patients.[21]

## Multicystic Dysplastic Kidney

In multicystic dysplasia normal renal parenchyma is replaced by a randomly shaped cluster of fluid-filled cysts of variable size with the pelvis and the ureter partially or totally atretic (Fig 2). Dysplasia can involve the whole kidney or an obstructed upper moiety of a duplicated system. The cysts are variable in size and are lined by low cuboidal epithelium. Primitive ducts (the hallmark of renal dysplasia), primitive ductules and glomeruli, cartilage islands, and a few mature golmeruli can be observed in the mesenchymal stroma interposed between the cysts. Islands of nonproliferative nodular renal blastema have been reported to occur in 2% to 5% of all multicystic kidneys (MCK).[22] The incidence of MCK is approximately 1 in 4300

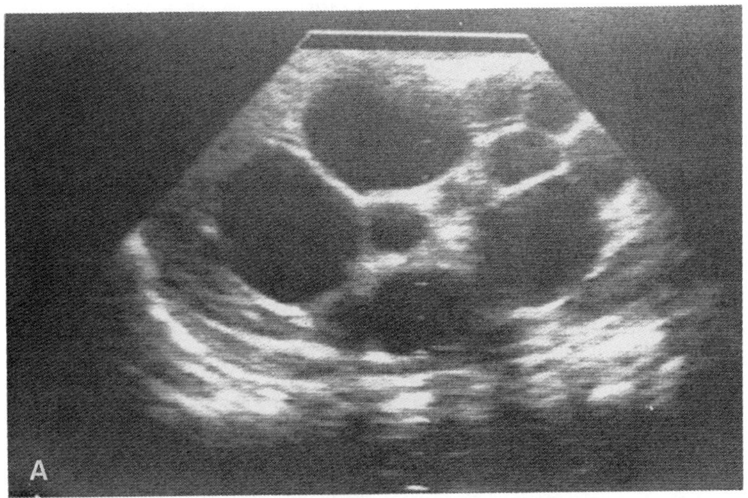


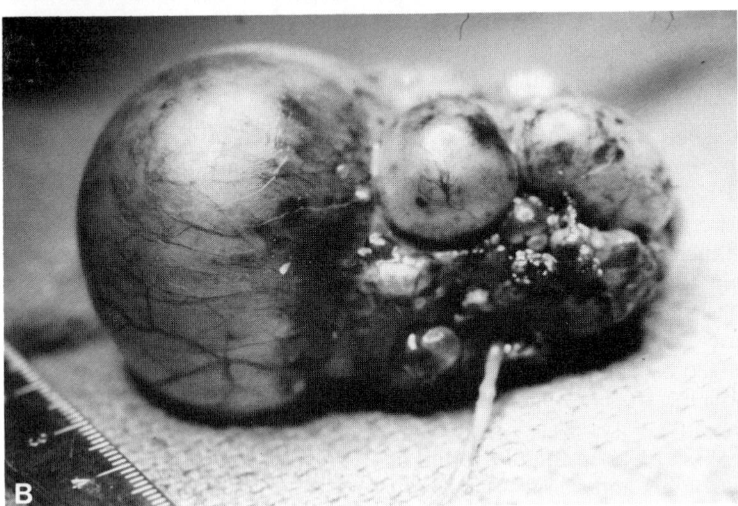


Fig 2. Male infant with prenatal diagnosis of multicystic kidney. **A,** sonogram showing multiple echolucent cysts of varying size with no discernible cortex; **B,** gross specimen of multicystic kidney.

live births and represents 10% of all fetal uropathies.[23] The contralateral kidney can be abnormal in 10% to 30% of cases, with ureteropelvic junction obstruction being the most commonly encountered anomaly. Bilateral MCK is rare and incompatible with life.

The pathogenesis of multicystic dysplasia is uncertain; controversy concerns whether fetal urinary tract obstruction can cause dysplasia or whether both ureteral obstruction and renal dysplasia are the consequence of a primitive insult to the developing urinary tract. Experimental results would suggest that fetal ureteral obstruction alone is not capable of inducing dysplasia in a normal blastema, whereas dysplasia can be produced by interfering with the normal interaction between ureteral bud and renal blastema; ureteral obstruction can further enhance the development of dysplasia.[24]

In recent years most MCKs are detected by prenatal ultrasound by the beginning of the third trimester of pregnancy,[7] but diagnostic accuracy is still rather low, about 53%.[25] The sonographic follow-up of nonoperated MCK has clarified the natural history of this disease: after birth the size of the cysts tends to decrease in most cases, leading to a small noncystic mass or even to a complete involution with inability to radiographically detect the dysplastic kidney.[26]

MCK is the most common abdominal mass in the newborn and in this group approximately 60% of MCK can be palpated as a firm mass with an irregularly lobulated surface.[27] In adults MCK is generally asymptomatic and can be incidentally found during investigations performed for other reasons, although in a few cases it has been reported to cause abdominal pain.

An abdominal mass in infants should be initially investigated by ultrasound; the sonographic criteria that identify MCK and allow differential diagnosis with hydronephrosis are the presence of interfacies between cysts with nonmedial location of the largest cyst and absence of an identifiable renal sinus. Multiplicity of cysts and absence of renal parenchyma are other confirmatory ultrasonic features[28] (Fig 2A). Differential diagnosis with hydronephrosis can be unclear in the rare ''hydronephrotic type'' of MCK in which the renal pelvis is present and dilated; in such cases intravenous urography or radionuclide imaging are mandatory. As a rule MCK is composed of nonfunctioning tissue, so it is not visualized during urography or renal scintigraphy; nevertheless a faint opacification on intravenous urogram or an uptake of DTPA on nuclear scan have both been reported in some occasional cases.[29,30]

Treatment today is highly controversial; in the past routine nephrectomy was considered to be necessary to confirm diagnosis; now newer imaging modalities have rendered ''diagnostic'' nephrectomy unnecessary. Nevertheless advocates of surgical removal of all MCK maintain that routine nephrectomy is still necessary to avoid future risks related to hypertension and to renal malignancies.[31,32]

Hypertension has been reported in nine patients with MCK and it responded to nephrectomy in only three cases.[33–35] Renal malignancy is even less common, with only seven reported cases. In four children a Wilms' tumor was found while in the other three patients (aged 15 to 68 years) the malignancy was a clear cell carcinoma.[23] It is our opinion that nephrectomy is justified when multicystic kidney is either symptomatic (respiratory embarrassment in the newborn, abdominal pain, hypertension) or if the presence of a ''mass'' causes great anxiety to the parents. Otherwise, the potential risks of leaving MCK are so low that routine nephrectomy in a healthy and asymptomatic child is not justifiable. MCK can be safely followed nonoperatively with serial ultrasounds.

## Other Cystic Diseases of the Kidney

### Genetically Transmitted Cystic Diseases

***Juvenile Nephronophthisis–Medullary Cystic Disease Complex.*** Juvenile nephronophthisis–medullary cystic disease complex (NMCD) comprises two genetically heterogeneous but clinically and pathologically similar cystic diseases of the kidney. Juvenile nephronophthisis is the autosomally recessive variety, associated with an array of nonrenal abnormalities.[36] A sixth of the patients have retinitis pigmentosa and the entity is then named renal-retinal syndrome; other ophthalmologic anomalies can occur, as well as mental retardation, cerebellar ataxia, skeletal abnormalities, and hepatic fibrosis. Nephronophthisis affects children, generally blond or red-haired, at approximately 10 years of age and is the most common cause of ESRD in adolescents.

Medullary cystic disease affects young adults (average age at onset 30 years), is not associated with other organ anomalies, and is inherited as an autosomal dominant trait. Both variants progressively lead to ESRD and the presentation is that of insidious onset of chronic renal failure: polyuria, polydipsia, severe anemia, and hypokalemia with muscular weakness secondary to renal salt wasting. Urinary concentrating defect, often causing nocturnal enuresis, usually precedes the onset of renal insufficiency. Kidneys are small and shrunken with severe tubulointerstitial fibrosis and small scattered cysts at the corticomedullary junction. Precise diagnosis relies mainly on renal biopsy. Ultrasound may reveal the small size of the kidneys with tiny medullary cysts and the absence of the corticomedullary differentiation. Due to renal insufficiency at the time of diagnosis intravenous urography is often unrewarding. Chronic hemodialysis and renal transplantation are the only specific treatments for NMCD.

***Renal Cysts Associated with Multiple Malformations Syndromes.*** Renal cysts in this group are associated with syndromes that can be classified according to the modalities of genetic transmission.[11] In chromosomal disorders such as trisomy 13 (Patau's syndrome), trisomy 18 (Edward's syndrome), trisomy 21 (Down syndrome), and trisomy C, large cysts are uncommon, but sometimes microscopic cysts of the glomerular space can be found.

In autosomal recessive syndromes such as Meckel's syndrome, Zellweger's or cerebrohepatorenal syndrome, and Jeune's or asphyxiating thoracic dystrophy syndrome, renal cysts are commonly found. Autosomal dominant syndromes such as Von Hippel–Lindau and tuberous sclerosis have extensive renal cystic involvement. Tuberous sclerosis is characterized by epilepsy, adenoma sebaceum, mental retardation, renal cysts and/or angiomyolipomas. Renal cysts can be large enough to compress normal renal parenchyma and distort the collecting system. Sonographically this can resemble DPK, and therefore, the diagnosis may be confirmed by a renal CT scan showing the presence of both renal cysts and angiomyolipomas. In Von Hippel–Lindau syndrome renal cysts are associated with cerebellar hemangiomatosis, renal angiomatosis, pheochromocytoma, renal cell carcinoma, and pancreatic cysts.

In X-linked dominant syndromes, such as *orofacio-digital syndrome type 1,* renal cysts occur later in the course of the disease and may resemble DPK.

***Congenital Nephrosis.*** Congenital nephrosis was originally described in Finland but many cases from other countries have been reported. It is inherited as an autosomal recessive disease and is characterized by microcystic dilatation of the proximal convolute tubule. Children present in the first year of life with edema, vomiting, failure to thrive, and massive proteinuria irresponsive to treatment, and death often ensues in the second or third year.

#### Nongenetically Transmitted Cystic Diseases

***Multilocular Renal Cyst (Cystic Nephroma).*** Multilocular cyst or cystic nephroma is a rare benign tumor of the kidney that occurs with equal frequency in children and in adults. It appears as a bulky, well-encapsulated, noninfiltrating cystic mass that can partially or totally replace the kidney, compressing the adjoining normal parenchyma.

Pathologic criteria for establishing diagnosis of multilocular cyst are a unilateral, solitary, multilocular cystic mass without communications between the cysts and the renal pelvis; cysts contain clear fluid and are lined by flat or cubic epithelium. The septa between the cysts are usually fibrous, but sometimes are myxomatous in children. Recently the presence of mature renal tissue in the septa has been considered to be compatible with diagnosis of cystic nephroma.[37]

When partially undifferentiated renal blastema is found in the septa, the lesion should be classified as a partially differentiated cystic nephroblastoma. This is probably a favorable histological variant of Wilms' tumor.

An abdominal mass is the usual presentation in children, whereas abdominal pain and hematuria are more common in adults. Ultrasound shows a cluster of fluid-filled cysts and CT scan usually reveals a thick-walled cystic mass compressing the adjoining kidney. Nephrectomy is the treatment of choice.

***Simple Renal Cysts.*** Simple renal cysts are extremely rare in children and their incidence increases with age. They are usually round, tense, and thin-walled fluid-filled cavities, whose diameter ranges from a few millimeters to several centimeters. Their pathogenesis is unknown and they are considered to be an acquired anomaly. Simple cysts are generally asymptomatic and are casually discovered at ultrasound or intravenous urography performed for other reasons.[38] Hypertension can rarely be the presenting sign in children.[39] Sonography shows an anechoic mass with a smooth posterior wall allowing an unequivocal diagnosis, but in equivocal cases CT scan can usually provide a better definition of the lesion. Differential diagnosis should be made with cystic Wilms' tumor, calyceal diverticulum, and pyeloureteric duplications.

When malignancy can be excluded with absolute certainty, simple cysts do not require any treatment except observation; otherwise ultrasonically guided cyst puncture with aspiration of the fluid and microscopic observation of sediment should be performed. If the cyst fluid is blood-stained or sediment is suspect, surgical exploration is indicated.

***Medullary Sponge Kidney.*** In medullary sponge kidney (MSK) dilated collecting ducts form small cysts at the papillary tips of the renal pyramids. The disease is usually bilateral and its cause is still unknown, although hereditary factors are thought to play a role. In most cases renal function remains stable throughout life, unless pyelonephritis supervenes. The disease is generally discovered in young adults, but it is not uncommon in children. The presenting symptoms are renal colic (50–60%) due to passage of calcium stones, gross hematuria (10–18%), or urinary tract infections (UTIs) (20–30%).[40] About 60% of MSK patients form and pass calculi and most of them show intraductal calcifications in the renal pyramids, probably due to urinary stasis in the dilated collecting ducts. UTIs are generally severe but respond promptly to antibiotic treatment.

Microlithiasis can cause hyperechogenicity of the pyramids, but the cysts are generally too small to be seen on ultrasound. The mainstay of the diagnosis of MSK is the excretory urogram because the contrast medium pools in the dilated pyramidal tubules, where it stagnates after the calyces have emptied, giving typical radiologic pictures (Fig 3). The morphology of the pathologic cavities has been variously described as fan-shaped or as resembling a cluster of grapes or a bunch of flowers. In the plain abdominal films renal calcifications and calcium stones are often visible. Medical treatment is directed toward prevention of lithiasis and treatment of urinary infections, while surgery or endoscopy is seldom required to treat complicated stones.

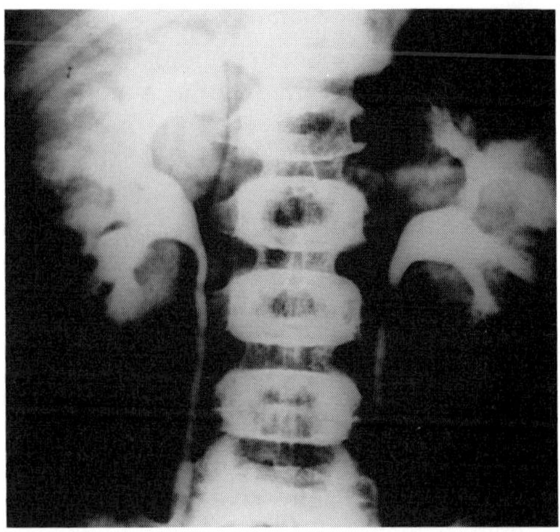

**Fig 3.** Excretory urogram of a 5-year-old boy with medullary sponge kidney. Characteristic puddling is visible, representing the contrast-filled dilated collecting tubules.

***Acquired Renal Cystic Disease.*** Patients in chronic hemodialysis often develop renal cysts that may cause intracystic or retroperitoneal hemorrhage when patients receive anticoagulants for hemodialysis. Renal tumors, most often benign and multiple, arise in 16.4% of acquired renal cystic disease patients.[41] The cysts generally tend to regress after renal transplantation.

## ANOMALIES OF ASCENT AND ROTATION

### Simple Renal Ectopia

By the end of the fifth week of gestation, the ureteral bud, originating from the Wolffian duct, acquires a cap of metanephric blastema in the region of the upper sacral somites. Through a combination of axial trunk lengthening, elongation of the ureter, intrinsic renal growth, and rotation, the metanephros ascends to a more cranial position. By the eighth week the kidney has reached its definitive retroperitoneal location, opposite the second lumbar vertebra and with the hilum facing medially. Elegant experimental work on the chick embryo demonstrated that when the caudal spine is interrupted mechanically, failure of renal ascent occurs.[42] Other factors that may contribute to abnormal ascent are failure of the ureteric bud to elongate, defective metanephric blastema, or genetic and teratogenic causes. The vascular supply to the kidney is locally derived until it reaches its final position, where the main renal arteries and veins develop. Whenever kidney occupies a position outside its normal location it is termed ectopic and represents a congenital developmental arrest. The reported incidence in an autopsy series averages about 1 in 900, without sex prevalence and with left side favored slightly.

**Pelvic Kidney.** Pelvic kidney is the most common type of simple ipsilateral renal ectopy, with its location overlying the bony pelvis and lumbosacral vertebrae. Further distinction is made between ''true pelvic'' if below the aortic bifurcation and ''lumbar'' if opposite the sacral promontory and anterior to the iliac vessels. The renal pelvis is usually anterior and its axis may be tilted or in a truly horizontal plane. The ureter is usually short and with a normal course, while the vascular supply is always anomalous and unpredictable. The pelvic kidney is more likely to be abnormal and frequently observed to be hydronephrotic either with true ureteropelvic junction obstruction or by nonobstructive dilatation due to vesicoureteric reflux or dysmorphism (Fig 4). Careful assessment must be made in these circumstances before the dilated kidney is assumed to be obstructed and treatment is instituted. The contralateral kidney may be abnormal in up to 50% of patients with a high incidence of contralateral agenesis, suggesting a teratogenic factor affecting both kidneys.[43] Associated anomalies are particularly common in up to 85% of patients, with an increased incidence (15–45%) of genital malformations including uni- or bicornuate uterus and duplication of the vagina in females and undescended testis, hypospadias, and duplication of the urethra in males.[44] Diagnosis may be missed on the excretory urogram due to poor visualization caused by pelvic bones or the overlying bowel. With impaired renal function, difficulty is further compounded. Enhanced visualization is seen with radionuclide DMSA scan or ultrasound with a full bladder as an acoustic window. CT may be of value when the kidney is suspected of harboring small stones.

In many cases the anomaly is asymptomatic and may remain unrecognized, but in clinical series up to 40% to 50% of patients are symptomatic.[45] Vague abdominal complaints, simulating gastrointestinal disease and related to obstruction or secondary to a stone, UTI, or an abdominal mass, is the most frequently described presenting symptom.

Ultimate prognosis depends on the contralateral kidney status and severity of the associated anomalies. Ectopic kidneys are at no greater risk for other renal diseases than normal kidneys. Concern has been expressed in female patients during pregnancy and delivery, but dystocia from a pelvic kidney has been very rarely reported.

**Thoracic Kidney.** Thoracic kidney is a very rare form of ectopia in which the kidney is cephalad to the normal lumbar position, protruding partially or completely in the thoracic cavity through the diaphragm. It is unclear whether the kidney continues to ascend intrinsically prior to closure of the diaphragm leaflets or if delayed closure of the leaflets allows for exaggerated renal ascent.[46] It is more common in males with a left side predominance and accompanied by eventration or herniation of the hemidiaphragm. Diagnosis is usually made on routine chest x-ray and confirmed by ultrasound or excretory urography. It is a morphologically normal and asymptomatic kidney and surgical treatment is not required.

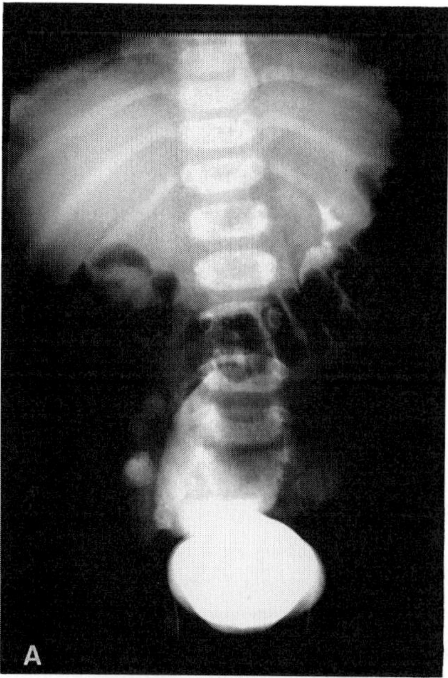


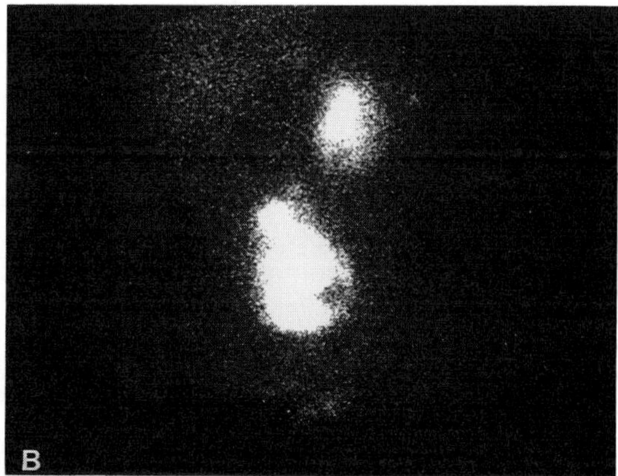


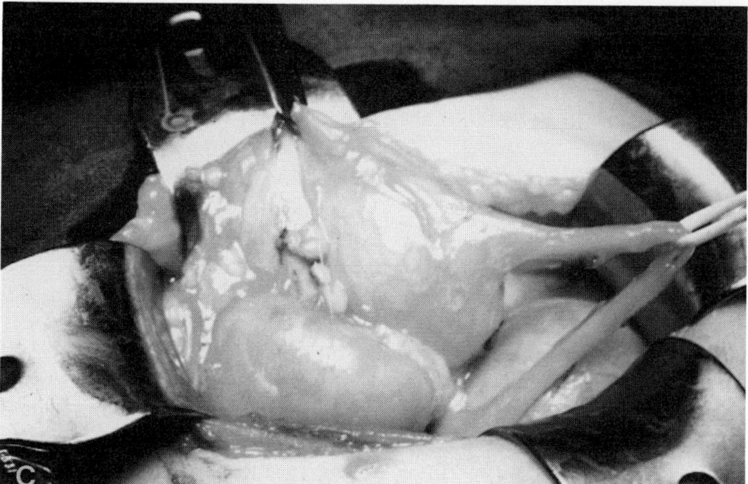


**Fig 4.** Two-year-old boy with history of recurrent UTI. **A,** excretory urogram showing severe hydronephrosis in a right pelvic kidney; **B,** MAG3 renal scan (anterior projection); **C,** intraoperative view demonstrating right ureteropelvic junction obstruction.

## Malrotation

Medial rotation of the collecting system occurs simultaneously with renal migration from the true pelvis and is concluded by the time that the ascent to the lumbar fossa is completed. Most often inappropriate orientation is found in conjunction with other renal anomalies such as ectopia with or without fusion. The true incidence is difficult to accurately calculate and involvement may be unilateral or bilateral. The kidney is usually rotated around its vertical axis and the pelvis can resume variable positions. The most common variant is the ventral, with the pelvis facing anteriorly as in the primitive embryonic position. Incomplete rotation may lead to an anteromedial orientation of the pelvis, while with hyperrotation it can become posterior or even lateral. It has been postulated that the abnormal rotation process is the result of unequal and excessive branching of successive orders of the ureteral tree.[47] The abnormal renal blood supply does not appear to be the cause but rather an effect, following the course of the malrotation. Dysmorphism of the pelvis and calyces is quite common, particularly when associated with ectopy and fusion anomalies. This can produce the appearance of hydronephrosis or of tumor compression and special diagnostic studies may be needed to establish the correct diagnosis. An excretory urogram or retrograde pyelogram will give the best anatomic definition, while isotope studies (DMSA, MAG3) will provide functional parenchymal evaluation. Rotational anomalies per se do not produce symptoms and rarely require any form of treatment. Hematuria, infection, and calculus formation may be related to impaired urinary drainage and should be treated accordingly.

## ANOMALIES OF FORM AND FUSION

In this group of anomalies are included kidneys that have migrated to become fused or contiguous with their contralateral mate. Two situations may occur: kidneys that have migrated together (horseshoe) or one kidney that has crossed the midline (crossed ectopia). This is a very early gestational event and several embryologic theories have been proposed to explain the exact etiology. These include faulty ureteral bud development, abnormalities of renal vasculature limiting renal ascent, and teratogenic and genetic factors.[48–50] A more recent and unified theory has been proposed, relating the position and fusion anomalies to abnormal variations in flexion and rotation of the entire hind end of the fetus.[51] In the horseshoe kidney excessive ventral flexion pushes the two blastemata together with midline fusion while they are still confined in the true pelvis. Exaggerated ventral and lateral flexion, with rotation of the tail, forces the ureteral bud and Wolffian duct to cross the midline in crossed ectopia, with or without fusion. Several variations in fusion anomalies may occur, the final morphology depending on the timing and extent of fusion, degree of renal rotation, and final location of the units. Malrotation is the rule and the orientation of each pelvis provides some evidence as to the embryologic timing of the fusion: an anteriorly placed pelvis indicates early fusion, while a medially directed pelvis suggests fusion after rotation was completed.

### Crossed Renal Ectopia

Crossed renal ectopia is a rare condition with an incidence of about 1 in 1000 individuals,[52] occurring twice as often in males as females and with left predominance. Four principal groups have been identified: crossed-fused, crossed nonfused, solitary crossed, and bilateral crossed.[53] The most common form involves fusion and six further categories are recognized with different morphologic appearances: superior or inferior fusion, sigmoid or S-shaped, lump, L-shaped, and disk kidneys. In crossed ectopia without fusion, the orthotopic unit is in its normal position and orientation, while the ectopic unit is usually caudal, incompletely rotated with an anteriorly directed pelvis (Fig 5). The vascular supply to each kidney is variable and even the normal orthotopic kidney frequently has an anomalous blood supply.[54] Ureteral ectopia is unusual, occurring in about 3% of patients, and involves predominantly the crossed unit. Urinary tract–associated anomalies, including reflux, multicystic dysplasia, and ureteropelvic junction obstruction, most commonly occur in the ectopic unit, although they are reported less frequently in the orthotopic unit (Fig 6).

The highest incidence of anomalies, both genitourinary and nonurinary, is with solitary crossed renal ectopia and seems more related to renal agenesis than to ectopy per se. Genital abnormalities are present in 50%, skeletal abnormalities in 25%, and imperforate anus in 20% of these patients.

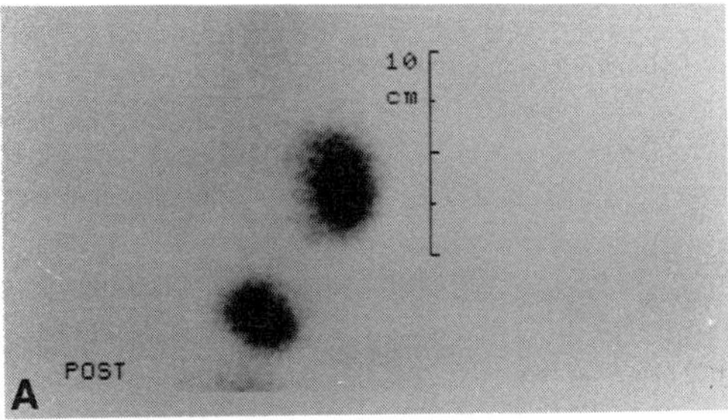


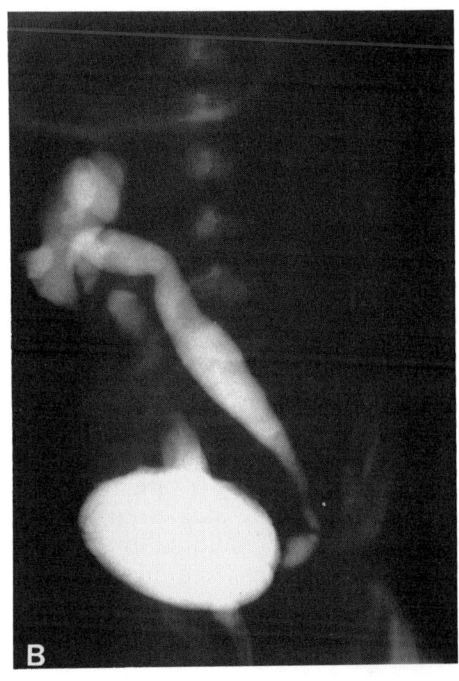


**Fig 5.** Female newborn with left crossed unfused ectopia. **A,** DMSA scan clearly shows left crossed ectopic kidney lying against the inferior pole of right orthotopic kidney; **B,** voiding cystourethrogram showing bilateral vesicoureteric reflux, with left ectopic crossed ureter demonstrated.

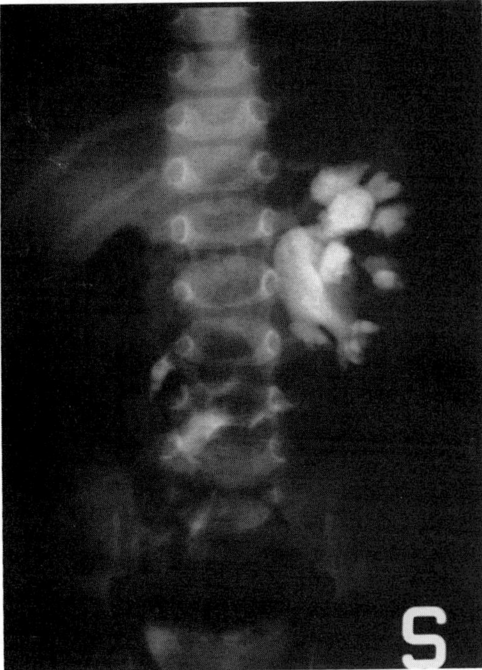


**Fig 6.** One-year-old boy with hypospadias: left hydronephrosis detected on screening ultrasound. Excretory urogram showing L-shaped right crossed fused ectopia, with left ureteropelvic junction obstruction.

Most of these cases remain asymptomatic or represent incidental findings during investigations for anorectal or cardiac malformations. In one third of the patients an asymptomatic abdominal mass may be the presenting sign.[52] Abdominal pain, hematuria, and urinary tract infection may present later in life in conjunction with hydronephrosis or renal calculi.

The diagnosis is usually made with ultrasound; excretory urogram and radionuclide studies (MAG3, DMSA) are all useful to locate and assess the function of the ectopic kidney. A voiding cystourethrogram should be included because of the high incidence of reflux. Most of these patients have a good prognosis, with surgery limited to obstruction relief or stone treatment.

## Horseshoe Kidney

Horseshoe kidney is the most common type of renal fusion anomaly with an incidence of 1 in 400 individuals and is twice as common in males as females.[55] Whatever the mechanism responsible for horseshoe formation, the abnormality occurs very early with fusion usually at the lower poles, prior to rotation and ascent of the two renal blastemata. The pelves are very rarely anteromedial, suggesting a later fusion after some rotation has occurred. There is great morphologic variation and in more than 90% there is lower pole fusion. This may be simply represented by fibrous bands, or, more commonly, by a thick mass of renal parenchyma with renal function. The migration as well is incomplete with a lower than normal position, presumably because the inferior mesenteric artery obstructs the isthmus, preventing further ascent. In most instances the isthmus lies anterior to the aorta and vena cava at the level of the fourth or fifth lumbar vertebra.

The vascular supply is variable and 30% of the kidneys have single renal arteries. More commonly multiple branches are present, originating from the aorta, common iliac, and at times from the hypogastric and middle sacral arteries.[56] The calyces are normal in number, but the axis of the collecting system shows lower pole inward deviation in most circumstances. The renal pelvis is more often anterior, with a high insertion of the ureter that crosses anteriorly over the isthmus as it descends toward the bladder.

Associated anomalies are common and can occur in at least one third of the patients involving skeletal, cardiovascular, and gastrointestinal systems. Many stillborn and neonatal death infants have horseshoe kidneys, but the kidney itself rarely contributes to death.[57]

Vesicoureteric reflux has been noted in approximately 50% of patients and ureteral duplication in 10% as well as an increase in cystic diseases, including multicystic dysplasia and polycystic disease. An increased incidence of genital anomalies is reported, with hypospadias and undescended testis in 4% of males and bicornuate uterus or septate vagina in 7% of females.[58] One third of these patients remain asymptomatic throughout life. When symptoms do develop, they are most commonly related to calculi, hydronephrosis, infection, or hematuria. Hydronephrosis has been reported as high as 80%, with ureteropelvic junction obstruction secondary to high insertion of the ureter in the renal pelvis being most common. Surgery may be more difficult because of the anomalous vascular supply. Isthmectomy is rarely felt to be necessary and both flap pyeloplasty or ureterocalicostomy have been proposed as primary procedures due to the anatomic variation of the horseshoe ureteropelvic junction.[59] Renal tumors have been reported with hypernephroma being the most common, and, in a significant number, arising from the isthmus.[60] There is also evidence of a 62-fold increase in Wilms' tumor during childhood.

Diagnosis can be made easily with excretory urography showing typical deviation of the renal axis and ureteral deviation by the isthmus. Radionuclide studies (DMSA and diuretic renogram) are very helpful for parenchymal definition and for

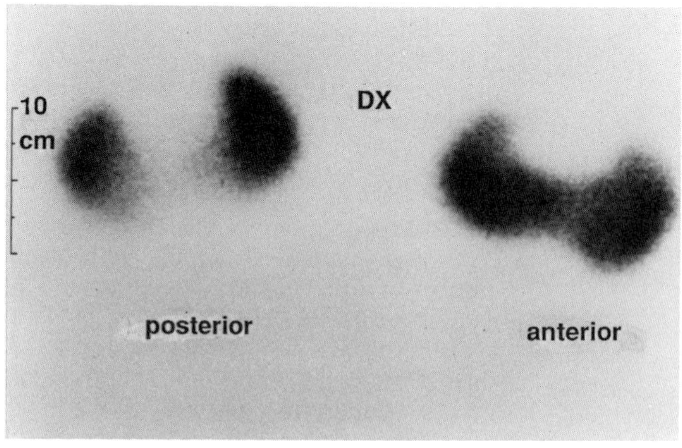

better evaluation of hydronephrosis (Fig 7). Voiding cystourethrogram should be added to document vesicoureteric reflux, which is frequently associated. If surgery is contemplated, angiographic study may be required for better definition of the variable arterial supply to the kidney. The presence of a horseshoe kidney does not adversely affect long-term survival and less than 25% of patients will ultimately require surgery for calculus or obstruction.[61] Pregnancy and delivery are not complicated by the presence of a normally positioned horseshoe kidney.[62]

## ANOMALIES OF THE RENAL COLLECTING SYSTEM

### Calyceal Diverticulum

The calyceal diverticulum is a cystic cavity peripherally located to an otherwise normal minor calyx. It is usually related to the upper calyx, but may be anywhere in the kidney and may be multiple. It communicates with the calyx through a narrow channel lined by transitional epithelium. The persistence of later generations of the dividing ureteral bud that fail to degenerate may explain the formation of a calyceal diverticulum.[63] The incidence in children and adults is similar and most cases are entirely asymptomatic or incidentally discovered. There is an increased frequency of stone formation, which may be responsible for secondary symptoms such as pain, infection, and hematuria.[64] Diagnosis is usually based on excretory urography (Fig 8) and rarely a retrograde study is required. Differential diagnosis should include other acquired abnormalities such as papillary necrosis, cortical abscess, and tuberculosis, all extremely rare in the pediatric age. Surgery is rarely required and consists of cyst marsupialization with calyceal neck division.[65]

### Hydrocalycosis

Hydrocalycosis is a condition in which there is obstruction of an individual calyx or group of calyces having a common infundibulum. The cause may be extrinsic or intrinsic and this entity is distinct from a calyceal diverticulum. Vascular compression (extrinsic) is usually an incidental finding in urograms, affecting the right kidney more commonly. Most cases are asymptomatic, although occasionally intermittent distention can produce pain, but surgery by infundiboloplasty is rarely necessary.[66] Intrinsic hydrocalycosis is extremely rare and is caused by infundibular or infundibolopelvic stenosis. In the latter variant multiple narrowed and obstructive infundibula drain variably dilated calyces into a poorly formed and abortive renal pelvis. The etiology is uncertain but the common association with renal dysplasia would suggest the result of anomalous branching of the ureteric bud.[67] Small or moderate size asymptomatic lesions require no treatment.

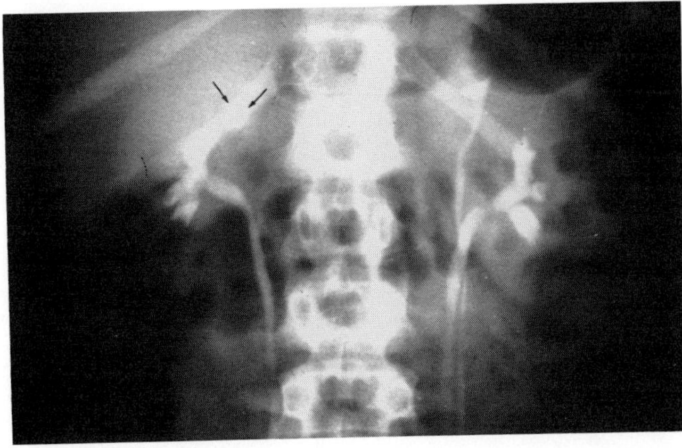

**Fig 8.** Excretory urogram in 9-year-old girl with hematuria demonstrating right-sided calyceal diverticulum (arrows) and left-sided duplication.

Intubated infundibulotomy is seldom justified but ureterocalycostomy may occasionally be helpful. Acquired infundibular stenosis is rare but may result from renal trauma, impaction of a stone, or tuberculosis.

## Megacalycosis

Megacalycosis is a nonobstructive condition with dilated and malformed calyces, often increased in number (polycalycosis). Males are more commonly affected than females and the presentation can be with hematuria, UTIs, or as an incidental finding with an asymptomatic course. Association with nonobstructive megaureter has been reported in 10% to 20% of adult patients.[68] The diagnosis can be made only in the true absence of an anatomically or functionally definable site of obstruction in the urinary tract. Congenital medullary hypoplasia[69] and transient fetal obstruction during the period of early parenchymal development[70] are the most accredited etiologic explanations. Differential diagnosis is with a true obstructive uropathy and from acquired conditions that may produce infundibular scarring and calyceal dilatation. As a nonobstructive deformity, treatment is usually not required and the overall prognosis is excellent.

## Bifid Pelvis

Bifid pelvis should be considered a variant of the normal anatomy, with the pelvis dividing prior to or just within its entrance at the renal hilus, where it forms two major calyces (Fig 9). It is present in approximately 10% of normal renal pelves and is an asymptomatic condition. Extremely rare is even further division of the pelvis, with subsequent triplication.

## Ureteropelvic Junction Obstruction

Ureteropelvic junction (UPJ) obstruction is the most common congenital obstruction of the urinary tract in childhood. Overall incidence is difficult to estimate and past data reported nearly 25% of cases within the first year of life and 50% before the age of 5 years.[71] With the increased use of prenatal ultrasound studies, fetal diagnosis of dilatation of the collecting system has become extremely common and the majority of children with UPJ obstruction can be diagnosed prenatally.[72] It occurs more commonly in males, especially in neonates, and in 60% of cases the lesion is on the left side. In approximately 20% of cases detected in the first year both kidneys are involved, whereas in older children bilaterality is less common (5%). Vesicoureteric reflux is present in nearly 15%[73] and the association of contralateral renal anomalies has been reported in up to 50%, including agenesis, duplication of the collecting system, malrotation, ectopia, and multicystic kidney.[74]

The cause of obstruction is variable and it may occur as a primary anomaly, with an intrinsic or extrinsic lesion, or as a sec-

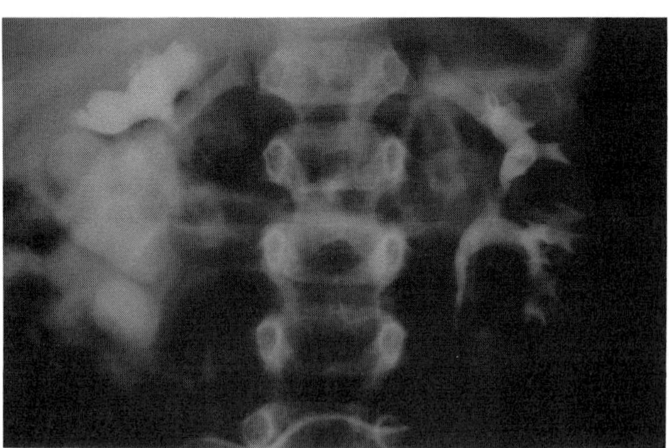

**Fig 9.** Excretory urogram of a 5-year-old boy with macrohematuria following minor blunt abdominal trauma showing a left bifid pelvis and right ureteropelvic junction obstruction of lower pole collecting system (incomplete duplication).

ondary phenomenon. Most congenital obstructions are intrinsic in nature but their exact pathogenesis remains obscure. Histologic examination by light and electron microscopy has found either a disorientation and deficiency of the circular and oblique muscular fibers surrounding the junction[75] or a relative increase in collagen fibers between the muscle bundles.[76,77] Another attractive proposed theory is failure of recanalization of the cephalic end of the developing ureter, which, between the fifth and sixth fetal week, goes through a solid phase.[78] Other intrinsic lesions include valves, polyps, and persistent ureteral folds that may produce a valve-like obstruction at the UPJ.[79] In the absence of obvious mechanical factors, obstruction may be caused by a functional disturbance in the ability of the pelvis to initiate, form, or conduct peristaltic waves across the UPJ.[80] Accessory lower pole renal vessels are the most common cause of extrinsic congenital obstruction, presenting in 15% to 30% of patients. Whether the anatomic relationship between these vessels and the UPJ is the cause or the result of obstruction is controversial. In many instances there may exist a primary intrinsic disturbance that produces pelvic overdistention and rotation and ultimately induces compression by lower pole vessels. This view is substantiated by the observation that dissection of the vessel and freeing of the ureteropelvic junction may not result in an unobstructed urine flow. Recent evidence suggests that the precise pathologic anatomy of the junction defines the pattern of flow across the obstruction and has important clinical implications.[81] Intrinsic abnormalities are characterized by a relatively fixed resistance, producing a constant degree of obstruction, while with extrinsic abnormalities there is a variable degree of resistance. The latter situation is often recognized clinically and defined as intermittent hydronephrosis. Secondary causes of UPJ obstruction are kinking and tortuosity of the ureter caused either by hydronephrosis from lower tract obstruction or by vesicoureteric reflux.

Clinical presentation with UPJ obstruction depends on the age of the patient. Without prenatal ultrasound detection, the most common sign in the newborn leading to diagnosis is the presence of a palpable abdominal mass.[82] Occasionally failure to thrive, feeding difficulties, fever, or sepsis secondary to urinary tract infection (present in 30%) are the presenting symptoms. In contrast, in the older children abdominal or flank pain simulating gastrointestinal disease, especially if intermittent and associated with vomiting, is the most common presentation.[83] Hematuria may occur spontaneously or following minor abdominal trauma, most probably due to the rupture of mucosal vessels in the dilated collecting system. Episodic intermittent flank pain, associated with increased fluid intake, is more common in the young adult and indicates sudden overdistention of the renal pelvis during diuresis. In the classic case in the neonate, the diagnosis can be easily confirmed by ultrasound and diuretic renal scan (MAG3, DTPA) (Fig 10). Functional assessment with nuclear scan is more accurate than excretory urogram, is not affected by bowel gas shadows, and exposure to radiation is reduced. A voiding cystourethrogram should also be done to exclude ipsilateral or contralateral reflux. Percutaneous nephrostomy and antegrade pyelography are useful to distinguish a poorly functioning kidney from a multicystic one. In the older child the excretory urogram is helpful and retains a unique role to provide additional anatomic features. The pelvicalyceal system is enlarged, contrast stops abruptly at the UPJ, and the ureter is usually not visualized (Figs 9 and 11). Delayed films are important and should always be obtained to determine the true level of obstruction. In equivocal cases additional diagnostic studies may be required to assess renal function and define obstruction, and include augmented renography and constant perfusion pressure flow testing.[84,85] With intermittent obstruction, evaluation performed during the acute episode of pain may be the only way to prove the diagnosis.[86]

Management strategies for infantile UPJ obstruction has undergone considerable evolution and timing of surgery remains a very controversial issue in the prenatally

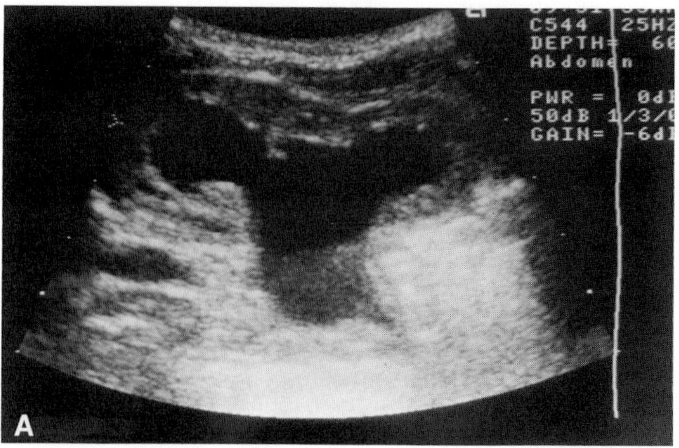


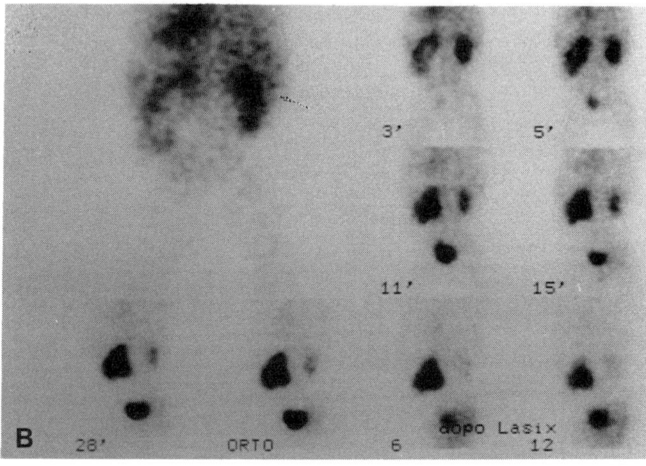


**Fig 10.** Male newborn with prenatal diagnosis of left hydronephrosis. **A,** renal ultrasound showing large pelvis communicating with clubbed calyces and cortical thinning; **B,** DTPA scan performed at 3 weeks showing left UPJ obstruction nonresponsive to furosemide.

diagnosed group. Our understanding of the natural history of unilateral asymptomatic hydronephrosis detected in utero has demonstrated that early neonatal pyeloplasty is seldom required.[87] The prognosis for obstructed kidneys is generally good when corrected in childhood, and, because of the unpredictable potential for renal recoverability in the pediatric patient, reconstructive surgery is almost always performed. The Anderson–Hynes dismembered anastomosis is the favored technique for pyeloplasty, with excision of the stenotic area and reduction of the excessive renal pelvis. Nephrectomy is rarely performed and reserved for the few cases in which radionuclide studies have demonstrated negligible renal function.

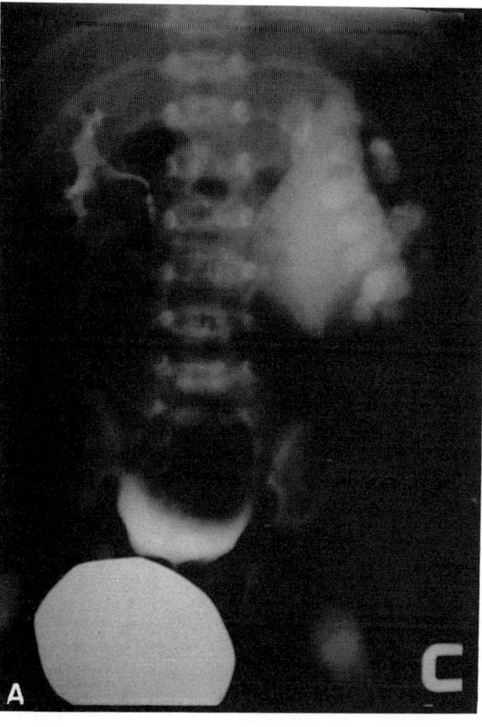


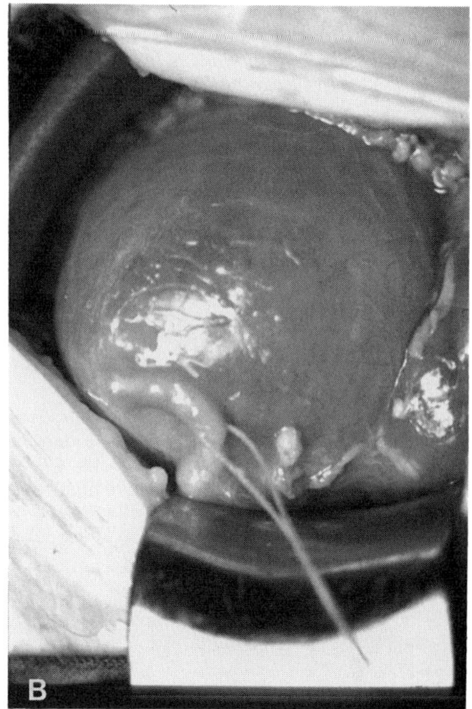


**Fig 11. A,** excretory urogram in 1-year-old boy with classic appearance of left UPJ obstruction. Note nonobstructive contralateral persistent ureteric folds (Ostling's valve); **B,** intraoperative view.

## REFERENCES


1. Potter EL. *Normal and Abnormal Development of the Kidney*. Chicago: Year Book; 1972.
2. Potter EL. Bilateral absence of ureters and kidneys. A report of 50 cases. *Obstet Gynecol.* 1965;25:3.
3. Roodhooft AM, Birnholz JC, Holmes LB. Familial nature of congenital absence and severe disgenesis of both kidneys. *N Engl J Med.* 1984;310:1341.
4. Ashley DBJ, Mostofi FK. Renal agenesis and dysgenesis. *J Urol.* 1960;83:211.
5. De Myer W, Baird I. Mortality and skeletal malformations from amniocentesis and oligohydramnios in rats: cleft palate, club foot, microstomia, adactyly. *Teratology.* 1969;2:33.
6. Hislop A, Hey E, Reid L. The lungs in congenital bilateral renal agenesis and dysplasia. *Arch Dis Child.* 1979;54:32.
7. Avni EF, Thoua Y, Laland B, et al. Multicystic dysplastic kidney: natural history from in utero diagnosis and postnatal follow up. *J Urol.* 1987;138:1420.
8. Emanuel B, Nachman R, Aronson N, et al. Congenital solitary kidney: a review of 74 cases. *J Urol.* 1974;111:394.
9. Cromie WJ. The remnant nephron hyperfiltration hypothesis: implications in pediatric urology. In: King LR, ed. *Urologic Surgery in Neonates and Young Infants*. Philadelphia: WB Saunders; 1988:132.
10. N'Guessan G, Stephens FD. Supernumerary kidney. *J Urol.* 1983;130:649.
11. Glassberg KI; Stephens FD, Lebowitz RL, et al. Renal dysgenesis and cystic diseases of the kidney: a report of the committee on terminology, nomenclature and classification. Section on Urology. American Academy of Pediatrics. *J Urol.* 1987;138:1085.
12. Resnick J, Vernier RL. Renal cystic diseases and renal dysplasia. In: Holliday MA, et al, eds. *Pediatric Nephrology*. 2nd ed. Baltimore: Williams and Wilkins; 1987:372.
13. Royer P, Habib R, Mathieu H, et al. L'hypoplasie renale bilaterale congenital avec redution du nombre et hypertrophie des nephrons chez l'enfant. *Ann Pediatr.* 1962;9:133.
14. Ask–Upmark E. Uber juvenile maligne nephrosklerose und ihr verhaltnis zu storungen in der nierenten wicklung. *Acta Pathol Microbiol Scand.* 1929;6:383.
15. Johnston JH, Mix LW. The Ask–Upmark kidney: a form of ascending pyelonephritis? *Br J Urol.* 1976;48:393.

16. Cussen LG, Stephens FD. Renal dysgenesis: a "urologic classification." In: Stephens FD, ed. *Congenital Malformations of the Urinary Tract*. New York: Praeger; 1983:463.
17. Reeders ST, Breuning MH, Davies KE, et al. A highly polymorphic DNA marker linked to adult polycystic disease of chromosome 16. *Nature*. 1985;317:542.
18. Kanwar YS, Carrone FA. Reversible changes of tubular wall and basement membrane in drug-induced renal cystic disease. *Kidney Int*. 1984;26:53.
19. Gabow PA, Ikle DW, Holmes JH. Polycystic kidney disease, prospective analysis of nonazotemic patients and family members. *Ann Intern Med*. 1984;101:238.
20. Glassberg KI, Filmer RB. Renal dysplasia, renal hypoplasia and cystic disease of the kidney. In: Kelalis PP, King RL, Belman AB, eds. *Clinical Pediatric Urology*. Vol 2. 2nd ed. Philadelphia: WB Saunders; 1985:941.
21. Sanfilippo FP, Vaughn WK, Peters TC, et al. Transplantation for polycystic disease. *Transplantation*. 1983;36:54.
22. Noe HN, Marshall JH, Edwards OP. Nodular renal blastema in the multicystic kidney. *J Urol*. 1989;142:486.
23. Thomas DFM. Diagnosis and management of the multicystic kidney. In: Gonzales ET, Roth D, eds. *Common Problems in Pediatric Urology*. St. Louis: Mosby; 1991:219.
24. Maizels M, Simpson SB. Primitive ducts of renal dysplasia induced by culturing ureteral buds denuded of condensed renal mesenchyma. *Science*. 1983;219:509.
25. Clarke NW, Gough DCS, Cohen S. Neonatal urological ultrasound diagnostic: inaccuracies and pitfalls. *Arch Dis Child*. 1989;64:578.
26. Pedicelli G, Jequier S, Bowen AD, et al. Multicystic dysplastic kidney: spontaneous regression demonstrated with ultrasound. *Radiology*. 1986;160:23.
27. Griscom NT. The roentgenology of neonatal abdominal masses. *Am J Roentgenol*. 1965:93(2):447.
28. Stuck KJ, Koff SA, Silver TM. Ultrasonic features of multicystic dysplastic kidney: expanded diagnostic criteria. *Radiology*. 1982;143:217.
29. Warshawsky AB, Miller KE, Kaplan GW. Urographic visualization of multicystic kidneys. *J Urol*. 1977;117:94.
30. O'Carey P, Howards SS. Multicystic dysplastic kidneys and diagnostic confusion on renal scan. *J Urol*. 1988;139:83.
31. Colodny AH. Management of multicystic dysplastic kidney. *Dial Ped Urol*. 1989;10(6):7.
32. King LR. The management of multicystic kidney and ureteropelvic junction obstruction. In: King LR, ed. *Urologic Surgery in Neonates and Young Infants*. Philadelphia: WB Saunders; 1988:140.
33. Javadpour N, Chelouhy E, Monlada L, et al. Hypertension in a child caused by a multicystic kidney. *J Urol*. 1979;104:918.
34. Ambrose SS, Gould RA, Trulock TS. Unilateral multicystic renal disease in adults. *J Urol*. 1982;128:336.
35. Chen YH, Stapleton FB, Shane R, et al. Neonatal hypertension from a unilateral multicystic dysplastic kidney. *J Urol*. 1985;133:664.
36. Waldherr R, Lennert T, Weber HP, et al. The nephronophtisis complex: a clinicopathologic study in children. *Virch Arch*. 1982;394:235.
37. Joshi VV, Beckwith JB. Multilocular cysts of the kidney (cystic nephroma) and partially differentiated nephroblastoma. *Cancer*. 1989;64:446.
38. Gordon RL, Pollack HM, Popky GL, et al. Simple renal cysts of kidney in children. *Radiology*. 1979;131:357.
39. Babka JC, Cohen MS, Sode S. Solitary intrarenal cyst causing hypertension. *N Engl J Med*. 1974;291:343.
40. Kuiper J. Medullary sponge kidney. In: Gardner KD Jr, ed. *Cystic Diseases of the Kidney*. New York: John Wiley and Sons; 1976:151.
41. Grantham JJ, Levine E. Acquired cystic disease: replacing one kidney disease with another. *Kidney Int*. 1985;28:99.
42. Maizels M, Stephens FD. The induction of urologic malformations. Understanding the relationship of renal ectopia and congenital scoliosis. *Invest Urol*. 1979;17:209.
43. Malek RS, Kelalis PP, Burke EC. Ectopic kidney in children and frequency of association of other malformations. *Mayo Clin Proc*. 1971;46:461.
44. Thompson GJ, Pace JM. Ectopic kidney: a review of 97 cases. *Surg Gynecol Obstet*. 1937;64:935.
45. Dows RA, Lane JW, Burns E. Solitary pelvic kidney. Its clinical implications. *Urology*. 1973;1:51.
46. Burke EC, Wenzel JE, Utz DC. The intrathoracic kidney. Report of a case. *Am J Dis Child*. 1967;113:487.
47. Weyrauch HM Jr. Anomalies of renal rotation. *Surg Gynecol Obstet*. 1939;69:183.
48. Wilmer HA. Unilateral fused kidney: a report of five cases and a review of the literature. *J Urol*. 1938;40:551.
49. Kelalis PP, Malek RS, Segura JW. Observations on renal ectopic fusion in children. *J Urol*. 1973;110:588.
50. Hildreth TA, Cass AS. Crossed renal ectopia with familial occurrence. *Urology*. 1978;12:59.
51. Cook WA, Stephens FD. Fused kidneys: morphologic study and theory of embryogenesis. *Birth Defects*. 1977;13:327.
52. Abeshouse BS, Bhisitko I. Crossed renal ectopia with and without fusion. *Urol Int*. 1959;9:63.

53. McDonald JH, McClellan DS. Crossed renal ectopia. *Am J Surg.* 1957;93:995.
54. Rubinstein ZJ, Hertz M, Shahin N, et al. Crossed renal ectopia: angiographic findings in six cases. *Am J Roentgenol.* 1976;126:1035.
55. Segura JW, Kelalis PP, Burke ET. Horseshoe kidney in children. *J Urol.* 1972;108:33.
56. Boatman DL, Cornell SH, Kollin CP. The arterial supply of horseshoe kidneys. *Am J Roentgenol.* 1971;113:447.
57. Zondek LH, Zondek T. Horseshoe kidney and associated congenital malformations. *Urol Int.* 1964;18:347.
58. Boatman DL, Kollin CP, Flocks RH. Congenital anomalies associated with horseshoe kidney. *J Urol.* 1972;107:205.
59. Mollard P, Braun P. Primary ureterocalycostomy for severe hydronephrosis in children. *J Pediatr Surg.* 1980;15:87.
60. Buntley D. Malignancy associated with horseshoe kidney. *Urology.* 1976;8:146.
61. Glenn JF. Analysis of 51 patients with horseshoe kidney. *N Engl J Med.* 1959;261:686.
62. Bell R. Horseshoe kidney in pregnancy. *J Urol.* 1946;56:159.
63. Timmons JW, Malek RR, Hattery RR, et al. Calyceal diverticulum. *J Urol.* 1975;114:6.
64. Middleton AW, Pfeister RD. Stone-containing pyelocalyceal diverticulum: embryogenic, anatomic, radiologic and clinical characteristics. *J Urol.* 1974;111:2.
65. Williams G, Blandy JP, Tresidder GC. Communicating cysts and diverticula of the renal pelvis. *Br J Urol.* 1969;41:163.
66. Johnston JH, Sandomirsky SK. Intrarenal vascular obstruction of the superior infundibulum in children. *J Pediatr Surg.* 1972;7:318.
67. Kelalis PP, Malek RS. Infundibulopelvic stenosis. *J Urol.* 1981;125:568.
68. Gittes RF. Congenital megacalyces. In: Stamey TA, ed. *1984 Monographs in Urology.* Princeton, NJ: Custom Publisher Service; 1984:1–19.
69. Puigvert A. Megacalycosis: diagnostico diferencial con la hidrocaliectasia. *Medicina Clinica* 1963;41:294.
70. Johnston JH. Megacalycosis: a burnt out obstruction? *J Urol.* 1973;110:344.
71. Williams DI, Kenawi MM. The prognosis of pelviureteric obstruction in childhood. A review of 190 cases. *Eur Urol.* 1976;2:57.
72. Elder JS, Duckett JW. Perinatal urology. In: Gillenwater JW, et al, eds. *Adult and Pediatric Urology.* St. Louis: Mosby; 1991:1717.
73. Bernstein GT, Mandell J, Lebowitz RL, et al. Ureteropelvic junction obstruction in the neonate. *J Urol.* 1988;140:1216.
74. Perlmutter AD, Retik AB, Bauer SB. Anomalies of the urinary tract. In: Walsh PC, et al, ed. *Campbell's Urology.* 5th ed. Philadelphia: WB Saunders; 1986:1665.
75. Murnaghan GF. Experimental aspects of hydronephrosis. *Br J Urol.* 1959;31:370.
76. Notley RG. Electron microscopy of the upper ureter and the pelviureteric junction. *Br J Urol.* 1968;40:37.
77. Hanna MK, Jeffs RD, Sturgess JM, et al. Ureteral structure and ultrastructure. 2. Congenital ureteropelvic obstruction and primary obstructive megaureter. *J Urol.* 1976;116:725.
78. Ruano-Gil D, Coca-Payeras A, Tejedo-Maten A. Obstruction and normal re-canalization of the ureter in human embryo: its relation to congenital ureteric obstruction. *Eur Urol J.* 1975;1:287.
79. Maizels M, Stephens FD. Valves of the ureter as a cause of primary obstruction of the ureter: anatomic, embryologic and clinical aspects. *J Urol.* 1980;123:742.
80. Costantinou CE, Djurhuus JC. Urodynamics of the multicalyceal upper urinary tract. In: O'Reilly PN, Gosling JA, eds. *Idiopathic Hydronephrosis.* New York: Springer-Verlag; 1982:16.
81. Koff SA, Hayden LJ, Cirulli C, et al. Pathophysiology of ureteropelvic junction obstruction: experimental and clinical observations. *J Urol.* 1986;136:336.
82. Murphy JP, Holder TM, Ashcraft KW, et al. Ureteropelvic junction obstruction in the newborn. *J Pediatr Surg.* 1984;16:642.
83. Snyder HM III, Lebowitz RL, Colodny AG, et al. Ureteropelvic junction obstruction in children. *Urol Clin North Am.* 1980;7:273.
84. O'Reilly PH, Testa HJ, Lawson RS, et al. Diuresis renography in equivocal urinary tract obstruction. *Br J Urol.* 1978;50:76.
85. Whitaker RH. Diagnosis of obstruction in dilated ureters. *Ann Roy Coll Surg Engl.* 1973;53:153.
86. Malek RS. Intermittent hydronephrosis: the occult ureteropelvic obstruction. *J Urol.* 1983;130:863.
87. Ransly PG, Dhillon HK, Gordon I, et al. The postnatal management of hydronephrosis diagnosed by prenatal ultrasound. *J Urol.* 1990;144:584.

# 48

# Anomalies of the Ureter

*Christopher W. Graham and*
*M. David Gibbons*

## EMBRYOLOGY OF THE URETER

In the developing embryo, the Wolffian body forms on the dorsal wall and gives rise to nephrogenic, gonadal, and Wolffian ductal structures. Where the Wolffian duct turns ventrally to meet the cloaca, a ureteric bud forms at day 28 that extends to meet the metanephric blastema. The ureteric bud then undergoes several divisions that ultimately develop into the renal pelvis, calyces, and collecting tubules. It is thought that the ingrowth of the ureteric bud into the nephrogenic tissue induces nephron development. By 8 weeks, the ureter is elongated as the kidney moves to its final position within the abdomen (Fig 1).

At the sixth week, the urorectal septum divides the cloaca transversely into a urogenital sinus anteriorly and the rectum posteriorly. The common excretory duct, which is the Wolffian duct distal to the ureteric bud, is absorbed by the developing bladder and becomes the trigone. As this takes place, the ureter loses its attachment to the Wolffian duct, moving laterally and cranially, while the Wolffian duct moves medially and caudally toward its final position in the proximal urethra (Fig 2). The Wolffian duct differentiates into the seminal vesicle, vas deferens, and epididymis in the male and Gartner's duct (a vestigial structure within the wall of the Mullerian duct) in the female. During this time, the muscular wall of the bladder forms and its epithelium becomes transitional.[1]

## URETERIC DUPLICATION

### Embryology

Abnormalities may occur during ureteric budding resulting in a variety of duplication anomalies, the most common of which is renal duplication, wherein two pelvocalyceal systems develop.[2] When two separate ureteric buds develop and intercept the metanephric blastema, complete duplication occurs, and the kidney is drained by two separate ureters (Fig 3). Rarely, one of the ureteric buds fails to induce renal growth and evolves into a blind-ending ureter. More frequently, ureteric anomalies arise during the process of ureteric branching. Normally, the early divisions occur adjacent to the nephrogenic tissue and produce the renal pelvis and calyceal system. When branching occurs early, a bifid ureter is formed. The earliest branching ureteric buds produce ureters that join near the bladder, while later branching ureteric buds produce bifid ureteric pelves.[3]

Two major embryologic consequences result from abnormal ureteric bud formation. A normal ureteric bud grows into the adjacent nephrogenic tissue, meeting the center of that tissue to produce the maxi-

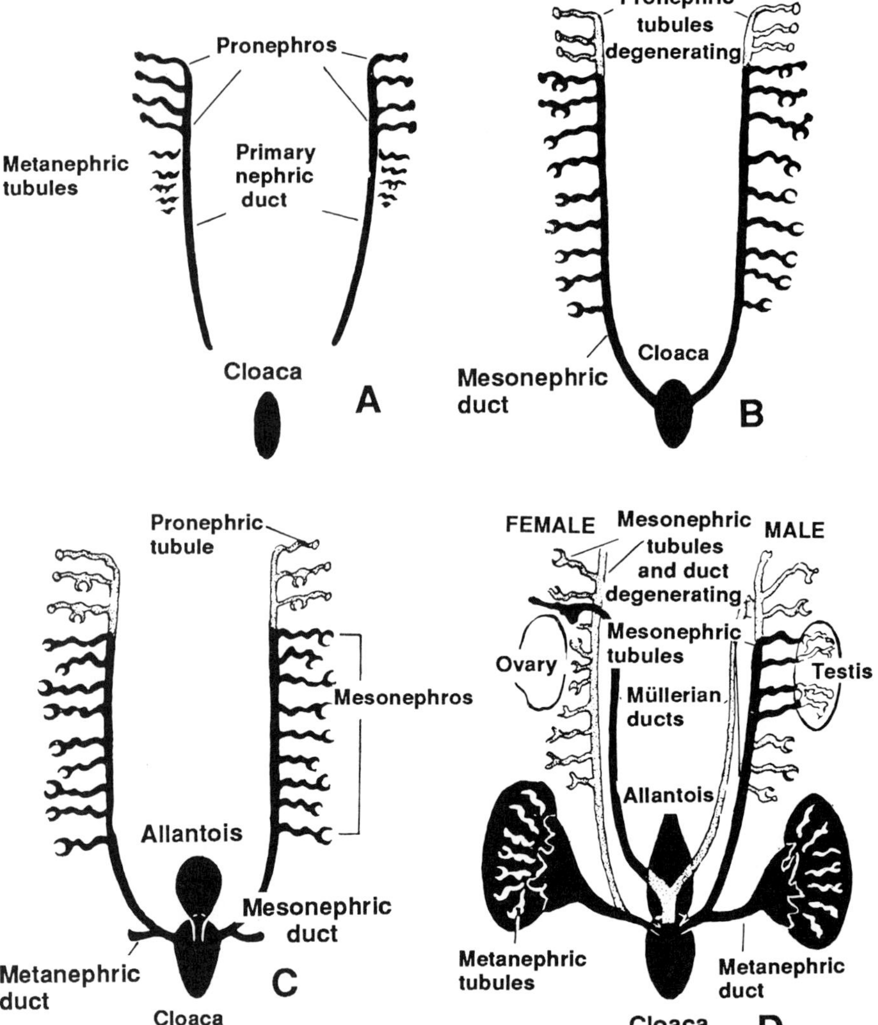


**Fig 1.** Diagrammatic representation of the pronephros, mesonephros, and metanephros during the development of the human kidney. **A,** the cephalically situated pronephros with tubules draining into the primary nephric duct; **B,** the pronephric tubules are degenerating and the mesonephric tubules have appeared and have ducts joining the mesonephric duct; **C, D,** the metanephric duct can be seen arising from the mesonephric duct and growing toward the metanephrogenic tissue to form the permanent kidney. Also the Mullerian ducts are shown **(D).** These later give rise to the oviducts, uterus, and vagina in the female. Note that the mesonephric and Mullerian ducts become vestigial in the male and the mesonephric ducts become vestigial in the female. [Adapted from Patten BM, *Human Embryology.* 3rd ed (New York: McGraw-Hill; 1968), with permission.]

mally functioning nephron mass. Mackie and Stephens[3] postulate that ureteric buds arising either too caudally or too cranially on the mesonephric duct contact the margin of the nephrogenic tissue, resulting in renal dysplasia (Fig 4). The lower pole ureter usually drains about two thirds of the kidney; the upper pole ureter is more likely to subtend dysplastic parenchyma. A single ectopic ureteric bud or one of the pair of

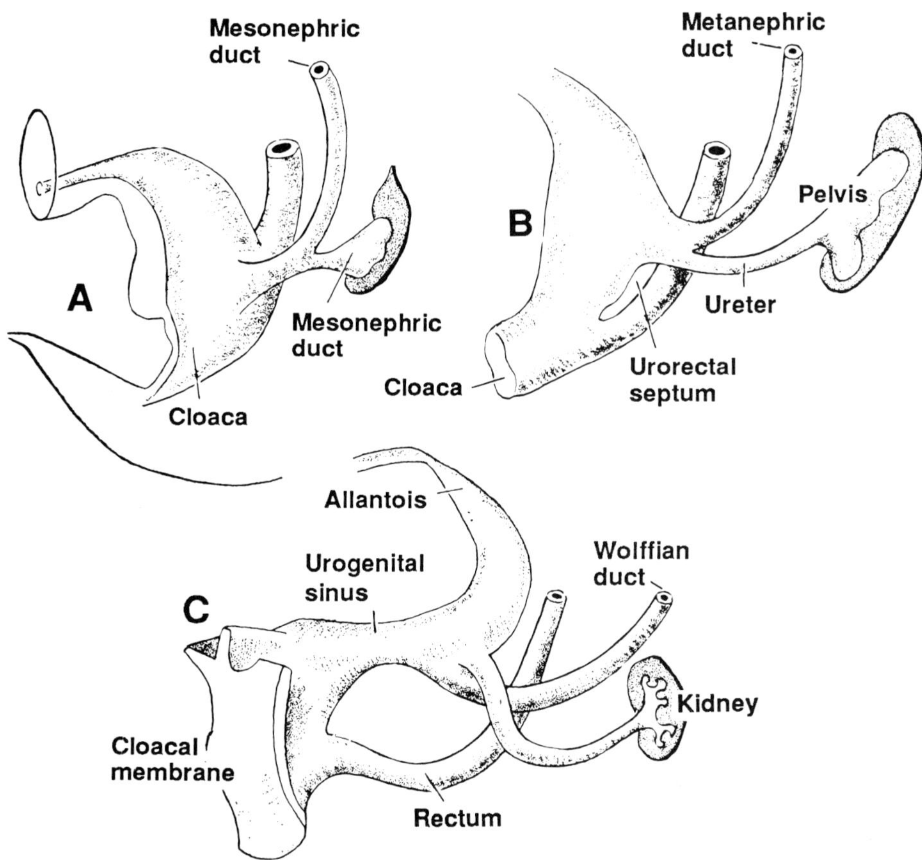


**Fig 2.** Development of the hindgut. **A,** the 11-mm embryo showing the relationship between the cloaca, rectum, and mesonephric ducts. The metanephric bud is shown growing into the metanephric tissue; **B,** a later stage of development in which the urorectal septum divides the cloaca into the ventral urogenital sinus and dorsal rectal parts; **C,** a further stage in the development of the cloaca showing the manner in which the mesonephric duct is absorbed into the urogenital sinus, causing the metanephric and mesonephric ducts (Wolffian duct) to open independently of each other. The former is more cephalad.

ureteric buds is likely to meet the nephrogenic tissue in this fashion.

The second consequence of abnormal position of the ureteric bud is the final position of the ureteric orifice. A normally positioned bud separates from the mesonephric duct as it meets trigone and migrates to a normal position on the trigone. A ureteric bud that forms caudally on the mesonephric duct subsequently reaches the trigone early; it then migrates too far laterally and cranially. These ureteric orifices tend to allow vesicoureteral reflux because of a deficiency in intramural tunnel length. Conversely, a cranial ureteric bud arrives late and then fails to migrate normally. These ectopic ureteric orifices are positioned medially and caudally and can be found on the distal trigone, at the bladder neck, or in the posterior urethra. They are usually obstructed, resulting in ureteric dilatation. If the ureteric bud fails to separate from the mesonephric duct completely, an ectopic ureter may terminate in a Wolffian structure (eg, ejaculatory duct, seminal vesicle, or vas deferens).

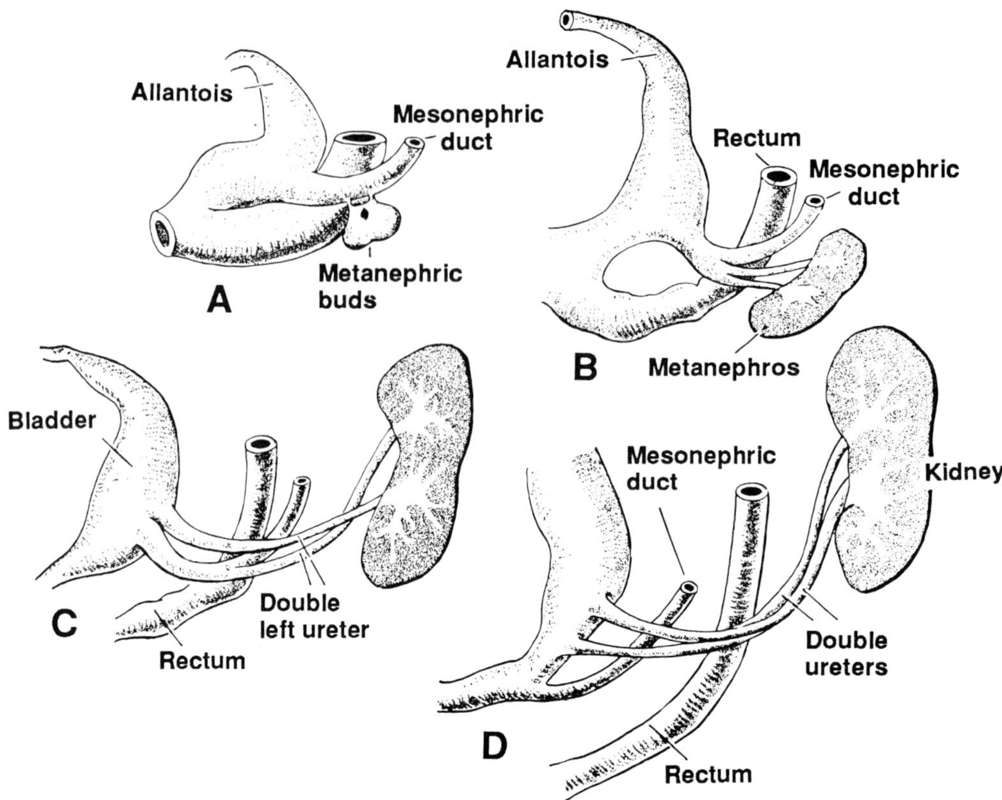


**Fig 3.** Embryology of complete duplicated ureters. **A, B,** two metanephric buds arising from the mesonephric duct grow into the metanephros; **C, D,** the ureter from the lower pole of the kidney is absorbed into the bladder before that from the upper pole, which therefore opens lower down.

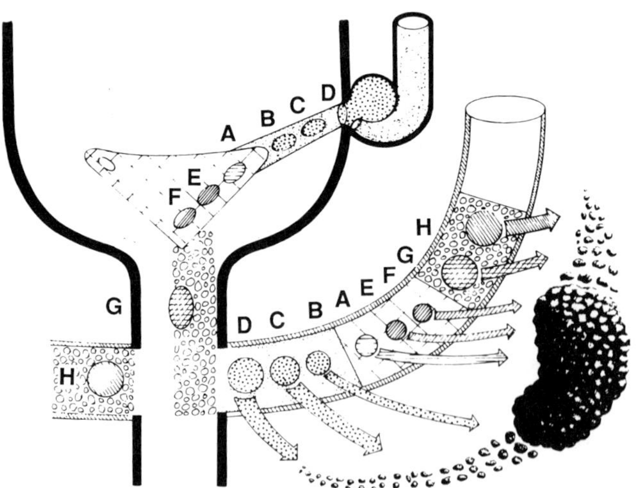


**Fig 4.** Relationship of position of ureteral bud on Wolffian duct (middle of figure) to nephrogenic blastema (bottom) and to final position of ureteral orifice in bladder or urethra (above and to left). [From Mackie.[3]]

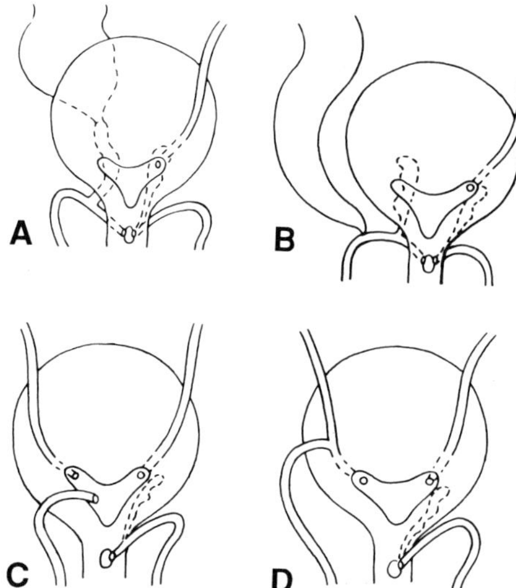


**Fig 5.** Classification of vas-ureteral ectopia in boys. Common mesonephric duct in ureteral ectopia with H position orifice into **A,** seminal vesicle and **B,** vas deferens. Proximal vas precursor in vas ectopia; **C,** vasovesical—vas drains into ipsilateral side of bladder. Orthotopic ureteral orifice in **A** position. Ectopic ureteral orifice in cranio-displaced and caudo-displaced positions; **D,** vasoureteral—vas drains into ipsilateral ureter. Orthotopic ureteral orifice in **A** position. Ectopic ureteral orifice in cranio-displaced and caudo-displaced positions. Complete ureteral duplication; vas drains into upper pole ureter. [From Gibbons, et al.[5]]

If the ureteric bud originates from the proximal vas precursor portion of the Wolffian duct, the vas may insert ectopically into either the ureter or the urinary bladder.[4] Ectopia of the vas deferens is a distinctly different entity than ectopia of the ureter into the vas. Ectopia of the vas deferens is usually associated with vesicoureteral reflux into the ipsilateral ureter but is also usually associated with adequate function of the ipsilateral kidney. Ectopia of the ureter into vas usually results in a nonfunctioning kidney that is small and dysplastic (Fig 5).

Duplex ureters originate and migrate from the ureteric bud in a fashion similar to that of single-system ureters. The Meyer–Weigert rule describes this relationship: the caudal ureteric bud from the Wolffian duct intercepts the inferior aspect of the metanephric blastema, becoming the lower pole ureter, and migrates to the lateral and cranial position on the trigone. This ureter is more likely to be involved with vesicoureteral reflux. The cranial ureteric bud from the Wolffian duct intercepts the upper portion of the developing metanephric blastema, migrating to the inferomedial aspect of the trigone or bladder neck. This orifice is more likely to be obstructed and to subtend dysplastic renal parenchyma. The migration of these ureteric buds follows Stephens's ectopic pathway.[2,6] Figure 6 illustrates ureteric budding

**Fig 6.** Embryology of the duplex system. The position of each ureteral bud along the mesonephric duct predetermines the architecture of the kidney and the collecting system in the child along with the associated clinical entity. The chart illustrates these relationships. [Figure courtesy of FD Stephens, MD.]

| Clinical Entity | Wolffian Duct | Ureteric Orifice | Parenchyma |
|---|---|---|---|
| Normal, complete duplex | Normal budding position | Both normal | Normal |
| Lower pole reflux | Caudal zone | Lower pole ectopia | Atrophic lower pole |
| Upper pole ectopic ureterocele | Cranial zone | Upper pole ectopic ureterocele | Atrophic, dysplastic |
| Lower pole reflux | Caudal zone | Lower pole reflux | Atrophic |
| Upper pole ectopic ureterocele | Cranial zone | Upper pole ectopic ureterocele | Atrophic, dysplastic |
| Upper and lower pole reflux | Caudal zone (two) | Lower and upper pole lateral ectopia | Atrophic, dysplastic |

The position of each ureteral bud along the mesonephric duct predetermines the architecture of the kidney and the collecting system in the child along with the associated clinical entity. The diagram illustrates these relationships.

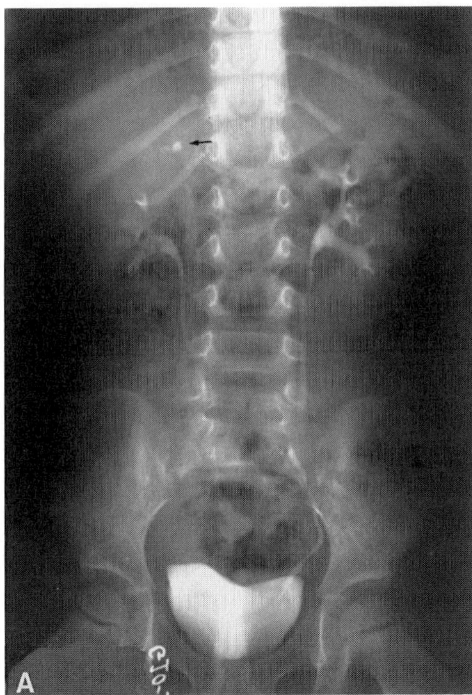

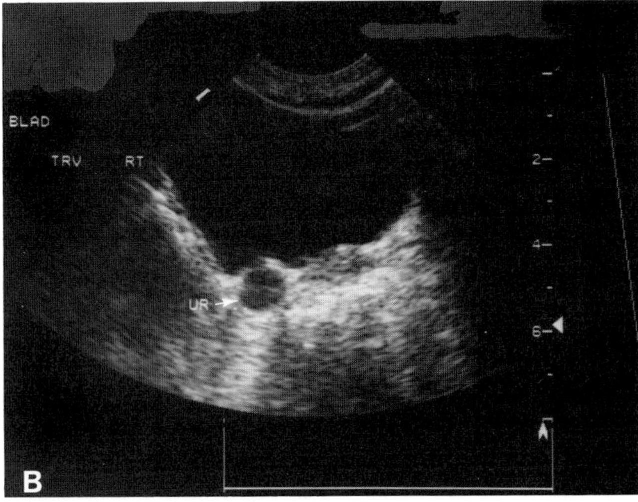


Fig 7A, B. A, a 2-year-old girl has experienced continually damp underpants. An intravenous urogram demonstrates a duplex right kidney with a small upper pole calyx (arrow); B, a dilated right ureter (UR) is seen posterior to the bladder on sonography.

zones from Wolffian duct, orifice position, and morphology and parenchymal quality.

## Incomplete Ureteric Duplication

A bifid ureteric pelvis is present in 10% of the population and is considered a normal variant. Incomplete ureteric duplications occur less frequently, and the ureters may join at any level. While the majority of these duplications are silent, dilatations of the ureters above the junction have been noted in up to 40%. This is thought to be the consequence of the "yo-yo phenomenon," in which discoordination of peristalsis between the segments allows urinary boluses from one segment to fill the relaxed proximal portion of the other ureteric seg-

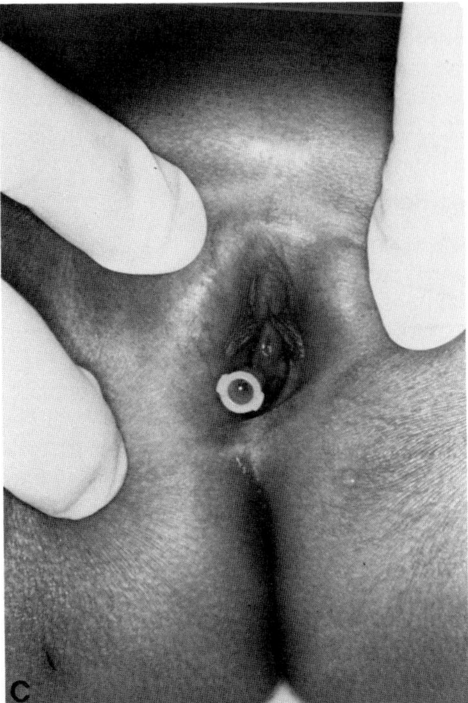


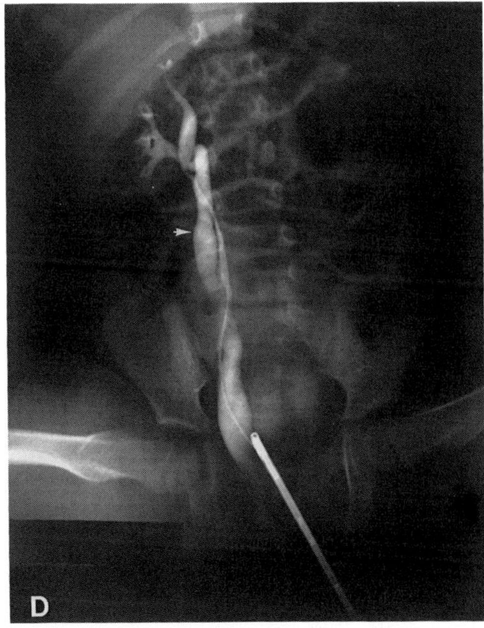


**Fig 7C, D. C,** on careful examination under anesthesia, a ureteral orifice located at the 7 o'clock position with respect to the urethral meatus is cannulated; **D,** after retrograde contrast injection of the ectopic ureter (arrow), a retrograde pyelogram of the orthotopic ureter demonstrates the anatomy of the lower pole system.

ment. Systems with distal ureteric junctions are at greater risk of the yo-yo effect, but it does not occur when the junction is within the Waldeyer sheath.[7]

When symptomatic, either from chronic pain or frequent infection, ureteropyelostomy (anastomosing ureters more proximally) or a common sheath reimplantation of both ureters (creating a complete, nonrefluxing ureteric duplication) corrects the problem.

## Complete Ureteric Duplication

Complete ureteric duplication in autopsy studies have shown an incidence of 0.7%. However, it is a finding in 4% of intravenous urogram studies, indicating that these anomalies can become clinically evident, most frequently on evaluation of urinary tract infections.[2] Hydronephrosis and scarring are identified in 27% of duplex kidneys, which is nine times more common than is seen in single-system kidneys on intravenous urogram. While duplication is only slightly more common in females than males, it is clinically evident two to three times as often in females. Bilateral duplex anomalies occur in 17% to 33% of cases.[2] In complete ureteric duplication, the lower pole system may be associated with vesicoureteral reflux or, less commonly, ureteropelvic junction obstruction. In both instances, dilatation of the lower pole moiety may be seen. On the other hand, the upper pole may be a poorly functioning segment with hypoplasia or dysplasia, with accompanying obstruction of the upper pole orifice. In these instances, the termination of the upper pole ureter is usually ectopic or associated with an ectopic ureterocele (Fig 7). Occasionally the small size of the upper pole and its poor function render it virtually "invisible" on standard radiographic studies. The "occult duplex" kidney is discussed under ureteric ectopia.

Surgical correction of symptomatic complete ureteric duplication must be individualized. When the upper pole segment is minimally functional and/or dysplastic, partial nephrectomy with excision of the proximal ureter is indicated. Ureteropyelostomy (preserving the upper pole segment) allows drainage of the functional, obstructed segment.[2,8] It should be noted that these upper pole segments occasionally bear nodular renal blastemata, raising the question of possible malignant predisposition.[4] However, recent flow cytometric DNA evaluation of upper pole dysplastic segments showed diploid ploidy, mitigating against this premalignant potential.[9]

When vesicoureteral reflux is present, implantation of both ureters in their common sheath will correct the reflux without compromising the blood supply to either ureter.[10,11] When there is disparity in caliber of completely duplex ureters, careful tailoring of the lower pole ureter, away from the common wall shared by both ureters, is possible.[2]

## VESICOURETERAL REFLUX

### Etiology

Under normal conditions, urine being stored in the urinary bladder cannot reenter the ureter, even during micturition. The ureter joins the bladder laterally and obliquely at the bladder muscular hiatus and courses beneath the bladder epithelium before ending at the ureteric orifice. Stephens's microdissection studies demonstrated longitudinal muscle fibers in the intravesical ureter and postulated that contraction of these fibers co-opts the opposing walls of the ureter when the ureter is appropriately fixed to the trigone. Ureteric peristalsis temporarily relaxes this valve mechanism to allow passage of urine into the bladder.[5]

Primary vesicoureteral reflux (VUR) occurs when there is a deficiency in subepithelial tunnel length, muscular backing, or both. Classically, the orifice is laterally positioned. Secondary VUR may result from some pathologic bladder problem (eg, bladder diverticulum, bladder outlet obstruction, and so forth) or altered pathophysiology of the bladder resulting in abnormally high intravesical pressures (eg, neuropathic bladder, dysfunctional voiding, and so forth).

### Incidence

Vesicoureteral reflux is most commonly discovered during the evaluation of urinary tract infections in children, where it has been found in 30% to 50%. It is seen most commonly in the infant, as VUR most often resolves with elongation of the subepithelial ureter with differential growth.[12] The incidence is substantially higher in girls than in boys and in Caucasian children than in black children. While the overall incidence of VUR is probably less than 1% of normal children, screening of siblings of children with VUR has revealed an incidence of 26% to 32%. Three quarters of siblings are asymptomatic.[13]

### Pathophysiology

Pyelonephritis is the most serious consequence and complication in children with primary or secondary VUR. The immature kidney, particularly in infants and children under the age of 5, is most at risk for renal scarring. The incidence of renal scarring following acute pyelonephritis may be as high as 30% to 50% in children with VUR[14] (Fig 8). Although most children with renal scarring following acute pyelonephritis have VUR, pyelonephritis may occur without VUR.[15] The polar areas of the kidney are most at risk for scarring because of the presence of compound renal papillae in these areas. Unlike the simple papilla, compound papillae allow intrarenal reflux of urine in the fused portion of the papilla. Thus, urine within the renal pelvis of kidneys with compound papillae may pass (through pyelotubular backflow) through these compound papillae and enter the renal parenchyma.[16]

Vesicoureteral reflux into an abnormal ureteric orifice allows a pathway for bacterial entry into the ureter and collecting system, introducing the risk of pyelonephritis. Ransley has postulated that the in-

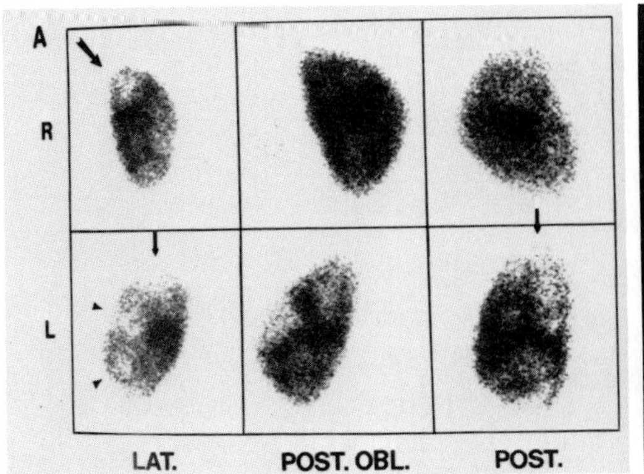


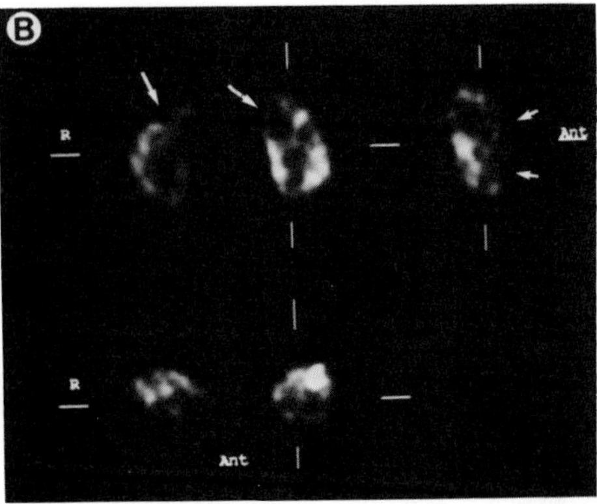


**Fig 8.** One year after a febrile urinary tract infection, a 16-month-old girl with bilateral vesicoureteric reflux (grade II/V) is reevaluated. She has had several urinary tract infections not associated with fever. **A,** pinhole images show defects of lateral and posterior aspects of left upper pole (small arrows) and possible defects of lateral aspect of left mid- and lower pole regions (arrowheads). Decreased activity of the right upper pole (large arrow), seen exclusively in the lateral view, is believed to represent liver attenuation; **B,** SPECT images reveal moth-eaten appearance of both renal units illustrating the diffuse nature of the disease process. Bilateral upper pole defects (large arrows) are seen, as well as defects in anterior aspect of left kidney (small arrows). [From Tarkington, et al.[22]]

itial episode of pyelonephritis may permanently damage all of the nephrons susceptible to infection, and subsequent infections may also result in further scarring.[16] Additionally, the role of sterile reflux in renal scar development is constantly being questioned and challenged, but most authorities feel that high-pressure, sterile VUR is injurious to renal parenchyma.

The development of pyelonephritic scar may occur in the presence of VUR, intrarenal reflux, and a bacterial urinary tract infection, due to fimbriated or nonfimbriated organisms. Prevention of the first febrile urinary tract infection is theoretically the most optimal scenario. Identification of VUR antenatally (hydronephrosis or upper urinary tract dilatation on fetal ultrasound) or screening of siblings at risk for VUR preempts the first infection, thereby avoiding the morbidity of acute pyelonephritis and renal scarring.

## Diagnosis

Voiding cystourethrography (VCUG) is highly recommended in the evaluation of the infant or younger child following a documented urinary tract infection. Contrast VCUG under fluoroscopy combines high sensitivity, superior anatomic definition of the urinary bladder, and accuracy in grading of the VUR (Fig 9). Isotope cystography is more sensitive than contrast cystography and uses 100 times less radiation than contrast VCUG.[17] Precise anatomic detail with grading is not possible with the isotope cystogram. We employ contrast cystography in our initial evaluation of children presenting with urinary tract infections or upper tract dilatation, and isotope cystography in the follow-up of children with VUR. The initial cystogram is delayed until the sterile urine culture is obtained.

## Classification

Vesicoureteral reflux may be classified and quantified. This is possible, based on contrast cystography, using the International Reflux Study Committee grading system (Fig 10).

The rate of VUR (calculated in milliliters per minute) is available with isotope cystography. This provides some quantification of the volume of refluxed urine. We have found that rates of VUR less than 10 to 12 mL/min generally have good prognoses with respect to subsequent, natural resolution (unpublished data).

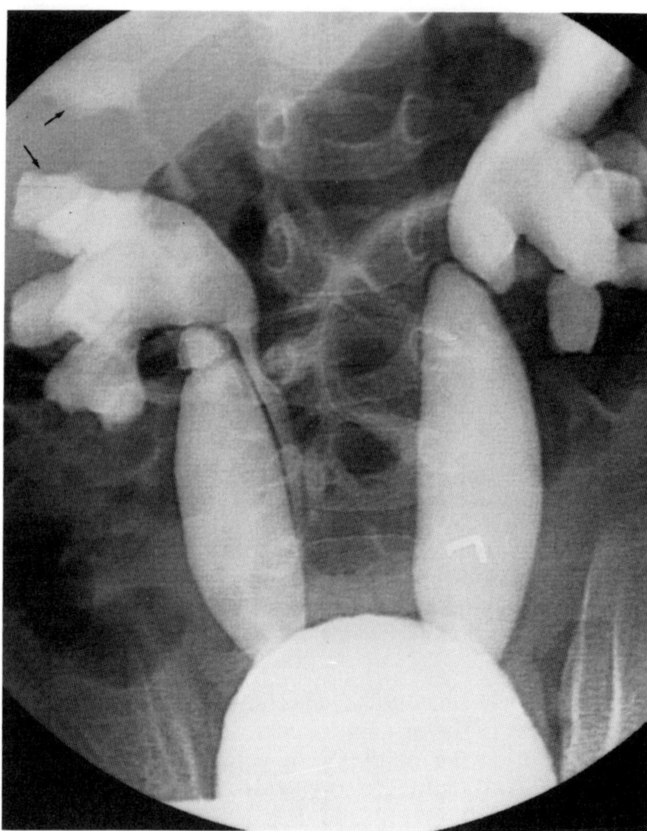

**Fig 9.** Bilateral grade V vesicoureteric reflux on voiding cystourethrogram. This represents the megaureter-megacystis syndrome and complete duplication of the right collecting system (arrows).

## Evaluation

There is little role for the intravenous urogram in the *functional* renal evaluation of kidneys associated with VUR. Of greater aid in renal functional evaluation is dimercaptosuccinic acid (DMSA) isotope scintigraphy[7,14,18,19] in evaluating (1) the child with an acute febrile urinary tract infection[15,20,21] and (2) the child with documented VUR.[22] The three-dimensional single photon emission computed tomography (SPECT) DMSA renal scan greatly improves anatomic resolution and spatial orientation both in the evaluation of acute pyelonephritis[21] and in the detection of reflux nephropathy and renal scarring.[22] SPECT imaging provides enhanced diagnostic accuracy and imaging capability when compared with two-dimensional pinhole techniques[22] (Fig 8).

Cystourethroscopy has a minor role in the evaluation of VUR. The anatomy of the involved ureteric orifice can be evaluated, particularly in instances of duplex systems. Associated bladder pathology (eg, diverticula) may also be assessed. Grossly abnormal ''golf-hole'' orifices or the presence of a large periureteric diverticulum are highly correlated with failure of VUR to resolve. Likewise, no other cystoscopic finding correlates with the outcome of VUR.[14]

## Treatment

The development of a renal scar is dependent on the presence of intrarenal reflux (IRR), VUR, and bacteriuria (UTI) (fimbriated or nonfimbriated). The equation VUR + UTI + IRR = scar is valid. The long-term sequelae of reflux nephropathy (global renal scarring) include chronic renal failure, hypertension, and proteinuria.

Medical therapy is directed at eliminating bacteriuria in order to reduce the risk of renal scarring. Long-term low-dose an-

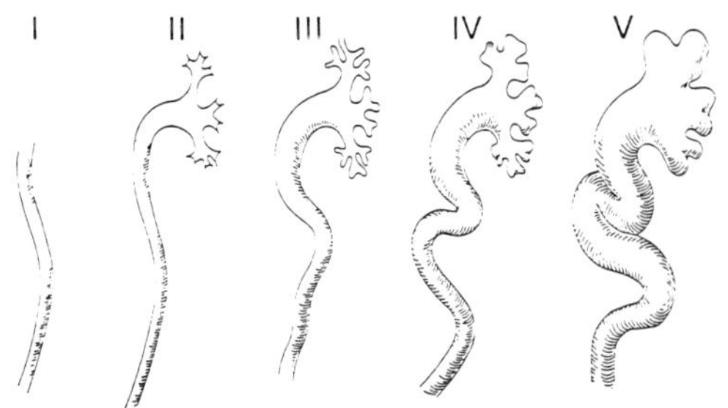


**Fig 10.** International classification of reflux. [From the United States Collaborative Study on Reflux.]

timicrobial prophylaxis is useful in maintaining urine sterility. This is attempted with the knowledge that the rate of natural resolution of VUR is high (80%) with maturation of the ureterovesical junction.[23] Edwards demonstrated the success of medical therapy in 121 renal units followed for 7 to 18 years.[23] Only two of these kidneys had further scarring while on antimicrobial prophylaxis, and both children had breakthrough infections. Continuous low-dose prophylaxis is far superior to intermittent therapy for infections only. This fact is illustrated in Lenaghan's study showing new scars in 21% and progression of existing scars in 66% when therapy is intermittent and not continuous.[24] VUR resolves at a rate of 20% to 30% per year. Bellinger showed an average time to resolution of 1.8 to 3.9 years.[14]

Medical management is continued until VUR resolves. In the preadolescent age group with persistent, nonresolving VUR, an antireflux procedure is indicated. The incidence of bacterial urinary tract infections increases dramatically in adolescence. The morbidity of recurrent pyelonephritis can be avoided with an expeditious antireflux procedure at this time. Young women with preexisting reflux nephropathy are at high risk for progression to end-stage renal disease during pregnancy.[25] It is our practice to recommend an antireflux procedure in children with primary VUR at the age of 9–10 or after failure of medical management.

Surgical management is indicated for unresolving reflux, breakthrough bacterial urinary tract infections, resistant organisms, or antibiotic intolerance or poor compliance. The high success rate associated with ureteric implantation[18] is reassuring. Duckett reported an overall success rate of 96% using several techniques. Failures from distal ureteric obstruction in 2% and persistent reflux in 2% were seen.[2] Ureters implanted using the Politano–Leadbetter technique (Fig 11) occasionally had postoperative reflux while postoperative stenosis of the ureteric orifice occurred occasionally with the Cohen–Ahmed transtrigonal technique[10,18] (Fig 12). Unilateral or bilateral implantations are performed, the latter being used when bilateral reflux is present or if a history of bilateral reflux is present. Distal ureteric tailoring

**Fig 11.** Politano–Leadbetter ureteroneocystostomy. The submucosal tunnel is lengthened by relocating the detrusor hiatus superolaterally and the ureteral orifice inferomedially. [From Fowler JE, ed, *Mastery of Surgery: Urology Surgery* (Boston: Little, Brown; 1992), with permission.]

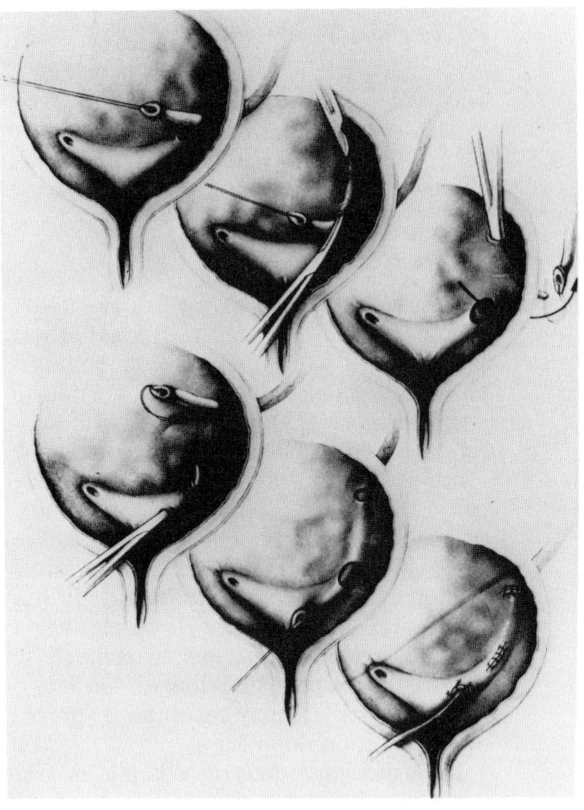

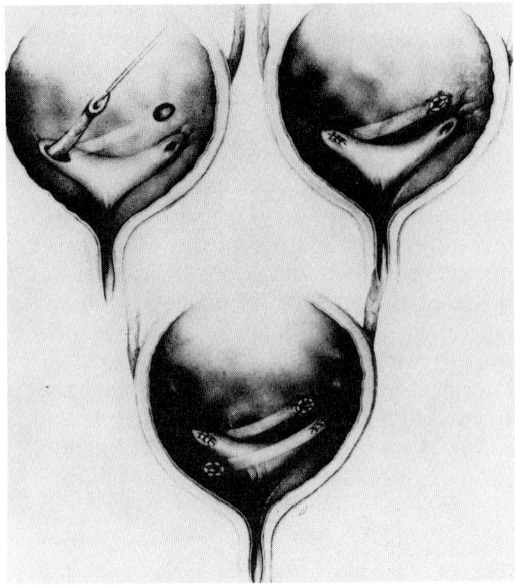

**Fig 12.** Cohen–Ahmed ureteroneocystostomy. The submucosal tunnel is lengthened by relocating the ureteral orifice across the midline of the bladder. [From Fowler JE, ed, *Mastery of Surgery: Urology Surgery.* (Boston: Little, Brown; 1992), with permission.]

may be necessary with grade IV to V reflux, usually to ensure that a 5 : 1 ratio of ureteric tunnel length to ureteric diameter is achieved.[11,26,27]

## URETERIC ECTOPIA

Ureteric ectopia occurs when the ureter terminates in an abnormal position. Ectopia is associated with single and duplex systems. Ectopia lateralis frequently results in a deficient subepithelial tunnel with subsequent VUR. When the orifice is in the ectopic pathway, the ureteric meatus may be on the trigone (usually nonobstructed), or at the bladder neck or distal to the bladder neck (obstructed)[1] (Fig 4). The terminal portion of the ectopic ureter is usually stenotic, preventing reflux. However, when ureteric obstruction is due to sphincteric constriction (sphincterostenotic orifices), paradoxical VUR may result with sphincteric relaxation on voiding.

In males, the ureteric ectopia is frequently associated with single systems. In duplex systems, the orifice may also be in the Wolffian ductal system (ejaculatory duct, seminal vesicle, or vas deferens) (Fig 5).

In females, the ectopic orifice is associated with duplex systems in 80% of cases, draining the upper pole moiety. The ectopic ureter most often terminates in the vaginal vestibule in a periurethral meatal position, followed closely in frequency by termination in the urethra, bladder neck, vagina, cervix, and uterus[28] (Figs 6 and 7).

In the male, the ureter always inserts proximal to the external sphincter, and thus incontinence is not present. The ureter may empty into any metanephric structure, including the seminal vesicle, vas deferens, or epididymis.[3] Epididymoorchitis in the infant or younger child is strongly suggestive of ureteric ectopia.

### Diagnosis

Incontinence is a common presentation in young girls since the ureter drains distal to the sphincter. However, ureters passing through the sphincteric mechanism proximal to the meatus may maintain continence until adulthood, at which time they present with incontinence, usually with a history of multiparity. As most of these ureters are partially obstructed, infection is common. Fever, flank pain, abdominal mass, and irritative voiding symptoms may also be associated with ureteric ectopia.

The clinical history often alerts the physician to the possibility of ureteric ectopia. Most of these ureters are partially obstructed; thus ultrasonography demonstrates dilatation of the involved ureter and renal collecting system to some degree.[29] The kidney (with single-system ectopia) or upper pole moiety (with duplex ectopia) may be hyperechoic on ultrasound, suggesting dysplasia. An adjacent lower pole moiety may be dilated secondary to vesicoureteral reflux or obstruction from compression by the upper pole ureter on the orthotopic (lower pole) ureter.

### Evaluation

In the older child, an intravenous urogram will demonstrate the ectopic moiety

**TABLE 1. Intravenous Urogram Findings Suggestive of an Occult Duplex Kidney with Ectopia**

Drooping lily sign—dilated upper pole segment displaces the visualized lower pole inferiorly and laterally.
Lateral displacement of the lower pole ureter.
Superior calyceal abnormalities:
- Paucity of calyces
- Infundibula shortened
- "Missing calyx" that should drain the uppermost kidney

Visualization of dilated, distal ectopic ureter on postvoid film.

if renal function is adequate for concentration of the contrast agent. If not, indirect evidence of duplication supports the diagnosis (Table 1). Computerized tomography and magnetic resonance imaging provide excellent anatomical definition of the anatomy but are rarely necessary.

Renal scintigraphy is helpful for several reasons. Assessment of the degree of function and obstruction is important in developing a management plan. A technetium diethylene triamine pentacetic acid (DTPA) or MAG-III renal scan will assess the degree of function and obstruction in single as well as duplex systems. Even minimally functioning upper pole segments can be seen on the DTPA or MAG-III scan. Alternatively, the SPECT DMSA renal scan (triad, three-dimensional) may be very helpful in the instance of an occult duplex anomaly, revealing the "absent apex sign"[30] in which the upper pole of the kidney appears flattened.

A VCUG is mandatory as half of ectopic ureters demonstrate VUR. A second or third void may be required before filling of the distal ureteric segment is adequate for visualization. Finally, examination under anesthesia and cystourethroscopy may help to identify the ectopic orifice if it has not been previously identified. Cannulation of the orifice in retrograde contrast studies confirm ectopia (Fig 7).

### Treatment

Upper pole partial nephrectomy and ureterectomy is the treatment of choice for poorly functioning upper pole segments in duplex systems. An anteromedial muscle splitting incision is used to remove the upper pole and nearly all of the upper pole ureter. Ureteropyelostomy can also be performed should upper pole function appear adequate. When lower pole VUR is associated with a functioning upper pole segment, common sheath reimplantation is definitive. Ectopic single systems are treated with nephrectomy or ureteric implantation.

## MEGAURETER

A megaureter is a dilated ureter. Classification according to etiology (Table 2) has gained wide acceptance, and treatment is dependent on the underlying cause of the dilatation.

### Evaluation

Megaureters may be identified by antenatal ultrasound or during the evaluation of urinary tract infections, abdominal masses, or abdominal pain. Recently, abdominal ultrasound has replaced the intravenous urogram in the initial evaluation of these conditions, demonstrating the course and extent of the dilated ureter as well as the renal and bladder anatomy. Calyceal and renal pelvic dilatation is variable. A VCUG is important as part of the evaluation to exclude VUR.

Once VUR has been excluded in evaluating the dilated ureter, a MAG-III or DTPA renal scan should be performed. The results of this study will delineate an obstructive from a nonobstructive megaureter. The diuretic drainage time ($T_{1/2}$) is helpful to evaluate emptying of the terminal aspect of the dilated ureter (Fig 13). Adequate hydration, a weight-related dose of furosemide, and bladder catheter drainage are important. Normal values have been defined previously.[31]

A primary obstructed megaureter results from a defective segment of distal ureter that fails to propagate peristaltic contractions. Histologically, this segment contains (1) an increase in collagenous tissue, (2) muscular hypoplasia, (3) smooth muscle arranged predominantly in a circular fashion, or (4) normal findings.[32] Only part of

**TABLE 2. Classification of Megaureter**

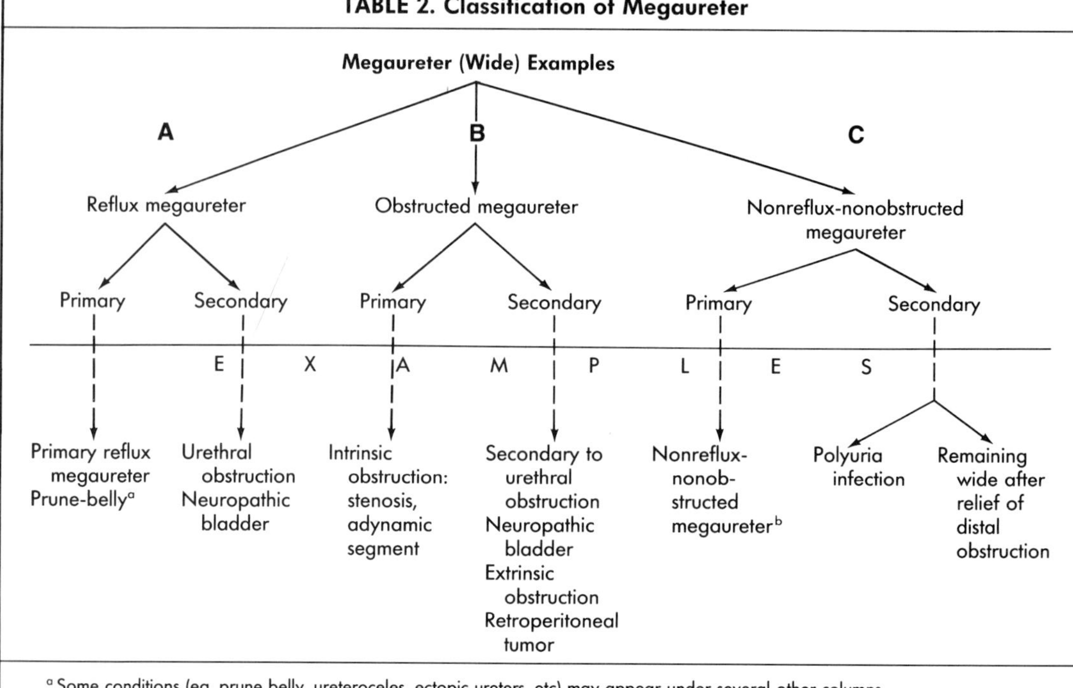


[a] Some conditions (eg, prune belly, ureteroceles, ectopic ureters, etc) may appear under several other columns.
[b] As proved not to be obstructed.
*Note:* An occasional megaureter may show reflux and apparent obstruction.
From Smith ED, et al. Report of working party to establish an international nomenclature for the large ureter. In Bergsma D, Duckett JW Jr, eds. *Birth Defects* (original article), 1977;13(5):3. Reproduced with permission from March of Dimes.

the urine bolus passes this "functional obstruction" despite a patent lumen. The remaining urine leads to a chronically dilated ureter proximal to this point.

A male predominance of 4:1 and a left-sided predominance of 2:1 exists in obstructed megaureter. Bilaterality occurs in 7% to 34%. Unlike the refluxing megaureter, which is often tortuous, the obstructed megaureter is usually relatively straight.

## Treatment

Management of primary obstructed megaureter is evolving at present. Indications for surgical correction include impaired renal function, large abdominal mass, and frequent or severe urinary tract infections. When renal function is not impaired, however, the choice of therapy is controversial. Newborns with antenatally diagnosed obstructive megaureters evaluated in the immediate newborn period can initially be managed nonoperatively. To illustrate this, Keating et al reported 20 antenatally diagosed megaureters, all followed without surgery, in which renal function remained stable.[33] However, in the event of impaired renal function, progressive renal deterioration, flank pain, or pyelonephritis, tailored ureteric reimplantation is the preferred modality of management.[26,34]

The primary refluxing megaureter results from severe VUR (grades IV and V). Ureteric wall changes produced by reflux can result in a poorly draining ureter that appears marginally obstructed as well. When discovered in infants, the involved kidney may have minimal function because of either severe hydronephrosis or renal dysplasia. Micturition can be impaired because large volumes of urine reflux during bladder contraction. This leads to the megacystis-megaureter syndrome[18,35] in which a large, smooth-walled urinary bladder is associated with a refluxing megaureter (Fig 9). When indicated, operative correction includes ureteric tailoring and implantation[26] (Fig 14). In our experience, tailoring seems superior to imbrication (Starr) or folding (Kalicinski), as the latter techniques create a bulky terminal ureter that may create problems arising from edema following implantation.

The primary nonrefluxing nonobstructed megaureter occurs occasionally but its cause is not known. It may represent a mild form of primary obstructed megaureter in which urine flow across the obstructed segment is adequate to preserve the intrarenal collecting system. Diuretic renography demonstrates the characteristic nonobstructed pattern. Management is medical but follow-up studies to ensure preservation of renal function are indicated. Bacterial urinary tract infections should be managed with prophylaxis and any tendency to acute pyelonephritis may be an indication for ureteric implantation.

Secondary megaureter is usually associated with other physiologic or anatomic conditions (diabetes insipidus, neuropathic bladder, posterior urethral valves, and so on). Management should be directed at the primary underlying problem. Only when the primary problem has been addressed should any attempt be made to manage the megaureter surgically, if indicated as a function of impaired renal function, pain, or infection.

## URETEROCELE

A ureterocele is a dilation of the intravesical portion of the ureter (Fig 15). Ureteroceles are of variable shape and configuration, and several classification systems have been developed. The simplest of these describes only its position: an "intravesical ureterocele" is one situated entirely within the bladder, while an "ectopic ureterocele" has at least one fixed point at the level of the bladder neck or urethra. The orifice of the ectopic ureterocele may be located anywhere on its surface.

Caldamone reviewed 58 cases of ureterocele; 90% were identified prior to age 3 with 25% seen in neonates. Fifty percent presented with urinary tract infections, of which half had developed urosepsis. A palpable flank mass, irritative bladder symptoms, and prolapse of the ureterocele at the urethral meatus in females were less frequent presentations.[36] The majority of ureteroceles discovered in children are at the terminus of upper pole ureters of duplex kidneys. Girls are affected four times more commonly than boys, and in girls 95% are ectopic ureteroceles. Up to 66% of ureteroceles in boys are associated with single-system kidneys.[37,38]

### Diagnosis

On ultrasonic evaluation of the bladder, ureteroceles can be seen directly as a cystic mass protruding into the bladder from its posterior, lateral side. Renal dysplasia of the upper pole is often seen, as is dilation of the ureter. Findings in the lower pole system are variable and may include dilation of the collecting system if VUR is present.

The intravenous urogram is usually not performed as the initial imaging study in children with suspected urinary tract abnormalities. Rather, the intravenous urogram is often helpful in better defining the anatomy in a child known to have a ureterocele. Table 2 describes the indirect intravenous pyelogram (IVP) findings of a nonfunctioning, often dysplastic upper pole segment. Small ureteroceles are seen as laterally placed filling defects in the bladder on earlier films in the study. Larger ureteroceles may replace the majority of the bladder. If the associated renal segment functions well enough to excrete contrast, the classic "cobra head" appearance is created by contrast on either side of the ureterocele wall (Fig 16). Ipsilateral lower pole function is delayed in 75% of patients. The contralateral kidney is often duplicated or hydronephrotic.[36,38]

Further evaluation should include a VCUG, as VUR into the ipsilateral lower pole ureter is present in 50% of patients. This occurs either because of lateral ectopia or because the ureterocele distorts the trigone and shortens the intramural ureter of the adjacent ureter. Contralateral reflux occurs in 8% of patients.[38] A DTPA renal scan will document the percent function of the associated renal segment, helping to determine whether or not a parenchyma-sparing repair should be performed. A SPECT DMSA scan may be helpful if the upper pole moiety is nondilated, in the instance of an occult duplex system.[30]

Finally, cystoscopy may be necessary to better define the ureterocele, but findings may be confusing. With irrigation, the ureterocele may decompress and essentially disappear or mimic a diverticulum. Large ureteroceles and bilateral ureteroceles can completely obscure normal landmarks. When necessary, a fine needle at the end of a ureteric catheter can be used to puncture the ureterocele and inject contrast material for a retrograde ureterogram.

## Treatment

The less common intravesical ureteroceles, usually associated with a single-system kidney and preservation of renal function, respond well to ureterocele excision

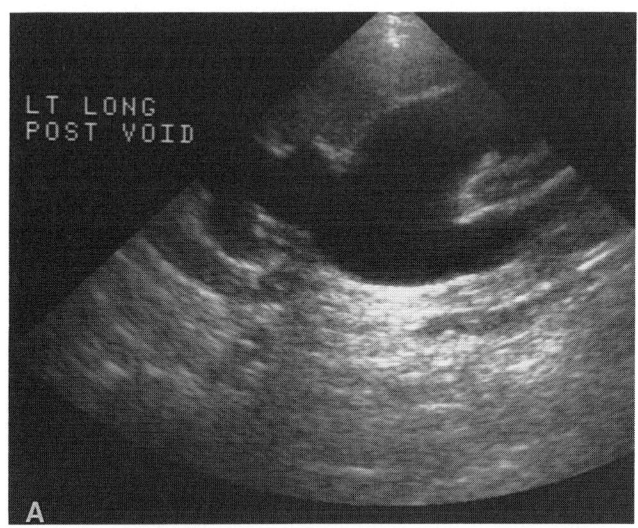


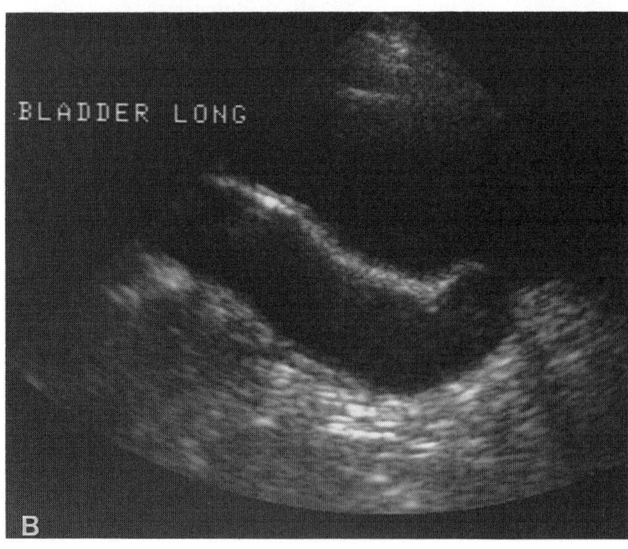


**Fig 13A, B. A,** sonography of a 9-month-old boy with a recent urinary tract infection demonstrates dilation of the left renal collecting system and ureter; **B,** the distal left ureter is dilated to the ureterovesical junction;

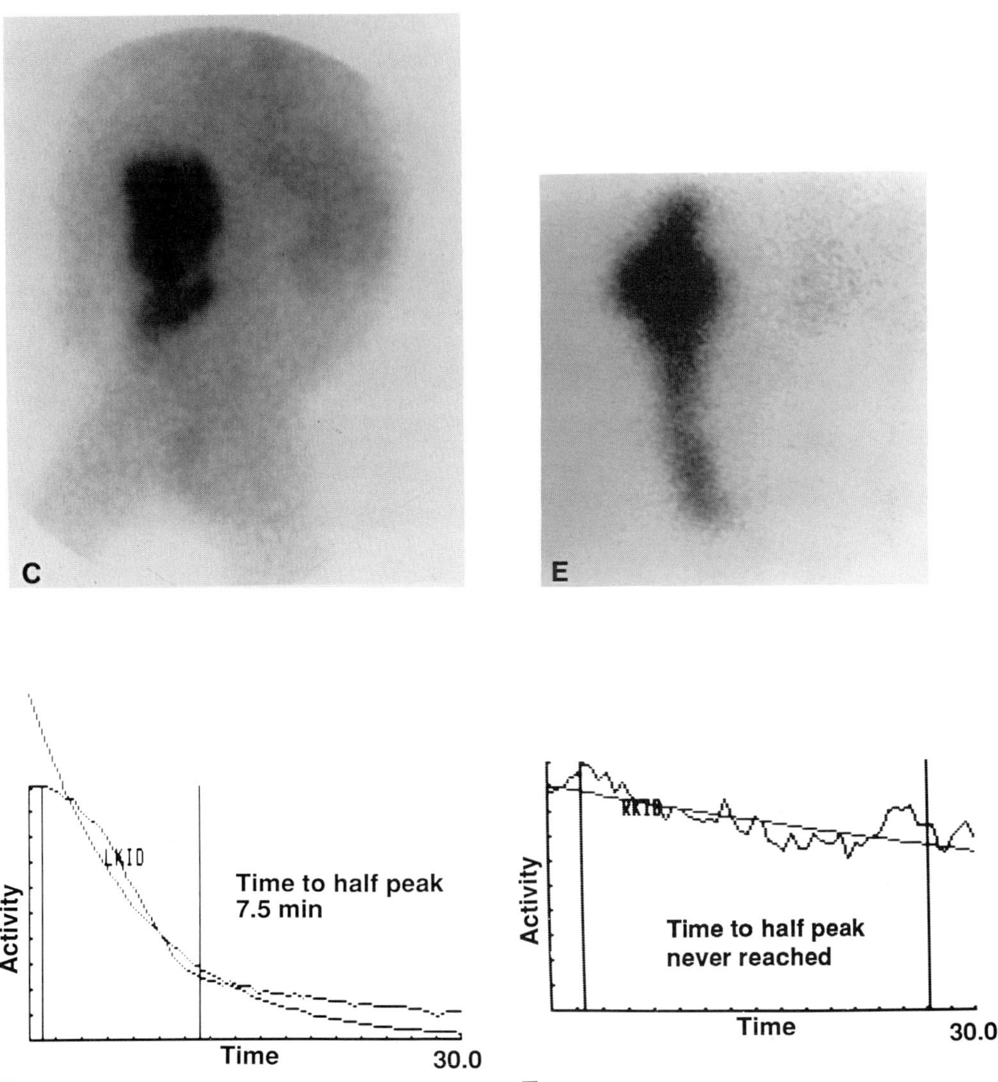


**Fig 13C, D. C,** on $TC^{99m}$ MAG-III renal scan, radiotracer pools in the left renal pelvis and ureter. The differential function of the left kidney is 56%; **D,** after furosemide, radiotracer readily washes out of the dilated portions of the ureter with a half-time of 7.5 minutes, confirming a nonobstructed megaureter; **E,** in a 4-month-old boy with a dysplastic right kidney, left hydronephrosis, and a left megaureter, $TC^{99m}$ MAG-III again fills the dilated segments; **F,** failure to wash out after furosemide is indicative of obstruction in the distal ureter.

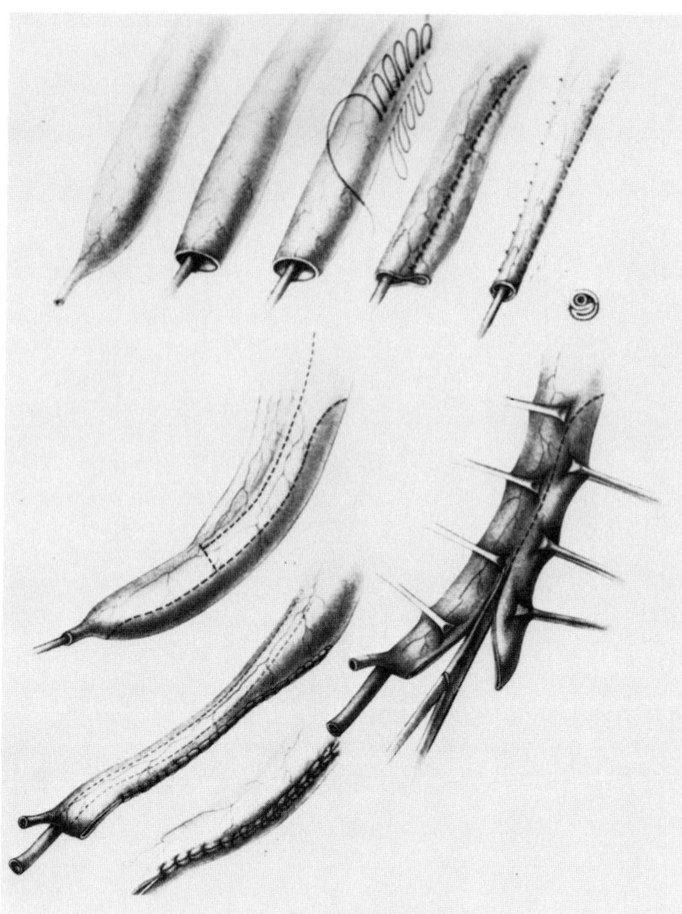

**Fig 14.** Remodeling of the dilated ureter by the plication technique (top) and the excisional tapering technique (bottom). Note that interrupted sutures are used to close the distal ureter after excisional tapering so that the ureter can be trimmed without disrupting the entire suture line. [From Fowler JE, ed, *Mastery of Surgery: Urology Surgery.* (Boston: Little, Brown; 1992), with permission.]

and ureteral reimplantation. Some bladder reconstruction may be necessary at the hiatus if the muscular wall supporting the ureterocele is attenuated. Alternatively, endoscopic incision may be attempted.[8]

Ectopic ureteroceles associated with duplication present a more challenging picture, and management options are controversial. As poor function of the renal segment associated with the dysplasia or long-standing obstruction is the rule, both the kidney and the bladder must be managed.

The least invasive option involves trans-

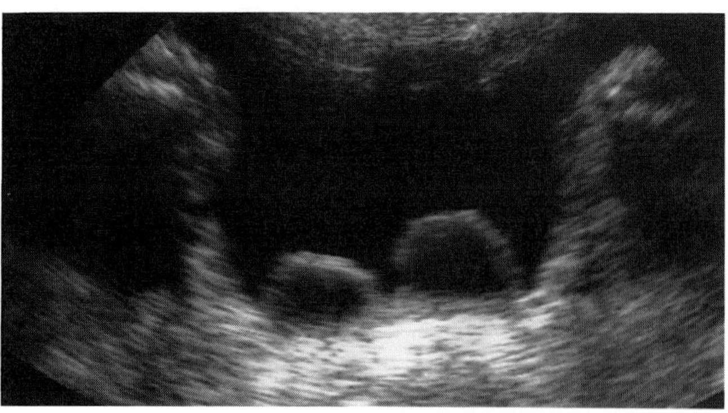

**Fig 15.** Bilateral ureteroceles are shown sonographically to be intraluminal cystic structures on the posterior wall of the bladder.

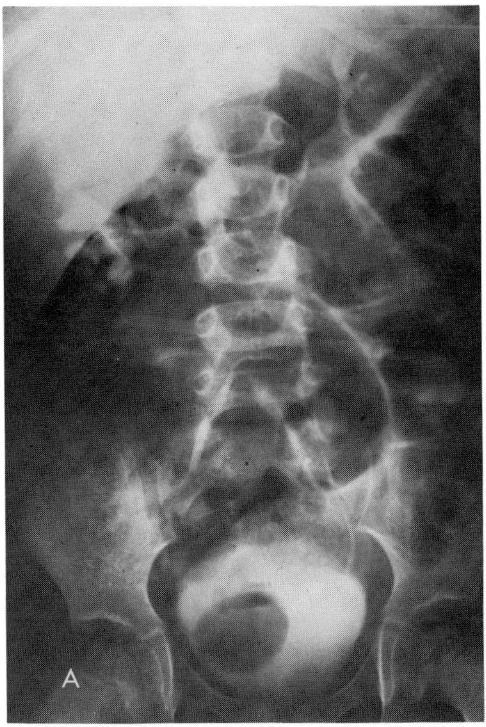


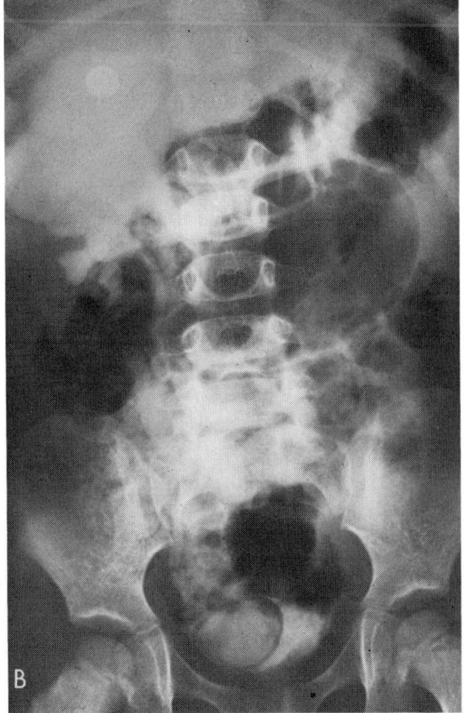


**Fig 16.** Intravenous urogram in a 2-year-old girl who presented with a history of recurrent urinary tract infections. **A,** a 10-minute exposure demonstrates a round filling defect in the bladder representing a simple ureterocele associated with a ureter draining the upper pole of a right duplex system; **B,** a radiograph 30 minutes later demonstrates filling of the ureterocele with contrast.

urethral incision of the ureterocele. This can be performed either as the initial step of a staged reconstruction that allows decompression of pyonephrosis or a dilated ureter,[37,39–41] or as the definitive procedure.[6,8] We have also employed percutaneous nephrostomy decompression in neonates with urosepsis and obstructing ureteroceles.[42] Assessment of renal function can be delayed until after distal obstruction is relieved. As a definitive modality of therapy, transurethral incision of the ureterocele is most successful in single-system ureteroceles, where preservation of renal function without postoperative VUR was accomplished in five of seven children.[40] Tank found that renal function improved in 50% of kidneys after transurethral incision of ureteroceles.[41] Furthermore, these children were spared nephroureterectomy, and only 10% required additional surgical management of multiple infections associated with VUR. However, VUR is a frequent complication of simple ureterocele incision.

In the few children with ectopic ureteroceles or ectopic ureters whose upper pole segment has adequate function as documented by IVP or renal scan, it is reasonable to preserve the renal parenchyma. Ureteropyelostomy or ureteroureterostomy with distal ureterectomy can be performed.[8] Some advocate ureterocele excision and dual ureteric implantation to prevent the possible complications associated with leaving the decompressed ureterocele unresected.[8]

Heminephrectomy is indicated in the majority of children who have nonfunction or minimal function of the upper pole segment. Several options exist for managing the ureterocele itself. Scherz and associates perform a single-staged, two-incision heminephrectomy, ureterectomy, ureterocele marsupialization, and lower pole ureteral reimplantation. Reoperation is necessary in 14% for persistent VUR.[38]

Alternatively, heminephrectomy and ureterectomy to the level of the iliac vessels is accomplished initially. This decompresses the distal ureter and ureterocele. Only in the setting of persistent reflux into the lower pole or contralateral ureter, symptomatic reflux into the upper pole ureteral stump, or bladder outlet obstruction from the decompressed ureterocele would a second procedure be accomplished. The need to reoperate has been reported to be as low as 20% (for bladder outlet obstruction and VUR), but rates of 47% to 60% have been reported, predominantly for persistent reflux.[36–38] Although this approach requires a second operation, previous decompression of the ureterocele simplifies the bladder repair. While this is the most popular approach currently, the treatment of ureteroceles must be individualized, and each of these options is valuable in selected patients.

## REFERENCES


1. Maizels M. Normal development of the urinary tract. In: Retik AB, Stamey TA, Vaughn ED, eds. *Campbells Urology*. Philadelphia: WB Saunders; 1992: chap 32.
2. Caldemone MD. Duplication anomalies of the upper urinary tract in infants and children. *Urol Clin North Am*. 1985;12(1).
3. Mackie GG, Stephens FD. Duplex kidneys: a correlation of renal dysplasia with position of the ureteral orifice. *J Urol*. 1975;114:274.
4. Gaddy CD, Gibbons MD, Gonzales ET, Finegold MJ. Obstructive uropathy, renal dysplasia and nodular renal blastemata: is there a relationship to Wilms' tumor? *J Urol*. 1985; 134:330–334.
5. Gibbons MD, Cromie WC, Duckett JW Jr. Classification of ectopic vas deferens. *J Urol*. 1978;120:597–604.
6. Stephens DF. *Congenital Malformations of the Urinary Tract*. New York: Praeger; 1983:286–306.
7. Rink RC, Adams MC, Mitchell ME. Ureteral abnormalities. In: Ashcraft KW, ed. *Pediatric Urology*. Philadelphia: WB Saunders; 1990: chap 6.
8. Reitelman C, Perlmutter AD. Ureteropyelostomy and ureteroureterostomy. In: Fowler J, ed. *Mastery of Surgery: Urology Surgery*. Boston: Little, Brown; 1992;218–220.
9. Lobos M, Horan JJ, Azumi N, Blair O, Gibbons MD. Flow cytometric evaluation of solid renal dysplasia. American Urological Association, Washington, DC, 1992, Abstract 257.
10. Dunne EF, Gibbons MD. Ureteroneocystostomy. In: Fowler J, ed. *Mastery of Surgery: Urology Surgery*. Boston: Little, Brown; 1992:194.
11. Rabinowitz R, Barkin M, Schillinger JF. Primary massive reflux in children. *Urology*. 1979;13:248–252.
12. Levitt SB, Weiss RA. Vesicoureteral reflux. In: Kelalis PP, King LP, Belman AB, eds. *Clinical Pediatric Urology*. 2nd ed. Philadelphia: WB Saunders; 1985:335.
13. Jerkins GR, Noe HN. Familial vesicoureteral reflux: a prospective study. *J Urol*. 1982; 128:774.
14. Bellinger MF. The management of vesicoureteral reflux. *Urol Clin North Am*. 1983;12(1):23–30.
15. Rushton HG, Majd M, Jantausch B, Wiedermann B, Belman AB. Renal scarring following reflux and nonreflux pyelonephritis in children: evaluation with 99-m technetium-dimercaptosuccinic acid scintigraphy. *J Urol*. 1992; 147:1327–1332.
16. Ransley PG. Vesicoureteral reflux: continuing surgical dilemma. *Urology*. 1978;12:246.
17. Conway JJ, King LR, Belman AB, Thurston T. Detection of vesicoureteral reflux with radionuclide cystography. *Am J Radiol*. 1972; 115:720.
18. Gibbons MD, Gonzales ET. Complications of antireflux surgery. *Urol Clin North Am*. 1983;10:489–501.
19. Rushton HG, Majd M, Chandra R, Yim D. Evaluation of 99-technetium dimercaptosuccinic acid renal scans in experimental acute pyelonephritis in piglets. *J Urol*. 1988;140:1169–1174.
20. Fildes R, O'Conner K, Levin K, Garra B, Newsome J, Harkness B, Sesterhan I, Gibbons MD. Advanced renal imaging in the diagnosis of acute pyelonephritis in the piglet. Society for Pediatric Research, Baltimore; 1992.
21. Giblin J, Gibbons MD, Fildes R, Levin K, O'Conner K, Harkness B, et al. Acute pyelonephritis in the piglet: SPECT DMSA scintigraphy—a pathologic correlation. American Academy of Pediatrics, San Francisco; 1992, Abstract 40.
22. Tarkington MA, Fildes RD, Levin K, Zeissman H, Harkness B, Gibbons MD. High resolution single photon emission computerized tomography (SPECT) 99-m technetium dimercaptosuccinic acid renal imaging: a state of the art technique. *J Urol*. 1990;144:598–600.
23. Edwards D, Normand ICS, Poseod N. Disappearance of vesicoureteral reflux during long-term prophylaxis of urinary tract infections in children. *Br J Med*. 1977;2:285–288.

24. Lenaghan D, Whitaker JG, Jensen F, Stephens FD. The natural history of reflux and long-term effects on the kidney. *J Urol.* 1976;115:728.
25. Becker GJ, Ihle BU, Fairley KF. Effect of pregnancy and moderate renal failure in reflux nephropathy. *Br Med J.* 1986;292:796.
26. Pfeffer DM, Caldamone AA. Management of the dilated ureter in children. In: Fowler J, ed. *Mastery of Surgery: Urology Surgery*. Boston: Little, Brown; 1992:221–227.
27. Glassberg KI. The management of primary reflux to the massively dilated upper urinary tract. In: Johnson JG, ed. *Management of Vesicoureteric Reflux*. Baltimore: Williams and Wilkins; 1984:137–145.
28. Malek RS, Kelalis PP, Stickler GB, Burke EC. Observations on ureteral ectopy in children. *J Urol.* 1972;107:308.
29. Nussbaum AD, Durst JP, Jeffs RD. Ectopic ureter and ureterocele: their varied sonographic appearance. *Radiology.* 1986;159:227.
30. Young R, Gibbons MD. SPECT DMSA scintigraphy: an adjunct in the identification of the occult duplex anomaly. Unpublished data, 1992.
31. Dejter SW, Gibbons MD. Delayed management of neonatally detected hydronephrosis. *J Urol.* 1988;140:1305–1309.
32. Hanna MK, Jeffs RD, Sturgess JM, Barkin M. Ureteral structure and ultrastructure. II. Congenital ureteropelvic junction and primary obstructive megaureter. *J Urol.* 1976;116:725.
33. Keating MA, Escala J, Snyder HMcC, Heyman S, Duckett, J.W. Changing concepts in the management of primary obstructive megaureter. *J Urol.* 1989;142:636–640.
34. Hendren WH. Operative repair of megaureter in children. *J Urol.* 1969;101:491.
35. Burbige KA, Lebowitz RL, Colodny AH, Bauer SB, Retik AB. The megacystis-megaureter syndrome. *J Urol.* 1984;131:1133.
36. Caldamone AA, Snyder HMcC, Duckett JW. Ureteroceles in children: followup of management with upper tract approach. *J Urol.* 1984;131:1130–1132.
37. Decter RM, Roth DM, Gonzales ET. Individualized treatment of ureteroceles. *J Urol.* 1989;142:535.
38. Scherz HC, Kaplan GW, Packer MG, Brock WA. Ectopic ureteroceles: surgical management with preservation of continence—review of 60 cases. *J Urol.* 1989;142:538.
39. Montfort G, Morrison-Lacombe G, Coquet M. Endoscopic treatment of ureteroceles revisited. *J Urol.* 1985;133:1031.
40. Rich MA, Keating MA, Snyder HMcC III, Duckett JW. Low transurethral incision of single system intravesical ureteroceles in children. *J Urol.* 1990;144:186.
41. Tank ES. Experience with endoscopic incisions and open unroofing of ureteroceles. *J Urol.* 1986;136:241–242.
42. O'Brien W, Matsumoto AH, Grant EG, Gibbons MD. Percutaneous nephrostomy in infants. *Urology.* 1990;36:269.

# 49

# Anomalies of the Bladder

*Dennis S. Peppas and John P. Gearhart*

## BLADDER EXSTROPHY

### History

Bladder exstrophy exists as part of a spectrum of anomalies that includes cloacal exstrophy at one extreme and glanular epispadias at the other. Exstrophy was first described on an Assyrian tablet from 2000 BC preserved in the British Museum in London. The next written description was in 1597 by Scheuke von Graffenberg, more than 3500 years after its initial description.[1]

In the 1850s, urinary diversion for bladder exstrophy was first employed in its treatment, but with little success.[2] Successful diversion via ureterosigmoidostomy began with Coffey.[3] However, because of severe complications (including infection and acidosis), it was not until the mucosa-to-mucosa anastomosis by Nesbit in 1949[4] and later the contributions of Leadbetter that ureterosigmoidostomy became popular, and remains so in parts of the world.[5]

In 1942 Hugh Hampton Young described the first continent female patient after bladder closure,[6] and in 1948 Michon reported the first success in the male.[7] Despite this initial success, many surgeons preferred treating bladder exstrophy with cystectomy and urinary diversion well into the 1950s.[8,9]

Osteotomy was introduced in 1958 by Schultz.[10] He performed bilateral iliac osteotomies and 2 weeks later bladder closure was performed with symphyseal approximation. A female patient thus treated became continent after removal of her catheter. By approximating the pubic bones into their normal position, it was felt that continence was improved at the level of the urogenital diaphragm.

Despite progressing success with bladder closure in the 1950s and 1960s, success with urinary continence was difficult to achieve. Dees's[11] modification of the Young bladder neck reconstruction, as well as the further improvements made by Leadbetter, resulted in improved dry intervals.[12] This was especially true for the group with epispadias, but those with exstrophy tended to do more poorly in terms of continence.[13,14]

However, over the past three decades, the acceptance of the staged reconstruction in exstrophy management has done much to improve the overall outcome of these children.[15,16] Closure within the first few days of life, with or without osteotomy, epispadias repair to help increase eventual bladder capacity by increasing urethral resistance, and bladder neck reconstruction at a time when bladder capacity has increased have all resulted in increased socialization and activity of these patients.[17,18]

### Incidence

Classical bladder exstrophy has an estimated incidence of between 1 in 10,000 and 1 in 50,000 live births.[19–21] The male-to-female ratio is approximately 2.3 : 1.[22] There appears to be an increased incidence in children of patients with exstrophy or epispadias. In a review by Shapiro et al,[23] the risk of exstrophy of the bladder in offspring of individuals with exstrophy of the bladder or epispadias was 1 in 70 live births, an almost 500-fold greater incidence than in the general population. There is also an increased risk of having a second family member with this condition. Nine affected siblings were found in 2500 indexed cases, giving a 3.6% overall risk to this group.

Epispadias occurs much less frequently than exstrophy. The incidence is approximately 1 in every 112,000 male and 1 in every 412,000 female births.[24] A recently completed review of 262 patients with exstrophy-epispadias complex seen at The Johns Hopkins Hospital between 1975 and 1992 revealed 195 with classic bladder exstrophy, 38 with complete epispadias, 14 with a variant of bladder exstrophy or epispadias, and 15 with cloacal exstrophy. The male-to-female ratios in this group were 0.5 : 1 for cloacal exstrophy with 4 males raised in the female sex, 3.1 : 1 for classical bladder exstrophy, 2.4 : 1 for complete epispadias, and 1.7 : 1 for exstrophy variants.

## Embryology

Normal genitourinary development occurs between the 4th and 12th weeks of gestation.[25] Therefore, an interference with the normal developmental processes must be responsible for this spectrum of anomalies.

During the 2nd and 3rd weeks of gestation, the tail attains a ventral position from its original dorsal location.[26] As this occurs, the common cloaca is formed which is separated from the amniotic space by the cloacal membrane, which is formed from an inner endodermal layer and an outer ectodermal layer. This cloacal membrane is then bordered laterally by two mesenchymal projections and cranially by the primordia of the genital tubercles. Normally, mesenchymal ingrowth between the layers of the cloacal membrane results in the formation of the lower abdominal muscles and pelvic bones. The division of the common cloaca begins at approximately 5 weeks gestational age, by the caudad growth of the urorectal septum, and the lateral infoldings that occur simultaneously. Thus, by the end of the 7th week, the cloaca is divided into a dorsal rectum and a ventral bladder and urogenital sinus.[25,26] The remaining portion of the cloacal membrane, after division of the cloaca into bladder and rectum, will then rupture to become the urethral groove in the male and the vestibule of the vagina in the female.[25,27] Bladder exstrophy would thus occur if rupture of the cloacal membrane occurred after completion of the urorectal septum but prior to ingrowth of the mesenchyma forming the abdominal wall. Furthermore, cloacal exstrophy (in which the bladder and hindgut are exposed) would thus occur if membrane rupture occurred before descent of the urorectal septum.[27]

In contrast to exstrophy, the embryology associated with epispadias appears to result from a persistence of the cloacal membrane cephalad to the genital tubercles.[29] Therefore, the paired genital tubercles and associated mesenchyma would fail to fuse in the midline resulting in an abnormal communication between the urogenital portion of the cloaca and the amniotic cavity, leading to this malformation.[28,29]

## Clinical Presentation

Despite the apparent anomaly seen by the parents soon after delivery, the abnormalities seen in bladder exstrophy are relatively confined to the abdomen and perineum, bladder, upper urinary tract, genitalia, spine, and bony pelvis (Fig 1). The area bounded by the umbilicus, rectus abdominis muscles, and anus forms a diamond into which the most apparent anomalies are located. There is foreshortening of the umbilical–anal distance, with the anus being located further anterior than normal. The rectus abdominis muscles are laterally displaced, inserting into the pubic tubercles. As a result of the lateral displacement of the rectus muscles, the internal inguinal canals are widened, placing the internal inguinal ring just beneath the

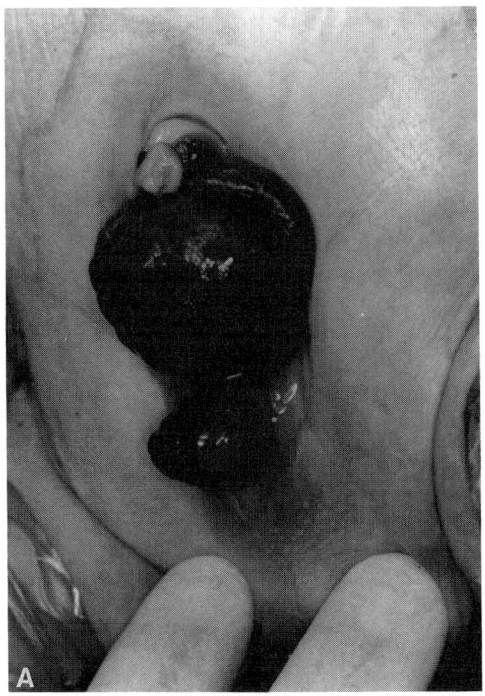


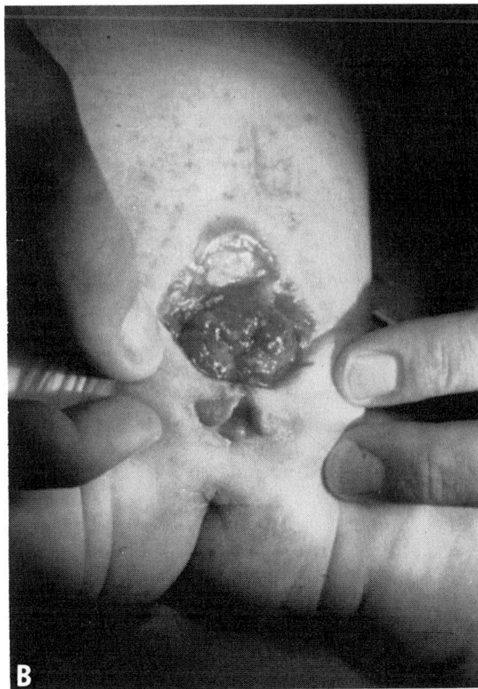


**Fig 1. A,** classic bladder exstrophy in male infant. Note the foreshortened appearance of the phallus; **B,** classic bladder exstrophy in female infant.

external inguinal ring. Therefore, indirect inguinal hernia is common, occurring in approximately 85% of the population.[30–32]

Imperforate anus is infrequently associated with bladder exstrophy; however, several cases have been reported.[30] Rectal prolapse is seen in untreated patients and in those with failed initial closures. This is associated with poor support by the displaced anal sling mechanism and the Valsalva pressures that occur during crying and grunting.[33] However, rectal prolapse is almost never seen after successful bladder closure.

The exposed bladder can vary in size from a very small patch with an estimated capacity of less than 5 $cm^3$ to one with significant capacity. The epithelium is very sensitive and develops a progressively worsening polypoid appearance as the bladder mucosa remains exposed. Polypoid changes occur as a result of mucosal irritation from salves or clothing (Fig 2). Shortly after birth, microscopic changes in the transitional epithelium can progress to squamous or adenomatous metaplasia that can later lead to squamous cell carcinoma or adenocarcinoma.[34–37] There are some data to suggest that in the unclosed exstrophy patient the epithelium is at a primitive stage and thus may predispose these patients to malignant changes.[38]

The blood supply to the exstrophied bladder is normal. The exstrophied bladder appears to be capable of normal neuromuscular activity and therefore should demonstrate normal detrusor activity once bladder closure has been successfully accomplished.[39] There are, however, at least two studies that suggested poor detrusor function in these bladders.[40]

The ureters course deeply through the bony pelvis and exit into the bladder with markedly shortened submucosal tunnels. As a result, a very large percentage of these patients demonstrate primary vesicoureteral reflux after successful bladder closure.[41] Ureteral activity appears to be normal.[42] The urethra is most commonly completely exposed, but may be covered

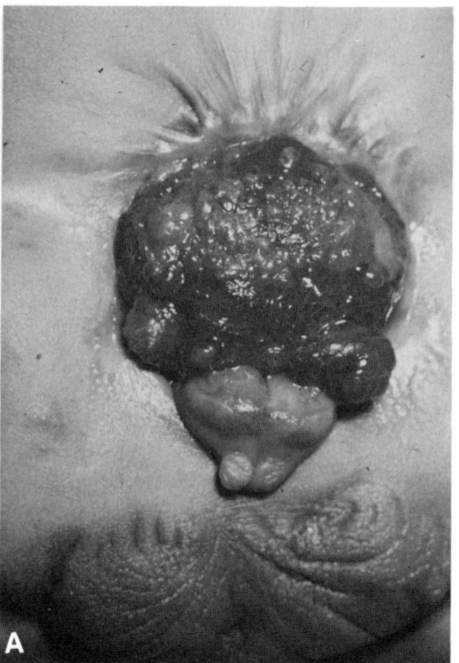


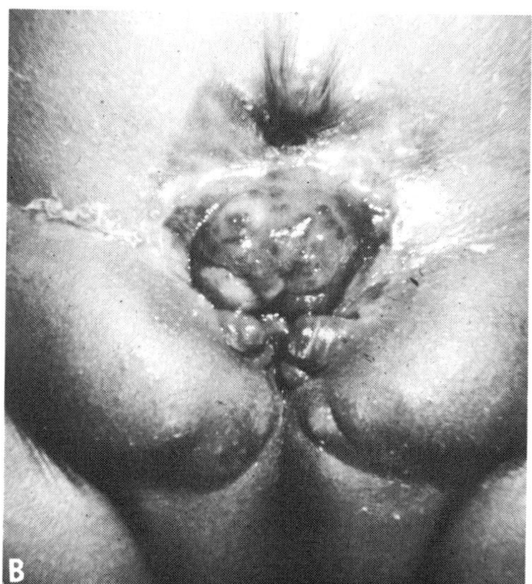


**Fig 2.** Exstrophic bladder in the male (**A**) and female (**B**). Note there are marked polypoid and epithelial changes present.

to the base of the symphysis pubis. In some exstrophy variants, there may be an incomplete epispadias or a normal urethra. Dorsal chordee is the rule.

The male phallus almost always appears shortened. This is due to the widely separate pubic bones, preventing the corpora cavernosa from joining in the midline in their usual position near the base of the pubis. As previously mentioned, dorsal chordee is almost always present, and there is often shortening of the urethral groove. Absence of a cavernosal body, rudimentary corpora, or diphallia may be present, but this occurs more frequently in cloacal exstrophy.

In contrast to the normal phallus, the neurovascular bundles that control erectile function in the epispadiac phallus are laterally displaced.[43] In patients with cloacal exstrophy, the corpora are more laterally displaced.[44] Despite the lateral deviation of the neurovascular bundles in exstrophy patients, most patients are capable of having satisfactory erections.

The structures derived from the mesonephric (Wolffian) duct are normal. Retrograde ejaculation and epididymitis are not uncommon in those patients with an open or dysfunctional bladder neck. The reason for this may be the location of the verumontanum and the ejaculatory ducts after successful bladder closure and bladder neck reconstruction. However, there have been reports of exstrophy patients fathering children.[45] Cryptorchidism has been reported to occur with a tenfold higher incidence compared to the normal population. The incidence of undescended testes in our patient population is low, occurring in 23 of 145 male patients treated for classical exstrophy at The Johns Hopkins Hospital.

In the female there is a hemiclitoris usually present on each side. There may be vaginal duplication, with the orifice or orifices easily seen just inferior to the exposed urethra. Uterine duplication may also be present. The ovaries and fallopian tubes are generally normal.

Virtually all patients with exstrophy or epispadias have pubic diastasis. There is usually outward rotation of the hips. Few if any long-term hip or gait problems result. There has been at least one report of a higher incidence of vertebral malformation in patients with exstrophy.[46] The incidence is certainly higher in those with cloacal exstrophy.[47]

## Diagnosis

With the advent of routine antenatal ultrasound, the diagnosis of exstrophy of the bladder in utero is possible.[48,49] The diagnosis is suspected if on ultrasound the bladder is never seen to fill throughout the study. In addition, the identification of an anterior abdominal mass and/or low-set umbilicus can suggest the diagnosis of bladder exstrophy. Serial ultrasound examinations must be performed, however, because of the low specificity and sensitivity of this test.

Postnatally, the diagnosis of bladder exstrophy is obvious. However, in the spectrum of anomalies thus far discussed, further evaluation may be required prior to treatment. This is especially true in a child with cloacal exstrophy where there is a higher incidence of myelomeningocele, renal anomalies, and where sex of rearing determinations need to be made.[50]

If the child is to be referred to a specialized center for the treatment of exstrophy, the bladder is to be covered with a square of clear plastic wrap (such as Saran) rather than a piece of moist gauze or a diaper. Also to be avoided are salves or petroleum jelly because any of these may dry and denude the epithelium.

The bladder is closely inspected. This is especially important in cases of cloacal exstrophy, where portions of hindgut are usually interposed between the hemibladders. Close inspection for the ureteral orifices is also made.

Phallic length in the male needs to be assessed. This is important not only for the child with cloacal exstrophy who may have his sex of rearing altered because of deficient corporal tissue or diminutive size of phallus, but also for the child with classical exstrophy. This is because (as will be discussed later) the decision as to whether to use paraexstrophy flaps will be based on the length of the urethral groove and the phallus.

## Treatment

Ultimately, bladder closure is performed in the first 24 to 48 hours after birth. If transfer to a medical center familiar with the care of exstrophy patients is to occur, then care in providing an adequate dressing for the open bladder is required.

It is of utmost importance that the parents of the child understand that the treatment of this condition is a staged surgical approach, requiring at a minimum two to three major surgical procedures over a period of several years. They should also understand prior to treatment that despite the numerous procedures required for the correction of this defect, their child can be expected to lead a normal life.[51]

With close attention to detail and a staged approach to reconstruction, few if any patients need be diverted.[52–55] In 72 children treated exclusively at The Johns Hopkins Hospital for classical bladder exstrophy, only one child was diverted initially for what was felt to be inadequate bladder capacity. Children with extremely small bladder capacities have demonstrated good bladder growth following primary closure and epispadias repair.[56]

The initial operative procedure is bladder closure with or without osteotomy. The argument against osteotomy stems from the persistence of maternal relaxin after delivery, lasting up to 72 hours after delivery. Optimally, closure is performed within the first 24 to 48 hours of life. The argument for osteotomy is that it allows for an unhurried closure, thereby increasing the likelihood of an initial successful closure.

In the male, epispadias repair is performed at approximately 2 years of age. In both males and females, the children are closely observed and regular assessments of bladder capacity under anesthesia are made. At a time when bladder volume exceeds 60 mL, bladder neck reconstruction can take place.[57,58] This normally occurs at approximately 3½ to 5 years of age.

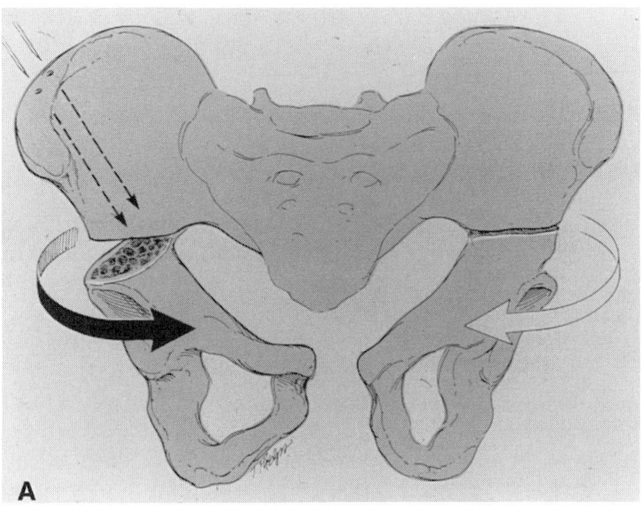


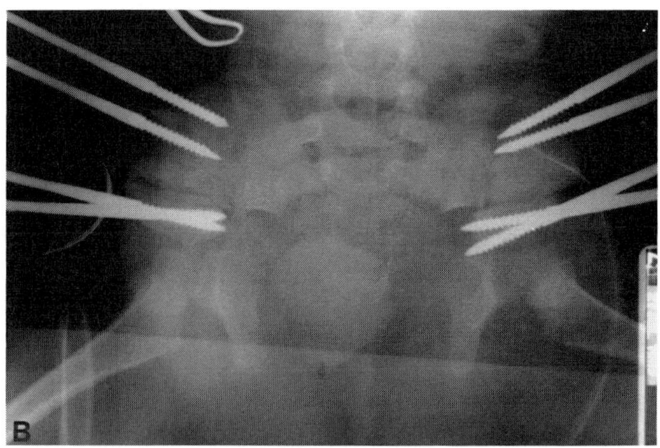


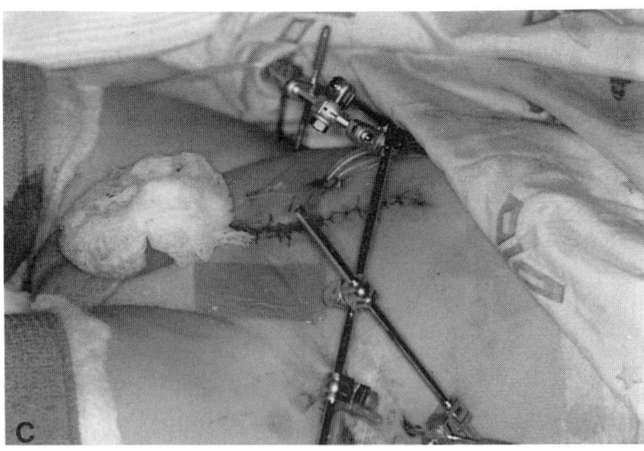


**Fig 3. A,** diagrammatic representation of anterior innominate osteotomy; **B,** intraoperative radiograph to verify proper pin placement; **C,** post external fixator placement.

## Operative Procedures

It is important to recognize that at the time of primary bladder closure the goals of the procedure are closure of the bladder, displacement to a posterior position deep within the pelvis, approximation of the pubic symphysis, and provision of free urethral drainage. Penile lengthening, if needed, should be performed at the same time.

In some cases, if the bladder is closed within the first 24 to 72 hours of life, osteotomy may not be needed. However, if the pubic diastasis is wide or the pelvis is not malleable, either posterior iliac or anterior innominate osteotomy should be performed at the time of initial closure.

In our experience, anterior innominate osteotomy is preferred over posterior (iliac) osteotomy.[59] The advantage of the anterior approach is that there is better pelvic mobilization and both the osteotomy and bladder closure can be completed with the patient in the supine position. In addition, placement of interfragmentary stabilizing pins across the osteotomy fixes the bone fragments and allows excellent callus formation. The pins are then held in place with an external fixator that is placed at the end of the abdominal closure (Fig 3). In the younger patient, modified Bryant's traction is used instead of an external fixator.

**Bladder Closure.** Prior to performing an incision for bladder closure, any polypoid areas on the bladder mucosa must be excised (Fig 2). An incision is then made beginning superior to the umbilicus (following osteotomy, if indicated), using the bladder as a template for the incision (Fig 4). The incision is carried down to the level of the verumontanum in males and to the vaginal orifice in females.[60] Squamous epithelium should not be incorporated into the bladder closure since this may result in squamous metaplasia, which may foster chronic infection. If the phallus in male patients is extremely small the consideration for genitoplasty and conversion to the female sex of rearing may be entertained. This is performed more frequently in the cloacal exstrophy patient and less frequently in classical bladder exstrophy. If the urethral plate is found to be short and there is significant dorsal chordee, then paraexstrophy flaps (the shiny skin adjacent to the area of the bladder neck) may be used to lengthen the urethral plate.[61] If paraexstrophy flaps are used, then the corporal bodies may also be dissected from the body of the pubis by bringing the proximal corpora together in the midline and thus increasing the apparent length of the penis.[61,62]

The bladder is then widely mobilized from the rectus muscles. The peritoneum is bluntly dissected from the posterior wall of the bladder so that the bladder can drop into the pelvis. The dissection is carried laterally to the level of the pubis. At this point, the fibromuscular attachments to the pubis are dissected away from the bone, separating the prostatic and membranous urethra from the pubis. In this manner the urethra will achieve a more posterior position after symphyseal approximation.

In the female, paraexstrophy flaps may also be used to allow further lengthening of the urethra. As opposed to the male, the entire female urethra can be reconstructed at the time of bladder closure. By deepithelializing the medial aspects of the clitoral halves, the clitoris can be brought together and approximated, leading to a more normal appearance.

Feeding tubes are then used to cannulate the ureters bilaterally. The bladder is then closed in two layers with absorbable sutures. Prior to completion of the bladder closure, a suprapubic catheter is placed through a separate stab incision. As one proceeds toward the bladder neck area, it is closed over a sound or catheter (14 French), large enough to provide an outlet for urine drainage but small enough to allow some resistance for bladder growth and to prevent bladder prolapse. Urethral catheters should not be used postoperatively. These have been shown to cause necrosis, erosion of the pubic suture, and, most importantly, failure of initial closure.[63]

Prior to skin closure, the symphysis pubis is reapproximated. A horizontal mattress suture using no. 2 nylon is our suture of choice. The rectus abdominus muscles

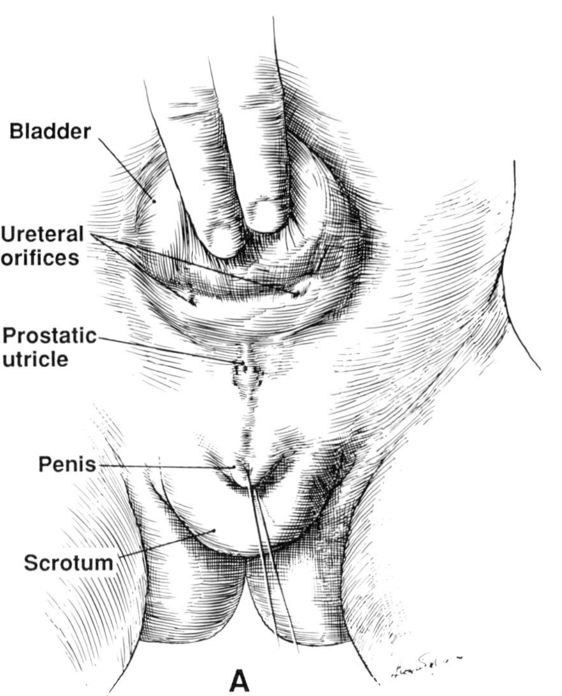


**Fig 4.** Primary bladder closure (if osteotomy is indicated, it is performed prior to bladder closure). **A–D,** Incision begun above umbilicus and carried around bladder to level distal to verumontanum. The urethral plate is not incised if there is adequate length of the urethral groove.

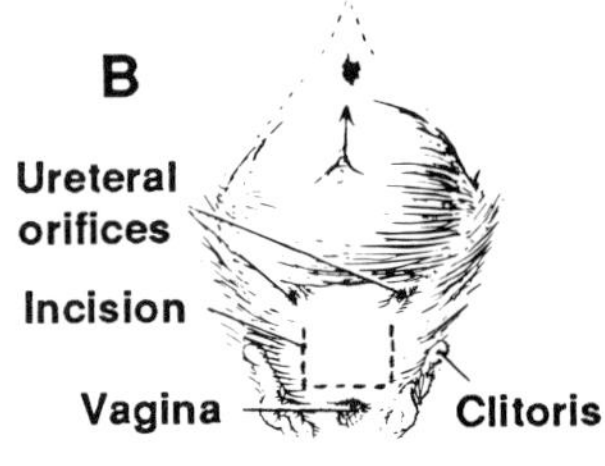


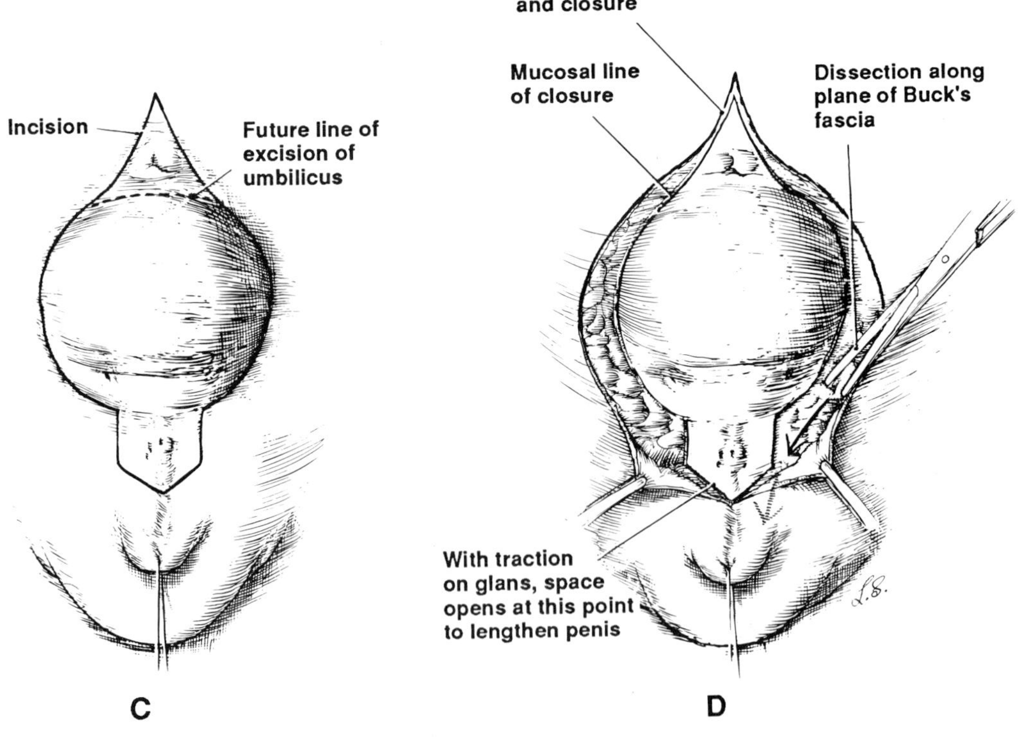

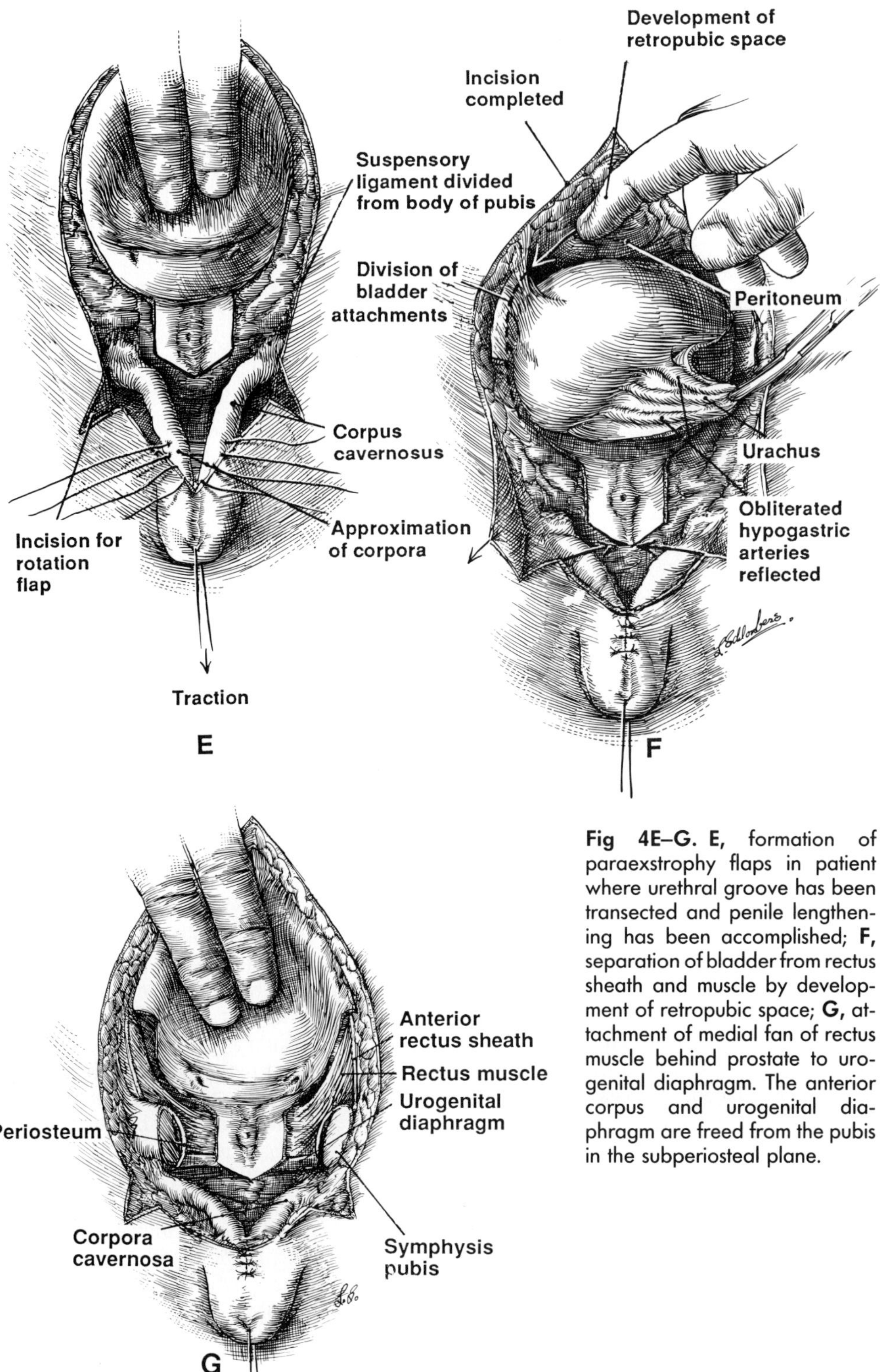


**Fig 4E–G. E,** formation of paraexstrophy flaps in patient where urethral groove has been transected and penile lengthening has been accomplished; **F,** separation of bladder from rectus sheath and muscle by development of retropubic space; **G,** attachment of medial fan of rectus muscle behind prostate to urogenital diaphragm. The anterior corpus and urogenital diaphragm are freed from the pubis in the subperiosteal plane.

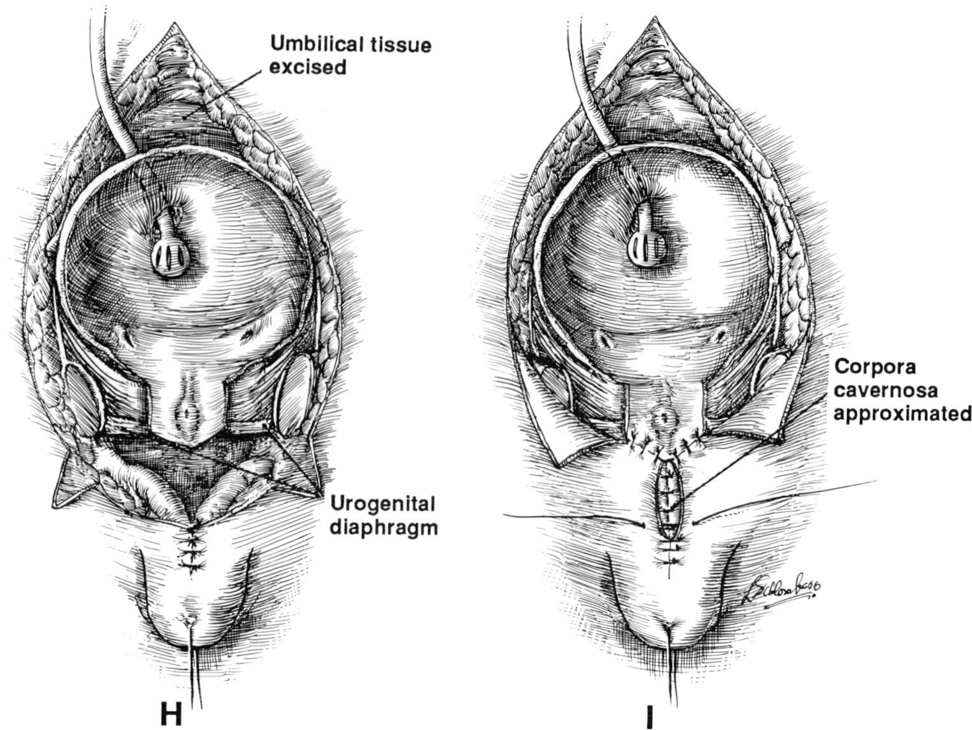


**Fig 4H–I.** After placement of a suprapubic catheter and ureteral feeding tubes, the paraexstrophy skin is anastomosed to the prostatic plate, and bladder closure in two layers is performed.

are brought together in the midline and the abdominal wall closure is completed.

If osteotomy had been performed prior to bladder closure, then the type of immobilization would be dependent on the type of osteotomy. If anterior innominate osteotomy was performed, an external fixator is placed, insuring against separation of the pubis.[59] If posterior iliac osteotomy has been performed, then a modified Bryant traction is placed. A Bryant traction is also used in those children who have not undergone osteotomy prior to bladder closure, and in younger patients who have undergone anterior innominate osteotomy, due to the lack of sufficient ossification of the pelvic bones as a site for pin fixation prior to 6 months of age.

***Incontinent Interval.*** Follow-up is essential after bladder closure and begins with calibration of the bladder outlet prior to discharge. Assessment of upper tract drainage by either excretory urography or ultrasound may be performed to rule out hydronephrosis. Since the majority of these children have vesicoureteral reflux, the development of hydronephrosis may indicate stenosis of the bladder neck area.[64] Routine urine cultures are performed at 2-month intervals to rule out any urinary tract infections. If urinary infection occurs, then an evaluation to include cystoscopy is undertaken to look for stones, squamous metaplasia, or, more commonly, suture erosion into the posterior urethra.

Most males will undergo an epispadias repair prior to an operation for continence. In our experience the bladder volume must be at least 60 mL for bladder neck reconstruction to be performed. Studies performed at The Johns Hopkins Hospital have demonstrated that after epispadias repair, bladder volume is further increased in anticipation of bladder neck reconstruction.[56,65] This appears to be true even for

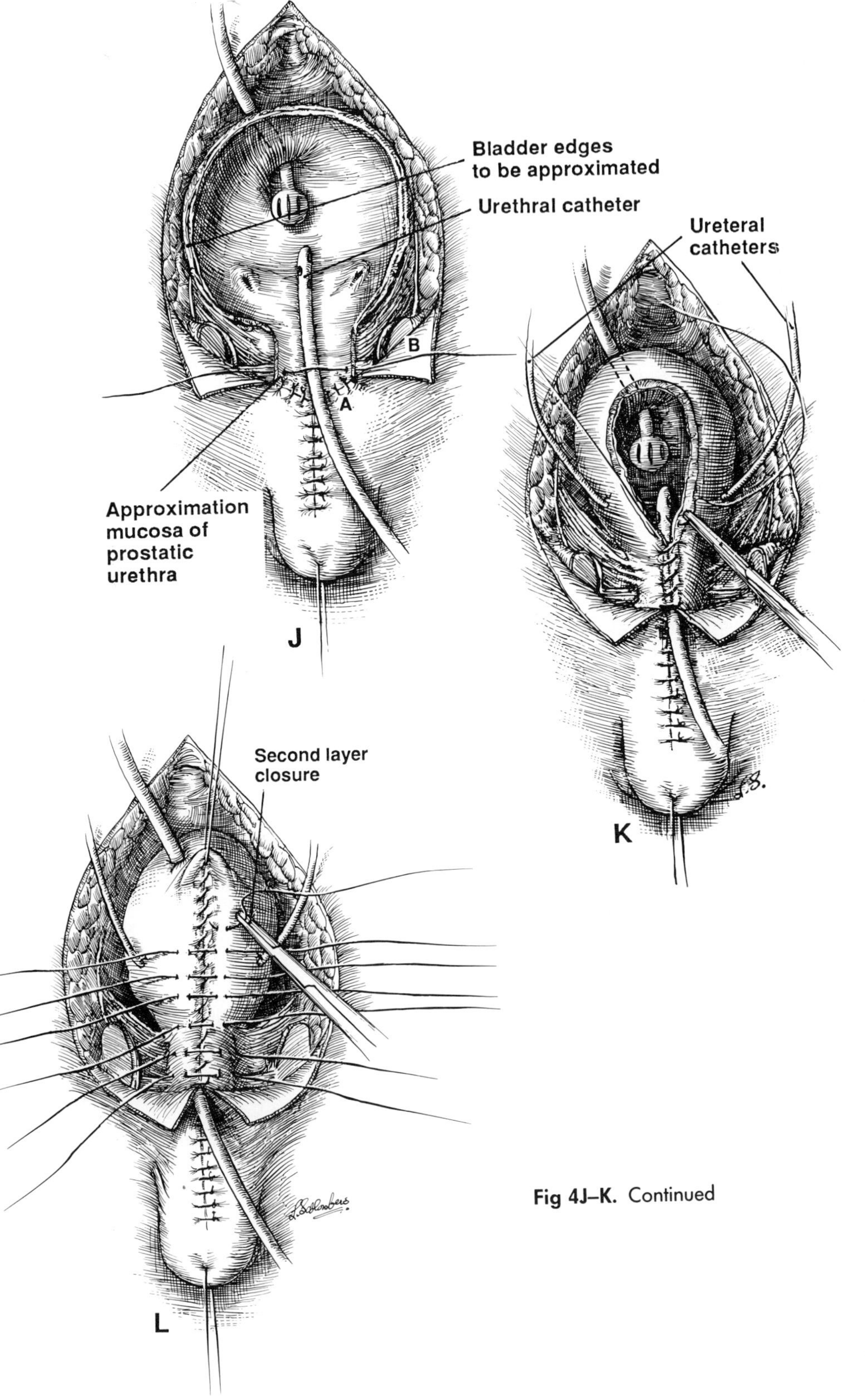


Fig 4J–K. Continued

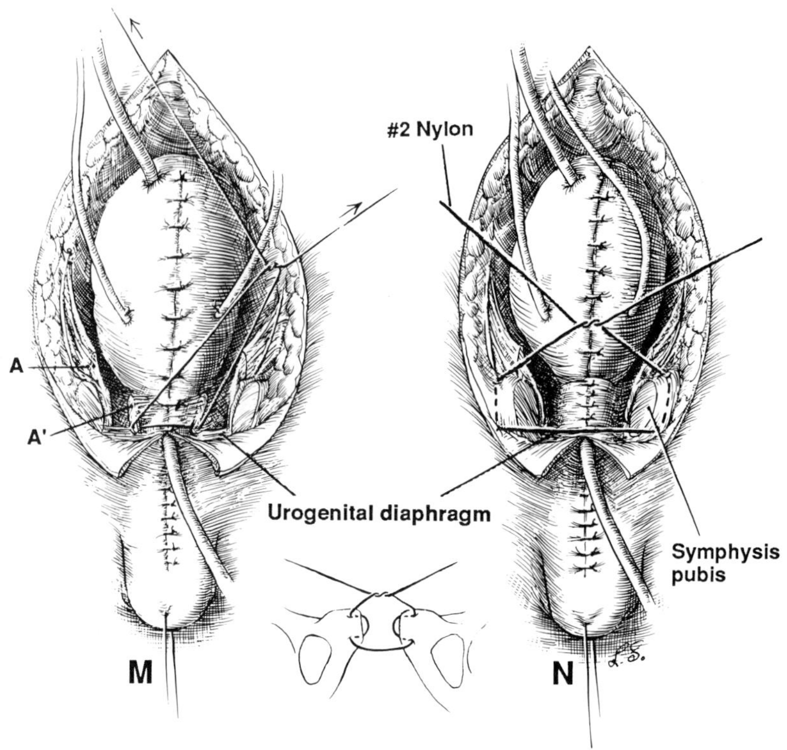


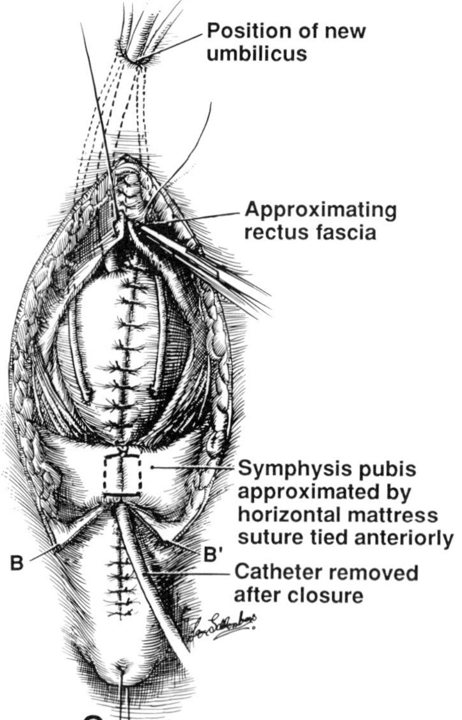


**Fig 4M–O. M,** if possible, the urogenital diaphragm is approximated; **N,** with medial rotation of the greater trocanters, the symphysis pubis is brought together using a horizontal mattress suture; **O,** creation of a neoumbilicus and abdominal wall closure, to include approximation of the skin at B to B′. This provides the anterior step from penile closure to abdominal wall closure. [Drawings by Leon Schlossberg and used with permission by WB Saunders Co.]

those children who at the time of initial closure may have had a small-capacity bladder and thus were considered for early diversion.

**Epispadias Repair.** The goals of epispadias repair are to lengthen and straighten the penis. In addition, it should provide an adequate urethra for normal voiding. Along with the creation of a neourethra, the persistent dorsal chordee also needs to be addressed. Preoperatively, because of the short penile length, testosterone is given intramuscularly to help increase corporal length and availability of penile skin.[66] Usually testosterone enanthate in oil, 2–3 mg/kg, is given intramuscularly 5 weeks and 2 weeks before epispadias repair. Many different procedures for creation of a neourethra have been proposed.[67] In our experience, the Ransley[68] modification of the Cantwell[69] procedure is the repair of choice (Fig 5).

The procedure is begun by placing a glans-holding suture. A strip along the urethral plate (approximately 1.5 cm in width) is then marked from the glans to the base of the penis. An Ipgam procedure may be performed at this point. The urethral plate is then incised along the axis of the markings. The ventral phallus is degloved in a manner similar to a hypospadias repair. However, care must be taken not to interrupt the leash of vessels that enter the urethral plate proximally between the corpora. The corporal bodies and the urethral plate are widely mobilized. The urethra is then closed over a soft catheter with a running absorbable suture. After formation of glandular wings, the neourethra is completed. The soft catheter is then sutured to the glans. By rotating the corporal bodies medially, the urethra assumes a more normal position in the penis and dorsal chordee is corrected.[70] The fistula rate is also reduced with this procedure.[71]

**Bladder Neck Reconstruction.** The goal of bladder neck reconstruction is to allow for voluntary voiding with continence. The prerequisites for bladder neck reconstruction include the ability of the child to communicate and a bladder capacity of at least 60 mL. Patience on the part of both the parents and the physician is imperative during this period as the child learns to recognize the sensation of a full bladder and learns to adequately empty the bladder when full. Initial or repeat osteotomy may need to be performed at the time of bladder neck reconstruction if there is a persistently wide pubic diastasis or a soft interpubic bar is present. Continence appears to be improved if osteotomy is used.[72,73]

Figure 6 illustrates bladder reconstruction. The skin is opened through a Pfannenstiel incision, and the bladder is opened vertically. Since the majority of these children have vesicoureteral reflux, ureteroneocystostomy is performed.[74] A cephalotrigonal reimplantation is usually performed allowing a larger portion of the trigone to be incorporated into the bladder neck reconstruction.[75]

A Young–Dees–Leadbetter bladder neck reconstruction is then performed.[67,76,77] Optimally a 30-mm-long × 15-mm-wide strip is outlined. This strip is marked beginning at the penile urethra and proceeding in a cranial direction. The epithelium lateral to the strip is excised. The strip is then rolled over an 8 French catheter into a tube. In a vest-over-pants fashion, the deepithelialized detrusor muscle is then closed over the tube. The final layer of sutures is left long in order to perform a bladder neck suspension. By suspending the bladder neck, increased urethral pressure can be achieved.[78] A suprapubic catheter and ureteral catheters are brought through separate stab incisions out of the bladder. The bladder is then closed in two layers. A Penrose drain is also placed. Again, as in initial bladder closure, no urethral stents or catheters are left in postoperatively.

## Results

**Bladder Closure.** In the years 1975 to 1992, 315 patients with exstrophy were seen. Of these, 72 children with classical bladder exstrophy were referred to The Johns Hopkins Hospital for initial treatment. Of the 72 patients, one child underwent a diversion because of what was felt to be a small bladder at the time of initial consultation.

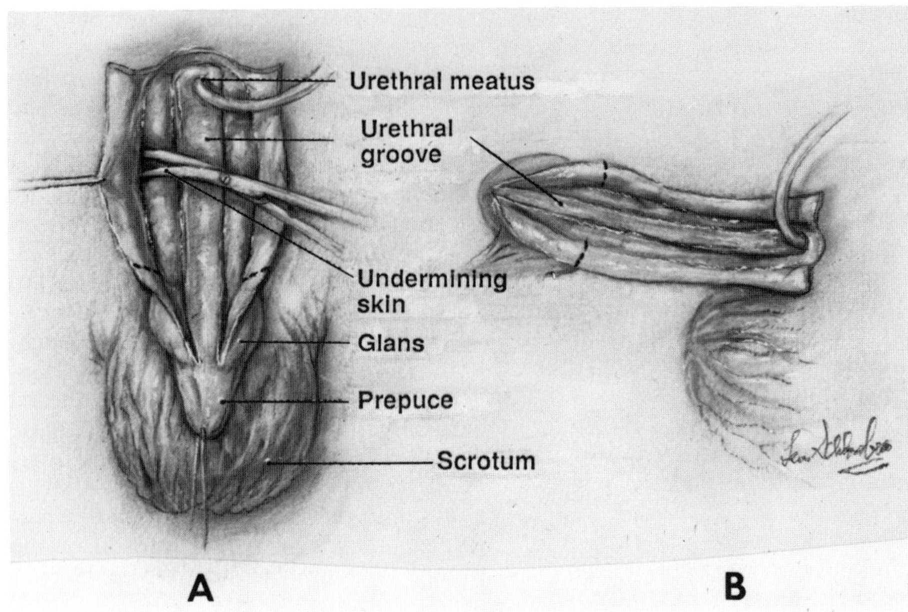


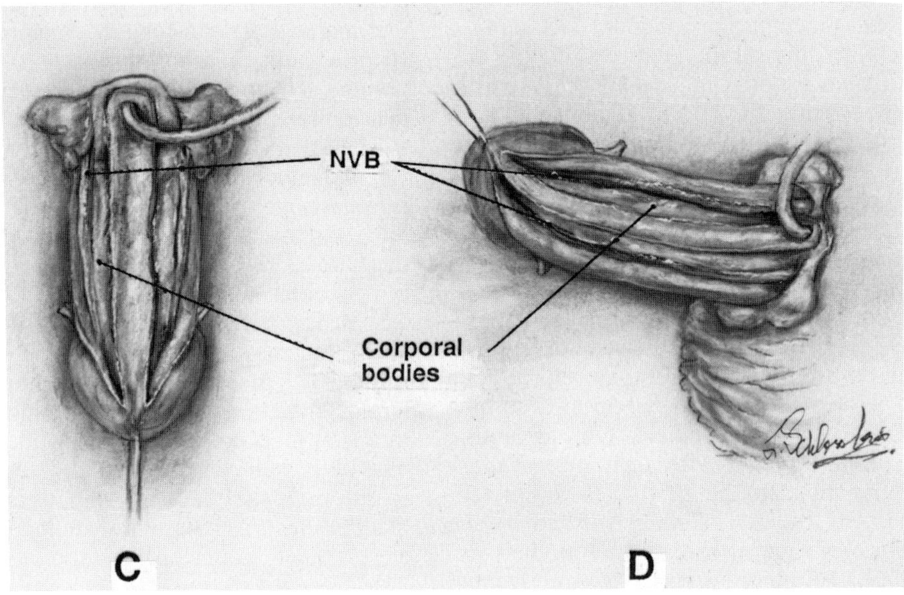


**Fig 5.** The Cantwell–Ransley epispadias repair. **A, B,** after placement of a glans suture, the urethral groove is marked and incised. The penile skin is then mobilized; **C, D,** extension of the incision into the glans and exposure of the laterally deviated neurovascular bundles (NVB).

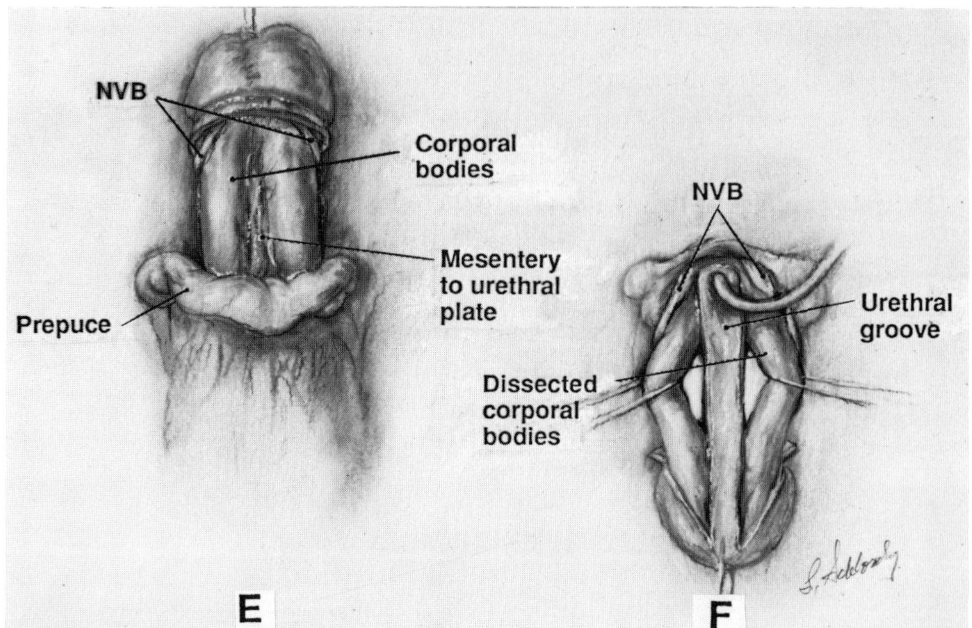


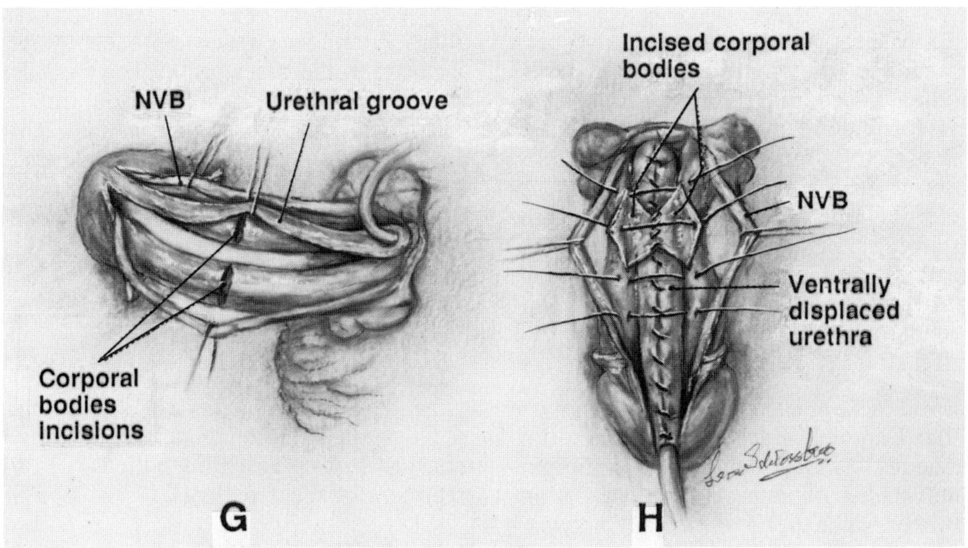


**Fig 5E–H. E, F,** beginning proximally, the urethral groove is separated from the corpora; **G,** the neurovascular bundles are mobilized and the corpora are incised; **H,** the corporal incisions are then approximated following closure of the urethral groove, displacing the urethral ventrally. Additional corporal sutures further bury the urethra under the corpora.

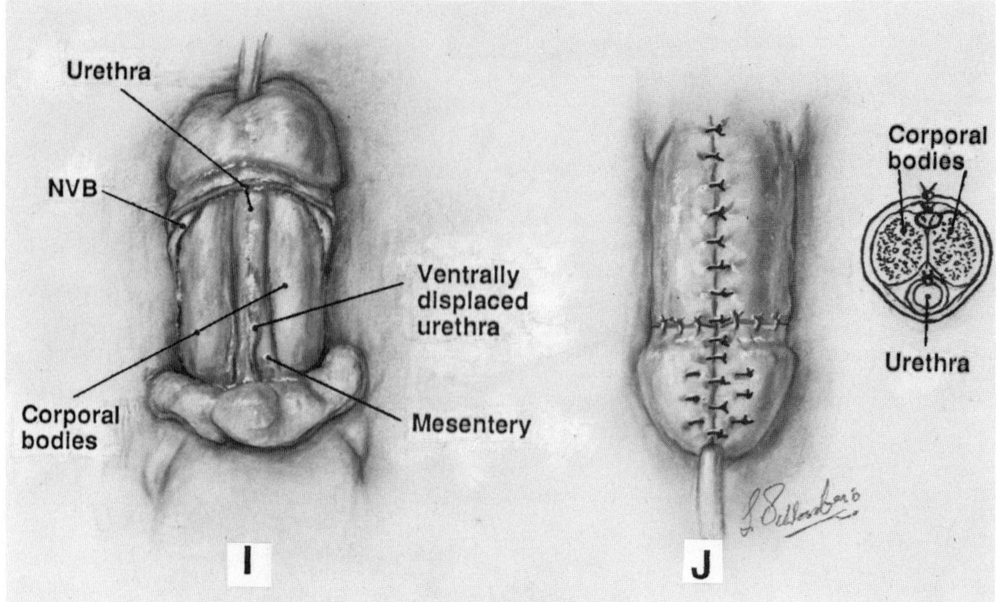


**Fig 5I–J. I,** completed repair with urethra now in ventral location (note inset); **J,** penile skin closure. [Drawings by Leon Schlossberg and used with permission by WB Saunders Co.]

In retrospect, that child would have been a candidate for initial closure. Of the 71 children closed initially at The Johns Hopkins Hospital, 53 underwent either bilateral iliac osteotomy or anterior innominate osteotomy at the time of their closure. Only two of the remaining 26 children had bladder prolapse postoperatively, requiring reclosure. Three children developed calculi, and two patients developed upper tract hydronephrosis requiring augmentation cystoplasty.

**Epispadias Repair.** Prior to the routine use of the Cantwell–Ransley repair, urethrocutaneous fistulas occurred in approximately 30% of our patient population. However, since the advent of the Cantwell–Ransley repair, only three fistulas out of 38 patients were noted, and two of these closed spontaneously without any further surgery.

**Bladder Neck Reconstruction.** Of the 71 patients treated exclusively at The Johns Hopkins Hospital, 45 have undergone bladder neck reconstruction. Stratifying children between the ages of 5 and 10 and 10 and older, continence rates approaching 90% are seen in the older group (Fig 7).[51] The reason for this is unclear. It is doubtful that the increase in size of the prostate at the time of puberty contributes any increased resistance to urine outflow.[79] It is postulated that these children over the age of 10 mature to the point of learning to use their continence.[51]

## Failed Staged Repair

Complications can occur during any stage of the reconstructive effort. Once again, strict attention to detail and persistent follow-up is essential to the successful treatment of these patients.

**Failed Initial Closure.** Children who have experienced dehiscence of the bladder or bladder prolapse have had a failed initial closure. Dehiscence can occur because of infection, or, more commonly, as a result of pubic separation. Bladder prolapse can result from either partial wound separation or failure to create a tight enough bladder neck outlet.[80]

If bladder size is adequate, then a second

closure of the bladder 4 to 6 months after initial attempt can be performed. Repeat closure should be performed with osteotomy or repeat osteotomy. Since 1980, 38 patients with failed initial bladder closure were seen at The Johns Hopkins Hospital. All of these children underwent reclosure with osteotomy. To date, there have been no complications from the repeat closure. However, despite the success of repeat closure, the continence rate is less than those with successful initial closures.[80,81]

**Failure to Gain Capacity.** A few patients, despite successful initial closure and epispadias repair, fail to gain bladder capacity suitable for bladder neck reconstruction. The development of hydronephrosis and recurrent urinary tract infections may preclude the development of adequate bladder volume. Bladder augmentation with bladder neck reconstruction, or augmentation cystoplasty with bladder neck transection and a continent abdominal stoma may be good options in these children.[80]

**Failed Bladder Neck Reconstruction.** If a continent interval does not develop within 2 years after bladder neck reconstruction, continence is a rare occurrence.[81,82] Repeat

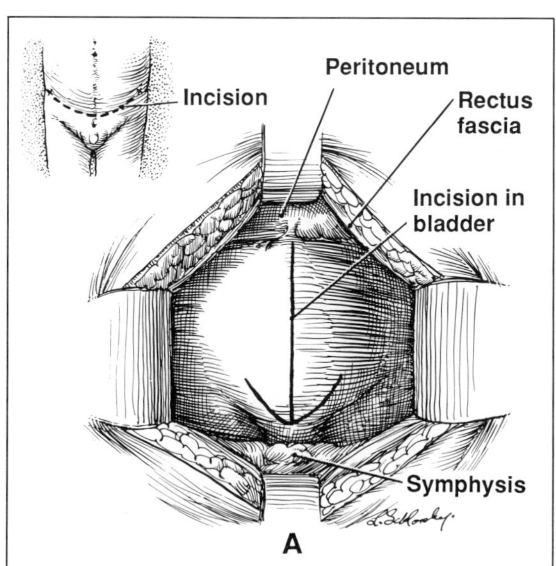


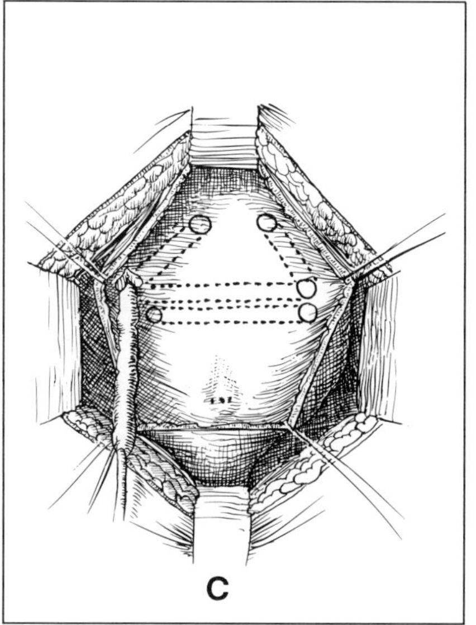


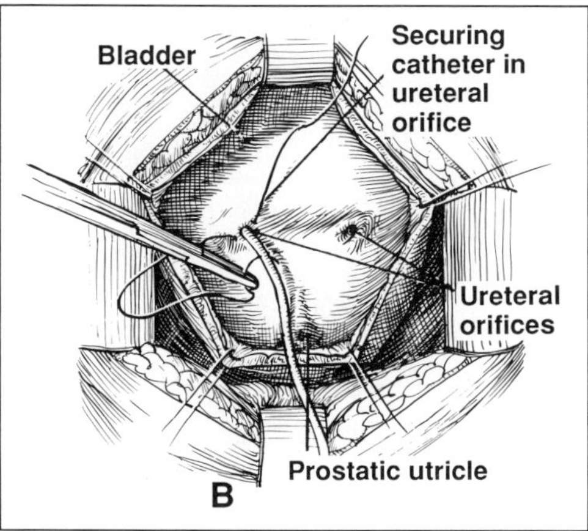


**Fig 6.** Bladder neck reconstruction with Cohen transtrigonal or cephalotrigonal reimplantation. **A,** area of incision in the bladder; **B, C,** ureteral mobilization with either transtrigonal or cephalotrigonal reimplantation.

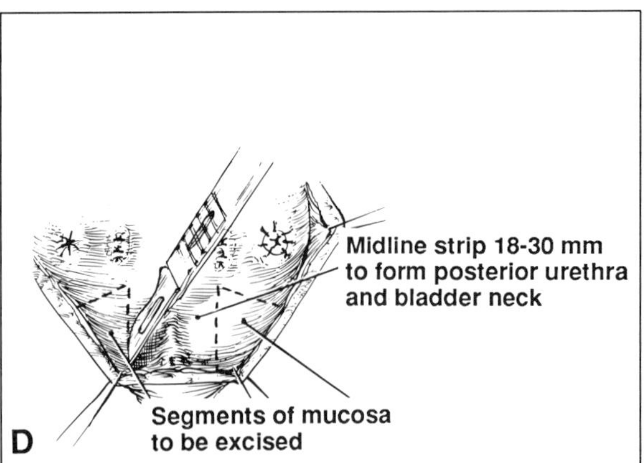


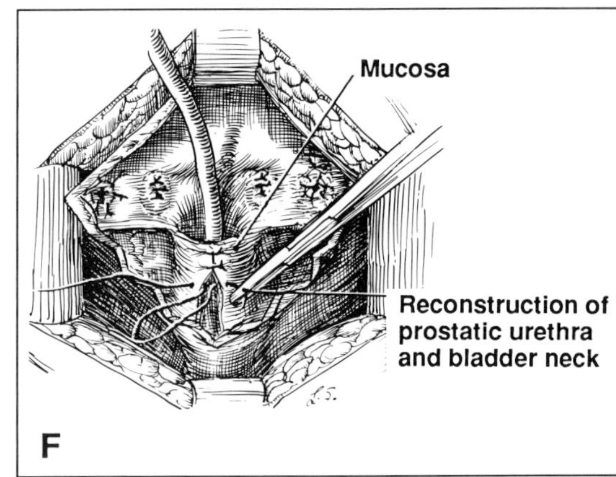


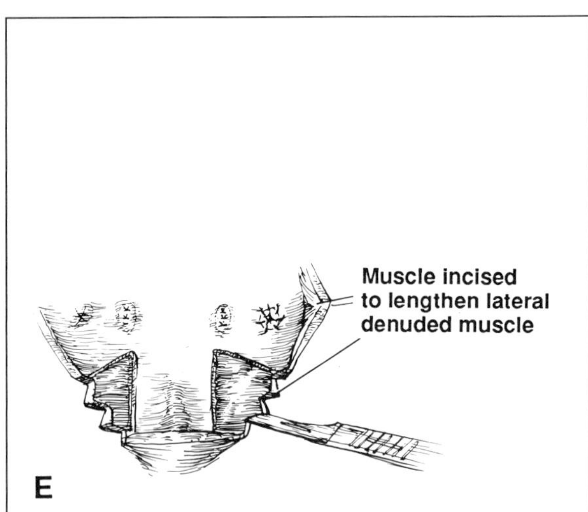


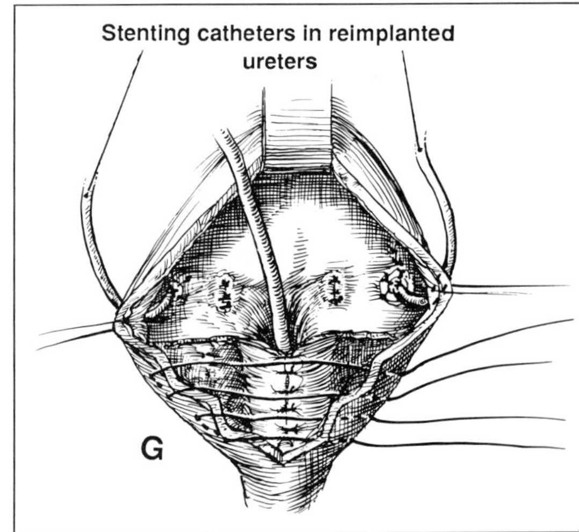


**Fig 6D, E.** After reimplantation is completed, the mucosal strip is marked (**D**) and the mucosa excised lateral to the strip (**E**); **F,** approximation of the mucosa over an 8 French catheter to form the bladder neck and prostatic urethra; **G,** the double-breasted approximation of detrusor muscle; **H,** completing reconstruction of the bladder neck.

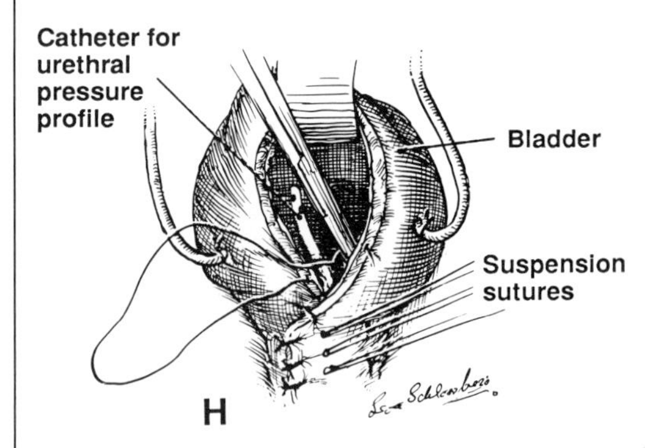

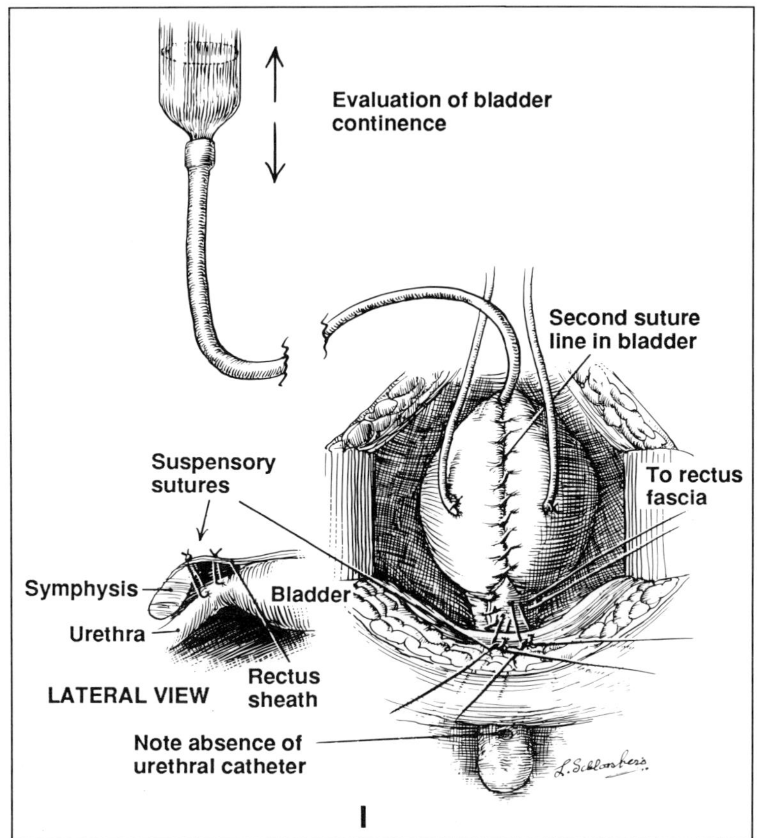


**Fig 6. I,** following bladder neck suspension (and possibly urethral profile measurements, if desired), the bladder is closed and the urethral catheter is removed. [Drawings by Leon Schlossberg and used with permission by WB Saunders Co.]

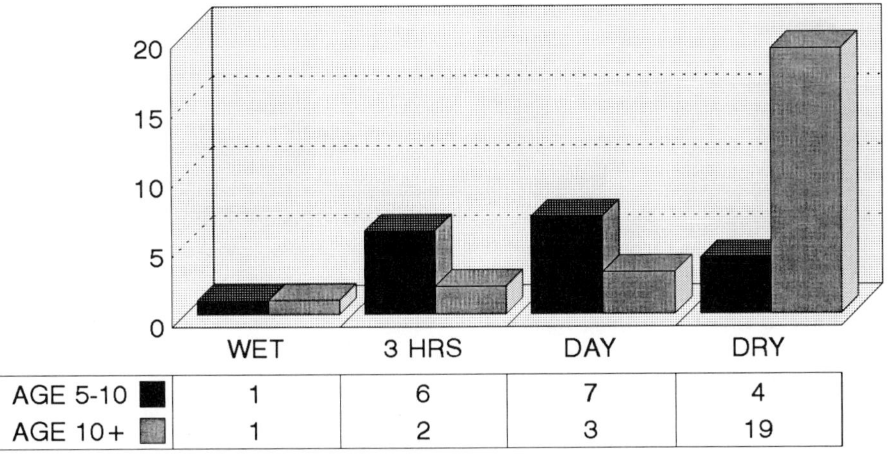


| | WET | 3 HRS | DAY | DRY |
|---|---|---|---|---|
| AGE 5-10 | 1 | 6 | 7 | 4 |
| AGE 10+ | 1 | 2 | 3 | 19 |

**Fig 7.** Breakdown of the 43 patients older than 5 years of age who have undergone bladder neck reconstruction following initial closure at the Johns Hopkins Hospital. The percentage of children greater than 10 years of age with daytime and both daytime and nighttime continence approaches 90%. It is anticipated that as the younger children get older their continence will likewise improve.

bladder neck plasty can be performed in these patients if the capacity seems adequate. In addition to repeat bladder neck reconstruction, bladder augmentation or placement of an artificial urinary sphincter can be performed. Alternatively, bladder neck transection and creation of a continent abdominal stoma with augmentation cystoplasty can also be performed.[83–92]

### Long-Term Outcome

**Quality of Life.** Many patients who have undergone treatment for bladder exstrophy have been followed into adulthood. Many have successful lives as businesspersons, scholars, athletes, physicians, and happily married parents.[93] Survival rates of the patients today far exceed the 40% and 70% expected survival rates in 1925[94,95] and 1947.[96]

**Malignancy.** The vast majority of tumors in these patients are adenocarcinoma. Adenocarcinoma occurs approximately 400 times more commonly in the exstrophy population than in the normal population. This information is derived from a review of those patients with untreated exstrophy.[97–99] Chronic irritation with transformation of the urothelium to cystitis glandularis and later to malignant degeneration has been postulated.[99] To date, no reports of adenocarcinoma in those patients undergoing closure at birth have been reported. Other tumors can also occur in the bladder exstrophy population.[99] These include squamous cell carcinoma, rhabdomyosarcoma, and undifferentiated urothelial carcinoma. The long-term results in those patients undergoing successful staged closure are yet to be determined.

**Genital Function and Fertility.** Many patients who have undergone staged reconstruction can be expected to have satisfactory sexual relations. Erections adequate enough for sexual function were reported in at least 70% of patients in one series.[54] As a population, males with bladder exstrophy are less fertile than the normal population.[93] Retrograde ejaculation as well as epididymitis can be a problem in these patients.

As a rule, fertility is not a problem in the female patient. In a review of over 2500 exstrophy patients, only 38 males fathered children, whereas 131 females gave birth to 156 offspring.[23]

## CLOACAL EXSTROPHY

Cloacal exstrophy, also known as vesicointestinal fissure, ileovesical fistula, or exstrophia splanchnica, is the most severe defect in the formation of the ventral abdominal wall. The incidence of cloacal exstrophy is estimated to be between 200,000 and 400,000 live births annually. There does not appear to be a sex predominance (Fig 8).

### Embryology

Two main theories exist regarding the embryology of this condition. The Patten and Barry theory proposes that the paired primordia of the genital tubercles are caudally displaced. This permits a persistence of a more cephalad cloacal membrane. Thus, if there is incomplete urorectal septal division and disintegration of the unstable cloacal membrane, then both exstrophied bladder and bowel would be on the ventral abdominal surface.[100] The Marshall and Muecke theory suggests that the cloacal membrane is overly developed. This prevents migration of the mesenchymal layer between the inner endodermal and outer ectodermal layers. As previously stated, this unstable membrane ruptures, and if this occurs before fusion of the genital tubercles and prior to descent of the urorectal septum, then the ventral abdominal wall defect arises.[28]

### Clinical Presentation

On examination the child is noted to have an omphalocele. There is usually a right and left hemibladder that are separated by a hindgut remnant (ileocecal area) (Fig 9). The superior portion of the exstrophied bowel contains an orifice usually composed of ileum. There may or may not be appendiceal duplication that would be present

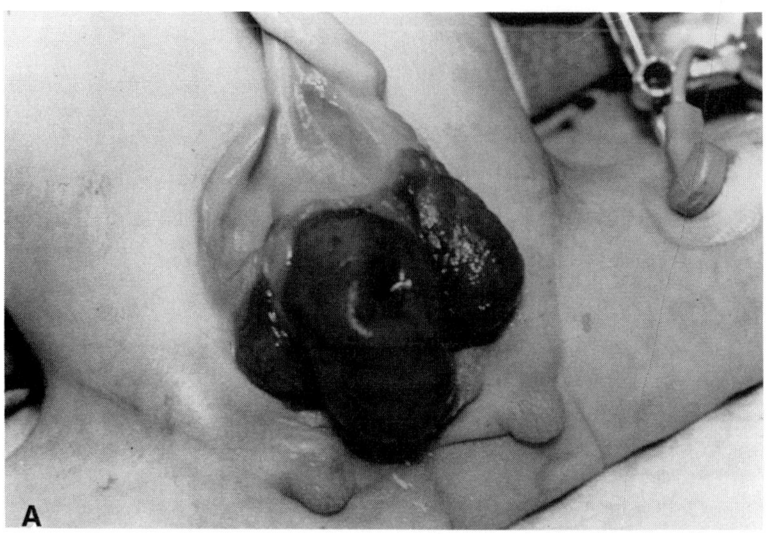


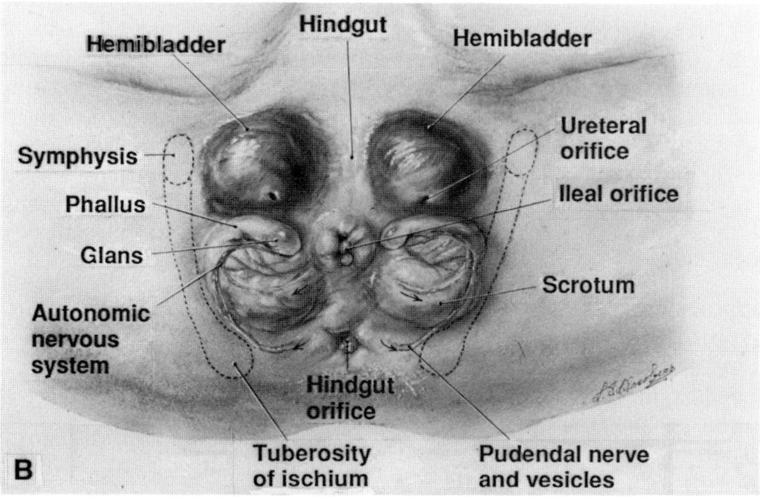


**Fig 8. A,** cloacal exstrophy without omphalocele; **B,** diagrammatic representation of child with cloacal exstrophy, without omphalocele, showing the gastrointestinal and genitourinary defects.

approximately midway between the upper bowel orifice and the most inferior bowel orifice. Inferiorly, there is usually a blind-ending short colonic segment. The penis is usually bifid in the male and may be rudimentary. In these children strong consideration must be given to gender conversion to female. Females may have a bifid vagina and even uterine abnormalities.

Associated abnormalities include myelodysplasia. The incidence of myelodysplasia approaches 50%. Included in this are myelomeningoceles and lipomeningoceles. A large percentage of these children will have an omphalocele. There is also a higher probability of a double vena cava. In addition to the spinal or neural tube defects noted previously, there is also a higher incidence of other skeletal anomalies.[101] There is a higher incidence of renal anomalies in children with cloacal exstrophy.

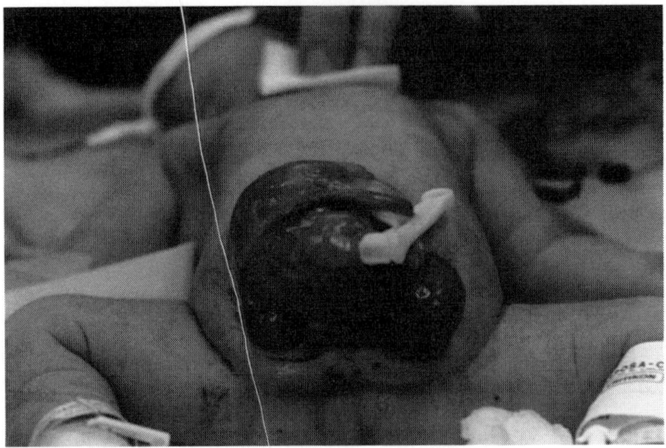

**Fig 9.** Newborn with cloacal exstrophy and omphalocele, prolapsed ileum, and asymmetric bladder halves.

These include renal agenesis, renal ectopia, ureteral ectopia, and ureterovesical junction obstruction.[50]

Because of the severe genital defects associated with this condition, including small or rudimentary corporal bodies, undescended testes, bifid scrota, and glans abnormalities, strong consideration must be given to gender reassignment in these patients.

### Treatment

A team approach including pediatric anesthesiology, pediatric general surgery, pediatric urology, pediatric neurosurgery, pediatric orthopedics, and specialized nursing care is required for the treatment of these children. The omphalocele should be closed primarily. This is the preferred method of treatment. However, if the omphalocele is unduly large, staged abdominal closure with the use of a silastic pouch or silo may be needed.[50]

If feasible, the entire distal colon should be preserved, creating an end colostomy. In 1960, Rickham demonstrated that the preservation of the ileocecal segment was important in the management of these children in preventing the problems associated with ileostomy.[102] The formation of ileostomy may lead to a short-bowel syndrome, thereby requiring these children to go on long-term hyperalimentation.[50]

The goals of bladder management are separation of the hemibladders from the bowel and then their reapproximation. Optimally, bladder closure should be performed. However, this may not be possible in all patients.

Since approximately 50% of these patients will have a form of myelodysplasia, involvement by a pediatric neurosurgeon is necessary. In addition, because many children with myelodysplasia have orthopedic difficulties, a pediatric orthopedic surgeon must be involved in the management of these children as well, in addition to the need for osteotomy.

## URACHAL ANOMALIES

The first reported description of a patient with a urachal anomaly was in 1550 by Bartholomaeus Cabrolius. He described a patent urachus in an 18-year-old female who was able to void from both the urethra and the umbilicus.[103] The first report of a urachal cyst was made in 1883 by Tail.[104] Urachal anomalies are certainly rare and they usually present in childhood. Four main anomalies have been described including patent urachus; urachal cyst, sinus, or both; alternating urachal sinus; and vesicourachal diverticulum.

### Embryology

The embryo is attached to the chorion by the body stalk. The body stalk contains the umbilical arteries and veins and the allantois, which is a projection of the yolk sac that opens into the cloaca. After division of the cloaca into an anterior bladder and a posterior rectum, this projection of the yolk sac normally closes. As the bladder enlarges it retains the attachment to the allantois, which becomes the urachus. The urachus eventually closes after birth, becoming a fibrous cord between the transversalis fascia and the peritoneum, called the median umbilical ligament.

The urachus is composed of three histologic layers. There is an outer smooth muscle layer, a submucosal tissue layer, and an inner cuboidal or transitional cell layer.[105–107]

Four anatomic variants of urachal termination have been described, which are based on the differential growth rates of the urachus and the abdominal wall as well as bladder descent.[108] In type I there is failure of the urachus to atrophy. The urachal attachment to the dome of the bladder persists. If the urachus fails to obliterate, then a patent urachus is the result. If the urachus remains patent only through part of its length, an umbilicourachal sinus results. In type II there is fusion of the urachus and one of the umbilical arteries continuing as a single cord to the umbilicus. In type III there is fusion of both umbilical arteries to the urachus continuing as a single structure to the umbilicus. As a result of their blind umbilical termination, a urachal cyst, sinus, or vesicourachal diverticulum may result from either a type II or a type III variant. In type IV, the urachus ends prior to fusing with the umbilical arteries.

## Patent Urachus

Failure of the urachus to obliterate results in a communication between the bladder and the umbilicus. This may be due to bladder outlet obstruction. However, outlet obstruction is an infrequent etiology for this condition. Normally, the urachus will be obliterated by the 4th to 5th month of gestation, whereas urine formation begins around the 10th week of gestation. Therefore, the timing of the obstruction is critical for obstruction to be the cause of the urachal patency.[109,110] The reported incidence is 1 to 2.5 per 100,000 births. There is an increased incidence in males with prune belly (triad) syndrome.[111]

The child will often present with a wet umbilicus (Fig 10).[112] The drainage may be continuous or intermittent. The drainage can be accentuated with crying, straining, voiding, or placement of the child in the prone position. There may be an associated umbilical hernia. Examination of the fluid for creatinine or blood urea nitrogen usually will confirm the diagnosis. A voiding cystourethrogram should be performed. This will help to identify possible bladder outlet obstruction as well as the fistulous tract. It may be necessary to perform a fistulogram in order to demonstrate the communication to the bladder. Patent urachus may also be confirmed by instillation of methylene blue into the bladder or the tract.[113]

If the etiology of the patent urachus is due to bladder outlet obstruction, then correction of the obstruction may result in spontaneous closure of the urachus. If, however, spontaneous closure does not occur and/or no evidence of bladder outlet obstruction exists, then excision of the urachus is indicated. The entire tract should be excised along with a small cuff of bladder.[110,112,114,115]

## Urachal Cyst

Since the innermost layer of the urachus is composed of cuboidal or transitional cells and obliteration is caused by desquamation of the epithelium, a urachal cyst may develop. A urachal cyst may therefore develop from a type II, III, or IV urachal variant. Most urachal cysts develop in the distal third of the urachus because of umbilical obliteration. However, in type IV variants the urachal cyst will occur in the proximal third of the urachus, due to degeneration of part of the plexus of Luschka.[116]

Urachal cysts normally present in adult life, with only one third discovered during infancy or childhood.[117] Infection is the usual presentation, with symptoms of fever, suprapubic pain, a palpable suprapubic mass, and possibly bladder irritative voiding symptoms.[112,117] Rupture of a urachal cyst can occur into the peritoneum and may result in fistula or abscess formation.[118–120] Evaluation should include ultrasound, ex-

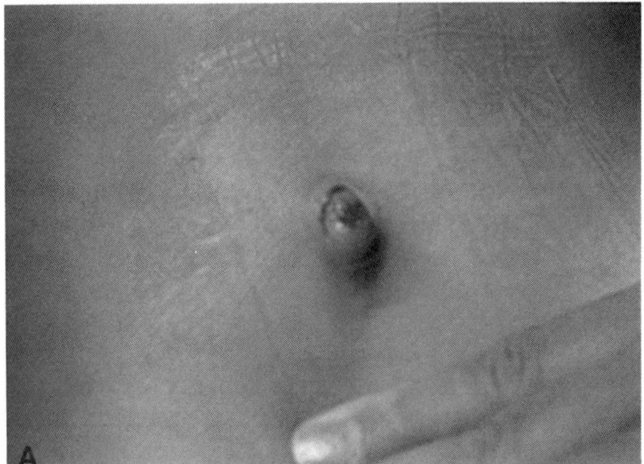


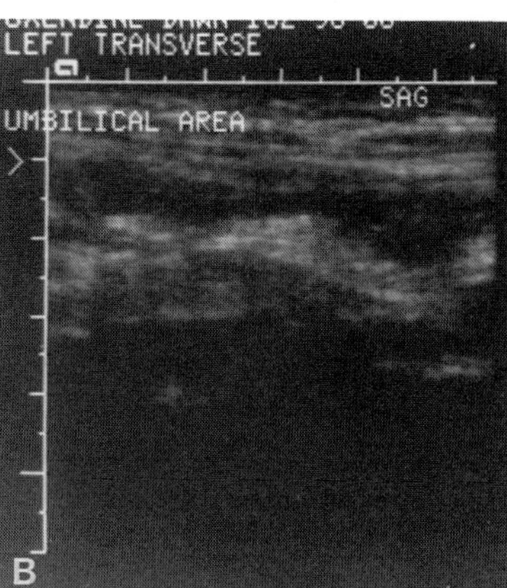


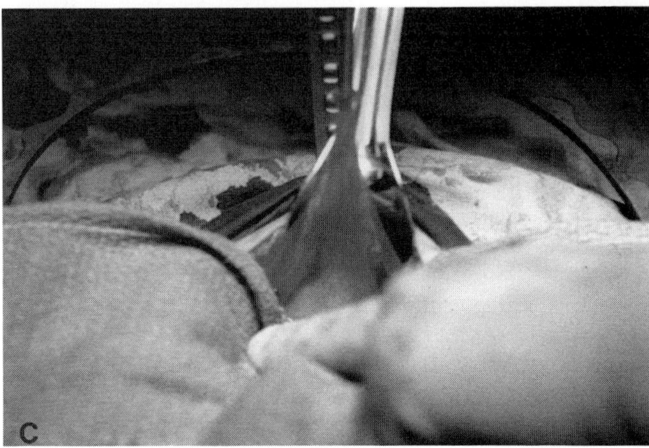


**Fig 10.** Child with patent urachus. **A,** umbilical sinus; **B,** ultrasound demonstrating patent urachus in area of umbilicus; **C,** surgical exposure prior to excision of anomalous tissue.

cretory urography with lateral views, and cystoscopy. Computerized tomography may also help in further defining the cyst.[112]

The goal of the initial treatment should be decompression of the cyst. This may be performed by incision and drainage, percutaneous drainage, or marsupialization. At a later date, the excision of the cyst can be undertaken after inflammation has subsided.

## Urachal Sinus

A urachal sinus is a urachal cyst that drains via the umbilicus. It may also drain into the bladder. Presenting symptoms are periumbilical or suprapubic pain and possibly the presence of umbilical drainage.[112] There is typically inflammation around the area of the umbilicus with the presence of granulation tissue. As in the urachal cyst, treatment should be directed to first treating the inflammatory process followed by complete excision.[112,121]

## Vesicourachal Diverticulum

A vesicourachal diverticulum is formed when the communication between the bladder and the urachus fails to become obliterated. These can be seen in bladder outlet obstruction and are commonly seen in prune belly syndrome.[120] In the majority of patients there is adequate drainage of the vesicourachal diverticulum into the bladder and treatment is not necessary. However, if a diverticulum has a narrow neck, then stagnation can ensue with possible calculus formation and/or urinary tract infection, and thus may require excision.

## REFERENCES


1. Hall EG, McCandles AD, Rickham PP. Vesicointestinal fissure with diphallus. *Br J Urol.* 1953:25:219.
2. Syme J. Ectopia Vesicae. *Lancet.* 1852;2:568.
3. Coffey RC. Physiological implantation of the severed ureter as common bioduct into intestine. *JAMA.* 1911;56:397.
4. Nesbit RM. Ureterosigmoid anastomosis by direct elliptical connection: a preliminary report. *J Urol.* 1949;61:728.
5. Leadbetter WF. Consideration of problems incident to performance of ureteroenterostomy: report of a technique. *J Urol.* 1955;73:67.
6. Young HH. Exstrophy of the bladder: the first case in which a normal bladder and urinary control have been obtained by plastic operation. *Surg Gynecol Obstet.* 1942;74:729.
7. Michon L. Conservative operations for exstrophy of the bladder, with particular references to urinary incontinence. *Br J Urol.* 1948;20:167.
8. Gross RE, Cressen SL. Exstrophy of the bladder; observations from 80 cases. *JAMA.* 1952;149:1640.
9. Higgins CC. Exstrophy of the bladder: Report of 158 cases. *Am Surgeon.* 1962;28:99.
10. Schultz WG. Plastic repair of exstrophy of bladder combined with bilateral osteotomy of ilia. *J Urol.* 1958;79:453.
11. Dees JE. Epispadias with incontinence in the male. *Surgery.* 1942;12:621.
12. Leadbetter GW Jr. Surgical correction of total urinary incontinence. *J Urol.* 1964;91:261.
13. Megalli M, Lattimer JK. Review of the management of 140 cases of exstrophy of the bladder. *J Urol.* 1973;109:246.
14. Williams DI, Keeton JE. Further progress with reconstruction of the exstrophied bladder. *Br J Surg.* 1973;60:203.
15. Jeffs RD. Exstrophy and cloacal exstrophy. *Urol Clin North Am.* 1978;5:127.
16. Jeffs RD, Guice SL, Oesch I. The factors in successful exstrophy closure. *J Urol.* 1982;127:974.
17. Lattimer JK, Beck L, Yeaw S, et al. Long term follow up after exstrophy closure: late improvement and good quality of life. *J Urol.* 1978;119:664.
18. Woodhouse CRJ, Ransley TC, Williams DI. The exstrophy patient in adult life. *Br J Urol.* 1983;55:632.
19. Rickham PP. Vesicointestinal fissure. *Arch Dis Child.* 1960;35:97.
20. Rickham PP. The incidence and treatment of ectopia vesicae. *Proc Roy Soc Med.* 1961;54:389.
21. Lattimer JK, Smith MJK. Exstrophy closure: a follow up on 70 cases. *J Urol.* 1966;95:356.
22. Jeffs RD. Exstrophy of the urinary bladder. In: Welch KJ, Randolph JG, Ravitch MM, O'Neill JA, Rowe MI, eds. *Pediatric Surgery.* Chicago: Yearbook Medical; 1986:1217.
23. Shapiro E, Lepor H, Jeffs RD. The inheritance of classical bladder exstrophy. *J Urol.* 1984;132:308.
24. Dees JE. Genital epispadias with incontinence. *J Urol.* 1949;62:513.
25. Moore KL. *The Developing Human: Clinically Oriented Embryology.* Philadelphia: WB Saunders; 1988:255–297.
26. Ambrose SS. The anterior body wall. In: Gray SW, Skandalakis JE, eds. *Embryology for Surgeons.* Philadelphia: WB Saunders; 1972:387–441.
27. Patten JF, Barry A. The genesis of exstrophy of the bladder and epispadias. *Am J Anat.* 1952;90:35–57.
28. Muecke EC. The role of the cloacal membrane in exstrophy: the first successful experimental study. *J Urol.* 1964;92:659.
29. Marshall VF, Muecke EC. Variations in exstrophy of the bladder. *J Urol.* 1962;889:766.
30. Gross RE, Cressen SL. Exstrophy of the bladder: observations from 80 cases. *JAMA.* 1952;149:1640.
31. Husmann DA, McLorie GA, Churchill BM, Ein SH. Inguinal pathology and its association with classical bladder exstrophy. *J Pediatr Surg.* 1990;25:332.
32. Connolly J, Peppas DS, Gearhart JP, Jeffs RD. The incidence of inguinal hernia in the exstrophy population. *J Urol.* 1992 (in press).
33. Pearl RH, Ein SH, Churchill B. Posterior sagittal anorectoplasty for pediatric recurrent rectal prolapse. *J Pediatr Surg.* 1989;24:1100.
34. Goyanna R, Emmett JL, McDonald JR. Exstrophy of the bladder complicated by adenocarcinoma. *J Urol.* 1951;65:391.
35. Culp DA. The histology of the exstrophied bladder. *J Urol.* 1964;91:538.
36. Gunge RG. Adophlin in treatment of human adenocarcinoma of the bladder. *J Urol.* 1952;68:475.
37. Engel RM, Wilkinson HA. Bladder exstrophy. *J Urol.* 1970;104:699.
38. Clark MA, O'Connell, KJ. Scanning and transmission of electron microscopic studies of an exstrophic human bladder. *J Urol.* 1983; 110:481.
39. Shapiro E, Jeffs RD, Gearhart JP, Lepor H. Muscarinic cholinergic receptors in bladder

exstrophy: insights into surgical management. *J Urol.* 1985;134:308.

40. Hollowell JG, Hill PD, Duffy PG, Ransley PG. Bladder function and dysfunction in exstrophy and epispadias. *Lancet.* 1991;338:926.
41. Nisonson I, Lattimer JK. How well can the exstrophied bladder work? *J Urol.* 1972; 107:664.
42. Maloney PK Jr, Gleason DM, Lattimer JK. Ureteral physiology and exstrophy of the bladder. *J Urol.* 1965;93:588.
43. Woodhouse CRJ, Kellett MJ. Anatomy of the penis and its deformities in exstrophy and epispadias. *J Urol.* 1984;132:1122.
44. Schlegel PN, Gearhart JP. Neuroanatomy of the pelvis in an infant with cloacal exstrophy: a detailed micro dissection with histology. *J Urol.* 1989;141:583.
45. Woodhouse CRJ, Ransley PG, Williams DI. The patient with exstrophy in adult life. *Br J Urol.* 1983;55:632.
46. Loder RP, Dayioglu MM. Association of congenital vertebral malformations with bladder and cloacal exstrophy. *J Pediatr Ortho Ped.* 1990;10:389.
47. Diamond DA, Jeffs RD. Cloacal exstrophy: a 22 year experience. *J Urol.* 1985;133:779.
48. Mirk P, Calisti A, Fileni A. Prenatal sonographic diagnosis of bladder exstrophy. *J Ultrasound Med.* 1986;5:291.
49. Jaffe R, Schoenfeld A, Ovadia J. Sonographic findings in the prenatal diagnosis of bladder exstrophy. *Am J Obstet Gynecol.* 1990; 162:675.
50. Howell C, Caldamone A, Snyder H, et al. Optimal management of cloacal exstrophy. *J Pediatr Surg.* 1983;18:365.
51. Peppas DS, Gearhart JP, Jeffs RD. The treatment of bladder exstrophy: a recipe for success. *J Urol.* 1992 (in press).
52. Canning DA, Oesterling JE, Gearhart JP, Jeffs RD. A computerized review of exstrophy patients managed during the past 13 years. *J Urol.* 1989;141:224A.
53. Connor JP, Hensle TW, Lattimer JK, Burbige KA. Long term follow up of 207 patients with bladder exstrophy: an evolution in treatment. *J Urol.* 1989;142:793.
54. Mesrobian HJ, Kelalis PP, Kramer SA. Long term follow up of 103 patients with bladder exstrophy. *J Urol.* 1988;139:719.
55. Merguerian PA, McLorie GA, McMullin ND, Khoury AE, Husmann DA, Churchill BM. Continence in bladder exstrophy: Determinants of success. *J Urol.* 1991;145:350.
56. Gearhart JP, Jeffs RD. Bladder exstrophy: increase in capacity following epispadias repair. *J Urol.* 1989;142:525.
57. Jeffs RD. Exstrophy and cloacal exstrophy. *Urol Clin North Am.* 1978;5:127.
58. Jeffs RD, Guice SL, Oesch I. The factors in successful exstrophy closure. *J Urol.* 1982; 127:974.
59. Sponseller PD, Gearhart JP, Jeffs RD. Anterior innominate osteotomies for failure or late closure of bladder exstrophy. *J Urol.* 1991; 146:137.
60. Lepor H, Shapiro E, Jeffs RD. Urethral reconstruction in boys with classical bladder exstrophy. *J Urol.* 1984;131:512.
61. Duckett JW. Use of paraexstrophy skin pedicle graphs for correction of exstrophy and epispadias repair. *Birth Defects.* 1977;13:175.
62. Johnston JH. The genital aspects of exstrophy. *J Urol.* 1975;113:701.
63. Husmann DA, McLorie GA, Churchill BM. Closure of the exstrophic bladder: an evaluation of the factors leading to its success and its importance on urinary continence. *J Urol.* 1989;142:522.
64. Gearhart JP, Peppas DS, Jeffs RD. The management of the failed initial exstrophy closure. *J Urol.* 1992 (in press).
65. Peters CA, Gearhart JP, Jeffs RD. Epispadias and incontinence: The challenge of the small bladder. *J Urol.* 1988;140:1199.
66. Gearhart JP, Jeffs RD. The use of parenteral testosterone therapy in genital reconstructive surgery. *J Urol.* 1987;138:1077.
67. Young HH. An operation for the cure of incontinence associated with epispadias. *J Urol.* 1922;7:1.
68. Ransley PG, Duffy PG, Wollin M. Bladder exstrophy closure and epispadias repair. In: Spitz L, Nixon HH, eds. *Operative Surgery.* London: Butterworths; 1988:620–632.
69. Cantwell FV. Operative treatment of epispadias by transplantation of the urethra. *Ann Surg.* 1895;22:689.
70. Koff SA, Eakins M. The treatment of penile chordee using corporeal rotation. *J Urol.* 1984;131:931.
71. Gearhart JP, Leonard MP, Burgers JK, Jeffs RD. Epispadias repair using the Cantwell–Ransley technique. *J Urol.* 1992;148:851–854.
72. Lepor H, Jeffs RD. Primary bladder closure and bladder neck reconstruction in classical bladder exstrophy. *J Urol.* 1983;130:1142.
73. Gearhart JP, Jeffs RD. State of the art reconstructive surgery for bladder exstrophy at the Johns Hopkins Hospital. *Am J Dis Child.* 1989;143:1475.
74. Cohen SJ. Ureterozystoneostomie eine neue antirefluxtechnik. *Aktuel Urol.* 1975;6:1.
75. Canning DA, Gearhart JP, Jeffs RD. The cephalotrigonal reimplant in bladder neck reconstruction for patients with exstrophy or epispadias. *J Urol.* 1990;143:276A.
76. Dees JE. Epispadias with incontinence in the male. *Surgery.* 1942;12:621.

77. Leadbetter GW Jr. Surgical correction of total urinary incontinence. *J Urol.* 1964;91:261.
78. Gearhart JP, Williams KA, Jeffs RD. Urethral pressure profilometry as an adjunct to bladder neck reconstruction. *J Urol.* 1986;136:1055.
79. Gearhart JP, Yang A, Jeffs RD, Zerhouni EA. Prostate size and configuration of adult men with classic bladder exstrophy. *J Urol.* 1992 (in press).
80. Gearhart JP, Peppas DS, Jeffs RD. The failed exstrophy closure: strategy for management. *Br J Urol.* 1992 (in press).
81. Oesterling JE, Jeffs RD. The importance of a successful initial bladder closure in the surgical management of classical bladder exstrophy: analysis of 144 patients treated at the Johns Hopkins Hospital between 1975 and 1985. *J Urol.* 1987;137:258.
82. Arap A, Giron AM, Goes GM. Initial results of the complete reconstruction of bladder exstrophy. *Urol Clin North Am.* 1980;7:477.
83. Gearhart JP, Jeffs RD. Augmentation cystoplasty in the failed exstrophy reconstruction. *J Urol.* 1988;139:790.
84. Kramer SA. Augmentation cystoplasty in patients with exstrophy-epispadias. *J Pediatr Surg.* 1989;24:1293.
85. Hanna MK. Artificial urinary sphincter for incontinent children. *Urology.* 1981;18:370.
86. Light JK, Scott FB. Treatment of the epispadias-exstrophy complex with the AS792 artificial urinary sphincter. *J Urol.* 1983;129:738.
87. Dector RM, Roth DR, Fishmen IJ, et al. Use of the AS800 device in exstrophy and epispadias. *J Urol.* 1988;140:1202.
88. Quinlan DM, Leonard MP, Brendler CB, Gearhart JP, Jeffs RD. Use of the Benchekroun hydraulic valve as a catheterizable continence mechanism. *J Urol.* 1991;145:1151.
89. Aliabadi H, Gonzalez R. Success of the artificial urinary sphincter after failed surgery for incontinence. *J Urol.* 1990;143:987.
90. Mitchell ME, Piser JA. Intestinocystoplasty and total bladder replacement in children and young adults: followup in 129 cases. *J Urol.* 1987;138:579.
91. Gonzalez R, Nguyen DH, Koleilat N, Sidi AA. Compatibility of enterocystoplasty and the artificial urinary sphincter. *J Urol.* 1989;142:502.
92. Leonard MP, Gearhart JP, Jeffs RD. Continent urinary reservoirs in pediatric urological practice. *J Urol.* 1990;144:330.
93. Lattimer JK, Beck L, Yeaw S, et al. Long-term follow-up after exstrophy closure: late improvement and good quality of life. *J Urol.* 1978;119:664.
94. Gross SD. *System of Surgery: Pathological, Diagnostic, Therapeutic, and Operative.* Philadelphia: Blanchard and Lea; 1862:270–272.
95. Mayo CH, Hendricks WA. Exstrophy of the bladder. *Surg Gynecol Obstet.* 1926;43:129.
96. Harvard BM, Thompson GJ. Congenital exstrophy of the bladder: late results of treatment by the Coffey–Mayo method or uretero-intestinal anastomosis. *J Urol.* 1951;65:223.
97. Mostofi FK. Potentialities of bladder epithelium. *J Urol.* 1954;71:705.
98. Kandzari SJ, Majid A, Orteza AM, Milam DF. Exstrophy of urinary bladder complicated by adenocarcinoma. *Urology.* 1974;3:496.
99. Krishmansetty RM, Rao NK, Hines CR, et al. Adenocarcinoma in exstrophy and dysfunctional ureteral sigmoidostomy. *J Kentucky Med Assoc.* 1988;86:409.
100. Patten BM, Barry A. The genesis of exstrophy of the bladder and epispadias. *Am J Anat.* 1952;90:35.
101. Soper RT, Kiljer K. Vesicointestinal fissure. *J Urol.* 1964;92:490.
102. Rickham TP. Vesicointestinal fissure. *Arch Dis Child.* 1960;35:97.
103. Atcheson DW. Patent urachus with a report of 2 additional cases. *J Urol.* 1944;51:424.
104. Rees HI. Infected urachal cysts. *Br Med J.* 1953;2:184.
105. Begg RC. Urachus: its anatomy, histology and development. *J Anat.* 1930;64:170.
106. Langman J. *Medical Embryology.* Baltimore: Williams & Wilkins; 1963:117–128.
107. Blickert-Toft M, Koch F, Nielson OV. Anatomic variations of the urachus related to clinical appearance and surgical treatment of urachal disorders. *Surg Gynecol Obstet.* 1973; 137:51.
108. Bauer SB, Retik AB. Urachal and related umbilical disorders. *Urol Clin North Am.* 1978; 5:195.
109. Gray SW, Skandalakis JE. *Embryology for Surgeons.* Philadelphia: WB Saunders; 1972:525.
110. Nix JT, Menville JG, Albert M, Wendt DL. Congenital patent urachus. *J Urol.* 1958; 79:264.
111. Lattimer JK. Congenital deficiency of the abdominal musculature and associated genito-urinary anomalies: a report of 22 cases. *J Urol.* 1958;79:263.
112. Nagasaki A, Sumitomo K, Iwanaga M, Oshgami H, Suita S, Yakabe S. Remnants of urachus in infants and children: the problems of diagnosis and treatment. *Jpn J Surg.* 1991; 21:167.
113. Perlmutter AD. Urachal disorders. In: Harrison JH, Gittes RF, Perlmutter AD, et al, eds. *Campbell's Urology.* 4th ed. Philadelphia: WB Saunders; 1978:883.
114. Himman F Jr. Surgical disorders of the bladder and umbilicus of urachal origin. *Surg Gynecol Obstet.* 1967;113:605.
115. Berman SM, Tolia BM, Laor R, Reid RE, Schweizerhof SP, Freed SZ. Urachal remnants in adults. *Urology.* 1988;31:17.

116. Brodie N. Infected urachal cysts. *Am J Surg.* 1945;69:243.

117. Boyle G, Rosenberg HK, O'Neill J. An unusual presentation of an infected urachal cyst. Review of urachal anomalies. *Clin Ped.* 1988;27:130.

118. Nunn LL. Urachal cysts and their complications. *Am J Surg.* 1952;84:252.

119. Akintan B, Adelkunle A. A fatal case of ruptured infected urachal cyst. *Int Urol Nephrol.* 1985;17:133.

120. Caldamone AA. Anomalies of the bladder and cloaca. In: Gillenwater JY, Grayhack JT, Howards SS, Duckett JW, eds. *Adult and Pediatric Urology.* Chicago: Yearbook Medical; 1987:1812–1815.

121. Retik AB, Bauer SB. Bladder and urachus. In: Kelalis PP, King LR, Belman AB, eds. *Clinical Pediatric Urology.* Philadelphia: WB Saunders; 1976:544–571.

# 50

# Anomalies of the Urethra

*Thomas E. Kingston, Michael A. Keating, and Anthony A. Caldamone*

## INTRODUCTION

Anomalies of the urethra comprise a wide variety of lesions that range from often asymptomatic, embryologic abnormalities found only incidentally to those causing severe obstruction with resultant hydroureteronephrosis, renal dysplasia, and chronic renal failure. Symptoms such as daytime or nighttime wetting, urinary tract infection, urinary obstruction, dysuria, or hematuria often herald occult intrinsic urethral abnormalities. Prenatal ultrasonography has allowed earlier diagnosis of the more obstructing lesions of the urethra thereby facilitating earlier intervention, particularly in patients with posterior urethral valves. Overall, the vast majority of these urethral lesions are successfully treated transurethrally, by open reconstruction, or often by simple observation.

Obstruction of the urethra occurs mostly in males and is most often due to posterior urethral valves. Other urethral anomalies causing obstruction include urethral polyps, urethral strictures, anterior urethral valves, and Cowper's gland duct cysts. Refined radiologic techniques, particularly in the areas of voiding cystourethrography, and improved pediatric endoscopic equipment have allowed dramatic improvement in diagnostic and therapeutic approaches to these lesions.

## URETHRAL MEATAL STENOSIS

Congenital stenosis of the distal urethral meatus in boys is a clinically recognized entity but is exceedingly rare. Most presently feel that congenital meatal stenosis has been overdiagnosed as a cause of childhood obstructive uropathy. Allen et al. used bougie à boule to calibrate the urethras of 100 consecutive newborn boys. Seventy-five percent had meatuses that were 8 or 9 Fr and approximately 9% had meatuses measuring 4 Fr with 10% measuring 6 Fr. They concluded that those with a urethral meatus of 4–6 Fr had meatal stenosis and those with a 6 Fr meatus had questionable stenosis.[1] None of these asymptomatic infants was evaluated radiographically to determine whether obstructive uropathy existed in association with or because of meatal stenosis. Morton and Litvak et al. subsequently measured meatal size in two large series of asymptomatic boys.[2,3] These data demonstrated that the normal size urethral meatus could be divided into three age groups. These studies defined the lower limit of normal for meatal size at 8 Fr in boys less than 4 years of age and less than 10 Fr in boys over 10 years. Despite a multitude of studies, however, there is little correlation between observation of the urinary stream and actual calibration. In addition, calibration studies have yet to be found useful for predicting clinically significant meatal stenosis.

### Embryology/Etiology

The embryologic basis for neonatal urethral meatal stenosis is considered to be a failure of the urethral membrane to canalize completely.[4] Partial canalization results in stenosis. Acquired stenosis in the circumcized male usually comprises a membranous web across the ventral portion of the meatus and is often associated with a history of meatitis or perimeatal balanitis.

### Diagnosis/Treatment

Significant neonatal meatal stenosis with resultant obstructive uropathy has only rarely been documented. Visual inspection of the meatus is notoriously unreliable. Noe and Dale reported on 280 patients admitted to the hospital for evaluation of meatal stenosis. All had an intravenous pyelogram and cystoscopy and most had a voiding cystourethrogram. Less than 1% of patients diagnosed with meatal stenosis by visual inspection were found to have a clinically significant finding such as reflux or hydronephrosis. Five percent of all patients had findings of significance on voiding cystourethrogram and all had evidence of urinary tract infection.[5] Current studies simply do not uphold previous implications that meatal stenosis can cause severe hydroureteronephrosis. In the hypospadiac urethra, however, stenosis has been well documented and can be associated with dysuria, frequency, meatal ulceration, and proximal urethral dilatation. Acquired stenosis will often present with dorsal deflection of the urinary stream and a very fine, forceful, long-distance stream is characteristic. Mothers will often complain of poor aim with wet bathrooms secondary to missed toilet bowls. The pendulous urethra can be seen to bulge ventrally at times and burning, frequency, hematuria, or bloody spotting may lead to the finding of a small meatus but may not be necessarily attributable to true meatal stenosis. Incomplete emptying of the obstructed urethra can result in stasis and infection as well as bulbous urethritis.

Neither cystoscopy nor radiographic evaluation is required for evaluation of simple meatal stenosis. A meatotomy is the treatment of choice for urethral meatal stenosis. This can be done by crushing the ventral web or dorsal aspect of the meatus and dividing this tissue for a short distance. The parents are then instructed to dilate the meatus with a lubricant and small eye dropper or ophthalmic antibiotic applicator twice daily for 2 weeks. This may prevent recurrence of the meatal stenosis. Sutures are occasionally needed for bleeding but are not used routinely.

## URETHRAL PROLAPSE

### Presentation

Circular prolapse of the urethral mucosa is a relatively rare condition, usually found in black prepubertal girls.[6] The common presentations include mild vaginal bleeding manifested as blood spotting on the underwear, painless vaginal mass, and occasional hematuria or dysuria.[7]

Physical examination reveals an interlabial mass that is circular with a central orifice (doughnut-shaped) (Fig 1). The mass is usually smooth and erythematous. It is usually nontender and bleeds easily. The differential diagnosis includes sarcoma botryoides, prolapsed ureterocele, imperforate hymen, condyloma accuminatum, or paraurethral cyst. The key to diagnosis is finding the urethral orifice in the center of the mass.[8] Intravenous pyelogram and/or cystoscopy has been recommended by some[9] and others feel that endoscopic examination alone is indicated as part of the evaluation.[10,11]

### Etiology

The exact etiology and pathophysiology of urethral prolapse remains obscure. Numerous hypotheses regarding the etiology have been described including perineal muscle weakness secondary to neuromuscular disorder, congenital deformity in the mucosa at the terminal urethra, fascial defects, poor bladder support, submucosal weakness, and deficiency in elastic tissue.[12–14] In addition, predisposing factors such as trauma (straddle injuries, catheter-

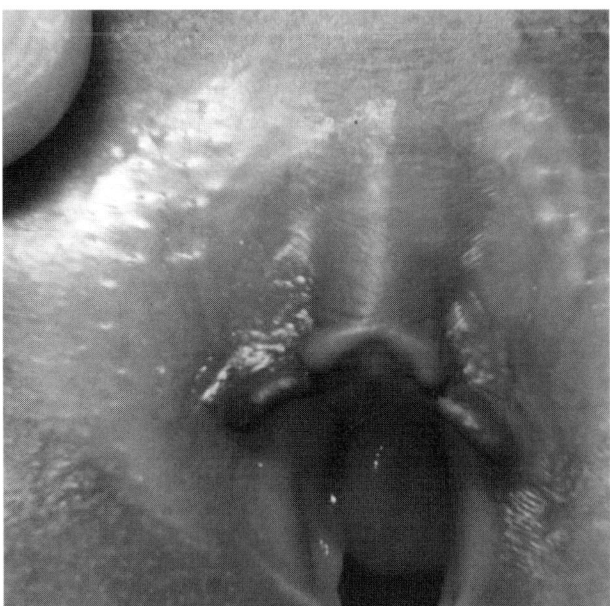

**Fig 1.** Urethral prolapse in a young black female. A circular mass of edematous mucosa with a central orifice can be seen.

ization), poor nutrition, stress with coughing, and constipation have been implicated as contributing to urethral prolapse.[15,16] Most recently, Lowe et al. proposed that urethral prolapse results from poor attachments between the longitudinal and circular-oblique smooth muscle layers of the urethra in association with superimposed episodes of increased intraabdominal pressure.[11]

### Treatment

Treatment recommendations in the literature include nonoperative treatment with antibiotics and local application of estrogens with Sitz baths, reductions of the prolapse and placement of an indwelling catheter, suture ligation around a catheter, cauterization, and suprapubic anterior urethropexy.[17–21,26] Most authors agree that little success is achieved with nonoperative management although two series report high success rates with this treatment.[20,21] Similarly, reduction of the prolapse with a catheter or finger has met with little success and has been found to be quite difficult and painful.[21] Some still advocate placement of a suture ligature over the prolapsed mucosa around a Foley catheter. The balloon is deflated and as the tissue undergoes ischemic necrosis the catheter is removed spontaneously. This usually takes 2–5 days and is less popular due to the prolonged catheter drainage and hospital stay. The anterior urethropexy technique, popularized by Hepburn, has largely been replaced by excisional techniques. This technique of urethral suspension is seemingly excessive to correct a benign local condition. Cauterization as well has largely been abandoned due to reports of urethral stricture associated with excision of the prolapse in this manner.[22,23] The vast majority of authors today advocate simple, circumferential, sharp excision (circumcision) of the prolapse with a catheter in place.[11,24,25] Four quadrant sutures are placed as the mucosa is excised, suturing urethral mucosa to mucosa of the introitus. Additional sutures are then placed between the quadrant sutures. Cystoscopy is performed prior to excision.

## DORSAL DIVERTICULUM OF THE FOSSA NAVICULARIS (LACUNA MAGNA)

### Presentation

Some young boys may present with hematuria and/or dysuria that is due to a dorsal urethral diverticulum of the fossa na-

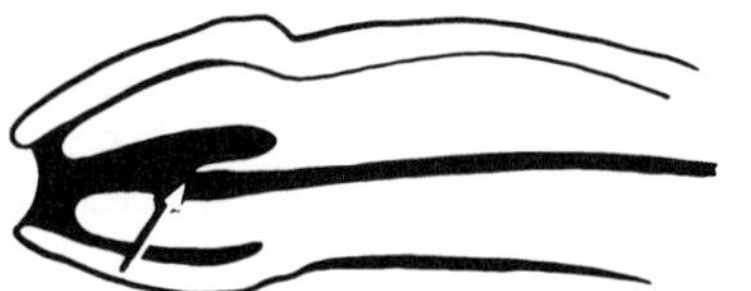

**Fig 2.** Diagrammatic representation of a dorsal diverticulum of the fossa navicularis (lacuna magna). Division of the septum generally results in resolution of the patient's symptoms.

vicularis. Symptoms appear to be related to overdistention of the lacuna magna, the largest of numerous outpouchings or lacunae of the fossa navicularis (Fig 2). This was first described by Morgagni, and Gray and Skandalakis further defined the septum between the lacuna magna and urethral lumen as the valve of Guerin.[4]

### Embryology

Embryologically, the ectodermal ingrowth at the center of the glans normally canalizes in a distal-to-proximal direction to meet the penile urethra, thereby completing urethral continuity. This process results in the formation of the fossa navicularis and urethral meatus; a diverticulum of the lacuna magna may form if the ectodermal ingrowth is abnormally long and/or the junction with the glanular urethra is not end-on.

### Diagnosis

While most patients will have sudden onset of dysuria or hematuria as presenting symptoms, occasionally patients will be asymptomatic. The diagnosis can be suspected on voiding cystourethrogram when a distended spherical diverticulum on the dorsal urethra at the junction of the penile shaft and glans is seen. Care must be taken when interpreting the films as drops of contrast on the external surface of the glans or surrounding towels may lead to misdiagnosis. Confirmation of the diagnosis is done by probing the urethra with a lacrimal duct probe or by examining the urethra with a urethroscope. Occasionally, the orifice of the diverticulum may be difficult to see on urethroscopy due to its proximity to the meatus.

### Treatment

The treatment for this lesion is simple dorsal incision of the valve of Guerin. The patient's symptoms will generally resolve after division of this septum.

## MEGALOURETHRA

### Etiology

Megalourethra is a rare congenital anomaly of the anterior urethra first described by Nesbitt in 1959.[27] Dorairajan and Stephens described the anomaly as a diffuse elongated expansion of the penile urethral lumen and differentiated it from an anterior urethral diverticulum.[28,29] The dilation of the urethra is not secondary to distal obstruction but rather to poor development of the corpus spongiosum. Kester postulated, however, that if the saccular dilatation becomes marked, the distal lip of the sac can press against the dorsal urethra and may produce mechanical obstruction resulting in secondary upper tract dilation.[30]

The etiology of megalourethra is not known. The possibility of an in utero vascular accident has been suggested although no support for this is available.[31] Additionally, no hereditary pattern has been demonstrated and maternal drug ingestion has not been implicated as an etiology.

### Embryology

Embryologically, megalourethra results from the failure of differentiation of the mesoderm in the urethral folds with subsequent failure of migration of spongy tissue formed from the inner genital folds. Between 6 and 10 weeks gestation the normal penile urethral groove will close from the urogenital diaphragm distally with concomitant ectodermal ingrowth of the glanular urethra. The urethra is then invested with vascular sinusoids and connective tissue of mesenchymal origin, thereby forming the corpus spongiosum. In the scaphoid type a failure of these mesenchymal elements to invest the urethra results in inadequate ventral support of the urethra. The dorsal aspect of the urethra remains firmly fixed by generally normal corpora cavernosa (they may be somewhat elongated), which causes the penis to deflect superiorly during voiding thereby decreasing the force of the urinary stream and giving the penis the characteristic scaphoid appearance. The more severe defect seen in the fusiform type results from the failure of the mesoderm in the urethral folds to form any erectile tissue. This results in urethral epithelium being laid on a fibrous wall of tunica albuginea.[28] Histopathologic examination of megalourethral specimens demonstrates normal but attenuated urethral tissue, Buck's fascia and penile skin and sinusoidal tissue are absent.[29]

There is a strong association between megalourethra and other congenital anomalies, particularly of the upper urinary tract and anterior abdominal wall. Shrom et al. reported an association between the fusiform type of megalourethra and other diffuse mesenchymal disorders including renal dysplasia-hypoplasia, vesicoureteral reflux, large bladder, atretic or stenotic posterior urethra, imperforate anus with rectovesical fistula, and undescended testes (Fig 3). In addition, they reported that 13 of 26 patients in their series with scaphoid megalourethra had recognizable prune belly syndrome.[32] Megalourethra has also been reported to be associated with posterior urethral valves,[33] urethral duplication,[34] and impotence in adults.[35] Wilson and Walker reported 11 patients with hypospadias and associated scaphoid megalourethra.[36]

**Fig 3.** DPTA renal scan demonstrating nonfunctioning right kidney (multicystic dysplastic kidney) in a patient with prune belly syndrome and scaphoid megalourethra.

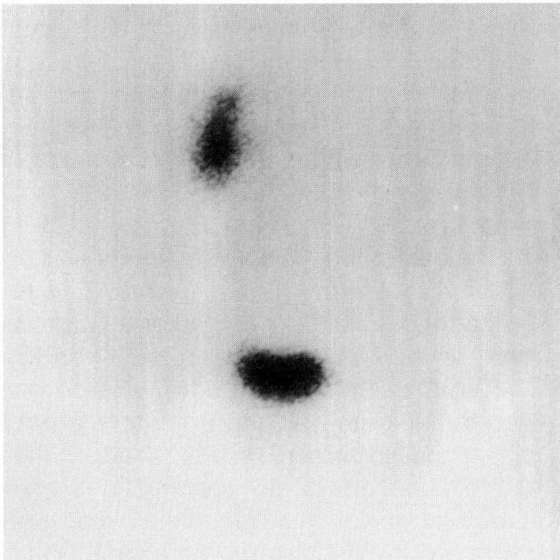

To date 45 cases of megalourethra have been reported in the literature.[30] It is generally believed that the fusiform type of megalourethra is associated with more severe secondary congenital anomalies. Recently this has become somewhat controversial.

Kelalis et al. reported on the initial eight patients with fusiform megalourethra, all of whom had associated congenital anomalies incompatible with life.[37] Later Shrom et al. reported a 20% mortality among patients with scaphoid megalourethra, mostly from renal failure with or without sepsis.[32] Appel and Kaplan, however, subsequently reported that 7 of 10 reported patients with fusiform megalourethra and 19 of 31 reported patients with scaphoid megalourethra were azotemic or dead, suggesting that the associated anomalies and ultimate outcome of the two groups were similar.[31]

As a corollary to this controversy several authors dispute the arbitrary distinction between the scaphoid and fusiform types of megalourethra.[29,34] They believe the disorder is more appropriately viewed as a spectrum rather than two distinct entities. Still other authors argue that this anomaly exists in three distinct forms (scaphoid, fusiform, and a middle form with localized absence of the corpus spongiosum and small saccular diverticulum).[38] This was also supported by Wilson and Walker, who reported 11 cases of hypospadias in association with a middle form of megalourethra in the apparent spectrum of mesodermal deficiencies of the penis.[36] Finally, Chehval and Mehan reported a case that demonstrated features of both a scaphoid and fusiform megalourethra, lending further support to the spectrum of mesodermal deficiency theory.[39]

## Diagnosis

The diagnosis of megalourethra is generally made by simple observation. The

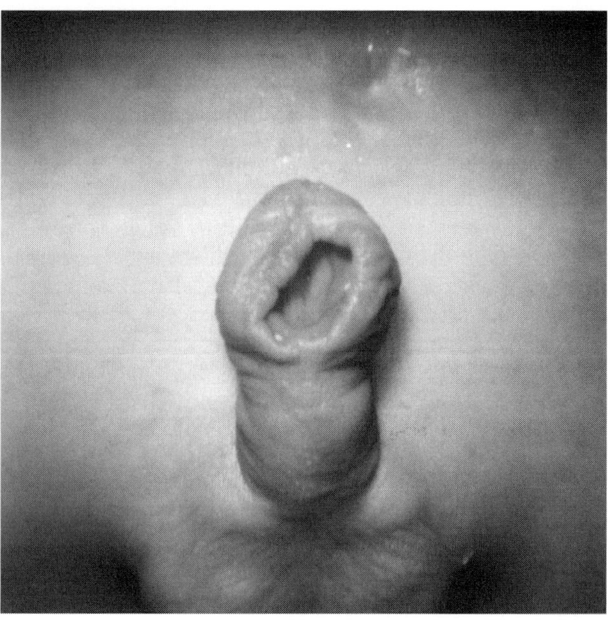

**Fig 4.** Scaphoid megalourethra in a patient with prune belly syndrome.

high incidence of associated upper urinary tract anomalies warrants full upper tract evaluation in all patients. An excretory urogram with follow-up voiding film should be the first diagnostic test. Sepsis following radiographic instrumentation has been well documented and most authors recommend avoiding studies that require catheterization.[32] Antegrade studies by way of percutaneous bladder puncture are an alternative means to study these patients and probably significantly reduce the chance of sepsis. Systemic antibiotics are generally recommended for this evaluation. The megalourethra is susceptible to bacterial colonization as a result of stasis and meatal contamination; suppressive antibiotics are generally indicated for long-term management, particularly if other genitourinary anomalies are present.

## Classification

Classically, megalourethra is divided into two basic types: scaphoid (incomplete) and fusiform (complete). These can be distinguished by their clinical and radiographic appearance. The scaphoid type of megalourethra is more common and the less severe form of this anomaly. A localized deficiency of the corpus spongiosum in the anterior urethra facilitates the formation of a ventral saccular diverticulum that balloons during voiding. In the fusiform type, the corpora cavernosa and the corpus spongiosum are absent, resulting in an elongated sac-like penis that distends markedly when filled with urine (Fig 4).

## Management

Nesbitt originally treated a large scaphoid megalourethra by circumcision and excision of the redundant urethra with reapproximate of the urethral skin over a catheter stent.[27] After making a circumscribing incision at the corona and degloving the penis, a ventral incision is made in the midline of the redundant ventral aspect of the urethra. The excess urethra is excised from the lateral flaps and a new urethra created by suturing over a catheter. The redundant penile skin is then excised and tailored to the cylindric form of the phallus. The skin is then resutured at the corona thereby covering the urethroplasty in order to prevent urethrocutaneous fistula. Alternatively, Shrom et al. recommended marsupialization of the megalourethra ventrally to prevent stasis and infection.[32]

Then a second procedure is done to close the defect when the child is older.

In the case of fusiform megalourethra, repair is complicated by lack of supporting structures and minimal corpora cavernosa as well as by excessive length of the penis. No cases of repair have been reported and consideration is often given to gender reassignment in these cases.[29] No cases of gender reassignment have been reported, however, most likely because of the severity of associated anomalies and low survival.

## ANTERIOR URETHRAL VALVES/DIVERTICULA

Anterior urethral valves are a rare cause of infravesical obstruction in boys. The majority of these valves are actually the distal lip of an anterior urethral diverticulum. These diverticuli occur in two different forms. The narrow-necked or globular type with a small sac that communicates with the bulb of the urethra does not cause obstruction but rather is associated with stasis and calculus formation. The wide-necked or saccular diverticulum usually has a much larger sac and often presents with obstruction due to the distal lip of the diverticulum that acts as a flap valve and is pushed up against the dorsal wall of the urethra on voiding.

Urethral diverticula have been reported in young girls as well but are exceedingly rare. None have been associated with obstruction and most present with urinary tract infection, vaginal introital mass, or urethral discharge.[38] Excision of the diverticulum or incision and drainage generally is adequate surgical therapy for these lesions.

Anterior urethral valves or ''folds'' without associated diverticula have been reported. Some have attempted to differentiate ''true'' anterior urethral valves from obstructing diverticula of the anterior urethra while others believe that these entities represent a spectrum disorder.[38] Many raise the question of whether the pathology is primarily an obstructing valve with subsequent diverticular formation or a diverticulum with secondary formation of an obstructing distal lip.[40]

Scherz et al. reported valves that appear as diaphanous to thick bands of tissue on the ventral aspect of the urethra, assuming an iris-like, semilumar, or cusp-like appearance.[41] Golimbu et al. reported on 25 known cases of these types of valves and found 46% to be cusp-like, 31% to be iris-like, and 23% to be semilumar.[42] While most will agree that the majority of anterior valves are found in association with saccular diverticula, Firlit and King reported 13 cases and only 4 were noted to be associated with diverticula.[43]

Anterior urethral diverticula/valves can be found anywhere distal to the membranous urethra but the majority are found in the bulbous urethra or at the penoscrotal junction. Golimbu et al. reported that 40% are found in the bulbous urethra, 30% at the penoscrotal junction, and 30% in the penile urethra.[42] Scherz et al. reported three cases located in the fossa navicularis.[41] The narrow-necked nonobstructing diverticula are found almost exclusively in the bulbous portion of the urethra.

### Etiology

The origin of anterior urethral valves/diverticula is unclear. All are located on the ventral aspect of the urethra and many theories to explain these lesions exist. Cystic dilatation of normal or accessory urethral glands that eventually communicate with the urethra has been suggested as a possible cause of urethral diverticula. Kaufman proposed a faulty union between the glandular and penile urethra that appears to account for the fossa navicularis diverticula as described by Scherz et al., but does not account for the majority of diverticula in the bulbous or proximal anterior urethra.[41,44] Voillemier proposed that the diverticula originate in an area of the urethra with partial deficiency of spongy tissue[45] and Depaoli believed that the defect was primary focal atrophy of the ventral urethral wall with minimal support from surrounding corpus spongiosum.[46] Boissonnat and Duhamel believed that originally a distal congenital obstructing membrane existed that subsequently disappeared after the formation of a proximal diverticulum.[47]

The most continuously accepted theory is one of a local defect in the development of the corpus spongiosum. There is a focal arrest in the differentiation of periurethral mesenchymal tissue into erectile tissue. Lack of an effective tissue buttress leads to urethral dilatation in the area of the deficiency and results in the formation of a diverticulum.

Histologically, the diverticular walls lack the supportive elements of the corpus spongiosum and are lined by epithelium and a thin, fibrous capsule.

## Presentation

Obstruction of the anterior urethra by a valve is variable and often the age at which the diagnosis is made depends on the degree of obstruction present. The more severe obstructions are generally found in neonates and younger children, and symptoms may include failure to thrive, acidosis, azotemia, massive hydronephrosis, megacystis, trabeculation of the bladder, or severe urosepsis or other symptoms of chronic renal failure. More commonly there may be a poor, dribbling stream, penile mass, or ballooning of the penile urethra during voiding. Pressure on such a diverticulum after voiding will result in further emptying of urine. Older children may present with enuresis, dribbling, blood staining of underclothes, or complaints of an enlarging penis during voiding, as well as frequency, dysuria, or a firm penoscrotal mass. Often observation of the patient's stream will reveal dribbling and diminished force or ballooning. In all cases, accurate diagnosis requires a high index of suspicion.

In the case of the nonobstructing narrow-mouthed diverticulum, patients may present with symptoms of infection due to stasis in the diverticulum or local pain secondary to stone formation.

## Diagnosis

The most accurate test to diagnose these lesions is the voiding cystourethrogram. This study will often reveal trabeculation of the bladder with dilatation of the urethra proximal to the diverticulum with the distal urethra appearing somewhat narrow. A sharp valvular distal lip of the wide-mouthed diverticulum can also often be seen (Fig 5). Vesicoureteral reflux may or

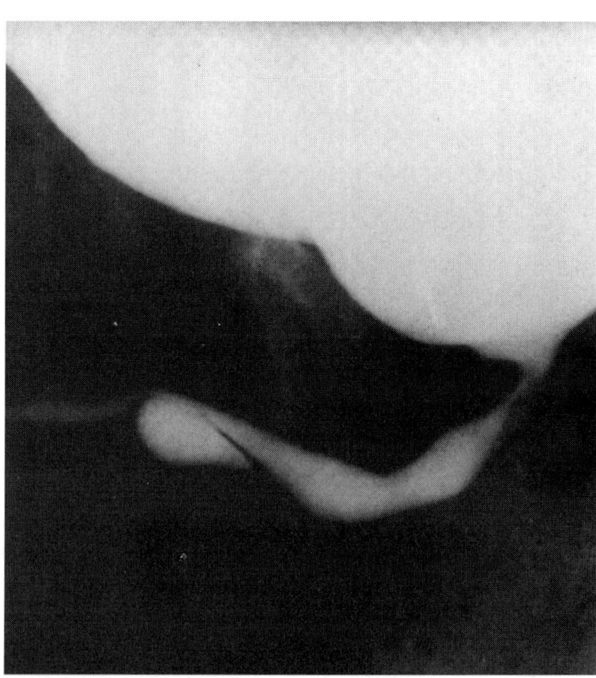

**Fig 5.** Anterior urethral diverticulum (valve) demonstrated by voiding cystourethrogram in a young boy.

may not be present. For accurate diagnosis, it is important that the area between the membranous urethra and the external urethral meatus be included in the voiding portion of the study.

Firlit et al. classified the radiographic findings with anterior urethra valves into four types based on the severity of the obstruction: (1) minimal proximal urethra distention; (2) proximal urethral diverticulum with normal bladder and normal upper tracts; (3) similar to type 2 but associated with bladder distention, trabeculation, and minimal ureterectasis; and (4) obstruction with severe hydroureteronephrosis.[40]

Simple cystography may not only fail to reveal the etiology of the obstruction in the urethra, but may also erroneously suggest a primary bladder neck obstruction. This results because, as in posterior urethral valves, there is proximal urethral dilatation making the bladder neck appear as a relative constriction. Golimbu et al. reported that in their series of 13 patients the cystogram revealed bladder trabeculation universally and reflux (generally bilateral) in 35% of cases. Intravenous pyelography, while not useful in making the diagnosis, indicated some degree of upper tract deterioration in 47% of cases. Voiding cystourethrogram revealed the obstructing lesion in greater than 95% of the Golimbu et al. series.[42]

The retrograde urethrogram is notoriously unreliable as a diagnostic radiologic study. Since ballooning of the diverticulum with concomitant obstruction by the valve may occur only with antegrade flow of urine, this study may demonstrate a normal urethra, particularly if the valve is flattened and the diverticulum small.

Endoscopy may be useful but, again, can be misleading; cystoscopy will often demonstrate the opening of the diverticulum if the urethra is adequately distended with irrigating fluid. However, often the full extent of the diverticulum is difficult to judge. Golimbu et al. found that cystoscopy was successful in diagnosing the valves in 41% of cases, but in many instances the cystoscope could not be passed beyond the obstruction.[42]

### Treatment

The treatment of anterior urethral valves includes simple disruption of the valve with a sound or cystoscope, transurethral resection or ablation of the distal lip, urethrotomy with excision of the valve only, and open excision with primary anastomosis. Most agree that the breakthrough method is the least desirable. Tank believes that all neonates are best served with an open repair rather than endoscopic resection whereas older children can be treated with endoscopic resection since the urethra is large enough for easy manipulation of the resectoscope.[48] Within the fossa navicularis Scherz et al. advocate sharp excision of the valve with an instrument since transurethral excision or ablation can be difficult because of the distal location.[41] Most commonly treatment is based on the size of the diverticulum; if there is an anterior valve without a significant diverticulum, endoscopic resection may be sufficient. If a large diverticulum is present, open excision with urethroplasty should be performed.

Rushton et al. recommend cutaneous vesicostomy as initial management of anterior valves particularly in patients with significant vesicoureteral reflux with associated renal failure due to the high complication rate associated with other types of management in these patients.[49]

## DUPLICATION OF THE URETHRA

Urethral duplication in males is a rare congenital anomaly. Female duplications are seen even less frequently and are usually complete duplications extending from the bladder to the perineum. In females they present with a short phallus without chordee and a patent phallic urethra along with a patent vaginal urethral meatus. The treatment includes clitoral relocation and vaginoplasty with or without excision of the accessory urethra. In males the vast majority of urethral duplications are dorsal-ventral and occur in the sagittal plane. Rare collateral types of urethral duplication are often seen in association with diphallus and duplications associated with bladder duplication have been described.

## Classification

Many classifications of urethral duplication exist. Most recently, however, authors have relied on two primary classification systems. Das and Brosman in 1977 proposed a simple classification of urethral duplication based on anatomic features.[50] In type I, the complete accessory urethra arises proximally from a separate or confluent opening in the bladder and extends distally to an external orifice. The accessory urethra is always dorsal to the main subcorporeal urethra. The accessory urethra meatus may be on the glans or in an epispadiac location on the shaft. In type II, the accessory urethra arises from the primary urethra and continues dorsally or ventrally with or without an external opening. This group includes patients with an accessory urethra with an external opening or variable length of urethra that ends blindly, as well as the so-called spindle urethra. In type III, a complete accessory urethra arises from a separate opening in the bladder neck from a dilated prostatic urethra and ended in the perineum anterior to the anal verge. The main urethra is normal or atretic.

Effman et al. proposed a different classification scheme around the same time. Many authors presently find this classification most complete, anatomically accurate, and clinically useful: type I, blind incomplete urethral duplication; type IIA, complete patent duplication with two urethral meatuses (type IIA-1, two noncommunicating urethras arising independently from the bladder. Type IIA-2, a second channel arising from the first and coursing independently to a second meatus); type IIB, patent urethral duplication with a single meatus (two urethras from bladder or posterior urethra uniting to form single distal channel); and type III, urethral duplication as a component of partial or complete caudal duplication.[51]

For the sake of discussion here, we will use the simple classification scheme proposed by Das and Brosman.

Of prime significance in all urethra duplications is the concept that regardless of where the two meatuses are, the lower or ventral urethra is the more functional one and generally contains the verumontanum, the sphincter, and the accessory glands. Partial (blind-ending) duplications (subgroup of type II) are much more common

**Fig 6.** Diagrammatic representation of a wide variety of urethral duplications.

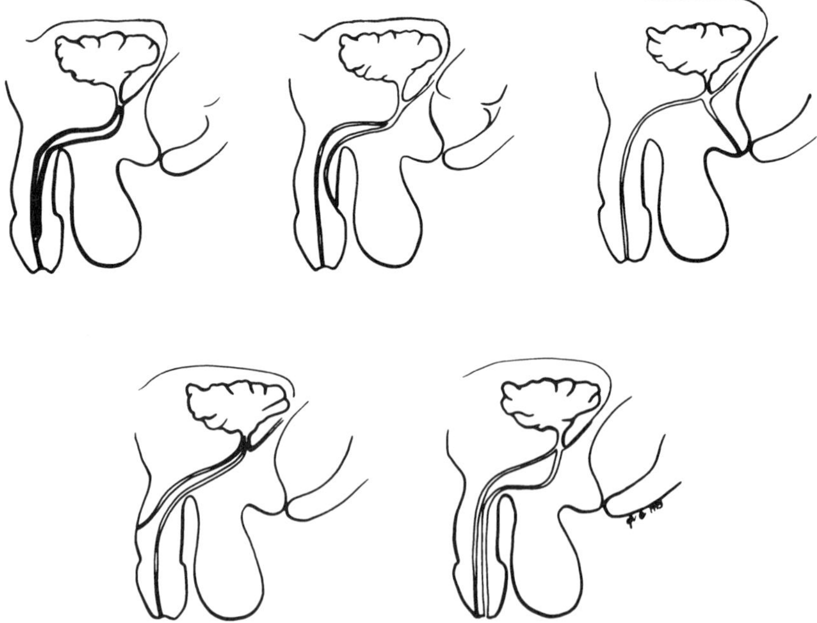

than other types and can often be seen in the distal form of hypospadias (Fig 6).

## Embryology

The exact embryology of urethral duplication is unknown although many theories have been proposed. No one hypothesis appears to explain the spectrum of anomalies that encompasses urethral duplication.

For type I duplications, Lowsley proposed that during the infolding of the genital ridge, the urogenital plate persists. This extends for the entire length of the penis with the urethra below and the urogenital penis above; if the plate fails to resorb or rupture, two urethras will form.[52] Johnson further elaborated that because of faulty fusion of the genital ridges, two separate channels are induced, one of endodermal origin (normal urethra) and one of ectodermal origin (accessory urethra).[53] Others have proposed that uncoordinated growth between the phallic segment of the urogenital sinus and the maturation of the urethral crest epithelium results in this particular anomaly. In cases in which the dorsal channel is in an epispadic position, the pubic symphysis is often found to be widened; the anomaly appears to be related to exstrophy of the bladder and true epispadias. Both of these anomalies are felt to be secondary to a lack of midline-mesodermal fusion. A partial failure or irregularity of lateral mesodermal growth between the ectodermal and endodermal layers of the cloacal membrane in the midline allows the phallic portion of the urogenital sinus to become associated with the dorsum of the phallus thereby creating the epispadias.

To explain type II or bifid urethral duplication, several authors believe that anomalous fusion of the genital folds causes bifurcation or complete sequestration of a part of the urethral anlage. The common accessory urethras, most frequently seen in hypospadias, is presumed to represent an ectodermal ingrowth from the glans that would normally communicate with the endodermal urethra.

Type III duplications are felt to be secondary to defective urorectal fold development. De Vries and Friedland felt that the separation of the cloacal membrane into anal and urogenital membranes was incomplete due to inhibition of growth of the terminal portion of the urorectal septum.[54] It has been suggested that these accessory channels may constitute fistulas rather than true urethral duplication. However, histologic evidence has revealed that these channels are urethral in origin.

## Presentation

Patients with complete patent urethral duplication (type I) can be asymptomatic or can present with a double stream, urinary incontinence, urinary tract infection, or outlet obstruction. Commonly patients with type I duplication present with a double stream, which can be annoying if the meatus is located proximally in the shaft. Often they will have varying degrees of incontinence that occurs mainly with stress and results from inadequate development of the proximal sphincter mechanism of the accessory urethra. The incontinence may be characterized by continual urinary flow, a narrow stream during voiding, or post-void dripping. Dorsal chordee can also be seen in type I patients due to the dorsal location of the ill-developed accessory urethra.

In type II duplications, the majority of patients are asymptomatic. Rarely, however, obstruction of the normal ventral urethra may result if the dorsal channel has stenosis that causes proximal distention and external compression of the adjacent urethra. This may result in dysuria and/or sepsis secondary to bladder outlet obstruction. Urinary tract infection can occur in up to one third of patients with type II duplications and is difficult to clear from the dorsal tract because of narrowness, tortuosity, and poor urinary washout. Persistent urethral discharge may also be a presenting symptom.

In type III duplication of the perineal urethra often appears to be more prominent anatomically and functionally (Fig 7). Generally, patients are continent of urine and void through the perineal tract. Recurrent lower urinary tract infections are common. In the case of blind-ending accessory urethras, most are asymptomatic and not noticed by the patient.

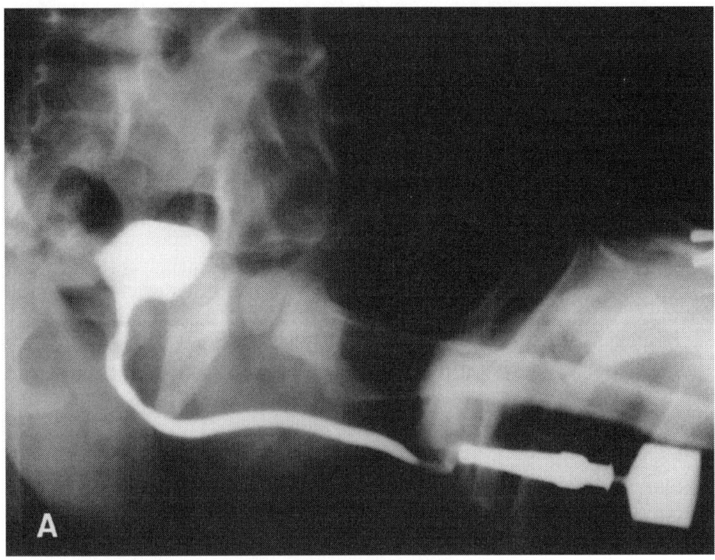


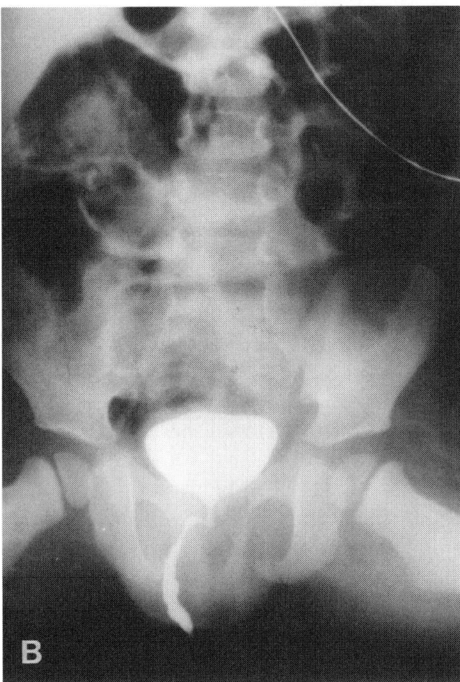


**Fig 7. A.** Retrograde urethrogram demonstrating the dorsal penile urethra in a type III urethral duplication in a 2-year-old boy. **B.** Voiding study in the same patient revealing the ventral urethra opening on the perineum.

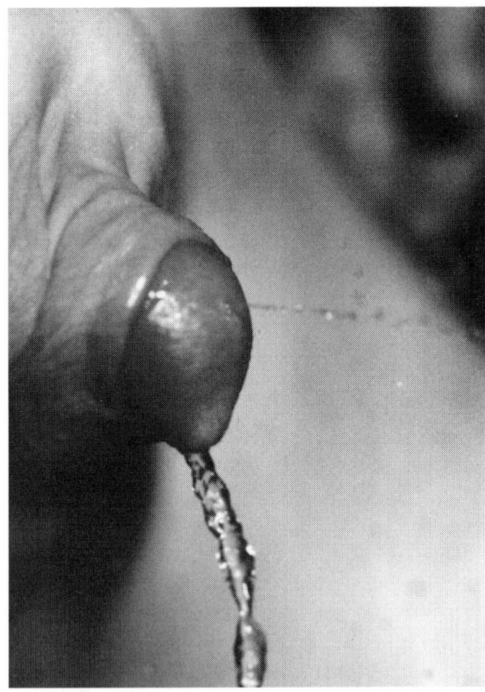

**Fig 8.** Voiding photograph of a patient with urethral duplication and both meatuses located on the glans.

Physical examination will often reveal two meatuses and nothing more (Fig 8). Type III anomalies are often found in association with undescended testes and patients with epispadiac duplication may have symptomatic chordee.

### Diagnosis

To confirm the diagnosis of urethral duplication a voiding cystourethrogram and retrograde urethrogram are often required. The evaluation of any patient referred with two meatal openings or double urinary stream is not complete until both urethral channels have been fully demonstrated.

Since the posterior urethra cannot be adequately evaluated by retrograde urethrogram and the anterior urethra cannot be completely visualized by voiding cystourethrogram, both studies are required to demonstrate the caliber and configuration of both channels of the duplication. In almost all cases, the ventrally positioned urethral channel, regardless of its meatal position, proves to be the more functional one and is generally more easily catheterizable (Fig 9).

This urethra will contain the verumontanum and opening of the genital ducts and will also contain the usual congenital anomalies that affect a single urethra, such as posterior urethral valves and anomalies of Cowper's ducts.[55]

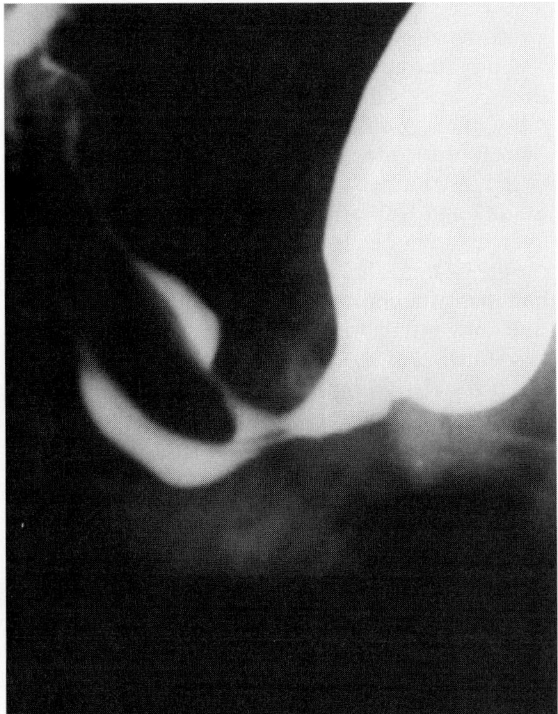

**Fig 9.** Voiding cystourethrogram of patient in Fig 8 revealing type II A-2 urethral duplication.

The use of endoscopic examination and the injection of contrast into the accessory channel is often useful to demonstrate the proximal connection in type II anomalies. The reports of associated upper tract anomalies have been variable but there are reports of renal agenesis, duplex systems, ectopia, and reflux.[56] All patients, therefore, should have a renal ultrasound or intravenous pyelogram.

Evaluation for anomalies in other organs—in particular, the internal genitalia, gastrointestinal tract, and lower spine—is indicated for all patients with type III urethral duplication. Also, in patients with a dorsal accessory channel with an epispadiac meatus, an abnormally wide (>1 cm) symphysis pubis has been noted.[57–59]

### Treatment

Various modalities of treatment have been used for urethral duplications. The treatment will depend on the type of duplication and clinical presentation. Those asymptomatic patients without evidence of occult bladder outlet obstruction warrant simple observation. For patients with recurrent infection, double stream, or incontinence, excision of the duplicated tract is generally indicated. Transurethral incision through the intraurethral septum has been reported with success in duplication where the meatuses are in close proximity.[60] Excision of the whole septum, thereby creating a single meatus, has also been reported.[61] Obliteration of the accessory channel with electrocautery or injection of sclerosants has also been reported but occasionally has been associated with corporal thrombosis or fibrosis.[50]

However, most authors recommend complete excision of the accessory tract, particularly when the tract lacks sphincter control.[51,62–64] The objective of excision is to remove the dorsal urethra with a minimum of postoperative fibrosis and no sphincter damage. Complete duplication (type I) may be excised by a combined retropubic and penile approach.[62] Urethrourethrostomy has also been used successfully to eliminate double streams and is often most suitable when one of the urethras is epispadiac or hypospadiac. Correction of dorsal chordee may have to be undertaken at the same time if present in epispadiac duplication as well as correction of hypospadias. Occasionally, the distal segment of the duplicated urethra can be used to form the new roof of a hypospadiac ventral urethra.

In the Y type of duplication (type III) with an anal or preanal meatus, the perineal urethra can sometimes be reconstructed and anastomosed to the penile portion of the dorsal urethra. Often, however, the penile urethra is atretic and fibrosed and does not allow this. Multiple-stage urethroplasty procedures have been recommended in the past, but presently a long bladder mucosal-grafted urethroplasty has been advocated after mobilizing the perineal urethral meatus.[55,65]

## URETHRAL STRICTURES

### Etiology

Urethral strictures in boys are not uncommon lesions. Kaplan and Brock stated that urethral strictures in boys are more common than the literature tends to suggest.[66] The causes of urethral strictures in childhood are iatrogenic, traumatic, inflammatory, and congenital. Iatrogenic stricture and trauma-induced stricture are the most common causes[66–68] and inflammatory strictures are rare, being most commonly associated with urethritis following an indwelling urethral catheter.[69] Nearly two thirds of all strictures are felt to be iatrogenic and are found following cystoscopy, traumatic urethral catheterization, or surgery such as fulguration of posterior urethral valves or hypospadias repair. Harshman et al. found that strictures following instrumentation are often due to inappropriate dilation or cystoscopy with an excessively large instrument.[68]

Traumatic bulbar strictures less commonly can be attributed to a straddle injury, a direct blow to the perineum, penetrating injury, or pelvic fracture. Scherz and Kaplan found that 19% of strictures were attributable to these types of injury.[69]

Inflammatory strictures result from urethritis. In the Scherz/Kaplan series these accounted for 7% of all strictures and all were associated with the use of indwelling latex catheters. They report no further inflammatory strictures after cessation of use of latex catheters.[69] Gonorrhea in the prepubertal child is very rare but the physician should be aware of the possibility when treating a stricture of the bulbar urethra, the common site of genoccocal-associated strictures. Nonspecific urethritis for which no causative agent could be found was described by Williams and Mikael in 17 boys (age 5–15 years).[70]

Congenital strictures are rare. Kaplan and Brock[66] reported 8 of 57 and Gibbons et al.[67] reported 4 of 22 urethral strictures to be congenital. Harshman et al., however, reported no cases of congenital strictures in a series of 25 patients; he purported that congenital strictures are a rare cause of urethral obstruction in boys and are grossly overdiagnosed.[68] He further recommended avoidance of the term *congenital urethral stricture* altogether.

Currarino and Stephens have suggested that Cowper's duct abnormalities may possibly play a role in these strictures and therefore for the present time should be labeled "strictures of unknown etiology."[71] Scherz and Kaplan strongly disagree, however, using an example of a patient treated on the second day of life and who had not had instrumentation at any time.[69] They define congenital stricture as any stricture that is identified at the time of an initial evaluation for the patient's presenting problem and in which there is no history of injury, inflammation, instrumentation, or surgery. These account for roughly 14% of the strictures they have observed.[69] The precise nature of congenital urethral strictures therefore remains somewhat controversial.

The vast majority of congenital urethral strictures occur in the proximal urethral bulb but they can occur anywhere in the anterior urethra.[66,72] The lesion is generally described as a soft circumferential mucosal membrane and some feel that this lesion may be synonymous embryologically with inframembranous type III urethral valves.[29,73,74] Most feel, however, that the etiology of this congenital membrane is attributable to failure of complete canalization of the urogenital membrane. Complete canalization as described by Stephens is done by ectodermal, genital fold, and endodermal urogenital sinus pits that meet and create the lumen through the membrane.[29] This process occurs at or near the junction of bulbous and membranous urethras and failure of this process results in a tight, stenotic mucosal aperture. This congenital membrane differs from inflammatory or traumatic strictures in that there is no deposition of abnormal tissue or periurethral fibrosis. Some consider this lesion embryologically analogous to the distal urethral ring seen in girls.[72]

Further evidence supporting the congenital nature of these strictures lies in their association with other congenital anomalies. Abnormalities of the cardiovascular, central nervous, and skeletal systems have been reported by Leadbetter and Leadbetter.[75] Redman and Fraiser reported congenital urethral strictures in two brothers[76] and English and Pryor reported strictures in a father and son.[77] Cobb et al. reported 38% of patients with congenital urethral stricture to have associated anomalies such as syndactyly, polydactyly, tetralogy of Fallot, cleft palate, myelomeningocele, and hypospadias.[72]

## Presentation

Symptoms of urethral stricture are similar to those in adults. Patients may present with acute urinary retention or urinary dribbling as well as poor stream, hematuria, hesitancy, frequency, enuresis, and urinary infection. Scherz and Kaplan found that when only nocturnal enuresis was present as a symptom, no improvement was noted with treatment of the stricture whereas 87% of patients with day and night time wetting improved with treatment.[69] Urethrocutaneous fistula with hypospadias repair also lends suspicion to the possible presence of a stricture.

## Diagnosis

The history and physical examination often will lead the examiner to suspect a urethral stricture. Observation of the patient while voiding may also be helpful. Radiologically, strictures are best diagnosed with an excretory urogram with subsequent voiding film. This can confirm the diagnosis without instrumentation but further evaluation may be necessary with either a voiding cystourethrogram or retrograde urethrogram. Uroflow rates will be found to be reduced and endoscopy can be used to directly examine the stricture.

## Treatment

Anterior urethral strictures can be treated by urethral dilatation, urethrotomy, or urethroplasty. The type of repair selected is dependent on a number of factors such as length, location, number and character of the stricture(s), as well as the presence of infection. The goal should be to select a repair that produces the best results with the least morbidity and requires the fewest surgical procedures. Dilatation is often the initial treatment but is often not permanently successful. Harshman et al. reported only 2 of 10 successful results with dilatation alone[68] and Kaplan and Brock reported a similar 28.6% overall success rate with dilation as the sole therapeutic modality.[66] Specifically, only two of four inflammatory, one of five congenital, one of five iatrogenic, and no traumatic strictures responded. Devereux and Williams were successful in seven of nine patients with single or infrequent dilation. They recommend that urethral dilation seems an appropriate initial treatment for short congenital strictures and strictures with hypospadias repair. They claim that in each of these instances 50% of patients will respond to a single dilation but they note recurrent problems up to 8–9 years later.[73] Repeated dilation, however, is not desirable. General anesthesia is usually required in children for dilation as children do not tolerate repeated dilation under local anesthesia in the office. Devereux and Burfield also noted that routine dilation in younger patients placed them at increased risk of having lower urinary tract complications.[78] This was supported by Blandy et al., who reported complications among 43% of patients who were doing well with routine dilation.[79] In addition, repeat dilations may be harmful because they increase associated fibrous tissue, thereby making subsequent surgical repair more difficult.

In infants, Scherz and Kaplan recommend a temporizing vesicostomy due to the historical evidence that urethral dilation in infants by itself can lead to stricture disease. He recommends avoiding manipulative modalities of treatment until the infant is older and better suited for certain forms of urethral repair.[69]

Direct-vision internal urethrotomy has been shown to be efficacious for congenital diaphragmatic strictures and short iatrogenic strictures in the bulbous urethra. Noe reported good short-term results (80% success)[80] and Scherz and Kaplan believe it to be as effective as urethral dilation for inflammatory and posthypospadias repairs although no data are available to support the efficacy of one over the other.[69] Steroid injections have been used as an adjunct to internal urethrotomy with mixed results.[81] Although reported in adults, there have been no reports on the use of balloon dilation or laser treatment of strictures in children. Electrosurgical urethrotomy has been used in the past but often results in increased stricture disease due to the thermal injury produced.

The strictures that do not respond to dilation or internal urethrotomy or strictures that are not deemed suitable for these modalities of treatment should be treated with formal urethroplasty. Staged operations have been used widely in the past but recently have fallen into disfavor. Kaplan and Brock report that five of eight patients required more than two procedures for a successful result.[66] Harshman et al. reported similar results with multistage repairs.[68] However, a multistaged approach may still be indicated if there is a great deal of inflammation around the stricture.

The preferable mode of therapy is generally felt to be a one-stage urethroplasty. If the stricture is short and in the penile or distal bulbar urethra, excision and reanastomosis has been shown to have excellent results. Harshman et al. reported successful outcomes in 100% of seven strictures treated in this manner.[68]

Alternatively, a full-thickness free patch graft of hairless penile skin may be used in a one-stage repair. Gibbons et al.[67] and Harshman et al.[68] report 100% and 75% success rate, respectively, with this technique. Scherz and Kaplan, however, feel that patch grafts are less suitable than vascularized pedicle flaps due to the reduced blood supply in the area of the stricture.[69] This would make the "take" of the graft less than one would expect. Vascularized pedicle flaps as a patch or tube have demonstrated good results.[61] It is important to avoid hair-bearing skin as well for a free patch graft or for vascularized grafts in order to avoid the later complications of infection and stones.

### Management

In general, the management of acute posterior urethral trauma remains controversial as in adults. The issue is immediate repair vs. initial suprapubic urinary diversion with delayed repair. Myers and DeWeerd reported good results in 20 of 22 patients treated by primary catheter realignment.[82] Waterhouse reported, however, that all nine of their patients treated by primary catheter realignment subsequently had strictures.[83] Morehouse and MacKinnon advocate initial suprapubic cystostomy with follow-up voiding study after 2–4 weeks. If the patient is able to void, the suprapubic tube is removed; if disruption exists, formal repair should be undertaken after tissue reaction has subsided (3–6 months).[84]

Many authors advocate the transpubic approach to repair of these strictures. The perineal approach in children is made technically difficult because the perineum is narrow and deep. Waterhouse reported excellent results in six of seven patients with traumatic membranous urethral disruption with the transpubic approach.[83]

Impotence following posterior urethral injuries has been reported from 0–78% of patients.[84–87] Waterhouse and Gross reported no cases among 32 children[88]; these data were supported by Malek et al.[89] and Bland et al.[90] who noted no impotence in 7 and 36 children, respectively. Urinary incontinence following posterior urethral disruption is reported to range from 0% to 33%.[84,89,90] Harshman et al. report four of seven patients with some degree of incontinence following urethral repair for disruption associated with severe pelvic fracture.[68]

## URETHRAL POLYPS

Urethral polyps occur exclusively in males and are a rare cause of urethral obstruction. They usually occur as single lesions arising in the area of the verumontanum (prostatic or posterior urethral polyps) or, less commonly, in the anterior urethra (anterior urethral polyps).[91] About 48 cases of posterior urethra polyps are reported in the literature[92] and only four cases of anterior urethral polyps have been reported.[93–95] The lesion is generally a 1- to 3-cm pedunculated mass arising on a long stalk generally from the verumontanum, although they have been noted to arise from the bladder neck or bulbous urethra.

### Etiology

Some speculation about the etiology of these lesions exists. Downs postulated that they represent a benign protrusion of the urethral wall[96] and Stephens believes they are simply congenital polyps.[29] Barrie and Simms suggested that the polyp is a response to urinary infection but most polyps do not occur in the setting that would support this hypothesis.[97] Kearney et al. felt that mesonephric derivatives form urethral polyps in boys just as they form polyps in the vagina and cervix in girls.[92] Microscopically, the lesions have a core of fibrous connective tissue with an outer lining of transitional epithelium. More than half will demonstrate some smooth muscle at the core. Islets of glandular tissue resembling Cowper's glands and nerve tissue can be found. Occasionally, the polyp will be covered by squamous metaplasia and glandular nests.

### Presentation

Patients may present with a history of intermittent obstruction or with acute urinary retention. Obstructive symptoms such as hesitancy and decreased urinary stream as well as dysuria, frequency, urgency, hematuria, enuresis, and urinary tract infection have been reported.

### Diagnosis

The most reliable means of diagnosis is a retrograde urethrogram or voiding cystourethrogram (Fig 10). This will generally demonstrate a filling defect that may vary in location (Fig 11). It may be within the bladder, at the bladder neck, in the posterior urethra, or in the bulbous urethra. Bladder diverticula and/or vesicoureteral reflux have been reported in association with these polyps; about half will be found to have upper tract changes.[74] An intravenous pyelogram may or may not demonstrate a polyp depending on the location of the polyp and the density of contrast material within the bladder. Sonography was also used in at least one reported case to

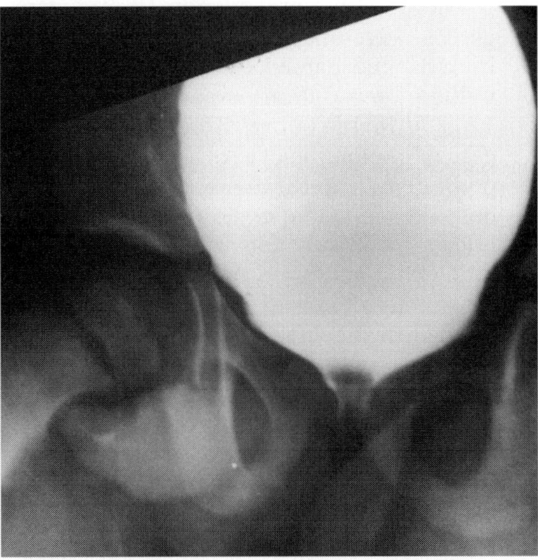

**Fig 10.** Urethral polyp seen as a filling defect at the bladder neck on a voiding study.

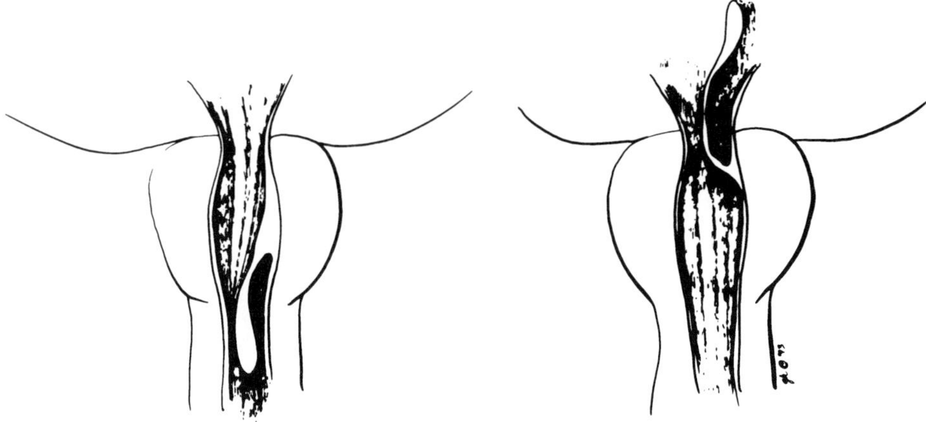

**Fig 11.** Diagrammatic representation of positional variability in a congenital urethral polyp.

identify a polyp arising on a stalk from the verumontanum.[91]

### Treatment

The current treatment is endoscopic resection.[92,98,99] It is important to excise the lesion completely at the base of the stalk since there have been two reports of recurrence of these polyps[56,100] which are felt to indicate incomplete removal.

## ABNORMALITIES OF COWPER'S DUCTS AND GLANDS

The bulbourethral glands, or Cowper's glands, were originally described by Mery in 1684 and named for Cowper after his written description was published in 1705.[101] In 1881 English reported the first case of a retention cyst of the duct of Cowper's gland; in 1886 Elbagen presented a detailed account of cysts arising in the bulbourethral glands and found an incidence of 2.3% in autopsied males.[102]

Although Cowper described only a single pair of diaphragmatic glands, there are actually two groups of periurethral glands.[103] One pair (the diaphragmatic glands) is situated in the transverse perineal portion of the urogenital diaphragm. Their ducts are directed distally through the substance of the bulb of the corpus spongiosum entering the ventral wall of the proximal bulbous urethra. They empty through minute orifices that open on either side of the midline of the ventral surface of the deep bulb. The other pair (bulbar glands), or the accessory glands, lies deep within the spongy tissue of the bulb itself. The presence of this second pair of glands helps account for the varied anatomic presentations (perineal vs. intraurethral) of lesions of Cowper's glands. These glands are considered accessory male sex glands and are the homologue of Bartholin's glands in the female.

### Embryology

Cowper's glands are evident in the 9-week-old male fetus as a pair of solid endodermal buds from the posterior wall of the urogenital sinus at the site of the future bulbous urethra. The ducts elongate backward, paralleling the urogenital sinus, and at 11 weeks acquire lumens. They terminate within the musculature of the urogenital diaphragm (or spongiosum in the case of the accessory glands). Differentiation into the mucus-secreting acini follows and they become functional at 4 months gestation. While the function of Cowper's glands has never been fully elucidated, it is known that they empty a clear alkaline mucus into the urethra during orgasm thereby adding their secretions to the spermatic fluid. In the rat, the secretions are known to be essential for the coagulation of semen,[104] and in man it is believed they act as a urethral lubricant and vehicle for spermatozoa.[105]

## Clinical and Radiologic Features

The true incidence of lesions of Cowper's glands is unknown. Many children with lesions of Cowper's ducts or glands are asymptomatic, and either a retention cyst or reflux into a dilated duct may be seen on films of the urethra during voiding in patients with no signs or symptoms of obstruction or other voiding abnormality. In children lesions are most commonly congenital while in adults lesions may be congenital or acquired (postinflammatory) or posttraumatic). Patients who are symptomatic may present with minor voiding complaints such as frequency, urgency, or dysuria or, depending on the size and location of the cyst, may have a diminished urinary stream, hematuria, urinary infection, or even urinary retention. If the diaphragmatic glands are obstructed resulting in retention cyst formation, they may enlarge posteriorly and present as perineal masses or abscesses.

## Classification

Several attempts have been made to classify these lesions. Muschat classified Cowper's duct cysts into those lesions that protrude into the urethral lumen compressing the urethra and producing signs of obstruction, and those that undergo extraurethral enlargement that becomes apparent as a bulging perineal mass.[106] Maizels and Stephens created a system in 1983 to classify each of the various appearances of these lesions based on urethrographic and endoscopic characteristics. This system appears useful for lesions that occur in children. They refer to dilated Cowper's ducts as syringoceles (Greek: *syringo,* tube; *cele,* swelling) and divide them into four groups:

1. Simple syringocele—minimally dilated duct
2. Perforate syringocele—bulbous duct that drains into the urethra via a patulous ostium and appears as a diverticulum
3. Imperforate syringocele—bulbous duct that resembles a submucosal cyst and appears as a radiolucent mass
4. Ruptured syringocele—the fragile membrane that remains in the urethra after a dilated duct ruptures.[107]

Several cases have been reported in newborns with severe obstruction resulting in complete urinary retention, hydroureteronephrosis, and hypertrophy of the bladder presumably secondary to a retention cyst; intrauterine and perinatal deaths have been reported as well.[108,109] In adults, calcification of Cowper's gland has been reported as well as several cases of mucinous adenocarcinomas.[110,111]

The radiologic findings are generally characteristic and unequivocal on the voiding phase of a cystourethrogram. A retention cyst of obstruction of the main duct will be seen as a filling defect on the floor of the bulbous urethra; if the cyst has decompressed spontaneously or by catheterization or instrumentation, filling of a dilated duct may be seen. The duct may also fill occasionally in a patient with distal urethral obstruction or no pathology at all. A large duct can be seen also when due to reflux into a patulous ostium. Cysts are best seen on a voiding study rather than retrograde urethrograms.

At endoscopy a spherical gray or blue translucent mass on the floor of the urethral bulb is seen in the case of an obstructed main duct or retention cyst. One or more openings in the floor of the bulbous urethra and/or the floor of the cyst may be seen if drainage has already occurred.

## Treatment

Asymptomatic patients with either retention cysts or dilated duct who do not require cystoscopy for other reasons do not need therapy as long as infection, obstruction, or voiding abnormalities do not develop. Symptomatic lesions that present intraurethrally are best treated by simple endoscopic unroofing with either a Bugbee electrode or a resectoscope (Fig 12). Follow-up urethrograms should show reflux into the dilated ducts.

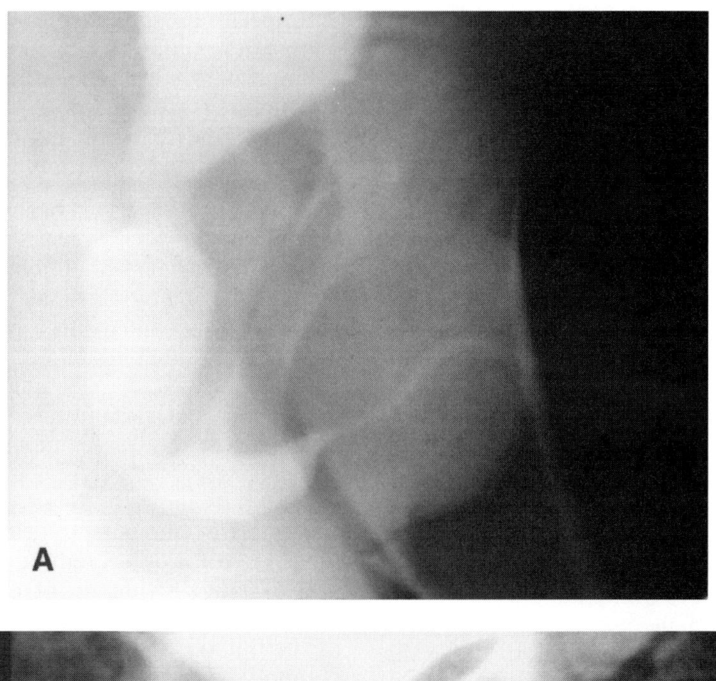


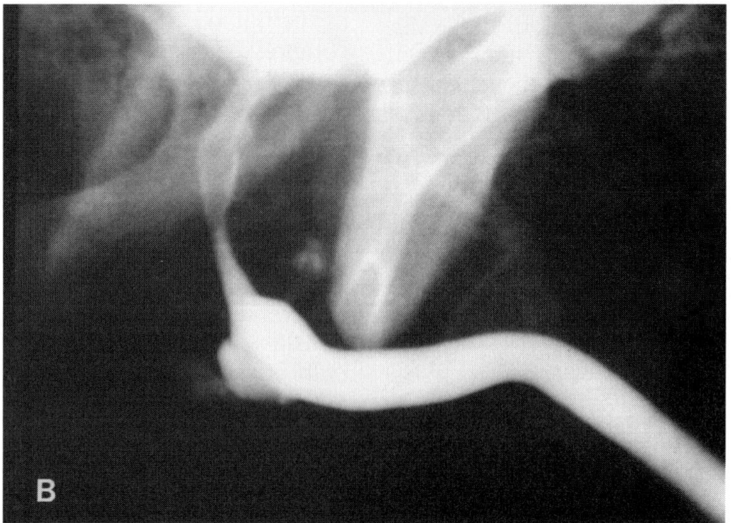


**Fig 12. A.** Voiding study demonstrating a large cyst of Cowper's duct in a 5-year-old boy. **B.** Follow-up voiding cystourethrogram in the same patient following endoscopic unroofing of Cowper's duct cyst. Note the residual reflux into the cystic remnant.

Lesions presenting perineally are often much larger and may require open surgical excision although Redman and Rountree advocate transurethral unroofing initially if the lesion can be visualized endoscopically.[112]

The most common error in diagnosis may occur if only a dilated duct is seen on endoscopy or urethrogram; this may be misinterpreted as a partial duplication of the urethra, urethral diverticulum, persistent Mullerian duct remnant, or ectopic ureter. These errors might be followed by an unnecessary operation, ie, open resection for a lesion that does not usually require surgery.

## POSTERIOR URETHRAL VALVES

The most common cause of congenital urethral obstruction in boys is posterior urethral valves. The overall prognosis for patients with posterior urethral valves has improved dramatically in recent years for several reasons. Increasing awareness of the condition by obstetricians and neonatologists has resulted in earlier referral to pediatric urologists. Equally important, improvements in diagnostic imaging techniques, particularly ultrasound, anesthesia, instrumentation, and neonatal intensive care have provided optimum management for these often very sick neonates. Despite these advances, the long-term consequences of this obstructive process, including impaired renal function and infection, remain serious problems for some patients.

### Embryology/Etiology

Posterior urethral valves are congenital lesions and are generally not felt to have a genetic basis. They are very rarely encountered in the same family although isolated cases have been reported. Valves have been reported in twins but even in identical twins often only one twin is affected.[113]

The actual etiology of posterior urethral valves remains controversial. In 1870 Tolmatschew proposed that these valves were a result of simple hypertrophy of the normally present distinct bilateral folds (plicae colliculi) that arise at the lateral side of a midline ridge located at the distal end of the verumontanum (crista urethralis).[114]

However, Stephens believes that these normal folds result from the embryologic integration of the mesonephric (Wolffian) duct with the urogenital sinus. He proposed that abnormal formation or regression of the folds or plicae, perhaps because of abnormal insertion of the Wolffian ducts into the cloaca, results in obstructive thickened folds rather than the small thin mucosal folds normally present. Further, for type III valves he felt the represented persistence of the urogenital membrane.[29]

Lowsley,[115] however, believed that the values were a result of abnormal junction of the ejaculatory (Wolffian) duct and the prostatic utricle (Mullerian duct), whereas Watson proposed that valves represent the fusion of epithelium of the seminal collicules with the roof of the urethra (posterior urethral groove).[116]

### Classification

Posterior urethral valves were first described by Hugh Hampton Young in 1919.[117] On the basis of autopsy findings he proposed three types of valves. Type I valves are described as bicuspid sails—exaggerated plicae colliculi that originate just distal to the verumontanum on either side and attach to the anterolateral walls of the urethra. Type II valves are folds that run between the verumontanum and bladder neck where they divide into fin-like membranes. Type III valves occur just distal or proximal to the verumontanum and have a diaphragmatic appearance with a small central opening (Fig 13). While this classification system is widely used, many authors feel that only two types of valves truly exist (type I and type II).[109] Most series do not report on type II valves although Lowsley and McRae have reported obstructing type II valves.[107] The embryologic precursor of type II valves remains obscure; however, most feel intuitively that these leaflets that run from the verumontanum to the bladder in a longitudinal direction seen unlikely to be able to cause obstruction to urinary flow.

Stephens has described a type IV valve in the posterior urethra that is characterized as a deep infold of the anterior and anterolateral walls that overrides the lumen of the urethra and noted rarely in conjunction with the prune belly syndrome.[29]

Further, Robertson and Hayes proposed that based on prepared autopsy studies of urethras that all valves were truly diaphragms thereby raising the question whether Type I and Type III valves are variations of the same lesion.[118] Despite this, most authors today will report on type I and type III valves as separate entities. Approximately 95% of valvular obstructions are felt to be type I, which can consist of filmy, easily disruptible membranes or,

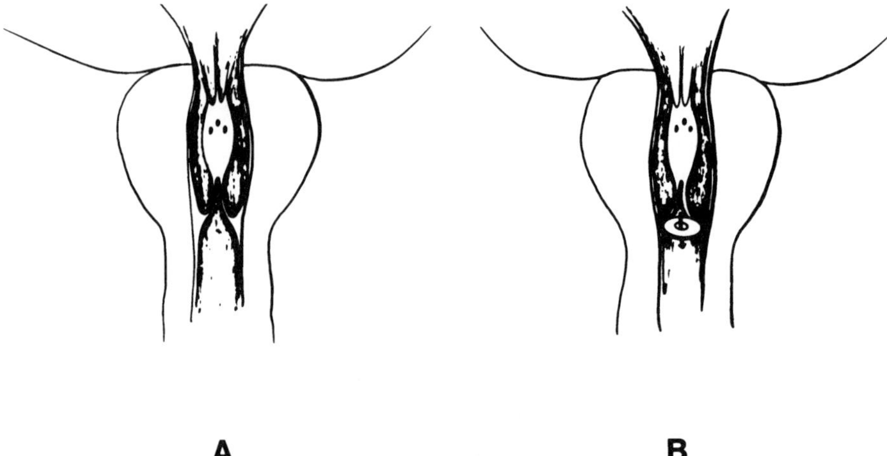


**Fig 13. A.** Graphic representation of a type I posterior urethral valve. The sail-like leaflets can be seen arising from the crista of the verumontanum to fuse at the 12 o'clock position anteriorly. **B.** Representation of a type III posterior urethral valve. The valve is diaphragmatic with a central small opening. Many authors doubt that type II valves actually exist.

in the worst case, a thickened layer of tissue with a small inferior opening. The remaining 5% of lesions are type III, being obstructing diaphragms with a central opening.

## Diagnosis

The diagnosis of congenital fetal urologic anomalies has increased dramatically in recent years due to frequent use of maternal ultrasonography. After ureteropelvic junction obstruction and primary obstructed megaureters, posterior urethral valves are the third most common urologic abnormality found on ultrasonography. The indication for the examination is often oligohydramnios since a severely obstructed bladder will make less urine than normal and, when oligohydramnios is present, more than 50% of the fetuses will have a severe urinary tract anomaly.[119] Presently, up to 80% of neonates with hydronephrosis will have had a prenatal ultrasound demonstrating hydronephrosis and 10% of these will have posterior urethral valves.[120]

Prenatal intervention to confirm the diagnosis of obstructive uropathy and to further treat the problem remains experimental and currently is only performed at a few select centers. Intrauterine contrast cystography to confirm the diagnosis has been reported, and some authors, however, feel justification for intervention is lacking for several reasons. Posterior urethral valves constitute less than 10% of anomalies in the total group with a prenatal diagnosis of urologic anomaly.[121] Only a small percentage of these will demonstrate obstructive hydronephrosis with significant oligohydramnios. The degree of oligohydramnios may be an indication of degree or obstruction in patients with moderate or severe oligohydramnios. Early intervention may be justified but very often these will be associated with severe pulmonary hypoplasia and renal dysplasia that is incompatible with life. Patients with incidentally discovered valves, ie, not on the basis of oligohydramnios, may have significantly better renal function and are perhaps best managed by prompt treatment at birth. Further, and perhaps most importantly, diagnostic errors of 30%–40% have been reported in several series and risks of injury to the mother and the fetus are not insignificant.[121] Nevertheless, urethral valves do represent a lesion that is not uncommonly lethal and intrauterine decompression does appear to be a reasonable way to limit the degree of renal damage.

### Presentation

Due to the use of ultrasound, far more cases of posterior urethral valves are diagnosed prenatally or at an earlier age than previously. Historically 40%–50% of patients with obstructive uropathy secondary to valves have presented in the first month of life with an additional 26% being diagnosed within the first year.[122] Boys with the worst degree of obstruction generally present the earliest and often will have a dribbling or weak stream or, occasionally, urinary retention. A good stream, however, does not preclude urethral obstruction by valves. The bladder of bilateral flank masses from hydronephrotic kidneys will often be palpable and occasionally patients will be acutely ill with sepsis or urinary tract infection. If the diagnosis is not made at or near birth, patients may become salt-depleted with severe acidosis due to renal failure or present with vomiting and failure to thrive. With renal failure and associated electrolyte disturbances, it is not unusual for such sick infants to be treated for respiratory distress syndrome or spontaneous pneumothorax for several days before the correct diagnosis is made. Most babies with true respiratory distress syndrome, however, are predominantly premature while babies with valves are full term and maybe have rapid respirations from the acidosis alone. Abdominal distention due to urinary ascites may also be a presenting sign and posterior urethral valves are the most common cause of urinary ascites.[123] The diagnosis can be confusing unless frank ascites is suspected since occasionally not much hydronephrosis may be detected by ultrasound or intravenous pyelogram.

The mechanism of urinary ascites in these patients is not well understood. Originally it was believed that ascites accumulated secondary to transudation through the dilated collecting system. This is now felt to be unlikely since the collecting system walls are thickened due to distal obstruction. The ascites is now felt to be leakage from the renal parenchyma or renal sinuses or rarely may be from bladder perforation.[124] The diagnosis can be made on clinical grounds and is confirmed by a plain x-ray of the abdomen that reveals the bowel "floating" in the midabdomen. It is felt by some that because some urine production continues despite obstruction, the immaturity of the renal lymphatics in a neonate, which in an adult would normally absorb this urine, could account for leaking of urine from the thinnest portion of the collecting system.[125] This remains unproven, however. In any case, a frank rupture of the collecting system generally cannot be demonstrated and it appears that the ascitic fluid reaches the abdominal cavity through the fornices and posterior parietal peritoneum. Adequate bladder decompression will prevent reflux and further ascites, but occasionally abdominal distention will be severe enough to compromise respiration and paracentesis must be performed. Although some advocate proximal diversion in patients with ascites, this is rarely necessary. Many consider extravasation of urine from the kidney to be a "popoff valve" type of phenomenon that allows for preservation of renal function much more than one would expect from the severity of the obstruction.[126]

Older infants and children present less acutely; they generally do not have ascites or flank masses. They often will have urinary tract infection, diurnal enuresis, or mild voiding abnormality. Very often they will have little if any hydronephrosis, no reflux, and good renal function, adding support to the dictum that valves have a spectrum of severity with the least severe presenting at an older age. Urethral valves may also present as hematuria in older boys, who may bleed from a hypertrophied bladder. Straining to void resulting in rectal prolapse or hernias may be found as well.

### Imaging

In the neonate, renal sonography will generally demonstrate bilateral hydronephrosis and a variable amount of renal dysplasia. This is manifested as increased echogenicity of the kidneys as well as renal cysts. The ureters are usually dilated and the bladder wall is usually thick. Posterior urethral dilatation can also be demon-

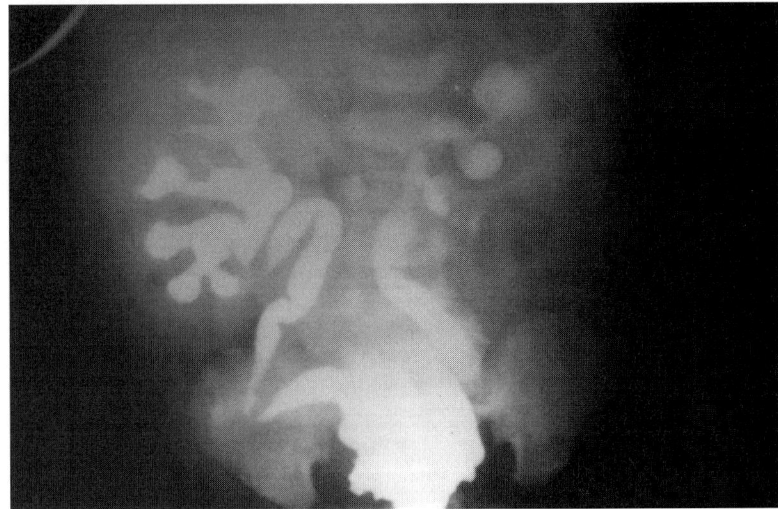

**Fig 14.** Voiding cystourethrogram in a patient with posterior urethral valves demonstrating significant bilateral hydroureteronephrosis with marked ureteral tortuosity and bladder trabeculation.

strated by ultrasound. The definite diagnosis is made by voiding cystourethrogram. This will demonstrate the characteristic features of posterior urethral obstruction, including an elongated, dilated urethra proximal to the valve and a trabeculated bladder with hypertrophy of the interureteric ridge and bladder neck (Fig 14). The valve itself may also be visualized (Fig 15). Cellules and occasionally frank

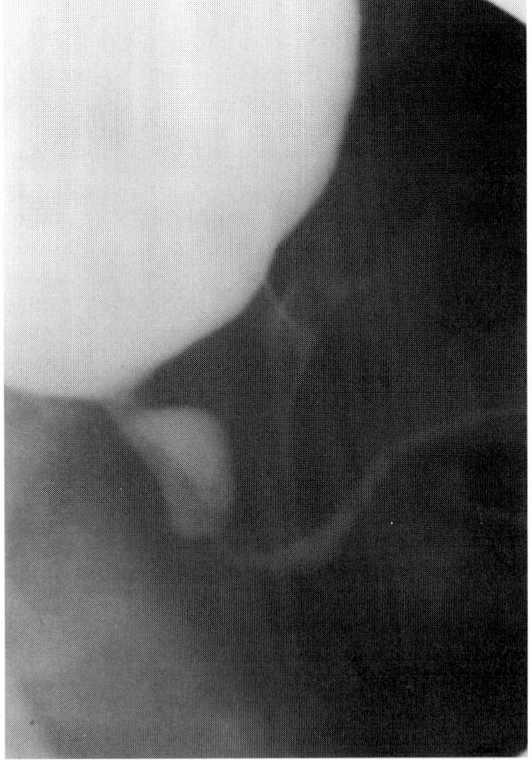

**Fig 15.** Voiding study revealing marked dilatation of the posterior urethra. Note that a valve leaflet is identifiable just distal to area of dilatation.

diverticula are often encountered. The bladder capacity may actually be significantly decreased and reflux into the genital ducts may be present. Vesicoureteral reflux may be unilateral or bilateral, and occurs in approximately 50% of cases at presentation.[127] An intravenous pyelogram should be performed with a catheter in the bladder if reflux is present to prevent the reflux from mimicking renal function. This may reveal poor function in addition to dilated collecting systems but a nuclear scan may give more definitive evidence of the presence or absence of renal function.

Older patients who present with mild voiding symptoms and who have so-called nonobstructing valves may have only a circumferential filling defect without a significant dilatation above the point of obstruction. Bladder abnormalities such as trabeculation are seldom noted but urodynamic evaluation may demonstrate elevated voiding pressures that have been reported to normalize after elimination of these small valves. Endoscopy is rarely needed in the neonate to confirm the diagnosis of valves but in the older child with equivocal findings on voiding cystourethrogram it is sometimes required to substantiate doubtful cases.

## Management

Initial treatment in neonates with posterior urethral valves should be based on the overall condition of the patient. In older patients without infections and with overall good health and renal function, effective treatment may require simple resection of the valves. A postoperative voiding cystourethrogram is essential to demonstrate that the valve leaflets have been adequately resected.

On the other hand, many neonates present with significant acidosis, hyperkalemia, azotemia, as well as sepsis. Resuscitation should be prompt and aggressive, and often effective bladder drainage with a small feeding tube (5 or 8 Fr) transurethrally may dramatically reverse the clinical course. A suprapubic catheter may also be used and may prevent any of the long-term sequelae of an indwelling urethral catheter. In addition, percutaneous nephrostomies as initial management to obtain maximal drainage in patients with urosepsis and impaired renal function have been used by some, although most often this is not necessary.[128,129]

A postoperative diuresis may occur with considerable salt and water loss after adequate drainage is established. Therefore, continued close management of electrolytes and other parameters is necessary. After stabilization of the neonate and correction of electrolyte imbalance, the valves should be surgically resected regardless of the degree of upper tract dilatation. Improved optics and smaller pediatric endoscopic equipment have allowed endoscopic valve ablation in the vast majority of patients. Usually an 8 Fr or 10 Fr endoscope will pass easily and care should be taken to avoid excessive dilatation of the anterior urethra in order to prevent later stricture formation. After clearly defining the external sphincter, the type I valve leaflets can be seen arising from the crista urethralis extending out laterally to fuse at the 12 o'clock position. Care is taken to avoid injury to the urethra or external sphincter when ablating the valves and although strictures have been reported by some authors, most feel this is not a significant problem. Some feel that inadequate ablation may occur up to 20%–30% of the time if destruction of the valve cusps is undertaken at the 5 and 7 o'clock positions rather than the 12 o'clock position.[130,131]

The infant resectoscope loop or cauterizing hook may also be used instead of the Bugbee electrode, but this may result in a higher incidence of stricture formation.[132] Success with the Nd:YAG laser has also been reported.[133] Prior to the development of smaller endoscopic equipment, perineal urethrotomy was used for access to the posterior urethra but this is seldom necessary today.

Type III valves can occasionally be definitively treated and ablated by dilatation with LeFort sounds (up to 10 Fr) but most agree that these should be fulgurated or incised at three points circumferentially.[134]

For the rare neonate whose urethra will

not accept a pediatric cystoscope or if such equipment is not available, cutaneous vesicostomy is an alternative. Further, the use of a Fogarty balloon catheter to rupture the valve has been reported in similar situations.[135] The use of the flexible or rigid endoscope in a percutaneous antegrade fashion has also been reported.[136]

After valve ablation or vesicostomy, the infant should be watched closely for infection and electrolyte abnormalities. If the child does not improve clinically within the first week or two, further assessment should be done with follow-up ultrasound and renography.

Patients with primary valve ablation may require cutaneous vesicostomy if upper tract drainage is inadequate. Patients with inadequate drainage with vesicostomy may further require high cutaneous ureterostomies or pyelostomies to ensure maximal renal recoverability. If ureterostomies are required, most clinicians advocate a simultaneous renal biopsy but many caution against the use of ureterostomies due to the high incidence of complications and difficulty encountered with eventual reconstruction.[127,137] These patients may do worse in terms of eventual renal function as well.[138]

Following relief of obstruction, bladder function will return to normal in many patients with decreased voiding pressures and regression of detrusor hypertrophy. Vesicoureteral reflux may improve or even disappear in up to 25% of patients with reflux. The urethra will be found to normalize almost immediately after ablation of valves and the hypertrophy and trabeculation of the bladder generally takes longer. The dilation and tortuosity of the ureters are slower to normalize. In patients where reimplantation eventually becomes necessary, surgery is technically much easier if the bladder hypertrophy and trabeculation is allowed to improve (over a year or two) and often tapering of the ureter will not need to be done with significant improvement in ureteral dilatation. In addition, in patients with cutaneous ureterostomies, urinary continuity should be reestablished prior to reimplantation since reimplantation into a dry bladder has been shown to have a high failure rate.

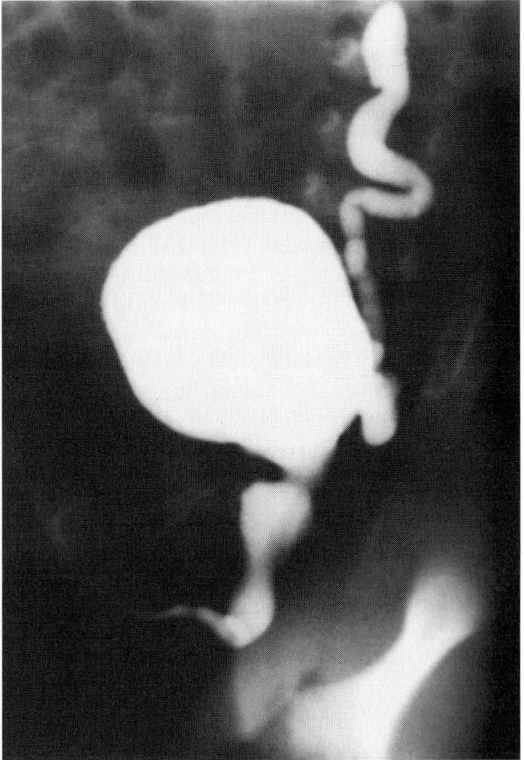

**Fig 16.** Voiding cystourethrogram in a patient with posterior urethral valves revealing the findings of the VURD syndrome (vesicoureteral reflux, renal dysplasia). Note the unilateral reflux to a dysplastic kidney which has acted as a "popoff" valve, thereby sparing the contralateral renal unit from the effects of severe reflux.

A small group of children with reflux have been found to have the VURD syndrome (vesicoureteral reflux, renal dysplasia). This is characterized by valves and unilateral reflux to a nonfunctioning kidney (Fig 16). This can act as a large, poorly functioning diverticulum and removal of this unit as a source of infection will also improve voiding dynamics.

## Full Valve Bladder Syndrome

Some children (25%) who were treated adequately at early ages will be found later to have persistent upper tract dilation without genuine obstruction by diuretic renography. This may result from elevated intravesical pressure even at low bladder volumes and this lack of bladder compliance may lead to a functional obstruction at the level of the ureterovesical junction. Voiding dysfunction may also be present and urodynamic evaluation usually reveals four abnormal patterns:

1. Absent bladder contractions
2. High filling and voiding pressures due to decreased bladder compliance
3. Persistent secondary bladder neck hypertrophy, and/or
4. Uninhibited detrusor contractions.[56]

It is necessary to rule out true ureterovesical junction obstruction or persistent urethral obstruction secondary to incompletely ablated valves or urethral stricture. The management of these patients can be difficult and some authors have demonstrated varying degrees of improvement with timed voiding (every 4 hr), clean intermittent catheterization, anticholinergic medication, or bladder augmentation.[139,141]

Urinary incontinence has also been a problem in some children. Many of these children were previously treated with bladder neck resection or Y-V plasty, but it is now known that the muscular hypertrophy at the bladder neck is related to the more inferior valvular obstruction and overall detrusor thickening. Stress incontinence may be due to the inability of the sphincter to coapt secondary to significant posterior urethral dilatation, which may actually improve with time. Most authors feel, however, that incontinence in these patients is due to bladder instability, polyuria secondary to a concentrating defect, or inadequate attempts to empty the bladder completely.[127,142] Generally, spontaneous overall improvement of incontinence occurs at puberty and this may be due to prostatic growth.[134]

## Prognosis

Many follow-up studies of these patients have attempted to determine outcome and prognostic features of these patients. Factors such as early presentation, presence of bilateral vesicoureteral reflux, and development of proteinuria were found to portend chronic renal failure in the Great Ormand Street study.[122] Later studies did not validate these findings, but Warshaw determined that children who had nadir neonatal creatinine values of 0.8 mg/dL or less at initial hospitalization maintained creatinine levels of 1.1 or less, while infants with higher levels developed chronic renal failure.[143] Similarly, measurement of glomerular filtration rate has been used and values of less than 50% of normal for age at diagnosis seems to forecast persistent chronic renal failure.[144] Renal transplantation has been performed for these patients although graft survival (50% at 5 years) appears to be worse than in other recipients. This may be secondary to altered bladder dynamics that may influence renal function in the transplanted kidney.[145]

Overall erectile potential in valve patients appears to be good, although fertility has been reported to be compromised because some may have a dribbling or absent ejaculate. Overall, semen quality is not good (high viscosity and pH) but sperm counts have been reported as normal.[146]

## REFERENCES

1. Allen JS, Summers JL. Meatal stenosis in children. *J Urol.* 1974;112:526.
2. Morton, HG. Meatus size in 1,000 circumcized children from two weeks to sixteen years of age. *J Fla Med Assoc.* 1963;50:137.
3. Litvak AS, Morris JD, McRoberts JW. Normal size of the urethral meatus in male children. *J Urol.* 1976;115:736.
4. Gray SW, Skandalakis JE. *Embryology for Surgeons.* Philadelphia: WB Saunders; 1972.
5. Noe HN, Dale GA. Evaluation of children with meatal stenosis. *J Urol.* 1975;114:455.
6. Owens SB, Morse WH. Prolapse of the female urethra in children. *J Urol.* 1968;100:171.
7. Klaus H, Stein RT. Urethral prolapse in young girls. *Pediatrics.* 1973;52:645.
8. Colodny AH. Disorders of the female genitalia. In: Kelalis P, King LR, Belman AB, eds. *Clinical Pediatric Urology,* 2nd ed. Philadelphia: WB Saunders; 1985.
9. King LR. Abnormalities of the urethra. In: Ravitch MM, et al., eds. *Pediatric Surgery,* 3rd ed. Chicago: Year Book; 1979.

10. Jerkins GR, Verheeck K, Noe HN. Treatment of girls with urethral prolapse. *J Urol.* 1984; 132:732.
11. Lowe FC, Hill GS, Jeffs RD, et al. Urethral prolapse in children: insights into etiology and management. *J Urol.* 1986;135:100.
12. Zeigerman JH. Prolapse of the female urethra in children. *J Urol.* 1968;100:171.
13. Epsteen A, Strauss B. Prolapse of the female urethra with gangrene. *Am J Surg.* 1937;35:563.
14. Mayers MM. A clinical consideration of the female urethra. *Urol Cutan Rev.* 1938;42:783.
15. Peters WA. Prolapse of the urethral mucosa. *Am J Obstet Gynecol.* 1962;84:862.
16. Parkes JR. Prolapse of the urethra in young Zulu girls. *S Afr Med J.* 1975;49:2011.
17. Livermore GR. The treatment of prolapse of the urethra. *Surg Gynecol Obstet.* 1931;32:99.
18. Owens SB, Morse WH. Prolapse of the female urethra in children. *J Urol.* 1968;100:171.
19. Devine PC, Kessel HC. Surgical correction of urethral prolapse. *J Urol.* 1980;123:856.
20. Redman JF. Conservative management of urethral prolapse in female children. *Urology.* 1982;19:505.
21. Richardson DA, Hajj SN, Herbst AL. Medical treatment of urethral prolapse in children. *Obstet Gynecol.* 1982;59:69.
22. Turner RW. Urethral prolapse in female children. *Urology.* 1973;2:530.
23. Ormond JK. Prolapse of the female urethra. *Am J Obstet Gynecol.* 1934;28:458.
24. Venable DD, Markland C. Urethral prolapse in girls. *S Med J.* 1982;75:951.
25. Esposito JM. Circular prolapse of the urethra in children: a cause of vaginal bleeding. *Obstet Gynecol.* 1968;31:363.
26. Hepburn TN. Prolapse of the female urethra. *Surg Gynecol Obstet.* 1920;31:83.
27. Nesbitt TE. Congenital megalourethra. *J Urol.* 1959;73:839.
28. Dorairajan T. Defects in spongy tissue and congenital diverticula of the penile urethra. *Aust N. Z. J. Surg.* 1963;32:209.
29. Stephens FD. *Congenital Malformations of the Rectum, Anus and Genitourinary Tract.* London: E. & S. Livingston Co; 1963.
30. Kester RR, Mooppan UMM, Ohm HK, et al. Congenital megalourethra. *J Urol.* 1990;143: 1213.
31. Appel RA, Kaplan GW, Brock WA. Megalourethra. *J Urol.* 1986;135:747.
32. Shrom SH, Cromie WJ, Duckett JW. Megalourethra. *Urology.* 1981;17:152.
33. Krueger RP, Churchill BM. Megalourethra with posterior urethral valves. *Urology.* 1981;18: 279.
34. Locke JR, Noe HN. Megalourethra: Surgical technique for correction of an unusual variant. *J Urol.* 1987;138:110.
35. Araki T, Ohmori H, Ohaski Y, et al. Surgical treatment of impotence caused by megalourethra. *Urology.* 1984;24:246.
36. Wilson JA, Walker RD. Megalourethra and hypospadias. *J Urol.* 1983;129:556.
37. Kelalis PP, King LR, Belman AB, eds. *Clinical Pediatric Urology.* Philadelphia: WB Saunders; 1976.
38. Burstein JD, Firlit CF. Obstructive uropathy (anterior urethra). In: Kelalis PP, King LR, Belman AB, eds. *Clinical Pediatric Urology,* 2nd ed. Philadelphia: WB Saunders; 1985:574.
39. Chehval MJ, Mehan DJ. Congenital megalourethra: report of a unique case. *J Urol.* 1980;123: 433.
40. Firlit CF. Urethral abnormalities. *Urol Clin North Am.* 1978;5(1):38.
41. Scherz HC, Kaplan GW, Packer MG. Anterior urethral valves in the fossa navicularis in children. *J Urol.* 1987;138:1211.
42. Golimbu M, Orca M, Al-Askari S, et al. Anterior urethral valves. *Urology.* 1978;12:343.
43. Firlit CF, King LR. Anterior urethral valves in children. *J Urol.* 1972;108:972.
44. Kaufman D. *Dtsch Chir.* 1886;8:123.
45. Voillemier LD. *Traite des maladies des voies urinares.* Paris: Masson; 1868.
46. Depaoli. Gaz med Ital Torino. *Obstr Zbl Chir.* 1885;12:905.
47. Boissonnat P, Duhamel B. Congenital diverticulum of the anterior urethra associated with aplasia of the abdominal muscles in a male infant. *Br J Urol.* 1962;34:59.
48. Tank ES. Anterior urethral valves resulting from congenital urethral diverticula. *Urology.* 1987;30:467.
49. Rushton HG, Parrot TS, Woodard JR, et al. The role of vesicostomy in the management of anterior urethral valves in neonates and infants. *J Urol.* 1987;138:107.
50. Das S, Brosman SA. Duplication of the male urethra. *J Urol.* 1977;117:452.
51. Effman EL, Lebowitz RL, Colodny AH. Duplication of the urethra. *Radiology.* 1976;119: 179.
52. Lowsley OS. Accessory urethra: a report of 2 cases with review of literature. *State J Med.* 1939;39:1022.
53. Johnson FP. The later development of the urethra in the male. *J Urol.* 1920;4:447.
54. De Vries PA, Friedland GW. Congenital ''H-type'' anourethral fistula. *Radiology.* 1974;113: 397.
55. Lorenzo RL, Turner WR, Bradford BF, et al. Duplication of the male urethra with posterior urethral valves. *Pediatr Radiol.* 1981;11:39.
56. Colodny AH. Urethral lesions in infants and children. In: Gillenwater JY, Grayhack JT, et al., eds. *Adult and Pediatric Urology,* 2nd ed. St. Louis: Mosby Year Book; 1991.

57. Muecke EC, Currino G. Congenital widening of the pubic symphysis. *AJR.* 1968;103:179.
58. Bramwit DN, Ziter FM. Accessory urethral channel. *Radiology.* 1970;94:359.
59. Weiss G, Becker JA, Berdon WE. Epispadias. *Radiology.* 1968;90:85.
60. O'Heeron MK, Webster FA. Report of two cases of double urethra in the male. *J Urol.* 1946;55:391.
61. Fellows GJ, Johnston JH. Incomplete urethral duplication and urinary retention. *Br J Urol.* 1974;46:449.
62. Gross RE, Moore TC. Duplication of the urethra. *Arch Surg.* 1950;60:749.
63. Naparstek S, Abrams HJ, Sutton AR, et al. Complete duplication of the male urethra in children. *Urology.* 1980;16:391.
64. Schmidt JD. Congenital urethral duplication. *J Urol.* 1971;105:397.
65. Belman AB. The repair of congenital H-type urethrorectal fistula using a scrotal flap urethroplasty. *J Urol.* 1979;118:659.
66. Kaplan GW, Brock WA. Urethral strictures in children. *J Urol.* 1983;129:1200.
67. Gibbons MD, Koontz WW, Smith MJV. Urethral strictures in boys. *J Urol.* 1979;121:217.
68. Harshman MW, Cromie WJ, Wein AJ, et al. Urethral stricture disease in children. *J Urol.* 1981;126:650.
69. Scherz HC, Kaplan GW. Etiology, diagnosis and management of urethral strictures in children. *Urol Clin N Am.* 1990;17(2):389.
70. Williams DI, Mikhael RB. Urethritis in male children. *Proc Soc Med.* 1971;64:133.
71. Currarino G, Stephens FD. An uncommon type of bulbar urethral stricture, sometimes familial, of unknown cause: congenital versus acquired. *J Urol.* 1981;126:658.
72. Cobb BG, Wolf JA, Ansell JS. Congenital stricture of the proximal urethral bulb. *J Urol.* 1968; 99:629.
73. Devereux MH, Williams DI. The treatment of urethral strictures in boys. *J Urol.* 1972;108: 489.
74. Duckett JW Jr, Snow BW. Disorders of the urethra and penis. In: Harrison JH, Gittes RF, Perlmutter AD, eds. *Campbell's Urology,* 5th ed. Philadelphia: WB Saunders; 1979.
75. Leadbetter GW Jr, Leadbetter WF. Urethral strictures in male children. *J Urol.* 1973;110: 599.
76. Redman IF, Fraiser LP. Apparent congenital anterior urethral strictures in brothers. *J Urol.* 1979;122:707.
77. English PJ, Pryor JP. Congenital bulbar urethral stricture occurring in a father and son. *Br J Urol.* 1986;58:732.
78. Devereux MH, Burfield GD. Prolonged follow-up of urethral strictures treated by intermittent dilation. *Br J Urol.* 1970;42:321.
79. Blandy JP, Wadhwa S, et al. Urethroplasty in context. *Br J Urol.* 1976;48:697.
80. Noe HN. Endoscopic management of urethral strictures in children. *J Urol.* 1981;125:712.
81. Hebert PW. The treatment of urethral strictures: transurethral injection of trancuolone. *J Urol.* 1972;108:745.
82. Myers RP, DeWeerd JH. Incidence of stricture following primary realignment of the disrupted proximal urethra. *J Urol.* 1972;107:265.
83. Waterhouse K. The surgical repair of membranous urethral strictures in children. *J Urol.* 1976;116:363.
84. Morehouse DD, MacKinnon KJ. Management of prostate membranous urethral disruption: 13-year experience. *J Urol.* 1980;123:173.
85. Gibson GR. Urologic management and complications of fractured pelvis and ruptured urethra. *J Urol.* 1974;111:353.
86. Chambers HL, Balfour J. The incidence of impotence following pelvic fracture with associated urinary tract injury. *J Urol.* 1963;89: 702.
87. Jackson DH, Williams JL. Urethral injury: a retrospective study. *Br J Urol.* 1974;46:665.
88. Waterhouse K, Gross M. Trauma to the genitourinary tract: a five-year experience with 251 cases. *J Urol.* 1969;101:241.
89. Malek RS, O'Dea MJ, Kelalis PP. Management of ruptured posterior urethra in childhood. *J Urol.* 1977;117:105.
90. Bland JP, Singh M, et al. The results and complications of scrotal flap urethroplasty for stricture. *Br J Urol.* 1971;43:52.
91. Williams DI, Abbassian A. Solitary pedunculated polyp of the posterior urethra in children. *J Urol.* 1966;96:483.
92. Kearney GP, Lebowitz RL, Retik AB. Obstructing polyps of the posterior urethra in boys. *J Urol.* 1979;122:802.
93. Redman JF, Robinson CM. Anterior urethral polyp in a child. *J Pediatr Surg.* 1977; 12:735.
94. Foster RS, Weigel JW, Mantz FA. Anterior urethral polyps. *J Urol.* 1980;124:145.
95. Falkowski WS, Cook A. Anterior urethral polyps: an unusual cause of hematuria in a child. *J Urol.* 1981;125:744.
96. Downs RA. Congenital polyps of the prostatic urethra: a review of the literature and report of two cases. *Br J Urol.* 1970;42:76.
97. Barrie HJ, Simms DC. Hydronephrosis resulting from obstruction of the urethra by a polyp of the verumontanum. *Am J Clin Pathol.* 1961; 36:356.
98. Aragona F, DiTonno F, Tuccitto G, et al. Congenital polyp of the prostatic urethra. *Urol Int.* 1988;43:113.
99. Zulian RA, Brito RR, Borges HJ. Transurethral resection of pedunculated congenital polyps of the posterior urethra. *Br J Urol.* 1982;54:45.

100. Frates R, DeLuca FG. Urethral polyps in male children. *Radiology.* 1967;89:289.
101. Firestone A. The neglected bulbo-urethral glands of Cowper. *Urol Cutan Rev.* 1937;41: 590.
102. Lowsley OS, Kirwin TJ. *Clinical Urology,* 2nd ed. Baltimore: Williams and Wilkins; 1944.
103. Moskowitz PS, Newton NA, Lebowitz RL. Retention cysts of Cowper's duct. *Radiology.* 1976;120:377.
104. Hart RG, Greenstein JS. A newly discovered role for Cowper's gland secretion in rodent semen coagulation. *J Reprod Fertil.* 1968;17:87.
105. Currarino G, Fugua F. Cowper's glands in the urethrogram. *AJR.* 1972;116:838.
106. Muschat M. Urethral and perineal cysts of the glands of Cowper. *J Urol.* 1929;22:239.
107. Maizels M, Stephens FD, King LR, et al. Cowper's syringocele: a classification of dilatations of Cowper's gland duct based upon clinical characteristics of 8 boys. *J Urol.* 1983;129:111.
108. Howell C, Lisansky ET, Scott E. Congenital cyst of the urethra in a three-week-old male infant causing pyelonephrosis and death. *Bull Univ Maryland.* 1942;26:241.
109. Abrams HJ, Joshi DP, Neier CR. Intrauterine urinary retention and electrolyte balance secondary to Cowper's gland cyst. *J Urol.* 1966; 95:565.
110. Bourque J-L, Charghi A, Gauthier G-E, et al. Primary carcinoma of Cowper's gland. *J Urol.* 1970;103:758.
111. Carpenter AA, Bernado JR. Adenoid cystic carcinoma of Cowper's gland. *J Urol.* 1971;106: 701.
112. Redman JF, Rountree GA. Pronounced dilatations of Cowper's gland duct manifest as a perineal mass: a recommendation for management. *J Urol.* 1988;139:87.
113. Gonzales ET Jr. Valves in twins, presented at annual meeting, American Academy of Pediatrics, 1983.
114. Tolmatschew Von N. Ein fall von semi lunaren klappen der harniohre and von vergrosserter vesicula prostatica. *Virchows Arch (Path).* 1870;49:348.
115. Lowsley OS. Congenital malformation of the posterior urethra. *Am Surg.* 1914;60:733.
116. Watson EM. The structural basis for congenital valve formation in the posterior urethra. *J Urol.* 1922;7:371.
117. Young HH, Frontz WA, Baldwin JC. Congenital obstruction of the posterior urethra. *J Urol.* 1919;3:289.
118. Robertson WB, Hayes JA. Congenital diaphragmatic obstruction of the male posterior urethra. *Br J Urol.* 1969;41:592.
119. Sivit CJ, Hill MC, Larsen JW, et al. The sonographic 30 weeks gestation. *AJR.* 1986;146: 1277.
120. Brown T, Mandell J, Lebowitz RL. Neonatal hydronephrosis in the era of sonography. *AJR.* 1987;148:959.
121. Turnock RR, Shawis R. Management of fetal urinary tract anomalies detected by prenatal ultrasonography. *Arch Dis Child.* 1984; 59:962.
122. Frank JD. Congenital disorders of the urethra. In: *Textbook for Genitourinary Surgery,* Whitfield HN, Hendry WF, eds. London: Churchill Livingstone; 1985.
123. Mitchell ME, Garrett RA. Perirenal urinary extravasation associated with urethral valves in infants. *J Urol.* 1980;124:688.
124. Trulock TS, Finnerty DP, Woodard JR. Neonatal bladder rupture. *J Urol.* 1985;133:271.
125. King LR. Posterior urethra. In: Kelalis RR, King LR, Belman AB, eds. *Clinical Pediatric Urology,* 2nd ed. Philadelphia: WB Saunders; 1985.
126. Rittenberg MH, Hulbert WC, Snyder HM III, Duckett JW. Protective factors in posterior urethral valves. *J Urol.* 1988;140:993.
127. Hulbert WC, Duckett JW. Current views on posterior urethral valves. *Ped Am.* 1988;17:1.
128. Williams DI, Cramie WJ. Ring ureterostomy. *Br J Urol.* 1975;47:789.
129. Churchill BM, Krueger RP, Hardy BE, et al. Complications of posterior urethral valve surgery and their prevention. *Urol Clin North Am.* 1983;10:519.
130. Cass AA, Stephens FD. Posterior urethral valves, diagnosis and management. *J Urol.* 1974;112:519.
131. Perlmutter AD. Temporary urinary diversion in the management of the clinically dilated urinary tract in children. In: *Reviews in Pediatric Urology,* p. 447.
132. Noe HN. Complications and management of childhood urethral stricture disease. *Urol Clin North Am.* 1983;10:531.
133. Ehrlich RM, Shanberg A, Fine RN. Neodymium: YAG laser ablation of posterior urethral valves. *J Urol.* 1987;138:959.
134. King LR. Obstructive uropathy (posterior urethra). In: Kelalis PP, King LR, Belman AB, eds. *Clinical Pediatric Urology,* 2nd ed. Philadelphia: WB Saunders; 1985.
135. Diamond DA, Ransley PG. Fogarty balloon catheter ablation of neonatal posterior urethral valves. *J Urol.* 1987;137:1209.
136. Zaontz MR, Gibbons MD. An antegrade technique for ablation of posterior urethral valves. *J Urol.* 1984;132:982.
137. Lane LY, Howat JM, Williams DI. The temporarily defunctionalized bladder in children. *J Urol.* 1972;108:469.
138. Parkhouse HF, Barratt TM, Dillon MJ, et al. Longterm outcome of boys with posterior urethral valves. *Br J Urol.* 1988;62:59.

139. Glassberg KI. Current issues regarding posterior urethral valves. *Urol Clin North Am.* 1985; 12:175.

140. McGuire EJ, Weiss RM. Secondary bladder neck obstruction in patients with urethral valves: treatment with phenoxybenzamine. *Urology.* 1975;5:756.

141. Mitchell ME. Persistent ureteral dilatation following valve resection. *Dialogues Pediatr Urol.* 1982;5:8.

142. Bauer SB, Dieppa RA, Labib KK, et al. The bladder in boys with posterior urethral valves: a urodynamic assessment. *J Urol.* 1979;121: 769.

143. Warshaw BL, Hymes LC, Woodard JR, et al. Prognostic features in infants with obstructive uropathy due to posterior urethral valves. *J Urol.* 1985;133:240.

144. Scott JE. Management of congenital posterior urethral valves. *Br J Urol.* 1985;57:71.

145. Reinberg Y, Gonzalez R, Fryd D, et al. The outcome of renal transplantation in children with posterior urethral valves. *J Urol.* 1988; 140:1491.

146. Woodhouse CRJ, Reilly JM, Bahadur G. Sexual function and fertility in patients treated for posterior urethral valves. *J Urol.* 1989;142:586.

# 51

# Current Concepts in the Management of Hypospadias

*Michael A. Keating and Anthony A. Caldamone*

## INTRODUCTION

Hypospadias remains one of the most challenging problems in the field of urology. Its incidence, which has been estimated at 1 in 300 live births,[1] assures every urologist of seeing a number of different anomalies during training and after entering clinical practice. Nearly 300 urethroplasties and their modifications have been described for its correction. This large number underscores a general dissatisfaction with many earlier repairs. However, each bears testimony to the surgical ingenuity of our predecessors, and, regardless of its success, contributes in some small way to the evolution of the art and science of modern *hypospadiology*. The cosmetic results of urethroplasty appear to be constantly improving and complications are reportedly on the decline. Nevertheless, recent additions to the literature serve as a constant reminder that the hypospadiologist's ultimate goal, to devise a procedure yielding maximal correction with minimal morbidity, is still being sought and may never be achieved. Other than technical shortcomings, the failures of our surgical solutions stem largely from the nature of the anomaly being addressed.

Like many other problems in urology, hypospadias should be regarded as a spectrum. Every variant presents its own peculiar anatomic nuances, each requiring a different technical response. Successful urethroplasties are obviously influenced by experience and ability but technique selection is probably the factor most crucial to maximizing surgical results. What has been increasingly borne out with time is that *no single method of urethroplasty is applicable to every hypospadias seen*. The hypospadiologist must be able to draw on a variety of treatment options in order to meet these different challenges once in the surgical suite. Maximizing the outcome of the repair and being able to offer surgical flexibility are contingent on having a thorough understanding of the problem.

## EMBRYOGENESIS

### Normal Development

Formation of the primordial genitalia becomes evident by the end of the first month of gestation. Testosterone production from the fetal testes is initiated and continues through the first trimester under the influence of chorionic gonadotropin. The androgen, converted to its active form in the developing external genitalia by 5α-reductase, causes the genital tubercle to take shape in the midline above the anterior margins of the cloacal membrane, which is destined to become the urogenital mem-

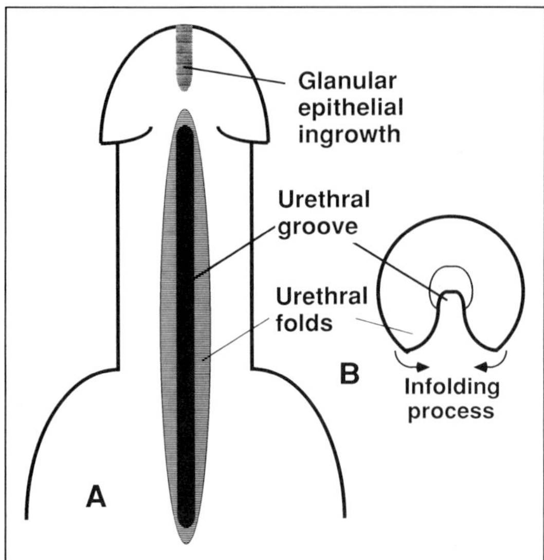


**Fig 1.** Normal urethral development. **A,** infolding process is responsible for urethral development to the level of the corona where distal epithelial ingrowth is met; **B,** cross-section of penis depicts infolding process.

brane. The tubercle is flanked on either side by two genital swellings that eventually migrate inferiorly and meet to become the scrotum. Further elongation of the tubercle induces the appearance of a longitudinal groove, the so-called urethral gutter, on its ventral surface. Continuity with the proximal urogenital sinus and future bladder are established after breakdown of the urogenital membrane. Genital folds, which emanate from either side of the gutter, ultimately fuse in the midline above the trough to create an isolated tubular urethra (Fig 1).

The infolding process is, in theory, responsible for creating the bulbar-pendulous urethra from the urogenital sinus, which has evolved from the cloaca, to the level of the coronal sulcus. Distally, the glanular urethra is excavated by an epithelial ingrowth that projects proximally to meet the newly developed penile urethra at the coronal sulcus. Synchronous midline fusion of the labial-scrotal folds creates the median raphe, extending that structure from the perineum to the corona. The penis is fully developed by the end of the first trimester and continues to grow through the remainder of gestation under the influence of testosterone, now driven by the fetal pituitary-gonadotropin axis. Further penile development is marked by differentiation of the spongiosum and the adjacent corpora in the early second trimester. Preputial development commences during the late first trimester and is contingent on prior formation of a normal penis and urethra in most cases. Beginning as a cuff of tissue that circumferentially extends from the margins of the sulcus, continued growth sees the prepuce gradually envelope and fuse to the glans penis.

### Dysgenesis

The stigmata of hypospadias (described below) are presumably brought about by errors affecting glanular epithelial ingrowth (yielding distal variants) or arresting the infolding process (resulting in more proximal variants). The union of these two at the sulcus, which represents the last step in urethral development, would account for the increased incidence of variants found at this position. A variety of different etiologies have been proposed for the chordee found with hypospadias including foreshortening by the anlage of the affected corpus spongiosum, tethering by the rudimentary urethral plate, and an abnormal growth differential between the dorsal and ventral penis.[2,3] Urethra maldevelopment also affects the ventral formation of the prepuce. One exception in this regard are the megameatus intact prepuce (MIP) variants. These unusual hypospadias are accompanied by a glans with an exaggerated cleft, widened distal urethra, and a complete foreskin. Chordee is not present. A defect that spares the prepuce yet injures the corpus spongiosum has been postulated.[4]

## ETIOLOGY

The source of the error(s) in embryogenesis that affect the developing tubercle cannot usually be defined. Hypospadias occurs in association with a number of syndromes that are summarized in Table 1. Other than these, deficiencies in the hor-

**TABLE 1. Syndromes and Congenital Anomalies Associated with Hypospadias**

| |
|---|
| **Frequent Associations** |
| Aniridia–Wilms' tumor association |
| Cryptophthalmos syndrome |
| Laurence–Moon–Biedl syndrome |
| Opitz's syndrome |
| Smith–Lemli–Opitz syndrome |
| 4p syndrome |
| 13q syndrome |
| Robinow's syndrome |
| **Common Associations** |
| Aarskog's syndrome |
| Beckwith-Wiedemann syndrome |
| Fanconi's pancytopenia |
| Fetal hydantoin effects |
| Russell–Silver syndrome |
| Popliteal web syndrome |
| Trisomy 18 (Edwards's syndrome) |
| XXY (Klinefelter's) syndrome |
| XYY syndrome |

Data from Rabinowitz.[5]

monal milieu are suggested in certain instances. Placental insufficiency and concomitant decreases in chorionic gonadotropin probably explain the eightfold increase of the anomaly seen with monozygotic twins, where the placenta may not be able to meet the gonadotropin demands required of two male fetuses. End-organ deficiencies of 5α-reductase have also been identified, but currently identifiable endocrinopathies are not felt to be prevalent. Novel research that examines deficiencies in androgen receptors at the cytoplasmic level may change our thinking in this regard.

Familial tendencies and genetic factors also exist. Bauer's review of over 300 children with hypospadias found 8% of fathers afflicted along with their sons. When one child is already affected, the risk of another son having the anomaly rises to 14%, which, if the father is also affected, rises still further to 26%.[6] A large amount of parental guilt accompanies any genital anomaly, but the parents should be reassured that perinatal teratogens are rarely implicated with hypospadias. One exception in this regard may be diethylstilbestrol (DES), whereby an increased incidence of hypospadias and other abnormalities of the penile urethra have been shown in a large group of women taking the medication.[7]

## CLASSIFICATIONS

A variety of different schema have been proposed for the classification of hypospadias. The large majority offer categorizations based on preoperative or clinical meatal position. Unfortunately, the implications of chordee and/or urethral maldevelopment for the actual technical severity of the anomaly cause these to be of little more than historical interest. It is not uncommon to encounter a phallus with the facade of a relatively innocuous distal hypospadias that belies a more challenging proximal variant (Fig 2). This masquerade often becomes apparent only at the time of surgery with the correction of chordee or revision of a dysgenetic urethra. Adaptability is key. An inexperienced urologist's decision to "correct only minor hypospadias" while in practice may not be acting in the patient's best interest. Each surgeon's armamentarium should include repairs that address more proximal variants for exactly these reasons. The perioperative classification proposed by Barcat,[8] which relates meatal position after correction of curvature, provides a logical standard for the comparison of series of hypospadias from different institutions and should be employed (Fig 3).

## ELEMENTS OF THE PROBLEM

In general, the stigmata of hypospadias consists of the following (Fig 4):

1. *A dystopic meatus located at a subcoronal position.* Meatal stenosis is more common with distal variants although voiding symptoms or proximal obstructive changes are rare occurrences in the younger child. The more proximal urethra should be of normal caliber but varying degrees of deficiency of the ventral shaft skin and urethral investing layers will occur that may require revision.

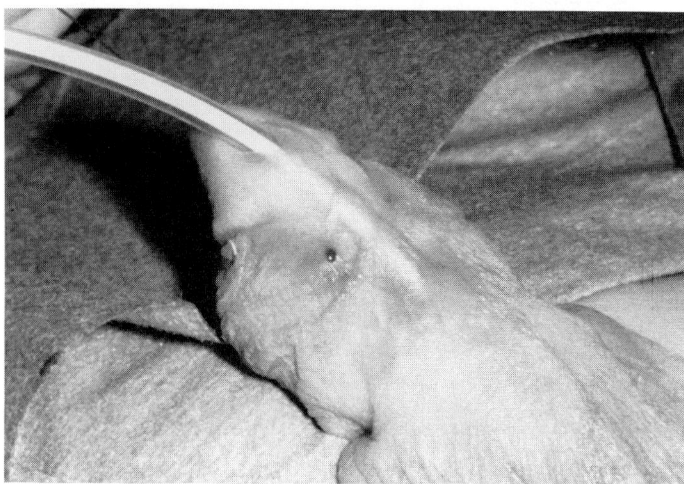

**Fig 2.** Maldevelopment of the urethra and its investing layers seen with distal hypospadias. Urethral revision will cause reclassification as more proximal variant.

2. *The "urethral plate" comprising the ventral shaft skin distal to the dystopic meatus.* This often takes a V-shaped configuration. With many distal and some proximal variants, a transverse web of tissue exists across the plate distal to the meatus that can cause deflection of the urinary stream and should be corrected in any repair. A glans cleft or groove is located beyond the web and a periurethral duct (or ducts) that courses dorsal to the true urethra is commonly found in the base of the cleft. The latter, perhaps remnants of ill-fated glanular urethral development, have variable length but are not clinically significant and need not be removed or closed at the time of surgery.

**Fig 3.** Distribution of hypospadias with classification scheme relating meatal position after correction of penile curvature.

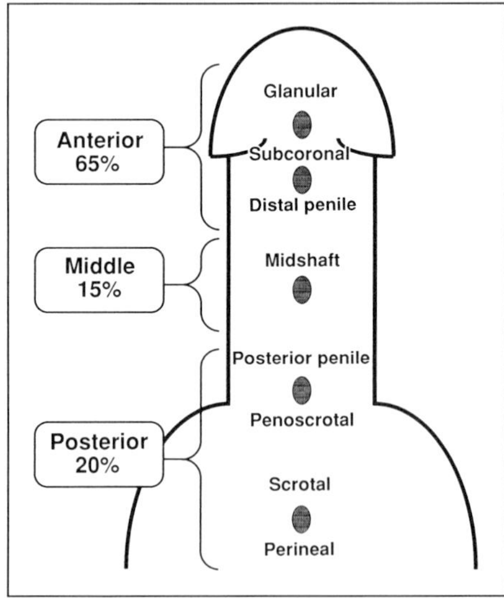


3. *A dorsally hooded foreskin.* The prepuce is absent ventrally and the origins of the remaining foreskin emanate from either side of the urethral plate. Here they commonly contribute to tilting of the glans and penile curvature. Surgery alleviates their tethering effects with takedown of the penile shaft skin. A normally developed circumferential foreskin can be found in 2% to 3% of hypospadias.[4,9]
4. *A glans configuration that is deficient and flattened ventrally.* The coronal ring of the glans is usually absent in the ventrum. When pinched together around the existing cleft, a normal, conically shaped glans can be envisioned. Exceptions occur with proximal variants that sometimes have nearly normal glanular configuration sans meatus.
5. *Chordee of varying degrees present with more than 50% of the cases.* The large majority of these are caused by superficial skin tethering in combination with the abnormal insertions of the prepuce that cause glans tilt. The resulting curvature can be impressive but often

will be corrected after the penile skin is freed from the underlying shaft.

## ASSOCIATED ANOMALIES

*Torsion of the shaft of the penis* is seen in about 15% of patients. This almost always occurs to the left and is accompanied by a raphe that is eccentric to the right of the midline and projects to the lateral extent of the preputial hood. Concomitant meatal deviation to the right sometimes also occurs.

*Enlargement of the utricle* (or the utriculus masculinus), a Müllerian duct remnant that also appears to be influenced by androgen deficiencies, is associated with hypospadias in direct relationship to the severity of the anomaly (Fig 5). In one study, 30% of scrotal-perineal variants demonstrated the vestigal organ; conversely, utricles were found in only 3% of glanular cases.[10] With an ostium usually positioned above the external sphincter, most utricles are rarely clinically significant. Recurrent urinary tract infections or calculi formation occasionally warrant removal. When this is the case, a midline transvesical approach is preferred to minimize damage to the perivesical neurovascular supply.

*Penoscrotal transposition* presumably results from incomplete migration of the genital swellings below the abnormal pubic tubercle. When severe, the scrotal engulfment that results can give the penis a diminutive and unusual appearance. Surgical correction is simply done by circumferentially mobilizing the scrotum from the base of the penis and employing V-Y advancements to a more inferior position. These rearrangements should not be performed in concert with primary urethroplasties with consideration to the blood supply of the adjoining tissues.

*Cryptorchidism* is commonly associated with hypospadias, and, like utricular enlargement, has an incidence directly related with the severity of the anomaly. An overall incidence of 9% was found in one series with undescended testes occurring with over 30% of proximal hypospadias and only 5% of distal variants.[11] Cryptorchidism that occurs in concert with hypospadias requires further evaluation to rule out an intersex state. This association is an uncommon one with anterior hypospadias but should still be considered. *Mixed gonadal dysgenesis* is the most common diagnosis when intersex has been discovered. Other inguinal pathology also occurs with hypospadias where a 10% incidence of associated hernias has been described.

*Ambiguous genitalia* and gender assignment are often questioned in the presence of a diminutive phallus and an evaluation to rule out an intersex state is sometimes required. In most instances, the presence of palpable gonads within the scrotum is a reassuring sign that the child is a genetic male. If sex assignment remains in doubt because of an unusually small phallus, hormonal stimulation should be used to assess penile response to androgens, a prognosticator of its future growth during puberty. Gonadotropin is given initially as an impetus to testicular androgen production, and, in most neonates, will induce phallic growth. When the testicular response is inadequate, exogenous testosterone can be given to assess end-organ responsiveness. Testosterone is also a useful preoperative adjunct to the repair of hypospadias with the smaller penis (testosterone propionate, 2 mg/kg IM 5 and 2 weeks before surgery). Given routinely in some institutions, selective administration is preferred by most clinicians because the majority of infant penises are large enough to correct without needing additional growth. The consequent neovascularity brought on by androgens may potentially aid in healing but also brings increased risks of perioperative bleeding and hematoma formation.

## PREOPERATIVE EVALUATION

### The Examination

A thorough history and physical is performed on every patient. The details of any previous genital surgeries, including circumcision, may have significant implications for the surgical options at the time of repair. Assessments of the size of the penis, glans configuration, and level and quality of the hypospadiac meatus and shaft skin

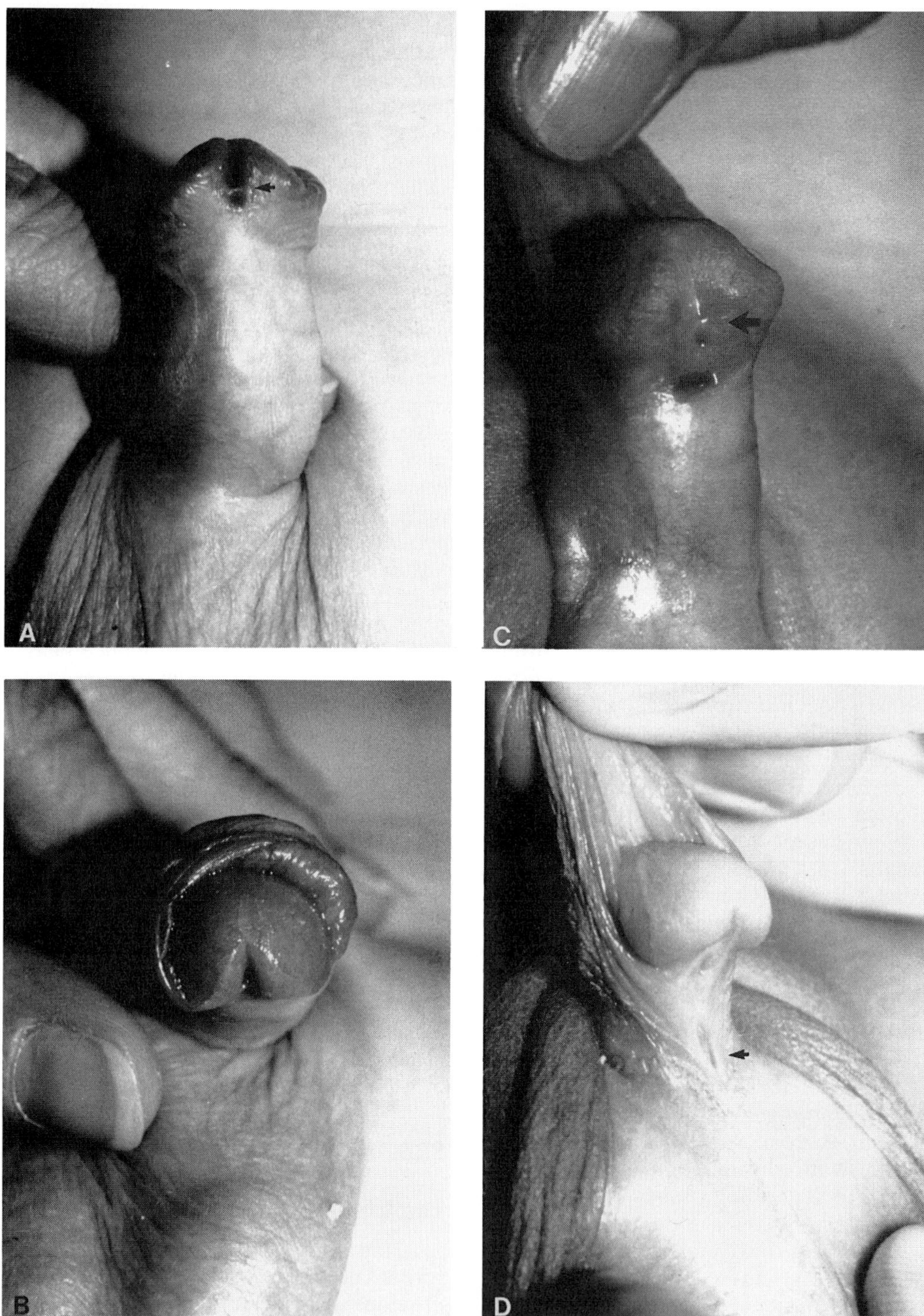


**Fig 4A–D.** Hypospadias presents spectrum. **A,** glanular variant demonstrates aberrant raphe and web beyond dystopic meatus (arrow); **B,** same penis shows dorsally hooded prepuce and flattened ventral glans; **C,** generous meatus, flattened urethral plate, and periurethal duct (arrow) found with subcoronal hypospadias; **D,** classic proximal hypospadias having deficient urethral plate, chordee, and penoscrotal meatus (arrow).

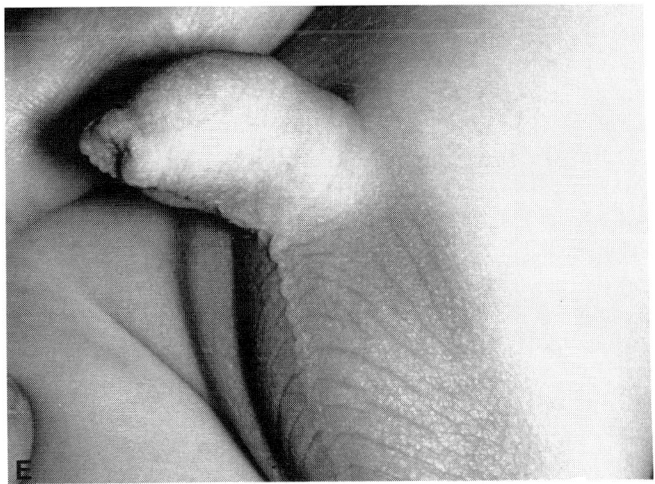


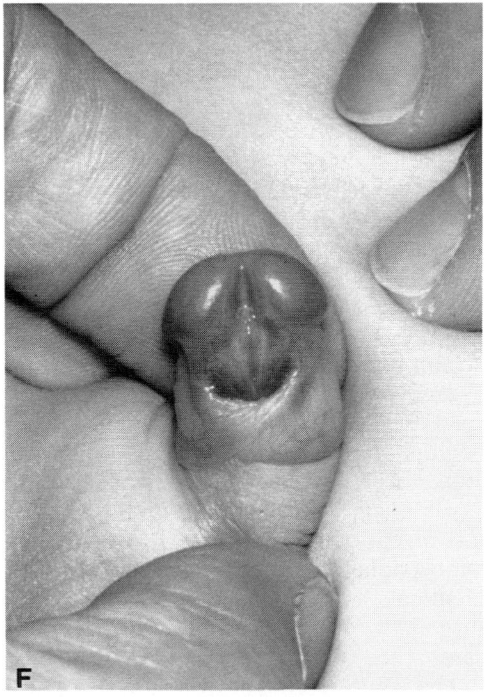


**Fig 4E, F. E,** complete prepuce seen with megameatus intact prepuce (MIP) variant; **F,** same penis, prepuce retracted.

are done. Elements of the patient's anomaly requiring simultaneous repair including chordee, meatal stenosis, and penile torsion or those that require secondary surgeries such as penoscrotal transposition are also discussed with the parents. The presence of an undescended testicle warrants further investigation through karyotyping.

## Additional Studies

Other than routine preoperative blood work and a urinalysis, no additional diagnostic studies are routinely recommended, although there are some exceptions. Evaluations of the upper urinary tract (usually with ultrasound) are obtained in

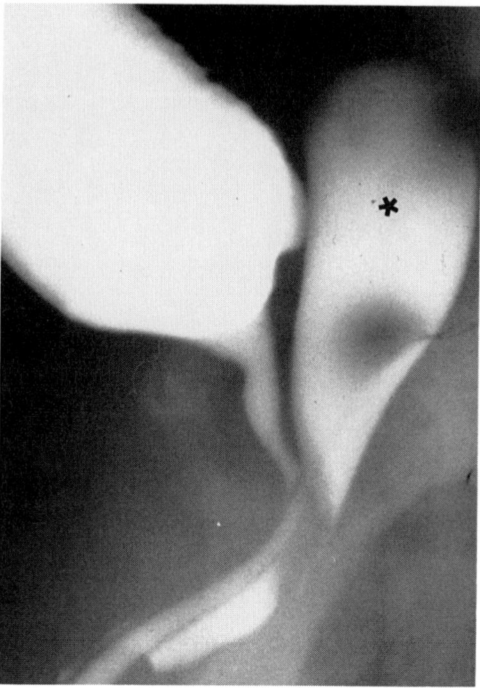


**Fig 5.** Large utricle (asterisk) found with penoscrotal hypospadias in child having recurrent urinary tract infections.

boys having hypospadias in concert with abnormalities affecting other organ systems.[12] The latter suggest a global insult that has occurred early in development and has potentially affected the kidneys and/or ureters. Otherwise routine radiologic surveys are unnecessary. The incidence of clinically significant upper tract abnormalities found with isolated hypospadias of any severity is no greater than that in the general population.[13,14] After considering the timing in embryogenesis of the external genitalia, which occurs much later than that of the upper urinary tract, this lack of an association is not surprising. Studies of the lower urinary tract can be of some benefit in patients with scrotal-perineal hypospadias. Here enlarged prostatic utricles can pose technical problems with catheterization at the time of repair. Ultrasonography usually gives adequate screening but voiding cystourethrography or retrograde genitograms are sometimes necessary to provide anatomic definition.[15]

## WHO NEEDS SURGERY?

It has always been an easy decision to recommend surgery for the child with proximal hypospadias who would ultimately have to sit to void. However, the large majority of hypospadias (60% to 70%) are of the glanular and coronal variety, and many children with distal hypospadias would remain functionally normal if surgery were deferred. No operation is without its attendant morbidity. When, then, does "mild" or "grade 1" hypospadias require correction? Concerned parents and referring physicians should not be given exaggerated descriptions of potential functional problems with distal hypospadias. Deflection or spraying of the urinary stream can often be managed by redirecting the penis and significant chordee having implications for intercourse is not a uniform occurrence. However, determination of which child will be affected by his hypospadias is entirely unpredictable. In addition, the cosmetic drawbacks of these anomalies, especially the unusual hooded prepuce and flattened, tilted glans, are very real and probably largely responsible for the psychological sequelae of hypospadias noted in many afflicted boys (see below). A number of adolescents are encountered every year who have uncorrected hypospadias yet want to "look normal" or are beginning to experience functional problems. Each would have been much more easily managed as an infant. In this regard, it is revealing that fathers with uncorrected hypospadias who have sons with nearly identical abnormalities commonly seek surgery for their progeny, even in milder cases.

The objectives set for contemporary urethroplasties, regardless of the severity of the primary malformation, now include:

1. Repositioning of the neomeatus to the tip of the penis
2. Creation of a symmetric glans and penile shaft
3. Complete straightening of the penis
4. Construction of a hairless urethra having a uniform caliber
5. Most importantly, normalization of voiding and erections

In short, the intention of today's hypospadiologist is to reconstruct a "normal" penis (Fig 6). The decision to recommend surgery rests with the surgeon's experience and judgment. When functional drawbacks (voiding symptoms, meatal stenosis, or chordee) are present or anticipated and cosmetic advantages could be envisioned, surgery is recommended without hesitation. In the hands of a well-trained hypospadiologist, the benefits of urethroplasty should far outweigh its risks in all but the very mildest forms of the anomaly.

## TIMING OF SURGERY

Refinements in microsurgical technique and improvements in anesthesia have allowed the performance of hypospadias repairs in progressively younger patients. This trend has been fortuitous as reconstructive urologists continue to gain insight into the psychological implications of genital surgery in children. With considerations to sexual orientation, genital awareness, body image, and bonding, the optimal time for hypospadias surgery appears to occur between 6 and 12 months of age.[16,17] In the otherwise healthy infant, anesthetic risks are minimized and the penis is usually large enough to enable cosmetic and functional results analogous to those attained previously in older children.[18,19] Parental acceptance of this approach has been excellent. Much parental anxiety or guilt is quickly allayed. In addition, the younger child is more easily managed and appears to have amnesia for the operation through subsequent development.

Historically, psychosexual consequences have burdened the male with hypospadias addressed in the prior era of surgery at a later age done in multiple stages. Lower self-esteem, lack of confidence about masculinity, and decreased capacity for interpersonal relations were prevalent.[20] In one series of adults (mean age 27 years) whose hypospadias were corrected at a mean age of 5, minimal or no sexual activity was commonplace (38%).[21] The long-term implications of today's altered approach in timing will not become apparent for years to come. However, it is hoped and strongly suspected that surgical corrections at an early age will make a significant difference in this regard.

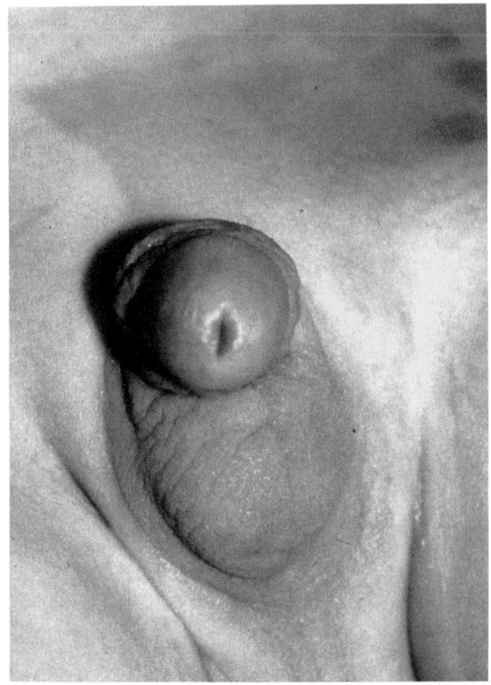

**Fig. 6.** Configuration of normal penis sets the standard for contemporary hypospadias repairs.

## PRINCIPLES IN TECHNIQUE

The best surgical results with primary or reoperative urethroplasties are achieved by applying plastic surgical instruments and that discipline's principles of tissue management.

### Basic Instruments

Castroviejo needle holders, fine iris-type scissors, skin hooks, delicate (0.5) forceps, and optical magnification are very helpful. Loupes are preferred but an operating microscope has been advocated by some.

### Tissue Handling

A "minimal-touch" technique is emphasized, reducing trauma to delicate tissues by using traction sutures or skin hooks whenever possible. Fine hemostats that grasp individual vessels and allow selective

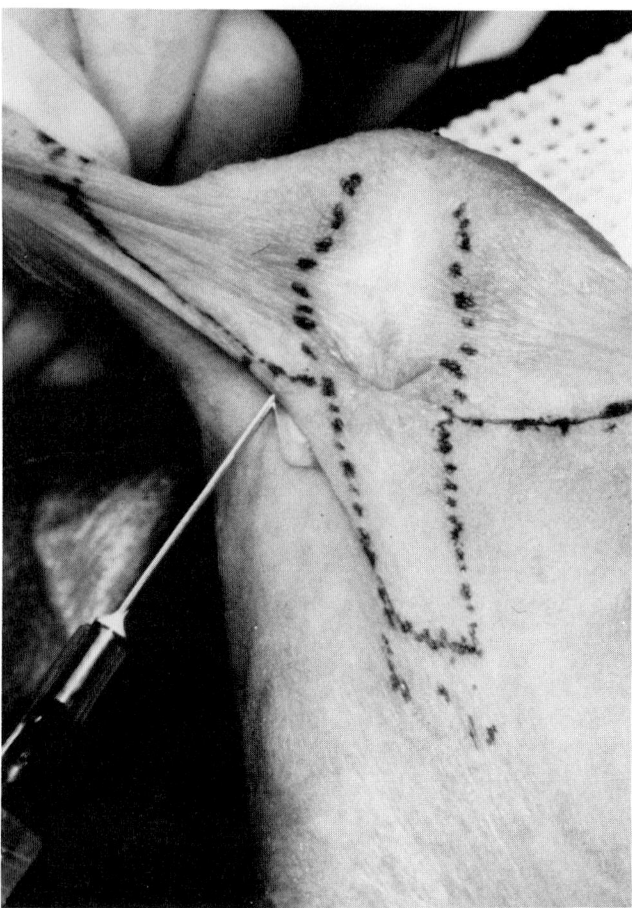

**Fig 7.** Epinephrine injected into the glans and along lines of incision provides a useful adjunct for hemostasis.

low-current electrocautery helps minimize ischemia. Cautery should not be used near tissues intended for construction or coverage of the neourethra. A dry field is helpful during this type of surgery but not to the detriment of an overabundance of tissue damage and vascular thrombosis, which both risk infection. When ischemia is questioned during surgery, the suspect tissue should be trimmed back until its revised edges bleed. Perioperative fluorescein has also been used by some clinicians to assess the viability of tissues.[22]

## Hemostasis

Epinephrine (1 : 100,000, maximum dosage 5 mg/kg) is an invaluable aid to perioperative hemostasis and is injected with a 25-gauge needle into the subcutaneous tissues of the proposed lines of incision and into the glans itself (Fig 7). Concern about penile ischemia should be nonexistent with proper dosing of the solution. Epinephrine has virtually eliminated the need for elastic tourniquets and rebound bleeding or tissue loss has not been a problem. Bleeding that occurs in the latter stages of longer cases usually stems from a full bladder, causing compromised venous return rather than loss of epinephrine's vasoconstrictive effects. Most minor bleeding stops with application of the dressing, but if a hematoma is appreciated beforehand, it should be evacuated. When concerns about bleeding persist, a small Penrose drain or Mini-Vac suction drain can be left in the subcutaneous space.

## Sutures—Skin

Fine chromic (6–0 or 7–0) is preferred for skin and at the meatus because it is quickly absorbed. Tension-free reapproximation minimizes ischemia. *Running mattress sutures* evert skin edges, provide excellent cosmetic results, and exit the incision within a few days. Epithelialized suture tracts (leading to so-called penile blackheads) have become less of a problem now that multiple interrupted stitches are used less frequently.

## Sutures—Neourethra

Polyglycolic or polydiaxanone (6–0 or 7–0) is preferred for their minimal reactivity in repairs where a neourethra is constructed. Urethral suture lines are meant to be urine-tight and are inverted luminally whenever possible. Eversion has been shown to be the risk factor for fistula formation.[23]

## Neourethra and Glans Construction

Construction of the neourethra and glans is critical to the success of any repair. Urethroplasties that utilize flaps or tubularized tissues are fashioned along an understandably fine line between luminal stenosis leading to stricture formation and urethral redundancy, whose turbulence poses a risk factor to subsequent fistula formation. The reconstructed neourethra is projected to have a circumference of 12 to 15 mm in the youngest babies and 18 to 20 mm in older boys. Frequent calibration with bougie-à-boules is used during the case as a useful gauge of patency.

The refashioned glans can represent a very real threat to the underlying neourethra. In the past, the glans tunnel technique was often recommended for use with tubularized neourethras. When the glans and cleft have an appearance worth salvaging, a generous buttonhole of epithelium and deeper spongiosal tissue should be removed to create an uncompromising hiatus. These instances are rare and instead a glans split is now recommended for most variants. Here the lateral wings are widely mobilized by defining the plane between the glans cap and the corpora (Fig 8). In some cases, it is helpful to excise some of the wings' deeper midline tissue before reconstructing the glans in two layers. Proximally circumferential anastomoses are spatulated to minimize stenosis and the running suture lines of tubularized neourethras are placed against the shaft of the penis to maximize their coverage.

## Avoiding Fistulas

Multiple layers of healthy tissue are an invaluable aid to minimizing the incidence of fistula by eliminating crossing suture lines and optimizing vascularization. Additional coverings for the urethroplasty can be obtained from redundant portions of a preputial pedicle, deepithelialized shaft skin,[24] or even the tunica vaginalis of an adjacent gonad[25] (Fig 9). Secondary coverage can often salvage a repair where skin loss has developed and the neourethra is placed at jeopardy. The importance of

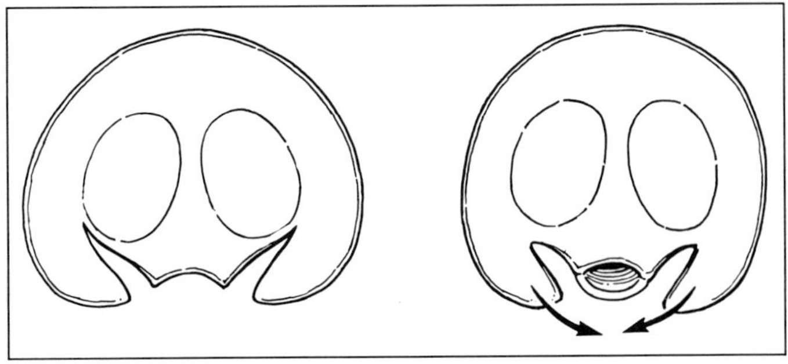

**Fig 8.** Generous glans mobilization is required to avoid compromise of neourethra. Shown here in repair that has preserved the urethral plate.

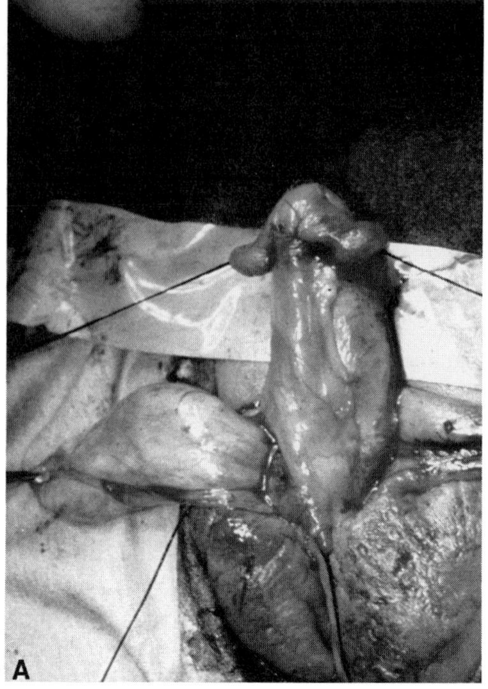


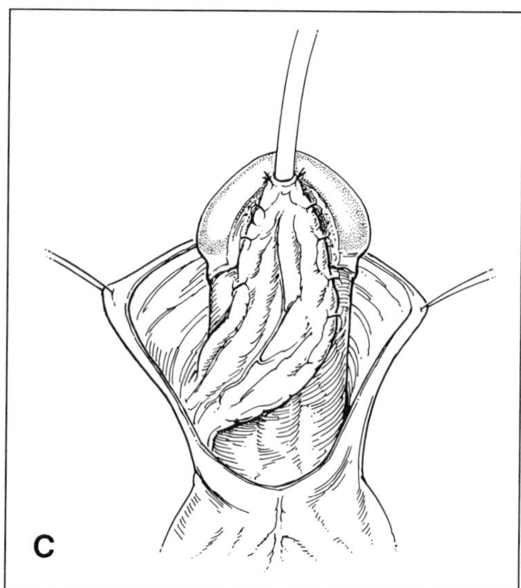


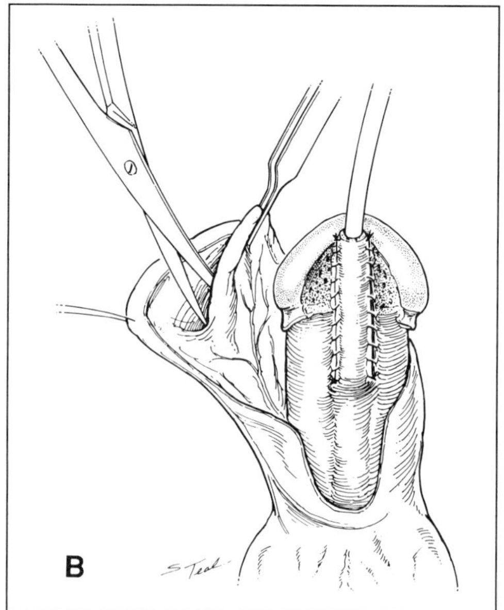


**Fig 9.** Additional layers of neourethral coverage. **A,** tunica vaginalis blanket from adjacent gonad; **B,C,** preputial subcutaneous tissue mobilized to cover meatal-based flap urethroplasty.

multiple-layered closures to urethroplasty has been dramatically emphasized by Kass and Bolong, who recently reported one fistula in 206 primary repairs using a double-layered closure of the neourethra.[26]

## Penoplasty

With most urethroplasties, adequate amounts of shaft skin remain to allow a midline ventral realignment to the level of

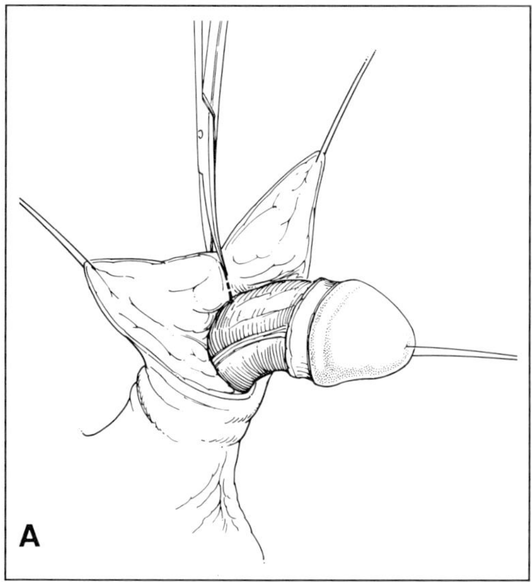


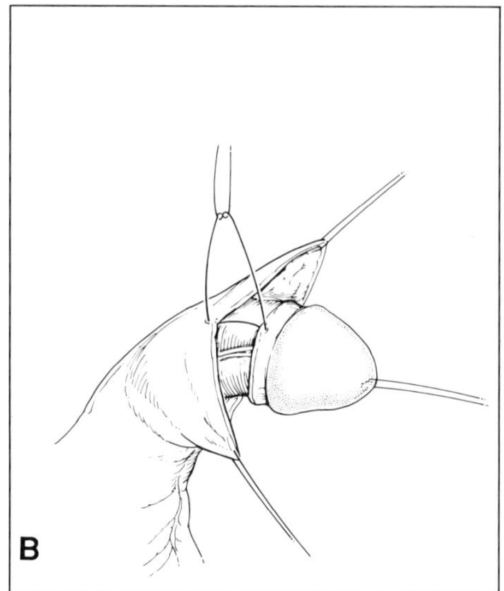


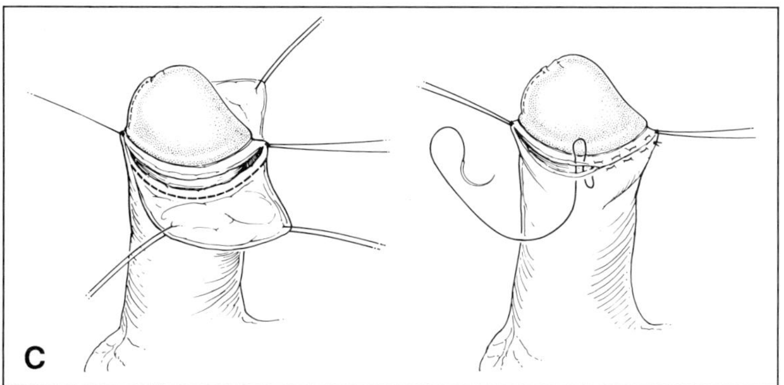


**Fig 10.** Ventral skin closures are possible after most urethroplasties. **A,** dorsal relaxing incision enables transfer of lateral distal shaft skin; **B,C,** after dorsal reapproximation and ventral realignment to cover any defect, excess prepuce excised and repair completed.

the corona. A dorsal relaxing incision of the hooded prepuce is made that releases the lateral shaft skin and enables its ventral transfer (Fig 10). Coverage of most defects resulting from the release of superficial chordee is usually possible and a raphe is recreated. This technique had been avoided in the past for fear of causing recurrent chordee. However, chordee has not been a problem and the cosmetic results of this "sleeve" reapproximation have been excellent and anatomically correct. In some instances, significant ventral deficits remain that require flap coverage using the effective but cosmetically less pleasing Byars method.[27] More complex Z-plasties tend to disrupt normal vascular patterns, increase the risks of skin loss, and should be avoided whenever possible.

## MANAGING CHORDEE

*Chordee,* or penile curvature, presents its own surgical challenges, and, as such, warrants discussion as an isolated entity. Interestingly, ventral curvature is a normal finding in fetal penile development.[2] This phenomenon, of an unclear etiology, typ-

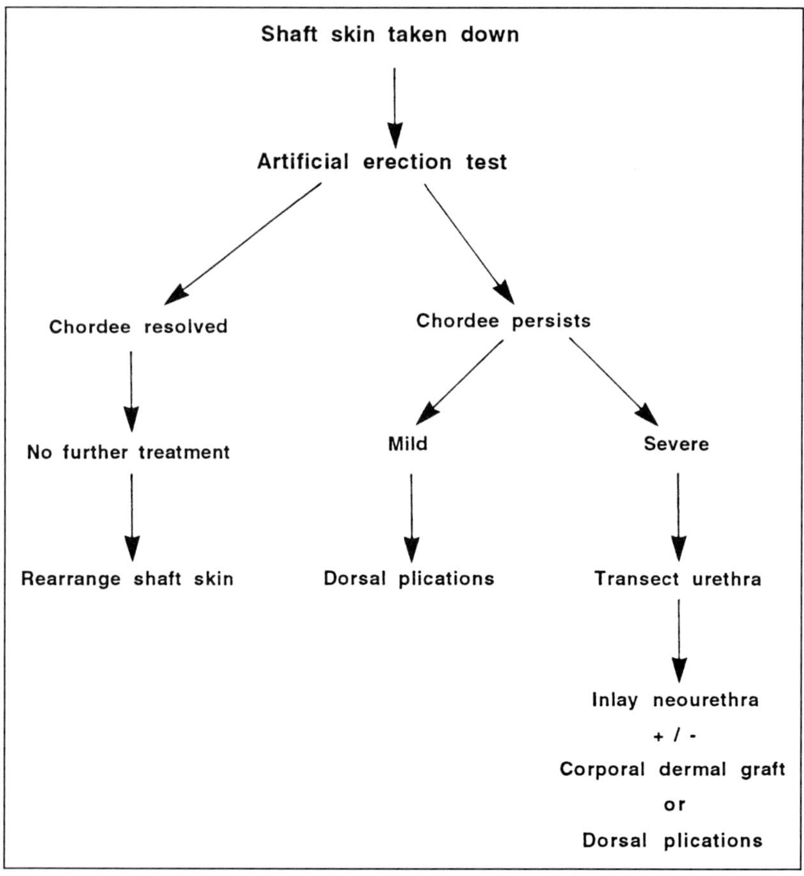


**Fig 11.** Management of chordee without hypospadias. Most are superficial and resolve with takedown of shaft skin.

ically resolves by term although postnatal resolution has also been noted, especially in premature infants. Curvature that persists is usually found in association with hypospadias, but chordee without hypospadias does occur. The anatomic basis of chordee without hypospadias mimics that seen with hypospadias with the exception of its urethral continuity. Tethering can occur at the skin, urethral, and corporal levels. Many chordee without hypospadias can be corrected by simply releasing the shaft skin alone. When curvature persists, subsequent management is dictated by the development of the urethra and its investing corpora spongiosum.[28,29] An algorithm that summarizes the management of chordee without hypospadias is shown (Fig 11).

The large majority (perhaps 90%) of curvature associated with hypospadias is caused by superficial or skin chordee. The shaft skin is taken down sharply to the base of the penis in nearly every case. Marked degrees of curvature can result from the tethering effects of dysgenetic ventral skin combined with the aberrant insertions of the hooded prepuce (Fig 12). Adequate straightening and removal of any remaining tethering tissues is confirmed before proceeding with construction of a primary neourethra. This is done by placing an elastic tourniquet at the penile base and injecting normal saline through a 25-gauge needle (the Gittes test) that has been placed through the glans into one corporal body.[30]

Chordee that persists after release of the penile skin can be caused by either a dysgenetic urethral plate, intrinsic corporal

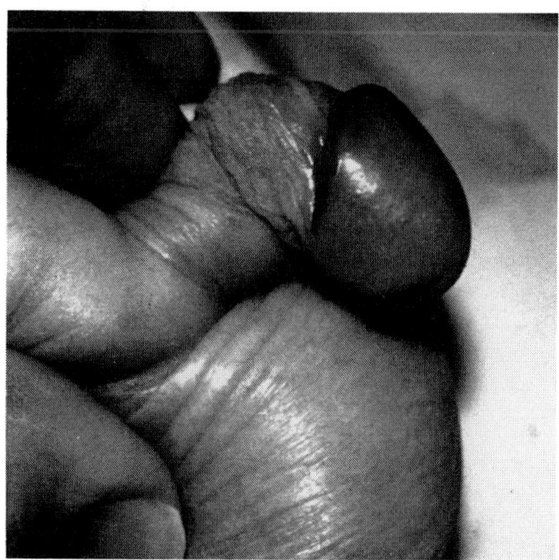

**Fig 12.** Distal hypospadias with marked curvature largely caused by glans tilt from aberrant preputial insertions.

scarring, or corporal disproportion. In the past, chordee that persisted after degloving of the penis was uniformly attributed to the plate. We now recognize that this is not always the case. Where the urethral plate is healthy, soft, and pliable, corporal problems have been increasingly implicated. In instances where the plate is fibrotic and inelastic, it should be removed and its tissues sharply excised. Distally, fibrotic plaque is excised from the ventral corpora with the dissections extending into the glans itself if necessary. Proximally, healthy urethra should be released from the tunica albuginea to enable removal of any tethering tissues beneath. This understandably alters the categorization of the hypospadias and the type of urethroplasty required for its correction.

Chordee that continues to persist after excision of the urethral plate can be corrected by placement of a ventral inlay graft of dermis[31] or tunica vaginalis[32] or dorsal plication sutures.[33] The long-term effects of dermal and tunica grafts in infants remain unclear and there have been concerns voiced with regard to the disruption of juvenile erectile tissues. Dorsal plications risk injury to the neurovascular bundle, but, if done carefully, have provided an effective solution to persistent chordee that has withstood the test of time. Our method of plication consists of initially identifying and elevating the dorsal neurovascular bundles by lateral to medial dissections of Buck's fascia. Two transverse parallel incisions are spaced 8 to 10 mm apart on the dorsolateral aspect of each corpora. Positioned at 10 and 2 o'clock, they should be made opposite the point of greatest penile curvature. Nonabsorbable sutures reapproximate the tunica (Fig 13). 4–0 braided Tevdek or Ticron is preferred for its relatively innocuous knots. Neurologic complications have not been a problem using this technique. Critics of dorsal plications

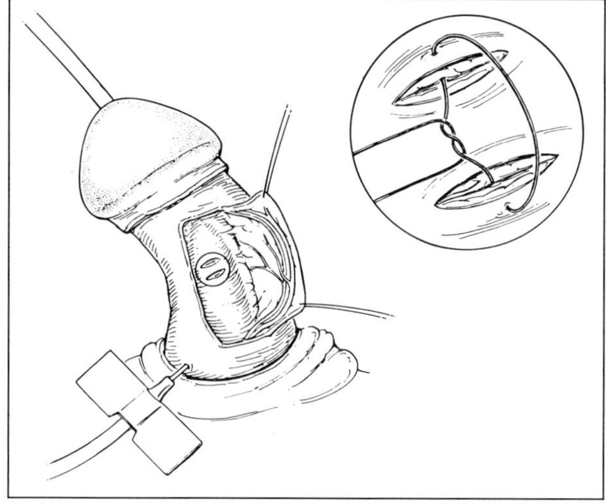

**Fig 13.** Technique of dorsal plications. Neurovascular bundles elevated with Buck's fascia. Nonabsorbable sutures (inset) approximate parallel incisions in tunica of corpora.

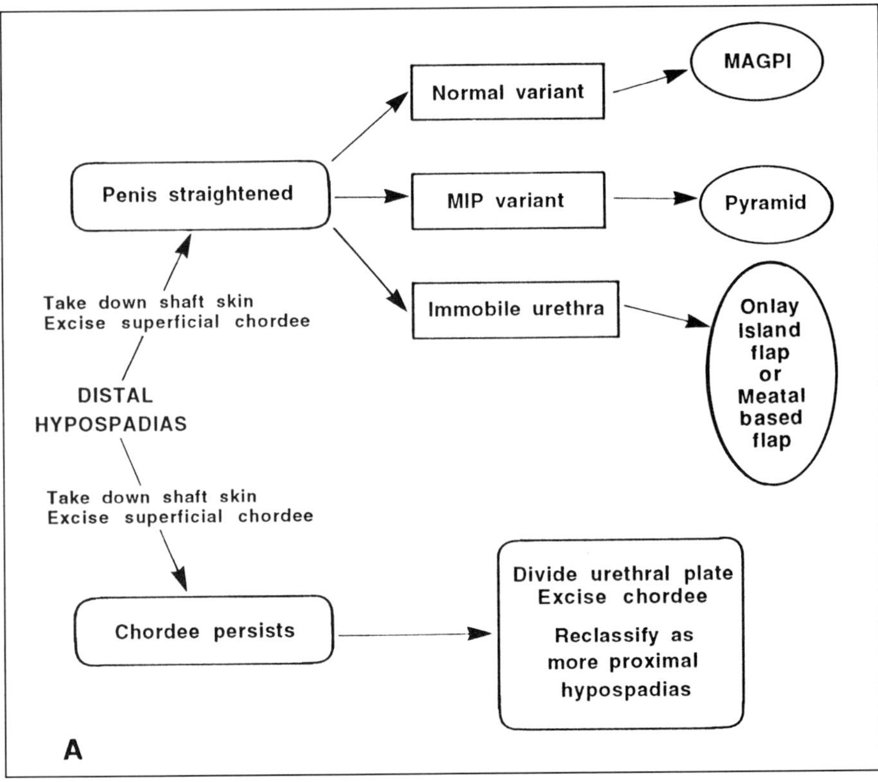


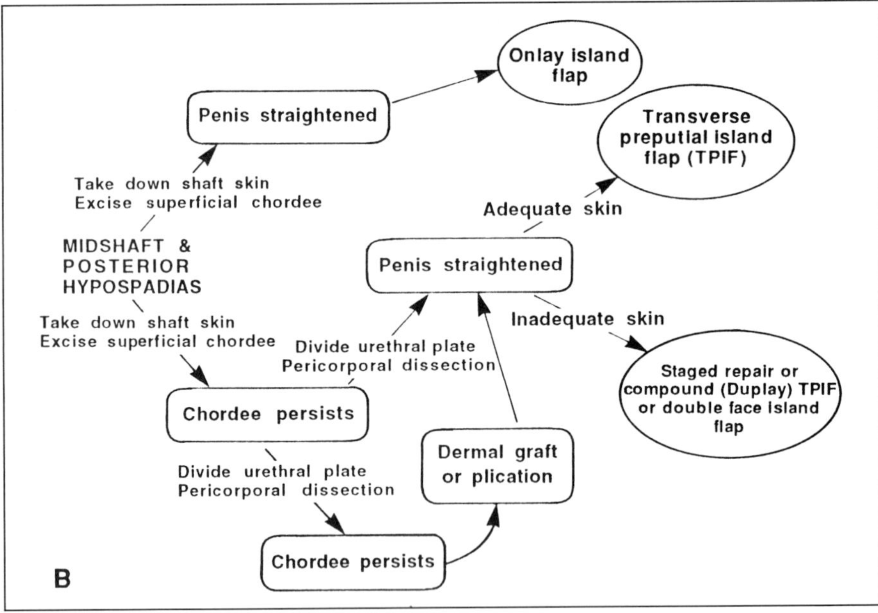


**Fig 14. A,** algorithm for repair of distal hypospadias. When chordee persists, reclassification is made to more proximal variant; **B,** algorithm for repair of midshaft and proximal hypospadias. MAGPI, meatal advancement and glanuloplasty; OIF, onlay island flap; TPIF, transverse preputial island flap.

have exaggerated the sacrifice of penile length that occurs with plications which in actuality amounts to less than 1 cm in all but the most severe cases. Where corporal disproportion has been the cause of chordee, this may even be a benefit. Dermal grafts are reserved for phalluses that are shorter and have more severe curvature. *Persistent glans tilt* without ventral chordee can be corrected by placing fine permanent sutures that hitch the dorsal glans to the corporal body, being careful to avoid the neurovascular bundles.

## TECHNIQUE SELECTION

Many of the complications of hypospadias surgery are caused not only by faulty technique but also by errors in design and application. Selecting a urethroplasty properly tailored to the individual's anatomy assumes primary importance to maximizing one's surgical results. *Adaptability is key*. Application of a "favorite repair" providing excellent results for one anomaly might concede inevitable complications to another. The surgical armamentarium should include a variety of repairs and familiarity with the limitations of each. Algorithms for hypospadias repair are shown in Figure 14.

### Meatal Advancement and Glanuloplasty

Briefly, for many distal (glandular and coronal) hypospadias without chordee the meatal advancement and glanuloplasty (MAGPI) repair is ideal.[34] The simplicity of the MAGPI belies the complex sequence of tissue transfers that are required of the technique. The technique is certainly not the "optical illusion" it was initially labeled. The decision to apply the standard MAGPI depends on the respective mobilities of the dorsal urethral plate and the ventral urethra as well as the pliability of the glans. Urethral immobility or attempts to apply the technique to subcoronal hypospadias invites urethral retrusion as an inevitable consequence of tension. When urethral mobility is a problem, an onlay island flap (OIF) or meatal-based flap should be chosen as an alternative repair. Variants having a wide-mouthed meatus or noncompliant glans are also unsuitable candidates. Here glans breakdown is predictable and the Pyramid or King-type repair is more appropriate. Any dissatisfaction with the MAGPI probably stems from its application in exactly these types of unsuitable candidates. When properly deployed, the cosmetic and functional results of this simple technique are excellent (Fig 15). A complication rate of less than 1% was cited in a recent report of over 1000 cases.[35]

### Onlay Island Flap

Midshaft and proximal hypospadias without chordee or most distal variants not amenable to the MAGPI are ideal candidates for the Onlay Island Flap (OIF) urethroplasty. Perimetal-based flaps (the Mathieu or the so-called flip-flap) have been a popular alternative for these types of hypospadias in many institutions. Flip-flaps are effective for hypospadias having a generous meatus as well as healthy ventral shaft skin. However, a preference for the OIF has evolved because of a vascular supply to the neourethra that is predictable and dependable; its adaptability to even more proximal variants; and its preservation of the ventral shaft skin, which, in most cases, allows a midline closure (Fig 16). In contradistinction, meatal-based flaps rely on vascularity from perimeatal tissues that are sometimes deficient, have their length and application in proximal hypospadias limited by the hair-bearing penoscrotal junction, and can cause significant ventral skin defects requiring more complex flap coverage. Harvesting preputial flaps becomes relatively simple with continued experience. Otherwise the technical challenges and principles of the two operations are very similar. The OIF was also shown to have a slightly lower complication rate than the perimeatal-based flap when applied to similar types of hypospadias (8% versus 10%).[36]

### Transverse Preputial Island Flap

For hypospadias at any position with chordee, the tubularized transverse pre-

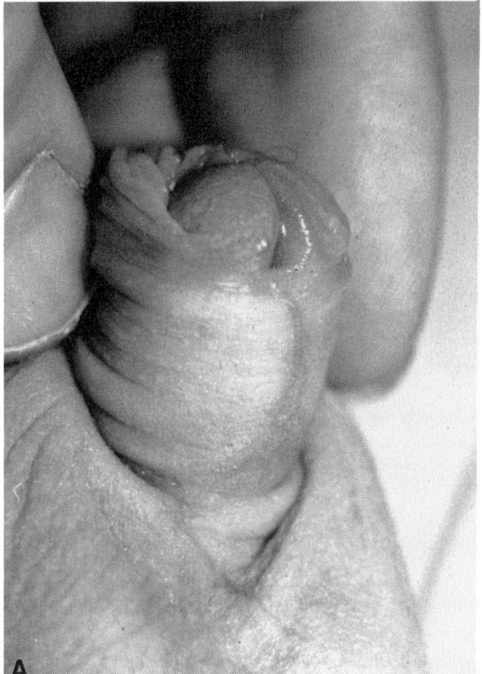


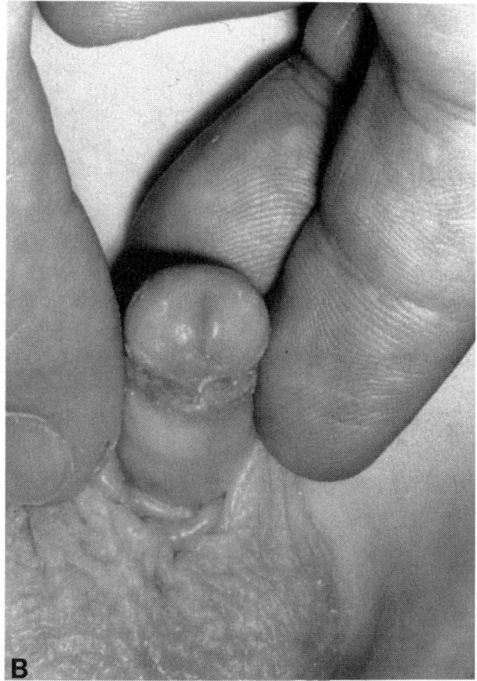


**Fig 15.** MAGPI repair provides excellent results when properly applied but determining preoperative suitability is difficult. **A,** typical distal hypospadias found to have adequate urethral and glanular mobility; **B,** postoperative appearance essentially normal.

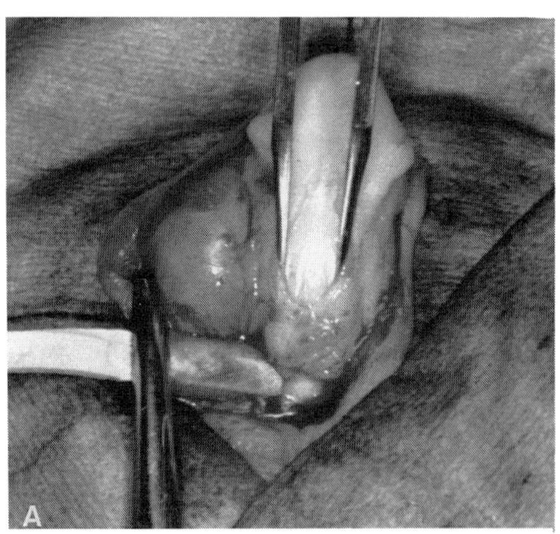


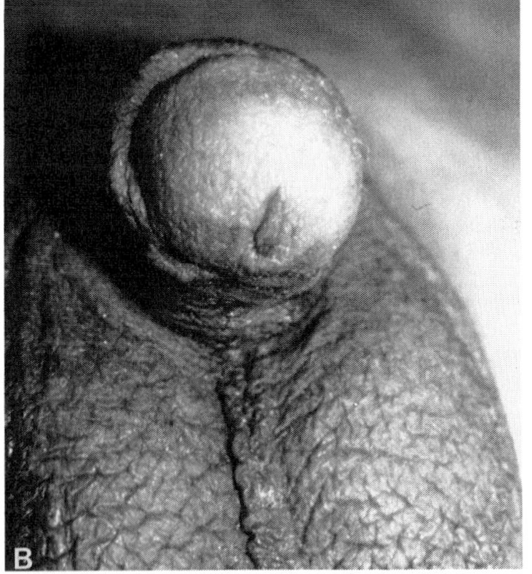


**Fig 16. A,** healthy urethral plate preserved in midshaft hypospadias variant without chordee; **B,** postoperative appearance after onlay island flap urethroplasty essentially normal.

putial island flap (TPIF) or Duckett procedure[37] remains the urethroplasty of choice. However, the decision to apply the tubularized TPIF is not made until other surgical options have been considered. In the past, once the presence of chordee was confirmed by a preincision artificial erection, the urethroplasty was commenced by skin incisions that methodically circumscribed the urethra and divided the urethral plate. Tubularized neourethras were then constructed by necessity. Our contemporary realization that severe curvature often results from superficial chordee rather than tethering by the urethral plate has since altered this approach (see "Managing Chordee"). Virtually every hypospadias repair is now begun by preserving the ventral urethral plate, taking down the shaft skin, and only then performing an artificial erection to assess the presence or absence of persistent chordee. Chordee tissue lateral to the plate can be resected from the corpora but the plate is left undisturbed to preserve its blood supply. Using these maneuvers, if the penis can be effectively straightened and the tissues of the urethral plate appear healthy and well developed, the OIF rather than its tubularized forebearer can be applied to more proximal hypospadias variants.

Advantages of the onlay when compared to the more technically challenging TPIF include:

1. Ease in sizing of the neourethra and simplification in its construction
2. Immobilization of the base of the neourethra which minimizes the kinking and tortuosity sometimes seen with the TPIF
3. Elimination of circumferential anastomoses at the original and new meatus, making stricture and stenosis less likely

The OIF has maintained a significantly lower complication rate than the TPIF when used to repair more proximal hypospadias (10% versus 15%).[36] Despite these technical benefits, the concomitant use of dorsal plications to correct chordee, preserve the urethral plate, and apply the OIF should probably be discouraged for the present time. When chordee persists, the plate should be divided and the urethra mobilized to clear the corpora of any offending tissues. Unfortunately, pericorporal dissections may not make a difference when corporal disproportion or intrinsic corporal fibrosis are its cause (Fig 17). It is this very circumstance that has clouded the recommendations for mild and moderate degrees of chordee found with a healthy urethral plate that does not appear to be contributing to chordee. Here, the OIF in concert with dorsal plications may become a very real alternative with continued experience and understanding of the natural history and identification of these types of anomalies.[38]

In summary, nearly every hypospadias can now be corrected with one of three standard urethroplasties: MAGPI, OIF, and TPIF. These three assume a position in a rational technical sequence based on their incisions, degree of difficulty in performance, and the severity of hypospadias to which they apply. Each repair predisposes to the next without "burning" any technical or anatomic bridges. Other less commonly used urethroplasties provide solutions for variants that are not amenable to one of the three. Once the position of each urethroplasty is properly understood within the algorithm of management, successful repairs hinge on technical detail and perioperative management.

## METHODS

### The MAGPI Procedure

Suitability for the MAGPI can be judged only at the time of the performance of its dorsal and ventral urethral advancements. However, the anatomy of certain hypospadias is not conducive to the tissue transfers required for successful MAGPI. Gibbons and Gonzales identified variants having an inelastic or wide-mouthed meatus and others with flat, noncompliant urethral plates as presenting anatomic barriers to tension-free glans approximations around the distally advanced urethra.[39] Marginally mobile ventral urethras also invite problems. To perform the MAGPI in these settings risks breakdown of the repair and its sequelae, the retrusive meatus—a

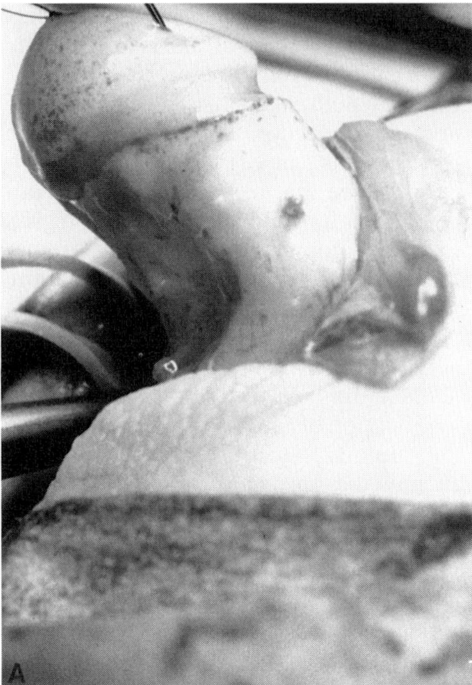


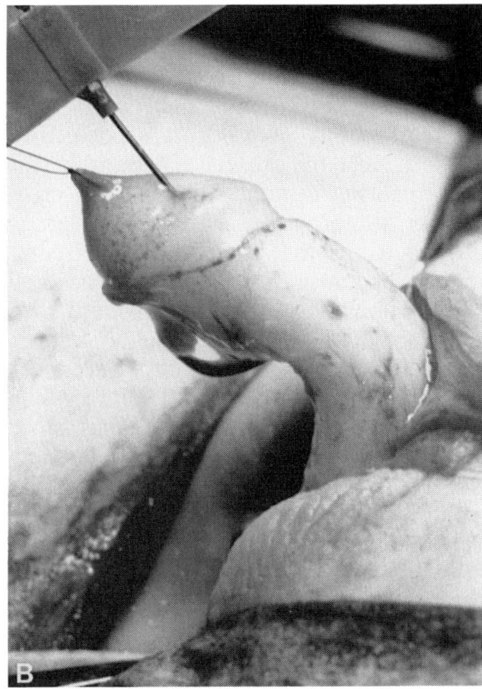


**Fig 17.** Chordee with hypospadias. **A,** urethral plate preserved; **B,** persistent chordee after division of plate and pericorporal dissections. This type of unpredictable occurrence clouds the recommendations for management of similar variants.

largely avoidable occurrence that is often worse than the original anomaly.

### Technique

***Preparation and Dissection.*** A traction suture placed in the glans facilitates handling. A circumferential incision is made approximately 5 to 7 mm from the coronal edge that is carried proximal to the meatus and the shaft skin is taken down (Fig 18A). Extreme caution is required during the ventral part of this dissection where the skin is often thin and fused to the underlying urethra and a deficient corpus spongiosum (Fig 18B). It is helpful to define initially the better developed tissue planes of the proximal shaft by bluntly spreading the scissors. The adherent tissues adjacent to the meatus can then be more easily appreciated and separated sharply by working distally. An 8 French feeding tube in the urethra is helpful during this part of the dissection.

Inadvertant urethrotomies occasionally occur and can be repaired using fine inverting absorbable sutures. However, the risks of fistula formation increase markedly with such an event and for more than the most minor urethrotomy it is probably advisable instead to revise the injured urethra and reconstruct its ventrum with an onlay flap of healthy prepuce.

***Meatal Advancement.*** The web of tissue between the meatus and the distal glanular groove is defined by lateral traction. A wedge of the web is removed by making two cuts from its lateral edges which meet in the midline and join the dorsal edge of the meatus to the glans groove (Fig 18C,D). This enlarges the meatus, flattens the dorsal urethral plate, and eliminates dog ears. The diamond-shaped defect in the urethral plate that results is closed transversely in Heinecke–Mikulicz fashion using 7–0 interrupted polyglycolic sutures, effectively advancing the dorsal urethra

(Fig 18E). Meatal stenosis and deflection of the stream are both eliminated by this maneuver.

Some dorsal urethras are not sufficiently mobile to allow these types of distal advancements. As a consequence, the more forgiving glans tip must be pulled proximally to meet the immobile urethra and bridge the defect. The result is an unsightly depressed glans tip. Urethral mobility can be tested using fine forceps, and, if immobility is suspected, the standard MAGPI should be deferred.

*Glanuloplasty.* Redundant tissues usually remain on either side of the glans wings after the skin incision (just proximal to the ventral meatal edge), remnants of the preputial insertions. For cosmetic purposes, these are excised so that the glans itself can be approximated. In Firlit's modification, the initial circumferential skin incision is carried more proximally below the coronal sulcus and preserves mucosal-type tissue for its ultimate ventral transfer and reapproximation in the midline beneath the glans.[40] However, excess skin usually continues to present a problem and must be revised. Gentle traction on a stay suture or fine skin hook placed at the meatal lip completes the urethral advancement ventrally. This allows the ventral glans edges to rotate together in the midline to create a more anatomic conical shape. The glans is closed without tension in two layers over the advanced urethra (Fig 19). Deeper glanular tissue is approximated with one or two 6–0 polyglycolic sutures. Fine interrupted chromic stitches are used to reapproximate the skin. After completion of the glanuloplasty, the meatus should allow the passage of a 10-French bougie-à-boule in all but the smallest penises. Extensive dissections beneath the lateral glans wings should not be required to access deeper tissues or achieve glanular mobility. This risks bleeding, and, if proven necessary, is probably an indication that the patient is an unsuitable candidate for the MAGPI.

*Penoplasty.* A midline sleeve reapproximation of the shaft skin completes most repairs. Preservation of the prepuce is occasionally requested and is possible with the MAGPI.

## The Pyramid Procedure

The pyramid procedure was initially offered as a solution for the MIP variant alone but its principles can be extended to any hypospadias with a generous glans cleft provided it is wide enough.[4] The megameatus variants can be of the most challenging hypospadias to address. The unusual configuration of the fish-mouthed meatus and glans groove presents a formidable barrier to the glanuloplasty of the MAGPI and its widened distal urethra provides a difficult challenge in tailoring when preparing the urethral plate and glans for an island onlay or meatal-based flap urethroplasty. In addition, the absence of chordee in combination with an intact prepuce frequently causes the anomaly to go unrecognized until after circumcision, thus eliminating flaps from consideration. The results with conventional urethroplasties had often been unsatisfactory. The pyramid technique, a variant of the King repair that historically constructed a neourethra to the level of the sulcus,[41] evolved from the experience with balanic epispadias whose findings mirror those of the MIP. The pyramid label was chosen in description of its exposure, which allows for a simple and safe dissection and reconstruction of the megameatus and urethra in both the circumcised and uncircumcised child. Successful results with the pyramid procedure or others like it, including the GAP (glans approximation procedure), another variation of the King procedure,[42] are contingent on a deep glans groove, which, when flattened, mobilized, and closed ventrally can be tubularized to an adequate size for age (Fig 20). Caution in selection must be exercised. The widespread application of these types of repairs to most distal hypospadias should probably be discouraged due to concern for long-term urethral caliber and patency.

### Technique

*Incisions and Dissection.* A tennis racquet-shaped incision extending from

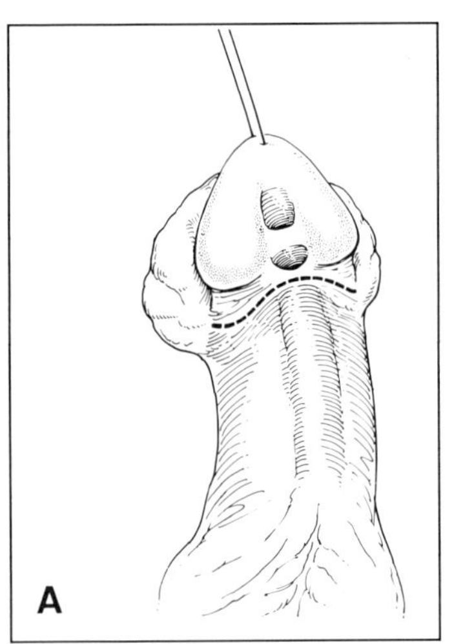


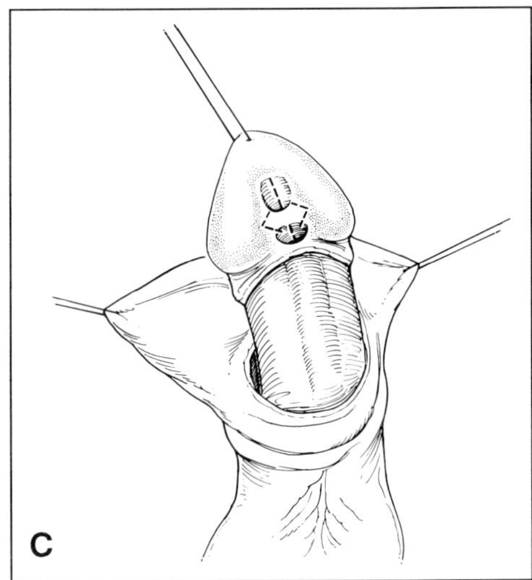


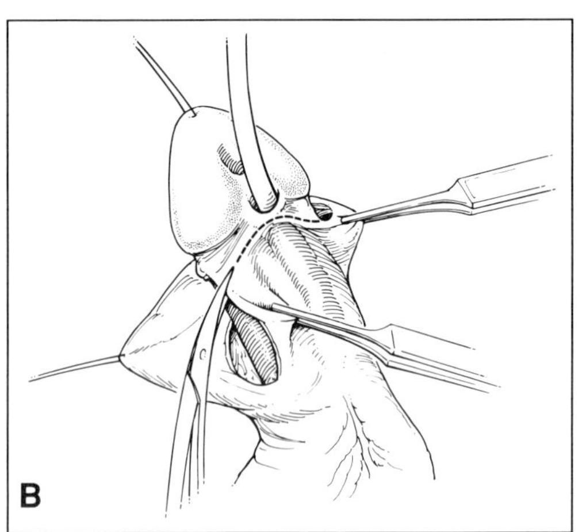


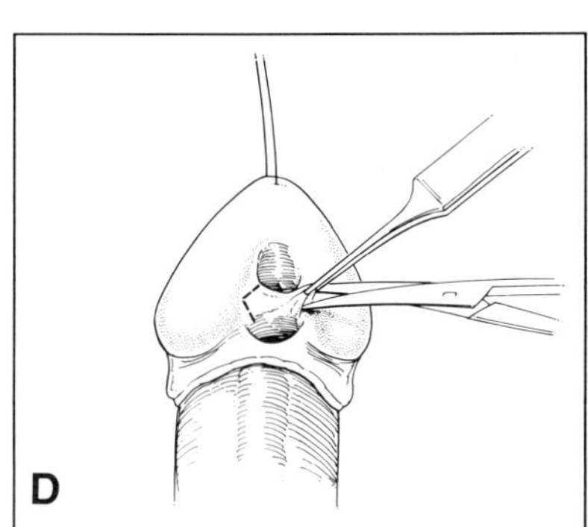


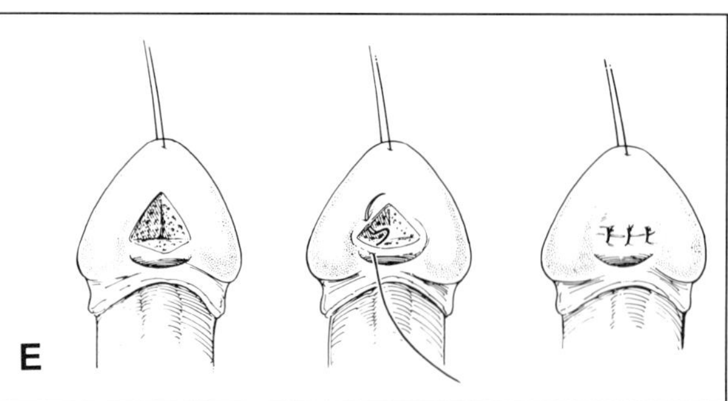


**Fig 18A–E.** MAGPI repair. **A,** lines of incision; **B,** care is taken when addressing the shaft skin overlying the urethra where fusion often occurs during maldevelopment; **C,D,E,** wedge resection of distal meatal web and reapproximation completes dorsal urethral advancement.

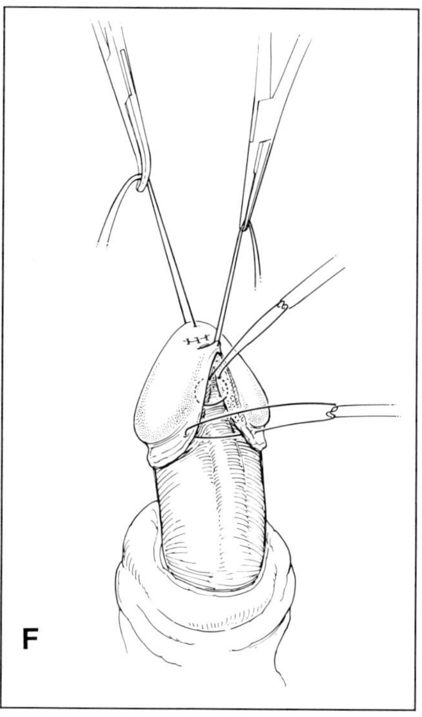


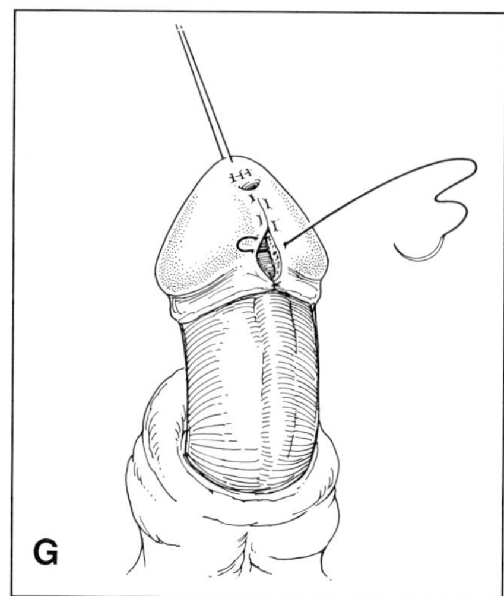


**Fig 18F,G.** Traction enables ventral urethral advancement as glans is reapproximated behind it.

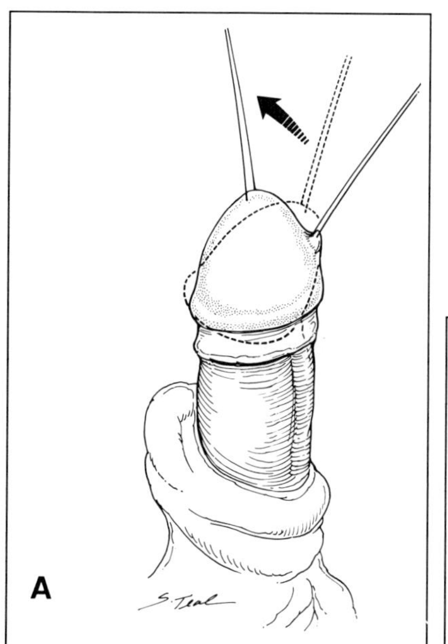


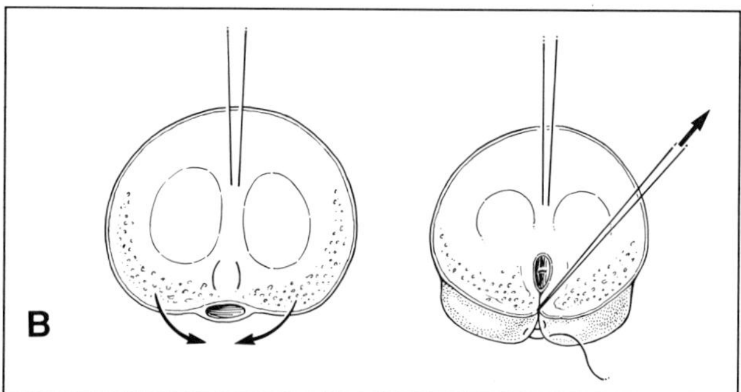


**Fig 19.** Successful MAGPI (**A**) effectively eliminates glans tilt with its urethral advancements and (**B**) provides a tension-free glans wrap of the urethra.

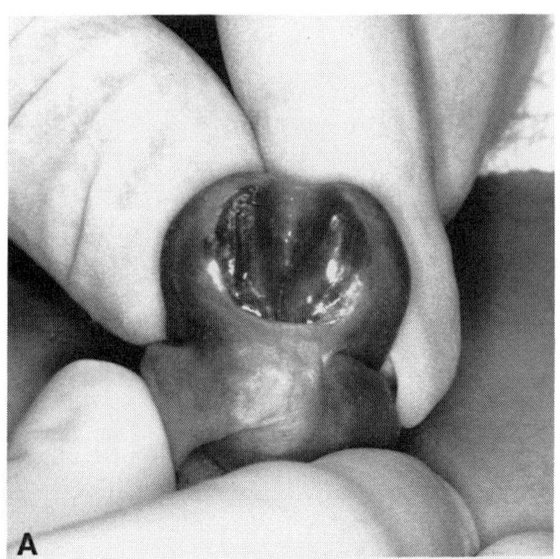


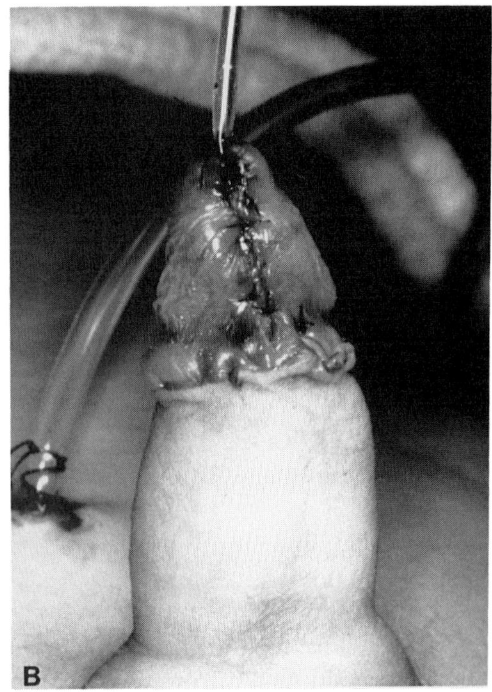


**Fig 20. A,** megameatus hypospadias variant; **B,** immediate perioperative result after pyramid repair. Success depends on a wide, deep glans groove.

the tip of the penis is carried around the edges of the megameatus (Fig 21A,B). Four traction sutures define the megameatus, forming the base of the pyramid (Fig 21C,D). This defines the urethral plate, which is kept wide (12 to 15 mm) and intact dorsally. Laterally, the edges of the glanular groove are deepened to mobilize the glans wings from the adjacent plate.

***Urethroplasty.*** Proximally, the widened distal urethra is detached from the overlying shaft skin, being careful to avoid entering the urethra. Taking down the remainder of the shaft skin is not required if chordee is absent. The urethra is tailored in continuity with the urethral plate by removing a wedge of ventral tissue as far proximal as necessary (Fig 21E). Both can then be tubularized to form the neourethra over a 12 or 14 French catheter, which serves as a useful template for size.

***Glans and Penoplasty.*** The glans wings are approximated in the midline in two layers. A sleeve approximation of the shaft skin completes the repair (Fig 21F).

## The Onlay Island Flap Urethroplasty

The island onlay provides the logical technical progression for distal hypospadias where a MAGPI has been considered but is found to be unsuitable at the time of surgery. In addition, its applications can be extended to more proximal variants when chordee does not present a problem after preservation of the urethral plate (see above).

### Technique

***Incisions and Dissection.*** The urethral plate is kept intact by making two parallel incisions (width 5 to 7 mm) that extend from around the meatus to the glans tip (Fig 22A). The circumferential skin incision meets these 5 mm proximal to the corona and the shaft skin is taken down by sharply defining the plane between Buck's fascia and the corporal bodies. Identifying the proper plane is crucial to preservation of the pedicle of the proposed flap. The glans wings are mobilized by sharp definition of the plane between the tips of the corpora and glans cap, with care taken not to undermine the plate.

***Urethroplasty.*** The urethra is revised by ventral spatulation and excision back to healthy spongiosal tissue (Fig 22B). The length of the defect to be bridged is measured.

***Harvesting the Flap.*** A transverse preputial flap of appropriate length and width is mobilized by developing its midline subcutaneous vascular pedicle completely to the base of the penis (Fig 22C,D,E). The width of the flap depends on the width of the urethral plate. The combined widths should total 12 to 15 mm. Exact sizing of the flap is unnecessary at this juncture since it will be tailored to size during the urethroplasty. Lateral dissections narrow and release the pedicle to help avoid penile torsion after the flap is transferred ventrally.

***Urethroplasty and Completion.*** After its ventral rotation, the onlay is approximated to one side of the urethral plate with a simple running suture. Interrupted sutures mature the flap at the revised proximal meatus and any excess of the onlay is trimmed appropriately (Fig 22F). A running subcuticular inverting stitch is used to close the flap's remaining side. A 10 or 12 French catheter serves as a useful template for gauging size during tailoring of the flap. Redundant subcutaneous tissues of the pedicle provide an additional layer of coverage. After reapproximating the glans wings, midline shaft skin coverage completes the repair (Fig 22G).

### The Perimeatal-Based Flap (Mathieu Procedure)

Perimeatal-based flaps remain a viable option for the repair of distal hypospadias accompanied by a flattened ventral glans and healthy distal shaft skin overlying the urethra. Meatal stenosis is a relative contraindication to the repair. The correction of stenosis, which requires a dorsal meatotomy and advancement, presents technical difficulties during closing of the two adjacent suture lines of the urethroplasty.

#### Technique (Fig. 23)

***Preparation of Plate and Flap.*** The distance from the meatus to the tip of the penis will determine the desired flap length. The plate is defined by making two parallel incisions 5 to 7 mm apart from the tip of the penis to the meatus. These incisions are extended down the penile shaft at the previously determined length and widened somewhat to create the flap. Less width should be taken from the plate to facilitate the subsequent glans wrap (with flap width again determined by the width of the plate, which together should total 12 to 15 mm). The urethral plate is further defined and glans wings mobilized by dissection of the plane between corpora cavernosum and glans cap (Fig 23A).

***Harvesting the Flap.*** Mobilization of the flap is done sharply. Caution is required near the flap elbow at the meatus where the tissues may thin precariously. Traction sutures on the flap and a catheter in the urethra facilitate this dissection. Care should be taken to preserve the vascular subcutaneous tissues adjacent to the meatus that supply the flap.

***Completing the Repair.*** The flap is "flipped" distally to form the ventral neourethra. No tension should be present when it is sutured to the distal extent of the urethral plate. Two layers of running subcuticular sutures are then used to close each side. The glans is reconstructed in two layers and shaft coverage completes the repair (Fig 23B,C). The Byars method is often required to cover the ventral skin defect.

### Transverse Preputial Island Flap (Duckett Procedure)

The transverse island flap (TPIF) remains the procedure of choice for mid- and proximal hypospadias whose chordee persists with the urethral plate intact. Vacularized flaps have been chosen with a preference for transferring and using tissues with their native blood supply whenever possible. The blood supply to the prepuce is reliable, easily delineated, and not as tenuous as some have written. Flaps avoid the crucial process of imbibition and inosculation required of grafts. However, it should be noted that the experience with tubularized free preputial grafts has been excellent in some hands.[43] Grafts can be a reliable alternative if healthy, well-vascularized skin coverage is available. Some hypospadiologists have voiced concerns about the potential for devascularization of the dorsal penile skin with the TPIF, especially skin that is destined to be transferred ventrally for use as skin coverage. However, if the takedown of the flap pedicle is done carefully, skin loss should not pose a problem.[44] Free grafts or the double-faced preputial island flap should be con-

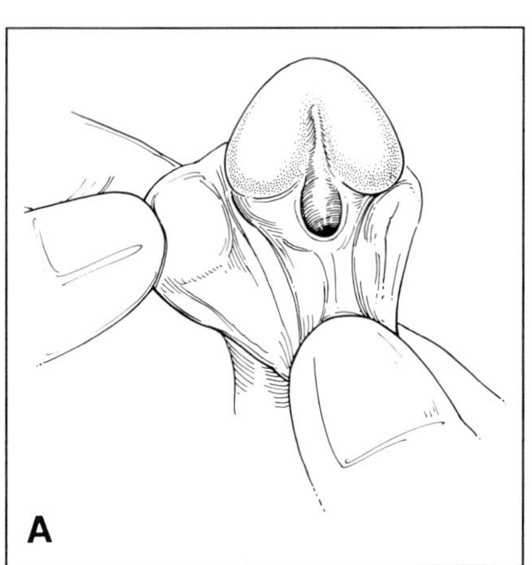


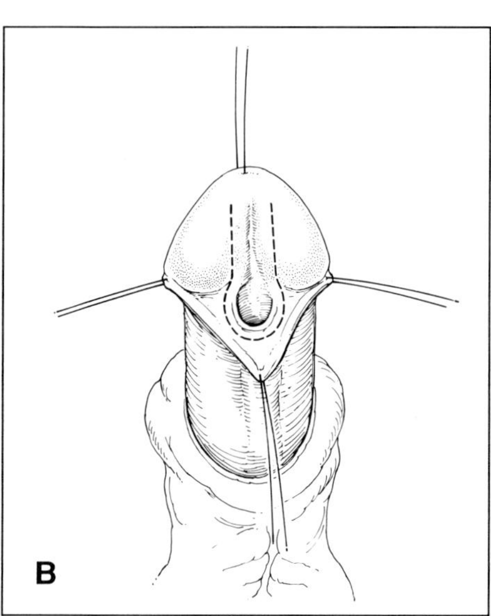


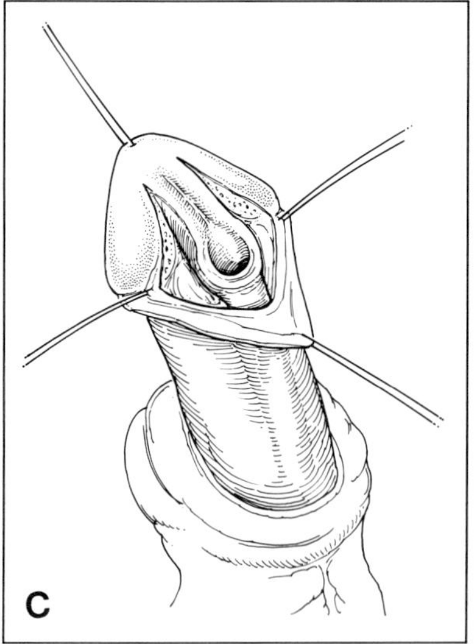


**Fig 21A–C.** Pyramid procedure. **A,** megameatus variant with widely clefted glans and complete prepuce; **B,** tennis racquet incision outlines meatus and urethral plate; **C,** four traction sutures define the base of "pyramid" used for periurethral dissection and urethral mobilization.

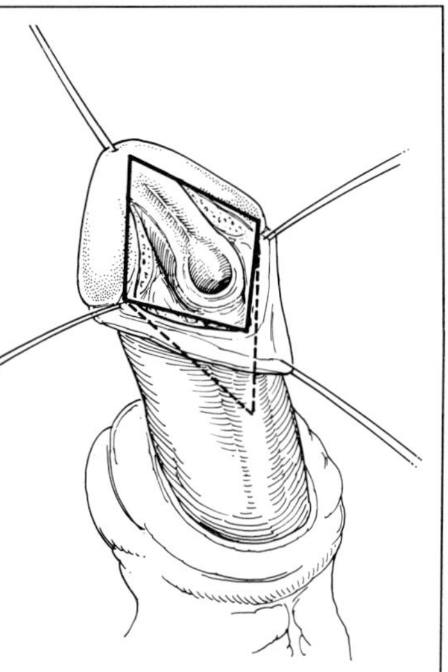

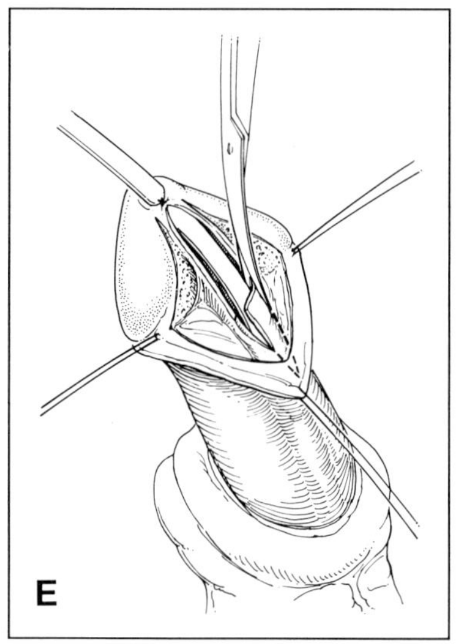


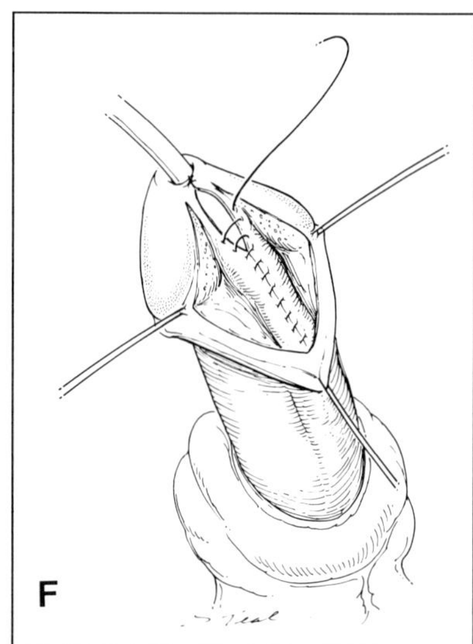


**Fig 21D–F. D,** pyramid shown; **E,** widened distal urethra is tailored to same size as urethral plate by removing its ventral wedge; **F,** proximal urethra tubularized in continuity with urethral plate with running subcuticular suture. Two-layer glans closure and skin cover complete the repair.

sidered when the subcutaneous pedicle to the inner preuce is thin and viability of the shaft skin questionable if a pedicle flap were to be harvested.

#### Technique

***Incisions and Dissection.*** Once the decision to perform the TPIF has been made, the urethra is completely circumscribed by dividing across the urethral plate. The corpora is cleared of any fibrous chordee and additional techniques (plications or corporal grafts) are completed (Fig 24A–E).

***Urethroplasty.*** The now mobilized urethra is spatulated back to healthy tissue and tacked back on the corpora at a more proximal level with interrupted sutures (Fig 24F). This helps to avoid kinking of the future anastomosis. The length of the defect that must be bridged by the new urethra is measured.

***Harvesting the Flap.*** A transverse preputial flap of appropriate length and width is defined on the mucosal (shiny) surface of the prepuce with tacking sutures. After the rectangle is incised, it is helpful to tubularize the flap over an appropriately sized red rubber catheter before its mobilization. Two layers of running subcuticular polydiaxanone are used for its closure, although interrupted sutures are left at each end to allow for any tailoring in length that might become necessary. The completed neourethra is then mobilized, using the catheter for gentle traction, by developing its midline subcutaneous vascular pedicle to the base of the penis. Lateral dissections narrow and release the pedicle to help avoid penile torsion after the flap has been transferred.

***Completing the Repair.*** After ventral rotation and placement of its running suture line against the corpora, the proximal anastomosis of the neourethra can be completed with either an interrupted or running suture. Redundant pedicle is fanned out to cover this area with a second layer of tissue. Distally, the new urethra is positioned between the glans wings where its meatus is matured with fine interrupted chromic sutures (Fig

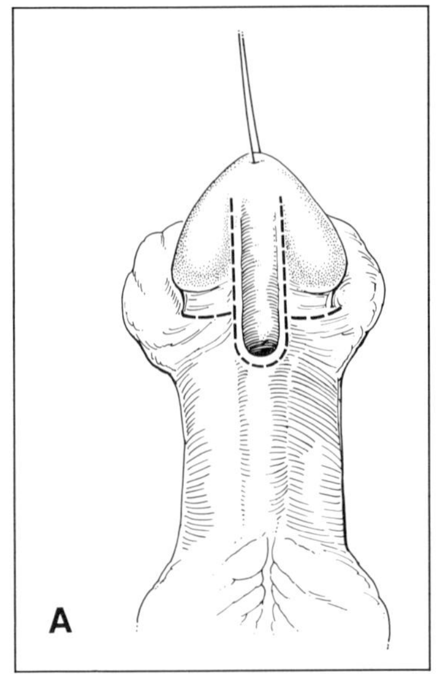


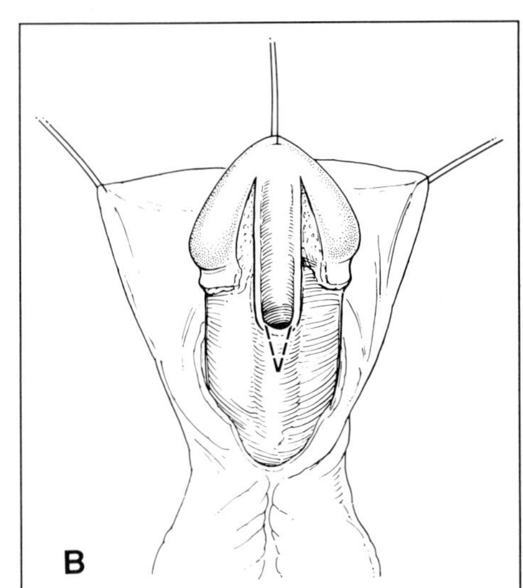


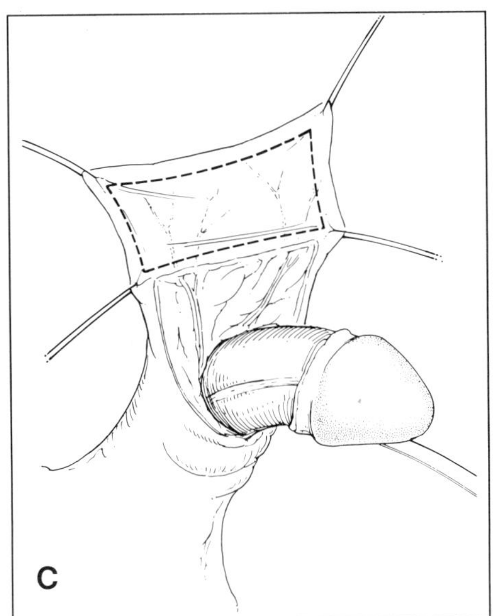


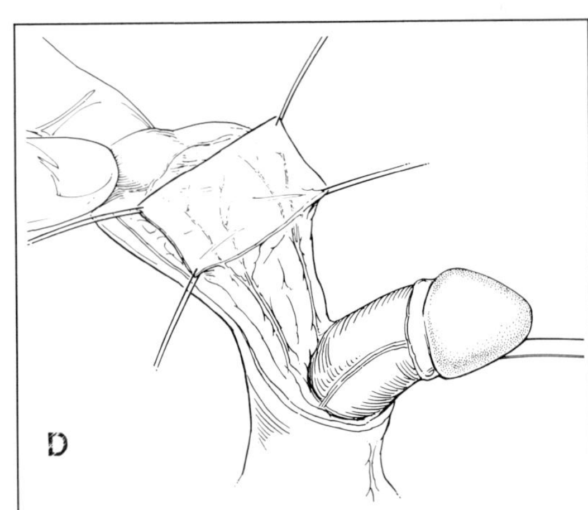


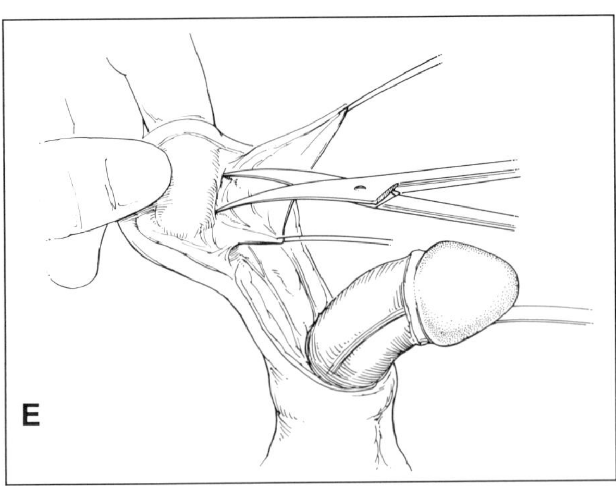


**Fig 22A–E.** OIF technique. **A,** lines of incision define urethral plate; **B,** urethra is spatulated after takedown of the shaft skin; **C,D,E,** island flap harvested from inner prepuce using traction sutures and sharp dissection.

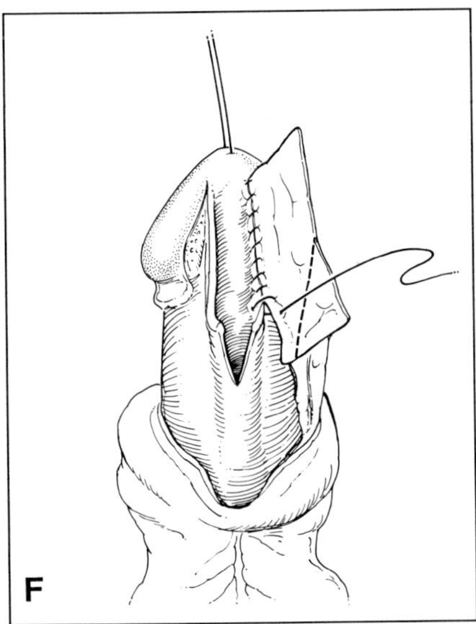


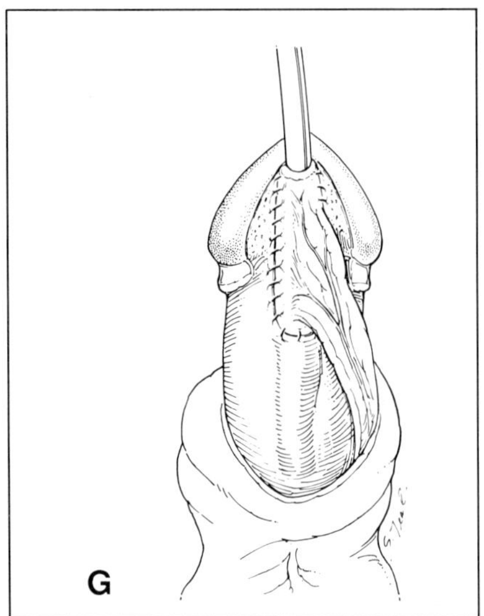


**Fig 22F,G.** After being swung ventrally, the island is tailored and anastomosed to the urethral plate. A two-layer glans closure and coverage of the shaft complete the repair.

24G). Ventral reapproximation of the glans is performed in two layers and skin coverage is completed using either the sleeve or the Byars method.

## Two-Stage Repair

Two-stage urethroplasties continue to have a place in the current management of hypospadias. In the past these repairs were unable to meet the objectives of the modern urethroplasty because of their inability to project the neourethra to the glans tip. However, within the revised framework of generous glans wing mobilization and coverage with transposed foreskin, the cosmetic results achieved with two-stage techniques mimic those of single-stage urethroplasties. The two-stage repair is especially useful for proximal hypospadias found in concert with a small penis or for cases where the available penile skin is insufficient to both reconstruct and cover a neourethra.

### Technique

***First Stage.*** The shaft skin is taken down and the penis straightened. Urethral mobilization, spatulation, and reattachment should be performed in a manner similar to the TPIF if chordee or meatal stenosis is present. The glans is opened in the midline and its wings generously mobilized on either side. The prepuce is split in the dorsum to the level of the sulcus (Fig 25A). Sharply separating its inner and outer layers permits distal extension and unfurls the tissues that ultimately compose the reconstructed urethral plate. A Byars transfer allows the prepuce to meet in the midline and cover the denuded ventral shaft and glans using fine interrupted chromic sutures (Fig 25B).

***Second Stage.*** The repair is completed 6 months later. Two parallel incisions are made 12 to 15 mm apart on the ventral shaft that extend from the tip of the penis proximal to the meatus where they join. The plate is mobilized by dissecting perpendicular to but not beneath its tissues, preserving vascularity. Distally, the glanular portion of the neourethra can be carefully detached and advanced between the glans wings to give a better cosmetic result but extensive detachment should be avoided. Tubularization is completed with two layers of subcuticular polydiaxanone (Fig 25C). A tunica vaginalis flap from an

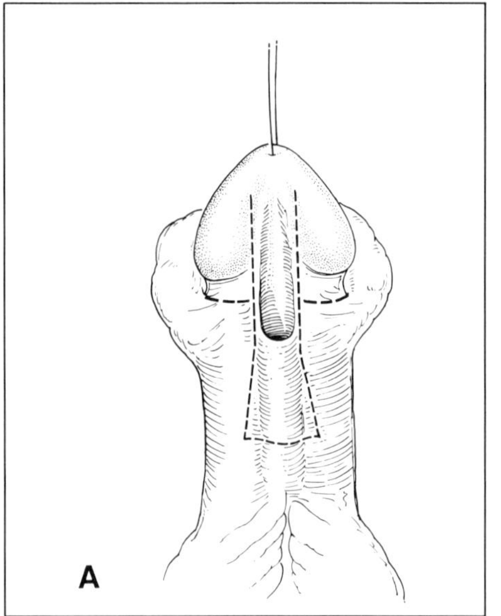


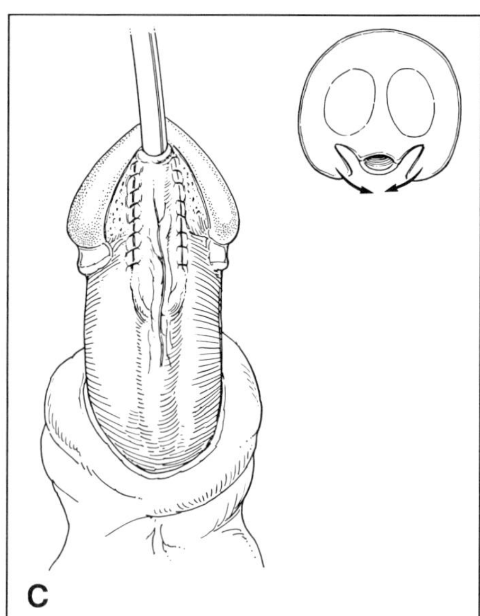


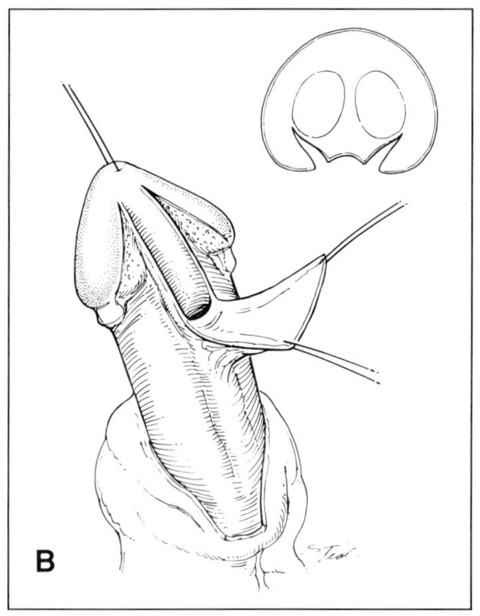


**Fig 23.** Flip-flap (Mathieu) repair. **A,** lines of incision define urethral plate and proximal flap which becomes ventral neourethra; **B,C,** flap mobilized, "flipped" distally, and reanastomosed to urethral plate. Glans wings (insets) must be well mobilized from the plate in this repair and the OIF to enable tension-free anastomosis above neourethra. Glans closure and shaft skin coverage complete the repair.

adjacent gonad provides useful coverage. The remainder of the shaft skin, which has been previously detached from the penile shaft, can be reapproximated over the neourethra with a sleeve or Byars-type repair (Fig 25D).

## Double-Faced Preputial Island Flap

The double-faced preputial flap can be used in cases where skin coverage presents a potential problem. In the double-faced technique tubularization of the mucosal layer of the prepuce is done without isolating the tissue from the outer preputial skin. Instead, the dorsal shaft skin is incised below the prepuce at the coronal level and the entire prepuce is mobilized with its subcutaneous pedicle to the base of the penis. After ventral rotation, the inner layer of the flap is tubularized to create the neourethra and the outer layer serves as coverage for the ventral penile shaft. Coverage of the repair is excellent but the flap rearrangements can be challenging and the cosmetic results of the repair are often less acceptable than those of the TPIF.

## DRAINS, DRESSINGS, AND DISPOSITION

Hypospadias, like so many other surgeries, has seen significant alterations in its management during recent years with the aim of cost containment. Virtually every primary repair is now performed on an outpatient basis but no noticeable increase in morbidity has resulted. Preoperative parental teaching and improvements in drainage and dressings have been instrumental in this regard. With the evolution of operations being performed on increasingly younger children, their management has become simplified and parental anxieties have been greatly assuaged.

Urinary diversion is used for every primary urethroplasty, with the exception of the MAGPI repair. Premature voiding through the reconstructed urethra, especially in the face of distal swelling and obstruction, poses a very real risk factor for fistula formation. A 6 French silastic tube (reinforced ventriculoperitoneal shunt tubing) is positioned across the neourethra and lies proximal to the external sphincter. This soft tube, which is stitched to the glans with 5–0 polypropylene on a tapered needle, provides for continual urinary drainage and has been very effective for younger boys. Bladder spasms are not usually a problem although belladonna and opiate (B & O) suppositories are occasionally required. Acetaminophen for infants or acetaminophen plus codeine is usually sufficient treatment for discomfort.

Diapers and open drainage can be unacceptable for many older patients. In these cases a suprapubic tube or a 13 French urethral splent[45] that lies across the repair but is left distal to the external urethra provides adequate drainage by allowing spontaneous voiding. If the boy can be taught to expect the discomfort that occurs with voiding, the splent is generally well tolerated. However, the experience with this form of diversion in infants and younger children, where discomfort seems inordinately severe, has been unsatisfactory.

There has been a recent trend toward disbanding totally with urinary diversion for midshaft and distal hypospadias repairs where the native urethra has been reconstructed. However, this form of management generally results in infants who experience considerable discomfort with voiding. In addition, some of these children have returned a few years later with fistulas that could only be appreciated once they became toilet-trained and were observed voiding. Whether these would have occurred regardless of drainage can be debated. However, the benefits of diversion continue to outweigh its drawbacks and for the time being is continued for 7 to 10 days, depending on the extensiveness of the repair and interval assessments of its healing.

A broad-spectrum antibiotic (cephalosporin) is given at the beginning of every case and trimethoprim-sulfamethoxazole is maintained as suppression for open urinary drainage. The medication is continued a few days after the tube is removed to cover any residual infection/colonization. Pubertal males should also be instructed on preoperative antiseptic showers to lower colonization counts of the perineal flora. Finally, erections occasionally present a problem for the older boy immediately after surgery but can usually be controlled with amyl nitrate inhalers or diazepam sedation.

The penile dressing after any repair accomplishes three functions: (1) immobilization of the penis and its drainage tube; (2) protection of delicate suture lines; and (3) containment of edema while providing hemostasis. A transparent, permeable dressing such as Op-Site is ideal in this regard and applies adequate compression to the penile shaft and glans without causing undue tension (Fig 26). Maximal penile swelling and edema generally begin to subside 48 to 72 hours after surgery. The repair is kept dry for 3 to 5 days when soaking in a warm bath is initiated. This loosens the adhesive dressing and facilitates its removal at home. The child returns a few days later for postoperative evaluation and

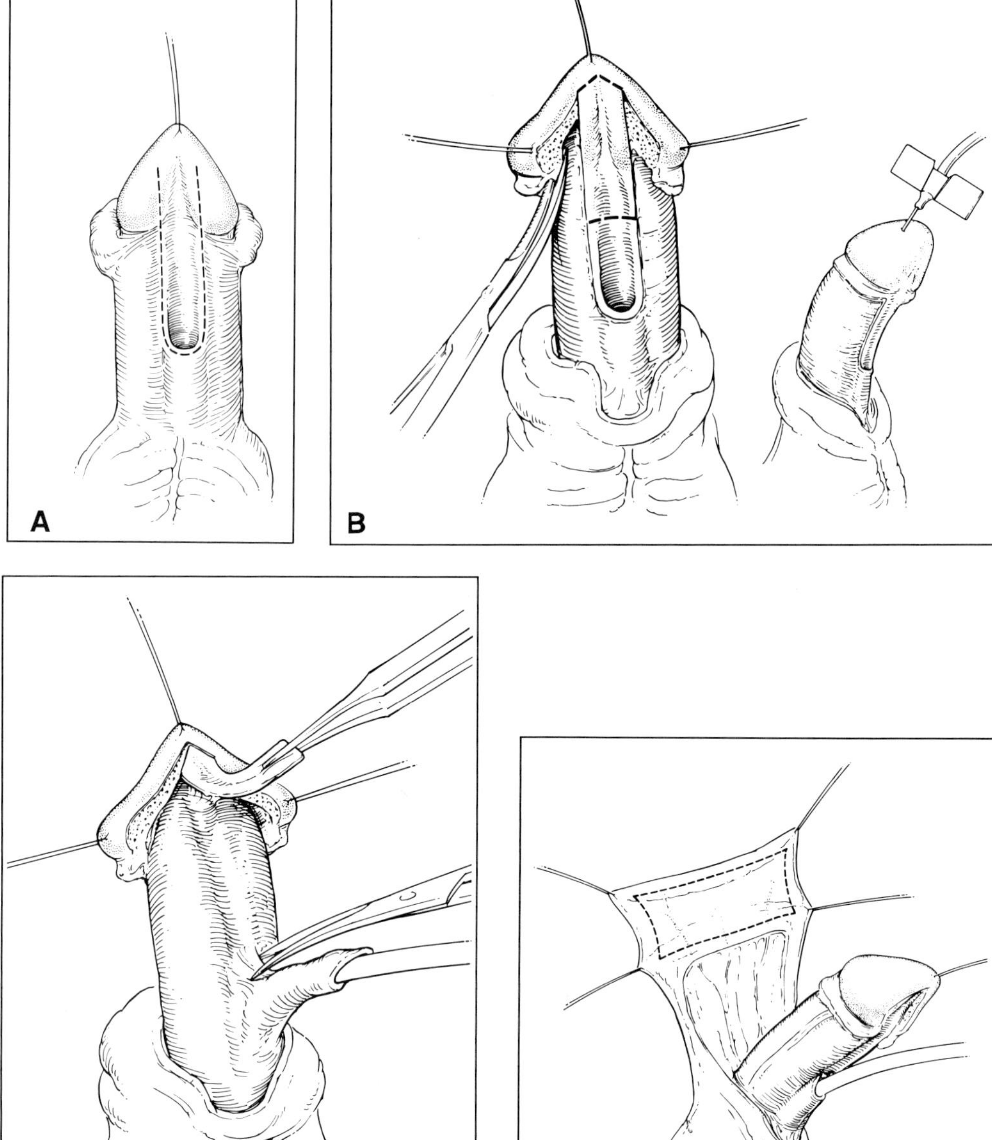


**Fig 24A–D.** TPIF (Duckett) repair. **A,** lines of incision outline and preserve urethral plate; **B,C,** saline erection documents persistent curvature with plate intact requiring its excision (dotted lines) and urethral mobilization; **D,** after correction of chordee, inner preputial flap proposed for tubularization is outlined. Mobilization is done in similar fashion to Figure 22C–E, p. 28.

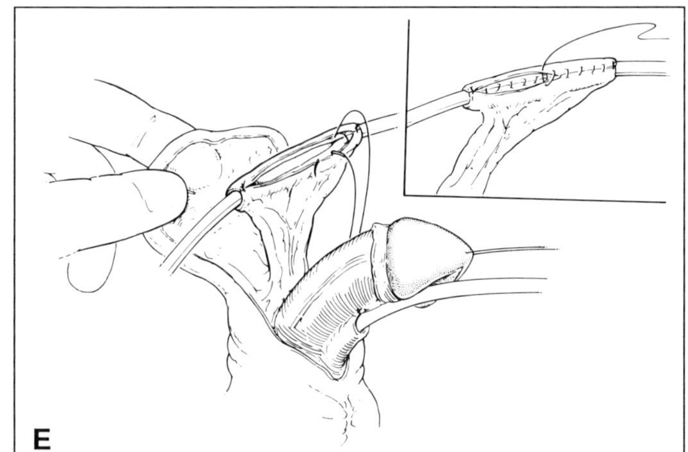


**Fig 24E–G. E,** flap is tubularized in two layers (inset); **F,** native urethra is tacked back to the corpora and spatulated before anastomosing the neourethra; **G,** preputial tube matured without tension to the penile tip between widely splayed glans wings. Two-layer glans closure and skin reapproximation complete the repair.

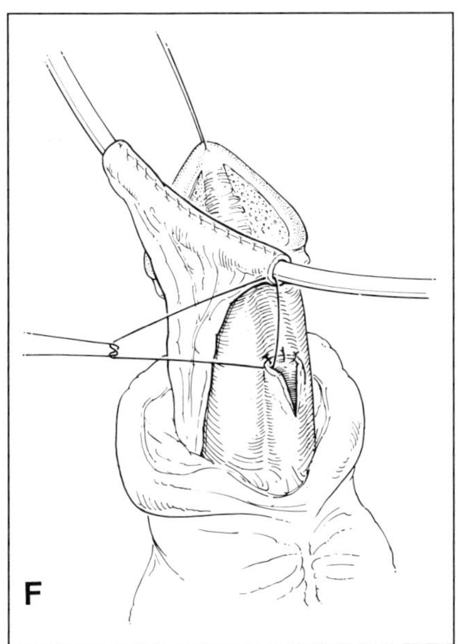


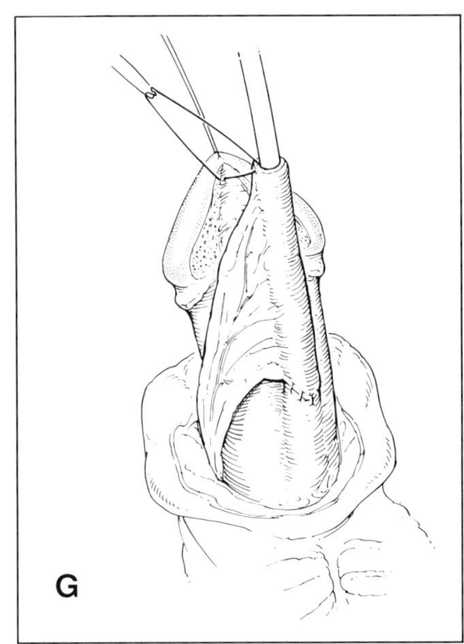


removal of his drainage tube when one has been left. Induration and swelling are anticipated but this should resolve during the next few weeks unless complications have occurred. A return visit is planned for 6 weeks and 6 months later unless there are problems in the interim. Parents are asked to gauge the quality of the stream and erections if possible. Routine dilatations or urethral calibrations are not routinely done unless a complication is suspected.

## MANAGEMENT OF EARLY COMPLICATIONS

Minor problems during the early postoperative period commonly occur. Fortunately, the penis is a relatively forgiving organ and the majority of problems with healing require no more than supportive measures. *Hematomas,* which first become apparent after the dressing is removed, usually organize and resolve but serial checks

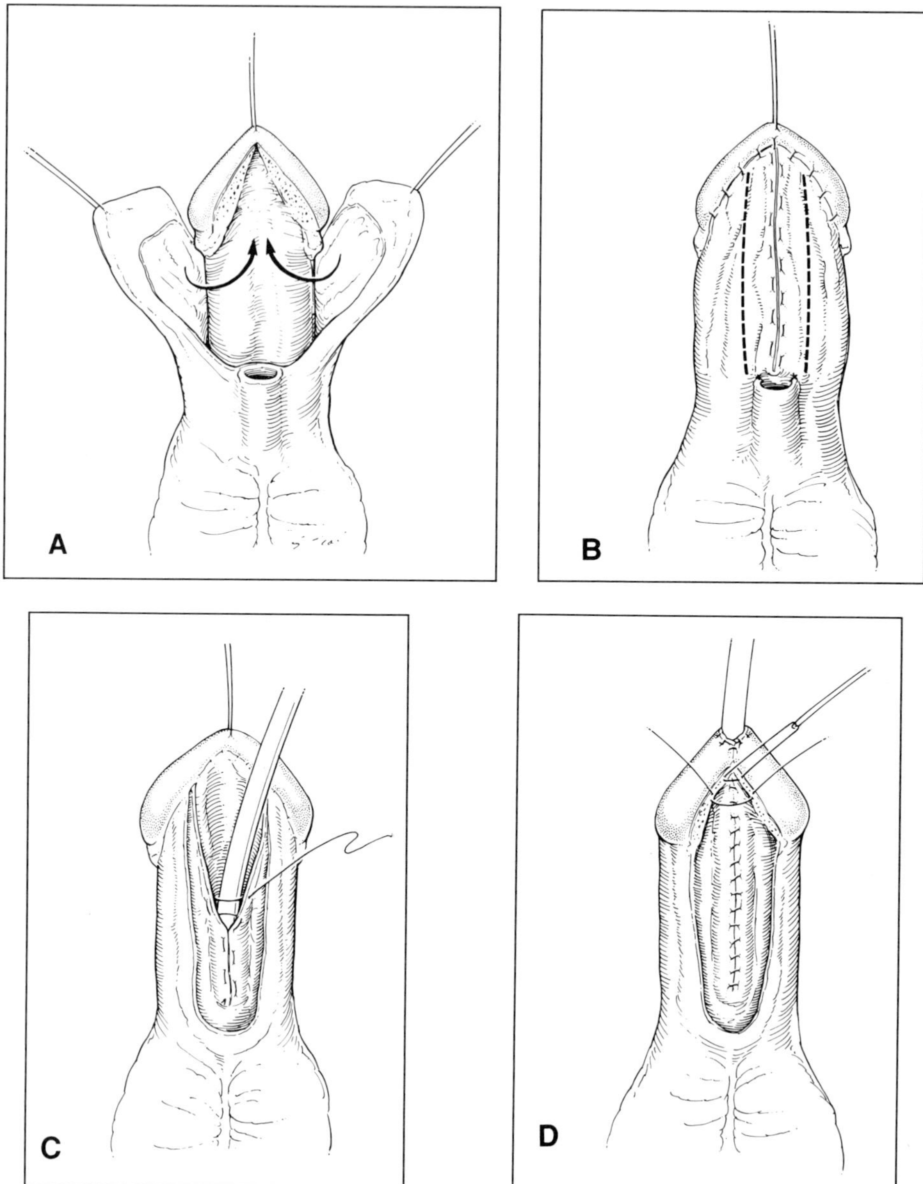


**Fig 25.** Two-stage repair. **A,** paucity of penile skin after chordee corrected. The glans is split and preputial skin unfurled and swung ventrally after dorsal relaxing incision; **B,** available skin covers ventral shaft and glans recreating urethral plate in anticipation of second-stage tubularization (dotted lines) 6 months later; **C,** second stage. Urethral plate incised, mobilized, and tubularized; **D,** mobilized glans wings reapproximated over tubularized neourethra.

are required lest they become infected. *Skin loss* results from tissue ischemia. Risk factors include hematoma, excessive tension, constrictive dressings, or vascular compromise during harvest of a preputial flap. In cases where skin loss or wound separation has occurred, the defect usually fills in with granulation tissue. Grafts are unnecessary since healthy reepithelialization with little scarring usually occurs. Multiple layers of

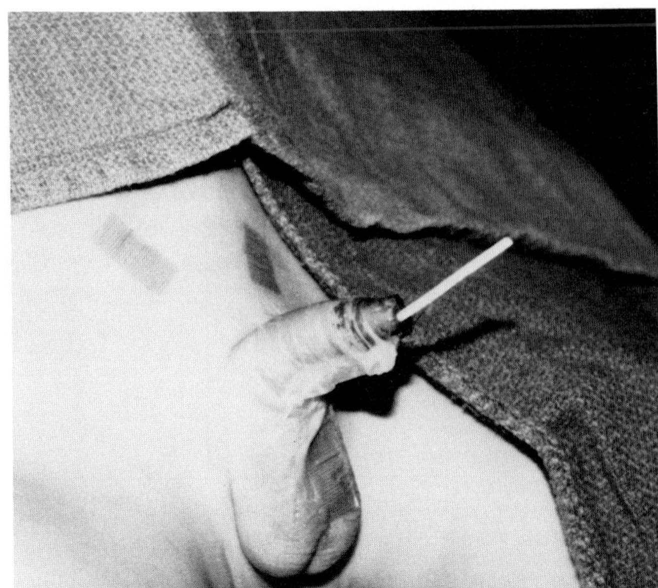

**Fig 26.** Bio-occlusive dressing and Silastic stent provide effective immobilization and drainage after repair of proximal hypospadias.

underlying urethral coverage assume additional importance to neourethral salvage in cases where skin viability is questioned. *Wound infections* are largely superficial and usually respond to local measures including frequent warm tub baths and topical antibiotics. If a more serious infection is suspected, the wound should be opened to establish drainage and a culture sent. Systemic antibiotics are given to stem the local progression of the process while tissue debridement is also occasionally necessary.

*Urethral fistulas* are typically the most ominous problem encountered early after surgery. While an exact etiology can never be defined, one or more of the three risk factors cited above can usually be implicated in their formation. Acutely, fistulas usually become evident upon discontinuation of urinary diversion when leakage along the ventral suture line becomes apparent, usually at the site of the original meatus. The affected penis exhibits an impressive amount of induration and swelling during the early stages of fistula maturation. This should be expected and the family assured that the child's cosmetic appearance will improve dramatically as the reaction subsides. Urinary drainage can be reestablished using a suprapubic tube, transurethral feeding tube, or Foley catheter but rarely resolves the problem. Secondary blowouts of proximal suture lines are common causes of fistula formation and the meatus should be checked for stenosis, edema, or plugging with dried secretions. If distal obstruction can be managed with periodic dilatation, spontaneous closure sometimes occurs.

## SURGICAL APPROACH TO PERSISTENT COMPLICATIONS

Adherence to the principles in technique and urethroplasty selection discussed above serve to minimize the incidence of complications and need for reoperative surgery. Nevertheless, complications occur in even the best of hands. A reapplication of those very principles will optimize subsequent surgical results. One of the commonest errors observed in referred cases is in the timing of corrective surgery for complications, especially fistulas. Other than local care, the initial management of most complications usually entails patience alone. This can be a frustrating recommendation for all the parties involved. Nevertheless, *no attempt at corrective surgery* should be made until penile induration and edema have completely resolved and the surrounding tissues are healthy, soft, and pliable.

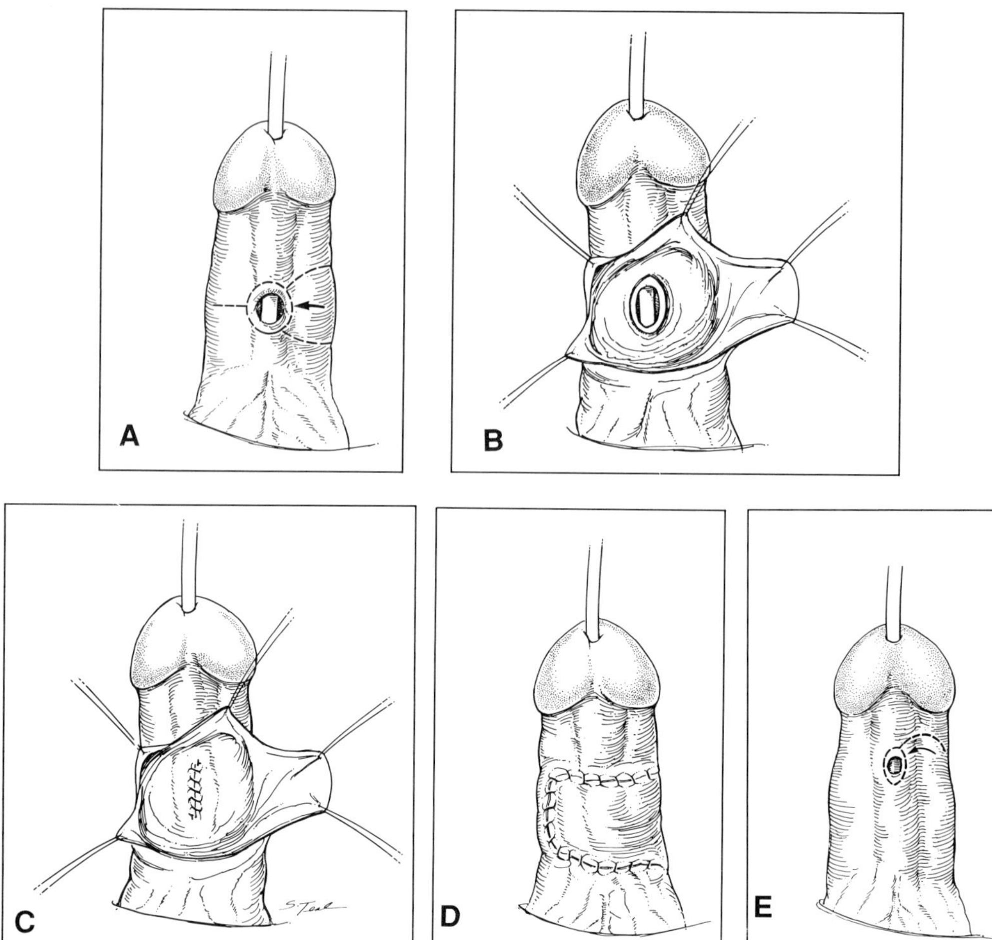


**Fig 27.** Urethral fistula. **A,** fistula outlined in continuity with flaps proposed for skin coverage; **B,C,** after mobilization and revision, running suture gives water-tight closure; **D,** skin flaps provide additional layers of healthy coverage; **E,** rotational flaps are also effective.

Maximal healing usually occurs by 6 months but reoperations should be deferred for up to a year in patients who have had a number of previous surgeries.

## Urethrocutaneous Fistulas

Urethrocutaneous fistulas represent the most common complication of hypospadias surgery. Most can be managed with simple excision and closure, although the position, size, and number of fistulas will influence the preference in repair. Before addressing the fistula or fistulas, stenosis or strictures of the distal urethra and meatus must be ruled out. The urethra can be adequately assessed for valve-like flaps or diverticula by calibrating the urethra with a bougie-à-boule and assessing the course of the fistulas using a lacrimal duct probe. Cystoscopy is traumatic and provides little additional information. When distal obstruction is present and must be addressed, it is usually appropriate to defer correcting the fistula for a later date. Operating on both ends of the urethra simultaneously appears to increase morbidity. The swelling and obstruction that inevitably results from distal manipulations jeopardize the more proximal fistula repair with higher urethral voiding pressures and a potential blowout recurrence.

Identification of any occult fistulas can be made by occluding the proximal urethra using the finger and injecting saline into the urethra with a feeding tube. After circumscribing the ostium, the fistulous tract is sharply dissected to its confluence with the urethra. A 3 French feeding tube, which is placed in the tract and sutured to its rim, provides traction. After mobilization, the tract is excised flush with the urethra. Any adjoining urethral redundancy or diverticulum that is present should also be revised. The edges of healthy urethra are inverted using fine (6–0 or 7–0) polydiaxanone sutures. Additional layers of adjacent subcutaneous tissues and skin are mobilized to help buttress the area. Minor rotational flaps or Y-V advancements of the penile shaft skin provide useful coverage of most fistulas and help eliminate overlapping suture lines (Fig 27) where a success rate of 95% to 98% should be expected.

Certain types of fistulas demand special attention. *Fistulas at the urethral meatus* or the coronal sulcus, regardless of size, can be the most challenging to repair. The adjacent tissues are often unhealthy and difficult to mobilize, and sloughs of the bridge of skin existing between the tract and the meatus are commonplace when simple closures are attempted. Instead, these fistulas should be brought in continuity with the meatus by incising the skin bridge. The resulting defect can then be repaired by tubularizing the defect in a manner similar to the pyramid procedure or by using a perifistula-based flap or onlay of redundant shaft skin. For *larger fistulas* simple Johannsen-type turn-ins can be effective but risk urethral narrowing at the site of fistula closure unless carefully performed. If the potential for luminal compromise exists, an onlay of adjacent penile skin or redundant skin from elsewhere along the penile shaft can be employed (see below). This maneuver is especially helpful when fistulas are associated with adjacent distal urethral strictures that must also be repaired. Finally, when *multiple fistulas* are found in close proximity, individual closures are difficult and can jeopardize the repair of adjoining tract(s). As an alternative, it is often better to incise the tissue between the different tracts. This creates one large fistula that can be repaired using a Johannsen repair or the onlay flap technique.

### Urethral Strictures

Strictures are seen at any position along a repair but usually occur in the region of the original meatus. Prior errors implicated in later stricture formation at this level include inadequate spatulation of the meatus and angulation of a tubularized pedicle flap. In other instances infection, fistulization, ischemia, or inadequate sizing can lead to neourethral narrowing. Late presentations, which include a decreased force in stream and straining to void, are common.

The results of treatment using "less invasive" techniques are somewhat unpredictable. In one series, a 65% success rate was cited with a single urethral dilatation under anesthesia[46] and gentle dilatation represents a reasonable initial step in management. When the stricture is more extensive or has recurred, direct visual urethrotomy can also be effective. The long-term success rates with visual urethrotomy for childhood strictures are reportedly as high as 80%[47] but the experience with urethrotomy for postoperative strictures has not been as encouraging. Repeated urethrotomies should be avoided to minimize secondary corporal fibrosis.

Dilatation or urethrotomy may provide temporary relief of symptoms but recalcitrant or extensive strictures usually require formal urethroplasty. This should not be done in the setting of any type of recent manipulation. Instead, urinary diversion employing a suprapubic tube or even perineal urethrostomy is recommended to allow for healing of the affected tissues. Primary excision with reanastomosis can be attempted for small strictures but mobilization and revision of previous urethroplasties is usually difficult or impossible. As an alternative, vascularized flaps are preferred whenever they can be harvested from redundant penile skin (Fig 28). Onlays that preserve the urethral plate can be used for smaller strictures and complete

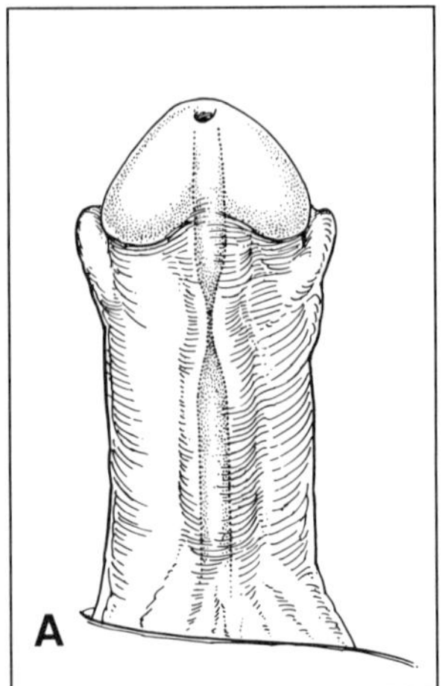

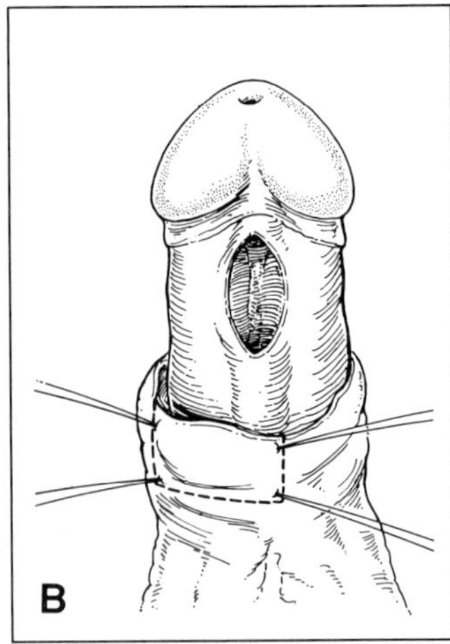

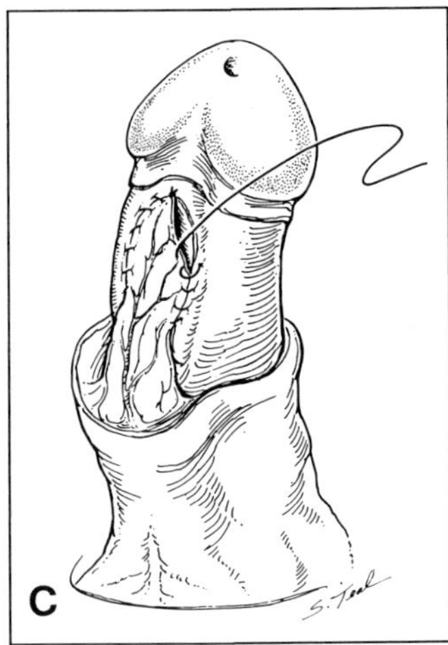


**Fig 28. A,** urethral stricture; **B,** after widely spatulating the stricture to healthy tissue on each end, a flap of redundant shaft skin is harvested with its pedicle; **C,** patch-graft urethroplasty using flap completes the repair.

tubularized flaps are used to bridge more extensive defects when longer strictures must be excised. Otherwise, the two-stage Johanssen procedure remains a useful alternative for extensive or recurrent strictures.[48] Here the stricture urethra is opened along its length and its ventral edges are matured to the adjacent penile skin. Six months later, the ventral plate is mobilized and tubularized in continuity with the proximal urethra and distal urethra, which has been kept intact.

## Meatal Stenosis

The distalmost manifestation of stricture, meatal stenosis, can be caused by transient edema, neourethral ischemia with scarring, or a poorly constructed glans tunnel or wrap. When stenosis is suspected, the meatus can be calibrated by passing an 8 or 10 French taper-tipped Hodgson sound.[49] Daily meatal dilations using the tip of the sound, an ophthalmic ointment tube, or fine feeding tube has provided a solution for many patients. For others a formal meatoplasty is required. The scarred meatus is incised dorsally or ventrally, depending on its position relative to the tip of the glans. The defect that is created in the cicatrix is closed by reapproximation of the urethral mucosa to the skin in a Heinecke–Mikulicz fashion, in effect advancing the urethra. In rare instances, distal stenosis involves the entire glanular neourethra. When this is the case the glans must be filleted open, its wings mobilized, and an onlay island or meatal-based flap used to augment the distal urethra.[50]

## Persistent Chordee

Persistent penile curvature can usually be attributed to an inadequate release of chordee at prior surgery. Successful correction can be attained by following the sequence in management outlined for primary chordee without hypospadias, although recurrent postsurgical chordee presents a more difficult problem. Attempts at mobilizing the urethra are usually futile. Transection, with hopes of salvaging the distal portion of a repair, risks neourethral viability but can be attempted if the glanular configuration is acceptable and the urethra appears healthy. Instead, for milder degrees of chordee, it is sometimes simpler and more effective to perform dorsal plications. Otherwise, the urethra should be discarded and a total urethral and glanular reconstruction performed after the chordee is corrected. In these cases a bladder mucosal graft is often necessary in the face of inadequate penile skin.

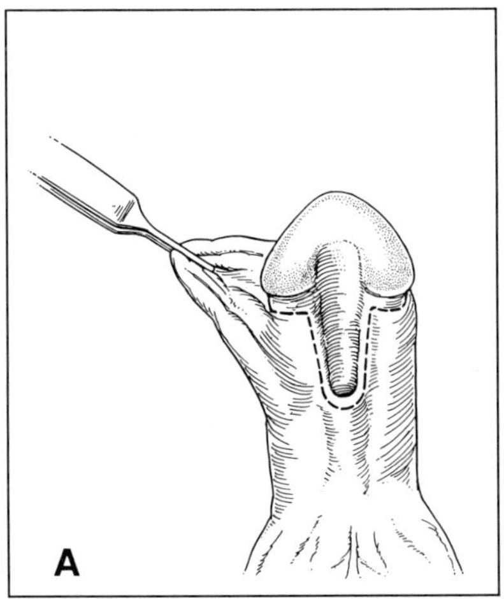


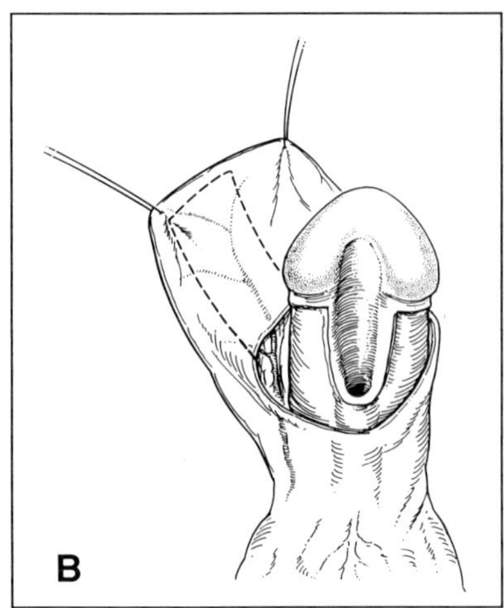


**Fig 29.** Retrusive meatus. **A,** urethral plate outlined. After breakdown, redundant shaft skin usually remains in continuity with its original blood supply; **B,** flap is mobilized and used in onlay-type repair after spatulating urethra.

## Miscellaneous Conditions

The hair-bearing potential of genital and extragenital skin is difficult to assess in the younger child. When follicles have been incorporated in an earlier urethroplasty, pubertal males will present with hair protruding from the meatus (the so-called bearded meatus) or recurrent urinary tract infections from the formation of intraurethral calculi on hair. Local measures such as cystoscopic depilation have been attempted with equivocal success. However, if the symptoms persist, excision and replacement of the involved urethra becomes necessary.

The *retrusive meatus* is an avoidable sequelae of an improperly applied MAGPI urethroplasty but can also occur with other repairs where problems in healing of the distal neourethra or its overlying glans has occurred. Symptoms are not usually a problem but the cosmetic drawbacks of this complication usually warrant its correction. Minor degrees of retraction can be approached by repeating the MAGPI sequence with good results if the urethral mobility and glanular quality are acceptable. More proximal retractions are best managed using pedicled onlay or perimeatal-based flaps to reconstruct the ventral neourethra (Fig 29).

*Urethral diverticula* are probably more common than generally supposed and in one series were seen in 30% of referred failures of hypospadias repair.[51] Urinary tract infection, a decreased force of stream, and postvoid dribbling are common presentations. The latter occurs as pooled urine slowly drains from the diverticulum. Ballooning of the urethra can be appreciated during voiding, and stones, the product of urinary stasis, are occasionally palpable. As a temporizing measure, the patient can be taught to "milk" the diverticulum using digital compression. Definitive correction consists of a ventral penile incision that allows excellent exposure of the involved urethra. Diverticula can be revised in a variety of ways after excision of their redundancy and use of the excess tissue to reconfigure the urethra.[52] A heightened suspicion and treatment of associated fistulas, strictures, and distal obstruction is also required in the management of diverticula.

## The Onlay Island Principle in Failed Urethroplasties

Successful correction of failed hypospadias repairs is contingent on a well-conceived utilization of "all the available material." Because of the nature of many

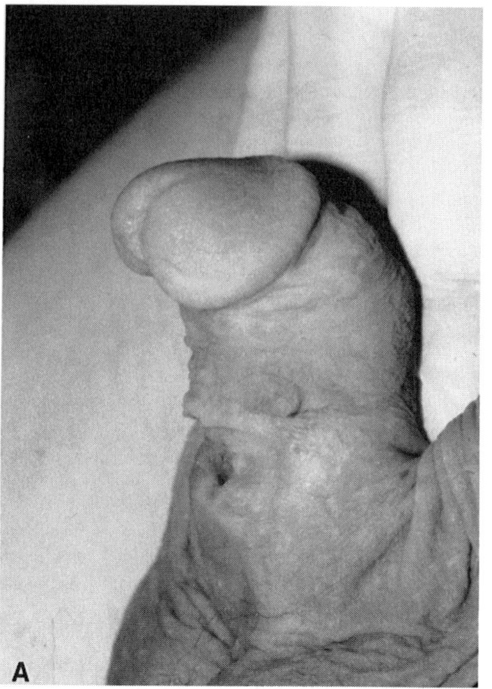


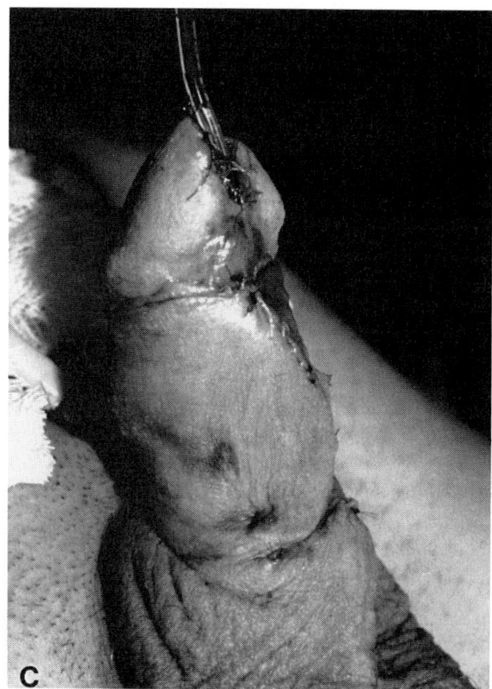


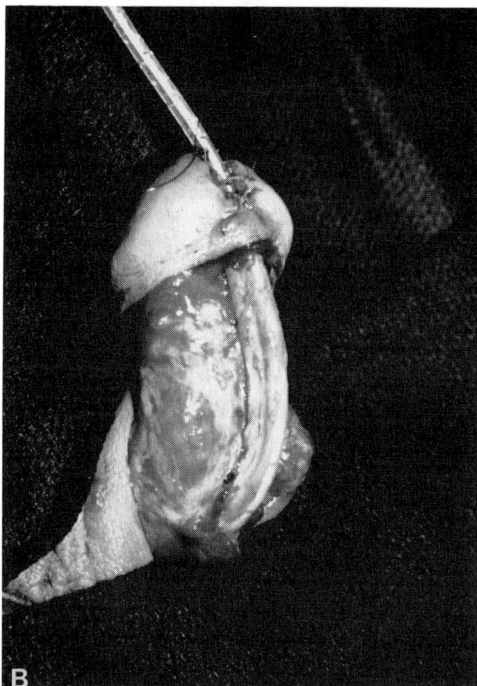


**Fig 30.** Bladder mucosal graft urethroplasty. **A,** preoperative appearance shows severe complications of multiple prior hypospadias repairs including persistent chordee and proximal meatus; **B,** bladder mucosal graft in place and chordee corrected; **C,** previously degloved shaft skin provides excellent coverage of repair.

complications and their antecedant urethroplasties, excess shaft skin is often present that remains in continuity with its original vascular pedicle at the distal extent of the external pudendal artery. These randomly located vascular flaps can be safely mobilized to serve as onlays after being tailored to fit the urethral plate, which is usually intact, healthy, and well vascularized. Little or no chordee must be present in order to apply the onlay island principle effectively. Ideal candidates include patients with the retrusive meatus, urethral stricture, or who present with a lengthy urethral defect between the proximal meatus and patent glanular urethra.

## COMPLEX REDO HYPOSPADIAS

Patients who arrive with a variety of different complications from prior hypospadias surgery were formerly known as hypospadias cripples. The classification of *complex redo hypospadias* has since been adopted for the patient's sake. Past histories are typically replete with a multitude of previous "minor" procedures that attempted to alleviate an evolving mixture of problems including stricture, fistulas, and chordee. As is often the case, usually only a more aggressive surgical solution will resolve the patient's dilemma. The key is replacing the involved urethra, which is typically scarred and unhealthy. Whenever possible, genital skin should be used for correction of these problems. However, the excess shaft skin in these cases is usually deficient or unsuitable for urethral reconstruction. In the future, grafts of autologous cultured skin might provide the solution to this tissue deficiency.[53] However, until these are proven to be a more viable alternative, the bladder mucosal graft urethroplasty provides a logical solution to the problem (Fig 30). The characteristics of bladder mucosa closely approximate those of native urethra. The tissue should not suffer from the effects of chronic exposure to urine and its thinness is conducive to the establishment of neovascularity. Disadvantages include the tissue's pliability and tendency to shrink, making fashioning of any neourethra an inexact science. Proliferative tendencies also occur at the tip of the penis for reasons that remain unclear. Despite these drawbacks, the performance of bladder mucosal grafts has been commendable when one considers the problems being addressed.[54]

### Bladder Mucosal Graft Technique

**Preparing the Graft Bed.** A circumferential incision is made proximal to the coronal sulcus and the shaft skin is taken down to the base of the penis. The skin should be left as thick as possible to provide viable coverage of the repair. The damaged urethra is discarded and taken back proximally to healthy tissue. Distally, removal is facilitated by extending an incision in the ventral midline and circumferentially dissecting the urethra from the surrounding glans cap. After preparing the graft bed, the penis is wrapped in moist sponges and set aside while the graft is harvested. In occasional cases, the recipient penile graft bed is extensively scarred and may not provide adequate neovascularity for a free graft. If vascular suitability is questionable, a two-stage approach should be used to maximize the chances of graft take. The penis is straightened, available shaft skin rearranged on its ventral surface, and a proximal urethrostomy matured until a later date.

**Harvesting the Graft.** The bladder is exposed through a transverse Pfannenstiel incision and the graft retrieved by one of two approaches (Fig 31A,B). The bladder can be entered immediately and an appropriately sized strip of mucosa sharply excised from one of its lateral walls. Alternatively, the muscularis alone is incised and its plane with the underlying mucosa defined by blunt and sharp dissection, creating the "dome cyst." Stay sutures help to define the limits of the graft before the mucosa is incised and the bladder is decompressed. Additional length can be obtained by extending the dissection superiorly into and around the dome (Fig 31C,D). The bladder mucosa should be moistened frequently and handled with fine forceps to minimize trauma.

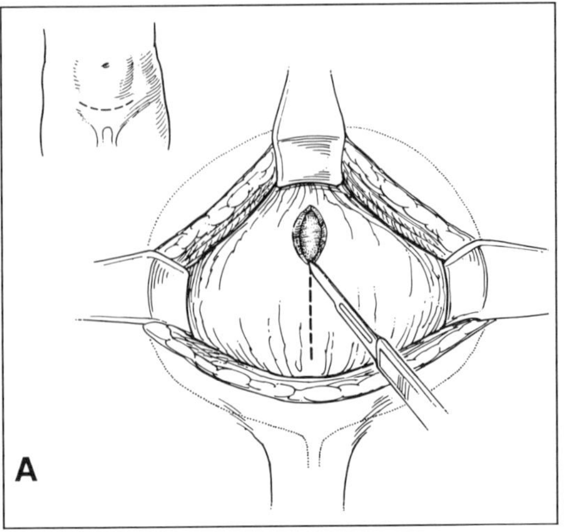


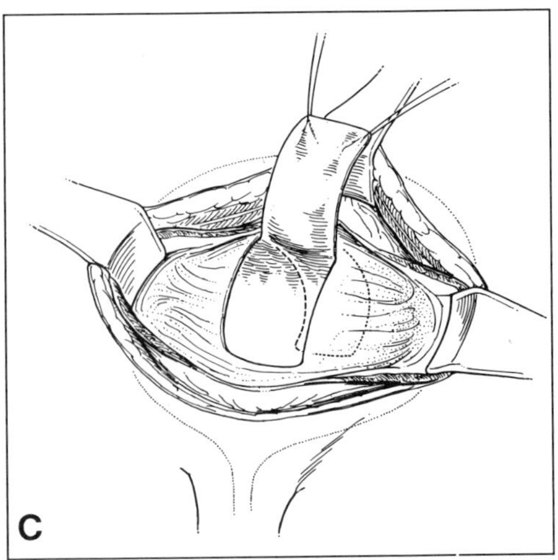


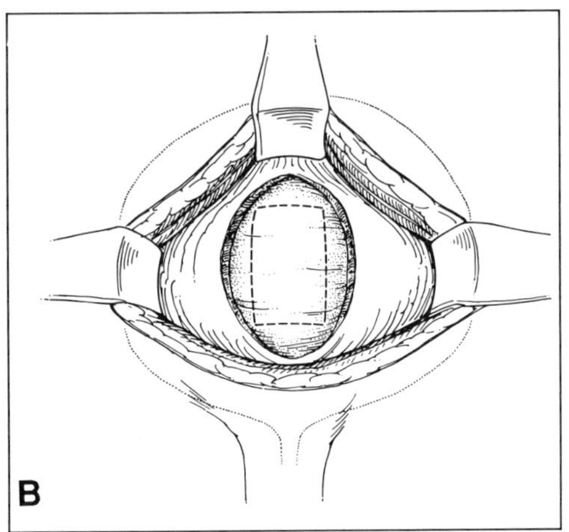


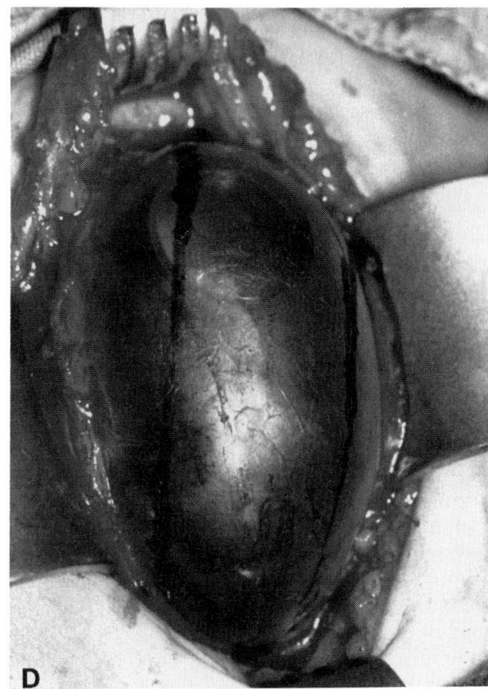


**Fig 31.** Harvesting bladder mucosal graft. **A,** muscularis of bladder incised after making Pfannenstiel incision; **B,** bladder mucosa exposed and graft marked out; **C,** additional length can be obtained from the bladder dome; **D,** dome mucosal cyst.

**Tailoring the Graft.** Bladder mucosal grafts contract but not as much as reconstructive urologists assumed from their earlier experiences with the tissue. Although the recommendations are empirical, a 20 to 24 French urethra is planned for an adult by tailoring the graft to a stretched width of approximately 30 mm. In smaller children a 17-mm-wide graft ideally translates to a 12 French urethra. Bladder mucosa is highly elastic and should be gently stretched when being measured. However, when errors are made in this understandably inexact portion of the technique, an excess is preferable to a paucity. The mucosa is tubularized with two layers of run-

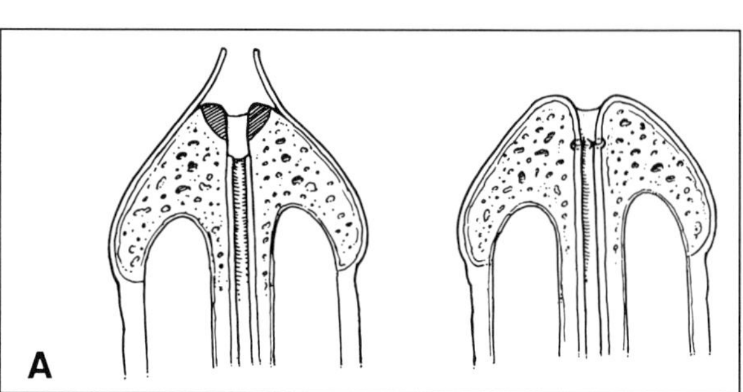


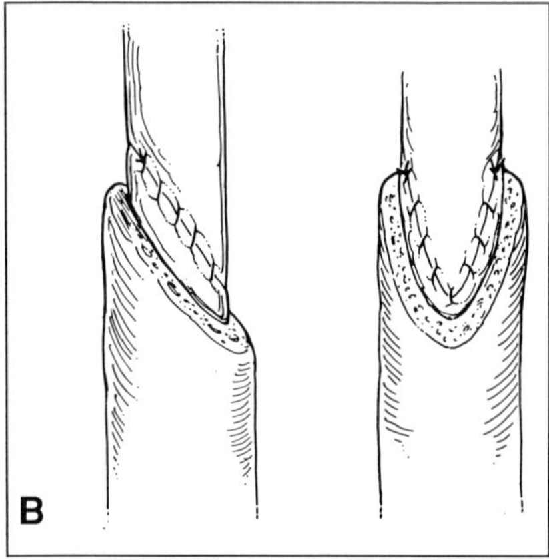


**Fig 32.** **A,** mucosa-to-mucosa anastomosis of graft to native urethra may help minimize stenosis; **B,** bladder mucosa graft recessed at glans tip in hopes of eliminating meatal reaction of the tissue.

ning polydiaxanone suture over an appropriately sized red rubber catheter that serves as a template for size.

**Completing the Repair.** The completed graft is positioned between the generously mobilized glans wings and matured at the meatus. Performing this portion of the repair initially allows the graft to be stretched down to the proximal anastomosis and minimizes any redundancy in length, perhaps lessening the risks of meatal prolapse. Proximally, a widely spatulated anastomosis is created and a few millimeters of spongiosum is resected on the borders of the urethra to assure a mucosal-to-mucosal anastomosis. Glans tissue is also resected from beneath the epithelium at the meatus in the hope of recessing the graft and minimizing stenosis[55] (Fig 32). Placing a skin graft at the end of the tubularized bladder mucosa has been suggested as a means of avoiding meatal problems with bladder mucosa but has not been successful in most cases.

**Postoperative Management.** A suprapubic tube provides adequate urinary drainage. Subcutaneous drains are not routinely used. A multifenestrated 8 French silicone stent is positioned distal to the external sphincter and across the graft to allow for the drainage of secretions. Its tip is liberally coated with antibiotic ointment to prevent encrustations. Complete bedrest for 3 to 4 days maximizes immobilization of the graft and protects fragile microcapillary ingrowth. The penile dressing is removed on the fifth postoperative day and warm soaks are begun. On the tenth postoperative day, the urethral stent is removed and a voiding trial given by clamping the suprapubic tube.

**Results.** An overall 40% complication rate has been cited in the literature with nearly two thirds of these classified as minor, requiring little or no revision. Problems at the neomeatus have been by far the most common complications seen. The cause of the poor performance of the tissue at this position remains unclear but daily meatal dilation for approximately 6 months has provided an effective solution to the problem. Other less common complications of bladder mucosal graft urethroplasties, including fistulas, strictures, etc., can be managed in a fashion similar to that described above for more standard urethroplasties. In the worst case scenario, that of complete graft failure, harvesting one bladder mucosal graft does not preclude the option of taking another at a later date for a second attempt at reconstruction.

## REFERENCES


1. Sweet RA, Scrott HG, Kurland R, et al. Study of the incidence of hypospadias in Rochester, Minnesota 1940–1970, and a case control comparison of possible etiologic factors. *Mayo Clin Proc.* 1974;49:52–59.
2. Kaplan GW, Lamm DL. Embryogenesis of chordee. *J Urol.* 1975;114:769–772.
3. Bellinger MF. Embryology of the male external genitalia. *Urol Clin North Am.* 1981;8:375–382.
4. Duckett JW, Keating MA. Technical challenge of the megameatus intact prepuce (MIP) variant: the pyramid procedure. *J Urol.* 1989;141:1407–1409.
5. Rabinowitz R. General considerations of congenital anomalies. In: Gillenwater JY, Grayhack JT, Howards JT, Duckett JW, eds. *Adult and Pediatric Urology.* Chicago: Year Book Medical; 1987:1506–1507.
6. Bauer SB, Retik AB, Colodny AH. Genetic aspects of hypospadias. *Urol Clin North Am.* 1981;8:559–564.
7. Henderson BE, Benton R, Cosgrove M, et al. Urogenital tract abnormalities in sons of women treated with diethylstilbesterol. *Pediatrics.* 1976;58:505–507.
8. Barcat J. Current concepts of treatment. In: Horton CE, ed. *Plastic and Reconstructive Surgery of the Genital Area.* Boston: Little, Brown; 1973:249–263.
9. Juskiewenski S, Vaysse P, Guitard J, et al. Traitment des hypospadias anterieurs. *Chir Pediatr.* 1983;24:75–79.
10. Shima H, Ikoma F, Terakawa T, et al. Developmental anomalies associated with hypospadias. *J Urol.* 1979;122:619–621.
11. Khuri FJ, Hardy BE, Churchill BM. Urologic anomalies associated with hypospadias. *Urol Clin North Am.* 1981;8:565–571.
12. Avellan L. The incidence of hypospadias in Sweden. *Scand J Plast Reconstr Surg.* 1975;9:129–138.
13. Cerasaro TS, Brock WA, Kaplan GW. Upper urinary tract anomalies associated with congenital hypospadias: is screening necessary? *J Urol.* 1986;135:537–542.
14. Shelton TB, Noe HN. The role of excretory urography in patients with hypospadias. *J Urol.* 1985;135:97–100.
15. Rozenman J, Hertz M, Boichis H. Radiographic findings of the urinary tract in hypospadias: a report of 110 cases. *Clin Radiol.* 1979;30:471.
16. Kass EJ, Kogan SJ, Manley C, Wacksman JA. Timing in elective surgery on the genitalia of male children with particular reference to hypospadia. In: Preliminary Report of the Action Committee on Surgery on the Genitalia of Male Children of the American Academy of Pediatrics, 1991.
17. Schultz JR, Klykylo WM, Wacksman JA. Timing of elective hypospadias repair in children. *Pediatrics.* 1983;71:342–351.
18. Belman AB, Kass EJ. Hypospadias repair in children less than 1 year old. *J Urol.* 1982;128:1273–1274.
19. Manley CB, Epstein ES. Early hypospadias repair. *J Urol.* 1981;125:698–700.
20. Berg R, Berg G. Penile malformation, gender identity and sexual orientation. *Acta Psychiatr Scand.* 1983;68:154.
21. Berg G, Svensson J, Astrom G. Social and sexual adjustment of men operated for hypospadias during childhood: a controlled study. *J Urol.* 1981;125:313.
22. McCraw JB, Myers B, Sanklin KD. The value of fluorescein in predicting the viability of arterialized flaps. *Plast Reconstr Surg.* 1977; 60:710.
23. Everingham WJ, Horton CE, Devine CJ. Studies of urethral healing in dogs. *Plast Reconstr Surg.* 1973;51:312.
24. Retik AB, Keating MA, Mandell J. Complications of hypospadias repair. *Urol Clin North Am.* 1988;15:223.
25. Snow BW. Use of tunica vaginalis to prevent fistulas in hypospadias. *J Urol.* 1986;136:861.
26. Kass EJ, Bolong D. Single stage hypospadias reconstruction without fistula. *J Urol.* 1990; 144:520–522.
27. Byars LT. Technique of consistently satisfactory repair of hypospadias. *Surg Gynecol Obstet.* 1955;100:184–190.
28. Nesbit RM. Operation for correction of distal penile curvature with and without hypospadias. *Trans Am Assoc Genitourin Surg.* 1966;58:12–14.
29. Kramer SA, Aydin G, Kelalis PP. Chordee without hypospadias in children. *J Urol.* 1982; 128:559–561.
30. Gittes RF, McLaughlin AP III. Injection techniques to induce penile erection. *Urology.* 1974;4:473.
31. Horton CE, Devine CJ. Peyronie's disease. *Plast Reconstr Surg.* 1973;52:503.
32. Das, S. Pyronie's disease. Excision and autografting with tunica vaginalis. *J Urol* 1980;124:818–819.
33. Nesbit R. Operation for correction of distal penile ventral curvature with and without hypospadias. *Tran Am Assoc Genitourin Surg.* 1966; 58:12–14.
34. Duckett JW. MAGPI (meatoplasty and glanduloplasty): a procedure for subcoronal hypospadias. *Urol Clin North Am.* 1981;8:513–520.
35. Duckett JW Jr, Snyder HM, Blyth B, Keating MA. Hypospadias repair: results of one thousand one hundred eleven meatal advancement and glanuloplasties. Abstract 135, presented at the American Urological Association Meeting, Toronto, June 2–6, 1991.

36. Hollowell JG, Keating MA, Synder HM, et al. Preservation of the urethral plate in hypospadias repair: Extended applications and further experience with the onlay island flap urethroplasty. *J Urol.* 1990;143:98–101.
37. Duckett JW. The island flap technique for hypospadias repair. *Urol Clin North Am.* 1981; 8:503–511.
38. Keating MA. Update, onlay island flap urethroplasty. In: Shapiro S, ed. Hypospadias repair: update and Controversies. *Dialogues in Pediatric Urology.* 1990;13(10).
39. Gibbons MD, Gonzales ET Jr. The subcoronal meatus. *J Urol.* 1983;130:739–742.
40. Firlit CF. The mucosal collar in hypospadias surgery. *J Urol.* 1987;137:80–85.
41. King LR. Hypospadias: a one-stage repair without skin graft based on a new principle: chordee is sometimes produced by the skin alone. *J Urol.* 1970;103:660–662.
42. Zaontz MR. The GAP (glans approximation procedure) for glanular/coronal hypospadias. *J Urol.* 1989;141:359.
43. Devine CJ Jr, Horton CE. A one-stage hypospadias repair. *J Urol.* 1961;85:166–172.
44. Duckett JW. Transverse preputial island flap technique for repair of severe hypospadias. *Urol Clin North Am.* 1980;7:423–431.
45. Mitchell ME, Kulb TB. Hypospadias repair without a bladder catheter. *J Urol.* 1986;135:321.
46. Barraza MA, Roth DR, Terry WJ, et al. One-stage reconstruction of moderately severe hypospadias. *J Urol.* 1987;137:714–715.
47. Noe HN. Complications and management of childhood urethral stricture disease. *Urol Clin North Am.* 1983;10:531.
48. Johanssen B. Reconstruction of the male urethra in stricture. *Acta Chir Scand (Suppl).* 1953:176.
49. Hodgson NB. Urethral sounds. *Soc Pediatr Urol Newslett.* May 16, 1986.
50. Jordan GH. Reconstruction of the fossa navicularis. *J Urol.* 1987;138:102.
51. Hinderer JT. Secondary repair of hypospadias failures. *Plast Reconstr Surg.* 1972;50:13.
52. Winslow BH, Vorstman B, Devine CJ Jr. Urethroplasty using diverticular tissue. *J Urol.* 1985;134:552.
53. Romagnoli G, De Luca M, Faranda F, Bandelloni R, Franzi AT, Cataliotti F, et al. Treatment of posterior hypospadias by the autologous graft of cultured urethral epithelium. *N Engl J Med.* 1990;323:527–530.
54. Keating MA, Cartwright PC, Duckett JW. Bladder mucosa in urethral reconstructions. *J Urol.* 1990;144:827.
55. Mollard P, Mouriquand P, Bringeon G, Bugmann P. Repair of hypospadias using bladder mucosal graft in 76 cases. *J Urol.* 1989; 142:1548.

# 52

# Abnormalities of the Testis and Groin

*Julian Wan, David A. Bloom, and Johannes Pohl*

## EMBRYOLOGY OF THE TESTIS AND INGUINAL CANAL

The early precursors of the testis, primordial germ cells of endodermal origin, are located caudal to the cloacal membrane and near the allantois in the third fetal week. Migration to the genital ridge produces a distinct bulge by the fifth week and an undifferentiated gonad is formed within another week. Sex cords develop from the genital ridge epithelium and invade the gonad to form seminiferous tubules and Sertoli cells. A recognizable and functional testis is present by week eight, lying high in the retroperitoneum. Testosterone produced by Leydig cells allows the mesonephric ducts to differentiate into rete testes, vas deferens, seminal vesicles, and ejaculatory ducts. Müllerian inhibitory substance (MIS), produced by the Sertoli cells, causes regression of the paramesonephric (Müllerian) ducts in the tenth week.[1] During the fourth through seventh gestational months, a peritoneal outpouching, the processus vaginalis, lies ventral to the gubernaculum and slowly extends toward the scrotum. At the seventh month the processus vaginalis rapidly elongates into the scrotum and the gonad follows. After descent the cranial portion of the processus vaginalis obliterates. Hutson hypothesized that testicular descent occurs in two stages: the abdominal phase may be mediated by MIS and is completed by the seventh month, and the inguinoscrotal phase may be mediated by testosterone and the genitofemoral nerve, which supplies the gubernaculum.[2]

## ABNORMALITIES OF TESTICULAR STRUCTURE AND NUMBER

### Agenesis/Monorchia

True agenesis of a testis is a rare phenomenon that is probably related to failure of germinal ridge development. The persistence of some Müllerian structures should accompany true agenesis because no MIS would be available to cause their involution. A more common explanation for testicular absence is fetal or perinatal loss of a testis, perhaps from vascular accident; most absent testes are not associated with ipsilateral Müllerian persistence. Gonadal absence is present in 4% of patients with undescended testis and in 40% of patients with a nonpalpable gonad.[3,4] The predisposition of the left side in unilateral testicular absence may reflect a fetal vascular vulnerability.[5,6] Testicular absence must be distinguished from a nonpalpable testis. Surgical exploration, venography/arteriography, and laparoscopy can make the distinction: one must find blind-ending spermatic vessels to declare testicular absence. Erroneous declaration of absence may leave behind an occult abdominal testis with its attendant risk of malignancy.[7]

Bilateral testicular absence, anorchia, is a tragic condition that has been called the vanishing testis syndrome.[8] The reported frequency is 1/20,000 males. The prime differential diagnosis is bilateral nonpalpable testes. Boys with absence of both testes have no rise in serum testosterone after stimulation by human chorionic gonadotropin (HCG). Follicular secretion hormone (FSH) and luteinizing hormone (LH) levels are high. Laparoscopy usually reveals hypoplastic spermatic vessels that end blindly either proximal to or at the internal inguinal ring and extraordinary Müllerian remnants are absent. Testicular prostheses should be placed in infancy for without them the scrotum is flat and hypoplastic. Testosterone shots are commenced at the anticipated time of puberty initiation and continued throughout life.

## Polyorchidism

Polyorchidism is the presence of more than two testes. This very rare phenomenon usually involves a single supernumerary testis that is intrascrotal or undescended. Most accessory testes are intrascrotal and are discovered at exploration for a testicular mass.[9] Transverse testicular ectopia is the primary differential diagnosis. Sixty percent of polyorchid testes are on the left side. Undescended testis, inguinal hernia, and torsion of the spermatic cord have been associated with polyorchidism.[10] Bilateral accessory testes have been reported.[11] Intrascrotal accessory testes should be biopsied and anchored in the scrotum.[12] Dysplastic or hypoplastic accessory testes, particularly if suprascrotal, are preferably removed with care to preserve the vascular integrity and vas of the dominant ipsilateral gonad.

## Structural Hypogonadism

The testis grows only modestly between the first year of life and puberty. Ninety percent of testicular volume consists of spermatic tubules.[13] Diminished volume may occur with undescended testes, varicocele, trauma, torsion, functional hypogonadism, inflammatory orchitis, chemotherapy, radiation, or sickle cell disease. Structural hypogonadism can be associated with excess, insufficient, or normal gonadotropin levels. Klinefelter's syndrome is the classic form of hypergonadotropic hypogonadism and patients have small to low-normal testes that fail to have a pubertal growth spurt. Other congenital syndromes that include small testes are the Noonan, Kallmann, Laurence–Moon–Biedl, Prader–Willi, and Del Castillo syndromes in addition to the XX male syndrome. Hypogonadotropic hypogonadism results from an FSH or LH deficiency due to a defect in hypothalamic or pituitary function. Testes may be normal at birth but remain immature after puberty due to a lack of gonadotropin stimulation. Defective androgen action, as occurs in several forms of male pseudohermaphroditism such as Reifenstein's syndrome, also results in small testes.[14]

## Macroorchidism

A macroorchid testis exceeds the age-related range for normal length and volume, ie, before puberty length exceeds the 95th percentile and after puberty testicular volume is in excess of 30 mL. The prime differential diagnosis is testicular malignancy. A testis that is apparently large may simply be larger in comparison with a hypoplastic contralateral mate. Compensatory hypertrophy, perhaps caused by FSH oversecretion, occurs in some boys with a contralateral absent or undescended testis.[15] Unilateral macroorchidism is evaluated by physical examination and testicular ultrasound. A patient with unilateral testicular macroorchidism and a normal testicular ultrasound may not need surgical exploration.[16] Bilateral prepubertal macroorchidism may be evidence of precocious puberty from congenital adrenal hyperplasia, adrenal cortical tumor, juvenile hypothyroidism, fragile X syndrome, or isosexual precocity. Extramedullary leukemia, particularly the acute monocytic variant, may also present with testicular enlargement.[17]

### Splenogonadal Fusion

Splenogonadal fusion takes one of two forms. In *continuous fusion* the gonad is attached to the orthotopic spleen by a cord of fibrosplenic tissue. In *discontinuous fusion* ectopic rests of accessory spleen are attached to the testis. Walther et al identified 93 cases in the literature, 51 being continuous and 42 discontinuous. Usually it is the left side that is involved. Occasionally the anomaly is symptomatic and frequently the patients have concomitant problems such as inguinal hernia, undescended testis, micrognathia, and limb deformities.[18]

### Testicular Tumors

Testicular tumors have a bimodal distribution. Most occur in the age range from 18 to 40 years of age and usually are seminomatous or nonseminomatous germ cell tumors. A much smaller group of tumors occur in the first few years of life, typically around 2 years of age. These are almost always nonseminomatous germ cell tumors (yolk cell tumors).[19,20] Paratesticular rhabdomyosarcoma may also be mistaken for a testicular mass.

Carcinoma in situ of the testis came to attention in 1972 when Skakkebaek observed embryonal carcinoma developing in two subfertile men whose previous biopsies showed atypical intratubular germ cells.[21] Since then evidence has accumulated suggesting that these cells (carcinoma in situ) are precursors to invasive germ cell tumors. Patients with undescended testis, intersex disorders, infertility, and past or present germ cell testis tumors have an increased risk for carcinoma in situ. For example, among 295 men with a history of undescended testis, 5 had carcinoma in situ on biopsy at age 24–26 years. Their orchidopexies had been performed at age 10–13 years. Curiously, 4 of the 5 patients had undergone right orchiopexy; the carcinoma in situ was present in 5 out of 5 right testes but in none of the left testes. As a result of the biopsies, orchiectomy was performed in all 5 patients.[22] Table 1 lists other miscellaneous tumors of the testis.

## ABNORMALITIES OF TESTICULAR POSITION

### Undescended Testes, Cryptorchidism

Testicular descent culminates in a scrotal position by the end of the 28th gestational week. Scorer and Farrington's data indicate that descent is incomplete or erroneous in 30% of premature infants, in 3% of full-term infants, in 1.8% of 1-year-olds, and in 1.8% of adults.[23] From these data it is evident that the chance of descent after 1 year of age is negligible. There are three primary clinical situations of cryptorchidism: nonpalpable testis (NPT), palpable undescended testis (UDT), and retractile

**TABLE 1. Miscellaneous Tumors of the Testis and Epididymis**

| Type | Malignant? | Comment |
|---|---|---|
| Adrenal rest | No | Mimics testicular torsion |
| Dermoid cyst | No | Only two germ cell layers |
| Epidermoid cyst | No | Confused with teratoma |
| Hemangioma | No | Observe to prevent hematomas |
| Lymphangioma | No | Watch for lymphangitis |
| Meconium | No | Usually can be left untreated |
| Neuroblastoma | Yes | Look for primary in retroperitoneum |
| Neurofibromatosis | Yes, potentially | Other neural crest problems can be nearby |
| Papillary cystadenoma of epididymis | No | Associated with Von Hippel–Lindau disease |
| Tunic cyst | No | Caused by trauma? |

testis (RT). Most "undescended testes" have in fact descended through the internal and external inguinal rings, but have become fixed in an ectopic location, ie, a superficial inguinal pouch that lies above the external ring between Scarpa's fascia and the external oblique fascia. The primary point of gubernacular fixation is proximal to the scrotum, often at the inguinoscrotal or inguinofemoral creases (Fig 1). Jackson's data give a typical distribution of positions for UDTs.[24] Physical examination may indicate position. Usually a high testis can be felt on supine exam by milking down from the internal ring toward the external ring and scrotum. A thin film of lubricant (liquid soap, jelly) applied to the groin may help detect an elusive gonad by reducing tactile friction; on occasion reexamination in the cross-legged position is necessary to find a testis. In 20% of patients with a UDT the gonad is nonpalpable. Testes are nonpalpable for three main reasons: testicular absence (usually with blind-ending spermatic vessels), intra-abdominal position, or occult low-lying testes that remain hidden in spite of careful examination (these are often hypoplastic and bilateral). Retractile testes are usually differentiated by careful and sometimes repetitive examinations. Occasionally testes that were believed to be normally descended upon careful examination subsequently prove to be undescended. Belman describes these as ascended testes.[25]

Undescended testicles are susceptible to a host of problems. When fixed in the superficial pouch anterior to the pubic rami they are more likely than a free-hanging gonad to be damaged by blunt trauma. The warmer core body temperature may interfere with the normal structural changes that should occur in puberty. Undescended testes have increased risk for malignancy. Even if they are palpable, adequate self-examination is not possible.

The use of hormones to inspire testicular descent once seemed logical, but objective data fail to substantiate their value.[26] Anyone who has ever dissected a testis sharply from the superficial inguinal pouch must wonder how hormones can accomplish the same feat. Some centers advocate the use of gonadotropins to help prime a testis in conjunction with orchidopexy.[27]

In most instances a prepubertal boy with a UDT should be explored, a concomitant patent processus vaginalis is closed, and

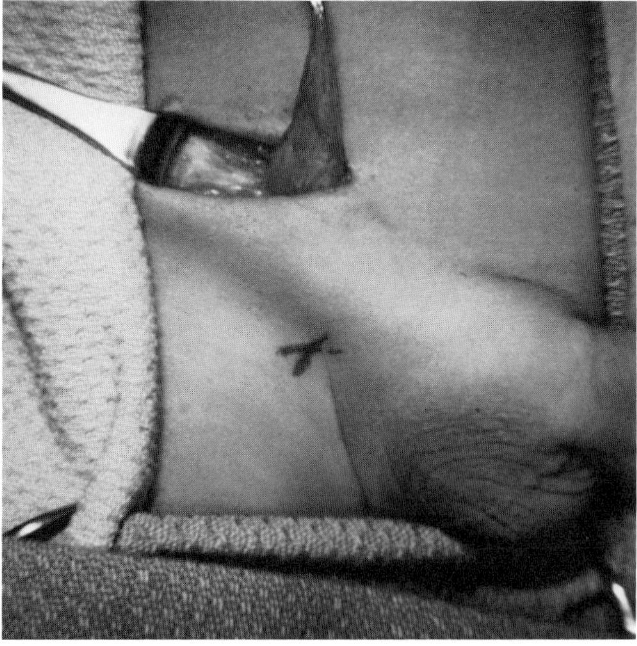

**Fig 1.** Abnormal attachment of the gubernaculum in a patient with an undescended testicle is demonstrated here by tugging gently on the spermatic cord. The X marks the point of fixation.

the testis is mobilized and relocated into a scrotal pouch. Hinman suggests that youngsters with disabilities such as Down syndrome do not need orchiopexy, but this opinion is debatable.[28] The NPT requires certainty of its presence or absence. The duty of a physician vis-à-vis the NPT is to locate and appropriately manage the gonad (with orchiectomy or orchidopexy) or to declare absence with a reasonable degree of confidence. An NPT can be evaluated by HCG stimulation, ultrasound, CT, or magnetic resonance imaging (MRI) scan. Open surgical exploration has been the usual definitive means of locating and managing the NPT. Laparoscopy (peritoneal endoscopy) is a useful alternative to imaging and hormonal evaluation and is the ideal first operative step, permitting localization of an NPT and determination of the next step. If blind-ending spermatic vessels are identified, there is likely no distal or proximal gonad (Fig 2). Inguinal exploration is therefore not indicated, but like Harris and Kogan we believe contralateral fixation should be performed under the same anesthetic to minimize the chances for subsequent torsion of the solitary testis.[6,29] If spermatic vessels go into the internal ring or if a patent processus vaginalis is present, inguinal exploration is indicated. One will find either a missed and usually hypoplastic testis or blind-ending vessels distal to the internal ring. If an intra-abdominal testis is found at endoscopy, the management is dictated by the specific clinical circumstances. For example, a dysmorphic small intra-abdominal testis in a boy with a normal contralateral gonad in the scrotum argues for orchiectomy. This can be performed endoscopically or expeditiously through a small, precisely directed incision. A peeping testis hovering around the internal inguinal ring with a long and lax spermatic vessel leash might be amenable to conventional orchidopexy with or without the Fowler–Stephens maneuver. Bilateral high intra-abdominal testes with short vascular pedicles have a high likelihood of salvage with two-step orchiopexy.[30,31] Any undescended testis, particularly the high variants, has significant malignant potential. Lifelong follow-up is mandatory and self-examination techniques must be taught after puberty.

**Fig 2.** Blind-ending gonadal vessels found during laparoscopy for nonpalpable testes. They come to an abrupt end before crossing the internal ring.

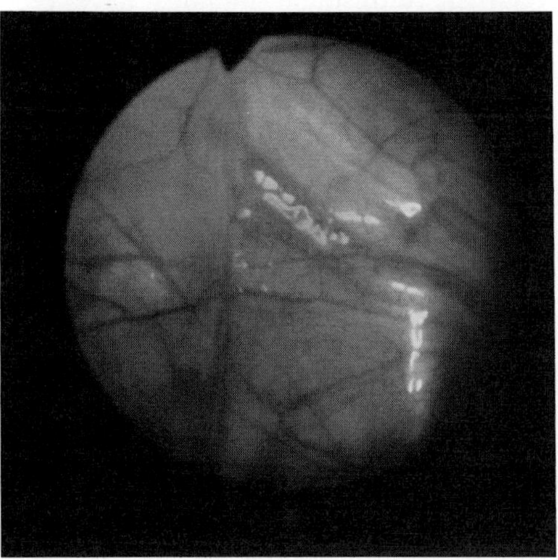

### Transverse Testicular Ectopia and Other Ectopic Locations

Transverse or crossed testicular ectopia (TTE) is a very rare form of gonadal ectopia (Fig 3). One testis crosses the midline to join its opposite mate at the internal inguinal ring, inguinal canal, or hemiscrotum so that two testes of contralateral origin come together at a single location. The ectopic gonad is defined as the one that crosses the midline and has a slight right-sided predominance.[32] The testes are usually not fused but remain distinct. They may be identical and normal, or the ectopic gonad may be smaller and dysmorphic. No simple embryologic explanation is accepted.[33,34] Transverse testicular ectopia usually presents as a nonpalpable testis with a contralateral normal testis and inguinal hernia. Differential diagnoses include testicular or paratesticular tumor, splenogonadal fusion, adrenal rest, polyorchidism, spermatocele, cord hydrocele, or any disorder responsible for a nonpalpable testis. Additional genitourinary anomalies including hypospadias, seminal vesical cyst, renal agenesis, horseshoe kidney, uretero-

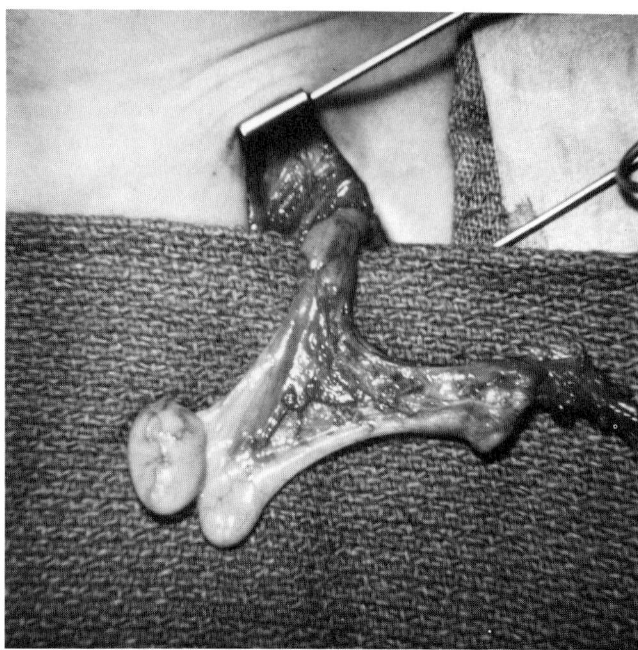

**Fig 3.** Transverse ectopic testis. Seen here are two testes found on a dissection of the right inguinal canal. The smaller of the two has crossed over from the left side.

pelvic junction obstruction, pseudohermaphroditism, and inadequate Müllerian regression occur in a fifth of patients.[32,35,36] Malignancy has developed in six patients.[37] Transverse testicular ectopia is usually discovered intraoperatively. If the ectopic testis is normal and high it should be brought into the most convenient hemiscrotum, but if both testes are already in a single hemiscrotum it is best to leave them alone. Persisting Müllerian structures can be removed so long as vasal integrity is maintained.

One of the most unusual ectopias is exstrophy of the testis, which is due to a defect in the scrotal wall. This anomaly is obvious at birth and is managed by orchiopexy unless the testis is terribly abnormal.[38] Gongaware et al introduced the term scrotoschisis to describe this strange anomaly.[39]

## Testicular Torsion and Trauma

Three major varieties of gonadal torsion occur in boys. Extravaginal torsion of the spermatic cord consists of rotation proximal to the attachment of the tunica vaginalis, either in the inguinal canal or just below it. Perinatal spermatic cord torsion is rare, probably contributing only 1 case per 100 intravaginal torsions, but may be a common cause for monorchidism. Because monorchid patients preferentially lack a left testis and because perinatal torsion seems to have equivalent prevalence on either side, torsion alone cannot explain all cases of monorchidism. Bilateral extravaginal torsion is even less common than unilateral and may be a cause of the vanished testis syndrome. Perinatal torsion presents as an asymptomatic scrotal swelling. Characteristic ultrasound findings have been described, but diagnosis is usually obvious on physical exam.[40] Bilateral involvement occurs in 12% of cases.[41] Perinatal torsion is a *prenatal* event (occurring in utero and manifest at birth) in 72% and a *postnatal* event (within the first 30 days of life) in 28%. Testicular salvage is very unlikely in prenatal torsion. Salvage is a possibility, although slim, in postnatal torsion if recognized promptly and explored immediately. The main point in operating for either type of perinatal torsion is prophylactic anchoring of the solitary remaining gonad. An inguinal incision is preferable because of the high site of cord torsion and the possibility of concomitant hernia. Spermatic vessels, vas deferens, and testicular parenchyma must be spared during orchiopexy; sutures are placed in paratesticular structures and subcutaneous scrotal fascia.[42] A necrotic testis should be removed. Testicular infarction, such as has been reported in association with polycythemia, may present similarly to torsion.[43]

Torsion of the spermatic cord distal to the attachment of tunica vaginalis (intravaginal torsion) is the more common cord twist. A bell-clapper deformity and horizontal testicular lie may predispose to this condition[44] (Fig 4). Patients are usually 3 to 20 years of age (and two thirds are between 12 and 18 years) and familial torsion has been reported.[45] The risk for torsion of testis or an appendage by age 25 years is about 1 in 160. One series found testicular torsion to be six times as common as appendiceal torsion. Intravaginal torsion has a very slight left-sided predominance and is bilateral in 2%.[46] It is exquisitely symptomatic and promptly results in loss of the testis unless spontaneous or surgical reduction occurs within 6 hours.[47] In a review of 52 patients with torsion, those under 18 years of age had a median delay of diagnosis of 20 hours, whereas the older patients had a median delay of 4 hours.[48] Pain may be accompanied by nausea and vomiting. Physical signs are scrotal edema, erythema, loss of the cremasteric reflex, and bloody hydrocele fluid.[49,50] The differential diagnoses include testicular trauma, acute hydrocele, inguinal hernia, Henoch–Schönlein purpura (HSP), epididymitis, funiculitis, and testicular tumor. Patients with scrotal trauma or HSP can also have concomitant torsion.[51] Scrotal edema and erythema from peritonitis can mimic torsion.[52] Manual detorsion and narcotic analgesia can relieve the crisis, although the definitive treatment of spermatic cord torsion is surgical exploration. Testes usually twist with an inward, or medial, rotation and can be detorsed with two or three lateral, or outward, rotations.[53] Inadequate reduction of torsion and the possibility of recurrence argue against reduction as a definitive treatment.[54] A Doppler stethoscope may confirm restoration of flow after manual detorsion.[55] The Doppler, however, is not fail-safe: Nasrallah et al had 4 patients with surgically proven torsion in spite of symmetric Doppler flow readings.[56] Preoperative cooling with ice packs improves salvage rates.[57,58] Necrotic testes should be

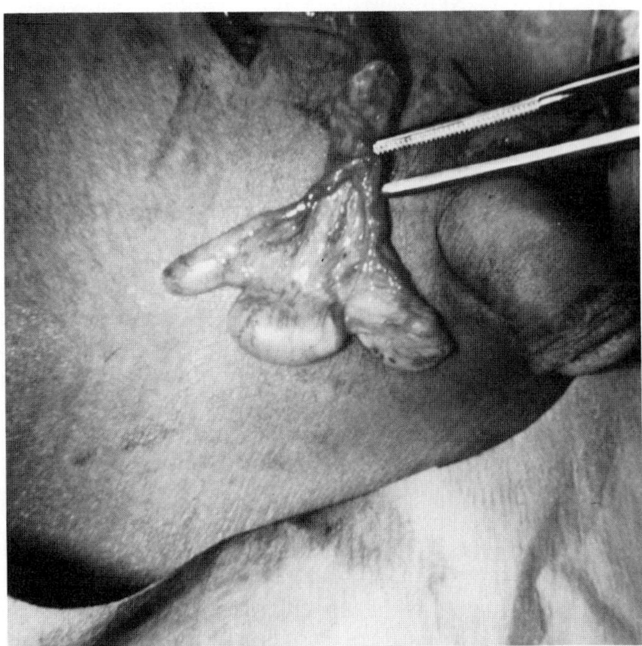

**Fig 4.** An example of the "bell-clapper" tranverse lie.

removed, but potentially viable gonads are retained. Sympathetic orchiopathia has been observed in laboratory models but not in humans.[59,60] Gonadal dysfunction, particularly damage to spermatogenesis, is likely after torsion.[61] A damaged but not destroyed testis still is of value. Normal contralateral testicular volume or compensatory hypertrophy has been documented up to 20 years after torsion.[62] Contralateral orchiopexy is mandatory in our opinion and that of others.[63] A contrary point of view was developed from a 15-year experience with 31 patients analyzed by chart review and questionnaire; the authors concluded that surgical fixation was unnecessary for either the torsed or contralateral testis. In the absence of any scientific data, we would ascribe the favorable outcome at that regional center more to luck than design and we still would subscribe to fixation techniques.[64] Diagnosis of torsion is difficult when trauma is involved.[65] Ultrasonography is helpful in defining normal structures in addition to demonstrating that the tunica albuginea is intact or that no testicular mass is present. Nuclear scans have been advocated for the diagnosis of torsion but are a poor substitute for competent history, physical examination, and clinical judgment. Nuclear scans cannot help but detour a patient from immediate operation and may also miss a torsion that spontaneously detorses.[66]

Episodic testicular pain of acute onset and brief duration, with or without scrotal edema and erythema, occurs in some young men. These episodes may occur sporadically several times in a year but may culminate in an episode of prolonged pain and surgical diagnosis of torsion. If a history compatible with intermittent torsion (torsion-detorsion) is obtained, elective orchiopexy should be offered.[67] Torsion occurs in undescended testes and abdominal gonads are not exempt.[68] It can also occur in spite of previous orchidopexy or genital surgery.[69]

The third variant of gonadal torsion involves an appendix testis or appendix epididymis. These appendages are vestigial structures usually at the upper pole of the testis or epididymis. Appendiceal torsion can be as symptomatic as torsion of the spermatic cord. It is usually a unilateral phenomenon, but bilateral appendiceal torsion and simultaneous torsion of appendiceal and epididymal appendages have occurred.[70] Identification of a specific point tenderness or "blue dot sign" at the upper pole of the testis is pathognomonic of appendiceal torsion. The diagnosis of appendiceal torsion, however, must be certain if a nonoperative course is taken. If recognition is delayed more than a day or so and if operation is performed, a diffuse peritesticular fibrinous inflammation and a serous hydrocele will be found.

Testicular trauma may be blunt or penetrating. Penetrating injuries are usually explored surgically whereas blunt injuries often are observed. The indications for exploring blunt testicular trauma include testicular rupture (disruption of the tunica albuginea), expanding hematoma, purulence, or the possibility of torsion. On occasion trauma may be related to torsion or difficult to distinguish from it. Some forms of trauma could conceivably impart a spin to the testis.

## EPIDIDYMAL AND VASAL ABNORMALITIES

In the sixth fetal week mesonephric tubules contact the rete testis and form the ductuli efferentes. In males the mesonephric (Wölffian) duct persists whereas the paramesonephric (Müllerian) duct atrophies except for the cranial and caudal portions that become the appendix testis and prostatic utricle, respectively. Vas deferens forms from a portion of mesonephric duct and the seminal vesicle buds out from the tail of the epididymis. The ejaculatory duct develops caudal to the seminal vesicle. The ureter originates as an outgrowth of the mesonephric duct during the fourth week. This ureteral bud quickly extends cephalad to penetrate the metanephric tissue. It dilates and branches into the renal pelvis and calyces. As the cloaca divides into the rectum and urogenital sinus the caudal mesonephric duct is absorbed into the urogenital (bladder) wall. Ureteric orifices come to lie in the bladder, separate from the mesonephric ducts that terminate adjacently in the prostatic urethra as the ejaculatory ducts.[71]

## Absent or Dysplastic Vas Deferens

Unilateral vasal agenesis or hypoplasia occurs in 0.5% to 1.0% of males and favors the left side with a ratio of 4 to 1.[72] Three percent of herniorrhaphy patients have an absent vas.[73] A caput epididymidis is usually present in patients with absent vas.[74] Patients with absence of a single vas should be evaluated for ipsilateral renal agenesis or dysplasia.[73] A combined anomaly is not surprising given that a small portion of the caudal mesonephric duct is the source of both vas deferens and ureteric bud.[72] In spite of an absent vas the ipsilateral seminal vesicle may be present.[75] Bilateral agenesis of vas deferens is common in cystic fibrosis.[72,73]

## Iatrogenic Injuries of the Vas Deferens

Herniorrhaphy and other operative procedures in the inguinal canal can injure the vas and jeopardize future fertility. In many instances the injury may not be recognized. If, however, the injury is visible, early repair may be advantageous. Pedersen studied postpubertal boys who had prepubertal herniorrhaphy and found significant titers of circulating antisperm antibodies in relationship to occult uncorrected vasal injury.[76] Correction of childhood vasal injury, even bilateral, can permit fertility.[77] The risks of routine exploration of a normal contralateral groin after herniorrhaphy may be underestimated.

## Ectopic Vas Deferens

The mesonephric duct is the common embryologic source of vas deferens and ureter. Anomalies of the two often coexist. For example, an ectopic vas deferens is likely to insert into a ureter to form a unified duct which then enters the bladder. Vordermark called this the persisting mesonephric duct syndrome.[78] There are two main embryologic explanations for this. An excessively cranial origin of the ureteral bud diminishes the normal separation between ureter and vas when the mesonephric duct is absorbed into the bladder and a single (persistent) common duct results. An alternative hypothesis is that the ureteral bud originates in the normal position but that the common excretory duct elongates excessively thereby preventing normal bladder absorption and separation.[79] Epididymitis and recurrent urinary tract infection are the usual clinical presentations of persistent mesonephric duct syndrome and intravenous urography (IVU) or voiding cystourography (VCUG) usually demonstrate the anomaly.[80–82] Associated problems include imperforate anus, renal dysplasia, hypospadias, cryptorchidism, and crossed testicular ectopia.[83,84]

## Cystic Fibrosis and Other Vasal Disorders

Cystic fibrosis (CF) is an autosomal recessive condition characterized by abnormally thick secretions from mucous glands and it occurs once in a thousand live births.[85] Pancreatic dysfunction and chronic obstructive pulmonary disease are the predominant disabilities. Males are infertile because of abnormal vas deferens development.[86,87] Mild cases of CF can be asymptomatic until the second decade of life; therefore discovery of an absent vas deferens during orchiopexy or herniorrhaphy should suggest the possibility of CF.

Diffuse or nodular thickening of the vas may result from bacterial or tuberculous inflammation. Occasionally, vasitis will present as an acute suppurative process.[88] Vasitis nodosa usually occurs after vasectomy or prostatectomy, but can simulate vasal tuberculosis and is unlikely to occur in childhood.

## Seminal Vesicle Lesions

The seminal vesicle forms from the caudal mesonephric duct in the fourth gestational month. Defective differentiation can result in cysts. Ipsilateral renal dysgenesis (agenesis, dysplasia, and hypoplasia) is likely when a seminal vesicle is absent or abnormal.[89,90] Absence can be diagnosed by transrectal ultrasound.[91] Testicular or perineal pain may occur after puberty when secretions have accumulated in the cyst. A large cyst can compress bladder and rectum. Ultrasonography, IVU, CT scan, and seminal vesiculography will all image these lesions. Seminal vesicle cysts are paramedial as compared to midline Müllerian duct cysts.[92] Combined cysts of ejaculatory ducts and seminal vesicles were described by Elder and Mostwin.[93] Suprapubic transvesical drainage and excision is the usual method of management, although transrectal aspiration, transurethral unroofing, and excision by perineal, retropubic, transsacral, and transrectal routes can be effective.[94] Papillary adenocarcinoma of the seminal vesicle in a 19-year-old presented with urethralgia, perineal pain, and dysuria.[95]

### Epididymal Anomalies and Other Lesions

Epididymal abnormalities are described in 24% to 63% of patients with undescended testicles.[96–101] The variability reflects the lack of uniform definitions to describe this anomaly. Toth found epididymal abnormalities in 23.6% of 1171 undescended testicles and described a distribution of anomalies using as a reference their points of attachment: 19.5% had head and tail attachment, 7.3% had isolated head attachment, 2.7% had tail only attachment, and 4.1% had complete separation of the testis and epididymis. In 197 consecutive cases of cryptorchidism Mininberg found 63% had unfurled epididymides distal to testis in the inguinal canal. These anomalies may help explain the enhanced potential for fertility problems in patients with cryptorchidism regardless of orchiopexy.[102,103]

Infertility evaluation may also uncover epididymal abnormality. Hendry discovered congenital testicular obstructions as well as iatrogenic injuries among 370 subfertile men. Incomplete epididymes were more likely to be iatrogenic than congenital, whereas epididymal obstructions result from infection.[104] Epididymal cysts are acquired rather than congenital.[105] Hemorrhagic infarction of an epididymal cyst in a 13-year-old has been reported.[106]

Epididymal tumors are very rare, particularly in children. Melanotic neuroectodermal tumor and fibrous dysplasia of the epididymis and aberrant epididymal tissue are rare epididymal lesions.[107–109]

### Epididymitis

Epididymitis and orchitis are unusual in prepubertal males and require investigation for a predisposing anomaly. In addition to urinary tract infection, epididymitis can result from trauma, chemical irritation, autoimmune disease, granulomatous disease, vasculitides, and secondary spread from meningitis.[110,111] Unusual infectious processes include hemophilus influenza, brucellosis, and cytomegalovirus.[112–114] Despite the many noninvasive procedures for evaluating an acute scrotum, surgical exploration is still frequently necessary to distinguish torsion from inflammation. Indeed, surgical exploration may be the safest and most cost-effective measure for suspected torsion, offering simultaneous diagnosis and treatment. Forty-seven percent of the prepubertal boys with epididymitis and 75% of the infants in one review had underlying anomalies such as ectopic vas deferens, ectopic ureter, urethral strictures, myelodysplasia, and rectourethral fistulae. A negative urine culture usually ruled out structural abnormality, but a positive culture did not confirm an occult anomaly.[115] A contradicting study rarely found structural abnormalities in boys with prepubertal epididymitis.[116] Nevertheless, infants and young children with epididymal orchitis are more likely to have underlying structural abnormalities than adolescents, and aggressive urinary tract imaging in prepubertal males with epididymal orchitis remains standard practice.

Treatment of pediatric epididymitis is initiated only if torsion is completely eliminated as a diagnostic possibility. Initial therapy is empiric, pending urine culture and sensitivity, although in many cases no organism is identified. For bacterial epididymitis the usual oral antimicrobials are successful, although a septic patient or a very hot epididymitis is preferably managed by parenteral agents. See et al showed that acute inflammation in a rat model enhances antibiotic penetration.[117]

## SCROTAL ABNORMALITIES

Mesenchymal cells in the third fetal week gather about the opening of the cloaca to form a pair of cloacal folds. These folds are joined at their cranial and caudal ends and a mound of tissue at the cranial end becomes the genital tubercle. The cloaca has divided into the urogenital sinus and the anorectal canal by the sixth week. The cloacal folds follow suit and subdivide into the anterior urethral folds and the posterior anal folds. Parallel ridges of tissue, the genital swellings, develop lateral to the cloacal folds. With elongation of the phallus, urethral folds are pulled forward and inward, forming a groove. The urethral groove closes gradually and is complete by the end of the third month. The genital swellings and cloacal folds move caudally in the fourth month and fuse in the midline to become the scrotum.

### Scrotal Anomalies

Bifid scrotum, penoscrotal transposition, and ectopic scrota are the principal anomalies. Usually these are associated with hypospadias or errors of caudal regression. Bifid scrotum occurs if the individual genital swellings fail to fuse at the midline and this occurs in patients with intersex, severe hypospadias, or penoscrotal transposition (PST). Isolated bifid scrotum is uncommon. PST results from defective genital tubercle formation and is associated with a delay in the midline fusion of the urethral folds thereby retarding caudal migration and fusion of the genital swellings. This is associated with severe major urinary, gastrointestinal, and/or cardiovascular anomalies.[118–120] PST was first described in 1922 in an adult with mild hypospadias and chordee.[121] It is often a fatal anomaly. In a recent review of 23 cases, 3 babies were stillborn and 5 had concomitant lethal conditions.[120] Ninety-one percent of the patients had urogenital anomalies (hypospadias, chordee, and agenesis of one or both upper urinary tracts) and 30% had additional gastrointestinal lesions (predominantly imperforate anus). Severe cardiovascular anomalies are less common.[122] Genital transposition occurs with caudal regression, XX/XY mosaicism, giant genital hemangiomas, and has familial tendencies.[123–125] Variants of penoscrotal transposition independent of a urethral anomaly include shawl, donut, and prepenile scrotums. All of these can be corrected with rotational scrotal flaps.[126–130] Severe instances of transposition require more complex repairs. Single-stage repair of PST, chordee, and hypospadias has become a litmus test of courage and skill in pediatric urology, but it is still often appropriate to perform these procedures in separate discrete steps.

Cleavage or abnormal migration of the genital swellings produces accessory and ectopic scrota in a variety of locations, ranging from the perineum and inguinal canal to the medial thigh.[131–133]

Scrotal hypoplasia is associated with testicular undescent or anorchism (Fig 5). The flat and poorly developed scrotum lacks normal rugal folds, but normal enlargement usually occurs after orchidopexy. Testicular prostheses appropriate for age should be placed in anorchid infants and replaced with larger units after puberty.

Scrotal cysts can occur along the raphe. These are usually dermoid cysts that result from cell rests left during the fusion of the genital swellings. They present as anterior scrotal swellings distinct from the underlying structures and may become infected or form calculi.[134]

### Acute Scrotum Sans Torsion

Acute scrotal swelling usually requires urgent surgical evaluation if spermatic cord torsion is suspected. Other lesions that produce scrotal swelling include epididymal orchitis, incarcerated hernia, intrascrotal tumors, traumatic hematocele, acute idiopathic scrotal edema, parasitic infection, lymphedema, and HSP.

Acute idiopathic scrotal edema typically presents with a sudden onset of edema with or without erythema. Tenderness is vari-

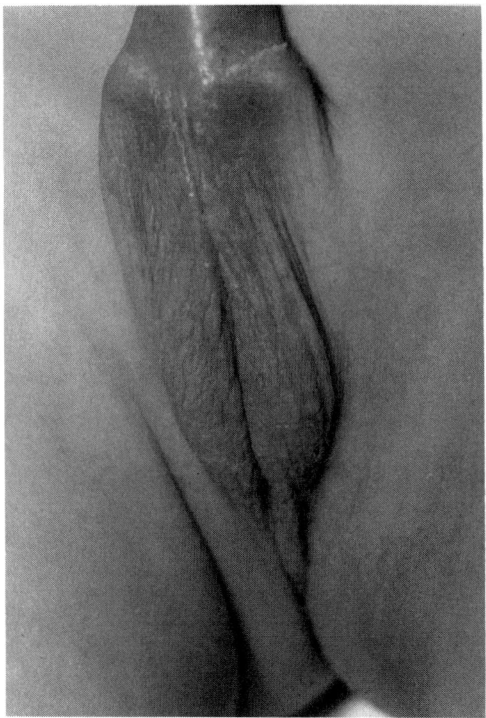

**Fig 5.** The flat scrotum in a child with bilateral undescended testicles.

able and patients are usually afebrile. Urinalysis and white blood cell count are normal. Urethrography, wound cultures, and testicular biopsies are normal.[135] Patients are usually between 4 and 10 years of age.[136] Edema may start on one side and spread to the entire scrotum with resolution after several days. Perianal infection, streptococcal cellulitis, allergic reactions, contact dermatitis, insect bites, and angioneurotic edema have been implicated as causes in individual cases. Scrotal edema usually resolves with rest and reassurance, although antihistamines may be beneficial. Acute idiopathic penile edema may be a variant of acute idiopathic scrotal edema. Lau and Ong report three cases of children ages 2.5 to 8 with gross penile swelling.[137] Temperature, urinalysis, white blood counts, and cultures were normal. The children had no evidence of trauma, allergic reaction, insect bite, or urine extravasation, and the condition subsided within 72 hours.

Child abuse and sexual abuse in particular have specific genitourinary manifestations. Children present with a wide variety of complaints including enuresis, encopresis, recurrent urinary tract infections, failure to thrive, irregular bruising, urinary retention, and constipation. Occult healed multiple long-bone fractures may be seen on x-rays. Acute scrotal swelling in the absence of direct scrotal trauma may be evidence of intra-abdominal injury.[138,139] Anogenital trauma and patterns of contusion may be strong evidence for abuse; however, most abused children, even victims of sexual abuse, show no physical evidence of abuse.

Parasitic infections of the scrotum occasionally occur in the United States. *Taenia solium,* the pork tapeworm, caused tender left scrotal swelling in a 9-year-old.[140] *Sparganum mansoni,* which normally cycles between the water flea *Cyclops* and canine and feline hosts, can sometimes infect humans after cyst ingestion. *S. mansoni* lodges in the subcutaneous tissue of the torso, limbs, and scrotum, requiring surgical removal.[141]

Primary or idiopathic lymphedema results from lymphatic abnormality or insufficiency that may present at birth, but more often develops after puberty. Extremity or genital lymphatics become increasingly incompetent during general somatic growth and swelling occurs in the involved regions. Nonsurgical management consists of scrotal elevation to decrease swelling and good skin care to decrease the risk of ulceration. Idiopathic lymphedema may require excision of involved skin and subcutaneous tissue with replacement by split thickness skin grafts. Grafting can be avoided by extensive excision of the subcutaneous tissue leaving behind thin skin flaps.[142]

Henoch–Schönlein purpura (HSP) is a systemic vasculitis with nonthrombocytopenic purpura in addition to skin, joint, intestinal, and genitourinary involvement. It is also called anaphylactoid purpura. Urinary manifestations include renal parenchymal involvement, ureteritis, renal pelvis bleeding, and acute painful swelling of spermatic cord and scrotum. A third of patients have scrotal involvement.[143–146] Most patients are younger than 7 years of age and the disease is self-limited with an average duration of 5 weeks.[147] Symptoms include a purpura; arthralgia; localized edema of the hands, feet, scalp, and facies; colicky abdominal pain; vomiting; bloody diarrhea; melena; hematemesis; gross and microscopic hematuria; and proteinuria. Renal involvement usually occurs after the presentation of other signs and symptoms and is more likely to occur in older patients.[147] The principal diagnostic problem is differentiation from testicular torsion. This can be easily made if the onset of the characteristic rash and other symptoms develop well before the acute scrotum. Torsion and HSP occasionally coexist.[148–150] If torsion cannot be unequivocally ruled out, surgical exploration is justified. Corticosteroids will relieve abdominal pain but not renal and skin involvement. Continued abdominal pain despite medical therapy is suggestive of a bowel lesion, particularly intussusception.

Focal fat necrosis or panniculitis may occur in obese children after physical activity and can mimic torsion.[151] The etiology is unknown and the treatment conservative.[152] Scrotal pneumatocele can result from a perforated viscus, such as Meckel's diverticulum.[153]

### Fournier's Gangrene

Necrotizing fasciitis of the perineum, known as Fournier's gangrene, occasionally occurs in infants and children. It is more prevalent in adults and rarely occurs in females. Predisposing factors include diabetes mellitus, trauma, cutaneous infection, injury by instrumentation, urethral stricture, and inguinal surgery.[154–156] Specific pediatric risk factors include severe diaper rash, phimosis/posthitis, perianal skin abscesses, scalds, insect bites, and circumcision.[157,158] The most common organisms identified are *Staphylococcus aureus, Streptococcus, Bacteroides fragilis, Escherichia coli,* and *Clostridium welchii.*[159–161] These spread through subcutaneous tissues and cause obliterative endarteritis in the branches of the internal pudendal artery and the superficial and deep external pudendal branches of the femoral artery leading to ischemic necrosis of the scrotum. The testicle and spermatic cord are usually spared because the testicular artery is unaffected.

Signs and symptoms of tachycardia, fever, erythema, local tenderness, and swelling develop rapidly. Mortality rates range up to 45%.[161] Treatment consists of urgent and aggressive debridement, drainage, and parenteral antibiotics. Extension of the gangrene to the penis, perineum, and lower abdomen may require suprapubic cystostomy. Frequent dressing changes and whirlpool debridement are advantageous and hyperbaric oxygen has been advocated.[161,162]

## INGUINAL CANAL ABNORMALITIES

The inguinal canal originates in the third fetal month as a protrusion of the peritoneal sac at the lower abdominal wall. The protrusion becomes a tube and follows the gubernaculum into the scrotum. The testicle uses this tube, the processus vaginalis, to transit the abdominal wall in the eighth fetal month. The processus usually occludes by birth or early infancy. Persistence of the processus, in its entirety or in part, results in an indirect inguinal hernia or hydrocele.

### Hernia

An inguinal bulge or scrotal mass in a child is usually a hernia or hydrocele. Most pediatric inguinal hernias are of the indirect type, such that peritoneal fluid, omentum, or viscera extend distal to the internal inguinal ring via a patent processus vaginalis. The majority of spermatic cords of undescended testes have a patent processus vaginalis. The inguinal or scrotal mass may be asymptomatic or painful. Bowel incarceration within the hernia sac and ischemic injury to the testis are potential but rare complications of indirect inguinal hernia. Direct inguinal hernia, due to a weakness in the inguinal floor, is uncommon in children.

Inguinal hernias usually can be reduced by firm distal traction and proximal pressure on the bulge. Herniorrhaphy can be deferred for convenience if reduction is easy, but if reduction is difficult the possibility of ischemic bowel argues for exploration without delay. Unsuccessful reduction, redness, pain, or evidence of bowel obstruction suggests intestinal incarceration. Radiologic diagnosis of inguinal hernia by intraperitoneal contrast injection is not difficult, but it is not necessary in the management of most patients.

Until this century pediatric inguinal hernia was usually treated by truss. Before 1940, Gross recommended that children under 2 years of age be managed by truss in preference to surgery given the greater operative and anesthetic risks of infants. He subsequently changed his opinion after improvements in anesthesia permitted operation on "even the smallest babies."[163]

Contralateral inguinal exploration is controversial. Some advocate routine exploration of an asymptomatic contralateral inguinal canal, particularly in infants.[164,165] Recent reports, however, suggest that the risk for contralateral hernia is small, although the possibility of injury to vas or spermatic vessels on the normal side is real.[166]

Inguinal hernia repair can be complicated by intra-abdominal shunts, sliding hernias, giant hernias, or recurrent hernias. The surgeon must additionally be prepared for the unexpected because a hernia sac will occasionally harbor extraordinary contents. The familiar denizens of the canal include isolated cord hydrocele, gonad of the appropriate sex, fallopian tube, omentum, lipoma, hematocele, and intestine. Lateral bladder wall may transiently protrude into the inguinal canal. This phenomenon is sometimes seen on voiding cystography and is described as bladder ears, which usually have no clinical significance.[167] If an unwary surgeon fails to recognize bladder within an inguinal hernia, the result can be catastrophic, ranging from occult bladder injury to subtotal cystectomy requiring urinary diversion.[168,169] Shaw and Santulli described 2 infants with bladder injury among 2378 consecutive children undergoing inguinal hernia repair.[170]

## Hydrocele

Hydrocele is a fluid collection within the tunica vaginalis of the testicle or along the spermatic cord. Hydroceles are common in newborns, most likely due to persistence of a tiny communication through the occluding processus vaginalis. Most neonatal hydroceles resolve. Surgical correction is indicated when a hydrocele has intermittent change in size (evidence of an enduring patency of processus vaginalis) or if it persists after 2 years of age. In some children a hydrocele may remain isolated in the spermatic cord, without communication to peritoneal cavity above or scrotum below it.

Because of the likelihood of a patent processus vaginalis, pediatric hydroceles are approached through inguinal incisions. Even if there is no obvious communication, the spermatic cord should be gently inspected for a tube of processus vaginalis, which can exist concomitantly with an isolated scrotal hydrocele. If no communication is present, the scrotal inlet is enlarged and testis is delivered into the operative field. The tunics are then opened and the presence of a communication with a patent processus vaginalis can be ascertained from below. The testis is measured and its epididymal configuration is described for the operative record. Genital appendices are removed. The testis is replaced within scrotum. Fixation is desirable if the gonad has a transverse lie, a bell-clapper configuration, or if it is solitary. The best solution is placement of the testis in a subcutaneous scrotal pouch.

Acute hydrocele may result from trauma, torsion, or tumor. If torsion is suspected exploration is performed urgently. In instances of trauma or suspicion of tumor, scrotal ultrasound provides good visualization of the gonad and permits informed decision making regarding operation or observation.

Inflammatory hydrocele can be due to epididymitis or parasitic disease. There are a number of named hydroceles including Dupuytren's hydrocele (bilocular hydrocele of tunica vaginalis), encysted hydrocele (cysts outside tunica vaginalis testis), hydrocele feminae (involving round ligament of female), funicular hydrocele (hydrocele of spermatic cord, but not extending down to testis), and hydrocele muliebris (hydrocele of the canal of Nuck in female).

Children with preexisting asymptomatic hernias or hydroceles occasionally develop acute painful scrotal enlargement that mimics incarcerated hernia. In these instances the communication between the inguinal portion of the hernia sac and the scrotal hydrocele is generally very small, if demonstrable at all, and acute presentation most likely occurs when such a marginally communicating hydrocele becomes noncommunicating. Lockwood in 1896 described an 18-year-old with pedunculated cysts within a hernia sac.[171] The illustrations in that report reveal a nonobstructive partial distal intussusception of the patent processus vaginalis. In 1974, Esho et al described protrusion and torsion of an inguinal hernia sac in a 10-year-old boy and we have seen similar occurrences in three children.[172] This problem may be an acute hydrocele variant wherein intra-abdominal pressure transmitted through a patent processus vaginalis causes inflammation, polyps, or intussusception at the inguinal-scrotal transition. Squire and Gough suggest a similar pathogenesis for abdominal scrotal hydrocele.[173]

## Other Unusual Findings in the Inguinal Canal and Scrotum

Minor structural variations of the vas deferens, testis, and epididymis are frequently observed during herniorrhaphy and orchiopexy.[174,175] Aside from recording gonadal dimensions and configurations for the operative record, nothing further can or need be done with most structural anomalies of the genital ducts. Nodules and cysts of the epididymis are nearly always benign and should be excised or biopsied with great care, lest an injury to the genital ducts occur. Epididymal cysts have been found in 13% to 14% of the boys born to mothers treated with gestational diethylstilbestrol.[175] Tunica albuginea cysts occur occasionally in postpubertal children and young adults and are of no clinical importance.[176,177] True testicular cysts are a rare benign finding.[178] Aberrant epididymal tissue has been associated with cystic fibrosis, Von Hippel–Lindau disease, and maternal diethylstilbestrol exposure. It may be found in the paratesticular area or intimately associated with the hernia sac. Vasal-epididymal anomalies and cryptorchidism has been associated with congenital rubella.[179] Donohue and Fauver called attention to unilateral absence of the vas deferens as a clue to possible ipsilateral renal agenesis.[180] Duplication of the vas may have significant medical-legal implications, particularly when identified in a resected hernia sac.

When inguinal exploration brings a testis into view it must be examined for the unlikely possibility of occult malignancy. We had a case of rhabdomyosarcoma in a youngster that was detected almost serendipitously, as the paratesticular erythema and induration were not dramatic and one might have considered these findings secondary to a hydrocele, when in fact the converse was the situation. Other types of malignancies have been described in the testis, epididymis, other paratesticular structures, and in the cord (Table 1).

Epididymal tumors are uncommon in adults and are almost unheard of in children. Sarcomas of the spermatic cord, including malignant fibrous histiocytoma, occur more frequently in adults, but in children rhabdomyosarcoma is the significant cord or adnexal malignancy.[181] The report of Pozza et al regarding a cord liposarcoma in a 16-year-old is a rare exception.[182] Similarly, extraordinary adult malignancies of tunica albuginea or tunica vaginalis, such as malignant mesothelioma, are almost singular occurrences in children.[183,184]

Primary and metastatic malignancies are more likely among the unpleasant surprises of adult hernia sacs, although an occasional metastatic cancer to the spermatic cord and testis in the pediatric age range has been reported.[185,186] Histologic diagnosis of any unusual finding in a hernia sac is therefore mandatory, whatever the age of the patient.

The classic surprise encountered during

inguinal exploration is the finding of reproductive organs of the opposite sex. In a male the presence of a fallopian tube, uterus, and testis was termed hernia uteri inguinale when first described in 1939 by Nilson.[187] Today's usage favors the term *persistent Müllerian duct syndrome.*[188,189] This familial disease probably involves a fetal MIS deficiency due to a Sertoli cell defect. Such patients are genetic and phenotypic males with a normal penis, but have unilateral or bilateral undescended testis and inguinal hernia. Testicular biopsy may be necessary to confirm the diagnosis and orchidopexy should be performed because these patients are potentially fertile without a particularly high risk for gonadal malignancy. Whether the Müllerian structures should be removed is debatable. Some authorities suggest that they be left alone, pointing to the risk of damage to vas deferens and gonadal vascularity from dissection of the adjacent fallopian tube and uterus.[190]

The analogous discovery of a normal testis in the hernia sac of a girl during inguinal herniorrhaphy is usually due to testicular feminization. Such gonads are usually removed after puberty, but if they are removed before then, exogenous estrogens must be administered for successful feminization.

Other unusual encounters have been reported in inguinal and scrotal explorations. On some occasions an appendix may pop out when one opens a hernia sac. In general, the best way to handle this is to simply replace the appendix in the peritoneum, back through the internal ring, and then proceed with high ligation of the sac. Acute appendicitis can first present itself within the inguinal canal and scrotum.[191] Other intraperitoneal catastrophes, such as ruptured spleen, may similarly become apparent by scrotal enlargement.[139]

Inspection of a hydrocele sac sometimes reveals free-floating whitish nodules that may be remnants of previous meconium peritonitis or torsed gonadal appendages.[192] Ventriculoperitoneal shunts may uncover an occult hernia or the shunt itself may insinuate into a hernia sac.[193,194] Acute diverticular disease or other intraperitoneal inflammations may extend down a patent processus vaginalis and present as an acute intrascrotal inflammation.[195] Testicular infarction in an incarcerated hernia is rediscovered periodically.[196]

## REFERENCES

1. Joss N. Physiology of sex differentiation: a guide to the understanding and management of the intersex child. *Pediatr Adolesc Endocrinol.* 1981;8:1.
2. Scott JES. The Hutson hypothesis: a clinical study. *Br J Urol.* 1987;60:74.
3. Levitt SB, Smith RB, Ship AG. Iatrogenic microphallus secondary to circumcision. *Urology.* 1976;8:472.
4. Bloom DA, Ayers JWT, McGuire EJ. The role of laparoscopy in management of nonpalpable testis. *J d'Urologie.* 1988;94:465.
5. Oesch I, Ransley PG. Unilaterally impalpable testis. *Eur Urol.* 1987;13:324.
6. Kogan SJ, Gill B, Bennett B, et al. Human monorchism: a clinicopathological study of unilateral absent testes in 65 boys. *J Urol.* 1986;135:758.
7. Brothers LR III, Weber CH Jr, Ball TP Jr. Anorchism versus cryptorchidism: the importance of a diligent search for intra-abdominal testes. *J Urol.* 1978;119:707.
8. Green AA. Congenital bilateral anorchia in childhood: a clinical, endocrine, and therapeutic evaluation of 21 cases. *Clin Endocrinol.* 1976;5:381.
9. Hancock RA, Hodgins TE. Polyorchidism. *Urology.* 1984;24:303.
10. Thum G. Polyorchidism: case report and review of the literature. *J Urol.* 1991;145:370–372.
11. Snow BW, Tarry WF, Duckett JW. Polyorchidism: an unusual case. *J Urol.* 1985; 133:483.
12. Kale N, Basaklar AC. Polyorchidism. *J Pediatr Surg.* 1991;26:1432.
13. Odell WD, Swerdloff RS. Male hypogonadism. *West J Med.* 1976;124:446.
14. Castro-Magaña M, Bronsther B, Angulo MA. Genetic forms of male hypogonadism. *Urology.* 1990;35:195.
15. Laron A, Ailka G. Compensatory hypertrophy of the testicle in unilateral cryptorchidism. *J Clin Endocrinol Metab.* 1969;29:1409.
16. MacMahon RA, Cussen LJ. Unilateral enlargement of the testis in childhood: does it need exploration? *J Pediatr Surg.* 1991;26:68.
17. Roberts JP, Atwell JD. Testicular enlargement as a presenting feature of monocytic leukemia in an infant. *J Pediatr Surg.* 1989;24:1306.
18. Walther MM, Trulock TS, Finnerty DP, et al. Splenic gonadal fusion. *Urology.* 1988;32:521.

19. Bloom DA, Wan J. Testicular tumors in children. In: Crawford ED, Das S, eds. *Current Genitourinary Cancer Surgery*. Philadelphia: Lea & Febiger; 1990:429–438.
20. Kay R. Unpublished data. Prepubertal Testicular Tumor Registry Report to Executive Committee, Section of Urology, American Academy of Pediatrics, 1992.
21. Skakkebaek NE. Abnormal morphology of germ cells in two infertile men. *Acta Pathol Microbiol Scand*. 1972;80:374.
22. Giwercman A, Bruun E, Frimodt-Moller C, Skakkebaek NE. Prevalence of carcinoma in situ and other histopathological abnormalities in testes of men with a history of cryptorchidism. *J Urol*. 1989;142:998.
23. Scorer CG, Farrington GH. *Congenital Deformities of the Testis and Epididymis*. New York: Appleton-Century Crofts; 1971:212.
24. Jackson MB, Ansell P, Gough MH. The ascending testis: anatomical obstruction to descent at orchiopexy. *Br J Urol*. 1987;60:181.
25. Belman AB. Acquired undescended (ascended) testis: effects of human chorionic gonadotropin. *J Urol*. 1988;140:1189.
26. DeMuinck Keizer-Schrama SM, Hazebroek FW, Drop SL, Degenhert HJ, Molenaar JC, Visser HK. Hormonal evaluation of boys born with undescended testes during their first year of life. *J Clin Endocrinol Metab*. 1988;66:159.
27. Hadziselimovic F. Treatment of cryptorchidism with GnRH. *Urol Clin North Am*. 1982;9:413.
28. Hinman F Jr. Alternatives to orchiopexy. *J Urol*. 1980;123:548.
29. Harris BH, Webb HW, Wilkinson AH Jr, Stevens PS. Protection of the solitary testis. *J Pediatr Surg*. 1982;17:950.
30. Ransley PG, Vordermark JS, Caldamone AA, Bellinger MF. Preliminary ligation of the gonadal vessels prior to orchidopexy for the intra-abdominal testicle. A staged Fowler–Stephens procedure. *World J Urol*. 1984;2:266.
31. Bloom DA. Two step orchiopexy with pelviscopic clip ligation of the spermatic vessels. *J Urol*. 1991;145:1030.
32. Golladay ES, Redman JF. Transverse testicular ectopia. *Urology*. 1982;19:181.
33. Berg AA. Transverse ectopy of the testis. *Ann Surg*. 1904;40:223.
34. Kimura T. Transverse ectopy of the testis with masculine uterus. *Ann Surg*. 1918;68:420.
35. Gauderer MWL, Grisoni ER, Stellato TA, et al. Transverse testicular ectopia. *J Pediatr Surg*. 1982;17:43.
36. Mouli K, McCarthy P, Ray P, et al. Persistent müllerian duct syndrome in a man with transverse testicular ectopia. *J Urol*. 1988;139:373.
37. Fujita J. Transverse testicular ectopia. *Urology*. 1980;16:400.
38. Heyns CF. Exstrophy of the testis. *J Urol*. 1990;144:724.
39. Gongaware RD, et al. Scrotoschisis as a mechanism for extracorporeal testicular ectopia. *J Pediatr Surg*. 1991;26:1430.
40. Zerin JM, DiPietro MA, Grignon A, et al. Testicular infarction in the newborn: ultrasound findings. *Pediatr Radiol*. 1990;20:329.
41. Das S, Singer A. Controversies of perinatal torsion of the spermatic cord: a review, survey and recommendations. *J Urol*. 1990;143:231.
42. Bellinger MF, Abromowitz H, Brantley S, Marshall G. Orchiopexy: an experimental study of the effect of surgical technique on testicular histology. *J Urol*. 1989;142:553.
43. Jung AL, McGaughey HR, Matlak ME. Neonatal testicular infarction and polycythemia. *J Urol*. 1980;123:781.
44. Corrierre JN Jr. Horizontal lie of the testicle: a diagnostic sign in torsion of the testis. *J Urol*. 1981;126:410.
45. Stewart JOR, Maiti AK. Familial torsion of the testicle. *Br J Urol*. 1985;57:190.
46. Williamson RCN. Torsion of the testis and allied conditions. *Br J Surg*. 1976;63:465.
47. Donohoe RE, Utley WL. Torsion of the spermatic cord. *Urology*. 1978;11:33.
48. Barada JH, Weingarten JL, Cromie WL. Testicular salvage. *J Urol*. 1984;142:746.
49. Rabinowitz R. The importance of the cremasteric reflex in acute scrotal swelling in children. *J Urol*. 1984;132:89.
50. Morgenlander HL, Wise GJ. Scrotal aspiration. *Urology*. 1974;4:686.
51. Loh HS, Jala OM. Testicular torsion in Henoch–Schönlein syndrome. *Br Med J*. 1974; 2:96.
52. Lynch DF Jr, Peterson NR, Powell RW. Pseudotorsion of testis. *Urology*. 1983;21:68.
53. Frazier WJ, Buch JG. Manipulation of torsion of the testicle. *J Urol*. 1975;114:410.
54. Haynes BE, Haynes VE. Manipulative detorsion: beware the twist that does not turn. *J Urol*. 1987;137:118.
55. Betts JM, Norris M, Cromie WJ, Duckett JW. Testicular detorsion using Doppler ultrasound monitoring. *J Pediatr Surg*. 1983;18:607.
56. Nasrallah PF, Manzone D, King LR. Falsely negative Doppler examinations in testicular torsion. *J Urol*. 1977;118:194.
57. Boyarsky S. Scrotal cooling and testicular torsion. *J Urol*. 1989;141:960.
58. Miller DC, Peron SE, Keck RW, Kropp KA. Effects of hypothermia on testicular ischemia. *J Urol*. 1990;143:1046.
59. Wallace DMA, Gunter PA, Landon GV, et al. Sympathetic orchiopathia: an experimental and clinical study. *Br J Urol*. 1982;54:765.

60. Turner TT. On unilateral testicular and epididymal torsion: no effect on the contralateral testis. *J Urol.* 1987;138:1285.

61. Fisch H, Laor E, Reid RE, et al. Gonadal dysfunction after testicular torsion: luteinizing hormone and follicle-stimulating hormone response to gonadotropin-releasing hormone. *J Urol.* 1988;139:961.

62. Puri P, Barton D, O'Donnell B. Prepubertal testicular torsion: subsequent fertility. *J Pediatr Surg.* 1985;20:598.

63. Feins NR. To pex or not to pex. *J Pediatr Surg.* 1983;18:697.

64. Mizrahi S, Shtamler B. Surgical approach and outcome in torsion of the testes. *Urology.* 1992;39:52–54.

65. Dimpoulos C, Giannopoulos A, Doikas J, et al. Unusual presentation of testicular torsion: a review of 40 cases. *Eur Urol.* 1976;2:179.

66. Valvo JR, Caldamone AA, O'Mara R, Rabinowitz R. Nuclear imaging in the pediatric acute scrotum. *Am J Dis Child.* 1982;136:831.

67. Cass AS. Elective orchiopexy for recurrent testicular torsion. *J Urol.* 1982;127:253.

68. Nistal M, Regadera J, Redondo E, et al. Cystic intra-abdominal testicular torsion in an infant. *J Urol.* 1985;133:481.

69. Hulecki SJ, Crawford JP, Broecker B. Testicular torsion after orchiopexy with nonabsorbable sutures. *Urology.* 1986;28:131.

70. Redman JF, O'Donnell PD. Simultaneous ipsilateral torsion of the appendices testis and epididymis. *J Urol.* 1977;117:255.

71. Langman J. *Medical Embryology.* 4th ed. Baltimore: Williams and Wilkins; 1981:234–267.

72. Deane AM, May RE. Absent vas deferens in association with renal abnormalities. *Br J Urol.* 1982;54:298–299.

73. Lukash F, Zwiren GT, Andrews HG. Significance of absent vas deferens at hernia repair in infants and children. *J Pediatr Surg.* 1975; 10:765.

74. Van Wingerden JJ, Franz I. The presence of a caput epididymides in congenital absence of the vas deferens. *J Urol.* 1984;131:764–766.

75. Goldstein M, Schlossberg S. Men with congenital absence of the vas deferens often have seminal vesicles. *J Urol.* 1988;140:85–86.

76. Pedersen J, Rubenson A. Occurrence of sperm antibodies in postpubertal boys operated upon for inguinal hernia in infancy or childhood. In: Pedersen J, ed. *Prefertile vas lesion as a cause of sperm antibody formation.* Pedersen, Goteberg, Sweden: University of Goteberg Press; 1987:2–11.

77. Weber CH. Successful restoration of fertility twenty-nine years after bilateral vasal injury in infancy. *Urology.* 1986;28:299–300.

78. Vordermark JS Jr. The persisting mesonephric duct syndrome; the description of a new syndrome. *J Urol.* 1983;130:958.

79. Schwarz R, Stephens FD. The persisting mesonephric duct: high junction of vas deferens and ureter. *J Urol.* 1978;120:592.

80. Ayyat F, Palmer MD, Tingley JO. Ectopic vas deferens communicating with lower ureter. *Urology.* 1982;19:423.

81. Boles ET Jr, Lobe TE, Hamoudi A. Congenital vas deferens–ureteral connection. *J Pediatr Surg.* 1978;13:41.

82. Alfert HJ, Gillenwater JY: Ectopic vas deferens communicating with lower ureter: embryological considerations. *J Urol.* 1972;126:172.

83. Hicks CM, Skoog SJ, Done S. Ectopic vas deferens, imperforate anus, and hypospadias: a new triad. *J Urol.* 1989;141:586–588.

84. Miura T, Takahashi G. Crossed ectopic testis with common vas deferens. *J Urol.* 1985; 134:1206–1208.

85. Holsclaw DS, Perlmutter AD, Jockin H, Shwachman H. Genital abnormalities in male patients with cystic fibrosis. *J Urol.* 1971; 106:568.

86. Kaplan E, Shwachman H, Perlmutter AD, Rule A, Khaw KT, Holsclaw DS. Reproductive failure in males with cystic fibrosis. *N Engl J Med.* 1968;279:65.

87. Valman HB, France NE. The vas deferens in cystic fibrosis. *Lancet.* 1969;2(620):566.

88. Ryan SP, Harte PJ. Suppurative inflammation of vas deferens: an unusual groin mass. *Urology.* 1988;31:245–246.

89. Steers WD, Corriere JN Jr. Case profile: seminal vesicle cyst. *Urology.* 1986;27:177–178.

90. Roehrborn CG, Schneider H-J, Rugenorff EW, Hamann W. Embryological and diagnostic aspects of seminal vesicle cysts associated with upper urinary tract malformation. *J Urol.* 1986;135:1029–1032.

91. Patel MR, Dulabon D, Roth R. Case profile: absent seminal vesicle diagnosed by transrectal ultrasound. *Urology.* 1987;29:332.

92. Shabsigh R, Lerner S, Fishman IJ, Kadmon D. The role of transrectal ultrasonography in the diagnosis and management of prostatic and seminal vesicle cysts. *J Urol.* 1989;141:1206–1209.

93. Elder JS, Mostwin JL. Cyst of the ejaculatory duct/urogenital sinus. *J Urol.* 1984;132:768–770.

94. Donohue RE, Denes K, Surya BV, Washecka R, Glasser J, Johanson KE. Cysts of the seminal vesicles: diagnosis and management. *Br J Urol.* 1988;62:491–493.

95. Kawahara M, Matsuhhashi M, Tajima M, et al. Primary carcinoma of the seminal vesicle. *Urology.* 1988;32:269–272.

96. Mininberg DT. The epididymis and testicular descent. *Eur J Pediatrics.* 1987;146(Suppl 2):S28–S30.

97. Johansen TEB. Anatomy of the testis and epididymis in cryptorchidism. *Andrologia.* 1987;19:565.

98. Gill B, Kogan S, Starr S, Reda E, Levitt S. Significance of epididymal and ductal anomalies associated with testicular maldescent. *J Urol.* 1989;142:556.

99. Marshall FF, Shermeta DW. Epididymal abnormalities associated with undescended testis. *J Urol.* 1979;121:341.

100. Heath AL, Man DWK, Eckstein HB. Epididymal abnormalities associated with maldescent of the testis. *J Pediatr Surg.* 1984;19:47.

101. Toth MMJ. Testicular-epididymal fusion abnormality in undescended testis. *Int Urol Neph.* 1987;19(2):179.

102. Cendron M, Keating MA, Huff DS, et al. Cryptorchidism, orchiopexy and infertility: a critical long-term retrospective analysis. *J Urol.* 1989;142:559.

103. DePalma L, Carter D, Weiss RM. Epididymal and vas deferens immaturity in cryptorchidism. *J Urol.* 1988;140:1194–1196.

104. Hendry WF. Testicular obstruction. *Br J Urol.* 1988;62:471.

105. Hellstrom P, Tammela T, Kontturi M, Lukkarinen O. Ethanolamine oleate as a sclerosant for testicular hydroceles and epididymal cysts. *Br J Urol.* 1988;62:445–448.

106. Hedelin H, Eddeland A, Johansson S, Mark J. Torsion of a large epididymal mass. *Br J Urol.* 1986;58:560–561.

107. Murayama T, Fujita K, Ohashi T, Matsushita T. Melanotic neuroectodermal tumor of the epididymis in infancy: a case report. *J Urol.* 1989;141:105–106.

108. Bloom DA, DiPietro MA, Gikas PW, McGuire EJ. Extratesticular dermoid cyst and fibrous dysplasia of epididymis. *J Urol.* 1987;137:996.

109. Wollin M, Marshall FF, Fink MP, Malhotra R, Diamond DA. Aberrant epididymal tissue: a significant clinical entity. *J Urol.* 1987; 138:1247–1250.

110. Waldman LS, Kosloske AM, Parsons DW. Acute epididymo-orchitis as the presenting manifestation of hemophilus influenzae septicemia. *J Pediatrics.* 1977;90:87.

111. Cervia JS, Tosi MF. Cellulitis of the scrotum with bacteremia caused by Haemophilus influenzae type b. *Ped Infec Dis.* 1988;7(7):517.

112. Greenfield SP. Type B Hemophilus influenzae epididymo-orchitis in the prepubertal boy. *J Urol.* 1986;136:1311.

113. Khan MS, Humayoon MS, Al Manee MS. Epididymo-orchitis and brucellosis. *Br J Urol.* 1989;63:87–89.

114. Randazzo RF, Hulette CM, Gottleib MS, Rajfer J. Cytomegaloviral epididymitis in a patient with the acquired immune deficiency syndrome. *J Urol.* 1986;136:1095–1097.

115. Siegel A, Snyder H, Duckett JW. Epididymitis in infants and boys: underlying urogenital anomalies and efficacy of imaging modalities. *J Urol.* 1987;138:1100–1103.

116. Gislason T, Noronha RFX, Gregory JG. Acute epididymitis in boys: a 5-year retrospective study. *J Urol.* 1980;124:533.

117. See WA, Taylor TO, Mack LA, Tartaglione TA, Opheim KE, Berger RE. Bacterial epididymitis in the rat: a model for assessing the impact of acute inflammation on epididymal antibiotic penetration. *J Urol.* 1990;144:780–784.

118. Lamm DL, Kaplan GW. Accessory and ectopic scrota. *Urology.* 1977;9:149.

119. Anlar B, Ayabakan S. Transposition of the external genitalia: a case with cardiovascular malformations and polycystic kidneys. *Eur J Pediatrics.* 1986;145:161.

120. Miller SF. Transposition of the external genitalia associated with the syndrome of caudal regression. *J Urol.* 1972;108:818.

121. Appleby LH. An unusual arrangement of the external genitalia. *Can Med Assoc J.* 1922; 13:514.

122. Berry SA, Johnson DE, Thompson TR. Agenesis of the penis, scrotal raphe, and anus in one of monoamniotic twins. *Teratology.* 1984; 29:173.

123. Sakamoto K, Kuroki Y, Fujisawa Y, et al. XX/XY chromosomal mosaicism presenting a chordee without hypospadias associated with scrotal transposition. *J Urol.* 1978;119:841.

124. Datta NS, Singh SM, Reddy AVS, et al. Transposition of penis and scrotum in 2 brothers. *J Urol.* 1971;105:739.

125. Lage JM, Driscoll SG, Bieber FR. Transposition of the external genitalia associated with caudal regression. *J Urol.* 1987;138:387.

126. Laing AG. Penoscrotal inversion and its management. *Br J Urol.* 1983;36:124.

127. Nakajima T, Yoshimura Y, Naide Y. Surgical correction of complete bifid scrotum using subcutaneous pedicle flaps: a report of two cases. *Br J Pediatr Surg.* 1989;42:328.

128. Paramo PG, Hinderer U, San Antonio J, et al. Prepenile scrotum. *Eur Urol.* 1981;7:246.

129. Mori Y, Ikoma F. Surgical correction of incomplete penoscrotal transposition associated with hypospadias. *J Pediatr Surg.* 1986;21:46.

130. Glenn JF, Anderson EE. Surgical correction of incomplete penoscrotal transposition. *J Urol.* 1973;110:603.

131. Tripathi FM, Khanna S. Accessory scrotum: a case report. *Br J Plas Surg.* 1983;36:127.

132. Mininberg DT, Richman A. Bilateral scrotal testicular ectopia. *J Urol.* 1972;108:652.

133. Yokokawa K, Nakano E, Takaha M. Accessory scrotum: a case report. *J Urol.* 1986;135:593.

134. Gupta SK, Gupta S, Khann S. Dermoid cyst of scrotal raphe containing calculi. *Br J Urol.* 1974;46:348.

135. Kaplan GW. Acute idiopathic scrotal edema. *J Pediatr Surg.* 1977;12:647.

136. Evans JP, Snyder HM. Idiopathic scrotal edema. *Urology.* 1977;9:549.

137. Lau JTK, Ong GB. Acute idiopathic penile edema: a separate clinical entity? *J Urol.* 1981;126:704.

138. Sujka SK, Jewett TC Jr, Karp MP. Acute scrotal swelling as the first evidence of intraabdominal trauma in a battered child. *J Pediatr Surg.* 1988;23:380.

139. Skoog SJ, Belman AB. The communicating hematocele: an unusual presentation for blunt splenic trauma. *J Urol.* 1986;136:1092–1093.

140. Andrews R, Mason W. Cysticercosis presenting as acute scrotal pain and swelling. *Pediatr Infec Dis J.* 1987;6:942.

141. Crewe W, Haddock DRW. *Parasites and Human Disease.* New York: John Wiley and Sons; 1985:99–100.

142. Feins NR. A new surgical technique for lymphedema of the penis and scrotum. *J Pediatr Surg.* 1980;15:787.

143. Fitzsimmons JS. Uncommon complication of anaphylactoid purpura. *Br Med J.* 1968;4:431.

144. Sahn DJ, Schwartz AD. Schonlein–Henoch syndrome: observations on some atypical clinical presentations. *Pediatrics.* 1972;49:614.

145. Clark WR, Kramer SA. Henoch–Schonlein purpura and the acute scrotum. *J Pediatr Surg.* 1986;21:991.

146. Kahn AU, Williams TH, Malek RS. Acute scrotal swelling in Henoch–Schonlein syndrome. *Urology.* 1977;10:139.

147. Allen DM, Diamond LK, Howell DA. Anaphylactoid purpura in children (Schonlein–Henoch syndrome). *Am J Dis Child.* 1960; 99:833.

148. Loh HS, Jalan OM. Testicular torsion in Henoch–Schonlein syndrome. *Br Med J.* 1974; 2:96.

149. Naiman JL, Harcke T, Sebastianelli J, Stein BS. Scrotal imaging in the Henoch–Schonlein syndrome. *J Pediatrics.* 1978;92:1021.

150. Stein BS, Kendall AR, Harke T, Naiman JL, Karafin L. Scrotal imaging in the Henoch–Schonlein syndrome. *J Urol.* 1980;124:568.

151. Hinman F Sr, Johnson CM. Differential diagnosis of acute fat necrosis in the scrotum. *J Urol.* 1939;41:726.

152. Nemoy NJ, Rosin S, Kaplan L. Scrotal panniculitis in the prepubertal male patient. *J Urol.* 1977;118:492.

153. Coppes MJ, Roukema JA, Bax NMA. Scrotal pneumatocele; a rare phenomenon. *J Pediatr Surg.* 1991;26:1428.

154. Mabry RM, Harwood AL. Fournier's disease: necrotizing gangrene of the male genitalia. *J Emer Med.* 1983;1:133.

155. Spirnak JP, Resnick MI, Hampel N, Persky L. Fournier's gangrene: report of 20 patients. *J Urol.* 1984;131:289.

156. Rothberg M, Klingman RR, Montag M, Redlan R, Fitzgibbons R Jr. Fournier's syndrome: an unusual case presentation. *Infec Surg.* 1989; 8:325.

157. Adeyokunnu AA. Fournier's syndrome in infants. *Clin Pediatrics.* 1983;22:101.

158. Sussman SJ, Schiller RP, Shashikumar VL. Fournier's syndrome: report of three cases and review of the literature. *Am J Dis Child.* 1978;132:1189.

159. Chaviano AH. Fournier's gangrene in children. *Infec Urol.* 1989;2:137.

160. DiFalco G, Guccione C, D'Annibale A, Ronsisvalle S, Lavesso P, Fregonese D, et al. Fournier's gangrene following a perianal abscess. *Dis Colon Rectum.* 1986;29:582.

161. Eltorai IM, Hart GB, Strauss MB, Montroy R, Juler GL. The role of hyperbaric oxygen in the management of Fournier's gangrene. *Int Surg.* 1986;71:53.

162. Ziser A, Girsh Z, Gozal D, Melamed Y, Adler M. Hyperbaric oxygen therapy for Fournier's gangrene. *Crit Care Med.* 1985;13:773.

163. Gross RE. *The Surgery of Infancy and Childhood.* Philadelphia: WB Saunders; 1953:453.

164. Moss RL, Hatch EI Jr. Inguinal hernia repair in early infancy. *Am J Surg.* 1991;161:596.

165. Rathauser F. Historical overview of the bilateral approach to pediatric inguinal hernias. *Am J Surg.* 1985;150:527.

166. Given JP, Rubin SZ. Occurrence of contralateral inguinal hernia following unilateral repair in a pediatric hospital. *J Pediatr Surg.* 1989; 24:963.

167. Allen RP, Condon VR. Transitory extraperitoneal hernia of the bladder in infants (bladder ears). *Radiology.* 1961;77:979–982.

168. Colodny AH. Bladder injury during herniorrhaphy. *Urology.* 1974;3:89–90.

169. Redman JF, Jacks BW, O'Donnell PD. Cystectomy: a catastrophic complication of herniorrhaphy. *J Urol.* 1985;133:97–98.

170. Shaw A, Santulli TV. Management of sliding hernias of the urinary bladder in infants. *Surg Gynecol Obstet.* 1967;124:1314–1316.

171. Lockwood CB. Pedunculated cysts within a hernial sac. *Trans Pathol Soc London.* 1896; 47:61–64.

172. Esho JO, Vitko RJ, Cass AS. Protrusion and torsion of an inguinal hernia sac inside a hydrocele of the scrotum. *J Pediatr Surg.* 1974; 9:423.

173. Squire R, Gough DCS. Abdominoscrotal hydrocele in infancy. *Br J Urol.* 1988;61:347–349.

174. Marshall FF, Shermeta DW. Epididymal abnormalities associated with undescended testes. *J Urol.* 1979;121:341.

175. Whitehead ED, Leiter E. Genital abnormalities and abnormal semen analysis in male patients exposed to diethylstilbesterol in utero. *J Urol.* 1981;125:47–50.

176. Schmidt SS, Minckler TM. Pseudocysts of the tunica albuginea: benign invasion by testicular tubules. *J Urol.* 1987;138:151.

177. Heetderks DR Jr, Hommerson HJ. Complex tunica albuginea cysts: a review of the literature. *J Urol.* 1988;139:1318–1320.

178. Altadonna V, Snyder HM, Rosenberg HK, Duckett JW. Simple cysts of the testis in children: preoperative diagnosis by ultrasound and excision with testicular preservation. *J Urol.* 1988;140:1505–1507.

179. Priebe CJ Jr, Holahan JA, Ziring PR. Abnormalities of the vas deferens and epididymis in cryptorchid boys with congenital rubella. *J Pediatr Surg.* 1979;14:834–838.

180. Donohue RE, Fauver HE. Unilateral absence of the vas deferens, a useful clinical sign. *JAMA.* 1989;261:1180.

181. Williamson JL, Johnson JD, Lamm DL, Tio F. Malignant fibrous histiocytoma of the spermatic cord. *J Urol.* 1980;123:785–788.

182. Pozza D, Masci P, D'Ottavio G, Zappvigna D. Spermatic cord liposarcoma in a young boy. *J Urol.* 1987;137:306–308.

183. Stein N, Henkes D. Mesothelioma of the testicle in a child. *J Urol.* 1986;135:794.

184. Velasco AL, Ophoven J, Priest JR, Brennom WS. Paratesticular malignant mesothelioma associated with abdominoscrotal hydrocele. *J Pediatr Surg.* 1988;11:1065–1067.

185. Lewis LG, Goodwin WE, Randall WS. Carcinoma of the spermatic cord and epididymis extension from primary carcinoma of the stomach. *J Urol.* 1944;51:75–80.

186. Yoell JH. Surprises in hernial sacs. Diagnosis of tumors by microscopic examination. *Cal Med.* 1959;91:146–148.

187. Nilson O. Hernia uteri inguinalis berm manne. *Acta Chir Scand.* 1939;83:231.

188. Sloan WR, Walsh PC. Familial persistent Müllerian duct syndrome. *J Urol.* 1976;115:459–461.

189. Beheshti M, Churchill BM, Hardy BE, Bailey JD, Weksberg R, Rogan GF. Familial persistent Müllerian duct syndrome. *J Urol.* 1984;131:968–969.

190. Rajfer J. *Urologic Endocrinology.* Philadelphia: WB Saunders; 1986:28–34.

191. Alvear DT, Rayfield MM. Acute appendicitis presenting as a scrotal mass. *J Pediatr Surg.* 1976;11:91–92.

192. Fries JW, Talbot BS. Scrotal calcification due to meconium peritonitis. *J Urol.* 1955;73:1059–1068.

193. Moazam F, Glenn JD, Kaplan BJ, Talbert JL, Mickle JP. Inguinal hernias after ventriculoperitoneal shunt procedures in pediatric patients. *Surg Gynecol Obstet.* 1984;159:570–572.

194. Ram Z, Findlet G, Guttman I, Cherniak R, Knoller N, Shacked I. Ventriculoperitoneal shunt malfunction due to migration of the abdominal catheter into the scrotum. *J Pediatr Surg.* 1987;11:1045–1046.

195. Kanzer B, Rosenberg RF. Unusual contents in inguinal hernia sacs. *New York State J Med.* Sept 1983:1055–1056.

196. Colodny AH. Testicular infarction. *Soc Ped Urol Newslett.* December 24, 1988:51.

# 53

# Myelomeningocele and Neuropathic Bladder

*Mark F. Bellinger*

## INTRODUCTION

The normal function of the lower urinary tract, its neurological control, and the stepwise development of normal control in the infant and child represent extremely complex processes. These processes involve the interaction of many distinct components that must come to function as a coordinated whole in order to produce normal urinary continence. Dysfunction of any component of this system may not only result in incontinence, but also jeopardize renal function. Children with neurovesical dysfunction challenge the urologist to provide stability of the upper tracts, ensure preservation of renal function, and implement a plan for urinary continence.

## PHYSIOLOGY OF THE LOWER URINARY TRACT

### Functional Anatomy

The lower urinary tract serves two functions: low-pressure storage and periodic voluntary elimination of urine. The bladder, composed of a mesh of smooth muscle bundles lined by mucosa and covered with an adventitium of connective tissue, is divided into two functionally distinct areas: the detrusor and the trigone or bladder base.[1] The trigone can be divided into two embryologically and anatomically distinct components: the deep trigone, considered to be a continuation of the musculature of the detrusor and the superficial trigone, a continuation of the longitudinal musculature of the distal ureter and Waldeyer's sheath.[2] At the bladder neck the smooth muscle fibers of the detrusor and trigone coalesce, although no anatomically distinct sphincter is found. The exact nature of the anatomic continuity of bladder and urethral smooth muscle remains a subject of debate. The more popular concept is that the longitudinal layer of the superficial trigone extends beyond the bladder neck to contribute to the musculature of the posterior portion of the male urethra (to the level of the verumontanum) and most of the urethral musculature in the female.[3] The urethra in both sexes has an inner longitudinal layer of smooth muscle and, although descriptions vary, is generally considered to have a thin outer circular layer.

The elements that make up the striated muscle component of the bladder outlet (the "external sphincter") have been given various anatomic descriptions by several authors, and their anatomy and function remain the subject of controversy.[4–6] Striated muscle fibers contribute to two components of the sphincter mechanism. The first, or intrinsic, component is made up of fibers that are intimately associated with the urethra and variously described as spiral, oblique, or circular in configuration. These fibers interdigitate with the smooth muscle of the outer layer of urethral musculature of the posterior urethra in the male and the entire portion of the female urethra located above the urogenital diaphragm. The extrinsic component of the striated sphincter corresponds to the classical anatomic external sphincter and is located between the leaves of the urogenital diaphragm, attached to the ischiopubic rami and encircling the membranous portion of the urethra. The fibers are tapered posteriorly in the male and are significantly more deficient in the female. Most contemporary descriptions in the male show striated muscle incorporated within the prostate and prostatic capsule, as if the primordia of the prostate thinned out the outer muscular sheath of the urethra during expansion from its urethral anlagen.[7] In the female, fibers of striated muscle surround the urethra and vagina, with a component that attaches to the ischiopubic rami and swings across the ventral urethra to act as a compressor muscle.

Although muscle fibers form the bladder reservoir and its anatomic sphincters, the function of the lower urinary tract is dependent on and regulated by the nervous system. Three separate groups of peripheral nerves are responsible for lower genitourinary tract function: somatic nerves (pudendal) and two sets of autonomic nerves, the sacral parasympathetics (pelvic nerves) and the thoracolumbar sympathetics (hypogastric nerves and sympathetic chain)[8] (Fig 1). Parasympathetic fibers originate from spinal cord segments S2–S4, exit via the ventral roots, and form the pelvic nerves. Efferent sympathetic fibers originate from the T11-L2 cord segments and pass via the lumbar sympathetic chain and superior hypogastric plexus to the right and left hypogastric nerves which, together

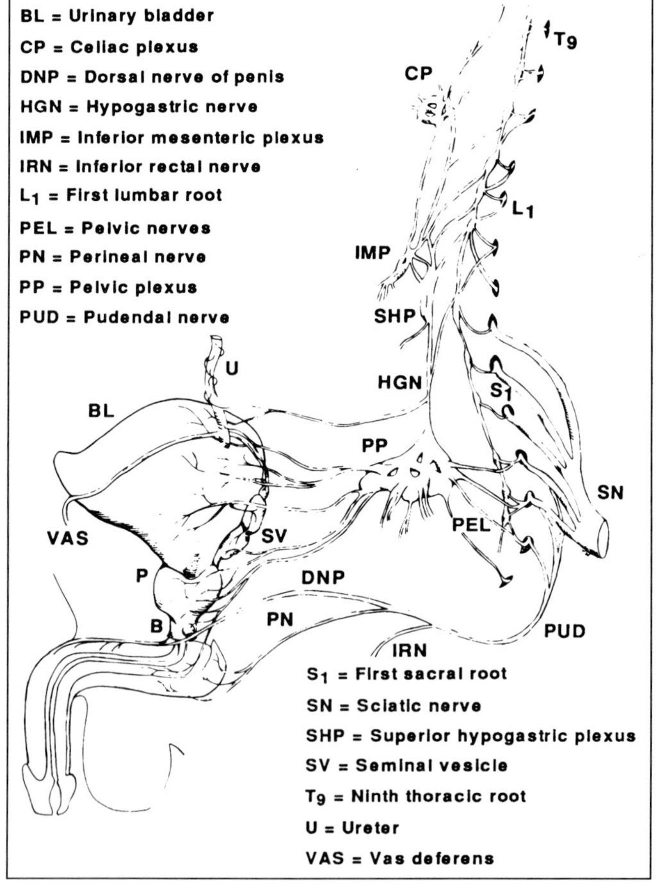


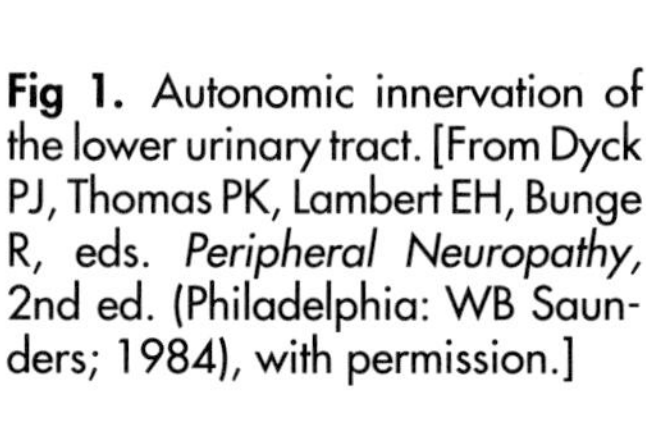
**Fig 1.** Autonomic innervation of the lower urinary tract. [From Dyck PJ, Thomas PK, Lambert EH, Bunge R, eds. *Peripheral Neuropathy,* 2nd ed. (Philadelphia: WB Saunders; 1984), with permission.]

with the pelvic nerves, form the pelvic plexus. The innervation of the striated sphincter is debated, although most authors agree that the sacral cord segments, via the pudendal nerve, provide the primary efferent input. Afferent fibers from submucosal and muscular fibers pass via the hypogastric, pelvic, and pudendal nerves through dorsal and ventral roots to the lumbosacral cord.[6]

Normal function of the lower urinary tract requires coordinated activity of this entire neuromuscular apparatus, such that the normal response to bladder filling at physiologic rates is a negligible rise in intravesical pressure, combined with increased urethral pressure. Micturition is initiated by outlet relaxation, followed by detrusor contraction.[8]

## NEUROVESICAL DYSFUNCTION

Alteration of the normal function of the lower urinary tract may result from both congenital and acquired lesions. The result of dysfunction may be expressed clinically as urinary retention, frequency, urgency, strangury, interrupted urination, or incontinence. Urodynamic findings may include urinary retention, incomplete bladder emptying, detrusor hyperreflexia, elevated intravesical pressures, nonrelaxing or incompetent bladder neck, or detrusor-sphincter dyssynergia. Hydronephrosis or vesicoureteric reflux (VUR) may be the end result, particularly in the face of elevated intravesical pressure.[9] The complex nature of neurovesical dysfunction and many approaches to its management have occasioned the proposal of several schemes for classification of neurovesical disease, each with proponents and detractors. Since classification and terminology seem to creep into any discussion of neurovesical disease, a superficial review of the most widely used schemes may be helpful to the clinician.

Bors and Comarr proposed the first widely accepted classification, based primarily on the clinical manifestations of patients with spinal cord injury.[10] They categorized neurologic lesions as affecting sensory neurons, motor neurons, or both; as being neurologically complete or incomplete; and as located either above or below the sacral reflex arc (upper or lower neuron lesion). They also noted whether the bladder was ''balanced'' (small residual urine volume as compared to bladder capacity) or ''unbalanced'' (greater than 10%–20% postvoid residual, implying detrusor-outlet dyssynergy). The Bors–Comarr classification is most applicable to patients with complete spinal cord injury.

Lapides outlined what has become perhaps the most widely utilized system for classification of neurovesical dysfunction: sensory neurogenic, motor paralytic, uninhibited neurogenic, reflex neurogenic, and autonomous neurogenic bladder dysfunction.[11] These categories of dysfunction, although highly descriptive, are rarely found in the pure state in clinical practice since most patients are found to possess characteristics of more than one group and demonstrate lesions of variable severity. The Lapides classification provides a bridge between the neurologic emphasis of the Bors and Comarr and the purely urodynamic classification later described by Krane and Siroky (which classifies the detrusor as hyperreflexic, normoreflexic, or areflexic, and subclassifies sphincter function as coordinated, dyssynergic, or nonrelaxing).[12] Similarly, the International Continence Society classifies detrusor function (normal, overactive, underactive), urethral function (normal, overactive, incompetent), and sensation (normal, hypersensitive, hyposensitive).[13]

On a purely functional basis, several authors have endorsed a simple classification system: failure to store vs. failure to empty.[14] This system can be expanded by subclassification of each category using functional characteristics described by Krane and Siroky[12] or the International Continence Society.[13]

## EVALUATION OF THE CHILD WITH NEUROVESICAL DYSFUNCTION

### History

The urologist may be asked to evaluate a child with known, suspected, or unrecognized neurovesical dysfunction. Presenting symptoms may include urinary tract infection; urinary retention; incontinence; hematuria; urgency, frequency, or other dysfunctional voiding pattern; or renal failure. In addition, young infants may demonstrate failure to thrive due to urinary tract infection or renal failure. When neurovesical dysfunction is known to exist, the medical history should include a review of all prior surgical procedures and previously attempted programs or therapies for bladder and bowel management (including medications prescribed in the past as well as the effects and side effects of each medication). Changes that have occurred in the general neurologic processes affecting the child and in bowel and bladder function in particular should be recorded. It is important to obtain the results of past urodynamic and radiographic evaluations.

If neurovesical disease is suspected but not proven, historical aspects take on a slightly different character, but with equal importance. A thorough voiding history should be obtained, beginning in infancy. It is important to know whether a period of "normal" urinary control existed prior to the development of the current symptom complex, whether changes in the pattern of urinary control have been rapid, gradual, or intermittent, and whether they are associated with other symptoms that might add further concern about neurologic dysfunction (constipation, fecal incontinence or other changes in bowel habits, spasticity, gait change, seizures, or back pain). Since incontinence may be a presenting complaint in many types of pediatric urologic disease, historical aspects take on an important role in the urologist's assessment of both the potential nature and seriousness of the complaint, and may influence the course of diagnostic evaluation and therapy. Incontinence may be primary or secondary, and thus a symptom of either congenital or acquired neurovesical disease. Secondary nocturnal enuresis is most commonly associated with either urinary tract infection or stress-related factors. Urge incontinence may be associated with uninhibited bladder activity and may be seen in neurovesical disease of several etiologies, but may also be a symptom of urinary tract infection or stress-related phenomenon. Dribbling or total incontinence may be a symptom of an ectopic ureter in a girl and may also be representative of sphincteric incompetence, detrusor hyperreflexia, overflow, or a combination of factors. Since emotional, behavioral, psychological, and stress factors are known to be a cause of extremely disordered voiding dynamics in children (see the section on Hinman–Allen Syndrome), and since the presentation of this syndrome may be difficult clinically to distinguish from both neurovesical dysfunction and infravesical obstruction, social factors and family dynamics should be surveyed as a part of the medical history. All aspects of the medical, developmental, social, and voiding history of children with proven or suspected neurovesical dysfunction should be taken into consideration during the initial evaluation and follow-up.

### Physical Examination

Physical examination may confirm evidence for the suspicion of neurovesical disease provided by the medical history. A complete physical examination should include an assessment of muscular development, gait and balance, and general neuromuscular function. Reflexes should be tested for symmetry and the presence of hyperreflexia. Rectal sphincter tone should be assessed, the presence of hard stool or impaction noted, and the bulbocavernosus reflex tested. The abdominal examination should seek evidence of bladder distension or a colon palpably distended with stool, and whether the crede maneuver results in the expression of urine from the bladder. The genitalia should be examined for skin excoriation or fecal soiling as evidence of incontinence. In the male meatal stenosis, hypospadias, and cryptorchidism should be noted, and in the female labial adhesions or introital or perineal anomalies may be of significance. The back should be examined for unusual sacral dimples, hair patches, or other cutaneous lesions (such as hemangiomas) that may indicate underlying spinal dysraphism (Fig 2).

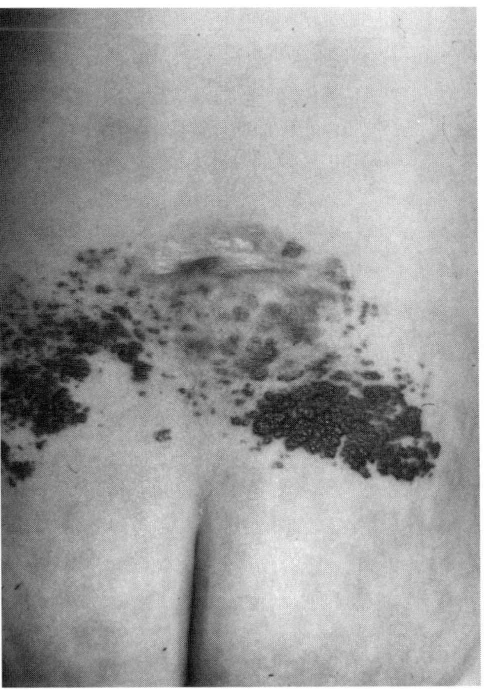

Fig 2. Sacral hemangioma associated with tethered spinal cord.

## Laboratory Examination

Laboratory examination of the child with neurovesical dysfunction includes urinalysis and urine culture and sensitivity. If neurovesical dysfunction is documented, baseline renal function studies should be obtained. If renal cortical damage is present, creatinine clearance determination by timed urine collection or determination of glomerular filtration rate by a radionuclide clearance technique should be carried out.

## Urinary Tract Imaging

Diagnostic ultrasound is the imaging modality most suited for screening and periodic reevaluation of the urinary tract in children with neurovesical dysfunction. Information that is most useful from ultrasound examination includes renal length, presence and degree of hydronephrosis, bladder wall thickness, and postvoid residual urine determination.

Voiding cystourethrography provides a great deal of anatomic and functional information. The plain film should be examined for evidence of spinal anomalies and constipation (Figs 3 and 4). Contrast studies offer information about bladder size and configuration (wall thickness and trabeculation), outlet competence (both internal and external sphincters), and the presence of paraureteric weakness or diverticula and the presence and severity of VUR (Fig 5). A voiding cystourethrogram (VCUG) should be performed in the neonate and any child with new-onset hydronephrosis (to rule out VUR). Children with VUR require periodic reevaluation. This is best carried out by nuclear voiding cystourethrography, a technique that exposes the child to less radiation. The routine VCUG, especially when performed with the child in the upright or semiupright position, provides information about the competence of the bladder neck that will be useful later in childhood when a plan for bladder management is being developed.

Radionuclide renal imaging may play a role in the evaluation and management of the child with neurovesical dysfunction in

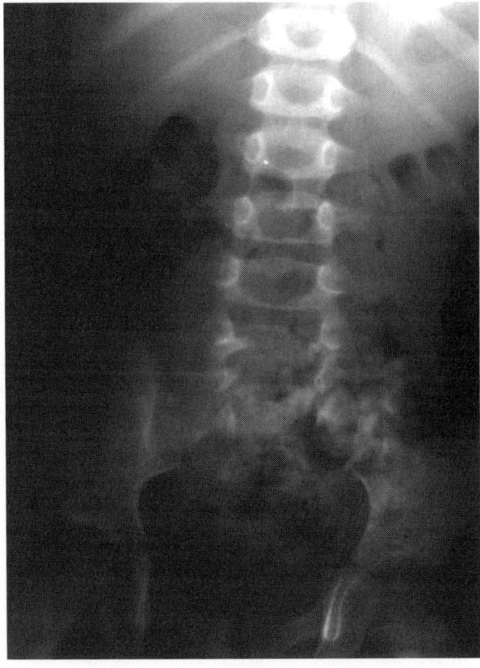

Fig 3. Widened lumbosacral spine with no external findings. Patient had tethered spinal cord.

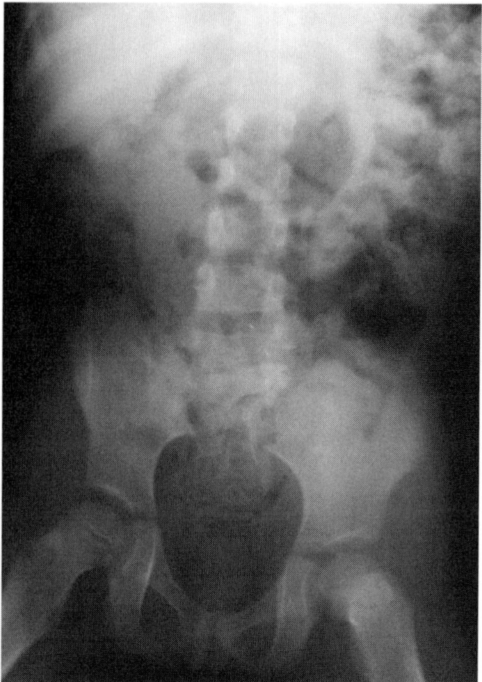

**Fig 4.** Anomalous lumbosacral spine and pelvis in a patient with imperforate anus and tethered spinal cord.

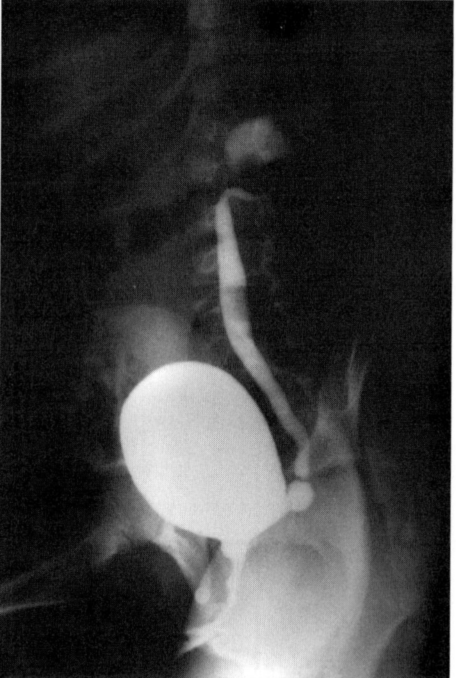

**Fig 5.** Voiding cystourethrogram showing left vesicoureteric reflux in a girl with a paraureteric diverticulum.

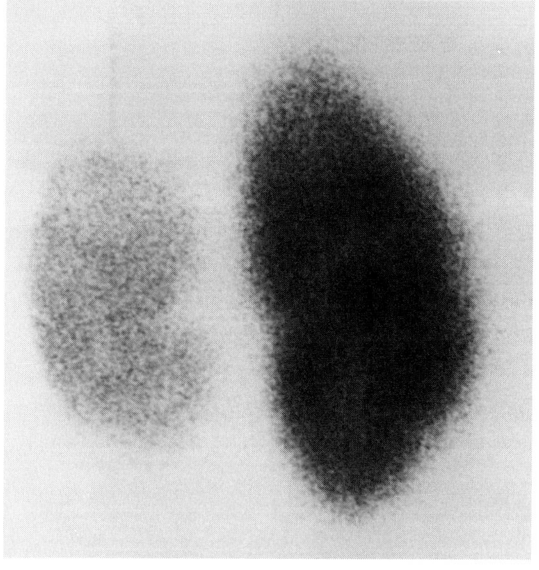

**Fig 6.** DMSA image of normal right kidney *(posterior view)*. Left kidney is barely seen out of the field of imaging.

specific instances. Static imaging with technetium-99m dimercaptosuccinic acid (DMSA) may be helpful in assessing differential renal size and function in the child with severe scoliosis, which makes ultrasound imaging technically difficult (Fig 6).[15] This imaging technique is especially valuable as an accurate tool for the diagnosis of acute pyelonephritis, which is demonstrated as a parenchymal filling defect (Fig 7).[16] In the child who is managed with chronic intermittent catheterization and who has a chronically colonized lower urinary tract, the presence of a fever may be a difficult diagnostic problem, and often the urinary tract is blamed for the fever solely because of the presence of bacteriuria. The DMSA scan, however, allows an accurate diagnosis of pyelonephritis. Similarly, the child with recurrent urinary tract infection and/or VUR may be studied to assess whether chronic renal parenchymal scarring has occurred (Fig 8). The diuresis renogram, a computer-assisted technique for assessing differential renal function and the washout or drainage of a dilated upper urinary tract, may be a valuable asset when the obstructive significance of a hydronephrotic renal unit is questioned.[18] When

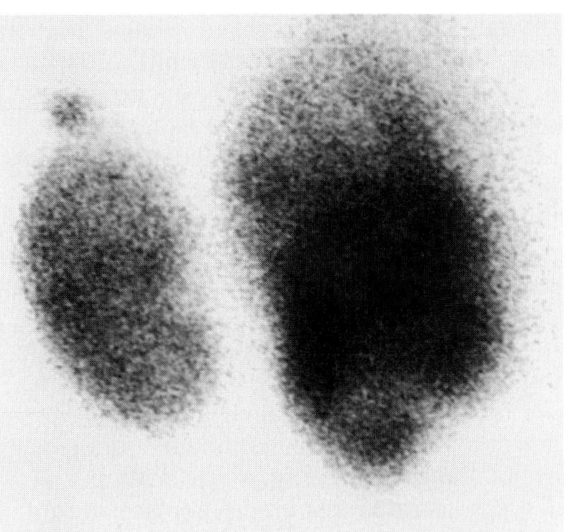

**Fig 7.** DMSA image of right kidney with acute pyelonephritits involving the upper pole and a small portion of the lower pole, seen as diminished uptake of radionuclide. Left kidney is barely seen out of the field of imaging.

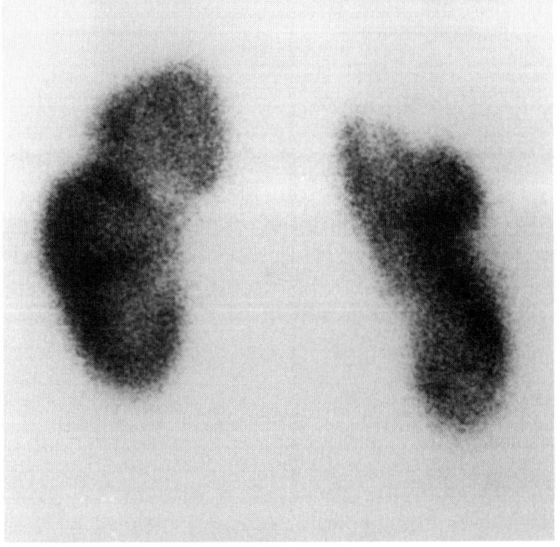

**Fig 8.** DMSA image *(posterior view)* of both kidneys with severe chronic parenchymal scarring.

performing diuresis renography in a child with neurovesical disease, a bladder catheter should be used to keep the bladder continually empty during the study. A full bladder, especially if poorly compliant with elevated intravesical pressure, may adversely affect ureteral drainage and create a false impression of obstruction.

## Urodynamic Evaluation

Urodynamic evaluation of children must be tailored to the information required and the age and ability of the child to cooperate with testing procedures. The physician must recognize that urodynamics in children may be time consuming, require a great deal of patience from all involved parties, and fail to provide as much basic information as might be obtained from comparable testing in an adult. In some cases, urodynamic testing may be abandoned or judged to be valueless if the child is unwilling to cooperate. In these cases, it may be necessary to infer the state of the bladder from the results of other examinations (VCUG and ultrasound) and a diary of the child's voiding habits or catheterization regimen. Noninvasive urodynamic information may be obtained by uroflow or uroflow/electromyographic (EMG) studies. Uroflow studies by themselves are appropriate for screening purposes or follow-up of urethral obstruction, while uroflow/EMG studies may offer more information about the mechanisms of micturition, ie, if the patient has evidence of abdominal straining or discoordinated closure of the pelvic floor. Studies can be carried out using external patch electrodes on the perineum and/or abdomen,[17] although more precise assessment of the pelvic floor musculature can be obtained using fine-needle or wire electrodes. Significant artifact can be introduced into pediatric uroflow/EMG studies, which require a great deal of cooperation on the part of the patient. The physician must interpret the results of testing cautiously and in concert with the results of other urodynamic, radiographic, and clinical information.

Cystometry in children likewise requires a great deal of patience and patient preparation, especially because of the necessity for urethral catheterization. Study of a child who balks at catheterization or is uncooperative will not likely provide useful information. Cystometry may be performed using water or gas. Gas cystometry is faster, but slow-fill water cystometry is more physiologic. The rate of fill should approximate 10%–20% of bladder capacity per minute and body temperature water should be used. To rule out artifact, abdominal pressure should be subtracted using a rectal catheter. Perineal floor EMG may be measured simultaneously.

An extensive urodynamic assessment can be obtained by combining urodynamic and radiographic studies in a video urodynamic evaluation. The ability to monitor urodynamic parameters while visualizing the bladder outlet and its response to bladder filling provides an unparalleled assessment of the function of the lower urinary tract.

### Management Concerns

The child with neurovesical dysfunction presents the urologist with several concerns: preservation of renal function, prevention of the complications of urinary tract infection, and establishment of a satisfactory program for bowel and bladder control. In this scheme of management, it is obvious that there are two separate levels of concern for the urologist: medical and social. The differentiation between the two sometimes blurs, but the concepts of bladder management are identical regardless of the goal. However, the intensity with which one pursues a program of bladder management may vary depending on whether the goal is social dryness or prevention of VUR and renal scarring. It should also be kept in mind that the developmental, cognitive, and social abilities of children with neurovesical dysfunction vary. In designing a bladder program, especially for social dryness, individual abilities and expectations of what is considered socially acceptable may vary greatly from child to child and family to family. These expectations may impact greatly on a plan of action. The following discussion of urologic management for the child with neurovesical dysfunction uses the child with myelomeningocele as a model.

## SPINA BIFIDA (MYELOMENINGOCELE AND RELATED DISORDERS)

### Neonate

The neonate with spina bifida should receive a full urologic evaluation in the first few weeks of life. Prior to discharge from the neonatal hospitalization, renal sonography is performed to document the status of the upper tracts. Voiding cystourethrography and urodynamic study either prior to hospital discharge or in the neonatal period provide valuable information that may influence bladder management in the infant.

The optimal initial bladder regimen for each infant should be individualized based on the results of the above-mentioned testing. In most cases, the infant who is voiding spontaneously and who has normal upper tracts may be managed in diapers. We prefer to avoid the crede maneuver in favor of spontaneous voiding, since Barbalias et al. demonstrated that crede increases intravesical pressure in most patients.[19] If VUR is present, management may depend on the urodynamic state of the bladder. In a very compliant bladder with low pressures, antibiotic prophylaxis may suffice with frequent follow-up evaluation. If reflux is of a moderate grade, intermittent catheterization with or without anticholinergic therapy may be appropriate, and if high-grade reflux is present, especially with poor bladder compliance or a social situation that fails to allow a proper catheterization regimen, cutaneous vesicostomy may be indicated for upper tract decompression.

Urodynamic evaluation of the infant with spina bifida is prognostic of the potential for upper tract deterioration. The most gross reflection of an improper bladder management routine is the presence of hydronephrosis, which may represent either VUR or poor ureteral emptying due to high intravesical pressure. McGuire et al. showed that an intravesical pressure of over 40 cm $H_2O$ is associated with a significant incidence of upper tract dilation, while in a group of patients with leak point pressures lower than 40 cm $H_2O$, no patient had VUR and only 9% of patients had ureteral dilation.[20] The prognostic significance of urodynamics in infants with neurovesical dysfunction was confirmed by Bauer et al., who studied neonates after sac closure.[21] They found that a relaxed pelvic floor was associated with upper tract deterioration in only 11% of patients, while the group with detrusor–sphincter dyssynergy eventually had a 72% incidence of deterioration over 18–48 months of follow-up.

In a subsequent study, they prospectively placed infants at risk for upper tract deterioration on a program of prophylactic intermittent catheterization and anticholinergic therapy. Hydronephrosis developed in less than 10% of these patients.[22] Whether one uses urodynamic evidence of low vesical compliance and elevated leak point pressure as an indication for instituting prophylactic intermittent catheterization or urethral dilation, or merely as a warning that the infant has a high potential for upper tract deterioration and must be watched more carefully than other children, the importance of urodynamics in the infant cannot be overestimated. It must also be noted that a great deal of artifact can be introduced into these studies, and that the VCUG may give a great deal of information about the characteristics of the bladder and the bladder outlet when urodynamic information is not readily available.

## The Older Infant and Child

Periodic urologic assessment is one of the most important aspects of care of the child with spina bifida, and a lifelong plan for urologic follow-up must begin in infancy. The frequency and intensity of reassessment will be determined by both the result of the child's initial urodynamic and radiographic evaluation and whether urodynamic and radiographic deterioration or urinary tract infections occur. If the initial urodynamic and radiologic assessment is favorable, follow-up ultrasonography should be performed at 3–6 months of age, at 1 year, and yearly thereafter. The ideal program of bladder management should be designed to prevent the development of complications. However, if urinary tract infection or upper tract fullness is found on routine follow-up, VCUG and urodynamic studies are indicated. If VUR, hydronephrosis, or urinary tract infection develops or progresses, the current bladder management program must be reassessed and altered to reverse the upper tract deterioration and prevent complications of infection. Whether pharmacotherapy, intermittent catheterization, a combination of the two, urethral dilation, cutaneous vesicostomy or other surgical intervention, electrical bladder stimulation, rhizotomy, and so on will be appropriate depends on the severity of the concern, the general condition and cooperation of the child, the family or caretaker's resources and commitment, and the experience and concern of the urologist. In all cases, the optimal management for each child must be individualized and the effect of each new intervention repeatedly evaluated to ensure that an optimal urodynamic result has been achieved. In many cases, one intervention will be found to be insufficient and subsequent changes will be necessary to achieve success.

A child who maintains sterile urine and nondilated upper tracts throughout childhood will require urodynamic and radiographic evaluation when urinary continence becomes a concern. There is no single chronological age at which a bladder program designed to alleviate incontinence is appropriate. Factors that must be taken into concern include the child's desire for continence and his or her manual dexterity, and family dynamics, resources, and commitment. It is important to realize that not all families and children share the same concept of continence. For some, absolute dryness is important, and for others, an adequate diaper system that does not allow leaking and visible wetness will suffice. It is also important to note that even a well-designed and executed plan for bladder control will not free a child from diapers if an adequate bowel program is not in place. A basic bowel training regimen is best begun in early childhood and modified to fit the child's developing needs.

## Urinary Continence

A small percentage of children with spina bifida will attain continence and void normally. For the remainder, continence usually requires intermittent catheterization, in most cases with the addition of pharmacotherapy, surgery, or other intervention. Although sterile catheterization may be required in certain clinical situations, nonsterile self-catheterization is the optimal goal of most bladder regimens. Such a regimen places a great burden of responsibility on the child, and not all children are ready to accept either the goal of continence or the responsibility for self-catheterization at the same age. In many cases, physical handicaps make self-catheterization a difficult if not impossible task to master without significant intervention on the part of parents, therapists, nurses, and physicians.

Nonsterile self-catheterization (clean intermittent catheterization, or CIC) is associated with chronic bacteriuria, but a significant chance of achieving upper tract stabilization and a low incidence of pyelonephritis unless VUR is present. Plunkett and Braren found bacteriuria in 80%, pyelonephritis in 6%, stable upper tracts in 82%, and improved upper tracts in 15% of children on a program of CIC.[23] This data was confirmed by Cass, who documented upper tract stability in 87.5% and improvement in 12.5%, although only 34% of children attained dryness.[24] The ability of a program of CIC to provide total dryness between catheterizations varies in reported series from 24% to 49%, with an additional group of patients in each series being "damp." In some cases, wetness is unavoidable even with a well-managed bladder program, while in other cases patient or family compliance to the prescribed regimen is suboptimal. In addition to being realistic about the expectations for continence when a program is begun, the physician must design a regimen that is compatible with the lifestyle of the patient. Being dry is a reasonable goal, but if it requires catheterization every 2 hr, continence may be impractical and hardly worth the effort.

Pharmacotherapy may be used alone or in conjunction with CIC or surgical intervention to modify the function of the bladder and bladder outlet. Children are frequently more sensitive than adults to the potential side effects of pharmacologic agents, so it is important to begin with small doses and gradually titrate up to a full dose or to a desired effect. Combinations of drugs are commonly used, and additive effects may be noted (Table 1).

Transurethral electrical bladder stimulation (TEBS) was first used for the treatment of neurovesical dysfunction secondary to spinal cord injury in the late 1950s, and a report of the results in a group of children with myelodysplasia was published in 1975.[25] TEBS has been used in the U.S. for neurovesical dysfunction, primarily in the pediatric myelomeningocele group, for approximately 10 years.[26] The postulated mechanism of action is through stimulation of intramural receptors. Although clinical experience with TEBS has been limited to a small group of patients at a few centers, the results of therapy have been encouraging. Reported beneficial effects have included improvement of bladder sensation, stimulation of detrusor contraction, increase in bladder capacity, and the establishment of urinary continence. Therapy is initiated after urodynamic evaluation and an initial test stimulation. Stimulation is performed by filling the bladder to one-half capacity with saline via a special electrode catheter. Electrical impulses

**TABLE 1. Commonly Used Pharmacotherapeutic Agents**

| Drug | Route | Maximum dose | # Doses/d |
|---|---|---|---|
| *Anticholinergic* | | | |
| Propantheline | Oral | 1.5 mg/kg/d | 3–4 |
| Oxybutynin | Oral | 0.2 mg/kg/dose | 3–4 |
| | Intravesical | 5–7.5 mg in 30 mL water | 2–3 |
| Dicyclomine | Oral | 5–10 mg/dose | 3–4 |
| Hyoscyamine | Oral | 0.75 mg/d | 4 |
| | Sublingual | 0.75 mg/d | 4 |
| *Sympathomimetic* | | | |
| Ephedrine | Oral | 1 mg/kg/dose | 3–4 |
| Phenylpropanolamine | Oral | 2.5 mg/kg/dose | 2–3 |
| *Combination* | | | |
| Imipramine | Oral | 0.7 mg/kg/dose | 2–3 |

are passed through the saline and are varied by alteration of the frequency, intensity, duration, and waveform of the impulse to produce an optimal result (detrusor contraction). Therapy is time consuming. Each patient may require up to 120 sessions (one 90-min session per day) in order to reach a desired effect. The therapy may then progress to biofeedback training that can be carried out at home.

Lyne and Bellinger recently reported on a series of 17 patients who had undergone a total of 618 sessions of TEBS.[27] All patients demonstrated detrusor contraction and 88% had some sensation of the contractions. Six patients showed a significant increase in bladder capacity during therapy, but in half of these a return to near-baseline capacity was noted after therapy was completed.

Surgery may be necessary to provide continence for patients in whom intermittent catheterization and pharmacotherapy prove inadequate. Depending on urodynamic findings, intervention may be needed to improve either outlet resistance or bladder capacity and compliance. Frequently, a combination of effects is desired. Augmentation of bladder volume may be achieved in several ways (Fig 9). Classically, small or large bowel has been the material of choice for bladder augmentation.[28] Intestinal disturbances, electrolyte imbalance, and incontinence due to mass contractions of the bowel segment have been reported after enterocystoplasty, but these complications have not been a major deterrent to the continued use of these bowel segments. Mucus production is a minor nuisance that necessitates daily irrigation of the bladder, a problem not seen in patients with gastrocystoplasty, a newer technique for enterocystoplasty that has been advocated to minimize electrolyte imbalance and urea reabsorption especially in patients with chronic renal failure, but which is itself not free from metabolic and local complications.[29] Ureterocystoplasty has recently been reported as a new technique applicable to a small number of patients.[30] The advantage of this technique is that it uses no extraurinary mucosal surface.

A growing body of literature has documented both delayed ''spontaneous'' bladder rupture and malignancy arising in the bowel patch after enterocystoplasty. Filmer and Spencer cited 14 reported cases of malignancy in augmented bladders, 10 arising in the bowel segment.[31] Bauer et al. re-

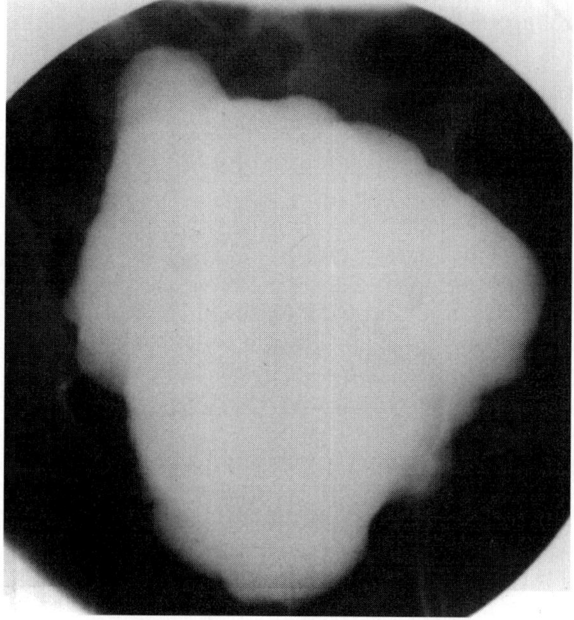

**Fig 9.** Cystogram after colocystoplasty in a child with tethered cord syndrome.

ported 15 spontaneous perforations in 12 of 264 children who underwent enterocystoplasty using small bowel, large bowel, and stomach.[32] All sites of rupture have been located in the bowel itself, at or near the junction of the bladder and the enteral patch. Ischemic necrosis is thought to play a role in the mechanism of rupture. A significant percentage of patients suffering spontaneous rupture have died. Recommendations for management include daily bladder irrigation and prevention of overdistension, especially in patients who have a competent bladder outlet or who have undergone surgical procedures to increase outlet resistance.

Diminished bladder outlet resistance is frequently present in children with myelomeningocele and other forms of neurovesical dysfunction. Surgical correction of this problem has been addressed for decades, and the fact that a perfect continence mechanism has not been developed is attested to by the fact that new procedures are being developed and reported on a regular basis. Proposed procedures have included Young-Dees Leadbetter urethropexy,[33] several variations of bladder neck sling,[34] artificial urinary sphincter implantation,[35] the Kropp method of tunneled urethral reimplantation,[36] and injection procedures for the bladder neck using Teflon paste or collagen.[37]

## HINMAN–ALLEN SYNDROME

In 1915 Beer described a group of children with hydronephrosis, reflux, and absence of neurologic signs who appeared to have a ''disharmony'' between the detrusor and sphincter muscles, and whom he felt to have occult neurologic processes responsible for the bladder changes.[38] Williams and Taylor and Paquin et al.[39,40] reported similar cases in which neither anatomic obstruction nor neurologic processes could be documented. The etiology of these changes was proposed to be neurologic in nature, and most authors considered the ''occult neuropathic bladder'' to be a diagnosis of exclusion. In 1971, Hinman described 14 boys with ''nonneurogenic neurogenic bladder'' dysfunction who had radiographic changes, incontinence, and urinary tract infection.[41] He proposed that the demonstrated abnormalities were behavioral in origin. In 1973, Hinman and Baumann reported further on these boys, strongly concluding that the etiology of the changes was functional,[42] a conclusion also reached by Allen.[43] The boys were described as having in common a ''failure'' personality: quiet, timid, shy, many with anxiety or depression. Thirteen of the 14 boys had resolution of symptoms and improvement in the radiologic appearance of the urinary tract after treatment of constipation, suggestion therapy and/or hypnosis, and short-term anticholinergic therapy. Ochoa recently reported on a group of similar patients with the additional finding of ''inversion of the facial expression,'' such that, upon smiling, the child appears to grimace. He postulated that lesions of the reticular formation of the brainstem might influence both micturition and facial expression.[44]

It has now been widely accepted that acquired dysfunctional voiding patterns may mimic neurovesical disease and that a broad spectrum of this symptom complex exists. In fact, most practitioners report seeing larger numbers of children with extreme daytime urinary frequency, termed the frequency syndrome of childhood.[45] This stress-related symptom complex is representative of the most benign and yet symptomatically bothersome end of the spectrum of voiding dysfunction, since upper tracts are normal and urine is uninfected. It may be this type of voiding pattern, however, that can become pathologic and lead to the true Hinman–Allen bladder. The pathologic voiding patterns that lead to severe upper tract deterioration mimic the dysfunctional neuropathic process of detrusor–sphincter dyssynergia. Hinman outlined the functional changes that result in this picture as the following: failure to inhibit the detrusor reflex and overcompensation by the external sphincter, usually in response, at least initially, to uninhibited detrusor contractions.[46] Children with documented Hinman–Allen syndrome are a group who share a few basic clinical and radiologic characteristics that closely mimic neurovesical dysfunction: day and night wetting, encopresis, urinary tract infection, reflux, and hydronephrosis. Prior to diagnosis, many will have undergone multiple radiographic and urologic procedures, and may have failed previous attempts at urologic surgical procedures, in particular ureteral reimplantation.

A consideration of dysfunctional voiding and the Hinman–Allen syndrome should be entertained in any child who presents with the above-mentioned symptom complex. A thorough voiding, medical, and social history should be obtained, particularly focusing on stressors, labile emotions, and family/school/social situations that might be a source of anxiety and result in alteration in voiding habits. Family and social aspects of development and rearing should be investigated. In particular, stressful situations such as separation, divorce, change in school, move to a new home, and any of a number of seemingly insignificant factors should be considered as possibly playing a role in triggering dysfunctional voiding. The attitude and behavior of the child and parent or caretakers should be noted. An overly shy or timid child, a hyperactive and noncompliant child, or an angry or vindictive parent who lacks understanding should raise a red flag. It is extremely important to assess family dynamics and be aware of the reaction of parents and the child's peers to wetting, soiling, and other dysfunctional symptoms, since punishment and ridicule may reinforce the chlid's sense of insecurity and anxiety. School performance may also suffer, particularly if ridicule for wetness is a part of the daily routine.

Physical findings may be minimal and may include a palpably distended bladder or colon. Lower extremity reflexes should be evaluated, and an examination of the lower back should rule out sacral dimples or hair patches suggestive of dysraphism. Rectal examination should assess sphincter tone and the presence of hard stool or fecal impaction. In all cases, neurosurgical consultation should be obtained to rule out a tethered cord. In some cases, the neurosurgical consultant may recommend magnetic resonance imaging (MRI) of the lumbosacral spine to conclusively rule out a tethered cord (Fig 10). Ultrasound examination in approximately 70% of children will re-

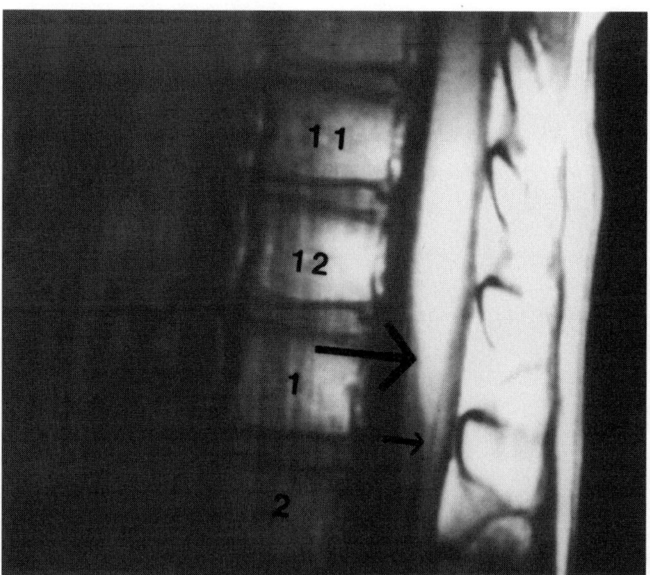


**Fig. 10.** Normal lateral MRI scan of lumbosacral spine in a girl with Hinman–Allen syndrome. The conus *(small arrow)* is at the level of the first lumbar vertebra. The conus in 98% of normal patients lies above the L2,3 level.

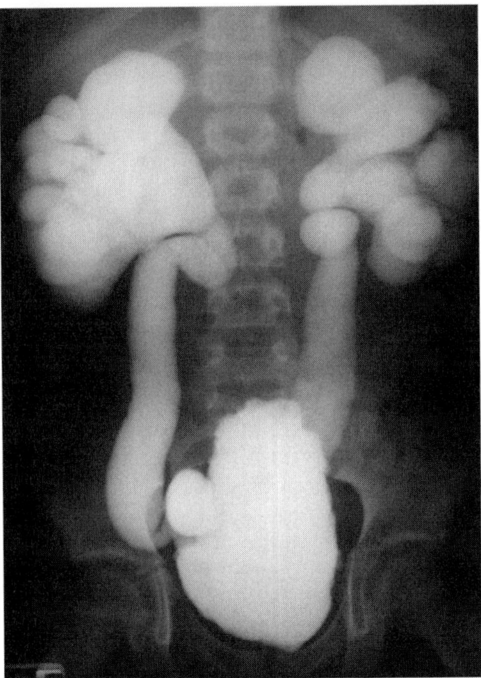

Fig 11. Severe bilateral vesicoureteral reflux in a boy with Hinman–Allen syndrome.

veal hydronephrosis, which is usually bilateral. Postvoid bladder ultrasonography will allow a noninvasive assessment of bladder emptying and residual urine determination, and may be repeated after double and triple voiding. Voiding cystourethrography demonstrates VUR in 50%–57% of cases (Fig 11), and fluoroscopy during micturition will show persistent or intermittent narrowing at the level of the external sphincter, with an interrupted urinary stream (Figs 12 and 13). Uroflow/EMG studies may be performed with surface or wire electrodes, and will show failure of relaxation or increased perineal floor activity during micturition (Fig 14). Cystometric findings may vary and will be influenced by the presence or absence of VUR, which may dampen bladder pressures and create a false impression of bladder capacity and compliance.

Once voiding dysfunction has been confirmed and neurovesical disease ruled out, treatment must be highly individualized. Therapy has two parallel treatment arms, treating both the bladder and the psychosocial and behavioral dysfunction that is at the core of the problem. Depending on the

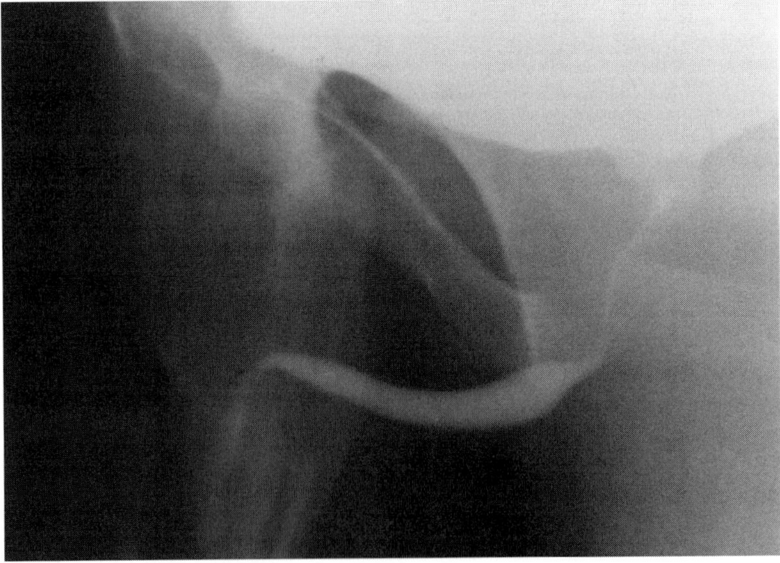

Fig 12. Voiding cystourethrogram in a boy with Hinman–Allen syndrome. Note the spasm of the external sphincter and posterior urethra that occurred intermittently during voiding.

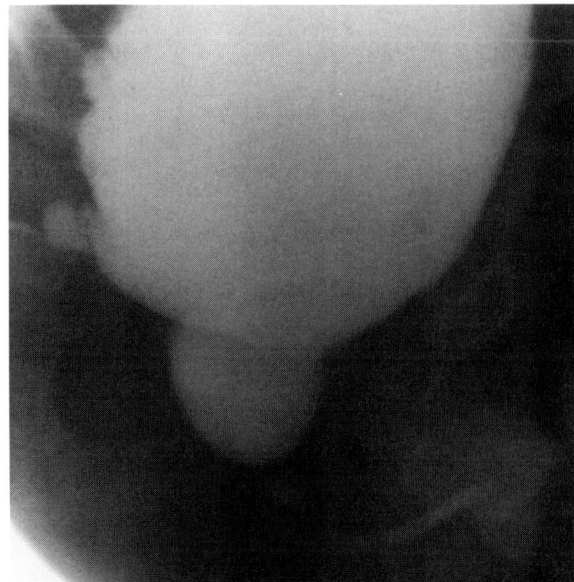

**Fig 13.** Voiding cystourethrogram in a boy with Hinman–Allen syndrome. Severe external sphincter spasm during voiding suggested posterior urethral valves. Cystoscopy was normal.

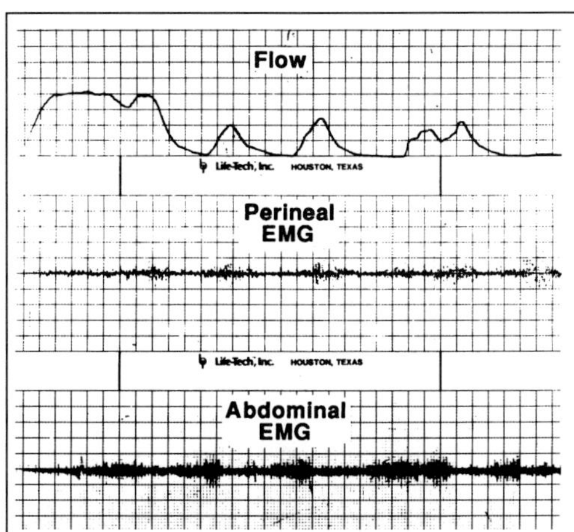


**Fig 14.** Uroflow/EMG study in a boy with Hinman–Allen syndrome. External patch electrodes were used. Note the interrupted urinary flow that begins after abdominal straining (increased abdominal EMG activity) and diminishes as the perineal EMG activity increases.

severity of the upper tract changes, the presence of infection, and renal functional impairment, the bladder may be managed variably. Timed voiding, using a timer to allow more relaxed voiding, and double and triple voiding are techniques that may be used to diminish residual urine and reinforce an appropriate voiding pattern. Biofeedback training can be carried out using perineal EMG monitoring to reinforce relaxation of the pelvic floor musculature during micturition. This can be a worthwhile but time-consuming therapy that may be effective if the child is receptive and the examiner patient. Constipation must be managed by stool softeners, dietary fiber, and in many cases by initiating a bowel cleanout with enemas. When upper tract deterioration is severe, intermittent catheterization may be necessary. Many children are uncooperative with catheterization, and temporary cutaneous vesicostomy may be necessary to stabilize the upper tracts. Counseling, stress reduction, psychological intervention, family therapy, and hypnosis have all been used in treating children with Hinman–Allen syndrome. In some cases, inpatient psychiatric therapy may be warranted, and intense family intervention may play a very important role. Whatever the severity of voiding dysfunction, antireflux surgery should be avoided unless a stable bladder function and social milieu can be documented. Long-term follow-up and periodic reevaluation of the child's urinary tract is important to guard against relapse.

## REFERENCES


1. El Badawi A, Schenk EA. Dual innervation of the mammalian urinary bladder: a histochemical study of the distribution of cholinergic and adrenergic nerves. *Am J Anat.* 1966;119:405.
2. Tanagho EA. The ureterovesical junction: anatomy and physiology. In: Chisolm GD, Williams D, eds. *Scientific Foundations of Urology.* Chicago: Year Book; 1982:295–404.
3. Tanagho EA, Smith DR. Mechanism of urinary continence. I. Embryologic, anatomic, and pathological considerations. *J. Urol.* 1968;100: 640.
4. Gosling JA, Chilton, CP. The anatomy of the bladder, urethra, and pelvic floor. In: Mundy AR, Stephenson TP, Wein AJ, eds. *Urodynamics: Principles, Practice and Applications.* London: Churchill Livingstone; 1984:3–13.
5. Tanagho EA. Anatomy of the lower urinary tract. In: Walsh PC, Gillen RF, Perlmutter AD, eds. *Campbell's Urology.* Philadelphia: WB Saunders; 1986:46–74.
6. Wein AJ, Levin RM, Barrett DM. Voiding function and dysfunction. In: Gillenwater JY, Grayhack JT, Howards SS, Duckett JW, eds. *Adult and Pediatric Urology,* 2nd ed. St. Louis: Mosby Year Book; 1991;933–999.
7. Oelrich TM. The urethral sphincter muscle in the male. *Am J Anat.* 1980;158:229.
8. DeGroat WC, Booth AM, Yoshimura Y. Neurophysiology of micturition and its modification in animal models of human disease. In: Maggi CA, ed. *Autonomic Nervous System.* Vol. 3. Cher, Switzerland: Harwood Academic; 1993: 227–290.
9. McGuire EJ, Woodside JR, Borden TA, et al. Prognostic value of urodynamic testing in myelodysplastic patients. *J Urol.* 1981;126:205.
10. Bors E, Comarr AE. *Neurological Urology.* Baltimore: University Park Press; 1971.
11. Lapides J. Neuromuscular, vesical and ureteral dysfunction. In: Campbell MF, Harrison JH, eds. *Urology.* Philadelphia: WB Saunders; 1970: 1343–1379.
12. Krane RJ, Siroky MB. Classification of voiding dysfunction: value of classification systems. In: Barrett DM, Wein AJ, eds. *Controversies in Neuro-Urology.* New York: Churchill-Livingstone; 1984:223–238.
13. International Continence Society Standardization Committee. Fourth report on the standardization of terminology of lower urinary tract function. *Br J Urol.* 1981;53:333.
14. Wein AJ. Classification of voiding dysfunction: a simple approach. In Barrett DM, Wein AJ (eds), *Controversies in Neuro-Urology.* New York: Churchill-Livingstone; 1984;239–250.
15. Taylor A. Delayed scanning with DMSA: a simple index of relative renal plasma flow. *Radiology.* 1980;136:449.
16. Verboven M, Ingels M, Delree M, Piepsz A. 99m Tc-DMSA scintigraphy in acute urinary tract infection in children. *Pediatr Radiol.* 1990;20:540.
17. Society for Fetal Urology and Pediatric Nuclear Medicine Council. The ''well-tempered'' diuretic renogram: a standard method to examine the asymptomatic neonate with hydronephrosis or hydroureteronephrosis. *J Nucl Med.* 1992;33: 2047.
18. Maizels M, Firlit CF. Pediatric urodynamics: clinical comparison of surface versus needle pelvic floor/sphincter electromyography. *J Urol.* 1979;122:518.
19. Barbalias GA, Klauber GT, Blaivas JG. Critical evaluation of the crede maneuver: a urodynamic study of 207 patients. *J Urol.* 1983;130:720.
20. McGuire EJ, Woodside JR, Borden TA, et al. Prognostic value of urodynamic testing in myelodysplastic patients. *J Urol.* 1981;126:205.
21. Bauer SB, Hallett M, Shoshbin S, et al. Predictive value of urodynamic evaluation in newborns with myelodysplasia. *JAMA.* 1984;252:650.
22. Kasabian NG, Bauer SB, Dyro FM, et al. The prophylactic value of clean intermittent catheterization and anticholinergic medication in newborns and infants with myelodysplasia at risk of developing urinary tract deterioration. *Am J Dis Child.* 1992;146:840.
23. Plunkett JM, Braren V. Clean intermittent catheterization in children. *J Urol.* 1979;121: 469.
24. Cass AS. Urinary tract complications in myelomeningocele patients. *J Urol.* 1976;115:102.
25. Katona F, Berenyi M. Intravesical transurethral electrotherapy in myelomeningocele patients. *Acta Paediatr Hung.* 1975;16:363.
26. Kaplan W, Richards I. Intravesical transurethral electrotherapy for neurogenic bladder. *J Urol.* 1986;136:243.
27. Lyne CJ, Bellinger MF. Early experience with transurethral electrical bladder stimulation. *J Urol.* 1993;150:697.
28. Smith RB, Van Cangh P, Skinner DG, et al. Augmentation cystoplasty: a critical review. *J Urol.* 1977;118:35.
29. Adams MC, Mitchell ME, Rink RC. Gastrocystoplasty: an alternative solution to the problem of urological reconstruction in the severely compromised patient. *J Urol.* 1988;140:1152.
30. Bellinger MF. Ureterocystoplasty: a unique method for vesical augmentation in children. *J Urol.* 1993;149:811.
31. Filmer RB, Spencer JR. Malignancies in bladder augmentations and substitutions. *J Urol.* 1990; 143:671.
32. Bauer SB, Hendren WH, Kozakewich H, et al. Perforation of the augmented bladder. *J Urol.* 1992;148:699.
33. Rink RC, Mitchell ME. Bladder neck/urethral re-

construction in the neuropathic bladder. *Dial Ped Urol.* 1987;10:5.

34. Elder JS. Periurethral and puboprostatic sling repair for incontinence in patients with myelodysplasia. *J Urol.,* part 2 1990;144:434.
35. Bosco PJ, Bauer SB, Colodny AH, et al. The long-term results of artificial sphincters in children. *J Urol.* 1991;146:396.
36. Belman AB, Kaplan GW. Experience with the Kropp anti-incontinence procedure. *J Urol.* 1989;141:1160.
37. Wan J, McGuire EJ, Bloom DA, Ritchey ML. The treatment of urinary incontinence in children using glutaraldehyde cross-linked collagen. *J Urol.* 1992;148:127.
38. Beer E. Chronic retention of urine in children. *JAMA.* 1915;65:1709.
39. Williams DI, Taylor JS. A rare congenital uropathy: vesico-urethral dysfunction with upper tract anomalies. *Br J Urol.* 1969;41:307.
40. Paquin AJ, Marshall VF, McGovern JH. The megacystis syndrome. *J Urol.* 1960;83:634.
41. Hinman F Jr. Non-neurogenic neurogenic bladder. Read at annual meeting of Americal Urological Association, Chicago, May 16–20, 1971.
42. Hinman F, Baumann FW. Vesical and ureteral damage from voiding dysfunction in boys without neurologic or obstructive disease. *J Urol.* 1973;109:727.
43. Allen TD. The non-neurogenic neurogenic bladder. *J Urol.* 1977;117:232.
44. Ochoa B. The urofacial (Ochoa) syndrome revisited. *J Urol.* 1992;148:580.
45. Zoubek J, Bloom DA, Sedman AB. Extraordinary urinary frequency. *Pediatrics* 1990;85: 1112.
46. Hinman F Jr. Nonneurogenic neurogenic bladder (the Hinman syndrome)—15 years later. *J Urol.* 1986;136:769.

# 54

# Intersex Disorders

*David A. Diamond*

## NORMAL SEXUAL DIFFERENTIATION

Under normal circumstances, sexual differentiation is a beautifully orchestrated process in which, according to the Jost paradigm, chromosomal sex determines gonadal sex, which in turn determines phenotypic sex.[1] Interference with this highly ordered process at any step can result in a disorder of sexual differentiation.

### Chromosomal Sex

Early work on the chromosomal basis of sexual differentiation, based on studies of *Drosophila,* suggested that sex was determined by an individual's X chromosomes.[2] The Y chromosome was thought to impart no genetic information until karyotyping of mammalian chromosomes, developed in the 1960s, demonstrated that the Y chromosome specified development of the testis.[3]

Further study of Y chromosomes suggested that the genetic information responsible for maleness was on the short arm of the chromosome, near the centromere. This theory was supported by experiments of nature, in which the short arm of the Y was lost and only the long arm remained, which resulted in a female phenotype.

What remains unknown is the molecular basis by which the responsible gene, or genes, promotes testicular differentiation. One recent theory proposes that the Y chromosome regulates the production of a cell-surface antigen, which in turn mediates transformation of the indifferent gonad into a testis.[4] This so-called H-Y antigen was first identified in 1955, when male-to-female skin grafts were rejected in a strain of mice that was able to accept female-to-male skin grafts.[5] It was theorized that rejection of the male-to-female graft was due to a histocompatibility gene located on the Y chromosome—the histocompatibility Y or H-Y gene. Subsequently, male-specific antibodies were detected in sera of female mice with male skin grafts, and assays for quantifying H-Y antigen were developed. Using these assays, it was discovered that the presence of a testis resulted in serologically detectable levels of H-Y antigen. This was confirmed in normal and intersex patients, as well as in males of other species. Thus it was believed that the H-Y gene was the testis-determining gene.[4]

Problems with the H-Y antigen theory have developed, however, raising the question as to whether the H-Y antigen is, in fact, the testis-determining factor. A number of women with 45 X gonadal dysgenesis have been found to be H-Y antigen positive.[6] And one patient reported to have a 45 X/46 XY karyotype and bilateral intraabdominal testes was H-Y antigen negative.[7] In addition, a mouse model for the male sex reversal syndrome (XX male) has been studied in which mice have two X chromosomes and testes, because a fragment of Y is translocated onto one of the X chromosomes. These mice are H-Y antigen negative and azoospermic. On the basis of this work, it has been suggested that the H-Y antigen does not determine testis formation, but may play a role in spermatogenesis.[8]

Research is currently ongoing to localize the testis-determining factor by genetic analysis of a series of XX males. It has been determined that the majority of XX males studied have evidence of Y-linked DNA material, and that a specific portion of the Y chromosome is common to all XX males studied. In addition, studies of a series of XY females have been carried out to determine which portion of the Y chromosome was deleted in these patients without testes. Based on these studies, it appears that the testis-determining factor is located distally on the short arm of the Y chromosome, within segment 1A (the H-Y transplant antigen has been located on the proximal portion of the long arm of the Y, near the centromere).[9]

A recently identified gene, known as SRY, has been located within a 35 kb sequence of DNA adjacent to the X/Y pairing zone on the short arm of the Y chromosome.[10] In other mammals, matching DNA segments which seem to be responsible for testis determination have been noted. Thus, it is likely that SRY will prove to be the testis-determining factor.

## Gonadal Sex

The formation of the gonadal blastema is completed by the fifth or sixth week of gestation. The rudimentary, indifferent gonad is composed of three cell types: 1) germ cells, 2) supporting cells from the coelomic epithelium that become Sertoli cells of the testis and granulosa cells of the ovary, and 3) stromal cells from the original mesenchymal gonadal ridge.

The gonad destined to become a fetal ovary demonstrates no characteristic changes until 2 to 3 months. But at 6 to 7 weeks, the male gonad exhibits evidence of sexual differentiation by the development of primordial Sertoli cells. The initial endocrine function of the fetal testis is the secretion of MIF (Müllerian inhibiting factor) by the Sertoli cells at 7 to 8 weeks of gestation.[11] MIF, one of the two hormones necessary for male sexual differentiation, acts locally to produce Müllerian regression. Although the mechanism of action remains unclear, MIF appears to alter cell surface proteins in the manner of an epidermal growth factor. The secretion of testosterone begins soon after differentiation of the spermatogenic cords, and occurs concomitantly with Leydig cell differentiation, at 9 to 10 weeks (Fig 1).

Jost clearly demonstrated that androgens are essential for virilization of Wolffian duct structures, the urogenital sinus, and the genital tubercle.[12] Testosterone (T), the major androgen secreted by the testis, enters target tissues by passive diffusion. In some cells, such as those in the urogenital sinus, T is converted to dihydrotestosterone (DHT) by intracellular 5$\alpha$-reductase. T, or DHT, then binds to a high-affinity intracellular receptor protein and this complex enters the nucleus, where it binds to acceptor sites on DNA, stimulating the production of new mRNA and protein synthesis (Fig 2). The androgen receptor has been characterized as a high-affinity receptor that mediates the action of T and DHT in all androgen-dependent tissues. In disorders of the androgen receptor, such as testicular feminization, T production is normal but the hormone is unable to reach the nucleus and interact with DNA. Various defects in the androgen receptor result in a spectrum of phenotypic abnormalities in the genetic male. Because gonadal females have androgen receptors within their tissues, administration of exogenous androgens produces virilization.

It has been well established that, while T-receptor complexes mediate Wolffian duct development, DHT receptor complexes mediate the development of the male external genitalia.[13] The role of DHT has been substantiated clinically in patients with 5$\alpha$-reductase deficiency and pseudovaginal perineoscrotal hypospadias.[14]

Unlike the testis, which functions primarily as a fetal endocrine organ, the ovary has primarily exocrine activity. Under the influence of elevated gonadotropins, ovarian germ cells proliferate to reach a maximum endowment of 7 million by week 20

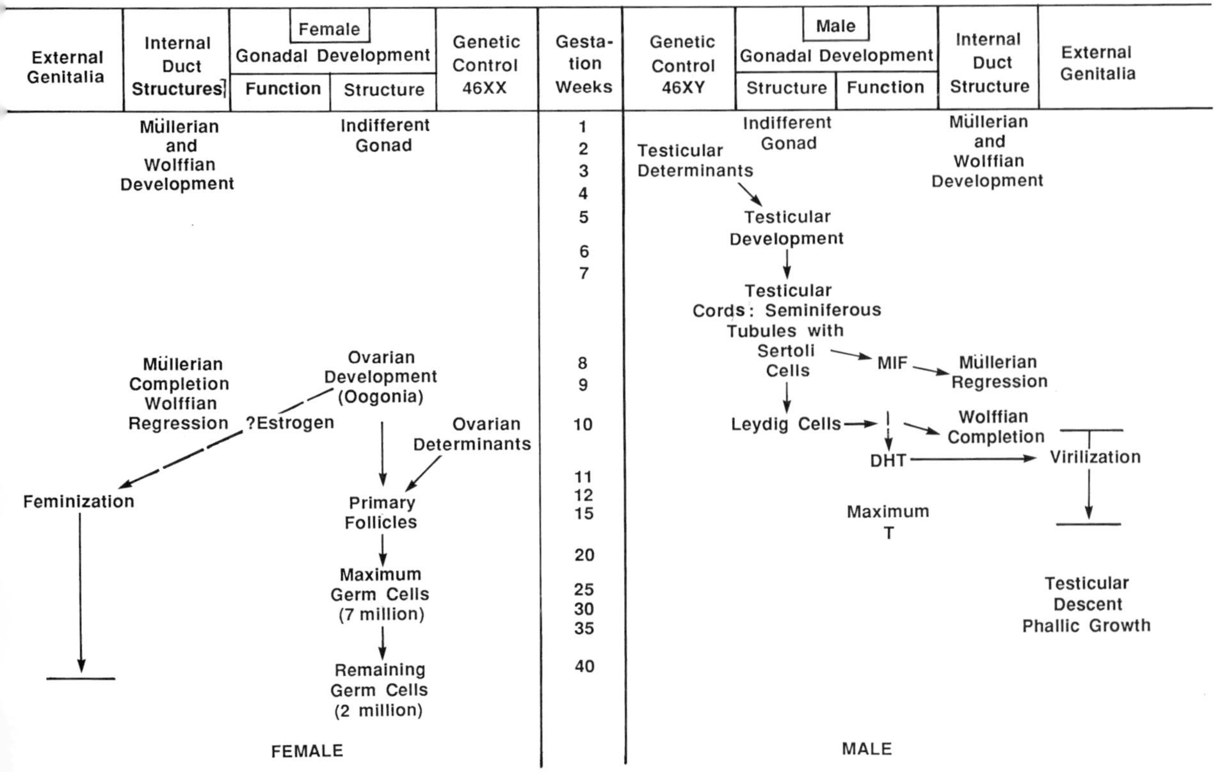

External Genitalia
Internal Duct Structures
Female
Gonadal Development
Function
Structure
Genetic Control 46XX
Gesta-tion Weeks
Genetic Control 46XY
Male
Gonadal Development
Structure
Function
Internal Duct Structure
External Genitalia
Müllerian and Wolffian Development
Indifferent Gonad
1
2
3
4
5
6
7
Indifferent Gonad
Testicular Determinants
Müllerian and Wolffian Development
Testicular Development
Testicular Cords: Seminiferous Tubules with Sertoli Cells
MIF
Müllerian Regression
Müllerian Completion Wolffian Regression
Ovarian Development (Oogonia)
8
9
?Estrogen
Ovarian Determinants
10
Leydig Cells
Wolffian Completion
DHT
Virilization
11
12
15
Feminization
Primary Follicles
Maximum T
20
Maximum Germ Cells (7 million)
25
30
35
Testicular Descent Phallic Growth
40
Remaining Germ Cells (2 million)
FEMALE
MALE

**Fig 1.** Timetable of normal sexual differentiation. [Adapted from Reindollar RH, Tho SPT, McDonough PG, *Clin Obstet Gynecol* (1987;30:699–700), with permission.]

LH
Gonadotropin regulation
Sexual differentiation
Testis
T
T
T
TR
TR*
+R
D
DR
DR*
Wolffian stimulation
External virilization
E
E
Sexual maturation at puberty
Target cells

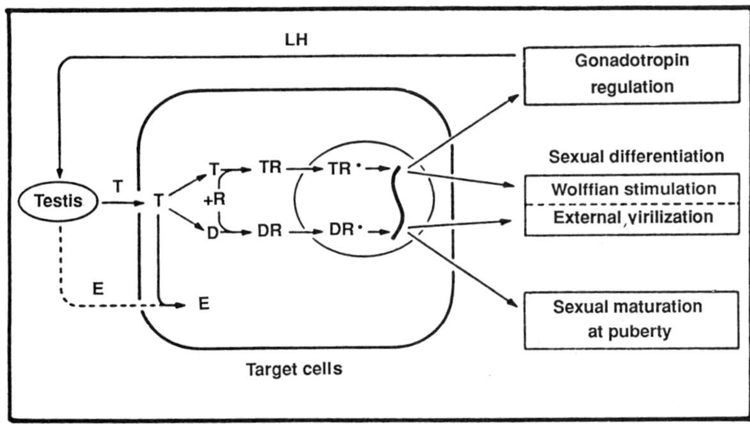

**Fig 2.** Model for androgen action; T = testosterone; D = dihydrotestosterone; E = estradiol; R = androgen receptor; R* = transformed androgen receptor; LH = luteinizing hormone (from Wilson[45]).

of gestation. The majority of these germ cells die, however, without the development of a protective surrounding mantle of follicular cells and stroma. This critical protective step in ovarian development is controlled by ovarian-determining genes. Usually, approximately 2 million germ cells remain viable at birth. The role of hormones in female development remains unclear. In the absence of T production,

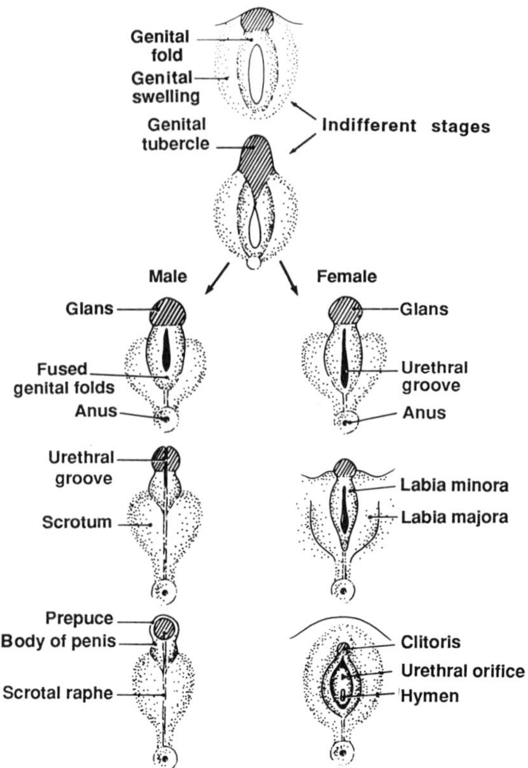


**Fig 3.** Formation of external genitalia in male and female from common anlagen (from Wilson[34]).

the fetus is exposed only to the maternal "sea" of hormones. Yet if one attempts to alter the maternal hormonal milieu in the mammalian model, placental dysfunction and abortion occur. Recent studies in marsupial species, however, suggest that estrogen has an active role in differentiation of the female genitalia.[15]

## Phenotypic Sex

Prior to the eighth week of gestation, the urogenital tract is identical in the two sexes. Both the Wolffian and Müllerian duct systems are present as anlagen of the internal accessory organs of reproduction. In addition, at this stage, the anlagen of the external genitalia of both male and female embryos are indistinguishable.

The first sign of male phenotypic differentiation is degeneration of the Müllerian ducts adjacent to the testis, which occurs as a result of MIF secretion by the Sertoli cells. Next, the genital tubercle elongates and the urethral folds fuse from posterior to anterior over the urethral groove. The urogenital swellings migrate posteriorly to the genital tubercle and fuse to form the scrotum (Fig 3). Formation of the penile urethra is completed within the first trimester, with closure of the elongated urogenital cleft. Under the influence of androgens secreted by the fetal testis, penile growth and testicular descent occur in the third trimester.

In the female, the internal reproductive tract is formed from the Müllerian ducts. The cephalic ends are anlagen of the fallopian tubes; the caudal ends fuse to form the uterus (Fig 4). Contact of the Müllerian ducts with the urogenital sinus induces formation of the uterovaginal plate, which ultimately forms the lumen of the vagina. The proximal two thirds of the vagina is contributed by the Müllerian ducts while the distal third is contributed by the urogenital sinus.

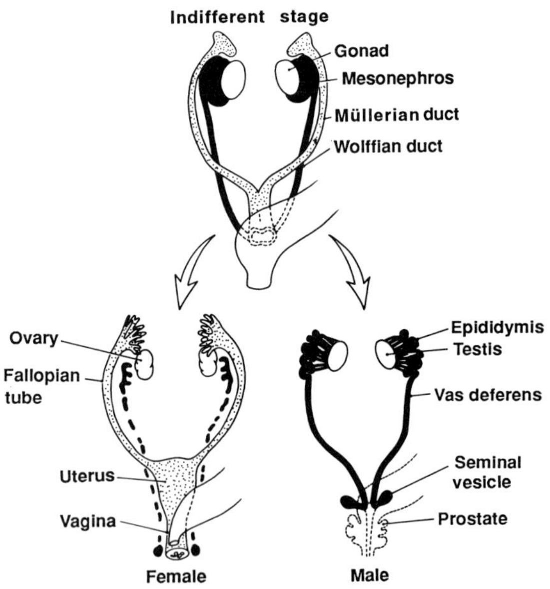


**Fig 4.** Differentiation of the Wolffian and Müllerian ducts and urogenital sinus in the male and female (from Wilson[34]).

## DISORDERS OF CHROMOSOMAL SEX

### Klinefelter Syndrome and Sex Reversal Syndrome (XX Male)

Klinefelter syndrome represents the most common major abnormality of sexual differentiation. By definition, males with at least one Y chromosome and at least 2 X chromosomes have the Klinefelter syndrome. The classic 47XXY complement arises as a result of nondisjunction during meiosis, and occurs in one of eight hundred live-born males. But the phenotype is also associated with 47 XY/47 XXY, 48 XXYY, and 49 XXXY. The most characteristic features of the syndrome are seminiferous tubular dysgenesis, androgen deficiency, and eunuchoidism.[16]

In 47 XXY adults, seminiferous tubules degenerate and are replaced with hyaline. As a result, testes are small and firm, and are rarely greater than 2 cm at the widest diameter. Leydig cells appear hyperplastic, because other testicular elements are deficient, but the absolute volume of Leydig cells is not increased. Serum T levels are approximately half those of normal men, and gonadotropins are elevated. The vast majority of patients are azoospermic; the presence of sperm suggests 46 XY/47 XXY mosaicism.

The decreased androgen production in patients with Klinefelter syndrome prevents normal secondary sexual development. Muscle development is poor and the fat distribution takes a more female than male pattern. Normal amounts of pubic and axillary hair may be present, but facial hair is sparse (Fig 5). Fifty percent to 75% of 47 XXY patients have increased parenchymal breast tissue, although visually obvious gynecomastia is less common. Patients with Klinefelter syndrome develop breast carcinoma 20 times more frequently than normal males. In addition, they are predisposed to developing malignant neoplasms of extragonadal germ-cell origin.[17,18]

Management options for patients with Klinefelter syndrome are limited to careful androgen supplementation in select males to improve libido, and surgical treatment of gynecomastia.

The sex reversal syndrome (XX male) probably represents a variant of the Klinefelter syndrome. The patients are clinically indistinguishable from those with Klinefelter syndrome[19] and although they lack a Y chromosome, the vast majority have detectable Y DNA.[19] In a recent study of 26 XX males performed at the Whitehead Institute, 24 were noted to have Y DNA material upon chromosomal analysis.[20] Thus, these patients possess the genetic information necessary for the formation of testes in addition to two X chromosomes, much like patients with Klinefelter syndrome. Management of patients with sex reversal syndrome is comparable to that of the Klinefelter syndrome patient.

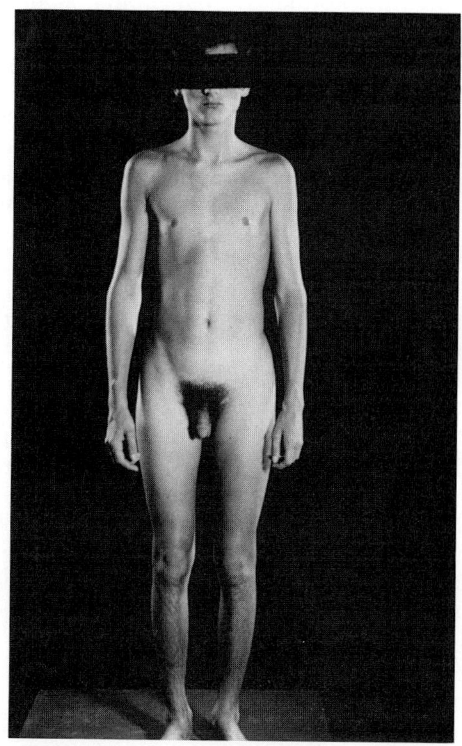

**Fig 5.** Male with Klinefelter syndrome exhibiting relatively poor muscle development and sparse facial hair. [From Diamond D, Intersex disorders: parts 1 & 2, *AUA Update Series* (Houston, Tex: American Urological Assoc. Office of Education; 1990;IX:lessons 9, 10), with permission.]

## Gonadal Dysgenesis (Turner's Syndrome)

This term applies to patients with bilateral streak gonads, sexual infantilism, short stature, and certain other somatic anomalies. Due to a loss of an X chromosome through nondisjunction in gametogenesis or an error in mitosis, 50% of patients with gonadal dysgenesis have a 45 X complement, and 25% have sex chromosomal mosaicism (45 X/46 XX). The remainder have either a structurally abnormal X or Y, or no detectable chromosomal abnormality.[21]

In the 45 X patient, the normal gonad is replaced by a white fibrous streak, 2 to 3 cm long and approximately 0.5 cm wide, located in the broad ligament. Histologically the streak possesses interlacing waves of dense fibrous stroma, which is devoid of oocytes but is otherwise indistinguishable from normal ovarian stroma. Both estrogen and androgen are decreased and follicle-stimulating hormone (FSH) and luteinizing hormone (LH) levels are elevated. Secondary sexual development does not, as a rule, occur. Pubic and axillary hair fail to develop in normal abundance, and the well-differentiated external genitalia, vagina, Müllerian derivatives, and breasts remain small. Turner's syndrome is the most common cause of primary amenorrhea, and the diagnosis is frequently made because pubertal development never occurs.

Individuals with Turner's syndrome are usually short (mean height = 141 cm) and have certain characteristic somatic anomalies. These include webbed neck, shield chest, coarctation of the aorta, lymphedema of the hands and feet, and epicanthal folds (Fig 6). Renal anomalies occur in 60% of 45 X patients; horseshoe kidney is most common.

It is well established that, for patients with Turner's syndrome, puberty can be induced by the administration of estrogen at the appropriate time. Recent studies indicate that the use of biosynthetic human growth hormone may also accelerate short-term growth in patients with Turner's syndrome contributing to the psychosocial well-being of these patients.[22]

The probability that a gonadal tumor (gonadoblastoma or dysgerminoma) will arise in a patient with a 45 XO karyotype and gonadal dysgenesis is relatively low. But if an XY cell line is demonstrated, the incidence increases to approximately 30%, with nearly twice this incidence in familial cases.[17] In a series of 119 patients with tumors secondary to gonadal dysgenesis, 91% of tumors were found in patients with Y chromosomal material.[23] Gonadoblastomas comprised two thirds of the tumors. Development of gonadoblastoma in 9% of patients without clearly detectable Y chromosomal material suggests mosaicism, which is sometimes difficult to detect. This raises the possibility that even those patients without obvious Y chromosomal material are at some risk for tumor formation. Thus, any patient with Turner's syndrome and clear evidence of a Y cell line should

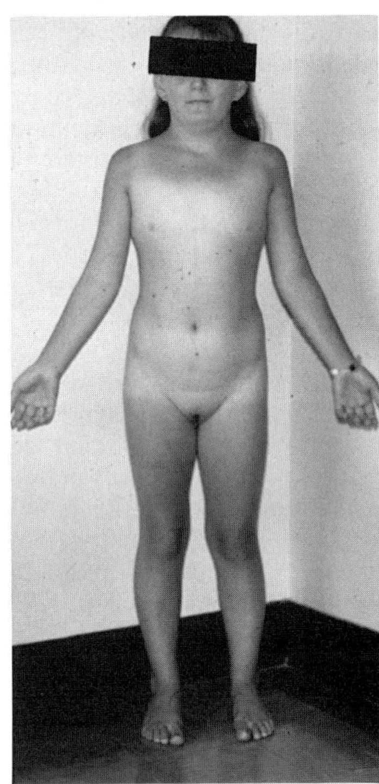

**Fig 6.** Patient with Turner's syndrome exhibiting short stature, low-set ears, webbed neck, shield chest, and widely-spaced, hypoplastic nipples. [From Diamond D, Intersex disorders: parts 1 & 2, *AUA Update Series* (Houston, Tex: American Urological Assoc. Office of Education; 1990; IX:lessons 9, 10), with permission.]

undergo bilateral streak gonadectomy. Given the potential risk for gonadoblastoma development, it seems advisable for patients with a 45 X karyotype to be considered for bilateral streak gonadectomy as well. At the very least, a thorough attempt should be made to rule out occult mosaicism in these patients.

## Mixed Gonadal Dysgenesis

Mixed gonadal dysgenesis is characterized by a unilateral testis, which is often intraabdominal, a contralateral streak gonad, and persistent Müllerian structures, associated with varying degrees of inadequate masculinization. Most patients with mixed gonadal dysgenesis have a 45 XO/46 XY karyotype, which is most likely the result of anaphase lag during early mitosis. Occult mosaicism is considered likely in those patients without the classic karyotype.

The vast majority of patients with mixed gonadal dysgenesis have ambiguous genitalia with varying degrees of phallic enlargement, a urogenital sinus and labioscrotal fusion, along with an undescended testis. In virtually all patients, a uterus, vagina, and fallopian tube are present. One third will exhibit somatic stigmata of Turner's syndrome and one half will be less than 148 cm tall. Two thirds of mixed gonadal dysgenesis patients are raised as females.

The potential mechanism by which the abnormal phenotype results in mixed gonadal dysgenesis is fascinating, in that the testes respond to gonadotropins and secrete T in normal quantities at puberty. Histologically, the testes lack germinal elements, and infertility is the rule. Yet despite normal postpubertal endocrine function, it is postulated that fetal testicular endocrine function is either deficient or delayed, resulting in persistence of Müllerian structures and inadequate masculinization.[24]

Patients with mixed gonadal dysgenesis are at increased risk for both gonadal and Wilms' tumors. The risk of developing a gonadal tumor (gonadoblastoma and dysgerminoma being the most common) is approximately 20%.[17] Patients with the closely related disorder, dysgenetic male pseudohermaphroditism (characterized by bilateral dysgenetic testes, persistent Müllerian structures, cryptorchidism, and inadequate virilization) are at similar risk. Rajfer found that of 100 patients with both intersex disorders and Wilms' tumor, 50% had mixed gonadal dysgenesis.[25] He postulated the presence of a genetic or teratogenic defect involving the urogenital ridge, the common embryonic anlage of both the kidney and gonad. The presence of glomerular disease in some of these patients is consistent with the Drash syndrome. This syndrome, recognized in 1970, is characterized by sexual ambiguity, Wilms' tumor, hypertension, proteinuria, and progressive renal failure.[26] One of the two patients originally described by Drash, and subsequent patients reported with this syndrome, have been found to have mixed gonadal dysgenesis.[27]

It is recommended that patients with mixed gonadal dysgenesis be reared as females. This allows for removal of the gonads and avoidance of their malignant potential. As males, they would be infertile, relatively short, and require urethral reconstruction. These patients should be screened regularly for Wilms' tumor and their renal function should be closely monitored.

## True Hermaphroditism

The true hermaphrodite has histologic evidence of both ovarian and testicular tissue, which may take the form of one ovary and one testis or, more often, one or two ovotestes. Forty percent of these patients have unilateral hermaphroditism (ovotestis on one side and testis or ovary on the other side); 20% bilateral (ovotestes on both sides); and 40% have lateral hermaphroditism (a testis on one side and ovary on the other).

Approximately two thirds of true hermaphrodites have a 46 XX karyotype, however, 46 XX/46 XY, 46 XX/47 XXYY mosaicism and 46 XY have been reported. The etiology of true hermaphroditism is somewhat unclear and may be heterogeneous. The 46 XX/46 XY cases probably result from chimerism, the presence in an indi-

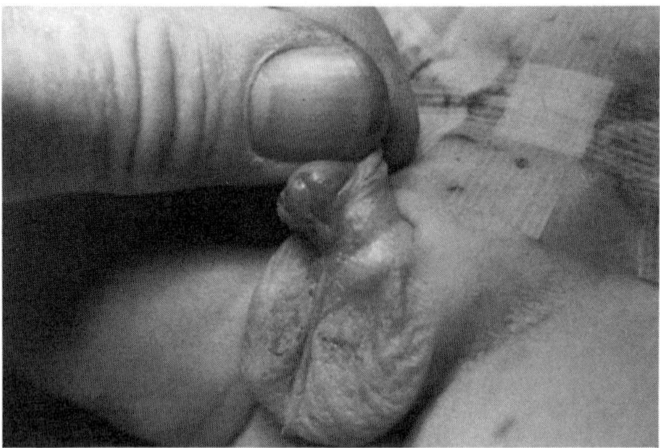

**Fig 7.** Infant with penile hypospadias, chordee, and bilaterally undescended testes found to have true hermaphroditism. [From Diamond D, Intersex disorders: parts 1 & 2, *AUA Update Series* (Houston, Tex: American Urological Assoc. Office of Education; 1990;IX:lessons 9, 10), with permission.]

vidual of cells derived from two zygotes. In 46 XX true hermaphrodites, the presence of testicular tissue has been postulated to result from: 1) translocation of testicular determinants from the Y chromosome to an X chromosome or autosome, 2) undetected mosaicism or chimerism, and 3) single sex-reversal gene mutations. The immunologic detection of H-Y antigen in almost all 46 XX true hermaphrodites supports the concept that a Y-chromosomal translocation too small for cytologic detection accounts for testicular differentiation.[28]

Both the external genitalia and internal duct structures of true hermaphrodites display gradations between male and female. In most patients, the external genitalia are masculinized to some extent and two thirds of true hermaphrodites are raised as male. Among those reared as males, 80% have hypospadias and over 50% have labioscrotal fusion (Fig 7). Among those raised as females, two thirds will have clitoromegaly. Virtually all patients have a urogenital sinus, and in most cases a uterus is present (Fig 8). The ovary is found in a normal location, but the testis or ovotestis may reside at any point along the path of testicular descent.[29]

The most important aspect of management of true hermaphrodites is gender assignment. Such decisions should be based upon the adequacy of the phallus and findings at laparotomy. Unlike mixed gonadal dysgenesis, patients with true hermaphroditism have the potential for fertility, which has been reported in a small number of females and males. Thus, the patient with an adequate phallus and testis which can be brought to the scrotum should be raised as a male. The patient with an ovary and normal Müllerian duct structures on one side should be raised as a female. Because 80% of ovotestes have testicular and ovarian elements juxtaposed end-to-end, the possibility of preserving the desired half of an ovotestis has been proposed. However, deciding upon the proper plane of cleavage intraoperatively is usually very difficult. Following gender assignment, all contradictory gonads and internal duct structures should be removed. Gonadoblastomas are rare in the absence of an XY cell line and thus are uncommon in true hermaphrodites, the majority of whom are 46 XX. However, two cases of gonadoblastoma arising in 46 XX true hermaphrodites have been described.[17]

## DISORDERS OF GONADAL SEX

### Pure Gonadal Dysgenesis

The syndrome of pure gonadal dysgenesis is characterized by the presence of

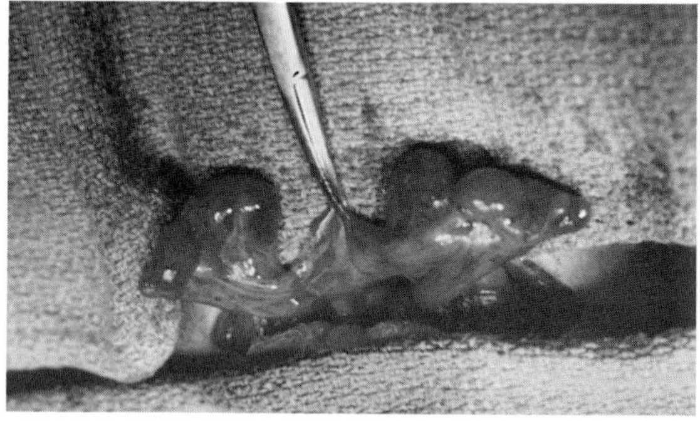

**Fig 8.** Laparotomy findings from true hermaphrodite noted in Fig 7; clamp on uterus with bilateral, fimbriated Fallopian tubes and bilateral ovotestes. [From Diamond D, Intersex disorders: parts 1 & 2, *AUA Update Series* (Houston, Tex: American Urological Assoc. Office of Education; 1990;IX:lessons 9, 10), with permission.]

bilateral streak gonads in phenotypic females with sexual infantilism and a 46 XX or 46 XY karyotype. The gonadal lesion is identical to that which accompanies Turner's syndrome (gonadal dysgenesis), but is unassociated in these patients with the short stature and other somatic stigmata of Turner's syndrome. In this respect, the gonadal dysgenesis is "pure." Because, by definition, pure gonadal dysgenesis is unassociated with chromosomal anomalies, it is considered a disorder of gonadal sex.[30]

The etiology of pure gonadal dysgenesis is not entirely clear. In 46 XY gonadal dysgenesis, it has been proposed that the testis-determining genetic information is absent because of a single mutation, which results in dysgenetic gonads. Interestingly, among patients with XY gonadal dysgenesis, some have been found to be H-Y antigen positive while others are H-Y antigen negative,[28] which may support the concept that the H-Y antigen is not the testis-determining factor. It now seems well accepted that XY gonadal dysgenesis results from an X-linked recessive or male-limited autosomal-dominant gene. XX gonadal dysgenesis is also thought to result from a single gene mutation with autosomal recessive inheritance. In either event, the absence of functional gonads reproduces the Jost model, such that independent of karyotype, a female phenotype results.

Clinically, patients are phenotypic females of normal or tall stature with bilateral streak gonads. The internal and external genitalia are entirely female, but remain infantile. Occasionally, clitoromegaly is noted. Sexual maturation, including the development of breasts and axillary and pubic hair is absent or markedly retarded.

The management of patients with pure gonadal dysgenesis is similar to that of those with Turner's syndrome, in that long-term estrogen therapy should be instituted at the expected time of puberty. However, the management of these two syndromes differs because neoplastic transformation of the dysgenetic gonad is far more likely to occur in those with pure gonadal dysgenesis, predominantly in those with an XY cell line. The probability that a gonadal tumor (gonadoblastoma or dysgerminoma) will arise in a patient with XY gonadal dysgenesis is approximately 30%, making routine gonadectomy in these patients mandatory (Fig 9). Among patients with XX gonadal dysgenesis, gonadal tumors are rare, and only three have been reported to date.[17]

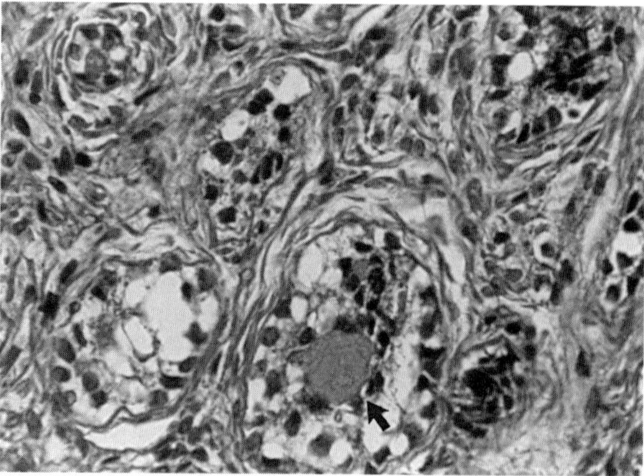

**Fig 9.** Histologic section of gonadoblastoma, with characteristic nests composed of germ cells and immature sex cord elements with hyaline bodies (black arrow). [From Diamond D, Intersex disorders: parts 1 & 2, *AUA Update Series* (Houston, Tex: American Urological Assoc. Office of Education; 1990;IX:lessons 9, 10), with permission.]

## Bilateral Vanishing Testes Syndrome

The syndrome of bilaterally vanishing testes or embryonic testicular regression is characterized by patients with a 46 XY karyotype and absent or rudimentary testes, in whom there is clear evidence of testicular function at some point during embryogenesis. The syndrome entails the presence of testes which "vanish" during embryogenesis and thus is distinguishable from pure gonadal dysgenesis, in which there is no evidence of in utero testicular function.[31]

The etiology of this disorder is unclear. It is possible that regression of the testes in utero is due to a genetic mutation, a teratogen, or bilateral torsion. The finding of familial instances of XY agonadism, which might be consistent with a rare recessive trait, supports the possibility of a genetic etiology. Thus far, chromosomal anomalies have not been identified in patients with this syndrome.[32]

Clinically, the syndrome encompasses a spectrum of phenotypes, ranging in severity from complete female through varying degrees of genital ambiguity to a male phenotype with development of a microphallus and empty scrotum. The diagnosis can be made on the basis of a 46 XY karyotype and castrate levels of T despite persistently elevated serum LH and FSH levels. In the most severe form of the disorder, agonadism is discovered in a 46 XY phenotypic female with no internal genital structures. This picture is presumed to result when a testis has elaborated MIF, but vanishes at approximately day 60 to 70 of gestation, prior to the elaboration of androgen. In this setting, a belated Jost model is created, and the individual goes on to develop a sexually infantile female phenotype, but lacks any internal ductal structures. At an intermediate point in the clinical spectrum is the 46 XY patient with absent gonads and internal ductal structures but with ambiguous genitalia due to incomplete elaboration of androgen by the vanishing testes. Finally, patients may present as agonadal XY phenotypic males with fully developed Wolffian structures, but an empty scrotum, absent prostate, and microphallus. This represents testicular regression following complete anatomical development of the male external genitalia within the first trimester.

Vasa are usually identified upon surgical exploration of these patients; biopsy of the distal ends demonstrates no recognizable testicular tissue histologically. Atrophic epididymal remnants may be observed, occasionally.

The management of patients with bilateral vanishing testes syndromes is dictated by their position in the clinical spectrum of the disorder. Sexually infantile phenotypic females require estrogen supplementation at the time of expected puberty for development of secondary sexual characteristics, and may require vaginoplasty. Similarly, phenotypic males require long-term androgen replacement, beginning at the time of expected puberty. A study of 21 males so treated has demonstrated that replacement therapy started at the correct time caused a normal pubertal growth spurt with development of normal secondary sex characteristics, including penile growth, together with normal bone maturation.[33] In addition, such male patients may benefit from placement of testicular prostheses. Patients with ambiguous genitalia require individualized assessment to determine the optimal sex of rearing.

## DISORDERS OF PHENOTYPIC SEX

### Female Pseudohermaphroditism

Female pseudohermaphroditism is a disorder of phenotypic sexual development in which 46 XX individuals with ovaries have a partially masculinized phenotype and ambiguous genitalia. By far the most common cause of female pseudohermaphroditism is congenital adrenal hyperplasia (CAH), which is the most common cause of ambiguous genitalia in the newborn (Fig 10). Two very rare causes of female pseudohermaphroditism include the maternal ingestion of androgens and virilizing tumors, such as arrhenoblastoma, in the mother.

**Congenital adrenal hyperplasia (CAH).** The adrenogenital syndrome due to CAH is a

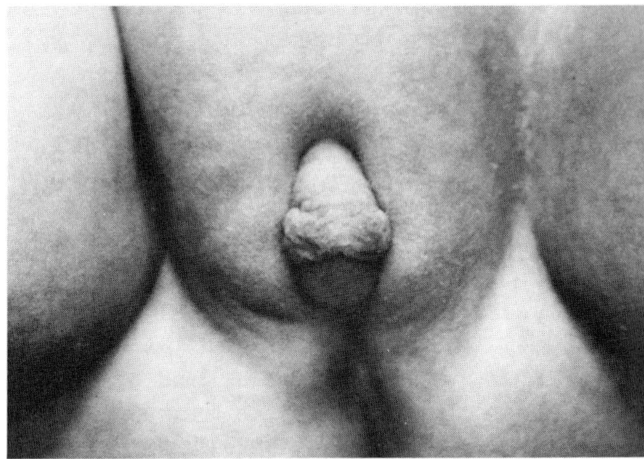

**Fig 10.** Genitalia of female pseudohermaphrodite with congenital adrenal hyperplasia demonstrating marked virilization with phallic enlargement and labioscrotal fusion. [From Diamond D, Intersex disorders: parts 1 & 2, *AUA Update Series* (Houston, Tex: American Urological Assoc. Office of Education; 1990;IX:lessons 9, 10), with permission.]

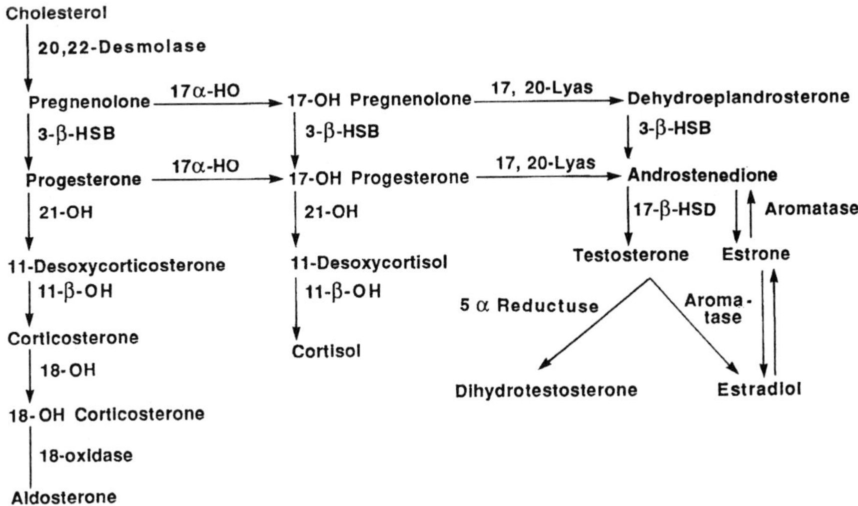


**Fig 11.** Enzymatic defects in synthesis of cortisol (congenital adrenal hyperplasia) and in synthesis of testosterone (male pseudohermaphroditism). HSD = hydroxysteroid dehydrogenase; OH = hydroxylase (courtesy of AM DiGeorge, MD).

classic example of an inborn error of metabolism—in this case an error involving cortisol synthesis. A defect in any one of the five enzymes involved in the cortisol biosynthetic pathway (20, 22-desmolase, 3-β-hydroxysteroid dehydrogenase, 17-hydroxylase, 21-hydroxylase, and 11-hydroxylase) may result in CAH (Fig 11). But the most commonly recognized syndromes result from a deficiency of one of the terminal two enzymes of glucocorticoid synthesis (21- or 11-hydroxylase). As a result of deficiency of either terminal enzyme, formation of hydrocortisone is impaired, causing a compensatory increase in adrenocorticotrophic hormone (ACTH) secretion. This increase enhances formation of adrenal steroids proximal to the enzymatic defect and a secondary increase in the formation of T, the active androgen in CAH.[34]

Deficiency in 21-hydroxylase occurs with an incidence ranging from 1 in 5,000 to 1 in 15,000 in the United States and Europe, and accounts for 95% of patients with CAH. 21-hydroxylase is a cytochrome P450 enzyme, whose gene locus is on the short arm of chromosome 6 within the HLA complex. It is transmitted in an autosomal recessive pattern.[29]

The majority of patients with CAH secondary to 21-hydroxylase deficiency exhibit one of the two classic forms of the disease—half present with salt wasting and half with simple virilization.

In the female with the simple virilizing form of the disorder, female pseudohermaphroditism results. Because the impaired steroidogenesis begins early in life—at the time of formation of the external genitalia (beginning at 10 weeks' gestation)—there is virtually always evidence of some degree of masculinization at birth. This is manifested by enlargement of the clitoris and varying degrees of labial fusion. In addition, the vagina and urethra open into a common urogenital sinus. The enlargement of the clitoris may be so dramatic as to make it appear to be a hypospadiac penis with bilateral cryptorchidism, and cases of complete formation of a masculinized urethra to the tip of an enlarged clitoris have been reported. The severity of the virilization is generally greater in infants who experience salt wasting. The Müllerian structures in these patients are typically normal.

After birth there is progression of masculinization of the untreated female; pubic and axillary hair develop prematurely, acne appears, and the voice deepens. There is rapid somatic maturation, resulting in premature epiphyseal closure and short adult stature. Although the internal genitalia are female, breast development and menstruation do not occur unless the excessive androgen production is suppressed by adequate steroid therapy.

In the male without salt wasting, the chief clinical manifestations are those of isosexual precocity. The infant appears normal at birth, but signs of sexual and somatic precocity appear within the first 2 to 3 years of life. Although the testes remain normal in size, enlargement of the penis, scrotum, and prostate occur, with the appearance of pubic hair, acne, and deepening of the voice. The musculature is well developed and bone age is more advanced than appropriate for the chronologic age.

In both males and females with the salt-losing variant, symptoms begin within the first few weeks after birth, with failure to regain birth weight, progressive weight loss, and dehydration. Vomiting is prominent, and may be so extreme that a mistaken diagnosis of pyloric stenosis may be made, particularly in the male.

In classic 21-hydroxylase deficiency, plasma levels of progesterone and 17-hydroxyprogesterone are markedly elevated. Urinary 17-ketosteroids and pregnanetriol are elevated. One may make the diagnosis biochemically using either radioimmunoassay of plasma steroid levels or a 24-hour urine collection of pregnanetriol.

A deficiency of 11-β-hydroxylase accounts for roughly 5% of cases of CAH. Both classic and mild forms have been recognized. Unlike 21-hydroxylase, 11-β-hydroxylase is not HLA-linked. Hypertension is a common finding in patients with this type of CAH, and is believed to be secondary to elevated serum levels of deoxycorticosterone (DOC). While the majority of patients are hypertensive, some are normotensive and others only experience intermittent hypertension. Virilization occurs in all patients, and is as severe as in those with the 21-hydroxylase defect.

At present, the most exciting aspect of CAH is the capability of diagnosing and treating the disorder prenatally. Prenatal diagnosis of CAH in the at-risk fetus is possible during the first trimester by HLA typing or by DNA analysis of genes within the HLA complex in cells obtained by chorionic villus sampling. By treating the mother with dexamethasone, which crosses the placenta, the fetal secretion of ACTH may be suppressed, thereby preventing virilization of the genitalia.[35] There are certain complexities to this form of management, however. The diagnosis of CAH in the fetus can be determined on chorionic villus cells at 8 to 10 weeks or on cells from amniotic fluid obtained at 16 to 17 weeks. However, treatment should be instituted at 5 to 6 weeks of gestation, prior to initial development of the external genitalia. Therefore, it is not possible to determine the diagnosis prior to initiating therapy. Because virilization is not a concern with the male fetus and three of four female fetuses at risk will be unaffected given the autosomal recessive pattern of inheritance, seven of eight fetuses may be treated unnecessarily.[36] Thus one goal is earlier diagnosis to avoid unnecessary therapy. Finally, reported series suggest that there are three groups of CAH infants born to mothers treated with dexamethasone.[37] In roughly one third of neonates, there is no evidence of masculinization, suggesting totally successful therapy. In another third, there seems to be milder masculinization than that noted in an affected sibling, suggesting partial success. In a final third there appears to be no recognizable effect of therapy whatsoever. This heterogeneity of response to therapy raises intriguing questions about the mechanisms involved in virilization of the CAH fetus.

The treatment of affected children with hydrocortisone achieves a number of goals, and as noted by Bongiovanni, is useful: "to supply the deficient hormone; to suppress pituitary ACTH secretion and hence adrenal androgens and clinical virilization; to forestall abnormally rapid somatic growth and osseous advance; to permit normal gonadal development; to correct salt-water loss or hypertension in the complicated forms; and to avoid side reactions of administered steroids in unnecessarily large doses.''[38] The recommended daily oral doses of hydrocortisone are 10-15 mg for the child younger than 5 years, 15-20 mg for children between the ages of 5 and 12 years, and 20-30 mg for children over age 12. The effectiveness of therapy may be assessed by measuring morning plasma 17-hydroxyprogesterone levels.

Those children with the salt-losing form of the disease require increased salt intake and mineralocorticoid treatment in addition to hydrocortisone therapy. After control of electrolytes and blood pressure have been achieved in the acute setting, maintenance therapy with the fluorohydrocortisone (0.05-0.10 mg daily) should be instituted.

The administration of hydrocortisone and, when required, fluorohydrocortisone are continued indefinitely in all patients. Increased doses are indicated during stressful events such as surgery or infection.

In the majority of children (who will not have been diagnosed and treated prenatally), it is appropriate to perform feminizing genitoplasty at 6–12 months of age, when a well-established course of medical therapy has been instituted, the risks of anesthesia have become minimal, and the child has grown large enough to make the procedure technically feasible.

## Male Pseudohermaphroditism

Male pseudohermaphroditism describes 46 XY individuals with testes who exhibit varying degrees of feminization phenotypically. It can result from a defect in either androgen synthesis, T metabolism (5α-reductase deficiency), androgen action, or Müllerian-duct regression. As a result of advances in biochemical techniques, our understanding of this particular group of disorders has progressed significantly over the past decade.

**Disorders of androgen synthesis.** The decrease in T biosynthesis in patients with male pseudohermaphroditism is due to a defect in one of the five enzymes required for the conversion of cholesterol to T. These include 20,22-desmolase, 3-β-OH steroid dehydrogenase, 17-hydroxylase, 17,20-desmolase, and 17-β-hydroxysteroid dehydrogenase. A defect in one of the first three enzymes listed results in cortisol as well as T deficiency, and is thus a form of CAH. A defect in either 17,20-desmolase or 17-β-hydroxysteroid dehydrogenase primarily affects T biosynthesis by the testis. In all cases low androgen levels result in incomplete virilization of the male fetus during embryogenesis.

Patients with defects involving 17,20-desmolase or 17-β-hydroxysteroid dehydrogenase are usually identified as female at birth. Subsequently, they may be found to have inguinal or abdominal testes, a blind-ending vagina, and absence of Müllerian tissue. Gonadotropin levels are elevated, baseline T is low, and the biochemical precursors before the enzyme block are high. At puberty, virilization occurs in the previously unrecognized patient.[32]

Management of these patients with severe defects is usually straightforward, as they are most appropriately raised as females, and entails early gonadectomy and reconstructive surgery if necessary, and estrogen replacement at the time of expected puberty. In less severe cases a male phenotype may be appropriate, although fertility has not been reported. These male patients must be assessed individually with regard to their need for supplemental androgen at puberty.

### Abnormalities in testosterone metabolism

***5α-reductase deficiency.*** The disorder of 5α-reductase deficiency is one of the most distinctive forms of male pseudohermaphroditism. The clinical presentation of this enzyme disorder was actually predicted in 1972, prior to the description of such patients in 1974.[39] This is an autosomal recessive defect which results in impaired intracellular conversion of T to DHT in target tissue. Thus, involved individuals have a 46 XY karyotype with normal T levels and normal male Wolffian structures, but predominantly female development of the urogenital sinus and external genitalia, which results in an external female phenotype.

Wilson's group has demonstrated that the 5α-reductase deficiency is actually a heterogeneous disorder that may result from a variety of distinct mutations.[40] Fibroblasts from most patients have very low or undetectable 5α-reductase activity and appear to form an enzyme with reduced affinity for T, leading to decreased conversion of T to DHT. In other pedigrees, the enzyme has been shown to be synthesized in normal or slightly decreased amounts, but to be inherently unstable in vitro under certain conditions. A third pedigree has been demonstrated, and confers intermediate levels of activity and stability of 5α-reductase. Phenotypically, these three varieties are indistinguishable.

Clinically, patients are born with markedly ambiguous genitalia, and are usually raised as female. Typically, they have an enlarged clitoris, a urogenital sinus with separate vaginal and urethral openings, and labioscrotal fusion (Figs 12–14). The vaginal pouch is blind ending and short. Testes and epididymides are located in the labia, inguinal canals, or abdomen, and the vasa terminate in the blind-ending vaginal pouch.

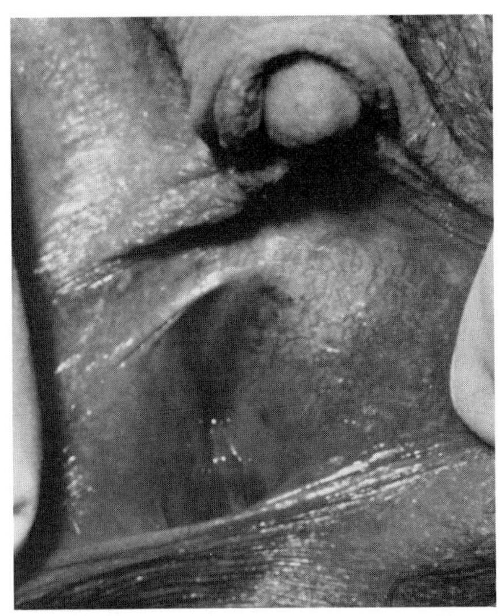

**Fig 13.** Intraoperative view of urogenital sinus in patient with 5α-reductase deficiency; note enlarged clitoris, urogenital sinus with separate urethral and vaginal openings, and posterior labioscrotal fusion. [From Diamond D, Intersex disorders: parts 1 & 2, *AUA Update Series* (Houston, Tex: American Urological Assoc. Office of Education; 1990;IX:lessons 9, 10), with permission.]

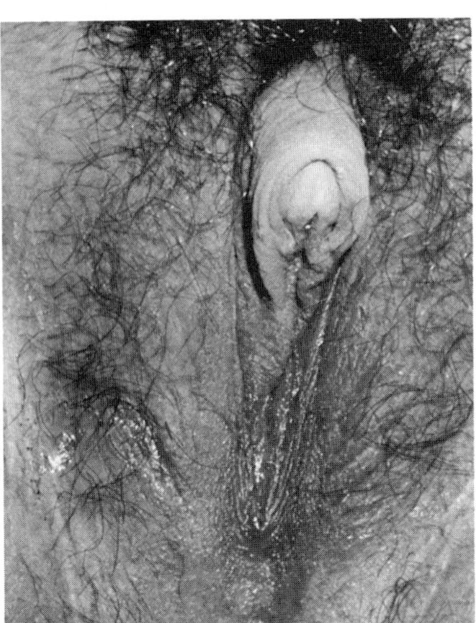

**Fig 12.** External genitalia from patient with 5α-reductase deficiency. Note cliteromegaly with marked labioscrotal fusion and small vaginal introitus. [From Diamond D, Intersex disorders: parts 1 & 2, *AUA Update Series* (Houston, Tex: American Urological Assoc. Office of Education; 1990;IX:lessons 9, 10), with permission.]

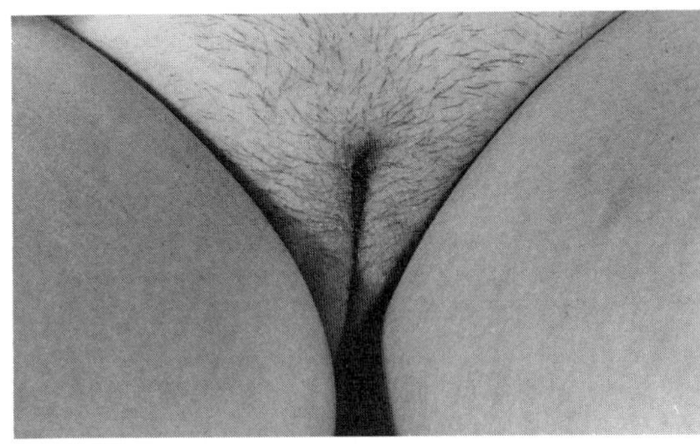

**Fig 14.** Postoperative result in patient from Fig 13 with 5α-reductase deficiency following clitoral recession and vaginoplasty. [From Diamond D, Intersex disorders: parts 1 & 2, *AUA Update Series* (Houston, Tex: American Urological Assoc. Office of Education; 1990;IX:lessons 9, 10), with permission.]

At puberty, partial masculinization occurs, probably as a result of small amounts of 5α-reductase, so that the phallus enlarges, erections occur and a male body habitus develops. As a result, the pedigree studied by Imperato-McGinley in the Dominican Republic underwent gender reversal at puberty, and were known within the community as "guavedoces" (penis at 12).[41]

The endocrine characteristics of 5α-reductase deficiency include normal male plasma levels of T before and after human chorionic gonadotropin (hCG) stimulation, and a deficient DHT response leading to a markedly increased T/DHT ratio. Fibroblasts cultured from genital skin exhibit deficient 5α-reductase activity.[42]

The management of 5α-reductase deficiency is primarily dependent upon the phenotypic findings and gender at the time of diagnosis. Given the severe defect of the external genitalia, most individuals are properly raised as females. For these patients, gonadectomy should be performed early—certainly well before puberty—to prevent masculinization. Estrogens should be administered at the time of expected puberty. Vaginoplasty and clitoral reduction should be performed within the first year of life, in the face of a severe defect, to provide for a normal appearance and to allay parental anxiety. If the diagnosis is made in infancy and the phallus is of acceptable size, one can consider raising such a child as male. Although these patients are infertile, their testes would serve as a lifelong source of T. A recent study of four men with 5α-reductase deficiency demonstrated that administering supraphysiologic doses of T resulted in long-term enhancement of virilization, with enlargement of the penis, increase in erectile potency and ejaculatory volume, and an increase in muscle bulk, with no improvement in spermatogenesis.[43]

### Abnormalities of Androgen Action

***Disorders of androgen receptor function.*** Patients with disorders of androgen receptor function characteristically have a 46 XY karyotype and testes and present with a spectrum of phenotypic abnormalities which vary from complete external feminization (syndrome of testicular feminization), to ambiguous genitalia (Reifenstein syndrome), to the phenotypically normal infertile male. While the clinical presentations of these disorders differ according to the severity of the receptor disorder, the pathophysiology is similar.

The essential problem in all of these patients is resistance to androgen action because of deficient or defective intracellular androgen receptor protein. This disorder was first recognized and most thoroughly studied in patients with testicular feminization, in whom a complete absence of the cytosol-located androgen binding sites in cultured skin fibroblasts from androgen-resistant male pseudohermaphrodites was discovered. However, subsequent studies demonstrated that a significant number of patients with testicular feminization have normal or even higher than normal concentrations of intracellular androgen receptors, indicating the wide molecular heterogeneity of this disorder.[44] In these patients, as well as in those with partial androgen insensitivity syndromes, qualitatively abnormal receptors, as a result of thermolability or abnormal binding, have been found to be the most common form of androgen receptor defect.[45] In addition, other patients with partial androgen insensitivity syndromes have been noted to have decreased amounts of apparently normal androgen receptor.[46]

In all of these patients, serum T levels are normal and the rate of testicular production of T is normal or elevated. Gonadotropins are elevated (accounting for the high T production) as a result of resistance to androgen at the hypothalamic–pituitary level. The high gonadotropin level increases estradiol production by the testis. The variable severity of androgen resistance and enhanced testicular production of estradiol results in different degrees of defective virilization and feminization noted in the syndromes of defective androgen receptor function.

Patients with testicular feminization (complete androgen insensitivity syndrome) have a normal female phenotype with the exception of diminished axillary and pubic hair. Their breast development and body habitus are feminine in character and their external genitalia are unequivocally female, although the vagina is short and has a blind end. Because the fetal testes secrete MIF, however, internal genitalia are absent, with the exception of the testes, which may be found in the labia, inguinal canal, or abdomen. These patients are diagnosed most commonly as a result of primary amenorrhea or when a testis is discovered at herniorrhaphy. Histologically, the testes exhibit incomplete or absent spermatogenesis with normal or hyperplastic Leydig cells. In two thirds of patients, there is a positive family history consistent with X linkage. Ten percent of patients with testicular feminization have an incomplete form of the disorder in which there is partial virilization with partial labioscrotal fusion, normal pubic hair, and identifiable but rudimentary Wolffian duct-derived tissue. These patients feminize at puberty.[40]

The treatment of patients with testicular feminization relates primarily to the optimal timing of gonadectomy. Because the testes produce estradiol, which results in the appropriate pubertal changes for the female phenotype, it is considered preferable to leave the testes in situ until puberty is complete. Exceptions to the approach of delayed gonadectomy occur in the presence of palpable testes or testes associated with a hernia. A competing concern is the potential for malignant degeneration of the retained testis. In patients with testicular feminization who reach adulthood with the retained testis, the risk of developing a testis tumor—usually a seminoma—is thought to be 2% to 5%, only slightly higher than in a standard cryptorchid testis.[17] Prior to adulthood, the risk is extremely low, and therefore delayed gonadectomy following puberty is believed to be safe.

The syndromes of partial androgen insensitivity, which were originally thought to be separate entities (Reifenstein, Gilbert-Dreyfus, Rosewater, and Lubs syndromes), now fall under the heading of Reifenstein syndrome.[40] These are X-linked disorders of incomplete male pseudohermaphroditism which are all believed to represent a single gene mutation that produces an abnormal androgen receptor. The classical phenotype is that of a man with perineoscrotal hypospadias, cryptorchidism, rudimentary Wolffian duct derivatives, gynecomastia, and infertility. However, the phenotypic spectrum can range from hypospadias and a pseudovagina to gynecomastia and azoospermia. The endocrine profile of Reifenstein syndrome is similar to that of testicular feminization.

The management of these patients must be individualized depending on the degree of genital ambiguity. This involves issues of cryptorchidism, reconstruction of external genitalia, and management of gynecomastia, when present. Price's report of one adult male with Reifenstein syndrome who responded impressively to supraphysiologic doses of T with increased penile size and increased erectile potency suggests that certain androgen receptor defects may be amenable to pharmacologic therapy.[43]

The most recently discovered and mildest form of androgen receptor abnormality is that of the infertile male syndrome. While these men are believed to be azoospermic on the basis of an androgen receptor defect, they are phenotypically normal in all respects and thus do not represent a true intersex disorder.

***Post-receptor defect of androgen resistance.*** Ten percent to 15% of patients with clinical and endocrinologic evidence of androgen resistance have been found to have normal intracellular levels and molecular behavior of androgen receptor. While the majority of these patients have had syndromes of partial androgen insensitivity, a recent report described a number of patients with evidence of complete androgen insensitivity and normal receptor.[47]

The phenotypes within this category may span the identical clinical spectrum noted in patients with androgen receptor defects. Indeed, Wilson points out that further study of these patients, with increasingly sophisticated biochemical techniques, is likely to uncover subtle qualitative abnormalities in androgen receptor function.

The management of these patients is identical to those with abnormal androgen receptors and similar phenotypes.

### Defects in Müllerian regression

***Persistent Müllerian duct syndrome (hernia uteri inguinale).*** Persistent Müllerian duct syndrome, or hernia uteri inguinale, the term originally used by Nilson,[48] characteristically describes a group of normal male patients in whom female internal genitalia are present. Typically, these phenotypic males have unilateral or bilateral undescended testes, bilateral fallopian tubes, a uterus, and an upper vagina draining into the prostatic utricle. The condition is commonly diagnosed when Müllerian tissue is encountered during inguinal herniorrhaphy.

Persistent Müllerian duct syndrome is thought to be due to an isolated defect in the fetal testicular production of MIF by the Sertoli cells in quantity or timing during embryogenesis, or due to end-organ insensitivity to the action of MIF. The condition is inherited as an autosomal-recessive or X-linked recessive mutation.

The treatment of persistent Müllerian duct syndrome is relatively straightforward, in that all patients are phenotypic males who require orchiopexy. The one treatment caveat relates to handling of the rudimentary Müllerian structures. Sloan and Walsh noted the close proximity of the vasa deferentia to the uterus and vagina, and recommended preserving these Müllerian structures to avoid damage to the vas, thus preserving fertility potential.[49] This potential is likely to be quite limited, as clear documentation of fertility in patients with this syndrome is lacking. However, because a malignancy has never been reported in the retained Müllerian structures in these patients, this approach seems reasonable.

## EVALUATION OF THE NEWBORN WITH AMBIGUOUS GENITALIA

The evaluation and initial management of the newborn with ambiguous genitalia must be regarded as a medical emergency and must be handled with great sensitivity toward the family. One's goal should be to make a precise diagnosis of the intersex disorder and to assign a proper sex of rearing based on this diagnosis and the status of the child's anatomy. Of paramount importance in considering a male sex of rearing is the adequacy of the phallus.

The family history is often unrevealing, but specific questions may reap large rewards. A history of infant death within the family would suggest the possibility of CAH, and infertility, amenorrhea, or hirsutism might also suggest possible familial patterns of intersex states. Certainly, maternal ingestion of medication during the pregnancy is of importance. Two delicate areas of relevance would be a history of maternal drug abuse during the pregnancy, as cocaine has been associated with genital ambiguity, and, finally, consanguinity. Familial feelings of guilt run high in this setting and thus the proper timing and wording of such inquiries is important.

The critical finding on physical examination is that of one or two gonads. This finding rules out female pseudohermaphroditism. As ovaries do not descend, a distinctly palpable gonad along the pathway of descent is suggestive of a testis. The patient with bilaterally impalpable testes or a unilaterally impalpable testis and hypospadias should be regarded as having an intersex disorder until proven otherwise. Rajfer and Walsh noted the presence of an intersex disorder among 27% of phenotypic males with cryptorchidism and hypospadias.[50]

An additional, important finding on physical examination is that of a uterus, which presents as an anterior midline, cordlike structure on rectal examination. Further definition of Müllerian anatomy can be achieved nicely with ultrasound examination.

The determination of chromosomal sex by means of a karyotype should be performed routinely, although the test requires 4 to 5 days for completion. While a buccal smear may provide immediate information regarding chromosomal sex, its inaccuracy limits its usefulness.

Following a history and physical examination, the first evaluation should be biochemical, to rule out CAH (where no gonad is palpable) particularly the salt-wasting form of CAH, which could be life threatening. Thus, one should determine the plasma 17-hydroxyprogesterone level or begin a 24-hour urine collection to measure 17-ketosteroids and pregnanetriol. In the absence of palpable testes, the presence of testicular tissue should be determined by means of an hCG stimulation test. In addition to ruling out anorchia, the study can enable one to diagnose 5α-reductase deficiency (by virtue of an increased T/DHT ratio) and help distinguish between impaired T synthesis (deficient response to hCG) and androgen insensitivity (normal response to hCG).

Anatomical definition of the urogenital sinus and ductal structures contributes to the correct diagnosis and is certainly necessary prior to any surgical intervention. The urogenital sinus is well imaged by retrograde contrast injection, which also opacifies duct structures, defines the entry of urethra and vagina into the sinus, and outlines the cervical impression within the vagina. Endoscopy can define these relationships more precisely, but is usually not necessary until surgical considerations become imminent.

Laparotomy and gonadal biopsy is usually the final clinical step required when a firm diagnosis based on all of the aforementioned data is impossible. It is conceivable that a laparoscopic approach would yield comparable information with less morbidity; thus, laparoscopy may become more widely utilized in this setting.

Finally, sophisticated biochemical studies on cultured genital skin fibroblasts may define the precise cellular abnormality responsible for a given intersex disorder—be it abnormal androgen receptor or an enzyme abnormality. These studies should be performed in specialized laboratories where normal values are well established. Rarely do they impact on one's initial decision regarding the sex of rearing.

## REFERENCES


1. Jost A. Problems of fetal endocrinology: the gonadal and hypophyseal hormones. *Recent Prog Horm Res*. 1953;8:379.
2. Vogel F, Matulsky AG. *Human Genetics*. Berlin: Springer–Verlag; 1979.
3. Davis RM. Localization of male determining factors in man: a thorough review of structural anomalies of the Y chromosome. *J Med Genet*. 1981;18:161–195.
4. Wachtel SS, Ohno S, Koo GC, Boyse EA. Possible role of H-Y antigen in the primary determination of sex. *Nature*. 1975;257:235–236.
5. Eichwald EJ, Silmser CR. Untitled Communication. *Transplant Bull*. 1955;2:148.
6. Wachtel SS. *H-Y Antigen and the Biology of Sex Determination*. New York: Grune and Stratton; 1983.
7. Lieber E, Wachtel SS, Aftalion B, Zaslav A. Diagnostic applications of H-Y serology: H-Y negative phenotype in cells from 45,X/46,XY fetus with testes. *Clin Genet*. 1986;30:366–373.
8. Burgoyne PS, Levy ER, McLaren A. Spermatogenic failure in male mice lacking H-Y antigen. *Nature*. 1986;320:170–172.
9. Volata G. Maleness pinpointed on Y chromosome. *Science*. 1986;234:1076–1077.
10. Sinclair AH, Berta P, Palmer MS, et al. A gene from the human sex-determining region encodes a protein with homology to a conserved DNA-binding motif. *Nature*. 1990;346:240.
11. Josso N, Picard JY, Tran D. The anti-Müllerian Hormone. *Recent Prog Horm Res*. 1977;33:117.
12. Jost A. The role of fetal hormones in prenatal development. *Harvey Lect*. 1961;55:201–226.
13. Siiteri PK, Wilson JD. Testosterone formation and metabolism during male sexual differentiation in the human embryo. *J Clin Endrocrinol Metab*. 1984;38:113–125.
14. Walsh PC, Madden JD, Harrod MJ, Goldstein JL, MacDonald PC, Wilson JD. Familial incomplete male pseudohermaphroditism, type 2. Decreased dihydrotestosterone formation in pseudovaginal perineoscrotal hypospadias. *N Engl J Med*. 1974;291:944–949.
15. Fadan BM, Tesoriero JV. Inhibition of testicular development and feminization of the male genitalia by neonatal estrogen treatment in a marsupial. *Biol Reprod*. 1986;34:771–776.
16. Klinefelter HF Jr, Reifenstein EC Jr, Albright F. Syndrome characterized by gynecomastia, aspermatogenesis without A-leydigism, and increased excretion of follicle stimulating hormone. *J Clin Endocrinol*. 1942;2:615.
17. Verp MS, Simpson JG. Abnormal sexual differentiation and neoplasia. *Cancer Genet Cytogenet*. 1987;25:191–218.
18. Arens R, Mareus D, Engelberg S, Findler D, Goodman RM, Passwell JH. Cerebral germinomas and Klinefelter syndrome. *Cancer*. 1988;61:1228–1231.
19. de la Chapelle A. Nature and origin of males with XX sex chromosomes. *Am J Hum Genet*. 1972;24:71.
20. Page D. Personal Communication.

21. Simpson JL. Abnormal sexual differentiation in humans. *Ann Rev Genet.* 1982;16:193–224.
22. Milner RDG. Current views on the treatment of Turner's Syndrome. *Acta Paediatr Scand.* 1987;331(suppl):53–58.
23. Troche V, Hernandez E. Neoplasia arising in dysgenetic gonads. *Obstet Gyn Surv.* 1986; 41:74–79.
24. Davidoff F, Federman DD. Mixed gonadal dysgenesis. *Pediatrics.* 1973;52:725–742.
25. Rajfer J. Association between Wilms' tumor and gonadal dysgenesis. *J Urol.* 1981;125: 388–390.
26. Drash A, Sherman F, Hartmann WH, Blizzard RM. A syndrome of pseudohermaphroditism, Wilms' tumor, hypertension, and degenerative renal disease. *J Pediatr.* 1970;76:585–593.
27. Gallo GE, Chemes HE. The association of Wilms' tumor, male pseudohermaphroditism and diffuse glomerular disease (Drash Syndrome). *Pediatr Pathol.* 1987;7:175–189.
28. Simpson A, Saenger P. Abnormal sexual differentiation: male pseudohermaphroditism and abnormal steroid synthesis metabolism and action. *Prog Clin Biol Res.* 1985;171:175–206.
29. Griffin JE, Wilson JD. Disorders of sexual differentiation. In: Walsh PC, Gittes RF, Perlmutter AD, Stamey TA (eds.). *Campbell's Urology.* ed 5. Philadelphia: WB Saunders; 1986:chap 41.
30. Sohval AR. The syndrome of pure gonadal dysgenesis. *Am J Med.* 1965;38:615–624.
31. Edman CD, Winters AJ, Porter JC, Wilson JD, MacDonald PC. Embryonic testicular regression: a clinical spectrum of XY agonadal individuals. *Obstet Gynecol.* 1977;49:208–217.
32. Wilson MD, Walsh PC. Disorders of sexual differentiation. In: Harrison JH, Gittes RF, Perlmutter AD, Stamey TA, Walsh PC (eds). *Campbell's Urology.* ed. 4. Philadelphia: WB Saunders; 1979:chap 42.
33. Aynsley-Green A, Zachman M, Illig R, Rampini S, Prader A. Congenital bilateral anorchia in childhood: a clinical, endocrine and therapeutic evaluation of 21 cases. *Clin Endocrinol.* 1976;5:381–391.
34. Camacho AM, Migeon CJ. Testosterone excretion and production rate in adults and in patients with congenital adrenal hyperplasia. *J Clin Endocrinol.* 1966;26:893–896.
35. Pang S, Pollack MS, Marshall RN, Immken L. Prenatal treatment of congenital adrenal hyperplasia due to 21-Hydroxylase deficiency. *N Engl J Med.* 1990;322:111–115.
36. Migeon CJ. Comments about the need for prenatal treatment of congenital adrenal hyperplasia due to 21-Hydroxylase deficiency. *J Clin Endocrinol.* 1990;70:836–837.
37. Speiser PW, Laforgia N, Kato K, et al. First trimester prenatal treatment and molecular genetic diagnosis of congenital adrenal hyperplasia. *J Clin Endocrinol.* 1990;70:838–848.
38. Bongiovanni AM, Root AW. The adrenogenital syndrome. *N Engl J Med.* 1963;268:1391–1399.
39. Wilson JD. Recent studies on the mechanism of action of testosterone. *N Engl J Med.* 1972; 287:1284–1291.
40. Griffin JE, Wilson JD. Syndromes of androgen resistance. *Hosp Pract.* 1987;22:99–114.
41. Imperato-McGinley J, Guerrero L, Gauthier T, et al. Steroid 5 Alpha-reductase deficiency in man: An inherited form of male pseudomaphroditism. *Science.* 1984;186:1213–1215.
42. Wilson JD. Disorders of androgen action. *Clin Res.* 1987;35:1–12.
43. Price P, Wass JAH, Griffin JE, et al. High dose androgen therapy in male pseudohermaphroditism due to 5 Alpha-reductase deficiency and disorders of the androgen receptor. *J Clin Immunol.* 1984;74:1496–1508.
44. Perez-Palacios G, Chavez B, Mendez JP, et al. The syndromes of androgen resistance revisited. *J Steroid Biochem.* 1987;27:1101–1108.
45. Evans BAJ, Jones TR, Hughes IA. Studies of the androgen dispersed fibroblasts: investigation of patients with androgen insensitivity. *Clin Endocrinol.* 1984;20:93–105.
46. Brown T, Migeon C. Androgen receptors in normal and abnormal male sexual differentiation. *Adv Exp Med Biol.* 1986;196:227–255.
47. Gottlieb B, Kaufman M, Pinsky L, et al. Extracellular correction of the androgen-receptor transformation defect in two families with complete androgen resistance. *J Steroid Biochem.* 1987;28:279–284.
48. Nilson O. Hernia uteri inguinalis beim Manne. *Acta Chir Scand.* 1939;83:231.
49. Sloan WR, Walsh PC. Familial persistent Müllerian duct syndrome. *J Urol.* 1976;115:459–461.
50. Rajfer J, Walsh PC. The incidence of intersexuality in patients with hypospadias and cryptorchidism. *J Urol.* 1976;116:769–770.

# 55

# Operative Correction of Intersex Problems

*William J. Cromie*

Disorders of sexual differentiation have fascinated basic scientists and clinicians alike, but the development of a satisfactory management philosophy has long been hindered by a lack of understanding of the basic mechanisms underlying the intersex states. In the past, decisions were often based more on the clinical appearance of the child rather than on an understanding of the pathophysiologic process resulting in the disorder. Significant advances in the understanding of the biochemistry of intersex as well as increased awareness of the activity of the H-Y antigen (1) have provided new insights into the nature of these disorders. Despite these advances, the impact of ambiguous genitalia on the family and those patients affected has changed little. Articles by Allen (2) and Walsh (3) review in detail the current concepts of normal and abnormal sexual differentiation, classifying these disorders, as well as outlining a philosophy of management; our goal will be to discuss those intersex states requiring therapy, with recommendations toward appropriate gender assignment.

## NORMAL SEXUAL DIFFERENTIATION

Normal sexual differentiation is divided essentially into these phases:

1. Differentiation of the gonads based on chromosomal sex
2. Development of internal ductal structures
3. Differentiation of the external genitalia

Briefly, at 3 to 5 weeks of intrauterine life, the gonad differentiates into testis or ovary based on the appropriate chromosomal message. In a male the H-Y antigen is felt to be the testis determining factor on the Y chromosome that accounts for gonadal differentiation. Once the testis is formed, two hormones are secreted which have a significant effect on the second phase or the development of the internal ductal structures. The first hormone is müllerian-inhibiting substance, which is derived from the Sertoli cells, and the second is testosterone, which is derived from the Leydig cells. The activity of these hormones together accounts first for the regression of müllerian duct structures and second for stimulation of the wolffian ducts to produce the ejaculatory ducts, vas, and epididymis. Based on the classical experiment of Jost (4), the opposite occurs in the female, where under ovarian stimulation and in the absence of müllerian-inhibiting substance, the fallopian tubes, uterus, and upper one third of the vagina develop. In addition, in the absence of testosterone, the wolffian duct structures regress. Of significance in these events is the fact that hormones secreted by the testis act locally and ipsilaterally.

During the third stage, the external genitalia differentiate along the lines dictated by the chromosomal and gonadal sex. At 10 to 15 weeks gestation, the genital tubercle, folds, swellings, and urogenital sinus of the fetus are undifferentiated. In the female, the urogenital sinus becomes the lower third of the vagina, the genital tubercle becomes the clitoris, the genital folds become the labia minora, and the genital swellings, the labia majora. In the male, under the stimulation of testicular androgen and due to the activity of dihydrotestosterone, the urogenital sinus becomes the prostatic urethra, the genital tubercle becomes the glans penis, the genital folds become the urethra and shaft of the penis, and the genital swellings, the scrotum (5). On the basis of this information, it is clear that the testis is the major force in sexual differentiation. It exerts its influence primarily through the elaboration of testosterone, which causes masculinization of the wolffian ducts and, after conversion to dihydrotestosterone, masculinization of the external genitalia. In addition, the activity of müllerian-inhibiting substance is responsible for involution of the müllerian system. Errors in production or utilization of these hormones are responsible for a majority of the intersex disorders in genetic males, while excess of androgens mimicking the activity of testosterone results in ambiguity in genetic females. Thus, intersex is the result of any disturbance during embryogenesis that inappropriately alters the hormonal milieu, such as:

1. Chromosomal anomalies resulting in abnormal gonadal differentiation (true hermaphroditism, mixed gonadal dysgenesis)
2. Excessive androgen production in the female (female pseudohermaphroditism)
3. Defective androgen production or action in the male (male pseudohermaphroditism)

By excluding those patients in whom phenotypic sex is firmly established such as those with Kleinfelter's or Turner's syndrome, we are left with four conditions most commonly producing ambiguous genitalia in the newborn: 1) true hermaphroditism, 2) mixed gonadal dysgenesis, 3) male pseudohermaphroditism, and 4) female pseudohermaphroditism.

## TRUE HERMAPHRODITISM

A true hermaphrodite by definition possesses both ovarian and testicular tissue. Less than 10% of the total patients presenting with intersex are hermaphrodites. The cause is unknown except for those few cases of XX/XY chimeras that appeared to be the result of a double fertilization. Over half of the true hermaphrodites in the literature have had 46, XX chromosomal complement, indicating that there may be other factors at work in the cause of this disorder (6).

The appearance of the external genitalia of true hermaphrodites is extremely variable but has a tendency toward maleness as evidenced by the fact that a majority of the patients have been raised as males (5). The most common appearance is a large phallus associated with varying degrees of labioscrotal fusion. Gonadal tissue is often palpable in the labioscrotal fold or groin, on one or both sides. As a rule, testicular tissue will descend but in some cases, ovotestis and even ovaries have been found in the scrotum (7).

Internally, the ductal structures usually reveal a fully formed uterus with fallopian tubes present on the side of an ovary or ovotestis. As a rule, the genital ducts develop in accordance with the gonad present on that side. Thus, if a testis is present, there is a vas and if an ovary is present, a fallopian tube. Most true hermaphrodites are classified into three specific types: 1) lateral type (testis plus ovary), 2) unilateral type (testis or ovary plus an ovotestis), and 3) bilateral type (ovotestis plus ovotestis).

Histologically, the ovaries are often normal, but testicular tissue tends to be abnormal after puberty regardless of whether it is intraabdominal or scrotal in position (6).

Many factors have to be considered in the management of the true hermaphrodite. First, the changes at puberty are unpredictable and depend primarily on the character and quality of the gonads. Although some degree of virilization may occur, breast development is also common and some patients have been found to be fertile. Despite disordered histology and ectopic locations of the gonads, tumors have rarely been reported (8). Bearing this in mind, the key factor in the management of the true hermaphrodite is early recognition and corrective surgery. Only through surgical exploration and gonadal biopsy can the diagnosis be established, as there are no distinctive chromosomal or biochemical features of this disorder (2). Sex assignment is totally dependent on the appearance of the external genitalia and the ease with which reconstruction can be carried out. Once gender assignment has been made, all structures inconsistent with the assigned phenotypic sex, including dysgenetic gonads, should be removed. In most cases, the males will have some form of hypospadias which will require correction.

## MIXED GONADAL DYSGENESIS

Mixed gonadal dysgenesis is second only to congenital adrenal hyperplasia as a cause of ambiguous genitalia in the neonate. Sohva (9) characterized a group of patients with this syndrome based on the presence of a testis and a companion gonad called a streak in view of its similarity to the gonadal streak of Turner's syndrome. Histologically, the streak gonad is composed of whorls of connective tissue reminiscent of ovarian stroma but lacking ovocytes. In addition to this specific gonadal pattern, mixed gonadal dysgenesis has a characteristic karyotype most commonly presented as XO/XY mosaicism (10). There are many other variations in karyotype; however, the constancy of the XO component is significant. Another very constant feature of this disorder is persistence of müllerian duct structures internally. Most patients have an infantile uterus and cervix with fallopian tubes. A fallopian tube invariably is present on the side of the gonadal streak but may be present on the testis side as well. Wolffian duct structures, if present at all, are generally seen on the side of the testis (11). In view of the failure of the testis to suppress müllerian derivatives, it is questionable whether they are adequate histologically, as spermatogenesis is exceedingly rare even in a descended testis. The external genitalia show great variability from labioscrotal separation with a small phallus and separate openings for the urethra and vagina to complete fusion of the scrotum with a prominent phallus and unilateral testicular descent (2).

Sex assignment in mixed gonadal dysgenesis, as in a patient with true hermaphroditism, in the past was largely determined by the appearance of the external genitalia. However, certain considerations must be borne in mind. First, these patients are usually short in stature, as are most individuals with the XO component in their karyotype, favoring a female assignment. Although the presence of a testis and the possibility for secretion of testosterone would appear to be advantageous for raising the child as a male, in most patients the seminiferous tubules lack all germinal elements, leaving only Sertoli cells (10). In addition, 25% of patients reared as males have developed testicular gonadoblastomas. Interestingly, when both testicular and streak material have been identified in patients with a gonadal tumor, the tumor has generally involved the testis rather than the streak; however, fully descended testis appear to be involved with tumor (2).

Although these patients will undoubtedly be infertile, most have internal ductal structures compatible with a female gender assignment, if detected in the neonatal period. While puberty comes at a normal age and is characterized by a degree of virilization compatible with the gonad present, it is our philosophy that overall these patients are probably best raised as females, due to the problems with stature and potential gonadal neoplasia. In those patients already fixed in the male gender, it would seem appropriate to remove any gonad which appeared dysgenetic or which could not be readily placed within the scrotum

## MALE PSEUDOHERMAPHRODITISM

Male pseudohermaphroditism is a disorder in which genetic males with bilateral testis differentiate partially or completely as phenotypic females. The pathophysiologic mechanisms of this disorder include four basic etiologic factors:

1. A deficiency of müllerian-inhibiting substance
2. Inadequate testosterone production
3. Incomplete conversion of testosterone to dihydrotestosterone
4. Insufficient androgen-binding protein at the target cells (12)

*Insufficiency of a müllerian-inhibiting substance*, otherwise known as hernia uteri inguinalis, is an extremely rare occurrence with less than 100 cases in the literature. The major feature is persistent müllerian structures in an otherwise normal XY male (13). The standard occurrence is to find an inguinal hernia with a normal testicle and an absent contralateral testicle. At the time of exploration, however, a uterus with fallopian tubes in addition to the remaining testicle is present within the hernia sac. Obviously, all the ductal systems inconsistent with a male phenotype should be removed and the testis preserved if an adequate vas and blood supply is present.

In the subsequent disorders of testosterone production, conversion and binding, management decisions are more difficult. In the case of *defective testosterone synthesis*, most patients have a female phenotype and may present with salt-wasting or hypertension in the neonatal period (2). Early diagnosis can only be made after finding an XY karyotype, and the presence of palpable gonads in an otherwise phenotypic female. In view of the rarity of these disorders as well as the underlying adrenal pathology, these patients are best placed in the female gender assignment. Internal ductal structures are usually solely of the wolffian system and can be removed at an elective date, followed by estrogen replacement at puberty.

*Defective testosterone conversion* results in an entity called *pseudovaginal perineoscrotal hypospadias* (Fig 1). This fascinating syndrome, described by Simpson (14) in 1963, reveals a neonate with clitoral enlargement and labioscrotal fusion, with separate openings for the urethra and vagina. A testis, however, may be palpable in the groin, and the internal ducts are solely of wolffian origin. At puberty, full virilization occurs with deepening of the voice, muscular development, clitoral enlargement, and a masculine hair pattern. To describe this paradox, Walsh and associates (15) showed that the external genital tissues of these patients were unable to convert testosterone to dihydrotestosterone because of a deficiency in 5$\alpha$-reductase. Thus, while dihydrotestosterone is critical for genital development in utero, the internal genitalia appear to be responsive directly to testosterone and differentiate in a normal fashion. It also appears that at the onset of puberty, again the genitalia are responsive to testosterone, accounting for their masculinization.

In most patients, the diagnosis has seldom been suspected before the female sex has been assigned. The patients have undergone orchidectomy followed by vaginoplasty at puberty. It is interesting to speculate whether or not it would be possible to maintain the child as a male if the diagnosis could be made in the neonatal period. Imperato-McGinley et al (16), in follow-up of their original reported series in the Dominican Republic, have found that while these children were in the female gender prior to puberty, at puberty they opted for a male gender role and began to dress and act as males, both physically and sexually. Thus, the intriguing possibility exists that patients fixed in the male gender with this syndrome could be functional as fertile males in adult life. Before a decision of this magnitude could be made, assessment of androgen action in cultured fibroblast cultures along with plasma and urinary steroid excretion patterns would be essential (3).

*Defective testosterone utilization* is the

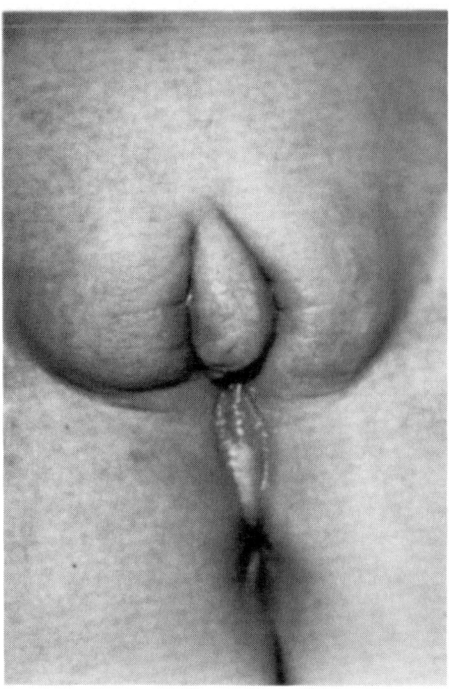

A

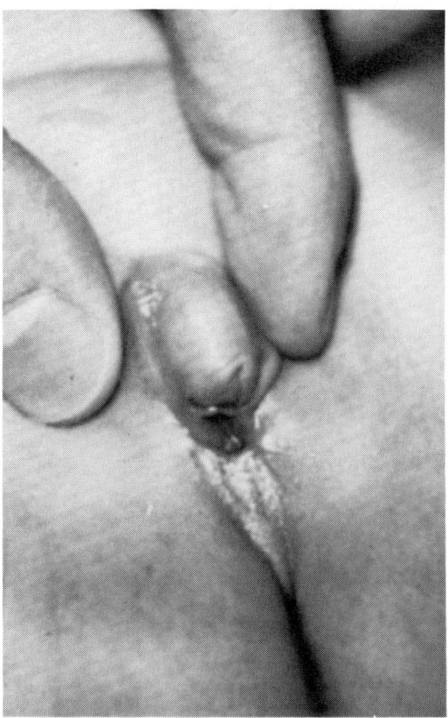

B

**Fig 1.** *A* and *B*. Pseudovaginal perineoscrotal hypospadias or 5α-reductase deficiency.

most frequent form of male pseudohermaphroditism and is commonly referred to in its complete form as the *testicular feminization syndrome*. Morris (17) was the first to detect this abnormality with the principal features of a testis normally responsive to gonadotropin producing normal or increased levels of testosterone but with complete insensitivity of end organs to both the virilizing and anabolic effects of the hormone. Patients are strikingly female with a eunuchoid body habitus and excellent breast development in response to adrenal estrogen at puberty. In these patients, the gonads are normal in size and may be present anywhere along the course of descent of the normal testis. A hernia with a gonad present in the sac is found in 78% of patients. In 50% of patients, there may be some wolffian structures present. These are usually histologically poorly developed. Studies reveal that this disorder is inherited as an X-linked recessive or X-limited dominant (2). The mechanism of the defect appears to involve the transfer of dihydrotestosterone receptor complex from the cytoplasm to the nucleus of the cell where nucleic acid induction occurs, resulting in an inadequate conversion of testosterone to dihydrotestosterone. (18).

Children with testicular feminization syndrome of course should be assigned as females. Some have proposed that the gonads be left in place until after puberty to permit a more physiologic menarche. (19). However, in today's sophisticated medical climate, retaining gonads for this period of time and explaining away the phenomenon when the individual is teenaged may be more difficult than in the past. It is certainly reasonable to remove the gonads and repair the hernias in the first year of life, and with the availability of sequential progesterone and estrogen compounds, a smooth menarche is also possible. If the gonads are retained, they certainly should be removed ultimately as there is an increased incidence of gonadal malignancy in these testes.

In addition to testicular feminization, there are many male pseudohermaphrodites with varying degrees of ambiguity of the external genitalia (Fig 2). Classically, a strong family history of involvement is found due to an X-linked recessive pattern. There is inadequate virilization in the absence of any evidence of abnormal steroidogenesis and routinely gynecomastia appears at puberty. In fact, this diagnosis is suspect whenever one encounters a male pseudohermaphrodite who has gynecomastia himself or who has relatives with genital ambiguity and gynecomastia. The diagnosis is confirmed in the postpubertal patient by the paradox of an elevated serum LH in the face of a normal or elevated serum testosterone (2). The spectrum of this disorder includes:

1. Lubs syndrome (20). This is the most feminine of the spectrum, with a large number of the patients being raised in the female gender. There is partial wolffian duct development with posterior labioscrotal fusion, a small phallus, and a single urogenital sinus for the urethra and vagina. At puberty, these individuals develop a eunuchoid to feminine body habitus with gynecomastia; however, the muscularity of their shoulders and thighs is more nearly masculine in appearance.
2. Gilbert-Dreyfus syndrome (21). In this case, the general body habitus is male.

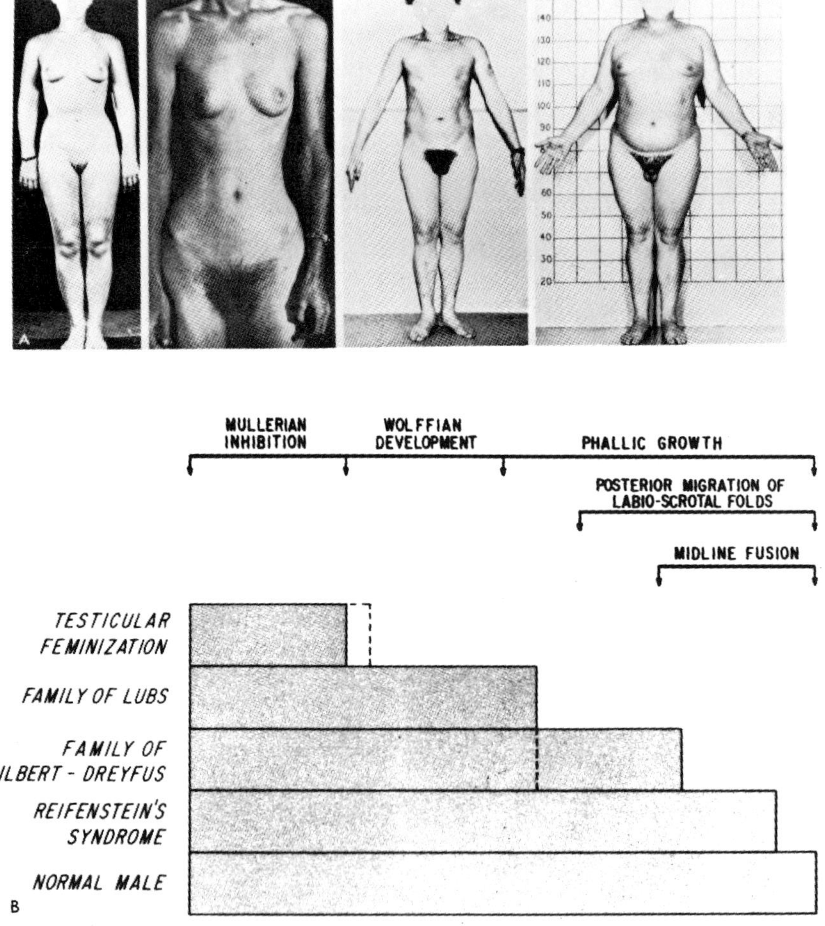


**Fig 2.** *A*. Spectrum of phenotypes associated with androgen insensitivity from classic testicular feminization to Reifenstein's syndrome. *B*. Stage at which virilization is influenced in each syndrome. (From Federman D: Abnormal Sexual Development. Philadelphia: Saunders, 1967, with permission.)

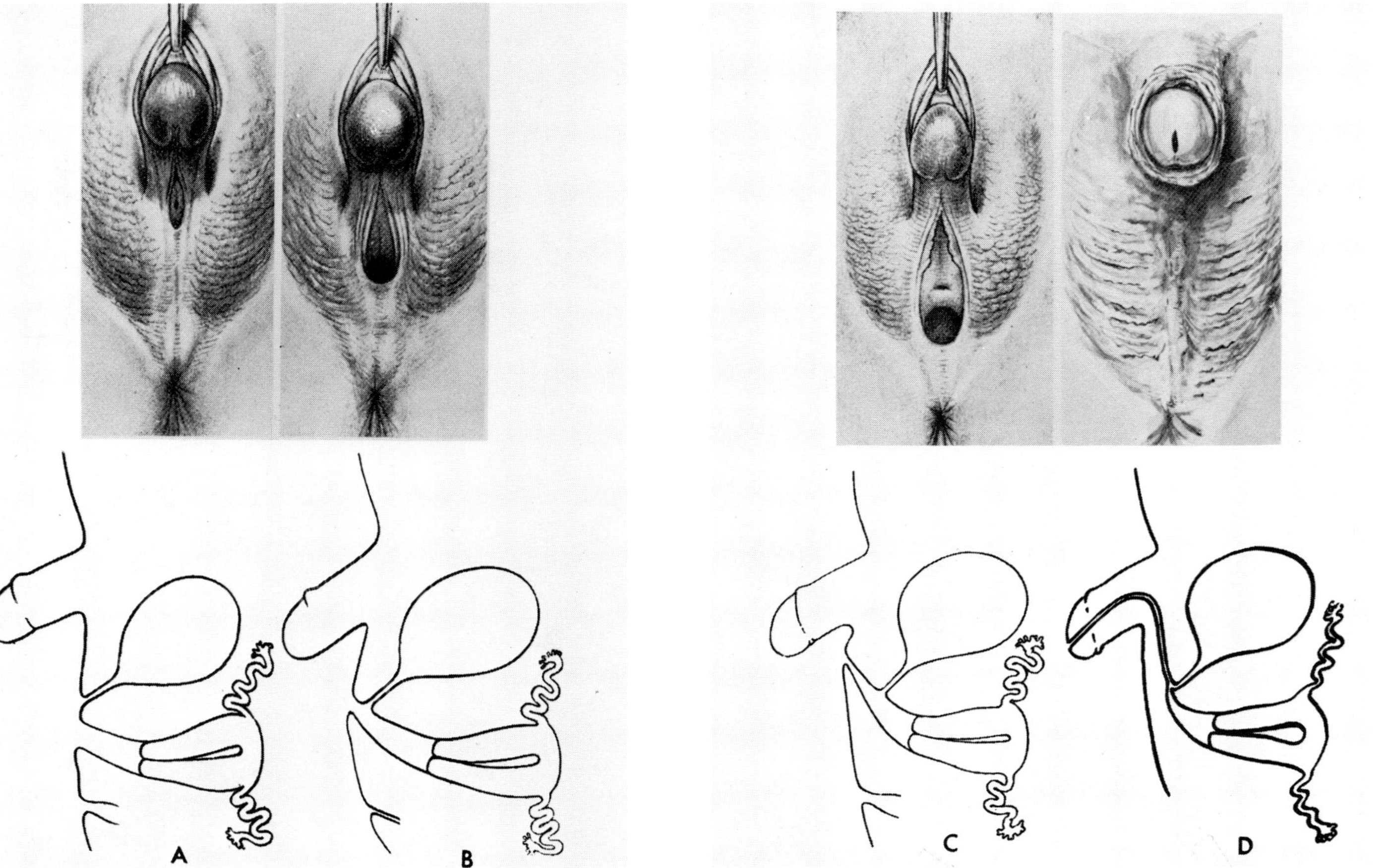


**Fig 3.** Spectrum of masculinization that may occur secondary to exogenous or endogenous androgen production in the female child. (From Federman D: Abnormal Sexual Development. Philadelphia: Saunders, 1967, with permission.)

There are incomplete wolffian structures, slightly more phallic enlargement with hypospadias, but again the onset of gynecomastia at puberty.

3. Reifenstein syndrome (22). This is the most common of the incomplete types. There is enough virilization that most patients are raised as males. Hypospadias is the cardinal manifestation with variable degrees of incomplete fusion of the labioscrotal folds. Gynecomastia again occurs at puberty.
4. Rosewater syndrome. This is the mildest form of the spectrum. All patients are well-virilized males with only gynecomastia and infertility.

The sex assignment is based primarily on the degree of masculinization of the external genitalia. Fertility has never been documented nor has gonadal malignancy, although there is every indication that this could occur as in any other patient with an undescended testis. Hypospadias and chordee can be managed at a time convenient to the patient and family, but preferably well before puberty.

## FEMALE PSEUDOHERMAPHRODITISM

The female pseudohermaphrodite is a genetically normal female with masculinized external genitalia due to exogenous or endogenous androgen exposure during fetal development. Masculinization of the external genitalia in children resulting from adrenal cortical hyperplasia ac-

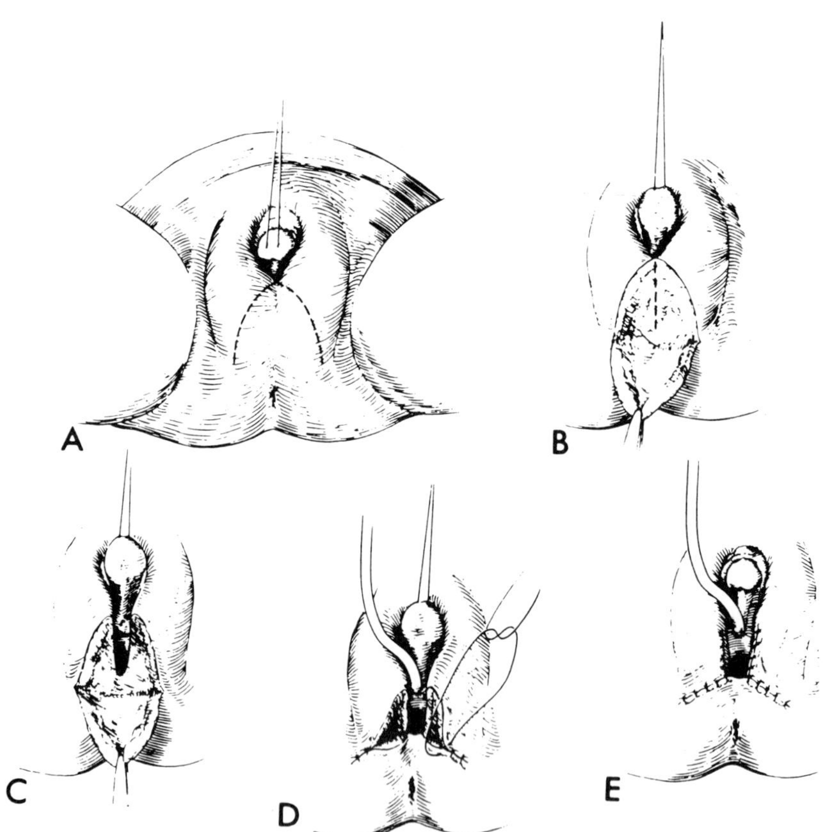


**Fig 4.** Vaginoplasty. *A*. Outline of flap on perineum. *B*. Incision. *C*. Opening of posterior vagina. *D*. Suturing of flap to posterior vaginal incision. *E*. Closure with catheter in place. (From Allen TD: Clinical Pediatric Urology. Philadelphia: Saunders, 1977, vol 2, with permission.)

counts for more than 60% of children presenting with intersex (5, 11, 19). The symptom complex otherwise known as the adrenogenital syndrome results from an enzyme defect, most commonly at the 21- and 11-hydroxalase positions in cortisol synthesis, preventing the full elaboration of hydrocortisone. This results in an overproduction of androgenic steroids under the excessive production of ACTH by the pituitary gland. The child is therefore masculinized (Fig 3), and precocious growth is stimulated. A female infant with this condition is born with an enlarged phallus with closure of the labioscrotal folds to give the appearance of hypospadias. The uterus, fallopian tubes, and ovaries are normal, and the vagina enters the urethra at a variable level, most often at a position corresponding to the membranous urethra. Because of the biochemical disturbance, 30% to 60% of these infants will suffer a salt-losing syndrome which is life threatening, requiring salt replacement and steroid therapy (23). To make the diagnosis at the appropriate time before the child becomes threatened by the enzyme deficiency, it is critical to assess the following points: On physical examination while the child has ambiguous genitalia, no gonads are usually palpable, indicating absence of testicular tissue. On standard serum electrolytes, a small fall in the $CO_2$ content coupled with the genital ambiguity should prompt further testing. Routinely, the urinary 17-ketosteroids as well as pregnanetriol values will be elevated with androsterone and etiocholanolone, the principal 17-ketosteroids excreted. Plasma cortisol values may be low or normal depending on whether or not the block is compensated, but low cortisol is usually associated with the salt-losing features of the syndrome (2, 9). In most cases, the diagnosis of adrenogenital syndrome can be established

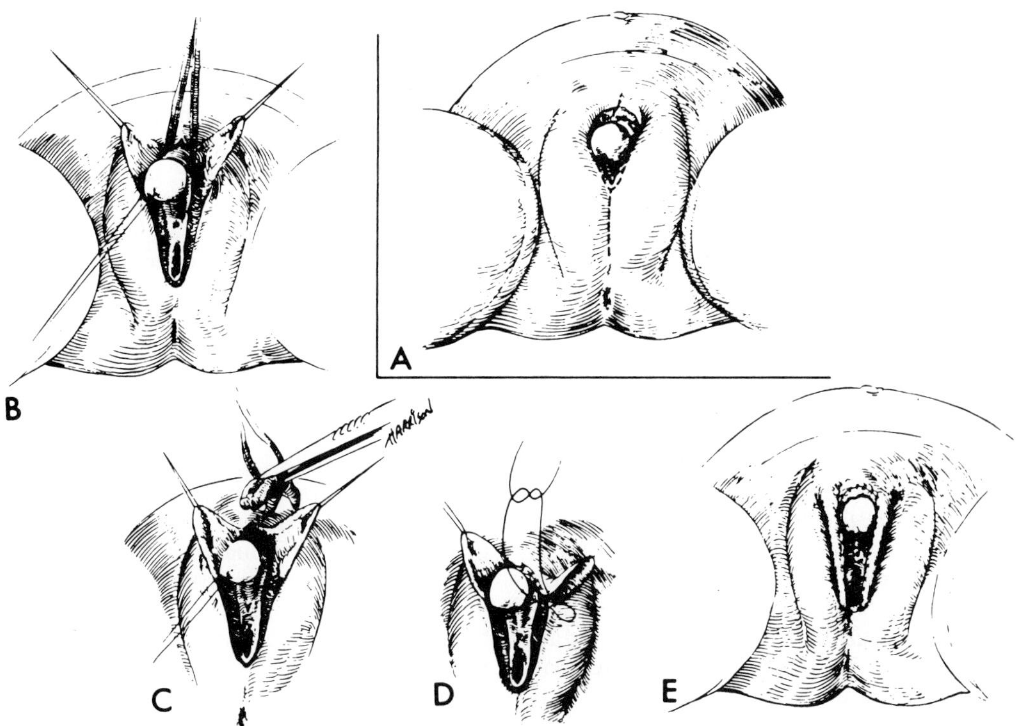


**Fig 5.** Combined clitoral reduction and vaginoplasty. *A.* Outline of skin incision. *B.* Dissection of phallic shaft. *C.* Excision and ligation of midportion of corporal bodies. *D.* Separation of dorsal skin into two flaps. *E.* Closure of lateral incisions. (From Allen TD: Clinical Pediatric Urology. Philadelphia: Saunders, 1977, vol 2, with permission.)

clinically by the karyotype and appropriate biochemical data, obviating surgical exploration. Once stable electrolyte balance is established, genital reconstruction can be carried out between 6 and 18 months of age.

Virilization of the female genitalia may also result from maternal hormonal influences secondary to administration of progestational compounds during pregnancy. Ethisterone and norethindrone are compounds which are most structurally related to testosterone, but many other agents have been implicated. Masculinization is limited to the external genitalia, with clitoral enlargement tending to be less than is usually seen with the adrenogenital syndrome (5). Fusion of the labioscrotal folds occurs when the androgenic compounds are given prior to the 12th week of gestation and may result in extensive masculinization even to the point of forming a phallic urethra. Virilizing tumors in the mother are another unusual cause of masculinization of the female fetus. The two most common neoplasms are arrhenoblastoma and the luteoma of pregnancy which usually regresses postpartum. It is possible that unrecognized tumors of this type may account for cases of female pseudohermaphroditism that arise without suitable explanation. (2).

The diagnosis of nonadrenal female pseudohermaphroditism should be considered whenever an XX karyotype and normal urinary 17-ketosteroids and pregnanetriol are found in a child with ambiguous genitalia. In many cases, the ambiguity is minimal and no surgery is required. However, in more severe degrees of virilization, the reconstruction is identical to those children with adrenogenital syndrome.

Following biochemical stabilization, the operative procedure in female pseudohermaphroditism is designed to produce the optimal female appearance. The goals of the procedure are to reduce the size of the phallus while retaining its maximum tactile sensations, in addition to opening the vagina to allow menstruation and subsequently intercourse. Various procedures have been advocated for the phallus which aim at preserving the glans with its special sensation. Some have suggested obliterating or tying down the corpora cavernosa so that none of the clitoris is excised, but this produces painful erections at puberty. Others remove a section of corpora cavernosa but preserve the urethral strip and the dorsal neurovascular bundle with the entire glans. In many cases, the glans itself is very large, particularly in older children, and if left at this size would obviate normal female appearance. In this case, some attenuation of the blood supply is considered. Some surgeons in the past have advised a simple amputation of the clitoris, but this leaves an ugly scar and is an unnecessarily destructive procedure (24).

On the basis of the presenting anatomy, we have divided the surgical technique into three specific groups. First, the child with a minimal degree of clitoral hypertrophy but an obliterated vaginal opening, producing reflux of urine into the vagina and causing recurrent urinary tract infections. The second procedure is a combined clitoroplasty and vaginoplasty with similar indications; however, the child has clitoromegaly. In the third case, there is a high vaginal opening off the urethra requiring a more technical vaginoplasty. In all of these patients as far as possible, vaginoplasty should be undertaken at the initial procedure although it is recognized that some revisions may be required at the start of sexual activity.

For the first type mentioned, a technique of vaginoplasty was described by Fortunoff (25) (Fig 4) using an inverted U-shape flap of skin from the perineum to be sutured to the posterior vaginal wall. The flap is outlined on the perineum, and an incision is carried down to the opening of the urogenital sinus with development of the flap. It is important to open the posterior vagina, with care being taken to avoid injury to the anal sphincter or rectum. Following this, the flap is sutured to the posterior vaginal incision and the skin edges are closed. A Foley catheter is left in the urethra for 1 to 2 days, with a small pack in the vagina.

In patients with combined clitoromegaly and labioscrotal fusion, we use a tech-

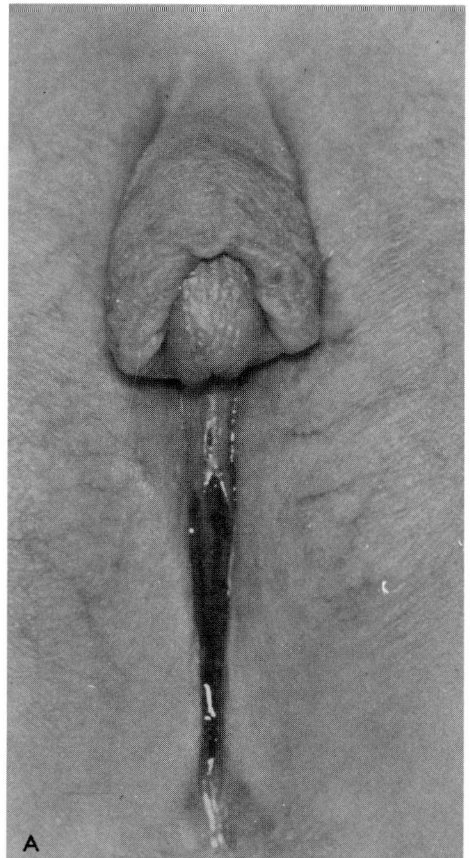


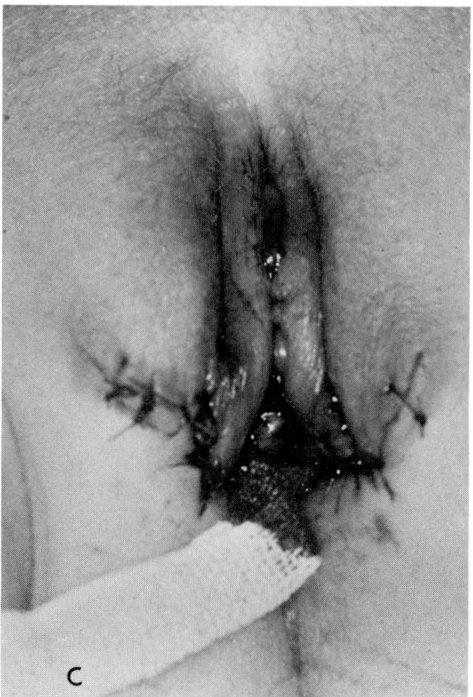


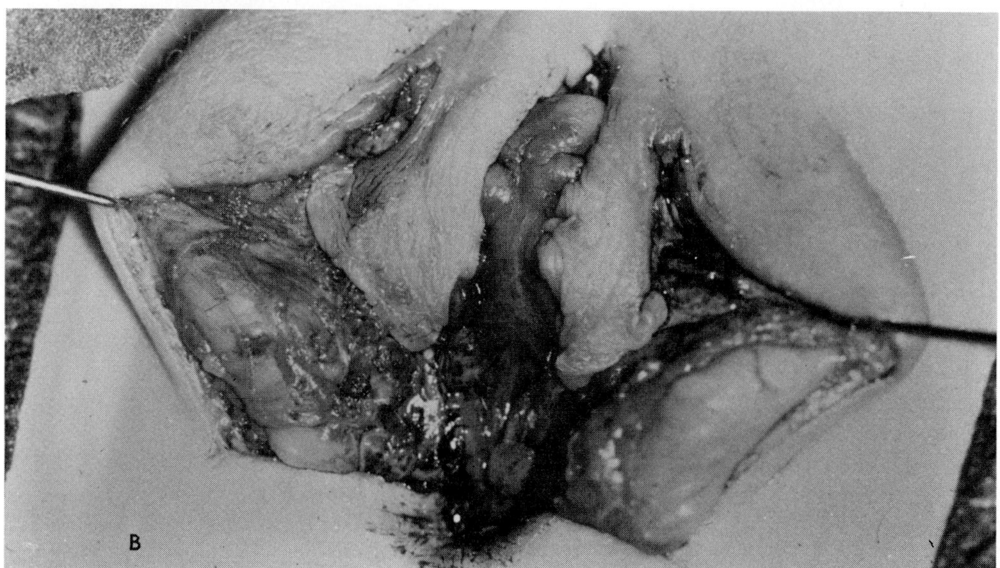


**Fig 6.** *A.* Clitoromegaly in congenital adrenal hyperplasia. *B.* Resection of the corporal bodies and formation of labia minora. *C.* Postoperative appearance.

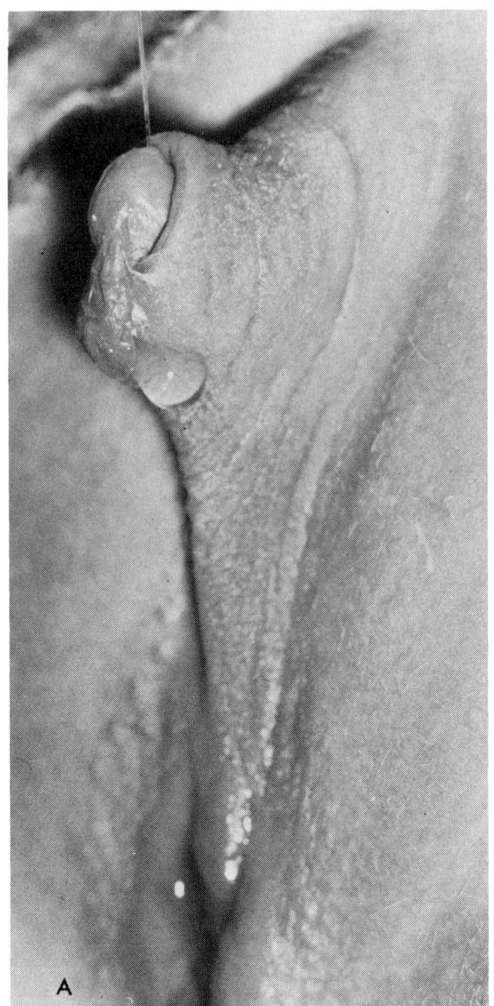


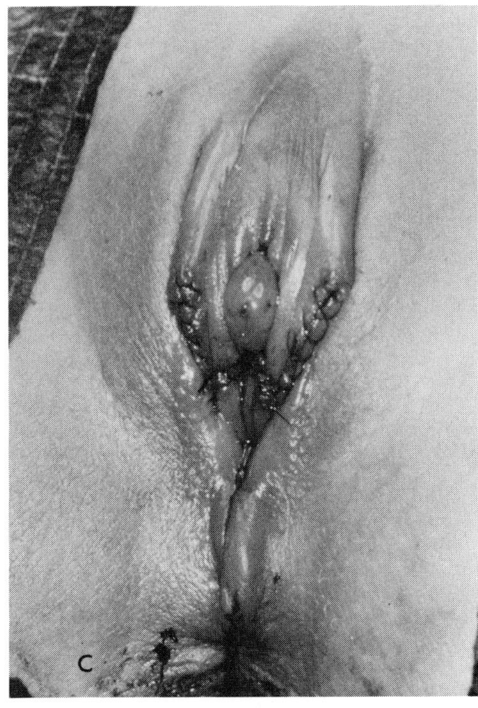


**Fig 7.** *A*. Clitoromegaly with a phallic urethra. *B*. Corporal dissection. *C*. Postoperative appearance.

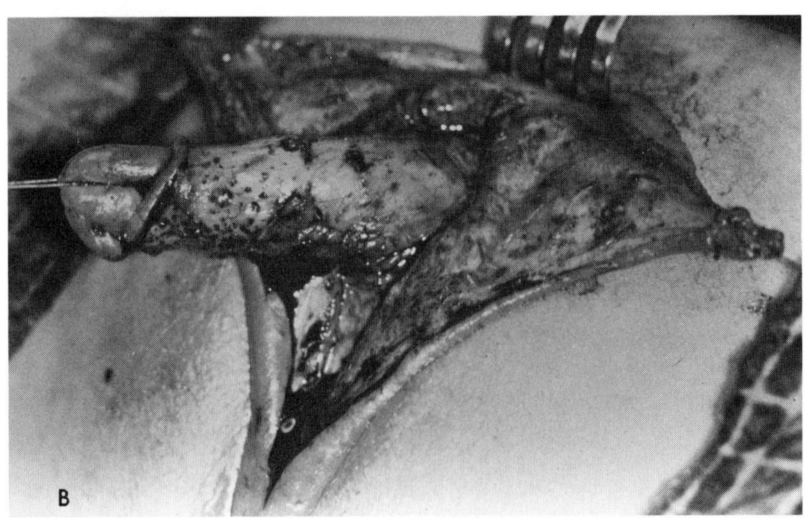

nique similar to that described by Marberger (24) (Fig 5). The skin incision is outlined at the corporal-shaft junction circumferentially around the phallus. If a simple cut-back vaginoplasty is possible, a vertical incision is made in the labioscrotal fusion. If, prior to the procedure the vagina is judged to be higher on urethroscopy and vaginoscopy, our initial incision with the vaginoplasty is similar to that seen in Figure 4, *A* to allow adequate vaginal reconstruction. Following the initial incision, the phallic shaft is dissected free from its surrounding attachments, leaving a ventral bridge of skin intact to the vagina and urethra, if possible. The glans is preserved and the neurovascular bundle along the dorsum of the shaft of the corpora is also dissected free to maintain nerve and blood supply. Following this, the midportion of the corporal bodies is excised and the base ligated with 3-0 silk sutures. Next, the dorsal skin is separated into two flaps which will be used to create the labia minora and the lateral incisions are closed, giving the child very feminine-appearing external genitalia. An example of this procedure can be seen in Figure 6 through 8. On occasion, advanced degrees of masculinization have been described. In the patient in Figure 7, *A* the phallic urethra developed to such a degree that a small urinary stream can be seen from the meatus. This could only be

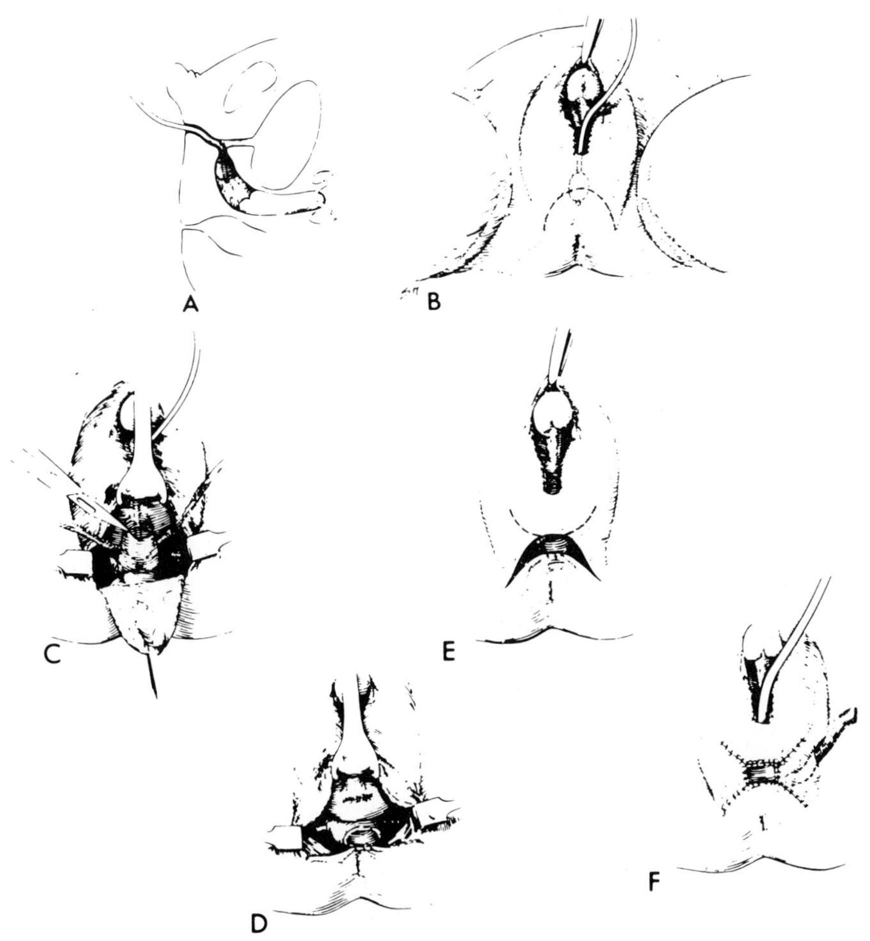


**Fig 8.** High perineal vaginoplasty. (From Allen TD: Clinical Pediatric Urology. Philadelphia: Saunders, 1977, vol 2, with permission.)

reproduced under anesthesia with excessive credé, and the child had a well-formed urogenital sinus, albeit somewhat posteriorly displaced. In view of this anatomic arrangement, the phallus was dissected free from its surrounding attachments using the previously described incisions (Fig 7, *B*) and placed in a more inferior location with development of labia minora and majora, making no attempt to excise the corporal portion of the phallus (Fig 7, *C*).

In other children with advanced masculinization, the development is manifested by the vagina entering the urethra quite high, often at or just above the external sphincter. Hendren and Crawford (26) found that the usual incision into the vagina from below injured the sphincter, resulting in some degree of stress incontinence. They advocate passing a Fogarty catheter into the vagina endoscopically and then approaching it through a perineal incision (Fig 8). With its communication to the urethra identified, the vagina is opened and urethra is closed. The vagina is then exteriorized by suturing it to the perineal skin which can be advanced into the wound. In those rare patients who have total absence of a vagina, a variety of techniques can be devised, including the use of isolated segments of intestine or full-thickness skin grafts sutured around a foam rubber mold (24). All of these procedures should be carried out at puberty, at a time when the patient can cooperate by keeping the vagina open with a stent, or at the assumption of intercourse.

## EVALUATION OF THE CHILD WITH AMBIGUOUS GENITALIA

Having reviewed the most common conditions that produce ambiguous genitalia, it is important to briefly outline the proper steps for investigation of these patients.

### History and Physical Examination

As many of these disorders are familial, a family history of abnormal sexual development, unexplained deaths during infancy, gynecomastia occurring in adolescence, or primary amenorrhea are important historical points. When a child presents with masculinization, the mother should be questioned about symptoms of virilization or ingestion of androgen or progestational agents during pregnancy. On physical examination, the single most important finding is the presence of a gonad in the labioscrotal fold or scrotum. As ovaries rarely descend, the presence of a palpable gonad virtually excludes the diagnosis of female pseudohermaphroditism. Any child with bilateral cryptor-

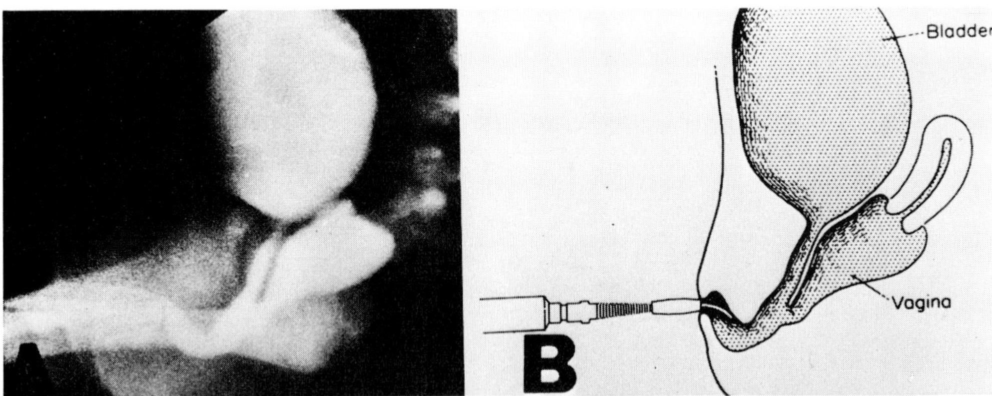


**Fig 9.** *A*. Genitogram. *B*. Technique of genitography. (From Parrott TS: Urologic implications of imperforate anus. Urology 10:407, 1977, with permission.)

chidism or unilateral cryptorchidism associated with hypospadias should be considered to have an intersex problem until proved otherwise (3). Finally, the size of the phallus and the location of the meatus should be carefully documented and the contents of any hernia found should be examined carefully.

### Evaluation of Genetic Sex

The time-honored buccal smear for the presence of chromatin clumps on the nuclear membrane is still a very valuable test. The Barr body, which represents the second X chromosome is found in 20% or more of nuclei of normal females and in less than 2% of cells of normal males (24). A more direct and accurate means of determining chromosomal sex involves culturing peripheral leukocytes to obtain a karyotype. It is hoped that in the future techniques will be available for measuring H-Y antigen to detect the presence of testis-determining factors in intersex children (1).

### Biochemical Evaluation

Measurement of the urinary excretion of 17-ketosteroids and pregnanetriol continues to be the most valuable aid in diagnosing congenital adrenal hyperplasia. In rare forms of the disorder, other plasma precursors may have to be measured to elucidate the specific enzymatic blockage. In cases in which estrogen levels need to be determined, an examination of the vaginal cytology, when possible, can be helpful. Urinary gonadotropins are available by radioimmune assay, and serum studies of cortisol, testosterone, and gonadotropins also may be readily obtained.

### Genitography and Endoscopy

One of the most useful examinations in the early neonatal period to outline the internal ductal structures of a child with ambiguous genitalia is genitography (Fig 9). With the use of a blunted syringe, contrast material is slowly injected under fluoroscopy, with selected spot films to

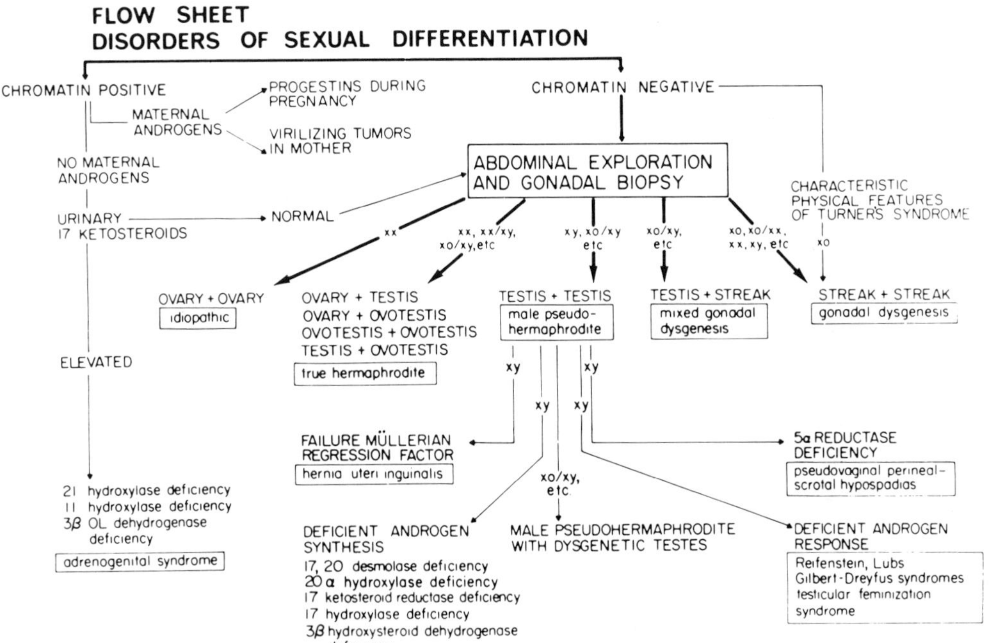


**Fig 10.** Flow sheet. (From Allen TD: Disorders of sexual differentiation. Urology 7[suppl]:1, 1976, with permission.)

delineate the anatomy of the urogenital sinus and outline any internal ductal structures (27). Following this, should the anatomy need to be further clarified, endoscopy can document the presence of a cervix, prostatic utricle, or a high vaginal take-off in a urogenital sinus.

### Exploratory Laparotomy and Gonadal Biopsy

Laparotomy in the newborn is indicated only if gonadal biopsy will influence the sex of rearing. For this reason, it is unnecessary in females with adrenogenital syndrome, female pseudohermaphrodites with proved maternal ingestion of androgen, individuals with Turner's syndrome, and male pseudohermaphrodites with a documented biochemical defect. In establishing the gender assignment, the major consideration should be achievement of functional genitalia. At the time of laparotomy, all structures contrary to the assigned sex should be removed.

Bearing all this information in mind, the flow sheet depicted in Figure 10 is a rational stepwise approach to the child with ambiguous genitalia.

In spite of the enormous amount of new information available in delineating the abnormalities that account for intersex, the problem is by no means simplified. Because of the potential life-threatening nature of some of these disorders and the expertise involved in their surgical management, referral to a major medical center is recommended. Great care and kindness must be exercised in the initial dealings with the parents and family of these unfortunate patients. Suspicion of parental guilt must be allayed and a clear exposition of the facts carried out when the information is available.

In our institution when problematic cases occur, the patient and family are seen by the chiefs of pediatric urology, pediatric surgery, pediatric endocrinology, and psychiatry. After this series of meetings, an assignment decision most beneficial to the child is reached and the appropriate therapy is begun.

## REFERENCES


1. Wachtel SS, et al: Serologic detection of a Y-linked gene in XX males and XX true hermaphrodites. N Eng J Med 295:750, 1976
2. Allen TD: Disorders of sexual differentiation. Urology 7(suppl):1, 1976
3. Walsh PC: Differential diagnosis of ambiguous genitalia in the newborn. Urol Clin North Am 5:1, 213, 1978
4. Jost A: A new look at the mechanisms controlling sex differentiation in mammals. Johns Hopkins Med J 130:38, 1972
5. Federman DD: Abnormal Sexual Development: A Genetic and Endocrine Approach to Differential Diagnosis. Philadelphia: Saunders, 1967
6. Butler LJ, et al: True hermaphroditism of gonadal intersexuality: Cytogenic and gonadal analyses of 5 new examples related to 67 known cases studied cytogenetically. Arch Dis Child 44:666, 1969
7. Josso N, et al: True hermaphroditism with XX/XY mosaicism, probably due to double fertilization of the ovum. J Clin Endocrinol Metab 25:114, 1965
8. Overzier C: Intersexuality. New York: Academic Press, 1963
9. Sohval AR: Mixed gonadal dysgenesis: A variety of hermaphroditism. Am J Hum Genet 15:155, 1963
10. Davidoff R, Federman DD: Mixed gonadal dysgenesis. Pediatrics 52:725, 1973
11. Jones HW, Jr, Scott WW: Hermaphroditism, Genital Anomalies and Related Endocrine Disorders, ed. 2. Baltimore: Williams & Wilkins, 1971
12. Wilson JD, MacDonald PC: Male pseudohermaphroditism due to androgen resistance: Testicular feminization and related syndromes. In Stanbury, Wyngaarden, Fredricksen DS: Metabolic Basis of Inherited Disease, ed. 4. New York: McGraw-Hill, 1977
13. Binns JH, Cross RM; Hernia uteri inguinalis in a male. Br J Surg 54:541, 1967
14. Simpson JL, New M, Peterson RE, German J: Pseudovaginal perineoscrotal hypospadias in sibs. Birth Defects 7:140, 1971
15. Walsh PC, et al: Familial incomplete male pseudohermaphroditism, type 2: Decreased dihydrotestosterone formation in pseudovaginal perineoscrotal hypospadias. N Eng J Med 291:944, 1974
16. Imperato-McGinley J, Guerrero L, Gautier T, Peterson RE: An unusual inherited form of male pseudohermaphroditism, a model of 5-alpha reductase deficiency in man. J Clin Invest 53:35, 1974
17. Morris JM: The syndrome of testicular feminization in male pseudohermaphrodites. Am J Obstet Gynecol 65:1192, 1953

18. Judd HL, et al: Androgen and gonadotropin dynamics in testicular feminization syndrome. Am J Obstet Gynecol 34:229, 1972
19. Wilkins LM: The Diagnosis and Treatment of Endocrine Disorders in Children and Adolescence. Springfield, IL: Thomas, 1950, p 271
20. Lubs HA, Jr, Vilar O, Bergenstal DM: Familial male pseudohermaphroditism with labial testes and partial feminization, endocrine studies and genetic aspects. J Clin Endocrinol Metab 19:1110, 1959
21. Gilbert-Dreyfus S, Sebaoun, CA, Belaisch J: Etude d'un cas familial d'androgyroidisme avec hypospadias grave, gynecomastric et hyperestrogenic. Ann Endocrinol 18:93, 1957
22. Reifenstein EC, Jr: Hereditary familial hypogonadism. Proc Am Fed Clin Res 3:86, 1947
23. Bongiovanni AM, Eberlein WR, Goldman AS, New M: Disorders of adrenal steroid biogenesis. Recent Prog Horm Res 23:375, 1967
24. Allen TD: Reconstruction of the female with ambiguous genitalia. In Kelalis P, King L (eds): Clinical Pediatric Urology. Philadelphia: Saunders, 1977, pp. 1023–1028
25. Fortunoff S, Lattimer JK, Edson M: Vaginoplasty technique for female pseudohermaphrodites. Surg Gynecol Obstet 118:545, 1964
26. Hendren WH, Crawford JD: Adrenogenital syndrome: The anatomy of the anomaly and its repair: Some new concepts. J Pediatr Surg 4:49, 1969
27. Cremin BJ: Intersex states in young children: The importance of radiology in making a correct diagnosis. Clin Radiol 25:63, 1974

# SUBJECT INDEX